www.harcourt-international.com

Bringing you products from all Harcourt Health Sciences companies including Baillière Tindall, Churchill Livingstone, Mosby and W.B. Saunders

- ◗ **Browse** for latest information on new books, journals and electronic products

- ◗ **Search** for information on over 20 000 published titles with full product information including tables of contents and sample chapters

- ◗ **Keep up to date** with our extensive publishing programme in your field by registering with eAlert or requesting postal updates

- ◗ **Secure online ordering** with prompt delivery, as well as full contact details to order by phone, fax or post

- ◗ **News** of special features and promotions

If you are based in the following countries, please visit the country-specific site to receive full details of product availability and local ordering information

USA: www.harcourthealth.com

Canada: www.harcourtcanada.com

Australia: www.harcourt.com.au

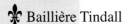 Baillière Tindall   CHURCHILL LIVINGSTONE 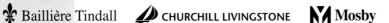 Mosby 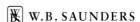 W.B. SAUNDERS

Paediatric
Cardiology
2nd Edition

Commissioning Editor: *Michael Houston*
Project Manager: *Scott Millar*
Design Direction: *Andy Chapman*

Paediatric Cardiology
2nd Edition

Edited by

Robert H Anderson
Joseph Levy Foundation Professor of
 Paediatric Cardiac Morphology
Cardiac Unit
Institute of Child Health
University College London
London, UK

Edward J Baker
Senior Lecturer and Consultant Paediatric
 Cardiologist
Department of Paediatrics
Guy's Hospital
London, UK

Rev Fergus J Macartney
(retired)
Formerly Vandervell Professor of Paediatric
 Cardiology and Honorary
Consultant Paediatric Cardiologist,
Great Ormond Street Children's Hospital
Great Ormond Street, London, UK

Michael L Rigby
Consultant Paediatric Cardiologist
Department of Paediatrics
Royal Brompton Hospital
London, UK

Elliot A Shinebourne
Consultant Paediatric Cardiologist
Department of Paediatrics
Royal Brompton Hospital
London, UK

Michael Tynan (retired)
Formerly Professor of Paediatric Cardiology
Evelina Department of Paediatrics (Cardiology)
Guy's Hospital
London, UK

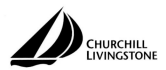
CHURCHILL
LIVINGSTONE

London • Edinburgh • New York • Philadelphia • St Louis • Sydney • Toronto 2002

Churchill Livingstone
An imprint of Harcourt Publishers Limited

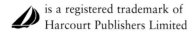
First edition published 1987

ISBN 0 443 07990 0

Cataloguing in Publication Data:
Catalogue records for this book are available from the British Library and the US Library
of Congress.

Note
Medical knowledge is constantly changing. As new information becomes available, changes in
treatment, procedures, equipment and the use of drugs become necessary. The editors, authors,
contributors and the publishers have, as far as possible, taken care to ensure that the information
given in this text is accurate and up to date. However, readers are strongly advised to confirm
that the information, especially with regard to drug usage, complies with the latest legislation and
standards of practice.

Printed by RDC Group in China

Contents

VOLUME 2

Colour Plate Section

General Paediatric Cardiological Disease

Risk Factors and Follow-up

Psychosociological Problems

Preface to First Edition

Ten years ago, when we started our collaboration concerning the naming of congenitally malformed hearts, a book such as this was in our minds. Initially it was conceived as a compilation of the work from several centres concerned with the diagnosis and treatment of childhood heart disease in the UK. When a publisher was found, it was decided that a comprehensive account would require a worldwide authorship. We have been most fortunate in obtaining the collaboration of many friends who are also leading authorities in their fields. All those invited accepted. We thank them for their efforts on our behalf.

A review of the table of contents will show that we have attempted to make the book comprehensive and applicable throughout the world. For example, we are happy to include a chapter on tropical heart disease, while our pleasure in incorporating an extensive chapter on rheumatic heart disease is clouded by the untimely death of its author, Professor I. P. Sukumar. Apart from innovations such as the chapter on ethical considerations, the general sections of the book follow the familiar pattern. Our major departure is in the organisation of the section dealing with congenital malformations. In this we have arranged the chapters in accord with our approach to nomenclature. We have felt this necessary since the study of congenital heart disease has moved on from 'syndromal' accounts to a more detailed and yet generalised understanding of the underlying anatomy and physiology. Although we have not yet achieved the ideal proposed by Moran Campbell (1977) of being able to ascribe causes to most of the individual malformations, our lnowledge even in this respect has deepened in the past decade. Our attempt to integrate the individual congenital anomalies in a sequential segmental fashion will, we hope, remove much of the confusion inherent in describing them as isolated syndromes.

The basis of our approach to diagnosis, description and treatment has been an understanding of the anatomy as it is observed. Here a major advance in the past decade has been the ability to study this three-dimensional anatomy in exquisite detail using cross-sectional echocardiography. We were fortunate that the technique arrived just before we began thinking about the book and has matured during its gestation. Today, this technique is the cornerstone of diagnosis. This is the first major textbook which has been able to accord it its rightful place.

The nomenclature found throughout the book reflects the renaissance of Old World thinking of which we have been major protagonists. We make no apologies for proposing these changes, radical though they may appear to those who were nurtured on more traditional works. The confusion which arises when scientific advances are not matched by complementary changes in nomenclature has been highlighted by Scadding (1967). That such confusion exists in the study of congenital heart diseases is undoubted. It is our hope that taking the naming of congenital lesions of the heart out of the arena of embryological and morphogenetic speculation will result in easier understanding for the clinician and will liberate embryologists and morphologists.

So much for the philosophy. Writing and editing a multiauthor textbook turned out to be a far more difficult task than any of us imagined, even in our worst nightmares. We cannot conclude this brief preface without a catalogue of thanks. First we thank all of our contributors. We edited their texts extensively but with their agreement. We give them credit for the strengths of the book, and take responsibility for any shortcomings. We thank our wives and families for their forebearance. Most of the chapters and references were compiled by Christine Anderson, Anne Kruger, Dorothy Lewis and Rachel Green. The considerable task of providing uniform illustrations was willingly undertaken by Siew Ywn Ho and Anita Hegerty. Throughout the preparation of our own chapters we drew heavily on ideas and contributions from or colleagues. In many cases these colleagues appear as co-authors. We sincerely thank all those who do not.

London, 1986

R. H.A.   F. J. M.
E. A. S.   M. T.

Campbell E J M 1977 The science of diagnosis. In: Phillips C I, Wolfe J N (eds) Clinical practice and econpmics. Pitman, London, pp 101–112
Scadding J G 1967 Diagnosis: the clinician and the computer. Lancet 2: 877–882

Preface

When we contracted with Churchill Livingstone to prepare a second edition of our textbook *Paediatric Cardiology*, we anticipated it would be very much simpler compared to the trials and tribulations of compiling the first edition. We could not have been more wrong. In truth, producing the second edition has been an even greater challenge. As with any convoy, a multi-authored textbook moves at the speed of the slowest ship, in this case the slowest author, and some of our contributors were tardy, but to those who delivered their material on time, we apologise. We owe a particular debt to those who stepped in and produced chapters at remarkably short notice.

Having made our apologies, we must then admit that we learnt a lot from producing the first edition. We are all that much older, and hopefully more experienced. We have also been joined by two new editors with expertise in the newer forms of non-invasive imaging. Thus, the focus of imaging is now very much on the display of the anatomic features of congenital cardiac malformations using cross-sectional formats. We also took note of the critical reviews we received following publication of the first edition, and we have given increased coverage to the aspects of cardiology in the young which have gained increasing importance over the past decade, notably molecular biology, molecular genetics, and transplantation. The essence of the book, nonetheless, remains the morphological, diagnostic, and therapeutic features of the various congenital lesions that make up the day-to-day practice of paediatric cardiology. At the same time, we have tried to cover the problems produced by acquired diseases, particularly those of importance in the emerging countries of the third world.

We have also done our utmost to produce the book using standardised spelling, punctuation, style, and syntax. Those who retain a conservative outlook may be disturbed by English plurals. Equally, they may be disturbed by lack of familiar Latin terminology. Increasingly, nonetheless, those attending symposiums in the United States of America find themselves walking round atriums in their hotels, which may be positioned close to stadiums. So why not atriums and infundibulums in the heart? And similarly, in our opinion, terms such as "dextrocardia" or "situs inversus" are better expressed as "heart in right chest", or "mirror-imaged arrangement", respectively, since both entities are then that much easier to understand, particularly for the patients or their parents. Classical terms, therefore, have been translated to their English equivalents.

The production of the book itself has not been made easier by the fact that our publishers themselves seem to have merged several times during its gestation. Throughout the difficult period of preparation and production, nonetheless, we have received constant support from Miranda Bromage. We thank her most sincerely for her unfailing confidence that the book would eventually appear. The fact that it has eventually appeared, nonetheless, owes much to Christine Anderson. Without her continual admonishments, careful administration, and excellent facilitation, we would have given up long since. In the final analysis, we think it has all been worthwhile, since we believe we have produced a good book. But only you, the reader, will be able to endorse or condemn our judgement. We hope, after all this time, that it will prove an endorsement.

London, August, 2001

Robert H. Anderson
Edward J. Baker
Fergus J. Macartney
Michael L. Rigby
Elliot A. Shinebourne
Michael Tynan

Contributors

Priscilla Alderson BA PhD
Reader in Childhood Studies
Social Science Research Unit
Institute of Education
University of London
London, UK

Lindsey D Allan MD FRCP FACC
Professor of Pediatrics in Obsterics and Gynecology
Department of Pediatric Cardiology
Babies and Childrens Hospital
Columbia University
New York, New York, USA

Mohamed Amrani MD PhD
Senior Lecturer and Consultant Cardiac Surgeon
Royal Brompton and Harefield NHS Trust
Harefield, UK

Page A W Anderson MD
Professor of Pediatrics
Department of Pediatric Cardiology
Duke University Medical Center
Durham, North Carolina, USA

Robert H Anderson BSc MD FRCPath
Joseph Levy Foundation Professor of Paediatric Cardiac Morphology
Cardiac Unit
Institute of Child Health
University College London
London, UK

Edward J Baker MA MD FRCP FRCPCH
Senior Lecturer and Consultant Paediatric Cardiologist
Department of Paediatrics
Guy's Hospital
London, UK

Paul J R Barton BSc PhD
Reader, Molecular Biology
Cardiothoracic Surgery
National Heart & Lung Institute
Imperial College School of Medicine
London, UK

Anton E Becker MD FACC FCCC
Head, Department of Cardiovascular Pathology
Central Medical Academy
Amsterdam, The Netherlands

Lee Beerman MD
Professor of Pediatrics
Division of Pediatric Cardiology
Children's Hospital of Pittsburgh
Pittsburgh, Pennsylvania, USA

Lee Benson MD
Department of Paediatrics (Cardiology)
Hospital for Sick Children
Toronto, Ontario, Canada

Edmond Bertrand MD
Professor of Cardiology
Hopital Nord Marseille
Marseille, France

Eugene H Blackstone MD
Professor
Thoracic and Cardiovascular Surgery
Cleveland Clinic Foundation
Cleveland, Ohio, USA

John Burn MD FRCP
Professor of Clinical Genetics
Institute of Human Genetics
University of Newcastle upon Tyne
Newcastle upon Tyne, UK

Andrew Bush, MBBS(Hons) MA MD FRCP FRCPCH
Reader in Paediatric Respirology
Royal Brompton & Harefield NHS Trust
London, UK

Julene S Carvalho
Department of Paediatrics
Royal Brompton Hospital
London, UK

Christopher L Case MD
Medical Director, Pediatric Cardiology
Fort Worth, Texas, USA

David S Celermajer MB BS MSc PhD FRACP
Department of Cardiology
Royal Prince Alfred Hospital
Camperdown, Australia

Sir Cyril Chantler MA MD FRCP
Chairman of the Board
Great Ormond St Hospital for Children
London, UK

Edward B Clark MD
Wilma T Gibson Presidential Professor
Chairman, Department of Pediatrics
University of Utah
Salt Lake City, Utah, UK

Richard W I Cooke MD FRCP FRCPCH
Professor of Neonatal Medicine
Institute of Child Health
Royal Liverpool Children's Hospital
University of Liverpool
Liverpool, UK

K N Cowan
Department of Paediatrics (Cardiology)
Hospital for Sick Children
Toronto, Ontario, Canada

John E Deanfield BA MB BChir FRCP
Consultant Cardiologist
Great Ormond Street Hospital for Children NHS Trust
Cardiothoracic Unit
London, UK

Gordon R Dunstan MA DD(Hon) LID(Hon) FRCP(Hon) FRCPCH
FRCGP(Hon) FRCOG(ad eondem)
Professor Emeritus of Moral and Social Theology
King's College Hospital
London, UK

Jose Ettedgui MD
Division of Paediatric Cardiology
University of Pittsburgh
Children's Hospital of Pittsburgh
Pittsburgh, Pennsylvania, USA

Donald R Fischer MD
Professor of Pediatrics
Pediatric Cardiology
Children's Hospital of Pittsburgh
Pittsburgh, Pennsylvania, USA

Robert M Freedom MD FRCP(C) FACC
Department of Paediatric Cardiology
The Hospital for Sick Children
Toronto, Ontario, Canada

Frederick J Fricker MD
Division of Pediatric Cardiologist
Health Science Center
University of Florida
Gainsville, Florida, UK

Helena Gardiner MD MRCP DCH FRCPCH
Senior Lecturer in Perinatal Cardiology
Department of Paediatric Cardiology
Royal Brompton Hospital
London, UK

Arthur Garson, Jr. MD MPH
Professor of Paediatrics
Baylor College of Medicine
Texas Childrens Hospital
Houston, Texas , USA

Michael A Gatzoulis MD PhD FACC
Director, Adult Congenital Heart Unit
Consultant Cardiologist
Royal Brompton Hospital
London, UK

Paul C Gillette MD
Cook County Arrhythmia
Medical Director, Pediatric Cardiology
Fort Worth, Texas, USA

Danya Glaser DCH MRCP
Consultant Child Psychiatrist
Great Ormond Street Hospital for Children NHS Trust
London, UK

Judith Goodship MD FRCP
Professor of Medical Genetics
Institute of Human Genetics
University of Newcastle upon Tyne, UK

Sheila G Haworth MD FRCPath FRCPCH FRCP FACC FMedSci
British Heart Foundation Professor of Developmental Cardiology
Vascular Biology and Pharmacology
Institute of Child Health
London, UK

Anthony M Heagerty MBBS MD FRCP FMedSci
Professor of Medicine
University Department of Medicine
Manchester Royal Infirmary
Manchester, UK

G William Henry
Department of Pediatric Cardiology
University of North Carolina
Chapel Hill, North Carolina, USA

Julien I E Hoffman BSc (Hons) MD FRCP
Emeritus Professor of Pediatrics
Department of Pediatrics
University of California
San Francisco, California, USA

Stewart Hunter MBChB(Abad) FRCP(Ed) FRCP(Glas) DCH(Glas)
Consultant in Paediatric Cardiology
Department of Paediatric Cardiology
The Freeman Hospital
Newcastle upon Tyne, UK

Ashley S Izzard BSc PhD
Research Associate
University Department of Medicine
Manchester Royal Infirmary
Manchester, UK

Ronald J Kanter MD
Department of Pediatrics
Duke University School of Medicine
Durham, NC, USA

Ashgar Khaghani
Cardiac and Thoracic Surgery
Harefield Hospital
London, UK

John W Kirklin MD
Professor Emeritus
Division of Cardiovascular Surgery
University of Alabama at Birmingham
Birmingham, Alabama, USA

Li Ling MB PhD
Cardiology Research Fellow
Institute of Human Genetics
University of Newcastle upon Tyne
Newcastle upon Tyne, UK

Walker A Long MD
Department of Pediatric Cardiology
University of North Carolina
Chapel Hill, North Carolina, USA

Rev Fergus J Macartney BA MB B.Chair FRCP (retired)
Formerly Vandervell Professor of Paediatric Cardiology and Honorary
Consultant Paediatric Cardiologist
Great Ormond St Children's Hospital
Great Ormond Street, London, UK

Dominique Metras MD
Professor of Thoracic and Cardiovascular Surgery
Department Cardiovascular Surgery
Children's Hospital la Timone
Marseille, France

Antoon F M Moorman
Experimental & Molecular Cardiology Group
Academic Medical Center
University of Amsterdam
Amsterdam, Netherlands

William H Neches MD
Director, Pediatric Cardiology
Children's Hospital of Pittsburgh
Pittsburgh, Pennsylvania, USA

Catherine A Neill MD FRCP(Lon)
Emeritus Professor of Paediatrics
Helen B Taussig Childrens Heart Center
Johns Hopkins Medical Institutions
Baltimore, Maryland, USA

Edgardo E Ortiz MD FPPS FPCC
Associate Professor of Pediatrics
Chief, Pediatric Cardiology
Department of Pediatrics
University of the Philippines College of Medicine
Philpine General Hospital
Manila, Philippines

Sang C Park MD
Professor of Pediatrics
University of Pittsburgh School of Medicine
Children's Hospital of Pittsburgh
Pittsburgh, Pennsylvania, USA

Daniel J Penny MD MRCPI
Director
Department of Paediatric Cardiology
Royal Melbourne Children's Hospital
Melbourne, Australia

Shakeel A Qureshi MBChB FRCP
Consultant Paediatric Cardiologist
Department of Congenital Heart Disease and Department of Radiology
Guy's Hospital
London, UK

Rosemary C Radley-Smith MBBS FRCP FRCPCH
Consultant Paediatric Cardiologist
Royal Brompton and Harefield NHS Trust
Harefield, Middlesex, UK

Andrew N Redington MD FRCP
Director
Department of Paediatric Cardiology
Hospital for Sick Children
Toronto, Canada

Christopher J D Reid MBChB MRCP(UK) FRCPCH
Consultant Paediatric Nephrologist
Department of Paediatric Nephrology and Urology
Guy's Hospital
London, UK

John F Reidy FRCR FRCP
Consultant Radiologist
Department of Radiology
Guy's Hospital
London, UK

Michael L Rigby MD FRCP FRCPCH
Consultant Paediatric Cardiologist
Department of Paediatrics
Royal Brompton Hospital
London, UK

Eric Rosenthal MD FRCP
Consultant Paediatric Cardiologist
Department of Paediatric Cardiology
Guy's Hospital
London, UK

Mark Rosenthal MBChB BSc MD FRCP FRCPH
Consultant Paediatrician
Royal Brompton Hospital
London, UK

Jeffrey F Smallhorn MBBS FRACP FRCP(C)
Professor of Paediatrics
Universirty of Toronto
Head, Section of Echocardiography
The Hospital for Sick Children
Toronto, Ontario, Canada

Norman H Silverman MD
Professor of Pediatrics and Radiology (Cardiology)
University of California
San Francisco, California, USA

Elliot A Shinebourne MD FRCP
Consultant Paediatric Cardiologist
Department of Paediatrics
Royal Brompton Hospital
London, UK

Michael de Swiet MBBChir MA FRCP FRCOG
Consultant Physician
Institute of Obstetrics & Gynaecology
Queen Charlotte's Hospital
London, UK

J M Tersak MD
Division of Hematology/Oncology and Bone Marrow
    Transplantation
University of Pittsburgh
Children's Hospital of Pittsburgh
Pittsburgh, Pennsylvania, USA

Jonathan R Tulip
Professor of Medicine
University Department of Medicine
Manchester Royal Infirmary
Manchester, UK

Michael Tynan MD FRCP (retired)
Formerly Professor of Paediatric Cardiology
Evelina Department of Paediatrics (Cardiology)
Guy's Hospital
London, UK

Steven Webber MBChB MRCP
Associate Professor of Pediatrics
Division of Cardiology
Children's Hospital of Pittsburgh
Pittsburgh, Pennsylvania, USA

Arnold C G Wenink MD PhD LLM
Associate Professor of Anatomy and Embryology
Department of Anatomy and Embryology
Lieden University Medical Center
Lieden, The Netherlands

James L Wilkinson MBChB FRCP FRACP FRCPCH FACC
Department of Cardiology
Royal Children's Hospital
Parkville, Victoria, Australia

Michael Wright MB MRCP
Consultant Clinical Geneticist
Institute of Human Genetics
University of Newcastle upon Tyne
Newcastle upon Tyne, UK

Sir Magdi H Yacoub
Department of Cardiothoracic Surgery
Professor of Cardiac Surgery
Royal Brompton Hospital
London, UK

Guangbin Zeng
Resident
Community and Family Medicine
Duke University School of Medicine
Durham, North Carolina, USA

James R Zuberbuhler MD
Professor of Pediatrics
University of Pittsburgh School of Medicine
Children's Hospital of Pittsburgh
Pittsburgh, Pennsylvania, USA

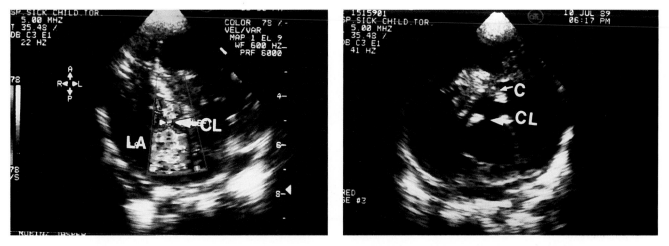

Plate 43.1. Short-axis view of the heart in a patient with an isolated cleft and associated regurgitation. Note the leak through the cleft.

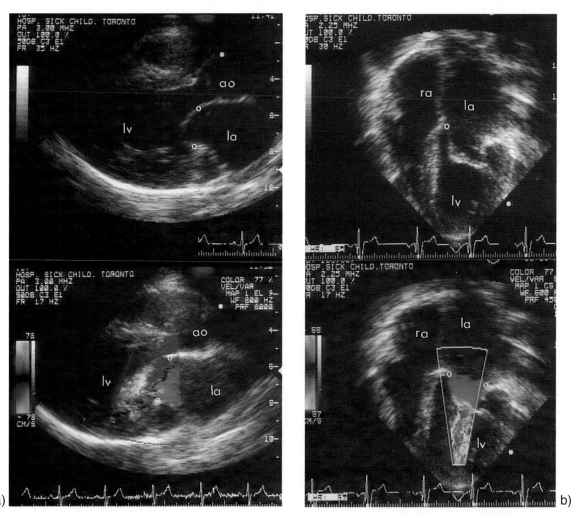

a)
b)

Plate 43.2. (a) Precordial long axis view in congenital mitral valvar stenosis, seen during diastole. Note the doming valve, with the colour flow disturbance occurring distal to the mitral annulus (outlined by the open circles). (b) Apical four chamber view demonstrating the doming thickened mitral valve, again with the disturbed flow starting below the annulus (outlined by the open circles). ao, aorta; la, left atrium; lv, left ventricle; ra, right atrium.

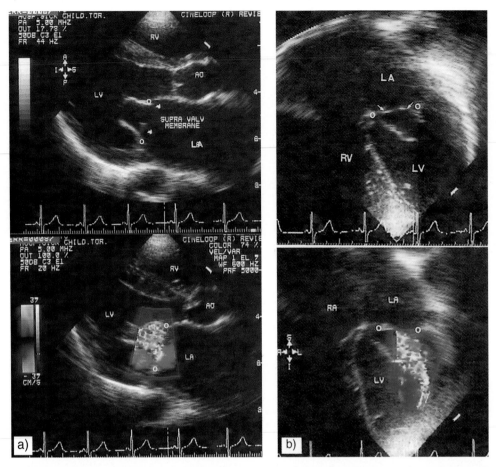

Plate 43.3. (a) Precordial long-axis view in a heart with mitral valvar stenosis in association with a supravalvar ring. Note the flow disturbance occurs at just above the annulus (compare with Plate 43.2a). (b) Note the supravalvar membrane in the upper panel, with the lower panel demonstrating the flow disturbance starting at a higher level than in Plate 43.2b (the open circles outline the annulus). AO, aorta; LA, left atrium; LV, left ventricle; RV, right ventricle.

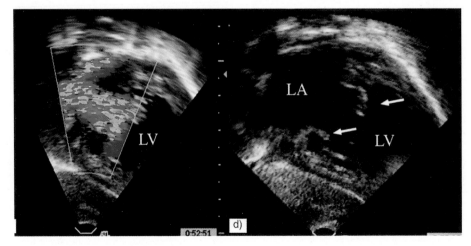

Plate 43.4. Montage demonstrating congenital mitral valve regurgitation in a baby secondary to isolated dysplasia of the mural leaflet. Note the poor coaption of the leaflets during systole as indicated by the arrow. The aortic leaflet is mobile (compare systole and diastole) with a relatively immobile mural leaflet. LA, left atrium; LV, left ventricle.

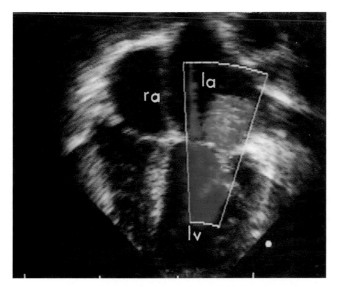

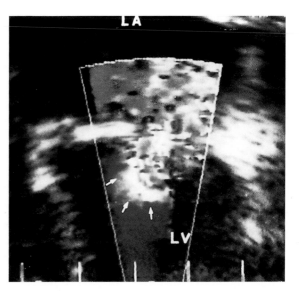

Plate 43.5. Apical four chamber view showing mild mitral valvar regurgitation. Note the area of the regurgitant jet is about 20% of the left atrial area in this view. la, left atrium; lv, left ventricle; ra, right atrium.

Plate 43.6. Expanded apical four chamber view in a heart with significant mitral valvar regurgitation, showing the phenomenon of PISA (proximal isovelocity surface area) calculations. LA, left atrium; LV, left ventricle.

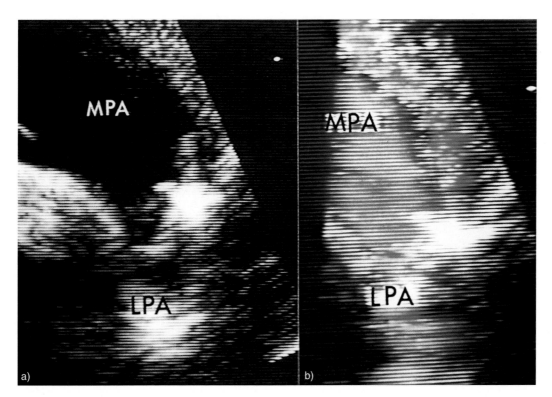

Plate 52.1. Ductal occlusion. Colour Doppler after ductal occlusion. The blue colour indicates blood flow in the aorta and pulmonary arteries. Note turbulent flow (yellow streak) of small residual shunt left to right. MPA, main pulmonary artery; LPA, left pulmonary artery.

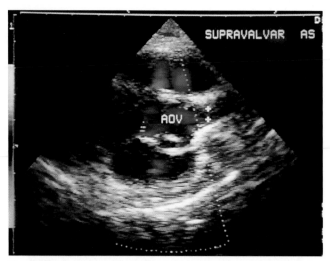

Plate 54.1. Parasternal long-axis view of supravalvar narrowing. AOV, aortic valve.

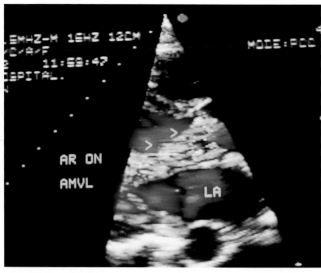

Plate 54.2. Colour flow mapping in left ventricular outflow tract with aortic regurgitation.

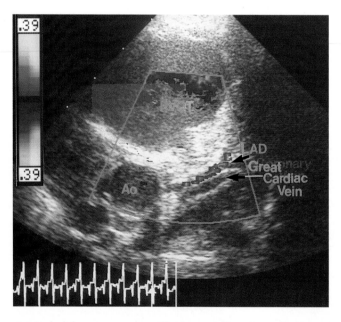

Plate 55.1. Doppler colour-flow mapping in the left coronary system. The great cardiac vein can be seen posterior to the left anterior descending aorta (LAD). Red, flow away from the aorta (Ao) towards the cardiac apex.

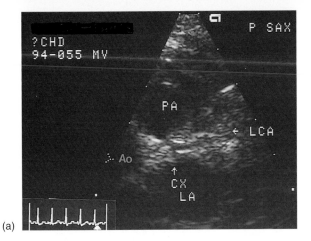

(a)

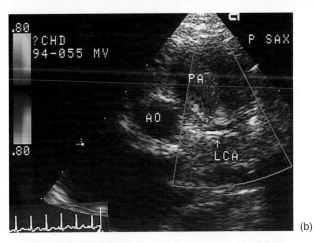

(b)

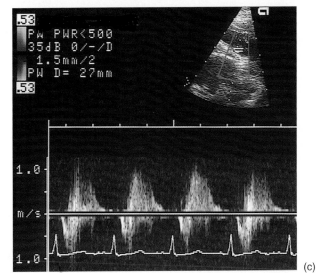

(c)

Plate 55.2. (a) Direct imaging of the anomalous origin of the left coronary artery (LCA) from the pulmonary trunk (PA) in the parasternal short-axis view. The left circumflex artery (CX) can also be seen just above the left atrium (LA). Ao, aorta. (b) With superimposition of the colour Doppler flow map on the artery, the resultant jet into the pulmonary trunk is seen from the abnormal coronary artery. (c) The pulsed Doppler flow signal shows the flow map coming towards the pulmonary trunk in early diastole. With these techniques, it is now possible to diagnose most patients who have this anomaly and successfully to exclude cardiomyopathy (compare with Plate 55.1).

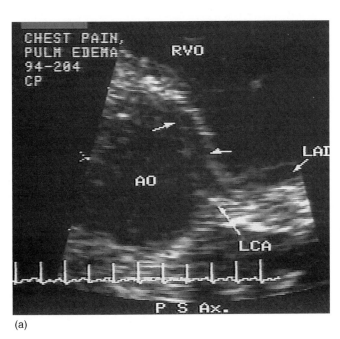

(a)

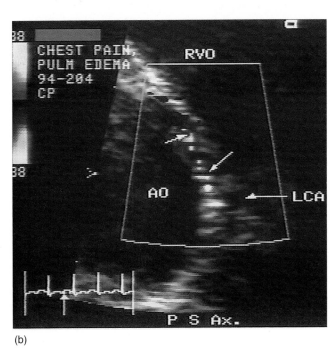

(b)

Plate 55.3. This parasternal short-axis view shows the left coronary artery arising from the right coronary sinus. (a) The course is through the wall of the aorta (intramural course; arrows). The artery exits from the usual position. Also displayed are the extramural course of the left coronary artery (LCA) and the left anterior descending coronary artery (LAD). The artery runs behind the right ventricular outflow tract (RVO). (b) Superimposition of the Doppler colour flow signal shows the origin of the flow within the artery, with aliasing as it courses intramurally through the aortic wall. This patient had chest pain and pulmonary oedema as presenting symptoms and underwent successful unroofing of the left coronary artery. (Published with permission from Poon C, Van Son J, Moore P, et al., 1999 *Pediatric Cardiology*, in press.)

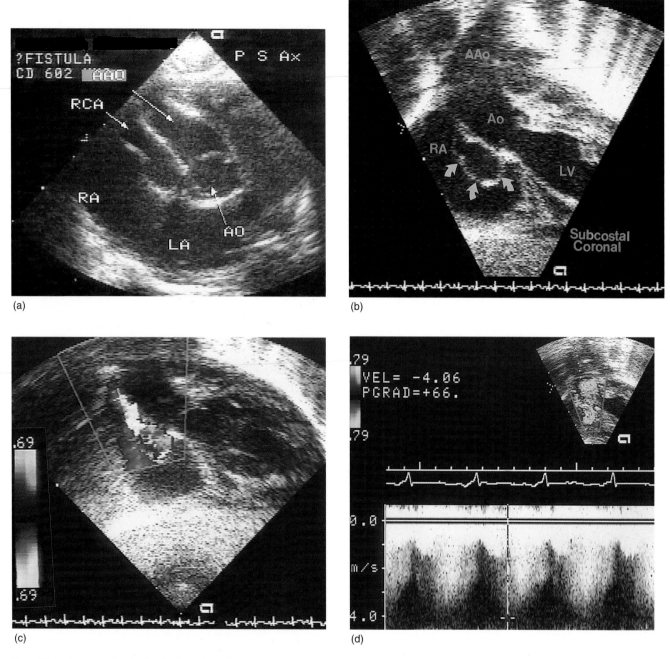

Plate 55.4. An example of a fistula from the right coronary artery (RCA) to the right atrium (RA) in a neonate presenting with cardiac failure showing the images using a variety of views and modalities. (a) In the parasternal short-axis view, the enlarged right coronary artery is seen to arise from the aortic root (AO). The descending aorta is only slightly larger than the ascending aorta (AAO). (b) This subcostal coronal frame shows the large aneurysmal connection of the fistula (arrows) with the right atrium. (c) This shows the superimposition of colour flow on the fistulous entry into the right atrium. (d) The continuous wave Doppler signal is shown across the area of the fistula. The velocity of flow is 4.06 m/s, corresponding to a pressure drop of 66 torr. LA, left atrium. (*Plate 55.4 (c) and (d) on next page.*)

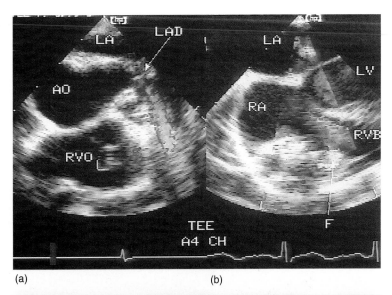

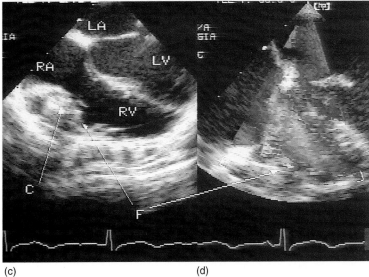

Plate 55.5. Echocardiographic recognition and monitoring of the embolization, shown angiographically in Figure 55.24. (a) The origin of the large left anterior descending coronary artery (LAD) is shown arising from the aortic root (AO). (b) Disturbed flow is seen across the entry into the right ventricle. (c, d) There is no flow after successful blocking of the fistula. C, site of the coils; F, position of the sealed fistula; LA, left atrium; LV, left ventricle; RA. right atrium: RV, right ventricle: RVB, right ventricular body.

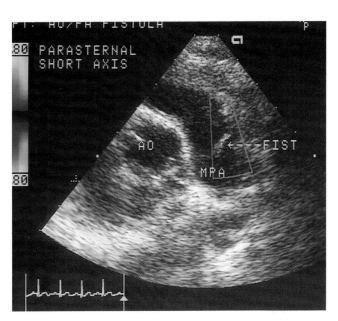

Plate 55.6. The Doppler colour flow signal found in the presence of a small fistula between a coronary artery and the pulmonary trunk (FIST). AO, aorta; MPA, pulmonary trunk.

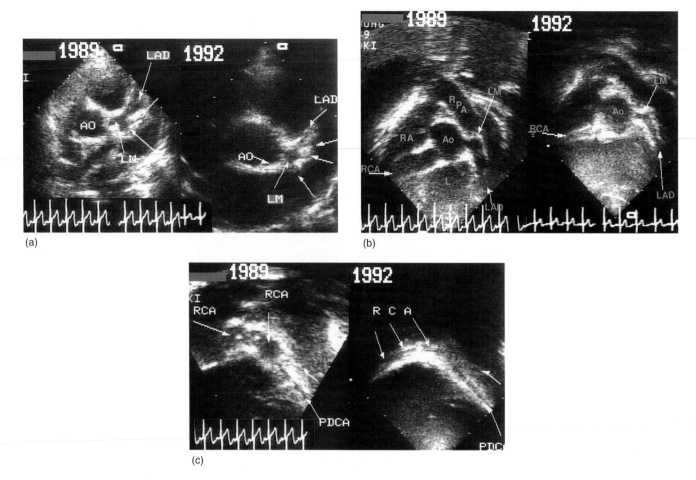

Plate 55.7. These series of frames were taken from the same patient with the mucocutaneous lymph node syndrome followed from 1989 (left frames) to 1992 (right frames). (a) Views taken in a parasternal short axis. The aorta (AO) is identified. The main stem (LM) of the left coronary artery divides into the left anterior descending (LAD), a marginal branch (arrow) and the circumflex coronary arteries. Note the difference in the size of the left anterior descending coronary artery. (b) Apically derived views show the left anterior descending artery and right coronary artery (RCA). (c) The right ventricle is shown posteriorly with the posterior portion of the right coronary artery shown to be enlarged and aneurysmal in 1989, whereas the posterior descending coronary artery (PDCA) is seen to be of normal size. In 1992, the right coronary artery no longer demonstrates aneurysms. RA, right atrium; RPA, right pulmonary artery.

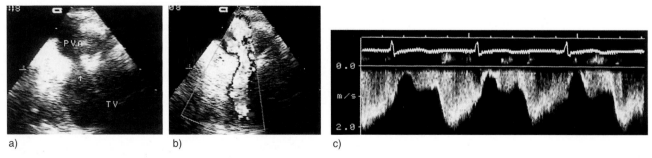

Plate 72.1. Transoesophageal echocardiographic pictures taken from a patient who has had a Mustard procedure for complete transposition with intact ventricular septum, but from whom only poor images could be obtained using standard transthoracic echocardiography. Mild narrowing of the pulmonary venous pathway can be seen (a) with turbulent colour flow Doppler in this region (b). (c) Pulsed Doppler signal is shown. These pictures are consistent with mild narrowing of the pulmonary venous pathway.

37

Ventricular septal defect

M. Tynan and R. H. Anderson

INTRODUCTION

Holes between the ventricles can occur as isolated anomalies or in association with many other defects. They are found as integral parts of entities such as the tetralogy of Fallot, double outlet ventricles and most cases of common arterial trunk. They occur as a component of atrioventricular septal defects and are frequently encountered in association with complete and congenitally corrected transposition. Even when found as so-called 'isolated' defects, then additional relatively minor complicating abnormalities are often encountered, such as persistence of the arterial duct, aortic or mitral valvar regurgitation or acquired subvalvar pulmonary stenosis. In this chapter, we will consider only the relatively isolated ventricular septal defect, but we will discuss the complications produced by other minor associations. Although holes between the ventricles have a long pedigree, it is with the name of Henri Roger (1879) that the anomaly is historically linked. It was Roger who recognized that an isolated ventricular septal defect produced a typical murmur and could be consistent with prolonged life and good health.

PREVALENCE

If we exclude aortic valves having two leaflets, and also exclude prolapse of the mitral valve (Roberts, 1984), then isolated ventricular septal defect is the most common congenital cardiac malformation. It is difficult to obtain an accurate assessment of prevalence, since most individuals with an isolated defect, being asymptomatic, are not candidates for cardiac catheterization and angiography. Consequently, in the past, there had been no objective proof of the presence of a defect. The advent of cross-sectional echocardiography, and colour flow Doppler, has changed all that. The known high rate of spontaneous closure (French, 1918; Weber, 1918; Evans et al, 1960; Krovetz, 1998) meant that postmortem data certainly underestimated the incidence of the defect. In series depending heavily on clinical observation, the estimated prevalence varied from 1.35 to 2.94 per 1000 live-births (Carlgren, 1959; Hoffman and Rudolph, 1965; Mitchell et al, 1971; Hoffman and Christianson, 1978). The most accurate clinical studies, backed up by postmortem data, are those derived from the populations of Bohemia (Šamanek et al, 1989), Merseyside in the United Kingdom (Jackson et al, 1996) and Malta (Grech, 1998). The prevalences at birth in Bohemia and Merseyside were 2.01 and 2.74 per 1000 births, respectively. That from the Maltese study, in contrast, was 3.94, a significant difference. This reflects the increased use of echocardiography in diagnosis. This trend is confirmed by data from the Baltimore–Washington Infant Study (Lewis et al, 1996), which also used echocardiographic techniques and showed a remarkable increase in the diagnosis of muscular defects, with a tenfold increase in prevalence. Ventricular septal defects accounted for one third of all cases identified in the infants of this study, and made up 44% of those seen in Malta. A particularly high prevalence of muscular defects has also been reported by those who scanned populations of neonates using colour flow imaging, noting subsequent spontaneous closure of many of the defects (Hiraishi et al, 1992; Du et al, 1996, 1998; Roguin et al, 1996). None of these studies, however, were population based (Dickinson, 1998).

MORPHOLOGY AND CLASSIFICATION

It is, perhaps, surprising that, as we start the 21st century, there is still no consensus concerning the best way to categorize and describe holes between the ventricles. Initially, systems ranged from the simple 'high' and 'low' (Lev, 1960), to exceedingly complex nosologies based on speculations concerning the developmental origins of the septal components (Goor et al, 1971). Throughout this period, it had also been popular to relate the defects to presumed components of the enigmatic crista (Rosenquist et al, 1973). Others had combined morphological and embryological features (Van Praagh et al, 1989) or had sought to establish a system considered to be of specific value to the surgeon (Kirklin et al, 1988). Over this same period, we had established (Soto et al, 1980) and refined (Anderson et al, 1986; Baker et al, 1988) an approach that we believed would satisfy all these needs. Subsequently, and even at the time, discussions suggested that we had not achieved this objective (Capelli et al, 1983; Soto et al, 1989). This set us to examine why there should be so many disagreements concerning such a relatively simple lesion.

One obvious problem is that the lesion is not always as simple as it first appears. For example, when associated with valvar overriding, there may be no consensus even on the plane in space that is chosen to represent the defect (Baker et al, 1988). Other disagreements stem from the fact that different schools choose different features on which to base their criterions for classification. The resolution of these various problems seems straightforward, at least to us. First, we must define clearly the plane of space that we choose to recognize as the defect. Then, having defined precisely the plane which represents our defect, we must account for all its various anatomical features. This will include its boundaries, its position relative to the landmarks and components of the ventricular septum (including the atrioventricular conduction axis), the description (if present) of valvar overriding and malalignment between the different septal components, and size. The system that has evolved to cater for all these features is applicable not only to the isolated defects, and those found in hearts with complete and corrected transposition (Anderson and Wilcox, 1992), but also to those seen in more complicated malformations such as tetralogy of Fallot or common arterial trunk (Anderson and Wilcox, 1993), and those in hearts with univentricular atrioventricular connection (Anderson et al, 1994).

WHAT IS THE DEFECT?

When there is a simple hole, punched as it were into the substance of the muscular ventricular septum, then there is no problem is defining its margins, nor in agreeing that the margins are exclusively muscular (Figure 37.1). Many holes, however, bordered by the crest of the muscular ventricular septum, abut directly upon the hingepoints of the leaflets of either the atrioventricular or the arterial valves, or both. Some of these lesions are associated with marked overriding of the valvar orifice (Figure 37.2). It is then much harder to define the precise borders and margins of the defect. This is because a cone of space, with an elongated base, is subtended from the attachments of the leaflets of the overriding valve to the crest of the muscular ventricular septum (Figure 37.3). Within this cone, any of a number of planes can justifiably be nominated to represent the defect. When viewed in a

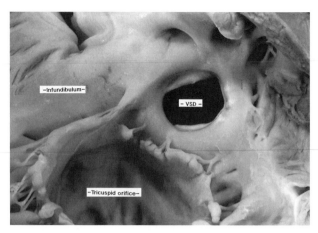

Figure 37.1. The hole in this heart is enclosed within the muscular septum. None would have difficulty in establishing the margins of the defect (VSD).

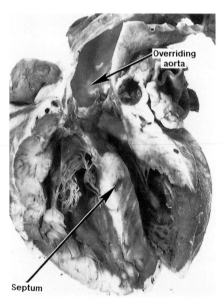

Figure 37.2. It is much more difficult to identify the precise plane of the defect in this heart, sectioned to replicate the four chamber plane incorporating the aortic root. The aorta is overriding the crest of the ventricular septum (see Figure 37.3).

single section, as seen by the echocardiographer, then at least three of these planes are important (Figure 37.4). One is the continuation of the long axis of the ventricular septum to the underside of the overriding valvar leaflets. Many choose this plane for nomination as the ventricular septal defect. This particular defect, however, exists only when the valvar leaflets are closed and is never the locus for placement of a patch by the surgeon during operative repair of an isolated defect. The second plane marks the boundary between the cone of space subtended beneath the overriding valve and the left ventricle. This plane is, effectively, the left ventricular outflow tract. It is an unequivocally important, but few, it any, would define it as the defect. The third plane is comparable to the second but marks the right ventricular borders of the

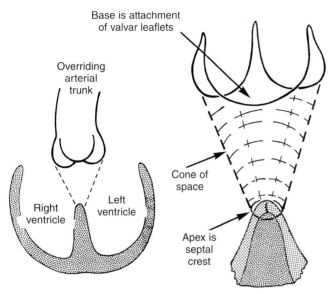

Figure 37.3. In hearts with overriding of an arterial trunk (see Figure 37.2), there is a cone of space subtended from the valvar leaflets to the crest of the ventricular septum. It is reasonable to nominate any plane within this cone as a ventricular septal defect, but three particular planes are of special importance (see Figure 37.4).

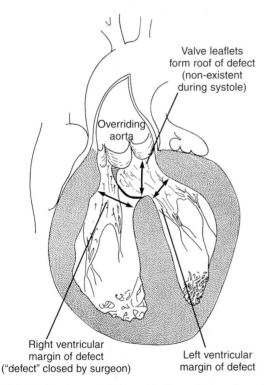

Figure 37.4. Within the cone illustrated in Figure 37.3, at least three planes are particularly important. We define the right ventricular margin closed by the surgeon as the defect requiring categorization.

cone of space. This plane is of equal, if not greater, importance since it is the border around which the surgeon will insert sutures to secure the patch placed to reconstitute the ventricular septum. It is this third plane that we choose as our focus when describing the margins

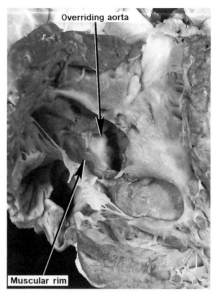

Figure 37.5. In this heart, the right ventricular margin of the hole between the ventricles, as viewed from the right ventricle, has exclusively muscular borders. The direct plane of the ventricular septum, however, would cut the undersurface of the aortic valve. Because we categorize according to the right ventricular margin, we nominate this heart as having a muscular outlet defect.

of ventricular septal defects (Figure 37.5). We then account for these margins as viewed from the morphologically right ventricle (Figure 37.6) or through the tricuspid valve, except when there is usual atrial arrangement and the atrioventricular connections are discordant, in which case the hole is viewed from the right-sided morphologically left ventricle (or through the mitral valve, see Chapter 49).

FEATURES OF THE DEFECT REQUIRING DESCRIPTION

We have already discussed how defects are either found within the muscular septum or at its margins, the latter septal deficiencies being related directly to the hinges of the valvar leaflets. As also indicated, it is an appreciation of these relationships as viewed from the right ventricle that we use as the primary criterion for description. In our experience, all defects can be placed into one of three groups when seen from the right ventricle according to the margins of the defect (Table 37.1). Those within the substance of the septum have exclusively muscular rims and are universally described as muscular defects (Figure 37.1). The second group are located along the inner curvature of the right side of the heart. In the normally structured heart, this is the area occupied by the so-called membranous part of the septum and the supraventricular crest. The membranous septum, on its left ventricular aspect, is directly continuous with the area of fibrous continuity between the leaflets of the aortic and mitral valves (Figure 37.7). The right end of this zone of continuity is

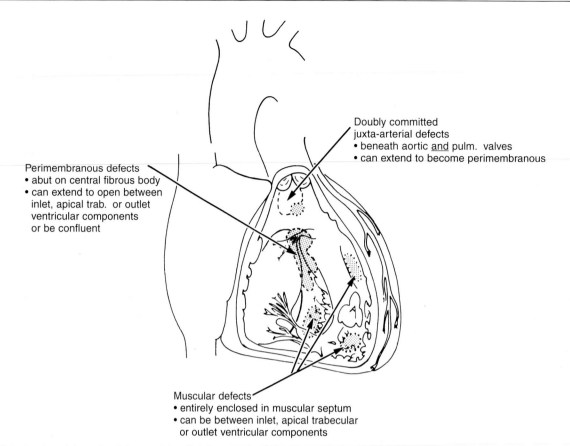

Perimembranous defects
• abut on central fibrous body
• can extend to open between inlet, apical trab. or outlet ventricular components or be confluent

Doubly committed juxta-arterial defects
• beneath aortic _and_ pulm. valves
• can extend to become perimembranous

Muscular defects
• entirely enclosed in muscular septum
• can be between inlet, apical trabecular or outlet ventricular components

Figure 37.6. As viewed from the right ventricle, all defects can be defined, according to the nature of their margins, as being perimembranous, muscular or doubly committed and juxta-arterial.

Table 37.1. Classification of the borders of ventricular septal defects

Defects abutting on area of continuity between atrioventricular and arterial valves (perimembranous)
    Opening into inlet of right ventricle
    Opening into outlet of right ventricle
    Confluent defects

Defects encased within musculature of ventricular septum (muscular)
    Opening between inlets
    Opening between apical components
    Opening between outlets
    Multiple
    Coexisting with perimembranous defect

Defects roofed by arterial valves in fibrous continuity (doubly committed and juxta-arterial)
    With muscular posteroinferior rim
    Extending to become perimembranous

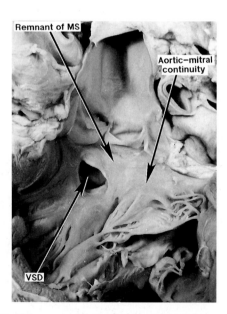

Remnant of MS

Aortic–mitral continuity

VSD

Figure 37.7. This ventricular septal defect (VSD) is shown from its left ventricular margin. Note that the posteroinferior margin is formed by fibrous continuity between the aortic and tricuspid valves through the remnant of the membranous septum (MS).

called the right fibrous trigone, and the fusion of trigone and membranous septum constitutes the central fibrous body. This entire area forms the fibrous root of the aorta and is continuous with the triangle of fibrous tissue ascending to occupy the space between the non-coronary and right coronary leaflets of the aortic valve. On the right side, the membranous septum itself is crossed by the hinge of the septal leaflet of the tricuspid valve, dividing it into atrioventricular and interventricular components. The axis of atrioventricular conduction tissue penetrates through this septum from the apex of the triangle of Koch (see Chapter 3); it then runs on the crest of the muscular septum, sandwiched between the fibrous and muscular septal components. In hearts with ventricular septal defects along the inner curvature, the septum can be considered to have sprung apart between the crest of the muscular septum and the membranous septum. This means that the posteroinferior margin of such defects, when seen from the right ventricle (or through the tricuspid valve), is formed by fibrous continuity between the leaflets of the aortic and tricuspid valves (Figure 37.8). In the past, such defects were often called membranous defects, since it was presumed that they existed because of a deficiency in the membranous septum. As Becu and his colleagues (1956) pointed out, this is unlikely, because the defects are always larger than the normal dimensions of the membranous septum. Furthermore, division of the membranous septum into its interventricular and atrioventricular components does not occur in fetal life until after the embryonic septum has already closed (Allwork and Anderson, 1979; Lamers et al, 1993). It is difficult, therefore, to account for presence of a defect on the basis of absence of a structure that is itself not formed until after normal closure of the embryonic interventricular communication. It seems far more likely that the defects persist because the muscular ventricular septum is deficient in the environs of the developing membranous septum. Because of this, our preference is to describe this group of defects as being perimembranous. Their anatomical hallmark in the otherwise normally constituted heart is the presence of fibrous continuity between the leaflets of the aortic and tricuspid valves.

There is then a third group of defects that are found in the region of the right ventricle, which in the normal heart is formed by the muscular subpulmonary infundibulum. In our initial description (Soto et al, 1980), we described this area as formed by the muscular outlet septum. We now know this to be incorrect, since the leaflets of the pulmonary valve, in the normal heart, are supported by a complete sleeve of free-standing infundibular musculature. A defect of the third type, therefore, characterized by fibrous continuity between the leaflets of the aortic and pulmonary valves (Figure 37.9), could not exist in the otherwise normally structured heart. This third type of defect, which we describe as being doubly committed and juxta-arterial, exists because of absence of not only the muscular outlet septum but also the septal components of the free-standing subpulmonary muscular infundibulum. Such a defect, when viewed from the right ventricle, most frequently has a muscular posteroinferior rim that separates the leaflets of the aortic and tricuspid valves (Figure 37.9). On occasions, nonetheless, the defect can extend so that its posteroinferior margin is formed by fibrous continuity between the aortic and tricuspid valvar leaflets, while its roof is made up of aortic–pulmonary valvar continuity. Defects with such margins are both doubly committed and juxta-arterial and, at the same time, perimembranous.

This third group of defects is also the group which, in the past, was held to be 'supracristal' (Rosenquist et al, 1973). There is no logic in this designation. Examination of the heart shown in Figure 37.9 shows that the defect

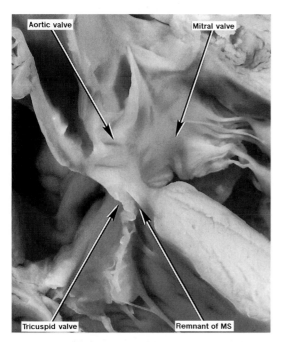

Figure 37.8. This simulated four chamber section shows the aortic-tricuspid valvar continuity that is the hallmark of the perimembranous nature of the ventricular septal defect. MS, membranous septum.

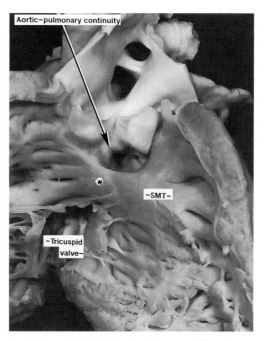

Figure 37.9. The roof of this defect is formed of fibrous continuity between the leaflets of the aortic and pulmonary valves, making it doubly committed and juxta-arterial. Note the muscular posteroinferior rim (star). The defect itself is between the limbs of the septomarginal trabeculation (SMT).

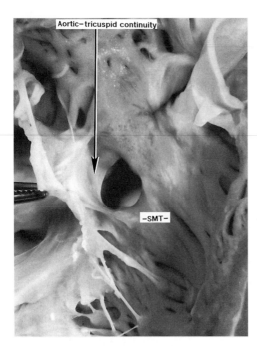

Figure 37.10. This defect, again between the limbs of the septomarginal trabeculation (SMT) when seen from the right ventricle, has fibrous continuity between the leaflets of the aortic and tricuspid valves in its posteroinferior rim. This feature makes the defect perimembranous.

is above the muscular structures formed by the limbs of the septomarginal trabeculation. But the so-called infracristal defect is also between the limbs of this structure (Figure 37.10). The difference between the two defects is that the roof of the so-called infracristal defect is the outlet septum supporting the free-standing subpulmonary infundibulum, whereas these muscular structures are absent in the so-called supracristal defect. Therefore, the defect does not move in relation to supposed components of the crista. Instead, the defining component (the outlet septum) is absent in one of the defects. It is because of this faulty logic, and similar problems that beset the description of tetralogy of Fallot (see Chapter 46), that we prefer to restrict description of the supraventricular crest (the 'crista') to the normally structured heart.

Having accounted for the margins of the defect, as viewed from the right side, and having used this as our primary criterion for definition, we then describe the location of the defect relative to the components of the right ventricle. In the past, we described defects as excavating into the inlet, outlet or apical trabecular components of the septum. For muscular defects, this system still holds good, and lesions can be recognized as being within the inlet, apical trabecular or outlet parts of the septum. The system is less accurate when used to describe perimembranous defects. This is because most of the septum, which, when viewed from the right side, seems to be an inlet structure, in reality separates the inlet of the right from the outlet of the left ventricle. It does this because of

the deeply wedged location of the normal subaortic outflow tract. Furthermore, in the normal heart, there is barely any part of the muscular septum that can readily be identified as a muscular outlet septum. As already discussed, this is because of the presence of the free-standing subpulmonary infundibulum. Consequently, when perimembranous defects open anteriorly towards the pulmonary valve, they do not excavate into the outlet septum. Instead, they open beneath the subaortic and subpulmonary outlets, thus permitting the outlet septum to be recognized as a muscular structure in its own right. Because of these features, we now describe perimembranous defects as opening into either the inlet or the outlet of the right ventricle, or else being sufficiently large to open between both inlet and outlet components, these last holes being described as confluent defects. The doubly committed and juxta-arterial defect is, of necessity, a defect that opens beneath both outlets because of the lack of the outlet septum and the septal components of the subpulmonary infundibulum.

The third important feature that requires description, when present, is valvar overriding, with its associated feature of malalignment of septal components. Many use the term 'malalignment' as their sole adjective for description of a ventricular septal defect. This is inadequate. In the presence of overriding of the aortic valve, for example, a defect with malalignment of the outlet septum can have either a muscular posteroinferior rim or a rim formed by fibrous continuity between the leaflets of the aortic and tricuspid valves. To distinguish these two defects, therefore, it is necessary additionally to state that one has the muscular rim (Figure 37.11a), while the other is perimembranous (Figure 37.11b). Furthermore, the outlet septum can be malaligned relative to the muscular septum so that it becomes a right ventricular structure (Figure 37.11) or, alternatively, a structure that obstructs the outflow tract of the left ventricle (Figure 37.12). There can also be malalignment between the muscular ventricular septum and the atrial septum, this being the feature of a particularly important defect characterized by overriding of the orifice of the tricuspid valve (Figure 37.13). There are, therefore, various types of malalignment, and all need to be described in addition to the other features of ventricular septal defects (Anderson et al, 1994).

Size is also important, in particular in determining the haemodynamic consequences of the various types of defect and in differentiating those defects most likely to diminish in size or close spontaneously. Size can be described according to taste, either using subjective adjectives such as large, medium or small, or by relating the different dimensions of the plane of space chosen to represent the defect to the diameter of the aortic root. The latter approach is more scientific but needs to be used in combination with the fact that, when associated with valvar overriding, several planes can be defined as the defect. Therefore, even though the

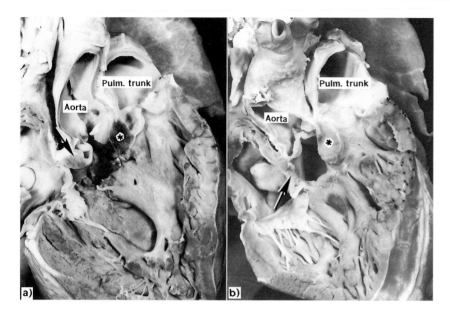

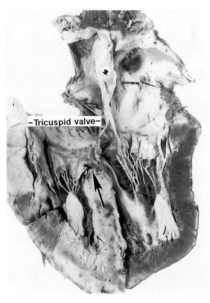

Figure 37.11. Both of these defects have malalignment of the muscular outlet septum (star) into the right ventricle, in association with overriding of the aortic valve. In (a), however, the posteroinferior margin is muscular (arrowed), while there is fibrous continuity at the arrowed point in the heart shown in (b), making this defect perimembranous.

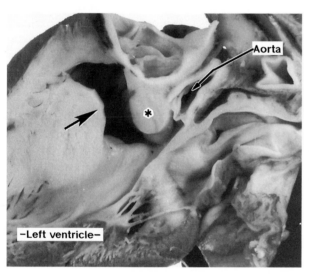

Figure 37.12. In this defect, the muscular outlet septum (star) is deviated posteriorly relative to the crest of the ventricular septum (arrowed), producing subaortic stenosis.

Figure 37.13. There is malalignment between the atrial (star) and ventricular (arrowed) septal structures in this heart, with straddling and overriding of the tricuspid valve.

right ventricular margin of the cone of space may be large, if the left ventricular margin is small, then problems will be produced should the right margin be closed at surgery.

PERIMEMBRANOUS VENTRICULAR SEPTAL DEFECTS

When a perimembranous defect extends to communicate mostly with the inlet of the right ventricle, then the aortic valve and central fibrous body form the anterosuperior part of the right ventricular margin of the defect. The posteroinferior part is roofed by a conjoined area of mitral to tricuspid valvar continuity. The area of atrioventricular muscular septum is correspondingly reduced.

When viewed from the right ventricle, the defect is curtained from view by the septal leaflet of the tricuspid valve. The medial papillary muscle is located anteriorly and cephalad to the defect (Figure 37.14). In the past, these defects were misleadingly termed the 'isolated atrioventricular canal' type (Neufeld et al, 1961). It is indeed the case that, on occasion, a defect opening between the ventricular inlets can be part of a heart having a common atrioventricular junction. The left atrioventricular valve will then have three leaflets, and the heart will show all the other features of an atrioventricular septal defect (see Chapter 36). Such a heart, therefore, truly has an atrioventricular septal defect with common atrioventricular junction, but with shunting occurring at ventricular level

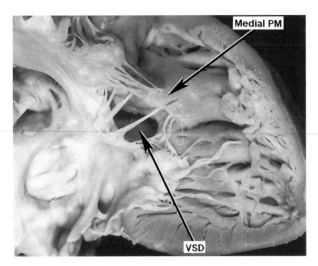

Figure 37.14. This perimembranous defect (VSD), with aortic–tricuspid valvar continuity in its posteroinferior rim, opens to the inlet of the right ventricle. Note the location of the medial papillary muscle (PM).

because the bridging leaflets of the valve guarding the common junction are firmly attached to the undersurface of the atrial septum. Straightforward perimembranous defects opening to the inlet of the right ventricle, in contrast, irrespective of their size, have separate atrioventricular junctions, with a mitral valve guarding the left junction even when it is cleft (Sigfùsson et al, 1995). The key to recognition is the separate nature of the right and left atrioventricular junctions. Such perimembranous inlet defects opening to the right ventricular inlet, therefore, should not be described as 'atrioventricular canal

defects'. The hearts already discussed with atrioventricular septal malalignment, and with the tricuspid valve straddling and overriding a defect between the ventricular inlets (Figure 37.13), should also be distinguished from hearts with atrioventricular septal defect and common atrioventricular junction. The defects found with overriding of the tricuspid valve constitute a particular subset of perimembranous defect, still possessing the feature of aortic–tricuspid valvar fibrous continuity, and once more having separate right and left atrioventricular junctions. However, because of the septal malalignment, there is an anomalous location of the atrioventricular conduction axis (Milo et al, 1979). Kirklin and his colleagues (1988) labelled such malformations the juxtacrux defect. We will deal with them in the chapter devoted to straddling atrioventricular valves (Chapter 41). This should not obscure the fact, however, that similar septal malalignment can be found in the setting of a common atrioventricular junction (see Chapter 36).

In those perimembranous defects that open to the inlet of the right ventricle, the septal leaflet of the tricuspid valve is frequently divided or deficient. If the two components of the abnormal leaflet are at all bound down to the margins, then shunting can occur from left ventricle to right atrium (Leung et al, 1986). Such shunting is frequently held to be caused by absence of the atrioventricular membranous septum (Gerbode et al, 1958) but this is a very unusual mechanism (McKay et al, 1989). It is the location of the hinge of the septal leaflet that is the key to differentiation between a perimembranous ventricular septal defect with atrioventricular shunting and a membranous atrioventricular septal defect (Figure 37.15).

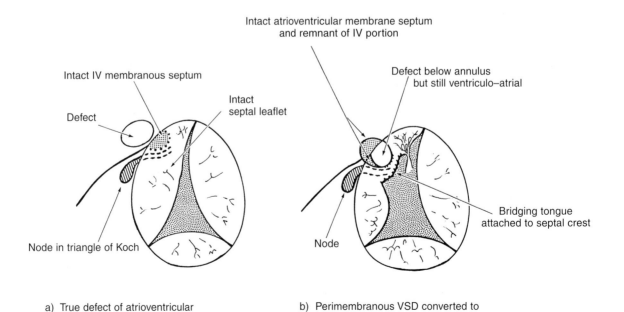

a) True defect of atrioventricular component of membranous septum

b) Perimembranous VSD converted to left ventricular–right atrial shunt

Figure 37.15. It is the relationship of defects to the hinge of the tricuspid valve that differentiates between a deficiency of the atrioventricular membranous septum (a) and a perimembranous defect shunting from left ventricle to right atrium because of an associated deficiency of the tricuspid valve (b). IV, interventricular.

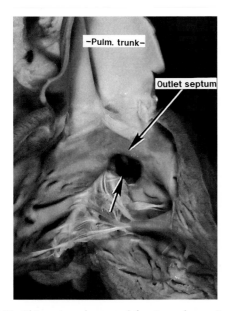

Figure 37.16. This perimembranous defect (note the aortic–tricuspid valvar continuity, arrowed) opens to the outlet of the right ventricle.

The other frequent type of perimembranous defect is the one that extends so as to open primarily beneath the ventricular outlets. The feature of these defects is that the medial papillary muscle is related to the posteroinferior rim and, more significantly, the outlet septum becomes recognizable as a discrete entity within the right ventricle (Figure 37.16), often being malaligned relative to the rest of the muscular septum (Figure 37.11b). When there is antero–cephalad malalignment of the outlet septum, then the orifice of the aortic valve overrides the muscular ventricular septum (Figure 37.11). Such malalignment defects opening between the outlets in the presence of aortic overriding are closely related to tetralogy of Fallot (see Chapter 46). The distinction between the two entities depends upon the presence or absence of muscular infundibular stenosis. The outlet septum can also be deviated posteriorly into the left ventricular outflow tract (Becu et al, 1955). This usually produces subaortic obstruction (Figure 37.12) and is almost always associated with obstructive lesions of the aortic arch, either severe tubular hypoplasia or interruption, the latter found most frequently between the brachiocephalic and common carotid arteries (Van Praagh and McNamara, 1968; Moulaert et al, 1976; Ho et al, 1983; Kutsche and Van Mierop, 1983). It was previously held that the pulmonary valvar orifice overrode the muscular ventricular septum in such defects. We now know that, because of the length of the free-standing subpulmonary infundibulum, valvar overriding is rare, usually being seen only when the defect is doubly committed and juxta-arterial (Al Marsafawy et al, 1995). In these defects with the outlet septum positioned towards the left ventricle, the abnormal location of the septum can be caused by angular septal malalignment as seen in the short-axis longitudinal deviation, or by a combination of the two.

Appreciation of these facts helps in the interpretation of the echocardiographic images (see below).

Irrespective of whether a perimembranous defect extends to open between the inlet or outlet ventricular components (or is confluent), the basic distribution of the axis for atrioventricular conduction is the same, although there are important subtle differences between the sub-types. In the normal heart, the penetrating component of the atrioventricular conduction axis passes through the central fibrous body, branching on the crest of the muscular ventricular septum. Since the central fibrous body forms the posteroinferior margin of perimembranous defects, this will be the site of penetration of the axis. The landmark of the atrioventricular node, as in the normal heart, is the apex of the triangle of Koch. When the defect opens to the right ventricular inlet, the triangle may itself be displaced posteriorly. Nonetheless, the apex of the triangle (and hence the site of the penetrating bundle) will be normally positioned. When the axis has penetrated through the central fibrous body, it is generally related to the posteroinferior rim of the perimembranous defect (Figure 37.17) (Truex and Bishof, 1958; Lev, 1960; Titus et al, 1963). The precise relationship of its non-branching component to the septal crest depends upon the location of the defect (Milo et al, 1980). It is much closer to the crest when a defect opens to the inlet, becoming more remote as the defect extends to open between the outlets. Very occasionally, the branching bundle may be positioned directly astride the septum in an outlet defect, but this is an exceptional finding (Titus et al, 1963; Anderson et al, 1977).

Because perimembranous defects are closely related to the septal leaflet of the tricuspid valve, there is always the possibility that they may be closed by plastering down of the leaflet across the defect (Figure 37.18). The most likely defects to close in this fashion are small ones opening to the right ventricular inlet. Defects between the outlet components, particularly when complicated by

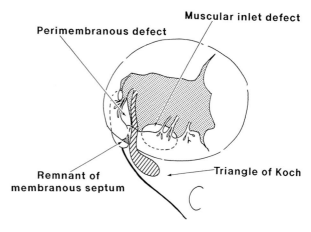

Figure 37.17. The atrioventricular conduction axis (hatched area), as viewed by the surgeon through the tricuspid valve, is to the right hand edge of a perimembranous defect, but to the left hand margin of a muscular defect opening to the inlet of the right ventricle.

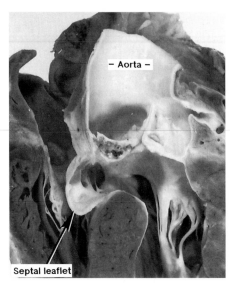

Figure 37.18. This perimembranous defect has been closed by plastering down of the septal leaflet of the tricuspid valve.

malalignment, are unlikely to close by this mechanism. Neither are extensive inlet defects. A closely related mechanism of closure is aneurysmal enlargement of fibrous tissue in the environs of the defect (Figure 37.19). Although often described as aneurysms of the membranous septum (Varghese and Rowe, 1969), it is unusual for the remnant of the membranous septum itself to be involved. In most cases, the grape-like lesions are sculpted from the underside of the leaflets of the tricuspid valve (Chesler et al, 1968). On occasion, the tags can be more extensive hammock-like lesions, with cordal attachments to the septum. In other cases, the aneurysmal tags can be found surrounding the defect (Figure

37.19). The defects most likely to be closed in this fashion are again small defects opening to the inlet (Somerville, 1979; Anderson et al, 1983; Beerman et al, 1985). The presence of tissue tags is known to indicate that defects have a better chance of spontaneous closure, a better clinical evolution and, hence, that there will be less necessity for surgical closure (Ramaciotti et al, 1986). On rare occasions, however, the tags can become sufficiently large as to balloon into the right ventricular outflow tract and produce subpulmonary obstruction (Bonvicini et al, 1982).

Aneurysmal prolapse of the right coronary leaflet of the aortic valve can be found in the setting of perimembranous defects, particularly those opening between the outlets when the outlet septum is markedly deficient. Prolapse of the non-coronary aortic leaflet has also been described (Van Praagh and McNamara, 1968; Tatsuno et al, 1973). Rarely, such valvar prolapse may produce partial or complete plugging of the defect and result in spontaneous closure (Moss and Siassi, 1970). In all of these possible mechanisms of closure or diminution in size, contraction and fibrosis around the edges of the defect are contributory factors.

MUSCULAR DEFECTS

Defects with entirely muscular rims can exist anywhere in the muscular septum. They, too, can be divided into those opening between the inlets, apical trabecular or outlet components (Figure 37.6). Muscular defects themselves can be multiple, particularly when in the apical trabecular septum, or can coexist with perimembranous or juxta-arterial defects. Muscular defects opening between the inlets are largely covered by the septal leaflet of the tricuspid valve (Figure 37.20). When they are towards the crux, there is no difficulty in distinguishing them from perimembranous defects opening to the inlet. When such a muscular defect is close to the central fibrous body, differentiation is more difficult. The key is that, in the muscular defect, a muscular bar (which may be quite small) interposes between the hingepoints of the leaflets of the mitral and tricuspid valves (Figure 37.20). The leaflets are in fibrous continuity when a perimembranous defect opens between the inlet components (Figure 37.8). This difference is crucial. In the muscular defect, the atrioventricular conduction axis passes above, or anterosuperior to, the defect (to the left hand as viewed by the surgeon). It is always beneath (or posteroinferior) a perimembranous defect (to the right hand as viewed by the surgeon; see Figure 37.17).

Muscular defects in the apical trabecular septum are frequently large holes that tend to be found to one or other side of the septomarginal trabeculation. Not infrequently, a single opening (as viewed from the left ventricular aspect) is crossed by trabeculations to produce two (or more) openings when viewed from the right ven-

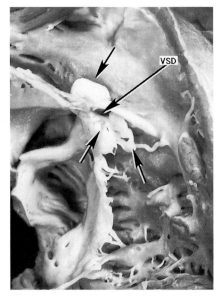

Figure 37.19. In this perimembranous defect, it is the formation of tissue tags from the leaflets of the tricuspid valve (arrowed) that virtually close the hole. The tags do not originate from the remnant of the interventricular membranous septum.

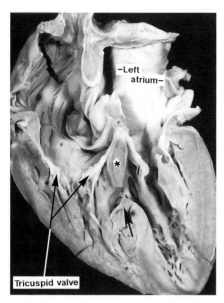

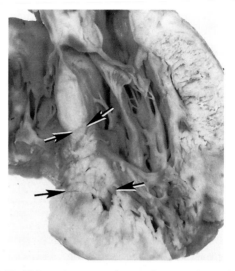

Figure 37.20. This simulated four chamber section shows a muscular inlet defect. The upper margin of the septum (star) produces off-setting of the leaflets of the atrioventricular valves. The arrow shows the ventricular septal crest.

Figure 37.22. This section across the apical septum shows the honeycomb arrangement between the arrows that produces the typical 'swiss-cheese' defects.

tricle (Figure 37.21). Multiple smaller muscular defects give the so-called 'swiss-cheese' septum. These may be particularly difficult to define in the postmortem specimen (Figure 37.22). Although the atrioventricular conduction axis is itself unrelated to muscular defects in the apical septum, the distal bundle branches may pass through the holes, producing 'pseudobifurcations' (Latham and Anderson, 1972). It is still unknown whether or not heart block could be produced by trauma at the defect and 'tracking' along the fibrous sheaths of the conduction fascicles to more proximal sites. It seems

unlikely, since there is no reported incidence of heart block following their repair.

Outlet, or infundibular, muscular defects are small and usually single (Figure 37.23). They can coexist with other defects. Their superior rim is the outlet septum (often attenuated) and the subpulmonary infundibulum, while the inferior muscular rim, which separates the defect from the membranous septum, is formed by fusion of the posterior limb of the septomarginal trabeculation with the ventriculo-infundibular fold. This muscle rim separates the conduction tissue axis from the crest of the septum, thus providing protection from surgical damage. This type of defect has previously been termed an intracristal defect (Rosenquist et al, 1973). Description of

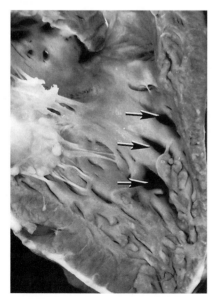

Figure 37.21. This heart has multiple muscular apical trabecular defects, but with a solitary opening within the left ventricle.

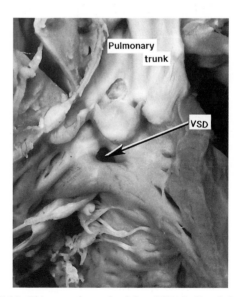

Figure 37.23. This muscular outlet defect (VSD) is directly beneath the hinge of the pulmonary valve but separated from it by the small muscular infundibulum.

the hole as having a muscular rim, and opening between the outlets, is more explicit. Small muscular defects probably close spontaneously simply by growth of the muscular structures surrounding them (Ferencz et al, 1993). They are almost certainly the most common defects undergoing spontaneous closure (Du et al, 1998; Krovetz, 1998).

DOUBLY COMMITTED JUXTA-ARTERIAL DEFECT

The defect is termed juxta-arterial because it is directly related to both aortic and pulmonary valves (Figure 37.9). It is because of this feature that both arterial valves frequently override the septum, giving a series of anomalies the end-point of which is double outlet left ventricle (Ueda and Becker, 1985). Such hearts with doubly committed juxta-arterial defects and overriding of both arterial valves have also been termed 'double outlet both ventricles' (Brandt et al, 1976). It is because the aortic valve is unsupported by the outlet septum that prolapse of its leaflets is so frequent with the juxta-arterial defect (Griffin et al, 1988). As discussed, nonetheless, aortic valvar prolapse can also lead to valvar insufficiency when a defect is perimembranous (Van Praagh and McNamara, 1968; Tatsuno et al, 1973). The relationship of the atrioventricular conduction axis depends on the posteroinferior margin. A well-formed muscular rim (Figure 37.9) protects the posteroinferior margin. In contrast, the atrioventricular bundle is more at risk when the doubly committed defect is also perimembranous (Figure 37.24).

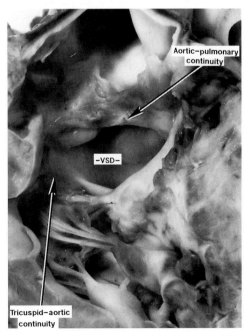

Figure 37.24. This doubly committed and juxta-arterial defect is also perimembranous because of the fibrous continuity between the leaflets of the aortic and tricuspid valves. VSD, ventricular septal defect.

MORPHOGENESIS

As described in Chapter 25, it is impossible to achieve normal closure of the embryonic interventricular communication until the right atrioventricular junction is connected to the right ventricle, and the subaortic outflow tract transferred to the left ventricle. Thereafter, the persisting interventricular communication is closed by tissue derived from various sources (see Chapter 21 for details). It is not closed specifically, however, by the interventricular membranous septum. When the interventricular communication is closed, the septal leaflet of the tricuspid valve has yet to be delaminated from the muscular septum (Lamers et al, 1995). There cannot, at this stage, be an interventricular component to the membranous septum. Perimembranous defects, therefore, cannot be explained simply on the basis of failure of closure of the embryonic interventricular communication by the interventricular component of the membranous septum. It is more likely that the muscular septum is deficient in the environs of the closing plug of tissue, which is a consequence of insufficient area or volume. Deficiency of the different parts of the muscular septum then accounts for the diversity in position and orientation of perimembranous defects.

The formation of muscular defects is more easily explained. It is now established that, at least in the chick, the muscular septum is produced by coalescence of embryonic trabeculations (Ben-Shachar et al, 1985). Muscular defects, therefore, likely result from failure of the trabeculations to coalesce. This produces the swiss cheese septum when extensive. Alternatively, there may be failure of fusion of the muscular septum with the free-standing septal component of the subpulmonary infundibulum, derived by muscularization of the outflow cushions. Such failure of fusion of the infundibulum with the muscular septum and the septomarginal trabeculation gives a good explanation for the muscular defect opening between the outlets. The doubly committed juxta-arterial defect, in contrast, is well explained simply on the basis of failure of formation of the muscular subpulmonary infundibulum. This defect, therefore, is closely related developmentally to common arterial trunk (see Chapter 51).

PATHOPHYSIOLOGY

The pathophysiology of ventricular septal defect is determined by the size of the defect and the state of the pulmonary vascular resistance. The site of the hole between the ventricles has little influence. Between them, size and resistance govern the direction and magnitude of flow through the defect, and thus the clinical features and symptomatology.

THE EFFECT OF SIZE

The size of the defect is dominant. Below a critical size, the defect itself presents a resistance to flow through it. This controls the magnitude but not the direction of the shunt. Above this critical size, there is no appreciable resistance to flow. Both magnitude and direction of flow are then determined by the level of pulmonary vascular resistance. There are few 'hard' data concerning this critical size. Some authorities (Rudolph, 1974; Graham et al, 1977) have made statements, unsupported by scientific investigation, to the effect that defects smaller than the aortic orifice are restrictive. In this respect, Sherman (1963), in his *Atlas of congenital heart disease*, pointed out that three quarters of the defects seen in hearts at postmortem from children are less than 75% of the diameter of the aorta. Perhaps more importantly, he noted that the smallest defects were observed in the oldest patients. Lucas et al (1961) attempted to quantify the critical size itself by comparing the diameter of the defect with body surface area. They found the critical size to be a defect with a diameter that was 1 cm/m^2 body surface area. This corresponds to an orificial area for the defect of approximately 0.8 cm^2/m^2. Defects having ratios smaller than this were restrictive and produced minor or no haemodynamic changes. This suggests that the critical size is smaller than the aortic orifice, since a normal aortic valvar orifice is calculated to be approximately 2.0 cm^2/m^2 body surface area. In practice, the judgement of size of the defect is generally made on haemodynamic grounds. When there is a left-to-right shunt, and no other associated anomalies such as pulmonary stenosis, a large defect is one that permits equalization of systolic pressures in the two ventricles. Such a defect is also unrestrictive. Since the right and left ventricles do not contract exactly simultaneously, there is always some inequality in the ventricular pressures. Consequently, throughout the greater part of systole, the pressure difference will promote left-to-right shunting. In 'isovolumic' relaxation, additional right-to-left shunting probably occurs. This is cleared by the subsequent diastolic left-to-right shunt unless right ventricular ejection is obstructed (Levin et al, 1967).

A restrictive defect, therefore, is one in which right ventricular and pulmonary arterial systolic pressures are lower than those in the left ventricle and aorta. The size of such defects may vary from those that are just restrictive (allowing some elevation of right-sided pressures) to small defects in which the right-sided pressures are normal. In effect, defects can be grouped into two categories: restrictive and unrestrictive. In the restrictive group, there is then a continuum of size between those large enough to allow a serious haemodynamic disturbance and those so small that there is only a small left-to-right shunt with normal right-sided pressures.

THE EFFECTS OF PULMONARY VASCULAR RESISTANCE

The effect of pulmonary resistance on the flow through restrictive defects is always secondary to size. The smaller the defect, the lower the flow through it. In unrestrictive defects, the pulmonary vascular resistance (and, to a lesser extent, systemic vascular resistance) is the controlling factor. When the pulmonary vascular resistance is low, the flow through the defect (and, therefore, pulmonary blood flow) will be high. Usually it is more than three times higher than systemic blood flow. Such a high pulmonary blood flow is not present at birth. It takes a finite time for the pulmonary resistance to fall from the high intrauterine to the normal postnatal levels. It is possible that the major fall is accomplished in the normal infant within the first 2 weeks of life (Dawes, 1968; Rudolph, 1970).

This fall may be delayed in infants with a large ventricular septal defect, and it may be limited in its extent. Contributory structural factors include limited postnatal growth of the lungs and limitation of the number of intra-acinar blood vessels. In addition, there is hypertrophy of the muscular coat of the intra-acinar arteries and veins (Wagenvoort et al, 1961; Naeye, 1966; Haworth et al, 1977; see Chapter 4). It is not entirely clear why growth of the lungs, and proliferation of pulmonary vessels, is limited. Muscular hypertrophy of the walls of the vessels, however, is probably secondary to the increased pulmonary flow. Such high pulmonary blood flow leads to increased left atrial pressure, which is known to cause pulmonary vasoconstriction in experimental animals (Rudolph, 1965). If the vasoconstriction is maintained, vascular muscular hypertrophy will presumably occur.

This delay in the fall of the pulmonary resistance means that the maximal haemodynamic effects of an unrestrictive defect may not be reached for some weeks after birth. The time and course, and the extent of the fall in pulmonary resistance, are all variable. The maximal flow through the defect is usually achieved between 1 and 6 weeks of age. This is usually enough to allow a very high pulmonary blood flow, but it may be so limited that little flow occurs through the defect. Such patients may escape detection until the effects of severe pulmonary vascular disease have become apparent.

Once it has fallen to its lowest value, pulmonary vascular resistance may increase again with the development of the pathological changes of pulmonary vascular disease (Haworth et al, 1977; Rabinovitch et al, 1978). This usually occurs only in patients in whom the pulmonary arterial pressure is high from birth; consequently it is almost entirely confined to those with an unrestrictive defect. As the resistance rises, flow across the defect decreases. When pulmonary vascular resistance exceeds that in the systemic circuit, the flow through the defect will change from left to right to a flow from right to left.

Thus, the level of resistance determines the direction of flow. Secondary effects of severe pulmonary vascular disease include enlargement of the right ventricle and the pulmonary trunk, and dilation of the infundibular attachments of the leaflets of the pulmonary valve. These may cause detectable, but usually haemodynamically insignificant, pulmonary regurgitation.

When defects are restrictive, there is wide spectrum of restrictiveness. In many, the defect is so small that the pulmonary vascular resistance has little or no effect on the magnitude of flow through it. In others, the defect is restrictive (not allowing equalization of pressures between the two ventricles) but is big enough to permit a significant elevation of right ventricular and pulmonary arterial pressures. In these defects, the level of pulmonary vascular resistance will play a significant (albeit subordinate) role in controlling the magnitude of flow of blood to the lungs. Between the two extremes of restrictive defects, there is a continuum of size and, therefore, of pathophysiological effects.

THE EFFECT OF OBSTRUCTION OF THE PULMONARY OUTFLOW TRACT

The above discussion has presumed an unobstructed pulmonary outflow tract. If there is coexisting obstruction within the right ventricular outflow tract (either valvar or subvalvar), then the resistance to ejection from the right ventricle will have a similar effect to elevation of the pulmonary vascular resistance. The flow through an unrestrictive defect (and thence pulmonary blood flow) will be limited in proportion to the severity of the obstruction. In restrictive defects, obstruction to the right ventricular outflow will result in elevation of right ventricular pressure, again in proportion to the severity of obstruction. The right ventricular pressure, in extreme cases, may come to exceed that in the left ventricle. As in unrestrictive defects, obstruction of the pulmonary outflow tract in the larger of the restrictive defects will also have a limiting effect on the magnitude of flow. There will be a reversal in the direction of the shunt in all cases where right ventricular pressure exceeds that in the left ventricle. Although pulmonary valvar obstruction may be present unequivocally from birth, subvalvar obstruction can be acquired.

THE CARDIAC RESPONSE TO VENTRICULAR SEPTAL DEFECT

The cardiac effects of a ventricular septal defect depend initially on the magnitude of pulmonary flow. With florid pulmonary flow (usually in non-restrictive defects), left atrial and left ventricular end-diastolic volumes are increased. Left ventricular muscle mass is always increased (Jarmakani et al, 1969). Studies of pressure and volume in the left ventricle demonstrate the marked increase in left ventricular work imposed by a large defect (Jarmakani et al, 1968). This necessitates left ventricular hypertrophy as a compensatory mechanism. With extreme pulmonary flow, there is also an increase in right ventricular dimensions. Because of the elevated right ventricular pressure, there will be an even more marked increase in right ventricular work. This results in additional right ventricular hypertrophy. This hypertrophic response may be one mechanism for the development of subvalvar pulmonary stenosis.

Left ventricular work is increased by restrictive defects in relation to the pulmonary flow, but the right ventricle is relatively spared. Consequently, there is left ventricular hypertrophy but little increase in right ventricular size or muscle mass. With elevation of pulmonary vascular resistance, or with development of right ventricular outflow obstruction, left ventricular work is diminished because of the decrease in pulmonary flow. The elevation of right ventricular pressure then results in right ventricular hypertrophy, which dominates the picture.

The pathophysiological effects of a ventricular septal defect can, in three situations, result in congestive cardiac failure. The first is an unrestrictive defect with high pulmonary blood flow, when the compensatory mechanisms are insufficient always to provide an adequate systemic flow. These mechanisms include recruitment of all sarcomeres to operate at their optimal end-diastolic length, muscular hypertrophy of right and left ventricles and increased catecholamine drive to the ventricles. Those circumstances are usually reached before the age of 6 months. The second situation occurs much later. It is encountered when the right ventricular myocardium has undergone degenerative changes as a consequence of long-term ejection against high resistance. This is found with pulmonary vascular disease and with prolonged and severe obstruction to the right ventricular outflow tract. The third situation is when a ventricular septal defect is complicated by aortic regurgitation. This imposes a further volume load on the left ventricle. It results in cardiac failure when the reflex is severe enough to outstrip the compensatory mechanisms as discussed above. It is most frequently seen in older children and adults.

CLINICAL FEATURES

PRESENTATION

The typical murmur of a ventricular septal defect is rarely heard at birth, since it takes time for the pulmonary vascular resistance to fall from the high levels of fetal life, which are sufficiently high to limit the flow through even an unrestrictive defect to levels insufficient to provide an audible murmur. Should there be any suspicion concerning the cardiac status, nonetheless, and should an ultrasonic examination be performed, then the diagnosis should be made. In fact, the diagnosis can now be made during fetal life by means of echocardiographic screening, albeit that a recent detailed study failed to detect three quarters of the cases seen within the population screened (Yagel et al, 1997). Even when cases are diagnosed during fetal life, it is necessary to exercise caution, since three quarters of those recognized in another study (Orie et al, 1994) subsequently closed spontaneously. Furthermore, very few, if any, of those diagnosed during fetal life will have the full clinical picture at birth. If diagnosis is made in the neonatal nursery, it is almost invariably during examination of the baby just prior to the mother's discharge. At the end of the first week of life, when any murmurs are detected, it is rare for the pulmonary vascular resistance to have fallen sufficiently for the patient to be symptomatic. Symptoms, when they occur, are related to the high pulmonary blood flow. Diminished lung compliance, and elevation of the left atrial pressure as a result of the high pulmonary blood flow, initially causes tachypnoea. This progresses with the onset of congestive cardiac failure to give dyspnoea on effort. This becomes obvious when the baby feeds. In a baby with a typical unrestrictive or large restrictive defect, the parents are likely to complain that feeds take progressively longer over the first month or two of life and lead to rapid exhaustion of the baby. Not only is the feeding prolonged, but it does not provide sufficient caloric intake for weight gain. With the development of severe cardiac failure, the baby will become obviously dyspnoeic even at rest. Intercostal, subcostal and supraclavicular recession are then readily seen. This increased work of respiration imposes an increased requirement for energy, which is not satisfied because of the difficulty of feeding. The vicious circle results in failure to thrive. Failure to thrive is, indeed, an alternative mode of presentation in infancy. It occurs in those babies with defects large enough to allow high pulmonary blood flow, but in whom the size of the defect, or the level of pulmonary vascular resistance, prevents the development of intractable congestive cardiac failure. Another association with high pulmonary blood flow is an increased susceptibility to respiratory infection. The parents may complain that their baby has frequent 'chesty' colds. It may be during such an episode that a murmur is noted, and that cardiac failure is precipitated.

A small and restrictive defect may be detected at any age by the discovery of a murmur. But such a defect will rarely, if ever, cause symptoms. When a defect is found in this fashion after the age of 1 year, it is highly unlikely that, in itself, it will ever cause congestive cardiac failure. No such assurance can be given when discovery occurs in early infancy.

There is a further small group of patients with ventricular septal defect who escape detection in infancy. They present with diminished effort tolerance and cyanosis during middle childhood or adolescence. These patients usually have severe pulmonary vascular disease. Even careful history-taking fails to elicit evidence of symptoms during infancy. It is probable that at no stage did their pulmonary vascular resistance fall to levels that permitted sufficient left-to-right shunting to allow recognition of the defect.

Another alternative, and rare, presentation is with respiratory symptoms from bronchial compression caused by the grossly enlarged pulmonary arteries. Typically, it is the right middle lobe bronchus that is compressed, but the left main and upper lobe bronchuses may also be involved (Stanger et al, 1969). This presentation is most frequently seen in patients with severe pulmonary vascular disease.

Ventricular septal defects, therefore, rarely present in the first days of life. In those with small restrictive defects, presentation is by the incidental discovery of a murmur, the patient remaining asymptomatic. In those with large but restrictive defects, and with unrestrictive defects, the initial finding may be a murmur, but symptoms rapidly ensue. It may be the symptoms of dyspnoea and failure to thrive that call attention to the heart. Presentation occurs only at the point of recognition of a right-to-left shunt in those rare patients with irreversible vascular disease, who may also present because of respiratory problems.

PHYSICAL EXAMINATION

The appearance of the patient is again dependent on the magnitude of flow through the defect. Those with small and restrictive defects are generally entirely normal. With large restrictive defects, but without frank congestive cardiac failure, patients tend to be small and thin for their age, with evidence of dyspnoea such as intercostal recession. Chronicity is suggested by a depression at the insertion of the diaphragm. This depression is at the site described by Harrison (a Lincolnshire general practitioner, 1766–1838) as a late effect of rickets (Bailey and Clain, 1954). There will also be bulging of the left chest, indicating cardiomegaly. In presence of large unrestrictive defects, similar appearance of more severe degree will be seen without the evidence of chronicity. Cyanosis will not be seen except in those older patients with severe pulmonary vascular disease or in those with severe obstruction within the right ventricular outflow tract.

A systolic thrill is felt in almost all patients, except those with tiny muscular or perimembranous defects. When a thrill is present, it is localized to the second, third and fourth intercostal spaces at the left sternal border. If the thrill is maximal in the first intercostal space or higher, and yet the auscultatory features are otherwise typical of a ventricular septal defect, the likelihood is that the defect is doubly committed and juxta-arterial (Steinfeld et al, 1972). There are usually no other palpable abnormalities in the presence of small restrictive defects. When the defect is large, with a high flow, the cardiac impulse will be hyperdynamic and the thrill may be more widespread. In presence of severe pulmonary vascular disease, the striking features are a localized left parasternal heave of right ventricular type and a palpable second sound. The peripheral pulses are normal. Abnormalities such as a pulse with high volume or absence of the femoral pulse should suggest an associated arterial duct or coarctation, respectively.

The most typical auscultatory finding, namely the loud pan-systolic murmur localized to the second and third left intercostal spaces, was not accepted as being caused by a ventricular septal defect at Roger's initial presentation to the Académie de Médicine (1879). This murmur is typical of many ventricular septal defects with a left-to-right shunt, even when they are small and restrictive. The murmur starts with the first sound and continues up to the second sound. If the murmur starts with the first heart sound but stops short of the second, the defect is likely to be a small muscular one closing in late systole. Large unrestrictive defects in infants sometimes give rise to a shortened ejection systolic murmur that is not accompanied by a thrill. It is said that a pan-systolic murmur may continue past the aortic component of the second heart sound (Harris et al, 1976). This is rarely appreciated by the ear. Similarly, the ear usually does not detect any variation in the intensity of the murmur, although phonocardiography does show that the murmur is loudest during mid-systole. When pulmonary flow is limited by pulmonary resistance, the systolic murmur is abbreviated and may be completely absent. In such cases, an early diastolic murmur of pulmonary regurgitation may be heard, as well as a pulmonary click. In patients who have an excessive pulmonary flow, the flow through the mitral valve is sufficient to produce a mid-diastolic murmur at the apex. The presence of this murmur is taken to indicate that pulmonary flow is more than twice the systemic flow. In patients with no other signs of pulmonary vascular disease, the appearance of a high-pitched early diastolic murmur is highly suggestive of the onset of aortic regurgitation.

In the absence of pulmonary vascular disease, the heart sounds appear normal. It is claimed that the second heart sound is widely split, with delay of its pulmonary component (Graham et al, 1977). In our experience, this is rarely appreciated on auscultation, although it is seen on phonocardiography. The pulmonary second sound is louder in patients with pulmonary hypertension. In severe hypertension, the increased intensity is easy to detect. In less severe cases, the fact that the second heart sound is audibly split at the apex indicates that the pulmonary component is louder than normal. Development of this finding during follow-up should alert to the possibility of development of pulmonary vascular disease. The second heart sound becomes single once severe pulmonary vascular disease has developed (Sutton et al, 1968).

INVESTIGATIONS

ELECTROCARDIOGRAPHY

The electrocardiographic features are not specific for ventricular septal defect. As may be expected, they do reflect the haemodynamic status. In patients with large unrestrictive defects presenting with a high pulmonary blood flow in infancy, there will be a normal sinus rhythm (probably with tachycardia), a frontal QRS axis within the normal range for age and biventricular hypertrophy. Finding a superior axis suggests multiple defects (Fox et al, 1978), that the lesion is the ventricular component of an atrioventricular septal defect or that an isolated perimembranous defect with separate atrioventricular junctions excavates extensively to open to the right ventricular inlet. Tall T waves over the right precordial leads in infancy strongly suggest that the right ventricular pressure is at systemic levels. Cardiac rhythm, and the QRS axis, is usually normal in large restrictive defects after the first few months of life. The QRS pattern is that of left ventricular dominance, with deep Q waves over the left chest leads indicating left ventricular volume overload. The electrocardiogram may be entirely normal in patients with small restrictive defects.

Serial electrocardiograms provide more prognostic information in the early months of life than does a single tracing. Large and unrestrictive defects maintain the biventricular QRS morphology, while the smaller defects show the normal diminution of right ventricular forces with age. At any age, the presence of pulmonary vascular disease, or severe obstruction to the right ventricular outflow tract, is reflected by right without left ventricular hypertrophy, and by right-axis deviation. Should aortic regurgitation complicate a small ventricular septal defect or, alternatively, occur in a patient with established obstruction of the right ventricular outflow tract, then the changes of left ventricular volume overload will come to dominate the picture.

RADIOLOGY

Once more, radiological findings reflect the haemodynamic state. The chest radiograph is usually entirely normal in the first days of life. With the development of left-to-right shunting, the lung fields become plethoric. When the pulmonary blood flow is large (as in unrestrictive defects), cardiomegaly is noted and pulmonary plethora is marked. The cardiac contour in such infants has no specific features. When defects are restrictive, with only mild elevation of the pulmonary blood flow, the chest radiograph may always appear normal.

The development and progression of pulmonary vascular disease is reflected in diminution of the peripheral pulmonary vascular shadows, leading to the classical 'pruning' of the peripheral pulmonary arteries, seen best in older children and adults. This is accompanied by progressive overall reduction in heart size as the pulmonary blood flow falls, but with characteristic enlargement of the pulmonary knob. When obstruction develops in the right ventricular outflow tract, there is reduction in both central and peripheral pulmonary arterial shadowing, but enlargement of the pulmonary trunk is rare. When complicated by aortic regurgitation, there will be progressive enlargement of the heart with the cardiac contour suggesting left ventricular dominance.

ECHOCARDIOGRAPHY

Cross-sectional echocardiographic examination (Bierman et al, 1980; Cheatham et al, 1981; van Mill et al, 1981; Sutherland et al, 1982; Capelli et al, 1983) is now recognized as the technique of choice for diagnosis (Driscoll et al, 1994). Not only does the technique show the presence of a defect, it also permits its accurate localization. Furthermore, because the defect should be identified in more than one plane, its size can be estimated. Perimembranous defects are recognized in long-axis, four chamber and short-axis views, with fibrous continuity between the leaflets of the tricuspid and mitral or aortic valves being the pathognomic feature. Perimembranous defects opening to the inlet of the right ventricle are recognized by cuts through the ventricular inlets (Figure 37.25). The four chamber sections will demonstrate tricuspid to mitral valvar continuity via the central fibrous body, with loss of the usual offsetting of the hingepoints of the leaflets. The key to recognition of defects opening between the outlets is recognition in the subcostal right oblique cut of the muscular outlet septum seen as an intracardiac structure immediately beneath the subpulmonary infundibulum (Figure 37.26). This is evidence of biventricular aortic connection (Alva et al, 1998).

The parasternal short-axis cut at the level of the aortic valve will similarly show this discrete outlet septum (Figure 37.27). When this feature is present, the parasternal long-axis section will usually demonstrate overriding of the aortic valve. For those outlet defects associated with posterior longitudinal deviation of the outlet septum, usually in the setting of aortic coarctation or interruption, the parasternal long-axis section will be the optimal plane for diagnosis. Muscular defects opening between the inlets are best seen in the four chamber cuts but retain the feature of atrioventricular valvar off-setting (Figure 37.28). Large trabecular muscular defects are identified in four chamber and short-axis planes (Figure 37.29), while outlet muscular defects are identified from long-axis or subcostal approaches. The best view with which to distinguish perimembranous from muscular outlet defects is the high parasternal short-axis section. This cut demonstrates the presence or absence of tricuspid–aortic valvar continuity. Small or multiple trabecular muscular defects are those least likely to be visualized without the aid of colour flow mapping. Doubly committed juxta-arterial defects are recognized because of the continuity of the leaflets of the aortic and pulmonary valves in the roof of the defect, with absence of much of the subpulmonary infundibulum. These features are seen in long-axis (Figure 37.30), short-axis and subcostal right oblique views (Figure 37.31). If present, prolapse of the aortic valvar leaflets will be visualized (Figure 37.32). By rotating the transducer to focus on the leaflets of the tricuspid valve, it is also possible to show whether a doubly committed juxta-arterial defect is perimembranous or is separated from the central fibrous body by a muscular rim. This feature will best be appreciated from the parasternal short-axis section across the aortic valve. Cross-sectional echocardiography also demonstrates the proximity of the defect to structures that may close it, such as aneurysmal formation of tricuspid tissue tags (Figures 37.19 and 37.33) or plastering of the tricuspid valvar leaflet tissue across the defect (Figure 37.18). Although transoesophageal echocardiography is not usually necessary in the delineation of ventricular septal defect in childhood, it may provide crucial information when there is straddling or overriding of the tricuspid valve (see Chapter 42). Identification of the site of the ventricular septal defect at initial examination will also provide hard evidence on the

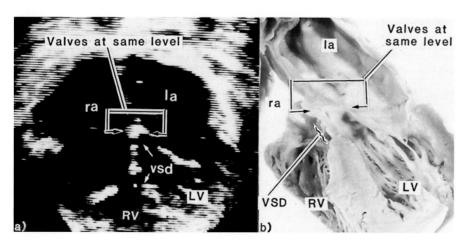

Figure 37.25. This cross-sectional echocardiogram, with a comparable specimen, shows the features of a perimembranous defect (vsd) opening to the inlet of the right ventricle. ra and la, right and left atriums, respectively; RV and LV, right and left ventricles, respectively.

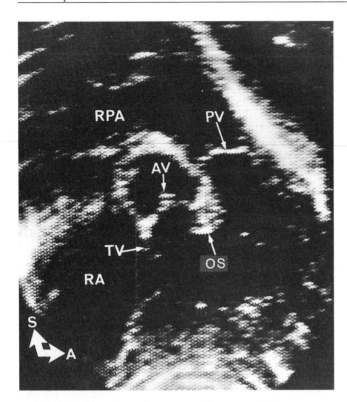

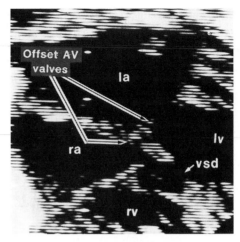

Figure 37.28. This echocardiogram, taken in long-axis four chamber section, shows the features of a muscular inlet defect. The hinges of the atrioventricular (AV) valves retain their normal off-set arrangement. Abbreviations as for Figure 37.25.

Figure 37.26. This echocardiogram in right anterior oblique section shows the features of a perimembranous defect opening to the outlet of the right ventricle with overriding of the aortic valve. OS, outlet septum; PV, pulmonary valve; RPA, right pulmonary artery; TV, tricuspid valve; AV, aortic valve; RA, right atrium.

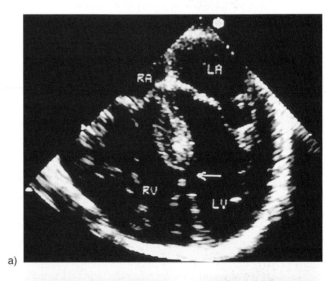

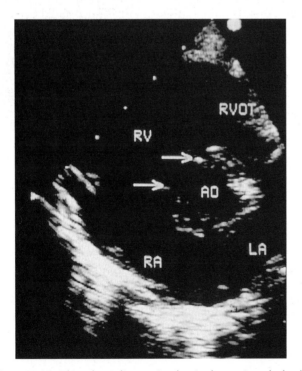

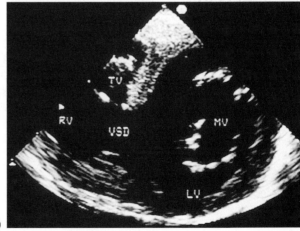

Figure 37.27. This echocardiogram is taken in short axis at the level of the aortic valve, showing a perimembranous defect (between arrows) opening to the outlet of the right ventricle (RVOT). Abbreviations as in Figures 37.25 and 37.26.

Figure 37.29. These sections, obtained in four chamber (a) and short-axis (b) cuts from the transoesophageal portal, illustrate the features of a muscular defect (VSD, arrow in a) opening between the apical trabecular components. Abbreviations as in Figure 37.25.

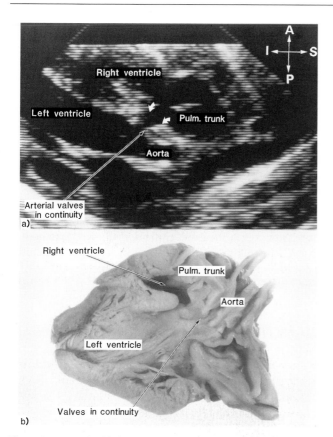

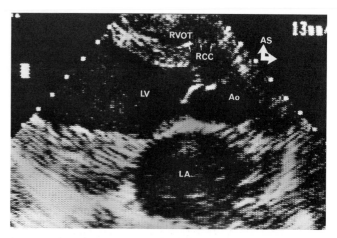

Figure 37.32. This parasternal long-axis section of a doubly committed juxta-arterial defect shows prolapse of the right coronary leaflet (RCC) of the aortic (Ao) valve into the right ventricular outflow tract (RVOT). LV, left ventricle; LA, left atrium.

Figure 37.30. A doubly committed juxta-arterial defect seen in long-axis parasternal section (a) with a comparable section in a heart from a different patient (b).

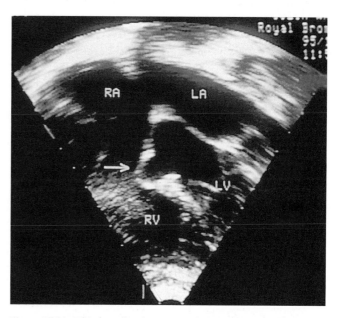

Figure 37.33. This four chamber section shows a fibrous tissue tag from the tricuspid valve (arrowed) partially closing a perimembranous ventricular septal defect. Abbreviations as in Figure 37.25.

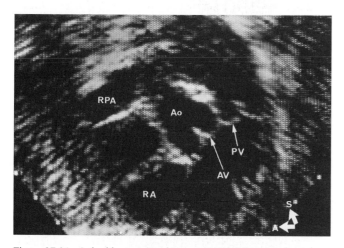

Figure 37.31. A doubly committed juxta-arterial defect seen in subcostal oblique paracoronal section. The aortic (AV) and pulmonary (PV) valves are seen in fibrous continuity, but the septum is not visualized. RPA, right pulmonary artery; RA, right atrium; Ao, aorta.

rate of spontaneous closure for different types of defect in different sites (Krovetz, 1998).

In addition to these specific diagnostic findings, the echocardiogram also reflects the haemodynamic state. Left atrial and left ventricular dilation are easily seen in infants with a high pulmonary blood flow, the left ventri-

cle being hyperdynamic. With large unrestrictive defects, there will be a concomitant increase in right ventricular dimensions, while in small restrictive defects the ventricular size and performance may be normal. Further insight into the physiological state is obtained by studying the motion of the leaflets of the pulmonary valve. With a high pulmonary flow, but a low pulmonary vascular resistance, the motion is normal. When there is a high pulmonary vascular resistance, the closure line of the leaflets is flattened and the a-dip disappears. The onset of aortic regurgitation is indicated by the appearance of diastolic vibration of the mitral valve, well-appreciated in earlier times on the M-mode tracing but now visualized directly with colour flow mapping. In this case, the cross-sectional echocardiogram should show the abnormalities of the aortic valve responsible for the regurgitation. For example, a prolapsing aortic valvar leaflet may be demonstrated (Figure 37.32); alternatively, perforations and vegetations associated with infective endocarditis may be identified.

As might be expected, all the advantages of cross-sectional echocardiography in diagnosis are accentuated when enhanced by three-dimensional reconstruction. Although such techniques are not yet generally available, the recently reported experience of Kardon and his colleagues (1998) points to their immense potential.

DOPPLER INTERROGATION

The complete evaluation of a ventricular septal defect includes not only an assessment of the size, site and number of defects, but also an estimate of the haemodynamic consequences. By using continuous wave Doppler ultrasound, it is possible to measure the velocity of blood flow across any ventricular septal defect. Then, by invoking the principles of the Bernoulli equation, it is possible to calculate the instantaneous peak systolic pressure drop between the right and the left ventricle. Assuming that the left ventricular peak systolic pressure is the same as the systolic blood pressure, the right ventricular systolic pressure can then be estimated. In the absence of any obstruction within the right ventricular outflow tract obstruction, this can be presumed to be equal to the pulmonary arterial systolic pressure. Infants and children with congenital cardiac defects, including those with a ventricular septal defect, frequently have mild tricuspid insufficiency. In this situation, it is possible to estimate the pressure drop across the tricuspid valve and, therefore, to estimate the right ventricular and pulmonary arterial systolic pressures. A potential source of error arises, however, when there is a shunt from left ventricle to right atrium through the defect via a deficiency in the septal leaflet of the tricuspid valve. In this situation, the regurgitant jet reflects the pressure drop between the left ventricle and right atrium.

Colour flow mapping has greatly facilitated the echocardiographic diagnosis of ventricular septal defect (Gatzoulis et al, 1997). Its most important uses include accurate alignment of the Doppler beam with the flow of blood, thus enhancing accurate quantification of velocity, the detection of multiple ventricular septal defects and the demonstration of shunting from left ventricle to right atrium. Colour flow mapping also plays a role in distinguishing innocent murmurs from those caused by very small ventricular septal defects.

Precordial cross-sectional echocardiography detects the vast majority of even small ventricular septal defects. In a small number of patients, especially older children, adolescents and adults, transoesophageal echocardio-graphy may be required for complete assessment. This technique may also be of particular value during the peri-operative period in the operating theatre and intensive care unit, especially to evaluate residual shunts. An important further use of transoesophageal echocardiography is to distinguish between a ruptured sinus of Valsalva and a perimembranous ventricular septal defect associated with aortic insufficiency. The technique is also indispensible when attempting closure of ventricular septal defects by interventional catheterization because it allows precise positioning of the paired umbrellas on either side of the defect. Three-dimensional echocardiography, at present, represents a growing area of research but is not yet a routine clinical tool. Reconstruction achieved in this fashion, nonetheless, can provide additional information about the morphological features of a ventricular septal defect.

MAGNETIC RESONANCE IMAGING

As may be anticipated, magnetic resonance imaging clearly shows the location and structure of defects (Figures 37.34 and 37.35). Hardly ever, however, is there a clinical indication for this investigation.

NUCLEAR ANGIOGRAPHY

First-pass studies in nuclear angiography demonstrate the presence of either a left-to-right or a right-to-left shunt and permit quantification of the ratios of systemic-to-pulmonary flow (Gates et al, 1973; Alderson et al, 1975).

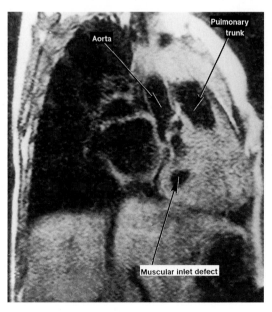

Figure 37.34. This resonance image, taken so as to be in the plane of the muscular ventricular septum, shows a muscular ventricular septal defect opening between the ventricular inlets.

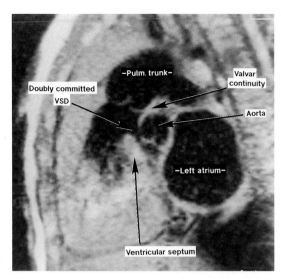

Figure 37.35. The features of a doubly committed and juxta-arterial defect are well seen in this magnetic resonance images.

Gated blood-pool scans allow assessment of left ventricular size and performance but do not differentiate the different sites or type of defect. These techniques are of value in long-term postoperative assessment, particularly when performed in association with an exercise or stress-testing protocol (Maron et al, 1973).

CARDIAC CATHETERIZATION

Prior to the advances made in cross-sectional echocardiography, catheterization was an essential part of the assessment of large restrictive and unrestrictive defects. It made possible the measurement of intracardiac pressures, particularly the pulmonary arterial pressure, along with quantification of pulmonary blood flow. From this information, it is possible to calculate the pulmonary vascular resistance. In addition, the technique provides confirmation of the interventricular location of the defect by the detection of a step-up in oxygen saturation at ventricular level, or by visualization of the passage of the catheter from right to left ventricle or to the aorta. If a ventricular septal defect is modified by abnormalities of the tricuspid valve to function as a shunt from left ventricle to right atrium, then the step-up in oxygen saturation is detected in the right atrium. This is also found, nonetheless, when a ventricular septal defect coexists with an atrial septal defect, or when there is an atrioventricular septal defect. Cardiac catheterization provided further information about the associated defects. Passage of the catheter from the pulmonary trunk to the descending aorta, for example, indicates the presence of a communication between these two arteries, usually an arterial duct.

The findings at catheterization reflect the pathophysiology. Unrestrictive defects with a high pulmonary blood flow have similar pressures in right and left ventricles. With an unobstructed right ventricular outflow tract, and a low pulmonary vascular resistance, the pulmonary arterial systemic pressure will be similar to that in the aorta. The diastolic and mean pulmonary arterial pressures, however, will be lower than aortic pressures. In such cases, a high pulmonary blood flow will be measured oximetrically or by dye dilution curves. In large but restrictive defects, the right ventricular and pulmonary arterial pressures will be lower than those in the left ventricle and aorta. At the end of the 1990s, the main indication for cardiac catheterization is to establish, beyond doubt, that a patient suspected to have pulmonary vascular disease does have an elevation of pulmonary vascular resistance so great as to render them inoperable.

ANGIOCARDIOGRAPHY

Although a case can still be made for performing catheterization in order to take measurements and calculate shunts and pressures, it is now rarely necessary to perform angiography. In the past, the technique was directed to anatomical delineation of the defect itself, and to the diagnosis or exclusion of associated abnormalities. Left ventricular angiocardiograms were best for anatomical diagnosis. If still performed, it is best to choose an axial oblique projection (Bargeron et al, 1977; Elliott et al, 1977; Soto et al, 1978; Green et al, 1981). The long-axis view is the best for demonstration of the different types of perimembranous defect (Figure 37.36; Santamaria et al, 1983). Doubly committed juxta-arterial defects will also be shown on this view, but demonstration of the lack of infundibular musculature separating the defect from the hingepoints of the leaflets of the pulmonary valve requires a right anterior oblique projection (Figure 37.37). The long-axis view is again best for demonstrating muscular defects in the apical trabecular septum (Figure 37.38). A muscular defect between the inlets is clearly demonstrated in the four chamber view (Figure 37.39a), while a muscular defect between the outlets is profiled in long-axial projection (Figure 37.39b). If there is doubt about the site of the defect, the long-axis view is helpful because defects opening to the right ventricular inlet appear behind the line of the anterior portion of the muscular septum. If performed, careful examination of the angiocardiograms should always be undertaken to exclude mitral regurgitation. In patients with pulmonary hypertension, a persistent arterial duct must always be excluded. This is frequently possible on the axial oblique left ventricular injection. When this is not the case, and echocardiography has not resolved the issues, aortography must be performed. A similar approach may also be necessary to exclude associated aortic coarctation. Retrograde aortography is important when aortic regurgitation is suspected. Right ventricular angiography is indicated when obstruction in the right

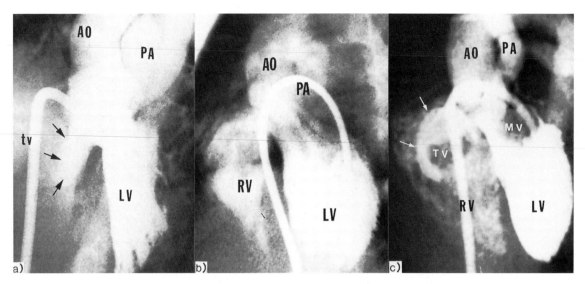

Figure 37.36. The different types of perimembranous defect as seen in long-axis projection of a left ventricular injection: (a) a defect opening to the inlet of the right ventricle; (b) a small trabecular defect; and (c) a defect extending to open into the right ventricular outlet. TV, tricuspid valve; MV, mitral valve; RV, right ventricle; LV, left ventricle; Ao, aorta; PA, pulmonary trunk. (Reproduced by kind permission of Dr B Soto, University of Alabama in Birmingham, USA.)

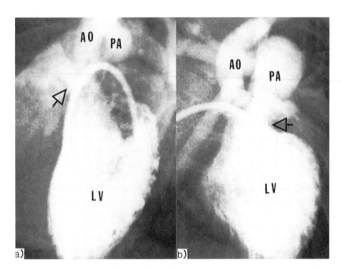

Figure 37.37. A doubly committed juxta-arterial defect (arrow) as seen in long-axis (a) and right anterior oblique (b) projections of a left ventricular injection. Abbreviations as in Figure 37.36. (Reproduced by kind permission of Dr B Soto, University of Alabama in Birmingham, USA.)

Figure 37.38. Long-axis projections of left ventricular injections showing a solitary (a) and multiple (b) muscular defects of the apical trabecular septum. Abbreviations as in Figure 37.36. (Reproduced by kind permission of Dr B Soto, University of Alabama in Birmingham, USA.)

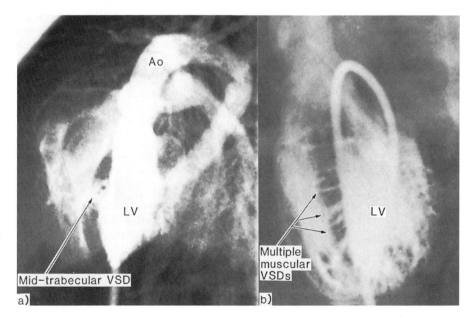

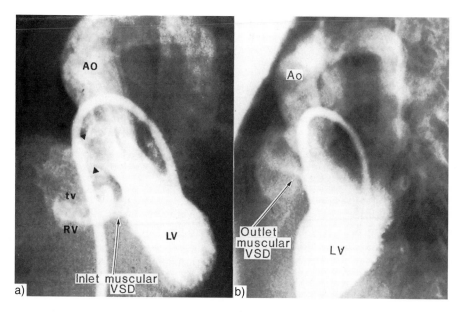

Figure 37.39. Left ventricular injections profiled (a) in four-chamber projection to show an inlet muscular and (b) in long axial projection to reveal an outlet muscular defect. Abbreviations as in Figure 37.36. (Reproduced by kind permission of Dr B Soto, University of Alabama in Birmingham, USA.)

ventricular outflow tract is found on cardiac catheterization (Pongiglione et al, 1982). This is best performed in the 45° head-up position using anteroposterior and lateral projections.

Left ventricular angiograms can be used for quantitative assessment of left ventricular function. Left ventricular end-diastolic volume is usually increased, and the ejection fraction is normal or increased. These indexes have prognostic significance but rarely, if ever, will the decision whether or not to opt for closure be influenced by these findings. Nowadays, it is rarely necessary to perform invasive studies in infants with ventricular septal defects. All the necessary information required to determine the need for surgical treatment is provided by non-invasive tests.

DIAGNOSIS

The definitive diagnosis of isolated ventricular septal defect no longer depends upon cardiac catheterization and angiocardiography but, as discussed above, is made with certainty in the majority of patients using cross-sectional echocardiography. In many instances, nonetheless, the diagnosis can also be made from purely clinical evidence supported by the electrocardiogram and the chest radiograph. Thus, in an asymptomatic child over the age of 1 year, the typical physical signs, taken together with the chest radiograph and electrocardiogram, permits a confident diagnosis. This is not the case in infancy, particularly during early infancy. In this setting, a ventricular septal defect is frequently a component of a more complex lesion. It may also be difficult on clinical grounds alone to be certain whether the defect is isolated. For example, when a ventricular septal defect occurs in the setting of complete transposition, the pulmonary blood flow may be so high that cyanosis is not

clinically apparent. Yet the thrill and murmur, and the radiographic and electrocardiographic features, may be compatible with an isolated lesion. In such patients, the response of blood gases to inhalation of 100% oxygen (Jones et al, 1976) may indicate that the malformation is a complex one. Occasionally this test is misleading, particularly when the ventricular septal defect is found in the setting of a common arterial trunk. Echocardiography is crucial in differentiating isolated defects from more complex anomalies and should, therefore, be performed in all infants suspected of having a ventricular septal defect (Danford et al, 1997). Although the clinical features may leave the diagnosis of isolated ventricular septal defect in doubt, the investigations when expertly performed leave little possibility of an alternative diagnosis. The only possible area of confusion is a ventricular septal defect so large that only a rim of septal tissue can be identified separating apical portions of the ventricles with distinctive right and left patterns. This condition is frequently misdiagnosed as double inlet to a solitary indeterminate ventricle. Although it may be suspected on angiocardiographic or echocardiographic grounds that a rim of ventricular septum is present, this can only be confirmed by direct inspection (see Chapter 38).

COURSE AND PROGNOSIS

The majority of patients live normal lives (Weidman et al, 1977a,b). It is difficult, if not impossible, to give accurate figures for the proportion of defects that close spontaneously. Studies from the 1970s cite 50–60% (Alpert et al, 1973; Corone et al, 1977). When account is taken of smaller defects now diagnosed echocardiographically, the proportion is almost certainly higher, perhaps as high as 80–90% (Krovetz, 1998). Closure usually happens during the first 5 years of life but can occur at any age. Indeed, many defects close during fetal life (Orie et al, 1994). As the defect becomes smaller, the murmur is said to lose its pansystolic nature, becoming shorter and decrescendo. These changes have value in predicting those defects that are about to close (Moss and Siassi, 1970). Even in the group of patients whose defects persist, most lead normal active lives with very little risk of a cardiac death before the age of 40 years (Corone et al, 1977).

A small number of infants, perhaps 10–15%, develop congestive cardiac failure requiring medical treatment (Keith, 1978). This almost invariably occurs during the first 6 months of life. Many of these children will not survive longer than 6 months unless surgical treatment is performed. Some, however, are adequately controlled on medical treatment and do not require surgery as a life-saving procedure. Such infants frequently have pulmonary hypertension as a consequence of their large defects and are at risk for the development of pulmonary vascular disease. They form the only reliably identifiable group of the 3–6% of all patients who develop this complication. Any infant with pulmonary hypertension persisting through the early months of life is likely to develop pulmonary vascular disease. This becomes established and irreversible in the majority before the age of 1 year. Patients who have experienced little or no fall in pulmonary vascular resistance after birth form the remainder of the subjects at high risk. Tragically, this latter group may escape detection until cyanosis supervenes. It is important, therefore, to recognize that irreversible and progressive pulmonary vascular disease is present in the affected patients long before they become cyanosed. The prognosis of patients with ventricular septal defect and pulmonary vascular disease is poor, but survival into adult life is common: death usually occurs before 40 years of age. In females with pulmonary vascular disease, pregnancy poses a particular risk. This is because blood loss of even moderate degree, as may occur at delivery, can precipitate an irreversible low output state. Women with this condition should be advised to avoid pregnancy. If they do not heed this advice, a difficult choice is necessary, since termination of pregnancy also carries a significant risk. On balance, unwanted pregnancies should be terminated. If the patient strongly wishes to continue, many can deliver safely with careful supervision (Szekely and Snaith, 1974), although the maternal mortality may be as high as 50%.

Two other complications of isolated ventricular septal defect may cause death before the age of 40 years. The first is development of aortic regurgitation (Keane et al, 1977). The reported incidence varies between 0.7 and 5% (Moss and Siassi, 1970; Frontera-Izquierdo and Caliegno-Huerta 1992). It occurs most usually either when the defect is doubly committed and juxta-arterial (where more than 70% may be affected (Ishikawa et al,

1994)) or when the defect is perimembranous (Van Praagh and McNamara, 1968). It can also occur in the presence of muscular outlet defects when the muscular outlet septum is hypoplastic (Tatsuno et al, 1973). Almost always it is the right coronary aortic leaflet that prolapses through the defect. In perimembranous defects, the non-coronary leaflet may also be involved. It is often recommended that surgical treatment be offered as soon as significant aortic regurgitation is recognized (Treasure et al, 1971). But it is now known that the condition is well tolerated during childhood in the majority of patients. It can occasionally precipitate heart failure refractory to medical treatment during childhood, but this complication is more frequently encountered during adult life.

The second complication is infective endocarditis. The incidence is approximately 1–2 per 1000 patient-years (Shah et al, 1966; Gersony and Hayes, 1977; Keith, 1978; Kidd et al, 1993). This represents a risk of approximately 1 in 10 of developing infective endocarditis before the age of 70 years (Keith, 1978). It is more likely, however, that infective endocarditis will be contracted after the age of 20 years rather than in childhood or adolescence. The size of defect has no influence on the incidence of the complication (Gersony and Hayes, 1977). Most patients who nowadays develop infective endocarditis are successfully treated. The lifetime risk of dying from infective endocarditis as a complication in the setting of isolated ventricular septal defect has been computed to be of the order of 2–3% (Keith, 1978). Surgical closure of defects does not eliminate the chance of contracting this infection. Indeed, it may initiate it (Gersony and Hayes, 1977; Keith, 1978). Avoidance of infective endocarditis cannot, therefore, be proposed as an indication for the surgical closure of ventricular septal defects (Moller et al, 1991). The problem also continues into adult life. In the study conducted by Neumayer and colleaques (1998), one tenth of patients had episodes of bacterial endocarditis. These were in adults with small defects.

MANAGEMENT

When a patient presents in early infancy, the outcome is always in doubt until a precise diagnosis has been made by echocardiography. For example, an asymptomatic infant presenting with a murmur at 1 month of age may be in intractable heart failure by the age of 3 months. Similarly, spontaneous closure of ventricular septal defect may occur even when the defect has been large enough to cause heart failure in infancy. The prognosis must always, therefore, be guarded during the first few months of life. Asymptomatic infants should be closely followed using echocardiography to assess the anatomy and the gradient from the left to the right ventricle. Those who remain asymptomatic, with no signs or investigations suggesting pulmonary hypertension, require no treatment. Nor should they take precautions other than prophylactic measures against infective endocarditis. These infants have small restrictive defects. Infants with congestive cardiac failure should be treated medically. If the heart failure is intractable to medical treatment, then surgical intervention is indicated. These infants usually have unrestrictive defects. Intractability of the heart failure can be deemed to be present when, despite maximal medical treatment with diuretics and afterload reduction, the infant requires nasogastric tube feeding.

Infants responding to medical treatment may have unrestrictive defects, but they usually have large restrictive ones. In either event, the pulmonary arterial pressure will be elevated in early infancy but may fall to normal by 6 months of age should the defect become smaller. Surgery is indicated in these patients if Doppler echocardiography fails to show a fall in right ventricular pressure to 50% of the left ventricular pressure by 5 to 6 months of age. This is because they are at risk for the development of irreversible pulmonary vascular disease. If the Doppler velocity indicates a lower right ventricular pressure, conservative management should be continued. A basic assumption behind this policy is that pulmonary vascular disease can be prevented or reversed in its early stages. It is not certain that this is possible in all cases. The above recommendations give the best chance of achieving this aim at present (Ikawa et al, 1995). It must be borne in mind that, in some patients, this policy will carry attendant surgical risks for closing defects which would have closed spontaneously (Blackstone et al, 1976). At present, the balance of the risks between corrective and expectant management appears to favour correction (Backer et al, 1993). If, and when, more precise ways of predicting reversibility and irreversibility of pulmonary vascular disease are developed, this policy will be modified accordingly.

It is rare for surgery to be required with an isolated defect after the age of 1 year. Occasional patients who have escaped detection, and who have a large left-to-right shunt and an enlarged heart, may need surgical closure in childhood. Recently this conservative policy has been questioned in the light of excellent surgical results, particularly with the prospect of possibly preventing aortic regurgitation (Backer et al, 1993). The question posed was 'should all defects be closed?' Despite cogent arguments of this type, most paediatric cardiologists and surgeons favour a conservative approach.

Aortic regurgitation, when it occurs, may be sufficiently severe to cause cardiomegaly or heart failure. In the latter instance, surgery should be performed at any age. If frank heart failure is not present, it is best, if possible, to defer surgery until adolescence or adult life, since it may be necessary to replace the aortic valve or to perform a Ross operation (see Chapter 54). Such delay is not advisable in the setting of significant left ventricular dilation. In this situation, we would recommend operation

on the basis of echocardiographic measurements. Therefore, if the end-systolic dimension is greater than 55 mm in adults, and greater then 29 mm/m^2 body surface area in children, surgery is indicated even in the absence of symptoms (Bonow et al, 1991). Severe obstruction of the right ventricular outflow tract develops in 5–10% of patients (Kaplan et al, 1963; Nadas and Fyler, 1968). It always requires surgical treatment. If possible, corrective surgery should be performed. The best results are probably obtained if the complication is treated as soon as it is recognized.

SURGICAL MANAGEMENT

When surgery is required as a life-saving procedure in early infancy, there are two options. The first is to perform a palliative operation (banding of the pulmonary trunk) followed by correction at a later age. The second is to perform primary closure. Banding of the pulmonary trunk is a safe and effective palliative procedure (Stark et al, 1970). But when assessing risk, account must be taken of the cumulative risk of palliation and subsequent correction. In the best hands, this was shown some time ago to be below 10% (Seybold-Epting et al, 1976; Sigmann et al, 1977; Turina, 1978), but this figure is now much too high when set against the excellent results of primary closure. Banding, furthermore, has its own complications, particularly the development of subvalvar pulmonary obstruction. This may contribute to the development of cyanosis with its attendant risks, which will make definitive surgery an even more complex undertaking. It is, therefore, advisable that the corrective operation should not be delayed beyond the second year of life. Patients with ventricular septal defect who have had banding of the pulmonary trunk also have an unduly high incidence of subaortic stenosis (Freed et al, 1973). It is not quite clear whether this is because the presence of the subaortic stenosis meant that banding was more likely to be needed or because banding has a tendency to cause subaortic stenosis. In most centres nowadays, nonetheless, banding is reserved for small infants with multiple ventricular septal defects and those with inlet defects where primary closure would carry a significant risk of damage to the atrioventricular valvar tension apparatus or the conduction axis. Banding is rarely, if ever, indicated nowadays in patients beyond the age of 6 months (Shore et al, 1995; Merrick et al, 1999).

Closure of an isolated ventricular septal defect can now be performed as a relative emergency in the first 6 months of life – with results in the best centres now approaching zero mortality (van den Heuvel et al, 1995). This is clearly superior to the best results of a two-stage approach. The operation can be performed using a ventriculotomy or by a transatrial approach. The applicability of the transatrial approach depends upon the site of the defect. Doubly committed juxta-arterial defects, and multiple defects, present particular difficulties. Nothing is lost, even in these patients, by carrying out an initial transatrial exploration, since this allows accurate placement and, therefore, limits the extent of the necessary ventricular incision (Lincoln, 1978). Multiple defects present a particular challenge. Apical left ventriculotomy has been proposed as the best approach (Singh et al, 1977; Griffiths et al, 1981). An alternative is to use a large dacron patch covering all the muscular defects (Serraf et al, 1992). Even with this approach, left ventriculotomy is not always avoidable, and the reported hospital mortality was 7.7%. The way forward is likely to be the combined use of surgery and catheter intervention. Closure of muscular defects has been achieved using the Clamshell umbrella device (Bridges et al, 1991). Unfortunately, this device suffered structural failure and has been withdrawn. The Rashkind PDA Occluder can be modified for occlusion of ventricular septal defects (Redington and Rigby, 1993). It can be used, singly or in numbers, to close muscular defects, providing each one is smaller than 8–9 mm in stretched diameter (Figure 37.40). The Amplatzer device also lends itself to closure of muscular defects and can likely cope with larger holes. We are also aware of one patient in which closure was achieved using coils (Latiff et al, 1999). The Rashkind occluder was also used for closure of perimembranous defects (Rigby and Redington, 1993) but with an undue incidence of complications. It may well be that devices designed specifically for closure of perimembranous defects may have a role in future, but at present we cannot recommended this procedure except in truly exceptional circumstances.

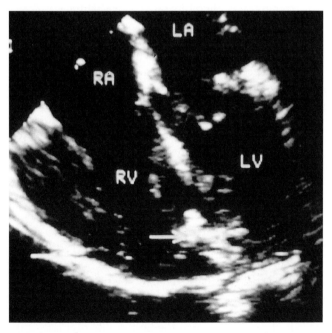

Figure 37.40. The echocardiographic image obtained in four chamber section from the transoesophageal window show how a Rashkind double umbrella (arrowed) has been inserted to close the muscular defect within the central part of the muscular septum shown in Figure 37.29. Abbreviations as in Figure 37.36.

Elective surgery for ventricular septal defect should aim to be corrective. Patients surviving the first 6 months of life with persisting pulmonary hypertension should have primary closure of the defect before the age of 1 year. The possible routes for closure are the same as those for emergency treatment. Similarly, those with a large left-to-right shunt who have escaped detection, or for other reasons have survived the first year of life, should be corrected at the first opportunity. In all patients, the only direct contraindication to surgery is the presence of established and severe pulmonary vascular disease. The initial assessment of pulmonary vascular disease is made from the haemodynamic data. Patients with a calculated pulmonary vascular resistance greater than 8 Wood units/m^2 are generally considered inoperable. In those with calculated resistances of between 4 and 8 Wood units/m^2, it is not possible to say whether the pulmonary vascular disease has become irreversible. More information must be provided to permit rational decisions in these patients. The administration of 100% oxygen during the cardiac catheterization nearly always produces a fall in calculated pulmonary vascular resistance. The greatest fall occurs in the patients with the highest pulmonary vascular resistance. When breathing room air, patients with undoubtedly severe pulmonary vascular disease retain measurable reactivity in their pulmonary vasculature (Morrison and Macartney, 1979). In the presence of severe pulmonary vascular disease, therefore, the demonstration of reactivity is not necessarily an index of operability. This casts doubt on the value of this test in the assessment of operability in patients with less severe elevation of pulmonary vascular resistance. Administration of 100% oxygen may be helpful in patients with pulmonary venous desaturation, since it should reverse the transient hypoxic vasoconstrictor response. Indeed, if such patients have a restrictive ventricular septal defect, administration of 100% oxygen can cause a prompt drop in pulmonary arterial pressure from systemic levels. More recently, inhalation of nitric oxide has been shown to cause a fall in pulmonary vascular resistance in patients with pulmonary hypertension of various causes, but it is not clear how useful this test is in differentiating those who are operable from those who are not (Adatia et al, 1995). In doubtful situations, a lung biopsy may provide useful information (Rabinovitch et al, 1978). In practice, perhaps because of the small and possibly unrepresentative sample, biopsy is prone to give misleading information. It is rarely used nowadays for clinical decision-making.

Elective surgery is also required when subvalvar pulmonary stenosis is present. Resection of the obstructing muscle will be necessary at the time of closure. The presence of aortic regurgitation poses greater problems. It has been suggested that closure of the defect in itself may limit the valvar regurgitation, this being most effective in doubly committed juxta-arterial defects (Keane et al, 1977). Indeed, there is a case to be made for closing all doubly committed juxta-arterial defects as soon as they are diagnosed, even in those rare instances where there is neither congestive cardiac failure nor high pulmonary arterial pressure. Once aortic regurgitation has developed, it is rarely possible in our experience to avoid a direct attack upon the aortic valve. Initially this may be conservative, and good results have been reported in the short and immediate term (Spencer et al, 1962; Trusler et al, 1973). Replacement of the aortic valve has been recommended as the best initial form of treatment, however, particularly when the valvar leaflets are deformed (Somerville et al, 1970). The balance of the evidence leads us to recommend an initial conservative approach wherever possible, with replacement only where this has failed or is impossible.

COURSE AFTER SURGERY

Subsequent to correction, the majority of patients live virtually normal lives and have normal exercise capacity (Meijboom et al, 1994). The clinical condition of almost nine tenths of the patients is graded as good or excellent on follow-up examination. Of the remaining patients, very few are still classified as poor, whereas such a classification is frequent prior to surgery (Weidman et al, 1977a,b). A significant cause of morbidity and mortality is pulmonary vascular disease. When this is established, it usually progresses inexorably despite a corrective operation. This complication is avoided by early corrective surgery (Meijboom et al, 1994). Late postoperative exercise testing confirms the improvement after correction, again pointing to the advantage of early surgery (Meijboom et al, 1994).

Disturbances of cardiac rhythm occur in a small proportion (approximately 5%) of patients following corrective surgery (Weidman et al, 1977a; Kidd et al, 1993), with some still suffering complete heart block. Even with precise knowledge of the conduction tissues, surgical heart block does still occur. This frequently requires the insertion of an artificial pacemaker, with its attendant morbidity (Ennker et al, 1985). Nonetheless, permanent pacing should certainly be provided if the patient remains in congestive cardiac failure with a slow heart rate. When Stokes–Adams attacks occur, or if 24-hour monitoring of the electrocardiogram demonstrates prolonged period of asystole, episodes of ventricular tachycardia, or ventricular fibrillation, then even if the patient is asymptomatic it is probably best to insert a pacemaker. In practice, a slow heart rate of 30–40 beats/min at any time of the day is frequently used as a relative indicator for pacing. Transient heart block after surgery may predispose to late sudden death (Moller et al, 1991), and the Second Natural History Study showed a higher prevalence of both serious arrhythmias and sudden death (Kidd et al, 1993). It follows that 24-hour tape monitoring is mandatory in all patients with heart block following surgery for ventricular septal defect, even when this resolves sponta-

neously. This investigation should be repeated periodically during follow-up. In the absence of symptoms, it should be performed at yearly or 6-monthly intervals. Monitoring should also be performed in patients with postoperative ventricular ectopic beats. There is some suggestive evidence that these, by triggering a life-threatening ventricular arrhythmia, may be responsible for sudden death (Gillette et al, 1977; Schuilenberg, 1981).

Intraventricular conduction disturbances are seen in the majority of patients who have had open heart surgery. Right bundle branch block is certainly seen following repair of ventricular septal defect, be this performed transatrially or by the ventricular route (Lincoln, 1978; Friedli, 1981). When this is an isolated phenomenon, it is not a prognostic sign. When it is associated with left-axis deviation and a prolonged PR interval (see Chapter 12), it may well be a precursor of late complete heart block, particularly when the postoperative period has been complicated by a period of transient complete heart block (Krongrad, 1978). In these patients, and in those where the right bundle branch block and left-axis deviation are not associated with a prolonged PR interval, intracardiac electrophysiological studies may assist in predicting the outcome (Friedli, 1981). The prognostic significance of all these changes for the occurrence of sudden unexpected death is at present uncertain (Schuilenberg, 1981). Close surveillance with 24-hour tape monitoring is a wise precaution. As with complete heart block, there are no generally accepted criterions for the insertion prophylactically of a pacemaker.

Crucial to the long-term outcome in patients with intraventricular conduction disturbances is the site of interference with the conduction tissues. If this is central, that is within the atrioventricular bundle, the risk of complete heart block is greater than if the damage is solely within the peripheral bundle branches. While intracardiac electrophysiological studies (see Chapter 17) have been suggested as being helpful, this is not always the case (Schuilenberg, 1981). Atrial arrhythmias may occur if there is damage to the sinus node (for instance, during cannulation), but these are a rare occurrence nowadays following surgery for correction of ventricular septal defect.

The other common complication is a residual ventricular septal defect (Weidman et al, 1977a). In general, such residual defects are of little haemodynamic significance (Meijboom et al, 1994). Occasionally they will be large enough to permit a considerable residual left-to-right shunt. When this results in congestive, or persistent, cardiac failure, revision of the operation is indicated. The presence of a residual ventricular septal defect reinforces the need for lifelong prophylactic measures against infective endocarditis. These measures should be continued even when the operation appears to have been totally successful.

Patients undergoing surgery for ventricular septal defect are at risk for all the complications associated with open heart surgery performed for any reason, including brain damage, renal damage, postpericardotomy syndrome, pulmonary complications and so on. The majority of patients, however, suffer no ill-effects, are improved and go on to lead normal lives. This they should be encouraged to do. Although it is too early to predict the ultimate lifespan of such patients, organizations such as the armed services and the police force can be prevailed upon to accept recruits who have undergone surgical repair of ventricular septal defect. It is also the case, nonetheless, that those who survive into adulthood without the need for surgery can continue to pose a problem. In the population of patients studied by Neumayer and colleagues (1998), although half had no complications over many years, and spontaneous closure occurred in one tenth, serious complications were encountered in one quarter. The malformation, therefore, is not entirely benign.

REFERENCES

Adatia I, Perry S, Lanzeberg M, Thompson J E, Wessel D L 1995 Inhaled nitric oxide and hemodynamic evaluation of patients with pulmonary hypertension before transplantation. Journal of the American College of Cardiology 25: 1656–1664

Alderson P O, Jost R G, Strauss A W, Boonvisut S, Markham J 1975 Radionucleotide angiography improved quantitation of left-to-right shunts using area ratio techniques in children. Circulation 51: 1136–1143

Allwork S P, Anderson R H 1979 Developmental anatomy of the membranous part of the ventricular septum in the human heart. British Heart Journal 41: 275–280

Al-Marsafawy H F M, Ho S Y, Redington A N, Anderson R H 1995 Relationship of the outlet septum to the aortic outflow tract in hearts with interruption of the aortic arch. Journal of Thoracic and Cardiovascular Surgery 109: 1225–1236

Alpert B S, Mellitis E D, Rowe R D 1973 Spontaneous closure of small ventricular septal defects; probability rates in the first five years of life. American Journal of Diseases of Childhood 125: 194–196

Alva C, Rigby M L, Ho S Y, Anderson R H 1998 Overriding and biventricular connection of arterial valves. Cardiology in the Young 8: 150–164

Anderson R H, Wilcox B R 1992 The surgical anatomy of ventricular septal defects. Journal of Cardiac Surgery 7: 17–35

Anderson R H, Wilcox B R 1993 The surgical anatomy of ventricular septal defects associated with overriding valvar orifices. Journal of Cardiac Surgery 8: 130–142

Anderson R H, Monro J L, Ho S Y, Smith A, Deverall P B 1977 Les voies de conduction auriculo-ventriculares dans le tetralogie de Fallot. Coeur 8: 793–807

Anderson R H, Lenox C C, Zuberbuhler J R 1983 Mechanisms of closure of perimembranous ventricular septal defect. American Journal of Cardiology 52: 341–345

Anderson R H, Becker A E, Tynan M 1986 Description of ventricular septal defects–or how long is a piece of string? International Journal of Cardiology 13: 267–278

Anderson R H, Ho S Y, Wilcox B R 1994 The surgical anatomy of ventricular septal defects with univentricular atrioventricular connection. Journal of Cardiac Surgery 9: 408–426

Backer C L, Winters R C, Zales V R et al 1993 Restrictive ventricular septal defect: how small is too small to close. Annals of Thoracic Surgery 56: 1014–1018

Bailey H, Clain A 1954 Demonstration of physical signs in clinical surgery. Wright, Bristol, p 149–150

Baker E J, Leung M P, Anderson R H, Fischer D R, Zuberbuhler J R 1988 The cross-sectional anatomy of ventricular septal defects. British Heart Journal 59: 339–351

Bargeron L M, Elliott L P, Soto B, Bream P R, Curry G C 1977 Axial cineangiography in congenital heart disease. Section I. Concept, technical and anatomical considerations. Circulation 56: 1075–1083

Becu L M, Tauxe W N, DuShane J W, Edwards J E 1955 A complex of congenital cardiac anomalies: ventricular septal defect, biventricular origin of the pulmonary trunk and subaortic stenosis. American Heart Journal 50: 901–911

Becu L M, Fontana R S, DuShane J W, Kirklin J W, Burchell H B, Edwards J E 1956 Anatomic and pathologic studies in ventricular septal defect. Circulation 14: 349–364

Beerman L B, Park S C, Fischer D R et al 1985 Ventricular septal defect associated with aneurysm of the membranous septum. Journal of the American College of Cardiology 5: 118–123

Ben-Shachar G, Arcilla R A, Lucas R V, Manasek F J 1985 Ventricular trabeculations in the chick embryo heart and their contribution to ventricular and muscular septal development. Circulation Research 57: 759–766

Bierman F Z, Fellows K, Williams R G 1980 Prospective identification of ventricular septal defects in infancy using subxiphoid two dimensional echocardiography. Circulation 62: 807–818

Blackstone E H, Kirklin J W, Bradley E L, DuShane J W, Appelbaum A 1976 Optimal age and results in repair of large ventricular septal defects. Journal of Thoracic and Cardiovascular Surgery 72: 661–679

Bonow R O, Lakatos E, Maron B J, Epstein S E 1991 Serial long-term assessment of the natural history of asymptomatic patients with chronic aortic regurgitation and normal left ventricular systolic function. Circulation 84: 1625–1635

Bonvicini M, Piovaccari G, Picchio F M 1982 Severe subpulmonary obstruction caused by an aneurysmal tissue tag complicating an infundibular perimembranous ventricular septal defect. British Heart Journal 48: 189–191

Brandt P W T, Calder A L, Barratt-Boyes B G, Neutze J M 1976 Double outlet left ventricle. Morphology, cineangiography, diagnosis and surgical treatment. American Journal of Cardiology 38: 897–909

Bridges N D, Perry S B, Keane J F et al 1991 Preoperative transcatheter closure of congenital muscular ventricular septal defects. New England Journal of Medicine 324: 1312–1317

Capelli H, Andrade J L, Somerville J 1983 Classification of the site of ventricular septal defect by 2-dimensional echocardiography. American Journal of Cardiology 51: 1474–1480

Carlgren L E 1959 The incidence of congenital heart disease in children born in Gothenburg 1941–1950. British Heart Journal 21: 40–50

Cheatham J P, Latson L A, Gutgesell H P 1981 Ventricular septal defect in infancy: detection with two dimensional echocardiography. American Journal of Cardiology 47: 85–89

Chesler E, Korns M E, Edwards J E 1968 Anomalies of the tricuspid valve, including pouches, resembling aneurysms of the membranous ventricular septum. American Journal of Cardiology 21: 661–668

Corone P, Doyen F, Gaudeau S et al 1977 Natural history of ventricular septal defect. A study involving 790 cases. Circulation 55: 908–915

Danford D A, Martin A B, Fletcher S E et al 1997 Children with heart murmurs: can ventricular septal defect be diagnosed reliably without an echocardiogram? Journal of the American College of Cardiology 30: 243–246

Dawes G S 1968 Fetal and neonatal physiology. Year Book Medical, Chicago, IL, p 95–96

Dickinson D F 1998 Ventricular septal defect–not another epidemic? Cardiology in the Young 8: 423–424

Driscoll D, Allen H A, Atkins D L et al 1994 Guidelines for evaluation and management of common congenital cardiac problems in infants, children and adolescents Circulation 90: 2180–2188

Du Z-D, Roguin N, Barak M, Bihari S G, Ben-Elisha M 1996 High prevalence of muscular ventricular septal defect in preterm neonates. American Journal of Cardiology 78: 1183–1185

Du Z-D, Roguin N, Wu X-J 1998 Spontaneous closure of muscular ventricular septal defect identified by echocardiography in neonates. Cardiology in the Young 8: 500–505

Elliott L P, Bargeron L M, Bream P R, Soto B, Curry G C 1977 Atrial cineangiography in congenital heart disease. Section II. Specific lesions. Circulation 56: 1084–1093

Ennker J, Stegman T H, Luhmer I, Oelert H 1985 Risks and benefits of cardiac pacing in children. International Journal of Cardiology 8: 125–134

Evans J R, Rowe R D, Keith J D 1960 Spontaneous closure of ventricular septal defects. Circulation 22: 1044–1054

Ferencz C, Loffredo C A, Correa-Villaseñor A, Wilson P D 1993 Perspectives in pediatric cardiology vol 5. Genetic and environmental risk factors of major cardiovascular malformations. The Baltimore–Washington Infant Study 1981–1989. Futura, Armonk, NY, p 149–163

Fox K M, Patel R G, Graham G R, Taylor J F N, Stark J, de Leval M, Macartney F J 1978 Multiple and single ventricular septal defects. A clinical and haemodynamic comparison. British Heart Journal 40: 111–146

Freed M D, Rosenthal A, Plauth W H Jr, Nadas A S 1973 Development of subaortic stenosis after pulmonary artery banding. Circulation 47–48 (suppl III) 7–10

French H 1918 The possibility of a loud congenital heart murmur disappearing when a child grows up. Guy's Hospital Gazette New Series 32: 87

Friedli B 1981 Prognostic significance of ventricular conduction abnormalities and extrasystoles after open heart surgery. In: Becker A E, Losekoot T G, Marcelletti C, Anderson R H (eds) Paediatric cardiology, vol 3. Churchill Livingstone, Edinburgh, p 150–159

Frontera-Izquierdo P, Cabezuelo-Huerta G 1992 Natural and modified history of ventricular septal defect: a 17-year study. Pediatric Cardiology 13: 193–197

Gates G F, Orme H W, Dore E K 1973 Cardiac shunt assessment in children with macroaggregated albumin technetium-99m. Radiology 112: 649–653

Gatzoulis M A, Li J, Ho S Y 1997 The echocardiographic anatomy of ventricular septal defects. Cardiology in the Young 7: 471–484

Gerbode F, Hultgren H, Melrose D, Osborn J 1958 Syndrome of left ventricular-right atrial shunt, successful surgical repair in five cases with observation of bradycardia on closure. Annals of Surgery 148: 433–466

Gersony W M, Hayes C J 1977 Bacterial endocarditis in patients with pulmonary stenosis, aortic stenosis or ventricular septal defect. Circulation 50: 1184–1187

Gillette P C, Yeoman M A, Mullins C E, McNamara D G 1977 Sudden death after repair of tetralogy of Fallot. Electrocardiographic and electrophysiologic abnormalities. Circulation 56: 566–571

Goor D A, Lillehei C W, Edwards J E 1971 Ventricular septal defects and pulmonic stenosis with and without dextroposition. Anatomic features and embryologic implications. Chest 60: 117–128

Graham T P, Bender H W, Spach M S 1977 Defects of the ventricular septum. In: Moss A J, Adams F H, Emmanouilides G C (eds) Heart disease in infants, children and adolescents, 2nd edn. Williams & Wilkins, Baltimore, MD, p 140–161

Grech V 1998 Epidemiology and diagnosis of ventricular septal defect in Malta. Cardiology in the Young 8: 329–336

Green C E, Elliott L P, Bargeron L M Jr 1981 Axial cineangiographic evaluation of the posterior ventricular septal defect. American Journal of Cardiology 48: 331–335

Griffin M L, Sullivan I D, Anderson R H, Macartney F J 1988 Doubly committed subarterial ventricular septal defect: new morphological criteria with echocardiographic and angiocardiographic correlation. British Heart Journal 59: 474–479

Griffiths S P, Tori G K, Ellis K et al 1981 Muscular ventricular septal defects repaired with left ventriculotomy. American Journal of Cardiology 48: 877–886

Harris A, Sutton G, Towers M 1976 Ventricular septal defect. In: Physiological and clinical aspects of cardiac auscultation. Medi-Cine, London, p 108

Haworth S G, Shuer U, Buhlmeyer K, Reid L 1977 Development of the pulmonary circulation in ventricular septal defect: a quantitative structural study. American Journal of Cardiology 40: 781–788

Hiraishi S, Agata Y, Nowatari M et al 1992 Incidence and natural history of trabecular ventricular septal defect: two dimensional echocardiography and colour Doppler flow imaging study. Journal of Pediatrics 120: 409–415

Ho S Y, Wilcox B R, Anderson R H, Lincoln J C R 1983 Interrupted aortic arch–anatomical features of surgical significance. Thoracic and Cardiovascular Surgeon 31: 199–205

Hoffman J I E, Christianson R 1978 Congenital heart disease in a cohort of 19 502 births with long term follow up. American Journal of Cardiology 42: 641–647

Hoffman J I E, Rudolph A M 1965 The natural history of ventricular septal defects in infancy. American Journal of Cardiology 16: 634–653

Ikawa S, Shimazaki Y, Nakano S, Kobayashi J, Matsuda H, Kawashima Y 1995 Pulmonary vascular resistance during exercise late after repair of large ventricular septal defects. Relation to age at the time of repair. Journal of Thoracic and Cardiovascular Surgery 109: 1218–1224

Ishikawa S, Morishita Y, Sato Y, Yoshida I, Otaki A, Otani Y 1994 Frequency and operative correction of aortic insufficiency associated with ventricular septal defect. Annals of Thoracic Surgery 57: 996–998

Jackson M, Walsh K P, Peart I, Arnold R 1996 Epidemiology of congenital heart disease in Merseyside – 1978–1988. Cardiology in the Young 6: 281–290

Jarmakani M M, Edwards S B, Spach M S et al 1968 Left ventricular pressure–volume characteristics in congenital heart disease. Circulation 37: 879–889

Jarmakani M M, Graham J P Jr, Canent R V Jr, Spach M S, Capp M P 1969 Effect of site of shunt on left heart-volume characteristics in children with ventricular septal defect and persistent ductus arteriosus. Circulation 40: 411–418

Jones R W A, Baumer J H, Joseph M C, Shinebourne E A 1976 Arterial oxygen tension and response to oxygen breathing in differential diagnosis of congenital heart disease in infancy. Archives of Disease in Childhood 51: 667–673

Kaplan S, Dauod G I, Benzing G, Devine F J, Glass I H, McGuire J 1963 Natural history of ventricular septal defect. American Journal of Diseases in Childhood 105: 581–587

Kardon R E, Cao Q L, Masani N et al 1998 New insights and observations in three-dimensional echocardiographic visualization of ventricular septal defects. Circulation 98: 1307–1314

Keane J F, Plauth W H, Nadas A S 1977 Ventricular septal defect with aortic regurgitation. Circulation 56(suppl I): 72–77

Keith J D 1978 Ventricular septal defect. In: Keith J D, Rowe R D, Vlad P (eds) Heart disease in infancy and childhood. 3rd edn. Macmillan, New York, p 321–379

Kidd L, Driscoll D J, Gersony W M et al 1993 Second natural history study of congenital heart defects. Results of treatment of patients with ventricular septal defects Circulation 87(Suppl I): 38–51

Kirklin J W, Kirklin J K, Soto B, Blackstone E A, Bargeron L M Jr 1988 Ventricular septal defects: a surgical viewpoint. In: Anderson R H, Neches W H, Park S, Zuberbuhler J R (eds) Perspectives in Pediatric Cardiology, Futura Publishing, Mount Kisco, NY, p 91

Krongrad E 1978 Prognosis for patients with congenital heart disease and postoperative intraventricular conduction defects. Circulation 57: 867–870

Krovetz L J 1998 Spontaneous closure of ventricular septal defect. American Journal of Cardiology 81: 100–101

Kutsche L M, Van Mierop L H S 1983 Pulmonary atresia with and without ventricular septal defect: a different

etiology and pathogenesis for the atresia in the 2 types. American Journal of Cardiology 51: 932–935

Lamers W H, Wessels A, Verbeek F J et al 1993 New findings concerning ventricular septation in the human heart. Circulation 86: 1194–1205

Lamers W H, Virágh S, Wessels A, Moorman A F M, Anderson R H 1995 Formation of the tricuspid valve in the human heart. Circulation 91: 111–121

Latham R A, Anderson R H 1972 Anatomical variations in atrioventricular conduction system with reference to ventricular septal defects. British Heart Journal 34: 185–190

Latiff H A, Alwi M, Kardhavel G, Samion H, Zambahari R 1999 Transcatheter closure of multiple muscular ventricular septal defects using Giantures cerils. Annals of Thoracic Surgery 68: 1400–1401

Leung M P, Mok C K, Lo R N S, Lau K C 1986 An echocardiographic study of perimembranous ventricular septal defect with left ventricular to right atrial shunting. British Heart Journal 55: 45–52

Lev M 1959 The pathologic anatomy of ventricular septal defect. Diseases of the Chest 35: 533–545

Lev M 1960 The architecture of the conduction system in congenital heart disease. III. Ventricular septal defect. Archives of Pathology 70: 529–549

Levin A R, Spach M S, Canent R V Jr et al 1967 Intracardiac pressure–flow dynamics in isolated ventricular septal defect. Circulation 35: 430–441

Lewis D A, Loffredo C A, Correa-Villaseñor A, Wilson D, Martin G R 1996 Descriptive epidemiology of membranous and muscular ventricular septal defects in the Baltimore–Washington Infant Study. Cardiology in the Young 6: 281–290

Lincoln C 1978 Transatrial versus ventricular closure of isolated ventricular septal defect. In: Anderson R H, Shinebourne E A (eds) Paediatric cardiology 1977. Churchill Livingstone, Edinburgh, p 155–162

Lucas R V Jr, Adams P Jr, Anderson R C, Meyne N G, Lillehei C W, Varco R L 1961 The natural history of isolated ventricular septal defect. A serial physiologic study. Circulation 24: 1372–1387

Maron B J, Redwood D R, Hirshfeld J W, Goldstein R E, Morrow A G, Epstein S E 1973 Postoperative assessment of patients with ventricular septal defect and pulmonary hypertension. Response to intense upright exercise. Circulation 73: 864–874

McKay R, Battistessa S A, Wilkinson J L, Wright J P 1989 A communication from the left ventricle to the right atrium: a defect in the central fibrous body. International Journal of Cardiology 23: 117–123

Meijboom F, Szatmari A, Utens E, Deckers J W, Roelandt J R, Hess J 1994 Long-term follow-up after surgical closure of ventricular septal defect in infancy and childhood. Journal of the American College of Cardiology 24: 1358–1364

Merrick A F, Lal M, Anderson R H, Shore D F 1999 Management of ventricular septal defect: a survey of practice in the United Kingdom. Annals of Thoracic Surgery 68: 983–988

Milo S, Ho S Y, Macartney F J, Wilkinson J L, et al 1979 Straddling and overriding atrioventricular valves: morphology and classification. American Journal of Cardiology 44: 1122–1134

Milo S, Ho S Y, Wilkinson J L, Anderson R H 1980 The surgical anatomy and atrioventricular conduction tissues of hearts with isolated ventricular septal defects. Journal of Thoracic and Cardiovascular Surgery 79: 244–255

Mitchell S C, Korones S B, Berendes H W 1971 Congenital heart disease in 56 109 births. Incidence and natural history. Circulation 43: 323–332

Moller J H, Patton C, Varco R L, Lillehei C W 1991 Late results (30 to 35 years) after operative closure of isolated ventricular septal defect from 1954 to 1960. American Journal of Cardiology 68: 1491–1497

Morrison G W, Macartney F J 1979 Effects of oxygen administration, bicarbonate infusions, and brief hyperventilation on patients with pulmonary vascular obstructive disease. British Heart Journal 41: 584–593

Moss A J, Siassi B 1970 Natural history of ventricular septal defect. Cardiovascular Clinics 2: 140–154

Moulaert A, Bruins C C, Oppenheimer-Dekker A 1976 Anomalies of the aortic arch and ventricular septal defects. Circulation 53: 1011–1015

Nadas A S, Fyler D C 1968 Ventricular septal defect. A review of current thoughts. Archives of Disease of Childhood 43: 268–282

Naeye R L 1966 The pulmonary arterial bed in ventricular septal defect. Anatomic features in childhood. Circulation 34: 962–983

Neufeld H N, Titus J L, DuShane J W, Burchell H B, Edwards J E 1961 Isolated ventricular septal defect of the persistent common atrioventricular canal type. Circulation 23: 685–696

Neumayer U, Stone S, Somerville 1998 Small ventricular septal defects in adults. European Heart Journal 19: 1573–1582

Nihill M R, Mullins C E, McNamara D G 1978 Visualisation of the pulmonary arteries in pseudotruncus by pulmonary vein wedge angiography. Circulation 58: 140–147

Orie J, Flotta D, Sherman F S 1994 To be or not to be a VSD. American Journal of Cardiology 74: 1284–1285

Pongiglione G, Freedom R M, Cook D, Rowe R D 1982 Mechanism of acquired right ventricular outflow tract obstruction in patients with ventricular septal defect: an angiocardiographic study. American Journal of Cardiology 50: 776–780

Rabinovitch M, Haworth S G, Castaneda A R, Nadas A S, Reid L M 1978 Lung biopsy in congenital heart disease: a morphometric approach to pulmonary vascular disease. Circulation 58: 1107–1121

Ramaciotti C, Kered A, Silverman N N 1986 Importance of pseudoneurysms of the ventricular septum in the natural history of isolated perimembranous ventricular septal defects. American Journal of Cardiology 57: 268–272

Redington A, Rigby M L 1993 Novel uses of the Rashkind ductal umbrella in adults and children with congenital heart disease. British Heart Journal 69: 47–51

Roberts W C 1984 The 2 most common congenital heart diseases. [Editorial] American Journal of Cardiology 53: 1198

Roger H 1879 Recherches cliniques sur la communication congenitale des deux coeurs, par innoclusion de septum interventriculaire. Bulletin de l'Académie de Médecine 8: 1077–1085

Roguin N, Du Z D, Barak M, Nasser N, Hershkowitz S, Milgram E 1996 High prevalence of muscular ventricular

septal defect in neonates. Journal of the American College of Cardiology 26: 1545–1548

Rosenquist G C, Sweeney L J, Stemple D R, Christianson S D, Rowe R D 1973 Ventricular septal defect in tetralogy of Fallot. American Journal of Cardiology 31: 749–754

Rudolph A M 1965 The effects of post-natal circulatory adjustments in congenital heart disease. Paediatrics 36: 763–772

Rudolph A M 1970 The changes in the circulation after birth: their importance in congenital heart disease. Circulation 41: 343–359

Rudolph A M 1974 Congenital Diseases of the Heart. Year Book Medical, Chicago, IL, p 206

Šamanek M, Slavik Z, Voriskova M et al 1989 The incidence of heart defects in children. Casopis Lekaru Ceskych 128: 422–424

Santamaria H, Soto B, Ceballos R, Bargeron L M Jr, Coghlan H C, Kirklin J W 1983 Angiographic differentiation of types of ventricular septal defects. American Journal of Radiology 141: 273–281

Schuilenberg R M 1981 Mechanisms of abnormal impulse formation and conduction. In: Becker A E, Losekoot T G, Marcelietti C, Anderson R H (eds) Paediatric cardiology, vol 3. Churchill Livingstone, Edinburgh, p 107–121

Serraf A, Lacour-Gayet F, Bruniaux J et al 1992 Surgical management of isolated multiple ventricular septal defects. Logical approach in 130 cases. Journal of Thoracic and Cardiovascular Surgery 103: 437–442

Seybold-Epting W, Reul G J, Hallman G L, Cooley D A 1976 Repair of ventricular septal defect after pulmonary artery banding. Journal of Thoracic and Cardiovascular Surgery 71: 392–397

Shah P, Singh W S A, Rose V, Keith J D 1966 Incidence of bacterial endocarditis in ventricular septal defects. Circulation 34: 127–131

Sherman F E 1963 An atlas of congenital heart disease. Lea & Febiger, Philadelphia

Shore D F, Rigby M L, Anderson R H 1995 Surgical for ventricular septal defect. In: Yacoub M, Pepper J (eds) Annual of cardiac surgery, 8th edn. Current Science, New York, p 147–156

Sigfùsson G, Ettedgui J A, Silverman N H, Anderson R H 1995 Is a cleft in the anterior leaflet of an otherwise normal mitral valve an atrioventricular canal malformation? Journal of the American College of Cardiology 26: 508–515

Sigmann J M, Perry B L, Behrendt D M, Stern A M, Kirsh M M, Sloan H E 1977 Ventricular septal defect: results after repair in infancy. American Journal of Cardiology 39: 66–71

Singh A K, de Leval M, Stark J 1977 Left ventriculotomy for closure of muscular ventricular septal defects. Annals of Surgery 186: 577–580

Somerville J 1979 Congenital heart disease – changes in form and function. British Heart Journal 41: 1–22

Somerville J, Brandao A, Ross D N 1970 Aortic regurgitation with ventricular septal defect. Circulation 41: 317–330

Soto B, Coghlan C H, Bargeron L M Jr 1978 Angiography of ventricular septal defects. In: Anderson R H, Shinebourne

E A (eds) Paediatric cardiology 1977. Churchill Livingstone, Edinburgh, p 125–135

Soto B, Becker A E, Moulaert A J, Lie J T, Anderson R H 1980 Classification of ventricular septal defects. British Heart Journal 43: 332–343

Soto B, Ceballos R, Kirklin J W 1989 Ventricular septal defects: a surgical viewpoint. Journal of the American College of Cardiology 14: 1291–1297

Spencer F C, Bahnson H T, Neil C A 1962 The treatment of aortic regurgitation associated with a ventricular septal defect. Journal of Thoracic and Cardiovascular Surgery 43: 222–233

Stanger P, Lucas P V Jr, Edwards J E 1969 Anatomic factors causing respiratory distress in acyanotic congenital cardiac disease: special reference to bronchial obstruction. Pediatrics 43: 760–769

Stark J, Tynan M, Tatooles C J, Aberdeen E, Waterston D J 1970 Banding of the pulmonary artery for transposition of the great arteries and ventricular septal defect. Circulation 41(Suppl II): 16–129

Steinfeld L, Dimich I, Park S, Baron M G 1972 Clinical diagnosis of isolated subpulmonic supracristal ventricular septal defect. American Journal of Cardiology 30: 19–24

Sutherland G R, Godman M J, Smallhorn J F et al 1982 Ventricular septal defects. Two dimensional echocardiographic and morphologic correlations. British Heart Journal 47: 316–328

Sutton G, Harris A, Leatham A 1968 Second heart sound in pulmonary hypertension. British Heart Journal 30: 743–756

Szekely P, Snaith L 1974 Ventricular septal defect. In: Heart disease and pregnancy. Churchill Livingstone, Edinburgh, p 157

Tatsuno K, Konno S, Sakakibara S 1973 Ventricular septal defect with aortic insufficiency. Angiographic aspects and a new classification. American Heart Journal 85: 13–21

Titus J L, Daugherty G W, Edwards J E 1963 Anatomy of the atrioventricular conduction system in ventricular septal defect. Circulation 28: 72–81

Treasure R L, Hopeman A R, Jahne E J, Green D C, Czarnecki S W 1971 Ventricular septal defect with aortic insufficiency. Annals of Thoracic Surgery 12: 411–418

Truex R C, Bishof J K 1958 Conduction system in human hearts with interventricular septal defects. Journal of Thoracic Surgery 35: 421–439

Trusler G A, Moes C A F, Kidd B S L 1973 Repair of ventricular septal defect with aortic insufficiency. Journal of Thoracic and Cardiovascular Surgery 66: 394–403

Turina M 1978 Early closure versus two-stage treatment for ventricular septal defect. In: Anderson R H, Shinebourne E A (eds) Paediatric cardiology 1977. Churchill Livingstone, Edinburgh, p 147–154

Ueda M, Becker A E 1985 Classification of hearts with overriding aortic and pulmonary valves. International Journal of Cardiology 9: 353–360

van den Heuvel F, Timmers T, Hess J 1995 Morphological, haemodynamic, and clinical variables as predictors for management of isolated ventricular septal defect. British Heart Journal 73: 49–52

van Mill G J, Moulaert A, Harinck E 1981 Two-dimensional echocardiographic localisation of isolated ventricular septal defects. In: Hunter S, Hall R (eds) Echocardiography I. Churchill Livingstone, Edinburgh, p 249–265

Van Praagh R, McNamara J J 1968 Anatomic types of ventricular septal defect with aortic insufficiency. American Heart Journal 75: 604–619

Van Praagh R, Geva T, Kreutzer J 1989 Ventricular septal defect: how shall we describe, name and classify them? Journal of the American College of Cardiology 14: 1298–1299

Varghese P J, Rowe R D 1969 Spontaneous closure of ventricular septal defects by aneurysmal formation of the membranous septum. Journal of Pediatrics 75: 700–703

Wagenvoort C A, Neufeld H N, DuShane J W, Edwards J E 1961 The pulmonary arterial tree in Ventricular septal defect. A quantitative study of anatomic features in fetuses, infants and children. Circulation 23: 740–748

Weber F P 1918 Can the clinical manifestations of congenital heart disease disappear with the general growth and development of the patient? British Journal of Childhood Diseases 15: 113

Weidman W H, Blount S G, DuShane J W, Gersony W M, Hayes C J, Nadas A S 1977a Clinical course in ventricular septal defect. Circulation 56(suppl I): 56–69

Weidman W H, DuShane J W, Ellison R C 1977b Clinical course in adults with ventricular septal defect. Circulation 56(suppl I): 78–79

Yagel S, Weissman A, Rotstein Z et al 1997 Congenital heart defects. Natural course and in utero development. Circulation 96: 550–555

38
Double-inlet ventricle
D. J. Penny and R. H. Anderson

INTRODUCTION

Knowledge of the diagnosis and appropriate surgical treatment of patients in whom both atriums are connected to the same ventricle has been hampered by lack of a unifying nomenclature or definition for the morphology involved. Therefore, while the classically described entity of 'single ventricle with outlet chamber' has been generally recognized as being the same thing as double inlet left ventricle, there has been no agreement as to whether hearts with double inlet right ventricle should be analysed in the same group, or whether it is appropriate to include other patients who simply have a huge ventricular septal defect. Since the mid-1990s, light has begun to emerge at the end of the tunnel for functionally univentricular hearts. Clarification has come with the realization that, in terms of atrioventricular connections, all congenitally malformed hearts can be divided basically into two groups (Anderson et al, 1984a,b). In the larger of these groups, each of the patient's atriums has a separate connection to one of two ventricles. Those are the patients with concordant, discordant and ambiguous atrioventricular connections. The second, much smaller, group is unified because the atriums are joined to only one ventricle. Where a second ventricle exists, it must of necessity be incomplete and, hence, rudimentary. Understanding of this second group has been clouded by an illogical desire to describe lesions falling within it as univentricular hearts, neglecting to recognize that their unifying feature is the univentricular atrioventricular connection (Anderson et al, 1983b, 1984a). For clinical purposes, three large divisions of patients stand out within this overall generic term, which we use only for the purpose of grouping and never in isolation as a descriptive term. They are the patients with double-inlet atrioventricular connection, to be discussed in this chapter; those with classical tricuspid atresia, discussed in Chapter 39; and those with absence of the left atrioventricular connection, who are considered in Chapter 49.

MORPHOLOGY

Morphologists have long shown interest in hearts with double inlet atrioventricular connection, particularly because the most common examples of such hearts, those with double inlet left ventricle, are conveniently interpreted as being a consequence of arrested normal development. It has been the desire to interpret the malformations in terms of embryogenesis that has underscored much of the controversy and disagreement which surround them. Of necessity, different views of morphogenesis result in different interpretations of the structure of the definitive heart. To avoid such hazards, we now prefer to ignore considerations of morphogenesis when classifying and describing hearts with double inlet ventricle. In their place, we use the anatomy as it is observed. It would be inappropriate, nonetheless, to ignore previous classifications and terminologies for the malformation that, for some considerable time, has been the paradigm of the functionally single ventricle, even though very few hearts within the group possess a truly solitary ventricular chamber.

Traditionally, the malformation was termed 'cor triloculare biatriatum'. This acknowledged the presumption that the malformed heart had two atriums but only one ventricle, and distinguished it from 'cor biloculare', which was reputed to have only one atrium and one ventricle (Mann, 1907; Mills, 1923; Wood and Williams, 1928; Favorite, 1934; Brodie, 1945; Rogers and Edwards, 1951; Harley, 1958). Even during this period, nonetheless, it was recognized that most examples of cor triloculare biatriatum possessed two chambers within the ventricular mass, rendering the logic of the Latin terminology less than perfect. Taussig (1939) had accepted this traditional approach when she used the term 'single ventricle with diminutive outlet chamber' for such a heart with one big and one small ventricle. This usage, in turn, led to the distinction of 'single ventricle with outlet chamber' from 'common ventricle', the latter label being applied to hearts with a truly solitary ventricle (Gasul et al, 1966). Over the same period, others (Elliott et al, 1962, 1964) had used the adjectives 'single' and 'common' interchangeably when describing the presumptive solitary ventricle. This led to confusion. Van Praagh and colleagues (1964) highlighted the literal deficiencies of these terms in a seminal paper. They demonstrated the morphological variability of the dominant ventricle to which the atriums were connected in the presence of double inlet. They distinguished four possibilities, arguing that the atriums could be connected to a left ventricle (type A), a right ventricle (type B), a mixed ventricle (type C) and an indeterminate ventricle (type D). Although this new convention was accepted by many, others continued to espouse the distinction between 'single' and 'common' ventricles (Lev et al, 1969). They pointed out that, as they interpreted morphogenetic events, the 'single' ventricle was equivalent to the primitive ventricle of the developing heart tube. Following this, still others used the term 'double inlet left ventricle' to describe this type of atrioventricular connection (Van Mierop and Gessner, 1972). This term had a long pedigree, having been used by Peacock in 1855. It had been devalued to some extent by its subsequent use to distinguish hearts with straddling valves from those with true double inlet, the latter being dubbed 'single ventricle' (Mehrizi and McMurphy, 1966; Tandon et al, 1974).

When we first studied hearts with double inlet, we initially attempted to resolve the problems as we saw them by following the lead of Lev and his associates (1969) and using embryological concepts. Therefore, we tried to expand their concept of 'primitive ventricle' to account for all hearts with double inlet, at the same time incorporating those with absence of one atrioventricular connection. Our concept depended upon whether or not a second rudimentary ventricle was present (Anderson et al, 1976; Wilkinson et al, 1976). At that time, we denied ventricular status to the second chamber, which we considered to represent the embryonic bulb. The concept foundered when we encountered hearts with double inlet right ventricle in the presence of a rudimentary left ventricle (Keeton et al, 1979). We then tried to categorize the hearts on the basis of their ventricular morphology (Anderson et al, 1979a; Wilkinson et al, 1979a), but we continued to deny ventricular status to the chamber considered rudimentary, irrespective of its morphology.

This fuelled rather than doused the flames of controversy, since those who had initially popularized the concept of double inlet as the criterion of single ventricle (Van Praagh et al, 1964) now recanted. Instead, they denied that hearts with double inlet right ventricle could be considered univentricular because of the presence of the second chamber of unequivocally left ventricular morphology (Van Praagh et al, 1979). This was despite the fact that double inlet had only then become widely

accepted as the criterion of 'single ventricle' (Edwards, 1977; Ellis, 1977). Indeed, Van Praagh and his colleagues (1982) then pointed to the acceptance of double inlet as the paradigm of 'single ventricle' as being the major flaw in our whole concept for description of functionally univentricular hearts (Anderson et al, 1979a).

In this concept, we had argued that all hearts with double inlet atrioventricular connection were unified because the atriums were connected to only one ventricle. A second ventricle, if present, of necessity lacked any connection with the atriums. It seemed, to us, illogical to describe this structure as an outlet chamber when there was double inlet left ventricle, yet to call the morphologically comparable structure a right ventricle in the setting of classical tricuspid atresia (Anderson et al, 1979b). We had recognized that we were using the term 'single ventricle', or rather its synonym 'univentricular heart', in illogical fashion when describing congenitally malformed hearts that unequivocally possessed two chambers within their ventricular mass. We attempted to correct this semantic deficiency by constructing formidable conventions that distinguished 'ventricles' from 'non-ventricles'. At the same time, we compounded our illogicality by accepting that our non-ventricles could be of right or left ventricular morphology! As was pointed out (McGoon, 1981; Van Praagh et al, 1982), this system produced major problems when applied to hearts with overriding and straddling atrioventricular valves. This was because a non-ventricle connected to 49% of an overriding atrioventricular junction suddenly became a ventricle when it was connected to 51% of the junction. We subsequently realized that our efforts to resolve in this fashion the controversy of functionally univentricular hearts were misplaced. The unifying feature of the hearts with double inlet, and those with absence of one atrioventricular connection, is not the univentricular nature of their ventricular mass. Instead, it is the univentricular connection of the atrium and ventricles across the atrioventricular junctions (Anderson, 1983; Anderson et al, 1983b, 1984a).

This is not to say that we now describe any individual heart as having a univentricular atrioventricular connection. The term is a generic one, which simply emphasizes the nature of the atrioventricular junction. It is equally important to draw attention to the differences in the hearts within this grouping. Indeed, not all appreciated the thrust of our argument when we highlighted the similarities between hearts with double inlet left ventricle and those with classical tricuspid atresia. Bharati and Lev (1979a), and Rao (1982) inferred that we suggested the lesions to be identical. This was never our intention. We simply pointed out that the entities are comparable in that both have univentricular atrioventricular connection to a dominant left ventricle. They certainly differ in that one lacks the right atrioventricular connection, while the other has double inlet ventricle. The ones with double inlet left ventricle resemble all other hearts with double inlet by virtue of their comparable atrioventricular connection but differ according to the nature of their ventricular morphology. In this chapter, we describe only those hearts that have double inlet connection, but we include all the morphological variants. Consequently, the atriums can be connected to a dominant left ventricle, a dominant right ventricle, or a solitary and indeterminate ventricle. Only the last variant is an example of a univentricular heart. The others possess second chambers within their ventricular mass, but chambers to which we no longer deny ventricular status. Rudimentary and incomplete right ventricles are found in hearts with double inlet to a dominant left ventricle, while rudimentary and incomplete left ventricles are found when there is double inlet to a dominant right ventricle. We include hearts with straddling valves in this chapter as long as the majority of the overriding junction is connected to the dominant ventricle; the overall group of hearts with straddling valves is discussed in Chapter 41.

The different prototypes of double inlet connection resemble, in terms of ventricular morphology, their counterparts with absent atrioventricular connection (Deanfield et al, 1982). We recognize fully, nonetheless, the major difference imparted by the absence of one atrioventricular connection. Those latter lesions, together with their 'close cousins' that have imperforate atrioventricular valves, are, therefore, described in the chapters devoted to tricuspid atresia (Chapter 39), hypoplastic left ventricle (Chapter 45) and left atrioventricular valvar atresia with patency of the subaortic outflow tract Chapter 40).

DOUBLE INLET LEFT VENTRICLE

By far the majority of hearts with double inlet connection have both atriums connected to a dominant left ventricle in the presence of a rudimentary and incomplete right ventricle (Figure 38.1). In the past, it was claimed that the dominant ventricle was of neither right nor left morphology (Bharati and Lev, 1979b). The smooth septal surface, combined with the pattern of the apical trabeculations, leaves little doubt that it is a left ventricle (Figure 38.2), although the apical trabeculations are often coarser than those of the normal left ventricle. It is also suggested that the rudimentary right ventricle is no more than an infundibulum (Van Praagh et al, 1979). The observed morphology again militates strongly against this contention. In all cases, it is possible to recognize the right ventricular nature of the apical trabeculations. This is most obvious when the ventriculo-arterial connections are concordant (Figure 38.3a), the trabecular portion being less prominent in those with discordant ventriculo-arterial connections (Figure 38.3b). Any doubt concerning the make-up of the ventricles in hearts with double inlet left ventricle is resolved by examination of hearts with double inlet to and double out from the dom-

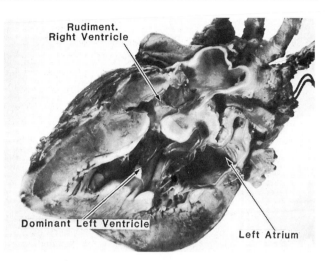

Figure 38.1. Double inlet ventricle exists, as in this heart, when both atrioventricular valves are tethered in the same ventricle, in this case the left ventricle. Very rarely, however, do such hearts have a solitary ventricle. As seen in this example, a rudimentary ventricle is found anterosuperiorly within the ventricular mass. See Figures 38.2 and 38.3 for the features of the dominant and rudimentary ventricles, respectively.

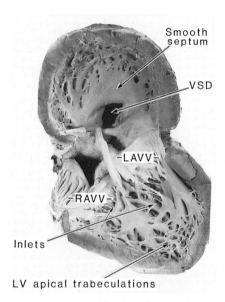

Figure 38.2. This heart with double inlet left ventricle is opened in clam-like fashion to show the structure of the dominant ventricle. The fine apical trabeculations, and the smooth septal surface, identify the ventricle as being morphologically left (LV). RAVV and LAVV, right and left atrioventricular valves, respectively; VSD, ventricular septal defect.

inant ventricle (Figure 38.4). If the 'outlet chamber' was only an infundibulum, it would not exist in such hearts with both outlets connected to the left ventricle. In reality, it is an easy matter to recognize complimentary ventricles of left and right ventricular morphology separated by the apical muscular ventricular septum, the true interventricular nature of this septum being validated by the fact that it carries the atrioventricular conduction axis (Lamers et al, 1992).

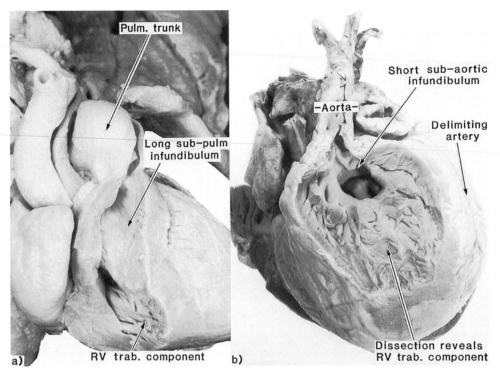

Figure 38.3. Rudimentary and incomplete right ventricles, when found with double inlet left ventricle, are always positioned anterosuperiorly. Their structure varies in the presence of concordant (a) and discordant (b) ventriculo-arterial trabeculations (trab.), but the coarse apical trabeculations identify the rudimentary and incomplete ventricle as being of right ventricular (RV) morphology. Pulm, pulmonary. (Reproduction of (a) is with kind permission of Dr J. R. Zuberbuhler, Children's Hospital of Pittsburgh.)

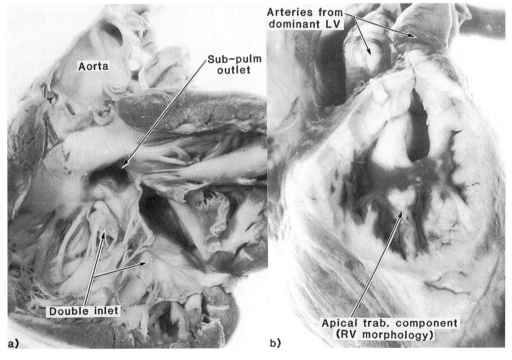

Figure 38.4. In this heart with double inlet left ventricle (a), both arterial trunks are also supported within the dominant left ventricle (LV). The rudimentary and incomplete right ventricle (b) is represented only by its apical trabecular (trab.) component, but the coarseness of the trabeculations show that this is, indeed, of right ventricular (RV) morphology.

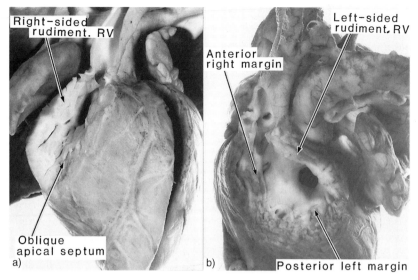

Figure 38.5. Rudimentary (rudiment.) right ventricles (RV), in the setting of double inlet left ventricle, are always found anterosuperiorly within the ventricular mass. They can be positioned directly anteriorly, as in Figure 38.36, but more usually they are either found to the right (a) or the left (b) sides of the dominant ventricle. In both of these hearts, the ventriculo-arterial connections are discordant.

In hearts with double inlet left ventricle, the rudimentary right ventricle is always found in basically an antero-superior position, with the apical ventricular septum never extending to the crux. The rudimentary right ventricle, nonetheless, may be right or left sided (Figure 38.5). As with any heart with double inlet, the atriums may have appendages arranged in usual, mirror-imaged or isomeric pattern. With double inlet left ventricle, however, it is rare to find other than usually arranged atrial appendages. The major subdivision of these hearts depends on the ventriculo-arterial connections. Most frequently, there are discordant ventriculo-arterial connections. The rudimentary ventricle and the aorta are then usually to the same

side, but not always. When the ventriculoarterial connections are discordant, the rudimentary right ventricle has a short infundibulum, and the ventricular septal defect is close to the aortic valve (Figure 38.5). Stenosis or atresia at the level of the ventricular septal defect (Figure 38.6) leads to subaortic obstruction and is associated with coarctation and/or hypoplasia or interruption of the aortic arch. Stenosis or atresia of the subpulmonary outflow tract from the dominant left ventricle is also frequent. This can have various causes. Most common is deviation of the outlet septum into the left ventricle, widening the aorta at the expense of the pulmonary trunk. Less common are valvar stenosis, anomalous insertion of

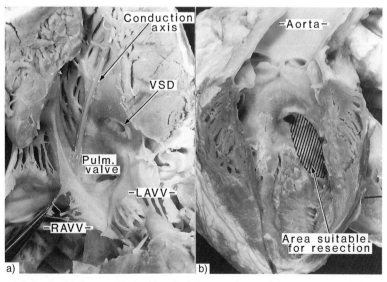

Figure 38.6. The ventricular septal defect in this heart with double inlet left ventricle is tightly restrictive. (a) The dominant ventricle opens in clamshell fashion (compare with Figure 38.2), and a catheter has been glued in the location of the ventricular conduction axis. (b) The right ventricle is opened from the front and the cross-hatching shows the apical wedge of septum that can be safely removed to enlarge the septal defect without damaging the conduction axis. Abbreviations as in Figures 38.2 and 38.3.

atrioventricular valvar tension apparatus across the outflow tract or aneurysms of fibrous tissue tags into the outflow tract from adjacent valvar or fibrous structures. When the outflow tract is atretic, there is usually no evidence of formation of the pulmonary valve. The pulmonary trunk then ends blindly, giving single outlet via the aorta with pulmonary atresia.

It is less common, but by no means infrequent, to find concordant ventriculo-arterial connections. Hearts of this type are often termed 'Holmes hearts' (Holmes, 1824; Marin-Garcia et al, 1974a; Anderson et al, 1983b, Dobell and Van Praagh, 1996). Usually in this combination, the apical component of the rudimentary right ventricle is on the opposite side from the subpulmonary infundibulum and the ventricular septal defect is a good distance from the pulmonary valve (Figure 38.3a). It is in these cases that the resemblance of the right ventricle to that seen in classical tricuspid atresia is most obvious (compare with Figure 38.10). Less frequently, the sub-pulmonary infundibulum and the right ventricular apical component are to the same side of the ventricular mass (Figure 38.7). Stenosis or obstruction of the ventricular septal defect is also frequent with concordant ventriculo-arterial connections, but then results in subpulmonary stenosis. Double outlet from the rudimentary right ventricle can occur but is infrequent. More frequent is double outlet from the dominant left ventricle. Then, as discussed above, the right ventricle is made up of no more than the apical trabecular component (Figure 38.4). Single outlet can also occur, most frequently owing to a single aortic trunk with pulmonary atresia, as already discussed, but either a common trunk or a solitary pulmonary trunk with aortic atresia are potential ventriculo-arterial connections.

Irrespective of the ventriculo-arterial connections, abnormalities of the atrioventricular valves are frequent (Quero Jimenez et al, 1975, 1979; Girod et al, 1984). Both the valves characteristically resemble a mitral valve (Figure 38.7). Although usually they possess separate papillary muscles and are frequently separated on the posteroinferior ventricular wall by a prominent posterior ridge, the two valves can share papillary muscles. Then there is no cleavage plane between them. Where one or other arterial valve is connected to the left ventricle, both atrioventricular valves are usually in continuity with it, although either, or rarely both, may be separated from it by persistence of the ventriculo-infundibular fold. Either the right or the left atrioventricular valve may be imperforate (Figure 38.8), stenotic, or may straddle or override the ventricular septum. When there is straddling, usually the right valve straddles into a right-sided rudimentary ventricle, but exceptions do occur. Providing more than half of the overriding junction is connected to the left ventricle, we continue to categorize the connection as double inlet. As a rule, the greater the override, the larger the right ventricle (Chapter 41). The atrioventricular conduction axis is grossly abnormal (Anderson et al, 1974; Bharati and Lev, 1975; Wenink, 1978; Essed et al, 1980; Anderson and Becker, 1983). The pattern is dictated by the lack of any ventricular septum at the crux. Because

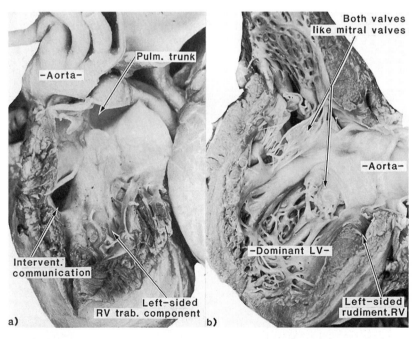

Figure 38.7. A less common arrangement of hearts with double inlet left ventricle and concordant ventriculo-arterial connections has the concordantly connected pulmonary trunk arising from a left-sided rudimentary and incomplete right ventricle (a). Opening the dominant left ventricle (b) reveals that both atrioventricular valves have the structure of the normal mitral valve. The typical arrangement is shown in Figure 38.3a. Abbreviations as in Figures 38.2 and 38.3. (Photographed and reproduced by kind permission of Dr J. R. Zuberbuhler, Children's Hospital of Pittsburgh.)

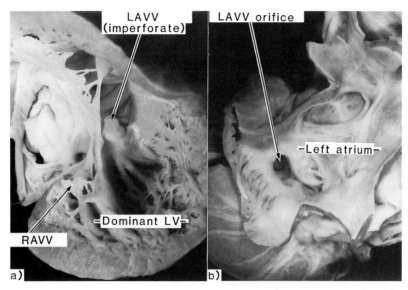

Figure 38.8. Double inlet left ventricle can be found when one atrioventricular valve is imperforate, in this case the left valve. This produces an unusual variant of mitral atresia. The heart is seen from its ventricular (a) and left atrial (b) aspects. Abbreviations as in Figure 38.2.

of this, the regular atrioventricular node in the atrial septum is unable to make contact with the atrioventricular conduction tissues positioned astride the apical muscular ventricular septum. Instead, an anomalous atrioventricular node is found in the anterior quadrant of the right atrioventricular orifice. From this node, the conduction axis penetrates the atrioventricular fibrous plane and ramifies as the ventricular conduction tissues. The precise course of the non-branching bundle depends on the position of the rudimentary right ventricle. When the right ventricle is right sided, the bundle is able to descend directly onto the septum and is unrelated to the pulmonary outflow tract (Figure 38.9). When the rudimentary ventricle is left sided, the bundle extends anterosuperiorly

round the pulmonary valvar orifice to reach the septum (Figure 38.10). Irrespective of the position of the rudimentary ventricle, the relation of conduction tissue and the ventricular septal defect is the same when viewed from the right ventricular aspect (Figure 38.11). The bundle branches on the left ventricular aspect of the septum and is well below the septal crest. Only the right bundle branch extends upwards, piercing the septum to ramify in the apical right ventricular trabecular component. Differences in disposition as perceived by the surgeon relate to different surgical approaches (Figure 38.12). The basic disposition is always the same. It is dictated by the orientation of the ventricular septum. The septum joins the atrioventricular junction more parietally when the

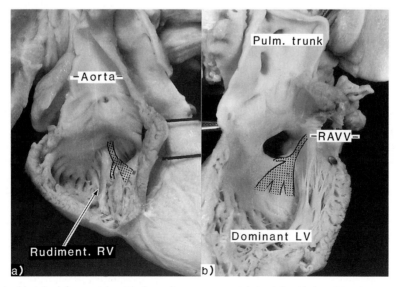

Figure 38.9. This heart with double inlet left ventricle with the rudimentary ventricle in right-sided position is prepared to show the course of the atrioventricular conduction axis (stippled area) as seen from the rudimentary right ventricle (a) and from the dominant left ventricle (b). The left valve has been removed to display the septal surface of the dominant left ventricle. Abbreviations as in Figures 38.2 and 38.3.

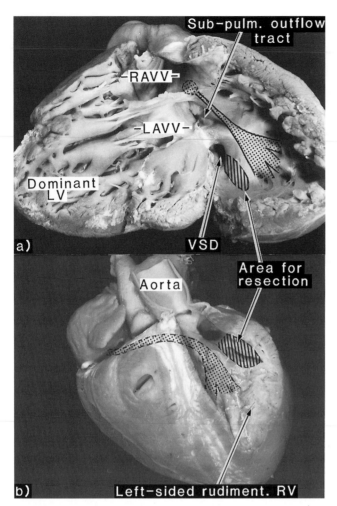

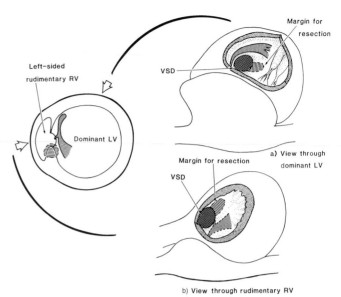

Figure 38.10. In this heart with double inlet left ventricle (a) the rudimentary right ventricle (b) is positioned anteriorly and to the left. The stippled area shows the course of the conduction axis, which passes anterosuperiorly to the ventricular septal defect when seen from the dominant ventricle (a) but is posteroinferior when seen from the rudimentary ventricle (b). The cross-hatched area shows the 'safe' segment of the septum that can be removed for surgical enlargement of the ventricular septal defect. Abbreviations as in Figures 38.2 and 38.3.

Figure 38.12. The conduction axis (fine cross-hatching) assumes an apparently different orientation relative to the ventricular septal defect (VSD) when viewed from the dominant left ventricle (LV) (a) than when viewed from the rudimentary right ventricle (RV) (b). The more coarsely cross-hatched area shows the segment of septum which can safely be resected. The conduction axis is on the *left ventricular* aspect of the septum.

right valve straddles. Because of this, the node and penetrating bundle are formed posterolaterally in the right atrioventricular orifice (Chapter 41).

The ventricular myocardium is rarely normal in hearts with double inlet left ventricle. Frequently the dominant left ventricle is thick and muscle-bound. The studies of Freedom and his colleagues (1977) have shown that banding of the pulmonary trunk can rapidly exacerbate this thickening, with increasing stenosis of the ventricular septal defect; hence subaortic obstruction can occur when the ventriculo-arterial connections are discordant.

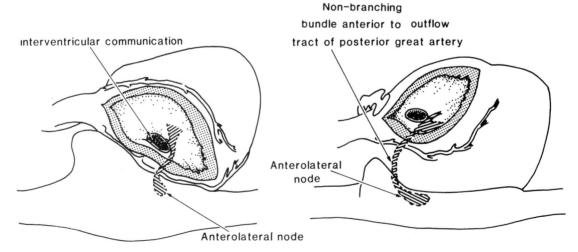

Figure 38.11. The double inlet left ventricle in surgical orientation shows the basically similar disposition of the atrioventricular conduction axis relative to the interventricular communication (ventricular septal defect) as viewed from the rudimentary and incomplete right ventricle (RV) irrespective of whether that chamber is right or left sided.

Comparable diminution in size of this defect to give pulmonary stenosis is a naturally occurring feature in hearts with concordant ventriculo-arterial connections (Somerville et al, 1975).

DOUBLE INLET RIGHT VENTRICLE

Hearts with double inlet right ventricle are almost always found with a rudimentary left ventricle located in postero-inferior position, usually to the left (Figure 38.13) but rarely to the right. In this setting, the ventricular septum does extend to the crux. As with double inlet left ventri-cle, hearts with a dominant right ventricle can be found with any atrial arrangement, but the usual arrangement and right isomeric patterns are found most frequently (Keeton et al, 1979; Soto et al, 1979). Hearts with strad-dling atrioventricular valves are categorized as double inlet right ventricle when less than half the overriding orifice is connected to the rudimentary left ventricle (Figure 38.14). We have only seen the left valve strad-dling into a left-sided left ventricle or the right valve into a right-sided left ventricle. In all cases, the straddling valve resembled a mitral valve and the non-straddling valve a tricuspid valve. Common valves committed exclusively or predominantly to the right ventricle are

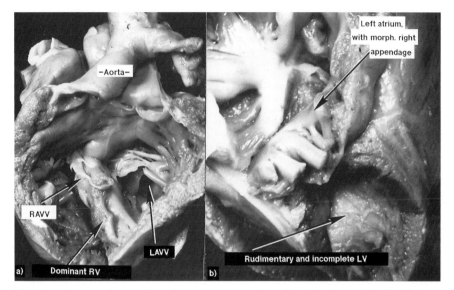

Figure 38.13. (a) The double inlet right ventricle seen through two atrioventricular valves. (b) The apical trabecular component of the left ventricle forms a slit-like rudimentary chamber in the posteroinferior wall of the ventricular mass (b). This heart had right isomerism and pulmonary atresia. Abbreviations as in Figure 38.2.

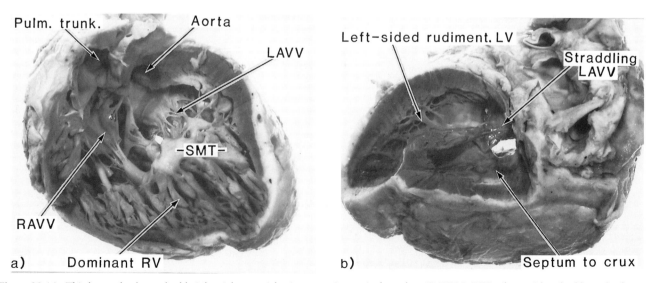

Figure 38.14. This heart also has a double inlet right ventricle via two atrioventricular valves (RAVV, LAVV), along with a double outlet from the dominant right ventricle (a). Note the septomarginal trabeculation (SMT) on the septal surface of the right ventricle. The left-sided rudimentary and incomplete left ventricle is much bigger in this heart because of the straddling of part of the tension apparatus of the left atrioventricular valve (b). Abbreviations as in Figures 38.2 and 38.3.

frequent, particularly when there is right isomerism. Malformations of the atrioventricular valves, excluding straddling and overriding, are less frequent than in double inlet left ventricle. When there are two valves, however, they frequently share the same papillary muscles. The rudimentary left ventricle tends to be bigger when there is straddling and overriding of an atrioventricular valve (compare Figures 38.13 and 38.14). The other feature that contributes to the morphology of the rudimentary ventricle is the ventriculo-arterial connection. Most frequently this is double outlet from the dominant right ventricle or single outlet with pulmonary atresia, the aorta arising from the right ventricle. The rudimentary left ventricle then consists only of its apical trabecular component (Figure 38.13), being larger when there is a straddling valve (Figure 38.14). In the presence of concordant or discordant ventriculo-arterial connections, the rudimentary ventricle has an outlet component, the aorta being connected to the left ventricle in all the hearts we have seen in this type. There is then aortic-atrioventricular valvar continuity in the roof of the ventricular septal defect (Figure 38.15). Discordant ventriculo-arterial connections should be anticipated, and double outlet from the rudimentary left ventricle must not be discounted. Stenosis can occur in either outflow tract, most frequently in the subpulmonary position. Because of the ventriculo-arterial connections, this stenosis is usually found at infundibular level.

The disposition of the conduction tissue is determined in part by the septal orientation and in part by the ventricular topology. Hearts with left-sided rudimentary ventricles show a right-handed pattern of ventricular topology. Then, because the septum extends to the crux, the connecting node is in its anticipated regular position. The penetrating bundle is posterior and branches either astride the trabecular septum or, rarely, runs on a prominent trabeculation within the dominant right ventricle (Wilkinson et al, 1979b). When the rudimentary left ventricle is right sided, the ventricular topology is left handed. This is then the dominant feature in determining the location of the conduction tissue, over and above the fact that the septum reaches to the crux (Anderson and Becker, 1983). In the only heart of this type we studied histologically, there was a sling of conduction tissue between anterior and regular nodes. The ventricular conduction tissue descended on a trabeculation within the right ventricle (Essed et al, 1980).

DOUBLE INLET INDETERMINATE VENTRICLE —

Hearts are rarely found with double inlet to a solitary ventricle of indeterminate morphology (Figure 38.16; Van Praagh et al, 1964; Anderson et al, 1979a). Usually the ventricle is particularly coarsely trabeculated, although prominent posterior trabeculations may on occasion simulate a ventricular septum (Figure 38.17). More significantly, it is usually criss-crossed by prominent free-standing apical muscle bundles that support the atrioventricular valvar tension apparatus. Sometimes it is difficult to differentiate the ventricle from a right ventricle solely on the basis of its apical trabeculations. In all the hearts we studied that might have had a solitary right ventricle, we were able to

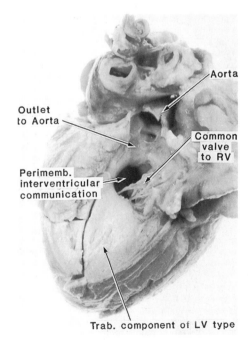

Figure 38.15. In this heart, with double inlet right ventricle (RV) through a common atrioventricular valve, the rudimentary and incomplete left ventricle (LV) gives rise to the aorta (concordant ventriculo-arterial connections). The ventricular septal defect (interventricular communication) is perimembranous (Perimemb.).

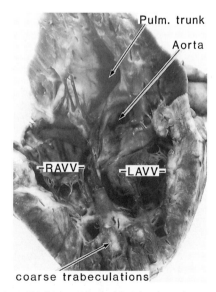

Figure 38.16. In this heart with double inlet through two atrioventricular valves (RAVV, LAVV) and double outlet, there is a truly solitary ventricle of indeterminate apical morphology. Note the coarse trabeculations throughout the apical regions. Abbreviations as in Figures 38.2 and 38.3.

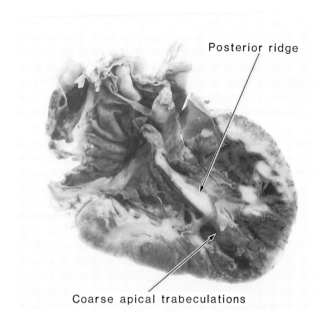

Figure 38.17. This simulated four chamber section is from the heart shown in Figure 38.16. At first sight, there is an 'inlet' septum. In reality, this is a prominent trabeculation that has had its surface sliced away. Again note the coarse trabeculations to either side of the apical region.

recognize the septomarginal trabeculation on the postero-inferior free wall of the ventricle. Guided by its limbs, further dissection revealed a tiny rudimentary left ventricle within the ventricular wall. Such a second ventricle has been absent in all those hearts we studied that truly possessed indeterminate ventricles.

Double inlet to an indeterminate ventricle is found most frequently with usual or isomeric atrial appendages

but may be found with mirror-imaged arrangement. There may be two atrioventricular valves or a common valve, but straddling valves cannot exist since there is no apical muscular septum. The two valves, when present, frequently have shared papillary muscles. Because of the solitary ventricle, the potential ventriculo-arterial connections are limited to either double outlet or single outlet of the heart. A bilateral infundibulum is a frequent finding in the hearts with double outlet. Arterial stenosis, if present, is usually at infundibular level. The free-standing muscle bundles can obstruct one or other outflow and may also produce the spurious appearance of an anterior rudimentary ventricle.

Because there is no apical trabecular septum, there cannot be a normal conduction system. Most frequently in our experience, there has been an anterior node with the bundle descending onto a free-standing muscle bar. The bundle can also descend in the parietal ventricular wall or else drop from a regular node (Wilkinson et al, 1979b). Slings of conduction tissue have been found in the posterior ventricular wall in patients with right isomerism (Dickinson et al, 1979).

HUGE VENTRICULAR SEPTAL DEFECTS

Hearts also exist in which most of the ventricular septum is absent, but an apical muscular rim persists dividing the ventricular mass into right ventricular and left ventricular components (Figure 38.18; Van Praagh et al, 1964). Because of the apical septum, the atrioventricular valves are committed to separate trabecular components. More importantly, in most cases but not all, it is usual to find a rim of inlet septum running between the apical septum

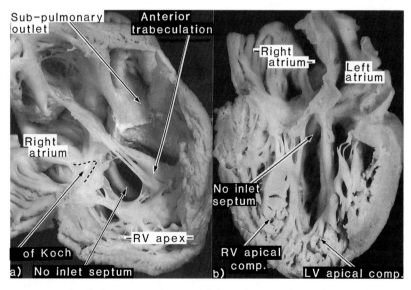

Figure 38.18. This specimen is an example of a huge ventricular septal defect. The apex of the right ventricle (a) is coarsely trabeculated, in comparison to the more finely trabeculated left ventricle (b) revealed by a four chamber section. Although there is an apical septum, there is no inlet septum present, which is unusual. The conduction axis descended from an anomalous node onto the anterior trabeculation (a), there being no muscular structure beneath the regular atrioventricular node located within the triangle of Koch.

and the crux. In our experience, this rim has always carried the non-branching bundle from a regularly positioned node. Morphologically, therefore, the hearts are readily distinguished from those with double inlet atrioventricular connection. We prefer to categorize them as huge ventricular septal defects, while recognizing some affinity with the other hearts described within this chapter.

MORPHOGENESIS

The problems arising with morphogenesis relate as much to terminology of the embryonic heart tube as they do to positive disagreements. From the standpoint of the occurrence of double inlet atrioventricular connection, the important feature is that, initially, the entire atrioventricular junction was connected to the inlet part of the primary heart tube, while the arterial pedicles were supported by the outlet component (Figure 38.19). As described in Chapter 20, the apical component of the developing left ventricle is derived from the inlet part of the primary tube, while that of the developing right ventricle is derived from the outlet part. The formation of the two trabecular components occurs concomitant with development of the apical trabecular septum. If the two pouches did not grow separately, but rather there was formation of a general trabecular component from the primary heart tube, then a solitary ventricle of indeterminate morphology would be produced (Figure 38.19, left

hand panel). Whether this exists with two valves or a common atrioventricular valve depends on the partitioning of the atrioventricular junction. Should the pouches form in normal fashion, but the atrioventricular junction remain connected only to the inlet part of the ventricular loop, then the end result would be double inlet left ventricle. The hypoplastic trabecular component derived from the outlet part of the loop would form the basis of the rudimentary right ventricle (Figure 38.19, lower right hand panel). Again, the arrangement of the atrioventricular valves would depend upon the mode of development of the atrioventricular junction. The ventriculo-arterial connections present would depend on the development of the outlet portions. The position of the rudimentary right ventricle would probably be determined by the initial looping of the primary tube, but equally it could be influenced by rotation of the entire heart.

Double inlet right ventricle probably results from transfer of the entire inlet part of the primary heart tube to the apical trabecular component, which is derived from the outlet, this process occurring subsequent to formation of the left ventricular apical component (Figure 38.19, upper right hand panel). This rudimentary trabecular component will then be the basis of the posteroinferior left ventricle. Valvar morphology and ventriculo-arterial connections will again depend on the development of the other parts of the heart tube. The position of the rudimentary ventricle will depend on the initial direction of ventricular looping. Rightward

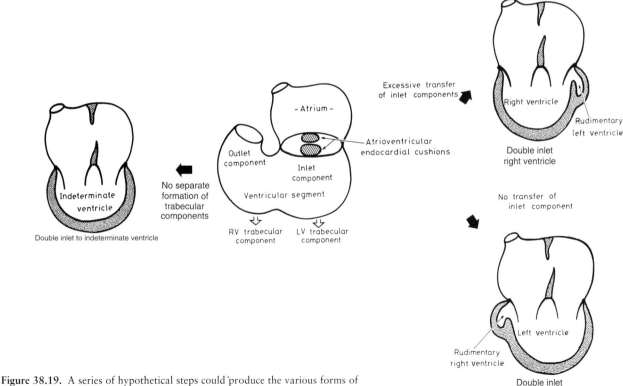

Figure 38.19. A series of hypothetical steps could produce the various forms of double inlet ventricle from the basic heart tube shown in the centre of the panel.

looping will give a left-sided rudimentary left ventricle, while leftward looping will result in a right-sided left ventricle. The morphogenesis of straddling and overriding valves is discussed in Chapter 41.

PREVALENCE

Double inlet ventricle comprised 1.5% of patients with congenital heart disease seen at the Hospital for Sick Children, Toronto between 1950 and 1973. The ratio of males to females was 1.25 to 1 (Kidd, 1978). Difficulties in diagnosis, particularly in the days before cross-sectional echocardiography, cast some doubt on the reliability of this figure. In an analysis by Scott et al (1984) of infants presenting to the Royal Brompton Hospital in the 10-year period to November 1983, 4.3% had double inlet ventricle. Weigel and co-workers (1989) studied the occurrence of congenital heart disease in 378 siblings of patients with double inlet ventricle. The overall incidence of congenital heart disease was 2.8%. Although numbers were small, the occurrence of congenital heart malformations in the siblings of patients with left isomerism appeared to be higher (28%; two of seven siblings).

PATHOPHYSIOLOGY

The major consequence of the double inlet atrioventricular connection is obligatory mixing of the atrial streams in the dominant ventricle, irrespective of its morphology. When there is a common atrioventricular valve, there will also be an ostium primum defect, and the valve itself will frequently be regurgitant.

Regurgitation of either of two separate valves is uncommon. When encountered, it is usually caused by arrhythmias, ruptured tension apparatus (Somerville, 1979) or bacterial endocarditis. Stenosis of one or other atrioventricular valve has been reported in about a third of cases at postmortem (Quero Jimenez et al, 1979), the left atrioventricular valve being more commonly affected than the right. Postmortem series invariably select more severe abnormalities. In clinical series, the incidence of atrioventricular valvar anomalies is much lower. The effect of these obstructive and regurgitant lesions is much the same as in hearts with biventricular atrioventricular connections.

MIXING OF BLOOD

Pulmonary and systemic venous streams tend to mix within the dominant ventricle, but this mixing is complete in only a third of patients (Rahimtoola et al, 1966; Macartney et al, 1976; Mocellin and Sauer, 1979). It is only guaranteed to be complete if one cardiac valve is imperforate (Macartney et al, 1976). Most patients have favourable streaming, with the systemic arterial being higher than pulmonary arterial saturation. Preferential streaming does not appear to be affected by obstruction of the subpulmonary outflow, but it is strongly influenced in those with double inlet left ventricle by the position of the rudimentary right ventricle. Consequently, patients with usual atrial arrangement and a right-sided or anterior rudimentary right ventricle tend to have favourable streaming in the presence of concordant ventriculo-arterial connections, and unfavourable streaming or complete mixing with discordant ventriculo-arterial connections. This is because the systemic venous blood preferentially enters the rudimentary right ventricle. In contrast, if the rudimentary right ventricle is to the left and connected to the aorta, it is closer to the left atrioventricular valve and, therefore, preferentially receives pulmonary venous blood (Macartney et al, 1976; Mocellin and Sauer, 1979).

Though the difference between pulmonary and systemic arterial oxygen saturations may be as high as 24% (Macartney et al, 1976; Ritter et al, 1979), streaming plays a relatively small part in determining systemic arterial oxygen saturation. This is highest when systemic blood flow is lowest and pulmonary blood flow is highest. Since systemic blood flow is usually maintained at or above normal levels (Macartney et al, 1976), this means that a high systemic arterial oxygen saturation (which may reach 96%) is bought at the cost of a considerably increased volume overload on the ventricle.

VENTRICULAR FUNCTION

The assessment of ventricular function in patients with univentricular atrioventricular connections is hampered by the non-uniformity of ventricular shape characteristic of these conditions. These limitations not withstanding, the assessment of their ventricular function has attracted much attention. Radionuclide studies by Parikh and co-workers (1991) demonstrated a reduced ejection fraction, with no significant difference between hearts with dominant right or left ventricles. Biplane cineangiographic studies of Sano and co-workers (1989), in contrast, had also demonstrated a reduction in ejection fraction, but one which was most profound in those with dominant right ventricles. Ventricular stress at end-systole was also higher in patients than in controls, and particularly high in those with dominant right ventricles. They concluded that the more profound reduction in ejection fraction in patients with dominant right ventricles was related to elevated afterload, rather than to specific differences in contractility.

There has also been interest in the assessment of ventricular diastolic function, following the report that patients with ventricular hypertrophy were at higher risk of death after the Fontan operation (Kirklin et al, 1986). In this respect, marked changes in ventricular relaxation were observed in the immediate postoperative period after a Fontan operation. These reflect the abrupt volume unloading of the previously overloaded dominant ventricle (Penny et al, 1992).

Regional abnormalities of ventricular contraction and relaxation have also been demonstrated both before and after the Fontan operation (Gibson et al, 1979; Penny et al, 1991a,b). Fogel and co-workers (1995) used magnetic resonance tagging to demonstrate regional variation in ventricular wall motion and strain. Data from Rigby and co-workers (Rigby et al, 1981; Rigby, 1983) may explain some of the functional abnormalities. They found a rather high incidence of abnormal levels of amplitude in the myocardium of patients with double inlet ventricle when they were studied by amplitude-processed echocardiography. These findings, suggestive of myocardial fibrosis, were limited to patients over the age of 8 years and were most common in patients with double inlet right ventricle.

STATUS OF THE VENTRICULAR SEPTAL DEFECT

The ventricular septal defect, which is usually muscular, has a tendency to become obstructive with increasing age. If the aorta originates from the rudimentary right ventricle, this will result in subaortic obstruction (Somerville et al, 1974). While it has been suggested that this tendency is increased by banding of the pulmonary trunk (Freedom et al, 1977), it remains unclear whether the relationship is coincidental, rather than causal.

When the pulmonary trunk arises from the rudimentary right ventricle, then progressive reduction in the size of the defect causes subpulmonary obstruction (Somerville et al, 1975).

EXERCISE CAPACITY

Exercise capacity is markedly reduced in all patients, particularly those with a low resting arterial oxygen saturation and a high haematocrit. For a given ratio between real and predicted maximal consumption of oxygen, the ratio of minute ventilation and maximal voluntary ventilation is much higher in patients with univentricular atrioventricular connection than in controls (Driscoll et al, 1984).

PRESENTATION AND CLINICAL SYMPTOMATOLOGY

Clinical symptomatology is independent of ventricular morphology but strongly related to associated lesions. Patients with stenosis of the left atrioventricular valve tend to present in infancy with congestive heart failure and pulmonary congestion. Apart from this, the mode of presentation is almost entirely dependent on the degree of pulmonary stenosis. At one extreme are patients with pulmonary atresia. They present with severe cyanosis without heart failure on the first day of life. If no pulmonary stenosis is present, infants present in the first month or two of life with severe heart failure, often without clinically evident cyanosis. The heart failure is exacerbated by the coexistence of interruption of the aortic arch or coarctation, which occurs in about a third of postmortem cases of double inlet left ventricle with discordant ventriculo-arterial connections (Marin-Garcia et al, 1974b; Van Praagh et al, 1979). It is much rarer if there are concordant ventriculo-arterial connections (Marin-Garcia et al, 1974a). These aortic arch anomalies are frequently associated with obstruction of a subaortic ventricular septal defect. Occasionally this obstruction is functionally complete (Macartney and Anderson, 1978). Exceptionally, there is aortic valvar atresia (Marin-Garcia et al, 1974b; Van Praagh et al, 1979). Acquired obstruction of the ventricular septal defect may lead to cyanotic spells if pulmonary blood flow is occluded (Somerville et al, 1975). Angina pectoris can occur if aortic blood flow is occluded (Somerville et al, 1974).

In between the Scylla of severe cyanosis and the Charybdis of flooded lungs lies just the right amount of pulmonary stenosis. Patients in this favourable category may present as asymptomatic children, or even as adults with murmurs detected at routine physical examination.

CLINICAL FINDINGS

Just over half of the patients with double inlet ventricle are cyanotic from birth and four-fifths become so by the end of the first year of life. About 5% are never clinically cyanotic, and 65% present without signs of heart failure (Marin-Garcia et al, 1974a,b). The degree of mixing of pulmonary and systemic venous blood means that patients who are severely cyanosed tend not to be in heart failure and vice versa.

The peripheral pulses are normal unless there is aortic stenosis or an obstructive abnormality of the aortic arch. The jugular venous pulse is usually not elevated, but the A wave is dominant.

The precordium is active if pulmonary blood flow is excessive, and a systolic thrill is palpable in about a third of patients. The first heart sound is usually normal, but the second heart sound is single in half the patients. In the remainder, physiological splitting is present and pulmonary valvar closure may be accentuated in some patients with pulmonary hypertension.

A long ejection systolic murmur is present in almost all patients, being particularly loud in those with moderate pulmonary stenosis. Patients with excessive pulmonary blood flow, and many of those with left atrioventricular valvar stenosis, also have apical mid-diastolic rumbles. Patients with severe pulmonary vascular obstructive disease may develop high-pitched early diastolic murmurs of pulmonary incompetence together with ejection clicks caused by pulmonary arterial dilation. If the second heart sound is split, with accentuation of pulmonary closure, this certainly indicates pulmonary hypertension. By comparison, a loud single second heart sound can indicate pulmonary vascular disease, proximity of the aortic valve to the chest wall with a posterior pulmonary valve, or subvalvar or valvar pulmonary stenosis.

INVESTIGATIONS

ELECTROVECTORCARDIOGRAPHY

In theory, electrovectorcardiography should be very helpful, given the highly abnormal position of the conduction system in double inlet left and indeterminate ventricle. One would expect, for example, some kind of correlation between the direction of the initial QRS vector and the orientation of the ventricular septum. Thus, in double inlet left ventricle with a right anterior rudimentary right ventricle, the initial forces would be expected to resemble those in a normal heart, whereas if the rudimentary ventricle were to the left, the initial forces would be expected to resemble those in hearts with discordant atrioventricular connections (Chapter 49). Guller and colleagues (1975), however, concluded that vectorcardiograms did not usefully distinguish patients with double inlet ventricle from those with large ventricular septal defects and comparable ventriculo-arterial connections. Contrasting results were found by Rigby (1983). He divided the electrocardiograms of patients known to have double inlet into four groups: those with right ventricular dominance, corresponding to the normal infant progression of precordial leads; those with left ventricular dominance, corresponding to the normal adult progression of precordial leads; those with balanced ventricular forces, namely a dominant R wave both in right and left precordial leads; and those with a dominant S wave in all precordial leads. Patients very rarely changed from one group to another with advancing age. Among patients with double inlet left ventricle, 83% of those with a right-sided rudimentary right ventricle had a pattern of left ventricular dominance and 95% had a mean frontal QRS axis to the right. By contrast, 77% of those with a left-sided right ventricle had a pattern other than left ventricular dominance and 98% had a leftward frontal QRS axis. Whereas right ventricular dominance was seen in only 3% of patients with double inlet left ventricle, it was present in 94% of patients with double inlet right ventricle. This high incidence of right ventricular dominance had also been reported previously (Quero Jimenez et al, 1973; Shinebourne et al, 1980).

Consequently, it is possible to make sense of the electrocardiogram or vectorcardiogram when the diagnosis is known. Making the diagnosis from the electrocardiogram, in contrast, is much more difficult. Two rough rules of thumb may be worth remembering. First, whenever the tracings suggest discordant atrioventricular connections, think of double inlet ventricle (Davachi and Moller, 1969). Second, whenever a child appears to have a straightforward condition, but the electrocardiogram is atypical, again consider the possibility of double inlet ventricle.

One important abnormality to watch for in following patients with known double inlet ventricle is inversion of the T waves and depression of the ST segment in the left precordial leads. This may indicate subaortic obstruction owing to a restrictive ventricular septal defect (Barber et al, 1984).

CHEST RADIOGRAPHY

The abnormalities present on a plain chest radiography are the consequence of the relatively high incidence of malposition of the heart (Van Praagh et al, 1964; Lev et al, 1969), the relatively high incidence of isomerism, the high incidence of discordant ventriculo-arterial connections or abnormally related great arteries, and the tendency toward complete mixing of blood in the dominant ventricle. This last feature implies a straightforward relationship between overall size of the heart and the degree of pulmonary vascularity. For example, if pulmonary vascularity is only mildly increased, yet the heart is greatly enlarged and the child is markedly cyanotic, markedly unfavourable streaming of blood within the heart would be suggested. This makes the diagnosis of double inlet ventricle rather improbable. If pulmonary vascularity is decreased in double inlet ventricle because of pulmonary stenosis, the heart will be normal in size or mildly enlarged. If pulmonary vascularity is greatly increased, then the size of the heart will also be greatly increased. Only when pulmonary vascular obstructive disease supervenes is one likely to see a combination of modest cardiomegaly and gross enlargement of proximal pulmonary arteries. In this case, peripheral pruning should also be evident. Left-sided rudimentary right ventricles occasionally protrude from the left border of the heart with double inlet left ventricle in a very characteristic fashion, which is almost pathognomonic (Elliott and Gedgandas, 1964). We have also observed this pattern in hearts with concordant atrioventricular connections and criss-cross ventricular relationships. In these hearts, an often hypoplastic right ventricle is also carried on the left shoulder of the heart.

POSITION OF HEART AND ORGANS

Bronchial isomerism, if present, may be seen on penetrated chest radiograph, or better, by filtered beam radiography. The heart may be central or in the right chest.

POSITION OF GREAT ARTERIES

Left-sided rudimentary right ventricles in the presence of double inlet left ventricle usually give rise to the aorta. If the 'head' of the rudimentary ventricle is also to the left, the aorta will ascend on the left border of the vascular pedicle, thus mimicking congenitally corrected transposition (Chapter 49). The smaller the thymus and left pulmonary artery, the more obvious is this abnormality. There is no particular association between a right aortic arch and double inlet ventricle.

The pulmonary trunk may be displaced rightward when the ventriculo-arterial connections are discordant. It then comes to lie in front of the spine. Consequently, even when it is greatly enlarged, it is usually not seen on the standard chest radiograph. This combination of peripheral pulmonary plethora with absence of a bulge caused by the pulmonary trunk is similar to that seen in complete transposition (Chapter 48).

TRANSTHORACIC ECHOCARDIOGRAPHY ────

M-MODE TRACINGS

Considerable attention was directed to the inferential echocardiographic diagnosis of double inlet ventricle using M-mode techniques (Beardshaw et al, 1977; Mortera et al, 1977; Bini et al, 1978; Seward et al, 1977). These studies remain of historical interest, but since the advent of cross-sectional techniques, M-mode is no longer used to delineate the anatomy of these hearts.

CROSS-SECTIONAL ECHOCARDIOGRAPHY

The salient echocardiographic features of double inlet ventricle have been described by several groups (Rigby et al, 1981; Smallhorn et al, 1981b; Sahn et al, 1982). As in any congenital cardiac lesion, accurate echocardiographic diagnosis is facilitated by use of the segmental approach.

Having inferred the atrial arrangement from the relationships between the abdominal great vessels, the examination proceeds to the delineation of the atrioventricular connections. The key to the diagnosis lies in the demonstration of two atrioventricular valves (Figure 38.20), one of which may be imperforate (Figure 38.21), or a common valve, opening into one ventricle. This is best demonstrated from the subcostal or apical windows with the transducer orientated so as to demonstrate both atriums and both atrioventricular valves (Figure 38.20). This is the cut that would normally produce a four chamber section. The relations between the atrioventricular junction and the ventricular septum should be assessed for overriding. If this exists, biventricular connections must be distinguished from a univentricular connection by applying the 50% rule. It is sometimes difficult to see both junctions in the same plane, particularly from the subcostal position, but slight rocking of the transducer from side to side so as to bring first one valve and then the other into view while recording continuously will normally produce the necessary information. Sometimes, precordial short-axis cuts demonstrate the double inlet connection well. An imperforate valve (Figure 38.21) appears as a thin mobile echo between one or other atrium and the dominant ventricle, sometimes with tension apparatus inserting into it (Rigby et al, 1981). If this is suspected, it is important to scan from front to back of the heart to ensure that it is not the valvar annulus that is being misinterpreted as an imperforate valve. A common valve appears quite different from a single valve to the experienced observer, resembling closely the common atrioventricular orifice of

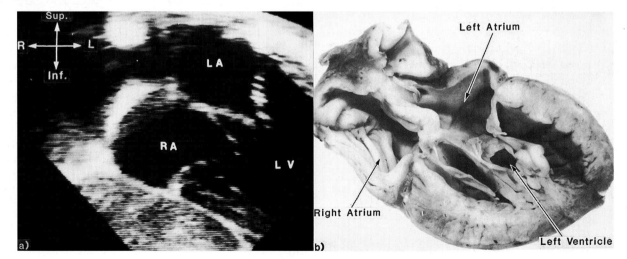

Figure 38.20. (a) This cross-sectional echocardiogram, in four chamber projection, shows a double inlet ventricle through two atrioventricular valves. The left ventricular (LV) nature of the dominant ventricle could only be determined once it was shown that the heart possessed also an anterosuperior ventricle of right morphology, not seen in the four chamber section. (b) A comparable morphological section is shown from a different heart. RA, right atrium; LA, left atrium. (Echocardiogram reproduced by kind permission of Drs M. Carminati and M.L. Rigby.)

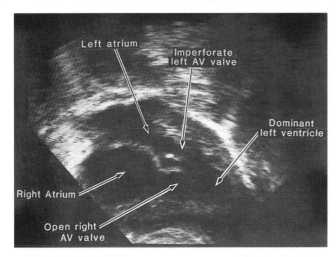

Figure 38.21. This four chamber section shows a double inlet left ventricle with an imperforate left atrioventricular (AV) valve. The cut is taken during ventricular diastole, but only the right valve is open. (Reproduced by permission of Prof. G. Sutherland.)

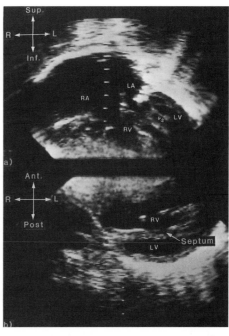

Figure 38.23. These sections in parasternal four chamber plane (a) and short axis (b) show double inlet to a dominant right ventricle (RV). Note the hypoplasia of the left atrioventricular valve. The short-axis section shows that the left ventricle (LV) is posteroinferiorly located, with the septum (vs) positioned behind both atrioventricular valves. RA, right atrium.

atrioventricular septal defects. The easiest way to recognize a common atrioventricular junction, however, is to identify the ostium primum defect, which has always been present in cases described so far (Smallhorn et al, 1981b).

In hearts with one big and one small ventricle, the displaced muscular ventricular septum separating them should be readily identified (Figures 38.22 and 38.23). If not, it should be searched for assiduously in short- and long-axis scans both from subcostal and precordial windows. Such cuts also demonstrate well the relation of the rudimentary to the dominant ventricle. These spatial relationships in the long-axis (Figure 38.22) and short-axis (Figures 38.23 and 38.24) planes are most useful in

inferring the morphology of the ventricles. In hearts with double inlet left ventricle, the rudimentary right ventricle is always carried on the anterosuperior shoulder of the dominant left ventricle (Figure 38.24). In contrast, in hearts with dominant right ventricles, the rudimentary left ventricle will occupy a posteroinferior position (Figure 38.23). If no rudimentary ventricle is identified,

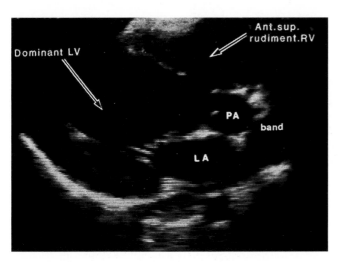

Figure 38.22. This parasternal long axis echocardiogram shows how the left atrioventricular valve is attached posteriorly relative to the remnant of the muscular ventricular septum, which divides the dominant left (LV) from the rudimentary right ventricle (RV). LA, left atrium; PA, banded pulmonary trunk. (Reproduced by permission of Drs M. Carminati and M.L. Rigby.)

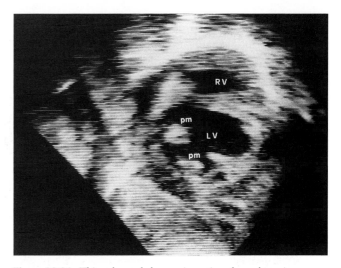

Figure 38.24. This subcostal short-axis section shows how, in a double inlet left ventricle, the rudimentary and incomplete right ventricle (RV) is always located in anterosuperior position. Note the papillary muscles (pm) of the valves in the dominant left ventricle (LV).

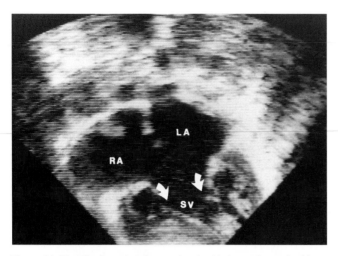

Figure 38.25. The four chamber section in this heart shows double inlet via a common atrioventricular valve (arrows) to a solitary and indeterminate ventricle (SV). Note the coarse apical trabeculations; the crucial feature in diagnosis was the inability to find a septum and a second, rudimentary, ventricle.

the ventricular morphology is presumed indeterminate (Figure 38.25). Once the existence and morphology of any rudimentary ventricle has been determined, the ventriculo-arterial connections can be established by tracing the arterial roots in subcostal or precordial long-axis cuts until they can be identified as either aorta or pulmonary trunk (Figures 38.26 and 38.27). Similar cuts will also demonstrate the nature of any subvalvar obstruction beneath the arterial valve or valves committed to the dominant ventricle.

Having established the basic anatomy, using the sequential approach, other features must be considered. Abnormalities of systemic and pulmonary venous return

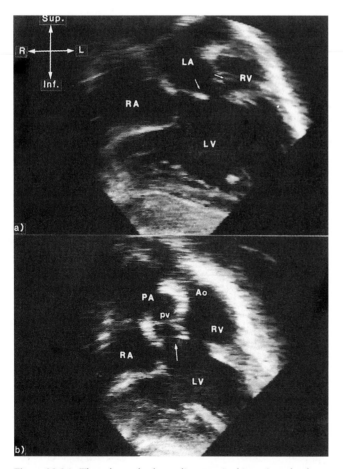

Figure 38.26. The subcostal echocardiograms in this patient clearly demonstrate the presence of a double inlet left ventricle (LV) with left-sided rudimentary right ventricle (RV), discordant ventriculo-arterial connections and straddling of the left atrioventricular valve (arrows). pv, pulmonary valve; PA, pulmonary trunk; Ao, aorta; LA, left atrium; RA, right atrium. (Reproduced with permission of Drs M. Carminati and M. L. Rigby.)

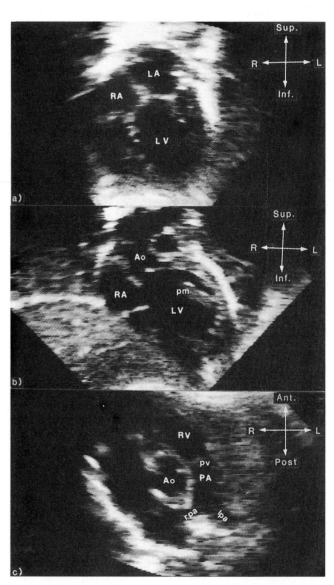

Figure 38.27. Echocardiographic features of a double inlet left ventricle with concordant ventriculo-arterial connections (the 'Holmes heart'). (a) Double inlet through two atrioventricular valves; (b) the aorta arising from the dominant left ventricle; (c) the normal position of the pulmonary trunk, arising from the rudimentary right ventricle, relative to the aorta and its right and left branches (rpa, lpa). Other abbreviations as in Fig 38.26. (Reproduced with permission of Drs M. Carminati and M.L. Rigby.)

can usually be readily identified from subcostal and suprasternal views. Identification of bilateral superior caval veins will assume greater importance in planning cavopulmonary shunts. Considerable attention should be directed to the assessment of the ventricular septal defect. The muscular, perimembranous, doubly committed or multiple nature of such defects can readily be identified (Bevilacqua et al, 1991; Shiraishi and Silverman, 1990). Measurements of the ventricular septal defect should be performed in two planes, usually taking the maximal diameters in both the short- and long-axis projections. These measurements can be used to calculate the area of the ventricular septal defect using the formula for a regular ellipse, which can be indexed to either body surface area (Matitiau et al, 1992) or to the cross-sectional area of the aorta. A close correlation has been demonstrated between these antemortem echocardiographic measurements and the dimensions of the ventricular septal defect assessed at postmortem (Matitiau et al, 1992). Because abnormalities of the atrioventricular valves have so frequently been described at postmortem, it is important to pay particular attention to their size and tension apparatus in multiple cuts. Recognition of interdigitating tension apparatus from the two atrioventricular valves is also important, since it constitutes a contraindication to septation. Doppler echocardiography has also been shown to be of value in detecting atrioventricular valvar regurgitation, though not yet stenosis, and stenosis and atresia of arterial valves (Bisset and Hirschfeld, 1983). Because there is no atrioventricular septum, there is no offsetting of the atrioventricular valves. At the same time, straddling of an atrioventricular valve (Smallhorn et al, 1981a) is readily revealed (Figure 38.26). A posterior ridge supporting valvar tension apparatus can frequently be identified in short-axis cuts (Sahn et al, 1982). This should not be confused with the muscular septum. A papillary muscle may also occasionally be confused at first with the apical ventricular septum, but not if insertion of tension apparatus into it is searched for.

The examination is modified accordingly when the heart is in the middle or to the right of the chest, but the basic principles of diagnosis remain the same.

FETAL ECHOCARDIOGRAPHY

Fetal ultrasonic scanning is now a routine part of antenatal care in many countries. Increasing numbers of fetal cardiac anomalies are being detected. Of 1735 fetuses in whom a definite diagnosis of congenital heart disease was demonstrated at Guy's Hospital, London in the period up to the end of 1996, double inlet ventricle was demonstrated in 30 (1.7%). Of these, one fetus had hydrops, while all had normal chromosomal analysis. Termination of pregnancy was performed in 18, there were two spontaneous intrauterine deaths and one postnatal death (G. Sharland, Guy's Hospital Trust, London, personal communication).

NUCLEAR IMAGING

Nuclear imaging is of no value in the diagnosis of double inlet ventricle.

MAGNETIC RESONANCE IMAGING

The recent widespread use of magnetic resonance imaging has provided exciting new insights into the anatomy and pathophysiology of double inlet ventricle. Magnetic resonance imaging can provide a complete sequential diagnosis in most patients (Figure 38.28), and is of particular utility in those in whom echocardiographic images

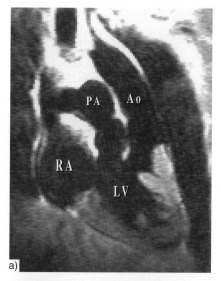

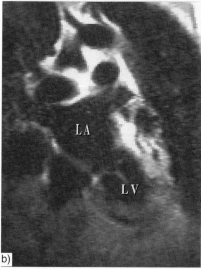

Figure 38.28. Resonance images show the long axis of the ventricular mass. (a) The right atrium (RA) connects to a dominant left ventricle (LV) in a heart with dominant left ventricle, rudimentary right ventricle and discordant ventriculo-arterial connections. (b) The left atrium (LA) also connects to the dominant left ventricle through a separate atrioventricular valve, confirming the diagnosis of double inlet left ventricle. PA, pulmonary trunk; Ao, aorta. (Reproduced by kind permission of Dr P. Kilner, Royal Brompton Hospital, London.)

are suboptimal. Its ability to demonstrate the distal pulmonary arteries may be of particular interest (Huggon et al, 1992). Magnetic resonance imaging has also been used to obtain information about the changes in the performance of the dominant ventricle in patients as they progress through staged palliative surgery (Fogel et al, 1995). It is unlikely, however, that the technique will, in the near future, entirely replace cardiac catheterization in the assessment of the patient prior to definitive palliation.

CARDIAC CATHETERIZATION

Despite advances in non-invasive investigative techniques, all patients being considered for definitive palliation in the current era require cardiac catheterization. This is principally because of the necessity of measuring pulmonary blood flow and resistance, but also because of the difficulty of recognizing mild degrees of subaortic obstruction in patients with double inlet left ventricle and discordant ventriculo-arterial connections. Cardiac catheterization will almost always be performed using a femoral approach, although, in patients after bidirectional cavopulmonary anastomosis, cannulation of the internal jugular vein will also be necessary if the cavopulmonary anastomosis is the only source of pulmonary blood flow. Angiograms should be performed in the brachiocephalic or superior caval vein(s) in order to delineate caval venous anatomy. Attempts should be made in all patients to enter the pulmonary venous atrium in order, first, to exclude stenosis of the atrioventricular valve and, second, to measure the transpulmonary pressure gradient. Fortunately, even if the atrial septum is intact, the capacious dominant ventricle permits easy looping of catheters within it and, hence, retrograde catheterization of the atrium. If it is not possible to enter the pulmonary venous atrium, an indirect measurement of the pulmonary venous atrial pressure from a catheter placed in the pulmonary arterial wedge position may be useful. The dominant ventricle is usually entered with ease through the right atrioventricular valve, although difficulties may be encountered entering the artery supported by it. Use of a flow-directed balloon catheter may be helpful. If not, retrograde arterial catheterization almost always succeeds when the catheter is passed through the aortic valve and looped in the dominant ventricle. It must be emphasized, however, that entry into the dominant left ventricle from a retrograde arterial approach must be performed with extreme caution in the patient with double inlet left ventricle and discordant ventriculoarterial connections, as it may result in subaortic obstruction or damage to the aortic valve. Careful withdrawals across the ventricular septal defect should be recorded to document any obstruction at that site.

The pulmonary arteries must always be entered in order to assess pulmonary vascular anatomy and physiology. If possible, measurements of the transpulmonary pressure gradient should be combined with measurements of cardiac output in order to derive pulmonary vascular resistance. In patients with double inlet left ventricle and discordant ventriculo-arterial connections, it is wise to give an intravenous infusion of isoprenaline (isoproterenol) to try to provoke a gradient across the ventricular septal defect while simultaneously measuring left ventricular and ascending aortic pressures. Careful withdrawal around the aortic arch will aid in the exclusion of obstruction within the arch.

ANGIOCARDIOGRAPHY

The investigator who can produce high-quality angiocardiograms in patients with double inlet ventricle will have no difficulty in any other field of angiocardiography. Excellent angiocardiograms have been published by Hallerman and colleagues (1966), by the group from Birmingham, Alabama (Soto et al, 1979, 1982; Bargeron L M Jr, 1987) and by Freedom and his associates (1997a,b). Although a detailed approach to establishing the diagnosis of double inlet ventricle using angiography has been published by Macartney et al (1979), advances in non-invasive imaging have now rendered this approach obsolete.

Injection into the dominant ventricle is performed in order to illustrate the ventricular septal defect and demonstrate the relationships between the two ventricles, to exclude incompetence of the atrioventricular valves and to opacify the systemic and pulmonary outflow tracts. Opacification of the volume-overloaded dominant ventricle usually requires injection of 1.8–2.0 ml/kg contrast medium. In all patients, biplane cineangiography should be performed, with one intensifier providing a lateral projection. Information obtained from the transthoracic echocardiogram may help in planning the optimal position of the second intensifier. In patients with double inlet right ventricle (Figure 38.29) or with double inlet left ventricle and a left-sided rudimentary right ventricle (Figure 38.30), an anteroposterior projection is chosen. These projections also serve to identify the solitary and indeterminate ventricle when the apical trabeculations are coarse and it is not possible to identify a second, rudimentary ventricle (Figure 38.31). In patients with double inlet left ventricle and a right-sided rudimentary right ventricle, a long-axial projection is usually best in profiling the ventricular septum. This demonstrates well the ventriculo-arterial connections (Figures 38.32 and 38.33) and also reveals the presence of a common valve (Figure 38.33). Injections into the rudimentary ventricle (Figures 38.30b and 38.34) can provide further imaging of the ventricular septal defect and demonstrate obstruction within the cavity of the rudimentary ventricle itself.

Pulmonary angiography should be performed in all patients prior to definitive palliation. The size of the

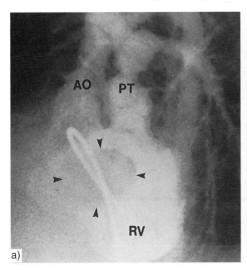

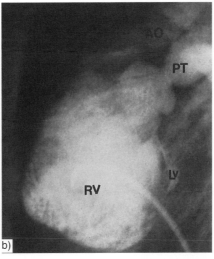

Figure 38.29. Angiograms profiled in frontal (a) and lateral (b) projections show double inlet right ventricle (RV) through a common atrioventricular valve (arrowheads). The morphology of the dominant right ventricle is confirmed by the lateral projection (b), which shows a slit-like posterior left ventricle (LV). There is a double outlet of the aorta (AO) and the banded pulmonary trunk (PT) from the dominant right ventricle.

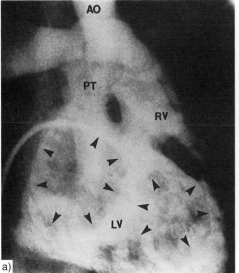

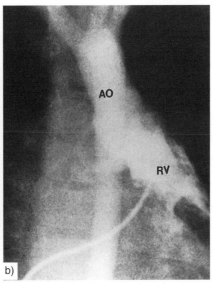

Figure 38.30. Angiograms profiled in frontal projection. (a) Double inlet through two atrioventricular valves (arrowheads) occurs into a dominant left ventricle (LV) with an anterior left-sided rudimentary left ventricle (RV). (b) The selective injection in the rudimentary ventricle confirms the presence of discordant ventriculo-arterial connections.

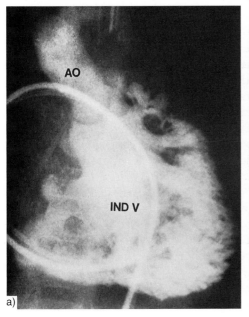

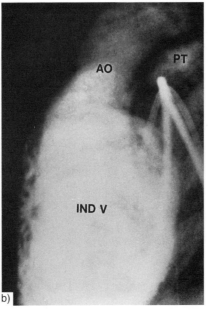

Figure 38.31. Angiograms profiled in frontal (a) and lateral (b) projections are from a postmortem-proven example of solitary and indeterminate (IND) ventricle (V). There are obvious coarse trabeculations within the ventricle, but the clinching diagnostic feature is the failure to show a rudimentary ventricle in the lateral projection (compare this with Figure 38.28b). Note the origin of the aorta (AO) from the ventricle with atresia of the pulmonary trunk (PT).

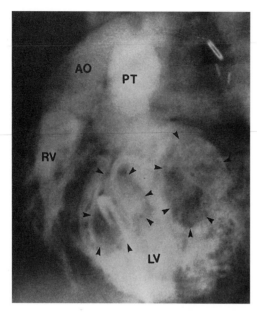

Figure 38.32. This angled long axis ventriculogram shows the essence of double inlet left ventricle through two atrioventricular valves (arrowheads) with rudimentary right ventricle and discordant ventriculo-arterial connections. Abbreviations as in Figure 38.29.

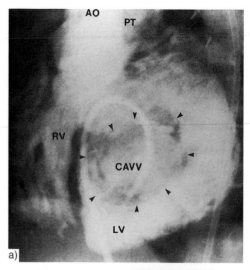

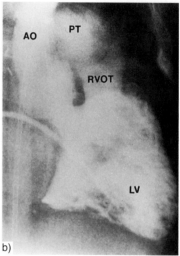

Figure 38.33. This long axis angled ventriculogram ((a) compare with Figure 38.32) shows double inlet left ventricle (LV) through a common atrioventricular valve (CAVV; arrowheads) but with concordant ventriculo-arterial connections: the pulmonary trunk (PT) arising from the rudimentary right ventricle (RV) above an extensive muscular outflow tract (RVOT). This is another example of the 'Holmes heart'. AO, aorta. The lateral projection (b) confirms the ventriculo-arterial connections as concordant.

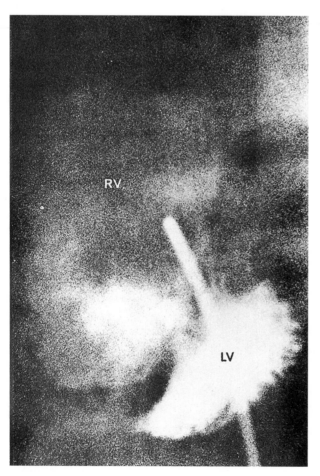

Figure 38.34. This selective injection fills a posteroinferior rudimentary and incomplete left ventricle (LV), composed exclusively of the apical trabecular component, in a heart with double inlet and double outlet from the dominant right ventricle (RV).

pulmonary arteries can be measured and indexed, using either the method of McGoon and co-workers (1975) or that of Nakata and co-workers (1984). Distortion of the pulmonary arteries, or pulmonary arterial stenoses, can be demonstrated and the pattern of pulmonary venous return delineated. In patients after staged palliation with either systemic-to-pulmonary arterial or cavopulmonary shunts, further angiograms are required to verify patency of the shunt, while in others, caval and/or aortic arch angiography will be necessary.

NATURAL HISTORY

The natural history of double inlet ventricle is easier to establish than that of most congenital heart defects, since surgical 'repair' is a relatively recent possibility. Against this, accurate diagnosis established early in life is also a relatively recent phenomenon. Of patients seen at the Hospital for Sick Children, Toronto, half had died within the first month of life, and three quarters within the first 6 months (Kidd, 1978). Even from the selected group of patients from the Mayo Clinic, where referrals during infancy are relatively uncommon, Moodie and colleagues (1984b) found that, in a series of patients who did not undergo surgery, only half those with a dominant left ventricle were alive after 14 years. The corresponding figure for patients with a solitary indeterminate ventricle was 50% at 4 years. There was no difference in survival between patients with and without pulmonary stenosis.

Franklin and co-workers (1991a) reviewed the outcome in 191 infants who presented to the Royal Brompton Hospital and Great Ormond Street Hospitals, London between 1973 and 1988. Actuarial survival without definitive repair was 57% at 1 year, 43% at 5 years and 42% at 10 years. Markers of increased risk of death included the presence of right isomerism, a common atrioventricular valve, pulmonary atresia, obstruction of the systemic outflow tract, and extracardiac anomalous pulmonary venous connection. Of 136 patients deemed potentially suitable for definitive repair at the time of presentation, only 78 were still alive and suitable 2 years later, with most deaths occurring secondary to 'low cardiac output' or palliative operations (Franklin et al, 1991b).

In another series of patients who had survived palliative surgery of one sort or another (Moodie et al, 1984a), 5-year survival was 68 ± 12% following banding and 72 ± 12% after a shunt procedure. Among patients with double inlet indeterminate ventricle who had received a shunt, survival was 54 ± 10% at 5 years. However, survival for 62 years without operation has been documented (Goldberg et al, 1983).

MANAGEMENT

MEDICAL MANAGEMENT

Neonates presenting with cyanosis, obstructed pulmonary circulation and duct-dependent pulmonary blood flow usually improve rapidly once ductal patency is re-established with an intravenous infusion of prostaglandin E_1 or E_2. A poor response to infusion of prostaglandin, particularly in the setting of right isomerism, may indicate obstructed pulmonary venous return. Supportive care with mechanical ventilation and correction of acidosis may provide temporary stability while awaiting urgent surgery.

Patients with obstructed systemic circulation and duct-dependent systemic blood flow may present in a critical condition, with poor peripheral pulses, acidosis and oliguria. Again, infusion of prostaglandin E_1 or E_2, combined with manoeuvres to augment pulmonary vascular resistance (see below), may be life saving.

The medical management of the patient with unobstructed pulmonary and systemic circulation is directed to optimizing the delicate balance between systemic and pulmonary blood flow. This is achieved by gentle systemic afterload reduction combined with manoeuvres to augment pulmonary vascular resistance, including positive pressure ventilation with a fraction of inspired oxygen of 0.21–0.25 and permissive hypercapnia to maintain the arterial tension of carbon dioxide between 5 and 6 kPa.

SURGICAL MANAGEMENT

INTERMEDIATE PALLIATIVE SURGERY

Intermediate palliative surgery is performed in order to allow survival in the short term and to set the scene for definitive palliation at low risk. This is achieved, first, by ensuring that pulmonary blood flows at low pressure through a low resistance, non-distorted pulmonary vascular bed, with no obstruction to pulmonary venous return. The second prerequisite is to prevent hypertrophy of the dominant ventricle related to volume or pressure overload. Intermediate palliative surgery, therefore, aims to augment pulmonary blood flow in those with pulmonary obstruction, limit it in those in whom pulmonary blood flow is excessive and to optimize systemic outflow in those with subaortic or aortic arch obstruction.

The results of 154 palliative operations that were performed in 121 of the 191 infants who presented to the Royal Brompton and Great Ormond Street Hospitals between 1973 and 1988 were reviewed by Franklin and co-workers. Survival after construction of a systemic-to-pulmonary arterial shunt was similar to that achieved after banding of the pulmonary trunk (84% and 77%, respectively, at 1 year; 62% and 45%, respectively, at 5 years). Patients who underwent surgery to relieve obstruction of the aortic arch fared particularly badly, with an actuarial survival of only 44% at 1 year and 22% at 5 years (Franklin et al, 1991c).

Banding of the pulmonary trunk in patients with excessive pulmonary blood flow

Banding of the pulmonary trunk is performed in order to reduce the volume load to the dominant ventricle, to reduce pulmonary blood flow and pressure, and to prevent the development of pulmonary vascular disease. The role of banding remains controversial because of the statistical association between this procedure and the development of acquired subaortic obstruction. It remains unclear, however, whether this relationship is a causal one or just reflects the natural history of the muscular ventricular septal defect.

Banding of the pulmonary trunk may be performed through a left thoracotomy or through a median sternotomy, with limited dissection between the aorta and pulmonary trunk, to reduce the risk of distal migration of the band producing stenosis of the pulmonary arterial branches. The size of the band can be predicted according to the method of Trusler and co-workers (Trusler and Mustard, 1972), although 'fine-tuning' of the size is usually performed according to systemic and pulmonary arterial pressures and systemic arterial oxygen saturation.

Systemic-to-pulmonary arterial shunts in the infant with inadequate pulmonary blood flow

The modified Blalock–Taussig shunt, in which a graft is interposed between the subclavian and pulmonary arteries, remains the procedure of choice. Pott's and Waterston's anastomoses are no longer performed because of their tendency to produce pulmonary arterial distortion and excessive pulmonary blood flow. Although traditionally the interposition graft has been placed through a thoracotomy, recently some groups have advocated use of a median sternotomy (Mayer, 1994). Potential advantages of this approach are, first, that the shunt can be placed more centrally, facilitating access during further procedures through the midline, and, second that entry to the pleural space is avoided.

Mayer (1994) reviewed the outcome in 63 infants who underwent systemic-to-pulmonary arterial shunts at the Children's Hospital, Boston between 1985 and 1991. There were 10 early (15.9%) and 12 late (19%) deaths. These figures compare closely with the data of Franklin and co-workers (Franklin et al, 1991c), who observed actuarial survival at 1 and 5 years of 84 and 62%, respectively, in 57 infants who underwent modified Blalock–Taussig shunt procedures in the setting of double inlet ventricle at the Royal Brompton and Great Ormond Street Hospitals between 1973 and 1988.

The bidirectional cavopulmonary shunt

In recent years, the classic Glenn shunt, which sacrifices the continuity between the right and left pulmonary arteries, has been replaced by the bidirectional cavopulmonary shunt, in which an end-to-side anastomosis is constructed between the superior caval vein and the undivided right pulmonary artery (Lamberti et al, 1990; Bridges et al, 1990a). The bidirectional shunt has now become widely used as a palliative procedure for all patients with univentricular atrioventricular connections. It is well established that the procedure can be performed with low operative risk (Pridjian et al, 1993; Cochrane et al, 1997), and it has been suggested that the bidirectional cavopulmonary shunt may reduce the risk of a subsequent Fontan operation in selected children (Cochrane et al, 1997). The physiological advantages of the bidirectional cavopulmonary shunt as a palliative procedure is that the volume load on the dominant ventricle is reduced, and often regurgitation of the atrioventricular valves is alleviated. One concern, however, is that the bidirectional cavopulmonary shunt may provide a suboptimal stimulus for subsequent growth of the pul-

monary arteries (Mendelson et al, 1994; Penny et al, 1995).

Although, traditionally, the tendency has been to avoid use of this shunt in young infants, recent data from San Francisco, where more than one third of all bidirectional cavopulmonary shunt procedures are performed in young infants (Reddy et al, 1997), showed an overall mortality of only 4.8% in patients who underwent this procedure before the age of 6 months. Nonetheless, in this series, an age of less than 1 month was a risk factor for death and the authors comment that their current preference is to defer this procedure until after the age of 2 months.

The operation, which involves a direct end-to-side anastomosis between the superior caval vein and the right pulmonary artery, has been performed without cardiopulmonary bypass, although most usually it is performed using a median sternotomy and cardiopulmonary bypass. In some centres, a physiologically similar operation, the so-called hemi-Fontan procedure, is performed; this more completely prepares the patient for a subsequent, simpler, complete Fontan operation (Jacobs and Norwood, 1992; Seshadri et al, 1993). It remains controversial whether accessory sources of pulmonary blood flow should be left in place when constructing a bidirectional cavopulmonary shunt (Mainwaring et al, 1995). Although systemic arterial oxygen saturation may be higher in patients in whom an accessory source of pulmonary blood flow is left in place (Webber et al, 1995), there have been some concerns regarding increased morbidity after this approach (Frommelt et al, 1995; Mainwaring et al, 1995).

Atrial septectomy

Atrial septectomy may be necessary to improve mixing or for palliation in patients with associated stenosis of the left atrioventricular valve. In the relatively old series reported from Birmingham, Alabama (Steffanelli et al, 1984), there were no deaths recorded in 14 patients, and 10-year actuarial survival was 76%.

Relief of obstruction produced by a subaortic ventricular septal defect

In the patient with double inlet left ventricle and discordant ventriculoarterial connections, the development of subaortic obstruction, related to restriction at the ventricular septal defect or within the cavity of the rudimentary right ventricle, is a major indicator of poor prognosis. In some, subaortic obstruction is overt at birth. When present, it is often associated with obstruction in the aortic arch and duct-dependent systemic circulation. In others, progressive restriction may develop during postnatal life. While many of these children will have undergone banding of the pulmonary trunk in early infancy, a causal relationship between this procedure and the development of subaortic obstruction remains unproven. Progressive subaortic obstruction will certainly occur in patients who have not undergone banding. It has been suggested that banding, by keeping the patient alive, allows the ventricular septal defect to manifest its natural tendency towards a reduction in size.

A number of surgical approaches to this problem have been described, suggesting that none is ideal. Direct relief has been achieved by enlargement of the ventricular septal defect combined with enlargement of the cavity of the rudimentary ventricle (Cheung et al, 1990; Ross et al, 1994). This procedure can be performed through the aortic valve or directly through the rudimentary ventricle. Ross and co-workers (1994) reported the extended experience at the Royal Brompton Hospital initially described by Cheung and colleagues (1990). The approach had been used in 16 patients by 1992; of these, four died early, death being related to aortic valvar insufficiency in three. Heart block was observed in two of those who survived in the medium term. Recurrence of the subaortic obstruction had not been observed since the technique was modified to include enlargement of the rudimentary ventricle with a synthetic patch.

An alternative approach used to alleviate subaortic obstruction in the neonate is to perform the arterial switch operation, leaving the restrictive ventricular septal defect to limit pulmonary blood flow (Lacour-Gayet et al, 1992). Because of differences in sizes of the arterial outflow tracts, the arterial switch is technically difficult in this setting. Furthermore, even minor degrees of pulmonary arterial distortion secondary to the arterial switch operation may assume greater significance in the patient in whom a Fontan operation is planned. Of 12 neonates with a univentricular atrioventricular connection in whom the arterial switch operation was performed at the Royal Children's Hospital, Melbourne (unpublished data), concomitant repair of the aortic arch was performed in 11. There were three early and one late deaths. Recurrence of subaortic obstruction or aortic valve incompetence was not observed at follow-up. Of the nine early survivors, six required construction of a modified Blalock–Taussig shunt because of increasing restriction at the level of the ventricular septal defect resulting in subpulmonary obstruction. Of the eight medium-term survivors, seven had progressed to more definitive palliation by means of cavopulmonary shunt procedures.

The creation of an anastomosis between the proximal pulmonary trunk and the ascending aorta, a modification of the procedure described by Damus (1975) for the palliation of complete transposition, is increasingly used as a means of alleviating subaortic obstruction in the patient with dominant left ventricle and discordant ventriculo-arterial connections. In such patients, pulmonary blood flow is ensured by constructing an interposition graft between the systemic and pulmonary arteries (Brawn et al, 1995). Alternatively, in the older infant, it is possible to achieve a cavopulmonary connection (Huddleston et al, 1993). The group from Ann Arbor, Michigan (Mosca et al, 1997) have adopted yet another approach.

They have treated these patients with a modification of the Norwood procedure, designed initially for the palliation of the hypoplastic left heart syndrome.

DEFINITIVE PALLIATION

Septation of the dominant ventricle

Septation of the dominant ventricle would seem the most logical approach to surgical repair since it preserves the patient's own tissues and their function as much as possible. Ventricular septation for double inlet ventricle was first accomplished in 1956 (McGoon et al, 1977). Isolated case reports, and 'series' of four patients or less, have appeared with some regularity (Hallman et al, 1967; Horiuchi et al, 1970; Sakakibara et al, 1972; Edie et al, 1973; Ionescu et al, 1973; Doty et al, 1979). Reasonably large series were then published by McGoon et al. (1977), McKay and colleagues (1982), and by Stefanelli and associates (1984). At the Mayo Clinic from 1973 to the time of the report by McGoon and his associates (1977), 30 patients with double inlet via two atrioventricular valves underwent septation using a transventricular approach, with 13 hospital deaths (43%). Ten developed complete heart block during surgery. The number of late deaths was also worrying. Of 24 survivors, eight died during follow-up. Of those continuing to survive, only 12 had a fair-to-good result (Feldt et al, 1981). McKay and colleagues (1982) considered only patients with double inlet left ventricle and an anterior left-sided rudimentary right ventricle. They reported a hospital mortality of 7 out of 16 patients (44%). Small heart size and obstruction of the ventricular septal defect were identified as incremental preoperative risk factors. In contrast to the Mayo Clinic group, these authors made no attempt to avoid heart block, which was induced in 10 out of 16 patients and treated with a pacemaker. Of the nine late survivors, all were in New York Heart Association class 1, though none performed normally on stress testing. Subsequent to these experiences, most centres throughout the world shifted to modifications of the Fontan procedure as the preferred means of definitive palliation in patients with double inlet ventricle. Despite this, several centres in Japan continued to favour the option of septation. Imai and co-workers (1994) performed septations in a series of 19 patients employing a transatrial approach. Many of these had contraindications to the Fontan approach, with 16 having a mean arterial pressure exceeding 16 mmHg, six a pulmonary vascular resistance index of more than 4, two a pulmonary arterial index of less than 250 mm²/m², seven a left ventricular ejection of less than 60%, and one with paroxysmal supraventricular tachycardia. Only one patient died within 30 days of surgery (5.3%), while three developed permanent and complete heart block at the time of operation. There were three further deaths within 100 days of surgery (16.7%; the overall survival at time of follow-up was 78%). Interestingly, in this series, neither preoperative mean pulmonary arterial pressure nor pulmonary vascular resistance were identified as incremental risk factors. Significant predictors of death were the presence of a high pressure gradient between the dominant ventricle and pulmonary arteries, a high peak systolic pressure, an elevated left ventricular end-diastolic pressure and a higher body surface area. Based on their experience, the authors suggested that septation should only be considered in patients in whom the combined volumes of the right and left ventricles at end-diastole exceeded 180 ml/m² body surface area, or approximately 250% of the expected normal left ventricular end-diastolic volume. Their current strategy for the care of patients with double inlet left ventricle and increased pulmonary blood flow consists of initial banding of the pulmonary trunk, followed by septation within the first year of life. Patients with reduced pulmonary blood flow are treated with the Fontan approach. Recent data from Osaka is also of interest (Uemura and Yagihara, 1998). Although early mortality after septation in their centre has been no more than 13% since 1983, a disturbing trend has been seen in the intermediate term, with five deaths occurring within 3 years of surgery in the 17 early survivors. Therefore, the results from Japan show that although septation can certainly be successfully performed in carefully selected patients, notably those with double inlet left ventricle, survival in the intermediate to long term is no better than for the Fontan procedure. Proper selection of patients, therefore, is crucial if results are to improve after septation. Endorsing the opinion of Imai and colleagues (1994) concerning the size of the dominant left ventricle, Uemura and Yagihara (1998) also point to the important feature of the structure and competence of the atrioventricular valves.

Ventricular exclusion

The introduction of the atriopulmonary anastomosis, and the demonstration of successful exclusion of a sub-pulmonary ventricle by Fontan and Baudet in 1971, has revolutionized the care of patients with univentricular atrioventricular connections, including those with double inlet ventricle. Since the original description of this approach, physiological insights and surgical technique have evolved in tandem. It was initially considered that the 'right atrial pump' might be important after ventricular exclusion. Because of this, application of the Fontan approach to those patients with double inlet ventricle necessitated closing the right atrioventricular valve in an attempt to maintain a subpulmonary atrium within the circulation (Yacoub and Radley-Smith, 1976; Kreutzer et al, 1981). Once the contribution of the subpulmonary atrium to pulmonary flow was questioned, the use of the total cavopulmonary connection, initially using an intra-atrial pathway (de Leval et al, 1988) or more recently an extra-cardiac tube (Nawa and Teramoto, 1988; Giannico et al, 1992; Petrossian et al, 1998), has gained increasing acceptance. Fenestration of the intra-atrial tunnel is increasingly used (Bridges et al, 1990b; Laks et al, 1991). It has been suggested that this approach may reduce the duration of hospital stay and pleural drainage (Cochrane et al, 1997). The original criterions for suitability formulated by Choussat and co-workers (1978) remain relevant, although they have been relaxed by most groups. In most centres, the Fontan operation can now be performed with low early mortality. Data from Melbourne (Cochrane et al, 1997) revealed an in-hospital mortality for patients who underwent Fontan operation between 1988 and 1995 of 1.8%. Nonetheless, concern remains about long-term outcome after this operation, particularly following publication of the combined experience from Bordeaux and Birmingham, Alabama, which demonstrated considerable late hazard in patients, even after the 'perfect' operation (Kirklin et al, 1990). Furthermore, although most patients are satisfied with their overall health and quality of life, less than one in five patients aged more than 18 years report no physical limitation (Gentles et al, 1997). The Fontan approach, therefore, must still be considered palliative rather than curative.

REFERENCES

Anderson R H 1983 Weasel words in paediatric cardiology. Single ventricle. International Journal of Cardiology 2: 425–429

Anderson R H, Ho S Y, Becker A E 1983 The surgical anatomy of the conduction tissues. Thorax 38: 408–420

Anderson R H, Arnold R, Thapar M K, Jones R S, Hamilton D I 1974 Cardiac specialized tissue in hearts with an apparently single ventricular chamber (double inlet left ventricle). American Journal of Cardiology 33: 95–106

Anderson R H, Becker A E, Wilkinson J L, Gerlis L M 1976 The morphogenesis of univentricular hearts. British Heart Journal 38: 558–572

Anderson R H, Becker A E, Freedom R M et al 1979a Problems in the nomenclature of the univentricular heart. Herz 4: 97–106

Anderson R H, Becker A E, Macartney F J, Shinebourne E A, Wilkinson J L, Tynan M J 1979b Is 'tricuspid atresia' a univentricular heart? Pediatric Cardiology 1: 51–56

Anderson R H, Lenox C C, Zuberbuhler J R, Ho S Y, Smith A, Wilkinson J L 1983a Double-inlet left ventricle with rudimentary right ventricle and ventriculoarterial concordance. American Journal of Cardiology 52: 573–577

Anderson R H, Macartney F J, Tynan M et al 1983b Univentricular atrioventricular connexion – the single ventricle trap unsprung. Pediatric Cardiology 4: 273–280

Anderson R H, Becker A E, Tynan M, Macartney F J, Rigby M L, Wilson J L 1984a The univentricular atrioventricular connection: getting to the root of a thorny problem. American Journal of Cardiology 54: 822–828

Anderson R H, Becker A E, Freedom R M et al 1984b Sequential segmental analysis of congenital heart disease. Pediatric Cardiology 5: 281–288

Barber G, Hagler D J, Edwards W D et al 1984 Surgical repair of univentricular heart (double inlet left ventricle) with obstructed anterior subaortic outlet chamber. Journal of the American College of Cardiology 4: 771–778

Bargeron L M Jr 1987 Angiography of double inlet ventricle. In: Anderson R H, Crupi G, Parenzan L (eds) Double inlet ventricle morphology, diagnosis and surgical treatment. Castle House Press, Tunbridge Wells, p 146–158

Beardshaw J A, Gibson D G, Pearson M C, Upton M T, Anderson R H 1977 Echocardiographic diagnosis of primitive ventricle with two atrioventricular valves. British Heart Journal 39: 266–275

Bevilacqua M, Sanders S P, Van Praagh S et al 1991 Double-inlet single left ventricle. Echocardiographic anatomy with emphasis on the morphology of the atrioventricular valves and ventricular septal defect. Journal of the American College of Cardiology 18: 559–568

Bharati S, Lev M 1975 The course of the conduction system in single ventricle with inverted (L-) loop and inverted (L-) transposition. Circulation 51: 723–730

Bharati S, Lev M 1979a The concept of tricuspid atresia complex as distinct from that of the single ventricle complex. Pediatric Cardiology 1: 57–62

Bharati S, Lev M 1979b The relationship between single ventricle and small outlet chamber and straddling and displaced tricuspid orifice and valve. Herz 4: 176–183

Bini R M, Bloom K R, Culham J A G, Freedom R M, Williams C M, Rowe R D 1978 The reliability and practicality of single crystal echocardiography in the evaluation of single ventricle. Angiographic and pathological correlates. Circulation 57: 269–277

Bisset G S III, Hirschfeld S S 1983 The univentricular heart: combined 2-dimensional-pulsed Doppler (Duplex) echocardiographic evaluation. American Journal of Cardiology 51: 1149–1154

Brawn W J, Sethia B, Jagtap R et al 1995 Univentricular heart with systemic outflow obstruction. Palliation by primary Damus procedure. Annals of Thoracic Surgery 59: 1441–1447

Bridges N D, Jonas R A, Mayer J E, Flanagan M F, Keane J F, Castaneda A R 1990a Bidirectional cavopulmonary anastomosis as interim palliation for high-risk Fontan candidates: early results. Circulation 82(suppl. IV): 170–176

Bridges N D, Lock J E, Castenada A R 1990b Baffle fenestration with subsequent transcatheter closure. Modifications of the Fontan operation for patients at higher risk. Circulation 82: 1681–1689

Brodie J 1945 Cor biatrium triloculare with transposition of the arterial trunks: a rare congenital malformation. Journal of Pathology and Bacteriology 57: 481–485

Cheung H C, Lincoln C, Anderson R H et al 1990 Options of surgical repair in hearts with univentricular atrioventricular connection and subaortic stenosis. Journal of Thoracic and Cardiovascular Surgery 100: 672–681

Choussat A, Fontan F, Besse P Vallot F, Chauve A, Bricaud H 1978 Selection criteria for Fontan's procedure. In: Anderson R H, Shinebourne E A (eds) Paediatric cardiology 1977. Churchill Livingstone, London, p 559–566

Cochrane A D, Brizard C P, Penny D J et al 1997 Management of the univentricular connection: are we improving? European Journal of Cardiothoracic Surgery 12: 107–115

Damus P S 1975 Letter to the editor. Annals of Thoracic Surgery 20: 724–725

Davachi F, Moller J H 1969 The electrocardiogram and vectocardiogram in single ventricle. Anatomic correlations. American Journal of Cardiology 23: 19–31

Deanfield J E, Tommasini G, Anderson R H, Macartney F J 1982 Tricuspid atresia: analysis of coronary artery distribution and ventricular morphology. British Heart Journal 48: 485–492

de Leval M R, Kilner P, Gewillig M, Bull C 1988 Total cavopulmonary connection: a logical alternative to atriopulmonary connection for complex Fontan operations. Journal of Thoracic and Cardiovascular Surgery 96: 682–695

Dickinson D F, Wilkinson J L, Anderson K R, Smith A, Ho S Y, Anderson R H 1979 The cardiac conduction system in situs ambiguus. Circulation 59: 879–885

Dobell A R, Van Praagh R 1996 The Holmes heart: historic associations and pathologic anatomy. American Heart Journal 132: 437–445

Doty D B, Schiehen R M, Lauer R M 1979 Septation of the univentricular heart. Transatrial approach. Journal of Thoracic and Cardiovascular Surgery 78: 423–430

Driscoll D J, Staats B A, Heise C T et al 1984 Functional single ventricle: cardiorespiratory response to exercise. Journal of the American College of Cardiology 4: 337–342

Edie R N, Ellis K, Gersony W M, Krongrad E, Bowman F O, Malm J R 1973 Surgical repair of single ventricle. Journal of Thoracic and Cardiovascular Surgery 66: 350–360

Edwards J E 1977 Discussion. In: Davila J C (ed.) 2nd Henry Ford Hospital international symposium on cardiac surgery. Appleton Century-Crofts, New York, p 242

Elliott L P, Gedgaddas E 1964 The roentgenologic findings in common ventricle with transposition of the great arteries. Radiology 82: 850–865

Elliott L P, Anderson R C, Adams P, Edwards J E 1962 Vectorelectrocardiogram in single ventricle. Circulation 26: 711

Elliott L P, Anderson R C, Edwards J E 1964 The common cardiac ventricle with transposition of the great vessels. British Heart Journal 26: 289–301

Ellis K 1977 Angiography in complex congenital heart disease: single ventricle, double inlet, double outlet and transposition. In: Davila J C (ed.) 2nd Henry Ford Hospital international symposium on cardiac surgery. Appleton-Century-Crofts, New York, p 222–224

Essed C E, Ho S Y, Hunter S, Anderson R H 1980 Atrioventricular conduction system in univentricular heart of right ventricular type with right-sided rudimentary chamber. Thorax 35: 123–127

Favorite G O 1934 Cor biatriatum triloculare with rudimentary right ventricle, hypoplasia of transposed aorta and patent ductus arteriosus, terminating by rupture of dilated pulmonary artery. American Journal of the Medical Sciences 187: 663–671

Feldt R H, Mair D D, Danielson G K, Wallace R B, McGoon D C 1981 Current status of the septation procedure for univentricular heart. Journal of Thoracic and Cardiovascular Surgery 82: 93–97

Fogel M A, Gupta K B, Weinberg P M, Hoffman E A 1995 Regional wall motion and strain analysis across stages of Fontan reconstruction by magnetic resonance tagging. American Journal of Physiology 269: H1132–H1152

Fontan F, Baudet E 1971 Surgical repair of tricuspid atresia. Thorax 26: 240–248

Franklin R C G, Spiegelhalter D J, Anderson R H et al 1991a Double inlet ventricle presenting in infancy I. Survival without definitive repair. Journal of Thoracic and Cardiovascular Surgery 101: 767–776

Franklin R C G, Spiegelhalter D J, Rossi Filho R I et al 1991b Double inlet ventricle presenting in infancy III. Outcome and potential for definitive repair. Journal of Thoracic and Cardiovascular Surgery 101: 924–934

Franklin R C G, Spiegelhalter D J, Anderson R H et al 1991c Double inlet ventricle presenting in infancy II. Results of palliative operations. Journal of Thoracic and Cardiovascular Surgery 101: 917–923

Freedom R M, Sondheimer H, Dische R, Rowe R D 1977a Development of 'subaortic stenosis' after pulmonary arterial banding for common ventricle. American Journal of Cardiology 39: 78–83

Freedom R M, Mawson J B, Yoo S-J, Benson L N 1997b Congenital heart disease: textbook of angiography. Futura, Armonk, NY, p 1201–1260

Frommelt M A, Frommelt P C, Berger S et al 1995 Does an additional source of pulmonary blood flow alter outcome after a bidirectional cavopulmonary shunt? Circulation 92(suppl II): 240–244

Gasul B M, Arcilla R A, Lev M 1966 In: Heart disease in children. Lippincott, Philadelphia, PA, p 869–881

Gentles T L, Gauvreau K, Mayer J E et al 1997 Functional outcome after the Fontan operation: factors influencing late morbidity. Journal of Thoracic and Cardiovascular Surgery 114: 392–403

Giannico S, Corno A, Marino B et al 1992 Total extracardiac right heart bypass. Circulation 86(suppl II): 110–117

Gibson D G, Traill T A, Brown D J 1979 Abnormal ventricular function in patients with univentricular heart. Herz 4: 226–231

Girod D A, Lima R C, Anderson R H, Ho S Y, Rigby M L, Quaegebeur J M 1984 Double inlet ventricle: morphological analysis and surgical implications in 32 cases. Journal of Thoracic and Cardiovascular Surgery 88: 590–600

Goldberg H L, Sniderman K, Devereux R B 1983 Prolonged survival (62 years) with single ventricle. American Journal of Cardiology 52: 214–215

Guller B, Mair D D, Ritter D G, Smith R E 1975 Frank vectorcardiogram in common ventricle; correlation with anatomic findings. American Heart Journal 90: 290–294

Hallerman F J, Davis G D, Ritter D G, Kincaid O W 1966 Roentgenographic features of common ventricle. Radiology 87: 409–423

Hallman G L, Gill S S, Bloodwell R D et al 1967 Surgical treatment of cardiac defects associated with corrected transposition of the great vessels. Circulation 35(suppl 1): 133–142

Harley H R S 1958 The embryology of cor triloculare biatriatum with bulber (rudimentary) cavity. Guy's Hospital Report 107: 116–143

Holmes A F 1824 Case of malformation of the heart. Transactions of the Medico-Chirurgical Society of Edinburgh 1: 252–259

Horiuchi T, Abe T, Okada Y et al 1970 Feasibility of total correction for single ventricle: a report of total correction in a six-year-old girl. Japanese Journal of Thoracic Surgery 23: 434–441

Huddleston C B, Canter C E, Spray T L 1993 Danus–Kaye–Stansel with cavopulmonary connection for single ventricle and subaortic obstruction. Annals of Thoracic Surgery 55: 339–346

Huggon I C, Baker E J, Maisey M N et al 1992 Magnetic resonance imaging of hearts with atrioventricular valve atresia or double inlet ventricle. British Heart Journal 68: 313–319

Imai Y, Hoshino S, Koh Y S et al 1994 Ventricular septation procedure for univentricular connection of left ventricular type. Seminars in Thoracic and Cardiovascular Surgery 6: 48–55

Ionescu M I, Macartney F J, Wooler G H 1973 Intracardiac repair of single ventricle with pulmonary stenosis. Journal of Thoracic and Cardiovascular Surgery 65: 602–607

Jacobs M L, Norwood W I 1992 Hypoplastic left heart syndrome. In: Jacobs M, Norwood W I (eds) Pediatric cardiac surgery: current issues. Butterworth, Stoneham, UK, p 182

Keeton B R, Macartney F J, Hunter S et al 1979 Univentricular heart of right ventricular type with double or common inlet. Circulation 59: 403–411

Kidd B S L 1978 Single ventricle. In: Keith J D, Rowe R D, Vlad P (eds) Heart disease in infancy and childhood, 3rd edn. Macmillan, New York, p 405–417

Kirklin J K, Blackstone E H, Kirklin J W, Pacifico A D, Bargeron L M 1986 The Fontan operation: ventricular hypertrophy, age and date of operation as risk factors. Journal of Thoracic and Cardiovascular Surgery 92: 1049–1064

Kirklin J W, Fernandez G, Costa F, Naftel D C, Tritto F, Blackstone E H 1990 Outcome after a 'perfect' Fontan operation. Circulation 81: 1520–1536

Kreutzer G, Schlichter A, Laura J P, Suarez J C, Vargas J F 1981 Univentricular heart with low pulmonary vascular resistances: septation vs atriopulmonary anastomosis. Arquivos Brasileiros de Cardiologie 37: 301–307

Lacour-Gayet F, Serraf A, Fermont L et al 1992 Early palliation of univentricular hearts with subaortic stenosis and ventriculoarterial discordance. The arterial switch option. Journal of Thoracic and Cardiovascular Surgery 87: 767–781

Laks H, Pearl J M, Heas G S et al 1991 Partial Fontan: advantages of an adjustable interatrial communication. Annals of Thoracic Surgery 52: 1084–1094

Lamberti J J, Spicer R L, Waldman J D et al 1990 The bidirectional cavopulmonary shunt. Journal of Thoracic and Cardiovascular Surgery 100: 22–30

Lamers W H, Wessels A, Verbeek F J et al 1992 New findings concerning ventricular septation in the human heart. Circulation 91: 111–121

Lev M, Liberthson R R, Kirkpatrick J R, Eckner F A O, Arcilla R A 1969 Single (primitive) ventricle. Circulation 39: 577–591

Macartney F J, Anderson R H 1978 Angiocardiography and haemodynamics of the univentricular heart with two atrioventricular valves or a common atrioventricular valve. In: Anderson R H, Shinebourne E A (eds) Paediatric cardiology 1977. Churchill Livingstone, Edinburgh, p 345–359

Macartney F J, Partridge J B, Scott O, Deverall P B 1976 Common or single ventricle. An angiocardiographic and hemodynamic study of 42 patients. Circulation 53: 543–554

Macartney F J, Daly K, Wilkinson J L, Anderson R H 1979 Angiocardiography in the preoperative evaluation of patients with univentricular hearts. Herz 4: 213–219

McGoon D C 1981 Discussion on Chapters 34–37. In: Becker A E, Losekoot G, Marcelletti C, Anderson R H (eds) Paediatric cardiology, vol 3. Churchill Livingstone, Edinburgh, p 443

McGoon D C, Baird D K, David G D 1975 Surgical management of large bronchial collateral arteries with pulmonary stenosis or atresia. Circulation 52: 109–118

McGoon D C, Danielson G K, Ritter D G, Wallace R B, Maloney J D, Marcelletti C 1977 Correction of the univentricular heart having two atrioventricular valves. Journal of Thoracic and Cardiovascular Surgery 74: 218–226

McKay R, Pacifico A D, Blackstone E H, Kirklin J W, Bargeron L M Jr 1982 Septation of the univentricular heart with left anterior subaortic chamber. Journal of Thoracic and Cardiovascular Surgery 84: 77–87

Mainwaring R D, Lamberti J J, Uzark K, Spicer R L 1995 Bidirectional Glenn: is accessory pulmonary blood flow good or bad? Circulation 92(suppl II): 295–297

Mann J D 1907 Cor triloculare biatriatum. British Medical Journal 1: 614–616

Marin-Garcia J, Tandon R, Moller J H, Edwards J E 1974a Common (single) ventricle with normally related great vessels. Circulation 49: 565–573

Marin-Garcia J, Tandon R, Moller J H, Edwards J E 1974b Single ventricle with transposition. Circulation 49: 994–1004

Matitiau A, Geva T, Colan S D et al 1992 Bulboventricular foramen size in infants with double-inlet left ventricle or tricuspid atresia with transposed great arteries: influence on initial palliative operation and rate of growth. Journal of the American College of Cardiology 19: 142–148

Mayer J E 1994 Initial management of the single ventricle patient. Seminars in Thoracic and Cardiovascular Surgery. 6: 2–7

Mehrizi A, McMurphy D M 1966 Syndrome of double inlet left ventricle. Angiographic differentiation from single ventricle with rudimentary outlet chamber. Bulletin of the Johns Hopkins Hospital 119: 225–267

Mendelsohn A M, Bove E L, Lupinetti F M, Crowley D C, Lloyd T R, Beekman R H III 1994 Central pulmonary artery growth after the bidirectional Glenn procedure. Journal of Thoracic and Cardiovascular Surgery 107: 1284–1290

Mills E S 1923 Cor triloculare biatriatum with coarctation of the aorta and anomaly of the coronary arteries. Journal of Medical Research 44: 257–262

Mocellin R, Sauer U 1979 Haemodynamic studies in patients with univentricular hearts. Herz 4: 242–247

Moodie D S, Ritter D G, Tajik A H, McGoon D C, Danielson G K, O'Fallon W M 1984a Long-term follow-up after palliative operation for univentricular heart. American Journal of Cardiology 53: 1648–1651

Moodie D S, Ritter D G, Tajik A J, O'Fallon W M 1984b Long-term follow-up in the unoperated univentricular heart. American Journal of Cardiology 53: 1124–1128

Mortera C, Hunter S, Terry G, Tynan M 1977 Echocardiography of primitive ventricle. British Heart Journal 39: 847–855

Mosca R S, Hennein H A, Kulik T J et al 1997 Modified Norwood operation for single left ventricle and ventriculoarterial discordance. An improved surgical technique. Annals of Thoracic Surgery 64: 1126–1132

Nakata S, Imai Y, Takanishi Y et al 1984 A new method for the quantitative standardization of cross-sectional areas of the pulmonary arteries in congenital heart diseases with decreased pulmonary blood flow. Journal of Thoracic and Cardiovascular Surgery 88: 610–619

Nawa S, Teramoto S 1988 New extension of the Fontan principle: inferior vena cava–pulmonary artery bridge operation. Thorax 43: 1022–1023

Parikh S R, Hurwitz R A, Caldwell R L, Girod D A 1991 Ventricular function in the single ventricle before and after Fontan surgery. American Journal of Cardiology 15: 1390–1395

Peacock T B 1855 Case of malformation of the heart. Both auricles opening into the left ventricle, and transposition of the aorta and pulmonary artery. Transactions of the Pathological Society of London 6: 117–119

Penny D J, Rigby M L, Redington A N 1991a Abnormal patterns of intraventricular flow and diastolic filling after the Fontan operation: evidence for incoordinate ventricular wall motion. British Heart Journal 66: 375–378

Penny D J, Redington A N 1991b Angiographic demonstration of incoordinate motion of the ventricular wall after the Fontan operation. British Heart Journal 66: 456–459

Penny D J, Lincoln C, Shore D F, Xiao H B, Rigby M L, Redington A N 1992 The early response of the systemic ventricle during transition to the Fontan circulation: an acute hypertrophic cardiomyopathy? Cardiology in the Young 2: 78–84

Penny D J, Pawade A, Wilkinson J L, Karl T R 1995 Pulmonary artery size after bidirectional cavopulmonary connection. Journal of Cardiac Surgery 20: 32–36

Petrossian E, McElhinney D B, Reddy V M, Thompson L D, Hanley F L 1998 The role of the extracardiac conduit as a cavopulmonary anastomosis in the evolution of the Fontan procedure. In Redington A N, Brawn W J, Deanfield J E, Anderson R H (eds) The right heart in congenital heart disease. Greenwich Medical Media, London, p 149–156

Pridjian A K, Mendelsohn A M, Lupinetti F M et al 1993 Usefulness of the bidirectional Glenn procedure as staged reconstruction for the functional single ventricle. American Journal of Cardiology 71: 959–962

Quero Jimenez M, Perez Martinez V M, Maitre Azcarate M J, Merino Batres G, Moreno Granados F 1973 Exaggerated displacement of the atrioventricular canal towards the bulbus cordis (rightward displacement of the mitral valve). British Heart Journal 35: 65–74

Quero Jimenez M, Perez Martinez V M, Sarrion Guzman M, Rodiquez Alonso M, Perez Diaz L 1975 Alterations des valvules auriculo-ventriculaires dans les ventricules uniques et anomalies similaires. Archives des Malodies du Couer et des Vaisseaux 68: 823–832

Quero Jimenez M, Cameron A H, Acerete F, Quero-Jimenez C 1979 Univentricular hearts: pathology of the atrioventricular valves. Herz 4: 161–165

Rahimtoola S H Ongley P A, Swan H J C 1966 The hemodynamics of common (or single) ventricle. Circulation 34: 14–23

Rao P S 1982 Terminology: tricuspid atresia or univentricular heart. In: Rao P S (ed.) Tricuspid atresia. Futura, Mount Kisco, NY, p 3–6

Reddy V M, McElhinney D B, Moore P, Haas G S, Hanley F L 1997 Outcomes after bidirectional cavopulmonary shunt in infants less than 6 months old. Journal of the American College of Cardiology 29: 1365–1370

Rigby M L 1983 The univentricular atrioventricular connexion: cross-sectional echocardiography, amplitude processing of the echocardiographic image, and electrocardiography. MD thesis, University of Leeds

Rigby M L, Anderson R H, Gibson D, Jones O D H, Joseph M C, Shinebourne E A 1981 Two dimensional echocardiographic categorisation of the univentricular heart. Ventricular morphology, type, and mode of atrioventricular connection. British Heart Journal 46: 603–612

Ritter D G, Seward J B, Moodie D, Danielson G 1979 Univentricular heart (common ventricle): preoperative diagnosis. Herz 4: 198–205

Rogers H M, Edwards J E 1951 Cor triloculare biatriatum: an analysis of the clinical and pathological features of nine cases. American Heart Journal 41: 299–310

Ross D B, Cheung H C, Lincoln C 1994 Direct relief of subaortic obstruction in patients with univentricular atrioventricular connection and discordant ventriculoarterial connection: intermediate results. Seminars in Thoracic and Cardiovascular Surgery 6: 33–38

Sahn D J, Harder J R, Freedom R M et al 1982 Cross-sectional echocardiographic diagnosis and subclassification of univentricular hearts: imaging studies of atrioventricular valves, septal structures and rudimentary outflow chambers. Circulation 66: 1070–1077

Sakakibara S, Tominaga S, Imai Y, Uehara K, Matsumuro M 1972 Successful total correction of common ventricle. Chest 61: 192–194

Scott D J, Rigby M L, Miller G A H, Shinebourne E A 1984 The presentation of symptomatic heart disease in infancy based on 10 years' experience 1973–1982: implications for the provision of services. British Heart Journal 52: 248–257

Sano T, Ogawa M, Taniguchi K et al 1989 Assessment of ventricular contractile state and function in patients with univentricular heart. Circulation 79: 1247–1256

Seshadri M, Jagaannath B R, Koppula A S, Desai R, Balakrishnan K R 1993 A new technique to simplify the Fontan procedure after a previous bidirectional Glenn shunt. Journal of Thoracic and Cardiovascular Surgery 106: 569–570

Seward J B, Tajik A J, Hagler D J, Giuliani E R, Gau G T, Ritter D G 1977 Echocardiogram in common (single) ventricle: angiographic–anatomic correlation. American Journal of Cardiology 39: 217–225

Shinebourne E A, Lau K-C, Calcaterra G, Anderson R H 1980 Univentricular heart of right ventricular type: clinical, angiographic and electrocardiographic features. American Journal of Cardiology 46: 439–445

Shiraishi H, Silverman N H 1990 Echocardiographic spectrum of double inlet ventricle: evaluation of the interventricular communication. Journal of the American College of Cardiology 15: 1401–1408

Smallhorn J F, Tommasini G, Macartney F J 1981a Detection and assessment of straddling and overriding atrioventricular valves by two-dimensional echocardiography. British Heart Journal 46: 254–262

Smallhorn J F, Tommasini G, Macartney F J 1981b Two-dimensional echocardiographic assessment of common atrioventricular valves in univentricular hearts. British Heart Journal 46: 30–34

Somerville J 1979 Changing form and function in one ventricle hearts. Herz 4: 206–212

Somerville J, Becu L, Ross D N 1974 Common ventricle with acquired subaortic obstruction. American Journal of Cardiology 34: 206–214

Somerville J, Ross D N, Yacoub M, Radley-Smith R 1975 Primitive ventricle with acquired sub-pulmonary stenosis. European Journal of Cardiology 3: 193–203

Soto B, Bertranou E G, Bream P R, Souza A, Bargeron L M Jr 1979 Angiographic study of univentricular heart of right ventricular type. Circulation 60: 1325–1334

Soto B, Pacifico A D, Di Sciascio G 1982 Univentricular heart: an angiographic study. American Journal of Cardiology 49: 787–794

Stefanelli G, Kirklin J W, Naftel D C et al 1984 Early and intermediate-term (10-year) results of surgery for univentricular atrioventricular connection ('single ventricle'). American Journal of Cardiology 54: 811–821

Tandon R, Becker A E, Moller J H, Edwards J E 1974 Double inlet left ventricle; straddling tricuspid valve. British Heart Journal 36: 747–750

Taussig H B 1939 A single ventricle with a diminutive outlet chamber. Journal of Technical Methods 19: 120–128

Trusler G A, Mustard W T 1972 A method of banding the pulmonary artery for large isolated ventricular septal defect, with and without transposition of the great arteries. Annals of Thoracic Surgery 13: 351–355

Uemura H, Yagihara T 1998 Ventricular septation in patients with double inlet left ventricle. In: Redington A N, Brawn W J, Deanfield J E, Anderson R H (eds). The right heart in congenital heart disease. Greenwich Medical Media, London, p 163–167

Van Mierop L H S, Gessner I H 1972 Pathogenetic mechanisms in congenital cardiovascular malformations. Progress in Cardiovascular Diseases 15: 67–85

Van Praagh R, Ongley P A, Swan H J C 1964 Anatomic type of single or common ventricle in man. Morphologic and geometric aspects of 60 necropsied cases. American Journal of Cardiology 13: 367–386

Van Praagh R, Plett J A, Van Praagh S 1979 Single ventricle. Pathology, embryology, terminology and classification. Herz 4: 113–150

Van Praagh R, David I, Van Praagh S 1982 A question of definition. What is a ventricle? The single ventricle trap. Pediatric Cardiology 2: 79–84

Webber S A, Horvath P, LeBlanc J G et al 1995 Influence of competitive pulmonary blood flow on the bidirectional superior cavopulmonary shunt: a multi-institutional study. Circulation 92(suppl II): 279–286

Weigel T J, Driscoll D J, Michels V V 1989 Occurrence of congenital heart defects in siblings of patients with univentricular heart and tricuspid atresia. American Journal of Cardiology 64: 768–771

Wenink A C G 1978 The conduction tissues in primitive ventricle with outlet chamber: two different possibilities. Journal of Thoracic and Cardiovascular Surgery 75: 747–753

Wilkinson J L, Anderson R H, Arnold R, Hamilton D I, Smith A 1976 The conducting tissues in primitive ventricular hearts without an outlet chamber. Circulation 53: 930–938

Wilkinson J L, Becker A E, Tynan M et al 1979a Nomenclature of the univentricular heart. Herz 4: 107–112

Wilkinson J L, Dickinson D F, Smith A, Anderson R H 1979b Conducting tissues in univentricular heart of right ventricular type with double or common inlet. Journal of Thoracic Cardiovascular Surgery 77: 691–698

Wood R H, Williams G A 1928 Primitive human hearts. Cor biloculare and triloculare; report of cases. American Journal of Medical Sciences 175: 242–255

Yacoub M H, Radley-Smith R 1976 Use of valved conduit from the right atrium to pulmonary artery for 'correction' of single ventricle. Circulation 54(suppl III): 63–70

39
Tricuspid atresia and the Fontan operation
M. L. Rigby and R. H. Anderson

INTRODUCTION

There is a group of patients who have in common the feature that the only egress for systemic venous blood from the morphologically right atrium is through an interatrial communication. This is because there is no direct communication across the atrioventricular junction between the right atrium and the ventricular mass. As we will see, in the majority of cases fitting this definition, there is no direct communication because the junction itself, and the inlet component of the morphologically right ventricle, are absent. The clinical picture can also be produced, nonetheless, by an imperforate valvar membrane blocking a formed right atrioventricular junction. This anatomical heterogeneity within what is, essentially, a clinical entity has led to considerable controversy, particular concerning the 'univentricular' nature of the commonest anatomical variant, characterized by absence of the right atrioventricular connection (Anderson et al, 1977; Bharati and Lev, 1979; Rao, 1992; Orie et al, 1995). Rashkind (1982), in an excellent historical review, pointed out that the term 'atresia' for this condition was first used by Schuberg (1861). Schuberg had described what can be considered the 'classical' anatomical pattern, that with atresia of the right venous ostium in the setting of a dominant left ventricle and a rudimentary and incomplete right ventricle. Complete obstruction of the right atrioventricular valvar orifice had been described as early as 1817 by Kreysig, although he had not used the term atresia. Between that time and Schuberg's account, several other descriptions had been given, most of which are recognizable as examples of the anomaly now termed simply 'tricuspid atresia'. As Rashkind indicates, the use of this description in the English literature has been a 20th century event. All these early accounts, however, were imprecise concerning the anatomy of the atrioventricular junction. This lack of precision has continued through the last decade of the 20th century (Rao, 1990, Weinberg, 1992), in part because of the anatomical heterogeneity seen in a malformation recognized on the basis of its clinical features.

If we were to use strictly anatomical definitions, then it would be justified to include in this chapter an account of those malformations with absence of the left-sided atrioventricular connection in which the junction, had it been formed, would have been guarded by a morphologically tricuspid valve. In these hearts, however, it is the pulmonary venous return that has no direct egress to the ventricular mass. A similar clinical situation is produced by an imperforate tricuspid valve in the setting of discordant atrioventricular connections. The first of these anatomical entities is included within the category of tricuspid atresia by Rao (1982a). While recognizing the embryological justification for such an inclusion, we find this approach potentially confusing for those wishing to understand the clinical manifestations. Those hearts with atresia of the exit from the morphologically left atrium, but without hypoplastic left heart syndrome, will be considered in Chapter 40. In this chapter, we will consider only those malformations in which the morphologically right atrium, in other words the systemic venous atrium, has no direct communication with the ventricular mass. Included in our grouping will be some hearts that the purist would argue are examples of mitral atresia. These rare anomalies are produced by either an imperforate right-sided valve or absence of the right-sided atrioventricular connection in the setting of left hand ventricular topology. We do not contest the fact that, anatomically, these entities are examples of 'mitral' atresia. The clinical picture, nonetheless, is that of tricuspid atresia. Because of this, they will be included in this chapter, although we will emphasize their specific morphology. In all variants of tricuspid atresia as thus defined, there is still further variability in the downstream anatomy, particularly in terms of the different ventriculo-arterial connections, which modify the physical derangement. These differences, when coupled with the degree of flow of blood to the lungs, were the basis of a popular alpha-numerical classification (Edwards and Burchell, 1949). While of great value in the past, the sophistication of modern diagnostic techniques has made such categorizations unduly procrustean. In this chapter, therefore, we will concentrate upon the specific morphology that underscores the important clinical manifestations of the clinical entity in which the systemic venous return has no direct ventricular exit from the morphologically right atrium.

──────INCIDENCE AND AETIOLOGY──────

Tricuspid atresia is a rare anomaly. Estimates of its frequency vary from 0.3% of all congenital cardiac malformations (Storstein et al, 1964) to 5.3% (Donzelot and D'Allaines, 1954). As is usually the case with serious lesions, the higher incidence is found in postmortem series. Leaving aside these extremes, other estimates cluster around 1 to 2.5% in both postmortem and clinical series (Abbott, 1936; Gibson and Clifton, 1938; Edwards and Burchell, 1949; Sommers and Johnson, 1951; Mitchell et al, 1971; Nadas and Fyler, 1972; Kenna et al, 1975). Rao (1982b) suggests that a figure of between 1.3 and 1.7% is a close approximation, with little racial or geographical variation. This results in an incidence of tricuspid atresia of 1 in every 10 000–20 000 births (Kenna et al, 1975; Drew et al, 1977; Rosenthal, 1977).

There is little sex difference in the incidence. If anything, there is minimally higher incidence in boys (Rao, 1982b). Tricuspid atresia with discordant ventriculoarterial connections occurs more frequently in boys (Dick et al, 1975; Bharati et al, 1976; Rao, 1982b). In the majority, no specific aetiological factor can be demonstrated but the condition has been reported following ingestion of thalidomide (Lenz and Pliess, 1963). It has also been seen as part of the 'cat eye' syndrome (Freedom and Gerald, 1973).

──ANATOMY AND MORPHOGENESIS──

The feature that underpins the understanding of the anatomy of tricuspid atresia is the differentiation of an imperforate valve from absence of one of the two atrioventricular connections (Figure 39.1). These two anatomical entities have the same physiological effect, but the morphology is totally different. An imperforate valve (Figure 39.2a) can only be formed in the setting of a discrete atrioventricular junction. With this arrangement, the parietal myocardium of the atrium is continuous with the parietal ventricular wall (Figure 39.2b). Hence the cavities of the atrium and the underlying ventricle are in potential communication. When the atrioventricular connection is absent (Figure 39.3a), this is not the case. The parietal walls of the right atrium and of the ventricle have no direct continuity, but instead they meet at the central fibrous body, with the fibrofatty tissues of the atrioventricular groove occupying the space between the adjacent layers of atrial and ventricular myocardium (Figure 39.3b). Since the imperforate valve modifies the morphology of the atrioventricular connection, it can be

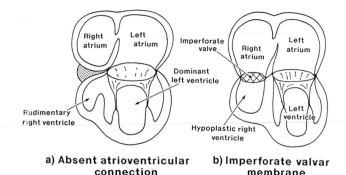

a) Absent atrioventricular connection   **b) Imperforate valvar membrane**

Figure 39.1. The fundamental anatomical difference is shown between atresia produced by absence of one atrioventricular connection (a) and the arrangement that is the consequence of an imperforate valvar membrane (b). Absent connection is illustrated as seen in the most common form of tricuspid atresia (see Figure 39.3), while the imperforate valve is shown as seen rarely when there is coexisting pulmonary atresia and the ventricular septum is intact (see Figure 31.14).

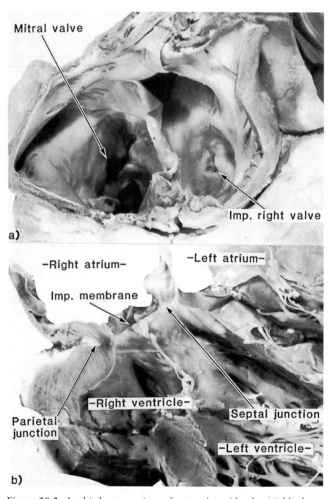

Figure 39.2. In this heart, an imperforate tricuspid valve (a) blocks the vestibule of the right atrium. A simulated four chamber section (b) shows that the imperforate (Imp.) valvar membrane is preventing flow across a formed right atrioventricular junction and overrides the crest of the ventricular septum, with tension apparatus from the imperforate valve attached to the septal crest.

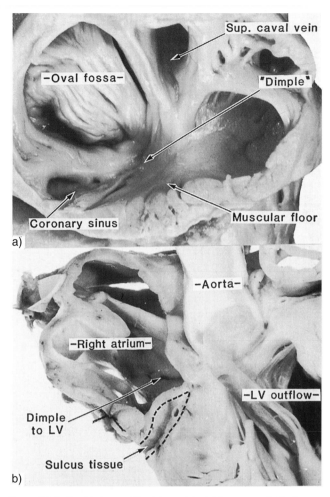

a)

b)

Figure 39.3. In this heart, the right atrium (a) has an exclusively muscular floor, with no evidence seen of either the vestibule or the tricuspid valve. The simulated four chamber section (b) shows that there is absence of the right atrioventricular connection, with the fibrofatty tissue of the atrioventricular groove interposed between the muscular floor of the atrium and the parietal wall of the ventricular mass.

found with concordant, discordant or double inlet atrioventricular connections (Figure 39.4). Any of these combinations will produce the obligatory admixture of systemic and venous returns that is the unifying physiological derangement of the entity described in clinical circumstances as tricuspid atresia. As we have discussed, in some of these instances, the imperforate valvar membrane involved is not morphologically part of the tricuspid valve. To a large extent, this fact is academic, since the examples produced by an imperforate atrioventricular valve account for only a small percentage of cases diagnosed clinically as tricuspid atresia. Furthermore, all of those we have seen thus far have been morphologically tricuspid valves, or imperforate right valves in the setting of double inlet left ventricle. The possibility of finding an imperforate right-sided mitral valve in hearts with discordant atrioventricular connections and left hand ventricular topology, nonetheless, must always be borne in mind.

Variability in terms of the ventricular mass is also to be found in those more common cases characterized by absence of the morphologically right atrioventricular connection. This particular arrangement (Figure 39.3) is a type of atrioventricular connection its own right. Self-evidently, since the usual exit from the atrium is absent, it produces exactly the same physiological effect as an imperforate valve (Figure 39.2). In fact, although previous textbooks often illustrated tricuspid atresia as being caused by an imperforate valve, and there are still some who subscribe to this notion (Rao, 1990), the majority of cases seen clinically have absence of the morphologically right atrioventricular connection, with the left atrium connected to a dominant left ventricle (Orie et al, 1995). Very rarely, hearts will be encountered when the right atrioventricular connection is absent and the left atrium is connected either to a dominant right ventricle

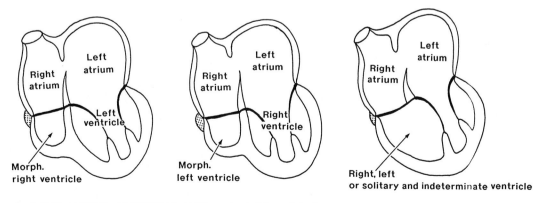

a) Concordant atrioventricular connections   b) Discordant atrioventricular connections   c) Double inlet connection

Figure 39.4. An imperforate valvar membrane can block the exit from the morphologically right atrium in hearts with (a) concordant, (b) discordant or (c) double inlet atrioventricular connections. When the connection is double inlet, the dominant ventricle can be of left, right or indeterminate morphology. All arrangements would produce the same haemodynamic disturbance, but only the one with concordant connections could strictly be considered 'tricuspid' atresia. An imperforate right atrioventricular valve can also be found when there is isomerism of the atrial appendages.

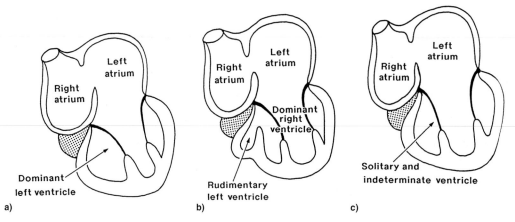

Figure 39.5. Absence of one atrioventricular connection leads to several combinations (compare with Figure 39.4). The chamber to which the left atrium is connected can be a dominant left ventricle (a), in which case the rudimentary and incomplete right ventricle would be positioned anterosuperiorly (see Figure 39.7); a dominant right ventricle (b); or, very rarely, a solitary ventricle of indeterminate morphology (c).

or, even more rarely, to a solitary and indeterminate ventricle (Figure 39.5).

As indicated, by far the most common variant is that initially recognized by Schuberg (1861), with absence of the morphologically right atrioventricular connection and with the left atrium connected to a dominant left ventricle in presence of an anterosuperior rudimentary right ventricle (Figure 39.3). Most of the anatomical description, therefore, will be devoted to this entity, which is the usual variant of tricuspid atresia. Brief consideration will be given, nonetheless, to the rarer segmental arrangements that we have encountered.

CLASSICAL TRICUSPID ATRESIA

The outstanding feature of classical tricuspid atresia is that there is no sign whatsoever of the vestibule and leaflets of the tricuspid valve on opening the morphologically right atrium (Figure 39.6). This, of course, is because there is complete absence of the right atrioventricular connection (Figure 39.3b). The atrium has a complete muscular floor, which is the lateral wall of the appendage. A muscular dimple is frequently seen anterosuperior to the orifice of the coronary sinus. This is often presumed to be the site of the right atrioventricular orifice. Sectioning through this dimple, however, shows that it overlies the atrioventricular membranous component of the central fibrous body (Figure 39.3). It points to the outflow tract of the morphologically left ventricle. The right atrial blood exits to the left atrium through an interatrial communication, usually within the oval fossa (Figures 39.6 and 39.7a). The left atrium is then connected through a morphologically mitral valve to a dominant left ventricle (Figure 39.7b). This ventricle, in turn, empties to a rudimentary right ventricle, which possesses apical trabecular and outlet components but lacks any inlet component (Figure 39.7c).

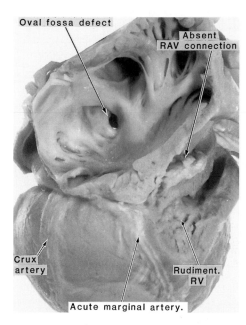

Figure 39.6. This example of classical tricuspid atresia is seen from right oblique and posterior position. Note the muscular floor of the right atrium, the absence of any vestibule or atrioventricular valvar tissue (absent RAV connection), and the deficiency of the atrial septum in the oval fossa. The artery delimiting the posteroinferior extent of the muscular ventricular septum descends at the acute margin of the ventricular mass, and not at the crux. The rudimentary and incomplete right ventricle (RV) is positioned anterosuperiorly.

The muscular ventricular septum, of necessity, has only apical trabecular and outlet components. It extends to the acute point of the atrioventricular junction, not reaching the crux as in a heart with biventricular atrioventricular connections (Figure 39.6). Its posteroinferior extent is marked, therefore, by the descent of the acute marginal branch of the right coronary artery (Deanfield et al, 1982). The rudimentary right ventricle is carried on the anterosuperior shoulder of the ventricular mass,

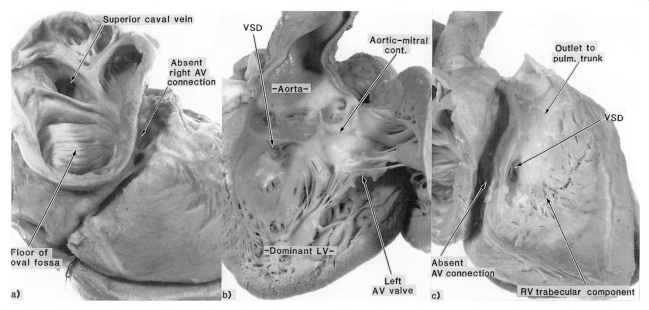

Figure 39.7. This series of pictures of the same heart shows the anatomy of classical tricuspid atresia with concordant ventriculo-arterial connections. (a) The muscular floor of the blind-ending right atrium can be seen; the floor of the oval fossa is perforate, providing access to the left atrium. (b) Here the dominant left ventricle (LV) and the morphologically mitral valve can be seen; with the aorta arising from the dominant ventricle. (c) The rudimentary right ventricle gives rise to the pulmonary (pulm.) trunk. The ventricular septal defect (VSD) is restrictive.

almost always with its trabecular component to the right (Figure 39.7c); rarely it can be directly anterior or, sometimes, even in left-sided position (Anderson et al, 1977). The anatomy described thus far is relatively constant for almost all examples of classical tricuspid atresia. Variability is mostly related to the ventriculo-arterial connections, and to the presence of stenosis or atresia of the ventricular outflow tracts.

Categorizing classical tricuspid atresia on the basis of obstruction to pulmonary blood flow was first suggested by Kuhne (1906). The refinement of this approach, which still enjoys wide popularity, is that of Edwards and Burchell (1949). They divided tricuspid atresia into subgroups with concordant ('normally related', type I) or discordant ('transposed', type II) ventriculo-arterial connections. Each of these subgroups was described with the potential for totally obstructed (type A), decreased (type B) or increased (type C) flow of blood to the lungs. This already complicated alpha-numeric classification was then further elaborated by Vlad (1978) to encompass hearts with discordant ventriculo-arterial connections in which the transposed aorta was left-sided (type III) but, importantly, with the right atrium still being the blind-ending atrial chamber. This rare entity, which certainly exists, fits also within our own definition of tricuspid atresia. Confusion was introduced in the alpha-numeric classification by Tandon and Edwards (1974), who included hearts with absence of the morphologically left atrioventricular connection as 'tricuspid atresia type III'. The right atrium in these hearts, however, is connected to a dominant left ventricle, with a left-sided rudimentary right ventricle supporting a discordantly connected left-sided aorta. Although fitting the anatomical definition of

tricuspid atresia, these present clinically as 'mitral atresia' (see Chapter 40). Furthermore, alpha-numeric systems always give problems when instances are encountered that do not fit the initial categorization. Such is the case with tricuspid atresia, since the initial system takes no account of double outlet from either the dominant left or the rudimentary right ventricle (Figure 39.8), nor the existence of common arterial trunk. The system itself, of course, can be expanded to accept these cases, or other variations as suggested by Rao (1980). To our mind, such expansion simply increases the unwieldness of the system and detracts from its value. We, therefore, recommend a descriptive approach to categorization.

Most usually, classical tricuspid atresia is found with concordant ventriculo-arterial connections, and with the aorta posterior and to the right of the pulmonary trunk ('normal relations': Figure 39.8a). Then there is usually an extensive right-sided apical trabecular component in the rudimentary right ventricle, the outlet portion swinging upwards and leftwards to the pulmonary trunk, which is supported by the extensive free-standing subpulmonary infundibulum. Most frequently, the ventricular septal defect, surrounded on all its margins by muscle, opens between the outlet and trabecular components and is stenotic (Figure 39.7c). The defect can be larger, but still restrictive (Figure 39.9a), or occasionally widely open (Figure 39.9b). On other occasions, the communication can be atretic, either as a primary event or because of secondary closure (Rao, 1977; Sauer and Hall, 1980). When the defect is stenotic, then a second stenotic area may be found at the proximal extent of the right ventricular trabecular component (Figure 39.10). Irrespective of the presence of a restrictive ventricular septal defect, the

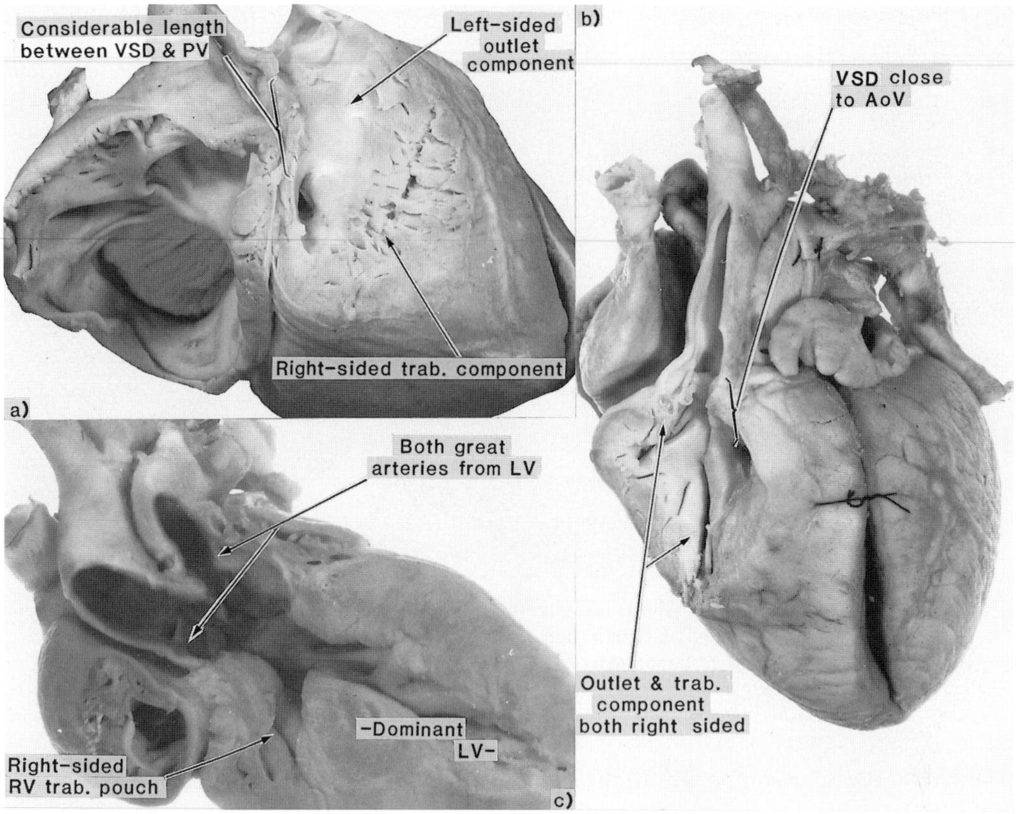

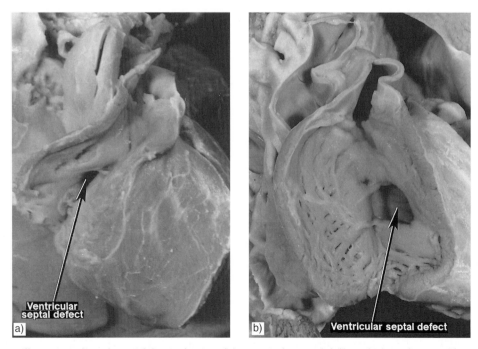

Figure 39.8. The morphology of the rudimentary right ventricle (RV) varies with the ventriculo-arterial connections, seen here in the setting of (a) concordant, (b) discordant and (c) double outlet variants. In the heart with double outlet from the dominant left ventricle (LV) (c), the rudimentary right ventricle is no more than an apical trabecular (trab.) pouch, but its apical trabeculations identify it as a right ventricle. AoV, aortic valve; PV, pulmonary valve.

Figure 39.9. These two illustrations show the variability in the size of the ventricular septal defect, which is of reasonable size but restrictive in (a), and large and unrestrictive in (b). Both hearts have concordant ventriculo-arterial connections, with the right ventricle supporting the pulmonary trunk.

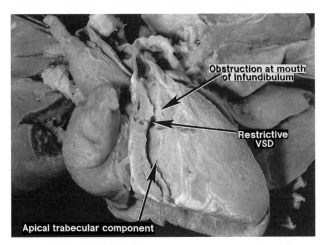

Figure 39.10. Most usually, when the ventriculo-arterial connections are concordant, restriction to pulmonary flow is found at the level of the ventricular septal defect (VSD). In this heart, a second level of restriction is found between the apical and infundibular components of the rudimentary and incomplete right ventricle.

rudimentary right ventricle is usually of reasonable size when the great arteries are 'normally related'. This is not to say it is of normal size. Because it is rudimentary and incomplete, it should be expected to be somewhat hypoplastic. But almost without exception, the apical trabecular component is well represented, even when the outflow tract is atretic. It is demarcated by the delimiting coronary arteries (Deanfield et al, 1982; Scalia et al, 1983). Not surprisingly, the smallest rudimentary right ventricles are found in association with pulmonary atresia. They may then be mere slits, requiring sectioning for demonstration. Except in these circumstances, the pulmonary valve is usually normal. Even when bicuspid, it is rarely stenotic. It is the exception to find obstruction to pulmonary flow at valvar or supravalvar level. Obstruction can be found, nonetheless, between the apical and infundibular components of the right ventricle (Figure 39.10).

Rarely, concordant ventriculo-arterial connections may exist when the rudimentary right ventricle and the pulmonary trunk are both right sided, with the aorta arising from the left ventricle above a muscular infundibulum and in anterior left-sided position. This arrangement is called anatomically corrected malposition (Freedom and Harrington, 1974; Anderson et al, 1975). Often it is associated with left juxtaposition of the atrial appendages and with pulmonary atresia. The rudimentary right ventricle is smaller than that found with 'normally related' great arteries.

The second most frequent type of ventriculo-arterial connection is discordant (Figure 39.8b). The trabecular component of the rudimentary right ventricle is less well developed, and the subaortic infundibulum (usually on the same side as the trabecular component) is much shorter (Scalia et al, 1983). The ventricular septal defect, therefore, tends to be in immediately subvalvar position. If stenotic, it produces subaortic obstruction, almost always with concomitant coarctation and isthmal hypoplasia. Subpulmonary obstruction is less frequent when the ventriculo-arterial connections are discordant, as is subaortic obstruction with concordant connections. When found, the lesion can be caused by either deviation of the outlet septum into the left ventricle or by 'tissue tags'. Rarely, the aorta can be directly anterior or left sided when the ventriculo-arterial connections are discordant (Anderson et al, 1977; Vlad, 1978). Other types of ventriculo-arterial connection are rare but do exist. For example, double outlet connections can be found, usually from the dominant left ventricle (Figure 39.8c), but rarely from the rudimentary right ventricle. Single outlet through a common arterial trunk also exists but is exceedingly rare, as is solitary pulmonary trunk with aortic atresia. Pulmonary atresia with a solitary aortic trunk is more common. In this setting, at least in anatomical specimens, the atretic pulmonary trunk can usually be traced to the grossly hypoplastic rudimentary right ventricle. The connections, therefore, can be established as being potentially concordant. With pulmonary atresia, the pulmonary blood flow is almost always duct dependent.

Most of the associated malformations that complicate classical tricuspid atresia have already been discussed, notably the atrial septal defect, the ventricular septal defect and the substrates of obstruction in the ventricular outflow tracts. Any malformation must, however, be anticipated to exist. Anomalies of systemic venous return are found, particularly persistence of the left superior caval vein draining to the coronary sinus. The valves of the systemic venous sinus, the Eustachian and Thebesian valves, also tend to be well formed. It is also possible for the mitral valve to straddle and override the crest of the ventricular septum. This rare associated malformation (Figure 39.11) gives a uniatrial but biventricular connection.

Of considerable surgical significance is the site and course of the conduction tissues. The sinus node will be in its expected site within the terminal groove, except when there is juxtaposition of the atrial appendages. Then the node tends to be closer to the atrioventricular junction than normal (Ho et al, 1979). The atrioventricular node is in its anticipated site at the apex of the triangle of Koch (Figure 39.12a). It is a large structure, spilling over and around the dimple (Dickinson et al, 1979). The atrioventricular conduction axis penetrates through the atrioventricular septal component of the central fibrous body. It then branches behind and inferior to the muscular margins of the ventricular septal defect. When seen from the rudimentary right ventricle, therefore, the penetrating and non-branching segments of the conduction axis are distant from the defect, being carried on the dominant left ventricular aspect of the septum. As seen by the surgeon, the axis is posteroinferior to the typical ventricular septal defects but would be anterosuperior to an apical muscular communication between the ventricles (Figure 39.12b).

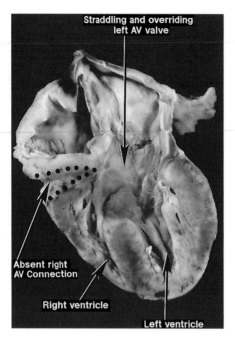

Figure 39.11. This simulated four chamber section shows unequivocal absence of the right atrioventricular (AV) connection, with the atrioventricular groove interposed between the floor of the right atrium and the ventricular mass. The left atrioventricular valve straddles and overrides the crest of the ventricular septum, being attached within both the dominant left and the rudimentary right ventricle.

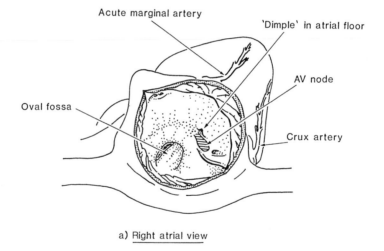

a) Right atrial view

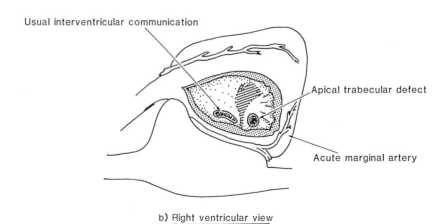

b) Right ventricular view

Figure 39.12. The disposition of the atrioventricular conduction tissues in classical tricuspid atresia as it might be viewed at operation through the right atrium (a) and through the rudimentary and incomplete right ventricle (b). Note that in (b) the axis is shown coursing between the typical ventricular septal defect and an apical trabecular defect.

It would be inappropriate to conclude this section without referring to the controversy concerning the relationship between classical tricuspid atresia and 'single ventricle', or the 'univentricular heart'. The morphological similarity of the ventricular mass in hearts with tricuspid or mitral atresia to those with double inlet had already been recognized by investigators such as Taussig (1939) and Edwards (1960). Emphasis of the association was continued by Elliott et al (1964). It was Van Praagh et al (1964) who, on purely arbitrary grounds, excluded the valvar atresias from their grouping of single ventricle. We subsequently attempted to show that the difference in morphology between these entities was in the atrioventricular connection and not in ventricular morphology, the latter being comparable in the two (Anderson et al, 1977, 1979). Our attempt to convey this fact was obscured by our use of the adjective univentricular to describe the ventricular mass in these hearts. There is no doubt that the ventricular mass in classical tricuspid atresia contains two ventricles (Figure 39.3), but so does the ventricular mass in classical single ventricle, as typified by double inlet left ventricle! The kernel of our argument, therefore, is better expressed by stating that it is the atrioventricular connection in both anomalies that is univentricular (Anderson et al, 1983, 1984). In tricuspid atresia, this is because the right atrioventricular connection is absent. In double inlet, self evidently it is directly to the left ventricle. Therefore, both classical tricuspid atresia and double inlet left ventricle have univentricular atrioventricular connection to a dominant left ventricle in presence of a rudimentary right ventricle that lacks its inlet portion (Deanfield et al, 1982; Anderson, 1983). Polemics concerning the 'univentricular' nature of tricuspid atresia, such as promoted by Rao (1982a, 1990), are unproductive, since our discussion has never related to the solitary nature of the ventricular mass.

VARIANTS OF TRICUSPID ATRESIA

The existence of an imperforate valve as a substrate of tricuspid atresia was discussed briefly by Van Praagh et al (1971) and subsequently enlarged upon by Ando and his colleagues (1980). They refer to this variant as the 'membranous' form of atresia. They have considered this possibility, however, only in the setting of concordant atrioventricular connections, when the imperforate valve is seen most frequently in the setting of Ebstein's malformation (Figure 39.13). This pattern was well described by Rao and colleagues (1973). An imperforate right valve can also be found at the normally positioned atrioventricular junction, typically when there is associated pulmonary atresia and the ventricular septum is intact (Figure 39.14). This combination is a variant of pulmonary atresia with intact ventricular septum (Chapter 44). Such valves at the normally positioned junction can also be found overriding the crest of the ventricular septum

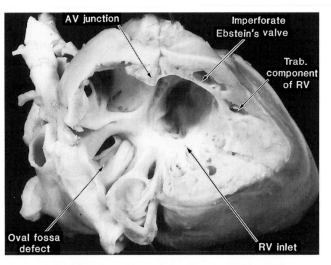

Figure 39.13. Ebstein's malformation with an imperforate right atrioventricular (AV) valve producing tricuspid atresia in the setting of concordant atrioventricular connections. RV, right ventricle; Trab., trabecular.

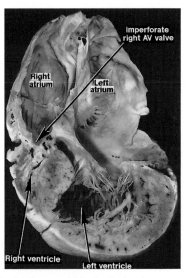

Figure 39.14. In this heart, which also had pulmonary atresia, the ventricular septum is intact and an imperforate valve blocks the right atrioventricular (AV) connection.

(Figure 39.2). Imperforate right valves have also been found when there is double inlet connection to a dominant left ventricle. They must be anticipated with double inlet right or indeterminate ventricles, or with discordant atrioventricular connections (see Figure 39.4). In the variant of imperforate valve associated with Ebstein's malformation, the right atrioventricular junction is unguarded because of displacement of the tricuspid valvar tissue to the junction of the inlet and apical trabecular components of the right ventricle. A further variant of tricuspid atresia can be found that has much in common with this pattern. Again the atrioventricular connections are concordant, and the right atrioventricular junction is unguarded (Figures 39.15a,b). However, in this type, the

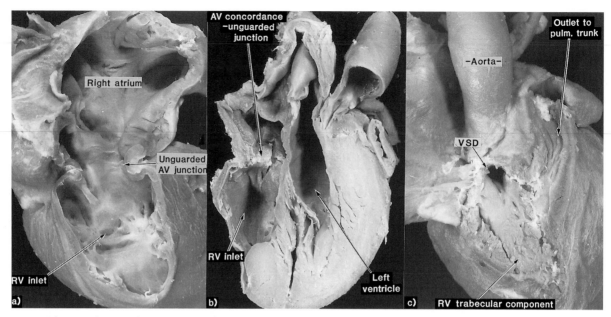

Figure 39.15. A heart with concordant atrioventricular connections, an unguarded right atrioventricular (AV) orifice and an imperforate partition between the inlet and the remainder of the right ventricle. (a) The right ventricular inlet is in free communication with the right atrium. (b) A four chamber cut through the inlet portions shows concordant atrioventricular connections. (c) The distal components of the morphologically right ventricle are fed from the left ventricle through the ventricular septal defect. Note the similarity to the rudimentary right ventricle of 'classical' tricuspid atresia (Figure 31.7c).

atresia is produced by a muscular partition between the inlet component and the remainder of the morphologically right ventricle, the latter having the typical appearance of the rudimentary and incomplete right ventricle seen in classical tricuspid atresia (Figure 39.15c) (Zuberbuhler et al, 1979; Scalia et al, 1983).

Absence of the right atrioventricular connection can also be found when the left atrium is connected to a dominant right ventricle (Shinebourne et al, 1980), or to

a solitary and indeterminate ventricle (Figure 39.5). Although infrequent in terms of reported cases, this is possibly because such variants have only rarely been recognized. Of those reported, the most common type is that in which the left-sided atrioventricular valve straddles the septum between the left-sided morphologically right ventricle and a right-sided rudimentary and in complete morphologically left ventricle (Figure 39.16) (Otero Coto et al, 1981; Ho et al, 1982). As with straddling of the left-

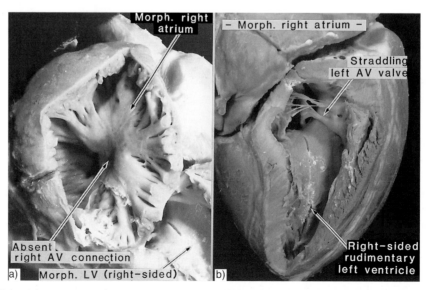

Figure 39.16. Absence of the right atrioventricular (AV) connection (a) with the left atrium (b) connected to a dominant right ventricle in presence of a right-sided rudimentary left ventricle (left hand ventricular topology). There is straddling of a small part of the tension apparatus of the left atrioventricular valve into the rudimentary ventricle. Note that the right atrium is indistinguishable from the arrangement seen in classical tricuspid atresia (Figure 39.3). Morph., morphologically.

sided valve and dominance of the left ventricle, this arrangement produces a uniatrial but biventricular atrioventricular connection (Chapter 40). When the dominant ventricle is of right ventricular morphology, both great arteries usually take origin from it. These hearts have a left hand pattern of ventricular topology, and a particularly bizarre disposition of their atrioventricular conduction tissues (Ho et al, 1982; see Chapter 40).

MORPHOGENESIS

Many conflicting views exist concerning the mode of development of tricuspid atresia, much of the argument centring upon the univentricular or biventricular nature of the lesion. All are speculative since, as Gessner (1982) has indicated in an excellent review, no-one has yet succeeded in producing tricuspid atresia in an experimental model. The concepts are, therefore, based upon presumptions of normal embryogenesis, coupled with deductions based on knowledge of the anatomy of the definitive lesion. One thing is certain. No single embryologic insult produces all the variants of tricuspid atresia as described above, and no unifying developmental hypothesis can explain the heterogeneous group of malformations that result in blood being unable to leave the right atrium other than via an interatrial communication.

It seems reasonable to us to propose a different morphogenetic background for, on the one hand, those hearts having an imperforate atrioventricular valve and, on the other hand, those with absence of an atrioventricular connection. It is much easier to provide a plausible explanation for imperforate valve membranes. It is known that development of the valvar leaflets is a late event, occurring after the establishment of the connections between the atriums and the ventricles (Bernays, 1876). Fusion of the leaflets during or subsequent to their formation would produce an imperforate valve. This could occur in any given segmental combination.

Absence of one atrioventricular connection is much harder to explain. Any offered hypothesis must account for the known anatomical facts, namely that the left atrium in this setting can be connected to a morphologically left, right or indeterminate ventricle, and that the right atrial anatomy in each is indistinguishable. Our own preference is to consider that the atrioventricular connection developed as though to produce double inlet connection, but for some reason the right atrioventricular orifice failed to develop. Indeed, examination of the developing human heart has shown that a stage exists early in its formation which is remarkably similar to absence of the atrioventricular connection, albeit prior to formation of the atrial septum (Lamers et al, 1992).

Those who argue against this concept, quoting the usual association between tricuspid atresia with concordant ventriculo-arterial connections and double inlet left ventricle with discordant ventriculo-arterial connections,

miss a crucial point. Both tricuspid atresia and double inlet left ventricle can exist with any ventriculo-arterial connection. When like is compared with like, the anatomical arrangements of the morphologically right ventricle are virtually indistinguishable (Deanfield et al, 1982). The dominant left ventricle is not identical in the two entities, being connected only to the left atrium in tricuspid atresia but to both atriums in double inlet. In this respect, the fact that the 'dimple' points to the left ventricular outflow tract is vital (Rosenquist et al, 1970; Anderson et al, 1977; Gessner, 1982). This suggests to us an initial connection of the blind-ending right atrium to the dominant left ventricle via the atrioventricular junction, as seen in the early developing heart (Lamers et al, 1992). The concept of the absent connection developing subsequently in an initial setting of double inlet ventricle accounts also for the rarer variants in which the left atrium is connected to a dominant right ventricle or a morphologically indeterminate ventricle. Almost certainly the embryological insult preventing formation of the second atrioventricular connection occurs much earlier during development than that which results in an imperforate atrioventricular valve.

PATHOPHYSIOLOGY

In hearts with tricuspid atresia, the only egress for systemic venous return from the right atrium is across an atrial septal defect or patent oval foramen to the left atrium. Unless there is a large atrial septal defect, the pressure in the right atrium is elevated compared with that in the left, and the right atrium enlarges. Of necessity, the left atrium receives both systemic and pulmonary venous return. Hence, common mixing occurs and desaturated blood flows from the left atrium to the left ventricle and then to the aorta and pulmonary trunk, where the saturations of oxygen will be equal. Because the left ventricle receives both systemic and pulmonary venous return, it is larger than normal in terms of both cavity size and muscle mass.

In the neonate with a large ventricular septal defect and either concordant or discordant ventriculo-arterial connections, cyanosis is evident at birth. As the pulmonary vascular resistance falls during the first month of life, the cyanosis becomes less marked, but the increasing flow of blood to the lungs usually results in symptoms of congestive cardiac failure. When there is pulmonary stenosis, either because of a restrictive ventricular septal defect in the presence of normally related great arteries or because of muscular subpulmonary stenosis with discordant ventriculo-arterial connections or double outlet left ventricle, the degree of cynaosis becomes greater with increasing severity of pulmonary stenosis, becoming most profound in the presence of pulmonary atresia. Therefore, the degree of central cyanosis, or the development of congestive cardiac failure, is a result of the interplay of various factors. These include the size of the ventricular septal defect, the presence or absence of pulmonary stenosis or atresia, patency of the arterial duct and the pulmonary and systemic vascular resistances. The lower the magnitude of pulmonary blood flow, the greater will be the degree of cyanosis. In contrast, increased flow of the blood to the lungs is associated with the development of the symptoms of congestive cardiac failure, and enlargement of the left atrium and left ventricle. Further modification of the clinical presentation will occur when there is aortic coarctation, usually in the setting of discordant ventriculo-arterial connections and restrictive ventricular septal defect. The increased pulmonary flow and diminished flow to the lower body will result in the early development of congestive cardiac failure and metabolic acidosis. As a result, it is common to encounter left ventricular dysfunction, which will further aggravate the symptoms of congestive cardiac failure and low cardiac output.

CLINICAL FEATURES

Although the vast majority of patients with tricuspid atresia present in the neonatal period or early infancy, the timing and exact clinical presentation will always be dictated by the associated anomalies and their severity. When there is severe obstruction to flow of blood to the lungs, presentation is usually in the neonatal period with a duct-dependent pulmonary circulation. Cyanosis will be present at birth and will become more severe with impending closure of the arterial duct. There will be a single second heart sound, a short ejection systolic murmur of pulmonary stenosis at the upper left sternal edge and sometimes a soft continuous murmur. When there is pulmonary atresia, there will also be a single second heart sound and frequently a continuous murmur from the arterial duct. In contrast, an infant with tricuspid atresia associated with discordant ventriculo-arterial connections and aortic coarctation will exhibit weak or absent femoral pulses, mild central cyanosis, and symptoms of high pulmonary blood flow, including tachypnoea, enlargement of the liver and feeding difficulties. Similarly, although the infant with a large ventricular septal defect will usually be symptom-free at birth, by the beginning of the second month of life the pulmonary vascular resistance will have fallen sufficiently for the symptoms and signs of high pulmonary blood flow to develop. In contrast, the infant with balanced systemic and pulmonary flows because of moderate pulmonary stenosis will be well, with mild central cyanosis and a pansystolic murmur heard best at the lower left sternal edge. As the ventricular septal defect becomes relatively smaller, and the degree of subpulmonary outflow tract obstruction increases, so cyanosis becomes more obvious and cyanotic spells might develop. When there is severe aortic coarctation, or aortic interruption, presentation may be with cardiogenic shock during the early neonatal period.

INVESTIGATIONS

CHEST RADIOGRAPHY

There is a close correlation between the size of the heart and the volume of flow to the lungs. With diminished pulmonary flow, the heart size remains normal, but it increases following construction of a systemic-to-pulmonary arterial shunt. In the absence of pulmonary stenosis, cardiomegaly is the rule when pulmonary blood flow is increased. There is no particular configuration of the cardiac outline that typifies tricuspid atresia. A prominent right heart border owing to right atrial distension is sometimes seen, particularly in the presence of a restrictive atrial septal defect. In the presence of pulmonary stenosis with pulmonary hypoplasia, there may be a pulmonary arterial bay. When the ventriculo-arterial connections are discordant, a narrow pedicle is commonly encountered. The pulmonary vascular markings again reflect the amount of pulmonary flow; as a result, pulmonary oligaemia is encountered when there is severe pulmonary stenosis, normal pulmonary vascular markings are evident when there is a balanced situation of relatively equal systemic and pulmonary blood flows, and increased pulmonary vascular markings may be found in the absence of pulmonary stenosis or when pulmonary stenosis or atresia is associated with a large arterial duct or other source of excessive pulmonary blood flow. We have encountered a right-sided heart with normal atrial arrangement in 3% of patients, and a right aortic arch in 8%.

ELECTROCARDIOGRAPHY

Typically, the standard surface electrocardiogram reveals a left superior axis between 0° and −90° in more than four fifths of patients. It is associated with a superior counter-clockwise frontal vector loop. An electrical axis between 0° and +90° occurs in less than one tenth of patients and is associated with an inferior counter-clockwise frontal vector. It is found more frequently, but not exclusively, when the ventriculo-arterial connections are discordant. Right-axis deviation with an electrical axis above +90° is unusual. The precordial leads almost always reveal a normal adult pattern of RS progression of the QRS and T waves. The T waves are inverted in leads V_5 and V_6 in up to half of patients. Right ventricular hypertrophy is associated with unusual anatomical arrangements, including those with tricuspid atresia in which the morphologically left atrium connects to a dominant right ventricle. A relatively short PR interval is encountered frequently, together with evidence of right or biatrial hypertrophy.

ECHOCARDIOGRAPHY

Cross-sectional echocardiography will almost always permit the diagnosis of the various forms of tricuspid atresia and the associated anomalies (Seward et al, 1978; Rigby et al, 1981, 1982). The subcostal and parasternal four chamber sections allow the most common form of tricuspid atresia, in which there is absence of the right atrioventricular connection, to be distinguished from those types in which there is an imperforate right atrioventricular valve. With absent connection, the fibrofatty tissue of the groove is seen interposing between the floor of the right atrium and the ventricular mass (Figure 39.17). In contrast, an imperforate valve will be seen ballooning into the morphologically right ventricle when there are concordant atrioventricular connections (Figure 39.18), and into the left ventricle when the atrioventricular connection is double inlet (Figure 39.19). Rudimentary tensor apparatus can sometimes be identified when there is an imperforate valve, but never when there is absence of the atrioventricular connection. In the typical forms of tricuspid atresia, the four chamber sections will show a small and rudimentary right ventricle to the right of the dominant morphologically left ventricle (Figure 39.17), with a solitary left atrioventricular valve guarding the junction between the left atrium and left ventricle.

The characteristics of the dominant and rudimentary ventricles in tricuspid atresia are identified with subcostal, parasternal and apical long and short-axis sections. In the common variant, the rudimentary right ventricle is anterior and to the right of the dominant left

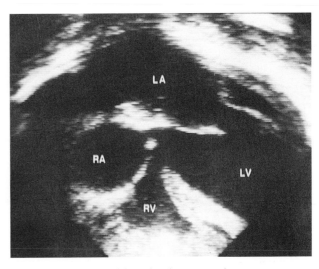

Figure 39.18. Parasternal four chamber section demonstrates an imperforate tricuspid valve, which interposes between the right atrium (RA) and right ventricle (RV). The left atrium (LA) connects to the left ventricle (LV) through a morphologically mitral valve and there is a small ventricular septal defect.

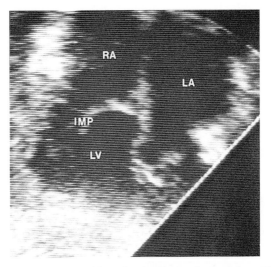

Figure 39.19. Parasternal four chamber section from a heart with double inlet left ventricle and an imperforate left atrioventricular valve (IMP), which separates the right atrium (RA) from the left ventricle (LV). The left atrium (LA) connects to the left ventricle through a patent left-sided atrioventricular valve.

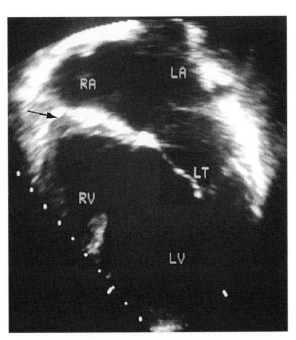

Figure 39.17. Parasternal four chamber section in classical tricuspid atresia. The atrioventricular groove interposes between the right atrium (RA) and right ventricle (RV). The left atrium (LA) connects to the left ventricle (LV) through the left atrioventricular valve (LT). There is a large ventricular septal defect.

ventricle (Figure 39.20). In those much rarer cases in which the left atrium connects to a dominant morphologically right ventricle, the rudimentary left ventricle will be posterior. Indeed, it is the position of the rudimentary and hypoplastic ventricle that is the most reliable echocardiographic guide to ventricular morphology. In practice, it is difficult to establish the morphology of the dominant ventricle by any other means, although, in classical tricuspid atresia, the left ventricle usually has smooth apical trabeculations (Figure 39.17), two papillary muscles and an atrioventricular junction guarded by a bileaflet valve. The infrequently encountered dominant

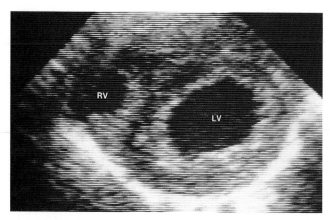

Figure 39.20. Parasternal short-axis section in classical tricuspid atresia showing that the rudimentary right ventricle (RV) is anterior and to the right of the dominant left ventricle (LV).

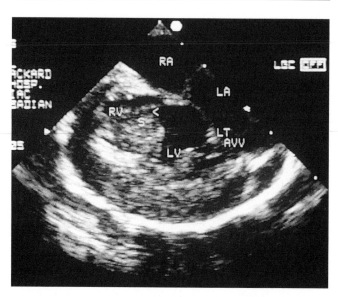

Figure 39.22. Transoesophageal echocardiogram in classical tricuspid atresia with a small and restrictive ventricular septal defect (arrow). The atrioventricular groove is seen interposing between the right atrium (RA) and right ventricle (RV), while the left atrium (LA) connects through the left atrioventricular valve (LTAVV) to the dominant left ventricle (LV). S, septum.

right ventricle, in contrast, is coarsely trabeculated with at least three groups of papillary muscles; it has an atrioventricular valve with three leaflets and cords inserting into the ventricular septum. Hearts can also very rarely be encountered with a solitary and indeterminate ventricle (Figure 39.21). The echocardiographic diagnosis of the variant is based upon extremely coarse trabeculations and absence of any second rudimentary ventricle.

One of the most important aspects of the evaluation of the ventricular mass is the visualization of the ventricular septal defect. The defects are usually solitary and muscular; they vary from being large (Figure 39.17) to extremely small (Figure 39.22). Multiple defects can also be encountered.

The approach to establishing the ventriculo-arterial connections and the morphology of the infundibulums is the same as that described in Chapter 13. Discordant ventriculo-arterial connections (Figure 39.23) may be associated with a restrictive ventricular septal defect, subaortic stenosis, aortic hypoplasia, aortic coarctation or even interruption of the aortic arch. When the ventriculo-arterial connections are concordant, and there is severe subpulmonary stenosis or pulmonary atresia, the pulmonary arteries can be extremely hypoplastic and difficult to identify by cross-sectional echocardiography; consequently, cardiac catheterization and angiography might be required.

An extremely unusual variant of tricuspid atresia, which is readily diagnosed by four chamber cross-sectional echocardiographic sections, is that in which the solitary atrioventricular valve overrides and straddles the ventricular septum; here both ventricles may be of similar size (Figure 39.24). The atrioventricular connection in this variant is uniatrial and biventricular. In order to identify this variant, the fibrofatty tissue of the right atrioventricular groove must be seen to extend to the interatrial septum, ruling out the possibility of common atrioventricular junction with double outlet left atrium. A second unusual variant that we have encountered is when tricuspid atresia is associated with isomerism of the atrial appendages.

A combination of cross-sectional and Doppler imaging is essential for the diagnosis of a restrictive atrial septal defect, the measurement of gradients across the ventricular septal defect or ventricular outflow tracts, and the demonstration of any atrioventricular valvar regurgitation or flow across an arterial duct. In older patients

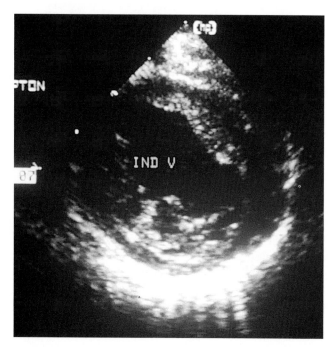

Figure 39.21. Parasternal short-axis section showing a solitary indeterminate ventricle (IND V) in the setting of tricuspid atresia.

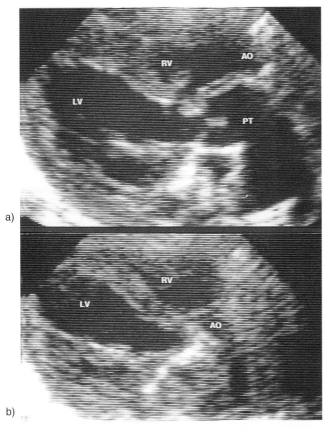

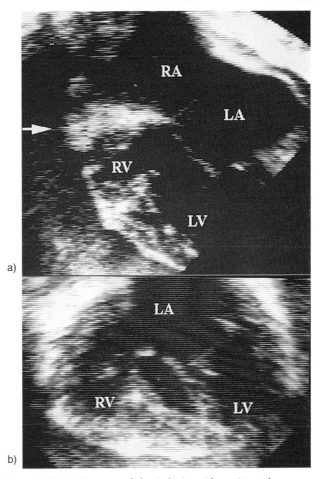

Figure 39.23. Parasternal long-axis sections in tricuspid atresia with a discordant ventriculo-arterial connection and a restrictive ventricular septal defect. A large pulmonary trunk (PT) arises from the morphologically left ventricle (LV), and a rather hypoplastic aorta (AO) arises from the anterior rudimentary right ventricle (RV). The right ventricle communicates with the left ventricle through a very small and restrictive ventricular septal defect.

Figure 39.24. (a) Features of classical tricuspid atresia can be seen with an atrioventricular groove interposing between the right atrium (RA) and the right ventricle (RV). (b) The left atrium connects to both the right-sided right ventricle and left ventricle (LV) through an atrioventricular valve, which has tensor apparatus within the right and left ventricles and is clearly straddling and overriding the ventricular septum.

with tricuspid atresia, it is not unusual to discover regurgitation across the left atrioventricular valve, often associated with systolic and diastolic abnormalities of left ventricular function.

Transoesophageal echocardiography is rarely required for precise diagnosis in children with tricuspid atresia, although it does have a role in patients with a poor precordial window, especially adolescents and adults. Horizontal sections can be used to demonstrate the absence of the right atrioventricular connection (Figure 39.25), and the anterior and right-sided rudimentary right ventricle. Vertical sections allow visualization of the ventricular outflow tracts and ventriculo-arterial connections. Similarly, although magnetic resonance imaging can be used in diagnosis, in day-to-day clinical practice it is rarely required, with the occasional exception in older patients.

CARDIAC CATHETERIZATION AND ANGIOGRAPHY

In the majority of infants with tricuspid atresia, the diagnosis is based on echocardiographic evaluation. Cardiac

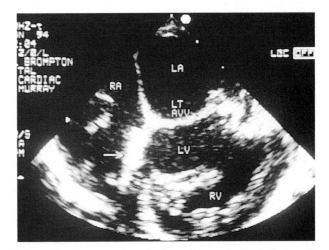

Figure 39.25. Transoesophageal echocardiogram in classical tricuspid atresia with a large ventricular septal defect. The atrioventricular groove (arrow) interposes between the right atrium (RA) and the ventricular mass. The left atrium (LA) connects through the left atrioventricular valve (LTAVV) to the dominant left ventricle (LV); the rudimentary right ventricle (RV) is seen anterior to the left ventricle.

catheterization is rarely undertaken early in life, and only then to identify unusual morphological features of the aorta and arch, hypoplastic pulmonary arteries, unusual sources of pulmonary blood supply, and to permit the measurement of pulmonary arterial pressure prior to a bidirectional Glenn operation (or later in life prior to a Fontan operation). It is our practice usually to perform balloon atrial septostomy to prevent the later development of a restrictive atrial septal defect. This procedure is carried out on the intensive care unit, guided by precordial or transoesophageal echocardiographic monitoring.

At cardiac catheterization, there will be evidence of right-to-left shunting at atrial level, common mixing of systemic and pulmonary venous blood within the ventricular mass, and varying degrees of systemic arterial oxygen desaturation. Mean atrial pressures will be similar when the interatrial communication is large, but there will be a mean pressure gradient, or an a wave gradient from right to left atrium, with a restrictive atrial septal defect.

In many instances, only right heart catheterization is required because the catheter can be readily advanced into the left and right ventricles, aorta and the pulmonary arteries. When there are concordant ventriculo-arterial connections, the systolic pressures in the left ventricle and aorta are equal. In the majority of patients, the right ventricular systolic pressure will be lower than that in the left ventricle because of the small size of the ventricular septal defect. When there is extreme hypoxia, it may not be possible to enter the pulmonary arteries. A good estimate of pulmonary arterial pressure can then be gained from a pulmonary venous wedge pressure. Following a modified Blalock–Taussig shunt, it is important to measure the pulmonary arterial pressure directly. A retrograde arterial approach from the femoral artery usually allows the shunt to be entered with a preshaped catheter.

Selective angiography is rarely required in the right atrium (Figure 39.26) because the atrioventricular junction is best demonstrated by cross-sectional echocardiography. When left ventricular angiography is performed with left oblique and craniocaudal angulation, it is almost always possible clearly to demonstrate the rudimentary right ventricle, the ventricular septum, any ventricular septal defects and the precise ventriculo-arterial connections (Figures 39.27–39.29). If the morphology of the pulmonary arteries is unclear, either from echocardiographic studies or following selective angiography, it may be necessary to perform pulmonary venous wedge angiography. The major role of cardiac catheterization, nonetheless, is not to demonstrate the morphological features of tricuspid atresia but to assess the outcome of previous palliative operations and to determine suitability for a bidirectional Glenn or Fontan operation. Of particular importance are the measurements of pulmonary arterial pressure, ventricular end-diastolic pressure and atrial pressures. If the mean pulmonary arterial pressure exceeds 15 mmHg, the pulmonary vascular resistance should be measured.

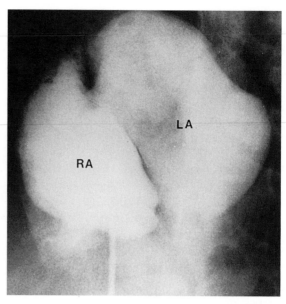

Figure 39.26. Right atrial angiogram performed in four chamber exposure showing contrast flowing from right atrium (RA) to left atrium (LA). The floor of the right atrium can be seen clearly, together with the interatrial septum.

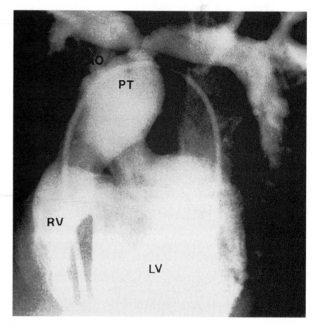

Figure 39.27. Four chamber left ventriculogram in classical tricuspid atresia. Contrast is seen to flow from the left ventricle (LV) to the right-sided rudimentary right ventricle (RV) through a relatively large ventricular septal defect. The pulmonary trunk (PT), which has been banded, arises from the rudimentary right ventricle.

The systolic gradient across the ventricular septal defect should be determined if the ventriculo-arterial connections are discordant. Angiography is designed to demonstrate the size and morphology of the pulmonary arteries (Figure 39.27), with particular attention paid to any naturally occurring or iatrogenic stenoses or distortions. It is also important to identify additional sources of

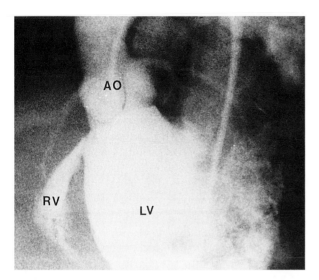

Figure 39.28. Left ventricular angiogram in classical tricuspid atresia with pulmonary atresia and a restrictive ventricular septal defect. Contrast flows from the left ventricle (LV) to the right ventricle (RV) through a small ventricular septal defect. There is no evidence of the pulmonary arteries, but the aorta (AO) is seen arising from the left ventricle.

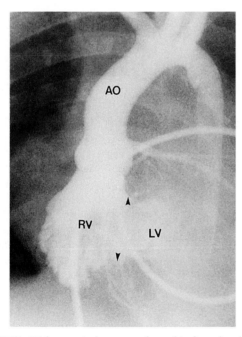

Figure 39.29. Right ventriculogram performed in four chamber projection in tricuspid atresia with discordant ventriculo-arterial connections. The arrowheads demonstrate a large ventricular septal defect between the rudimentary right ventricle (RV) and the dominant left ventricle (LV). The aorta (AO) can be seen arising entirely from the rudimentary right ventricle.

pulmonary blood flow, such as aortopulmonary collateral arteries, which might be suitable for coil embolization.

Left ventricular volume measurements derived from angiograms have demonstrated increased size and reduced ejection fraction in these patients compared with values in the normal heart, although such measurements are

not usually part of the preoperative evaluation by cardiac catheterization (Nishioka et al, 1981; Rigby and Redington, 1987).

NATURAL HISTORY

There is now little opportunity to study the natural history of patients with tricuspid atresia. Most information is from studies undertaken in the 1970s and early 1980s (Dick et al, 1975; Moodie et al, 1984). In general terms, the natural history is determined in early life by the presence and severity of obstruction to pulmonary blood flow, by the presence of aortic coarctation, or later by the left ventricular dysfunction that develops in response to volume overload. In tricuspid atresia with concordant ventriculo-arterial connections, obstruction at subpulmonary level is commonly encountered and gives rise to moderate-to-severe cyanosis. The relative reduction in size of the ventricular septal defect during infancy means that flow of blood to the lungs diminishes still further (Freedom, 1987). Because of this, and other factors nine tenths of patients will have died by the end of the first year (Vlad, 1978).

When pulmonary blood flow is normal or increased, life expectancy is better. Some patients can die in early infancy of congestive cardiac failure secondary to the excessive flow of blood to the lungs. Much more frequently, spontaneous narrowing of the ventricular septal defect and the progression of infundibular pulmonary stenosis produce a more balanced flow of systemic and pulmonary flows during later infancy. Nevertheless, if left untreated, nine tenths of these patients will have died by the age of 10 years (Vlad, 1978). A few patients will survive to the second and third decades of life and beyond without surgery, although the chronic volume overload of the left ventricle, and the development of ventricular dysfunction and functional mitral incompetence, eventually cause death from low cardiac output.

In general terms, the natural history for patients with tricuspid atresia and discordant ventriculo-arterial connections is worse than for those with concordant connections. As the ventricular septal defect becomes smaller, so the pulmonary blood flow increases, and the secondary subaortic stenosis reduces systemic blood flow. A number of these patients will have aortic coarctation and die during the early neonatal period. Even in the absence of coarctation or aortic interruption, the majority of patients will have died by the age of 1 year. Some patients with discordant ventriculo-arterial connections have mild-to-moderate muscular subpulmonary stenosis, usually associated with a large ventricular septal defect. The early prognosis is then better, although only one tenth of patients will survive beyond the age of 7 years.

The left ventricle in tricuspid atresia will always receive both systemic and pulmonary venous return. Thus, left ventricular myocardium is always subjected to volume overload to some degree, and to continuing hypoxia and polycythaemia. During the first decade of life, there will be increasing left ventricular volume and muscle mass, with diminishing ejection and shortening fractions (Nishioka et al, 1981; Rigby and Redington, 1987). It is the chronic volume overload that will result in the functional mitral regurgitation so commonly encountered during the second and third decades of life.

MANAGEMENT

MEDICAL MANAGEMENT

Nowadays, the diagnosis of tricuspid atresia is usually made during fetal life, the neonatal period or early infancy. Unless there are balanced pulmonary and systemic flows because of moderate pulmonary stenosis, palliative surgical treatment is usually required in early infancy. Intravenous prostaglandin E_1 is used to re-establish or preserve ductal patency when there is severe hypoxia. This can be because of pulmonary stenosis or atresia or when systemic flow is inadequate because of aortic coarctation or interruption; both these aortic anomalies are usually associated with a restrictive ventricular septal defect and subaortic stenosis. Almost always, it is possible to correct the acidosis that accompanies severe hypoxia or reduced systemic flow prior to initial surgery. When tricuspid atresia presents with congestive cardiac failure and mild hypoxia during the second month of life, the initial treatment is with diuretics and vasodilators. Occasionally, a restrictive atrial septal defect is manifest by low cardiac output and marked enlargement of the liver. Balloon atrial septostomy should then be performed. We generally perform balloon atrial septostomy for the majority of patients to prevent the late development of a restrictive atrial septal defect, but otherwise cardiac catheterization is rarely required in early infancy, the precise diagnosis almost always being made by cross-sectional echocardiography alone.

INITIAL SURGICAL MANAGEMENT

When there is inadequate flow of blood to the lungs because of severe pulmonary stenosis or atresia, a systemic-to-pulmonary arterial shunt is created to increase pulmonary supply. A modified Blalock–Taussig shunt is preferred, using a 3.5 or 4.0 mm polytetrafluroethylene graft. This operation is usually undertaken through a lateral thoracotomy, although more recently some have advocated the use of a midline sternotomy (Jonas, 1994). As a general rule, it is preferable, but not essential, to place the shunt on the same side as the superior caval vein. This is because shunts in this position will be easier to control and to take down at any subsequent operation.

When there is excessive pulmonary blood flow, banding of the pulmonary trunk is performed through a left

lateral thoracotomy. It is important to place the band sufficiently proximal on the pulmonary trunk to avoid distortion of the branches of the pulmonary arteries, at the same time taking care to avoid damage to the pulmonary valvar leaflets. Excessive pulmonary flow may be found when there is a large ventricular septal defect and either concordant or discordant ventriculo-arterial connections, but it also occurs with obstruction to aortic flow. This last situation is usually found when the ventriculo-arterial connections are discordant, coupled in most cases with a restrictive ventricular septal defect, subaortic stenosis, aortic coarctation or interruption, together with varying degrees of hypoplasia of the ascending aorta and arch. A variety of surgical protocols have been used to deal with these problems (Neches et al, 1973; Freedom et al, 1980; Doty et al, 1981; Barber et al, 1984; Jonas et al, 1985; Lin et al, 1986; Cheung et al, 1990; Danielson, 1991; Huddleston et al, 1993). The first is to repair the aortic coarctation and band the pulmonary trunk via a left thoracotomy, followed, usually within 3 to 4 months, by enlargement of the ventricular septal defect or creation of an aortopulmonary window via a midline sternotomy using deep hypothermia and circulatory arrest. Alternatively, correction can be undertaken in one stage by repairing the aortic coarctation or interruption, enlarging the ventricular septal defect and rudimentary right ventricle, and banding the pulmonary trunk in the early neonatal period via a midline sternotomy, again using deep hypothermia and circulatory arrest. Another approach is to repair the coarctation or interruption and to anastamose the pulmonary trunk to the ascending aorta. Flow of blood to the disconnected right and left pulmonary arteries is provided by a Blalock–Taussig shunt. Another surgical strategy is to perform an arterial switch operation and repair the aortic coarctation or interruption via a midline sternotomy, once more using deep hypothermia and circulatory arrest.

At the Royal Brompton Hospital, we have chosen enlargement of the restrictive ventricular septal defect and patch enlargement of the right ventricle as our preferred option in the majority of patients (Cheung et al, 1990), providing that the ventricular septal defect is not crossed by atrioventricular valvar leaflets or cords. The advantage of this technique is that the patient remains with a banded pulmonary trunk rather than a systemic-to-pulmonary arterial shunt. In theory, flow of blood to the lungs then occurs only during systole. Aortic diastolic blood pressure, therefore, is likely to be higher, with better flow of blood into the coronary arteries than in the patient with a systemic-to-pulmonary arterial shunt.

MANAGEMENT FOLLOWING EARLY PALLIATION

It is important following early palliation to ensure that patients will be suitable candidates for Fontan-like repair. Early management is directed at the control of congestive heart failure with diuretics, and the use of inhibitors of angiotensin-converting enzyme when there is ventricular dysfunction. It is important to identify problems such as recurrent obstruction in the aortic arch, progression of subaortic stenosis, distortion of the pulmonary arteries, deterioration of ventricular function or the development of atrioventricular valvar insufficiency. Some of these problems may contribute to poorly controlled congestive heart failure. Because of this, it helps to perform frequent echocardiographic examinations. It is also wise to perform cardiac catheterization at about the age of 6 to 8 months in order to measure the pulmonary arterial pressure and resistance, identify any distortion of the pulmonary arteries and localize any significant collateral communications between the systemic and pulmonary circulations that might be suitable for coil embolization prior to any further surgery.

The subsequent surgical management of the infant with tricuspid atresia is designed to minimize ventricular pressure and volume overload. This is achieved, on the one hand, by relieving any subaortic or aortic arch stenosis and, on the other hand, by avoiding excessive flow of blood to the lungs. The bidirectional cavopulmonary shunt, or Fontan-type operations, will achieve the goal of relieving volume overload on the ventricle, but the respective roles of these two operations is not always clear cut (Jonas, 1994). When there is a significant risk factor in infancy for a subsequent Fontan-type repair, however, such as pulmonary arterial distortion, pulmonary vascular resistance greater than 2 wood units, mean pulmonary arterial pressure greater than 15 mmHg, atrioventricular valvar regurgitation, ventricular dysfunction or poorly controlled congestive heart failure, an early bidirectional cavopulmonary shunt should be constructed (Bridges et al, 1990a; Chang et al, 1993). This can then be used in conjunction with other operations, particularly relief of subaortic stenosis. A subsequent Fontan-like operation can then be performed at any time from 2 years onwards, taking into account the clinical condition of the patient and the findings on echocardiography, cardiac catheterization and angiography. It would be unusual in the current era to advise construction of a contralateral Blalock–Taussig shunt. Such a procedure might increase the risk of any subsequent Fontan-like operation (Mietus-Snyder et al, 1987).

SUBSEQUENT SURGICAL MANAGEMENT

THE BIDIRECTIONAL SUPERIOR CAVOPULMONARY SHUNT

The bidirectional superior cavopulmonary shunt is a palliative operation in which the right superior caval vein is anastamosed to the superior aspect of the right pulmonary artery, the distal portion of the superior caval vein being closed (Bridges et al, 1990a). Thus, blood from the superior caval vein, or from bilateral superior caval veins, is diverted to the pulmonary arteries, with preservation of continuity between right and left pulmonary arteries. Other sources of pulmonary blood flow, either through the pulmonary trunk or via a surgically created systemic-to-pulmonary arterial shunt, are usually interrupted. The advantage of maintaining pulsatile flow from the ventricular mass through the pulmonary trunk (Kobayashi et al, 1991) is that there may be a reduction in the frequency of development of pulmonary arterio-venous malformations, these lesions being a well-recognized complication of the Glenn operation. When there is no plan to interrupt other sources of pulmonary blood flow, the procedure can be carried out without cardiopulmonary bypass via a right lateral thoracotomy, although a midline thoracotomy and cardiopulmonary bypass is sometimes preferred. There are also advocates for performing a classical Glenn operation via a right thoracotomy and maintaining other sources of flow to the left pulmonary artery.

HEMI-FONTAN OPERATION

The hemi-Fontan operation is similar to the bidirectional superior caval cavopulmonary shunt, but it carries the advantage of more completely preparing the heart for any subsequent Fontan operation (Douville et al, 1991). Both ends of the divided superior caval vein are connected to the right pulmonary artery, and a patch is placed within the right atrium at the entrance of the superior caval vein. If this approach is used, completion of a subsequent total cavopulmonary connection simply involves removal of the patch at the junction of the superior caval vein and the right atrium, and placement of an intra-atrial lateral tube to divert inferior caval blood to the superior caval venous orifice.

THE FONTAN OPERATIONS

The original Fontan operation (Fontan and Baudet, 1971) as first used in the management of tricuspid atresia has undergone a variety of modifications. Nowadays, the term Fontan operation can be considered a generic term that encompasses all the modifications described (Kreutzer et al, 1973; de Leval et al, 1988; Driscoll et al, 1992), some of which have now been abandoned. Whatever modification is now used, the basic principle remains to divert all systemic venous blood directly to the pulmonary circulation. The ideal patient will be in sinus rhythm, from 3–12 years of age, with a mean pulmonary arterial pressure of less than 15 mmHg and a pulmonary vascular resistance less than 2 resistance units. The size of the distal pulmonary arteries should be within the normal range, any major distortion of central pulmonary arteries should already have been repaired, and left ventricular ejection fraction measured by echocardiography should be at least 50%. The most commonly used modification is now the total cavopulmonary connection.

This consists of a superior bidirectional cavopulmonary shunt combined with an intra-atrial lateral tunnel used to baffle blood from the inferior caval vein to the inferior aspect of the right pulmonary artery. This procedure is held to provide a hydrodynamic advantage because energy losses resulting from turbulence are minimized (de Leval et al, 1988). Dilation of the right atrium is also avoided, with concomitant avoidance of late atrial arrhythmias and compression of the distal pulmonary venous pathways.

Under some circumstances, and particularly for so-called higher-risk patients, the total cavopulmonary connection can be fenestrated (Bridges et al, 1990b). In essence, a small atrial septal defect is created in the lateral tube using a 4 or 5 mm aortic punch. The disadvantage of this procedure is that it produces a right-to-left shunt at atrial level and, as a result, the patient becomes cyanosed, sometimes severely so. But fenestration may reduce early mortality and shorten both the duration of stay on the intensive care unit in the immediate post-operative period and the total period of hospitalization. Quite often the fenestration closes spontaneously during a period of several months. In patients who remain cyanosed, it is our practice to close the intra-atrial communication at cardiac catheterization using an appropriate device delivered through a long transvenous sheath. Alternatively, the fenestration can be adjusted in the early postoperative period following the technique described by Laks and his associates (1995).

Another variation of the total cavopulmonary connection, described independently in 1988 by Humes et al and Nawa and Teromoto, is to take an external tube from the inferior caval vein to the inferior aspect of the right pulmonary artery (Marcelletti et al, 1990). This procedure minimizes the need for cardiopulmonary bypass, being achieved using partial cardiopulmonary bypass and continued ventilation to maintain perfusion of the pulmonary circulation via the bidirectional Glenn anastomosis. An essential component of the extracardiac conduit, therefore, is prior construction of a bidirectional superior cavopulmonary shunt. During the operation, ventricular and pulmonary vascular function are preserved by avoiding aortic cross-clamping, cardioplegic arrest and hypothermia. A polytetrafluoroethylene or allograft conduit is anastomosed inferiorly to the transected end of the inferior caval vein where it had joined the right atrium, and superiorly to the underside of the right atrium. Alternatively, an extracardiac lateral tunnel can be used in the manner described by Laschinger and colleagues (1997). To minimize the risk of obstruction to the conduit, the patient should weigh at least 15 kg, and the diameter of the tube should be at least 20 mm. Fenestration of an extracardiac conduit or external lateral tunnel may be performed if required. It is not known whether or not the use of an external tube will prevent late arrhythmias. The major concern about the use of extracardiac conduits in children in general is that they frequently degenerate or

become occluded and require replacement. Obstruction of the conduit used in early modifications of the Fontan operation was a major problem (Fontan and Baudet, 1971; Kreutzer et al, 1973; Fernandez et al, 1989). This remains a potential problem when an extracardiac conduit forms part of the Fontan circulation. So far, however, obstruction has not been described for extra-cardiac conduits (Petrossian et al, 1998).

The Fontan operation achieved by means of direct right atriopulmonary arterial connection remains an alternative to the total cavopulmonary connection (Mair et al, 1990). It can be performed with or without the creation of an interatrial fenestration but carries the disadvantages of producing severe dilation of the right atrium with risk of late atrial arrhythmias (Weber et al, 1989; Balaji et al, 1991; Gewillig et al, 1992; Peters and Somerville, 1992), obstruction of the pulmonary venous pathways and formation of thrombus (Dobell et al, 1986; Fyfe et al, 1991). For patients developing atrial arrhythmias some years after direct atriopulmonary anastomosis, conversion to a total cavopulmonary connection has been considered as a potential treatment, but recent studies have failed to demonstrate that this variant prevents the late development of atrial arrhythmias (Pearl et al, 1991; Kao et al, 1994; Kreutzer et al, 1996). The use of a non-valved or valved connection from the right atrium to the right ventricle was limited to patients with tricuspid atresia, or those with double inlet left ventricle and concordant ventriculo-arterial connections. It is now largely obsolete.

When Tam and co-workers (1989) analysed the fate of those patients with tricuspid atresia presenting in infancy to the Hospital for Sick Children, Toronto, during the early Fontan era, they found that, for various reasons, almost two fifths were excluded from 'corrective' surgery. The most common of reasons for these exclusions were hypoplasia of the pulmonary arteries, more than one early palliative operation, discordant ventriculo-arterial connections requiring banding of the pulmonary trunk and the development of subaortic stenosis. The combined experience of the Royal Brompton Hospital and the Hospital for Sick Children, Great Ormond Street, London of 237 infants with tricuspid atresia was studied by Franklin and co-workers (1993). Almost half of these patients died before the Fontan operation could be undertaken or they became unsuitable for the procedure. There was an actuarial survival of 72% at 1 year, 53% at 5 years and 46% at 10 years. The univariate analysis of risk factors revealed that poor survival included patients with discordant ventriculo-arterial connections, pulmonary atresia, subaortic stenosis and obstruction of the aortic arch. These two important studies emphasize the importance of good early palliation in patients with hypoplastic pulmonary arteries; subaortic stenosis and obstructed aortic arches; they also show that, however good the early palliative management may be, there will always be a significant minority of infants who will never be suitable for eventual Fontan repair. Far fewer patients are likely to be excluded nowadays, however, than in the era covered by these studies.

RESULTS OF THE FONTAN OPERATION IN PATIENTS WITH UNIVENTRICULAR ATRIOVENTRICULAR CONNECTIONS

EARLY OUTCOME

Following the first report of the surgical repair of tricuspid atresia by Fontan and Baudet in 1971 and by Kreutzer and colleagues in 1973, various advances in selection of patients, palliation in infancy, operative techniques and postoperative management have been accompanied by an improvement in reported early mortality from over 25% to appreciably less than 10% (Kawashima et al, 1984; Matsuda et al, 1987; de Leval et al, 1988; Bridges et al, 1989; Mair et al, 1990; Cohen et al, 1991; Driscoll et al, 1992; Mayer et al, 1992; Weber et al, 1992). This improvement in early survival has taken place despite the trend in some series to include patients at higher risk. Nevertheless, no matter how carefully selected and expert the surgery, early postoperative complications are frequently encountered. This, in part, may be a result of the anatomical and functional changes in the systemic ventricle, which occur almost immediately. There is remodelling of the ventricular mass, with an immediate reduction in end-diastolic volume and an increase in wall thickness (Penny et al, 1992). The changes in diastolic ventricular function include altered filling patterns, prolongation of the time constant of relaxation, incoordinate ventricular relaxation and possible increased myocardial stiffness (Penny et al, 1991). The early complications include recurrent pleural effusions, ascites, pericardial effusions, supraventricular tachyarrhythmias, heart block, pulmonary embolism secondary to formation of right atrial thrombus and low cardiac output and death.

The most important immediate complication of the Fontan operation is low cardiac output, this being the major cause of early death. In every patient, therefore, the early postoperative management is designed to minimize pulmonary and systemic vascular resistance. The general principles include the use of systemic vasodilating agents such as nitroprusside and amrinone, pulmonary vascular dilators such as epoprostenol (prostacyclin) and nitric oxide, the avoidance when possible of agents that cause peripheral vasoconstriction and the elimination of positive end-expiratory pressure in ventilated patients. An improvement in cardiac output can also be achieved by hyperventilation to an arterial tension of carbon dioxide of 25 mmHg. Of particular importance is the prompt treatment of tachyarrhythmias, and the early detection and drainage of pleural and pericardial effusions and ascites, all of which are common complications contributing to low cardiac output.

It is important to recognize that, despite the most careful selection, there are a few patients who cannot tolerate the physiological changes associated with the Fontan operation (Knott-Craig et al, 1995; Gentles et al, 1997a). Manifestations of failure of the operation include persistent elevation of the systemic venous pressure to greater than 18 mmHg, persistent low cardiac output with low mixed venous saturations, oliguria, poor peripheral perfusion and persisting metabolic acidosis. When a fenestrated Fontan operation has been performed, the warning signs will include severe systemic arterial desaturation without severe elevation of the right atrial pressure. If the left atrial pressure is elevated to within 5 mmHg of the right atrial pressure, ventricular dysfunction is a likely cause of the poor clinical state. If cross-sectional echocardiography and cardiac catheterization fail to demonstrate residual and correctable anomalies, there should be no hesitation in proceeding to take down the Fontan procedure and convert to a bidirectional cavopulmonary shunt. The exception is the patient with poor ventricular function, for whom cardiac transplantation might be the only remedy.

LATE OUTCOME

There is a growing concern, however, about the late outcome of the Fontan operation, and the continuing hazard for late death because of chronically low cardiac output, ventricular dysfunction, the development of atrial flutter and other tachyarrhythmias, venous thrombosis and pulmonary embolism, protein-losing enteropathy (Rothman and Snyder, 1991; Davis et al, 1994), chronic ascites, hepatic congestion and cirrhosis. All of these complications can develop even in those patients who initially have a good functional result. Some patients will also develop cyanosis because of pulmonary arteriovenous fistulous communications or because collateral vessels permit right-to-left shunting from systemic veins to the left atrium. In others, there is an increase in the flow of blood of the lungs because of development of aortopulmonary collateral vessels (Triedman et al, 1993).

Many reports have emphasized that the early survival after the Fontan operation has been better in patients with tricuspid atresia than in those with other anatomical variants (Fontan et al, 1990; Cohen et al, 1991; Driscoll et al, 1992). The initial mortality, including patients with a bidirectional superior cavopulmonary anastomosis or fenestrated Fontan operation, has been as low as 5%. Analysis of survival after the so-called 'perfect' Fontan operation, however, under pre- and perioperative circumstances that can be considered ideal, has indicated that a late, albeit slowly rising, phase of hazard is still present. Under these ideal circumstances, the 15-year survival is predicted to be 73% (Fontan et al, 1990). It may be that the Fontan circulation itself is the cause of the late hazard, along with its various but frequent complications.

Many retrospective reviews have attempted to identify factors that influence the early and late outcome of the Fontan operation. Early survival has gradually improved (Mayer et al, 1992). When, within a few hours of surgery, the haemodynamic state of the patient is so poor that the probability of survival seems low, take down of the Fontan operation to a bidirectional Glenn is likely to result in a superior survival than take down to a systemic-to-pulmonary arterial shunt. Predictors of early failure often include the calendar year, with outcome improving with increased experience (Kirklin et al, 1986). In the current era, the poorest outcome is in those patients with hypoplastic left heart syndrome, or other variants of mitral atresia (Caspi et al, 1990). Patients with a common atrioventricular valve, usually associated with isomerism of the atrial appendages (Culbertson et al, 1992) or a dominant right ventricle (Matsuda et al, 1987), are additionally at risk of early failure. When the aorta arises from the rudimentary right ventricle, it is frequent to encounter a restrictive ventricular septal defect and concomitant subaortic stenosis. These patients will usually have undergone banding of the pulmonary trunk (Freedom, 1987). Unrelieved subaortic stenosis and left ventricular hypertrophy are forerunners of poor outcome. Early relief of subaortic stenosis, combined with a bidirectional Glenn operation, should always be performed prior to any Fontan procedure. Although direct atriopulmonary anastomosis carries a higher early mortality than total cavopulmonary connection (Pearl et al, 1991), this probably reflects the learning curve, with the total cavopulmonary connection being a more recent innovation. Early mortality is also associated with a preoperative mean pulmonary arterial pressure of more than 15 mmHg (and certainly more than 19 mmHg), according to one recent extensive review (Gentles et al, 1997a). Younger age at operation does appear to be a risk factor for death or early take down (Kirklin et al, 1986). The risk of death begins to rise as the age of operation is reduced to 3 years and then rises more steeply as age at operation is reduced to less than 2 years. Nevertheless, good results can be obtained when surgery is performed in children under 2 years of age, although a mortality of 55% was reported for patients under 4 years of age by Meyer and colleagues (1992). It has been shown that right and left atrial pressures measured on the day of operation are important indicators of early outcome. A right atrial pressure equal to or greater than 17 mmHg, or a left atrial pressure equal to or greater than 11 mmHg, is associated with early death. Although small size of central pulmonary arteries has been considered a risk factor for early death, if the small size is limited to the prebranching portions of the right and left pulmonary arteries, and these are enlarged at the time of repair, there is then little relationship with eventual outcome (Fontan et al, 1989). While some groups have reported improved survival and a reduction in the prevalence of prolonged pleural effusions without the use of fenestration, others have shown that the major advantage of fenestration is in the improvement of early outcome, independent of other variables related either to the patients or the procedures (Bridges et al, 1990b; Mayer et al, 1992).

Consequently, it appears that those risk factors for early death related to the patient include younger age at operation; certain morphological diagnoses, including hypoplastic left heart syndrome, mitral atresia, and isomerism; the use of an atriopulmonary anastomosis; ventricular hypertrophy in patients with discordant ventriculo-arterial connections (Seliem et al, 1989; Akagi et al, 1992) and restrictive ventricular septal defect; pulmonary arterial distortion; an elevated pulmonary arterial pressure and pulmonary vascular resistance; and, in some reports, absence of fenestration. The early results of the Fontan operation incorporating an extracardiac conduit have been extremely promising, with very low reported rates of mortality (Petrossian et al, 1998).

The symptoms and continuing hazard for late death after the Fontan operation are, in essence, the result of the persistently elevated right atrial and systemic venous pressures. Surprisingly, more than nine tenths of patients consider themselves to be well and are in the first or second classes of the functional classification of the New York Heart Association during the early postoperative years. As the interval between operation and follow-up increases, less patients are in the first class, and up to two thirds are receiving diuretics, digoxin, vasodilators or antiarrhythmic drugs. The incidence of limitation to exercise appears to be related to the length of follow-up. Poor functional state is also associated with a primary diagnosis of left atrioventricular valvar atresia and/or the hypoplastic left heart syndrome, a previously restrictive ventricular septal defect with discordant ventriculo-arterial connections, and isomerism of the atrial appendages (Driscoll et al, 1992). Even for patients without symptoms, exercise capacity and cardiac output are subnormal, being worse in those with an atriopulmonary anastomosis than in the group with total cavopulmonary connection (Rosenthal et al, 1995).

The high resting right atrial pressure after the Fontan procedure increases on exercise, and pulmonary blood flow increases with inspiration but is severely curtailed during a Valsalva manoeuvre. Progressive right atrial enlargement is an inevitable consequence of a direct atriopulmonary connection, which presents a significant risk of late atrial arrhythmias, obstruction of pulmonary venous pathways and formation of thrombus and pulmonary embolism. Supraventricular arrhythmias such as atrial flutter, however, have not been abolished by the use of the lateral tunnel or external conduit. On the whole, atrial arrhythmias are poorly tolerated, giving rise to symptoms of low cardiac output in most patients. There is an increased risk of venous thrombosis, intra-atrial thrombus and pulmonary embolism. The tachycardias may be abolished by surgical or ablative division of potential pathways for anomalous conduction (Swatz et al, 1994; Cox et al, 1995). The surgical approach can conveniently be used while converting an atriopulmonary anastomosis to a total cavopulmonary connection. There has been limited experience with implantable atrial defibrillators following the Fontan procedure (Cooper et al, 1997).

Protein-losing enteropathy is a well-recognized and distressing late complication of the Fontan operation (Rothman and Snyder, 1991; Davis et al, 1994); it has been documented to occur in 2–3% of patients (Gentles et al, 1997b). Excessive loss of protein from the gastrointestinal tract results in hypoalbuminaemia of such degree that generalized oedema, ascites and even pleural effusions develop in patients who may have previously been completely well. There is no satisfactory treatment for the condition, apart from regular infusions of albumin when required. Some patients are improved by the creation of an atrial fenestration; this allows right-to-left shunting but often results in significant cyanosis. Alternative strategies are to convert the Fontan circulation to a bidirectional Glenn shunt or to undertake cardiac transplantation.

Other late complications of the Fontan circulation include mild elevation of liver enzymes, including aspartate transaminase and alanine transaminase, cirrhosis of the liver, and the production of the procoagulation factor protein C. Because of the increased risk of thromboembolic complications, many units advocate routine anticoagulation therapy for all patients. There is no general consensus, however, about the need for anticoagulation and what type of anticoagulant should be advised. Given that thromboembolic complications may be unpredictable and fatal, there is a strong case for anticoagulation therapy in all patients. Certainly at a minimum aspirin should be prescribed for every patient; with the onset of atrial arrhythmias, this should be replaced by warfarin. Alternatively, every patient should receive warfarin from the outset. Jahangiri and colleagues (1997) reviewed coagulation factor abnormalities after the Fontan procedure and concluded that deficiency in protein C, protein S and factor VII partly account for the prevalence of thromboembolism. The authors recommended that the reduction in these factors should be regarded as a risk for thromboembolism and such patients should be treated with anticoagulants.

The occurrence of pulmonary arterio-venous fistulas is an important late complication following a classical Glenn anastomosis, with a reported incidence of up to one quarter (Moore et al, 1989). In contrast, fistulous communications following the bidirectional cavopulmonary anastomosis are low. The exception to this is patients with isomerism of the left atrial appendages, in whom a bidirectional cavopulmonary anastomosis directs all venous return to the lungs, except for the venous return from the heart and liver. Recent studies have shown a high incidence of fistulas in patients with left isomerism (Srivastava et al, 1995). In most patients reported in the literature, the common anatomical feature is the exclusion of normal hepatic venous flow from the affected lung. It is postulated that a biochemical product of normal hepatic metabolism prevents the formation of fistulas. This seems to be confirmed by the reversibility of fistulous formation after re-routing the flow of hepatic blood to the pulmonary circulation (Knight and Mee, 1995). Isomerism of the atrial appendages may be associated not only with pulmonary arterio-venous fistulas but also with veno-venous fistulas (Gatzoulis et al, 1995). The mechanism for development of all of these is unclear, but their effect is to cause profound hypoxia. The outcome of occlusion of fistulous communications by transcatheter insertion of devices is often disappointing (Hayes et al, 1994), with the patients showing a tendency to the development of additional fistulous channels.

In summary, although many patients benefit immensely from the Fontan operation, and it has transformed the outlook for those born with tricuspid atresia and other malformations with one functioning ventricle, later complications are almost inevitable, resulting from the high systemic venous pressure and low cardiac output. The concept of the Fontan operation as a corrective procedure is flawed. It can never be more than a palliative procedure, which, in an increasing number of instances, serves as a bridge to eventual cardiac transplantation. Nevertheless, when complications develop, it is important to exclude any obstruction in the Fontan circulation (and to identify other problems that can be remedied) using cardiac catheterization and angiography. The recent report from Gentles and colleagues (1997a) has shown that one fifth of their patients had undergone late operations, of which the most common were insertion of pacemakers, revision or replacement of conduits, relief of subaortic stenosis, closure of residual intra-atrial defects and pericardiotomy. One quarter had required interventional cardiac catheterization, including closure of residual fenestration, coil embolization of aortopulmonary collateral arteries, closure of residual defects in the atrial baffle, implantation of systemic venous stents and balloon angioplasty for pulmonary arterial stenosis. These observations emphasize the need for continuing rigorous follow-up, with careful investigations in patients with functional deterioration, to identify treatable problems.

REFERENCES

Abbott M E 1936 Atlas of congenital heart disease. The American Heart Association, New York, p 61

Akagi T, Benson L N, Green M et al 1992 Ventricular performance before and after Fontan repair for univentricular atrioventricular connection: angiographic and radionuclide assessment. Journal of the American College of Cardiology 20: 920–926

Anderson R H 1983 Weasel words in paediatric cardiology. Single ventricle. International Journal of Cardiology 2: 425–429

Anderson R H, Becker A E, Losekoot T G, Gerlis L M 1975 Anatomically corrected malposition of the great arteries. British Heart Journal 37: 993–1013

Anderson R H, Wilkinson J L, Gerlis L M, Smith A, Becker A E 1977 Atresia of the right atrioventricular orifice. British Heart Journal 39: 414–428

Anderson R H, Becker A E, Macartney F J, Shinebourne E A, Wilkinson J L, Tynan M J 1979 Is 'tricuspid atresia' a univentricular heart? Pediatric Cardiology 1: 51–56

Anderson R H, Macartney F J, Tynan M et al 1983 Univentricular atrioventricular connexion–the single ventricle trap unsprung. Pediatric Cardiology 4: 273–280

Anderson R H, Becker A E, Tynan M, Macartney F J, Rigby M L, Wilkinson J L 1984 The univentricular atrioventricular connexion: getting to the root of a thorny problem. American Journal of Cardiology 54: 822–828

Ando M, Satomi G, Takao A 1980 Atresia of tricuspid or mitral orifice: anatomic spectrum and morphogenetic hypothesis. In: Van Praagh R, Takao A (eds) Etiology and morphogenesis of congential heart disease. Futura, Mount Kisco, NY, p 421–488

Balaji S, Gewillig M, Bull C et al 1991 Arrhythmias after the Fontan procedure. Comparison of total cavopulmonary connection and atriopulmonary connection. Circulation 84(suppl III): 162–167

Barber G, Hagler D J, Edwards W D et al 1984 Surgical repair of univentricular heart (double inlet left ventricle) with obstructed anterior subaortic outlet chamber. Journal of the American College of Cardiology 4: 771–777

Bernays A C 1876 Entwicklungsgeschichte der atrioventrikularklappen. Morphologische Jahrebook 2: 479–518

Bharati S, Lev M 1979 The concept of tricuspid atresia complex as distinct from that of the single ventricle complex. Pediatric Cardiology 1: 57–62

Bharati S, McAllister H A, Tatooles C J et al 1976 Anatomic variations in underdeveloped right ventricle related to tricuspid atresia and stenosis. Journal of Thoracic and Cardiovascular Surgery 72: 383–400

Bridges N D, Farrell P E Jr, Pigott J D Jr et al 1989 Pulmonary artery index. A nonpredictor of operative survival in patients undergoing modified Fontan repair. Circulation 80: 216–221

Bridges N D, Jonas R A, Mayer J E et al 1990a Bidirectional cavopulmonary anastomosis as interim palliation for high-risk Fontan candidates. Early results. Circulation 82(suppl IV): 170–176

Bridges N D, Lock J E, Castañeda A R 1990b Baffle fenestration with subsequent transcatheter closure. Modification of the Fontan operation for patients at increased risk. Circulation 82: 1681–1689

Caspi J, Coles J G, Rabinovitch et al 1990 Morphological findings contributing to a failed Fontan procedure in the current era. Circulation 82(suppl IV): 177–182

Chang A C, Hanley F L, Wernovsky G et al 1993 Early bidirectional cavopulmonary shunt in young infants. Postoperative course and early results. Circulation 88: 149–158

Cheung H C, Lincoln C, Anderson R H et al 1990 Options for surgical repair in hearts with univentricular atrioventricular connection and subaortic stenosis. Journal of Thoracic and Cardiovascular Surgery 100: 672–681

Cohen A J, Cleveland D C, Dyck J et al 1991 Results of the Fontan procedure for patients with univentricular heart. Annals of Thoracic Surgery 52: 1266–1271

Cooper R, Jojnson E E, Wharton J M 1997 Internal atrial defibrillation in humans. Improved efficacy of biphasic waveforms and the importance of phase duration. Circulation 95: 1487–1496

Cox J L, Boineau J P, Schuessler R B et al 1995 Modification of the maze procedures for atrial flutter and atrial fibrillation. Rationale and surgical approach. Journal of Thoracic and Cardiovascular Surgery 110: 473–484

Culbertson C G, George B L, Day R W et al 1992 Factors influencing survival of patients with heterotaxy syndrome undergoing the Fontan procedure. Journal of the American College of Cardiology 20: 678–684

Danielson G K 1991 Damus–Stansel–Kaye procedure: personal observations. Annals of Thoracic Surgery 47: 62–64

Davis C A, Driscoll D J, Perrault J et al 1994 Enteric protein loss after the Fontan operation. Mayo Clinic Procedures 69: 112–114

Deanfield J E, Tommasini G, Anderson R H, Macartney F J 1982 Tricuspid atresia: analysis of coronary artery distribution and ventricular morphology. British Heart Journal 48: 485–492

de Leval M R, Kilner P, Gewilig M et al 1988 Total cavopulmonary connection: a logical alternative to atriopulmonary connection for complex Fontan operations. Journal of Thoracic and Cardiovascular Surgery 96: 682–695

Dick M, Fyler D C, Nadas A S 1975 Tricuspid atresia: clinical course in 101 patients. American Journal of Cardiology 36: 327–337

Dickinson D F, Wilkinson J L, Smith A, Becker A E, Anderson R H 1979 Atrioventricular conduction tissues in univentricular hearts of left ventricular type with absent right atrioventricular connection ('tricuspid atresia'). British Heart Journal 42: 1–8

Dobell A R, Trusler G A, Smallhorn J F et al 1986 Atrial thrombi after the Fontan operation. Annals of Thoracic Surgery 42: 664–667

Donzelot E, D'Allaines F 1954 Traite des cardiopathies congenitales. Masson & Cie, Paris

Doty D B, Marvin W J J, Lauer R M 1981 Single ventricle with aortic outflow obstruction. Operative repair by creation of double outlet to the aorta and application of the Fontan principle. Journal of Thoracic and Cardiovascular Surgery 81: 636–640

Douville E C, Sade R M, Fyfe D A 1991 Hemi-Fontan operation in surgery for single ventricle: A preliminary report. Annals of Thoracic Surgery 51: 893–899

Drew J H, Parkinson P, Walstab J E, Beischer N A 1977 Incidences and types of malformations in newborn infants. Medical Journal of Australia 2: 945–949

Driscoll D J, Offord K P, Feldt R H et al 1992 Five-to-fifteen-year followup after the Fontan operation. Circulation 85: 469–496

Edwards J E 1960 Tricuspid atresia. In: Gould S E (ed.) Pathology of the heart. Charles C. Thomas, Springfield, IL, p 379

Edwards J E, Burchell H B 1949 congenital tricuspid atresia: a classification. Medical Clinics of North America 33: 1117–1119

Elliott L P, Anderson R C, Edwards J E 1964 The common cardiac ventricle with transposition of the great vessels. British Heart Journal 26: 289–301

Fernandez G, Costa F, Fontan F et al 1989 Prevalence of reoperation for pathway obstruction after Fontan operation. Annual of Thoracic Surgery 48: 654–659

Fontan F, Baudet E 1971 Surgical repair of tricuspid atresia. Thorax 26: 240–248

Fontan F, Fernandez G, Casta F et al 1989 The size of the pulmonary arteries and the results of the Fontan operation. Journal of Thoracic and Cardiovascular Surgery 98: 711–724

Fontan F, Kirklin J, Fernandez G et al 1990 Outcome after a 'perfect' Fontan operation. Circulation 81: 1520–1536

Franklin R C G, Spiegalhalter D J, Sullivan I D et al 1993 Tricuspid atresia presenting in infancy. Survival and suitability for the Fontan operation. Circulation 87: 427–439

Freedom R M 1987 The dinosaur and banding of the main pulmonary trunk in the heart with functionally one ventricle and transposition of the great arteries: a saga of evolution and caution. Journal of the American College of Cardiology 10: 427–429

Freedom R M, Gerald P S 1973 Congenital cardiovascular disease and the 'cat-eye' syndrome. American Journal of Diseases of Childhood 126: 16–18

Freedom R M, Harrington D P 1974 Anatomically corrected malposition of the great arteries. Report of 2 cases, one with congenital asplenia: frequent association with juxtaposition of atrial appendages. British Heart Journal 36: 207–215

Freedom R M, Williams W G, Fowler R S et al 1980 Tricuspid atresia, transposition of the great arteries, and banded pulmonary artery. Repair by arterial switch, coronary artery reimplantation, and right atrioventricular valved conduit. Journal of Thoracic and Cardiovascular Surgery 80: 621–628

Fyfe D A, Kline C H, Sade R M et al 1991 Transesophageal echocardiography detects thrombus formation not identified by transthoracic echocardiography after the Fontan operation. Journal of the American College of Cardiology 18: 1733–1737

Gatzoulis M A, Shinebourne E A, Redington A N et al 1995 Increasing cyanosis after cavopulmonary connection caused by abnormal systemic venous channels. British Heart Journal 73: 182–186

Gentles T L, Mayer J E, Gauvrea K et al 1997a Fontan operation in five hundred consecutive patients: factors influencing early and late outcome. Journal of Thoracic and Cardiovascular Surgery 114: 376–389

Gentles T L, Gauvreau K, Mayer J E et al 1997b Functional outcome after the Fontan operation: factors influencing late morbidity. Journal of Thoracic and Cardiovascular Surgery 114: 392–403

Gessner I H 1982 Embryology of atrioventricular valve formation and embryogenesis of tricuspid atresia. In: Rao P S (ed.) Tricuspid atresia. Futura, Mount Kisco, NY, p 83–111

Gewillig M, Wyse R K, de Leval M R et al 1992 Early and late arrhythmias after the Fontan operation: predisposing factors and clinical consequences. British Heart Journal 67: 72–79

Gibson S, Clifton W M 1938 Congenital heart disease: clinical and postmortem study of 105 cases. American Journal of Diseases of Childhood 55: 761–767

Hayes A M, Burrows P E, Benson L N 1994 An unusual cause of cyanosis after the modified Fontan procedure–closure of venous communications between the coronary sinus and left atrium by transcatheter techniques. Cardiology in the Young 4: 172–174

Ho S Y, Monro J L, Anderson R H 1979 Disposition of the sinus node in left-sided juxtaposition of the atrial appendage. British Heart Journal 41: 129–132

Ho S Y, Milo S, Anderson R H et al 1982 Straddling atrioventricular valve with absent atrioventricular connection. Report of 10 cases. British Heart Journal 47: 344–352

Huddleston C B B, Canter C E, Spray T L et al 1993 Damus–Kaye–Stansel with cavopulmonary connection for single ventricle and subaortic obstruction. Annals of Thoracic Surgery 55: 339–345

Humes R A, Feldt R H, Porter C J et al 1988 The modified Fontan operation for asplenia and polysplenia syndromes. Journal of Thoracic and Cardiovascular Surgery 96: 212–218

Jahangiri M, Shore D, Kakkar V et al 1997 Coagulation factor abnormalities after the Fontan procedure and its modifications. Journal of Thoracic and Cardiovascular Surgery 113: 989–993

Jonas R A 1994 Indications and timing for the bidirectional Glenn shunt versus the fenestrated Fontan circulation. Journal of Thoracic and Cardiovascular Surgery 108: 522–524

Jonas R A, Castañeda A R, Lang P 1985 Single ventricle (single-or double-inlet) complicated by subaortic stenosis: surgical options in infancy. Annals of Thoracic Surgery 39: 361–366

Kao J M, Alejos J C, Grant P W et al 1994 Conversion of atriopulmonary to cavopulmonary anastomosis in management of late arrhythmias and atrial thrombosis. Annals of Thoracic Surgery 58: 1510–1514

Kawashima Y, Kitamura S, Matsuda H et al 1984 Total cavopulmonary shunt operation in complex cardiac anomalies. A new operation. Journal of Thoracic and Cardiovascular Surgery 87: 74–81

Kenna A P, Smithells R W, Fielding D W 1975 Congenital heart disease in Liverpool: 1960–69. Quarterly Journal of Medicine 43: 2–44

Kirklin J K, Blackstone E H, Kirklin J W et al 1986 The Fontan operation. Ventricular hypertrophy, age, and date of operation as risk factors. Journal of Thoracic and Cardiovascular Surgery 92: 1049–1064

Knight W B, Mee R B 1995 A cure for pulmonary arteriovenous fistulas? Annals of Thoracic Surgery 59: 999–1001

Kobayashi J, Matsuda H, Nakano S et al 1991 Hemodynamic effects of bidirectional cavopulmonary shunt with pulsatile pulmonary flow. Circulation 84: 219–225

Knott-Craig C J, Danielson G K, Schaff H V et al 1995 The modified Fontan operation. An analysis of risk factors for early postoperative death or takedown in 702 consecutive patients from one institution. Journal of Thoracic and Cardiovascular Surgery 109: 1237–1243

Kreutzer G, Galindez E, Bono H et al 1973 An operation for the correction of tricuspid atresia. Journal of Thoracic and Cardiovascular Surgery 66: 613–621

Kreutzer J, Keane J F, Lock J E, et al 1996 Conversion of modified Fontan procedure to lateral atrial tunnel cavopulmonary anastomosis. Journal of Thoracic and Cardiovascular Surgery 111: 1169–1176

Kreysig F L 1817 Die Krankheiten des Herzens. Dritte Thiel, p 104. [Cited by Rashkind W J 1982]

Kuhne M 1906 Uber zwei Falle von kongenitaler Atresie des Ostium venosum dextrum. Jahrb Kinderheile. 63: 235–249

Laks H, Ardehali A, Grant P W et al 1995 Modification of the Fontan procedure. Superior vena cava to left pulmonary artery connection and inferior vena cava to right pulmonary artery connection with adjustable atrial septal defect. Circulation 91: 2943–2947

Lamers W H, Wessels A, Verbeek F J et al 1992 New findings concerning ventricular septation in the human heart. Circulation 86: 1194–1205

Laschinger J C, Redmond J M, Cameron D E et al 1997 Intermediate results of the extracardiac Fontan procedure. Annals of Thoracic Surgery 62: 1261–1267

Lenz W, Pliess G 1963 The pathology of thalidomide embryopathy and associated defects of the heart. In: Memorias del IV Congreso Mundial de Cardiologia, Congenitos hemodynamica, Mexico, vol 1A, p 150

Lin A E, Laks H, Barber G et al 1986 Subaortic obstruction in complex congenital heart disease management by proximal pulmonary artery to ascending aorta end to side anastomosis. Journal of the American College of Cardiology 7: 617–624

Mair D D, Hagler D J, Puga F J et al 1990 Fontan operation in 176 patients with tricuspid atresia: results and a proposed new index for patient selection. Circulation 82(suppl IV): 164–169

Mair D D, Hagler D J, Julsrud P R et al 1991 Early and late results of the modified Fontan procedure for double inlet left ventricle: the Mayo Clinic Experience. Journal of the American College of Cardiology 18: 1727–1732

Marcelletti C, Corno A, Giannico S et al 1990 Inferior vena cava–pulmonary artery extracardiac conduit. A new form of right heart bypass. Journal of Thoracic and Cardiovascular Surgery 100: 228–232

Matsuda H, Kawashima Y, Kishimoto H et al 1987 Problems in the modified Fontan operation for univentricular heart of the right ventricular type. Circulation 76(suppl III): 45–52

Mayer J E Jr, Bridges N D, Lock J E et al 1992 Factors associated with marked reduction in mortality for Fontan operations in patients with single ventricle. Journal of Thoracic and Cardiovascular Surgery 103: 444–452

Mietus-Snyder M, Lang P, Mayer J E et al 1987 Childhood systemic–pulmonary shunts: subsequent suitability for Fontan operation. Circulation 76: 39–44

Mitchell S C, Korones S B, Berendes H W 1971 Congenital heart disease in 56 109 births. Incidence and natural history. Circulation 43: 323–332

Moodie D S, Ritter D G, Tajik A H et al 1984 Long-term follow-up of unoperated patients with univentricular heart. American Journal of Cardiology 53: 1124–1128

Moore J W, Kirby W C, Madden W A et al 1989 Development of pulmonary arteriovenous malformations after modified Fontan operations. Journal of Thoracic and Cardiovascular Surgery 98: 1045–1050

Nadas A S, Fyler D C 1972 Pediatric cardiology, 3rd edn. WB Saunders, Philadelphia, PA, p 588–589

Nawa S, Teromoto S 1988 New extension of the Fontan principle: inferior vena cava–pulmonary artery bridge operation. Thorax 43: 1022–1023

Neches W H, Park S C, Lenox C C et al 1973 Tricuspid atresia with transposition of the great arteries and closing ventricular septal defect. Successful palliation by banding of the pulmonary artery and creation of an aorticopulmonary window. Journal of Thoracic and Cardiovascular Surgery 4: 538–542

Nishioka K, Kamiya T, Ueda T et al 1981 Left ventricular volume characteristics in children with tricuspid atresia before and after surgery. American Journal of Cardiology 47: 1105–1110

Orie J D, Anderson C, Ettedgui J A, Zuberbuhler J R, Anderson R H 1995 Echocardiographic–morphologic correlations in tricuspid atresia. Journal of the American College of Cardiology 26: 750–758

Otero Coto E, Calabro R, Marsico F, Lopez Arranz J S 1981 Right atrial outlet atresia with straddling left atrioventricular valve. A form of double outlet atrium. British Heart Journal 45: 317–324

Pearl J M, Laks H, Stein D G et al 1991 Total cavopulmonary anastomosis versus conventional modified Fontan procedure. Annals of Thoracic Surgery 52: 189–196

Penny D J, Rigby M L, Redington A N 1991 Abnormal patterns of intraventricular flow and diastolic filling after the Fontan operation: evidence for incoordinate ventricular wall motion. British Heart Journal 66: 375–378

Penny D J, Lincoln C, Shore D F et al 1992 The early response of the systemic ventricle during transition to the Fontan circulation: an acute hypertrophic cardiomyopathy. Cardiology in the Young 2: 78–84

Peters N S, Somerville J 1992 Arrhythmias after the Fontan procedure. British Heart Journal 68: 199–204

Petrossian E, McElhinney D B, Reddy V M et al 1998 The role of the extracardiac conduit as a cavopulmonary anastomosis in the evolution of the Fontan procedure, In: Redington A N, Brawn W J, Deanfield J E, Anderson R H (eds), The right heart in congenital heart disease. GMM, London 149–155

Rashkind W J 1982 Tricuspid atresia. A nineteenth century view. In Rao P S (ed.) Tricuspid atresia. Futura, Mount Kisco, NY, p 7–11

Rao P S 1977 Natural history of the ventricular septal defect in tricuspid atresia and its surgical implications. British Heart Journal 39: 276–288

Rao P S 1980 A unified classification for tricuspid atresia. American Heart Journal 99: 799–804

Rao P S 1982a Terminology: tricuspid atresia or univentricular heart. In: Rao P S (ed.) Tricuspid atresia. Futura, Mount Kisco, NY, p 3–6

Rao P S 1982b Demographic features of tricuspid atresia. In: Rao P S (ed.) Tricuspid atresia. Futura, Mount Kisco, NY, p 13–24

Rao P S 1990 Is the term 'tricuspid atresia' appropriate? American Journal of Cardiology 66: 1251–1254

Rao P S 1992 Tricuspid Atresia, 2nd edn. Futura, Mount Kisco, NY.

Rao P S, Jue K L, Isabel-Jones J, Ruttenberg H D 1973 Ebstein's malformation of the tricuspid atresia. Differentiation from isolated tricuspid atresia. American Journal of Cardiology 32: 1004–1009

Rigby M L, Redington A 1987 Assessment of ventricular function. In Anderson R H, Crupi G, Panenzan L (eds) Double inlet ventricle. Castle House, Tunbridge Wells, UK, p 133–145

Rigby M L, Anderson R H, Gibson D et al 1981 Two-dimensional echocardiographic categorisation of the univentricular heart. Ventricular morphology, type and mode of atrioventricular connection. British Heart Journal 46: 603–612

Rigby M L, Gibson D G, Joseph M C et al 1982 Recognition of imperforate atrioventricular valves by two-dimensional echocardiography. British Heart Journal 47: 329–336

Rosenquist G C, Levy R J, Rowe R D 1970 Right atrial–left ventricular relationships in tricuspid atresia. Position of the presumed site of the atretic valve as determined by transillumination. American Heart Journal 80: 493–497

Rosenthal A 1977 Tricuspid atresia. In: Moss A J, Adams F H, Emmanouilides G C (eds) Heart disease in infants, children and adolescents, 2nd edn. Williams & Wilkins, Baltimore, MD, p 289–301

Rosenthal M, Bush A, Deanfield J, Redington A N 1995 Comparison of cardiopulmonary adaptation during exercise in children after the atriopulmonary and total cavopulmonary connection Fontan procedures. Circulation 91: 372–378

Rothman A, Snyder J 1991 Protein-losing enteropathy following the Fontan operation: resolution with prednisone therapy. American Heart Journal 121: 618–619

Sauer U, Hall D 1980 Spontaneous closure or critical decrease in size of the ventricular septal defect in tricuspid atresia with normally connected great arteries: surgical implications. Herz 5: 369–384

Scalia D, Russo P, Anderson R H et al 1983 The surgical anatomy of hearts with no direct communication between the right atrium and the ventricular mass–so-called tricuspid atresia. Journal of Thoracic and Cardiovascular Surgery 87: 743–755

Schuberg W 1861 Beobachtung von Verkummerung des rechten Herzventikels in Folge von Atresie des Ost. venos. dextr.: Perforation des Herzscheidewand und dadurch Bildung eines Canales. der durch den rudimentaren rechten Ventrikel in die Art. pulmon. fuhrt. Virchow Archives of Pathology and Anatomy 20: 294–296. [Cited by Rashkind W J 1982]

Seliem M, Muster A J, Paul M H et al 1989 Relation between preoperative left ventricular muscle mass and outcome of the Fontan procedure in patients with tricuspid atresia. Journal of the American College of Cardiology 14: 750–755

Seward J B, Tajik A J, Hagler D J 1978 Echocardiographic spectrum of tricuspid atresia. Mayo Clinic Procedures 53: 100–108

Shinebourne E A, Lau K C, Calcaterra G, Anderson R H 1980 Univentricular heart of right ventricular type: clinical, angiographic and electrocardiographic features. American Journal of Cardiology 46: 439–445

Sommers S C, Johnson J M 1951 Congential tricuspid atresia. American Heart Journal 41: 130–143

Srivastava D, Preminger T, Lock J E et al 1995 Hepatic venous blood and the development of pulmonary arteriovenous malformations in congenital heart disease. Circulation 92: 1217–1222

Storstein O, Rokseth R, Sorland S 1964 Congenital heart disease in a clinical material. An analysis of 1000 consecutive cases. Acta Medica Scandinavica 176: 195–200

Swatz J F, Pellersels G, Silvers J et al 1994 A catheter based curative approach to atrial fibrillation in humans. Circulation 90: 335–342

Tam C K H, Lightfoot W E, Finlay C D et al 1989 Course of tricuspid atresia in the Fontan era. American Journal of Cardiology 63: 589–593

Tandon R, Edwards J E 1974 Tricuspid atresia. A re-evaluation and classification. Journal of Thoracic and Cardiovascular Surgery 67: 530–542

Taussig H B 1939 A single ventricle with a diminutive outlet chamber. Journal of Technical Methods 19: 120–128

Triedman J K, Bridges N D, Mayer J E et al 1993 Prevalence and risk factors for aortopulmonary collateral vessels after Fontan and bidirectional Glenn procedures. Journal of the American College of Cardiology 22: 207–215

Van Praagh R, Ongley P A, Swan H J C 1964 Anatomic types of single or common ventricle in man: morphologic and geometric aspects of sixty necropsied cases. American Journal of Cardiology 13: 367–386

Van Praagh R, Ando M, Dungan W T 1971 Anatomic types of tricuspid atresia: clinical and developmental implications. Circulation 45(suppl II): 115

Vlad P 1978 Tricuspid atresia. In: Keith J D, Rowe R D, Vlad P (eds) Heart disease in infancy and childhood, 3rd edn. Macmillan, New York, p 518–541

Weber H S, Hellenbrand W E, Kleinman C S et al 1989 Predictors of rhythm disturbances and subsequent morbidity after the Fontan operation. American Journal of Cardiology 64: 762–767

Weber H S, Gleason M M, Myers J L et al 1992 The Fontan operation in infants less that 2 years of age. Journal of the American College of Cardiology 19: 828–833

Weinberg P M 1992 Pathological anatomy of tricuspid atresia. In: Rao P S (ed.) Tricuspid Atresia, 2nd edn. Futura, Mount Kisco, NY, p 81–100

Zuberbuhler J R, Allwork S P, Anderson R H 1979 The spectrum of Ebstein's anomaly of the tricuspid valve. Journal of Thoracic and Cardiovascular Surgery 77: 202–211

40

Atresia of the morphologically left atrioventricular orifice

M. L. Rigby and R. H. Anderson

INTRODUCTION

In previous chapters of this book, we have discussed the problems that underscore the difficulty in providing a satisfactory anatomical definition for tricuspid atresia (Chapter 39) and the hypoplastic left heart syndrome (Chapter 45). These problems, in part, reflect the fact that the atrioventricular valves 'belong' to the ventricles rather than the atriums. Consequently, on occasions, an imperforate valve that is morphologically tricuspid can block completely the exit from the morphologically left rather than the right atrium. Similarly, hearts can be found in which all the evidence points to the fact that had a left-sided atrioventricular connection developed in a heart with a dominant left ventricle and left-sided rudimentary and incomplete right ventricle, it would have been guarded by a morphologically tricuspid valve. Absence of the connection, therefore, can be considered anatomically to represent tricuspid atresia. These hearts, with no direct exit from the left rather than the right atrium, however, do not present with the clinical features expected for tricuspid atresia. Instead, the haemodynamic pattern produced is that expected for mitral atresia. It is then the case that, while most hearts with mitral atresia are appropriately grouped under the heading of hypoplastic left heart syndrome, not all fit comfortably in this setting. This is because an integral part of the typical syndrome is severe obstruction to aortic flow. Yet a subset of hearts with unequivocal atresia of the mitral valve have patent subaortic outflow tracts that permit unobstructed flow. This morphology was recognized some time ago as a specific entity and called mitral atresia with patent subaortic outlet (Watson et al, 1960). The clinical profile of patients with this condition was highlighted by Mickell and his colleagues (1980), who shortly thereafter emphasized that this clinical grouping would include some of the hearts in which the left atrioventricular orifice was blocked by a morphologically tricuspid valve, or its embryological precursor was lacking. This overall group of patients are unified clinically because they have compete obstruction of the atrioventricular orifice of the morphologically left atrium but with a patent subaortic outflow tract from the ventricular mass. They form the subject of this chapter.

ANATOMY AND MORPHOGENESIS

ANATOMY

As emphasized above, the unifying morphological feature of the hearts under discussion is absence of direct communication from the morphologically left atrium to the ventricular mass. As with complete blockage of the atrioventricular orifice of the morphologically right atrium, this situation can be the consequence either of presence of an imperforate valvar membrane or of absence of the morphologically left atrioventricular connection (Figure 40.1). This clinical entity, of course, is necessarily confined to the morphologically left side of the heart. Therefore, in patients who have mirror-imaged atrial arrangement, the obstructed morphologically left atrioventricular orifice is a right-sided structure. Such patients are included within the group described in this chapter, although as yet we have not, ourselves, seen any examples. In contrast, we will not include here those other patients with mirror-imaged atrial arrangement who have otherwise 'classical' tricuspid atresia (Figure 40.2).

Amongst those who do fit the anatomical criterions for inclusion, there is marked variability according to the individual segmental connections. Taken together, these hearts are rare. Probably the most common examples are those in which there is usual atrial arrangement, right hand ventricular topology and double outlet from the morphologically right ventricle. This entity can be found with concordant atrioventricular connections and an imperforate mitral valve (Figure 40.3). It is also seen when the left atrioventricular connection is absent and

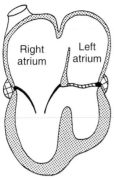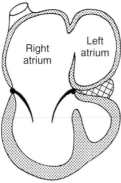

a) Imperforate valvar
membrane

b) Absent atrioventricular
connection

Figure 40.1. The fundamental difference can be seen between an imperforate valve blocking completely the egress from the morphologically left atrium (a) and absence of the left atrioventricular connection (b). Both result in the same haemodynamic disturbance. Various segmental combinations can be found with each of these patterns.

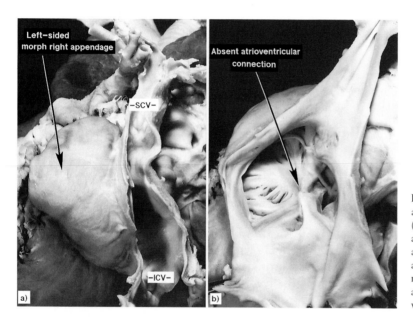

Figure 40.2. This heart has mirror-imaged atrial arrangement. (a) A left-sided right atrium can be seen. (b) There is complete absence of the left-sided atrioventricular connection, but this produces tricuspid atresia, as discussed in Chapter 39. In this chapter, we are concerned with atresia of the outlet from the morphologically (morph) left atrium, not the left-sided atrium. ICV, inferior caval vein; SCV, superior caval vein.

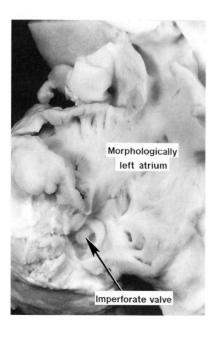

Figure 40.3. Blockage of egress from the morphologically left atrium in this heart is the consequence of an imperforate mitral valve. The atrioventricular connections were concordant, with double outlet from the right ventricle.

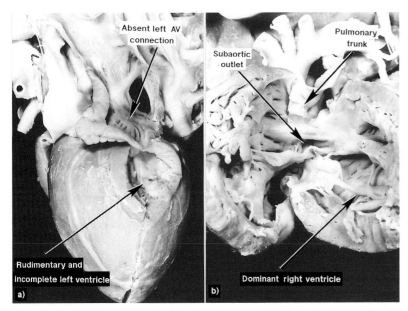

Figure 40.4. In this heart, there is complete absence of the left atrioventricular (AV) connection (a). The left ventricle is rudimentary and incomplete. The aorta, however, is patent because it and the pulmonary trunk arise from the right ventricle (b).

the right atrium is connected to a dominant right ventricle through a morphologically tricuspid valve (Figure 40.4). In either of these settings, there is usually a ventricular septal defect, and the left ventricle can sometimes approach its normal dimensions. Patients can also be encountered, nonetheless, in whom the ventricular septal defect is small or the ventricular septum is intact. The left ventricle can then be grossly hypoplastic. The lesions still do not fall into the category of classical hypoplastic left heart syndrome because of the patent subaortic outlet. In those examples with a ventricular septal defect, the arterial trunks are typically normally related. Frequently there is aortic-to-atrioventricular valvar continuity through the roof of the defect, emphasizing that both

arterial trunks can arise exclusively from the right ventricle in absence of bilateral infundibulums. Although less frequent, similar examples of this subset of mitral atresia can be found when the patent aorta arises exclusively from the left ventricle, either in the setting of absent atrioventricular connection (Figure 40.5a,b) or with an imperforate mitral valve (Figure 40.5c).

The second most common subset of hearts that fits the criterions for inclusion within this clinical heading is that in which the left atrioventricular connection is absent and the right atrium is connected through a morphologically mitral valve to a dominant left ventricle (Figure 40.6). Almost always in this setting, the rudimentary right ventricle is positioned anteriorly and to the left, and the

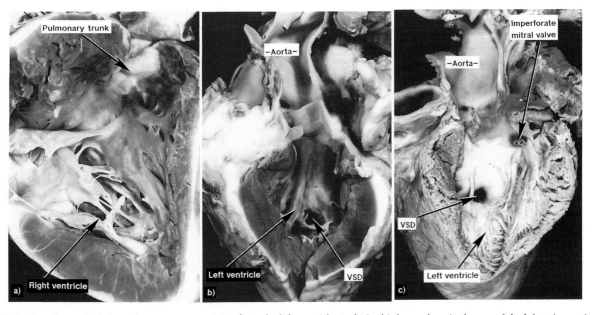

Figure 40.5. These hearts both have the patent aorta arising from the left ventricle. (a, b) In this heart, there is absence of the left atrioventricular connection. (c) In this heart, the mitral valve is imperforate in the setting of concordant atrioventricular connections. VSD, ventricular septal defect.

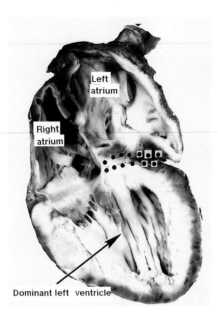

Figure 40.6. This simulated four chamber section shows absence of the left atrioventricular connection with the right atrium connected to a dominant left ventricle.

ventriculo-arterial connections are discordant (Figure 40.7). Without question, had the left atrioventricular connection developed in this setting of left hand ventricular topology, it would have been guarded by a morphologically tricuspid valve. The hearts represent 'close cousins' of congenitally corrected transposition (Chapter 49). Equally certain, nonetheless, is that the clinical presentation of such patients is that anticipated for mitral atresia. That is why we discuss them within this chapter.

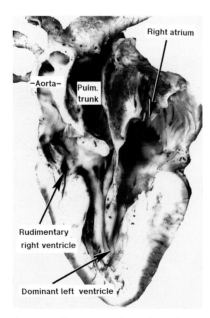

Figure 40.7. This cut, in long axis and at right angles to the section of the same heart shown in Figure 40.6, shows the anterior rudimentary and incomplete right ventricle together with discordant ventriculo-arterial connections. The muscular outlet septum is deviated posteriorly, producing subpulmonary stenosis. Pulm, pulmonary.

As with other hearts having a dominant left ventricle and discordant ventriculo-arterial connections, obstruction is frequent at the ventricular septal defect and produces subaortic obstruction. This is then associated with aortic coarctation, or even interruption. In this respect, the patients have many of the features of hypoplastic left heart syndrome, but self-evidently without any hypoplasia of the morphologically left ventricle. The atrioventricular conduction tissues are abnormally disposed, with the bundle arising from an anterior atrioventricular node beneath the mouth of the right atrial appendage. It then encircles the subpulmonary outflow tract as it courses to reach the anteriorly located ventricular septum. When viewed from the rudimentary right ventricle, as in all hearts with dominant left and rudimentary right ventricles, the conduction axis runs posteroinferiorly relative to the ventricular septal defect (Figure 40.8) (Cheung et al, 1990). As a variant of this pattern, some hearts can have double inlet left ventricle with left-sided rudimentary right ventricle and an imperforate left atrioventricular valve (Figure 40.9). These serve to demonstrate the affinity of all those hearts having univentricular atrioventricular connection to a dominant left ventricle.

The majority of hearts seen clinically fit into these two groupings, but in about one tenth of the hearts studied by Mickell and his colleagues (1983), there was no evidence of a second chamber within the ventricular mass. The solitary ventricle was particularly coarsely trabeculated throughout its apical regions. These were considered to represent solitary ventricles of indeterminate morphology. We have seen no postmortem examples of this combination but have no reason to doubt its existence. It is also to be anticipated that other segmental combinations will be encountered. Hearts with discordant atrioventricular connections may be encountered with an imperforate left-sided tricuspid valve, or even with imperforate tricuspid and aortic valves in the setting of congenitally corrected transposition. If found, the latter anomaly would have all the features of hypoplas-

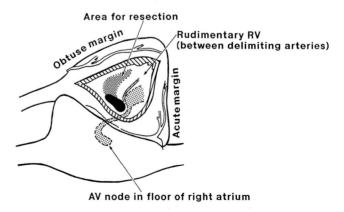

Figure 40.8. The surgeon's view of the rudimentary right ventricle (RV) in hearts with univentricular atrioventricular connection and dominant left ventricle. It shows the area in which the septum can safely be resected to enlarge the ventricular septal defect.

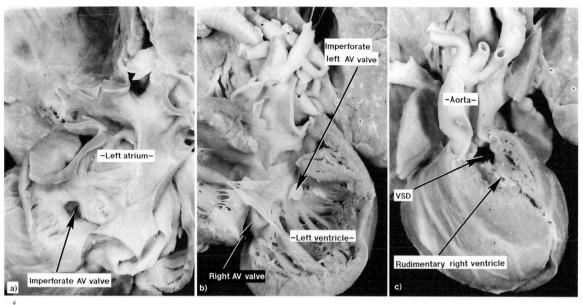

Figure 40.9. This heart has an imperforate left atrioventricular (AV) valve (a), but with both atrioventricular junctions connected in their entirety to the dominant left ventricle, a double inlet left ventricle (b). The right ventricle is rudimentary and incomplete, supporting the anterior and left-sided aorta (c). VSD, ventricular septal defect.

tic left heart syndrome, even though it would be the morphologically right ventricle that would be hypoplastic (Figure 40.10). Entities such as these are readily accounted for by sequential segmental analysis, even though they may not yet have been encountered. In similar fashion, hearts must be anticipated with double inlet right ventricle and imperforate left-sided atrioventricular valve, irrespective of whether the rudimentary and incomplete left ventricle is left or right sided. Significantly, we have seen hearts with absence of the left-

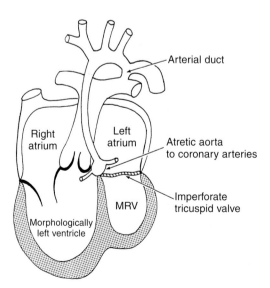

Figure 40.10. The hypothetical situation (at present) in which combined atresia of the left atrioventricular and arterial valves could produce the clinical picture of 'hypoplastic left heart' in the setting of discordant atrioventricular connections, but with hypoplasia of the morphologically right ventricle (MRV).

sided atrioventriclar connection (Figure 40.11a) in which the right-sided atrioventricular valve straddles and overrides the ventricular septum (Figure 40.11b). These hearts have uniatrial but biventricular atrioventricular connection (Chapter 41). Their clinical profile is dominated by the absence of any direct communication between the left atrium and the ventricular mass. They, too, fit within the clinical profile emphasized in this chapter. These rare entities must be anticipated with either right hand or left hand ventricular topology, although we have seen only the variant with right hand topology (Figure 40.11). There can also be marked variability in the size of the two ventricles.

The anatomical feature that unifies all the hearts falling within this grouping is the absence of direct outlet from the morphologically left atrium, whether the obstruction is caused by the muscular floor of the left atrium or an imperforate valvar membrane. The pulmonary venous return, therefore, enters the circulation by crossing the atrial septum, almost always through the oval foramen, which is most often restrictive or even aneurysmal towards the right atrium. Alternative routes for pulmonary venous return must be anticipated in this setting, such as fenestration of the coronary sinus, presence of a levoatrial cardinal vein or anomalous pulmonary venous connections. So far, we have never identified any of these possibilities.

MORPHOGENESIS

The anatomical heterogeneity encountered can readily be explained on the basis of what is already known concerning cardiac development. Indeed, the presumed

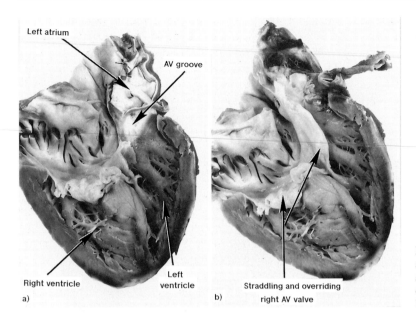

Figure 40.11. This heart has absence of the left atrioventricular (AV) connection (a), but with the right atrioventricular valve straddling and overriding the crest of the ventricular septum (b). This produces the uniatrial but biventricular connection (see also Chapter 41).

processes of cardiac development, with either rightward or leftward looping of the ventricular component of the primary heart tube, provide an entirely logical explanation of why either the right or the left atrium can be connected to the morphologically right ventricle. Equally, the evidence from examination of the hearts seen with various forms of straddling and overriding valves (Chapter 41) support strongly the concept that the atrioventricular junction, during development, can maintain its initial connection to the developing left ventricle, or it can become exclusively connected to the developing right ventricle. Growth of the atrial septum to exclude the left atrium from the developing atrioventricular junction, or subsequent closure of an initially perforate left atrioventricular valve, can be interpreted in the various potentials for formation of the heart itself; they then provide a rational explanation for all the entities described above.

CLASSIFICATION

It is clear from the previous morphological description that there are two major subsets of patients encountered in the setting of usual atrial arrangement. In the first, the morphologically right atrium connects directly to the morphologically right ventricle. There may be absence of the left atrioventricular connection; alternatively, an imperforate left atrioventricular valve may block potentially concordant or double inlet atrioventricular connections. There is also considerable variability in the ventriculo-arterial connections. With concordant connections and normally related great arteries, the aorta arising from the hypoplastic left ventricle itself often exhibits varying degrees of hypoplasia, with or without aortic coarctation. When there is double outlet right ventricle, the great arterial trunks are usually normally

related, although rarely the aorta can be found anterior and to the right of the pulmonary trunk.

The second subset of patients are those in which the morphologically right atrium is connected to the dominant morphologically left ventricle. Again, there may be variability in the type of atrioventricular connection; consequently, patients are encountered in whom there is absence of the left atrioventricular connection or, less frequently, an imperforate left atrioventricular valve, usually with double inlet left ventricle but, rarely, with discordant atrioventricular connections. In general terms, the ventriculo-arterial connections are less variable than in the first subset. Most commonly, discordant connections are found, with the aorta arising from a left-sided and hypoplastic morphologically right ventricle. In this situation, it is not uncommon to find a restrictive ventricular septal defect, often in association with hypoplasia of the ascending aorta and aortic coarctation

In each of these subsets, independent of the morphology of the dominate ventricle, patients are encountered in which there is muscular subpulmonary stenosis or valvar pulmonary stenosis, although unrestricted pulmonary blood flow is more frequent.

PATHOPHYSIOLOGY

In all the patients falling within this clinical grouping, irrespective of the morphological substrate for the valvar atresia, the only egress of pulmonary venous return from the left atrium is across an atrial septal defect or patent oval foramen to the right atrium. Restriction of the interatrial communication is frequent; this results in elevated pressure in the left atrium compared with that in the right. Of necessity, the right atrium receives systemic and pulmonary venous returns. Because of the obligatory common mixing, it is desaturated blood that flows from the right atrium to the ventricular mass, and thence to the aorta and pulmonary arteries, where the saturations of oxygen will be equal. Because the dominant ventricle receives both systemic and pulmonary venous returns, it is larger than normal in terms of both cavity size and muscle mass.

In the neonate with a restrictive atrial septal defect, there is effectively obstruction to pulmonary venous return. Consequently, the symptoms of acute pulmonary oedema may develop extremely rapidly, with profound tachypnoea and congestive cardiac failure. Severe cyanosis will be present. Alternatively, a restrictive inter-atrial communication can produce high pulmonary vascular resistance and low pulmonary blood flow; in this case, severe cyanosis is the predominant feature in the absence of symptoms of pulmonary oedema. In the neonate with a non-restrictive atrial septal defect, cyanosis will again be evident at birth. As the pulmonary vascular resistance falls during the first month of life, cyanosis becomes less marked, but the increasing flow of blood to the lungs produces the symptoms of congestive cardiac failure. When there is pulmonary stenosis, the degree of cyanosis increases with increasing severity of the stenosis, becoming most profound in the presence of pulmonary atresia. Therefore, the degree of central cyanosis, or the development of congestive cardiac failure, is the result of the interplay of various factors. These include the presence or absence of pulmonary stenosis, patency of the arterial duct, the resistances in the pulmonary and systemic circuits and the size of the interatrial communication. The lower the magnitude of pulmonary blood flow, the greater will be the degree of cyanosis; in comparison, large volumes of flow to the lungs are associated with the development of symptoms of congestive cardiac failure. Further modification of the clinical presentation will occur when there is aortic coarctation. The increased flow to the lungs, coupled with diminished flow to the lower body, will then result in the early development of congestive cardiac failure together with metabolic acidosis. The resulting ventricular dysfunction may further aggravate the symptoms of congestive cardiac failure and low cardiac output.

CLINICAL FEATURES

Although the majority of patients with mitral atresia present in the neonatal period or early infancy, the timing and exact clinical presentation will always be dictated by the associated anomalies and their severity. A crucial factor in the timing of presentation is the size of the inter-atrial communication. Frequently it is small. Then the left atrial and pulmonary venous pressures are raised, giving rise to acute pulmonary oedema and severe congestive cardiac failure, usually during the first week of life. This, in turn, results in tachypnoea and low cardiac output or,

alternatively, to reduced flow to the lungs and severe cyanosis, but without symptoms of pulmonary oedema. The infant with aortic coarctation will exhibit weak or absent femoral pulses, mild central cyanosis and symptoms of high pulmonary blood flow or of pulmonary oedema. These include tachypnoea, enlargement of the liver and difficulties in feeding. In a few patients who have severe obstruction to pulmonary blood flow, presentation is usually in the neonatal period with a duct-dependent pulmonary circulation. Cyanosis will be present at birth and will become more severe with impending closure of the arterial duct. There will be a single second heart sound, a short ejection systolic murmur of pulmonary stenosis at the upper left sternal edge and sometimes a soft continuous murmur. For those patients in whom the atrial septal defect is not restrictive, and in whom the right atrium connects to a dominant left ventricle with discordant ventriculo-arterial connections, symptoms may not develop until the second month of life. It is at this stage that pulmonary vascular resistance has fallen sufficiently for flow of blood to the lungs to increase. Occasionally, there is an absence of significant symptoms in the infant with balanced flows to the systemic and pulmonary circuits. This is either because of moderate pulmonary stenosis or because of a moderately restrictive atrial septal defect and moderate elevation of the pulmonary vascular resistance. Mild central cyanosis may then be the only obvious presenting feature. In many cases, nonetheless, it is the presence of aortic coarctation, or even aortic interruption, that governs the clinical presentation. In this setting, there is early development of congestive cardiac failure, often followed by cardiogenic shock during the first few days of life.

INVESTIGATIONS

CHEST RADIOGRAPHY

There is no particular configuration of the cardiac outline that typifies mitral atresia with patent subaortic outlet. There is a close correlation, however, between the size of the heart and the volume of flow to the lungs. With diminished pulmonary blood flow, because of pulmonary venous hypertension secondary to a restrictive atrial septal defect or secondary to pulmonary stenosis, the heart tends to remain of normal size. In the absence of pulmonary stenosis, when flow of blood to the lungs is increased, cardiomegaly is the rule. It is unusual for the left atrium to enlarge, even when the atrial septal defect is restrictive. The pulmonary vascular markings reflect the pressures in the left atrium and the pulmonary veins, along with the amount of pulmonary blood flow. Hence, pulmonary oedema is encountered when there is severe left atrial hypertension and increased pulmonary vascular markings in the absence of pulmonary stenosis, or when pulmonary stenosis or atresia is associated with a large arterial duct or another source of excessive pulmonary flow. Pulmonary oligaemia may be encountered when there is severe pulmonary stenosis or when there is high pulmonary vascular resistance secondary to left atrial hypertension. In patients with absence of the left atrioventricular connection, and with the right atrium connected to a morphologically left ventricle, the heart may be positioned in the right chest with its apex pointing to the right.

ELECTROCARDIOGRAPHY

There are no typical standard surface electrocardiographic features of patients with the clinical features of mitral atresia and patent subaortic outlet. In those with the right atrium connected to a dominant right ventricle, there is almost always a neonatal pattern of progression of the precordial RS complexes, with a dominant R wave in leads V_4R and V_1, and dominant S wave in leads V_5 and V_6. In the majority, the mean frontal QRS axis is between +90° and +180°. The features of left atrial hypertrophy are commonly encountered.

In the subset of patients with the right atrium connected to a dominant morphologically left ventricle, usually all the precordial leads demonstrate prominent R and S waves, and the T waves are commonly inverted in leads V_5 and V_6. The mean frontal QRS axis is extremely variable but is most commonly in the range 0 to +90°. The electrocardiographic features of left atrial hypertrophy are again frequently encountered.

ECHOCARDIOGRAPHY

Cross-sectional echocardiography will almost always permit the precise diagnosis of the various forms of left atrioventricular valvar atresia, along with all the associated anomalies (Freedom et al, 1982; Rigby et al, 1981; 1982). The subcostal and parasternal four chamber sections allow the most common form of mitral atresia, in which there is absence of the atrioventricular connection, to be distinguished from those types in which there is an imperforate left atrioventricular valve. With absent connection, the left atrioventricular groove can be seen interposing between the muscular floor of the left atrium and the ventricular mass (Figure 40.12). An imperforate valve, in contrast, blocks a formed atrioventricular junction and is seen ballooning into the hypoplastic ventricle when the atrioventricular connections are concordant (Figure 40.13) or discordant, or into the dominant ventricle when there is double inlet ventricle. Rudimentary tension apparatus can sometimes be identified supporting an imperforate valvar membrane, but never when there is absence of the atrioventricular connection. In the typical forms of left atrioventricular valvar atresia, the four chamber sections will show a small and rudimentary

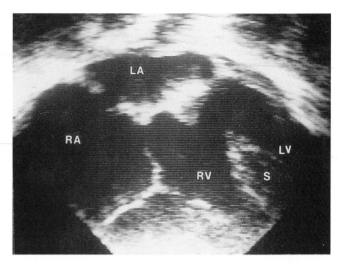

Figure 40.12. This parasternal four chamber section is from a patient with absence of the left atrioventricular connection and with the right atrium (RA) connected to a dominant right ventricle (RV). The ventricular septum (S) can be seen dividing the right from the left ventricle (LV). The fibrofatty tissue of the atrioventricular groove interposes between the floor of the left atrium (LA) and the ventricular mass. There is a large ventricular septal defect.

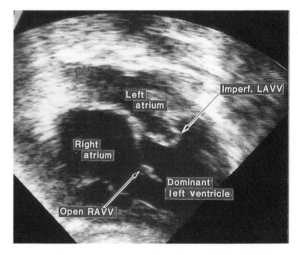

Figure 40.13. This patient has a double inlet left ventricle with an imperforate left atrioventricular valve shown through a parasternal four chamber section.

left ventricle to the left of the dominant morphologically right ventricle, and a solitary right atrioventricular valve guarding the junction between the right atrium and the right ventricle (Figure 40.12). Alternatively, a small and rudimentary right ventricle is seen to the left and anterosuperior relative to the dominant left ventricle, with a solitary right atrioventricular valve guarding the junction between the right atrium and the dominant left ventricle (Figure 40.14).

The characteristics of the dominant and rudimentary ventricles in left atrioventricular valve atresia are identified with subcostal, parasternal and apical long- and short-axis sections in exactly the same manner as all

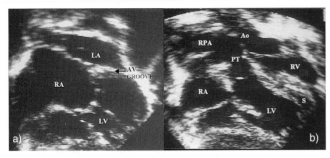

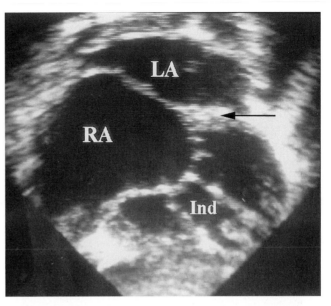

Figure 40.14. Left atrioventricular valvar atresia with dominant left ventricle. (a) A subcostal four chamber section shows the absence of the left atrioventricular (AV) connection and fibrofatty tissue of the atrioventricular groove interposing between the floor of the left atrium (LA) and the left ventricle (LV). There is direct communication between the right atrium (RA) and the left ventricle. (b) A subcostal outlet section that demonstrates the pulmonary trunk (PT) arising from the left ventricle and the aorta (Ao) arising from the left-sided rudimentary right ventricle (RV). RPA, right pulmonary artery; S, septum.

Figure 40.15. This four chamber echocardiographic section is from a patient with absence of the left atrioventricular connection and with the right atrium (RA) connected to a solitary and indeterminate ventricle (Ind). The fibrofatty tissue of the atrioventricular groove interposes between the floor of the left atrium (LA) and the ventricular mass.

other hearts with a univentricular atrioventricular connection. A rudimentary right ventricle will be antero-superior and to the left of the dominant left ventricle, whereas a rudimentary left ventricle will be posteroinferior and to the left of the dominant morphologically right ventricle. It is the position of the rudimentary and hypoplastic ventricle that is the most reliable echocardiographic guide to ventricular morphology. In practise, it is difficult to establish the morphology of the dominant ventricle by any other means, although a dominant left ventricle usually has smooth apical trabeculations while a dominant right ventricle is coarsely trabeculated. Occasionally, hearts are encountered in which atresia of the left atrioventricular valve is found in the setting of a solitary and indeterminate ventricle (Figure 40.15). The echocardiographic diagnosis is then based upon extremely coarse trabeculations, coupled with failure to identify any second rudimentary ventricle.

One of the most important aspects of the evaluation of the ventricular mass is the visualization of the communications between the ventricles. These defects are usually solitary and muscular. They vary from large to extremely small, but multiple defects may also be encountered. The approach to establishing the ventriculo-arterial connections, and the morphology of the infundibulums, is described in Chapter 13. Subaortic stenosis, aortic hypoplasia, and coarctation or interruption are frequent, irrespective of the morphology of the dominant ventricle and the ventriculo-arterial connections. In contrast, pulmonary stenosis or pulmonary atresia is encountered infrequently.

An unusual variant of left atrioventricular valve atresia, and one that is readily diagnosed by four chamber cross-sectional echocardiographic sections, is that in which the solitary atrioventricular valve overrides and straddles the ventricular septum. In this setting, that of uniatrial but biventricular connection (so-called

double outlet atrium), both the ventricles may be of similar size (Figure 40.16). When diagnosing this variant, it is crucial to exclude the presence of a common atrioventricular junction. This is done by tracing the fibrofatty tissues of the right atrioventricular groove to the location of the interatrial septum, the muscular inferior margin of the septum being continuous with the muscular floor of the left atrium. In the variant with atrioventricular septal defect and common atrioventricular junction, the egress from the left atrium is through a defect at the lower margin of the atrial septum (Chapter 36).

A combination of imaging and Doppler is essential to diagnose restriction at the level of the interatrial communication, to measure gradients across ventricular septal defects or across the subaortic or subpulmonary outflow tracts, and to demonstrate any atrioventricular valvar regurgitation or flow across an arterial duct.

CARDIAC CATHETERIZATION AND ANGIOGRAPHY

In the majority of infants with left atrioventricular valvar atresia, the diagnosis will be made exclusively from the echocardiographic evaluation. An essential part of the early management, nonetheless, will usually be cardiac catheterization to permit balloon atrial septostomy. This is because the interatrial communication will be restrictive in most patients. Septostomy, can also be carried out in the intensive care unit guided by precordial or transoesophageal echocardiographic monitoring. Cardiac catheterization is usually carried out again between the

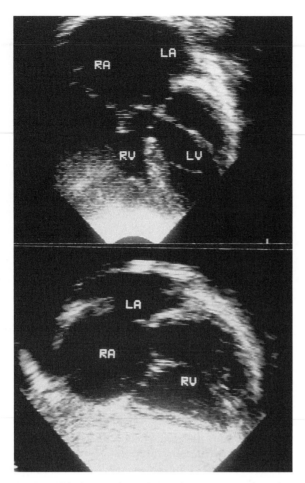

Figure 40.16. These two echocardiographic sections are from the same patient, who has absence of the left atrioventricular connection and straddling atrioventricular valve. Both show the atrioventricular groove interposing between the floor of the left atrium (LA) and the ventricular mass. (a) The right atrium (RA) is connected to both the left (LV) and right (RV) ventricles with the tension apparatus from the valve extending into both ventricles. (b) The atrial septum meets the left atrioventricular groove, confirming the absent left atrioventricular connection and excluding the presence of an atrioventricular septal defect with common atrioventricular junction.

ages of 3 and 6 months, following palliative surgery performed in the neonatal period. The primary objective is to measure the pulmonary arterial pressure prior to construction of a bidirectional Glenn shunt, to measure the left atrial pressure and to exclude any pulmonary venous stenoses.

At cardiac catheterization, there will be evidence of left-to-right shunting at atrial level, common mixing of systemic and pulmonary venous blood within the ventricular mass and varying degrees of systemic arterial oxygen desaturation. Mean atrial pressures will be similar when the interatrial communication is large, but there will be a mean pressure gradient, or an a-wave gradient, from left to right when the interatrial communication is restrictive. Catheterization of the right heart usually permits the measurement of pressures in the atriums, the ventricles, the aorta and pulmonary arteries,

and recording of a pulmonary arterial wedge pressure. Gradients should be sought between the ventricles and the aorta caused by restriction at the ventricular septal defect or in subaortic position.

The major role of cardiac catheterization, therefore, is not to demonstrate the morphological features but to assess the outcome of previous palliative operations and to determine suitability for a bidirectional Glenn operation and the Fontan procedure. Of particular importance are the measurements of pulmonary arterial pressure, ventricular end-diastolic pressure and atrial pressures. A comparison of left atrial and pulmonary arterial wedge pressures will also permit the identification of any pulmonary venous stenosis. If the mean pulmonary arterial pressure exceeds 15 mmHg, the pulmonary vascular resistance should be measured. Angiography (Soto et al, 1982) is designed primarily to demonstrate the size and the morphology of the aorta and the pulmonary arteries, with particular attention paid to any naturally occurring or iatrogenic stenoses or distortions. It is also important to identify additional sources of pulmonary blood flow, such as aortopulmonary collateral arteries, that might be suitable for coil embolization.

For those hearts in which the right ventricle is dominant, the lateral projection of the right ventriculogram will demonstrate a posterior rudimentary left ventricle (Thies et al, 1986) and any ventricular septal defect (Figure 40.17). When there is a dominant left ventricle, a frontal exposure of the ventriculogram will demonstrate the ventricular septal defect and the rudimentary right ventricle on the left shoulder of the heart (Figure 40.18). It is noteworthy that the angiographic and echocardio-

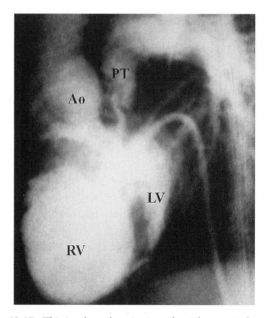

Figure 40.17. This is a lateral projection of a right ventricular angiogram, showing a rudimentary left ventricle (LV) posterior to a dominant right ventricle (RV). There is double outlet right ventricle with the anterior aorta (Ao) and the posterior pulmonary trunk (PT) both arising from the right ventricle.

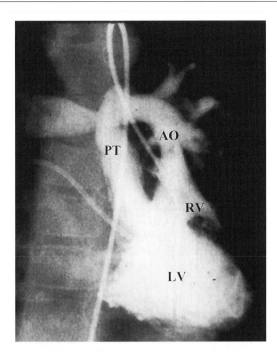

Figure 40.18. This is an anterior projection of the dominant left ventricle in a patient with absence of the left atrioventricular connection and the right atrium connected to a dominant left ventricle (LV). There is a left-sided rudimentary right ventricle (RV) and the ventriculoarterial connections are discordant, the aorta (AO) arising from the rudimentary right ventricle and pulmonary trunk (PT) arising from the left ventricle. The appearances of this angiogram are virtually identical to those found in double inlet left ventricle with a left-sided rudimentary right ventricle.

graphic appearances of the ventricular mass when left atrioventricular valve atresia is associated with the right atrium connected to the dominant left ventricle and left-sided rudimentary left ventricle (Figure 40.18) is indistinguishable from the appearances of double inlet left ventricle with left-sided rudimentary right ventricle (Thies et al, 1986). The lateral view of the left ventriculogram will demonstrate the anterior position of the rudimentary right ventricle and of the aorta.

NATURAL HISTORY

In general terms, the natural history for patients with atresia of the left atrioventricular valve but patency of the subaortic outflow tract is unknown. If untreated, death will usually occur in the neonatal period in the majority because of aortic coarctation or restriction of the interatrial communication, this giving rise to left atrial and pulmonary venous hypertension. The rare combination of a non-restrictive atrial septal defect and moderate pulmonary stenosis, with balanced flows to the systemic and pulmonary circuits, provides the best prognosis. In many cases, the aorta will arise from the rudimentary ventricle. As a consequence, there is always the risk of the development of subaortic stenosis because of a restrictive ven-

tricular septal defect. This is an additional factor that will influence the natural history in a fashion comparable to other examples of hearts with univentricular atrioventricular connection to a dominant left ventricle (Freedom et al, 1986).

MANAGEMENT

MEDICAL TREATMENT

The essential difference between atresia of the left atrioventricular valve associated with patent subaortic outlet and hypoplastic left heart syndrome is that, in the former, the aorta is sufficiently well developed to allow an adequate cardiac output. The diagnosis nowadays is almost always made during fetal life, the neonatal period or early infancy. Palliative surgical treatment is almost always required in early infancy. Intravenous prostaglandin E_1 is used to re-establish or preserve ductal patency when the systemic flow is inadequate because of aortic coarctation or interruption, both of which are often associated with a restrictive ventricular septal defect and subaortic stenosis. It is unusual to encounter severe hypoxia because of pulmonary stenosis or atresia. In this event, intravenous prostaglandins can also be used to re-establish or preserve ductal patency. If an increase in pulmonary blood flow is permitted, however, pulmonary oedema may result when the interatrial communication is small. Almost always, it is possible to correct the metabolic acidosis that accompanies reduced flow to the systemic circuit prior to initial surgery. The first step in medical management is to perform balloon atrial septostomy. Because of the small size of the oval foramen, coupled with the frequent extreme hypertrophy of the atrial septum, it is not always possible to create an adequate interatrial communication. Blade septostomy offers an alternative palliative option in this circumstance and is preferable to surgical septectomy (Chapter 16). Congestive cardiac failure should be treated with diuretics and vasodilators.

SURGICAL TREATMENT

When surgery is undertaken, attention should be paid to the need for atrial septectomy in the event of balloon or blade septostomy being inadequate. When there is excessive flow to the lungs, the pulmonary trunk is banded through a left lateral thoracotomy. It is important to place the band sufficiently proximal on the pulmonary trunk to avoid distortion of the pulmonary arterial branches, at the same time taking care to avoid damage to the pulmonary valvar leaflets. Excessive flow to the lungs is often associated with aortic coarctation, a restrictive ventricular septal defect and subaortic stenosis. Although a variety of surgical protocols can be used to deal with these problems, the best first option is probably to repair the aortic coarctation and band the pulmonary trunk via a left thoracotomy. When there is a restrictive ventricular septal defect, an alternative is to use a one-stage approach, repairing the aortic coarctation, enlarging the ventricular septal defect and banding the pulmonary trunk through a midline sternotomy using deep hypothermia and circulatory arrest. Alternatively, the pulmonary trunk can be anastomosed to the ascending aorta in a modification of the Norwood procedure, especially if subaortic stenosis is not the result of a restrictive ventricular septal defect.

MANAGEMENT FOLLOWING EARLY PALLIATION

It is important, following early palliation, to ensure that patients will be suitable candidates for Fontan-like repair. Early management, particularly when there is ventricular dysfunction, is directed to the control of congestive heart failure with diuretics and vasodilators. It is important to identify any potential problems, such as restriction at the interatrial communication, recurrent obstruction in the aortic arch, progressive subaortic stenosis, distortion of the pulmonary arteries, deterioration of ventricular function or the development of atrioventricular valvar insufficiency. Some of these problems can contribute to poorly controlled congestive heart failure. It is important, therefore, to perform regular echocardiographic examinations. It is also wise to perform cardiac catheterization when the child is between 3 and 6 months of age in order to measure the left atrial pressure, along with pulmonary arterial pressure and resistance. At the same time, it is possible to identify any distortion of the pulmonary arteries or aorta, and the presence of any significant collateral arteries between the systemic and pulmonary circulations. If identified, these can then be embolized prior to any further surgery. The subsequent surgical management is designed to minimize left atrial hypertension and pressure and volume overload on the ventricles. This is achieved, on the one hand, by ensuring that the interatrial communication is large and, on the other, by relieving subaortic stenosis and avoiding excessive flow to the lungs. Construction of a bidirectional cavopulmonary shunt will achieve the goal of relieving ventricular volume overload. The presence of left atrioventricular valvar atresia itself is probably a significant risk factor in infancy for the subsequent Fontan-type repair. Because of this, it is wise to perform an early bidirectional cavopulmonary shunt before the age of 6 months. This can be used in conjunction with other operations designed to relieve subaortic stenosis. Construction of the Fontan circulation can then be achieved at any time from 3 years of age onwards, taking into account the clinical condition of the patient and the findings on echocardiography and cardiac catheterization and angiography.

As indicated, atresia of the left atrioventricular valve has been identified as a risk factor for early death following the Fontan operation. This may not be a morphological risk factor in itself but rather a morphological arrangement that necessitated, until recently, the use of a complex baffle when partitioning the atrial chambers. Construction of such a baffle often resulted in some obstruction of the pulmonary venous pathway to the right atrioventricular valve. It may be that, rather than using one of various modifications of the Fontan operation for more complex anatomical situations (Gale et al, 1979; DeLeon et al, 1986; Mayer et al, 1986; de Leval et al, 1988; Stein et al, 1991), the use of some form of extracardiac conduit will be ideal in this situation (Marcelletti et al, 1990; Gundry et al, 1997). An alternative explanation for the reported poor outcome might be the effect of left atrial hypertension on the pulmonary vasculature, both in the fetus and in the neonate. Elevation of the mean pulmonary arterial pressure and vascular resistance have been shown to increase the risk of the Fontan operation in a number of studies, and it seems likely that, in general, pulmonary vascular resistance will be higher when there is atresia of the left atrioventricular valve than in patients with other forms of univentricular atrioventricular connection.

REFERENCES

Cheung H C, Lincoln C, Anderson R H et al 1990 Options for surgical repair in hearts with univentricular atrioventricular connection and subaortic stenosis. Journal of Thoracic and Cardiovascular Surgery 100: 672–681

DeLeon S Y, Ilbawi M N, Idriss F S et al 1986 Fontan type operation for complex lesions: surgical consideration to improve survival. Journal of Thoracic Cardiovascular Surgery 92: 1029–1037

de Leval M R, Kilner P, Gewillig M et al 1988 Total cavopulmonary connection: a logical alternative to atriopulmonary connection for complex Fontan operation – experimental studies and early clinical experience. Journal of Thoracic Cardiovascular Surgery 96: 682–695

Freedom R M, Picchio F, Duncan W J et al 1982 The atrioventricular junction in the univentricular heart: a two-dimensional echocardiographic analysis. Pediatric Cardiology 3: 105–117

Freedom R M, Benson L M, Smallhorn J F et al 1986 Subaortic stenosis, the univentricular heart, and banding of the pulmonary artery: an analysis of the courses of 43 patients with univentricular heart palliated by pulmonary artery banding. Circulation 73: 758–764

Gale A W, Danielson G K, McGoon D C et al 1979 Modified Fontan operation for the univentricular heart and complicated lesions. Journal of Thoracic Cardiovascular Surgery 78: 831–838

Gundry S R, Razzouk A J, del Rio M J et al 1997 The optimal Fontan connection: a growing extracardiac tunnel with pedicled pericardium. Journal of Thoracic Cardiovascular Surgery 114: 552–559

Marcelletti C, Corno A, Giannico S et al 1990 Inferior vena cava–pulmonary artery extracardiac conduit. A new form of right heart bypass. Journal of Thoracic Cardiovascular Surgery 100: 228–232

Mayer J E Jr, Hegalson H N D, Locke J E et al 1986 Extending the limits for modified Fontan procedures. Journal of Thoracic Cardiovascular Surgery 92: 1021–1028

Mickell J J, Mathews R A, Park S C et al 1980 Left atrioventricular valve atresia: clinical management. Circulation 61: 123–127

Mickell J J, Mathews R A, Anderson R H et al 1983 The anatomical heterogeneity of hearts lacking a patent communication between the left atrium and the ventricular mass ('mitral atresia') in presence of a patent aortic valve. European Heart Journal 4: 477–486

Rigby M L, Anderson R H, Gibson D et al 1981 Two-dimensional echocardiographic categorisation of the univentricular heart: ventricular morphology, type and mode of atrioventricular connection. British Heart Journal 46: 603–612

Rigby M L, Gibson D, Joseph M C et al 1982 Recognition of imperforate atrioventricular valves by two-dimensional echocardiography. British Heart Journal 47: 329–336

Soto B, Pacifico A D, Di Sciascio G 1982 Univentricular heart: an angiographic study. American Journal of Cardiology 7: 1099–1103

Stein D G, Laks H, Drinkwater D C et al 1991 Results of total cavopulmonary connection in the treatment of patients with a functional single ventricle. Journal of Thoracic Cardiovascular Surgery 102: 280–287

Thies W R, Bargeron L M J, Bini R M et al 1986 Spectrum of hearts with one underdeveloped and one dominant ventricle. Pediatric Cardiology 7: 129–139

Watson D G, Rowe R D, Conen P E, Duckworth J W 1960 Mitral atresia with normal aortic valve. Report of 11 cases and review of the literature. Pediatrics 25: 450–459

41

Straddling atrioventricular valves

R. H. Anderson and M. L. Rigby

INTRODUCTION

The entities to be considered in this chapter differ from all those others considered in this section of our book devoted to Specific lesions. This is because hearts with straddling and overriding atrioventricular valves represent a series of anatomical stages between the extremes of double inlet and biventricular atrioventricular connections. As such, therefore, straddling and overriding can involve the right or left atrioventricular valve, or a common atrioventricular valve, in the setting of either double inlet right or double inlet left ventricle. The other end of these various spectrums will then, self-evidently, depend upon the valve involved and the morphology of the ventricular mass. The structure of the individual heart itself will reflect the precise degree of straddling as opposed to overriding of the valvar structures. Because of this, it is not possible to approach the lesions in the same fashion as all others discussed in this section of our book. The clinical features will not only reflect the variations already discussed above but will also differ markedly according to the specific ventriculo-arterial connections present, and the associated malformations. The understanding of the malformations, and their correct diagnosis, depends on a thorough appreciation of their anatomical features. We will describe the different patterns, therefore, on the basis of their structure. This, in itself, requires that we define precisely our understanding of the nature of straddling and overriding, since the definition of these features, and the way in which they are described, has varied markedly.

DEFINITIONS

In the normally structured heart, each ventricle, which functions as the muscular pump driving its circulation, has competent valves guarding its inlet and its outlet. The functional components of these valves are the leaflets. Of necessity, if the heart is normal, these leaflets are attached exclusively within their own ventricle. There are subtle differences between the nature of the valvar attachments that are not strictly relevant to this chapter but worthy

of emphasis. The leaflets of the atrioventricular valves are normally attached in annular fashion, and their line of attachment is coincident with the anatomical atrioventricular junction (Figure 41.1). The leaflets of the arterial valves, in contrast, are attached in semilunar fashion, with their line of attachment crossing the anatomical ventriculo-arterial junction (Figure 41.2). Much more significant from the stance of our definitions for straddling and overriding is the nature of the free edge of the valvar leaflets. The atrioventricular valves close against the full force of ventricular systole. In order to retain valvar competence, therefore, the free edges of the leaflets are furnished with tension apparatus. In the normal ventricles, the entire tension apparatus for each valve, like the attachments of the leaflets at the atrioventricular

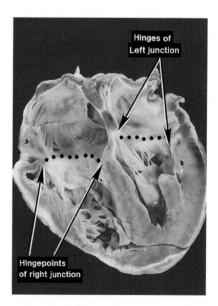

Figure 41.1. In the normal heart, each atrium is connected to its own ventricle, and the leaflets of the valve guarding the respective junction are exclusively connected within that ventricle, with the hinge of the valvar leaflet attached in annular fashion at the level of the junction, even though the right and left junctions themselves are at different levels.

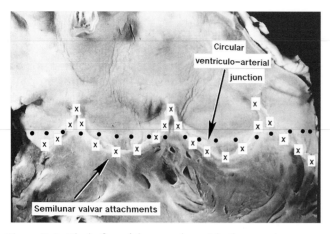

Figure 41.2. The leaflets of the normal arterial valves are also supported exclusively within their respective ventricles, but the semilunar level of attachment crosses the circular anatomical ventriculo-arterial junction.

junctions, is exclusively contained within its own ventricle. The arterial valves, in contrast, close in ventricular diastole. It is the force of the column of blood supported by the leaflets that ensures their competence. Arterial valves, therefore, lack any tension apparatus.

In malformed hearts, both the atrioventricular and ventriculo-arterial junctions can be shared between the two ventricles. Indeed, the sharing of an atrioventricular junction between the ventricles is an essential feature of most of the entities to be discussed in this chapter. But in most of the abnormal hearts to be discussed the tension apparatus is also attached not in one but in both the ventricles. In order to distinguish between the arrangement of the junctions and the structure of the tension appara-

tus, and also to produce a terminology that is applicable to both atrioventricular and ventriculo-arterial valves, we define separately the nature of these two independent features (Milo et al, 1979). We use the term 'overriding' to describe the situation in which a junction, either atrioventricular or ventriculo-arterial, is shared between the ventricles (Figure 41.3). We then reserve the term 'straddling' to describe the arrangement in which the valvar tension apparatus is attached to either side of the ventricular septum and, hence, tethers the valvar leaflets in both ventricles (Figure 41.4). Using these definitions, therefore, it follows that an atrioventricular valve can straddle and override (Figure 41.5a). Such an arrangement, in fact, is by far the most common encountered. It is also possible for an atrioventricular valve to straddle without overriding (Figure 41.5b) or to override in the absence of straddling of the tensor apparatus (Figure 41.5c). It also follows that, within our definitions, it is possible for an arterial valve to override but not to straddle, since arterial valves lack any tension apparatus.

The definitions that we have chosen also have major implications for the description of other features of the hearts that are malformed because of straddling and overriding atrioventricular valves. It is the degree of overriding of the abnormal valve that will determine the precise atrioventricular connections in the heart containing the valve. There are two ways of coping with this situation. The first is to consider straddling itself as a special case. This was the approach chosen by Liberthson et al (1971). This group, along with Mehrizi and his colleagues (1966), were among the first to emphasize the significance of straddling atrioventricular valves. The philosophy of considering the straddling valve as a

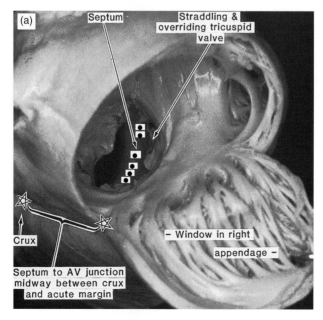

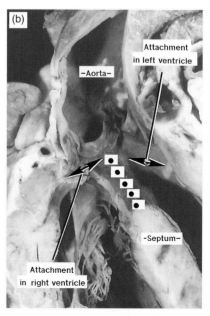

Figure 41.3. Both the atrioventricular (a) and the arterial (b) valves can override the crest of the muscular ventricular septum when their attachments are to both ventricles. The degree of overriding is determined by the position of the ventricular septum versus the junctional attachments. (Reproduction of (a) is by kind permission of Dr L.H.S. Van Mierop, Gainsville, FL.)

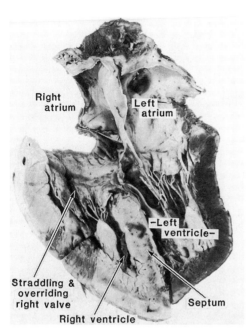

Figure 41.4. This cross-section of the atrioventricular junctions shows how an atrioventricular valve, in this case the tricuspid valve, straddles the ventricular septum when its tension apparatus is attached within both ventricles.

separate entity was also adopted by de la Cruz and Miller (1968), and then by Tandon et al (1974). Indeed, they described hearts with straddling and overriding of the tricuspid valve as exhibiting 'double inlet left ventricle'. They distinguished this entity at that time from those other hearts in which both atrioventricular valves were tethered exclusively in the left ventricle, since the latter lesion was then considered to represent 'single ventricle'.

Now, of course, it is recognized that double inlet left ventricle is a much more accurate descriptor for the entire group of hearts in which the greater part of both atrioventricular junctions are connected to the dominant left ventricle (see Chapter 38).

However, since the degree of overriding in hearts with straddling atrioventricular valves can also extend to include those with biventricular atrioventricular connections (Figure 41.6), then rather than considering all these markedly different spectrums as separate entities, we prefer to concentrate on the effect that the spectrum has on the connection and to divide it at its midpoint when categorizing the segmental arrangement (see Chapter 2). If the spectrum of straddling of the tricuspid valve is considered as an example, we would describe the hearts containing the straddling valve as exhibiting either double inlet ventricle or concordant or discordant atrioventricular connections according to their precise segmental make-up. This is the principle to be used throughout this chapter. It is, of course, much easier to divide this spectrum in theory than it is in practice.

When we first used this '50% rule' for the purpose of dividing the spectrum of override, we had problems in moving from 49% to 51% since, depending on our decision, a biventricular heart would suddenly become a 'univentricular heart'. This was when we also promoted the concept of 'univentricular hearts', illogically disqualifying from ventricular status those chambers which lacked an inlet component or, more specifically, half an inlet component (Anderson et al, 1979). Once we realised, prompted by Brandt and colleagues (Brandt, 1981) the lack of logic in this approach and observed that the atrioventricular connection rather than the ventricular mass in

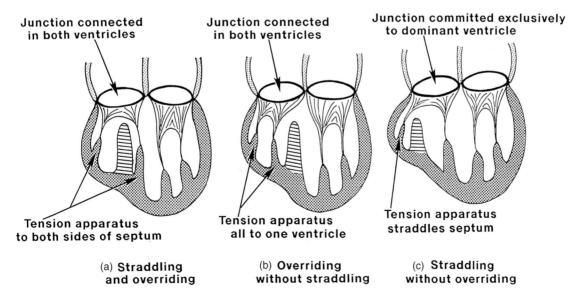

Figure 41.5. Sharing of the atrioventricular junction between the ventricles can occur in three ways. (a) In most situations in which the junction is shared between the ventricles to produce overriding, there is also straddling of the valvar tension apparatus. It is possible, however, within the definitions used, for a valve to straddle in the absence of override (b), or override without any straddling of the valvar tension apparatus (c).

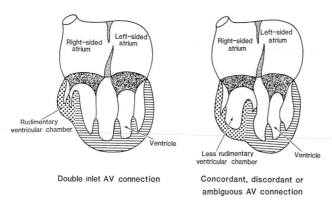

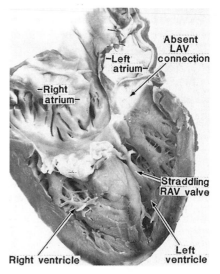

Figure 41.6. When the atrioventricular junction is shared between the ventricles (overriding), there is a series of anomalies produced depending on the precise connection of the overriding junction. The extremes of the spectrum are illustrated here, being either double inlet on the one hand (a), or concordant, discordant or ambiguous atrioventricular (AV) connections on the other (b). The precise type of biventricular connection depends upon the particular morphology of the chambers.

Figure 41.7. The distinction between double inlet and biventricular atrioventricular connections is made according to the proportion of the overriding junction connected in the right as opposed to the left ventricles. In this heart with straddling tricuspid valve, most of the junction is connected within the right ventricle, giving effectively concordant atrioventricular connections.

such hearts was effectively biventricular or univentricular, then the semantic problems disappeared (Anderson et al, 1984). The procedural problems, nonetheless, remained. It is still difficult precisely to adjudicate between 49% and 51% of overriding of an atrioventricular junction. Since the decision will no longer affect the description of the ventricles, it loses much of its force. As we will see, in clinical practice it is more important to describe the size of the ventricles in this setting. But, while this reflects to some extent the precise atrioventricular connection, it is certainly not the only determining feature. The degree of override, therefore, is determined with as much accuracy as is possible, splitting the spectrum on the basis of the proportion of the overriding junction attached within the two ventricles relative to the location of the ventricular septum (Figure 41.7).

There is then a second major point to consider in terms of definitions. This is when the valve that straddles and overrides is guarding a common atrioventricular junction rather than a separate right or left atrioventricular junction. The first problem here is in defining a common atrioventricular junction and distinguishing the common junction from the arrangement seen when one atrioventricular connection is absent and the other junction is itself straddling and overriding (Figure 41.8). We use the atrial septum as our defining feature. A common atrioventricular junction is defined as one which is common to both atriums and both ventricles, although the sharing of this junction does not have to be uniform between the four chambers. The exemplar of hearts with such a common junction is the entity usually described simply as an atrioventricular septal defect (Figure 41.9; see Chapter 36). In these hearts, the presence of the septal defect between the lower edge of the atrial septum and the crest of the ventricular septum serves to emphasize the common nature of the junction. In all hearts having

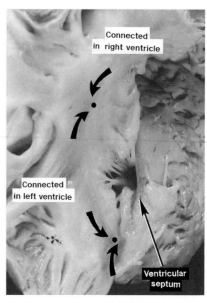

Figure 41.8. This anatomical section, in four chamber plane, shows the essence of a uniatrial but biventricular atrioventricular connection, here resulting from absence of the left atrioventricular connection and straddling of the right atrioventricular valve in the setting of right hand ventricular topology. Note that the atrial septum walls off the left atrium from the atrioventricular junction (compare with Figure 41.12).

such an atrioventricular septal defect and common atrioventricular junction, the common atrioventricular valve of necessity both straddles and overrides. By convention, such hearts are not discussed under the heading of straddling and overriding (Liberthson et al, 1971), although there is no reason why they should not be thus described, since the feature of leaflets being tethered in both

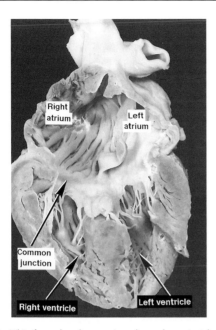

Figure 41.9. This four chamber section shows how, in 'classical' atrioventricular septal defect with common atrioventricular junction, the junction is shared more-or-less equally between the four chambers.

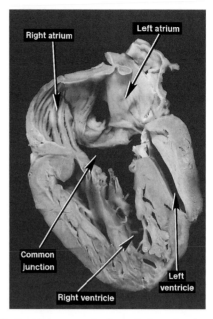

Figure 41.10. In this heart, again shown in four chamber section, there is a common atrioventricular junction, but one that is exclusively connected to the right ventricle because of double inlet atrioventricular connection (compare with Figure 41.9).

ventricles is found in both settings. Other hearts can have a common atrioventricular junction guarded by a common atrioventricular valve, in contrast, which are not usually described as atrioventricular septal defects. These are the hearts with double inlet ventricle with both atrioventricular junctions guarded by a common atrioventricular valve. In these hearts (Figure 41.10), the common atrioventricular valve self-evidently does not straddle and override. In between these extremes, however, there are further spectrums of malformations that reflect the precise degree of override of the common valve. These series of anomalies parallel the spectrums of overriding of the right or left valves that will be described in the body of this chapter. In such hearts with eccentric commitment of the common atrioventricular valve, it is again hard to make the distinction between double inlet and biventricular atrioventricular connections. Here, the decision reached could affect clinical decision-making, since the patient, depending on the decision made, will be categorized as having either double inlet ventricle or an atrioventricular septal defect with either right or left ventricular dominance (Figure 41.11). This could affect the options for univentricular as opposed to biventricular repair. From the morphological stance also, the decision is harder to make than when either the right or left valve is straddling, since it requires the use of a '75% rule' rather than a '50% rule' (Figure 41.11). In clinical terms, it is almost certainly the size of the ventricle that is most important in determining the feasibility of biventricular versus univentricular repair, but the precise atrioventricular connection is by no means insignificant. This is again made, therefore, on the basis of the perceived attachments of the overriding

junction, using the best information available to reach this decision. We will not consider further in this chapter those hearts with common valve that are intermediate between the extremes of atrioventricular septal defect and double inlet ventricle, but they exist in the same patterns of right and left hand ventricular topology that will be discussed for straddling and overriding of separate right and left atrioventricular valves.

Before leaving the topic of definitions, it is important to return to the problems that exist in distinguishing a common valve from a straddling solitary valve associated with absence of one atrioventricular connection (Figure 41.8). As already stated, we use the arrangement of the atrial septum as our arbiter. In almost all hearts in which one atrioventricular connection is absent, the atrial septum fuses with the parietal atrial wall in a way that separates the blind-ending atrial chamber from the patent atrioventricular junction. This arrangement is seen even when the valve guarding the right or left atrioventricular junction is itself straddling and overriding between the ventricles (Figure 41.8). This morphological pattern serves to distinguish these hearts in which one atrium is connected to both ventricles, in other words those with a uniatrial but biventricular atrioventricular connection (Figure 41.8), from other hearts with comparable connection of one atrium to both ventricles, so-called 'double outlet atrium', in which there is a common atrioventricular junction. In this last group, which unequivocally has straddling and overriding of an atrioventricular valve, the valve itself is common to both the atriums because the atrial septum has failed to fuse with the parietal atrioventricular junction (Figure 41.12).

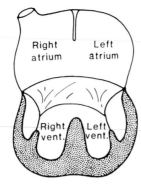

a) Common valve

straddling with equal commitment

– concordant connection

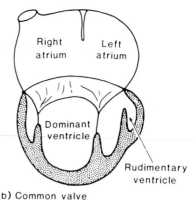

b) Common valve

total commitment to one chamber

no straddling

– double inlet ventricle

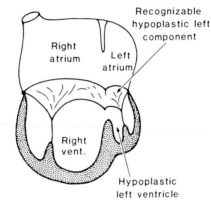

c) Common valve

straddling with unequal commitment

hypoplasia of left–sided component

–concordant connection with dominant RV

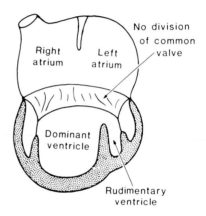

d) Common valve

straddling with unequal commitment

no division of right and left components

– double inlet ventricle

Figure 41.11. A common valve can be found in the setting of concordant atrioventricular connections (Figure 41.9 and (a)) or can be exclusively connected to one ventricle (Figure 41.10 and (b)). Any number of transitional forms exist between these extremes. Some of these result from hypoplasia of the right or left side of the heart, with (c) showing left-sided hypoplasia. Others, however, are analogous to the situation found with overriding of a right or left atrioventricular valve (d). In this setting, the atrioventricular connection is adjudicated on the basis of the '75% rule', with the illustrated example having double inlet ventricle.

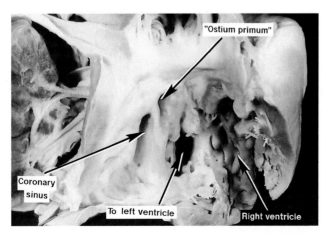

Figure 41.12. In some cases of atrioventricular septal defect with common atrioventricular junction, the junction is shared between the ventricles but committed exclusively to one atrium because of malalignment of the atrial septum. This produces one variant of double outlet atrium, with this heart showing double outlet right atrium. This entity is distinguished from absent connection with straddling valve (Figure 41.8) because the left atrial myocardium is continuous with the common junction through the 'ostium primum' defect. This heart also has a persistent left superior caval vein draining through the enlarged coronary sinus.

This, in turn, is the consequence of malalignment between the atrial and ventricular septums. The space between the malaligned atrial septum in these hearts and the atrioventricular junction is the 'ostium primum' defect. It can be argued that, in such a setting, this inter-atrial communication can become gradually smaller until it disappears and, therefore, the entities should be grouped together. In morphogenetic terms, there is much to commend such an approach. From the stance of strict morphology, however, the junction remains a common structure until the primary foramen, or the 'ostium primum', has closed. The hearts with common atrioventricular valves and double outlet atrium (Horiuchi et al, 1976) are discussed further in Chapter 36. Those with a uniatrial but biventricular atrioventricular connection (Figure 41.8) will receive further attention in this chapter and are also discussed in Chapter 40.

INCIDENCE AND AETIOLOGY

In that all atrioventricular septal defects with common orifice have a straddling valve as here defined, they should strictly be included in statistics concerning incidence. Because of problems of this kind, and because recognition of straddling and overriding is a recent event, it is difficult, if not impossible, to give precise figures. In a postmortem series of 1300 specimens with congenital heart disease, 10 cases were found with straddling valve. The estimate in a clinical series from the same centre was lower, making up only 0.20% of the patients seen (Quero-Jimenez and Otero Coto, 1981). In our experience, straddling valves are now recognized with much more frequency now that they are specifically sought, particularly in anomalies such as congenitally corrected transposition (Chapter 49), hearts with double inlet ventricle (Chapter 38) and in double outlet right ventricle with subpulmonary ventricular septal defect (Kitamura et al, 1974; Chapter 50). It is also significant that clinical recognition of straddling of atrioventricular valves, as opposed to overriding, was not possible before the development of cross-sectional echocardiography. The tensor apparatus could not be identified in detail using angiography; consequently, straddling could only be inferred from the demonstration of the valvar orifice overriding the ventricular septum. As either overriding and straddling can exist in isolation, there were obvious diagnostic limitations. Straddling valves in the context of congenital heart disease as a whole, therefore, are considered as rare but significant malformations.

In terms of aetiology, straddling mitral and tricuspid valves have been produced in rat fetuses exposed to nimustine (1-(4-amino-2-methyl-5-pyramidinyl)methyl-3(2-chlorethyl-3-nitrosourea hydrochloride)) (Mijagawa et al, 1988). Straddling tricuspid valve was also produced in the chick by mechanically preventing expansion of the right atrioventricular junction (Gessner, 1972).

MORPHOLOGY AND DIAGNOSIS

Although straddling right or left atrioventricular valves can be found with any segmental combination (Milo et al, 1979; Anderson and Ho, 1981), description and diagnosis is simplified if they are considered in five series of malformations (Figure 41.13). Four of the five concern straddling of either the right or left atrioventricular valve in the settings of right hand or left hand ventricular topology, respectively. As we have discussed, a common valve can also straddle and override with either right hand or left hand ventricular topology (upper and lower panels of Figure 41.13) and show all the extremes between double inlet and biventricular atrioventricular connections. As explained, however, these variants with common valve will not be further discussed in this chapter, although it would be entirely appropriate to include such details. The middle panel of Figure 41.13 is the lesion that has uniatrial but biventricular atrioventricular connection. As we will see, there are also several

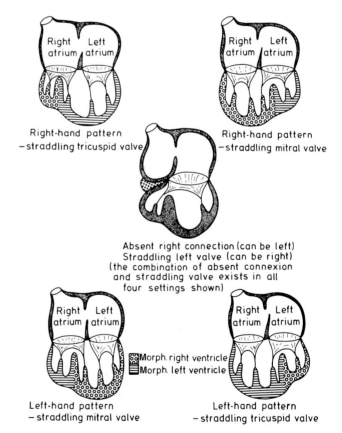

Figure 41.13. Overriding and straddling between the extremes of double inlet or biventricular atrioventricular connection can be found in various settings. This figure shows the settings that exist with usually arranged atrial chambers. The upper panels show straddling and overriding with right hand ventricular topology, while the lower panels show comparable arrangements with left hand topology. Similar variants with straddling of the right-sided and left-sided valves are found with mirror-imaged and isomeric atrial arrangements. There is still further variation for the option of a straddling valve coexisting with an absent atrioventricular connection (centre panel). The different settings for this combination are shown in Figure 41.32.

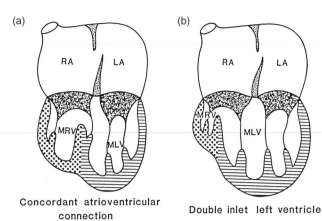

Concordant atrioventricular
connection

Double inlet left ventricle

Figure 41.14. When the right atrioventricular valve (tricuspid) straddles and overrides in the setting of usual atrial arrangement and right hand ventricular topology, the extremes of the spectrum for the atrioventricular connections are concordant (a) and double inlet left ventricle with right-sided rudimentary and incomplete right ventricle (b). RA, right atrium; LA, left atrium; MRV, morphologically right ventricle; MLV, morphologically left ventricle.

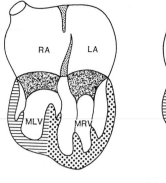

(a) Discordant atrioventricular connection

(b) Double inlet right ventricle (right-sided rudimentary LV)

Figure 41.15. The straddling and overriding of the right atrioventricular valve (mitral) with usual atrial arrangement and left hand ventricular topology can give rise to discordant atrioventricular connections (a) and double inlet right ventricle with right-sided rudimentary left ventricle. Abbreviations as in Figure 41.14.

morphological variants of this prototype depending on ventricular topology and the side of the absent connection. For the present, nonetheless, we are concerned with the four patterns in which either the right or left atrioventricular valve is straddling.

The first of these spectrums is straddling of the right (morphologically tricuspid) atrioventricular valve in the setting of right hand ventricular topology (Figure 41.3a). When the larger part of the overriding junction in this spectrum is committed to the dominant ventricle, the entity is best described as double inlet left ventricle with right-sided right ventricle and straddling right atrioventricular valve (Figure 41.14b). The other extreme in the spectrum is straddling tricuspid valve with concordant atrioventricular connections (Figure 41.14a). The second series comprises hearts in which the straddling valve is a right-sided morphologically mitral valve in a heart with left hand ventricular topology. The extreme connections are, on the one hand, discordant atrioventricular connections and, on the other, double inlet right ventricle with right-sided left ventricle (Figure 41.15). The third series places straddling of a left-sided morphologically mitral valve in a ventricular mass with right hand topology, with the extremes in terms of commitment of the overriding junction producing effectively concordant atrioventricular connections on the one hand, and double inlet right ventricle with left-sided morphologically left ventricle on the other (Figure 41.16). The fourth series involves the extremes of override of a straddling left-sided morphologically tricuspid valve in left hand ventricular topology between discordant atrioventricular connections (Figure 41.17a) and double inlet left ventricle with left-sided morphologically right ventricle (Figure

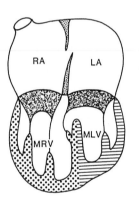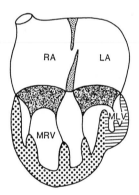

(a) Concordant AV connection   (b) Double inlet right ventricle

Figure 41.16. Straddling and overriding of the left atrioventricular valve (mitral) is shown in the setting of the usual atrial arrangement and right hand ventricular topology. Following the sequence in Figures 41.14 and 41.15, this can give rise to a spectrum from concordant atrioventricular connections (a) to double inlet right ventricle (b). Abbreviations as in Figure 41.14.

41.17b). Usual atrial arrangement has been presumed for each of these series, but all can exist with mirror-imaged atrial arrangement, as well as in hearts with isomeric atrial appendages. The ventricular topology will always be such that a given heart can be placed in one of the above series according to whether the straddling valve is right or left sided.

While it might appear self-evident that straddling of an atrioventricular valve implies the presence of a ventricular septal defect, hearts are found in which an overriding atrioventricular valve straddles the septum but the valvar

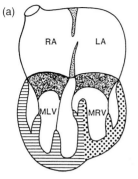

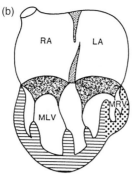

Discordant atrioventricular connection

Double inlet left ventricle (Left-sided rudimentary RV)

Figure 41.17. This completes the sequence for usual atrial arrangement shown in Figure 41.14–41.16 and illustrates the spectrum for straddling and overriding of the left-sided valve (tricuspid) with left hand ventricular topology from discordant atrioventricular connections (a) to double inlet left ventricle with left-sided rudimentary right ventricle (b). Abbreviations as in Figure 41.14.

leaflets are firmly adherent to the septal crest as they straddle (Isomatu et al, 1989). In such cases, a bridging tongue between the straddling leaflets usually creates two orifices within the overriding valve, with one valvar orifice then opening into each ventricle. This situation is comparable to the atrioventricular septal defect with common atrioventricular junction guarded by separate right and left atrioventricular valves (Chapter 36).

It is now well recognized that straddling atrioventricular valves are frequently associated with so-called 'criss-cross' hearts and superoinferior ventricles (Chapter 49; Aziz et al, 1979; Milo et al, 1979; Tabry et al, 1979; Rice et al, 1985; Robinson et al, 1985; Anderson et al, 1987; Geva et al, 1991). There is no justification, however, for grouping such hearts together into one separate category, since that would be to deny the whole point of the method of sequential chamber localization. No matter how bizarre the morphology of the heart, its sequential arrangement can always be determined, and the presence of straddling and overriding valves recognized within these combinations.

STRADDLING RIGHT (TRICUSPID) VALVE IN THE SETTING OF RIGHT HAND VENTRICULAR TOPOLOGY

The essence of the series of straddling right valve in the setting of right hand ventricular topology is that the valve usually overrides the posterior part of a ventricular septum that does not extend to the crux (Wenink and Gittenberger de Groot, 1982). When the atrioventricular connections are concordant, the septum joins the atrioventricular junction in its posteroinferior quadrant,

whereas when the connection is basically double inlet, the septum joins the junction more or less at the acute margin. When the degree of override is approximately equal, the septum joins the junction halfway between the crux and the acute margin (Figure 41.3a). Irrespective of the precise atrioventricular connection, the septum does not reach the crux and is malaligned relative to the atrial septum (Figure 41.18). Because of this, there is an abnormal atrioventricular conduction system (Milo et al, 1979; Anderson, 1990). The connecting atrioventricular node is always formed at the site where the ventricular septum joins the atrioventricular junction, the bundle branches being disposed astride the posteroinferior part of the septum (Figure 41.19). We have, on one occasion, seen straddling of a tricuspid valve through a muscular inlet defect in the absence of override of the atrioventricular junction in a heart with concordant atrioventricular connections. The conduction system then came from a regular atrioventricular node.

The size and morphology of the right ventricle depend in part on the degree of override. When the valve is connected mostly to the right ventricle, the ventricle tends to be of more-or-less normal morphology (Figure 41.20a). When the junction is mostly connected to the left ventricle, the right ventricular morphology is virtually identical to that found in hearts with double inlet left ventricle (Figure 41.20b). Various ventriculo-arterial connections can be found, and these also influence the size of the right ventricle. When the ventriculo-arterial connections are

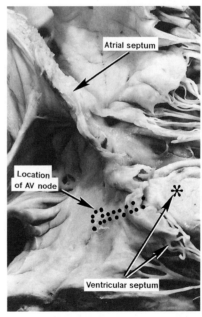

Figure 41.18. This heart has been sectioned in simulated four chamber projection. It shows how the pathognomonic feature of straddling and overriding of the tricuspid valve with right hand ventricular topology is malalignment between the atrial and muscular ventricular septums. In this heart, the atrioventricular connections are concordant, but because of the septal malalignment, the atrioventricular conduction axis arises from an anomalous posteroinferior atrioventricular node formed at the point where the ventricular septum meets the atrioventricular junction.

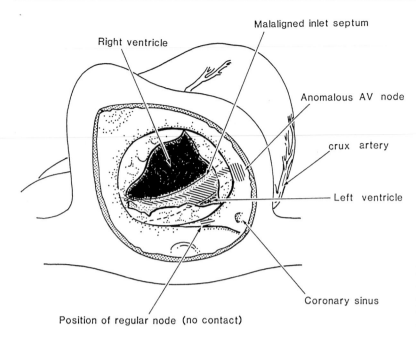

Figure 41.19. The disposition of the conduction tissue in straddling tricuspid valve with usual atrial arrangement and right hand ventricular topology (see Figure 41.18) is shown as it would be seen by the surgeon through a right atriotomy. AV, atrioventricular.

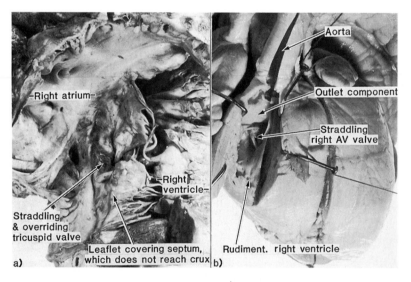

Figure 41.20. The morphologically right ventricle, when there is a straddling tricuspid valve in the setting of usual atrial arrangement and right hand ventricular topology (this heart is shown in sectional format in Figures 41.4 and 41.19), is comparable with the normal right ventricle when the atrioventricular connections are concordant (a), except of course for the straddling valvar leaflets. When the atrioventricular connection is effectively double inlet (b), however, the right ventricle is much more rudimentary and closely resembles that seen in 'classical' double inlet left ventricle.

concordant, it has been customary to describe the entity as an 'isolated ventricular septal defect of atrioventricular canal type' (Neufeld et al, 1961; Rastelli et al, 1968; LaCorte et al, 1976; Van Praagh et al, 1989). This is an inappropriate description since the left atrioventricular valve in hearts with straddling tricuspid valve is morphologically mitral. It does not guard part of a common atrioventricular junction as it does in the setting of an 'atrioventricular canal' (Smallhorn et al, 1981b; Anderson et al, 1998; see Chapter 36). Rarely, nonetheless, a common valve can override in a fashion analogous to the straddling tricuspid valve. This is found with marked malalignment between the atrial and ventricular septal structures, and with the common atrioventricular junction connected predominantly within the dominant left ventricle. The atrioventricular conduction tissues are then disposed in similar anomalous fashion (Pillai et al, 1984). Complete transposition, double outlet right

ventricle and Fallot's tetralogy can also be complicated by straddling of the tricuspid valve.

In terms of echocardiographic diagnosis, the most important feature is the malalignment between the atrial and ventricular septal structures (Figure 41.21; Smallhorn et al, 1981a). In the past, this feature made it possible to make the diagnosis using the M-mode technique, since the valvar leaflets of the right atrioventricular valve crossed the crest of the ventricular septum, meeting in diastole behind it (Seward et al, 1975). Such niceties are now of only historical interest, since cross-sectional examinations show the precise morphology present, particularly when conducted via the trans-oesophageal portal (Figure 41.21). In the great majority of cases, both atrioventricular valves are attached to the atrial septum at the same level. This is clearly seen in transthoracic subcostal and apical four chamber cuts (Smallhorn et al, 1981a, 1982). In those rare cases where

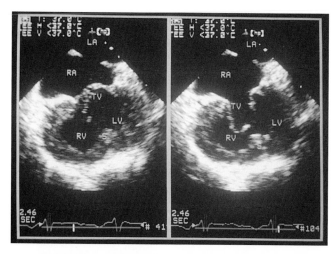

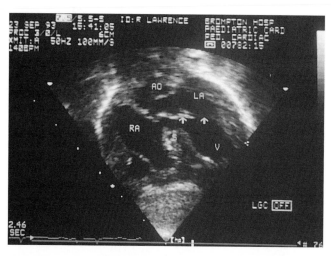

Figure 41.21. Cross-sectional echos in ventricular systole (left) and diastole (right) are taken from the transoesophageal portal and show overriding of the right atrioventricular junction in the setting of straddling tricuspid valve (TV) with effectively concordant atrioventricular connections. RV, right ventricle; LV, left ventricle; RA, right atrium; LA, left atrium.

Figure 41.22. This transthoracic subcostal echocardiogram shows straddling of the tension apparatus of the tricuspid valve (arrowed) in the absence of junctional overriding. The atrioventricular septal structures were intact in this patient; note the normal 'wedged' position of the aorta (AO). S, septum; V, left ventricle; other abbreviations as in Figure 41.21.

there is straddling but no overriding (Figure 41.22), the atrioventricular septum will be intact, producing normal offsetting of the atrioventricular valves (Smallhorn et al, 1981a). Overriding of the annulus is assessed according to the location of the ventricular septum. This is best done in a cut in which the overriding junction and the ventricular septum are visualized without showing the mitral annulus. A normal four chamber cut may be too anterior to detect the displacement of the posterior extent of the ventricular septum. This is important in the differentiation of straddling tricuspid valve from a simple perimembranous inlet defect (Smallhorn et al, 1982).

Suspicion should be raised of a straddling valve whenever one ventricle is found to be unexpectedly hypoplastic. This used to be of great value when angiography was the technique used for diagnosis (Figure 41.23; Shinebourne et al, 1983). Easy passage of the catheter from the right atrium to both ventricles was suggestive, but certainly not diagnostic, of a straddling valve. Much more suggestive was a right atrial injection that opacified both ventricles in two streams (Figure 41.24a; Liberthson et al, 1971). Most reliable was a ventricular injection profiled to demonstrate the ventricular septum in relation to the overriding valvar orifice (Figure 41.24b; Soto et al, 1985). Malalignment of the ventricular septum relative to the crux, however, and the tendency of the heart as a whole to be rotated or tilted in association with crisscross or superoinferior ventricles made it very difficult to predict the orientation of the ventricular septum using angiography. The accuracy of echocardiographic diagnosis now obviates the need for angiography, particularly when accompanied by flow mapping or when performed from the transoesophageal or transgastric windows (Figure 41.21).

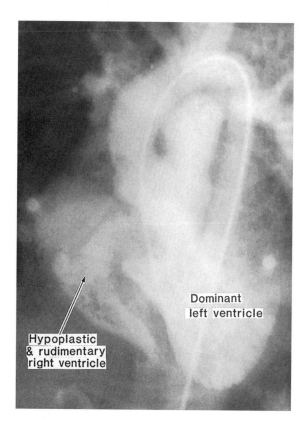

Dominant left ventricle

Hypoplastic & rudimentary right ventricle

Figure 41.23. Hypoplasia of the right ventricle as seen angiocardiographically in a patient with straddling tricuspid valve. The part of the right junction committed to the left ventricle is shown by unopacified blood (see also Figure 41.24). (Reproduced by kind permission of Dr R. M. Freedom, Hospital for Sick Children, Toronto.)

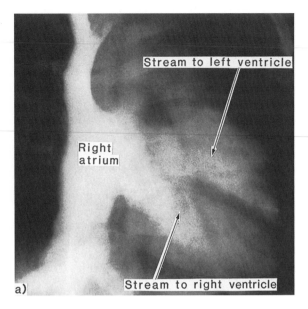

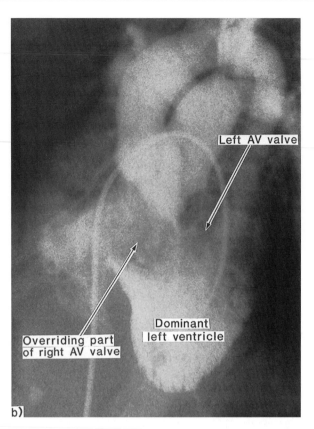

Figure 41.24. These angiograms show (a) splitting of the stream from the right atrium and (b) commitment of the junction to both ventricle in the setting of straddling and overriding of the tricuspid valve. (Reproduced by kind permission of Dr R. M. Freedom, Hospital for Sick Children, Toronto.)

STRADDLING RIGHT (MITRAL) VALVE IN THE SETTING OF LEFT HAND VENTRICULAR TOPOLOGY

In the setting of left hand ventricular topology, a straddling right valve (Figure 41.15), covers the anterior part of a septum that does extend to the crux (Sieg et al, 1977; Becker et al, 1980). When the overriding atrioventricular junction is connected mostly to the left-sided morphologically right ventricle, then the atrioventricular connection is effectively double inlet right ventricle. The right-sided morphologically left ventricle may than be no more than a posteroinferior slit, particularly as the ventriculo-arterial connection is almost always double outlet from the dominant right ventricle. Double outlet right ventricle is also the expected ventriculo-arterial connection when the atrioventricular connections are discordant rather than double inlet. Alternatively, there may be single outlet with pulmonary atresia, the aorta arising from the right ventricle. Concordant or discordant ventriculo-arterial connections are very rare. The disposition of the conduction tissues is dictated by the left hand pattern of ventricular topology. When the ventriculo-arterial connection is double outlet from the right ventricle, it is possible for both anterior and posterior atrioventricular nodes to make contact with the ventricular conduction tissues, giving a so-called 'sling'

(Monckeberg, 1913; Wenink, 1979; Becker et al, 1980). This is in contrast to the expected situation in congenitally corrected transposition, where only the anterior node makes contact with the ventricular conduction tissues (Anderson et al, 1974). Kurosawa and colleagues (1990), nonetheless, have described a heart with congenitally corrected transposition and straddling mitral valve in which there was only a regularly positioned node and bundle. There was an anterocephalic continuation of the bundle, which vanished into a 'dead-end tract'. Both the presence of a sling and the existence of a regular posterior node reflect the better alignment of the atrial and muscular ventricular septums in the presence of double outlet right ventricle (Figure 41.25b).

The presence of straddling of the mitral valve should always be suspected when clinical investigation suggests discordant atrioventricular connections but the morphologically left ventricle is small. Cross-sectional echocardiography is again the diagnostic technique of choice (Figure 41.26). Angiography, nonetheless, with injections into the right atrium, sometimes shows the division of the stream between the ventricles (Figure 41.25a). Ventricular angiograms taken in the appropriate projection should illustrate the degree of override of the atrioventricular junction, but this will be better quantified using echocardiography, particularly from the transoesophageal window.

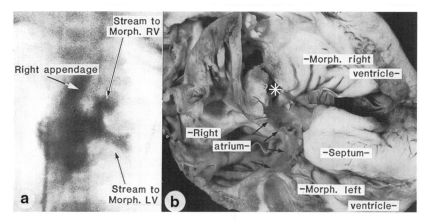

Figure 41.25. (a) Angiocardiogram shows splitting of the stream of right atrial contrast (compare with Figure 41.24a). (b) Postmortem specimen from the same patient showing straddling and overriding of the morphologically mitral valve in a heart with left hand ventricular topology and effectively discordant atrioventricular connections. Note the alignment of the atrial and ventricular septums, with the subpulmonary outflow tract (asterisk) connected in the right ventricle (double outlet right ventricle). Abbreviations as in Figure 41.21.

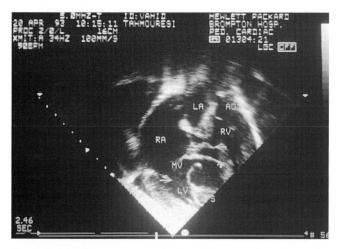

Figure 41.26. This cross-sectional echocardiogram, taken subcostally, shows straddling of the tension apparatus of the mitral valve (MV) in a patient with effectively discordant atrioventricular connections. AO, aorta; S, septum; other abbreviations as in Figure 41.21.

STRADDLING LEFT (MITRAL) VALVE IN THE SETTING OF RIGHT HAND VENTRICULAR TOPOLOGY

This, the straddling mitral valve in the setting of right hand ventricular topology (Freedom et al, 1978), is again encountered most frequently in association with double outlet right ventricle, be the atrioventricular connections concordant (Kitamura et al, 1974; Aziz et al, 1979; Muster et al, 1979) or double inlet right ventricle. The essence of the anomaly is that the mitral valve straddles and overrides the anterior part of the muscular ventricular septum. With this arrangement, nonetheless, the posterior part of the septum does extend to the crux (Figure 41.27). Because of this, the conduction tissues are located in their usual position for the normal heart irrespective of the atrioventricular connection (Milo et al, 1979). The leaflet of the mitral valve, which straddles into the right ventricle, is

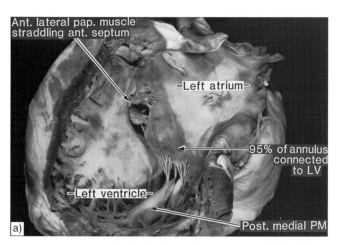

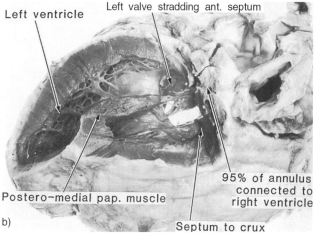

Figure 41.27. The extremes of overriding of a left-sided mitral valve as seen from the left ventricular aspect in the setting of usual atrial arrangement and right hand ventricular topology. (a) The atrioventricular connections are concordant. (b) Effective double inlet right ventricle is shown. In both cases, the valve straddles the outlet part of a septum, which continues to reach to the crux.

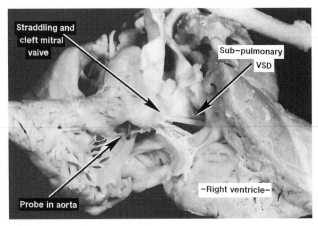

Figure 41.28. Overriding and straddling of a cleft mitral valve is shown from the right ventricle in a heart with effectively concordant atrioventricular connections. This is an example of the 'Taussig–Bing' malformation (see Chapter 50). VSD, ventricular septal defect.

itself frequently cleft (Figure 41.28; Soto et al, 1985). This feature emphasizes, in the setting of intact atrioventricular septal structures, the difference between a true cleft of a morphologically mitral valve and the zone of apposition between the bridging leaflets to be found in hearts with atrioventricular septal defect and common atrioventricular junction (Chapter 36).

Diagnosis of the anomaly using cross-sectional techniques, particularly combined with flow mapping and use of the transoesophageal window, is remarkably accurate (Figure 41.29). Though ventricular hypoplasia, when it occurs, usually affects the left ventricle, Geva and colleagues (1991) have described a small series of right-sided hearts with usual arrangement and straddling mitral valve with concordant atrioventricular connections and double outlet right ventricle. In the patients they encountered, diagnosed using cross-sectional echocardiography, it was the right ventricle that was hypoplastic, together

with tricuspid stenosis and hypoplasia, a large right ventricular outflow tract, an anterior ventricular septal defect and criss-cross atrioventricular relations.

A presumptive angiocardiographic diagnosis of straddling mitral valve can be made either directly following left atrial injection or by observing the flow of contrast-free blood through the annulus following a ventricular injection in the four chamber projection (Soto et al, 1985). As with the other entities discussed in this chapter, the need for angiographic investigation has now been obviated by the accuracy of cross-sectional echocardiography.

STRADDLING LEFT (TRICUSPID) VALVE IN THE SETTING OF LEFT HAND VENTRICULAR TOPOLOGY

In the series comprising straddling left (tricuspid) valve with left hand ventricular topograph, the straddling valve overrides the posterior part of the muscular ventricular septum, which does not extend to the crux. The two extremes of the series are congenitally corrected transposition with straddling tricuspid valve on the one hand (Figure 41.17a) and double inlet left ventricle with left-sided morphologically right ventricle on the other (Figure 41.17b). The ventriculo-arterial connections in either type are usually discordant, but other connections must be anticipated. Whatever the atrioventricular connections, the ventricular conduction tissues arise from an anterolateral node in the right atrioventricular junction. A long non-branching bundle encircles the pulmonary valvar orifice to reach and branch on the anterosuperior part of the muscular ventricular septum (Figure 41.30; Milo et al, 1979).

As with straddling tricuspid valve with right hand ventricular topology, it was possible to diagnose this variant with single-beam echocardiography because the two valves closed behind the septum during diastole. The diagnosis is made nowadays using cross-sectional

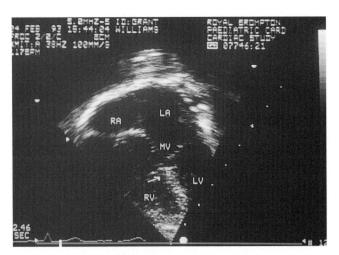

Figure 41.29. This four chamber echocardiographic cut taken subcostally shows straddling and overriding of the left (mitral) atrioventricular valve (MV) in the setting of usual atrial arrangement and right hand ventricular topology. Abbreviations as in Figure 41.21.

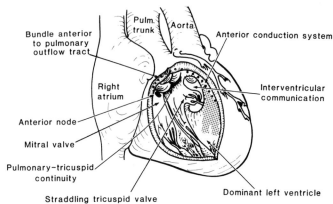

Figure 41.30. The disposition of the conduction tissues as seen through the morphologically left ventricle (right-sided) in a patient with usual atrial arrangement, left hand ventricular topology and straddling tricuspid (left-sided) valve.

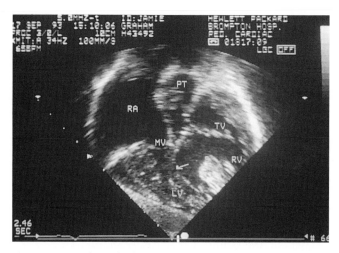

Figure 41.31. Subcostal echocardiogram in a patient with effectively discordant atrioventricular connections shows the tension apparatus of the tricuspid valve straddling through an inlet ventricular septal defect. MV, mitral valve; PT, pulmonary trunk; other abbreviations as in Figure 41.21.

techniques (Figure 41.31). This shows both the degree of override of the annulus and the precise attachments of the straddling valvar tension apparatus (Rice et al, 1985). The entity should be suspected whenever the morphologically right ventricle is unexpectedly small in patients thought to have congenitally corrected transposition, or unusually large when the working diagnosis is double inlet left ventricle with left-sided rudimentary right ventricle. As with all the other variants, angiography has been rendered obsolete by the excellence of cross-sectional echocardiography, particularly when carried out from the transoesophageal portal.

—— SURGICAL OPTIONS ——

In determining the surgical options, then both the precise connections of the overriding junction and the arrangement of the straddling tension apparatus are important, together with the size of the rudimentary ventricle (Tabry et al, 1979; McGoon et al, 1981). It is also important not to rule out palliative operations, since in the long run these may offer the best chance of success. Palliative procedures performed have included redirection of the circulations at either atrial or arterial levels, banding of the pulmonary trunk or release of a previously placed band, construction of systemic-to-pulmonary arterial shunts, or replacement of a regurgitant straddling valve and placement of a dacron graft to the pulmonary trunk in order to bypass pulmonary stenosis. In selected patients, more corrective surgery can be performed by using a variant of the Fontan procedure; alternatively, septation and biventricular repair can be achieved in those with the most favourable anatomy. This is particularly the case when valvar overriding exists in the absence of straddling. This presents only a minor problem to the surgeon, since any

patch placed to close a ventricular septal defect can be deviated to the plane that passes between the atrioventricular valves (McGoon et al, 1981). By contrast, straddling of an atrioventricular valve, or very rarely both valves, presents major problems. The key choice to be made, if opting for correction rather than palliation, is whether to settle for a univentricular repair, which will be some variant of the Fontan procedure, or to seek biventricular repair by opting for more complex septation. If one atrioventricular connection is absent, then biventricular repair is virtually impossible, although it may theoretically be possible to resect the atrial septum and divide the overriding valve if each ventricle is of substantial size and the ventriculo-arterial connections are concordant. If the arrangement of the straddling tension apparatus is such that the aberrant cords insert within 1 cm of the crest of the ventricular septum (Tabry et al, 1979), then the straddling can be dealt with by closing the defect in such a way as to leave the cords that were on the wrong side of the ventricular septum on the correct side of the patch. This is straightforward if the cords are straddling towards the surgeon, as would be the case in concordant atrioventricular connections with straddling mitral valve. It is not so simple when the straddling cords insert on the far side of the ventricular septum from the surgeon, as is the case with straddling tricuspid valve and right hand ventricular topology. The technical challenge of securing the patch on the 'wrong' side of the septum is then comparable with the technique used to avoid the conduction tissues in patients with discordant atrioventricular connections uncomplicated by straddling (de Leval et al, 1979). Sometimes it may be necessary to enlarge the defect in order to bring the straddling cords nearer its margin (Tabry et al, 1979; Piot et al, 1993). Further possibilities include, very occasionally, division of a single straddling cord attached to a limited amount of atrioventricular valvar tissue (Kirklin and Barratt-Boyes, 1993). Alternatively, the cords may be passed through a slot in the patch (Pacifico et al, 1979). The slot is then sutured to create the smallest possible residual defect consistent with free movement of the cord.

When the straddling tension apparatus is attached only to one papillary muscle, or to an area of the muscular ventricular septum in the inappropriate ventricle, then that muscle may be sectioned at its base if it has no other cordal attachments. The septal defect can then be closed and the papillary muscle reattached to the patch or the intraventricular tunnel thus created (Kirklin and Barratt-Boyes, 1993). This approach has been used extensively by the group of surgeons working at the University of California in San Francisco (Reddy et al, 1997).

With tension apparatus inserting on the muscular ventricular septum further than 1 cm from its crest, or inserting into the parietal wall of the dominant ventricle, the mortality of attempted biventricular repair was prohibitive and often involved replacing the straddling valve with a prosthesis (McGoon et al, 1981).

There is also the problem of avoiding the conduction tissues when attempting to close the ventricular septal defect or achieving septation in hearts with straddling atrioventricular valves. As we have described, the arrangement is frequently abnormal, even in hearts with straddling tricuspid valve and concordant atrioventricular connections (Figure 41.19). Indeed, in the series of cases reported by Pacifico et al (1979), surgically induced atrioventricular dissociation was a major complication. This was presumably because the ventricular conduction tissues were presumed to arise from the regular atrioventricular node located in the triangle of Koch. As we have emphasized, in this entity the node is formed at the point where the muscular ventricular septum makes contact with the atrioventricular junction. The group from Paris, nonetheless, achieved success in avoiding heart block simply by placing very fine sutures in the crest of the ventricular septum (Serraf et al, 1996). It would seem more prudent to us for surgeons to attempt to avoid the known site of the atrioventricular node. This is always abnormal in the group of hearts with straddling left valve in the setting of left hand ventricular topology and usually deviates from the normal when the right valve straddles in this setting (Anderson, 1997). These arrangements are already well recognized in patients with congenitally corrected transposition (Chapter 49).

All things considered, surgical repair of straddling valves is a daunting prospect. As McGoon et al (1981) suggested, the approach of choice for needful infants or small children remains a palliative one: banding or shunting as appropriate. When straddling is minimal, and the patient is larger, closure of the defect by deviating the patch is to be recommended. This may also be done in infancy when there is no valvar regurgitation. The recent excellent results reported by Serraf and colleagues (1996) and by Reddy and his associates (1997) point to the potential advantages of this approach. When the morphology precludes deviation of the patch, it is still possible to replace the straddling valve and close the ventricular septal defect once the patients have reached a suitable age. In all of these situations, nonetheless, many would consider the modified Fontan procedure a safer approach despite its long-term uncertainties. Russo and colleagues (1988) reported only two deaths after a modified Fontan operation in a group of 12 patients with double outlet right ventricle, three of whom had straddling mitral and nine straddling tricuspid valves. Both deaths were in the group with straddling tricuspid valve. Three of the patients described by Geva and colleagues (1991) have undergone successful repair using the modified Fontan approach, and several of the patients in the series reported from New Delhi were submitted for Fontan-type surgery because of the presence of straddling atrioventricular valves (Murari et al, 1998). With the renaissance of interest in transatrial septation (Kurosawa et al, 1990; Uemura and Yagihara, 1998), this procedure will provide another option for those with straddling valves and double inlet atrioventricular connection.

STRADDLING VALVES WITH ABSENT ATRIOVENTRICULAR CONNECTION

Hearts in which one atrioventricular connection is absent and the solitary atrioventricular valve straddles and overrides the ventricular septum are extremely rare and exceedingly complex anatomically (Ho et al, 1982). They form a specific subset of atrioventricular connections, giving an arrangement that is neither biventricular nor univentricular but which is uniatrial and biventricular (Anderson and Rigby, 1987; Anderson and Ho, 1997). This group is important for understanding the range of morphology to be found in congenitally malformed hearts, and it emphasizes the value of sequential segmental analysis. We have now seen examples with absence of either the right or left atrioventricular connections, and with either right hand or left hand ventricular topology (Figure 41.32). Furthermore, for each prototypic heart shown in Figure 41.32, there are two

Right–hand ventricular topology

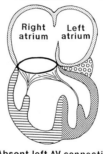
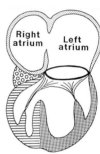

(a) **Absent left AV connection** Straddling right (tricuspid) valve

(b) **Absent right AV connection** Straddling left (mitral) valve

Left–hand ventricular topology

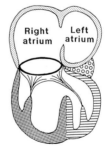
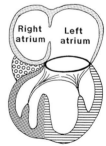

(c) **Absent left AV connection** Straddling right (mitral) valve

(d) **Absent right AV connection** Straddling left (tricuspid) valve

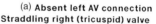

▭ Morph. right ventricle
▨ Morph. left ventricle

Figure 41.32. Absence of either the right or the left atrioventricular connection can coexist with straddling of the other atrioventricular valve in patients with usual atrial arrangement when there is either right hand (a,b) or left hand (c,d) ventricular topology. There is further variation in terms of the dominance of the ventricles, different ventriculo-arterial connection, and so on.

hearts, structure depending on which ventricle is dominant. This means that there are eight possible arrangements in all. All but one of these were described by Ho and colleagues in 1982. The missing one, as yet undescribed to the best of our knowledge, would have absence of the left connection with straddling right atrioventricular valve, probably of mitral morphology, a dominant right ventricle and left hand ventricular topology. Since the report of Ho et al (1982), further cases have been described of absent right connection with dominant left ventricle, with right hand ventricular topology in one (Aiello et al, 1990) and left hand topology in four (de Vivie et al, 1989; Shinpo et al, 1992). Shinpo and colleagues (1992) also described eight cases with usual atrial arrangement, absent left connection and straddling tricuspid valve with right hand ventricular topology.

The alert reader may notice the widespread description of ventricular topology when categorizing these hearts. Why should this be necessary? First, because it can be assumed that the disposition of the conduction system will depend on ventricular topology. Thus far, detailed histological study has only been carried out in two patients (Ho et al, 1982) but revealed unexpected findings. For example, when the right atrioventricular connection was absent and the left valve was straddling in the setting of left hand ventricular topology (Figure 41.33), a sling of conduction tissue was encountered, with the posterior node formed in the left-sided atrioventricular junction. This points again to the crucial feature of the junction between the muscular ventricular septum and the atrioventricular junction in determining the location of the atrioventricular node, along with the equally important facet of ventricular topology. Second, irrespective of how the heart is imaged, the result will be heavily dependent on the ventricular topology, even in hearts in which the blood goes round the same way physiologically. Third, from an embryological point of view, there is all the difference in the world between a heart with absent right connection in left hand and in right hand topology, just as there is a great difference between straddling mitral and straddling tricuspid valve. It is usually, but not always, possible to predict the valvar morphology from the ventricular topology, and vice-versa (Ho et al, 1982). Hence, it is best to establish both the morphology of the straddling valve and the ventricular topology. The latter, nonetheless, may be impossible to determine in some hearts (Aiello et al, 1990). If that proves to be the case, clear and unambiguous description is essential.

In the hearts with uniatrial but biventricular connection, the clinical picture will be dominated by the side of the absent connection and by other associated anomalies, such as those resulting in reduced pulmonary blood flow. The clue to diagnosis will be either finding a most unexpected ventricular morphology or else observing at echocardiography the finding of the straddling valve combined with the absent connection (Figure 41.34). During echocardiographic examination, it is important to assess the competence of the straddling valve, since regurgitation is common, at least in straddling of the morphologically tricuspid valve (Shinpo et al, 1992). Although, on some occasions, the ventricles are of comparable size (Figure 41.8), offering the theoretical option of septation should the ventriculo-arterial connections be favourable, the morphology is so complex that the operative options are unlikely ever to extend beyond those of palliation or a modified Fontan procedure.

One case has been reported of repair in a heart with usual atrial arrangement, absent right connection with

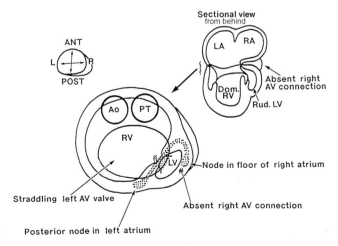

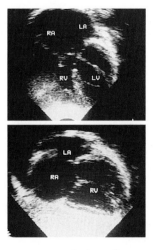

Figure 41.33. The location of a 'sling' of conduction system is shown as viewed from the atrial aspect in a heart with absent right atrioventricular (AV) connection and straddling left valve in the setting of left hand ventricular topology. The arrangement of the heart is shown in the sectional view from behind. AO, aorta; PT, pulmonary trunk; RV, right ventricle; LV, left ventricle; LA, left atrium; RA, right atrium; Dom., dominant; Rud., rudimentary.

Figure 41.34. These cross-sectional echocardiograms, obtained from the subcostal window, showing absence of the left atrioventricular connection (lower panel) with straddling and overriding of the solitary right atrioventricular valve into a ventricular mass with right hand topology (upper panel). Note how, in the lower panel, the atrial septum fuses with the atrioventricular junction (compare with Figure 41.8). Abbreviations as in Figure 41.21.

right hand ventricular topology and straddling of the left-sided morphologically mitral valve. Despite the straddling, the ventricular septal defect was restrictive and the pressure in the right ventricle was normal. It was necessary to perform a de Vega annuloplasty in order to limit incompetence of the cleft and straddling mitral valve. The septal defect was closed in such a way as to incorporate all cords in the left ventricle, and an atrioventricular conduit was connected to the large right ventricle (Gildein et al, 1990). A further repair using a Fontan procedure has been reported in a patient with usual atrial arrangement, absent right atrioventricular connection, left hand topology, straddling left-sided tricuspid valve and severe subvalvar and valvar pulmonary stenosis (Shinpo et al, 1992).

MORPHOGENESIS

The various series of hearts with straddling valves are readily explained on the basis of abnormalities of connection of the atrioventricular junctions to the ventricular trabecular components (Mehrizi et al, 1966; de la Cruz and Miller, 1968; Quero-Jimenez et al, 1973). During normal development with right hand ventricular looping (Figure 41.35a) the atrioventricular junction is initially committed exclusively to the developing left ventricle. With rightward expansion, and division, of the atrioventricular junction, the right-sided inlet becomes connected to the developing right ventricle (Lamers et al, 1995). Incomplete connection of various degree produces straddling right atrioventricular valve, while exaggerated commitment of the newly formed left atrioventricular junction to the developing right ventricle accounts for straddling and overriding of the left atrioventricular valve. The extreme of such exaggerated rightward commitment then explains pure double inlet right ventricle, the left ventricle remaining as the rudimentary and incomplete left-sided chamber. Exactly the same processes can occur with left hand ventricular looping, thus producing the other series of straddling valves (Figure 41.35b). Similar events, but with eccentric development of the atrial septum and fusion with the atrioventricular junction, will produce all the variants of straddling valve with absent atrioventricular connection. As we have discussed, straddling of an atrioventricular valve in the setting of absent atrioventricular connection produces one variant of double outlet atrium. The other variant is found in the setting of a common atrioventricular

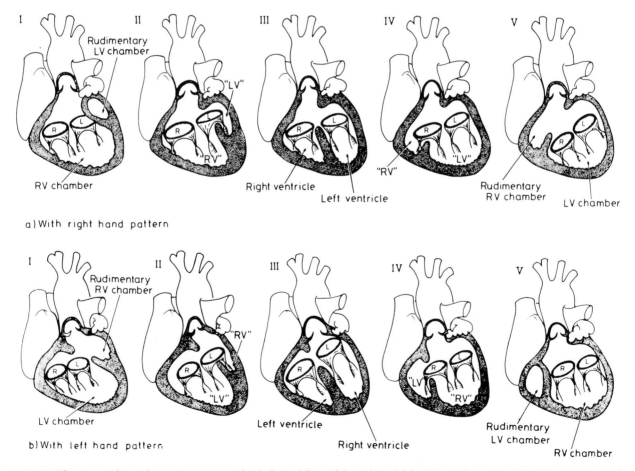

Figure 41.35. The suggested morphogenetic sequences that link straddling of the right and left valves in the setting of right hand (a) and left hand (b) ventricular topology. See text for further discussion. Abbreviations as in Figure 41.21.

junction with gross malalignment of the atrial septum (Horiuchi et al, 1976). This is well explained on the basis of eccentric formation of the atrial septum but failure of fusion with the atrioventricular junction. As we emphasized, it is the morphology of the atrial septum that serves to distinguish these lesions.

REFERENCES

Aiello V, Ho S Y, Anderson R H 1990 Absence of one atrioventricular connection associated with straddling atrioventricular valve: distinction of a solitary from a common valve and further considerations on the diagnosis of ventricular topology. American Journal of Cardiovascular Pathology 3: 107–113

Anderson R H 1990 Straddling valve. [Letter to the editor] Journal of Thoracic and Cardiovascular Surgery 100: 631

Anderson R H 1997 Surgical repair of straddling and overriding tricuspid valve. [Editorial] Cardiology in the Young 7: 122–128

Anderson R H, Ho S Y 1981 Straddling and overriding valves – segmental morphology. In: Wenink A C G (ed.) Boerhaave Series, vol. 21, The ventricular septum of the heart. Martinus Nijhoff, the Hague, p 157–173

Anderson R H, Ho S Y 1997 Sequential segmental analysis – description and categorization for the millenium. Cardiology in the Young 7: 98–116

Anderson R H, Rigby M L 1987 The morphologic heterogeneity of 'tricuspid atresia'. International Journal of Cardiology 16: 67–73

Anderson R H, Becker A E, Arnold R, Wilkinson J L 1974 The conduction tissues in congenitally corrected transposition. Circulation 50: 911–924

Anderson R H, Becker A E, Freedom R M et al 1979 Problems in the nomenclature of the univentricular heart. Herz 4: 97–106

Anderson R H, Becker A E, Tynan M, Macartney F J, Rigby M L, Wilkinson J L 1984 The univentricular atrioventricular connection: getting to the root of a thorny problem. American Journal of Cardiology 54: 822–828

Anderson R H, Smith A, Wilkinson J L 1987 Disharmony between atrioventricular connections and segmental combinations of 'crisscross' hearts. Journal of the American College of Cardiology 10: 1274–1277

Anderson R H, Ho S Y, Falcao S, Daliento L, Rigby M L 1998 The diagnostic features of atrioventricular septal defect with common atrioventricular junction. Cardiology in the Young 8: 33–49

Aziz K U, Paul M H, Muster A J, Idriss F S 1979 Positional abnormalities of atrioventricular valves in transposition of the great arteries including double outlet right ventricle, atrioventricular valve straddling and malattachment. American Journal of Cardiology 45: 1135–1145

Becker A E, Ho S Y, Caruso G, Milo S, Anderson R H 1980 Straddling right atrioventricular valves in atrioventricular discordance. Circulation 61: 1133–1141

Brandt P W T 1981 Cineangiography of atrioventricular and ventriculo-arterial connexions. In: Godman M J (ed.) Paediatric cardiology, Churchill Livingstone, Edinburgh, vol. 4, p 199–220

de la Cruz M V, Miller B L 1968 Double-inlet left ventricle. Two pathological specimens with comments on the embryology and on the relation to single ventricle. Circulation 37: 249–260

de Leval M, Bastos P, Stark J, Taylor J F N, Macartney F J, Anderson R H 1979 Surgical technique to reduce the risks of heart block following closure of ventricular septal defect in atrioventricular discordance. Journal of Thoracic and Cardiovascular Surgery 78: 515–526

de Vivie R, Van Praagh S, Bein G, Eigster G, Vogt J, Van Praagh R 1989 Transposition of the great arteries with straddling tricuspid valve. Report of two rare cases with acquired subaortic stenosis after main pulmonary artery banding. Journal of Thoracic and Cardiovascular Surgery 78: 205–213

Freedom R M, Bini R M, Dische R, Rowe R D 1978 The straddling mitral valve: morphological observations and clinical implications. European Journal of Cardiology 8: 27–50

Gessner I H 1972 Tricuspid valve in DILV. Naturally occurring in human. Experimentally produced in chick. Pediatric Research 1972; 6: 362–369

Geva T, Van Praagh S, Sanders S P, Mayer J E Jr, Van Praagh R 1991 Straddling mitral valve with hypoplastic right ventricle, double outlet right ventricle and dextrocardia: morphologic, diagnostic and surgical considerations. Journal of the American College of Cardiology 17: 1603–1612

Gildein H P, Ahmadi A, Fontan F, Mocellin F 1990 Special problems in Fontan type operations for complex congenital heart lesions. International Journal of Cardiology 29: 21–28

Ho S Y, Milo S, Anderson R H et al 1982 Straddling atrioventricular valve with absent atrioventricular connection. Report of 10 cases. British Heart Journal 47: 344–352

Horiuchi T, Saji K, Osuka Y, Sato K, Okada Y 1976 Successful correction of double outlet left atrium associated with complete atrioventricular canal and 1-loop double outlet right ventricle with stenosis of the pulmonary artery. Journal of Cardiovascular Surgery 17: 157–161

Isomatsu Y, Kurosawa H, Imai Y 1989 Straddling tricuspid valve without a ventricular septal defect. British Heart Journal 62: 222–224

Kirklin J W, Barratt-Boyes B G 1993 Cardiac Surgery, 2nd edn. Churchill Livingstone, London, p 814

Kitamura N, Takao A, Ando M, Imai Y, Konno S 1974 Taussig–Bing heart with mitral valve straddling: case reports and post-mortem study. Circulation 49: 761–767

Kurosawa H, Imai Y, Becker A E 1990 Congenitally corrected transposition with normally positioned atria, straddling mitral valve, and isolated-posterior atrioventricular node and bundle. Journal of Thoracic and Cardiovascular Surgery 99: 312–313

LaCorte M A, Fellows K E, Williams R G 1976 Overriding tricuspid valve. Echocardiographic and angiocardiographic features: 8 cases of ventricular septal defect of atrioventricular canal type. American Journal of Cardiology 37: 911–919

Lamers W H, Virágh S, Wessels A, Moorman A F M, Anderson R H 1995 Formation of the tricuspid valve in the human heart. Circulation 91: 111–121

Liberthson R R, Paul M H, Muster A J, Arcilia R A, Eckner F A O, Lev M 1971 Straddling and displaced atrioventricular orifices and valves with primitive ventricles. Circulation 43: 213–226

McGoon D C, Danielson G K, Wallace R B, Puga F J 1981 Surgical implications of straddling atrioventricular valves. In: Becker A E, Losekoot T G, Marcelletti C, Anderson R H (eds) Paediatric cardiology. Churchill Livingstone, Edinburgh, vol. 3, p 431–445

Mehrizi A, McMurphy D M, Otteson O E, Rowe R D 1966 Syndrome of double inlet left ventricle. Angiographic differentiation from single ventricle with rudimentary outlet chamber. Bulletin of the Johns Hopkins Hospital 119: 225–267

Milo S, Ho S Y, Macartney F J et al 1979 Straddling and overriding atrioventricular valves morphology and classification. American Journal of Cardiology 44: 1122–1134

Mijagawa S, Ando M, Takao A 1988 Cardiovascular anomalies produced by nimustine hydrochloride in the rat fetus. Teratology 38: 553–558

Monckeberg J G 1913 Zur Entwicklungsgeschichte des Atrioventrikularsystems. Verhandlungsband der Deutschen Gesellschaft für Pathologie 16: 228–249

Murari V, Sharma R, Airan B et al 1998 Morphology of hearts undergoing Fontan repair. Cardiology in the Young 8: 165–171

Muster A J, Bharati S, Aziz K U et al 1979 Taussig Bing anomaly with straddling mitral valve. Journal of Thoracic and Cardiovascular Surgery 77: 832–842

Neufeld H N, Titus J L, Dushane J W, Burchell H B, Edwards J E 1961 Isolated ventricular septal defect of the persistent common atrioventricular canal type. Circulation 23: 685–696

Pacifico A D, Soto B, Bargeron L M Jr 1979 Surgical treatment of straddling tricuspid valves. Circulation 60: 655–664

Pillai R, Ho S Y, Anderson R H, Shinebourne E A, Lincoln C 1984 Malalignment of the interventricular septum with atrioventricular septal defect: its implications concerning conduction tissue disposition. Thoracic and Cardiovascular Surgeon 32: 1–3

Piot J D, Rey C, Serraf A, Bruniaux J, Planché C 1993 Malformation de Taussing Bing avec straddling des 2 valves auriculo-ventriculaires. Description échocardiographique a propos d'un cas. Archives des Maladies du Coeur 86: 631–634

Quero-Jimenez M, Otero Coto E 1981 Straddling atrioventricular valves. Introduction. In: Becker A E, Losekoot T E, Marcelleti C, Anderson R H (eds) Paediatric cardiology. Churchill Livingstone, Edinburgh, vol. 3, p 399–401

Quero-Jimenez M, Martinez V M P, Azcarate M J M, Batres G M, Granados F M 1973 Exaggerated displacement of the atrioventricular canal towards the bulbus cordis (rightward displacement of the mitral valve). British Heart Journal 35: 65–74

Rastelli G C, Ongley P A, Titus J L 1968 Ventricular septal defect of atrioventricular canal type with straddling right atrioventricular valve and mitral valve deformity. Circulation 37: 816–825

Reddy V M, Liddicoat J R, McElhinney D B, Brrok M M, van Sohn J A M 1997 Biventricular repair of lesions with straddling tricuspid valves using techniques of cordal translocation and realignment. Cardiology in the Young 7: 147–152

Rice M J, Seward J B, Edwards W D et al 1985 Straddling atrioventricular valve: two-dimensional echocardiographic diagnosis, classification, and surgical implication. American Journal of Cardiology 55: 505–513

Robinson P J, Kumpeng V, Macartney F J 1985 Cross-sectional echocardiographic and angiocardiographic correlation in criss-cross hearts. British Heart Journal 54: 61–67

Russo P, Danielson G K, Puga F J, McGoon D C, Humes R 1988 Modified Fontan procedure for biventricular hearts with complex forms of double outlet right ventricle. Circulation 78(suppl. III): 20–25

Serraf A, Nakamura T, Lacour-Gayet F et al 1996 Surgical approaches for double-outlet right ventricle or transposition of the great arteries associated with straddling atrioventricular valves. Journal of Thoracic and Cardiovascular Surgery 111: 527–535

Seward J B, Tajik A K, Ritter D G 1975 Echocardiographic features of straddling tricuspid valve. Mayo Clinic Proceedings 50: 427–434

Shinebourne E A, Albuquerque A, Rigby M L, Anderson R H 1983 Angiography of double outlet right ventricle. In: Anderson R H, Macartney F J, Shinebourne E A, Tynan M (eds) Paediatric cardiology. Churchill Livingstone, Edinburgh, vol. 5, p 408–420

Shinpo H, Van Praagh S, Parness I, Sanders S, Molthan M, Castaneda A 1992 Mitral atresia with a large left ventricle and an underdeveloped or absent right ventricular sinus. Clinical profile, anatomic data and surgical considerations. Journal of the American College of Cardiology 19: 1561–1576

Sieg K, Hagler D G, Ritter D G et al 1977 Straddling right atrioventricular valve in crisscross atrioventricular relationships. Mayo Clinic Proceedings 52: 561–568

Smallhorn J F, Tommasini G, Macartney F J 1981a Detection and assessment of straddling and overriding atrioventricular valves by two dimensional echocardiography. British Heart Journal 46: 254–262

Smallhorn J F, Tommasini G, Macartney F J 1981b Two-dimensional echocardiographic assessment of common atrioventricular valves in univentricular hearts. British Heart Journal 46: 30–34

Smallhorn J F, Sutherland G, Anderson R H, Macartney F J 1982 Cross-sectional echocardiographic assessment of conditions with atrioventricular valve leaflets attached to the atrial septum at the same level. British Heart Journal 48: 331–341

Soto B, Ceballos R, Nath P H, Bim R M, Pacifico A D 1985 Overriding atrioventricular valves. An angiographic-anatomical correlate. International Journal of Cardiology 9: 327–340

Tabry I F, McGoon D C, Danielson G K, Wallace R B, Tajik A J, Seward J B 1979 Surgical management of straddling atrioventricular valve. Journal of Thoracic and Cardiovascular Surgery 77: 191–200

Tandon R, Becker A E, Moller J H, Edwards J E 1974 Double inlet left ventricle: straddling tricuspid valve. British Heart Journal 36: 747–759

Uemura H, Yagihara T 1998 Anatomic biventricular repair by intraventricular and interatrial rerouting in patients with discordant atrioventricular connections. In: Redington A N, Brawn W J, Deanfield J E, Anderson R H (eds) The right heart in congenital heart disease. GMM, London, p 237–242

Van Praagh R, Geva T, Kreutzer J 1989 Ventricular septal defects: how shall we describe, name and classify them? Journal of the American College of Cardiology 14: 1298–1299

Wenink A C G 1979 Congenitally complete heart block with an interrupted Monckeberg sling. European Journal of Cardiology 9: 89–99

Wenink A C G, Gittenberger de Groot A C 1982 Straddling mitral and tricuspid valves: morphologic differences and developmental background. American Journal of Cardiology 49: 1959–1971

42

Diseases of the tricuspid valve

D. S. Celermajer and J. E Deanfield

INTRODUCTION

The most common congenital lesions of the tricuspid valve are Ebstein's malformation and tricuspid valvar dysplasia, which are considered in this chapter together with acquired malformations afflicting the valve. Tricuspid valvar abnormalities, or abnormalities of the morphologically right atrioventricular valve, may also be associated with atrioventricular septal defects, ventricular septal defect with straddling valve, or pulmonary atresia with intact septum. These lesions are described in detail elsewhere. Uhl's anomaly, however, and fatty replacement of the wall of the right ventricle (or arrhythogenic right ventricular cardiomyopathy as it has become known), are so frequently discussed in the setting of Ebstein's malformation that we will give brief consideration to these two entities, even though they are not malformations of the tricuspid valve.

EBSTEIN'S MALFORMATION

Ebstein's malformation has an extremely variable natural history depending on the degree of abnormality of the tricuspid valvar apparatus, which may range from mild to severe (Lev et al, 1970; Anderson et al, 1979; Zuberbuhler et al, 1979). If the deformity of the tricuspid valve is severe, it may result in profound congestive heart failure in the neonatal period, or even in intrauterine death (Roberson and Silverman, 1989). At the other end of the spectrum, patients with a mild degree of displacement of the hinge of the valve away from the atrioventricular junction may remain asymptomatic until late adult life (Adams and Hudson, 1956) or may remain symptomless throughout life.

Ebstein's own description of this anomaly (Figure 42.1) detailed the anatomical findings of a single postmortem specimen (1866). The patient was Joseph Prescher, a 19-year-old labourer with cyanosis, who had been troubled with dyspnoea and palpitations since childhood. The premortem diagnosis had been 'congenital cardiac defect'. The first case described in the English literature was not published until 1900 (Mann and Lie, 1979). It was not until 1951 that the diagnosis was made during life, using angiocardiography (Soloff et al, 1951). By the 1950s, successful surgical palliation had been achieved (Engle et al, 1950), and the association with Wolff–Parkinson–White syndrome had been recognized (Gasul et al, 1959). In the 1960s came the first attempts at corrective surgery, including valvar replacement (Barnard and Schrire, 1963) and

repair (Hardy et al, 1964). Throughout the 1960s and the 1970s, the disease was thought to be extremely rare (Keith, 1978). At that time, diagnosis was based on clinical, electrocardiographic and angiocardiographic features. The malformation was considered to account for 0.3% of congenital heart disease (Rowe et al, 1981), giving an incidence of about 24 per million livebirths. In 1974, a retrospective review of all cases from 61 centres summarized data from only 505 patients (Waston, 1974). Of these, only 7% were aged less than 1 year at diagnosis.

With the advent of cross-sectional echocardiography (Shiina et al, 1984), it became much easier to make the diagnosis, particularly in fetal life (Sharland et al, 1991). These, and similar, experiences have shown that the malformation is more common than previously appreciated. The spectrum of disease seen by paediatric cardiologists, therefore, has changed. In a series of over 200 cases recently collected from hospitals in southeast England, the number of cases diagnosed had increased appreciably since the advent of echocardiography, and more than half of the patients were aged less than 1 year at diagnosis (Celermajer et al, 1994). Throughout the 1980s and 1990s, excellent surgical results have been reported in selected cases following use of innovative techniques for repair (Danielson and Fuster, 1982; Carpentier et al, 1988; Quaegebeur et al, 1991; Chauvaud et al, 1996, 1998; Augustin et al, 1997). Fontan procedures have been shown to be appropriate for others (Starnes et al,

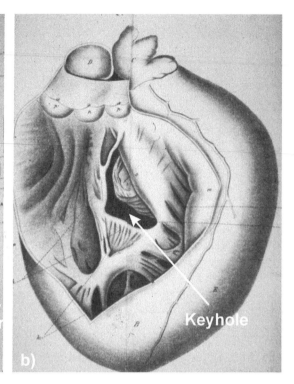

Figure 42.1. The illustrations from Ebstein's original description, made by Dr Weiss, have been scanned and re-labelled. When drawn from the atrial aspect (a), a gap is shown along the right atrioventricular junction, but with normal attachment of the hinge of the mural leaflet, albeit with grossly abnormal tethering of this leaflet. The septal leaflet is also shown with a normal hingepoint, but with a tongue extending to the abnormal anterosuperior leaflet. As drawn from the ventricular aspect (b), it can be seen that the valvar mechanism takes the form of a bifoliate 'keyhole' orientated towards the infundibulum. (Compare with Figures 42.3 and 42.4cb.)

1991), while cardiac transplantation is an option for the most severe cases (Mayer et al, 1990).

This chapter addresses Ebstein's malformation in hearts with concordant atrioventricular connections, with or without associated defects. The lesion is also frequently seen in patients with discordant atrioventricular connections, but this combination will be considered in Chapter 49.

ANATOMY

The essence of Ebstein's malformation is an abnormal location of some part of the annular attachment of the leaflets of the tricuspid valve away from the atrioventricular junction (Anderson and Ho, 1998). In Ebstein's own patient, the illustration made by Dr Weiss shows that only the septal leaflet has a proximal attachment at a distance from the atrioventricular junction, although both the mural and the anterosuperior leaflets are far from normally structured (Figure 42.1). It remains a fact that, in series studied at postmortem, hearts can be encountered in which only the septal leaflet is involved in the fundamental process underscoring the malformation, and then only to minimal degree (Figure 42.2). Unlike Ebstein's index case, these others involve exclusively the septal leaflet of the valve and are very much in the minority (Schreiber et al, 1999). It is unlikely that they produce typical symptomatology. It is also the case that problems exist during life in

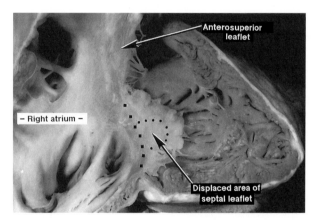

Figure 42.2. In this heart, the septal leaflet of the tricuspid valve was minimally dysplastic, and densely adherent to the ventricular septum over the area delimited by the dotted line. The remainder of the valve, however, is normally attached. Although qualifying as Ebstein's malformation within the definition of displaced annular attachment of part of the septal leaflet, it is highly unlikely that this type of lesion would produce problems during life. Clinical details were unavailable for this particular specimen.

distinguishing such minimal displacement of the septal leaflet from the typical valvar off-setting found in the normal heart. This has led to the construction of formulas to distinguish normal off-setting from 'micro-Ebstein's malformation' (Gussenhoven et al, 1980). The utility of such formulas has still to be established. In those cases coming to clinical attention, the entirety of the tricuspid

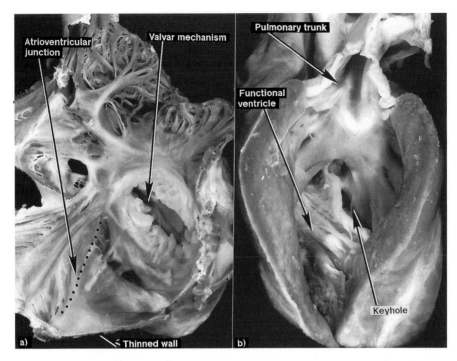

Figure 42.3. These views, showing the inlet (a) and outlet (b) aspects of a florid case of Ebstein's malformation, demonstrate formation of a potentially competent but stenotic orifice at the junction of the inlet component of the right ventricle with the 'functional' ventricle, the latter made up of the apical trabecular and the infundibular components. Note the thinned wall of the inlet component (anatomical atrialization), and the similarity between the outlet aspect and the original case of Ebstein (see Figure 42.1b). The valvar mechanism is bifoliate.

valvar apparatus is malformed, and obviously so. In almost all cases, nonetheless, it is only the septal and mural leaflets that have their annular attachment displaced from the atrioventricular junction, with sparing of the proximal attachment of the anterosuperior leaflet (Leung et al, 1988; Schreiber et al, 1999).

A major problem for the morphologist in analysing these cases coming to clinical attention is precisely to distinguish, in the abnormal valve, the boundaries between the mural and anterosuperior leaflets. In fact, there is a marked tendency for the valvar apparatus to assume a bifoliate configuration, with a plane of closure at the junction of the inlet and apical components of the right ventricle (Figure 42.3). It is the appreciation of this abnormal position and structure of the valve that is the key to subsequent analysis, and arguably to selection of appropriate treatment, rather than slavishly seeking to establish the degree of 'downward displacement' of the valvar leaflets.

Once the abnormal location of the abnormal valve has been appreciated relative to the components of the right ventricle (Figure 42.3), it must then be recognized that there is marked variation from patient to patient. In those coming to postmortem, this variability involves only to limited extent the location of the valvar annular attachments (Schreiber et al, 1999). Much more significant are the degree of formation of the septal leaflet and the nature of the distal attachments of the anterosuperior and mural leaflets. In the typical diseased valve as seen in the postmortem room, the septal leaflet is either represented by an array of verrucous remnants adherent to the

septum towards the ventricular apex (Figure 42.4a) or is formed as a tongue that joins the anterosuperior leaflet (Figure 42.4b). In either event, at first sight the leaflet may seem to be absent or, in rare cases (as in Ebstein's index case), represented by a solitary nodular remnant (Figure 42.4c). The result is to produce a bifoliate valvar orifice guarding the junction between the atrialized ventricular inlet (Figure 42.3a) and the functional right ventricle, the latter made up of the apical trabecular and infundibular components (Figure 42.3b). As already indicated, the mural and anterosuperior leaflets themselves tend to be combined as an abnormal curtain, which forms the parietal part of the abnormal bifoliate valve (Figure 42.3a). This part is attached to the atrioventricular junction along the supraventricular crest but moves increasingly away from the junction as the leaflet is attached along the diaphragmatic surface of the ventricular mass. This arrangement reinforces the impression that the mural leaflet is totally lacking (Figure 42.5). Oftentimes, when seen in the postmortem room, this arrangement seems to have produced a competent valve. In other cases, nonetheless, the valvar mechanism is clearly seen to be incompetent and, relative to the mass of the atrialized right ventricle, is frequently judged to be stenotic. In this setting, the upstream components of the right side of the heart, both the atrium and the right ventricular inlet, are dilated and thin walled. This produces 'anatomical' atrialization. Irrespective of the thickness of its wall, the inlet component of the ventricle is always at atrial pressures in haemodynamic terms simply because

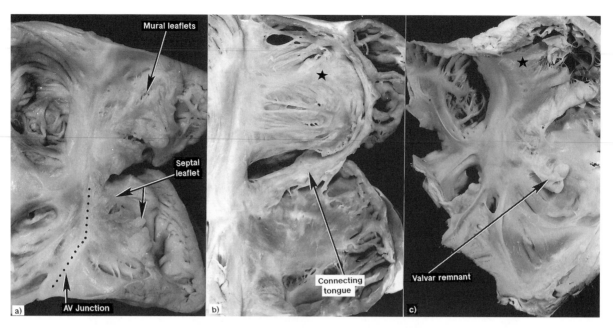

Figure 42.4. This series of specimens shows the degree of variation in formation of the abnormal septal leaflet. (a) The leaflet is represented by an array of verrucous nodules and angles away from the atrioventricular junction to be maximally displaced at the crux. Note the focal attachments of the anterosuperior leaflet, but the tethered mural leaflet. (b) Only the apical part of the leaflet is formed, which extends as a tongue to connect with the abnormal anteriosuperior leaflet, itself confluent with the linearly attached mural leaflet (star). (c) The septal leaflet is represented by a solitary nodule displaced away from the atrioventricular junction, comparable in some ways with Ebstein's index case (see Figure 42.1a). The anterosuperior leaflet is again attached in focal fashion, but the mural leaflet has a linear distal attachment.

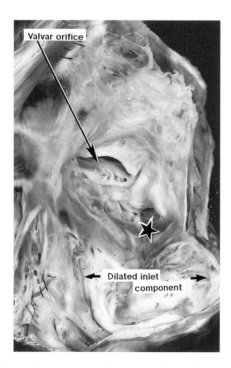

Figure 42.5. In this heart, the right atrium and the inlet of the right ventricle are grossly dilated. The valvar orifice is again formed at the junction of the atrialized inlet with the functional right ventricle (see Figure 42.3b). The maximum point of displacement of the leaflets is along the junction of the septum with the diaphragmatic inferior wall of the right ventricle (starred). Note the linear attachment of the anterosuperior leaflet. The outlet aspect of this heart is shown in Figure 42.6c.

of the abnormal location of the valvar hingepoints. Electrically, because the junction remains at its normal site, the atrialized component has ventricular potentials.

Further variation is then seen in the nature of the distal attachments of the mural and anterosuperior components of the valvar curtain, which are almost always additionally dysplastic (Becker et al, 1971). In some cases, the anterosuperior leaflet retains its focal attachment to the medial and anterior papillary muscles (Figure 42.6a). In the most florid cases, the entire leading edge of the anterosuperior leaflet is attached linearly to a muscular shelf formed between the inlet and apical trabecular components of the ventricle (Figure 42.6c). Between these extremes are found hearts in which the edge of the leaflet is attached in hyphenated fashion along the muscular shelf (Figure 42.6b). Further abnormal tetherings can be found between the ventricular aspect of the abnormal leaflets and the parietal ventricular wall (Figure 42.6b). Such tetherings serve to constrain still further the motion of the abnormal sail produced by the combined mural and anterosuperior leaflets. This reduced motion is of particular surgical importance (Chauvaud et al, 1996, 1998).

When the valvar mechanism is arranged as a bifoliate structure, then its opening is adjacent to the septum and is directed towards the ventricular outlet component (Figure 42.3b). There are then still more cases to be found in which this 'keyhole' becomes increasingly restricted and stenotic. When closure of the valvar mechanism is complete, the result is tricuspid atresia in the

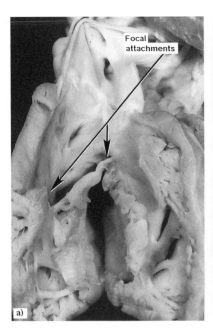
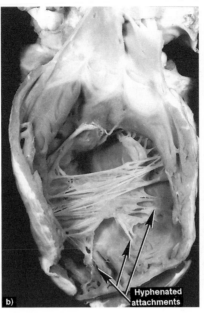
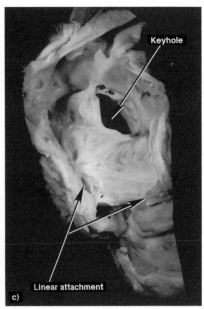

Figure 42.6. These specimens show the variability in distal attachment of the anterosuperior leaflet. (a) The heart here has focal attachment. (b) Hyphenated attachment is shown; the inlet aspect of this heart is shown in Figure 42.4b. (c) Linear attachment can be seen; the inlet aspect of this heart is shown in Figure 42.5. Compare the 'keyhole' with Ebstein's index case (Figure 42.1b).

setting of Ebstein's malformation (Figure 42.7). This variant is also known as the 'tricuspid sack' lesion. Therefore, the essence of symptomatic Ebstein's malformation is formation of an abnormal bifoliate valvar mechanism, with septal and parietal components, at the junction between the atrialized inlet part of the right ventricle and the 'functional' right ventricle, the latter comprising the apical and outlet components.

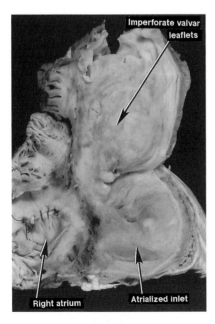

Figure 42.7. Fusion of the anterosuperior and the septal leaflets at the keyhole produces tricuspid atresia in the setting of Ebstein's malformation, or the so-called 'tricuspid sack'.

Although the annular attachments of the septal leaflet of the valve are displaced from the atrioventricular junction, the triangle of Koch continues to be the landmark for the atrial components of the atrioventricular conduction tissue axis (Anderson et al, 1979). Right bundle branch block is commonly found and may be caused by fibrosis in the distal conduction tissue (Lev et al, 1970). The frequent presence of accessory muscular pathways across the atrioventricular junctions results in a high incidence of pre-excitation (Schiebler et al, 1959; Watson 1974), this feature being found in up to one quarter of patients. The accessory pathways are often multiple and are usually found to the right of the inferior paraseptal space; or in the right free wall (Becker et al, 1978; Till et al, 1992; Cappato et al, 1996).

As we have already discussed, the abnormally located line of attachment of the valvar leaflets divides the right ventricle into proximal atrialized and distal functional portions. The proximal portion lies between the atrioventricular junction and the displaced attachments of the leaflets. This atrialized portion has muscular walls, but in symptomatic patients tends to be smooth, thin-walled and dilated, with the walls containing a high content of fibrous tissue. When very thin, it moves paradoxically during ventricular systole, and it may also expand during atrial systole. Its electrical potentials are ventricular, but its pressure pulse shows an atrial waveform.

The cavitary portion of the functional right ventricle is usually smaller than the normal ventricle. This feature, however, may be modified by dilation, which is a frequent finding. The functional portion consists of the infundibulum, the trabeculated apex and that portion of the ventricle beneath the distal attachments of the combined mural and anterosuperior leaflets. The walls of this functional ventricle, particularly when dilated, are also usually thinner than normal. They contain fewer than normal muscle fibres (Anderson and Lie, 1979) and more fibrous tissue (Celermajer et al, 1992a). There may be a congenital paucity of myocardial cells in the right ventricle in this disease; as a result, the dilation of both portions of the ventricle is a part of the developmental anomaly rather than entirely its haemodynamic consequences.

Left ventricular abnormalities, consisting of abnormal contraction and contour, are frequently present (Monibi et al, 1978; Ng et al, 1979). They can sometimes simply be the consequence of the gross dilation of the right-sided chambers. In severe cases, the left ventricular free wall also has an abnormally high content of fibrous tissue, although its thickness is usually normal (Celermajer et al, 1992a). The mitral valve is frequently nodular and thickened, and prolapse of the leaflets is commonly associated (Cabin and Roberts, 1981).

Associated cardiac defects are common, particularly in those diagnosed in fetal or neonatal life. Almost all patients have a coexisting interatrial communication at the oval fossa, usually a patent foramen. Any type of communication, nonetheless, may be present, including primum defects in the setting of a common atrioventricular junction. A large spectrum of other lesions has been described in addition to atrioventricular septal defects, including ventricular septal defects, tetralogy of Fallot, aortic coarctation and persistent arterial duct. The most common associated defect is pulmonary stenosis or atresia, which is found in up to one-third of those presenting in infancy (Celermajer et al, 1992b). It can be argued whether this is strictly 'Ebstein's malformation' (Becker, 1997). The abnormal annular attachment of the leaflets, nonetheless, is unequivocal. Obstruction of the right ventricular outflow tract is commonly associated with Ebstein's malformation when diagnosed in fetal life (Sharland et al, 1991). In this setting, it may be difficult to distinguish stuctural from functional pulmonary atresia using echocardiography, especially in the presence of severe tricuspid regurgitation (Yeager et al, 1988). In either case, the pulmonary valvar abnormality is probably secondary to the Ebstein's malformation, with hypoplasia of the outflow tract resulting from low anterograde flow through the right heart. When severe Ebstein's malformation is associated with fetal and neonatal distress, or death, both lungs are usually hypoplastic but otherwise normal. The hypoplasia is secondary to the gross cardiomegaly, itself caused by dilation of the right heart (Lang et al, 1991).

MORPHOGENESIS

As emphasized, the hallmark of Ebstein's malformation is annular attachment of the septal and mural leaflets within the right ventricle rather than at the atrioventricular junction. This results developmentally from failure of liberation of these leaflets from the ventricular wall. The anterosuperior leaflet, in contrast, has a different developmental origin (Lamers et al, 1995). Because of this, it retains its normal junctional hinge. It was well recognized late in the 19th century that formation of the leaflets was a relatively late embryologic event (Gegenbaur, 1885). At the time of closure of the embryonic interventricular communication, the septal and mural leaflets of the tricuspid valve have not begun to develop. These are produced subsequently by delamination of the superficial layer of the ventricular myocardium (Lamers et al, 1995). Ebstein's malformation is a consequence of failure of this delaminatory process.

It is also now well established that programmed cell death (apoptosis) plays an important part in normal cardiac morphogenesis (Pexeider, 1975). The microscopic findings of increased right ventricular fibrosis, and an absolute decrease in the number of myocytes in the right ventricle in hearts from neonates with Ebstein's malformation (Anderson et al, 1979; Celermajer et al, 1992a), lend credence to the notion that abnormal cell death during fetal life is important in the aetiology of the abnormality. It can be argued that abnormal right ventricular fibrosis seen in the malformation is caused by haemodynamic stress secondary to severe tricuspid regurgitation (Pexeider, 1975). The findings of increased fibrosis in the left ventricle, coupled with the absence of thinning of the left ventricular wall, or any difference between subendocardial and subepicardial fibrous content (Celermajer et al, 1992a), nonetheless, makes unlikely a haemodynamic explanation for the cell death and subsequent fibrosis. Instead, the markedly increased fibrous content of the left ventricle supports the concept of a genetic or chemical basis for the abnormal apoptosis. In this context, it may be relevant that there is also an association between some cases of Ebstein's malformation and use of lithium in pregnancy (Weinstein and Goldfield, 1975).

PATHOPHYSIOLOGY

The physiological effects of the malformation depend on whether the abnormally positioned valvar mechanism is stenotic or incompetent, or both stenotic and incompetent. Also important is the size and structure of the functional right ventricle. This may be very small and unable to provide effective propulsion to promote flow of blood to the lungs. The effective tricuspid valvar orifice, at the junction between the atrialized and functional parts of the right ventricle, is often the major site of obstruction. In the more severely affected hearts, in addition to the obstruction caused by the reduced size of the valvar orifice, the abnormal distal attachments of the parietal part of the bifoliate valvar curtain do not allow it to close completely. Since the leaflets are usually additionally dysplastic (Becker et al, 1971), a degree of tricuspid regurgitation is usual. When combined, tricuspid regurgitation and stenosis tend to lead to right atrial dilation and hypertrophy. Thus, when blood flow from the right atrium to the pulmonary circuit is obstructed, there is a right-to-left atrial shunt and consequent cyanosis. The shunt is enhanced in the presence of tricuspid regurgitation. When the valvar malformation is less severe, obstruction to pulmonary blood flow is also less marked. In the mildest malformation, there may be a bidirectional shunt through the atrial septal defect, which is almost always present, or even occasionally a left-to-right shunt.

The motion of the abnormal bifoliate tricuspid valve is grossly abnormal. In the severest forms, only the anterosuperior leaflet moves. Since it is usually 'tied' down by its abnormal tension apparatus, it has a billowing motion, in contrast to the opening and closing motion found in the normal valve. This billowing motion, well demonstrated echocardiographically, results in its delayed sound of closure (Crews et al, 1972), which is sometimes called the 'sail sound' (Fontana and Wooley, 1972).

Atrioventricular re-entry tachycardias commonly occur in patients with accessory conduction pathways between the atriums and the ventricles. Atrial fibrillation or flutter are also commonly found, usually related to right atrial dilation. Such tachycardias may further diminish pulmonary blood flow by shortening right ventricular filling time.

CLINICAL FEATURES

The clinical features, as with the pathophysiology, vary with the severity of the lesion. In the mildest forms, the anomaly may escape detection during a normal life span (Makous and van der Veer, 1966), particularly in those where the abnormality is restricted to the septal leaflet of the valve (Figure 42.2). More frequently, symptoms occur in the first months of life (Schiebler et al, 1959). The mode of presentation differs depending on the age at which the patient is first seen. In fetal life, most cases are diagnosed because of abnormal findings encountered during a routine ultrasonic study. Most neonates present with cyanosis, which may decrease in severity with the normal evolution of the pulmonary vasculature, only to return after some years (Engle et al, 1950). In infants, dyspnoea is frequent. It is a symptom of heart failure and is usually seen in those with severe tricuspid regurgitation. Presentation in childhood is most commonly as a result of an incidentally heard murmur; in contrast adolescents and young adults most often present with an arrhythmia.

Physical findings may include cyanosis and signs of increased venous pressure, such as distended veins in the neck and, in infants, hepatomegaly. Abnormalities of the pulse or blood pressure are rare. The most dramatic signs are the auscultatory ones. There is a systolic murmur in the majority, heard at the left sternal edge, sometimes accompanied by a thrill. The loudest and longest murmurs are heard in patients with severe tricuspid regurgitation. A low-pitched 'scratchy' diastolic murmur is frequently present and may be confused with a pericardial friction rub. Although first described in older patients (Wood, 1962), it can be heard at all ages. The first heart sound is widely split. Its second, tricuspid, component is loud and sharp. This is caused by the closing motion of the enlarged anterosuperior leaflet (Crews et al, 1972; Willis and Craige, 1983). The pulmonary component of the second heart sound may be delayed and soft. A loud third sound is also present, corresponding to the 'opening snap' of the anterosuperior leaflet. Occasionally, a fourth heart sound is also heard. The heart sounds may be difficult to analyse accurately in the newborn period. It may just appear that the heart is 'full of sounds' which alone may suggest the diagnosis.

INVESTIGATIONS

CHEST RADIOGRAPHY

The chest radiographic appearance may be dramatic, particularly in patients presenting in the neonatal period. Cardiomegaly may be so pronounced as to leave little of the lung fields visible. Indeed, such extreme cardiomegaly in a cyanosed neonate is almost diagnostic of Ebstein's malformation. The heart often has a rounded or box-like cardiac contour beneath a narrow pedicle (Figure 42.8).

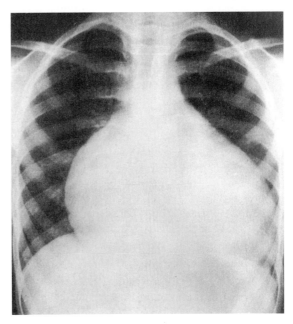

Figure 42.8. The frontal chest radiograph in a typical patient with Ebstein's malformation.

In the frontal view, the whole of the silhouette is then formed by right atrium and right ventricle. Because of the normal or oligaemic lung fields, the silhouette has a peculiarly sharp edge. As with other features of the disease, there is a wide variation in the size of the heart (Schiebler et al, 1959). In a few patients, it may remain normal; in most it is only moderately enlarged (Kumar et al, 1971). The left heart, aortic and pulmonary arterial shadows are not usually enlarged.

ELECTROCARDIOGRAPHY

The electrocardiogram is often unhelpful in diagnosis in the neonatal period, as QRS morphology may appear normal at this time. With increasing age, the electrocardiographic evidence of intraventricular conduction delay becomes more obvious, with widening of the QRS complex. In older children and adults, there may be characteristic electrocardiographic abnormalities. The classical picture is of right atrial enlargement, a prolonged PR interval, right bundle branch block and small QRS voltages over the right chest leads (van Lingen and Bauserfeld, 1955; Bialostozky et al, 1972). Inverted T waves in leads V_1 through V_4 are quite common. Evidence of ventricular pre-excitation is found in up to one quarter of patients, almost always of a right-sided (type B) Wolff–Parkinson–White pattern (Watson, 1974).

The relationship of the electrocardiogram to the severity of the pathological anomaly is not clear. The height of the P wave may reflect severity (Kumar et al, 1971). Although the magnitude of the R wave in V_1 is rarely greater than 7 mm, it appears that this feature is also, to some extent, inversely related to the severity of the anatomical malformation. Rarely the electrocardiogram may be normal (Taussig, 1960).

Supraventricular arrhythmia is commonly seen and may be paroxysmal and recurrent. Atrioventricular nodal re-entry tachycardia, atrial flutter and atrial fibrillation may all be found. Ventricular tachycardia is usually related to cardiac catheterization, but it may occur spontaneously (Celermajer et al, 1994).

ECHOCARDIOGRAPHY

Cross-sectional echocardiography, particularly with its Doppler and colour modalities, has changed the facility and accuracy of diagnosis, especially prenatally and neonatally. The diagnosis could be made using M-mode images, which demonstrated delayed closure of the tricuspid valvar leaflets and abnormal dimensions of the right heart (Farooki et al, 1976). This technique, of course, has now been superseded by cross-sectional examination (Rusconi et al, 1991). This allows precise anatomical visualization of the abnormal tricuspid valvar apparatus, assessment of the motion of the abnormal leaflets, recognition of stenosis and/or regurgitation, evaluation of both the right and left heart chambers and

recognition of any associated defects (Rigby and Mota, 1998). It is also possible to use ultrasound to assess the feasibility of repair rather than replacement of the valve (Shiina et al, 1984).

The malformation is recognized on the basis of the displaced attachment of the septal and mural leaflets (Figure 42.9). This is best seen in subcostal four chamber views, but the abnormal location of the septal leaflet is also well seen in parasternal sections, or their transoesophageal equivalent (Figure 42.10). The displacement of the effective valvar orifice to the junction between the atrialized inlet and the functional right ventricle also means that the tricuspid valve is seen in the standard parasternal long-axis and in the subcostal outlet views. Normally, it is not seen in these planes at all. Occasionally, the displaced leaflets can be visualized towards the outlet in the parasternal short-axis view. The sections permit recognition of the shape of the abnormal septal leaflet, particularly when it is attached in tube-like fashion (Figure 42.11) or arranged as a series of verrucous remnants (Figure 42.12). Attention to the anterosuperior leaflet shows its normal junctional attachment but also shows the nature of its distal attachments (Figure 42.13) and demonstrates its billowing motion (Figure 42.14).

Careful echocardiographic examination (Rigby and Mota, 1998), therefore, can define all the abnormalities of the valve recognized by the morphologist (Anderson and Ho, 1998). The size of the functional portion of the right ventricle can also be determined, particularly from the subcostal views. The thickness and motion of the

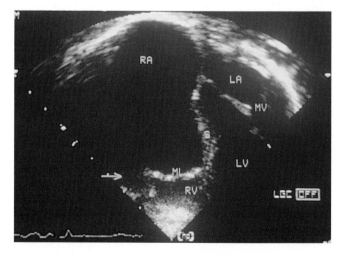

Figure 42.9. This cross-sectional echocardiogram, taken from the subcostal window, shows massive dilation of the right atrium (RA) and the atrialized part of the right ventricle (RV). Note the annular attachment of the septal and mural leaflets of the valve well away from the atrioventricular junction, with the functional right ventricle distal to the leaflets. The left atrium (LA), mitral valve (MV) and left ventricle (LV) are all normal. (From Rigby and Mota (1998); reproduced with kind permission of the authors and GMM publications.)

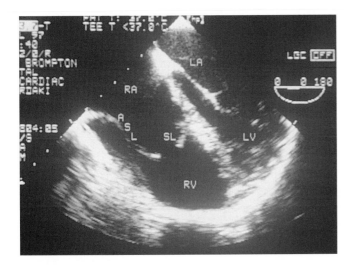

Figure 42.10. This transoesophageal horizontal section is comparable to the parasternal four chamber view. It shows the attachment of the septal leaflet (SL) away from the atrioventricular junction. Note the normal junctional attachment of the anterosuperior leaflet (ASL). Other abbreviations as in Figure 42.9. (From Rigby and Mota (1998); reproduced with kind permission of the authors and GMM publications.)

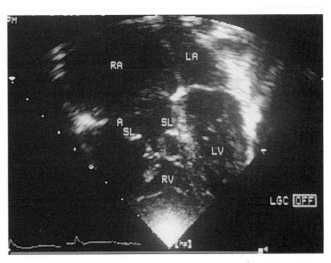

Figure 42.11. This parasternal four chamber section shows a tubular attachment of the abnormal septal leaflet. Abbreviations as in Figures 42.9 and 42.10. (From Rigby and Mota (1998); reproduced with kind permission of the authors and GMM publications.)

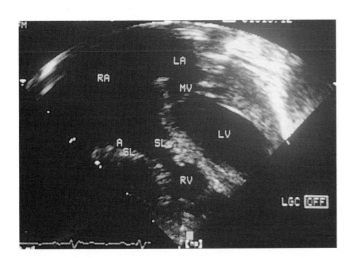

Figure 42.12. In this patient, shown again by a parasternal four chamber section, the septal leaflet (SL) is represented by a verrucous remnant. Abbreviations as in Figures 42.9 and 42.10. (From Rigby and Mota (1998); reproduced with kind permission of the authors and GMM publications.)

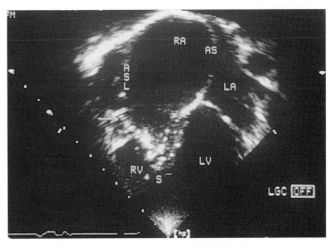

Figure 42.13. This parasternal four chamber section shows linear attachment of the distal edge of the anterosuperior leaflet to an abnormal apical muscular shelf (arrowed). AS, atrial septum. Other abbreviations as in Figures 42.9 and 42.10. (From Rigby and Mota (1998); reproduced with kind permission of the authors and GMM publications.)

atrialized portion, along with the dimensions of the right atrium (Figure 42.11) and the size, contour and function of the left ventricle can also assessed.

In children, there is no evidence as yet that the degree of 'downward' displacement of the leaflets is related to the clinical severity of the condition. In those presenting as neonates and infants, however, a grading system based on echocardiographic evaluation of the dilation of the right atrium and atrialized ventricular inlet has been shown to be of greater value (Celermajer et al, 1992b).

The grade is obtained by calculating the ratio of the combined area of the right atrium and atrialized right ventricle to that of the combined area of the functional right ventricle, left atrium and left ventricle. This is achieved using a four chamber view at end-diastole. Depending on the ratio, four grades of severity are defined: less than 0.5, 0.5–1.0, 1.0–1.49, and greater than 1.5. The indicated probability of survival for those presenting as neonates then permits prognostic stratification from an early age (Figure 42.15). (Celermajer et al, 1994).

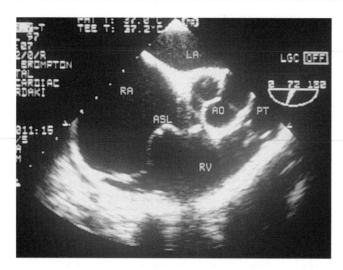

Figure 42.14. This transoesophageal section is taken in the short axis at the level of the aortic valve (AO). It shows the 'sail-like' motion of the large anterosuperior leaflet (ASL). PT, pulmonary trunk; other abbreviations as in Figure 42.9. (From Rigby and Mota (1998); reproduced with kind permission of the authors and GMM publications.)

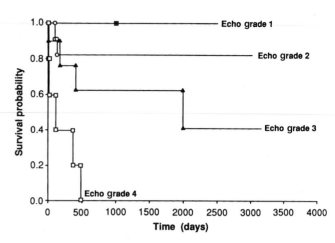

Figure 42.15. These curves show the probability of survival according to the echocardiographic grading in the patients seen by Celermajer and his associates (1994). See text for further discussion.

CARDIAC CATHETERIZATION AND ANGIOGRAPHY

The advent of cross-sectional echocardiography has replaced cardiac catheterization as the means of definitive diagnosis and, consequently, invasive studies are now only rarely required. The frequency of catheter-induced arrhythmias has long been appreciated, occurring in up to one third of cases. A number of deaths were reported, particularly in the early years of catheterization (Mayer et al, 1957; Wood, 1962).

If catheterization is performed, the large cavity of the right atrium and atrialized right ventricle will be easily visualized because of a large catheter loop. The mean right atrial pressure is frequently modestly elevated. This atrial wave form is also recorded in the atrialized portion of the right ventricle, which may be identified on the basis of its ventricular potentials by using an electrode catheter. The atrial pressure traces give some indication of the haemodynamic effects of the abnormal tricuspid valve. Stenosis is associated with a prominent A wave not transmitted to the distal ventricle; an incompetent valve is evidenced by a dominant V wave. In most cases, there is oximetric evidence of right-to-left atrial shunting, although occasionally a left-to-right shunt may be found. The presence of the latter finding suggests a coexisting atrial septal defect, with a relatively mild abnormality of the tricuspid valve.

Occasionally, it may prove difficult to enter the distal component of the right ventricle (Van Mierop et al, 1977) because of the abnormal attachments of the anterosuperior leaflet. The abnormal course through the tricuspid valve also increases the difficulty of entering the pulmonary trunk. When the right ventricle is entered,

the pressure is usually found to be normal or low, although hearts are found with increased pressure, which probably reflect an obstruction of the outflow tract coexisting with a competent tricuspid valve. Usually the right ventricular tracing has a normal contour. Tall A waves indicate increased end-diastolic pressure, in turn manifesting the usual increase in atrial systolic pressure, which may be transmitted onwards into the pulmonary trunk.

If angiocardiography is performed in the distal portion of the right ventricle (Figure 42.16a), it can demonstrate the size of the apical trabecular and outlet parts (Ellis et al, 1964). At the same time, it shows the separation of the effective valvar orifice away from the atrioventricular junction and reveals any regurgitation through the valve (Figure 42.16b). It also shows the state of the pulmonary circulation.

Left ventriculography is useful to show the contraction pattern of this chamber, which is often abnormal. Ventricular injections will also show the type and position of a ventricular septal defect when present.

ELECTROPHYSIOLOGICAL STUDIES

Detailed electrophysiology is indicated to diagnose the substrate for drug-refractory supraventricular arrhythmias or to study patients with arrhythmia or pre-excitation in whom surgery will be required on the tricuspid valve (Till et al, 1992). Accessory pathways are known to be frequent in patients with pre-excitation. They may be multiple and usually they are right sided (Smith et al, 1982; Till et al, 1992; Cappato et al, 1996). Left-sided accessory pathways have been found (Becker

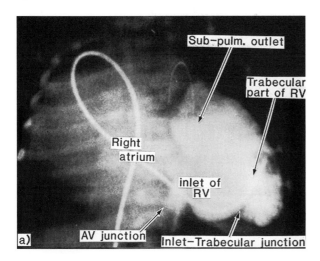
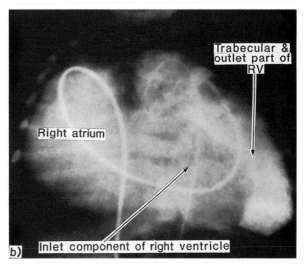

Figure 42.16. These angiograms are viewed in the frontal projection following an injection (a) in the functional component of the right ventricle (RV). Regurgitation across the valve (b) shows the size of the atrialized and functional components of the ventricle. AV, atrioventricular; sub-pulm., subpulmonary.

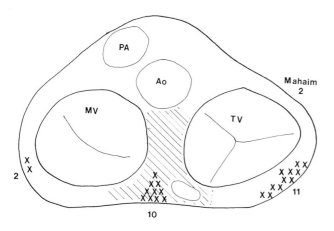

Figure 42.17. The crosses show the location of anomalous pathways (as encountered at the Royal Brompton Hospital and the Hospital for Sick Children, Great Ormond Street, London) producing Wolff–Parkinson–White syndrome in the setting of Ebstein's malformation. Two pathways produced the so-called 'Mahaim' variant, and these pathways were found at the acute margin of the right atrioventricular junction. The cartoon is based on viewing the atrial aspect of the atrioventricular junctions. MV, TV, mitral and tricuspid valves, respectively; PA, pulmonary trunk, Ao, aorta.

et al, 1978) but are rare (Figure 42.17). Radiofrequency ablation of accessory pathways may be undertaken at the time of the electrophysiological study. This procedure is often difficult because of the enlarged right atrium, distorted atrioventricular anatomical relations and the presence of multiple pathways. In skilled hands, nonetheless, the results of ablation are impressive (Cappato et al, 1996).

COURSE AND PROGNOSIS

Ebstein's malformation may present at any age, from fetal life to geriatric presentation. The incidence is

approximately equal in both sexes. Exceptionally, familial cases have been reported (Balaji et al, 1991).

Early presentation is usually a consequence of severe disease, the presence of associated cardiac defects or both these features. The prognosis is generally poor. In later life, the malformation is usually detected because of coexistent palpitations or arrhythmia, or an incidental murmur, and the outlook is much better. Morbidity and mortality mainly result from haemodynamic problems and arrhythmias.

Cyanosis appearing after the neonatal period tends to be slowly progressive, and survival is related to its severity (Giuliani et al, 1979). Severe cyanosis is associated with a 20% survival at 8 years, whereas patients with mild cyanosis have a 94% survival at this stage (Kumar et al, 1971). The onset of congestive heart failure is also a poor prognostic sign. Without surgery, death usually follows within 2 years (Watson, 1974). Heart failure may be precipitated by the onset of arrhythmia.

The true natural history of Ebstein's malformation is difficult to assess. Early studies, before the advent of cross-sectional echocardiography, included mainly older patients and so were inevitably biased towards factors favouring survival. More recent studies have included more neonates and infants, but the 'natural' history is difficult to determine as many undergo surgical intervention. Survival data have recently been calculated (Figure 42.18) from a cohort of 220 patients seen over a 30-year period in southeast England (Celermajer et al, 1994). Data was presented in three ways: the observed survival, the most optimistic case with the patients withdrawn as alive at the time of surgery, and the worst case with patients withdrawn as dead at the time of surgery. The true natural history lies between the curves for the observed and worst cases. It is probably closer to the line representing withdrawal as dead, since patients in our

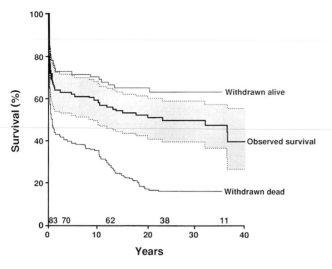

Figure 42.18. These curves illustrate the probability of survival for patients born with Ebstein's malformation and are based on the study of Celermajer et al (1994). Numbers above the *x* axis are the number remaining in the study. See text for discussion.

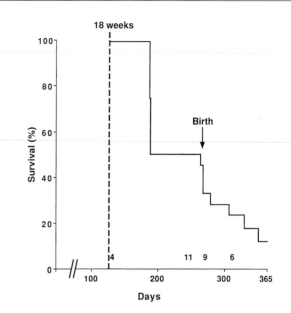

Figure 42.19. This graph shows the poor prognosis for those patients with Ebstein's malformation diagnosed during fetal life or as infants. (Data from Celermajer et al, 1994.)

series usually underwent surgery when they were severely symptomatic.

PRESENTATION IN FETAL LIFE

Severe examples of Ebstein's malformation may be detected on a prenatal scan because of gross right atrial dilation. This feature is readily appreciable in a standard four chamber view (Hornberger et al, 1991). Such views are now routinely included in the screening scan performed at 18–20 weeks of gestation. Other cases may be detected because of fetal tachyarrhythmia. In our experience, the outcome for those presenting during fetal life is poor (Figure 42.19). Of 21 fetuses reviewed, there were eight terminations, four intrauterine and six postnatal deaths and only three survivors. The survival at 1 year was no more than 15% (Celermajer et al, 1994). Not one fetus with an echocardiographic grading ratio of greater than unity survived. The ratio in those surviving was between 0.5 and unity, with no fetuses detected with a ratio lower than 0.5. One fetus with associated tachycardia was treated successfully with maternal flecainide.

PRESENTATION IN THE NEONATAL PERIOD

The most common mode of presentation of the neonate is with cyanosis, usually in the first 3 days of life. Associated cardiac defects occur in about half these patients, most commonly pulmonary stenosis or atresia. In a series of 50 consecutive neonates seen at our institution (Celermajer et al, 1992b), nine (18%) died in the first month of life: six with heart failure and/or pulmonary hypoplasia with respiratory insufficiency, two with ventricular arrhythmia and one at the time of

surgery. There was a continuing hazard for later death, with 15 children dying during follow-up. The causes of death were late haemodynamic deterioration in nine, often associated with left ventricular failure, sudden death in five and non-cardiac problems in one. Actuarial survival at 1 year was 76%, and at 10 years was 61% (Figure 42.20). The prognosis of those presenting as neonates is again closely associated with their echocardiographic grading at presentation (Figure 42.15). A common pattern amongst survivors was resolution of cyanosis over the first week of life, concomitant with the normal fall in pulmonary vascular resistance. Persistent cyanosis, particularly in those with associated obstruction of the right ventricular outflow tract, could be palliated surgically, and these patients have a good outcome in the medium term.

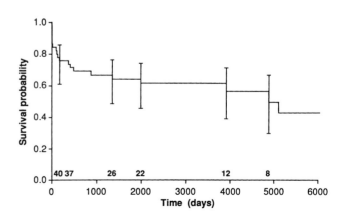

Figure 42.20. The actuarial survival curve for 50 consecutive neonates seen at the Hospital for Sick Children, Great Ormond Street London. (From Celermajer et al, 1992b.)

PRESENTATION IN INFANCY AND CHILDHOOD

The most common mode of presentation in infants is with heart failure. Approximately 20% have associated cardiac defects. Presentation beyond the neonatal period is associated with a lower risk of death. Children are usually diagnosed because of an incidentally heard murmur. Actuarial survival for asymptomatic presentation is 85% at 10 years, with a good outlook thereafter (Celemajer et al, 1994). Other possible modes of presentation are with cyanosis and/or palpitations, which may be caused by arrhythmia associated with accessory atrioventricular connections.

PRESENTATION IN ADOLESCENCE AND ADULT LIFE

Patients who do not present until adolescence or adult life generally have mild symptoms, are acyanotic, may have a normally sized heart on chest radiograph; the prognosis for these patients is good (Genton and Blount, 1967; Seward et al, 1979). Palpitation is the commonest presenting feature and is associated with pre-excitation, atrial flutter or fibrillation or, occasionally, supraventricular tachycardia without pre-excitation. Arrhythmias are often recurrent and difficult to treat medically. Occasionally, the onset of arrhythmia will precipitate heart failure in a previously well patient.

PREGNANCY

Pregnancy may be well tolerated by adults with Ebstein's malformation, although severe cyanosis is associated with a high risk of fetal loss (Somerville et al, 1992). Of 30 women aged 16 years or over observed in our recent series, 15 had been pregnant on a total of 23 occasions (Celermajer et al, 1994). The pregnancies resulted in 14 normal deliveries, eight miscarriages and one stillbirth. One of these children is known to have a ventricular septal defect.

MORBIDITY

Most adults with Ebstein's malformation are in excellent functional state and receive no medications. Despite this, there is a significant incidence of late heart failure, cyanosis and/or arrhythmia. Late haemodynamic deterioration can be caused by either progressive tricuspid regurgitation and/or right heart failure or important left ventricular dysfunction. Exercise tolerance measured objectively may be reduced even in asymptomatic patients, probably related to mild left ventricular dysfunction (Driscoll et al 1988; Saxena et al, 1991). The cause of left heart failure is not clear but may be a result of dilation of the right heart with abnormal ventricular septal motion, chronic cyanosis and/or left ventricular

fibrosis. Other rarer complications include paradoxical embolus and cerebral abscess. With routine antibiotic prophylaxis, endocarditis is rare. Survival with Ebstein's malformation has been reported up to age 85 years (Williams et al, 1980).

PRE-EXCITATION AND ARRHYTHMIA

Pre-excitation is found in up to one quarter of patients with Ebstein's anomaly and is frequently associated with supraventricular tachycardia, often in the first year of life. Supraventricular arrhythmia is more likely to occur in patients with pre-excitation compared with those without (Figure 42.21). Many arrhythmic types have been documented, including atrial and atrioventricular nodal re-entry tachycardia (Pressley et al, 1992; Smith et al, 1992). Such supraventricular tachycardias usually have a broad QRS complex of right bundle branch block morphology. More complex arrhythmias involving 'Mahaim' fibres and ventricular tachycardia or fibrillation have also been reported (Kastor et al, 1975; Sealy et al, 1978; Till et al, 1992; Cappato et al, 1996). Atrial flutter and fibrillation are often found in older patients with right atrial dilation and may compromise haemodynamic function. Bradyarrhythmia is usually only seen as a complication of cardiac catheterization or surgery. In some patients, more than one form of arrhythmia may occur.

MORTALITY

Congestive cardiac failure is the most common cause of death in those who die of cardiac problems with Ebstein's

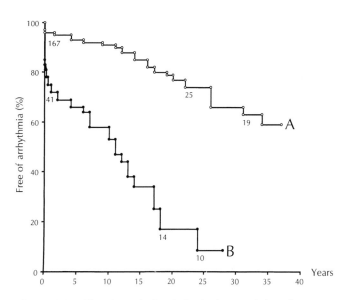

Figure 42.21. There is marked variation in the association of Ebstein's malformation with arrhythmias according to whether the patients do (A) or do not (B) have associated ventricular pre-excitation. (Data from patients seen at Great Ormond Street and Royal Brompton Hospitals.)

malformation (Kumar et al, 1971; Watson, 1974). Perioperative death is probably the next most common cause in the modern era; it accounted for one third of the deaths encountered in the review of Celermajer et al (1994). Sudden death in previously well patients is recognized and is almost certainly related to arrhythmia (Genton and Blount 1967; Gentles et al, 1992). Paradoxical embolus, cerebral abscess, endocarditis and catheter-related deaths are rare but reported terminal events (Genton and Blount, 1967; Mathews et al, 1983).

PREDICTORS OF OUTCOME

In our review of over 200 cases of Ebstein's malformation (Celermajer et al, 1994), we analysed the relationship between outcome and presenting features such as age, sex, era at diagnosis, cardiothoracic ratio, presence or absence or pre-excitation, echocardiographic grade of severity and presence or absence of associated cardiac defects. Univariate analysis for the whole group showed significant risk of death was associated with an echocardiographic ratio of greater than 1.5. The relative risk for these patients, compared with those with a ratio of less than 0.5, was 13.3 (95% confidence limits (CL) 1.6–111). Further risk factors, with their relative risks, were a cardiothoracic ratio greater than 60% (risk of 5.4 compared with those less than 60%; 95% CL 1.9–15), associated obstruction in the right ventricular outflow (risk of 2.5 compared with those with no obstruction; 95% CL 1.3–4.8) and presentation in fetal life (risk of 10.1 compared with presentation in childhood; 95% CL 2.3–44). All three subjects with a cardiothoracic ratio above 90% at presentation died. Pre-excitation was not a risk factor for mortality, nor was era at diagnosis. When the echocardiographic ratio was treated as a continuous variable, each incremental grade was associated with a relative risk of 2.7 (95% CL 1.6–4.6). On multivariate analysis, we found that significant risk of death was associated with presentation in fetal life relative to childhood (risk 6.9; 95% CL 1.6–9.5) and the presence of obstruction in the right ventricular outflow tract (risk 2.1; 95% CL 1.1–4.4). Gentles et al (1992) performed a similar analysis in 48 patients. They found that a cardiothoracic ratio greater than 65% and severely dysfunctional state were significant predictors of death.

TREATMENT

MEDICAL THERAPY

Treatment of the critically ill neonate with Ebstein's malformation involves use of prostaglandin E_1 to maintain patency of the arterial duct, and the use of pulmonary vasodilators. High levels of inspired oxygen, and occasionally epoprostenol (prostacyclin) or tolazoline, are also used. Many babies improve spontaneously as the pulmonary vascular resistance falls, with consequent improvement in forward flow through the tricuspid valve and right ventricular outflow, and reduced right-to-left shunting at atrial level. Intensive support, including ventilation, may be required during the first few days. If cyanosis is caused by associated structural obstruction of the right ventricular outflow tract, palliative surgery is indicated (see below).

Most older children and adults are asymptomatic and can be managed conservatively. Exceptions include those with palpitations or symptoms of heart failure. Arrhythmias in general are difficult to treat. Accurate diagnosis should be obtained by 12-lead or ambulatory electrocardiographic monitoring, or home telemetry devices if necessary. Drug-refractory patients, or those with syncope, should have detailed electrophysiological studies. In our experience, the most useful agents for control of tachyarrhythmias include flecainide and amiodarone. Despite this, over half the patients require a trial of two or more antiarrhythmic agents to obtain reasonable symptomatic control (Till et al, 1992). Digoxin is useful for controlling the response rate of the ventricles in those with atrial fibrillation but is contraindicated in patients with pre-excitation. Radiofrequency ablation may prove an effective alternative for those with accessory atrioventricular connections, although the procedure may be complicated by the presence of multiple pathways, the enlarged right atrium and the distorted anatomy of the tricuspid valve.

Heart failure may be treated with diuretics, and afterload reduction is appropriate for those with known left ventricular dysfunction. Antibiotic prophylaxis against endocarditis should be routinely prescribed. Oral anticoagulation is advisable for any patient with paroxysmal or chronic atrial fibrillation or flutter, except in those with a bleeding diathesis or other contraindication.

SURGERY

Palliative operations, such as construction of a systemic-to-pulmonary arterial shunt, a Glenn anastomosis or pulmonary valvotomy, may be required for neonates and infants with persistent cyanosis associated with structural pulmonary stenosis or atresia. In general, these procedures can be performed with low risk (Kirklin and Barratt-Boyes, 1992). Open heart surgery usually consists of an attempt to improve the function of the abnormal tricuspid valve by repair or replacement. Occasionally, surgery for repair of associated defects is indicated in isolation, such as closure of an atrial septal defect with left-to-right shunting, closure of ventricular septal defect or isolated surgery to cure arrhythmias.

The question remains as to which patients should have tricuspid valvar surgery. The great majority of patients reported in the various series have been in the worst functional classes at the time of operation, with symptoms of congestive heart failure and cyanosis. Giuliani et al (1979) inferred that one of the reasons for the poor results of surgery at that time was that the patients selected had entered the end-stage of the disease process. The prognosis of asymptomatic patients is good, none-theless, and operation carries a risk of death, even in the best reported series (Danielson and Fuster, 1982; Carpentier et al, 1988; Quaegebeur et al, 1991; Augustin et al, 1997; Chauvaud et al, 1998).

There is no evidence that successful surgery decreases the risk of late sudden death. We currently perform reparative surgery, therefore, only for symptomatic patients. The long-term effects of operation are still unknown. One possible concern is the potential problems from left ventricular dysfunction, which may not improve postoperatively (Ng et al, 1979).

The critical question in planning surgical amelioration of the haemodynamics is whether the functional right ventricle (in other words that part distal to the level of the 'effective' valvar orifice) is capable of supporting the entire cardiac output. If not, alternative procedures, such as creation of tricuspid atresia and Fontan-type operation (Starnes et al, 1991), should be undertaken (see below). Orthotopic cardiac transplantation may even be considered in such cases (Mayer et al, 1990). If the functional right ventricle is adequate, repair can usually be undertaken if the anterosuperior leaflet is not too abnormal or too adherent to the ventricular wall. In complex cases, replacement of the valve may be required. In either case, surgery to divide accessory pathways, guided by intra-operative mapping, may be performed at the same procedure. This is generally done before the valve is repaired or replaced, although ablation is frequently replacing surgery in this setting (Cappato et al, 1996). Successful results were also achieved using the combined surgical approach (Pressley et al, 1992).

The optimal technique for valvar reconstruction has yet to be established. The best tested method of repair is that used by Danielson and Fuster (1982), this being a modification of the initial approach of Hardy et al (1964). This involves transverse plication of the atrialized portion of the right ventricle (Figure 42.22), followed by creation of a competent 'monocusp' valve fashioned from the abnormal anterosuperior leaflet. The surgeons from the Deutches Herzzentrum have long used the monocusp approach, but without resort to plication of the atrialized inlet component (Augustin et al, 1997). Results of these procedures have been good for selected older children and adults, with a low perioperative mortality (5%). Excellent results, with slightly higher mortality (10%), have also been reported for the repair devised by Carpentier et al (1988), which involves longitudinal plication of the atrialized right ventricle and tricuspid annuloplasty, with or without placement of an annuloplasty ring (Chauvaud et al, 1998). A similar approach has been used by Quaegebeur and his colleagues (1991). Most survivors of repair achieve good functional status and have improved exercise performance (Melo et al, 1979; Silver et al, 1984). Most have a competent tricuspid valve.

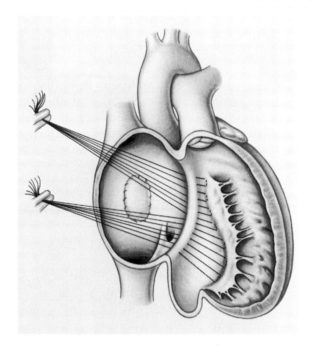

Figure 42.22. The basis of surgical repair of Ebstein's malformation according to the concept of Hardy and his colleagues (1964) is longitudinal plication of the atrialized portion of the right ventricle using sutures inserted along the septum. The concept of Carpentier and his colleagues (1988) is to achieve horizontal plication, parallel rather than at tight angles to the ventricular septum. The group from the Deutches Herzzentrum (Augustin et al, 1997) do not plicate the atrialized inlet.

Residual symptoms, when present, usually relate to late tachyarrhythmias (Westaby et al, 1982).

In a proportion of patients who come to surgery, the morphology or immobility of the anterosuperior leaflet is deemed to prevent repair, and replacement is required (Kirklin and Barratt-Boyes, 1992). The number of such patients often reflects the skill of the surgeons in reparative procedures, with less than 3% of those patients referred to Hôpital Broussais requiring valvar replacement (Chauvaud et al, 1998). When replacement is necessary, the abnormal leaflets are excised, taking care to preserve the area of the triangle of Koch in the region of the membranous septum. Many types of prosthesis have been used, including Dacron-mounted allograft pulmonary valves (Kirklin and Barratt-Boyes, 1992), dura mater prostheses (Barbero-Marcial et al, 1979), large heterograft valves or mechanical prostheses (in adults) (Charles et al, 1981). Bioprosthetic valves may be preferable in women of childbearing age, as oral anticoagulation can be avoided. Reoperation, however, is inevitable in these patients. When the atrialized right ventricle is thin walled and moves paradoxically, it is plicated during the procedure. Reported perioperative mortality in these patients is up to 15–20% (Kirklin and Barratt-Boyes, 1992). All mechanical prostheses inserted in the tricuspid position mandate lifelong anticoagulation.

In some neonates and infants, the malformation is so severe that the distal portion of the right ventricle is functionally useless. Results of valvar surgery for persistent cyanosis and heart failure in these patients have been poor. Because of this, Starnes et al (1991) devised an operation to abolish antegrade flow from the right atrium, and separately to establish a reliable source of pulmonary flow. This involves enlargement of the atrial septal defect, closing the tricuspid orifice with a pericardial patch and creating a systemic-to-pulmonary arterial shunt. The perioperative risk for children who can be stabilized preoperatively can be low (Starnes et al, 1991), and such children may be suitable for a later Fontan-type procedure.

———RELATED MALFORMATIONS———

The lesions to be described in this section do not have malformations of their tricuspid valves. Yet they are often discussed in relation to Ebstein's malformation. Although they should readily be distinguished, we will emphasize those features that might produce problems in separating them from Ebstein's malformation. The entities which might cause confusion are Uhl's anomaly, fatty replacement of the right ventricular myocardium, the so-called 'sausage-shaped' right ventricle, and idiopathic dilation of the right atrium.

UHL'S ANOMALY ————————————

The heart described by Uhl (1952) came from an infant aged 8 months at death. The characteristic feature was total absence of the myocardium throughout the parietal walls of the right ventricle, but with normal septal trabeculations and with normal structure of the tricuspid and pulmonary valves. The left side of the heart was also normal, thus distinguishing Uhl's case from Osler's famous 'parchment heart', described by Segall (1950), in which all four cardiac chambers were thin walled and dilated. Comparable examples of the entity described by Uhl are exceedingly rare, but we have one example within our postmortem collection (Figure 42.23). Vecht and his colleagues (1979) collected a series of hearts fitting the original description and, surprisingly, found that the patients presented at all ages from 1 day to 57 years, although nearly half had presented in the first year. Most had dyspnoea and tachypnoea, with cyanosis present in two thirds. Signs of congestive cardiac failure, including oedema, hepatomegaly and elevation of jugular venous pressures, were also common, particularly in the older patients. The chest radiography shows cardiomegaly because of the dilation of the right-sided chambers. Right atrial hypertrophy, and diminution of right ventricular forces, are the electrocardiographic features. Cross-sectional echocardiography should be diagnostic, showing the normal valvar anatomy in the setting of dilated right-sided chambers with uniformly paper-thin walls.

Most of those presenting in infancy have died in infancy. They are so rare that no centre has sufficient experience to propose any systematic approach to surgery. To us, it seems that the crucial factor is likely to be right atrial performance, since the total absence of parietal right ventricular myocardium means that the ventricle is no more than a passive but dilated conduit. If surgery is contemplated, the approach formulated by Starnes and his colleagues (1991) for Ebstein's

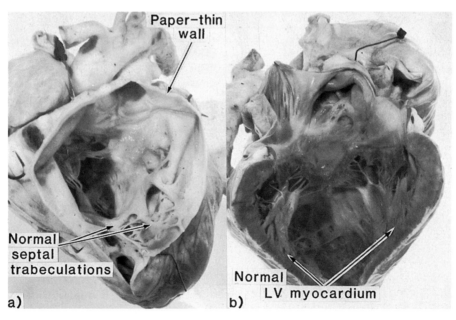

Figure 42.23. (a) The myocardium is completely absent from the parietal wall of the right ventricle in a postmortem example of Uhl's anomaly. Note the normal arrangement of the septal trabeculations and the leaflets of the tricuspid and pulmonary valves. (b) The left side of the heart is also normal.

malformation, with exclusion of the right ventricle and either construction of a systemic-to-pulmonary arterial shunt or use of the Fontan procedure, should offer the best chance of success. Transplantation is another option. O'Connor and his colleagues (1992) have described a patient with tricuspid atresia associated with partial total absence of the parietal right ventricular myocardium which they argue is a form of Uhl's malformation; however, the anatomical differences between the entities are obvious.

ARRHYTHMOGENIC RIGHT VENTRICULAR CARDIOMYOPATHY

It is now well established that arrhythmogenic right ventricular cardiomyopathy (see also Chapter 27) is caused by excessive deposition of fat in the interstices of the parietal right ventricular myocardium (Figure 42.24). Fat, of course, is a ubiquitous component of the normal right ventricular myocardium, and there are difficulties in some hearts in determining the borderline between 'lipomatosis cordis' and arrhythmogenic dysplasia (Fontaliran et al, 1998; Burke et al, 1998). The fatty infiltration, however, is very much a feature of ageing, whereas the cardiomyopathic form is found in adolescents and young adults, who present with palpitations, tachycardia and syncope, or even with sudden death. Furthermore, the familial nature of the arrhythmogenic variant, coupled with the frequent findings of scattered focuses of inflammation, lead to the conclusion that fatty infiltration is probably a separate entity (Burke et al, 1998). The arrhythmogenic form, and its association with right ventricular myocardial dysplasia, was first highlighted by Marcus and his colleagues (1982). They pointed to the significance of the 'triangle of dysplasia', with patchy fibrofatty lesions replacing the normal myocardium in the inlet, apical and infundibular parts of the right ventricle. The lesions are very characteristic, producing circumscribed areas of virtual absence of myocardium, which transilluminate when seen in the heart at postmortem (Figure 42.24). Histology confirms that the myocardium is replaced by adipose and fibrous tissue rather than simply being absent (Figure 42.25). The fibrofatty replacement is now known also to involve the left ventricle in up to half the patients (Fornes et al, 1998). It is the patchy area of the thinned myocardial lesions, and the preservation of strands of normal myocardium even within these abnormal areas, that serves to distinguish right ventricular dysplasia from Uhl's anomaly (Gerlis et al, 1993). The normal structure of the valves differentiates both these lesions from Ebstein's malformation. It is possible that the three entities might be linked aetiologically, since apoptosis has been invoked as a mechanism for all of them (James et al, 1996). The anatomy, nonetheless, and the genetic background (Fontaine et al, 1998) confirm that they should be analysed separately, with additional subsets found in the arrhythmogenic cardiomyopathic forms depending on the genetic make-up.

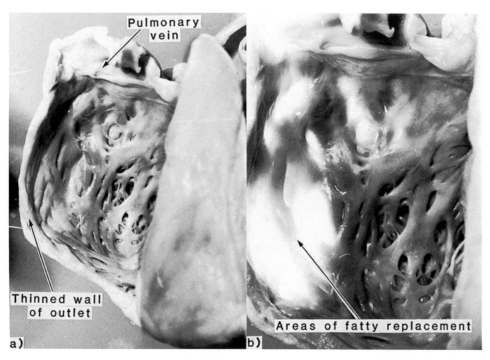

Figure 42.24. This heart has the typical morphological features of arrhythmogenic right ventricular cardiomyopathy. (a) The infundibulum has been opened to show the thinned areas of myocardium. (b) Transilluminated shows this thinning clearly. The myocardium is replaced by fibrofatty tissue (see Figure 42.25).

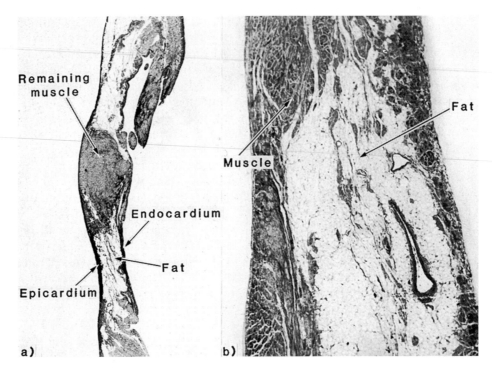

Figure 42.25. Histological sections across the thinned areas shown in Figure 42.24 reveal replacement by fibrous and adipose tissue. This distinguishes arrhythmogenic cardiomyopathy from Uhl's anomaly, in which the myocardium is completely absent, permitting apposition of the epicardium and endocardium.

HYPOPLASIA OF THE APICAL COMPONENT OF THE RIGHT VENTRICLE

First described by van der Hauwaert and his colleagues in 1971, hypoplasia of the atrial component of the right ventricle should give no problems in its distinction from Ebstein's malformation; similarly, it should not be confused with either Uhl's anomaly or arrhythmogenic right ventricular cardiomyopathy. The anatomy is characteris-

tic (Oldershaw et al, 1985). The inlet and infundibular components of the right ventricle are normal, as are the tricuspid and pulmonary valves. There is, however, effective absence of the apical trabecular component; consequently the ventricle is no more than a muscular tube connecting the two valves (Figures 42.26). The problem used to arise in clinical diagnosis. The patients can first be seen as infants but often do not present until middle age (Barboso Filho et al, 1983; Oldershaw et al, 1985).

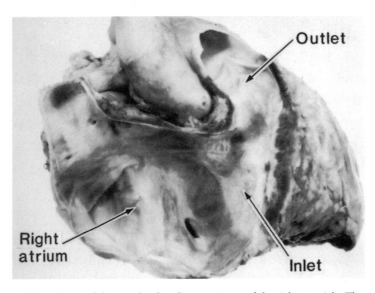

Figure 42.26. An example of isolated hypoplasia of the apical trabecular component of the right ventricle. The remaining ventricle forms a restricted fibromuscular conduit between the normal tricuspid and pulmonary valves.

Apart from cyanosis, which is not always present, physical examination is unremarkable. The chest radiography shows right atrial enlargement with diminished pulmonary vascularity. When diagnosis largely depended on catheterization, the haemodynamic findings were confusing (Haworth et al, 1975). The right ventricular and pulmonary arterial pressures were normal in the presence of an atrial shunt from right to left, with the only abnormality being minimal elevation of right atrial pressure. Cross-sectional echocardiography should be diagnostic and is in those for whom the condition is suspected, however, in several reported cases, admittedly prior to the era of sophisticated cross-sectional techniques, diagnosis was not made until postmortem (Barboso Filho et al, 1983; Oldershaw et al, 1985). In the context of this chapter, nonetheless, there should be no problems now in distinguishing right ventricular apical hypoplasia from Ebstein's malformation or the other lesions discussed above.

IDIOPATHIC DILATION OF THE RIGHT ATRIUM

Idiopathic dilation of the right atrium is a rare condition first described by Bailey in 1955. By the end of the 1980s, about 60 cases had been described, with most authors considering it to have a congenital origin (Terada et al, 1988), although it has been suggested that the dilation could represent an acute acquired event (Beder et al, 1982). Irrespective of such niceties, the potential problems in distinguishing the entity from Ebstein's malformation reflect the radiographic appearance, with marked dilation of the right border of the cardiac silhouette. Cross-sectional echocardiography reveals the normal annular attachments of the leaflets of the tricuspid valve at the atrioventricular junction (Ztot et al, 1998). The outcome amongst the published cases has varied. In most instances, it is a well-tolerated abnormality, but it can be a harbinger of arrhythmias or intra-atrial thrombus. Sudden death has been reported (Tenckhoff et al, 1969). Management has usually consisted of follow-up, with treatment of complications when appropriate, but surgical plication of the dilated atrium has been proposed for those presenting in infancy (Blaysat et al, 1997).

TRICUSPID VALVAR DYSPLASIA

Dysplastic valves are those which have normal proximal attachments at the anatomical atrioventricular junction, but with abnormalities of the leaflets and tension apparatus (Figure 42.27). The abnormalities are usually seen as nodular excrescences on the distal free margin and tension apparatus, but there may be deficiencies of the leaflet(s) themselves (Becker et al, 1971). Such lesions may occur in combination with almost any other congenital cardiac malformation (Kincaid et al, 1962; Sanyal

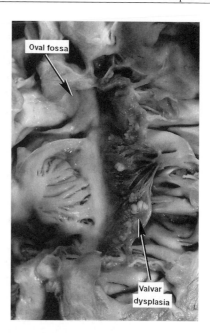

Figure 42.27. The right atrioventricular junction has been opened wide in this specimen to reveal marked dysplasia of all leaflets of the tricuspid valve, but with normal annular attachment at the atrioventricular junction.

et al, 1968; Barr et al, 1974). The incidence and aetiology of dysplastic valves are unknown, but the condition is rare, although it is now being seen with increasing frequency in fetal life (Lang et al, 1991).

The abnormality may escape detection in postnatal life when it is mild. When it is severe, presentation in the neonatal or, increasingly, the fetal period is usual. It is the 'wall-to-wall' heart that draws attention to the fetuses with this malformation. Patients have severe and progressive cyanosis and congestive cardiac failure. The outcome in those diagnosed in fetal life is particularly poor (Sharland et al, 1991). In those presenting postnatally, a systolic murmur is usually present, best heard at the lower left sternal edge. The second heart sound is single, the pulmonary component being inaudible. A mid-diastolic tricuspid murmur may be present.

The chest radiograph reveals gross cardiomegaly, the heart shadow obscuring the lung fields. The electrocardiogram reflects the right atrial enlargement with peaked P-waves. Cross-sectional echocardiography will demonstrate right atrial enlargement with normal junctional attachment of the dysplastic valvar leaflets. In addition, poor motion of a normal pulmonary valve may be seen. Peripheral contrast injection will demonstrate a right-to-left shunt to be at the atrial level. Little or no contrast may enter the pulmonary arteries. The problem of distinguishing functional from organic pulmonary atresia in this setting may be difficult to resolve even with cardiac catheterization (Freedom et al, 1978). The group from Toronto recommend retrograde aortography to opacify the pulmonary trunk via the duct. Regurgitation of contrast material into the right ventricle excludes organic atresia. This investigation may be performed in the neonate because such patients will usually be treated with prostaglandin E1 prior to invasive investigation. Medical management consists of prostaglandin and diuretic therapy. The surgical options for management of these sick infants include valvar replacement, creation of tricuspid atresia as described above, or cardiac transplantation.

ACQUIRED TRICUSPID VALVAR DISEASE

Older children and adolescents may rarely present with acquired problems of the tricuspid valve, most commonly functional tricuspid incompetence secondary to right ventricular dilation. This most often results from left-sided obstructive lesions with pulmonary hypertension. In these patients, the tricuspid annulus dilates and fails to shorten during systole (Ubago et al, 1983). The leaflets and tendinous cords, however, remain normal in appearance (Waller et al, 1986).

Tricuspid incompetence is also occasionally found in patients with dilated right ventricles after repair of tetralogy of Fallot with residual pulmonary regurgitation, or after intra-atrial repair for complete transposition. After the Mustard or Senning operations, the tricuspid valve is in the systemic circulation, and the development of tricuspid regurgitation is of concern. In a series from our institution of over 700 such patients, tricuspid regurgitation was almost always associated with right ventricular dysfunction and dilation rather than a structural abnormality of the tricuspid valve (J.E.N. Taylor personal communication).

Rheumatic tricuspid disease is rare in children (see Chapter 65) but may present in association with rheumatic involvement of the mitral and/or aortic valves. Tricuspid valvar endocarditis may complicate the use of indwelling central lines in any sick child; it is occasionally seen complicating intravenous drug abuse in adolescents. Tricuspid endocarditis is most commonly caused by *Staphylococcus epidermidis* or *S. aureus* (Stern et al, 1986), or rarely by *Candida* species. The organisms may form masses on the valve or destroy large portions of the leaflets and/or tendinous cords. Rarely, the tricuspid valve is involved in systemic lupus erythematosus (Gibson and Wood, 1955), metastatic carcinoid disease (Carpena et al, 1973) or hypereosinophilic syndromes (Chusid et al, 1975).

REFERENCES

Adams J C L, Hudson R 1956 A case of Ebstein's anomaly surviving to age 79. British Heart Journal 18: 129–131

Anderson K R, Lie J T 1979 The right ventricular myocardium in Ebstein's anomaly. A morphometric histopathologic study. Mayo Clinic Proceedings 54: 181–186

Anderson K R, Zuberbuhler J R, Anderson R H, Becker A E, Lie J T 1979 Ebstein's anomaly: a review of the pathologic anatomy. Mayo Clinic Proceedings 54: 174–180

Anderson R H, Ho S Y 1998 The anatomy of Ebstein's malformation. In: Redington A N, Brawn W J, Deanfield J E, Anderson R H (eds) The right heart in congenital heart disease GMM, London, p 169–176

Augustin N, Schmidt-Habelmann P, Wottke M, Meisner H, Sebening F 1997 Results after surgical repair of Ebstein's anomaly. Annals of Thoracic Surgery 63: 1650–1656

Bailey C P 1955 Surgery of the Heart. Lea & Febiger Philadelphia, PA, p 413

Balaji S, Dennis N R, Keeton B R 1991 Familial Ebstein's anomaly: a report of six cases in two generations associated with mild skeletal abnormalities. British Heart Journal 66: 26–28

Barbero-Marcial M, Verginelli G, Awad M, Ferreira S, Ebaid M, Zerbini E J 1979 Surgical treatment of Ebstein's anomaly. Early and late results in twenty patients subjected to valve replacement. Journal of Thoracic and Cardiovascular Surgery 78: 416–422

Barbosa Filho J, Monteiro de Melo J C, Siguera Lopes A, Buarque Benchimol C, Lacerda P R S, Bulamaqui Benchimol A 1983 Hipoplasia isolada do ventriculo direito. Revista Latina de Cardiologia 4: 193–204

Barnard C N, Schrire Y 1963 Surgical correction of Ebstein's malformation with a prosthetic tricuspid valve. Surgery 54: 302–308

Barr P A, Celermajer J M, Bowdler J S, Cartmill T B 1974 Severe congenital tricuspid incompetence in the neonate. Circulation 49: 962–967

Becker A E, Becker M J, Edwards J E 1971 Pathologic spectrum of dysplasia of the tricuspid valve. Archives of Pathology 91: 167–178

Becker A E, Anderson R H, Durrer D, Wellens H J J 1978 The anatomical substrates of Wolff–Parkinson–White syndrome; a clinicopathologic correlation in seven patients. Circulation 57: 870–879

Beder S D, Nihill M R, McNamara D C 1982 Idiopathic dilatation of the right atrium in a child. American Heart Journal 103: 134–137

Bialostozky D, Horwitz S, Espino-Vela J 1972 Ebstein's malformation of the tricuspid valve. American Journal of Cardiology 29: 826–836

Blaysat G, Villain E, Marçon F 1997 Prognostic et évolution de la dilatation idiopathique de l'oreillette droite chez l'enfant. Archives des Maladies du Coeur et des Vaisseaux 90: 645–648

Burke A P, Farb A, Tashko G, Virmani R 1998 Arrhythmogenic right ventricular cardiomyopathy and fatty replacement of the right ventricular myocardium: are they different diseases? Circulation 97: 1571–1580

Cabin H S, Roberts W C 1981 Ebstein's anomaly of the tricuspid valve and prolapse of the mitral valve. American Heart Journal 101: 177–180

Cappato R, Schluter M, Weiss C et al 1996 Radiofrequency current catheter ablation of accessory atrioventricular pathways in Ebstein's anomaly. Circulation 94: 376–383

Carpena C, Kay J H, Mendez A M, Redington J V, Zubiate P, Zucker R 1973 Carcinoid heart disease: surgery for tricuspid and pulmonary valve lesions. American Journal of Cardiology 32: 229–233

Carpentier A, Chauvaud S, Mace L et al 1988 A new reconstructive operation for Ebstein's anomaly of the tricuspid valve. Journal of Thoracic and Cardiovascular Surgery 96: 91–101

Celermajer D S, Dodd S M, Greenwald S E, Wyse R K H, Deanfield J E 1992a Morbid anatomy in neonates with Ebstein's anomaly of the tricuspid valve: pathophysiologic and clinical implications. Journal of the American College of Cardiology 19: 1049–1053

Celermajer D S, Cullen S, Sullivan I D, Spiegelhalter D J, Wyse R K, Deanfield J E 1992b Outcome in neonates with Ebstein's anomaly. Journal of the American College of Cardiology 19: 1041–1046

Celermajer D S, Bull C, Till J et al 1994 Ebstein's anomaly: presentation and outcome from fetal to adult. Journal of the American College of Cardiology 23: 170–176

Charles R G, Barnard C N, Beck W 1981 Tricuspid valve replacement for Ebstein's anomaly: a 19 year review of the first case. British Heart Journal 46: 578–580

Chauvaud S M, Milhaileanu S A, Gaer A R, Carpentier A C 1996 Surgical treatment of Ebstein's malformation – the 'Hôpital Broussais' experience. Cardiology in the Young 6: 4–11

Chauvaud S, Fuzellier J F, Berrebi A, Marino J P, Milaileanu S, Carpentier A 1998 Bidirectional cavopulmonary shunt associated with ventriculo and valvuloplasty in Ebstein's anomaly: benefits in high risk patients. European Journal of Cardiothoracic Surgery 13: 514–519

Chusid M J, Dale D C, West B C, Wolffe S M 1975 The hypereosinophilic syndrome: analysis of fourteen cases with review of the literature. Medicine (Baltimore) 52: 1–27

Crews T L, Pridie R B, Benham R, Leatham A 1972 Auscultatory and phonocardiographic findings in Ebstein's anomaly. Correlation of first heart sound with ultrasonic records of tricuspid valve movement. British Heart Journal 34: 681–687

Danielson G K, Fuster V 1982 Surgical repair of Ebstein's anomaly. Annals of Surgery 196: 499–504

Driscoll D J, Mottram C D, Danielson G K 1988 Spectrum of exercise intolerance in 45 patients with Ebstein's anomaly and observations on exercise tolerance in 11 patients after surgical repair. Journal of the American College of Cardiology 11: 831–836

Ebstein W 1866 Uber einen sehr seltenen Fall von Insufficient der valvula tricuspidalis, bedingt durch eine angedorenen hochgradige missbildung derselben. Archiv Für Anatomie und Physiologie, 328

Ellis K, Griffiths S P, Burris J O, Ramsey G C, Fleming R J 1964 Ebstein's anomaly of the tricuspid valve: angiocardiographic considerations. American Journal of Roentgenology 92: 1338–1351

Engle M A, Payne T P B, Bruins C, Taussig H B 1950 Ebstein's anomaly of the tricuspid valve: report of three cases and analysis of clinical syndrome. Circulation 1: 1246–1260

Farooki Z Q, Henry T G, Green E W 1976 Echocardiographic spectrum of Ebstein's anomaly of the tricuspid valve. Circulation 53: 63–68

Fontaine G, Fontaliran F, Frank R 1998 Arrhythmogenic right ventricular cardiomyopathies: clinical forms and main differential diagnoses. Circulation 97: 1532–1535

Fontaliran F, Arkwright S, Vilde F, Fontaine G 1998 Arrhythmogenic right ventricular dysplasia and cardiomyopathy. Clinical and anatomic-pathologic aspects, nosologic approach. Archives Anatomie Cytologie Pathologique 46: 171–177

Fontana M E, Wooley C F 1972 Sail-sound in Ebstein's anomaly. Circulation 46: 155–164

Fornes P, Ratel S, Lecomte D 1998 Pathology of arrhythmogenic right ventricular cardiomyopathy/dysplasia – an autopsy study of 20 forensic cases. Journal of Forensic Science 43: 777–783

Freedom R M, Culham G, Moes F, Olley P M, Rowe R D 1978 Differentiation of functional and structural pulmonary atresia: role of aortography. American Journal of Cardiology 41: 914–920

Gasul B M, Weinberg M Jr, Luan L L, Fell E H, Bicoff J, Steiger Z 1959 Superior vena cava–right main pulmonary artery anastomosis. Journal of the American Medical Association 171: 1797–1803

Gegenbaur C 1885 Lehrbuch der Anatomic des Herzen. Wilhelm Engelmann, Leipzig, p 639

Gentles T L, Calder A L, Clarkson P M, Neutze J M 1992 Ebstein's anomaly of the tricuspid valve: a clinical review with long-term follow-up. American Journal of Cardiology 69: 377–381

Genton E, Blount G 1967 The spectrum of Ebstein's anomaly. American Heart Journal 73: 395–425

Gerlis L M, Schmidt-Ott S C, Ho S Y, Anderson R H 1993 Dysplastic conditions of the right ventricular myocardium: Uhl's anomaly *v* arrhythmogenic right ventricular dysplasia. British Heart Journal 69: 142–150

Gibson R, Wood P 1955 The diagnosis of tricuspid stenosis. British Heart Journal 17: 552–562

Giuliani E R, Fuster V, Brandenburg R O, Mair D D 1979 Ebstein's anomaly. The clinical features and natural history of Ebstein's anomaly of the tricuspid valve. Mayo Clinical Proceedings 54: 163–173

Gussenhoven W J, Spitaels S E C, Bom N, Becker A E 1980 Echocardiographic criteria for Ebstein's anomaly of tricuspid valve. British Heart Journal 43: 31–37

Hardy K L, May I A, Webster C A, Kimball K G 1964 Ebstein's anomaly: a functional concept and successful definitive repair. Journal of Thoracic and Cardiovascular Surgery 48: 927–940

Haworth S G, Shinebourne E A, Miller G A H 1975 Right to left interatrial shunting with normal right ventricular pressure. A puzzling haemodynamic picture associated with some rare congenital malformations of the right ventricle and tricuspid valve. British Heart Journal 37: 386–391

Hornberger L K, Sahn D J, Kleinman C S, Copel J A, Reed K L 1991 Tricuspid valve disease with significant tricuspid valve insufficiency in the fetus: diagnosis and outcome. Journal of the American College of Cardiology 17: 167–173

James T N, Nichols M M, Sapire D W, Lopez S M 1996 Complete heart block and fatal right ventricular failure in an infant. Circulation 93: 1588–1600

Kastor J A, Goldreyer B N, Josephson M E et al 1975 Electrophysiologic characteristics of Ebstein's anomaly of the tricuspid valve. Circulation 52: 987–995

Keith J D 1978 Ebstein's disease. In: Keith J D, Rowe R D, Vlad P (eds) Heart disease in infancy and childhood, 3rd edn. Macmillan, New York, p 847–855

Kincaid O W, Swan H J C, Ongley P A, Titus J L 1962 Congenital tricuspid insufficiency: report of two cases. Proceedings of the Mayo Clinic 37: 640–650

Kirklin J W, Barratt-Boyes B G 1992 Ebstein's malformation. In: Cardiac surgery, 2nd edn. Churchill Livingstone, New York, p 1105–1130

Kumar A J, Fyler D C, Miettinen O S, Nadas A S 1971 Ebstein's anomaly. Clinical profile and natural history. American Journal of Cardiology 28: 84–95

Lamers W H, Virágh S, Wessels A, Moorman A F M, Anderson R H 1995 Formation of the tricuspid valve in the human heart. Circulation 91: 111–121

Lang D, Oberhoffer R, Cook A, Sharland G, Allan L, Fagg N, Anderson R H 1991 Pathologic spectrum of malformations of the tricuspid valve in prenatal and neonatal life. Journal of the American College of Cardiology 17: 1161–1167

Leung M P, Baker E J, Anderson R H, Zuberbuhler J R 1988 Cineangiographic spectrum of Ebstein's malformation: its relevance to clinical presentation and outcome. Journal of the American College of Cardiology 11: 154–161

Lev M, Liberthson R R, Joseph R H et al 1970 The pathologic anatomy of Ebstein's disease. Archives of Pathology 90: 334–343

Makous N, van der Veer J B 1966 Ebstein's anomaly and life expectancy. Report of a survival to over age 79. American Journal of Cardiology 18: 100–104

Mann R J, Lie J T 1979 The life story of Wilhelm Ebstein (1836–1912) and his almost overlooked description of a congenital heart disease. Mayo Clinic Proceedings 54: 197–204

Marcus F I, Fontaine G H, Guiraudon G et al 1982 Right ventricular dysplasia: a report of 24 adult cases. Circulation 65: 384–398

Mathews J L, Pennington W S, Isobe J H, Gaskin T A, Dumas J H, Kahn D R 1983 Paradoxical embolization with Ebstein's anomaly. Archives of Surgery 118: 1101

Mayer F E, Nadas A S, Ongley P A 1957 Ebstein's anomaly: presentation of ten cases. Circulation 16: 1057–1069

Mayer J E Jr, Perry S, O'Brien P, Perez-Atayde P, Jonas R A, Castañeda A R, Parness I R 1990 Orthotopic heart transplantation for complex congenital heart disease. Journal of Thoracic and Cardiovascular Surgery 99: 484–492

Melo J, Saylam A, Knight R, Starr A 1979 Long-term results after surgical correction of Ebstein's anomaly. Report of 2 cases. Journal of Thoracic and Cardiovascular Surgery 78: 233–235

Monibi A A, Neches W H, Lenox C C, Park S C, Mathews R A, Zuberbuhler J R 1978 Left ventricular anomalies associated with Ebstein's malformation of the tricuspid valve. Circulation 57: 303–306

Ng R, Somerville J, Ross D 1979 Ebstein's anomaly: late results of surgical correction. European Journal of Cardiology 9: 39–52

O'Connor W N, Cottrill C M, Marion M T, Noonan J A 1992 Defective regional myocardial development and vascularization in one variant of tricuspid atresia – clinical and necropsy findings in three cases. Cardiology in the Young 2: 42–52

Oldershaw P, Ward D, Anderson R H 1985 Hypoplasia of the apical trabecular component of the morphologically right ventricle. American Journal of Cardiology 55: 862–864

Pexeider T 1975 Cell death in the morphogenesis and teratogenesis of the heart. Advances in the Anatomy, Embryology and Cell Biology 51: 1–100

Pressley J C, Wharton M, Lang A S L, Lowe J E, Gallagher J J, Prystowsky E N 1992 Effect of Ebstein's anomaly on short-and long-term outcome of surgically treated patients with Wolff–Parkinson–White syndrome. Circulation 86: 1147–1155

Quaegebeur J M, Sreeram N, Fraser A G 1991 Surgery for Ebstein's anomaly: the clinical and echocardiographic evaluation of a new technique. Journal of the American College of Cardiology 17: 722–728

Rigby M L, Mota C 1998 Echocardiographic evaluation and diagnosis of Ebstein's malformation. In: Redington A N, Brawn W J, Deanfield J E, Anderson R H (eds). The right heart in congenital heart disease. GMM, London, p 177–184

Roberson D A, Silverman N H 1989 Ebstein's anomaly: echocardiographic and clinical features in the fetus and neonate. Journal of the American College of Cardiology 14: 1300–1307

Rowe R D, Freedom R M, Mehrizi A, Bloom K R 1981 The neonate with congenital heart disease, 2nd edn. Saunders, Philadelphia, PA p 515–528

Rusconi P G, Zuberbuhler J R, Anderson R H, Rigby M L 1991 Morphologic–echocardiographic correlates of Ebstein's malformation. European Heart Journal 12: 784–790

Sanyal S K, Bhargava S K, Saxena H M, Gosh S 1968 Congenital insufficiency of the tricuspid valve. A rare case of massive cardiomegaly and congestive cardiac failure in the neonate. Indian Heart Journal 20: 214–215

Saxena A, Fong L V, Tristam M, Ackery D M, Keeton B R 1991 Late noninvasive evaluation of cardiac performance in mildly symptomatic older patients with Ebstein's anomaly of tricuspid valve. Journal of the American College of Cardiology 17: 182–186

Schiebler G L, Adams P Jr, Anderson R C, Amplatz K, Lester R G 1959 Clinical study of twenty-three cases of Ebstein's anomaly of the tricuspid valve. Circulation 19: 165–187

Schrieber C, Cook A, Ho S Y, Augustin N, Anderson R H 1999 Morphology of Ebstein's malformation: revisitation relative to surgical repair. Journal of Thoracic and Cardiovascular Surgery 117: 148–155

Sealy W C, Gallagher J J, Pritchett E L, Wallace A G 1978 Surgical treatment of tachyarrhythmias in patients with both an Ebstein anomaly and a Kent bundle. Journal of Thoracic and Cardiovascular Surgery 75: 847–853

Segall H N 1950 Parchment heart (Osler). American Heart Journal 40: 948–950

Seward J B, Tajik A J, Feist D J, Smith H C 1979 Ebstein's anomaly in an 85-year-old man. Mayo Clinic Proceedings 54: 193–196

Sharland G K, Cita S K, Allan L D 1991 Tricuspid valve dysplasia or displacement in intrauterine life. Journal of the American College of Cardiology 17: 944–949

Shiina A, Seward J B, Edwards W D, Hagler D J, Tajik A J 1984 Two-dimensional echocardiographic spectrum of Ebstein's anomaly: detailed anatomic assessment. Journal of the American College of Cardiology 3: 356–370

Silver M A, Cohen S R, McIntosh C L, Cannon R O III, Roberts W C 1984 Late (5 to 132 months) clinical and hemodynamic results after either tricuspid valve replacement or anuloplasty for Ebstein's anomaly of the tricuspid valve. American Journal of Cardiology 54: 627–632

Smith W M, Gallagher J J, Kerr C R et al 1982 The electrophysiologic basis and management of symptomatic recurrent tachycardia in patients with Ebstein's anomaly of the tricuspid valve. American Journal of Cardiology 49: 1223–1234

Soloff L A, Stauffer H M, Zatuchni J 1951 Ebstein's disease: report of the first case diagnosed during life. American Journal of Medical Science 222: 554–561

Somerville J, Presbitero P, Stone S, Aruta E, Spiegelhalter D 1992 Pregnancy in cyanotic congenital heart disease: maternal complications and factors influencing successful fetal outcome. British Heart Journal 68: 96

Starnes V A, Pitlick P T, Bernstein D, Griffin M L, Choy M, Shumway N E 1991 Ebstein's anomaly appearing in the neonate. Journal of Thoracic and Cardiovascular Surgery 101: 1082–1087

Stern J H, Sisto D A, Strom J A, Soeiro R, Jones S R, Frater R W 1986 Immediate tricuspid valve replacement for endocarditis. Journal of Thoracic and Cardiovascular Surgery 91: 163–167

Taussig H B 1960 Congenital malformations of the heart, 2nd edn, vol 2. The Commonwealth Fund, Harvard University Press, Cambridge, MA, p 466–489

Tenckhoff L, Stamm S J, Beckwith J B 1969 Sudden death in idiopathic (congenital) right atrium enlargement. Circulation 40: 227–235

Terada T, Oiwake H, Nakanuma Y 1988 An autopsy case of idiopathic enlargement of the right atrium and a review of the literature. Acta Pathologica Japonica 38: 361–370

Till J, Celermajer D S, Deanfield J E 1992 The natural history of arrhythmias in Ebstein's anomaly. Journal of the American College of Cardiology 19(suppl A): 273A

Ubago J L, Figuero A, Ochoteco A, Colman T, Duran R M, Duran C G 1983 Analysis of the amount of tricuspid valve anular dilatation required to produce functional tricuspid regurgitation. American Journal of Cardiology 52: 155–158

Uhl H S M 1952 A previously undescribed congenital malformation of the heart: almost total absence of the myocardium of the right ventricle. Bulletin of the Johns Hopkins Hospital 91: 197–205

van der Hauwaert L G, Michaelson M 1971 Isolated right ventricular hypoplasia. Circulation 44: 466–474

van Lingen B, Bauersfeld S R 1955 The electrocardiogram in Ebstein's anomaly of the tricuspid valve. American Heart Journal 50: 13–23

Van Mierop L H S, Schiebler G L, Victorica B E 1977 Anomalies of the tricuspid valve resulting in stenosis or incompetence. In: Moss A J, Adams F H, Emmanoulides G C (eds) Heart disease in infants, children and adolescents, 2nd edn. Williams & Wilkins, Baltimore MD, p 262–274

Vecht R J, Carmichael D J S, Gopal R, Philip G 1979 Uhl's anomaly. British Heart Journal 41: 676–682

Waller B J, Moriarty A T, Ebie J N, Davey D M, Hawley D A, Pless J E 1986 Etiology of pure tricuspid regurgitation based on anular circumference and leaflet area: analysis of 45 necropsy patients with clinical and morphologic evidence of pure tricuspid regurgitation. Journal of the American College of Cardiology 7: 1063–1074

Watson H 1974 Natural history of Ebstein's anomaly of tricuspid valve in childhood and adolescence. British Heart Journal 36: 417–427

Weinstein M R, Goldfield M D 1975 Cardiovascular malformations with lithium use during pregnancy. American Journal of Psychiatry 132: 529–531

Westaby S, Karp R B, Kirklin J W, Waldo A L, Blackstone E H 1982 Surgical treatment in Ebstein's malformation. Annals of Thoracic Surgery 34: 388–395

Williams J B, Karp R B, Kirklin J W et al 1980 Considerations in selection and management of patients undergoing valve replacement with glutareldehyde-fixed porcine bioprostheses. Annals of Thoracic Surgery 30: 247–258

Willis P W IV, Craige E 1983 First heart sounds in Ebstein's anomaly: observations on the cause of wide-splitting by echophonocardiographic studies before and after operative repair. Journal of the American College of Cardiology 2: 1165–1168

Wood P 1962 Diseases of the heart and circulation. 2nd edn. Eyre & Spottiswoode, London, p 352–358

Yeager S B, Parness I R, Danders S P 1988 Severe tricuspid regurgitation simulating pulmonary atresia in the fetus. American Heart Journal 115: 906–908

Ztot S, Haddour L, Cherti M, Akoudad H, Arharbi M 1998 Idiopathic dilation of the right atrium. A case report. Cardiovascular Imaging 10: 101–103

Zuberbuhler J R, Allwork S P, Anderson R H 1979 The spectrum of Ebstein's anomaly of the tricuspid valve. Journal of Thoracic and Cardiovascular Surgery 77: 202–211

43

Mitral valvar anomalies and supravalvar mitral ring

J. Smallhorn and F. J. Macartney

INTRODUCTION

This chapter concerns congenital anomalies that affect the function of the morphologically mitral valve. Accessory mitral valvar tissue producing subaortic stenosis (Sellers et al, 1964), therefore, is dealt with in Chapter 54. Insufficiency of the left atrioventricular valve is so much a part of atrioventricular septal defect with common atrioventricular junction, and hearts with discordant atrio-ventricular connections, that these are considered, not here, but in Chapters 36 and 49. Left atrioventricular valvar abnormalities in double inlet ventricle are dealt with in Chapter 38. Straddling mitral valve is considered in Chapter 41. Supravalvar mitral ring is so commonly associated with congenital mitral stenosis, however, and mimics it so closely that it is covered in this section.

INCIDENCE AND AETIOLOGY

Congenital deformities of the mitral valve are rare, if those involving the left valve in hearts with common atrioventricular junction are excluded, with mitral stenosis occurring in 0.6% of postmortems and in 0.21–0.42% of clinical series (Collins-Nakai et al, 1977). Congenital mitral incompetence is even rarer. There is a male to female ratio of around 1.5:1 to 2.2:1 (Collins-Nakai et al, 1977; Ruckman and Van Praagh, 1978). Congenital mitral valvar anomalies are rarely isolated. The fully developed syndrome of so-called 'parachute mitral valve' (Shone et al, 1963) includes four obstructions within the left heart, namely the valvar lesion itself, supravalvar mitral ring, subaortic stenosis and aortic coarctation. Any of these obstructions may coexist with any congenital lesion afflicting the mitral valve, particularly coarctation. In a clinical series of patients with congenital mitral stenosis, excluding hypoplasia of the left heart, almost three-quarters had additional anomalies (Collins-Nakai et al, 1977). It is tempting to imagine that development of one abnormality upstream may, during morphogenesis, result in a series of more distal abnormalities owing to disturbance in the patterns of flow. Annular hypoplasia of the mitral valve is almost always associated with hypoplasia of the left ventricle and aortic stenosis or atresia (Chapter 45) (Macartney et al, 1976; Ruckman and Van Praagh, 1978). Ventricular septal defect is quite common in this setting, and double outlet right ventricle and tetralogy of Fallot occasionally occur. When the mitral valve is imperforate, left ventricular hypoplasia is inevitable unless there is an associated ventricular septal defect.

MORPHOLOGY

It is convenient to describe the abnormal morphology in terms of malformation of the various components of the mitral valve, remembering that, in functional terms, such derangement can result in stenosis, incompetence or both (Carpentier, 1983a, Chauvaud et al, 1997a,b). It is appropriate to commence by considering anomalies of the entire valvar apparatus.

MITRAL VALVAR DYSPLASIA AND HYPOPLASIA

Mitral valvar dysplasia and hypoplasia is defined in terms of abnormal development of the entire valvar apparatus (Becker, 1983; Daliento et al, 1991). The leaflets are thickened, the intercordal spaces often obliterated and the papillary muscles deformed, the last frequently extending as muscular strands directly into the leaflets (Figure 43.1). Usually such a valve shows global hypoplasia and is the most common lesion underscoring isolated congenital mitral stenosis (Ruckman and Van Praagh, 1978). When the free edges of the dysplastic valve leaflets are thickened and rolled, the valve may be incompetent as well as

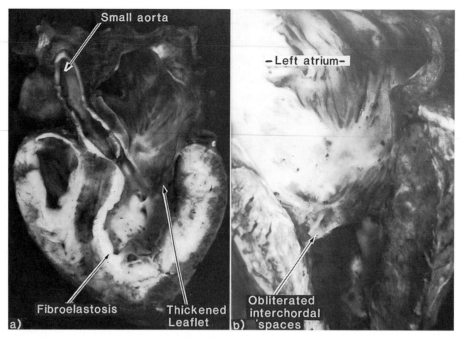

Figure 43.1. The typical stenotic mitral valve found in the setting of the hypoplastic left heart syndrome. (a) A stimulated long-axis section. (b) The fibroelastotic process has obliterated the intercordal spaces.

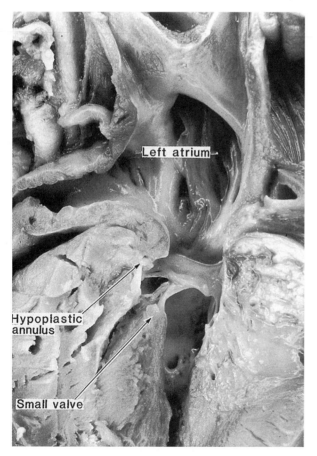

Figure 43.2. A stenotic mitral valve with miniaturization of all the components, including the atrioventricular junction. The leaflet tissue is more normal than that shown in Figure 43.1, however, and the intercordal spaces are preserved. (Specimen photographed and reproduced by kind permission of Dr J. R. Zuberbuhler, University of Pittsburgh.)

stenotic. Occasionally, mitral stenosis may be produced when the valve is miniaturized in its entirety but does not show dysplastic features (Figure 43.2). This is much rarer than the hypoplastic and dysplastic valve. Of more significance is the arrangement when only part of the valve is hypoplastic. This is typically seen when one papillary muscle, usually the anterolateral muscle, is grossly reduced in size or even, on occasions, totally absent. Then the anterolateral commissure either inserts directly to the left ventricular free wall or else is supported on the wall by a small papillary muscle. The tension apparatus then has a grossly eccentric appearance, effectively inserting into a solitary papillary muscle (Figure 43.3). This arrangement

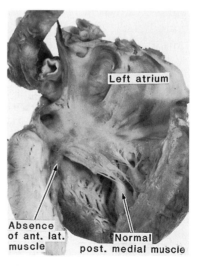

Figure 43.3. The so-called parachute arrangement produced by gross hypoplasia of the anterolateral papillary muscle (viewed from behind).

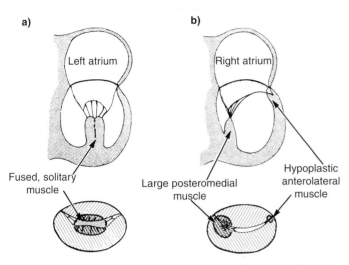

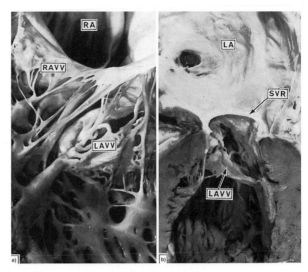

Figure 43.4. Diagrams comparing and contrasting the two mechanisms that can simulate so-called 'parachute' arrangement of the mitral valve.

Figure 43.5. In this heart with double inlet left ventricle, the left valve (LAVV) shows a 'parachute' arrangement resulting from hypoplasia of the lateral papillary muscle. In addition (b), there is a supravalvar ring (SVR) in the left atrium (LA). RA, right atrium; RAVV, right atrioventricular valve.

is the source of much confusion to the morphologist, since it is that illustrated by Shone and colleagues (1963) as a 'parachute mitral valve'. But the situation produced (Figure 43.4b) bears less resemblance to a parachute than does that in which the two papillary muscles are fused into a solid solitary structure that supports the tension apparatus from the entire valve (Figure 43.4a), and even this arrangement would produce a lethal parachute, since its canopy would be open! This confusing situation was highlighted by Rosenquist (1974), who described the arrangement with fused muscles and commented, 'The specimens could be classified as parachute mitral valves because there appeared to be only one papillary muscle'. In the account of Carpentier and colleagues (1976), designed to guide the surgeon, it is fused papillary muscles that are described as parachute valves. In the detailed study of Ruckman and Van Praagh (1978), however, such cases were specifically excluded, since they did not fit the original illustration of Shone and his colleagues (1963). The form with fused papillary muscles, nonetheless, is more likely to be chosen by clinicians as their paradigm for the parachute malformation. Furthermore, for the morphologist, an absent or hypoplastic papillary muscle is readily recognized and described as such. Similar precision is provided by cross-sectional echocardiography (Vogt et al, 1981). An echocardiographic–morphological correlation noted that many patients with aortic coarctation have altered positions of the left ventricular papillary muscles and narrowing of the interpapillary valley (Goldberg et al, 1995).

In this chapter, therefore, when we speak of 'parachute valves', we will specify whether we are discussing the variant produced by fusion of the papillary muscles into a solid mass, often additionally dysplastic, or whether there is hypoplasia or absence of one or other of the papillary muscles. Before leaving the topic, we must also mention the supravalvar stenosing ring, which was described by Shone and his colleagues (1963) as part of

the complex including the parachute valve. The best examples of truly supravalvar rings that we have seen were associated with double inlet left ventricle. The supravalvar ring in this setting was a concentric thickening of the left atrial endocardium immediately above the atrioventricular junction (Figure 43.5). In the clinical setting, in contrast, it seems that the so-called stenosing supravalvar ring is formed on the atrial aspect of the valvar leaflets (Sullivan et al, 1986). In reality, therefore, the more common variant of the lesion should be considered as involving the valvar leaflets (see below).

ANOMALIES OF THE LEAFLETS

The most extreme anomaly is an imperforate mitral valve. Such imperforate valves usually coexist with aortic atresia, forming part of the 'hypoplastic left ventricle syndrome'. For the anatomist, this entity is then distinguished from absence of the left atrioventricular connection, but this morphological distinction is rarely, if ever, of clinical significance (Anderson and Thiene, 1981; Thiene et al, 1981). Imperforate mitral valves can also be found without aortic atresia and are then part of the combination termed 'mitral atresia with patent aortic root' (Watson et al, 1960; Moreno et al, 1976). Often, the ventriculo-arterial connection is double outlet from the right ventricle but, in a signficant number of cases, the patent aorta arises from a good-sized left ventricle filled through a ventricular septal defect and separated from the left atrium by the imperforate valvar membrane with its own hypoplastic tension apparatus (Figure 43.6). The ventricular septal defect can be of varying morphology (Mickell et al, 1983).

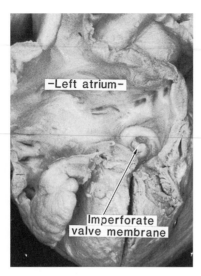

Figure 43.6. The left atrial aspect of a hypoplastic and imperforate left atrioventricular valve. (Reproduced by kind permission of Dr J. R. Zuberbuhler, University of Pittsburgh.)

Ebstein's malformation can rarely affect the morphologically mitral valve. A case was reported by Ruschhaupt and colleagues (1976), and we have seen several similar cases (Figure 43.7) (Leung et al, 1987). The feature of Ebstein's malformation when it involves the morphologically mitral valve is that the mural leaflet is plastered down onto the ventricular wall; consequently, its hinge is below the atrioventricular junction but there is no thinning of the atrialized inlet portion as is usually seen when it is the morphologically tricuspid valve that is deformed in the setting of concordant atrioventricular connections. Interestingly, nonetheless, lack of morphologic atrialization is also a feature of Ebstein's malformation in the

setting of discordant atrioventricular connections (see Chapter 49).

An isolated cleft of the mitral valve is also an anomaly confined to the leaflet, and one that primarily produces mitral incompetence. As pointed out by Becker (1983), the affected leaflet tends to be dysplastic, and its edges are usually rolled and thickened (Figure 43.8). It is important to distinguish an isolated cleft of the aortic leaflet of the mitral valve in hearts with separate atrioventricular junction from a so-called 'cleft' in the left valve of atrioventricular septal defects with common atrioventricular junction. The isolated cleft 'points' into the aortic outflow tract, often in association with a ventricular septal defect (Sigfusson et al, 1995), and the aortic leaflet is readily reconstituted by suture of its edges. In contrast, the so-called cleft in atrioventricular septal defects points to the septum. It is the space between the left ventricular components of the bridging leaflets guarding the common atrioventricular junction. Closure of the bridging leaflets cannot produce a left valve that, in any way, resembles a normal mitral valve (Smallhorn et al, 1982a,b; Sigfusson et al, 1995; Kohl and Silverman, 1996) (see Chapter 36).

Carpentier and his colleagues (1976) described an isolated anomaly of the valvar leaflets, which they termed a 'funnel-shaped valve'. It was characterized by thickened and retracted leaflet tissue with fused cords but was supported by normal papillary muscles. The funnel produces mitral stenosis. It is rare in postmortem collections. Much more common are valves with dual orifices. These can take two patterns. The most common is that in which a tongue of valvar tissue extends between the mural and aortic leaflets, dividing the valvar orifice into two components. Such an arrangement is frequently encountered in the left valve seen in atrioventricular septal defect with common atrioventricular junction. The rarer variant,

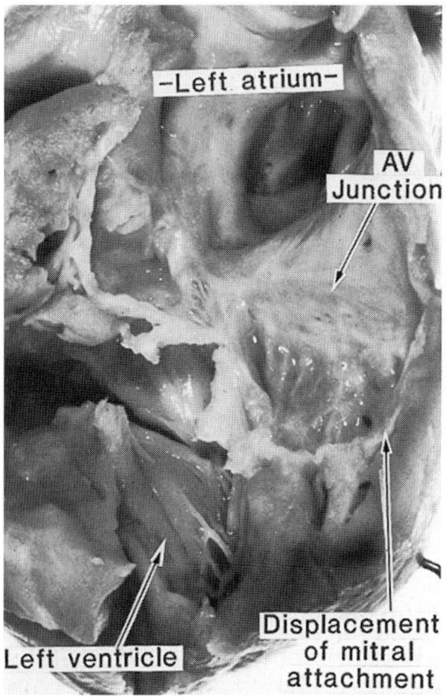

Figure 43.7. The rare arrangement in which an Ebstein-like lesion afflicts the normally located morphologically mitral valve.

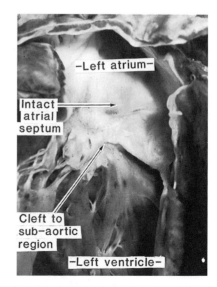

Figure 43.8. An isolated cleft in the aortic leaflet of the otherwise normal mitral valve (viewed from the posterior aspect). (Reproduced by kind permission of Professor A. E. Becker, University of Amsterdam.)

involving the otherwise normal mitral valve, shows duplication of the entire valvar structure; as a result, the left atrium is connected to the left ventricle by two valves, each with annulus, leaflets, cords and papillary muscles. This particular anomaly can exist in otherwise normal hearts, as well as in more complex anomalies such as tricuspid atresia (Bini et al, 1980) or double inlet ventricle. A rarer abnormality that can result in congenital mitral valve regurgitation is hypoplasia of the mural leaflet such that the valve leaflets cannot coapt normally during systole (Oberhansli et al, 1997).

ANOMALIES OF THE TENSION APPARATUS

Anomalies of the tension apparatus include the lesions variously referred to as mitral arcade (Layman and Edwards, 1967) or hammock valve (Carpentier et al, 1976). The abnormality is that the papillary muscles extend directly to the edges of the leaflets (Figure 43.9). In the most severe form, the muscles fuse on the leading edge of the aortic leaflet, forming the muscular arcade observed by the pathologist. When viewed from the atrial aspect, with the valve intact as seen by the surgeon, the intermixing of cords attached to the enlarged papillary muscle gives the appearance of a hammock.

STENOSIS VERSUS INCOMPETENCE

It is often difficult for the morphologist to predict from a specimen whether the observed pathology would have produced stenosis or incompetence. A much better appreciation is obtained by the surgeon (Carpentier et al, 1976; Chauvaud et al, 1997a,b). When insufficiency is the primary lesion, then this is most frequently the con-

sequence of problems with the leaflets and the annulus. Alternatively, insufficiency as a primary feature can be caused by subvalvar problems such as cordal retraction or elongation, papillary muscular hypoplasia or agenesis, and papillary muscular prolapse. When stenosis is the major problem, this is likely to be a result of commissural fusion in a dysplastic valve, a hammock lesion, parachute deformity or a funnel-shaped valve. Combined stenosis and insufficiency are related to commissural fusion of a dysplastic valve, a hammock valve, a parachute deformity or papillary muscular hypertrophy.

EFFECT ON THE HEART

Valvar pathology always affects the cardiac pump and, despite compensatory mechanisms, may lead to serious side effects in the myocardium and endocardium. Valvar pathology can also affect the pulmonary vascular bed, with pulmonary hypertension as a possible consequence (Becker, 1983).

PATHOPHYSIOLOGY

Supravalvar mitral ring and congenital mitral stenosis are, by and large, indistinguishable in their effects. Unless specific differences are mentioned, they may be assumed to behave in the same way. Pure mitral stenosis, or imperforate mitral valve, results in a diastolic pressure difference between the left atrium and left ventricle with a consequent elevation of left atrial pressure. Patients in sinus rhythm (the great majority) have a tall A wave in the left atrial trace. Coexistence of an interatrial communication results in decompression of the left atrium. This may be so profound as to obscure or eliminate the transmitral pressure difference, even when the mitral

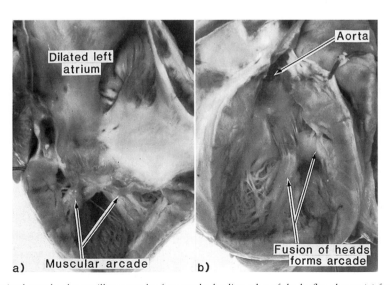

Figure 43.9. In the so-called mitral arcade, the papillary muscles fuse on the leading edge of the leaflet, shown (a) from the inlet and (b) from the outlet.

valve is imperforate. By contrast, excessive flow through the mitral valve, as may result from an associated ventricular septal defect, will exaggerate the transmitral diastolic pressure difference. Elevation of the left atrial pressure usually results in reflex pulmonary vasoconstriction, particularly if the development of pulmonary oedema results in ventilation–perfusion mismatch and pulmonary venous hypoxaemia. The combined effect is to produce pulmonary hypertension. In the presence of an associated duct or ventricular septal defect, this can result in right-to-left shunting at an earlier age than would be expected were mitral obstruction not present. The rise in pulmonary vascular resistance, and consequent fall in pulmonary blood flow, means that, on sequential cardiac catheterizations in individuals with mitral stenosis, the gradient is frequently found to fall (Collins-Nakai et al, 1977). This finding is similar to medical intervention using nitric oxide in patients with congenital mitral stenosis (Atz et al, 1996), where it was observed that the pulmonary vasoreactivity was greater than previously reported in adults. In the absence of pulmonary stenosis, and without any communication at great arterial or ventricular level, the pulmonary arterial systolic pressure may exceed systemic pressure. Right heart failure may then ensue. By contrast, severe pulmonary stenosis in the setting of a ventricular septal defect may mask entirely the effects of the valvar obstruction by reducing pulmonary blood flow. Left atrial pressure is bound to be lower than pulmonary arterial pressure however severe the mitral obstruction. Pure mitral insufficiency may cause left atrial hypertension with all the consequences already described. More commonly, considerable left atrial dilation occurs, with the result that left atrial hypertension is modest or non-existent. The rarity of this condition means that few systematic studies have been carried out. Our impression is that the haemodynamic effects of congenital mitral regurgitation in children are very similar to those described for pure mitral regurgitation (almost always rheumatic) described by Sulayman and associates (1975). Cardiac output is maintained with a normal left ventricular ejection fraction by a modest increase in left ventricular end-systolic volume and a marked increase in left ventricular end-diastolic volume. This is not as striking as the increase in left atrial volume. The regurgitant fraction may be as high as 83%. Associated obstructive lesions downstream obviously increase the severity of the mitral regurgitation. In contrast to rheumatic mitral disease, the congenitally malformed valve is usually either obstructed or regurgitant. An intermediate situation is produced in the rare case of mixed stenosis and incompetence. In rare instances, an anterior position of the single papillary muscle in the so-called parachute valve results in the aortic leaflet apposing the ventricular septum during systole, or else the large single papillary muscle divides the left ventricular chamber in two, particularly during systole. In either case, the result is functional subaortic obstruction mimicking hypertrophic obstructive cardiomyopathy (Simon et al, 1969; Macartney et al, 1974).

CLINICAL PRESENTATION AND SYMPTOMATOLOGY

Congenital disease of the mitral valve usually presents as a result of the associated abnormalities, such as coarctation or ventricular septal defect. In these lesions, the symptoms are exacerbated by the presence of the mitral valvar problem, but this may be too subtle to detect. As already mentioned, the effects of the valvar anomaly are more or less neutralized by pulmonary stenosis and an interventricular communication. So, whatever the associated anomaly, the result tends to be that mitral disease is masked and will not be recognized unless specially looked for. Collins-Nakai and associates (1977) found a considerable lag between the time of recognition of congenital heart disease and the diagnosis of mitral stenosis, the latter frequently not being found until surgery or postmortem. The presentation of isolated mitral valvar disease is largely determined by the height of the left atrial pressure. If this is normal, there are usually no symptoms at all. At most there will be fatigue after severe exertion. A high left atrial pressure is likely to result in poor feeding, sweating in infancy and failure to thrive. Patients with severe obstruction are likely to present in intractable cardiac failure in the first month or so of life. Orthopnoea is extremely rare, but patients frequently complain of a dry nocturnal cough. Wheezing and respiratory infections are frequent. Syncope, haemoptysis or aphonia owing to compression of the recurrent laryngeal nerve by an enlarged left atrium have occasionally been described (van der Horst and Hastreiter, 1967). Pure mitral stenosis is characterized by poor nourishment, tachypnoea and intercostal recession. There are normal-to-small peripheral arterial pulses, and the jugular venous pulse is also usually normal. If pulmonary hypertension is severe, a prominent A wave will reflect the raised right ventricular end-diastolic pressure. A systolic wave will demonstrate secondary tricuspid incompetence. Palpation of the heart will reveal either a normal impulse or right ventricular hypertrophy, and there may be an apical diastolic thrill. Pulmonary valvar closure will be palpable if pulmonary hypertension is severe. The first heart sound is either normal or loud and, in contrast to rheumatic mitral stenosis, an opening snap is only occasionally audible (van der Horst and Hastreiter, 1967; Collins-Nakai et al, 1977). Closure of the pulmonary valve is accentuated in patients with pulmonary hypertension. There is a loud low-pitched mid-diastolic murmur at the apex, usually with presystolic accentuation. Occasionally, no diastolic murmur is heard (Collins-Nakai et al, 1977). In severe untreated disease, an early diastolic murmur of pulmonary incompetence and a pan-systolic murmur of tricuspid incompetence may be heard, both resulting from pulmonary hypertension. Crepitations may be heard in the lung fields, but these are usually clear. Cyanosis is not seen unless there is severe pulmonary venous desaturation, or a right-to-left shunt through an associated defect.

PURE MITRAL INSUFFICIENCY

The occasional patient has a general appearance mimicking that of a patient with mitral stenosis. Most children are well nourished and in no distress. The peripheral pulses are usually normal, though sometimes jerky because of the predominant ejection of blood in early, rather than late, systole (Nichol et al, 1976). The jugular venous pulse is normally not elevated. On palpation of the heart, left rather than right hypertrophy is usually discovered. On auscultation, the first and second heart sounds are usually normal, except in the relatively rare case of pulmonary hypertension. There is a blowing pan-systolic murmur at the apex. The pan-systolic murmur of ventricular septal defect is much rougher, is maximal at the left sternal border and does not radiate to the axilla. If mitral regurgitation is more than mild to moderate, an apical third heart sound will be heard, followed by a diastolic flow murmur in severe cases. This diastolic murmur, particularly if it is accompanied by a third sound, does not necessarily indicate stenosis. When congenital mitral anomalies are associated with other cardiac defects, the physical signs are usually dominated by the other lesions. In particular, an imperforate mitral valve generates no direct physical signs, though evidence of pulmonary hypertension is almost invariable. The main clue to the presence of mitral stenosis in association with other defects is an inappropriately prominent mid-diastolic murmur (Macartney et al, 1974). A typical example would be that of a 6-month-old child who, in earlier life, had typical signs of ventricular septal defect and yet who now has all the signs of Eisenmenger's syndrome except an unexpected loud mid-diastolic murmur, often with presystolic accentuation. Care has to be taken with many children with aortic coarctation, and a few with discrete subaortic stenosis. Such patients may have short apical mid-diastolic murmurs, which, for reasons that are not obvious, disappear after resection of the obstruction.

INVESTIGATIONS

ELECTROCARDIOGRAPHY

Sinus rhythm is the rule in children, though first-degree heart block is common, particularly when the left atrium is greatly enlarged. Left atrial hypertrophy occurs in about 90% of patients, and right atrial hypertrophy is the rule in patients with pulmonary hypertension. In mitral stenosis, the mean frontal QRS is usually normal, or to the right and inferior, whereas it is generally normal in mitral incompetence (Talner et al, 1961). The pattern of ventricular hypertrophy reflects the underlying haemodynamics. Consequently, patients with mitral stenosis tend to have right ventricular hypertrophy, while those with mitral incompetence have left ventricular hypertrophy (Talner et al, 1961). All of these findings are modified by associated abnormalities. In patients with the physical signs of mitral regurgitation, the electrocardiogram provides important clues to the presence of atrioventricular septal defects with common atrioventricular junction (superior counter-clockwise QRS loop), and discordant atrioventricular connections (Q waves in the right and inferior precordial leads). Mitral regurgitation secondary to anomalous origin of the left coronary artery from the pulmonary trunk is suggested by a pattern of anterolateral infarction, and primary endocardial fibroelastosis by the severe left ventricular hypertrophy and 'strain' pattern, though this is not unique to fibroelastosis.

CHEST RADIOGRAPHY

Whatever the nature of the mitral abnormality, cardiac enlargement tends to be considerable. Splaying of the bronchuses by the enlarged left atrium is particularly prominent. Infants with imperforate mitral valve, or severe mitral stenosis, very occasionally show the ground-glass appearance of pulmonary oedema. More commonly, left atrial hypertension is manifested in older children by Kerley B lines and diversion of blood to the upper lobes. In infants, the pulmonary trunk and left atrial appendage do not form discrete bulges on the upper left cardiac border, which is consequently straighter than normal. In older children, prominence of the left atrial appendage is the rule and, in patients with pulmonary hypertension, the pulmonary trunk is prominent. These appearances may be profoundly modified by associated abnormalities. If the ascending aorta is seen on the left upper cardiac border and the patient has clinical features of mitral incompetence, then congenitally corrected transposition with tricuspid rather than mitral incompetence is the most likely diagnosis.

ECHOCARDIOGRAPHY

M-mode echocardiography provides non-specific evidence as to enlargement of chambers (left ventricle, left atrium, right ventricle), much as has been described above. It is unhelpful in diagnosing mitral incompetence. A number of features are suggestive of mitral stenosis, but none of them is invariably present. These include anterior movement of the mural leaflet in diastole (Figure 43.10) (Driscoll et al, 1978), a prolonged time to reach 20% of the peak rate in change of left ventricular dimensions and a reduced peak rate of these changes in dimension (Smallhorn et al, 1981).

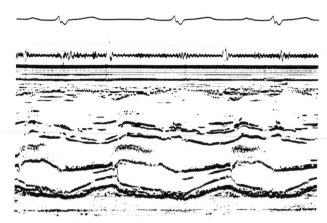

Figure 43.10. This M-mode examination of a patient with congenital mitral valve stenosis demonstrates fluttering of the valve leaflets, along with anterior motion of the mural leaflet.

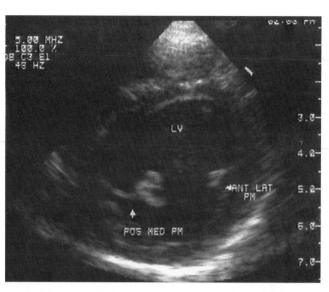

Figure 43.11. Precordial short-axis view demonstrating normal disposition of the papillary muscles. LV, left ventricle; ANT LAT PM, anterolateral papillary muscle; POST MED PM, posteromedial papillary muscle.

A flattening of the E–F slope is again suggestive (Lundstrom, 1972) but difficult to recognize in infants with tachycardia. The time from closure of the aortic valve to opening of the mitral, and from left ventricular minimum dimension to mitral opening, have proved unhelpful as indicators of congenital mitral stenosis (Smallhorn et al, 1981), though they are useful in assessment of acquired mitral valvar disease. There is dispute in the literature as to whether supravalvar mitral ring can be recognized by M-mode techniques (LaCorte et al, 1976; Driscoll et al, 1978; Snider et al, 1980). The presence of artefactual lines in the normal left atrium, and multiple echos from normal valvar leaflets, adds to the problems, as do other structures producing lines within the left atrium, such as the wall of an enlarged coronary sinus and the membrane of a partitioned left atrium (cor triatriatum) (LaCorte et al, 1976).

Cross-sectional examination of the mitral valve has made a major difference to the non-invasive understanding of pathology. Assessment usually consists of short-axis scans from the apex of the left ventricle to the left atrium, carried out from both subcostal and precordial windows. In such scans, the papillary muscles normally appear at 3 and 8 o'clock in the parasternal short-axis view (Figure 43.11) (Celano et al, 1984). In the parachute valve, the two muscles are usually fused into one (Figure 43.12) (Snider et al, 1980; Smallhorn et al, 1981; Vogt et al, 1981; Vitarelli et al, 1984). The alternative arrangement, with hypoplasia or absence of one papillary muscle, may also be observed, particularly in patients with associated coarctation (Celano et al, 1984). As the beam is moved towards the left atrium, so the mitral orifice appears. This is normally symmetrical but is frequently eccentric in patients with congenital mitral stenosis; consequently, standard cuts give little idea of the severity of stenosis (Smallhorn et al, 1981). If multiple sections are observed with varying degrees of obliquity, it does appear possible to obtain a cross-sectional area that correlates well with that calculated using the Gorlin formula from cardiac catheterization (Riggs et al, 1983).

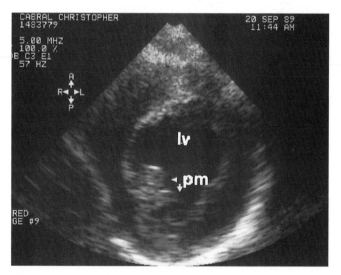

Figure 43.12. Precordial short-axis view demonstrating a single papillary muscle. lv, left ventricle; pm, papillary muscle.

This view is also of value for recognizing the anomalous mitral arcade (Pacileo et al, 1991). The most striking and important abnormality recognized in these short-axis sections is the isolated cleft of the aortic (anterior) leaflet. This appears as a splitting of the leaflet into two during diastole (Figure 43.13). The cleft points to the left ventricular outflow tract, not the septum (Smallhorn et al, 1982a) and is seen in normal short-axis planes (Di Segni et al, 1983) not the horizontal precordial plane, which best demonstrates the so-called 'cleft' in an atrioventricular septal defect with common atrioventricular junction (Figure 43.14) (Beppu et al, 1980). Cordal attachments from the edges of the cleft aortic leaflet can be observed in this setting (Figure 43.15 and Plate 43.1). In hearts

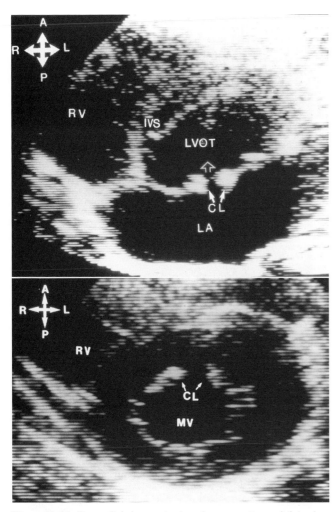

Figure 43.13. Precordial short-axis view demonstrating a cleft in the aortic leaflet of an otherwise normal mitral valve. The cleft points towards the left ventricular outflow tract. A, anterior; CL, cleft; IVS, interventricular septum; L, left; LA, left atrium; LVOT, left ventricular outflow tract; MV, mitral valve; P, posterior; R, right; RV, right ventricle.

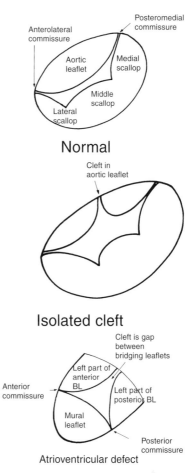

Figure 43.14. Schematic diagram outlining the differences between an isolated cleft and that seen in an atrioventricular septal defect, as seen by a surgeon. BL, bridging leaflet.

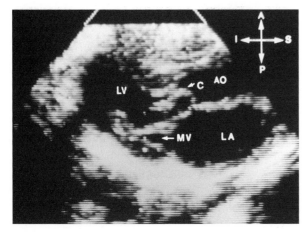

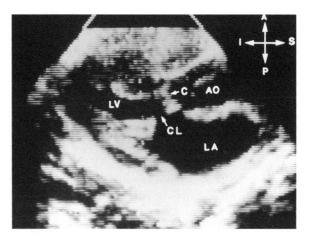

Figure 43.15. Precordial long-axis views of a heart with a cleft (CL) of the aortic (AO) leaflet and accessory cords (C) inserting into the left ventricular (LV) outflow tract. MV, mitral valve.

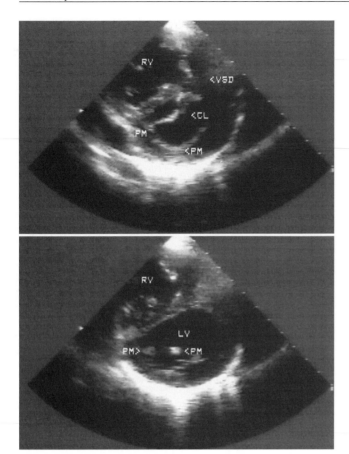

Figure 43.16. Precordial short-axis view in a patient with rotation of the anterolateral papillary muscle (PM) towards the posteromedial one, such that the cleft (CL) in the mitral valve points towards the anterolateral aspect of the left ventricle (LV). RV, right ventricle; VSD, ventricular septal defect.

with discordant ventriculo-arterial connections or double outlet right ventricle with subpulmonary ventricular septal defect (Coto et al 1984), particularly in the presence of a straddling mitral valve, we have observed that the cleft appears to be more asymmetrical, pointing towards the anterolateral aspect of the left ventricle. This, in turn, is often associated with medial rotation of the anterolateral papillary muscle (Figure 43.16). It has been questioned on embryological premises whether this represents a true cleft in the mitral valve as opposed to a commissure (Wenink et al, 1986). In functional terms, however, the space is not a usual zone of apposition between valvar leaflets, and it requires closure at surgery. The short-axis view also provides an excellent means for identifying dual orifices in the mitral valve, particularly when each orifice is supported by its own papillary muscle (Figure 43.17) (Di Segni et al, 1983; Rowe et al, 1984; Trowitzsch et al, 1985; Scardi et al, 1994).

Parasternal long-axis sections permit further assessment of texture and mobility of the leaflets. They frequently demonstrate crowding of the subvalvar apparatus (Smallhorn et al, 1981), with difficulty in differentiating between the leaflet and the tension apparatus to which it

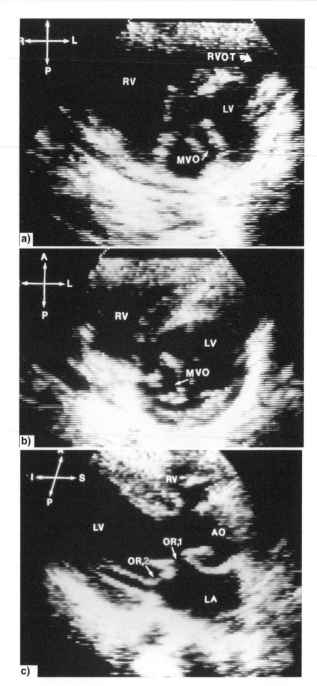

Figure 43.17. The heart in a patient with a double orifice mitral valve. (a,b) Precordial short-axis view. (b) Long-axis view shows the two orifices. AO, aorta; LV, left ventricle; MVO, mitral valve orifice; OR, 1, orifice 1; OR, 2, orifice 2; other abbreviations as in Figure 43.13.

is fused (Plate 43.2a). This is particularly valuable for detecting a supramitral ring, which is usually associated with valvar and subvalvar pathology. As emphasized, the ring is usually related intimately to the valvar leaflets (Snider et al, 1980; Celano et al, 1984; Glaser et al, 1984, Sullivan et al, 1986). The ring, which starts at the annulus, extends downwards onto the valve leaflets, such that at first glance the echocardiographer has the impression that it is a subvalvar structure.

It has been suggested that a mass in the cavity of the left ventricle attached to both aortic and mural leaflets is characteristic of anomalous mitral arcade (Parr et al, 1983). Normal values for mitral annular dimension as seen in parasternal long-axis and apical four chamber views have been published (Smallhorn et al, 1981; King et al, 1982; Riggs et al, 1983). In the great majority of patients with congenital mitral stenosis, this is normal (Figure 43.18) (Smallhorn et al, 1981). Occasionally, particularly in the presence of a ventricular septal defect, annular hypoplasia can be the main component of the mitral stenosis (Figure 43.19).

Four chamber sections, either from the apical or subcostal approach, complete the morphological picture, with the former providing the best position for Doppler assessment of valvar gradient. As in the parasternal long-axis view, the valve appears to be thickened, with evidence of doming during the cardiac cycle (Plate 43.2b). The presence of a supramitral ring is also appreciated in

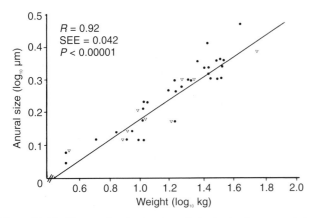

Figure 43.18. The annular size in congenital mitral valvar stenosis is usually with normal limits. Mitral stenosis ($\triangledown$) and controls ($\bullet$) from 41 subjects.

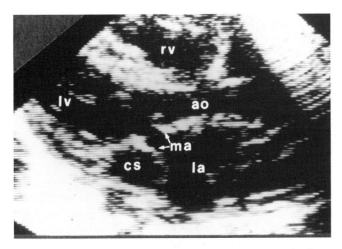

Figure 43.19. Precordial long-axis view in a heart with mitral valvar stenosis secondary to annular hypoplasia. This patient had an associated muscular ventricular septal defect. ao, aorta; cs, coronary sinus; ma, mitral annulus; lv, left ventricle; rv, right ventricle.

this position (Plate 43.3b). This position is also suitable for diagnosing Ebstein's malformation of the mitral valve and for assessing left atrial size. In this rare condition, the aortic leaflet of the mitral valve originates normally with respect to the tricuspid valve, but the mural leaflet is displaced downwards (Leung et al, 1987). Mitral regurgitation secondary to myocardial dysfunction is suggested by poor myocardial contractility and/or dyskinesis. It is essential to demonstrate origin of the left coronary artery from the aortic root in all patients with the clinical picture of pure mitral regurgitation, bearing in mind that, in patients with a pericardial effusion, the transverse sinus of the pericardium may be mistaken for the left coronary artery by the inexperienced observer (Robinson et al, 1984). If not diligently sought, anomalous origin or atresia of the left coronary artery may well be missed. With the advent of colour flow Doppler, in conjunction with a measurement of the right coronary artery (Koike et al, 1989; Karr et al, 1992), it is now rare to miss the diagnosis. Imperforate mitral valve may be recognized as a thin, sometimes mobile, membrane between the left atrium and left ventricle, which can usually, but not invariably, be distinguished from the thick wedge produced by the atrioventricular groove when the left atrioventricular connection is absent (Rigby et al, 1982). In other cases, the mitral valve regurgitation can be caused by dysplastic leaflets that are relatively immobile, thus preventing full coaption during systole (Plate 43.4). From personal experience, the mural leaflet seems to be involved more frequently in this process (Oberhansli et al, 1997).

PULSED AND CONTINUOUS WAVE DOPPLER ECHOCARDIOGRAPHY

Doppler echocardiography has had a major impact on the evaluation of mitral valvar disease, both in the areas of stenosis and regurgitation. With mitral valvar stenosis, a turbulent inflow jet is seen, both by pulsed (Stevenson, 1977; Grenadier et al, 1984; Veyrat et al, 1984) and continuous wave Doppler. The latter modality can be used to calculate the gradient across the valve and its area (Figure 43.20). In adults and older patients, the pressure half-time provides an accurate assessment of area, independent of cardiac output (Hatle et al, 1978). This same technique can be applied to children, although absolute areas calculated in this way are of little value because of the wide variation in body surface area (Banerjee et al, 1995). Mean gradients across the valve have traditionally been used in assessment of congenital heart disease, despite the limitation of its dependency on cardiac output (Banerjee et al, 1995). In our laboratory, we use a combination of pressure half-time, mean mitral gradient and left atrial size to assess the severity of congenital mitral valvar stenosis. This, in conjunction with an assessment of pulmonary arterial pressure, either resulting from tricuspid regurgitation or

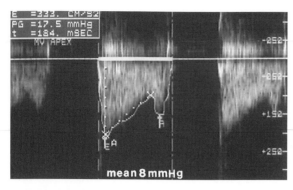

Figure 43.20. Doppler spectral trace in congenital mitral valvar stenosis, showing an increased pressure half time of 184 ms, with a mean gradient of 8 mmHg.

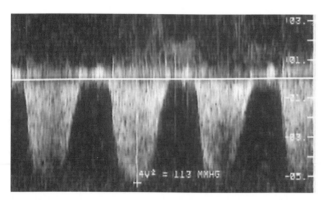

Figure 43.21. Doppler spectral trace of tricuspid valvar regurgitant velocity in congenital mitral valvar stenosis, demonstrating systemic right ventricular pressure (113 mmHg).

pulmonary insufficiency (Figure 43.21), completes the hemodynamic evaluation.

While pulsed Doppler flow mapping has fallen from grace in assessing the severity of mitral regurgitation, it still plays a small semiquantitative role through the use of pulmonary venous sampling. In general, reversed systolic flow is seen in hearts with more severe regurgitation (Passofini et al, 1995). A quantitative measurement of regurgitant volume and fraction can be obtained using pulsed Doppler techniques. This is achieved by calculating the difference between forward stroke volume through the aorta and that measured through the mitral valve, the latter consisting of normal pulmonary venous return plus the regurgitant volume (Enriques-Sarano et al, 1993).

The contribution of colour flow Doppler in this lesion is twofold. First, it excludes or establishes associated regurgitation and, second, it pinpoints the site of obstruction and the pattern of flow through the valve. In patients with an associated supramitral ring, the variance starts just above the annulus (Plate 43.3a). In the other forms, it starts below the level of the annulus (Plate 43.2a). This technique also provides valuable clues about the site of exit of the blood. In a parachute valve, for example, there appears to be a conical jet of

blood, whereas in those with two papillary muscles, the jet is more dispersed.

An assessment of mitral valvar regurgitation is well suited to the technology of colour flow Doppler (Yoshida et al, 1988). This technique permits an accurate assessment of the site of the regurgitant jet, for example from the edges of a cleft mitral valve (Plate 43.1) or at the site of prolapse in those with floppy leaflets (see below and Plate 43.7). It also provides information regarding the direction of the jet, along with the extent to which the velocity signal can be observed in the left atrium (Plate 43.5). (Mele et al, 1995). One of the major problems, however, is that mapping of flow provides only a semi-quantitative assessment of the severity of the regurgitation, as the echocardiographer measures velocity not volume. Despite this limitation, a reasonably reliable assessment of severity is possible, particularly if more than one plane is used. Limitations relate to depth, position of the jet in relationship to the atrial wall, gain settings, driving pressure and transmitted frequency (Cape et al, 1991; Simpson and Sahn, 1991; Chao et al, 1992). Similarly, in large populations of apparently normal subjects, physiological mitral regurgitation is encountered, with a rate of 38–45% (Yoshida et al, 1988). More recently, attempts have been made to assess the volume of flow by using other techniques, such as momentum analysis (Thomas et al, 1990) and 'PISA' (proximal isovelocity surface area) calculations (Utsunomiya et al, 1991; Pu et al, 1995; Simpson et al, 1996), and jet width (Mele et al, 1995). These are, potentially, the key to an accurate assessment of volume of flow, which can then be related to changes in left ventricular dimension (Plate 43.6). The problem, at present, is that it is unclear whether an increase in the size of a ventricle represents a deterioration in ventricular function or just an alteration to accommodate an increase in regurgitant volume (Cheitlin, 1991). As a result of problems in calculating absolute regurgitant volumes by Doppler echocardiography, some authors have concentrated on the relationship of end-systolic volume to outcome (Nakano et al, 1994). In adults, it appears that an end-systolic volume of greater than 100 ml/m^2 is predictive of a poor outcome after valvar surgery. Whether this can be applied to children is open to conjecture, although potentially it provides some objective data for timing of valvar replacement.

An assessment of left ventricular function and left atrial size are of paramount importance in these patients. In general, data from adults would dictate that a falling ejection fraction, in conjunction with an increasing left ventricular end-systolic dimension, points to the need for intervention (Reed et al, 1991). Unlike our colleagues dealing with adults, who have absolute dimensions to guide them, the technique is less reliable for assessment of children, where differing body surface areas hamper simple values.

The more recent advent of transoesophageal echocardiography has provided an additional tool for the evaluation of the congenitally abnormal mitral valve. Fortunately, apart form the older child or obese patient, this technique is unnecessary in most children. It is also apparent that transoesophageal colour flow mapping appears to be more sensitive than transthoracic assessment. Systematic overestimation of the severity of regurgitation is found when it is compared with standard transthoracic assessment (Mimo et al, 1991; Smith et al, 1991; Castello et al, 1992a). Despite this difference, both techniques provide a good correlation with angiography (Castello et al, 1992b). Transoesophageal and epicardial echocardiography have both been used extensively in making decisions during surgical repair of the mitral valve (Stewart et al, 1990; Maurer et al, 1991). Transoesophageal echocardiography also lends itself to three-dimensional reconstruction, providing much more detailed information about valvar morphology. So far, the technique has been used only in adults but has obvious potential benefits for assessment of congenital lesions, where more detailed morphological information could potentially aid in making decisions concerning surgical treatment.

RADIONUCLIDE ANGIOGRAPHY

Radionuclide angiography is of little practical value in congenital mitral valvar disease, apart from pure mitral regurgitation. Radionuclide gated cardiac blood pool imaging can be used to determine right and left ventricular stroke index, and hence stroke index ratio. This correlates well with angiocardiographically determined regurgitant fraction and returns to normal after valvar replacement. There is a wide range in the ratio of stroke index in patients without regurgitation, which means that the technique is useless in detecting mitral regurgitation. Furthermore, other workers have found that the method becomes highly inaccurate in patients with a depressed left ventricular ejection fraction (Lam et al, 1981).

MAGNETIC RESONANCE IMAGING

Magnetic resonance imaging is currently finding its role in the routine investigation of the child with congenital heart disease. So far, its strengths have revolved around the evaluation of the extracardiac anatomy, in particular the aortic arch and pulmonary arteries, where detailed structural information is available. The technique is equally suited to the evaluation of intracardiac structures, both static and dynamic. The mitral valve can be imaged in several planes, along with its supporting papillary muscles (Nazarian et al, 1987; Higgins et al, 1990; Raymond et al, 1990). Few data are available at present with regards to detailed anatomical descriptions of congenital anomalies. While this would be interesting, it is probably in the area of functional assessment that the

technique holds the greatest promise. The ability to assess mass and volume with a high degree of accuracy, in conjunction with the determination of regurgitant volumes (Higgins et al, 1991), is of great potential for the evaluation of the chronically regurgitant mitral valve. Mitral regurgitation causes a signal void in the left atrium in systole, with a high degree of sensitivity when compared with other imaging techniques. This technique also permits an assessment of regurgitant volume, by comparing the stroke volume of the left and right ventricles and then comparing it with the signal void, yielding a correlation coefficient of 0.84 (Higgins et al, 1991). Similarly it is possible to assess inflow gradients by utilizing velocity-encoded techniques (Mohiaddin et al, 1991).

CARDIAC CATHETERIZATION

The final arbiter of mitral obstruction is demonstration of a difference in diastolic pressures between the left atrium and ventricle. The Peter principle dictates that, when you most need to know the left atrial pressure, it is most difficult to obtain. The high left atrial pressure seems to seal the valvar mechanism of the oval foramen with remarkable effectiveness. Entry to the left atrium from the right, therefore, often demands trans-septal puncture (Roveti et al, 1962; Mullins, 1983). While this technique is remarkably safe, particularly in the hands of experts who practise it constantly, it is not to be recommended to the occasional operator. Retrograde passage of the catheter through the mitral valve (Morrison et al, 1977) is an alternative but is more difficult if the valve is stenotic. Suprasternal puncture of the left atrium is easier than it sounds, particularly when the left atrium is enlarged. Details of these techniques are given in Chapter 16. Before any of these techniques are used, efforts should be made to obtain a satisfactory pulmonary capillary wedge pressure simultaneous with the left ventricular pressure. The wedge pressure can be regarded as a reliable reflection of left atrial pressure if the wave form is undamped, fully saturated blood can be aspirated through the catheter and repeated measurements in different sites give the same pressure. Routine measurement of wedge pressures during cardiac catheterization goes a long way towards detecting otherwise masked mitral stenosis. Lynch and colleagues (1962) were able to diagnose supravalvar mitral ring by careful analysis of the pressure trace on withdrawal from left ventricle to left atrium. This success has not, to our knowledge, been repeated, presumably because of the close proximity of the mitral valve and supravalvar ring, and the high association between supravalvar ring and valvar stenosis (Collins-Nakai et al, 1977). The documentation of a pressure gradient between the pulmonary capillary wedge pressure and the left ventricular diastolic pressure only proves the existence of mitral stenosis or supravalvar ring if the pulmonary veins are normally connected to the left atrium and there is no partition, tumour or thrombus within it. All of these can be excluded by cross-sectional echocardiography supplemented, if necessary, by angiocardiography.

ANGIOCARDIOGRAPHY

Pulmonary arteriography is of little specific value, except that it demonstrates the normality of pulmonary veins and (almost always) the absence of a divided left atrium (cor triatriatum). Enlargement of the left atrium will be seen but will rarely surprise the operator. It is widely held that isolated mitral stenosis 'holds up' contrast medium in the left atrium, but we find this expression curious. Blood is not flowing through the mitral valve more slowly than through the aortic or pulmonary valves, and pulmonary blood flow is rarely decreased (Collins-Nakai et al, 1977). Pulmonary angiography is nothing but a special form of indicator dilution curve. If prolonged left atrial opacification is not the result of reduced pulmonary blood flow, it must be caused by an increased blood volume between the site of injection of contrast and the mitral valve – that is, enlargement of the left atrium and/or the intrapulmonary blood vessels. Such enlargement is undoubtedly present in mitral stenosis and explains the prolonged left atrial opacification. It is also present, for example, in pure mitral regurgitation. Demonstration of a curvilinear membrane running across

the mitral annulus convex to the valve is suggestive, but not diagnostic, of a supravalvar ring (Figure 43.22) (Macartney et al, 1974). Left atrial injections produce much the same information (or lack of it) as pulmonary arteriograms. They can only demonstrate the valvar leaflets during the first ventricular diastole. The contrast medium is then upstream but not downstream to the leaflets. Thereafter, the leaflets, unless they are extremely thickened, disappear because of equalization of the concentration of contrast medium on either side of them. The main advantage of left atrial injections is that they differentiate an imperforate mitral valve from extreme mitral stenosis with annular hypoplasia. These may give similar appearance on injection into the left ventricle. Left atrial injections are best made in left anterior oblique projections with caudocranial tilt, since this profiles the atrial septum. If the mitral valve is perforate, and the atrial septum is intact, contrast medium will be seen to traverse the mitral orifice. If there is an intact inferior rim of septum and contrast medium passes only to the right atrium, there is either an imperforate left atrioventricular valve or an absent left connection. These two conditions may give the same appearance (Figure 43.23a). If there is a primary ostium defect, the diagnosis is an atrioventricular septal defect with common atrioventricular junction and either a univentricular (see Chapter 38) or biventricular atrioventricular connections (usually with right ventricular dominance; see Chapter 36).

Left ventricular angiocardiography gives easily the best angiocardiographic demonstration of abnormal mitral valvar anatomy. This is because, throughout the injection, non-opacified blood traversing the mitral valve during diastole maintains a visible difference in concentration of contrast medium between blood on the atrial and ventricular sides of the leaflets (Macartney et al, 1976). Be the valve perforate or imperforate, the atrium produces a filling defect within the left ventricle bounded by the smoothly curved mitral annulus (Figures 43.24 and 43.25). Consequently, demonstration of the annulus does not indicate that the valve is perforate; only that it, and therefore the left atrioventricular connection, is present. Thus far, we are not aware of having been confused by downstream injections of contrast medium. Even when the imperforate mitral valve is extremely small, a smooth-bordered, elliptical left atrial filling defect is still seen in the lateral angiocardiogram (Figure 43.23b) (Macartney et al, 1979). If the valve is perforate, non-opacified blood can usually be seen to traverse the valve in diastole; however, occasionally the picture is confused by non-opacified blood entering from the right ventricle via a ventricular septal defect. Under these circumstances, left atrial injection is essential, though contrast echocardiography might be chosen in preference to angiocardiography.

Parachute mitral valve has frequently been diagnosed in the past on the basis of visualization of a single papillary muscle and cone-shaped valvar leaflets (Terzaki et al, 1968; Simon et al, 1969). Neither of these criterions is adequate,

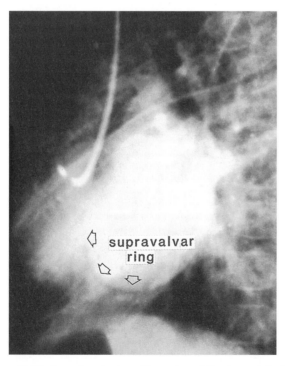

Figure 43.22. Lateral projection of laevophase following an injection into the left ventricle that has opacified the pulmonary circulation through a ventricular septal defect. A fine membrane, the supravalvar ring, is demonstrated in the vestibule of the left atrium, though this cannot be regarded as absolutely diagnostic.

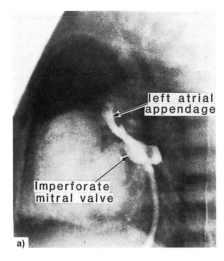

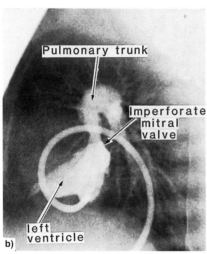

Figure 43.23. Imperforate mitral valve in lateral projection. (a) Injection in the left atrium shows a slightly curved structure that can be provisionally recognized as an imperforate valve, though it could simply be the left atrial free wall. (b) On injection into the left ventricle, it can be seen that there is an imperforate mitral valve, because the left ventricular outline fits precisely the curved floor of the left atrium identified in (a).

for cone-shaped leaflets are the rule in any form of mitral stenosis, and only one of the two papillary muscles is seen in almost half of high-quality left ventricular angiocardiograms. The key to the diagnosis is the combination of these two into the diastolic deformity in the shape of an hourglass or egg-timer formed by the leaflets converging on a single papillary muscle (Figure 43.26) (Macartney et al, 1974).

Anomalous mitral arcade may be suspected when there appears to be virtual continuity between the papillary muscles and leaflets (Figure 43.27) (Macartney et al, 1976). In general, since tendinous cords cannot be visualized, their abnormalities can only be inferred, not seen. Mitral regurgitation is easily identified by angiocardiography, though contrast echocardiography (see above) may be more reliable. 'Eye-balling' the degree of regurgitation correlates poorly with the quantitative estimate

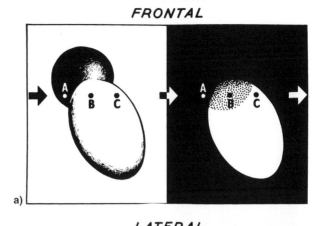

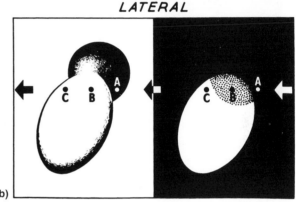

Figure 43.24. Diagram illustrating how the left atrial filling defect in the opacified left ventricle outlines the mitral annulus, whether the mitral valve is perforate or imperforate. To the left are pictures of the heart in frontal and lateral views, and to the right are the corresponding projections. At point A, there is no contrast medium, and the picture is of necessity black. At point B, there is contrast medium, but this is encroached upon by the left atrium, so an intermediate density is obtained. At point C, there is no left atrial filling defect, and opacification is, therefore, dense.

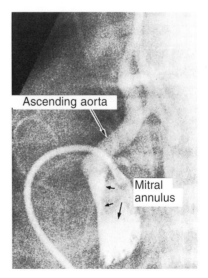

Figure 43.25. Imperforate mitral valve (proved at postmortem). In this lateral projection, the catheter has been advanced into the left ventricle through a ventricular septal defect. Note how well the mitral annulus is demonstrated, since this does not depend upon patency of the mitral valve.

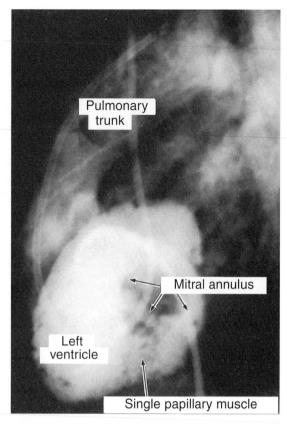

Figure 43.26. Lateral projection in patient with double outlet right ventricle with parachute mitral valve. Note how the mitral annulus and the single papillary muscle together form the hour-glass configuration.

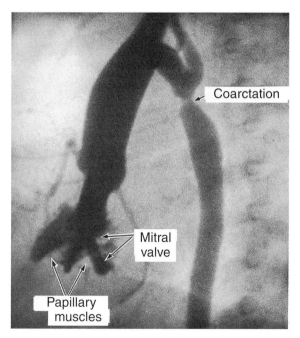

Figure 43.27. Anomalous mitral arcade (proved at postmortem). Note how, in the right anterior oblique projection, the mitral valve approaches closely the heads of the papillary muscles, suggesting that they insert directly into the free margin of the mitral valve.

of regurgitant fraction (Nichol et al, 1976). The anatomical substrate of incompetence is extremely elusive. Congenitally short cords and isolated mitral cleft are indistinguishable (Macartney et al, 1976). The coronary arteries should be demonstrated to originate from the aorta in patients with apparently pure mitral regurgitation. Aortography may be necessary if there is any suspicion of left ventricular dysfunction.

The ability to define the anatomical substrates of congenital mitral valvar anomalies has not been formally studied by comparing angiocardiography with cross-sectional echocardiography. Nonetheless, we have little doubt that the latter technique is superior for each variety, with the possible exception of imperforate mitral valve.

DIFFERENTIAL DIAGNOSIS

As already emphasized, the main problem lies in recognizing that a mitral anomaly is present when associated defects dominate the clinical picture. Careful clinical examination and echocardiography, coupled with a high index of suspicion in patients with other left-sided obstructive lesions, provide the best means of making the diagnosis. In secondary mitral regurgitation, left ventricular dysfunction usually dominates the clinical picture, whereas left ventricular function is usually normal in primary regurgitation. The possibility of silent mitral stenosis always haunts the clinician confronted with the patient with apparently severe and irreversible pulmonary vascular disease. In earlier days, it was our practice to rule this out by cardiac catheterization in each patient. We now tend to the view that careful auscultation, cross-sectional echocardiography and Doppler examination can rule out significant obstruction in all cases and that catheterization is unnecessary for diagnostic purposes in patients where high-quality noninvasive investigation is possible.

COURSE AND PROGNOSIS

Imperforate mitral valve is usually lethal in early infancy, as is absence of the left atrioventricular connection (see Chapter 39), except in those cases associated with a patent subaortic outflow tract (Mickell et al, 1983). Mitral stenosis has a slightly better, but still poor, prognosis. Collins-Nakai and colleagues (1977) found that actuarial survival was 40% at 10 years of age when patients were treated medically, and 56% at the same age for surgically treated patients. At the age of 18 years, survival was 18% in both groups. Mitral incompetence has the best prognosis. Even when associated with coarctation, most patients survive childhood. The degree of mitral regurgitation may remain static, or even decrease once the coarctation is resected (Freed et al, 1974). Prolonged and significant mitral regurgitation will eventually depress left ventricular function, though it is unclear whether it does so at a similar rate as in adults.

———— MANAGEMENT ————

MEDICAL MANAGEMENT AND TIMING OF INTERVENTION

For patients with congenital stenosis, medical management is frequently dictated by associated lesions. In those patients where it is isolated, treatment with diuretics may buy some time; although surgical repair is possible, the long-term results are disappointing (Collins-Nakai, 1977; Coles et al, 1987). Unfortunately, pulmonary hypertension is frequently encountered in these patients, thus forcing the hand of the cardiologist and surgeon. Until recently, surgery was the only option, but angioplasty has become a treatment of choice in those with rheumatic valvar disease (Zaibag et al, 1989), with encouraging results in a smaller population of children having congenital stenosis (Lock et al, 1985; Spevak et al, 1990; Grifka et al, 1992; Alday et al, 1994). This technique has been used in adults following previous surgical commissurotomy and promises great things for the ongoing treatment of children with this lesion (Davidson et al, 1992).

Regurgitation is generally managed medically until there is evidence of clinical symptoms that which are not improved by standard therapeutic regimens combined with a trial of afterload reduction. Afterload reduction has been shown to be of value in management of mitral incompetence in adults (Greenberg et al, 1978). Hydralazine and nitroprusside can also be shown to produce an acute increase in cardiac index and stroke index in children with left ventricular dysfunction or mitral regurgitation. A month of oral therapy is of proven benefit but, beyond that, recurrent heart failure is common (Beekman et al, 1984). Likewise, isosorbide dinitrate and nifedipine have been shown to have acute benefits in children with chronic mitral regurgitation (Kelbaek et al, 1996).

With the introduction of angiotensin-converting enzyme (ACE) inhibitors, which reduce the afterload on the left ventricle, morbidity and mortality have both been shown to improve in adults with left ventricular dysfunction (SOLVD Investigators, 1991, 1992; CONSENSUS Trial Study Group, 1987). Similar improvements in left ventricular ejection fraction, with a reduction in regurgitant fraction, have been demonstrated following the use of ACE inhibitors in symptomatic patients with chronic mitral valvar regurgitation (Schon et al, 1994; Seneviratne et al, 1994; Shimoyama et al, 1995; Levine and Gaasch, 1996). So far, however, no long-term benefits have been observed in asymptomatic patients with mitral valvar regurgitation.

SURGICAL MANAGEMENT

Imperforate mitral valve is, in theory, treatable by valvar replacement if the atrioventricular junction is of sufficient size. Such an operation has not yet been described. Alternative approaches that have proved successful in the short term in a very few patients include placement of a conduit from the left atrium to the left ventricle (Corno et al, 1986) and a 'reversed Fontan'. The latter operation is similar to that described for absent left connection (Shore et al, 1982). The atrial septum is excised and pulmonary venous blood is guided by a baffle through the tricuspid orifice. Continuity from the right atrium to the pulmonary arteries is then established with a conduit. It may also be necessary to create an unobstructed pathway from the right ventricle to the aorta. The success of this operation depends on the presence of a low pulmonary vascular resistance, which is, in the nature of the condition, rare. In a neonate with valvar regurgitation, where the annulus was too small for insertion of a prosthetic valve, the mitral valve was oversewn, an atrial septectomy performed, a ventricular septal defect created and the pulmonary trunk banded, with the aim of waiting until the mitral annulus grew and a prosthetic valve could be inserted (Westerman et al, 1987).

The poor long-term outlook of this condition means that the decision to undertake palliative measures in early infancy needs careful discussion with the parents. Those patients with severe mitral valvar stenosis who present in the neonatal period (and frequently have some degree of left ventricular hypoplasia and aortic valve stenosis) tend to be managed with the Norwood protocol. This includes creating an aortopulmonary anastomosis, an open atrial septectomy and constructing a shunt from the aorta to the pulmonary arteries, either centrally or peripherally (Norwood et al, 1983). Accurate determination of left ventricular size, along with the diagnosis of all associated anomalies, is of paramount importance in the decision-making process (Rhodes et al, 1991).

Outside the neonatal period, the best option is to attempt to repair the valve, if balloon angioplasty is not available, as valvar replacement in children is still fraught with problems. In earlier days, closed mitral valvotomy was practised, with occasional improvement (van der Horst and Hastreiter, 1967; Lundstrom, 1972). There are at least two reasons why it should not now be performed. First, if there is an undiagnosed supravalvar mitral ring, the result will be definitely suboptimal. Second, the lesion is rarely as seen in rheumatic mitral stenosis, namely a basically normal valve with fusion of the ends of the zone of apposition between the leaflets. Any and every combination of abnormalities of annulus, leaflets and tension apparatus may be present, each demanding an individual approach. The presence of intractable heart failure, severe pulmonary hypertension or pulmonary oedema means that the need for operation in infancy or early childhood is forced upon the management team. In contrast, in congenital mitral incompetence, the generally good prognosis with medical management means that operation can usually be postponed as long as possible. The exception to this conservative approach is that of isolated cleft of the aortic (anterior) leaflet, where the results of repair are so good as to justify surgery at any age if there is significant cardiomegaly (Smallhorn et al, 1982b). Supravalvar mitral ring is best treated by excision of the ring under direct vision. Small surgical series of repair without mortality, and with considerable symptomatic improvement, have been reported (Collins-Nakai et al, 1977; Neirotti et al, 1977; Coles et al, 1987; Stellin et al, 1988). Mitral valvotomy, even if performed under direct vision, almost always results in residual stenosis (Anabtawi and Ellison, 1965; Collins-Nakai et al, 1977; Coles et al, 1987; Stellin et al, 1988). Nevertheless, precious time is bought by this procedure, which can be carried out even in infancy. If, however, the supravalvar mitral ring is missed during repair of other associated anomalies, particularly tetralogy of Fallot, death is likely to result (Oglietti et al, 1976). Generally speaking, surgical management for both mitral stenosis and incompetence comes down to the choice between valvar replacement and valvar repair. Valvar replacement is currently under a cloud in children because of the high incidence of late fibrocalcific obstruction of glutaraldehyde-preserved valves (Geha et al, 1979; Kutsche et al, 1979; Fiddler et al, 1983), which may be accompanied by intravascular haemolysis (Weesner et al, 1981). Replacement of one bioprosthesis by another is no answer, since accelerated calcification seems to occur in the second (Fiddler et al, 1983). The great advantage of bioprostheses in children (the lack of need for anticoagulation) is more than neutralized by this problem (Deverall, 1983). Most large series of mitral valvar replacement in children have been predominantly for rheumatic heart disease and atrioventricular septal defects. Berry and colleagues (1974) reported six (23%) early and two late deaths from 26 replacements in children between 1962 and 1972, of whom the youngest was 18 months of age. Just under half of these patients had congenital mitral disease of the variety discussed in this chapter. A similar proportion was found in the 50 children undergoing mitral replacement reported by Williams et al (1981) between 1963 and 1980, the youngest being 8 months of age. Of these, 16 (32%) died early and actuarial survival at 5 years was only 50%. Of the 19 patients with isolated congenital mitral stenosis or insufficiency, five died early and four late. The rate of complications was as high with mechanical as with tissue valves, though the former were all at least anticoagulated with warfarin. More encouraging immediate results were reported from Johns Hopkins Hospital, with no early deaths in eight patients with congenital disease (Gardner et al, 1982). These authors also reported a low incidence of thromboembolism. Of 38 patients with aortic, mitral or tricuspid mechanical prostheses, only two had thromboembolic complications, though 13 had not been managed continuously with anticoagulants. The group from Mexico City inserted the Bjork–Shiley prosthesis in children below the age of 16 years, with operative survival of 92% and no clinical episodes of embolism in the survivors (Attie et al, 1986). A novel approach used by Adatia and colleagues (1997) is to insert the prosthesis in the supra-annular position in patients where the annulus is too small. Actuarial survival rates were 88% at 1 month, and 71, 62 and 53% at 1, 2 and 10 years, respectively. Large atrial v waves indicated left atrial hypertension in the absence of prosthetic valvar obstruction. Though most authors still advocate the use of anticoagulation therapy in children after valvar replacement, a number of reports describe apparently successful replacement without anticoagulation. Stansel and colleagues (1975) experienced one thromboembolic incidence per 35.7 years of patient follow-up in their series of 10 children receiving a Starr–Edwards valve. Similar low rates have been reported with the St Jude Medical valve (Pass et al, 1984). Sufficient doubt exists about the value of anticoagulants, therefore, to justify a controlled trial. If valvar replacement is successful, it causes a fall in pulmonary arterial pressure and resistance, a fall in pulmonary capillary wedge pressure, a rise in cardiac output and a fall in end-diastolic volume with no change in ejection fraction (Benmimoun et al, 1982).

Valvar repair is best exemplified by the work of Carpentier and colleagues (Carpentier, 1976, 1983a,b; Chauvaud et al, 1986). The mitral anatomy is carefully inspected at operation and the repair precisely tailored to the abnormality found. Reduction in annular size may be achieved by insertion of a Carpentier ring. Clefts are sutured. Regions with insufficient cordal support are plicated, and excessively long cords are partly buried in the tip of the associated papillary muscle, or else the papillary muscle is shortened by a sliding plasty operation. Fused commissures or tendinous cords are separated, and the single papillary muscle of a parachute valve split into two. Unnecessary obstructive cords are excised. All told, they have now performed operations on 135 children with valvar insufficiency, and 58 with valvar stenosis. Valvar replacement in their hands was needed in only six patients with regurgitant valves, and three with stenotic ones. Mortality was 4% for those with regurgitation, and 22% for those with stenosis. Symptoms were dramatically improved in the majority of patients, most becoming asymptomatic. In the hands of experts such as Carpentier and his colleagues, therefore, repair of the mitral valve appears to be an attractive alternative to valvar replacement, particularly because residual incompetence is usually well tolerated.

Other groups have reported similarly encouraging results for surgical repair of the mitral valve in children (Aharon et al, 1994; Uva et al, 1995; Zias et al, 1998). In an earlier series reported by Coles (1987), which included both stenotic and regurgitant lesions, the operative mortality decreased from 18% prior to 1975 to

2.9% up to 1986. Stellin and his colleagues (1988) had an overall mortality of 16.6%, with one late death; and all bar two of those who underwent repair were a-symptomatic 5 months to 15 years after operation. The results are best, nonetheless, in those undergoing repair for congenital regurgitation, with Okita and colleagues (1988) reporting only one death in 66 patients (1.9%). Actuarial survival was 93.1 ± 3.1% at 7 years and 88.4 ± 0.1% after 17 years, with a rate of freedom from failure of valvoplasty of 80 ± 6.7% after 5 years, 67 ± 7.2% after 10 years and 44 ± 11.9% after 15 years. In patients with hypoplasia of the mural leaflet as an isolated anomaly, repair has been successful by the use of a ring annuloplasty; this provides better coaption of the leaflets (Plate 43.4) (Oberhansli et al, 1997). Another approach to this anomaly is to detach the leaflet at the annulus, patch it with pericardium and then reattach it to the annulus, thus creating improved coaption of the leaflet without compromising potential annular growth in the small child.

— FLOPPY MITRAL VALVE SYNDROME —

It may well be that, since the mid-1970s, there have been more words written about floppy mitral valve syndrome than children who have suffered from it. We confess to the heretical view that the reason why so much of what has been written has been conflicting and confusing is that there has been a misunderstanding of the nature and use of diagnosis. In most of cardiology, and in paediatric cardiology in particular, the establishment of a diagnosis is a crucial step in the logical process that begins with presentation of the patient and ends with the institution of appropriate management. But this is only because the presence of an indubitable anatomical abnormality can be established with a high degree of certainty. For example, a newborn baby presents with severe cyanosis. The diagnosis of complete transposition can be established with certainty, and there is no possibility of confusion with a normal heart. Once the diagnosis is known, balloon atrial septostomy is performed and further management is carried out depending on associated physiological and anatomical abnormalities. The statement 'This patient has complete transposition' carries a great deal of both certainty and meaning (assuming agreement as to the definition of complete transposition). It has to be contrasted with two other types of diagnostic statement, of which examples are 'This patient has Marfan's syndrome' and 'This patient has systemic hypertension'. These only carry meaning in proportion to their certainty, which may not be high at all. We believe both of the last two statements mentioned to be analogous to the statement, 'This patient has floppy mitral valve syndrome'. The understanding of floppy valve can be enhanced by analogy to these other statements. Turning to the first, the problem with Marfan's syndrome as a diagnosis is pre-

cisely the same as with all other syndromes, namely that the definition consists of a constellation of different features, each of which may or may not be present. For all that has been written on the subject, there can be no logical answer to questions such as 'Is isolated annulo-aortic ectasia a forme fruste [atypical form] of Marfan's syndrome?'. Annulo-aortic ectasia is undoubtedly a feature of Marfan's syndrome. And whether one wishes to regard the presence of a single feature as diagnostic of the syndrome is an arbitrary matter. Such questions are only asked by those whose logical rigidity demands that the pathway from presentation to prognosis must pass through diagnosis, which it need not do. The correct question to ask is 'What is the prognostic significance of isolated annulo-aortic ectasia? For example, what is the risk of sudden death from dissecting aneurysm, both in the individual and in relatives?' Therefore, recognition of the presence of a syndrome is important not because it provides the grounds for futile discussion about the diagnosis of the syndrome, but because it enables appropriate questions about prognosis to be asked and even answered. If this is true of a well-defined entity such as annulo-aortic ectasia, how much more is it true of the floppy mitral valve syndrome! Ebel (1978), listed from the literature no fewer than 44 synonyms for this syndrome. This testifies to the diversity of opinion as to whether this is a disease or a syndrome, and to its hallmarks. We have chosen the name 'floppy mitral valve' precisely because it is not very specific. It, therefore, expresses the essential ambiguity of the present situation. The term 'mitral valve prolapse syndrome' is much less satisfactory, since it indicates that prolapse is the paradigm of the syndrome. This is a view expressed particularly strongly by cross-sectional echocardiographers (Morganroth et al, 1980). If so, it is not a syndrome but a specific disease. We have to approach the problem as we approach a syndrome rather than a disease simply because, in most patients, the prognosis is so benign that direct visualization of mitral valvar prolapse will never be achieved, and, therefore, prolapse will never be proved. In other words, we believe the appropriate questions to ask are not so much diagnostic as prognostic. When floppy mitral valve is regarded as a syndrome, one example of an appropriate question is 'What is the life expectancy of a 15-year-old female patient who has a mid-systolic click and late systolic murmur; is this altered if she also has inverted T waves in the left precordial leads?' We now make analogy with the second diagnostic statement: 'This patient has systemic hypertension'. Its essential meaninglessness is immediately evident because it begs other questions such as 'What precisely is the patient's blood pressure?' and 'What is your definition of hypertension?'. These questions arise not because of any difficulty in measurement but because patients with systemic hypertension merely constitute one end of a normal spectrum of blood pressure. Again, what is important about blood pressure is not that it enables a diagnosis to be made, but that a prognosis can be given and modified by appropriate treatment, if necessary. Turning to these considerations in the setting of the floppy mitral valve, it is clear from the literature that whether patients are studied by echocardiography, angiography, at surgery or at postmortem, there is a continuous spectrum between subjects with indubitably normal mitral valves and patients with florid prolapse of the valvar leaflets. When such a spectrum exists, the question 'Does this patient have floppy mitral valve syndrome?' has no more validity than 'Does he have systemic hypertension?'. Specifically, juggling with the precise criterions for diagnosis is a meaningless exercise, since the answer obtained depends upon whether you wish to believe that floppy mitral valve syndrome is common or rare. The important questions are again prognostic not diagnostic: for example, 'Can a relationship be established between the position of the mitral leaflets during systole and either life expectancy or the probability of developing severe mitral regurgitation?'. Until such questions can be answered, it seems to us that there is considerable merit in defining the syndrome in terms of auscultatory findings. In contrast to echocardiographic and radiographic criterions, the mid-systolic click and late systolic murmur are either present at some stage or not. Furthermore, really long-term follow-up information is currently available only for patients in whom the diagnosis was reached by auscultation and/or phonocardiography. We shall regard the presence at some point in the patient's history of a mid-systolic click, a late systolic murmur or both of these findings on auscultation as necessary for the diagnosis. This decision has been made in the interests of clarity. It is not intended as a denial of the existence of 'silent mitral valve prolapse' but as a plea for demonstration of the prognostic importance of this angiocardiographic (Jeresaty, 1973) or echocardiographic (Popp et al, 1974) finding. We shall endeavour to present the facts about the floppy mitral valve syndrome as we have defined it. This is not always possible, as floppy valves mean different things to different people. Some of the most interesting work on the subject has been done by workers who have chosen different diagnostic criterions from those we have adopted.

INCIDENCE AND AETIOLOGY

As already stated, we define the floppy mitral valve syndrome according to auscultatory findings. It is important, nonetheless, to know the relationship between the syndrome thus defined and the syndrome defined on other criterions. Up until the late 1970s, widespread overdiagnosis was rife. This resulted, first, from failure to define precisely the position of the mitral annulus by angiocardiography (Smith et al, 1977; Spindola-Franco et al, 1980) and, second, from failure to distinguish between the body and the free edge of the mitral leaflet by M-

mode echocardiography (Sahn et al, 1977). Incorrect angulation of the transducer can also result in pseudoprolapse (Weiss et al, 1975; Markiewicz et al, 1976). Now that angiocardiography is not used to make the diagnosis, the M-mode echocardiographic criterions for diagnosis have been improved, and cross-sectional and pulsed Doppler echocardiography is available, it appears that patients with echocardiographic prolapse form a virtual subset of those with the auscultatory syndrome, at least in adults. Therefore, if the presence of the auscultatory syndrome is taken as the standard, M-mode echocardiography has a sensitivity of 50% (Abbasi et al, 1983) to 85% (Haikal et al, 1982) and a specificity of 99% (Haikal et al, 1982). Cross-sectional echocardiography has a sensitivity of 68% and pulsed Doppler echocardiography of 72% (Abbasi et al, 1983). If the standard is the auscultatory syndrome combined with standard M-mode criterions, then the sensitivity of cross-sectional echocardiography is, hardly surprisingly, much higher (87%), with a specificity of 97% (Alpert et al, 1984). A survey of 12 050 black South African children from 2–18 years of age showed that 168 (1.4%) had either a non-ejection click (isolated in 73%) or a late systolic murmur and 22% had both (McLaren et al, 1976). The male to female ratio was 1:1.9. When 139 of the 168 were re-examined 4 years later (Cohen et al, 1978), 55% had no auscultatory abnormality, despite the fact that in an age- and sex-matched control group of 139 normal children, six had loud non-ejection clicks and 17 had soft ones. In all, 16.5% had non-ejection clicks, accompanied in about one third of children by a late systolic murmur. The increase in incidence of the auscultatory syndrome is striking, but probably resulted from the fact that, in the follow-up study, all patients were examined by one consultant cardiologist, who did not know whether patients were in the follow-up group or not. The object of the original survey had been to determine the incidence of rheumatic fever, not the click/murmur syndrome, and patients were examined by a number of observers with varying degrees of training. This evidence as to the transitory nature of the click/murmur syndrome means that it is difficult to be sure how much of the apparent increase in prevalence with age (Gingell and Vlad, 1978) indicates a real change, and how much is the effect of repeated auscultation, which increases the probability of detection of a transient anomaly. Independent evidence of the low incidence of the syndrome in children does, however, come from the study of relatives of patients with prolapse diagnosed by M-mode echocardiography. Of 143 adults, 51 exhibited the syndrome (43%), compared with 3 out of 36 children (8%) (Devereux, 1982). The prevalence of the auscultatory syndrome found in 1169 volunteer wives of US air force personnel aged 17–54 (mean 32 years) was 6.3% (Procacci et al, 1976). Using phonocardiography in the upright position with amyl nitrite inhalation, Markiewicz and colleagues (1976) were able to demonstrate a mid–late systolic click and/or a late systolic murmur in 17 of 100 healthy female paid volunteers. Had supine phonocardiography alone been used, the syndrome would have been found in only eight. Volunteers, it should be pointed out, may contain a greater proportion of patients with floppy mitral valves than the normal population, who are less anxious. Chandraratna and colleagues (1979), having originally screened 100 newborn girls with M-mode echocardiography, found three with mid-systolic clicks by auscultation. More recently, Nascimento and colleagues (1997) screened 1752 newborns using both auscultatory and cross-sectional echocardiography and reported no positive cases of prolapsing leaflets. In the Framingham study, where the diagnosis was based solely on M-mode echocardiographic findings, prolapse was found in 5% of adults. There was a striking decrease in prevalence in the female population, from 17% of those in their twenties to 1% of those in their eighties, whereas the prevalence in males was 2–4% throughout life (Savage et al, 1983). In marked contrast to these findings in life is a careful study of 1984 routine hospital necropsies, in which Davies and colleagues (1978) found only 3 hearts out of 155 (1.9%) in patients under 40 years that demonstrated any degree of expansion or prolapse of the leaflets (the incidence of frank prolapse beyond 40 was 5%, with a male to female ratio of 3:4). This postmortem evidence, together with the transitoriness of the auscultatory findings in some patients, indicates strongly that the click/murmur syndrome can exist without any valvar anomaly being recognizable in the non-beating heart. This would partly explain the high false-positive angiographic diagnosis in patients with atrial defects in the oval fossa reported by Somerville and colleagues (1978), correlating angiocardiographic with operative findings. Problems with angiocardiographic interpretation already alluded to could also have been responsible. These difficulties with diagnosis cast considerable doubt on the high association between other forms of congenital heart disease and prolapse reported by some observers (Rippe et al, 1979), particularly subaortic stenosis and lesions producing volume overload of the left ventricle. These may in themselves produce echocardiographic pseudo-prolapse (Sahn et al, 1977). There does, however, seem to be an unduly high incidence of floppy valves in patients with defects in the oval fossa (McDonald et al, 1971; Pocock and Barlow, 1971). Furthermore, in a postmortem (and therefore biased) study of patients with ventricular septal defect, Lucas and Edwards (1983) found an 18% incidence of floppy valves, which appeared independent of age and was also associated with floppy tricuspid, pulmonary and aortic valves. A large population based study (Flack 1999) using cross-sectional echocardiography addressed anthropometric and physiologic correlates of mitral valve prolapse. In a community based study of 4136 young adults definite mitral valve prolapse was only observed in 0.6%, with a similar frequency between the sexes and across ethnic groups. There is con-

siderable evidence that floppy mitral valve syndrome is often one manifestation of a wider connective tissue disorder. In most series of patients with the syndrome, the youngest have had Marfan's syndrome (Gooch et al, 1972; Gullotta et al, 1974). Perloff and Roberts (1972) illustrated florid prolapse of the leaflets of the mitral valve in 22 out of 26 children aged 2–18 years with the auscultatory syndrome; the dimensions of the aortic root exceeded the 95th percentile for surface area, though only five were thought to have Marfan's syndrome (Sahn et al, 1977). In a study of the family of a proband with type IV Ehler–Danlos syndrome, there was complete concordance of the auscultatory syndrome and abnormal production of type III collagen in skin biopsies (Jaffe et al, 1981). Myxomatous degeneration of the mitral valve has been described in osteogenesis imperfecta (Stein and Kloster, 1977). Patients with Duchenne's muscular dystrophy have a high incidence of non-ejection clicks (Sanyal et al, 1979). Mitral prolapse as detected by M-mode echocardiography was reported in 10 out of 14 patients with pseudoxanthoma elasticum (Lebwohl et al, 1982). The auscultatory syndrome with cross-sectional echocardiographic evidence of prolapse was found in 9 out of 15 patients with von Willebrand's syndrome (Pickering et al, 1981). This association can be explained on the basis of a common mesenchymal anomaly. Thoracic bony abnormalities, including loss of the normal thoracic kyphosis (straight back), pectus excavatum and scoliosis are commonly found (Bon Tempo et al, 1975; Cohen et al, 1978). Udoshi and colleagues (1979) reported a 31% incidence of mitral valve prolapse in a prospective study of 80 patients with a flat chest, pectus excavatum or a straight back. This may be an overestimate, since the main criterion for diagnosis was M-mode echocardiography. Prolapse has also been observed in patients who are dehydrated, with reversal to normal in some following rehydration (Lax et al, 1992; Aufderheide et al, 1995). Overdiagnosis of prolapse would be expected in the presence of a thoracic deformity because of uncertainty as to the precise position of the valve. In the Framingham study, subjects with prolapse were significantly leaner than those without (Savage et al, 1983). Further evidence to support the concept of a generalized disorder of connective tissue is the absence of the type III and AB collagens reported in a single patient with ruptured tendinous cords (Hammer et al, 1979) and the high incidence of tricuspid and even aortic prolapse in patients with mitral prolapse. In all these studies, prolapse was defined by cross-sectional echocardiography (see below) (Morganroth et al, 1980; Ogawa et al, 1982). Floppy mitral valve syndrome is frequently familial (Barlow and Bosman, 1966; Hunt and Sloman, 1969; Shell et al, 1969; Shappell et al, 1973; Weiss et al, 1975). It then appears to be transmitted as an autosomal dominant trait. Furthermore, the findings in a large study of relatives of probands with prolapse diagnosed by M-mode echocardiography were consistent with autosomal dominant inheritance with reduced penetrance in children and males (Devereux et al, 1982). This pattern of inheritance has been questioned (Wilcken, 1992), with the suggestion that, in those cases not associated with other lesions, the pattern of inheritance is polygenic. It has been claimed that there is an association with an increased number of arches in the fingerprints (Swartz et al, 1976), but this is disputed (Kramer-Fox et al, 1984). The rather low incidence of coronary arterial disease in those with floppy valves suggests that there is no aetiological link between the two conditions (Jeresaty, 1975). The original suggestion that the cause was, in part, rheumatic (Barlow et al, 1968) was later withdrawn after no progression was seen on follow-up of black children not given prophylaxis against rheumatic fever (Cohen et al, 1978). The Framingham study also showed no association between other forms of acquired heart disease and prolapse diagnosed by M-mode echocardiography (Savage et al, 1983). More recent data from the Framington study indicated that the incidence of mitral valve prolapse was 2.4% (84/3491) of which 47 (1.3%) had classic prolapse and 37 (1.1%) nonclassic prolapse. Classic prolapse was defined as displacement of more than 2 mm with a maximum thickness during diastasis of at least 5 mm, with nonclassic having a displacement of 2 mm and a maximal valve thickness of less than 5 mm.

ANATOMY AND MORPHOGENESIS

The problems concerning the pathology of prolapse of the mitral valve are as numerous as those concerning its clinical features. There is no unanimity concerning nomenclature or aetiology and, perhaps more important, no standard definition of what precisely constitutes prolapse of the leaflets. The morphologist is under considerable constraint in this respect, since he sees the valve only in its fixed postmortem state. He can only speculate what might have happened as the valvar leaflets moved from their open diastolic position to the closed systolic pattern unless the heart is fixed with pressure in the left ventricle so that the leaflets assume their systolic position (Figure 43.28). Nonetheless, much can be learnt concerning the mechanics of prolapse if we consider first the anatomy of the normal valve and then the morphology of valves that illustrate prolapse (or the condition usually described by the pathologist, namely a 'floppy' valve). Pathologists such as Davies (1980) use the term 'floppy valve' (Read et al, 1965) as though synonymous with a prolapsing leaflet. This is the convention we have followed (Becker and Anderson, 1983). The term prolapse was introduced by Criley and colleagues (1966) and was put forward as the optimal term by Abrams (1976) in his 'plea for unanimity'. Several pathological processes can produce a prolapsed leaflet as their end-point, such as ruptured tendinous cords secondary to ischaemic heart disease.

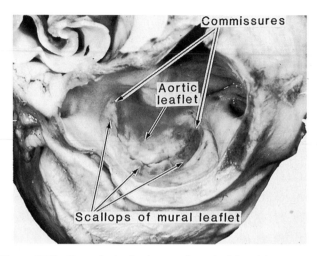

Figure 43.28. Normal mitral valve seen from the left atrial aspect with the heart fixed under pressure in the left ventricle to retain the systolic position of the leaflets. Note the way the mural leaflet curves round the aortic leaflet. (The heart was prepared and photographed by kind permission of Professor Michael Davies, St George's Hospital, London.)

The particular process we are concerned with in the click/murmur syndrome, nonetheless, is almost universally described by morphologists as a 'floppy valve'. As discussed above, it is also our preference to describe the auscultatory syndrome in terms of the purposefully vague 'floppy valve'. We will describe first its gross features and then the microscopic appearance of the afflicted valvar leaflets, this being significant when considering concepts of aetiology and morphogenesis.

ANATOMY OF THE NORMAL MITRAL VALVE

The mitral valve is typical of any mammalian atrioventricular valve in that it possesses an annulus, leaflets and tension apparatus. Equally significant in the make-up of the valve is the insertion of the left atrial musculature into the atrial aspect of the leaflets throughout their circumference and the attachment of the papillary muscles to the ventricular myocardium. All of these structures taken together constitute the valvar apparatus. This functions as a unit, the integrity of each of the subunits being essential for normal function (Perloff and Roberts, 1972).

The particular anatomy is typical for the mitral valve and permits its ready distinction from a morphologically tricuspid valve. About two thirds of the annulus is supported by a fibro-aerolar junction, which serves also to separate the parietal portion of the left atrial myocardium from the ventricular myocardium (Figure 43.29b). The remaining third of the ring is part of an extensive sheet of fibrous continuity with the leaflets of the aortic valve, strengthened at its ends by the left and right fibrous trigones (Figure 43.29a). This arrangement of the annulus conditions the formation of the leaflets. There are two so-called commissural areas within the valve, corresponding more or less to the areas of the fibrous trigones. The zone

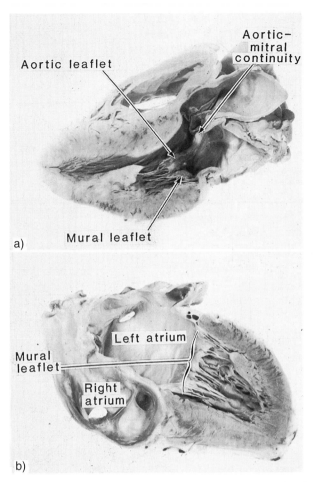

Figure 43.29. Normal mitral anatomy, displayed to correspond with echocardiographic planes. (a) Simulated parasternal long-axis section. (b) Simulated subcostal four chamber section, rotated counterclockwise and tilted posterior so as to eliminate the right ventricle from the picture.

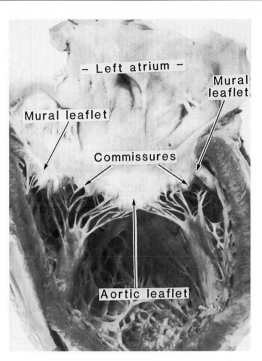

Figure 43.30. Normal mitral anatomy displaying, in particular, the so-called commissural cords.

of apposition between these areas delineates the two primary valvar leaflets. The more extensive leaflet is attached to the parietal part of the annulus. Although usually termed a 'posterior' leaflet, it is more accurate to describe this as the mural leaflet. It has relatively little depth; consequently, when the valve is closed, it is seen as a long rectangular structure (Figure 43.30). It is usually divided into subunits termed 'scallops' or 'commissural leaflets'. Although these are usually three in number, with a large central and smaller lateral and medial structures, there may be five or more scallops seen in some aged valves. There is little justification, therefore, for suggesting that the mitral valve has four rather than the traditional two leaflets (Yacoub, 1976). Indeed, as was emphasized by Victor and Nayak (1994), the best way of viewing the arrangement of the mural leaflet is on the basis of a series of slits within the overall skirt, analogous to pleats, enabling it to fit snugly against the much shorter aortic leaflet. This second major leaflet of the valve is attached along the area of aorto-mitral fibrous continuity. Although its overall shape is semicircular, it is much

squarer and more box-like than the long, rectangular mural leaflet (Figures 43.29b and 43.30). Often termed the 'anterior' leaflet, it is not strictly anterior in position. That is why we prefer to describe it as the aortic leaflet.

The tension apparatus of the valve consists of the tendinous cords and the papillary muscles. The tendinous cords have been categorized with exquisite precision by Lam and his colleagues (1970). We share the view of Frater (1976) that overemphasis on such categorization can give the impression of spurious accuracy. In essence, the important cords are those supporting the free edge of the leaflets, (notably the commissural fan-shaped cords), those supporting the rough zone (particularly the thick strut cords) of the aortic leaflet and the basal cords. The cords supporting the free edge are much more significant in support of the mural leaflet (Figure 43.31a). In contrast, the rough zone and strut cords are more significant in support of the aortic leaflet (Figure 43.31b). Although it is generally assumed that the 'normal' mitral valve, particularly its mural leaflet, has uniform support along the free edge, this is not the case. The study by Becker and de Wit (1979) showed considerable variation in normal hearts. As we will see, this finding could be of major significance in the context of prolapse. The papillary muscles of the mitral valve are relatively constant in position, although they, too, show marked variation in their detailed anatomy (Becker and de Wit, 1979). They are sited beneath the ends of the zone of apposition between the leaflets in posteromedial and anterolateral position and have a typical paired appearance (Figures 43.30 and 43.31). The axis of opening of the valve subtends a considerable angle relative to the inlet septum. The posterior extension of the subaortic

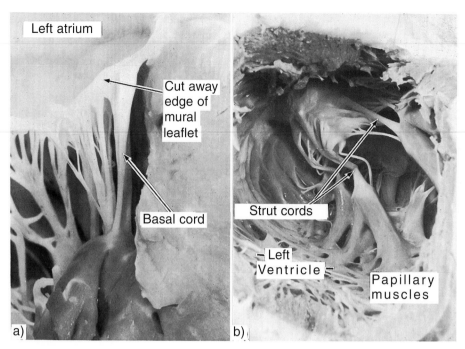

Figure 43.31. Normal mitral valves, arranged so as to display basal and strut cords.

outflow tract is deeply wedged into this angle, and it is significant that the leaflets of the mitral valve, unlike the septal leaflet of the tricuspid valve, are never attached by tendinous cords directly to the inlet component of the muscular ventricular septum.

The final anatomical feature of the normal mitral valve is its line of closure. This is on the atrial aspect of the valve and is about one third of the distance from the free edge of the leaflets to their annular attachment. This line is often accentuated by a zone of raised tissue on the atrial aspect. It is important to note, therefore, that the valve does not close at its free edge. The arrangement described gives quite some degree of safety in terms of the amount of dilation of the valvar orifice needed to produce regurgitation. But this does not mean that only the leaflets are significant in terms of regurgitation. As Perloff and Roberts (1972) emphasized, lesions of any one of the normal subunits can result in valvar incompetence.

GROSS ANATOMY OF FLOPPY LEAFLETS OF THE MITRAL VALVE

It is the mural leaflet that is most usually involved in floppy leaflets. The lesion may affect only one of its scallops, or the entire leaflet may be involved. The affected leaflets are hooded with their convexity to the left atrium. When the whole leaflet is involved, as is seen mostly in adult hearts, the arrangement of the domed leaflets with their elongated cords has been likened to a parachute (Pomerance, 1972). This is perhaps unfortunate in the setting of congenital heart disease because of the more well-known adjectival use of 'parachute' in the context of the mitral valve. When the leaflets are grossly prolapsed,

there is little difficulty in recognition (Figure 43.32a); such prolapse is now well recognized as affecting also the aortic leaflet of the mitral valve (Figure 43.32b). As with clinical experience, most floppy valves have been seen in adult patients. Shrivastava and colleagues (1977) have commented on the difficulty of distinguishing minimal prolapse from a variant of the normal arrangement of the mitral valve. This is significant since Becker and de Wit (1979) observed that, in some normal valves, parts of the mural leaflet were less well supported by free-edge cords than other parts. They suggested that such an arrangement might predispose to prolapse. Subsequent observations have shown that the prolapsed segments of an affected leaflet are less well supported than the non-prolapsed parts (Figure 43.33) (van der Bel Kahn et al, 1985). The affected leaflets are grossly thickened with myxomatous transformation of their atrial aspect. Dilation of the annulus is also found when careful measurements are performed. This feature was observed only in patients with prolapse or with Marfan's disease (Bulkley and Roberts 1975).

HISTOLOGICAL FEATURES OF AFFECTED LEAFLETS

As judged by gross examination, the thickening of the valve leaflet is seen mostly on the atrial aspect of the leaflet. When studied microscopically, this is reflected by obvious myxomatous proliferation of the spongy layer of the leaflet (Fernex and Fernex, 1958). There is an increased proliferation of acid mucopolysaccharides, and these impinge on the fibrous layer, with focal interruption. The end result is destruction of the fibrous core of the

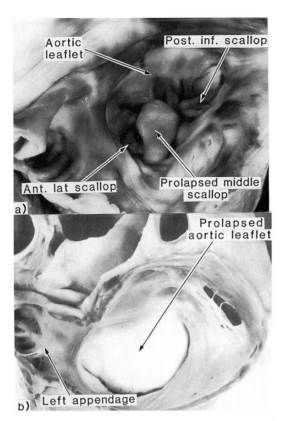

Figure 43.32. Prolapsed mitral valve, as displayed in pressure-fixed postmortem specimens. (a) Note the obviously prolapsed middle scallop. (b) Rather more unusually, the aortic leaflet in this specimen is prolapsed. And, anterior; inf, inferior; lat, lateral; Post, posterior. (Part (b) by kind permission of Professor Michael J. Davies.)

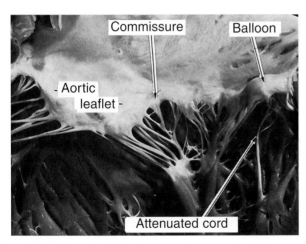

Figure 43.33. Postmortem specimen of a heart showing mild ballooning of the middle scallop of the mural leaflet of the mitral valve. This part is relatively unsupported. There is an attenuated cord as the sole support of the middle part of the scallop. (Reproduced by kind permission of Professor Anton E. Becker.)

valve, this being seen by Davies (1980) and King and colleagues (1982) as the essence of the lesion. There is, however, no appreciable inflammatory reaction. Indeed, absence of inflammatory changes and absence of any disease of the small coronary arteries are two of the car-

dinal features of mitral valvar prolapse (Jeresaty, 1979). Chesler and colleagues (1983) described aggregates of connective tissue, fibrin, platelets, leucocytes and red cells in the angle between left atrial wall and mural leaflet in three postmortem specimens. These could be the source of the cerebral emboluses that, in rare instances, have been associated with mitral prolapse (Cheitlin, 1979). A study by Marks et al (1989) indicated that those patients with the classic form with thickened leaflets and redundancy had a higher risk for developing infectious and haemodynamic complications than those with the non-classic form.

AETIOLOGY OF MITRAL VALVAR PROLAPSE

The two major morphological features of mitral valvar prolapse that bear upon pathogenesis are the accumulation of acid mucopolysaccharides with weakening of the fibrous core of the valve and the inequality of cordal support to the free edge of the affected valvar leaflet. A myocardial factor has been proposed by many authors but is probably not of significance (Jeresaty, 1979). The accumulation of acid mucopolysaccharide with weakening of the fibrous tissue and impaired collagen formation is seen typically in Marfan's syndrome. Indeed, prolapsed valvar leaflets are a well-recognized feature of this syndrome. The most obvious case we have seen in a child was in one suffering with Marfan's disease (Figure 43.32a). On the basis of these limitations, it has been suggested that prolapse is a forme fruste (atypical form) of Marfan's syndrome (Read et al, 1965). Furthermore, it has been proposed that the increase in ground substance is the underlying cause of the leaflet prolapse. Others have implicated congenital deficiency of collagen synthesis, and Davies (1980) has reported accumulated collagen precursors in affected valves. But as Roberts and colleagues (1973) have pointed out, it is very difficult to implicate these rather slight histological changes as the causative feature. This is particularly so since no detailed comparable information is available on the structure of normal valvar leaflets. Jeresaty (1979) has also reviewed the evidence and is sceptical of the suggested association. The possibility that the prolapse is caused by lack of cordal support of the free edge, as suggested by Becker and de Wit (1979), is much more appealing. This is more so since van der Bel Kahn et al (1985) have now observed cases of prolapsed leaflets with inadequate support (Figure 43.33). As with so many controversies, the truth may well prove to lie between the two extremes, with disorders of both biochemical make-up and cordal support contributing to production of the floppy leaflets.

PATHOPHYSIOLOGY

As Jeresaty (1975) has neatly argued, two main theories have been advanced to explain the floppy valve syndrome: one valvar and the other myocardial.

THE VALVAR THEORY

The valvar theory suggests that the primary abnormality, as described above, is redundancy of valvar tissue and cordal elongation owing to myxomatous degeneration of the spongy part of the valve. This may itself be caused by lack of cordal support, particularly to the mural leaflet. Initially, the only abnormality is excessive hooding of the leaflets, which does not prevent their normal apposition. With the passing of time, coaptation of the leaflets becomes more and more tenuous, until finally one leaflet slips back over the other into the left atrium during systole. Prolapse has occurred. As prolapse becomes more and more severe, so cordal rupture may result in a flail leaflet. Recent analysis of annular dimensions in patients with mitral prolapse suggests that this scheme may need slight modification, in that the annular area is often, but not always, abnormally great in patients with prolapse. Some patients with no more than an isolated click have annular areas greater than two standard deviations above the normal. It is tempting to suppose that these are at greater risk of progression to severe incompetence (Ormiston et al, 1982). Timed cineangiograms have shown that the event closest to the mid-systolic click is maximal expansion of the prolapsed leaflet and that the late systolic murmur coincides with mitral regurgitation (Criley et al, 1966). Echocardiographically, the timing of the click is closely correlated with the mid-systolic buckle. This corresponds to the onset of abrupt posterior movement of either or both of the leaflets (Winkle et al, 1975a). During interventions such as head-up tilt and amyl nitrate inhalation the timing of the click alters but it occurs at a rather constant ventricular dimension in individuals. Amyl nitrate tends to increase normalized maximal circumferential rate of shortening of the myocardial fibres without changing end-diastolic dimension, while head-up tilt tends to decrease end-diastolic dimension without altering normalized shortening. Hence, both contractility and volume influence the timing of the click (Mathey et al, 1976).

THE MYOCARDIAL THEORY

The myocardial theory is based upon the recognition of a variety of myocardial segmental contraction anomalies. These include abnormal systolic protrusion of the inferior aspect of the left ventricle (Grossman et al, 1968), non-contraction of (or late systolic expansion of) the inflow tract of the left ventricle (Liedtke et al, 1973) or a variety of patterns of left ventricular asynergy (Scampardonis et al, 1973). Echocardiographically determined ventricular contractility has also been found to be reduced in patients with the auscultatory syndrome compared with normal (Mathey et al, 1976). Endomyocardial biopsies in patients with floppy mitral valve syndrome and disabling chest pain have shown a markedly abnormal birefringence response to adenosine triphosphate (Malcolm et al,

1979). These abnormalities would produce mitral regurgitation by upsetting the delicate and precisely timed balance between the various components of the valvar apparatus required for normal valvar closure (Perloff and Roberts, 1972; Little, 1979). In particular, a myocardial abnormality might produce prolapse by interfering with contraction of the mitral apparatus, by causing papillary muscle dysfunction directly or by interfering with contraction of the left ventricular wall around the papillary muscles. This region is essential for normal papillary muscle function (Perloff and Roberts, 1972). It is difficult to ignore the considerable evidence from a wide variety of sources that some patients with mitral valve prolapse have an abnormal myocardium, in many cases not associated with coronary arterial disease. The very diversity of anomalies of left ventricular function described, however, suggests that these patients do not have a primary myocardial disorder with a floppy mitral valve as one of its consequences. As the title of this chapter indicates, we believe that an isolated valvar anomaly can explain the great majority of cases seen, certainly in children. Whatever the primary disorder, the end-result is first bowing of the mitral leaflets into the left atrium. Then, if this is sufficiently severe, there is regurgitation. In the majority of adults and all children (save some with Marfan's syndrome), this is so mild as to cause no significant haemodynamic disturbance (Jeresaty, 1973). In Marfan's syndrome, even though mitral regurgitation may be severe, its long-standing nature results in left atrial dilatation. Resting left atrial and left ventricular end-diastolic pressures, therefore, remain normal until a late stage in the disease. An attractive classification of this disease based upon the concept of progressive valvar disorder has been put forward by Barlow and Pocock (1985). They suggest that prolapse should imply failure of coaptation of the leaflets, and that excessive bowing should be termed 'billowing' rather than 'prolapse'. A flail leaflet is one with ruptured cords. The distinction between 'billowing' and 'floppy' in their classification is unclear. While this approach may clarify matters in the future, it cannot do so as long as it is impossible in life to distinguish all these entities.

PRESENTATION AND SYMPTOMATOLOGY ———

The majority of patients have no symptoms at all. They present with murmurs found on routine examination, usually in late adolescence or adulthood. Early presentation should raise the suspicion of Marfan's syndrome. A tiny but unforgettable subset (1%) present with murmurs ('honks') that can be heard not only by the patient but also by companions across the room. The intensity of the murmur (see below) usually is critically dependent on posture (Fiddler and Scott, 1980). A large minority of patients have other symptoms. The most common is chest pain, usually unrelated to activity, that is ill-defined, located to the precordial area, sharp and fleeting or more prolonged. This pain has been attributed to excessive cordal tension (Jeresaty, 1973). Other symptoms include dyspnoea, fatigue, light-headedness and palpitations. Patients with prolapse are often neurotic even before the diagnosis is made. This tendency, together with the rather non-specific symptomatology, has led to the interesting suggestion that the overall syndrome is nothing more than a reincarnation of the entity variously known as Da Costa's syndrome, soldiers' heart, effort syndrome or neurocirculatory asthenia (Wooley, 1976). These syndromes, as with mitral valvar prolapse, all seem to be associated with decreased parasympathetic and β-adrenergic tone and hypersensitivity to isoprenaline (isoproterenol) infusion (Gaffney et al, 1979; Boudoulas et al, 1980, 1983).

PHYSICAL SIGNS

The skeletal abnormalities already noted (flat chest, straight back, pectus excavatum) are frequently observed (Seliem et al, 1992). Peripheral arterial and venous pulses are normal. Palpation of the heart is usually normal, unless a 'honk' is present; this is usually accompanied by a thrill. Careful palpation in the left lateral decubitus position may permit detection of mid-systolic retraction (Devereux et al, 1976). Auscultation at the apex reveals either a mid-systolic click (which may be multiple), a late systolic murmur or both (Figure 43.34). The murmur must be heard to reach the second heart sound, if necessary by inching the stethoscope from the apex to the base (Leatham and Brigden, 1980). Clicks are sometimes only heard with the patient upright or in the left lateral decubitus position. It is apparent that not all mobile systolic clicks are associated with anatomical and echocardio-

graphic evidence of prolapsed leaflets. They can be generated by redundant tendinous cords in the absence of prolapse, or even be caused by redundant leaflets (Weis et al, 1995). As long as the murmur remains late systolic, the heart sounds can be normal. When the murmur is holosystolic, then a loud first heart sound indicates early prolapse. A soft first heart sound indicates flail leaflets (Tei et al, 1982). Manoeuvres that decrease left ventricular end-diastolic volume or increase the rate of left ventricular contraction (such as sitting or standing from supine, the strain phase of a Valsalva manoeuvre, tachycardia or administration of vasodilators such as amyl nitrate) all move the click and murmur closer to the first heart sound. Squatting, the release phase of the Valsalva manoeuvre, bradycardia and administration of vasoconstrictors, in contrast, all move the click and murmur towards the second heart sound and often make the murmur become fainter or disappear (Devereux et al, 1976). Pregnancy also may cause disappearance of the murmur.

With prolonged follow-up, the murmur does become pan-systolic in some adults (Allen et al, 1974; Mills et al, 1977). This finding is rare in children unless they have Marfan's syndrome. An early diastolic sound or, less often, an early diastolic murmur is occasionally heard or recorded by phonocardiography (Wei and Fortuin, 1981). This has been ascribed to recoaptation of the prolapsing leaflets but could also be caused by aortic prolapse (Morganroth et al, 1980).

INVESTIGATIONS

CHEST RADIOGRAPHY

Chest radiography usually gives normal results apart from the skeletal abnormalities already noted. If mitral valvar regurgitation is severe, there will be an increase in the cardiothoracic ratio and the size of the left atrium.

ELECTROCARDIOGRAPHY

About a fifth of children with the auscultatory syndrome have inverted T waves in II, III and aVF and, rather less commonly V_5 and V_6. These abnormalities may not be constant. Indeed they may be produced acutely by, for example, inhalation of amyl nitrite (Jeresaty, 1973). Pseudo-ischaemic ST changes can be induced by hyperventilation (Gardin et al, 1980). The ST and T abnormalities are rarely associated with coronary arterial disease, even in adults (Lobstein et al, 1973), and their cause is obscure. Prolongation of the Q–Tc interval occurs in 10–15% of all patients (Ebel, 1978). Among 75 children with isolated floppy mitral valves, most of whom had the auscultatory syndrome, two had ventricular tachycardia, two supraventricular tachycardia and four premature ventricular contractions on a standard

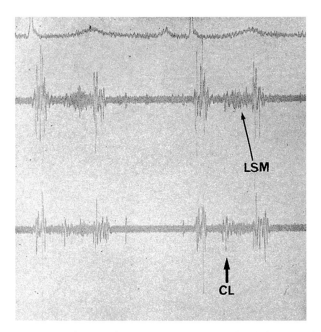

Figure 43.34. Phonocardiogram showing mid-systolic click (CL) and late systolic murmur (LSM) in a patient with floppy mitral valve.

electrocardiogram (Gingell and Vlad, 1978). Kavey and colleagues (1980) describe a wide variety of atrial arrhythmias on exercise and 24-hour ambulatory monitoring but seem unaware that, with the exception of one patient with supraventricular tachycardia, these are normal findings (Scott et al, 1980; Southall et al, 1981). The same group describe what they term 'potentially serious ventricular arrhythmias' in six patients (multi-focal premature beats, R-on-T). Despite this, the incidence of sudden death is very rare (Oakley et al, 1992). This emotive language becomes less impressive when it is appreciated that premature ventricular contractions in normal boys are usually multifocal (Scott et al, 1980), and R-on-T occurred in 3 out of 50 male medical students aged from 23 to 27 years who had no evidence of heart disease (Brodsky et al, 1977). One of these medical students even had a brief episode of ventricular tachycardia during sleep. These arrhythmias become more prevalent in older patients with floppy valves, as indeed they do in patients without. Winkle and colleagues (1975b) studied, with 24-hour electrocardiography, a group of 24 adults, 23 of whom had various clicks and murmurs documented by phonocardiography. Of these six (25%) had no premature ventricular contractions, six (25%) had less than 50 per 24 hours and 12 (50%) had more than 425 per 24 hours. In the last group, five patients had ventricular tachycardia. Premature atrial contractions occurred in 15 patients (62.5%) but did not segregate into distinct low- and high-frequency groups as did premature ventricular contractions. Paroxysmal supraventricular tachycardia occurred in seven patients (29%). More recently, signal-averaged electrocardiograms have been used to identify those patients who are at a potentially greater risk of paroxysmal supraventricular tachycardia (Banasiak et al, 1995). Spontaneously terminating ventricular fibrillation has been documented in a single patient (Campbell et al, 1976). Two alternative hypotheses have been put forward to explain the arrhythmias seen with prolapsing mitral valve. The first is high α-adrenergic tone (Boudoulas et al, 1980, 1983). The second comes from Perloff's (1982) interpretation of the demonstration that cardiac muscle inserting into the leaflets of the human mitral valve can initiate impulses and might be a site of origin of arrhythmias (Wit et al, 1979). The idea is that increased tension on the valve could somehow provoke supraventricular tachycardias.

ECHOCARDIOGRAPHY

When the cross-sectional echocardiographic appearances of prolapsing leaflets are appreciated, it becomes easier to understand the M-mode appearances, particularly the ways in which pseudo-prolapse may be produced. In short, cross-sectional echocardiography enhances the diagnosis of prolapse by enhancing the spatial configuration of the valvar leaflets (Feigenbaum, 1992; Malkowski et al, 1996). During diastole, the leaflets of the normal valve lie widely open and are more-or-less parallel, as seen in long-axis sections. With the onset of systole, the two leaflets (moving in opposite directions) coapt to give a funnel-shaped appearance. As systole continues, the line of coaptation moves anteriorly and lags behind the aortic root. The entire valvar apparatus then moves anteriorly and inferiorly. Both leaflets frequently arch slightly towards each other and become more horizontal, but no part of the leaflets appear above the atrioventricular junction (Gilbert et al, 1976; Sahn et al, 1977; Morganroth et al, 1980). Volume overload of the left ventricle from ventricular septal defect results in an increase in the total excursion of the mitral valve, and an even more horizontal position of the leaflets during ventricular systole (Sahn et al, 1977). In prolapsing valves, the mural or, less often, the aortic leaflet (or both) arch towards each other to an excessive degree and pass above the plane of the atrioventricular junction into the left atrium. The line of coaptation between the leaflets is displaced superiorly and posteriorly (Figure 43.35 and Plate 43.7) (Gilbert et al, 1976; Sahn et al, 1977). M-mode criterions for the floppy valve syndrome are mid-systolic buckling and pan-systole hammocking (Figure 43.36) (Shah and Gramiak, 1970; Popp et al, 1974). The usual C–D slope of the echocardiogram in normal individuals is positive throughout its duration (with the exception of the first 50 ms of systole), reflecting the anterior movement during this time. If the transducer is angled at all inferiorly, however, the effect of downward movement of the mitral valve may outweigh its anterior motion. The C–D slope will then show a prolonged initial negative component, giving rise to normal pan-systolic hammocking. If careful attention is not paid to angulation of the transducer, false-positive diagnoses are inevitable (Weiss et al, 1975; Devereux et al, 1976; Markiewicz et al, 1976). Just as incorrect angulation of the transducer may produce pseudo-prolapse, so may 'incorrect' angulation of the heart. Anything that makes the systolic position of the mitral valve more horizontal, such as volume overload, will increase the incidence of false-positive diagnoses (Sahn et al, 1977). This may be the sole explanation for the otherwise unexpected observation that the degree of mitral valvar prolapse as assessed from M-mode echocardiography is inversely related to the left ventricular end-diastolic dimension in patients with Marfan's syndrome (Lima et al, 1985). If records of motion are made from the body of the leaflets rather than from their free edges, about one in six normal patients will have pseudo-prolapse owing to holosystolic hammocking. Even mid-systolic buckling can be artefactually produced in patients with ventricular septal defect and normal mitral valves. Immobility of the aortic leaflet close to its hinge, as is seen in subaortic stenosis, means that the leaflet must buckle in order to permit systolic coaptation. This also gives rise to pseudo-prolapse (Sahn et al, 1977). In short, M-mode echocardiograms purporting to show mitral valvar prolapse in the presence of

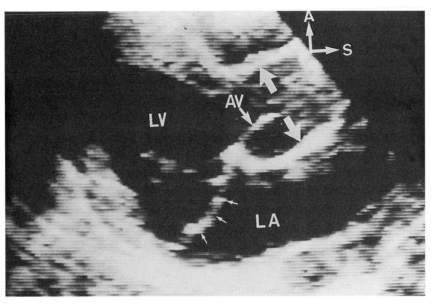

Figure 43.35. Mitral valve prolapse in Marfan's syndrome. Note that both leaflets (little white arrows) are bowed upwards into the left atrium (LA), and that the line of coaptation is superior to the annulus. There is also considerable dilation of the aortic root (large white arrows). The left ventricle (LV) is dilated because of mitral and aortic regurgitation. A, anterior; AV, aortic valve; S, superior.

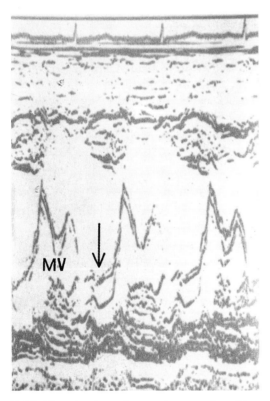

Figure 43.36. M-mode echocardiogram demonstrating mid-systolic buckling (arrow) of the mitral valve (MV). (Reproduced by kind permission of Dr M. Rigby.)

associated cardiac defects should be treated with extreme caution.

The depth of posterior motion of the leaflet after mid-systolic buckling can be artefactually produced in patients by means of the tensive cold pressor response (Pitcher et al, 1980). This test is particularly useful in patients with pan-systolic hammocking alone, since mid-systolic buckling is more specific. The place of apical four chamber sections in assessing prolapse in children is controversial. Bowing of one or other leaflet above the annulus was found to be 97% specific for the auscultatory syndrome in adults (Alpert et al, 1984). These authors pointed out that bowing could be produced by extreme caudal angulation of the transducer. By contrast, the prevalence of this finding in children without the auscultatory syndrome was found to increase dramatically with age, reaching 35% between the ages of 10 and 18 years (Warth et al, 1985). Since these same authors found a much lower prevalence of such bowing in parasternal long-axis cuts (3/193), their findings casts doubt concerning the validity of this view in the assessment of mitral valvar prolapse. Indeed, the observation that the valvar annulus is not perfectly circular but assumes a saddle shape, with one dimension being in a different plane to the other (Levine, 1987, 1988, 1989, 1992) provides an explanation for the discrepancy between findings obtained using the parasternal long-axis and four chamber views. Therefore, it has been suggested (Feigenbaum, 1992) that fairly reliable signs of mitral valvar prolapse include late systolic bulging as seen on M-mode tracings, displacement of the leaflets into the left atrium as seen in the parasternal long-axis view and thickening of the leaflets. Less reliable criterions include holosystolic prolapse as seen in M-mode tracings, displacement of the leaflets into the left atrium displayed in the apical four chamber view and late systolic regurgitation.

Regurgitation in the setting of prolapsing leaflets is best assessed by colour flow Doppler. Care must be taken if attempts are made to quantify the severity by means of the PISA phenomenon, since the amount of regurgitation is not constant throughout systole (Enriquez-Sarano et al, 1995).

CARDIAC CATHETERIZATION AND ANGIOCARDIOGRAPHY

Cardiac catheterization and angiocardiography are hardly ever indicated in children with floppy mitral valves. Most of our information on the subject comes from the era when it was necessary to prove that the mid-systolic click and late systolic murmur originated from the mitral valve. This was achieved by angiocardiography (Barlow et al, 1963) and intracardiac phonocardiography (Segal and Likoff, 1964; Ronan et al, 1965). Mitral valvar prolapse is best sought in the right anterior oblique projections of the selective left ventricular angiocardiogram (Figure 43.37), though the left anterior oblique projection is also useful. Since the essence of the prolapse is that the leaflets reach abnormally far towards the left atrium in relation to the atrioventricular junction, it is axiomatic that the junction must be clearly demonstrated. Unfortunately, though mitral regurgitation was first demonstrated in 1963 by Barlow and colleagues, it was not until 1980 that this seemingly elementary point was made in the literature (Spindola-Franco et al, 1980). Any information published prior to that date is immediately called into question. The atrioventricular junction can be identified with certainty only during diastole when relatively heavily opacified blood becomes trapped behind the leaflets. This most inferior point on the mitral annulus in the right anterior oblique projection is termed

the 'fulcrum' and probably corresponds to the position of the posteromedial scallop. The left ventricular free wall in this projection between the fulcrum and the base of the posterior papillary muscle corresponds to one length of the inlet portion of the left ventricle (Spindola-Franco et al, 1980). As shown in Figure 43.38, in normal individuals this part of the inlet may be smooth or notched and the fulcrum high (close to the aortic valve) or low. The same group defined prolapse of the mural leaflet as displacement of the leaflet beyond the fulcrum in an inferior and posterior direction. They argued that the normal mural leaflet may bulge posteriorly but not inferior to the fulcrum to give rise to pseudo-prolapse. This normal bulging was recognized in all patients except those with a high fulcrum and notched inlet. All 21 patients with angiocardiographic prolapse thus defined had M-mode echocardiographic evidence of prolapse, and 13 of those had the auscultatory syndrome (Cohen et al, 1979). By contrast, 20 out of 100 subjects with normal mitral valves studied by auscultation and echo-cardiography showed so-called pseudo-prolapse (Figure 43.38) (Spindola-Franco et al, 1980). The usual difficulties in separating normal from abnormal pertain; yet even in this very careful study, it appears that the auscultatory syndrome was overdiagnosed by angiocardiography. If so, the incidence of pseudo-prolapse is probably a conservative estimate. In particular, if the inferior part of the inlet is notched and the fulcrum low, the recess between the notched inlet and the mitral leaflet may be misinterpreted as prolapse. These conclusions are further supported by the study of Smith and colleagues (1977). According to their chosen criterions, they found silent

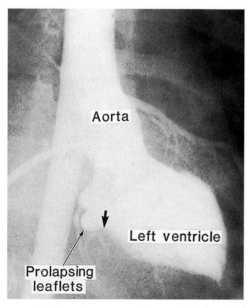

Figure 43.37. Shallow right anterior oblique projection of left ventriculogram. The position of the fulcrum (mitral annulus), established from the diastolic frame, is indicated by the solitary black arrow. As leaflet tissue is bulging inferior to this point, this is true prolapse.

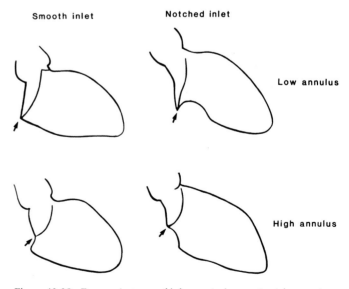

Figure 43.38. Four main types of left ventriculogram in right anterior oblique projection, according to Spindola-Franco and colleagues (1980). The upper row is intrinsically more likely to demonstrate pseudoprolapse than the lower row, because of the low position of the fulcrum (black arrow), which is the lowest portion of the mitral annulus. A notched inlet (fornix) is also liable to be mistaken for mitral valve prolapse.

prolapse in 40% of consecutive angiocardiograms. They concluded that 'the angiographic pattern by itself cannot be considered indicative of pathologic mitral valve function.' When a prolapsing valve is also severely regurgitant, the site of the prolapse can be identified with some accuracy (Ranganathan et al, 1973, 1976). In the right anterior oblique projection, the aortic and mural leaflets overlap. Hence, the prolapsed posteromedial scallop protrudes posterior and inferior to the fulcrum and the prolapsed anterolateral scallop protrudes anterior to the aortic root; the middle scallop is between the two. Prolapse of the aortic leaflet is much rarer than prolapse of the mural leaflet. It is distinct in the left anterior oblique projection, where the aortic leaflet, seen to be in continuity with the aortic valve in diastole, can be followed through to systole. If prolapse occurs, the valve is then seen to balloon superiorly and above the mural leaflet. When routine angiocardiograms are reviewed in the absence of regurgitation, there is a high degree of inter- and intraobserver variation as to both the presence and the site of prolapse (Kennett et al, 1981).

COURSE AND PROGNOSIS

Floppy mitral valve syndrome is an entirely benign condition in the great majority of patients. Allen and colleagues (1974) followed 62 patients with an isolated late systolic murmur (33 also had a click) for a period of 9 to 22 years (mean 13.8). Most had been known to have the murmur for much longer (mean 27 years; maximum 51 years). Patients with T wave abnormalities were excluded unless these only succeeded runs of premature contractions. Patients with multiple premature ventricular contractions were not excluded. Three patients died from irrelevant causes, one from bacterial endocarditis and one (at 75 years of age) from increasing mitral regurgitation. In one patient, cordal rupture necessitated valvar replacement. A further patient required treatment for bacterial endocarditis. In ten patients, there was slight deterioration, without development of symptoms, over a period averaging 11 years. No deterioration at all occurred in 41 patients (66%) over a mean of 13.8 years. Extremely similar findings were reported by Mills and colleagues (1977). One of their patients developed ventricular fibrillation requiring resuscitation following a previous self-limiting syncopal episode. One died suddenly after progressive cardiomegaly, atrial fibrillation, cardioversion and quinidine therapy. Five patients developed severe mitral regurgitation, the murmur becoming pan-systolic in each case. These authors did include, in their original 53 patients, 20 with electrocardiographic abnormalities. They also included 22 patients with an isolated click, three of whom had neither a click nor echocardiographic evidence of prolapse on follow-up. Whether or not these three patients were included, there was a highly significant difference in late complications between patients with a late systolic murmur with or

without a click, and those with a click alone, who had no complications at all. An abnormal electrocardiogram was not predictive of outcome, though the sudden death and ventricular fibrillation both occurred in patients with previously abnormal electrocardiograms, both of which showed T wave abnormalities. These results are extremely important because they define precisely two groups of patients at extremely low risk, namely those with isolated clicks and those with normal T waves and a normal QT interval on the electrocardiogram. Bacterial endocarditis has, however, been documented in two patients with an isolated systolic click (Le Bauer et al, 1967; Lachman et al, 1975). In a follow-up (mean 6.9 years) of 119 children with the auscultatory syndrome, two patients required antiarrhythmic medication for supraventricular tachycardia, one developed bacterial endocarditis and one had a cerebrovascular accident. There were no deaths, and mitral incompetence never increased (Bisset et al, 1980). Some of the very rare sudden late deaths recorded have been in adults with cardiomegaly, mitral regurgitation and atrial fibrillation (Mills et al, 1977). Others, however, have occurred in apparently normal patients with the click/murmur syndrome. Campbell and colleagues (1976) suggested that the patients with the auscultatory syndrome who were at high risk were those with left precordial or inferior T wave inversion or QT prolongation. In complete published papers in English, we have been able to find descriptions of 18 patients with the auscultatory syndrome and a documented electrocardiogram who died suddenly or developed ventricular fibrillation without dying (Hancock and Cohn, 1966; Barlow et al, 1968; Trent et al, 1970; Jeresaty, 1973, 1976; Gullotta et al, 1974; Shappell and Marshall, 1975; Campbell et al, 1976; Ritchie et al, 1976; Cobbs and King, 1977; Mills et al, 1977; Bharati et al, 1981; Salmela et al, 1981; Pocock et al, 1984). Of the 18 patients, 13 were female (assuming the extra patient of Shappell and Marshall was female). All of these patients fell into Campbell's (1976) group of patients at high risk except the patient described by Gullotta and colleagues for whom no T wave anomalies were described. This was the only patient of the 16 in whom there is any doubt about the auscultatory findings. She had mild mitral regurgitation, however, and must have had either a mid-systolic click and/or a late or pan-systolic murmur. One of the men described by Jeresaty (1976) had a pan-systolic murmur when first seen, with no click but massive angiocardiographic prolapse. Wei and colleagues (1978) described four further patients with the auscultatory syndrome who survived ventricular fibrillation, and Mair (1980) described three sudden deaths in young adult women (two of whom had the auscultatory syndrome and one of whom had a floppy valve at postmortem). It is impossible to tell from these papers whether QT or T abnormalities were present. At present, it is not possible to narrow down much further this rather large group of patients considered at high risk. Those with the familial syndrome may well be at high risk. A varying number of relatives of patients known to have the auscultatory syndrome died suddenly at ages varying from 12 to 40 (Barlow and Bosman, 1966; Shell et al, 1969; Shappell et al, 1973). It is not known whether the relatives also had the auscultatory syndrome. Furthermore, three patients dying suddenly and prematurely have been found to have relatives with the auscultatory syndrome. In two, the patient also had the auscultatory syndrome. In the third, a floppy mitral valve was found at postmortem (Hancock and Cohn, 1966; Marshall and Shappell, 1974). The sudden deaths and family histories are well summarized by Schwartz and colleagues (1977). T and QT abnormalities are strongly associated with ventricular arrhythmias such as R-on-T or multiform premature depolarizations, tachycardia and fibrillation (Campbell et al, 1976). The arrhythmias are also strongly associated with sudden death (Schwartz et al, 1977). Accordingly, 24-hour electrocardiography is likely to prove in the long run to be the best predictor of risk of sudden death.

MANAGEMENT

Patients with the click/murmur syndrome are often neurotic before the diagnosis is made. Given that the risk of sudden death and complications is so small, the last thing most of them need is either discussion of the risks of sudden death or the thoughtless but common combination of repeated reassurance and endless follow-up. 'If the doctor is not worried about me, why is he doing all this?' Some graded response in proportion to the risk involved is essential, which is inevitably arbitrary. We suggest the following regimen for children with normal T waves and QT interval and no evidence of Marfan's syndrome. Children with a click only should be reviewed in 5 years. It is not necessary to prescribe prophylaxis against bacterial endocarditis. Any benefit would be outweighed in the population as a whole by giving prophylaxis to patients whose click will have disappeared by the follow-up examination and who can then be discharged. Children with a late systolic murmur only should be advised concerning prophylaxis against bacterial endocarditis. There seems little doubt that the risk is greater in patients with prolapse than in those without (Clemens et al, 1982). They should be reviewed in 3 years. Children with T wave inversion in II, III, aVF, V_5 or V_6, or a prolonged QTc, and children with a family history of premature sudden death and the click/murmur syndrome, should have a 24-hour electrocardiogram, which must be compared against standards for normal individuals of their age (see Chapter 12). If this shows ventricular tachycardia or fibrillation (or if there are significant symptoms and an abnormally high incidence of premature ventricular contractions), then antiarrhythmic therapy (see Chapter 26) should be begun. The frequency of follow-up should be adjusted according to the response. If the 24-hour electrocardiogram is within normal limits, annual follow-up is instituted, repeating 24-hour monitoring only if indicated by symptoms such as dizziness or syncope or if the incidence of arrhythmias increases in the standard electrocardiogram. Prophylaxis against bacterial endocarditis should be as for patients with normal electrocardiograms. Parents of children with a persistent late systolic murmur should be advised of the small chance of progressive mitral regurgitation, which might necessitate surgery in adulthood. This has been observed to be more likely with advancing age, male sex, thickened leaflets and a holosystolic murmur (Rosen et al, 1994; Fukada et al, 1995; Zuppinoli et al, 1995). Successful replacement of floppy mitral valves has been reported in three of five children aged from 9 to 14 years in whom histology confirmed myxomatous degeneration. Three, including the two who died, also required replacement of the tricuspid valve because of floppy degeneration (Eguchi et al, 1976). It is not clear whether these patients ever had the click/murmur syndrome, or whether the mitral lesion was congenital or acquired.

REFERENCES

Abbasi A S, DeCristofaro D, Anabtawi J, Irwin L 1983 Mitral valve prolapse: comparative value of M-mode, two-dimensional and Doppler echocardiography. Journal of the American College of Cardiology 2: 1219–1223

Abrams J 1976 Mitral valve prolapse: a plea for unanimity. American Heart Journal 92: 413–415

Adatia I, Moore P M, Jonas R A, Colan S D, Lock J E, Keane J F 1997 Clinical course and hemodynamic observations after supraannular mitral valve replacement in infants and children. Journal of the American College of Cardiology 29: 1089–1094

Aharon A S, Laks H, Drinkwater D C et al 1994 Early and late results of mitral valve repair in children. Journal of Thoracic and Cardiovascular Surgery 107: 1262–1271

Alday L E, Juaneda E, Spillmann A, Ruiz E 1994 Early and late results of balloon dilation for congenital mitral stenosis. Cardiology of the Young 4: 122–125

Allen H, Harris A, Leatham A 1974 Significance and prognosis of an isolated late systolic murmur: a 9- to 22-year follow-up. British Heart Journal 36: 525–532

Alpert M A, Carney R J, Flaker G C, Sanfelippo J F, Webel R R, Kelly D L 1984 Sensitivity and specificity of two-dimensional echocardiographic signs of mitral valve prolapse. American Journal of Cardiology 54: 792–796

Anabtawi I N, Ellison R G 1965 Congenital stenosing right of the left atrioventricular canal (supravalvular mitral stenosis). Journal of Thoracic and Cardiovascular Surgery 49: 994–1005

Anderson R H, Thiene G 1981 The clinical morphology of mitral atresia. Atresia of the left atrioventricular valve. Giornale Italiano di Cardiologia 11: 1860–1870

Attie F, Lopez-Soriano F, Ovseyevits J et al 1986 Late results of mitral valve replacement with Bjork–Shiley prosthesis in children under 16 years of age. Journal of Thoracic and Cardiovascular Surgery 91: 754–758

Atz A M, Adatia I, Jonas R A, Wessel D L 1996 Inhaled nitric oxide in children with pulmonary hypertension and congenital mitral stenosis. American Journal of Cardiology 77: 316–319

Aufderheide S, Lax D, Goldberg S J 1995 Gender differences in dehydration-induced mitral valve prolapse. American Heart Journal 129: 83–86

Banerjee A, Kohl T, Silverman N H 1995 Echocardiographic evaluation of congenital mitral valve anomalies in children. The American Journal of Cardiology 76: 1284–1291

Barlow J B, Bosman C K 1966 Aneurysmal protrusion of the posterior leaflet of the mitral valve. An auscultatory–electrocardiographic syndrome. American Heart Journal 71: 166–178

Barlow J B, Pocock W A 1985 Billowing, floppy, prolapsed or flail mitral valves? American Journal of Cardiology 55: 501–502

Barlow J B, Pocock W A, Marchand P, Denny M 1963 The significance of late systolic murmur. American Heart Journal 66: 443–452

Barlow J B, Bosman C K, Pocock W A, Marchand P 1968 Late systolic murmurs and non-ejection ('mid-late') systolic clicks. British Heart Journal 30: 203–218

Becker A E 1983 Valve pathology in the paediatric age group. In: Anderson R H, Macartney F J, Shinebourne E A, Tynan M (eds) Paediatric cardiology, vol 5. Churchill Livingstone, Edinburgh, p 345–360

Becker A E, Anderson R H 1983 Cardiac pathology: an integrated text and colour atlas. Gower, London, p 4.8–4.11

Becker A E, de Wit A P M 1979 Mitral valve apparatus. A spectrum of normality relevant to mitral valve prolapse. British Heart Journal 42: 690

Beekman R H, Rocchini A P, Dick M II, Crowley D C, Rosenthal A 1984 Vasodilator therapy in children: acute and chronic effects in children with left ventricular dysfunction or mitral regurgitation. Pediatrics 73: 43–51

Benmimoun E G, Friedli B, Rutishauser W, Faidutti B 1982 Mitral valve replacement in children. Comparative study of pre- and postoperative haemodynamics and left ventricular function. British Heart Journal 48: 117–124

Beppu S, Nimura Y, Sakakibara H, Nagata S, Park Y, Baba K, et al 1980 Mitral cleft in ostium primum atrial septal defect assessed by cross-sectional echocardiography. Circulation 62: 1099–1107

Berry B E, Ritter D G, Wallace R B, McGoon D C, Danielson G K 1974 Cardiac valve replacement in children. Journal of Thoracic and Cardiovascular Surgery 68: 705–710

Bharati S, Granston A S, Liebson P R, Loeb H S, Rosen K M, Lev M 1981 The conduction system in mitral valve prolapse syndrome with sudden death. American Heart Journal 101: 667–670

Bini R M, Pellegrino P A, Mazzucco A et al 1980 Tricuspid atresia with double-outlet left atrium. Chest 78: 109–111

Bisset G S III, Schwartz D C, Meyer R A, James F W, Kaplan S 1980 Clinical spectrum and long-term follow-up of isolated mitral valve prolapse in 119 children. Circulation 62: 423–429

Bon Tempo C P, Ronan J A Jr, Leon A C D Jr, Twill H L 1975 Radiographic appearance of the thorax in the systolic click-late systolic murmur syndrome. American Journal of Cardiology 36: 27–31

Boudoulas H, Reynolds J C, Mazzaferri E, Wooley C F 1980 Metabolic studies in mitral valve prolapse syndrome. A neuroendocrine – cardiovascular process. Circulation 61: 1200–1205

Boudoulas H, Reynolds J C, Mazzaferri E, Wooley C F 1983 Mitral valve prolapse syndrome: the effect of adrenergic stimulation. Journal of the American College of Cardiology 2: 638–644

Brodsky M, Wu D, Denes P, Kanakis C, Rosen K M 1977 Arrhythmias documented by 24 hour continuous electrocardiographic monitoring in 50 male medical students without apparent heart disease. American Journal of Cardiology 39: 390–395

Bulkley B H, Roberts W C 1975 Dilatation of the mitral annulus. A rare cause of mitral regurgitation. American Journal of Medicine 59: 457–463

Campbell R W F, Godman M G, Fiddler G I, Marquis R M, Julian D G 1976 Ventricular arrhythmias in syndrome of balloon deformity of mitral valve. Definition of possible high risk group. British Heart Journal 38: 1053–1057

Cape E G, Yoganathan A P, Weyman A E, Levine R A 1991 Adjacent solid boundaries alter the size of regurgitant jets on Doppler color flow maps. Journal of the American College of Cardiology 17: 1094–1102

Carpentier A 1983a Mitral valve reconstruction in children. In: Anderson R H, Macartney F J, Shinebourne E A, Tynan M (eds) Paediatric cardiology, vol 5. Churchill Livingstone, Edinburgh, p 361–368

Carpentier A L 1983b Cardiac valve surgery – the French correction. Journal of Thoracic and Cardiovascular Surgery 86: 323–337

Carpentier A, Branchini B, Cour J C, et al 1976 Congenital malformations of the mitral valve in children. Pathology and surgical treatment. Journal of Thoracic and Cardiovascular Surgery 72: 854–866

Castello R, Lenzen P, Aguire F, Labovitz A 1992a Variability in the quantitation of mitral regurgitation by Doppler color flow mapping; Comparison of transthoracic and transesophageal studies. Journal of the American College of Cardiology 20: 433–438

Castello R, Lenzen P, Aguire F, Labovitz A J 1992b Quantitation of mitral regurgitation by transesophageal echocardiography with Doppler color flow mapping: correlation with cardiac catheterization. Journal of the American College of Cardiology 19: 1516–1521

Celano V, Pieroni D R, Morera J A, Roland J-M A, Gingell R L 1984 Two-dimensional echocardiographic examination of mitral valve abnormalities associated with coarctation of the aorta. Circulation 69: 924–932

Chandraratna P A N, Vlahovich G, Kong Y, Wilson D 1979 Incidence of mitral valve prolapse in one hundred clinically stable newborn baby girls: an echocardiographic study. American Heart Journal 98: 312–314

Chao K, Moises V A, Shandas R, Elkadi T, Sahn D J, Weintraub R 1992 Influence of the Coanda effect on color Doppler jet area and color encoding. In vitro studies using color Doppler flow mapping. Circulation 85: 333–341

Chauvaud S, Perier P, Touati G 1986 Long-term results of valve repair in children with acquired mitral valve incompetence. Circulation 74(suppl I): 104–109

Chauvaud S M, Milhaileanu S A, Gaer J A R, Carpentier A C 1997a Surgical treatment of congenital mitral valvar insufficiency: 'the Hopital Broussais' experience. Cardiology of the Young 7: 5–14

Chauvaud S M, Milhaileanu S A, Gaer J A R, Carpentier A C 1997b Surgical treatment of congenital mitral valvar stenosis: 'the Hopital Broussais' experience. Cardiology of the Young 7: 15–21

Cheitlin M D 1979 Editorial: thromboembolic studies in the patient with the prolapsed mitral valve. Has Salome dropped another vein? Circulation 60: 46–47

Cheitlin M D 1991 Valvular heart disease: management and intervention. Circulation 84(suppl I): 259–264

Chesler E, King R A, Edwards J E 1983 The myxomatous mitral valve and sudden death. Circulation 67: 632–639

Clemens J D, Horwitz R I, Jaffe C C, Feinstein A R, Stanton B F 1982 A controlled evaluation of the risk of bacterial endocarditis in persons with mitral-valve prolapse. New England Journal of Medicine 307: 776–781

Cobbs B W Jr, King S B III 1977 Ventricular buckling: a factor in the abnormal ventriculogram and peculiar hemodynamics associated with mitral valve prolapse. American Heart Journal 93: 741–758

Cohen M, Pocock W A, Lakier J B, McLaren M J, Lachman A S, Barlow J B 1978 Four year follow-up of black schoolchildren with non-ejection systolic clicks and mitral systolic murmurs. American Heart Journal 95: 697–701

Cohen M V, Shah P K, Spindola-Franco H 1979 Angiographic – echocardiographic correlation in mitral valve prolapse. American Heart Journal 97: 43–52

Coles J G, Williams W G, Watanabe T et al 1987 Surgical experience with reparative techniques in patients with congenital mitral valvular anomalies. Circulation 76(suppl III): 117–122

Collins-Nakai R L, Rosenthal A, Castaneda A R, Bernhard W F, Nadas A S 1977 Congenital mitral stenosis. A review of 20 years' experience. Circulation 56: 1039–1046

CONSENSUS Trial Study Group 1987 Effect of enalapril on mortality in severe congestive heart failure: Members of the cooperative North Scandinavin Enalapril Survival Study (CONSENSUS). New England Journal of Medicine 316: 1429–1435

Corno A, Giannico S, Leibovich S, Mazzera E, Marcelletti C 1986 The hypoplastic mitral valve. Journal of Thoracic and Cardiovascular Surgery 91: 848–851

Coto E O, Jimenez M Q, Deverall P B, Bain H 1984 Anomalous mitral 'cleft' with abnormal ventriculoarterial connection: anatomical findings and surgical implications. Pediatric Cardiology 5: 1–6

Criley J M, Lewis K B, Humphries J O, Ross R S 1966 Prolapse of the mitral valve: clinical and cineangiocardiographic findings. British Heart Journal 28: 488–496

Daliento L, Thiene G, Chirillo F et al 1991 Congenital mitral valve malformations: clinical and morphological aspects. Italian Journal of Cardiology 21: 1205–1216

Davidson C J, Bashmore T M, Mickel M, Davis K 1992 Balloon mitral commissurotomy after previous surgical commissurotomy. Circulation 86: 91–99

Davies M J 1980 Pathology of the cardiac valves. Butterworths, London, p 75–86

Davies M J, Moore B P, Braimbridge M V 1978 The floppy mitral valve. Study of incidence, pathology, and complications in surgical, necropsy, and forensic material. British Heart Journal 40: 468–481

Deverall P B 1983 Valve replacement in patients less than 15 years of age. In: Anderson R H, Macartney F J, Shinebourne E A, Tynan M (eds) Paediatric cardiology, vol 5. Churchill Livingstone, Edinburgh, p 369–376

Devereux R B, Perloff J K, Reichek N, Josephson M E 1976 Mitral valve prolapse. Circulation 54: 3–14

Devereux R B, Brown W T, Kramer-Fox R, Sachs I 1982 Inheritance of mitral valve prolapse: effect of age and sex on gene expression. Annals of Internal Medicine 97: 826–832

Di Segni E, Bass J L, Lucas R V Jr, Einzig S 1983 Isolated cleft mitral valve: a variety of congenital mitral regurgitation identified by 2-dimensional echocardiography. American Journal of Cardiology 51: 927–931

Driscoll D J, Gutgesell H P, McNamara D G 1978 Echocardiographic features of congenital mitral stenosis. American Journal of Cardiology 42: 259–266

Ebel T A 1978 Mitral valve prolapse. Advances in Pediatrics 25: 263–325

Eguchi S, Nakamura C, Asano K-I, Tanaka M 1976 Surgical treatment of floppy mitral valve syndrome in children. Journal of Thoracic and Cardiovascular Surgery 71: 899–903

Enriquez-Sarano M, Bailey K R, Seward J B, Tajik A J, Krohn M J, Mays J M 1993 Quantitative Doppler assessment of valvular regurgitation. Circulation 87: 841–848

Enriquez-Sarano M, Sinak L J, Tajik A J, Bailey K R, Seward J B 1995 Changes in effective regurgitant orifice throughout systole in patients with mitral valve prolapse. A clinical study using the proximal isovelocity surface area method. Circulation 92(10): 2951–2958

Feigenbaum H 1992 Echocardiography in the management of mitral valve prolapse. Australian and New Zealand Journal of Medicine 22: 550–555

Fernex M, Fernex C 1958 La degenerescence mucoide des valvules mitrales. Ses repercussions functionelles. Helvetica Medica Acta 25: 694–705

Fiddler G I, Scott O 1980 Heart murmurs audible across the room in children with mitral valve prolapse. British Heart Journal 44: 201–203

Fiddler G I, Gerlis L M, Walker D R, Scott O, Williams G J 1983 Calcification of glutaraldehyde-preserved porcine and bovine xenograft valves in young children. Annals of Thoracic Surgery 35: 257–261

Flack J M, Kvasnicka J H, Gardin J M, Gidding S S, Manolio T A, Jacobs D R Jr 1999 Anthropometric and physiologic correlates of mitral valve prolapse in a biethnic cohort of young adults: the CARDIA study. American Heart Journal 138: 486–492

Frater R 1976 Discussion. In: Kalmanson D (ed.) The mitral valve, a pluridisciplinary approach. Publishing Sciences Group, Acton, MA, p 41

Freed L A, Levy D, Levine R A et al 1999 Prevalence and clinical outcome of mitral – valve prolapse. New England Journal Medicine 341: 41–7

Freed M D, Keane J F, Van Praagh R, Castaneda A R, Bernhard W F, Nadas A S 1974 Coarctation of the aorta with congenital mitral regurgitation. Circulation 49: 1175–1184

Fukuda N, Oki T, Iuchi A et al 1995 Predisposing factors for severe mitral regurgitation in idiopathic mitral valve prolapse. American Journal of Cardiology 76(7): 503–507

Gaffney F A, Karlsson E S, Campbell W et al 1979 Automatic dysfunction in women with mitral valve prolapse syndrome. Circulation 59: 894–901

Gardin J M, Isner J M, Ronan J A Jr, Fox S M 1980 Pseudoischemic 'false positive' S–T segment changes induced by hyperventilation in patients with mitral valve prolapse. American Journal of Cardiology 45: 952–958

Gardner T J, Roland J M A, Neill C A, Donahoo J S 1982 Valve replacement in children. A fifteen-year perspective. Journal of Thoracic and Cardiovascular Surgery 83: 178–185

Geha A S, Laks H, Stansel H C Jr et al 1979 Late failure of porcine valve heterografts in children. Journal of Thoracic and Cardiovascular Surgery 78: 351–364

Gilbert B W, Schatz R A, Von Ramm O T, Behar V S, Kisslo J A 1976 Mitral valve prolapse. Two-dimensional echocardiographic and angiographic correlation. Circulation 54: 716–723

Gingell R L, Vlad P 1978 Mitral valve prolapse. In: Keith J D, Rowe R D, Vlad P (eds) Heart disease in infancy and childhood. Macmillan, New York, p 810–827

Glaser J, Yakirevich V, Vidne B A 1984 Preoperative echographic diagnosis of supravalvular stenosing ring of the left atrium. American Heart Journal 108: 169–171

Goldberg S J, Gerlis L M, Ho S Y, Penilla M B 1995 Location of the left papillary muscles in juxtaductal aortic coarctation. The American Journal of Cardiology 75: 746–750

Gooch A S, Vicencio F, Maranhao V, Goldberg H 1972 Arrhythmias and left ventricular asynergy in the prelapsing mitral leaflet syndrome. American Journal of Cardiology 29: 611–620

Greenberg B H, Massie B M, Brundage B H, Botvinick E H, Parmley W W, Chatterjee K 1978 Beneficial effects of hydralazine in severe mitral regurgitation. Circulation 58: 273–279

Grenadier E, Sahn D J, Valdes-Cruz L M, Allen H D, Lima C O, Goldberg S J 1984 Two-dimensional echo Doppler study of congenital disorders of the mitral valve. American Heart Journal 107: 319–325

Grifka R G, O'Laughlin M P, Nihill M R, Mullins C E 1992 Double-transseptal, double-balloon valvuloplasty for congenital mitral stenosis. Circulation 85: 123–129

Grossman H, Fleming R J, Engle M A, Levin A H, Ehlers K H 1968 Angiocardiography in the apical systolic click syndrome: left ventricular abnormality, mitral insufficiency, late systolic murmur, and inversion of T waves. Radiology 91: 898–904

Gullotta S J, Gulco L, Padmanabhan V, Miller S 1974 The syndrome of systolic click, murmur, and mitral valve prolapse – a cardiomyopathy? Circulation 49: 717–728

Haikal M, Alpert M A, Whiting R B, Ahmad M, Kelly D 1982 Sensitivity and specificity of M mode echocardiographic signs of mitral valve prolapse. American Journal of Cardiology 50: 185–190

Hammer D, Leier C V, Baba N, Vasko J S, Wooley C F,

Pinnell S R 1979 Altered collagen composition in a prolapsing mitral valve with ruptured chordae tendineae. American Journal of Medicine 67: 863–866

Hancock E W, Cohn K 1966 The syndrome associated with mid systolic click and late systolic murmur. American Journal of Medicine 41: 183–196

Hatle L, Brubakk A, Tromsdal A, Angelsen B 1978 Noninvasive assessment of pressure drop in mitral stenosis by Doppler ultrasound. British Heart Journal 40: 131–140

Higgins C B, Silverman N H, Kersting-Sommerhoff, Schmidt K G 1990 Congenital heart disease: echocardiography and magnetic resonance imaging. Raven Press, New York, p 62–71

Higgins C B, Wagner S, Kondo C, Suzuki J I, Caputo G R 1991 Evaluation of valvular heart disease with cine gradient echo magnetic resonance imaging. Circulation 84(suppl I): 198–207

Hunt D, Sloman G 1969 Prolapse of the posterior leaflet of the mitral valve occurring in eleven members of a family. American Heart Journal 78: 149–153

Jaffe A S, Geltman E M, Rodey G E, Uitto J 1981 Mitral valve prolapse: a consistent manifestation of type IV Ehler–Danlos syndrome. The pathogenetic role of the abnormal production of type III collagen. Circulation 64: 121–125

Jeresaty R M 1973 Mitral valve prolapse-click syndrome. Progress in Cardiovascular Diseases 15: 623–652

Jeresaty R M 1975 Etiology of the mitral valve prolapse-click syndrome. American Journal of Cardiology 36: 110–113

Jeresaty R M 1976 Sudden death in the mitral valve prolapse-click syndrome. American Journal of Cardiology 37: 317–318

Jeresaty R M 1979 Mitral valve prolapse. Raven Press, New York, p 9–18

Karr S S, Parness I A, Spevak P J et al 1992 Diagnosis of anomalous left coronary artery by Doppler color flow mapping: distinction from other causes of dilated cardiomyopathy. Journal of the American College of Cardiology 19: 1271–1275

Kavey R-E W, Sondheimer H M, Blackman M S 1980 Detection of dysrhythmia in pediatric patients with mitral valve prolapse. Circulation 62: 582–587

Kelbaek H, Aldershvile J, Skagen K, Hildebrandt P, Nielsen S L 1996 Pre and afterload reduction in chronic mitral regurgitation: a double-blind randomized placebo-controlled trial of the acute and 2 weeks effect of nifedipine or isosorbide dinitrate treatment on left ventricular function and the severity of mitral regurgitation. British Journal of Clinical Pharmacology 41: 493–497

Kennett J D, Rust P F, Martin R H, Parker B M, Watson L E 1981 Observer variation in the angiocardiographic diagnosis of mitral valve prolapse. Chest 79: 146–150

King B D, Clark M A, Baba N, Kilman J W, Wooley C F 1982 'Myxomatous' mitral valves: collagen dissolution as the primary defect. Circulation 66: 288–296

Kohl T, Silverman N 1996 Comparison of cleft and papillary muscle position in cleft mitral valve and atrioventricular septal defect. American Journal of Cardiology 77: 164–169

Koike K, Musewe N M, Smallhorn J F, Freedom R M 1989 Distinguishing between anomalous origin of the left coronary artery from the pulmonary trunk and dilated cardiomyopathy: role of echocardiographic measurement of the right coronary artery diameter. British Heart Journal 61: 192–197

Kramer-Fox R, Devereux R B, Brown T, Hatman N, Elston R C 1984 Lack of association between dermal arches and mitral valve prolapse: relation to anxiety. American Journal of Cardiology 53: 148–152

Kutsche L M, Oyer P, Shumway N, Baum D 1979 An important complication of Hancock mitral valve replacement in children. Circulation 60(suppl I): 98–103

Lachman A S, Bramwell-Jones D M, Lakier J B, Pocock W A, Barlow J B 1975 Infective endocarditis in the billowing mitral leaflet syndrome. British Heart Journal 37: 326–330

Lacorte M, Harada K, Williams R G 1976 Echocardiographic features of congenital left ventricular inflow obstruction. Circulation 54: 562–566

Lam J H C, Ranganathan N, Wigle E D, Silver M D 1970 Morphology of the human mitral valve. I. Chordae tendineae: a new classification. Circulation 41: 449–458

Lam W, Pavel D, Byrom E, Sheikh A, Best D, Rosen K 1981 Radionucleotide regurgitant index: value and limitations. American Journal of Cardiology 47: 292–298

Lax D, Eicher M, Goldberg S J 1992 Mild dehydration induces echocardiographic signs of mitral valve prolapse in healthy females with prior normal cardiac findings. American Heart Journal 124(6): 1533–1540

Layman T E, Edwards J E 1967 Anomalous mitral arcade. A type of congenital mitral insufficiency. Circulation 35: 389–395

Leatham A, Brigden W 1980 Mild mitral regurgitation and the mitral prolapse fiasco. American Heart Journal 99: 659–664

Le Bauer E J, Perloff K, Keliher T F 1967 The isolated systolic click with bacterial endocarditis. American Heart Journal 73: 534–537

Lebwohl M G, Distefono D, Prioleau P G, Uram M, Yannuzzi L A, Fleischmajer R 1982 Pseudoxanthoma elasticum and mitral-valve prolapse. New England Journal of Medicine 307: 228–231

Leung M, Rigby M L, Anderson R H, Wyse R K H, Macartney F J 1987 Reversed offsetting of the septal attachments of the atrioventricular valves and Ebstein's malformation of the morphologically mitral valve. British Heart Journal 57: 184–187

Levine H J, Gaasch W H 1996 Vasoactive drugs in chronic regurgitant lesions of the mitral and aortic valves. Journal of the American College of Cardiology 28: 1083–1091

Levine R A, Triulzi M O, Harrigan P, Weyman A E 1987 The relationship of mitral annular shape to the diagnosis of mitral valve prolapse. Circulation 75: 756–767

Levine R A, Stathogiannis E, Newell J B, Harrigan P, Weyman A E 1988 Reconsideration of echocardiographic standards for mitral valve prolapse: lack of association between leaflet displacement isolated to the apical four chamber view and independent echocardiographic evidence of abnormality. Journal of the American College of Cardiology 11: 1010–1019

Levine R A, Handschumacher M D, Sanfilippo A J et al 1989 Three-dimensional echocardiographic reconstruction of the mitral valve, with implications for the diagnosis of mitral valve prolapse. Circulation 80: 589–598

Levine R A, Weyman A E, Handschumacher M D 1992 Three-dimensional echocardiography: techniques and applications. American Journal of Cardiology 69: 121H–130H; discussion 131H–134H

Liedtke A J, Gault J H, Leaman D M, Blumenthal M S 1973 Geometry of left ventricular contraction in the systolic click syndrome. Characterization of a segmental myocardial abnormality. Circulation 47: 27–35

Lima S D, Lima J A C, Pyeritz R E, Weiss J L 1985 Relation of mitral valve prolapse to left ventricular size in Marfan's syndrome. American Journal of Cardiology 55: 739–743

Little R C 1979 The mechanism of closure of the mitral valve: a continuing controversy. Circulation 59: 615–618

Lobstein H P, Horwitz L D, Curry G C, Mullins C B 1973 Electrocardiographic abnormalities and coronary arteriograms in the mitral click–murmur syndrome. New England Journal of Medicine 289: 127–131

Lock J E, Khalilullah M, Shrivastava S, Bahl V, Keane J F 1985 Percutaneous catheter commissurotomy in rheumatic mitral stenosis. New England Journal of Medicine 313: 1515–1518

Lucas R V Jr, Edwards J E 1983 Floppy mitral valve and ventricular septal defect: an anatomic study. Journal of the American College of Cardiology 1: 1337–1347

Lundstrom N -R 1972 Echocardiography in the diagnosis of congenital mitral stenosis and in evaluation of the results of mitral valvotomy. Circulation 46: 44–54

Lynch M F, Ryan N J, Williams G R et al 1962 Preoperative diagnosis and surgical correction of supravalvular mitral stenosis and ventricular septal defect. Circulation 25: 854–861

Macartney F J, Scott P O, Ionescu M I, Deverall P B 1974 Diagnosis and management of parachute mitral valve and supravalvular mitral ring. British Heart Journal 36: 641–652

Macartney F J, Bain H H, Ionescu M I, Deverall P B, Scott O 1976 Angiocardiographic/pathologic correlations in congenital mitral valve anomalies. European Journal of Cardiology 4: 191–211

Macartney F J, Daly K, Wilkinson J L, Anderson R H 1979 Angiocardiography in the preoperative evaluation of patients with univentricular hearts. Herz 4: 126–9

Mair W J 1980 Sudden death in young females with floppy mitral valve syndrome. Australian and New Zealand Journal of Medicine 10: 221–223

Malcolm A D, Cankovic-Darracott S, Chayen J, Jenkins B S, Webb-Peploe M M 1979 Biopsy evidence of left ventricular myocardial abnormality in patients with a mitral leaflet prolapse and chest pain. Lancet i: 1052–1055

Malkowski M J, Boudoulas H, Wooley C F, Guo R, Pearson A C, Gray P G 1996 Spectrum of structural abnormalities in floppy mitral valve echocardiographic evaluation. American Heart Journal 132: 145–151

Markiewicz W, Stoner J, London E, Hunt S A, Popp R L 1976 Mitral valve prolapse in one hundred presumably healthy young females. Circulation 53: 464–473

Marks A R, Choong C Y, Chir M B, Sanfilippo A J, Ferre M, Weyman A E 1989 New England Journal of Medicine 320: 1031–1036

Marshall C E, Shappell S D 1974 Sudden death and the ballooning posterior leaflet syndrome. Detailed anatomic and histochemical investigation. Archives of Pathology 98: 134–138

Mathey D G, Decoodt P R, Allen H N, Swan H J C 1976 The determinants of onset of mitral valve prolapse in the systolic click–late systolic murmur syndrome. Circulation 53: 872–878

Maurer G, Siegel R J, Czer L S C 1991 The use of color flow mapping for intraoperative assessment of valve repair. Circulation 84(suppl I): 250–258

McDonald A, Harris A, Jefferson K, Marshall J, McDonald L 1971 Association of prolapse of posterior cusp of mitral valve and atrial septal defect. British Heart Journal 33: 383–387

McLaren M J, Hawkins D M, Lachman A S, Lakier J B, Pocock W A, Barlow J B 1976 Non-ejection systolic clicks and mitral systolic murmurs in black schoolchildren of Soweto, Johannesburg. British Heart Journal 38: 718–724

Mele D, Vandercoort P, Palacios I et al 1995 Proximal jet size by Doppler color flow mapping predicts severity of mitral regurgitation. Circulation 91: 746–754

Mickell J J, Mathews R A, Anderson R H et al 1983 The anatomical heterogeneity of hearts lacking a patent communication between the left atrium and the ventricular mass ('mitral atresia') in presence of a patent aortic valve. European Heart Journal 4: 477–486

Mills P, Rose J, Hollingsworth J, Amara I, Craige E 1977 Long-term prognosis of mitral-valve prolapse. New England Journal of Medicine 297: 13–18

Mimo R, Sparacino L, Nicolosi G L et al 1991 Quantification of mitral regurgitation: comparison between transthoracic and transesophageal color doppler flow mapping. Echocardiography 8: 619–626

Mohiaddin R H, Amanuma M, Kilner P J, Pennell D J, Manzara C, Longmore D B 1991 MR phase-shift velocity mapping of mitral and pulmonary venous flow. Journal of Computer Assisted Tomography 15: 237–243

Moreno F, Quero M, Diaz L P 1976 Mitral atresia with normal aortic valve. A study of eighteen cases and a review of the literature. Circulation 53: 1004–1010

Morganroth J, Jones R H, Chen C, Naito M 1980 Two dimensional echocardiography in mitral, aortic and tricuspid valve prolapse. The clinical problem, cardiac nuclear imaging considerations and a proposed standard for diagnosis. American Journal of Cardiology 46: 1164–1177

Morrison G W, Scott O, Macartney F J 1977 Retrograde left atrial catheterization in children with congenital heart disease. American Heart Journal 94: 333–335

Mullins C E 1983 Transseptal left heart catheterization: experience with a new technique in 520 pediatric and adult patients. Pediatric Cardiology 4: 239–245

Nakano S, Sakai K, Taniguchi K et al 1994 Relation of impaired left ventricular function in mitral regurgitation to left ventricular contractile state after mitral valve replacement. American Journal of Cardiology 73: 70–74

Nascimento R, Freitas A, Teixeira F et al 1997 Is mitral valve prolapse a congenital or acquired disease? American Journal of Cardiology 79: 226–227

Nazarian G K, Julsrud P R, Ehman R L, Edwards W D 1987 Correlation between magnetic resonance imaging of the heart and cardiac anatomy. Mayo Clinical Proceedings 62: 573–583

Neirotti R, Kreutzer G, Galindez E, Becu L, Ross D 1977 Supravalvular mitral stenosis associated with ventricular septal defect. American Journal of Diseases of Children 131: 862–865

Nichol P M, Boughner D R, Persaud J A 1976 Noninvasive assessment of mitral insufficiency by transcutaneous Doppler ultrasound. Circulation 54: 656–661

Norwood W I, Lang P, Hansen D D 1983 Physiologic repair of aortic atresia–hypoplastic left heart syndrome: New England Journal of Medicine 308: 23–26

Oakley C M 1992 Mitral valve palpitations. Australia and New Zealand Journal of Medicine 22: 562–565

Oberhansli I, Baldovinos A, Beghetti M, Friedli B, Faidutti B 1997 Hypoplasia of the posterior leaflet as a rare cause of congenital mitral insufficiency. Journal of Cardiac Surgery 12: 339–342

Ogawa S, Hayashi J, Sasaki H et al 1982 Evaluation of combined valvular prolapse syndrome by two-dimensional echocardiography. Circulation 65: 174–180

Oglietti J, Reul G J Jr, Leachman R D, Cooley D A 1976 Supravalvular stenosing ring of the left atrium. Annals of Thoracic Surgery 21: 421–424

Okita Y, Miki S, Kusuhara K 1988 Early and late results of reconstructive operation for congenital regurgitation in pediatric age group. Journal of Thoracic and Cardiovascular Surgery 96: 294–298

Ormiston J A, Shah P M, Tei C, Wong M 1982 Size and motion of the mitral valve annulus in man. II. Abnormalities in mitral valve prolapse. Circulation 65: 713–719

Pacileo G, Russo M G, Calabro R 1991 Anomalous arcade: echocardiographic and color flow findings. Echocardiography: American Journal of Cardiovascular Ultrasound and Applied Technology 8: 657–659

Parr G V S, Fripp R R, Whitman V, Bharati S, Lev M 1983 Anomalous mitral arcade: echocardiographic and angiographic recognition. Pediatric Cardiology 4: 163–165

Pass H I, Sade R M, Crawford F A, Hohn A R 1984 Cardiac valve prostheses in children without anticoagulation. Journal of Thoracic and Cardiovascular Surgery 87: 832–835

Passafini A, Shiota T, Depp M, Paik J, Ge S, Shandas R, Sahn D 1995 Factors influencing pulmonary venous flow velocity patterns in mitral regurgitation: an in vitro study. Journal of the American College of Cardiology 26: 1333–1339

Perloff J K 1982 Evolving concepts of mitral-valve prolapse. New England Journal of Medicine 307: 369–370

Perloff J K, Roberts W C 1972 The mitral apparatus. Functional anatomy of mitral regurgitation. Circulation 46: 227–239

Pickering N J, Brody J L, Barrett M J 1981 Von Willebrand syndromes and mitral-valve prolapse. Linked mesenchymal dysplasias. New England Journal of Medicine 305: 131–134

Pitcher D, Tynan M, Wainwright R, Curry P, Sowton E 1980 New intervention in mitral valve prolapse. Use of cold pressor test during echocardiography. British Heart Journal 44: 524–528

Pocock W A, Barlow J B 1971 An association between the billowing posterior mitral leaflet syndrome and congenital heart disease, particularly atrial septal defect. American Heart Journal 81: 720–722

Pocock W A, Bosman C K, Chester E, Barlow J B, Edwards J E 1984 Sudden death in primary mitral valve prolapse. American Heart Journal 107: 378–382

Pomerance A 1979 Pathology and valvular heart disease. British Heart Journal 34: 437–443

Popp R L, Brown O R, Silverman J F, Harrison D C 1974 Echocardiographic abnormalities in the mitral valve prolapse syndrome. Circulation 49: 428–433

Procacci P M, Savran S V, Schreiter S L, Bryson A L 1976 Prevalence of clinical mitral-valve prolapse in 1169 young women. New England Journal of Medicine 294: 1086–1088

Pu M, Vandervoort P M, Griffin B P et al 1995 Quantification of mitral regurgitation by the proximal convergence method using transesophageal echocardiography. Circulation 92: 2169–2177

Ranganathan N, Silver M D, Robinson T I et al 1973 Angiographic-morphologic correlation in patients with severe mitral regurgitation due to prolapse of the posterior mitral valve leaflet. Circulation 48: 514–518

Ranganathan N, Silver M D, Robinson T I, Wilson J K 1976 Idiopathic prolapsed mitral leaflet syndrome. Angiographic–clinical correlations. Circulation 54: 126–132

Raymond H W, Zwiebel W J, Harnsberger H R 1990 Magnetic resonance imaging in pediatric cardiac disease. Seminars in Ultrasound, Computed Tomography and Magnetic Resonance 11: 184–197

Read R C, Thai A P, Wendt V E 1965 Symptomatic valvular myxomatous transformation (the floppy valve syndrome): a possible forme fruste of the Marfan syndrome. Circulation 32: 897–910

Reed D, Abbott R D, Smucker M L, Kaul S 1991 Prediction of outcome after mitral valve replacement in patients with symptomatic chronic mitral regurgitation. Circulation 84: 23–34

Rhodes L A, Colan S D, Perry S B, Jonas R A, Sanders P 1991 Predictors of survival in neonates with critical aortic stenosis. Circulation 84: 2325–2335

Rigby M L, Gibson D G, Joseph M C et al 1982 Recognition of imperforate atrioventricular valves by two dimensional echocardiography. British Heart Journal 471: 329–336

Riggs T W, Lapin G D, Paul M H et al 1983 Measurement of mitral valve orifice area in infants and children by two-dimensional echocardiography. Journal of the American College of Cardiology 1: 873–878

Rippe J M, Sloss L J, Angoff G, Alpert J S 1979 Mitral valve prolapse in adults with congenital heart disease. American Heart Journal 97: 561–573

Ritchie J L, Hammermeister K E, Kennedy J W 1976 Refractory ventricular tachycardia and fibrillation in a patient with the prolapsing mitral leaflet syndrome: successful control with overdrive pacing. American Journal of Cardiology 37: 314–316

Roberts W C, Dangel J C, Bulkely B H 1973 Nonrheumatic valvular cardiac disease: a clinicopathologic survey of 27 different conditions causing valvular dysfunction. Cardiovascular Clinics 5: 334–446

Robinson P J, Sullivan I D, Kumpeng V, Anderson R H, Macartney F J 1984 Anomalous origin of the left coronary artery from the pulmonary trunk. Potential for false negative diagnosis with cross sectional echocardiography. British Heart Journal 52: 272–277

Ronan J A, Perloff J K, Harvey W P 1965 Systolic clicks and the late systolic murmur. Intracardiac phonocardiographic evidence of their mitral valve origin. American Heart Journal 70: 319–325

Rosen S E, Borer J S, Hochreiter C et al 1994 Natural history of the asymptomatic/minimally symptomatic patient with severe mitral regurgitation secondary to mitral valve prolapse and normal right and left ventricular performance. American Journal of Cardiology 74(4): 374–380

Rosenquist G C 1974 Congenital mitral valve disease associated with coarctation of the aorta. A spectrum that includes parachute deformity of the mural valve. Circulation 49: 985–993

Roveti G C, Ross R S, Bahnson H T 1962 Transseptal left heart catheterization in the pediatric age group. Journal of Pediatrics 61: 855–858

Rowe D W, Desai B, Bezmalinovic Z, Desai J M, Wessel R J, Grayson L H 1984 Two-dimensional echocardiography in double orifice mitral valve. Journal of the American College of Cardiology 4: 429–433

Ruckman R N, Van Praagh R 1978 Anatomic types of congenital mitral stenosis: report of 49 autopsy cases with consideration of diagnosis and surgical implications. American Journal of Cardiology 42: 592–601

Ruschhaupt D G, Bharati S, Lev M 1976 Mitral valve malformation of Ebstein type in absence of corrected transposition. American Journal of Cardiology 38: 109–112

Sahn D J, Wood J, Allen H D, Peoples W, Goldberg S J 1977 Echocardiographic spectrum of mitral valve motion in children with and without mitral valve prolapse: the nature of false positive diagnosis. American Journal of Cardiology 39: 422–431

Salmela P I, Ikaheimo M, Juustila H 1981 Fatal ventricular fibrillation after treatment with digoxin in a 27-year-old man with mitral leaflet prolapse syndrome. British Heart Journal 46: 338–341

Sanyal S K, Leung R K F, Tiemey R C, Gilmartin R, Pitner S 1979 Mitral valve prolapse syndrome in children with Duchenne's progressive muscular dystrophy. Pediatrics 63: 116–123

Savage D D, Garrison R J, Devereux R B et al 1983 Mitral valve prolapse in the general population. 1. Epidemiologic features: the Framingham study. American Heart Journal 106: 571–576

Scampardonis G, Yang S S, Maranhao V, Goldberg H, Gooch A S 1973 Left ventricular abnormalities in prolapsed mitral leaflet syndrome. Review of eighty-seven cases. Circulation 48: 287–297

Scardi S, Pandullo C, Poletti A 1994 Isolated double orifice mitral valve. Italian Journal of Cardiology 24: 1007–1010

Schon Hans-Rudiger, Schroter G, Blomer H, Schomig A 1994 Beneficial effects of a single dose of Quinapril for left ventricular performance in chronic mitral regurgitation. American Journal of Cardiology, 73: 785–791

Scott O, Williams G J, Fiddler G I 1980 Results of 24 hour ambulatory monitoring of electrocardiogram in 131 healthy boys aged 10 to 13 years. British Heart Journal 44: 304–308

Segal B L, Likoff W 1964 Late systolic murmur of mitral regurgitation. American Heart Journal 67: 757–763

Seliem M A, Duffy C E, Gidding S S, Berdusis K, Benson D W Jr 1992 Echocardiographic evaluation of the aortic root and mitral valve in children and adolescents with isolated pectus excavatum: comparison with Marfan patients. Pediatric Cardiology 13: 20–23

Sellers R D, Lillehei C W, Edwards J E 1964 Subaortic stenosis caused by anomalies of the atrioventricular valves. Journal of Thoracic and Cardiovascular Surgery 48: 289–302

Seneviratne B, Moore G A, West P D 1994 Effects of captopril on functional mitral regurgitation in dilated heart failure: a double blind placebo controlled trial. British Heart Journal 72: 63–68

Shah P M, Gramiak R 1970 Echocardiographic recognition of mitral valve prolapse. Circulation 42(suppl III): 45

Shappell S D, Marshall C E 1975 Ballooning posterior leaflet syndrome. Syncope and sudden death. Archives of Internal Medicine 135: 664–667

Shappell S D, Marshall C E, Brown R E, Bruce T A 1973 Sudden death and the familial occurrence of mid-systolic click, late systolic murmur syndrome. Circulation 48: 1128–1134

Shell W E, Walton J A, Clifford M E, Willis P W 1969 The familial occurrence of the syndrome of mid-late systolic click and late systolic murmur. Circulation 39: 327–337

Shimoyama H, Sabbah H N, Rosman H, Alam M, Goldstein S 1995 Effects of long-term therapy with enalapril on severity of functional mitral regurgitation in dogs with moderate heart failure. Journal of the American College of Cardiology 25: 768–772

Shone J D, Sellers R D, Anderson R C, Adams P Jr, Lillehei C W, Edwards J E 1963 The developmental complex of 'parachute mitral valve', supravalvular ring of left atrium, subaortic stenosis, and coarctation of aorta. American Journal of Cardiology 11: 714–725

Shore D, Jones O, Rigby M L, Anderson R H, Lincoln C 1982 Atresia of left atrioventricular connection. Surgical considerations. British Heart Journal 47: 35–40

Shrivastava S, Guthrie R B, Edwards J E 1977 Prolapse of the mitral valve. Modern Concepts of Cardiovascular Diseases 46: 57–72

Sigfusson G, Ettedgui J A, Silverman N H, Anderson R H 1995 Is a cleft in the anterior leaflet of an otherwise normal mitral valve an atrioventricular canal malformation. Journal of the American College of Cardiology 26: 508–515

Simon A L, Friedman W F, Roberts W C 1969 The angiographic features of a case of parachute mitral valve. American Heart Journal 77: 809–813

Simpson I A, Sahn D J 1991 Quantification of valvular regurgitation by Doppler echocardiography. Circulation 84(suppl I): 188–192

Simpson I A, Takahiro S, Gharib M, Sahn D 1996 Current status of flow convergence for clinical applications: Is it a leaning tower of 'Pisa'? Journal of the American College of Cardiology 27: 504–509

Smallhorn J, Tommasini G, Deanfield J, Douglas J, Gibson D, Macartney F 1981 Congenital mitral stenosis. Anatomical and functional assessment by echocardiography. British Heart Journal 45: 527–534

Smallhorn J F, De Leval M, Stark J et al 1982a Isolated anterior mitral cleft. Two dimensional echocardiographic assessment and differentiation from 'clefts' associated with atrioventricular septal defect. British Heart Journal 48: 109–116

Smallhorn J F, Sutherland G R, Anderson R H, Macartney F J 1982b Cross-sectional echocardiographic assessment of conditions with atrioventricular valve leaflets attached to

the atrial septum at the same level. British Heart Journal 48: 331–341

Smith E R, Fraser D B, Purdy J W, Anderson R N 1977 Angiographic diagnosis of mitral valve prolapse: correlation with echocardiography. American Journal of Cardiology 40: 165–170

Smith M D, Harrison M R, Pinton R, Kandil H, Kwan O L, DeMaria A N 1991 Regurgitant jet size by transesophageal compared with transthoracic Doppler color flow imaging. Circulation 83: 79–86

Snider A R, Roge C L, Schiller N B, Silverman N H 1980 Congenital left ventricular inflow obstruction evaluated by two-dimensional echocardiography. Circulation 61: 848–855

SOLVD Investigators 1991 Effect of enalapril on survival in patients with reduced left ventricular ejection fractions and congestive heart failure. New England Journal of Medicine 325: 293–302

SOLVD Investigators 1992 Effect on mortality and development of heart failure in asymptomatic patients with reduced left ventricular ejection fractions. New England Journal of Medicine 327: 685–691

Somerville J, Kaku S, Saravalli O 1978 Prolapsed mitral cusps in atrial septal defect. An erroneous radiological interpretation. British Heart Journal 40: 58–63

Southall D P, Johnston F, Shinebourne E A, Johnston P G B 1981 24-hour electrocardiographic study of heart rate and rhythm patterns in population of healthy children. British Heart Journal 45: 281–291

Spevak P J, Bass J L, Ben-Shachar G et al 1990 Balloon angioplasty for congenital mitral stenosis. American Journal of Cardiology 66: 472–476

Spindola-Franco H, Bjork L, Adams D F, Abrams H L 1980 Classification of the radiological morphology of the mitral valve. Differentiation between true and pseudoprolapse. British Heart Journal 44: 30–36

Stansel H C Jr, Nudel D B, Berman M A, Talner N S 1975 Prosthetic valve replacement in children. Archives of Surgery 110: 1397–1400

Stein D, Kloster F E 1977 Valvular heart disease in osteogenesis imperfects. American Heart Journal 94: 637–641

Stellin G, Bortolotti U, Mazzucco A 1988 Repair of congenitally malformed mitral valve in children. Journal of Thoracic and Cardiovascular Surgery 95: 480–485

Stevenson J G, Kawabori I, Guntheroth W G 1977 Differentiation of ventricular septal defects from mitral regurgitation by pulsed Doppler echocardiography. Circulation 56: 14–18

Stewart W J, Currie P J, Salcedo E E et al 1990 Intraoperative Doppler color flow mapping for decision-making in valve repair for mitral regurgitation (technique and results in 100 patients). Circulation 81: 556–566

Sulayman R, Mathew R, Thilenius O G, Replogle R, Arcilla R A 1975 Hemodynamics and annuloplasty in isolated mitral regurgitation in children. Circulation 52: 1144–1151

Sullivan I D, Robinson P J, de Leval M, Graham T P Jr 1986 Membranous supravalvular mitral stenosis: a treatable form of congenital heart disease. Journal of the American College of Cardiology 8: 159–164

Swartz M, Herman M V, Teichholz L E 1976 Dermatoglyphic patterns in patients with mitral valve prolapse: a clue to pathogenesis. American Journal of Cardiology 38: 588–593

Swartz M H, Teichholz L E, Donoso E 1977 Mitral valve prolapse: a review of associated arrhythmias. American Journal of Medicine 62: 377–389

Talner N S, Stern A M, Sloan H E Jr 1961 Congenital mitral insufficiency. Circulation 23: 339–349

Tei C, Shah P M, Cherian G, Wong M, Ormiston J A 1982 The correlates of an abnormal first heart sound in mitral-valve-prolapse syndromes. New England Journal of Medicine 307: 334–339

Terzaki A K, Leachman R D, Ali M K, Hallman G L, Cooley D A 1968 Successful surgical treatment for 'parachute mitral valve' complex: report of 2 cases. Journal of Thoracic and Cardiovascular Surgery 56: 1–10

Thiene G, Daliento L, Frescura C, De Tommasi M, Macartney F J, Anderson R H 1981 Atresia of left atrioventricular orifice. Anatomical investigation in 62 cases. British Heart Journal 45: 393–401

Thomas J D, Liu C M, Flachskampf F A, O'Shea J P, Davidoff R, Weyman A E 1990 Quantification of jet flow by momemtum analysis. Circulation 81: 247–259

Trent J K, Adelman A G, Wigle E D, Silver M D 1970 Morphology of a prolapsed posterior mitral valve leaflet. American Heart Journal 79: 539–543

Trowitzsch E, Bano-Rodrigo A, Burger B M, Colan S D, Sanders S P 1985 Two-dimensional echocardiographic findings in double orifice mitral valve. Journal of the American College of Cardiology 6: 383–387

Udoshi M B, Shah A, Fisher V J, Dolgin M 1979 Incidence of mitral valve prolapse in subjects with thoracic skeletal abnormalities – a prospective study. American Heart Journal 97: 303–311

Utsunomiya T, Ogawa T, Doshi R et al 1991 Doppler color flow 'proximal isovelocity surface area' method for estimating volume flow rate: effects of orifice shape and machine factors. Journal of the American College of Cardiology 17: 1103–1111

Uva M S, Galletti L, Gayet F L et al 1995 Surgery for congenital mitral valve disease in the first year of life. Journal of Thoracic and Cardiovascular Surgery 109: 164–176

Van der Bel Kahn J, Duren D R, Becker A E 1985 Isolated mitral valve prolapse: chordal architecture as an anatomic basis in older patients. Journal of the American College of Cardiology 5: 1335–1340

van der Horst R L, Hastreiter A R 1967 Congenital mitral stenosis. American Journal of Cardiology 20: 773–783

Veyrat C, Ameur A, Bas S, Lessana A, Abitbol G, Kalmanson D 1984 Pulsed Doppler echocardiographic indices for assessing mitral regurgitation. British Heart Journal 51: 130–138

Victor S, Nayak V M 1994 Definition and function of commissures, slits and scallops of the mitral valve: analysis in 100 hearts. Asia Pacific Journal of Thoracic and Cardiovascular Surgery 3: 10–16

Vitarelli A, Landolina G, Gentile R, Caleffi T, Sciomer S 1984 Echocardiographic assessment of congenital mitral stenosis. American Heart Journal 108: 523–531

Vogt J, Rupprath G, Grimm T, Koncz S, de Vivie E R, Beuren A J 1981 The diagnosis of parachute mitral valve complex (Shone4 complex) by two-dimensional sector-echocardiography. Zeitschrift für Kardiologie 70: 842–848

Warth D C, King M E, Cohen J M, Tesoriero V L, Marcus E, Weyman A E 1985 Prevalence of mitral valve prolapse in normal children. Journal of the American College of Cardiology 5: 1173–1177

Watson D G, Rowe R D, Coren P E, Duckworth J W A 1960 Mitral atresia with normal aortic valve. Report of 11 cases and review of the literature. Pediatrics 25: 450–467

Weesner K M, Rocchini A P, Rosenthal A, Behrendt D 1981 Intravascular hemolysis associated with porcine mitral valve calcification in children. American Journal of Cardiology 47: 1286–1288

Wei J Y, Fortuin N J 1981 Diastolic sounds and murmurs associated with mitral valve prolapse. Circulation 63: 559–564

Wei J Y, Bulkley B H, Shaeffer A H, Greene H L, Reid P R 1978 Mitral valve prolapse syndrome and recurrent ventricular tachyarrhythmias. A malignant variant refractory to conventional drug therapy. Annals of Internal Medicine 89: 6–9

Weis A J, Salcedo E E, Stewart W J, Lever H M, Klein A L, Thomas J D 1995 Anatomic explanation of mobile systolic clicks: implications for the clinical and echocardiographic diagnosis of mitral valve prolapse. American Heart Journal 129(2): 314–320

Weiss A N, Mimbs J W, Ludbrook P A, Sobel B E 1975 Echocardiographic detection of mitral valve prolapse. Exclusion of false positive diagnosis and determination of inheritance. Circulation 52: 1091–1096

Wenink A C G, Goot G D, Brom A G 1986 Developmental considerations of mitral valve anomalies. International Journal of Cardiology 11: 85–98

Westerman G R, van Devanter S H, Norton J B Jr, Readinger R I 1987 Congenital mitral valve stenosis in infancy: A different approach to a difficult problem. Journal of Thoracic and Cardiovascular Surgery 94: 305–307

Wilcken 1992 Genes, gender and geometry and the prolapsing mitral valve. Australian and New Zealand Journal of Medicine 22: 556–561

Williams W G, Pollock J C, Geiss D M, Trusler G A, Folwer R S 1981 Experience with aortic and mitral valve replacement in children. Journal of Thoracic and Cardiovascular Surgery 81: 326–333

Winkle R A, Goodman D J, Popp R L 1975a Simultaneous echocardiographic – phonocardiographic recordings at rest and during amyl nitrite administration in patients with mitral valve prolapse. Circulation 51: 522–529

Winkle R A, Lopes M G, Fitzgerald J W, Goodman D J, Schroeder J S, Harrison D C 1975b Arrhythmias in patients with mitral valve prolapse. Circulation 52: 73–81

Wit A L, Fenoglio J J Jr, Hordof A J, Reemtsma K 1979 Ultrastructure and transmembrane potentials of cardiac muscle in the human anterior mitral valve leaflet. Circulation 59: 1284–1292

Wooley C F 1976 Where are the diseases of yesteryear? Da Costa's syndrome, soldiers heart, the effort syndrome, neurocirculatory asthenia – and the mitral valve prolapse syndrome. Circulation 53: 749–751

Yacoub M 1976 Anatomy of the mitral valve chordae and cusps. In: Kalmanson D (ed.) The mitral valve, a pluridisciplinary approach. Publishing Sciences Group, Acton, MA, p 15–20

Yoshida K, Yoshikawa J, Shakudo M et al 1988 Color Doppler evaluation of valvular regurgitation in normal subjects. Circulation 78: 840–847

Zaibag M A, Ribeiro P A, Al Kasab S et al 1989 One-year follow-up after percutaneous double balloon mitral valvotomy. American Journal of Cardiology 63: 126–127

Zias E A, Mavroudis C, Backer C L, Kohr L M, Goteiner N L, Rocchini A P 1998 Surgical repair of the congenitally malformed mitral valve in infants and children. Annals of Thoracic Surgery 66: 1551–1559

Zuppiroli A, Rinaldi M, Kramer-Fox R, Favilli S, Roman M J, Devereux R B 1995 Natural history of mitral valve prolapse. American Journal of Cardiology 75(15): 028–1032

44

Pulmonary atresia with intact ventricular septum

F. J. Fricker and J. R. Zuberbuhler

INTRODUCTION

Pulmonary atresia occurs in three major settings: with an intact ventricular septum; with a ventricular septal defect in the setting of tetralogy of Fallot; and with complex cardiac malformations such as atrioventricular septal defect, double inlet atrioventricular connection with isomeric atrial appendages, or complete or corrected transposition. Only the first, pulmonary atresia with an intact ventricular septum, will be dealt with in this chapter.

Complete obstruction of the right ventricular outflow tract is always a very serious cardiac malformation, and in all types there must be some alternative source of pulmonary blood flow if the infant is to survive. Some varieties, however, are more likely than others to be lethal in the newborn period. Not all newborns with tetralogy of Fallot and pulmonary atresia are duct dependent, since some have systemic–pulmonary collateral arteries large enough to sustain life. This collateral flow tends to be stable. In contrast, individuals with pulmonary atresia and an intact ventricular septum hardly ever have such collateral arteries. The high early morbidity and mortality that occur in the absence of treatment in this variety of pulmonary atresia, therefore, can be explained by total dependence upon persistent patency of the arterial duct.

Although pulmonary atresia with an intact ventricular septum may seem the least complex form of complete right ventricular outflow tract obstruction, it is never an 'isolated' anomaly confined to an imperforate pulmonary valve. The right ventricle is always abnormal in some way. The cavity is usually hypoplastic, and infundibular atresia or severe stenosis is common. The tricuspid valve is also usually abnormal, being either small or dysplastic, or showing the features of Ebstein's malformation. Anomalies of the coronary arteries are also frequent, usually in hearts with a very small right ventricle, and myocardial abnormalities are often present, perhaps as a consequence of the coronary–cardiac fistulas.

The management of infants born with pulmonary atresia remains unsatisfactory. In some, the abnormalities afflicting the right ventricle are so severe as to preclude 'correction'; in this case, even construction of a systemic-to-pulmonary arterial shunt carries a rather high mortality. Even in those with relatively favourable anatomy, surgery is often not successful.

INCIDENCE

Freedom and Keith (1979) reported the incidence of this malformation to be 2.5% in a very large series of children with congenital heart disease seen at the Toronto Hospital for Sick Children. At the Children's Hospital of Pittsburgh, this variety of pulmonary atresia made up 2.4% of patients with congenital heart disease undergoing surgery in the 1980s (50 of 2064 operations). During a 12-year period, 4% of postmortems involving those with congenital heart disease showed this anomaly (25 of 627). There was a slight male predominance in this series.

CLASSIFICATION AND MORPHOLOGY

By definition, the central morphological abnormality is complete obstruction to right ventricular outflow in the presence of an intact ventricular septum. Other right heart structures are commonly abnormal as well. Hypoplasia of the right ventricle is usual, but there has been debate over whether the distribution of the right ventricular cavity size is bimodal or a continuum. Greenwold et al (1956) reported that the right ventricular cavity size could be classified as small or large, and Davignon et al (1961) and Celermajer et al (1968) concurred in this view. In contrast, Gersony et al (1967), Bowman et al (1971) and Murphy et al (1971) contended that the right ventricular size constituted a spectrum. Zuberbuhler and Anderson (1979) described the morphological features of a series of 37 specimens with pulmonary atresia and intact ventricular septum and devised a system for quantifying right ventricular size. Inlet and outlet dimensions of both right and left ventricles were measured, and then a ratio of the product of the right ventricular dimensions to the product of the corresponding left ventricular dimensions was calculated. This device permitted the estimation of right ventricular size relative to left ventricular size, each heart serving as its own control. The results were compared with those for 20 hearts from newborns dying of causes other than congenital heart disease. The series was eventually extended to 54 (Zuberbuhler et al, 1979b) and supported the view that there is a spectrum of right ventricular cavity size (Figure 44.1). The right ventricle was usually smaller than normal, although some fell into the normal range and a few were larger than normal (Figure 44.2). In every case, there was complete obstruction at the level of the pulmonary valve; infundibular obstruction was also common. Muscular atresia of the infundibulum correlated strongly with the presence of a tiny right ventricle, while infundibular stenosis was usual in hearts with a larger, but still diminutive, right ventricle. Occasionally, there was no subvalvar obstruction, the valve itself being an imperforate membrane. The right ventricular wall was almost always abnormally thick. Indeed, the cavitary right ventricular hypoplasia is related to this massive hypertrophy of the right ventricular wall (Bull et al, 1982). Right ventricular trabeculations were typically more shallow than normal, and right ventricular endocardial fibroelastosis was present

in almost one quarter of the cases. The extent of obliteration of the ventricular cavity by hypertrophy of the wall and its trabeculations is now used as a means of classifying patients for surgical treatment. (de Leval et al, 1982). The system proposed has also led to some confusion. In the initial study, de Leval and his colleagues (1982) observed that the mural hypertrophy occurred initially in the apical trabecular component, leaving the ventricular cavity represented only by its inlet and outlet components. In more severely affected infants, it seemed that the outlet component was also obliterated, leaving only the inlet to function as the ventricular cavity. Some then misinterpreted these findings to argue that some of the ventricular components were absent, and descriptions of 'unipartite' and 'bipartite' ventricles became commonplace. While a useful shorthand, this is an oversimplification of the anatomical situation. In reality; as explained, all three ventricular components are present in all cases. It remains a fact that the spectrum of anatomical abnormality can broadly be interpreted in terms of (with increasing severity) the muscular hypertrophy squeezing out first the apical component and then the infundibulum, leaving only the inlet as the effctive cavity (Anderson et al 1991). These observations continue to have value in determining the options for surgical treatment.

The tricuspid valvar apparatus is abnormal in most cases of pulmonary atresia with an intact ventricular septum (Freedom et al, 1978). A small tricuspid annulus is common. In the study of Zuberbuhler and Anderson (1979), the ratio of tricuspid to mitral annular diameter was compared with a similar ratio in a series of normal newborn hearts and was found also to constitute a spectrum. The size of the tricuspid annulus correlated strongly with right ventricular cavity size. Dysplasia of the tricuspid leaflets is common but does not correlate with right ventricular hypoplasia. A diminutive but normally formed tricuspid valve can be found associated with a very small right ventricle, while severe dysplasia is sometimes seen in hearts with a normal sized right ventricle. Except for dysplasia, Ebstein's malformation is the most common abnormality involving the tricuspid valve found associated with pulmonary atresia (Zuberbuhler et al, 1979a), occurring in 37% of the series reported by Anderson et al (1990). In some hearts, the abnormality consisted solely of adherence of the proximal portion of the septal leaflet to the septum, but in others the valve was more distorted, with near absence of the septal leaflet and fenestration of the anterosuperior leaflet. This latter type of valvar abnormality was associated with the largest right ventricles and must have resulted in severe tricuspid regurgitation. Ebstein's malformation may also be obstructive, with the anterosuperior leaflet of the tricuspid valve having a linear attachment to the junction of the lateral right ventricular wall and the septum; this will partially or completely subdivide the right ventricle into inlet and trabecular-outlet portions (Figure 44.3) (Zuberbuhler et al, 1979a).

The pulmonary trunk is usually of normal size, although it may, rarely, be small or even atretic. There is no

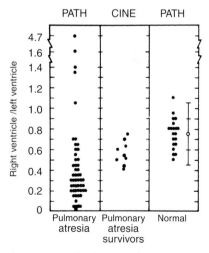

Figure 44.1 The spectrum of right ventricle (RV) size is demonstrated by area measurements made in pathological specimens (PATH) from infants with pulmonary atresia and intact ventricular septum and infants dying from causes other than congenital heart disease. Similar measurements were made from cineangiograms (CINE) of surviving infants illustrating relatively normal RV size.

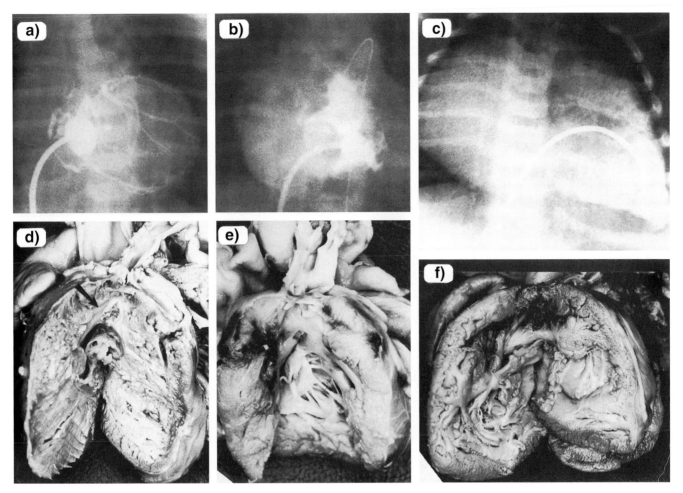

Figure 44.2 Cineangiographic and morphologic correlation of right ventricular size: tiny (a,d), small (b,e) and large (c,f) (see text).

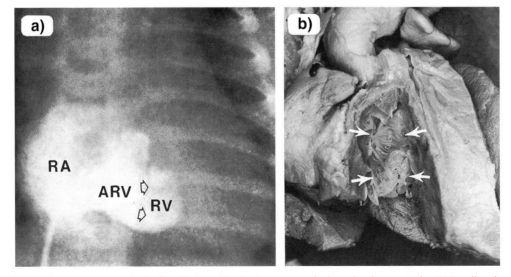

Figure 44.3 Attachment of the antero-superior leaflet of tricuspid valve (arrows) to the lateral right ventricular (RV) wall and septum seen in both the right ventriculogram (a) and the pathological specimen (b). This curtain of atrioventricular valvar tissue subdivides the right ventricle and may be obstructive. ARV, atrialized right ventricle; RA, right atrium.

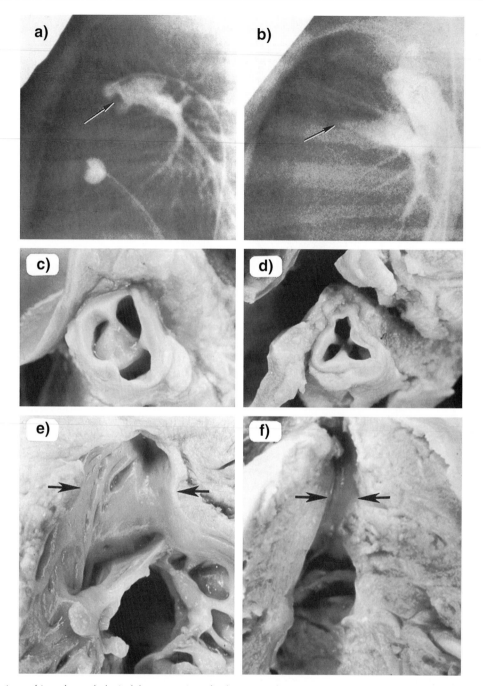

Figure 44.4 Cineangiographic and morphological demonstration of pulmonary valvar anatomy and associated status of the infundibulum (see text).

correlation with right ventricular cavity size, and a tiny right ventricle may be associated with a normally sized pulmonary trunk. There are two varieties of pulmonary valve in patients with pulmonary atresia and intact ventricular septum (Figure 44.4). In one, prominent commissural ridges meet at the centre of the pulmonary root. This type is associated with either infundibular atresia or with severe tricuspid regurgitation, the latter usually on the basis of Ebstein's malformation. In the other variety, there are peripheral raphes, but the central portion of the valve is smooth and dome shaped. This

type is associated with a patent infundibulum and probably results from high right ventricular pressure playing on the under-surface of the valve (Zuberbuhler and Anderson, 1979).

Coronary arterial abnormalities are common in pulmonary atresia with intact ventricular septum and are an important risk factor (Freedom and Harrington, 1974; O'Conner et al, 1982). Fistulous communications with the right ventricle have been reported to occur in about one third (Giglia et al, 1992) and are found exclusively in patients with a diminutive right ventricular cavity. In one series, there was a very strong correlation with muscular infundibular atresia (Anderson et al, 1991); in another, trabecular and infundibular portions of the right ventricle were noted to be 'absent', in such patients (Kasznica et al, 1987). Abnormalities of coronary arterial calibre are common in patients with fistulas; these include obstruction and segmental dilation (Burrows et al, 1990). Fistulous communications were noted in 60% of a postmortem series reported by Calder et al (1986), and all patient with fistulas had histological abnormalities of the coronary arteries. In 50%, there was severe narrowing or obliteration of at least one coronary arterial lumen. Abnormalities of origin also occur, including complete absence of proximal coronary arteries, all flow being via fistulous communications with the right ventricle (Lenox and Briner, 1972). Left ventricular endocardial fibroelastosis occurs but is less common than the right ventricular endocardial abnormality.

PATHOPHYSIOLOGY

The embryological genesis of this anomaly is unknown. It seems likely, however, that the central malformation is complete obstruction of the right ventricular outflow developing relatively late in fetal life, with the other right heart and coronary arterial abnormalities being secondary. The studies of Heymann and Rudolph (1972), and Shapiro et al (1973), are consistent with this hypothesis, since they showed that creation of pulmonary stenosis in fetal lambs resulted in a smaller than normal right ventricle. Since there is such a broad spectrum of right ventricular size, however, there must be other determinants of this variable, and tricuspid valvar morphology and function are likely candidates. In the series reported by Zuberbuhler and Anderson (1979), the largest right ventricles were found in hearts that had severe tricuspid regurgitation secondary to Ebstein's malformation of the tricuspid valve. (Also, during life, a murmur of tricuspid regurgitation is a good clinical marker of a relatively large ventricle; see below.) Conversely, in the above series, tricuspid stenosis or an obstructive Ebstein's malformation was found only in association with a very small right ventricle. Right ventricular inflow obstruction has also been reported to be a determinant of right ventricular growth after birth (Patel et al, 1980). Complete obstruction of the right ventricular outflow tract also may affect coronary arterial development. Fistulous communications between the right ventricle and the coronary arteries are common with pulmonary atresia and intact ventricular septum, presumably because the high right ventricular pressure causes persistence of communications between the right ventricular cavity and the coronary vessels in early embryologic life. Since fistulas are not found in pulmonary atresia with a normal sized right ventricle, or in severe valvar pulmonary stenosis (both situations where right ventricular pressure would be expected to be suprasystemic), it may be that both marked

right ventricular hypoplasia and coronary–cardiac fistulas are related to development of the atresia at a very early gestational age (Lenox and Briner, 1972; Kasznica et al, 1987). Cineangiographic studies have shown bidirectional flow through the abnormal coronary system, with flow from the aorta to the coronary arteries during diastole, and from the right ventricle to the coronary arteries during systole. It may be that perfusion of the myocardium with poorly oxygenated blood from the right ventricle is responsible for the left ventricular myocardial fibrosis seen in this anomaly (Harinck et al, 1977). Freedom and Harrington (1974) have shown that the fistulous communications may regress following surgical decompression of the right ventricle. Stenosis, or even interruption of a coronary artery proximal to a fistula connecting it to the right ventricle, may have no effect on flow and, therefore, on myocardial perfusion as long as the fistula is patent and right ventricular pressure is high. Right ventricular decompression produced by surgically opening the right ventricular outflow tract, or by occluding the tricuspid valve or rendering it incompetent, removes the contribution of the fistula to distal coronary flow. The resultant myocardial ischaemia may then have disastrous consequences (Burrows et al, 1990).

The alterations in fetal flow occasioned by pulmonary atresia also affect the aortic isthmus and the arterial duct. It is known that aortic coarctation is more frequent in situations where flow through the isthmus is reduced (such as left ventricular outflow obstruction); however, with pulmonary atresia, the entire cardiac output traverses the isthmus and coarctation is virtually unknown. Also, the duct is long and tortuous and joins the aorta at a more acute angle than normal (Santos et al, 1980). The oval foramen tends to be large, since all systemic venous return leaves the right atrium through it. The left atrium and left ventricle are invariably well developed.

CLINICAL FINDINGS

PRESENTATION

Infants with pulmonary atresia and intact ventricular septum almost always present with cyanosis in the neonatal period. The arterial duct is the sole source of pulmonary blood flow, and this rarely remains widely patent for more than a few hours or days. Very rarely, patients may be found with systemic-to-pulmonary collateral arteries (Mildner et al, 1997), but usually, as soon as the duct narrows, arterial oxygen desaturation increases and deep cyanosis results. Closure of the duct may be intermittent at first, and cyanosis may wax and wane. Infants with severe tricuspid regurgitation may also show signs of congestive heart failure; usually hypoxaemia, with its attendant cyanosis, tachypnoea and eventual acidosis, dominates the clinical picture.

PHYSICAL FINDINGS

The usual physical findings of pulmonary atresia can be explained by the abnormal morphology. Mention has already been made of cyanosis. Pulses and blood pressure are normal since cardiac output is not impaired. The jugular venous pulse is hard to evaluate in newborns and is not a useful diagnostic sign. Precordial motion is normal since a pure pressure overload of the right ventricle does not usually result in an exaggerated left parasternal lift. The second heart sound at the high left sternal border is invariably soft and single or is inaudible. The first heart sound is normal, and an ejection sound is not present. Several murmurs may be heard. The most common is a soft high-pitched continuous murmur at the high left sternal border. This murmur originates in the duct and is usually quite subtle. Occasionally, it may be heard only intermittently, disappearing when the duct narrows and cyanosis deepens, and appearing again as the duct opens and cyanosis lightens. Some infants with pulmonary atresia have a soft high-pitched systolic murmur of tricuspid regurgitation at the low left sternal border. The presence of this murmur correlates strongly with a relatively large right ventricle (Zuberbuhler, 1981), but lack of a murmur of tricuspid regurgitation does not rule out a normally sized right ventricle. When there is severe tricuspid regurgitation, there is often a soft, medium-pitched, mid-diastolic murmur at the low left sternal border, representing relative tricuspid stenosis. Such a murmur is not heard in those with severe tricuspid stenosis alone, since there is little or no flow across such a valve in the presence of pulmonary atresia. Some infants with pulmonary atresia have no murmur; in this situation, the only indication of congenital heart disease on physical examination is the severe cyanosis.

INVESTIGATIONS

ELECTROCARDIOGRAPHY

The electrocardiogram is usually abnormal and reflects the abnormal morphology. The frontal plane axis is less rightward than normal and usually falls between 30 and 90 degrees. Most newborns with pulmonary atresia have an 'adult' precordial pattern rather than the usual right ventricular hypertrophy (Figure 44.5). Less commonly, the pattern of right ventricular hypertrophy is present. It must be noted that the electrocardiographic patterns of right

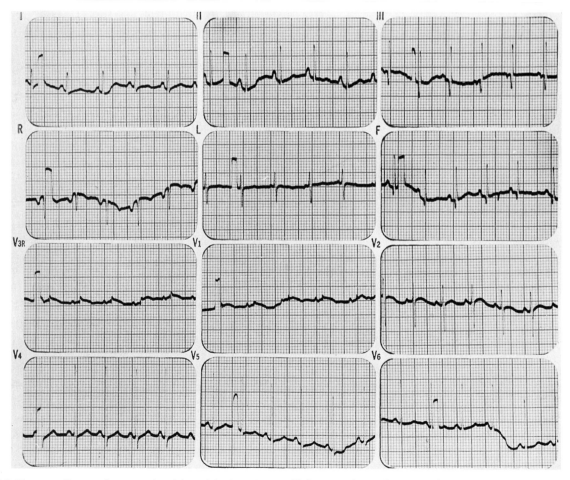

Figure 44.5 Electrocardiogram demonstrating right atrial enlargement and left ventricular predominance that is abnormal for a term newborn infant.

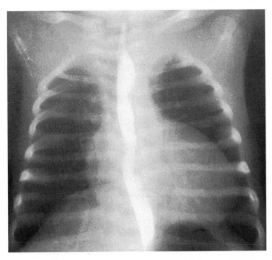
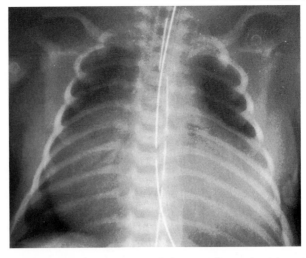

a)

b)

Figure 44.6 Chest radiographs in two patients with pulmonary atresia and intact ventricular septum. (a) Moderate cardiomegaly, right atrial enlargement and decreased pulmonary vascular markings. (b) Marked cardiomegaly in an infant with Ebstein's malformation of the tricuspid valve and severe tricuspid regurgitation.

ventricular hypertrophy, or of left ventricular predominance, do not reliably predict right ventricular size. ST–T wave changes suggestive of myocardial ischaemia are occasionally present and may be related to the abnormal coronary arteries (Freedom and Harrington, 1974). The tall peaked P waves of right atrial enlargement may be present.

CHEST RADIOGRAPHY

There is no characteristic radiographic appearance of pulmonary atresia with intact ventricular septum. The abdominal organs are normally positioned, and the heart is left sided. Bronchuses are normally lateralized, and the aortic arch is left sided. Pulmonary vascular markings are not increased, but the distinction between normal and decreased markings is difficult at best in the neonatal period, which is when most infants with pulmonary atresia present. The cardiac contour is not distinctive, and there is a wide range of cardiac size, from normal to 'wall-to-wall' (Figure 44.6). Although the very largest hearts occur when there is severe tricuspid regurgitation, heart size is not a reliable predictor of the size of the right ventricular cavity.

ECHOCARDIOGRAPHY

Cross-sectional echocardiography is now the primary technique in the diagnosis of pulmonary atresia with intact ventricular septum, and in the evaluation of right heart morphology (Figure 44.7). The degree of obliteration of the three components of the cavity of the right ventricle by mural hypertrophy can be shown, and the overall right ventricular cavity size assessed. Infundibular stenosis or atresia can be demonstrated in the subcostal oblique and short-axis views, and lack of antegrade flow

across the pulmonary valve confirmed by colour Doppler interrogation. In our experience, the right ventricular cavity may seem smaller echocardiographically than it appears cineangiographically, largely because the apical trabecular zone may seem completely obliterated when, in reality, there are intertrabecular spaces. This can be a very important distinction in selecting patients for surgical repair, since this portion of the right ventricular cavity may expand very substantially following relief of the obstruction in the right ventricular outflow tract. The tricuspid valvar annulus can be measured, and dysplasia of the tricuspid valvar leaflets identified. Ebstein's malformation of the tricuspid valve can usually be diagnosed. If there is tricuspid regurgitation, Doppler measurement of the velocity of the jet gives a good estimate of right ventricular pressure. The obligatory right-to-left flow across the patent oval foramen is also easily demonstrated.

CARDIAC CATHETERIZATION AND ANGIOGRAPHY

Despite the increased role of echocardiography, cardiac catheterization and angiography may still be helpful in the evaluation of an infant with pulmonary atresia, particularly in assessing the presence of fistulous communications. The usual approach is via the femoral vein, or by way of the umbilical vein if the study is undertaken in the early neonatal period. Oximetry is not particularly helpful, except to show right-to-left shunting at atrial level. Mean right atrial pressure is usually slightly higher than left atrial, but a large gradient is not expected since the oval foramen is usually large and widely patent. Right ventricular pressure is usually suprasystemic, although right ventricular pressure is low if tricuspid regurgitation is very severe. If the right ventricle is small, repeated probing with an end-hole catheter may be required to enter it.

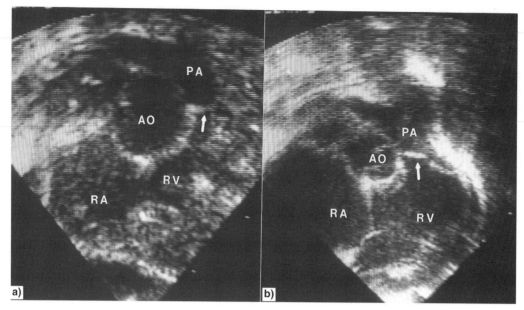

Figure 44.7 Echocardiograms in the subcostal view. The arrows indicate an atretic pulmonic valve. (a) A very small right ventricular cavity can be seen with a patent but stenotic infundibulum. Coronary-cardiac fistulas were present but not well visualized here. (b) A normal-sized right ventricle can be seen with a widely patent infundibulum and normal-sized tricuspid annulus. AO, aorta; PA, pulmonary trunk; RA, right atrium; RV, right ventricle.

The diagnosis of pulmonary atresia with intact ventricular septum can be made reliably by cineangiography. The right ventriculogram is the single most valuable study and, if the diagnosis is suspected, it should be done before an attempt is made to enter the pulmonary trunk from the right ventricle. The difficulties inherent in accurately measuring right ventricular size have been reported by Graham et al (1974) and Patel et al (1980). Relative right ventricular cavity size can be estimated by the method described above (in the section on morphology) since there is a high correlation between cineangiographic and morphological measurements in the same hearts (F.J. Fricker, unpublished data). Stenosis or atresia of the infundibulum can be diagnosed; if an imperforate pulmonary valve is present, it may be seen moving to and fro at the top of a patent infundibulum. Tricuspid regurgitation can be roughly quantified, since catheter-induced regurgitation is usually mild. Coronary–cardiac fistulas are also well demonstrated by right ventriculography (Figure 44.2a). Stenoses in, or interruption of, both right and left coronary arteries should be searched for; if there is doubt about the coronary arterial anatomy or distribution after the right ventriculogram, then aortic root injection should be performed. A left ventriculogram should also be performed, both for judging the relative right ventricular size and to visualize the duct and the pulmonary trunk. Simultaneous injection into the aorta and into the right ventricle may show the extent of the gap between the right ventricular cavity and the pulmonary trunk (Freedom et al, 1974).

Tricuspid and mitral orificial size can be estimated from the ventriculogram, and specific tricuspid valvar abnormalities can sometimes be diagnosed by right ventriculography. An example is an obstructing Ebstein's malformation, which partitions the right ventricle (Figure 44.3).

DIAGNOSIS

The diagnosis of pulmonary atresia and intact ventricular septum should be considered in any cyanotic neonate. In this setting, the differential diagnosis includes abnormalities of vascular connection, other valvar atresias and other varieties of obstruction of the right ventricular outflow tract. Certain findings on physical examination or on the electrocardiogram, chest radiograph or echocardiogram support the diagnosis of pulmonary atresia. In a cyanotic neonate, a continuous murmur localized to the high left sternal border almost always originates in a duct and indicates complete obstruction of the right ventricular outflow tract (Zuberbuhler et al, 1975), although it does not differentiate atresia with an intact ventricular septum from the other varieties of pulmonary atresia. A rare exception to this general rule is the venous hum, which may be heard with totally anomalous pulmonary venous connection to the left brachiocephalic vein (Keith et al, 1954). The hum tends to vary with respiration, particularly with straining, while the ductal murmur does not. In the clinical setting of a cyanotic newborn, a systolic murmur heard at the low left sternal border usually indicates tricuspid regurgitation, since a ventricular septal defect is silent in most malformations that cause cyanosis. With such a murmur, 'isolated' Ebstein's malformation must be considered, as well as pulmonary atresia with intact ventricular septum. A soft or inaudible second heart sound at the high left sternal border is consistent with either pulmonary atresia or severe pulmonary stenosis, while a loud or split second heart sound is inconsistent with these diagnoses. An early systolic ejection sound argues against the diagnosis of pulmonary atresia with an intact septum, being more consistent with tetralogy of Fallot and pulmonary atresia if heard at the apex, or with severe valvar pulmonary stenosis if heard at the base. Generally poor pulses, or a prominent left parasternal lift, are not signs of pulmonary atresia and are suggestive of severe left ventricular outflow tract obstruction (such as aortic atresia). Congestive heart failure is also far more common with other entities than with pulmonary atresia.

The pattern of left ventricular predominance seen in the precordial electrocardiographic leads suggests pulmonary or tricuspid atresia, but it may also be seen with double inlet atrioventricular connection. A superior axis suggests tricuspid rather than pulmonary atresia. A pattern of right ventricular hypertrophy is more consistent with pulmonary stenosis than atresia but is not conclusive, since some patients with pulmonary atresia have right ventricular hypertrophy and some with critical pulmonary stenosis (functional atresia) have left ventricular predominance.

Increased vascular markings on the chest radiograph suggest complete transposition, totally anomalous pulmonary venous connection or a left heart obstruction such as mitral or aortic atresia. A right aortic arch is not seen with pulmonary atresia with an intact ventricular septum, and points instead to tetralogy of Fallot, with or without pulmonary atresia. Abnormal arrangement of the abdominal organs, or symmetrical bronchuses, should raise the question of isomerism of the atrial appendages, with its associated complex cardiac malformations (Macartney et al, 1980).

A definitive diagnosis can usually be made echocardiographically if colour Doppler is included. Certain findings make the diagnosis untenable: a ventricular septal defect, hypoplasia of the left ventricle or ascending aorta, or absence of the right or left atrioventricular connection.

——— COURSE AND PROGNOSIS ———

Surgical intervention is always necessary early in the neonatal period. Since pulmonary atresia with intact ventricular septum is a duct-dependent anomaly, and since the duct almost invariably closes early in life, there is no chance of survival unless a stable source of pulmonary blood flow can be established. Prostaglandin given intravenously is a very effective, albeit temporary, means of preserving ductal patency until surgery can be carried out (Olley et al, 1976; Heyman and Rudolph, 1977). There is wide agreement that, if possible, continuity between the right ventricle and the pulmonary arteries should be established at the first surgical procedure. This can be accomplished by transventricular valvotomy (Hawkins et al, 1990; Shaddy et al, 1990), by open transpulmonary valvotomy or by patching the outflow tract (Cole et al, 1968; Moller et al, 1970; Trusler et al, 1976; de Leval et al, 1982; Steinberger et al, 1992). Any of these techniques is effective if the right ventricle is not too diminutive, and if there is not infundibular atresia or severe stenosis. Patching the outflow tract is probably the technique that is applicable to the widest range of morphology (Steinberger et al, 1992), but even this procedure is difficult or impossible to accomplish if there is a long segment of infundibular atresia and the right ventricle is very small. Transcatheter techniques for creating continuity between the right ventricle and the pulmonary arteries have been developed in recent years. Rosenthal and colleagues have described both laser and radiofrequency techniques for perforation of the atretic pulmonary valve (Rosenthal et al, 1993 a,b). This is usually performed by a venous approach, with the tip of the catheter placed immediately under the atretic valve. Heat generated by energy from the catheter tip results in perforation of the valve, and this is followed by serial dilation with balloons of increasing size. Complication rates with these techniques have been high, although these reports represent the first experiences with transcatheter techniques in this condition and, therefore, reflect the 'learning curve' for these new treatments. We can anticipate further clinical application of these methods over the next few years, hopefully in the setting of carefully designed clinical trials in a small number of centres.

Neonates with right ventricles that are normal or nearly normal in size and who do not have severe tricuspid regurgitation are sometimes able to maintain adequate pulmonary flow even after the duct is closed at operation, or closes spontaneously in the immediate postoperative period. In others, the right ventricle is so small or dysfunctional that other measures are required to support pulmonary blood flow. Several days, or even weeks, of intravenous prostaglandin therapy postoperatively may give the right ventricle time to grow and to develop better systolic and diastolic function. If this is ineffective, a systemic-to-pulmonary arterial shunt is constructed. In most centres, a modified Blalock–Taussig shunt is preferred, since there is less chance of pulmonary overcirculation or of pulmonary arterial distortion than with other shunts. In those with the smallest right ventricles, a shunt may be the preferred initial operation.

There is a strong tendency for the right ventricle and the tricuspid orifice to grow once continuity with the pulmonary arteries has been established and right ventricular pressure falls below systemic levels (Figure 44.8) (Freedom et al, 1983; Shaddy et al, 1990). This permits regression of right ventricular hypertrophy, allowing the right ventricular cavity to enlarge and right ventricular compliance to improve. The degree of tricuspid

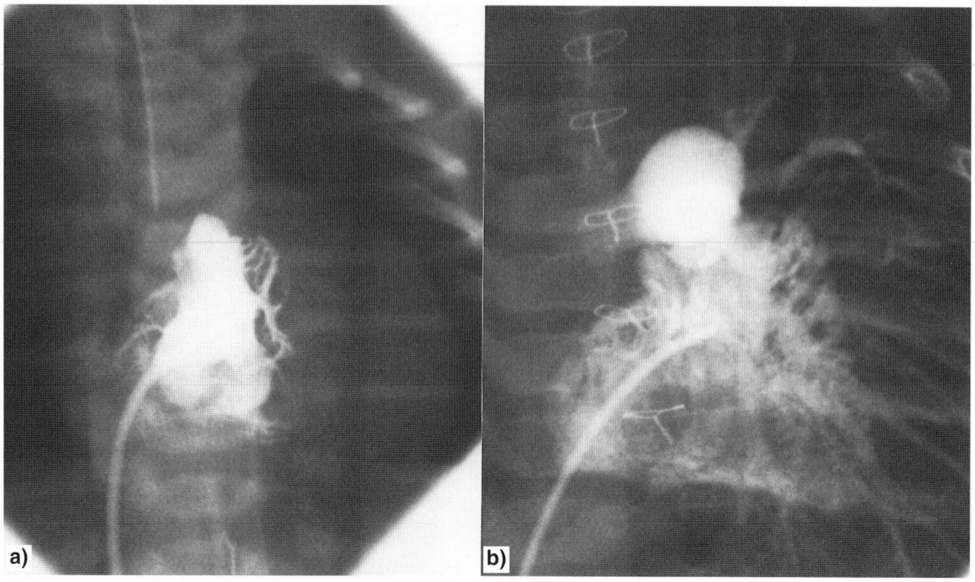

Figure 44.8 Right ventriculograms. (a) At 1 day of life, a small but well-formed right ventricle can be seen with a patent infundibulum and valvar atresia. (b) The same child scanned at $4\frac{1}{2}$ months of life following valvotomy as a newborn. The right ventricle is now of normal size. The right pulmonary artery is not well filled because of unopacified blood flowing through a right modified Blalock–Taussig shunt.

regurgitation also will decrease unless the valve is very dysplastic. Right ventricular growth takes place more slowly, or not at all, if such continuity is not established and if pulmonary flow is entirely via a systemic-to-pulmonary arterial shunt (F.J. Fricker, unpublished data).

Often there is residual obstruction within the right ventricular outflow tract following the initial operation. In some, balloon dilation is effective in reducing the gradient to tolerable levels (Leung et al, 1991), while in others a second surgical procedure is needed to reduce obstruction, often by patching the outflow tract.

Balloon atrial septostomy should not be done at the initial preoperative catheterization if there is any hope of establishing continuity between the right ventricle and the pulmonary arteries (Neches et al, 1973). The patent oval foramen is always large enough to permit adequate right-to-left shunting in the immediate postoperative period while the right ventricle is adjusting to its role as the pulmonary ventricle. A very large interatrial communication, which precludes an elevation in right atrial pressure, may inhibit right ventricular filling and, therefore, antegrade pulmonary blood flow. Eventually, after right ventricular forward flow is well established, an interatrial communication that permits any right-to-left flow or substantial left-to-right flow must be closed.

Coronary arterial anomalies are common in pulmonary atresia, especially in those with the smallest right ventricles, and these may complicate therapy (Anderson et al, 1991). If the right ventricle is relatively large and well developed, fistulous communications are almost never present, and preoperative evaluation by echocardiography is sufficient. With a smaller right ventricle, especially if muscular infundibular atresia is present, fistulous communications are very common, and cardiac

catheterization and angiographic visualization of the coronary arteries is mandatory prior to attempting any surgical procedure that is expected to reduce right ventricular pressure. Such procedures include the establishment of continuity from the right ventricle to the pulmonary arteries, and exclusion of a very diminutive right ventricle from the circulation. In a recently published study, Giglia et al (1992) reported a series of 16 patients with well-defined coronary arteries who underwent right ventricular decompression. There were no survivors among the three who had proximal stenosis of both right and left coronary arteries and two of six who had stenosis of one coronary artery failed to survive. There were no deaths in seven with fistulous communications but no stenosis. In a larger series, Coles et al (1989) reported that all seven patients who had fistulas and stenosis or interruption of the proximal left anterior descending coronary artery died at or shortly after right ventricular decompression. Williams et al (1991), reporting from the same institution, noted that five of twelve children who underwent thromboexclusion of the diminutive right ventricle died, and that each of the five had proximal stenosis or interruption of the left anterior descending coronary artery. There is no satisfactory treatment for the group of patients who have coronary circulation that is largely dependent upon right ventricular function. The right ventricle cannot safely be decompressed or excluded, and the continued presence of coronary perfusion with highly unsaturated right ventricular blood inevitably leads to myocardial fibrosis and congestive failure.

There is also no satisfactory therapy for the small subset of patients with a hugely dilated, thin-walled and low-pressure right ventricle. The genesis of these features is marked dysplasia of the tricuspid valve, usually with features of Ebstein's malformation, but occasionally with a congenitally unguarded tricuspid orifice (Anderson et al, 1990). There are even no short-term survivors in this subset of patients in our own series.

Long-term results following surgery for pulmonary atresia have been disappointing. In one very large surgical series extending from 1965 to 1987, actuarial survival was only 25% in 13 years (Coles et al, 1989). Mortality has decreased in more recent series, with 5-year survival of 79% (Steinberger et al, 1992) and 86% (Hawkins et al, 1990) in two studies. There were no early deaths in a selected series of 22 patients with a patent infundibulum who underwent patching of the right ventricular outflow tract (Shaddy et al, 1990). In spite of these encouraging reports, newborns with pulmonary atresia and intact ventricular septum continue to present a difficult challenge. For some subsets of patients, those with a coronary circulation that is dependent upon right ventricular function and those with a hugely dilated low-pressure right ventricle, no satisfactory therapy exists, other than the consideration of cardiac transplantation, itself arguably less than satisfactory.

For the more typical cases, some direction for the future has been provided by two multicentric studies. The Congenital Heart Surgeons Society prospectively studied 171 neonates presenting between 1987 and 1990 (Hanley et al, 1993). Variables in outcome were correlated with Z-scores for the tricuspid valve. Other morphological features were less well documented. Predictors of death after an initial procedure included low birthweight, presence of right ventricular dependency of the coronary circulation, and smaller tricuspid valvar Z-score. The last was a predictor of adverse outcome only when the initial procedure included a valvotomy or transannular patch. It did not affect outcome when the initial procedure was isolated construction of a systemic-to-pulmonary shunt. Probability of survival after the initial procedure was 81% at 1 month but was only 64% by 4 years. The United Kingdom and Eire Collaborative Study of Pulmonary Atresia with Intact Ventricular Septum is a unique population-based study of all infants born with this condition over a 5-year period from 1991 to 1995 (Daubeney et al, 1995a,b). Over this period, all 183 live-born infants with pulmonary atresia and intact ventricular septum born within the United Kingdom and Eire were enrolled into the study, and detailed morphological information was obtained on each infant. Overall survival was almost identical to that in the Congenital Heart Surgeons Society Study. An interesting feature of the study performed in the United Kingdom was the large number of patients undergoing initial palliation by transcatheter techniques using lasers or radiofrequency waves. An initial procedure attempted to establish continuity between the right ventricle and the pulmonary trunk without concomitant use of a systemic-to-pulmonary shunt in 67 of the 183 infants (37%). In 40 of these (60%), an attempt was made to establish this continuity by transcatheter perforation and dilatation of the atretic valve. The remaining 27 patients underwent surgical valvotomy, valvectomy or transannular patch. The need for reintervention to increase pulmonary blood flow within 6 weeks of the primary procedure was significantly greater in the group undergoing catheterization than in the group submitted to surgery. In most of this former group, this was the result of failure successfully to cross the pulmonary valve at the time of the initial intervention. Among the 24 infants in whom the atretic valve was successfully perforated and dilated, only five (21%) required reintervention, a figure comparable to that for the patients treated surgically (early reintervention was required in 32%). These results suggest that transcatheter techniques may prove to be an important new tool for initial management of selected patients with right ventricles of good size, providing the valve can be successfully crossed. In some patients, this may prove to be a definitive procedure. Ongoing recruitment into, and analysis of, these two major multi-institutional studies may resolve some of the many outstanding dilemmas in the clinical management of this difficult lesion.

REFERENCES

Anderson R H, Silverman N H, Zuberbuhler J R 1990 Congenitally unguarded tricuspid orifice: its differentiation from Ebstein's malformation in association with pulmonary atresia and intact ventricular septum. Pediatric Cardiology 11: 86–90

Anderson R H, Anderson C, Zuberbuhler J R 1991 Further morphologic studies on hearts with pulmonary atresia and intact ventricular septum. Cardiology in the Young 1: 105–113

Bowman F O, Malm J R, Hayes C J, Gersony W M, Ellis K 1971 Pulmonary atresia with intact ventricular septum. American Journal of Cardiology 61: 85–93

Bull C, de Leval M R, Mercanti C, Macartney F J, Anderson R H 1982 Pulmonary atresia and intact ventricular septum: A revised classification. Circulation 66: 266–272

Burrows P E, Freedom R M, Benson L N et al 1990 Coronary angiography of pulmonary atresia, hypoplastic right ventricle, and ventriculocoronary communications. American Journal of Roentgenology 154: 789–795

Calder A L, Co E E, Sage M D 1986 Coronary arterial abnormalities in pulmonary atresia with intact ventricular septum. Journal of Thoracic and Cardiovascular Surgery 59: 436–442

Celermajer J, Bowdler J D, Gengos D, Cohen D, Struckley D 1968 Pulmonary valve fusion with intact ventricular septum. American Heart Journal 65: 452–465

Cole R B, Muster A J, Lev M, Paul M H 1968 Pulmonary atresia with intact ventricular septum. American Journal of Cardiology 21: 23–31

Coles J G, Freedom R M, Lightfoot N E et al 1989 Long-term results in neonates with pulmonary atresia and intact ventricular septum. Annals of Thoracic Surgery 47: 213–216

Davignon A L, Greenwold W E, DuShane J W, Edwards J E 1961 Congenital pulmonary atresia with intact ventricular septum. Clinicopathologic correlation of two anatomic types. American Heart Journal 62: 591–602

Daubeney P E F, Delany D J, Slavik Z for the United Kingdom National Collaborative Study of Pulmonary Atresia with Intact Ventricular Septum 1995a Pulmonary atresia with intact ventricular septum: range of morphology in a population based study. Circulation 92(suppl I): 126

Daubeney P E F, Delany D J, Keeton B R for the United Kingdom National Collaborative Study of Pulmonary Atresia with Intact Ventricular Septum 1995b Pulmonary atresia/intact ventricular septum: early outcome after right ventricular outflow reconstruction by surgery or catheter intervention. Circulation 92(suppl I): 380

de Leval M, Bull C, Stark J, Anderson R H, Tayler J F N, Macartney F J 1982 Pulmonary atresia and intact ventricular septum: Surgical management based on a revised classification. Circulation 66: 272–280

Freedom R M, Keith J D 1979 Pulmonary atresia with normal aortic root. In: Keith J D, Rowe R D, Vlad P (eds) Heart disease in infancy and childhood. MacMillan, New York, p 506–517

Freedom R M, Harrington D 1974 Contributions of intramyocardial sinusoids in pulmonary atresia and intact ventricular septum to a right sided circular shunt. British Heart Journal 36: 1061–1065

Freedom R M, White R I Jr, Ho C S, Gingell R L, Hawker R E, Rowe R D 1974 Evaluation of patients with pulmonary atresia and intact ventricular septum by double catheter technique. American Journal of Cardiology 33: 892–895

Freedom R M, Dische M R, Rowe R D 1978 The tricuspid valve in pulmonary atresia and intact ventricular septum. Arch Pathol Lab Med 102: 28–31

Freedom R M, Wilson G, Trusler G A et al 1983 Pulmonary atresia and intact ventricular septum. A review of the anatomy, myocardium, and factors influencing right ventricular growth and guidelines with surgical intervention. Scandinavian Journal of Thoracic and Cardiovascular Surgery 17: 1–28

Gersony W M, Bernhard W F, Nadas A, Gross R E 1967 Diagnosis and surgical treatment of infants with critical pulmonary outflow obstruction. Study of thirty-four infants with pulmonary stenosis or atresia and intact ventricular septum. Circulation 35: 765–776

Giglia T M, Mandell V S, Connor A R, Mayer J E, Lock J E 1992 Diagnosis and management of right ventricle-dependent coronary circulation in pulmonary atresia with intact ventricular septum. Circulation 86: 1516–1528

Graham T P Jr, Bender H W, Atwood G F, Page D L, Sell C G R 1974 Increase in right ventricular volume following valvulotomy for pulmonary atresia or stenosis with intact ventricular septum. Circulation 50(suppl II): 67–79

Greenwold W E, DuShane J W, Burchell H B, Bruwer A, Edwards J E 1956 Congenital pulmonary atresia with intact ventricular septum: Two anatomic types. In: Proceedings of the 29th scientific sessions of the American Heart Association. p 51

Hanley F L, Sade R M, Blackstone E H, Kirklin J W, Freedom R M, Nanda N C 1993 Outcomes in neonatal pulmonary atresia with intact ventricular septum. Journal of Thoracic and Cardiovascular Surgery 105: 406–427

Harinck E, Becker A E, Gittenberger-de Groot A C, Oppenheimer-Derren A, Versprille A 1977 The left ventricle in congenital isolated pulmonary valve stenosis. British Heart Journal 39: 429–435

Hawkins J A, Thorne J K, Boucek M M et al 1990 Early and late results in pulmonary atresia and intact ventricular septum. Journal of Thoracic and Cardiovascular Surgery 100: 492–497

Heymann M A, Rudolph A M 1972 Effects of congenital heart disease on fetal and neonatal circulation. In: Friedman W F (ed.) Neonatal Heart Disease. Grune & Stratton, New York, p 51–79

Heymann M A, Rudolph A M 1977 Ductus arteriosus dilatation by prostaglandin E_1 in infants with pulmonary atresia. Pediatrics 59: 325–329

Kasznica J, Ursel P C, Blanc W A, Gersony W M 1987 Abnormalities of the coronary circulation in pulmonary atresia and intact ventricular septum. American Heart Journal 114: 1415–1420

Keith J D, Rowe R D, Vlad P, O'Hanley J H 1954 Complete anomalous pulmonary venous drainage. American Journal of Medicine 16: 23–38

Lenox C C, Briner J 1972 Absent proximal coronary arteries associated with pulmonic atresia. American Journal of Cardiology 30: 666–669

Leung M P, Lo R N S, Cheung H, Lee J, Mok C K 1991 Balloon valvuloplasty after pulmonary valvotomy for babies with pulmonary atresia and intact ventricular septum. Annals of Thoracic Surgery 53: 864–870

Macartney F J, Zuberbuhler J R, Anderson R H 1980 Morphological considerations pertaining to recognition of atrial isomerism. Consequences for sequential chamber localisation. British Heart Journal 44: 657–667

Mildner R J, Kiraly L, Sreeram N 1997 Pulmonary atresia, 'intact ventricular septum', and aortopulmonary collateral arteries. Heart 77: 173–175

Moller J H, Girod D, Amplatz K, Varco R L 1970 Pulmonary valvulotomy in pulmonary atresia with hypoplastic right ventricle. Surgery 68: 630–634

Murphy D A, Murphy D R, Gibbons J E, Dobell A R C 1971 Surgical treatment of pulmonary atresia with intact ventricular septum. Journal of Thoracic and Cardiovascular Surgery 62: 213–219

Neches W H, Mullins C E, McNamara D G 1973 Balloon atrial septostomy in congenital heart disease in infancy. American Journal of Diseases in Childhood 125: 371–375

O'Conner W N, Cottrill C M, Johnson G L, Noonan J A, Tood E P 1982 Pulmonary atresia with intact ventricular septum and ventriculocoronary communications: Surgical significance. Circulation 65: 805–809

Olley P M, Coccani F, Bodach E 1976 A new emergency therapy for certain cyanotic congenital heart malformations. Circulation 53: 728–731

Patel R G, Freedom R M, Moes C A F et al 1980 Right ventricular volume determinations in 18 patients with pulmonary atresia and intact ventricular septum. Circulation 61: 428–440

Rosenthal E, Qureshi S A, Kakadekar A P, Anjos R, Baker E J, Tynan M 1993a Technique of percutaneous laser-assisted valve dilatation for valvar atresia in congenital heart disease. British Heart Journal 69: 556–562

Rosenthal E, Qureshi S A, Chan K C, Martin R P, Skehan D J, Jordan S C, Tynan M 1993b Radiofrequency-assisted balloon dilatation in patients with pulmonary valve atresia and an intact ventricular septum. British Heart Journal 69: 347–351

Santos M A, Moll J N, Drumond C, Araujo W B, Roma N, Reis N B 1980 Development of the ductus arteriosus in right ventricular outflow tract obstruction. Circulation 62: 818–822

Shaddy R E, Sturtevant J E, Judd V E, McGough E C 1990 Right ventricular growth after transventricular pulmonary valvotomy and central aortopulmonary shunt for pulmonary atresia and intact ventricular septum. Circulation 82 (suppl IV): 157–163

Shapiro S, Lakir J, Rudolph A, Heymann M A 1973 Pulmonic stenosis in fetal lambs. Circulation 48(suppl IV): NI44

Steinberger J, Berry J M, Bass J L et al 1992 Results of right ventricular outflow patch for pulmonary atresia with intact ventricular septum. Circulation 86(suppl II): 167–175

Trusler G A, Yamamoto N, Williams W G, Izukawa T, Rowe R D, Mustard W T 1976 Surgical treatment of pulmonary atresia with intact ventricular septum. British Heart Journal 38: 957–960

Williams G W, Burrows P, Freedeom R M et al 1991 Thromboexclusion of the right ventricle in children with pulmonary atresia and intact ventricular septum. American Journal of Cardiology 101: 222–229

Zuberbuhler J R 1981 Clinical diagnosis in pediatric cardiology. Churchill Livingstone, Edinburgh, p 110

Zuberbuhler J R, Anderson R H 1979 Morphological variations in pulmonary atresia with intact ventricular septum. British Heart Journal 41: 281–288

Zuberbuhler J R, Lenox C C, Park S C, Neches W H 1975 Continuous murmurs in the newborn. In: Leon D F, Shaver J A (eds) Physiologic principles of heart sound and murmurs. American Heart Association, New York, p 209–214

Zuberbuhler J R, Allwork S P, Anderson R H (1979a) The spectrum of Ebstein's anomaly of the tricuspid valve. Journal of Thoracic and Cardiovascular Surgery 211: 77–202

Zuberbuhler J R, Fricker F J, Park S C et al (1979b) Pulmonary atresia with intact ventricular septum: morbid anatomy. In: Goodman M J, Marquis R M (eds) Paediatric cardiology, Vol 2. Heart disease in the newborn. Churchill Livingstone, Edinburgh, p 285

45

Hypoplastic left heart syndrome

R. Dhillon and A. N. Redington

INTRODUCTION

Rather than being a single lesion, the entity usually described as hypoplastic left heart syndrome is a group of conditions with characteristic anatomical, physiological and clinical properties. The earliest grouping of these features was made by Lev in 1952, but he described the syndrome as 'hypoplasia of the aortic tract'. As will be discussed below, the syndrome is not synonymous with aortic atresia or hypoplasia. This is because the aortic lesions can exist with a left ventricle of normal size, particularly when the abnormal aorta takes origin from the right ventricle. As far as we are aware, it was in 1958 that Noonan and Nadas first used the term 'hypoplastic left heart syndrome', and this is the term now generally accepted for description.

Although the combinations of anatomical lesions that constitute the syndrome are variable, the features of gross hypoplasia of the left ventricle in association with hypoplasia, stenosis or atresia of its inlet and outlet valves are unmistakable in 'classic' cases. This description includes virtually all cases of aortic atresia and most cases of left atrioventricular valvar atresia. As already stated, nonetheless, aortic atresia can rarely be found with a left ventricle of normal size (Freedom et al, 1976; Pellegrino and Thiene, 1976; Roberts et al, 1976; Perry et al, 1977; Thiene et al, 1979), usually with an associated ventricular septal defect. In these cases, the aorta may potentially be connected to the left ventricle. An atretic aorta with a normal or dominant left ventricle is also seen, but again rarely, in the setting of discordant ventriculo-arterial connections (McGarry et al, 1980). Aortic atresia coexisting with univentricular atrioventricular connections is typically seen with dominant left ventricle, but aortic atresia with hypoplastic left ventricle has been found with double inlet to and double outlet from the right ventricle (Keeton et al, 1979). In most of the cases of left atrioventricular valvar atresia with right hand ventricular topology, the left ventricle is usually hypoplastic. These fall within the group of classic cases, particularly when the ventricular septum is intact. When both arteries are connected to the right ventricle in this setting, nonetheless, the aorta may be of good size despite the left ven-

tricular hypoplasia. Furthermore, when the ventriculo-arterial connections are discordant, the left ventricle may again be hypoplastic, although to a lesser degree; however, it will then support the pulmonary trunk rather than the aorta. In the setting of intact ventricular septum, this combination has more in common with pulmonary atresia, although strictly representing also hypoplasia of the left heart. It is very rare. Other cases of left atrioventricular valvar atresia are unequivocally not examples of hypoplastic left heart, since the right atrium can be connected through a patent right atrioventricular valve to a dominant left ventricle. These examples are described in Chapter 40. Associated hypoplasia of the aortic valve and aorta are well described in this setting, albeit arising from the incomplete and rudimentary right ventricle (Tandon et al, 1974). The left ventricle, aortic valve and ascending aorta may all also be hypoplastic in the context of atrioventricular septal defect with so-called right ventricular dominance. In this setting, the greater part of the common atrioventricular junction is connected to the right ventricle (Barber, 1986; Barber et al, 1988). Significantly, in most of the cases initially studied by Noonan and Nadas (1958), aortic coarctation was the major anatomical feature, although the left ventricle was described as being hypoplastic. It is questionable whether such cases would nowadays be considered as examples of hypoplastic left heart syndrome. It follows from all the above discussion concerning morphological patterns that there are major difficulties in providing an all-encompassing anatomical definition for this syndrome. It is more realistic, therefore, to look at the unifying haemodynamic features. Physiologically, the hypoplastic left heart syndrome can be defined as the situation in which the systemic circulation is dependent on the right ventricle in the setting of atresia or severe hypoplasia of the aortic valve (Bove et al, 1996). This definition is clinically more robust. It should be stressed again, nonetheless, that aortic atresia in isolation does not necessarily represent the hypoplastic left heart syndrome. In aortic atresia with discordant ventriculo-arterial connections for example, the systemic circulation is dependent on the left ventricle. This combination self-evidently does not satisfy the haemodynamic definition proposed above and is excluded from our further considerations. For the purposes of this chapter, therefore, we will deal exclusively with those lesions with a small left ventricle, an intact ventricular septum and either atresia or critical stenosis of the aortic valve.

EPIDEMIOLOGY

Before fetal echocardiography routinely became a part of antenatal screening, the reported incidence of the hypoplastic left heart syndrome ranged from 0.16 to 0.36 per 1000 livebirths (Brownell and Shokeir, 1976; Fyler et al, 1980). Postmortem studies from this earlier era suggested that hypoplastic left heart syndrome accounted for 1.4–3.8% of cases of congenital heart disease (Abbott, 1936; Edwards, 1953). In many countries, cardiac four chamber screening is now routinely performed during antenatal ultrasonography, and the diagnosis of hypoplastic left heart syndrome is often made by the noncardiologist. Some parents learning of the diagnosis prior to 20 weeks of gestation will opt for termination of the pregnancy (Allan, 1993). This has contributed, in some areas of the world, to a decline in the number of newborns seen with hypoplastic left heart syndrome (Allan et al, 1991). Of those surviving to term, two thirds are male (Sinha et al, 1968; Roberts et al, 1976; Hawkins and Doty, 1984). It has been estimated that the risk of recurrence of hypoplastic left heart syndrome in siblings is 0.5%, with a risk of 2.2% for the occurrence of other forms of congenital heart disease (Holmes et al, 1974; Brownell and Shokeir, 1976; Nora and Nora, 1978).

Although the hypoplastic left heart syndrome is not a common form of congenital heart disease, it continues to account for a large proportion of the cardiovascular mortality occurring in the first month of life. In one series, a quarter of neonatal deaths resulting from congenital heart disease were attributable to hypoplastic left heart syndrome (Watson and Rowe, 1962), but this was prior to the introduction and successful development of palliative surgical programmes.

Hypoplastic left heart syndrome has been described in the setting of Turner's syndrome or its mosaic variant (Natowicz and Kelley, 1987; Lin, 1988; van Egmond et al, 1988). It has also been encountered in Noonan's syndrome (Antonelli et al, 1990), in the CATCH 22 syndrome (Consevage et al, 1996), Holt–Oram syndrome (Glauser et al, 1989), Edward's syndrome (Helton et al, 1986) and in a number of other chromosomal abnormalities, including 4q, 4p, 18p deletions, and in several cases of 11q deletion (Natowicz et al, 1988; Guenthard et al, 1994). Although hypoplastic left heart syndrome has been associated with different Mendelian syndromes, a consistent genetic abnormality remains to be elucidated (Ferencz et al, 1997).

Fetal echocardiography can be employed to ascertain the risk for recurrence of congenital heart disease, and this can be performed in early pregnancy. The rates of recurrence for major lesions are higher than those reported in postnatal studies, and this may reflect high fetal loss in these cases. In the study by Allan et al (1986) of 1021 mothers referred for fetal echocardiography with a family history of congenital heart disease, the rates for recurrence of obstructive lesions in the left heart were particularly high. Aortic valvar atresia was associated with a recurrence rate of 1 in 28, and aortic coarctation with a rate of 1 in 15, against an overall recurrence rate of 1 in 52 in those with a previously affected child. These observations support the case for a genetic predisposition to the development of such lesions.

Epidemiological evidence of a genetic contribution to the aetiology of hypoplastic left heart syndrome is provided by the Baltimore–Washington infant study (Ferencz et al, 1997). Six paediatric cardiology centres participated in this population-based analysis, which ascertained patients born between 1981 and 1989. In relation to hypoplastic left heart syndrome, there were seven families in whom a first-degree relative had congenital heart disease. Out of these, five had obstructive lesions in the left heart, namely hypoplastic left heart syndrome in one, bicuspid aortic valve in one and aortic coarctation in three. Furthermore, in the multivariate analysis of risk factors for hypoplastic left heart syndrome, family history was the strongest factor, with an odds ratio of 4.8, followed by maternal diabetes mellitus, with an odds ratio of 3.9.

AETIOLOGY

The aetiology of the hypoplastic left heart syndrome is unknown in most patients. In one North American series, two-fifths of fetuses with the hypoplastic left heart syndrome were found to have associated chromosomal or extracardiac defects (Blake et al, 1991). Although it is important to look for such associations, they are inconsistent and have failed to refine our understanding of the genetic precursor of the disease.

Current theories are based on the findings at postmortem, postnatal echocardiography and, importantly, fetal echocardiography. The last has enabled us to define the normal and abnormal development of the heart during gestation. Indeed, in hypoplastic left heart syndrome, there may be impaired left ventricular growth in the presence of diminished inflow or obstruction to outflow, although this may not become obvious until after 20 weeks of gestation (Allan et al, 1989; Sharland et al, 1991).

Mitral stenosis and imperforate mitral valve both exist as part of the hypoplastic left heart syndrome. In experiments with chick embryos, hypoplasia of the left ventricle has been produced following intervention to occlude the mitral valve (Harh et al, 1973). This is not a likely mechanism in the development of hypoplastic left heart syndrome in humans, however, as mitral stenosis occurring as a primary lesion results in enlargement of the left atrium. In the hypoplastic left heart syndrome, the left atrium is usually diminished in size. A popular theory for the development of the hypoplastic left heart syndrome is that of displacement of the primary atrial septum (Weinberg et al, 1986). This is said to reduce flow through the inferior caval vein via the oval foramen to the left atrium and left ventricle, resulting in left ventricular hypoplasia. There is no evidence, however, to show that the displaced septum is not itself a consequence of the disordered flow. Indeed, studies of fetal flow suggest that it is the ventricular problem that occurs first (Berning et al, 1996). Furthermore, Cook and colleagues at Guy's Hospital, London, have isolated viral particles from the myocardium of postmortem cases, suggesting that, for some at least, fetal viral myocarditis is the harbinger of decreased left ventricular growth (unpublished observations).

Obstruction to the left ventricular outflow tract is invariably present in the hypoplastic left heart syndrome and it, too, has been implicated as an aetiological factor (Bharati and Lev, 1984). The left ventricle is almost always hypoplastic in aortic atresia with an intact ventricular septum, and endocardial fibroelastosis is usually prominent, but only when the mitral valve is patent. In these patients, there can be little doubt that the high left ventricular pressure, particularly in diastole, is an important additional aetiological factor in the development of the endocardial ischaemia and scarring. In those rare cases associated with a large ventricular septal defect, nonetheless, the left ventricle may be of normal size and free of fibrosis, making a primary myocardial problem an unlikely precursor in this rare subgroup. In view of the varied anatomical findings in the syndrome, it is perhaps optimistic even to anticipate finding one unifying aetiological factor underlying its existence. The observation of familial occurrence of obstructive lesions in the left ventricular outflow tract and aortic arch is intriguing, nonetheless, and suggests that genetic advances in the near future will provide new aetiological insights.

ANATOMY

OVERALL STRUCTURE

Typically in the hypoplastic left heart syndrome, there is usual atrial arrangement with concordant atrioventricular and ventriculo-arterial connections (Figure 45.1). The main anatomical feature, of necessity, is hypoplasia of the left ventricle. There is usually obstruction to the left ventricular inflow and outflow, but this is variable. At the extreme, the left ventricular cavity may be almost nonexistent. In this setting, it may be left to the morphologist to demonstrate the presence of the vestigial ventricle (Figure 45.2). While the anatomist can discover small ventricles, however, it is almost impossible for the anatomist to determine precisely when the left ventricle should be considered hypoplastic in patients with aortic valvar stenosis rather than atresia. Some of these hearts show obvious fibroelastosis in the small ventricle and certainly fulfil the anatomic criterions for the syndrome

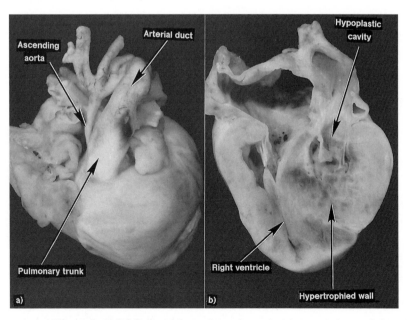

Figure 45.1. The typical arrangement of hypoplastic left heart syndrome is aortic atresia (a) or stenosis, coexisting with mitral stenosis (b) or atresia. Note the thread-like ascending aorta, which functions as a conduit for retrograde flow to the coronary arteries; the arterial duct, which takes the entire ventricular output; and the hypoplastic left ventricle, which despite its cavitary hypoplasia has grossly hypertrophic walls.

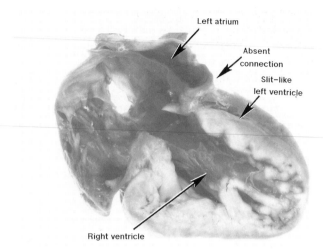

Figure 45.2. In this example of hypoplastic left heart with mitral atresia, there is complete absence of the left atrioventricular connection, and the rudimentary and incomplete left ventricle is no more than a slit in the posteroinferior wall of the ventricular mass.

(Figure 45.3). Under other circumstances, the ventricle may seem hypoplastic, but it is impossible for the morphologist to judge the ability of the ventricle to maintain an effective systemic circulation. The distinction of the physiological inadequacy of such a ventricle may then have been no easier in life, although diagnostic algorithms are being refined (see below).

Typically, the left ventricular walls are hypertrophied (Figure 45.1b), and the left ventricular mass may rarely be increased rather than decreased despite the cavitary hypoplasia. The left atrium is usually small. In typical cases, there can be hypertrophy of the left atrial walls, and

some patients can be seen with an enlarged atrium, particularly the appendage. Left atrial endocardial fibroelastosis is rare. In perhaps one tenth of patients, the atrial septum is intact, as judged at postmortem (Figure 45.4a). In some of these, while the pulmonary venous connections are normal, the pulmonary venous drainage can be abnormal (Lev et al, 1963; Schall and Dalldorf, 1984). Because of these findings, premature closure of the oval foramen has been implicated as a potential aetiological factor in the development of the syndrome (Lev et al, 1963). This ignores the fact that the oval foramen is patent in most patients (Figure 45.4b) and does not obstruct flow from left to right. It is much more likely that the intact septum is an occasional consequence of the left-sided hypoplasia, rather than its cause.

Anomalous pulmonary venous connections are seen in a small proportion of patients, with supracardiac drainage being most often encountered. When the atrial septum is intact, or the oval foramen is restrictive, there may also be abnormal pulmonary venous drainage via an anomalous channel often described as the laevoatrial cardinal vein (Figure 45.5). This channel usually passes from the left atrium to the brachiocephalic vein and is readily identified by cross-sectional echocardiography (Pinto et al, 1993). Although often described as a cardinal vein, it is unlikely that this channel represents persistence of the embryological cardinal venous system (Bernstein et al, 1995) but rather is a newly developed venous structure. The other route that may allow escape of pulmonary venous blood from the left atrium is 'unroofing' or fenestration of the coronary sinus (Figure 45.6) (Freedom et al, 1981; Suzuki et al, 1990; Seliem et al, 1992). This can be seen in association with persistence of the left superior

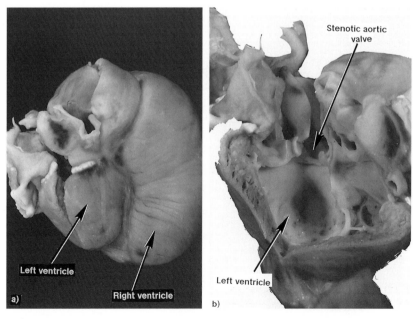

Figure 45.3. This heart is an example of critical aortic stenosis: note the dysplastic leaflets of the aortic valve (b); gross hypoplasia of the left ventricle (a) and fibroelastosis of the walls of the hypoplastic cavity of the left ventricle (b). When the size of the left ventricle is assessed relative to the right ventricle (a), this unequivocally falls within the category of hypoplastic left heart syndrome.

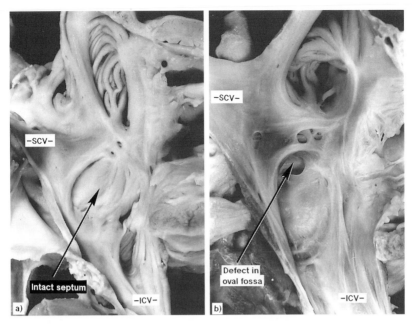

Figure 45.4. In a proportion of cases of hypoplastic left heart, the atrial septum is found to be intact at postmortem (a). Usually, however, the oval foramen is deficient or probe patent (b). SCV and ICV, superior and inferior caval veins, respectively.

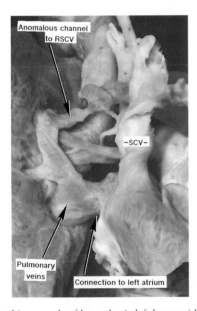

Figure 45.5. In this example of hypoplastic left heart with mitral atresia, the laevoatrial cardinal vein provides an anastomotic channel from the left atrium to the right superior caval vein (RSCV).

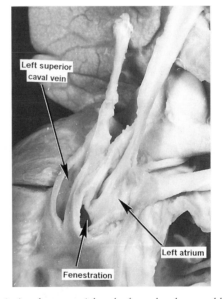

Figure 45.6. Another potential outlet from the obstructed left atrium in hypoplastic left heart, as shown in this specimen, is a fenestration between the left atrium and the coronary sinus, which in this case also drains a persistent left superior caval vein.

caval vein, which is truly a derivative of the cardinal venous system and, therefore, to be distinguished from the laevoatrial cardinal vein.

OBSTRUCTION OF INFLOW TO AND OUTFLOW FROM THE LEFT VENTRICLE

In almost all cases, the mitral valve is either stenosed (Ruckman and Van Praagh, 1978) or atretic (Thiene et al,

1981). In the presence of mitral stenosis, all components of the valve (the annulus, leaflets, tendinous cords and papillary muscles) may contribute to the obstruction (Figure 45.7). When atretic, the mitral valve may be imperforate (Figure 45.8a) or may be absent together with the left atrioventricular connection (Figures 45.2 and 45.8b). Left ventricular endocardial fibroelastosis is seen only when the mitral valve is perforate (Figure 45.1b). Obstruction of the left ventricular outflow tract is an invariable feature of the hypoplastic left heart syndrome. Aortic atresia, as with mitral atresia, can result

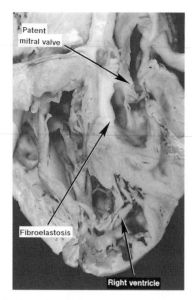

Figure 45.7. This four chamber section shows the typical structure of the hypoplastic left ventricle in the setting of mitral stenosis. The ventricular walls are fibroelastotic, and the mitral valve is miniaturized. All its components, that is the junction, leaflets, tendinous cords and papillary muscles, are involved.

from an imperforate valve (Figure 45.9a). Alternatively, there can be absence of the ventriculo-arterial connection. Complete absence of the connection, nonetheless, is rare. Most usually, the subaortic outlet is blocked by fibrous tissue (Figure 45.9b). The aortic root itself is usually markedly hypoplastic. When the outflow tract is patent, the aortic leaflets are thickened and dysplastic (Figure 45.3b). Rarely, they may be absent, with a stenosing ring seen at the ventriculo-arterial junction, similar to that observed in absent pulmonary valve syndrome

(Rossi et al, 1986). Hearts with absence of the leaflets of the arterial valves have recently been described in mice with knock-out of the transcription factor NF-ATc (de la Pompa et al, 1998; Ranger et al, 1998). The overall cardiac structure of the mice, however, shows no resemblance to known human syndromes, emphasizing the problems that still exist in correlating the genetic background with human disease. The aorta itself in typical hypoplastic left heart syndrome is often at its most narrow at the sinutubular junction, with the hypoplastic aortic root simply functioning as a conduit that feeds the coronary arteries (Figure 45.1a). This arrangement has, on occasion, been described as anomalous origin of the coronary arteries from the brachiocephalic artery in the setting of solitary pulmonary trunk! Not a diagnosis that would be made by the readers of this book!!

Further distally, aortic coarctation is common, occurring in over four fifths of patients, (Hawkins and Doty, 1984; Lang et al, 1985). The obstructive shelf is typically in preductal location (Figure 45.10a) but can be found paraductally (Figure 45.10b) Ductal tissue is not only incorporated into the stenosing shelf (Anderson et al, 1986) but also may extend proximally and distally (Machii and Becker, 1995). These findings may account for the relatively high incidence of recurrent coarctation following palliative surgery, including heart transplantation (Bailey and Gundry, 1990).

CORONARY ARTERIES AND CONDUCTION TISSUES

Abnormalities of the coronary arteries, such as ventriculocoronary fistulas and abnormal tortuosity, are more

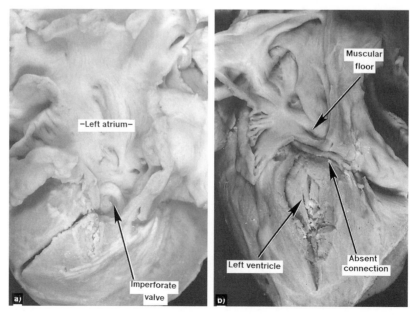

Figure 45.8. These hearts show mitral atresia as produced by an imperforate mitral valve in the setting of concordant atrioventricular connections (a) and by absence of the left atrioventricular connection (b). Both coexisted with unequivocal hypoplastic left heart syndrome.

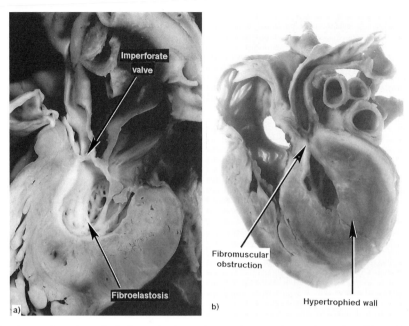

Figure 45.9. These four chamber sections through the hypoplastic aortic root show aortic atresia produced by an imperforate valvar membrane (a) and by an atretic fibromuscular segment of the subaortic outlet (b).

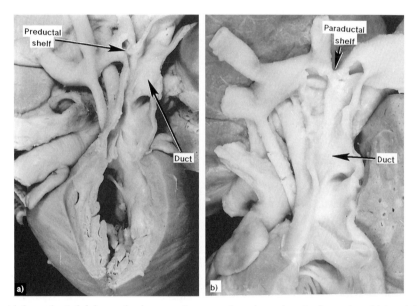

Figure 45.10. Most hearts with hypoplastic left heart also have aortic coarctation, shown here in the preductal (a) and the paraductal (b) position.

common in the subgroup of patients with mitral stenosis and aortic atresia (Sauer et al, 1989). In one study (Lloyd et al, 1986), nonetheless, there was no difference found in the diameter of the coronary arteries and their orifices when unselected patients and controls were studied at necropsy. Furthermore, myocardial fibrosis and necrosis was not found to correlate with diameters of the coronary arteries. In another postmortem study, coronary arterial fistulas were not seen to be associated with histological abnormalities of the right ventricle (Baffa et al, 1992).

The conduction tissues are in their expected location, albeit with miniaturization of the left bundle branch in keeping with the size of the left ventricle.

PHYSIOLOGY

As already emphasized, the most appropriate defining feature of the hypoplastic left heart syndrome is presence of a systemic circulation that is dependent on the right ventricle and, therefore, on patency of the arterial duct (Bove and Lloyd, 1996). Because the hypoplastic left ventricle is unable to support systemic blood flow, even in those hearts with forward flow across the mitral and aortic valves, pulmonary venous return must reach the right ventricle via the right atrium. The usual route is through an atrial septal defect or patent oval foramen. When the communication between the left and right atriums is restrictive, pulmonary venous congestion results. Clinical presentation may be within the first few hours of life, with a combination of pulmonary oedema, cyanosis and metabolic acidosis, reflecting the reduced pulmonary and systemic perfusion. Those patients that have had severely obstructed pulmonary venous return during fetal life represent the group at highest risk for surgical palliation, presumably because of secondary pulmonary changes owing to chronic pulmonary venous congestion.

Pulmonary and systemic venous blood mixes in the right atrium and passes to the right ventricle. It is the dominant right ventricle that supports flow not only into the pulmonary arteries but also, via the arterial duct, to the aorta. The ascending aorta and transverse aortic arch (and, therefore, the coronary arteries and brachiocephalic arteries) are then supplied retrogradely. In this situation, the systemic and pulmonary circulations are subtly balanced, being bridged by the arterial duct. The balance of flow across this bridge depends on the vascular resistance in the parallel circuits. While the resistances are balanced, so are flows of pulmonary and systemic blood. In those patients with a relatively low pulmonary vascular resistance, flow of blood to the lungs will be excessively high, and these infants have an inappropriately high arterial oxygen saturation. They will rapidly become acidotic because of impaired systemic perfusion. Rarely, the pulmonary vascular resistance is relatively high, and this results in marked cyanosis. These infants may also become acidotic, but because of impaired systemic delivery of oxygen (Barnea et al, 1994).

The ratio of pulmonary to systemic flows can be adjusted by altering the concentration of inspired oxygen and, in this way, the pulmonary vascular resistance. The therapeutic manipulation of the pulmonary vascular resistance is described in detail below but is ideally directed to maintain peripheral saturation of oxygen of approximately 75%. Assuming a mixed venous oxygen saturation of approximately 50%, and fully saturated pulmonary venous blood, this value reflects a ratio of pulmonary to systemic flows of unity.

CLINICAL FEATURES

Although they may present in the first few hours of life, as described above, it is rare for these babies to have symptoms at birth. The Apgar score will most often be normal, and most affected babies have a normal birthweight. This is because, during fetal life, oxygenation occurs through the placenta and there is a relatively high ratio of pulmonary to systemic resistance; consequently, oxygenated blood arriving in the right atrium will travel via the patent arterial duct into the descending aorta. Retrograde flow to the head and neck may be impaired by coarctation or hypoplasia of the aortic arch; as a result, cerebral blood flow may be lower than normal.

This may contribute to the relatively high incidence of micrencephaly and hypoplasia of the cerebral mantle, as well as other congenital anomalies of the brain seen in these patients (Glauser et al, 1990).

Clinical presentation, usually within 48 hours, is typically with features of congestive heart failure and acidosis. The usual cause is closure of the arterial duct, with concomitant reduction of systemic blood flow. If the duct remains open, the presenting features depend on the balance of pulmonary and systemic vascular resistances (Barnea et al, 1994). Increased pulmonary flow at the expense of systemic blood flow is the norm, but occasionally, if there is marked elevation of pulmonary vascular resistance (usually resulting from obstructed pulmonary venous return), cyanosis may be the dominant clinical feature. Rarely, the pulmonary and systemic flows remain balanced for weeks or months, the patient then presenting with secondary elevation of the pulmonary vascular resistance. There are isolated reports of individuals with hypoplastic left heart syndrome surviving without palliation. One child has been reported with survival to the age of 7 years (Ehrlich et al, 1986) and another surviving to adulthood (Vargas Barron et al, 1992).

INVESTIGATIONS

As with all forms of structural congenital heart disease, the mainstay of diagnosis nowadays is cross-sectional echocardiography. This modality may not be available, however, in the centre in which the baby is born. It should be remembered, therefore, that the relatively mundane techniques of electrocardiography and chest radiography provide important clues to the diagnosis, which, together with the clinical features, serve as the basis for a clinical diagnosis.

ELECTROCARDIOGRAPHY

The electrocardiogram is rarely normal, but the abnormalities are non-specific. In almost all cases there will be sinus rhythm. A rare exception is when there is isomerism of the left or right atrial appendages, in which case abnormalities of the P wave axis can be expected. Right atrial enlargement and right axis deviation of the mean frontal QRS axis are commonly seen. This may be accompanied by electrocardiographic evidence of right ventricular hypertrophy (Figure 45.11). Diminished left ventricular forces are to be expected and are usually manifest by an rS pattern in the left precordial leads (von Rueden and Moller, 1978). There is evidence of myocardial ischaemia in some patients, with abnormalities of the ST segment and T wave, reflecting reduced coronary arterial flow. This may be a consequence of ductal constriction, with reduced retrograde aortic flow. Alternatively, it

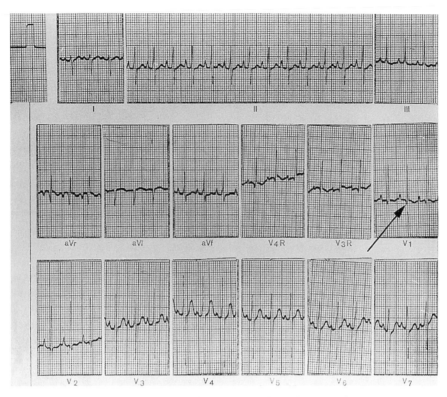

Figure 45.11. This electrocardiogram is from a neonate with combined aortic and mitral atresia. The QR progression in the right precordial leads (arrow) is consistent with gross right ventricular dominance.

may be caused by low arterial diastolic pressure and a 'steal' effect from the coronary circulation when the duct is widely patent and there is an inappropriately low pulmonary vascular resistance.

CHEST RADIOGRAPHY

As with electrocardiography, although there is no single diagnostic feature, this investigation is rarely normal. Usually the heart is in the left chest, with usual arrangement of the abdominal and thoracic organs. Cardiomegaly is characteristic, and there may be evidence of right atrial enlargement, with a prominent right heart border. The appearance of the pulmonary vascular markings is variable, usually normal within the first few hours of life, with progressive accentuation thereafter (Figure 45.12a). There may be intense pulmonary oedema in those patients with premature closure of the oval foramen (Figure 45.12b).

ECHOCARDIOGRAPHY

Echocardiography is now the major diagnostic modality, permitting delineation of all the significant anatomical and physiological characteristics (Bash et al, 1986). The diagnosis can be obvious, particularly when there is atresia of the mitral or aortic valves (Figure 45.13). The echocardiographic images then permit distinction of

mitral valvar atresia (Figure 45.14) and show whether this results from absence of the atrioventricular connection or an imperforate valve, although this is of no functional significance. In similar fashion, the images demonstrate complete obstruction of the subaortic outlet (Figure 45.15) from critical aortic stenosis with unequivocal hypoplasia of the left ventricle (Figure 45.16). In other situations, the diagnosis is less clear-cut. The differentiation of severe aortic stenosis with a hypoplastic left ventricle still capable of supporting the systemic circulation from the hypoplastic left heart syndrome, for example, depends on the precise measurements of the dimensions of the left-sided chambers. The echocardiogram also demonstrates clearly the degree of hypoplasia of the ascending aorta (Figure 45.17) and, with careful analysis, the presence or absence of coarctation at the junction of the duct with the isthmus and the descending aorta (Figure 45.18).

In an attempt to provide echocardiographic discriminators for the hypoplastic left heart syndrome, Ludman and colleagues (1990) studied prospectively 10 neonates with hypoplastic left heart syndrome, comparing their findings with 15 neonates with other causes of right ventricular volume overload and 15 normal controls. They examined the dimensions of the left and right ventricular cavities, the diameter of the aortic root at the sinuses of Valsalva and the sinutubular junction, the diameter of the ascending aorta as seen in the parasternal long-axis view and the diameter of the mitral valvar annulus in the

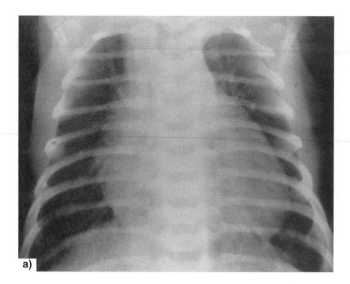

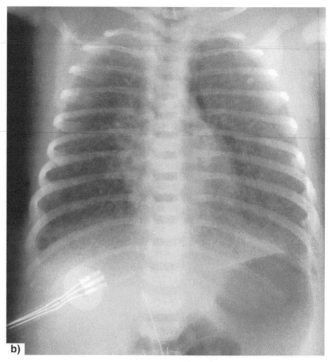

Figure 45.12. Frontal chest radiographs in hypoplastic left heart syndrome typically show cardiomegaly and a degree of pulmonary plethora (a). Pulmonary oedema can be intense, however, when there is premature closure of the oval foramen (b) (diagnosis confirmed at postmortem in this case).

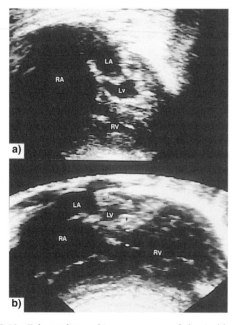

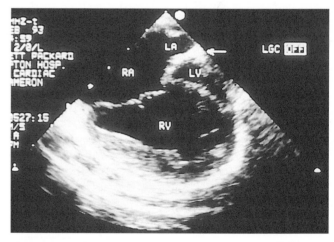

Figure 45.14. This cross-sectional echocardiogram shows absence of the left atrioventricular connection. Note the fibro-fatty tissue of the atrioventricular groove (arrow) between the left atrium and left ventricle. Abbreviations as in Figure 45.13.

Figure 45.13. Echocardiographic appearances of classical hypoplastic left heart syndrome with aortic valve atresia. The mitral valve is miniaturized (a) with marked hypoplasia of the left ventricular cavity and severe endocardial fibroelastosis (b). LA, left atrium; LV, left ventricle; RA, right atrium; RV, right ventricle.

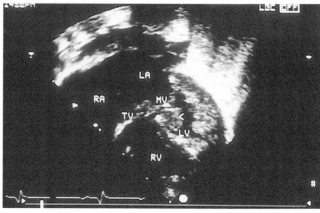

Figure 45.15. This cross-sectional echocardiogram in four chamber section shows hypoplastic left heart syndrome with complete obstruction of the subaortic outlet (arrowhead). MV, mitral valve, TV, tricuspid valve; other abbreviations as in Figure 45.13.

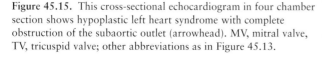

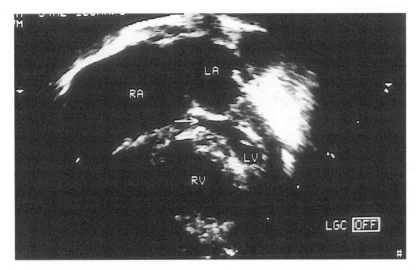

Figure 45.16. In this four chamber echocardiogram, there is obvious hypoplasia of the left ventricle, but with critical stenosis of a patent aortic valve (arrowed). Abbreviations as in Figure 45.13.

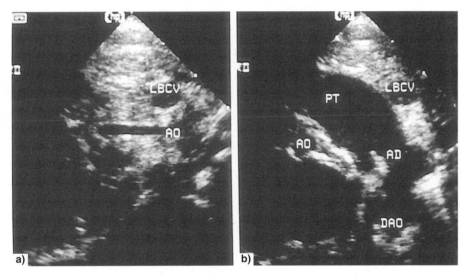

Figure 45.17. Echocardiographic parasternal sections showing (a) the diminutive ascending aorta and (b) large arterial duct continuous with the descending aorta. AO, aorta; LSCV, left superior caval vein: DAO, descending aorta; PT, pulmonary trunk; AD, arterial duct.

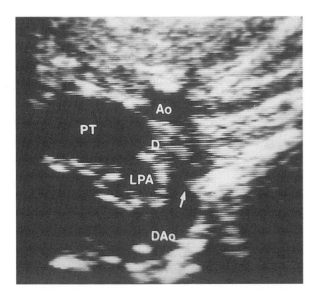

Figure 45.18. This cross-sectional echocardiogram shows discrete preductal coarctation (arrow) in a patient with classical hypoplastic left heart syndrome. Ao, aorta; DAo, descending aorta; LPA, left pulmonary artery; PT, pulmonary trunk.

apical four chamber view. The size of the left atrioventricular junction (when less than 36.3 mm/m²) was found to be the best single discriminator. There was considerable overlap, nonetheless, in measured variables between patients with hypoplastic left heart syndrome and other causes of right ventricular volume overload. Therefore, even with multiple and careful measurements (Latson et al, 1981; Mocellin et al, 1983) it is difficult to be sure when the left ventricle is sufficiently large to support the systemic circulation. In most cases, the subjective identification of hypoplasia of the left ventricle on cross-sectional echocardiography is all that is required for most patients (Figures 45.15 and 45.16). In more borderline cases, the 'bullet formula' can be applied.

The bullet formula is based on a geometric model of the left ventricle as a hemiellipse adjacent to a cylinder, shaped rather like a bullet. Hammon and colleagues (1988), studying patients undergoing surgical aortic valvotomy for critical aortic stenosis, found that all of those that died had end-diastolic volumes of the left ventricle as measured with the bullet formula of less than 20 ml/m². This value, therefore, is considered by some as a threshold for defining hypoplasia of the left ventricle. Survival following intervention for critical aortic stenosis, nonetheless, has now been examined by others in order to establish guidelines to suitability for biventricular repair. Rhodes and colleagues (1991) analysed retrospectively the echocardiographic and catheterization data from 65 infants undergoing biventricular repair with aortic valvotomy, balloon valvoplasty or a Norwood procedure. Although size of the left ventricular cavity was one discriminator for survival, it was not the best single measure. Survival was predicted with almost 90% accuracy when a formula was applied that incorporated the area of the mitral valve, the ratio of the left ventricular long axes and the size of the aortic root. A discriminating score of less than −0.35 was predictive of a fatal outcome following a two-ventricle repair. This study, although based on patients with critical aortic stenosis, is of particular relevance to the diagnosis of hypoplastic left heart syndrome. It reinforces the fact that, in borderline cases, size of the left ventricular cavity size is not the only factor determining the need for a Norwood procedure. Assessment of the inflow to and the outflow from the ventricle is also essential.

Echocardiography confirms that the right ventricle, tricuspid valve and pulmonary trunk are all enlarged. Right ventricular dysfunction is relatively common, particularly in those in whom systemic acidosis has been a feature. Primary abnormalities of the tricuspid valve are rare, but some degree of tricuspid regurgitation is common, again being more severe if there has been a prior haemodynamic insult. Assessment of the degree of tricuspid regurgitation is important, as its preoperative severity may be predictive of poor outcome after palliative surgery (Barber et al, 1988, 1989). Much physiological information will be obtained from assessment of the size of the oval foramen and arterial duct. In most patients, there

will be left-to-right flow across the oval foramen. When this is restrictive, Doppler interrogation will reveal an increased velocity of flow across the foramen. Isthmal hypoplasia, with a discrete shelf-like coarctation, was found in more than 80% of patients studied at postmortem, but this may be difficult to detect echocardiographically. Hypoplasia of the transverse aortic arch is relatively uncommon, but this, and even interruption, should actively be excluded. Spectral Doppler and colour flow mapping are particularly useful in assessing the patterns of systemic and pulmonary blood flows. Pulsed wave Doppler, with the sample gate within the arterial duct, will usually show bidirectional flow. This is from right to left in systole, and from left to right in diastole (Rychik et al, 1996). A subjective analysis of the balance of systemic and pulmonary flows can be obtained from the degree of antegrade and retrograde flow demonstrable more distally in the aorta.

FETAL ECHOCARDIOGRAPHY

Fetal echocardiography permits serial observation of the normal and abnormal development of the heart. Several clues pointing to potential development of the hypoplastic left heart syndrome can be elicited during fetal life. In addition to small or dysplastic left heart structures, the presence or potential for hypoplastic left heart syndrome in the fetus can be indicated by reversed or bidirectional flow across the oval foramen. Retrograde flow in the distal aortic arch is another indicator. In the study made by Hornberger et al (1995) of the developing fetal heart, these abnormalities of atrial and aortic flow were only observed in those fetuses subsequently found to be incapable of supporting a biventricular circulation. If such findings are noted, serial echocardiography must be performed to confirm the findings and chart the progress of the lesions.

CARDIAC CATHETERIZATION ———————

Cardiac catheterization has almost been replaced by echocardiography as a diagnostic tool. It will sometimes be required for intervention, for example balloon atrial septostomy or deployment of a stent in the arterial duct. The latter procedure permits maintenance of the patency of the arterial duct as a bridge to cardiac transplantation (Gibbs et al, 1993; Ruiz et al, 1993a,b; Slack et al, 1994). Stenting has secured systemic blood flow for up to 5 months in rare cases (Ruiz et al, 1993b).

An adequate interatrial communication is necessary for survival both before and after the Norwood procedure. In situations where the atrial septum is felt to be overly restrictive, balloon atrial septostomy is feasible (Gibbs et al, 1993). Some degree of restriction, however, is often beneficial, so this intervention is only rarely required. Indeed, by markedly lowering pulmonary arterial resistance, it may promote an inappropriately high preoperative pulmonary blood flow. Angiocardiography is now hardly ever needed to make the diagnosis. In skilled hands, nonetheless, it produces exquisite documentation of the state of the circulation in the ascending aorta and brachiocephalic artery (Figure 45.19). Aortography also demonstrates coarctation when present (Figure 45.20).

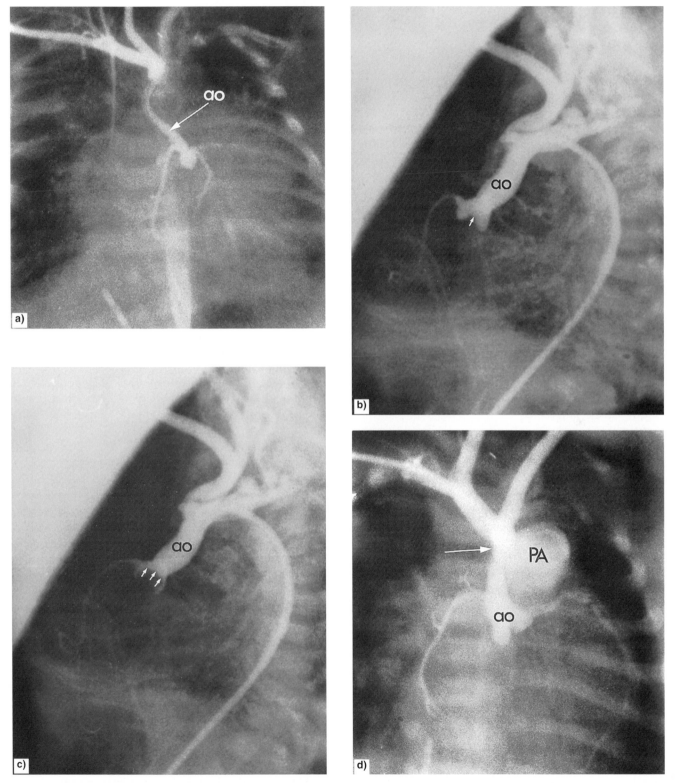

Figure 45.19. These examples of retrograde aortography reveal the variation in size of the ascending aorta in hypoplastic left heart syndrome. (a) A diminutive aorta (ao) can be seen. (b,c) A doming membrane, shown by the arrows, is produced by an imperforate valve. (d) The atretic aortic root is of almost normal size but the aorta tapers to its narrowest point at the origin of the brachiocephalic artery (arrowed). Note the contrast in the pulmonary trunk (PA).

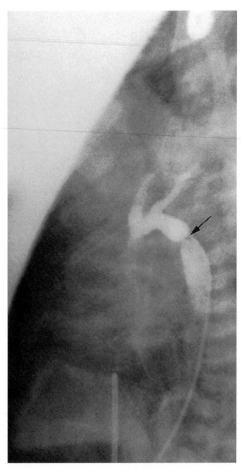

Figure 45.20. This retrograde aortogram reveals severe preductal coarctation (arrowed). There was aortic atresia.

LABORATORY INVESTIGATIONS

In view of the known association with chromosomal defects, karyotyping should be performed in all patients presenting with the hypoplastic left heart syndrome. These children may also have more subtle chromosomal abnormalities in the form of deletions and ring abnormalities (Natowicz et al, 1988; Glauser et al, 1989; Guenthard et al, 1994; Consevage et al, 1996). In one study, two fifths of fetuses with the hypoplastic left heart syndrome had chromosomal or extracardiac defects (Blake et al, 1991). Postnatally, extracardiac defects, predominantly cerebral and renal, are present in one eighth of children with hypoplastic left heart syndrome and should prompt a careful search, initially by cranial and renal ultrasound (Fyler et al, 1980).

Estimates of the incidence of microcephaly, which may be acquired, and other structural abnormalities of the brain in infants with hypoplastic left heart syndrome range from one third to three quarters (Rogers et al, 1995; Hagemo et al, 1997). In a postmortem study, Glauser and colleagues (1990) detected microcephaly in one third of babies with hypoplastic left heart syndrome, and structural malformations of the brain in three tenths. These included

absence of the corpus callosum, holoprosencephaly and abnormalities of the cortical mantle. Not surprisingly, cognitive maldevelopment has been found to be associated with poor cranial growth in the survivors of palliative surgery (Rogers et al, 1995; Hagemo et al, 1997).

DIFFERENTIAL DIAGNOSIS

The clinical syndrome of a sick newborn presenting with congestive cardiac failure, cyanosis, poor peripheral pulses and metabolic acidosis on analysis of blood gases may be present in more discrete forms of left heart obstruction, for example aortic coarctation, interrupted aortic arch, critical aortic stenosis or obstructed totally anomalous pulmonary venous connection. A similar clinical picture can result from non-structural cardiac disease. This includes supraventricular tachycardia, which may have been detected during fetal life, neonatal myocarditis, transient myocardial ischaemia and large systemic arterio-venous malformations (Fong et al, 1992). Rarely, cardiac neoplasms, for example rhabdomyomas, may produce significant obstruction of either the inflow to or the outflow from the left ventricle (Cooley, 1990). Non-cardiac diagnoses producing a very similar presentation include overwhelming septicaemia, for example group B streptococcal sepsis or congenital pneumonia, and inborn errors of metabolism (Kliegman and Behrman, 1992). The diagnosis of hypoplastic left heart syndrome, nonetheless, will be established rapidly by cross-sectional echocardiography.

MANAGEMENT

There are, at present, three approaches to treatment. These are staged palliative surgery, cardiac transplantation and, increasingly rarely, passive euthanasia. When surgical approaches are being considered, the preoperative management of the patient has a critical bearing on operative and postoperative results. It has been suggested that, when the diagnosis is made antenatally, transfer of the mother for delivery in a centre specializing in the surgical treatment of the hypoplastic left heart syndrome will produce better results (Chang et al, 1991). It is more difficult to demonstrate whether it is the transfer, or the expertise that is available in such centres, that counts. No matter where the baby is born, the best results from palliative surgery are obtained in those centres dealing with large numbers of patients. These superior results reflect focused and improved preoperative, operative and postoperative expertise.

PRESURGICAL THERAPY

As has been emphasized, the relative flow of blood to the systemic and pulmonary circulations can be manipulated

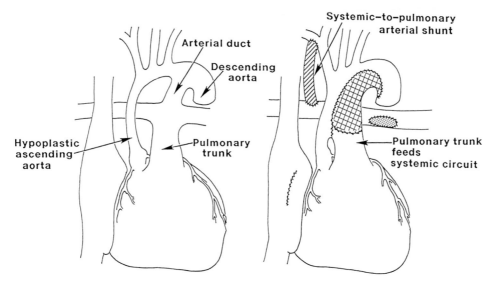

Figure 45.21. These diagrams show the arrangement of the circulations before and after the classical Norwood procedure, which is the first stage of palliative surgery.

by therapies to adjust their respective vascular resistances. In this respect, preoperative management, and that following the first stage of palliative surgery, are similar. Prior to surgery, the pulmonary and systemic circulations are bridged by the arterial duct. Following the first stage of palliative surgery (Figure 45.21), the bridge is a modified Blalock–Taussig shunt (Figure 45.22). Such a shunt is no longer amenable to the pharmacological manipulation with prostaglandins that markedly influences the duct (and may have secondary effects on the pulmonary vascular bed). The ratio of flows of systemic and pulmonary blood, nonetheless, still depends on vascular resistances on either side of the bridge. In general, systemic perfusion is optimized by preventing the development of an inappropriately low pulmonary vascular resistance. In practice, this is usually achieved by reducing the fraction of inspired oxygen. Supplemental oxygen is rarely required, room air being most appropriate. Some have taken this principle further, suggesting the use of a hypoxic environment obtained with inspiration of 18% oxygen to elevate the pulmonary vascular resistance (Barnea et al, 1994; Riordan et al, 1996). Relative hypercapnia is another method of maintaining an adequately high pulmonary vascular resistance. This can be effectively achieved only in the mechanically ventilated patient. The arterial tension of carbon dioxide is usually maintained at 5–7 kPa, either by adjusting the ventilation each minute or by supplementing inspired carbon dioxide, which is probably more desirable (Jobes et al, 1992). Inotropic agents are only indicated when there is severe right ventricular dysfunction, and only when the balance of pulmonary and systemic vascular resistances has been optimized. Systemic arterial vasodilators, such as sodium nitroprusside, may effectively lower the systemic vascular resistance. This makes subsequent management of the ratio of pulmonary and systemic flows more advantageous.

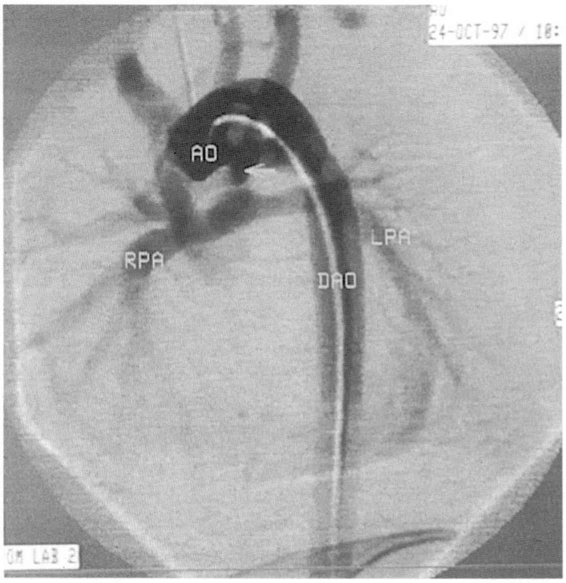

STAGED PALLIATIVE SURGERY

Surgical palliation of the hypoplastic left heart syndrome was first achieved by Norwood and his colleagues in 1983. The palliative procedures have now evolved in three stages, culminating in the construction of the Fontan circulation, usually by means of a total cavopulmonary connection. The first stage is now commonly referred to simply as 'the Norwood procedure'. It is performed during the neonatal period, often within the first

Figure 45.22. Following the first stage of palliative surgery, a modified Blalock–Taussig shunt (arrowed) provides the bridge between the aorta (AO) and the right and left pulmonary arteries (RPA, LPA). DAO, descending aorta.

week of life. Its key feature (Figure 45.21) is transsection of the pulmonary trunk proximal to the pulmonary bifurcation and its anastomosis with the hypoplastic ascending aorta, incorporating a triangular patch of homograft material to augment the ascending aorta, arch and distal aorta beyond the insertion of the duct. The atrial septum is resected to ensure adequacy of the interatrial communication. A modified Blalock–Taussig shunt is then fashioned on the right side using a 3–4 mm Gore-tex tube placed between the subclavian artery and the pulmonary artery, thus providing for, but also limiting, pulmonary flow. Further modifications have been described, for example one obviating the need for homograft material (Fraser and Mee, 1995). Their general principle remains the same as the initial procedure.

The management of the immediate postoperative phase is critical. As was the case prior to palliative surgery, there is a delicate balance between the flows of systemic and pulmonary blood, which is dependent on vascular resistances and driving pressure. The move towards placing a smaller sized shunt, which, in turn, has been made possible by the advent and earlier performance of the second stage, has markedly simplified postoperative management. Formerly, when it was the norm to construct shunts of 5 mm diameter, all efforts were directed towards maintaining a high pulmonary vascular resistance; sporadic acute increases in resistance were a common mode of death. Nowadays, with shunts that limit pulmonary flow, a more liberal management of the pulmonary vascular resistance can be allowed, and only rarely are measures required to increase pulmonary vascular resistance (see above). The child is initially ventilated with a mixture containing a low content of oxygen, and often in air.

At the age of approximately 3 to 6 months, the second palliative stage is performed. This comprises a bidirectional Glenn procedure, anastomosing end-to-side the superior caval vein to the right pulmonary artery. This approach, which is also performed in a somewhat modified form called the hemi-Fontan procedure (Douville et al, 1991; Jonas, 1991), has resulted in an improved outcome not only for patients with hypoplastic left heart syndrome but also for other forms of heart with a functionally univentricular circulation that will ultimately be palliated with a Fontan circulation (Bove and Lloyd, 1996; Jacobs et al, 1996). In patients with hypoplastic left heart syndrome, the third stage is the completion of a total cavopulmonary circulation using either a lateral atrial tunnel (de Leval et al, 1988) or an extracardiac conduit (Giannico et al, 1992); this is performed at approximately 18 to 36 months of age. The results of staged palliation for hypoplastic left heart syndrome differ markedly between centres. Bove and Lloyd (1996) reported 120 hospital survivors of 158 consecutive patients undergoing the first stage of surgery between 1990 and 1995. Actuarial survival in these patients was 58% at 5 years, although few patients had been followed

for this length of time. A mortality of 50% was found by Bando et al (1996) during the first postoperative year after the first stage of palliation. They followed 50 newborns undergoing surgery from 1989 to 1995. In another large series, the mortality reported in the first month after first-stage procedures performed in 212 patients between 1983 and 1993 was 46% (Forbess et al, 1995). A smaller series from a British centre reported 41% hospital mortality in 17 patients undergoing the Norwood procedure (Bu'Lock et al, 1995). In an earlier report, Meliones et al (1990) described how almost four fifths of 57 patients undergoing surgery from 1983 to 1989 died following the first stage of palliation, three quarters of these within the first 30 postoperative days.

On the whole, these results are not greatly encouraging. Indeed, a consortium of 40 hospitals in the USA reported an operative mortality of 53% for babies undergoing staged palliation from 1989 through 1995 (Gutgesell and Massaro, 1995). In one small series of 13 patients undergoing surgery during 1994 and 1995, nonetheless, there was only one operative death following a modified Norwood procedure, and no late deaths (Fraser and Mee, 1995).

Reported follow-up to later stages of palliation is limited, but it is clear that there is continued attrition between stages, mainly between the first and second stages. The results in terms of assessment of measures of outcome other than survival are also discouraging (Dhillon and Redington, 1997). In their study of neuropsychiatric outcome following completion of staged palliation, Hagemo et al (1997) analysed the entire Norwegian national experience to 1996. In this series, 52% of patients died, despite all patients being referred overseas in order that the surgery could be performed by the same experienced team. Of the 15 survivors, 12 had completed the full surgical programme and 10 of these underwent neuropsychiatric assessment. Only three patients had normal gross and fine motor function. Four had abnormal cognitive function and six had problems with attention. Only three children were assessed as having normal neurodevelopment and psychological function. Rogers et al (1995) also assessed neurodevelopment in 11 survivors of staged palliation, of whom seven had completed the full surgical protocol. They found that only 1 of these 11 patients was neurodevelopmentally normal, and even this patient had substantial functional disability. Although these studies have been derived from small numbers of patients, they do suggest that survivors of staged palliation for hypoplastic left heart syndrome have substantial neuropsychiatric morbidity, even in the presence of good haemodynamic results. In this respect, it should be noted that there is a high incidence of microcephaly in infants with hypoplastic left heart syndrome. In the study of Rogers et al (1995), 8 of 11 (73%) patients had acquired microcephaly, with cranial circumferences falling to below the 5th percentile. Cognitive maldevelopment was found to be associated with poor cranial growth, in that 8 of 9 patients with cognitive delay had acquired microcephaly. Hagemo et al (1997) detected microcephaly in 3 of their 10 patients when using the more stringent definition of a cranial circumference below the 2.5th percentile. As already discussed, Glauser et al (1990), in a postmortem study, detected microcephaly (a head circumference below the 2nd percentile) in one third of babies with hypoplastic left heart syndrome. As already emphasized, an additional three tenths of these patients had structural malformations of the brain, including absence of the corpus callosum, holoprosencephaly and abnormalities of the cortical mantle.

The available data for the results of staged palliation suggest a mortality of approximately 50% on intermediate follow-up. There is a striking comparability of statistics for survival amongst centres in the USA (Fraser & Mee, 1995; Forbess et al, 1995; Gutgesell and Massaro, 1995; Bando et al, 1996; Bove and Lloyd, 1996) and in the United Kingdom. It could be argued that referral to a surgical team with particular expertise would yield better results, but the overall mortality was 52% with just such a team in the series reported by Hagemo et al (1997), albeit that patients were transferred abroad for surgery.

CARDIAC TRANSPLANTATION

In general, there has been a lower early mortality following cardiac transplantation. The consortium of 40 university hospitals in the USA reported an operative mortality of 42%, although it is difficult to ascertain the ages at which the transplants were performed and whether any of the patients had previously undergone staged palliation (Gutgesell and Massaro, 1995). In a centre utilizing both staged palliation and transplantation, the mortality was 24% at 1 year for newborns undergoing transplantation between 1989 and 1995 compared with 50% early mortality following the first stage of surgical palliation (Bando et al, 1996).

Although the mortality for cardiac transplantation appears to be lower than that for staged palliation, this must be viewed in the context of limited availability of suitable donors for neonatal transplantation. In 1995, the median waiting time for infants listed for cardiac transplantation in the United States of America was 53 days (Gutgesell and Massaro, 1995). It has been recommended that, in the event of a donor being unavailable by the age of 30 days, there should be elective crossover to staged palliation, even though the survival with the latter approach is poor. It is also the case, however, that the results of transplantation after this time are substantially worse in most centres (Bando et al, 1996). Suitable donors are even harder to find in the Ubuted Kingdom. Stuart and colleagues (1991) identified a major shortfall in potential donors for patients with the hypoplastic left heart syndrome over the 8 years between 1983 and 1990. In the period to 1999, there had been 19 cardiac transplants performed as a primary treatment for hypoplastic left heart syndrome in the United Kingdom, of which only two have survived (data provided by the transplant coordinators of Harefield Hospital, London; Great Ormond Street Hospital, London; and Freeman Hospital, Newcastle-upon-Tyne).

Following transplantation, survivors are committed to life-long immunosuppression, with all its attendant risks. Chronic systemic hypertension is common (Olivari et al, 1990; Bando et al, 1996) and premature coronary arterial disease is beginning to be reported (Braunlin et al, 1991). In the series from Loma Linda, nonetheless, there was a gratifyingly low incidence of mental and psychomotor delay as assessed by the Bayley scales of infant development. Neurological deficit was found in only one tenth of patients, mainly dystonia (Razzouk et al, 1996). Survivors of cardiac transplantation, therefore, seem to exhibit fewer neurological problems than are seen after staged palliation. These are chiefly motor, with relatively little cognitive dysfunction (Lynch et al, 1994). It is difficult, however, to reconcile this observation with the reported incidence of congenital microcephaly and other abnormalities of the brain.

NON-SURGICAL THERAPY

Some clinicians have suggested that it is no longer ethical to abstain from surgical treatment for patients with hypoplastic left heart syndrome. It is worth re-emphasizing, nonetheless, that the currently available data can, at best, only be regarded as intermediate. Increasing concerns regarding the long-term viability of the Fontan circulation, even when performed under ideal circumstances, must add to the uncertainty with which we advise the parents of our patients (Fontan et al, 1990). The results presented by Hagemo et al (1997) and Rogers et al (1995) must prompt us to be more guarded in our expectations of staged palliation. Furthermore, this caution should extend to our counselling of the families of these infants. It is our responsibility to present the facts to parents as they exist today, rather than what we would hope them to be in the future. Whilst we await the results from larger cohorts, babies undergoing surgical palliation for hypoplastic left heart syndrome appear to have an uncertain neurodevelopmental outlook, even in those with currently satisfactory haemodynamic results.

Non-surgical therapy has been described as passive euthanasia (Storch, 1992). Many contemporary practitioners in the field of paediatric cardiology and cardiac surgery feel this approach to be nihilistic and non-progressive. A potent argument in their favour is the success of surgical approaches in other congenital cardiac defects, defects that in the past were themselves thought to be inoperable. This viewpoint must then be tempered by the known mortality and morbidity following existing surgical approaches and by the lack of knowledge concerning the long-term consequences in survivors of the Fontan circulation and cardiac transplantation. In some instances, it can be entirely appropriate to provide terminal supportive care for a baby with hypoplastic left heart syndrome for whom informed parents have decided not to opt for surgical therapy. Furthermore, it is important that parents are supported in such a decision in an environment that permits and encourages them to grieve. It should be suggested that parents in this situation, if they wish, take their child home. If this option is chosen, appropriate paediatric support should be provided in the community. All parents must be offered counselling, including genetic advice, together with detailed fetal echocardiographic screening in subsequent pregnancies.

REFERENCES

Abbott M E 1936 Atlas of Congenital Cardiac Diseases. American Heart Association, New York, p 48–61

Allan L D 1993 Fetal diagnosis of fatal congenital heart disease. Journal of Heart and Lung Transplantation 12: S159–S160

Allan L D, Crawford D C, Chita S K, Anderson R H, Tynan M J 1986 Familial recurrence of congenital heart disease in a prospective series of mothers referred for fetal echocardiography. American Journal of Cardiology 58: 334–337

Allan L D, Sharland G, Tynan M J 1989 The natural history of the hypoplastic left heart syndrome. International Journal of Cardiology 25: 341–343

Allan L D, Cook A, Sullivan I, Sharland G K 1991 Hypoplastic left heart syndrome: effects of fetal echocardiography on birth prevalence. Lancet 337: 959–961

Anderson R H, Ho S Y, Zuberbuhler J R, Moulton A L, Gerlis L M 1986 Surgical anatomy and definitions. Surgery for hypoplastic left heart syndrome: a fiction? In: Marceletti C, Anderson R H, Becker A E, Corno A, di Carlo D, Mazzera E (eds) Paediatric cardiology, vol 6. Churchill Livingstone, Edinburgh, p 111–126

Antonelli D, Antonelli J, Rosenfeld T 1990 Noonan's syndrome associated with hypoplastic left heart. Cardiology 77: 62–65

Baffa J M, Chen S L, Guttenberg M E, Norwood W I, Weinberg P M 1992 Coronary artery abnormalities and right ventricular histology in hypoplastic left heart syndrome. Journal of the American College of Cardiology 20: 350–358

Bailey L L, Gundry S R 1990 Hypoplastic left heart syndrome. Pediatric Clinics of North America 37: 137–150

Bando K, Turrentine M W, Sun K et al 1996 Surgical management of hypoplastic left heart syndrome. Annals of Thoracic Surgery 62: 70–76

Barber G 1986 The significance of preoperative tricuspid regurgitation in hypoplastic left heart syndrome. Circulation 74: II–36

Barber G, Helton J G, Aglira B A et al 1988 The significance of tricuspid regurgitation in hypoplastic left–heart syndrome. American Heart Journal 116: 1563–1567

Barber G, Chin A J, Murphy J D, Pigott J D, Norwood W I 1989 Hypoplastic left heart syndrome: lack of correlation between preoperative demographic and laboratory findings and survival following palliative surgery. Pediatric Cardiology 10: 129–134

Barnea O, Austin E H, Richman B, Santamore W P 1994 Balancing the circulation: theoretic optimization of pulmonary/systemic flow ratio in hypoplastic left heart syndrome. Journal of the American College of Cardiology 24: 1376–1381

Bash S E, Huhta J C, Vick G W 3, Gutgesell H P, Ott D A 1986 Hypoplastic left heart syndrome: is echocardiography accurate enough to guide surgical palliation? Journal of the American College of Cardiology 7: 610–616

Berning R A, Silverman N H, Villegas M, Sahn D J, Martin G R, Rice M J 1996 Reversed shunting across the ductus arteriosus or atrial septum in utero heralds severe congenital heart disease. Journal of the American College of Cardiology 27: 481–486

Bernstein H S, Moore P, Stanger P, Silverman N H 1995 The levoatriocardinal vein: morphology and echocardiographic identification of the pulmonary–systemic connection. Journal of the American College of Cardiology 26: 995–1001

Bharati S, Lev M 1984 The surgical anatomy of hypoplasia of aortic tract complex. Journal of Thoracic and Cardiovascular Surgery 88: 97–101

Blake D M, Copel J A, Kleinman C S 1991 Hypoplastic left heart syndrome: prenatal diagnosis, clinical profile, and management. American Journal of Obstetrics and Gynecology 165: 529–534

Bove E L, Lloyd T R 1996 Staged reconstruction for hypoplastic left heart syndrome. Contemporary results. Annals of Surgery 224: 387–394

Braunlin E A, Hunter D W, Canter C E et al 1991 Coronary artery disease in pediatric cardiac transplant recipients receiving triple-drug immunosuppression. Circulation 84 (Suppl III): 303–309

Brownell L G, Shokeir M H 1976 Inheritance of hypoplastic left heart syndrome (HLHS): further observations. Clinical Genetics 9: 245–249

Bu'Lock F A, Stumper O, Jagtap R et al 1995 Surgery for infants with a hypoplastic systemic ventricle and severe outflow obstruction: early results with a modified Norwood procedure. British Heart Journal 73: 456–461

Chang A C, Huhta J C, Yoon G Y et al 1991 Diagnosis, transport, and outcome in fetuses with left ventricular outflow tract obstruction. Journal of Thoracic and Cardiovascular Surgery 102: 841–848

Consevage M W, Seip J R, Belchis D A, Davis A T, Baylen B G, Rogan P K 1996 Association of a mosaic chromosomal 22q11 deletion with hypoplastic left heart syndrome. American Journal of Cardiology 77: 1023–1025

Cooley D A 1990 Surgical treatment of cardiac neoplasms: 32 year experience. Journal of Thoracic and Cardiovascular Surgery 38: 176–182

de la Pompa J L, Timmerman, L A, Takimoto H et al 1998 Role of the NF-ATc transcription factor in morphogenesis of cardiac valves and septum. Nature 392: 182–186 de Leval M R, Kilner P, Gewillig M, Bull C 1988 Total cavopulmonary connection: a logical alternative to atriopulmonary connection for complex Fontan operations. Journal of Thoracic and Cardiovascular Surgeon 96: 682–695

Dhillon R, Redington A 1997 Outcome of surgical approaches to the hypoplastic left heart syndrome. Cardiology in the Young 7: 242–244

Douville E C, Sade R M, Fyfe D A 1991 Hemi-Fontan operation in surgery for single ventricle: a preliminary report. Annals of Thoracic Surgery 51: 893–900

Edwards J E 1953 Pathology of the Heart Charles C Thomas, Springfield, IL, p 407

Ehrlich M, Bierman F Z, Ellis K, Gersony W M 1986 Hypoplastic left heart syndrome: report of a unique survivor. Journal of the American College of Cardiology 7: 361–365

Ferencz C, Loffredo C A, Correa-Villasenor A, Wilson P D 1997 Genetic and environmental risk factors of major cardiovascular malformations – the Baltimore–Washington infant study 1981–1989. In Anderson R H (ed) Perspectives in pediatric cardiology, vol 5. Futura, Armonk, NY, p 178–189

Fong L V, Lee S H, Salmon A P 1992 Diagnosis of cerebral arteriovenous malformation by colour Doppler examination. European Heart Journal 13: 414–417

Fontan F, Kirklin J W, Fernandez G et al 1990 Outcome after a 'perfect' Fontan operation. Circulation 81: 1520–1536

Forbess J M, Cook N, Roth S J, Serraf A, Mayer J E Jr, Jonas R A 1995 Ten-year institutional experience with palliative surgery for hypoplastic left heart syndrome. Risk factors related to stage I mortality. Circulation 92 (suppl II): 262–266

Fraser C D Jr, Mee R B 1995 Modified Norwood procedure for hypoplastic left heart syndrome. Annals of Thoracic Surgery 60: S546–S549

Freedom R M, Culham J A, Moes C A, Harrington D P 1976 Selective aortic root angiography in the hypoplastic left heart syndrome. European Journal of Cardiology 4: 25–29

Freedom R M, Culham J A, Rowe R D 1981 Left atrial to coronary sinus fenestration (partially unroofed coronary sinus). Morphological and angiocardiographic observations. British Heart Journal 46: 63–68

Fyler D C, Buckley L P, Hellenbrand W E, Cohn W E 1980 Report of the New England Regional Infant Cardiac Program. Pediatrics 65: 376–461

Giannico S, Corno A, Marino B et al 1992 Total extracardiac right heart bypass. Circulation 86(suppl II): 110–117

Gibbs J L, Wren C, Watterson K G, Hunter S, Hamilton J R 1993 Stenting of the arterial duct combined with banding of the pulmonary arteries and atrial septectomy or septostomy: a new approach to palliation for the hypoplastic left heart syndrome. British Heart Journal 69: 551–555

Glauser T A, Zackai E, Weinberg P, Clancy R 1989 Holt–Oram syndrome associated with the hypoplastic left heart syndrome. Clinical Genetics 36: 69–72

Glauser T A, Rorke L B, Weinberg P M, Clancy R R 1990 Congenital brain anomalies associated with the hypoplastic left heart syndrome. Pediatrics 85: 984–990

Guenthard J, Buehler E, Jaeggi E, Wyler F 1994 Possible genes for left heart formation on 11q23.3. Annals of Genetics 37: 143–146

Gutgesell H P, Massaro T A 1995 Management of hypoplastic left heart syndrome in a consortium of university hospitals. American Journal of Cardiology 76: 809–811

Hagemo P S, Rasmussen M, Bryhn G, Vandvik I H 1997 Hypoplastic left heart syndrome multiprofessional follow-up in the mid-term following palliative procedures. Cardiology in the Young 7: 248–253

Hammon J J W, Lupinetti F M, Maples M D et al 1988 Predictors of operative mortality in critical valvular aortic stenosis presenting in infancy. Annals of Thoracic Surgery 45: 537–540

Harh J Y, Paul M H, Gallen W J, Friedberg D Z, Kaplan S 1973 Experimental production of hypoplastic left heart syndrome in the chick embryo. American Journal of Cardiology 31: 51–56

Hawkins J A, Doty D B 1984 Aortic atresia: morphologic characteristics affecting survival and operative palliation. Journal of Thoracic and Cardiovascular Surgery 88: 620–626

Helton J G, Aglira B A, Chin A J, Murphy J D, Pigott J D, Norwood W I 1986 Analysis of potential anatomic or physiologic determinants of outcome of palliative surgery for hypoplastic left heart syndrome. Circulation 74(suppl I): 70–76

Holmes L B, Rose V, Child A H, Kratzer W 1974 Hypoplastic left heart. Evidence for possible autosomal recessive inheritance. [Comment] Birth Defects 10: 228–230

Hornberger L K, Sanders S P, Rein A J, Spevak P J, Parness I A, Colan S D 1995 Left heart obstructive lesions and left ventricular growth in the midtrimester fetus. A longitudinal study. Circulation 92: 1531–1538

Jacobs M L, Rychik J, Rome J J et al 1996 Early reduction of the volume work of the single ventricle: the hemi-Fontan operation. Annals of Thoracic Surgery 62: 456–461

Jobes D R, Nicolson S C, Steven J M, Miller M, Jacobs M L, Norwood W I Jr 1992 Carbon dioxide prevents pulmonary overcirculation in hypoplastic left heart syndrome. Annals of Thoracic Surgery 54: 150–151

Jonas R A 1991 Intermediate procedures after first-stage Norwood operation facilitate subsequent repair. Annals of Thoracic Surgery 52: 696–700

Keeton B R, Macartney F J, Hunter S et al 1979 Univentricular heart of right ventricular type with double or common inlet. Circulation 59: 403–411

Kliegman R M, Behrman R E 1992 Bacteremia and septicemia. In: Behrman RE, (ed.) Nelson textbook of pediatrics, 14th edn. Saunders, Philadelphiap, PA, 681–682

Lang P, Jonas R A, Norwood W I, Mayer J E Jr, Castaneda A R 1985 The surgical anatomy of hypoplasia of aortic tract complex. [Letter] Journal of Thoracic and Cardiovascular Surgery 89: 149–150

Latson L A, Cheatham J P, Gutgesell H P 1981 Relation of the echocardiographic estimate of left ventricular size to mortality in infants with severe left ventricular outflow obstruction. American Journal of Cardiology 48: 887–891

Lev M 1952 Pathological anatomy and interrelationship of hypoplasia of the aortic tract complexes. Laboratory Investigation 1: 61–70

Lev M, Arcilla R, Rimoldi H J A, Licata R H, Gasul B M 1963 Premature closure or narrowing of the foramen ovale. American Heart Journal 65: 638–647

Lin A E 1988 Turner syndrome and hypoplastic left-heart syndrome. [Letter] American Journal of Diseases in Childhood 142: 122–132

Lloyd T R, Evans T C, Marvin W J Jr 1986 Morphologic determinants of coronary blood flow in the hypoplastic left heart syndrome. American Heart Journal 112: 666–671

Ludman P, Foale R, Alexander N, Nihoyannopoulos P 1990 Cross sectional echocardiographic identification of hypoplastic left heart syndrome and differentiation from other causes of right ventricular overload. British Heart Journal 63: 355–361

Lynch B J, Glauser T A, Canter C, Spray T 1994 Neurologic complications of pediatric heart transplantation. Archives of Pediatric and Adolescent Medicine 148: 973–979

Machii M, Becker A E 1995 Nature of coarctation in hypoplastic left heart syndrome. Annals of Thoracic Surgery 59: 1491–1494

McGarry K M, Taylor J F, Macartney F J 1980 Aortic atresia occurring with complete transposition of great arteries. British Heart Journal 44: 711–713

Meliones J N, Snider A R, Bove E L, Rosenthal A, Rosen D A 1990 Longitudinal results after first-stage palliation for hypoplastic left heart syndrome. Circulation 82(suppl IV): 151–156

Mocellin R, Sauer U, Simon B, Comazzi M, Sebening F, Buhlmeyer K 1983 Reduced left ventricular size and endocardial fibroelastosis as correlates of mortality in newborns and young infants with severe aortic valve stenosis. Pediatric Cardiology 4: 265–272

Natowicz M, Kelley R I 1987 Association of Turner syndrome with hypoplastic left-heart syndrome. American Journal of Diseases in Childhood 141: 218–220

Natowicz M, Chatten J, Clancy R et al 1988 Genetic disorders and major extracardiac anomalies associated with the hypoplastic left heart syndrome. Pediatrics 82: 698–706

Noonan J A, Nadas A S 1958 The hypoplastic left heart syndrome. Pediatric Clinics of North America 5: 1029–1056

Nora J J, Nora A H 1978 The evolution of specific genetic and environmental counseling in congenital heart diseases. Circulation 57: 205–213

Norwood W I, Lang P, Hansen D D 1983 Physiologic repair of aortic atresia-hypoplastic left heart syndrome. New England Journal of Medicine 308: 23–26

Olivari M T, Kubo S H, Braunlin E A, Bolman R M, Ring W S 1990 Five-year experience with triple-drug immunosuppressive therapy in cardiac transplantation. Circulation 82(suppl IV): 276–280

Pellegrino P A, Thiene G 1976 Aortic valve atresia with a normally developed left ventricle. Chest 69: 121–122

Perry L W, Scott L P3, Shapiro S R, Chandra R S, Roberts W C 1977 Atresia of the aortic valve with ventricular septal defect. A clinicopathologic study of four newborns. Chest 72: 757–761

Pinto C A M, Ho S Y, Redington A, Shinebourne E A, Anderson R H 1993 Morphological features of the levoatriocardinal vein (or pulmonary-to-systemic collateral) vein. Pediatric Pathology 13: 751–761

Ranger A M, Grusby M J, Hodge M R et al 1998 The transcription factor NF-ATc is essential for cardiac valve formation. Nature 392: 186–190

Razzouk A J, Chinnock R E, Gundry S R et al 1996 Transplantation as a primary treatment for hypoplastic left heart syndrome: intermediate-term results. Annals of Thoracic Surgery 62: 1–7

Rhodes L A, Colan S D, Perry S B, Jonas R A, Sanders S P 1991 Predictors of survival in neonates with critical aortic stenosis. Circulation 84: 2325–2335 [Published erratum appears in Circulation 1995 92(7): 2005]

Riordan C J, Randsbeck F, Storey J H, Montgomery W D, Santamore W P, Austin E H 1996 Effects of oxygen, positive end–expiratory pressure, and carbon dioxide on oxygen delivery in an animal model of the univentricular heart. Journal of Thoracic and Cardiovascular Surgery 112: 644–654

Roberts W C, Perry L W, Chandra R S, Myers G E, Shapiro S R, Scott L P 1976 Aortic valve atresia: a new classification based on necropsy study of 73 cases. American Journal of Cardiology 37: 753–756

Rogers B T, Msall M E, Buck G M et al 1995 Neurodevelopmental outcome of infants with hypoplastic left heart syndrome. Journal of Pediatrics 126: 496–498

Rossi M B, Ho S Y, Tasker R C 1986 Absent aortic valve leaflets. International Journal of Cardiology 11: 235–237

Ruckman R N, Van Praagh R 1978 Anatomic types of congenital mitral stenosis: report of 49 autopsy cases with consideration of diagnosis and surgical implications. American Journal of Cardiology 42: 592–601

Ruiz C E, Gamra H, Zhang H P, Garcia E J, Boucek M M 1993a Brief report: stenting of the ductus arteriosus as a bridge to cardiac transplantation in infants with the hypoplastic left-heart syndrome. New England Journal of Medicine 328: 1605–1608

Ruiz C E, Zhang H P, Larsen R L 1993b The role of interventional cardiology in pediatric heart transplantation. Journal of Heart and Lung Transplantation 12: S164–S167

Rychik J, Gullquist S D, Jacobs M L, Norwood W I 1996 Doppler echocardiographic analysis of flow in the ductus arteriosus of infants with hypoplastic left heart syndrome: relationship of flow patterns to systemic oxygenation and size of interatrial communication. Journal of the American Society of Echocardiographers 9: 166–173

Sauer U, Gittenberger-de Groot A C, Geishauser M, Babic R, Buhlmeyer K 1989 Coronary arteries in the hypoplastic left heart syndrome. Histopathologic and histometrical studies and implications for surgery. Circulation 80(suppl I): 168–176

Schall S A, Dalldorf F G 1984 Premature closure of the foramen ovale and hypoplasia of the left heart. International Journal of Cardiology 5: 103–107

Seliem M A, Chin A J, Norwood W I 1992 Patterns of anomalous pulmonary venous connection/drainage in hypoplastic left heart syndrome: diagnostic role of Doppler color flow mapping and surgical implications. Journal of the American College of Cardiology 19: 135–141

Sharland G K, Chita S K, Fagg N L 1991 Left ventricular dysfunction in the fetus: relation to aortic valve anomalies and endocardial fibroelastosis. British Heart Journal 66: 419–424

Sinha S N, Rusnak S L, Sommers H M, Cole R B, Muster A J, Paul M H 1968 Hypoplastic left ventricle syndrome.

Analysis of thirty autopsy cases in infants with surgical considerations. American Journal of Cardiology 21: 166–173

Slack M C, Kirby W C, Towbin J A et al 1994 Stenting of the ductus arteriosus in hypoplastic left heart syndrome as an ambulatory bridge to cardiac transplantation. American Journal of Cardiology 74: 636–637

Storch T G 1992 Passive euthanasia for hypoplastic left heart syndrome. [Editorial] American Journal of Diseases in Childhood 146: 1426

Stuart A G, Wren C, Sharples P M, Hunter S, Hey E N 1991 Hypoplastic left heart syndrome: more potential transplant recipients than suitable donors. Lancet 337: 957–959

Suzuki K, Doi S, Oku K et al 1990 Hypoplastic left heart syndrome with premature closure of foramen ovale: report of an unusual type of totally anomalous pulmonary venous return. Heart and Vessels 5: 117–119

Tandon R, Becker A E, Moller J H, Edwards J E 1974 Double inlet left ventricle. Straddling tricuspid valve. British Heart Journal 36: 747–759

Thiene G, Gallucci V, Macartney F J, del Torso S, Pellegrino P A, Anderson R H 1979 Anatomy of aortic atresia. Cases presenting with a ventricular septal defect. Circulation 59: 173–178

Thiene G, Daliento L, Frescura C, de Tommasi M, Macartney F J, Anderson R H 1981 Atresia of left atrioventricular orifice. Anatomical investigation in 62 cases. British Heart Journal 45: 393–401

van Egmond H, Orye E, Praet M, Coppens M, Devloo Blancquaert A 1988 Hypoplastic left heart syndrome and 45X karyotype. British Heart Journal 60: 69–71

Vargas Barron J, Rijlaarsdam M, Romero Cardenas A et al 1992 Hypoplastic left heart syndrome: report of a case of spontaneous survival to adulthood. American Heart Journal 123: 1713–1719

von Rueden T J, Moller J H 1978 The electrocardiogram in aortic valvular atresia. Chest 73: 66–68

Watson D G, Rowe R D 1962 Aortic valve atresia. Report of 43 cases. Journal of the American Medical Association 179: 14–21

Weinberg P M, Chin A J, Murphy J D, Pigott J D, Norwood W I 1986 Postmortem echocardiography and tomographic anatomy of hypoplastic left heart syndrome after palliative surgery. American Journal of Cardiology 58: 1228–1232

46

Fallot's tetralogy

E. A. Shinebourne and R. H. Anderson

INTRODUCTION

Tetralogy of Fallot is a congenital cardiac anomaly recognized on the basis of its characteristic anatomy. All affected individuals have a large ventricular septal defect, muscular obstruction within the right ventricular outflow tract, rightward deviation of the aorta with biventricular connection of the valvar leaflets so that its orifice overrides the ventricular septum, and right ventricular hypertrophy. According to Marquis (1956), the malformation was first described by Nicholas Steno in 1673, but the lesion earned its eponym as a result of a series of papers published by Fallot in 1888, the diagnosis made in life being confirmed at postmortem. Precise definition of the anomaly remains difficult. As Lev and Eckner (1964) have stated, no two cases of tetralogy are exactly the same. It can be argued that Fallot's tetralogy is not a discrete entity, forming instead part of a spectrum of cardiac anomalies (Van Mierop and Wiglesworth, 1963; Goor et al, 1971). Consequently, when obstruction within the right ventricular outflow tract is minimal, distinction from ventricular septal defect with aortic overriding is hard to make, even using anatomical criterions (Oppenheimer-Dekker et al, 1985). When obstruction is complete, the condition represents the most common variant of pulmonary atresia with ventricular septal defect. All hearts with tetralogy of Fallot, nonetheless, are unified by the anatomical hallmark of subpulmonary infundibular narrowing owing to anterior and cephalad deviation of the septal insertion of the outlet (infundibular) septum relative to the septomarginal trabeculation, combined with hypertrophy of septoparietal trabeculations at the mouth of the subpulmonary infundibulum. The feature of deviation of the muscular outlet septum accounts both for the ventricular septal defect and a more rightward position of the aortic root than normal (Becker et al, 1975). The precise anatomy, nonetheless, and hence the haemodynamic consequences, vary considerably. Problems also exist when the muscular outlet septum and the septal components of the subpulmonary infundibulum are absent. Another spectrum of morphology exists in this respect whereby the outlet septum, usually prominent, becomes increasingly hypoplastic. At the end of this spectrum, when the outlet septum is absent, the hearts can self-evidently no longer satisfy the criterion of showing anterocephalad deviation of the muscular outlet septum. Yet patients in whom the subpulmonary infundibulum is deficient and the outlet septum is absent (this is particularly common in the Far East and South America (Ando, 1974; Neirotti et al, 1978)) are usually still classified within the spectrum of tetralogy (Becker, 1992). All of these morphologic conundrums will be explored in this chapter.

INCIDENCE, PREVALENCE AND AETIOLOGY

Of infants born with congenital heart disease, approximately 3.5% will have tetralogy of Fallot (Mitchell et al, 1971). Expressed in another way, there will be 0.28 per 1000, or 1 in 3600, livebirths. Males and females are equally affected. The frequency of tetralogy of Fallot compared with other forms of cyanotic congenital heart disease increases with age. This is largely because infants with more lethal cardiac anomalies tend to die, whereas many with tetralogy of Fallot will survive beyond infancy even without treatment.

As with many congenital cardiac anomalies, precise aetiology is unknown. The majority of cases are sporadic, although a few familial occurrences have been reported (Pitt, 1962; Ehlers and Engle, 1966). According to Nora et al (1970), the risk of recurrence in siblings is about 3% if there are no other affected first-degree relatives. Our experience suggests this view to be perhaps a little pessimistic. Rubella in the first trimester of pregnancy has been implicated in a small number of cases (Gibson and Lewis, 1952; Brinton and Campbell, 1953). Viruses have been isolated from patients with severe pulmonary arterial hypoplasia (Celermajer et al, 1969). Patterson et al (1974) have bred Keeshond dogs to produce a spectrum of inherited malformations of the ventricular outflow tracts that include anomalies similar to tetralogy of Fallot. Their experiments indicate a polygenic model of inheritance in which the genes act additively to produce the spectrum of maldevelopment. More recent studies have shown an unequivocal link between the morphologic entity of tetralogy and abnormal migration of cells from the neural crest. Dosage of rats with bisdiamine, known to inhibit migration from the neural crest when given at critical periods of development, produces tetralogy of Fallot in all its variants (Momma et al, 1990; Jackson et al, 1995). In a significant proportion of clinical cases, furthermore, there are microdeletions of the q11 region of chromosome 22. Di George syndrome and the velocardiofacial syndrome (also known as the conotruncal anomaly face syndrome) (Burn et al, 1993) are well known to be associated with this chromosomal anomaly, now known as Catch 22 syndrome. This relationship adds credence to the significance of abnormal migration of cells from the neural crest. In series of consecutive patients studied with tetralogy of Fallot, this microdeletion has been found in up to a quarter, irrespective of whether the patients have the typical dysmorphic features of the syndromes (Trainer et al, 1996; Webber et al, 1996). Therefore, there is a place for investigation of the genome using fluorescent in situ hybridization in all patients with tetralogy of Fallot. In this respect, a significant proportion of patients having tetralogy with pulmonary atresia rather than stenosis, and with pulmonary arterial supply through systemic-to-pulmonary collateral arteries, also have deletions in their chromosome 22, supporting still further the inclusion of these patients within the overall spectrum of tetralogy of Fallot (Digilio et al, 1996).

The majority of subjects with tetralogy of Fallot can now be expected to survive 'corrective surgery' and reach adult life. Women patients may well ask the question 'is it safe for me to become pregnant?', while both women and men will wish to know the risks of their progeny inheriting the condition. It has been known for some time that the incidence of congenital heart disease in children born to women with congenital heart disease is higher than in the normal population (Czeizel et al, 1982; Whittemore et al, 1982). Studies by Dennis and Warren (1981) and by Whittemore et al (1994) have shown no differences in the incidence of affected children whether the mother or father has tetralogy of Fallot. The latter group gives a figure of approximately 10%, slighter higher than previous studies (Zellers et al, 1990), for the offspring being affected, although this risk is for any congenital heart malformation, including minor lesions not requiring intervention. The risk is much higher, at above 40%, if the affected parent has a sibling with the same or a similar cardiac anomaly. It could well be that identification of patients with a microdeletion of chromosome 22q11 will allow refinement of these calculations for risk of recurrence.

ANATOMY

OVERALL DESCRIPTION OF THE OUTFLOW TRACT

The anatomical hallmark of tetralogy of Fallot is anterocephalad deviation of the insertion of the muscular outlet septum relative to the rest of the ventricular septum. This feature combines with hypertrophy of septoparietal trabeculations to produce narrowing of the subpulmonary infundibulum. Both are needed to provide the characteristic morphology. In the normal heart, the muscular outlet septum is an insignificant structure, inserted and buried between the limbs of the prominent septomarginal trabeculation. Indeed, it is so fully incorporated into the septum (Figure 46.1) that it is not possible to distinguish an 'outlet septal' area from the dominant component of the supraventricular crest, namely the free-standing subpulmonary infundibulum and its continuation as the ventriculo-infundibular fold. In tetralogy, however, outlet septum and ventriculo-infundibular fold are divorced from each other, and neither muscular structure is inserted between the limbs of the septomarginal trabeculation. Instead, the ventricular septal defect and the overriding component of the aorta are situated between, and bordered by, these various muscle bundles (Figure 46.2). The most noticeable and constant feature of their divorce is that the septal insertion of the outlet septum is either fused with, or is cephalad and anterior to, the anterior limb of the septomarginal trabeculation. The septal malalignment thus produced is one of the major architectural features of the infundibular stenosis. The other crucial feature is hypertrophy of the septoparietal trabeculations, the two together 'squeezing' the subpulmonary infundibulum. Both these features are needed to produce tetralogy (Figure 46.3a), since the outlet septum can be deviated in anterocephalad direction without there being subpulmonary stenosis (Figure 46.3b). This latter arrangement is known as the Eisenmenger complex (Oppenheimer-Dekker et al, 1985).

The simple fact that the outlet septum, the ventriculo-infundibular fold and the septomarginal trabeculation are separated and distinct from each other is at the root of much of the confusion and controversy that has bedevilled description of the abnormal outflow tracts. This is because each of these three structures, at various times and in various places, had been nominated as a component of the 'crista'. Consequently, when the crista was encountered in descriptions of tetralogy, it was difficult to be sure to which of the different structures it referred. It was against this background that we suggested that the term crista, or its translation as supraventricular crest, be reserved for description of the muscular structure separating the attachments of the leaflets of the tricuspid and pulmonary valves in the normal right ventricular outflow tract. In situations where the muscular structures making up the normal subpulmonary infundibulum are separated

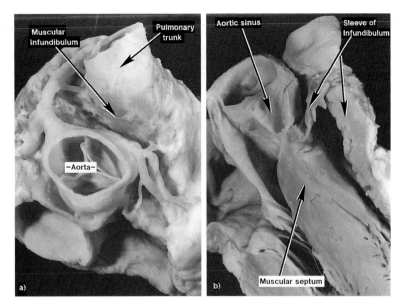

Figure 46.1. The normal heart. (a) The pulmonary trunk is supported on an extensive sleeve of free-standing subpulmonary musculature. (b) A long-axis section shows the tissue plane between the posterior wall of this infundibulum and the sinuses of the aortic root. There is no discrete muscular outlet septum in the normal heart.

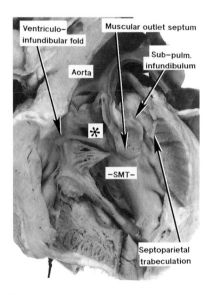

Figure 46.2. The essence of tetralogy is divorce of the hypertrophied outlet septum from the rest of the muscular ventricular septum. The outlet septum, which cannot be identified as such in the normal heart (compare with Figure 46.1) has septal and parietal extensions. The septal extension joins the rest of the muscular septum anterocephalad to the anterior limb of the septomarginal trabeculation (SMT), thus narrowing the subpulmonary infundibulum. Because of the overriding of the aortic valve, the ventriculo-infundibular fold now separates the attachments of the leaflets of the aortic and tricuspid valves. The star shows the ventricular septal defect.

one from the other, as is the case in tetralogy, we suggested that each structure be accounted for in its own right using descriptive and mutually exclusive terms (Anderson et al, 1977a). This is the basic convention to be followed here (Figure 46.4). Any muscular structure interposing between the subpulmonary and subaortic

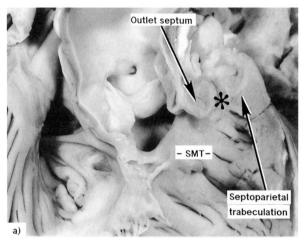

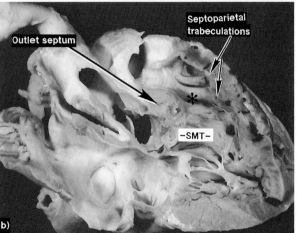

Figure 46.3. In addition to anterocephalad deviation of the muscular outlet septum, it is also necessary to have hypertrophy of septoparietal trabeculations (a) to produce tetralogy of Fallot. (b) This feature, which narrows the subpulmonary infundibulum (asterisk) is lacking in the so-called Eisenmenger defect.

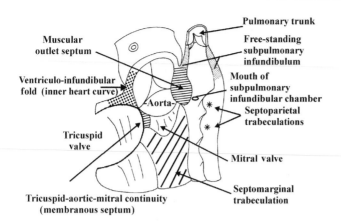

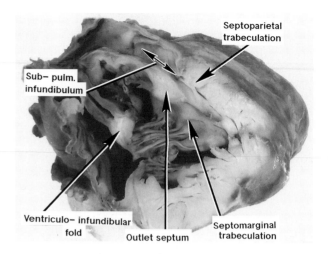

Figure 46.4. The terms to be used to describe the muscular components of the right ventricular outflow tract are illustrated here in the setting of a perimembranous ventricular septal defect (see text for further discussion).

Figure 46.5. The various muscular structures surrounding the interventricular communication are revealed by a cut simulating the right oblique subcostal echocardiographic projection. Sub-pulm., subpulmonary.

outflow tracts is called the 'outlet septum'. This septum has septal and parietal insertions and is contiguous with the sleeve of free-standing subpulmonary infundibular musculature. Any muscular structure separating the leaflets of an arterial from an atrioventricular valve is called the 'ventriculo-infundibular fold'. This represents the musculature of the inner heart curve. The extensive septal trabeculation of the morphologically right ventricle is called the 'septomarginal trabeculation'. It has a body together with anterior and posterior limbs, the latter components usually supporting the inferior margin of the ventricular septal defect. The moderator band arises apically from its body and crosses to the free ventricular wall. The moderator band is, however, only one of a series of muscle bars that extend to the parietal wall. The others are the septoparietal trabeculations (Goor and Lillehei, 1975). Using these terms, the different structures surrounding the ventricular septal defect can be described simply, and with less fear of causing confusion (Figure 46.5).

VARIABILITY IN THE VENTRICULAR SEPTAL DEFECT

The typical ventricular septal deficiency in tetralogy opens beneath the overriding aortic valvar orifice. It can thus be considered an outlet defect. The muscular outlet septum itself, however, is usually well formed but is malaligned relative to the rest of the muscular septum. Indeed, as already discussed, the essence of tetralogy is anterocephalad deviation of the septal insertion of the outlet septum such that it becomes a right ventricular rather than an interventricular structure, this deviation coexisting with hypertrophy of the septomarginal trabeculations (Figure 46.3a). It is this outlet septum, and its fusion with the anterior limb of the septomarginal trabeculation, that forms the anterior margins of the defect. The crest of the muscular ventricular septum is then reinforced by the limbs of the septomarginal trabeculation, and these two structures form the floor of the defect.

Because of the septal malalignment, the roof of the defect is formed by the attachments of the leaflets of the overriding aortic valve to the ventriculo-infundibular fold. Indeed, because of the overriding of the aortic orifice, problems exist simply in defining the nature of the ventricular septal defect. Any one of a host of planes within the cone of space subtended from the valvar leaflets to the crest of the septum can be nominated as a septal defect (Figures 46.6 and 46.7). We concentrate on the right ventricular margin of the cone, because this is where the surgeon places the patch to repair the malformation. With the defect defined in this fashion, the area that shows most anatomical variability is the posteroinferior quadrant. In about four fifths of patients (Rosenquist et al, 1973; Becker et al, 1975; Anderson et al, 1981), this margin is formed by fibrous continuity between the leaflets of the aortic, mitral and tricuspid valves (Figure 46.8). From this standpoint, the defect is identical to typical perimembranous defects opening to the outlet of the right ventricle in the absence of aortic overriding. In our view, it is unnecessary to consider the defect in tetralogy as a separate entity simply because it coexists with malalignment of the outlet septum. The defect is unequivocally perimembranous but is also associated with malalignment between the outlet septum and the remainder of the muscular ventricular septum. These anatomical features are reflected in the distribution of the atrioventricular conduction tissues. As in all other hearts with concordant atrioventricular connections, the guides to the location of the atrioventricular node are the landmarks of the triangle of Koch. The penetrating bundle perforates the central fibrous body through the area of aortic–mitral–tricuspid valvar continuity (Figure 46.9). Here, the bundle is frequently overlaid by a remnant of the interventricular membranous septum, which may on occasions become aneurysmal. The septal remnant itself,

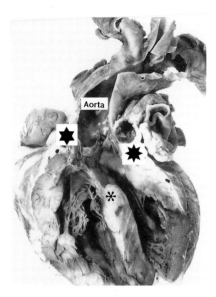

Figure 46.6. This simulated four chamber section shows how the aortic valvar orifice overrides the crest of the muscular septum (asterisk), with right ventricular (6-pointed star) and left ventricular (8-pointed star) entrances to the cone of space thus enclosed (see Figure 46.7).

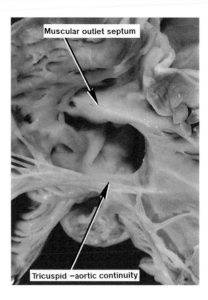

Figure 46.8. The typical defect in tetralogy of Fallot is bordered by extensive fibrous continuity between the leaflets of the aortic, mitral and tricuspid valves. It is, therefore, a perimembranous ventricular septal defect.

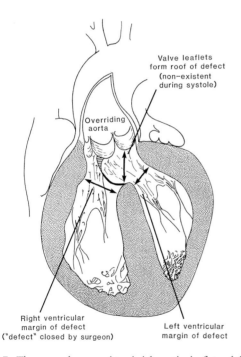

Figure 46.7. The cone of space subtended from the leaflets of the overriding aortic valve to the crest of the muscular ventricular septum.

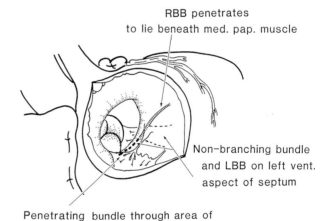

Figure 46.9. Drawings showing the surgeon's view through a right infundibulotomy of a perimembranous defect (upper) and a defect with a muscular posteroinferior rim (lower). The presence of the muscular rim modifies the location of the atrioventricular conduction axis. The usual arrangement is shown for a perimembranous defect in which the axis and left bundle branch (LBB) are carried on the left ventricular (vent.) aspect of the septum well below its crest. med. pap., medial papillary.

called the membranous flap, is safe tissue for anchorage of sutures (Kurosawa et al, 1988), but it lies directly superficial to the penetrating bundle (Howell et al, 1990). Deeply placed sutures in this area are liable to produce complete heart block (Anderson and Becker, 1975). It is safer, therefore, to place sutures through the leaflet of the tricuspid valve, which usually overlaps the membranous flap in this area of the defect. Having perforated, the non-

branching atrioventricular bundle enters the left ventricular part of the aortic outflow tract and almost always veers away from the septal crest. In most patients, therefore, the branching atrioventricular bundle is carried on the left ventricular aspect of the septum (Lev, 1959), staying remote from the septal crest. In a minority of hearts, the bundle may branch directly astride the septum (Titus et al, 1963; Anderson et al, 1977b). Such an arrangement places the bundle at risk should sutures be placed into the crest of the septum. In those cases in which the conduction axis branches astride the septum, the anterior fascicle of the left bundle branch is also at risk from sutures placed on the right ventricular aspect of the septum. In the more usual arrangement, the anterior part of the branching bundle remains well below the septal crest. The right bundle branch then penetrates the septum to descend towards the apex within the substance of the septomarginal trabeculation.

The second most common type of ventricular septal defect, occurring in about one fifth of patients, is characterized by interruption of the area of aortic–tricuspid–valvar continuity by a muscular fold (Figure 46.10). When viewed from the right ventricular aspect, the defect has a complete muscular rim, formed by fusion of the posterior limb of the septomarginal trabeculation with the ventriculo-infundibular fold. A normally formed membranous septum is then present between the muscle fold and the remaining atrioventricular septal structures. The atrioventricular conduction axis is posteroinferior to the membranous septum. As a result, the muscle bundle, together with the membranous septum, separates the conduction tissues from the crest of the ventricular septum (Figure 46.11). When the muscular fold is of good dimensions, as is usually the case, the entire muscular margins of the defect are suitable for anchorage of sutures, none of the rim being 'at risk'. On the left ventricular aspect, however, there is still aortic-to-mitral fibrous valvar continuity, as indeed there is in almost all other examples of tetralogy. Very rarely, nonetheless, hearts can be found with all the other features of tetralogy but in presence of a completely muscular subaortic infundibulum (Dickinson et al, 1982).

There is yet a third variety of the defect, but its existence in tetralogy gives problems in definitions. This is the

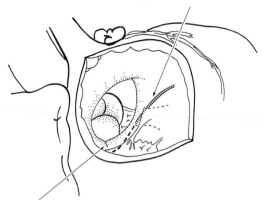

Ventriculo–infundibular fold

fuses with septomarginal trabeculation

– safe conduction axis

Figure 46.11. A similar view to that in Figure 46.9, showing protection of the conduction axis by a muscular posteroinferior rim.

doubly committed juxta-arterial defect, by far the least common in the Western World. This defect is both subaortic and subpulmonary as a consequence of absence of the outlet septum and failure of formation of a complete muscular subpulmonary infundibulum (Figure 46.12). Logically, when the outlet septum is absent, a case can be made for such hearts being excluded from the category of tetralogy, since the hallmark of the lesion has been defined as anterocephalad deviation of the outlet septum (Griffin et al, 1988). However, the anatomy otherwise is exactly that of tetralogy. If the muscular outlet septum were restored, along with the subpulmonary infundibulum, the hearts would be indistinguishable from tetralogy. It is usual, therefore, to include them as examples

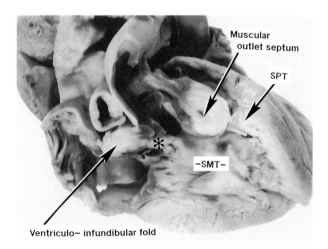

Figure 46.10. An example of a heart with a muscular posteroinferior rim (asterisk) produced by fusion of the posterior limb of the septomarginal trabeculation (SMT) with the ventriculo-infundibular fold. SPT, septoparietal trabeculation.

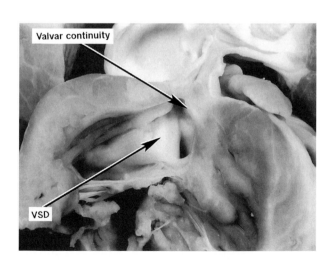

Figure 46.12. Complete absence of the muscular outlet septum, together with the 'septal' components of the subpulmonary infundibulum, produces a doubly committed juxta-arterial defect (VSD) which, in this heart, extends to become perimembranous. It is roofed by fibrous continuity between the leaflets of the aortic and pulmonary valves.

of tetralogy (Becker, 1992). Such defects can be found with aortic–tricuspid valvar continuity (perimembranous) or with a muscular posteroinferior rim, with the attendant implications concerning the location of the atrioventricular conduction tissues. They are much more common in the Far East (Ando, 1974) and South America (Neirotti et al, 1978).

The various types of defect normally present in tetralogy, which open between the outflow tracts, can coexist with defects elsewhere in the septum. Inlet defects are particularly important, be they muscular inlet defects that are discrete from the outlet defects, defects associated with straddling and overriding of the tricuspid valve (Figure 46.13) or perimembranous defects opening between the inlets, which become confluent with the outlet defect. Confluent perimembranous defects extending to open between the inlets can be found with normal atrioventricular septation or as part of an atrioventricular septal defect with common atrioventricular junction (Bharati et al, 1980). The combination of an atrioventricular septal defect with common atrioventricular junction and tetralogy poses additional problems to the surgeon, but these difficulties have now been overcome in centres of excellence (McElhinney et al, 1998). Almost always in tetralogy, the ventricular septal defect is large, approximating in size to the diameter of the aortic root. Rarely, it may be restrictive as a result of the presence of accessory fibrous tissue tags formed at the margins of the defect. Such tags may be derived in part from the tricuspid valve (Neufeld et al, 1960; Hoffman et al, 1960a; Faggian et al, 1983) or may extend from attachment of the tension apparatus of the mitral valve across the left ventricular aspect of the defect (Van Praagh et al, 1970a).

PULMONARY INFUNDIBULAR STENOSIS

The subpulmonary stenosis, which is an essential part of tetralogy, is caused principally by the 'squeeze' between the anterocephalad deviation of the outlet septum and the hypertrophied septoparietal trabeculations (Figures 46.3 and 46.5). Aortic overriding with valvar pulmonary stenosis in the absence of muscular subpulmonary stenosis should not be categorized as tetralogy. As indicated, the anterior component of the subpulmonary obstruction is usually formed from the hypertrophied septoparietal trabeculations extending onto the ventricular free wall (Figure 46.5). Additional hypertrophy of the moderator band, together with apical trabeculations, may produce more proximal stenosis. This gives the arrangement described as a two chambered right ventricle (Rowland et al, 1975). This obstruction is then within the apical trabecular component of the right ventricle and is superimposed on the muscular obstruction occurring at infundibular level (Alva et al, 1999). The subpulmonary infundibulum, distal to the squeeze between outlet septum and septoparietal trabeculations, can itself vary considerably in length. Van Praagh et al (1970b) stated that hypoplasia of the subpulmonary infundibulum was the essence of tetralogy. The measurements taken by Becker et al (1975) and confirmed by Howell et al (1990) showed that the subpulmonary infundibulum was significantly longer than usual when considered for tetralogy as a whole (Figure 46.14). In individual patients, nonetheless, the infundibulum may vary from being excessively long to very hypoplastic, or even to complete absence when the defect is doubly committed (Figure 46.12) (Anderson et al, 1981).

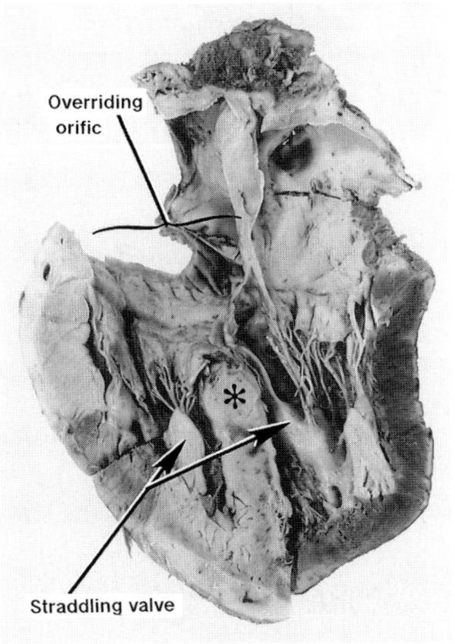

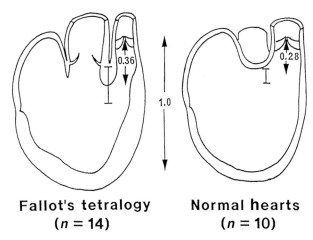

Figure 46.13. This heart shows straddling and overriding of the tricuspid valve in association with tetralogy of Fallot. Note the malalignment between the atrial septum and the muscular ventricular septum (asterisk). This produces an abnormal disposition of the atrioventricular conduction tissues (see Chapter 36).

Figure 46.14. The subpulmonary infundibulum in Fallot's tetralogy is significantly longer in the abnormal arrangement than it is in the normal heart (Becker et al, 1975).

AORTIC OVERRIDING

Because the normal aortic sinuses override the right ventricular infundibulum, some have described aortic overriding in the normal heart (Kleinert and Geva, 1993). In the normal heart, however, the leaflets of the aortic valve are attached exclusively within the left ventricle (Figure 46.1). Aortic overriding, in our opinion, exists only when the leaflets of the valve are attached in both right and left ventricles. Self-evidently, this requires the presence of a ventricular septal defect (Alva et al, 1998). Measurements made by Goor et al (1971) and by Becker et al (1975) showed unequivocally that not only was the aortic valve attached within both ventricles but also that true rightward deviation of the aorta was present. This has been confirmed by measurements from cross-sectional echograms (Isaaz et al, 1986). The precise degree of aortic override, judged according to the proportions of the leaflets supported by right or left ventricular structures, can vary between 5 and 100% (Anderson et al, 1981). This feature has surgical significance. A much larger patch will be required to connect to the left ventricle an aorta that originates predominantly from the right ventricle. Care must be taken to be sure that the patch is not placed so tightly as to obstruct the newly created left ventricular outflow tract.

The precise connections of the aortic valvar leaflets in right versus left ventricles also have implications for nomenclature. It is our convention to describe those hearts in which more than half of the circumferences of both great arterial valves are connected in the same ventricle as showing double outlet ventriculo-arterial connection. When, therefore, in the context of the lesion discussed in this chapter, more than half of the leaflets of the aortic valve are hinged from right ventricular structures, we continue to describe the lesion as tetralogy of Fallot but we categorize the ventriculo-arterial connection as double outlet. There is no reason why the two should not coexist. 'Double outlet' is simply one particular ventriculo-arterial connection. Tetralogy of Fallot is the consequence of abnormal morphology. The two features are not mutually exclusive (Wilcox et al, 1981; Edwards, 1981).

OTHER LESIONS OF THE PULMONARY CIRCULATION

Although the subpulmonary infundibulum is usually the narrowest part of the pulmonary outflow tract, other lesions are to be found elsewhere in the outflow tracts and the pulmonary arteries. Pulmonary valvar stenosis is a frequent accompaniment. This is sometimes caused by domed stenosis, more frequently to stenosis of a bicuspid valve or to stenosis of a valve with three leaflets. The valvar lesion is rarely the major cause of obstruction. In young infants, however, valvar stenosis has been found at surgery as the major obstructive lesion (Castaneda et al, 1977). Acquired valvar atresia can also occur. So-called 'absence' of the leaflets of the pulmonary valve is another important

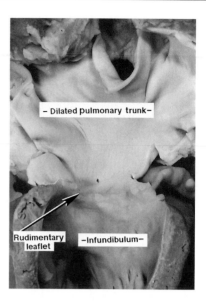

Figure 46.15. The typical morphology of tetralogy with so-called 'absence' of the pulmonary valve. The valvar leaflets are rudimentary, and the pulmonary arteries are grossly dilated.

lesion. Most usually, the valve is represented by an annular array of fibrous rudiments, usually found with marked dilatation of the pulmonary trunk (Figure 46.15). Stenoses within the pulmonary arteries themselves are of major surgical significance and usually occur at branching sites from the bifurcation outwards. Lack of origin of one pulmonary artery, typically the left, from the pulmonary trunk is by no means infrequent. The isolated pulmonary artery is almost always present, usually being connected by the arterial duct, or ligament, to some part of the system of aortic arches. Rarely, one pulmonary artery may arise directly from the ascending aorta, but then it tends to be the right one that is anomalously connected. Major systemic-to-pulmonary collateral arteries are sometimes present in association with tetralogy and pulmonary stenosis, but with normal right and left pulmonary arteries (Ramsay et al, 1985). Such arteries can be the sole source of pulmonary arterial flow when tetralogy coexists with pulmonary atresia (see Chapter 47).

ASSOCIATED ANOMALIES

Many other lesions can coexist with tetralogy. Patency of the oval foramen is common. An atrial septal defect may be present, a combination described by some as 'pentalogy of Fallot', but not by us. A second inlet muscular ventricular septal defect, straddling of the tricuspid valve, a common atrioventricular valve and anomalous origin of the anterior interventricular coronary artery from the right coronary artery (Figure 46.16) (Li et al, 1998) are all of great surgical importance. A right aortic arch, though not of functional importance, is common. When detected, it alerts to the diagnosis of tetralogy. Aortic incompetence is more common in older patients (Higgins and Mulder, 1972).

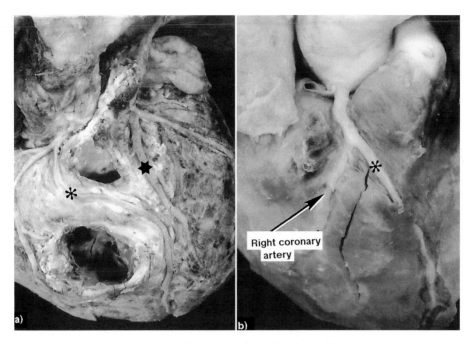

Figure 46.16. Examples of coronary arterial malformations found in tetralogy of Fallot. (a) An accessory anterior interventricular artery can be seen arising from the right coronary artery (asterisks). (b) The arrangement is shown in which the entire supply to the anterior interventricular septum is from the anomalous artery (asterisk) arising from the right coronary artery.

MORPHOGENESIS

The notion that tetralogy of Fallot reflects malseptation of the arterial segment of the developing heart dates back to von Rokitansky (1875). Like others (Peacock, 1867), he clearly illustrated the malformation prior to Fallot's classical paper. Von Rokitansky, in an elegant series of diagrams, showed that many other malformations could also be explained by unequal septation, together with connection of the great arteries to different ventricles. The malseptation hypothesis received considerable subsequent support, although other concepts were advanced. A popular recent theory, as proposed by Van Praagh et al (1970b), is that of incomplete growth of the subpulmonary 'conus'. The justification for this theory was that the pulmonary infundibulum was 'too short, too narrow and too shallow'. As we have described, a short subpulmonary infundibulum can occur but is far from a constant feature. Indeed, when the length of the infundibulum has been measured and compared with the normal (Figure 45.14), it is found to be significantly longer (Becker et al, 1975; Howell et al, 1990). It is difficult, therefore, to substantiate the hypothesis of inadequate growth of the subpulmonary infundibulum to account for all examples of tetralogy. The malseptation hypothesis, in contrast, is supported by observations concerning naturally occurring infundibular lesions in Keeshond dogs (Van Mierop et al, 1977). These animals show a spectrum of malformations ranging from absence of the medial papillary muscle, through ventricular septal defect, to a constellation of anomalies similar to tetralogy. Study of embryos in which developmental stages of these malformations were observed showed that the 'factory' for production of the lesions was within the ventricular outflow tracts. Specifically, abnormalities were found in the formation and position of the endocardial cushions, which normally fuse to septate the ventricular outlets. These observations have now been confirmed in rats closed with bisdiamine (Momma et al, 1990; Jackson et al, 1995). The findings from patients with Catch 22 syndrome strongly support the existence of a similar mechanism in humans and point to problems in migration of cells from the neural crest. Based on the anatomical findings, therefore, it can be said with some degree of certainty that there is malseptation of the ventricular outlets and the arterial pole of the heart at the expense of the pulmonary trunk, together with failure of normal incorporation of the aortic outflow tract into the morphologically left ventricle. These processes together account for the presence of the ventricular septal defect, the aortic overriding and the subpulmonary muscular stenosis. The right ventricular hypertrophy is a haemodynamic consequence of the anatomical lesions.

PATHOPHYSIOLOGY

HAEMODYNAMICS AND ITS CONSEQUENCE

The haemodynamic consequences of tetralogy of Fallot are dominated by the severity of obstruction within the subpulmonary right ventricular outflow tract, superimposed upon the presence of a large ventricular septal defect. In more than 99% of patients, the interventricular communication is large and non-limiting. This results in equalization of right and left ventricular systolic pressure, regardless of the severity of pulmonary stenosis (Vogelpoel et al, 1957). Normally, the right and left ventricles behave as a common ejectile chamber. They have similar, but not identical, pressure waveforms, except in the rare circumstances where either the septal leaflet of the tricuspid valve (Hoffman et al, 1960a; Neufeld et al, 1960; Faggian et al, 1983) or part of the mitral valvar apparatus (Van Praagh et al, 1970a) partially or completely occludes the defect. Even more rarely, especially in older untreated patients (Hoffman et al, 1960b), the defect may become limiting through to muscular contraction of the septum.

The relative flows in the pulmonary and systemic circuits depend on the relative resistances, or impedances, to emptying of the right and left ventricles. When right ventricular outflow obstruction is minimal, and the pulmonary vascular resistance is normal, pulmonary blood flow will exceed systemic blood flow. There will then be a dominant left-to-right shunt, and the clinical picture will resemble closely that of a ventricular septal defect. Under these circumstances, cyanosis will be absent. When obstruction to right ventricular emptying is similar to that provided by the systemic vascular resistance, a balanced situation exists. There will be no overall shunting in either direction, although transient small right-to-left and left-to-right shunts occur during each cardiac cycle. Pulmonary and systemic flows, at least at rest, will be equal. On exercise, however, a fall in systemic vascular resistance, with or without an increase in infundibular stenosis, will result in a right-to-left shunt with cyanosis. The systemic flow will then exceed the pulmonary flow. With increasing degrees of obstruction in the subpulmonary right ventricular outflow tract, a dominant right-to-left shunt develops. Cyanosis then becomes a constant feature. Such severe obstruction may be present from birth. More usually, increasing infundibular stenosis develops coincidentally with progressive right ventricular hypertrophy (Gasul et al, 1957). Cyanosis is dependent on the degree of pulmonary stenosis but is unrelated to the degree of aortic override (Brotmacher and Campbell, 1958).

Typically, the pulmonary arterial pressure is lower than normal, coincidental with reduced pulmonary blood flow. Pulmonary arterial systolic pressure, though lower than that in the right ventricle, may be higher than normal in the group with mild stenosis and increased pulmonary flow (Rowe et al, 1955). Right ventricular and aortic systolic pressures always remain the same. The right ventricular systolic pressure rises with systemic hypertension, or on administration of pressor agents such as phenylephrine (Vogelpoel et al, 1960). It falls in the presence of a vasodilator agent, such as amyl nitrite (Vogelpoel et al, 1959). The right ventricular pressure may also fall, along with aortic pressure, during (or particularly after) exercise when the systemic vascular resistance is decreased. As already indicated, a fall in systemic resistance, with no change in resistance to right ventricular emptying, will result in an increased right-to-left shunt.

HAEMATOLOGICAL EFFECTS OF CYANOSIS

The normal postnatal fall in haemoglobin levels that occurs in neonates will not occur if arterial desaturation is marked from birth, although relative anaemia in this situation develops by the third or fourth month of life (Rudolph et al, 1953). The bone marrow normally responds to hypoxia by increasing erythropoiesis, with an increase in red cell count, haemoglobin level and haematocrit. As iron stores in the fetus are limited, and the amount of iron in milk is low, a large number of red blood cells may be produced that are poorly filled with haemoglobin. Consequently, a large number of red blood cells (possibly more than 7×10^9 ml) may be found with a correspondingly raised haematocrit. There will, however, be a low mean corpuscular haemoglobin concentration and a low mean corpuscular volume, as found in typical iron-deficiency anaemia (Rudolph et al, 1953). The consequences of iron-deficiency anaemia in cyanotic heart disease are dire, either in infancy or later. It is the oxygen-carrying capacity of the blood far more than adjustments of ventilation that ensure adequate delivery of oxygen to the tissues (Husson and Otis, 1957). The tendency to develop metabolic acidosis, and hypercyanotic attacks, is exacerbated by the relative iron-deficiency anaemia. Similarly, with very high counts of red cell, blood viscosity is increased, and with it the tendency to cerebrovascular accidents. When the haematocrit is above 60%, further small increases produce large increments in viscosity (Kontras et al, 1970). At a haematocrit level of 70%, blood viscosity is so high that fluidity in small vessels becomes critical.

Some degree of secondary polycythaemia, however, is beneficial. First, the oxygen-carrying capacity of the blood is increased. Second, there is an increase in total blood volume because of the increase in red cell mass. Plasma volume, in contrast to 'polycythaemia rubra vera', is normal or reduced (Verel, 1961). Rosenthal et al (1971) have demonstrated that, at any given haematocrit, cardiac output is greater with increased than with normal blood volumes. If the haematocrit becomes too high, severe headaches and the risk of cerebrovascular accidents make its reduction important. If attempts are made to do this by phlebotomy, it is essential that the excessive volume is maintained by exchanging plasma, or 5% albumin, for blood. If blood viscosity is reduced in this way, which will not be the case if the patient is simply bled, there is an increase in systemic blood flow and decrease in apparent systemic vascular resistance (Rosenthal et al, 1970).

CLINICAL PRESENTATION

The clinical presentation is dominated by the degree of muscular obstruction of the right ventricular outflow tract (Shinebourne et al, 1975). This is sometimes modified by associated anomalies, such as persistent patency of the arterial duct or presence of large systemic-to-pulmonary collateral arteries.

PRESENTATION WHEN SUBPULMONARY OBSTRUCTION IS SEVERE FROM BIRTH

When the obstruction of the right ventricular outflow tract is severe at birth, presentation is in the neonatal period. Persistent cyanosis becomes apparent within the first few days of life. With severe arterial desaturation, a metabolic acidosis develops that is compensated by an increased respiratory rate. The concomitant fall in arterial content of carbon dioxide gives rise to a compensatory respiratory alkalosis. Intercostal or subcostal recession, however, is unusual. Cyanosis, which dominates the clinical picture, increases with crying, feeding or other activities. At least initially, the baby does not appear unduly distressed. Sometimes the pulmonary circulation is 'duct dependent'. In this setting, the degree of subpulmonary obstruction is so great that there is little antegrade flow, and virtually all pulmonary blood flow is derived from a left-to-right shunt via the arterial duct. Under such circumstances, spontaneous closure of the duct results in death. Maintenance of ductal patency, usually by infusion of prostaglandin E, is crucial (see below).

PRESENTATION WHEN SUBPULMONARY OBSTRUCTION IS MODERATE AT BIRTH

The majority of children with tetralogy of Fallot are acyanotic at birth. They present because a systolic heart murmur is detected within the first weeks of life. The development of cyanosis is dependent on increasing infundibular stenosis and not on the degree of aortic override (Brotmacher and Campbell, 1958). This usually occurs between 6 and 18 months of age. Development of cyanosis may rarely be delayed to late childhood. The systolic murmur, present in all patients other than those with very severe stenosis or acquired atresia, originates at the site of subpulmonary obstruction, and not because of flow across the ventricular septal defect (Vogelpoel and Schrire, 1960). At this stage, infants or children are asymptomatic. They may be diagnosed as having only a small ventricular septal defect. Indeed, physical examination may reveal findings identical with such an anomaly, such as a pan-systolic murmur at the lower left sternal edge, with a normal second heart sound.

Cyanosis is detectable when the concentration of reduced haemoglobin in systemic arterial blood is more than 5 g/100 ml. Minor degrees of arterial desaturation may not be detectable clinically, especially if the patient is anaemic. In the group with moderate subpulmonary obstruction, cyanosis is detected intermittently at first,

being apparent with crying, on exercise or on feeding. The magnitude of the right-to-left shunt is directly related to the severity of muscular obstruction and inversely related to the systemic vascular resistance. The former will tend to increase during exercise, because of increased sympathetic activity, while the latter falls. Both factors combine to exacerbate cyanosis on exertion. A reduction in exercise tolerance accompanies the onset of intermittent cyanosis. Breathlessness on exertion then becomes apparent, especially in toddlers who attack exercise as vigorously as they are able. In this group, and in the group with minimal obstruction, squatting and so-called hypercyanotic attacks, or 'spells', are important and highly characteristic features of the history. For this reason we will deal with them separately (see below).

PRESENTATION WHEN SUBPULMONARY OBSTRUCTION IS MINIMAL AT BIRTH

Some infants with tetralogy may uncommonly present at 4–6 weeks with features indistinguishable from those of a large ventricular septal defect (see Chapter 37). These babies are breathless, feed poorly, gain weight poorly and are not cyanosed. With increasing right ventricular hypertrophy, the subpulmonary obstruction becomes more marked and, as the shunt is reversed, the patients exhibit the signs and progression as described for the group with moderate obstruction.

PRESENTATION WITH 'ABSENT PULMONARY VALVE'

When tetralogy is complicated by so-called 'absence' of the leaflets of the pulmonary valve, which are usually present in rudimentary form (Figure 46.15), the presentation is characteristic yet different from the previously described groups. The majority with this complication present in infancy with respiratory symptoms of inspiratory and expiratory stridor, dyspnoea caused by lobar collapse or, at times, lobar emphysema. These features reflect compression of the bronchial tree by the grossly dilated proximal pulmonary arteries. While bronchial obstruction may lead to lobar collapse, and subsequent infection, partial obstruction may produce a ball-valve effect, resulting in emphysema. Because there is stenosis at the site of the rudimentary leaflets of the pulmonary valve, symptoms directly related to abnormal haemodynamics are unusual.

SQUATTING

Squatting, along with other postures, may alleviate the degree of cyanosis, dyspnoea or feeling of faintness induced by exercise. In 1784, Hunter reported a young adult with the condition we now recognize as tetralogy of Fallot who was able to alleviate symptoms of extreme cyanosis by lying on his left side. These observations were extended by Taussig (1947), who noted a spontaneous preference by patients for certain postures. The most dramatic was squatting, when the child was observed to sit down with the legs closely drawn up beneath the trunk. Taussig also noted patients sitting with the legs drawn up on the seat of a chair, and others who adopted a prone knee-chest position. Lurie (1953) added still further nuances. He noted that patients, when asked to stand, often crossed their legs and squeezed them together. Babies are sometimes soothed by being held with their legs flexed and knees squeezed well into their abdomen.

The means by which squatting alleviates the symptoms of cyanosis and dyspnoea have caused considerable debate. Certainly it prevents postural hypotension after exercise, which would otherwise result from the decrease in systemic venous return owing to venous pooling (Lurie, 1953). In normal subjects, squatting is known to produce increases in systemic blood pressure, vascular resistance and venous return, as well as an increase in oxygen saturation (Sharpey-Shafer, 1956). Brotmacher (1957) suggested that part of the increase in systemic vascular resistance was caused by kinking of the iliac arteries. This view was not supported by O'Donnell and McIlroy (1962), who concluded that squatting reduced the distending pressure of gravity on the vessels in the legs. These authors also demonstrated an increase in central blood volume, with a shift in circulating blood from the lower body. This resulted in an increased oxygen saturation and blood pressures in the upper body. A decrease in systemic venous return on squatting was demonstrated by Guntheroth et al (1968), which they suggested prevented more highly desaturated blood from leg veins reaching the heart. Analysis of their findings, however, shows that, initially at least, there is an increase, not a decrease, in inferior caval venous flow and systemic venous return.

Irrespective of the precise mechanisms, there is little doubt that squatting causes an abrupt increase in systemic venous return at a time when systemic vascular resistance is acutely increased. As we have emphasized, right-to-left shunting is decreased by an increase in systemic vascular resistance. Therefore, at a time when the volume of blood presenting itself to the right ventricle is increased, a higher proportion passes to the lungs, with immediate improvement in arterial oxygen saturation.

HYPERCYANOTIC ATTACKS

An important, and often dramatic, feature of patients with tetralogy is a history of 'turns' or blue spells, often accompanied by transient loss of consciousness (Wood, 1958). These episodes, which are most common between 6 months and 2 years of age (Morgan et al, 1965), are often alarming to the parents. They are also potentially dangerous, as they may lead to cerebral damage or death (Wood, 1958). The majority last between 15 and 60 minutes, but an individual spell may be of shorter duration or can last for several hours. They occur typically on waking in the morning but may be precipitated by crying, defecation, eating, exercise, hot weather (Morgan et al, 1965) or come out of the blue! Initial presentation of infants or children may be with a history of episodic loss of consciousness (Shinebourne et al, 1975) or convulsions, episodes of going 'floppy' or pale, transient vacant episodes or episodes of becoming deeply cyanosed followed by loss of consciousness or sleep. The episodes are usually sufficiently dramatic for parents to volunteer information concerning their presence. Sometimes, however, parents may not associate such episodes with a cardiac abnormality. Direct questioning will be necessary for their presence to be divulged. Another striking feature of these spells may be episodes of very rapid deep respiration or hyperpnoea, or a high-pitched abnormal cry.

It was Wood (1958) who postulated that the spells resulted from infundibular spasm or shutdown. He noted that, at the time of the 'spell', the loud systolic murmur typical of tetralogy became softer and frequently disappeared completely. Angiographic documentation of infundibular shutdown was provided by Honey et al (1964). They also demonstrated that some of the haemodynamic consequences of an increase in infundibular stenosis could be alleviated by β-adrenergic blockade. They postulated that an increase in the activity of the sympathetic nervous system, or circulating catecholamines, may have provoked infundibular spasm. An abrupt increase in infundibular stenosis produces a rapid fall in pulmonary blood flow, a massive right-to-left shunt and arterial hypoxaemia. This leads to systemic vasodilation, which further increases the right-to-left shunt. The abrupt fall in oxygen saturation, together with rapid development of metabolic acidosis because of poor delivery of oxygen to the tissues, results in hyperventilation from stimulation of the respiratory centre and chemoreceptors. If effective, this has the effect of blowing off carbon dioxide to compensate the rapidly developing metabolic acidosis. Because pulmonary flow is so reduced during a hypercyanotic attack, sampling of arterial blood typically shows low levels of oxygen, low pH and normal or increased values for carbon dioxide (Gootman et al, 1963).

To us, infundibular spasm is an adequate explanation for hypercyanotic attacks. Other explanations have been offered, especially to explain hyperventilation or the presence of spells in patients with tetralogy with pulmonary atresia, or in classical tricuspid atresia. The observation that hypercyanotic attacks occur typically after sleep prompted Guntheroth et al (1965) to suggest that altered sensitivity of the respiratory centre at such a time could render the subject particularly sensitive to alterations in arterial blood gases. None of their data, however, nor other reports in the literature, support the notion that the mechanism of hypercyanotic attacks is other than that of infundibular shutdown. Therefore, even in the case of a hypercyanotic attack being precipitated by supraventricular tachycardia (Young and Elbl, 1971), the reason for increased right-to-left shunting is liable to be an increase in obstruction to right ventricular emptying (King and Franch, 1971).

PHYSICAL EXAMINATION

The essential abnormal findings in the neonate with severe tetralogy of Fallot are cyanosis and, on auscultation, a single second heart sound. A murmur may or may not be present. The baby may be normally grown, although a higher proportion weigh less than would be expected by chance (Rowe et al, 1955). Pulses are almost always normal in all limbs, aortic coarctation being exceedingly rare in symptomatic neonates with tetralogy of Fallot (Rudolph et al, 1972; Shinebourne and Elseed, 1974). Central cyanosis is present, although overt clubbing of fingers and toes is typically not detected until 2 or 3 months of age. Nonetheless, erythema of the terminal digits is usual, hypoxia being associated with increased peripheral flow and opening up of distal arterio-venous anastomoses. The cardiac impulse may be normal, or the parasternal right ventricular impulse may be increased. The first heart sound is normal, but the second is single, closure of the pulmonary valve being inaudible. An aortic ejection click may sometimes be heard at the lower left sternal edge or at the apex (Zuberbuhler et al, 1975). This finding is the rule when there is acquired pulmonary atresia (Vogelpoel and Schrire, 1960). An ejection systolic murmur may be present, heard maximally at the second or third left intercostal space, but can be absent, especially when cyanosis is profound. Presumably this is because flow through the subpulmonary infundibulum is insufficient to produce audible turbulence, while flow from the right ventricle into the overriding aortic root is largely laminar. Another possible source of an ejection systolic murmur heard at the base is from left-to-right shunting across a persistently patent arterial duct. Usually the duct is narrow, and flow during diastole is insufficient to produce audible turbulence. The murmur is, therefore, systolic rather than continuous. When a loud continuous murmur is heard in the neonatal period, and clinical features are otherwise compatible with the diagnosis of tetralogy, it is more likely to originate from flow through large major systemic-to-pulmonary collateral arteries (Zuberbuhler et al, 1975). The patient is then likely to have coexisting pulmonary atresia. In these patients, cyanosis may not be so profound, since pulmonary blood flow is more adequately maintained through the multiple collateral arteries. Examination of the lungs reveals no abnormality. The liver, at least initially, will not be enlarged. Hepatomegaly

may occur as an early sign of congestive cardiac failure, which, although uncommon, is more likely to occur in this age group than in older children.

When subpulmonary obstruction is moderate at birth, cyanosis is not seen initially but has usually become apparent at rest by the end of the first year. It will have been present on crying for some months before. Clubbing of the fingers and toes is to be expected. This physical sign is retained in children who are desaturated but in whom severe anaemia prevents the clinical detection of cyanosis. Although growth may initially have been normal, cyanosed children grow less rapidly than normal (Lund, 1952). They are likely to be below their expected percentiles for height and weight (Mehrizi and Drash, 1962). There may be a normal or slightly increased parasternal impulse, indicating right ventricular hypertrophy, with a normal apical impulse. Pulses will be normal or possibly increased but equal in the arms and legs. Auscultation reveals a normal first heart sound and, if the patient is cyanotic, a second sound that is typically single. If acyanotic, the pulmonary component of the second sound may be audible but is soft and delayed. In previous times, when surgeons often created an excessively large systemic–pulmonary anastomosis (such as a Waterston or Pott's anastomosis), the pulmonary component of the second sound was often increased. Rarely, pulmonary closure may be accentuated, for example in the untreated adult who has developed thrombotic pulmonary vascular disease. A single second sound, however, is the rule. In contrast to patients having pulmonary stenosis with an intact ventricular septum (Leatham and Weitzman, 1957), pulmonary ejection sounds in the second or third intercostal space, or third and fourth heart sounds, are virtually never found in children with tetralogy. They have been reported in some adults with relatively mild stenosis (Martin et al, 1973). Even then, they reflect associated valvar pulmonary stenosis. Heart failure with an associated gallop rhythm is uncommon in children but will commonly be found in the untreated adult in their third or fourth decade (Higgins and Mulder, 1972).

A systolic murmur will be present in children with moderately severe tetralogy. The exception is during hypercyanotic attacks, when the murmur disappears (Wood, 1958). Since the murmur originates at the site of subpulmonary obstruction, and not at the ventricular septal defect (Vogelpoel and Schrire, 1960), it is hardly surprising that it disappears during infundibular shutdown. The presence of the ventricular septal defect does, however, influence the characteristics of the systolic murmur heard maximally at the third intercostal space just to the left of the sternum. When mild-to-moderate stenosis is present, the murmur has many of the characteristics of the typical pan-systolic murmur of isolated ventricular septal defect. It starts with the first heart sound and retains a similar intensity up to the second sound (or at least to the audible aortic component of the second sound). As the severity of infundibular stenosis increases, the murmur becomes more crescendo–decrescendo in character. When obstruction is severe, the murmur softens and finishes well before the second sound. This contrasts with the situation in isolated pulmonary stenosis, where, with increasing severity, the murmur becomes longer and peaks later in systole (Vogelpoel and Schrire, 1955, 1960; Leatham and Weitzman, 1957). Diastolic murmurs are not found in uncomplicated cases of tetralogy of Fallot except in those acyanotic patients with very mild pulmonary stenosis. In these, an increased pulmonary blood flow, and hence increased pulmonary venous return, results in an apical mid-diastolic flow murmur across the mitral valve. In patients who have not undergone surgery, early diastolic murmurs may be generated by associated aortic incompetence. The one situation characterized by a long loud early diastolic decrescendo murmur from pulmonary regurgitation is the 'absent pulmonary valve' syndrome (Miller et al, 1962; see below). Continuous murmurs may originate in a persistent arterial duct, or from systemic-to-pulmonary collateral arteries (Campbell and Deuchar, 1961; Ongley et al, 1966). The murmur from the duct is most commonly heard maximally at the second intercostal space on the side of the aortic arch. Continuous murmurs from systemic-to-pulmonary collateral arteries are often more widely transmitted and are heard easily at the back.

Children with tetralogy in whom subpulmonary obstruction is minimal or absent at birth exhibit tachypnoea, dyspnoea and intercostal or subcostal recession. This group has a large left-to-right shunt, with an increased pulmonary blood flow. A prominent parasternal impulse and hepatomegaly are present. On auscultation, the second sound is split, possibly with an accentuated pulmonary component. A pan-systolic murmur at the lower left sternal edge, and even an apical mitral diastolic flow murmur, completes the picture, which is that seen far more commonly in a large simple uncomplicated ventricular septal defect. There is usually an adequate clinical response to treatment of heart failure, with progressive improvement in symptoms over the next year. There are several possible reasons why a child with a large ventricular septal defect may improve symptomatically with time. The most obvious is that the defect is becoming smaller. Alternatively, pulmonary vascular disease may be developing. When there is tetralogy of Fallot, it is progressive infundibular stenosis that limits the magnitude of the left-to-right shunt.

Signs compatible with a diagnosis of tetralogy may be found with Down's syndrome. While such patients may have isolated tetralogy, a coexistent atrioventricular septal defect should always be considered.

INVESTIGATIONS

While the diagnosis of tetralogy of Fallot is usually made from clinical assessment, confirmation is now provided largely by cross-sectional echocardiography. This technique allows visualization of all features of the intracardiac anatomy, including associated anomalies such as straddling valves, additional ventricular septal defects or common atrioventricular junction. While the pulmonary trunk, along with the proximal right and left pulmonary arteries, can readily be imaged, peripheral stenoses may not be identified with certainty. The coronary arteries can also be visualized, nowadays usually with the certainty needed to exclude an anomalous vessel crossing the subpulmonary infundibulum (Sullivan, 1998). Systemic-to-pulmonary collateral arteries can be indicated by colour flow Doppler, but their extent cannot be determined echocardiographically. Before describing the echocardiographic features, however, we will discuss the plain chest radiograph and the electrocardiogram, as these are usually carried out as part of the general cardiac assessment of a child.

CHEST RADIOGRAPHY

In the young child with severe tetralogy of Fallot, the plain frontal chest radiograph may be so typical that any other diagnosis is unlikely (Figure 46.17). In the acyanotic patient with tetralogy, the plain chest radiograph may be normal. Most patients have the usual arrangement of thoracic and abdominal organs together with a left-sided heart, but tetralogy may occur with mirror-imaged arrangement, when the heart is usually right sided. With usual atrial arrangement, presence of a right-sided aortic arch in the condition we now know as tetralogy of Fallot was first described by Corvisart (1818). Up

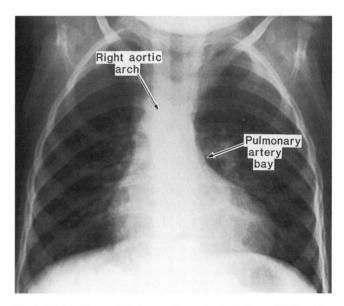

Figure 46.17. The typical chest radiograph of tetralogy of Fallot. The trachea is slightly compressed by the aorta arching to its right side. Instead of the normal convexity produced by the pulmonary trunk, a concavity, or pulmonary arterial bay, is present.

to 30% of patients with tetralogy have such a right aortic arch (Hastreiter et al, 1966). Of all subjects with a right aortic arch, three quarters have tetralogy of Fallot with or without pulmonary atresia. The diagnosis is more likely if there are reduced pulmonary vascular markings. Even in a patient with a right arch and increased vascular markings, it is wise to consider the diagnosis of tetralogy with minimal subpulmonary obstruction. When pulmonary plethora coexists with a right-sided aortic arch, however, a common arterial trunk or aortopulmonary window is more common (Lau et al, 1982). In addition to the aortic arch being right sided, the descending aorta, which may be dilated, is also frequently right sided.

Pulmonary vascular markings will be reduced in cyanotic patients, the lung fields being strikingly oligaemic in neonates when subpulmonary obstruction is severe. In contrast, vascular markings will be normal when infundibular stenosis is moderate. When subpulmonary obstruction is minimal, there will be pulmonary plethora, reflecting the left-to-right shunt. In typical tetralogy, however, pulmonary vascular markings are reduced. With increasing subpulmonary obstruction, especially in older patients, there is a tendency to develop multiple small bronchopulmonary collateral arteries, giving either a reticular appearance or that of multiple small nodular opacities (Campbell and Gardner, 1950). Major systemic-to-pulmonary collateral arteries, producing abnormal linear shadows on the plain chest radiogram, are much more common in tetralogy with pulmonary atresia. Such congenital collateral arteries rarely cause rib notching in patients not having undergone surgery; however, after a classical Blalock–Taussig shunt, rib notching may be found on the under surface of the third to ninth ribs on the side of the shunt (Kent, 1953). This results from flow of blood passing through collateral arteries from the lower part of the chest wall to the axilla and arm. The direction of blood flow is the opposite to that found in collateral vessels in aortic coarctation (Campbell, 1958). When the pulmonary valvar leaflets are rudimentary ('absent valve syndrome'), the proximal pulmonary arteries are aneurysmally dilated and the peripheral markings are reduced (Figure 46.18).

The heart is usually of normal size in tetralogy. Cardiomegaly may rarely be found in the small infant with functional tricuspid regurgitation, and in the adult with congestive failure (Higgins and Mulder, 1972). The cardiac contour should be analysed, eschewing imagination, according to whether each of the normal features are present. This is preferable to analysis in terms of whether the heart shadow looks wearable, edible or usable as a golf club. The upper right cardiac border may be prominent owing to displacement of the superior caval vein by a right aortic arch. The arch, when right sided, can be seen to deviate the trachea to the left. The lower right cardiac border will be normal. A pulmonary bay, or concavity, below the left-sided aortic arch reflects a

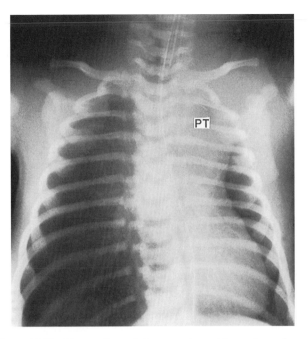

Figure 46.18. Chest radiograph from a patient with tetralogy of Fallot with rudimentary pulmonary valvar leaflets (so-called 'absent' valve). Note the grossly dilated pulmonary trunk (PT). Because of compression and partial obstruction of the right main bronchus, the right lung is overinflated, pushing the heart and mediastinum to the left.

small pulmonary trunk. The apex of the heart may be upturned, probably because the hypertrophied right ventricle forms the apex in the posteroanterior projection. There is no evidence to support the explanation that this appearance reflects hypoplasia of the left ventricle.

ELECTROCARDIOGRAPHY

The essential features of the electrocardiogram are a mean frontal QRS axis to the right of normal (Khoury et al, 1965) and right ventricular hypertrophy (Baker et al, 1949). Right atrial hypertrophy is present in about 20% of patients (evidenced by tall peaked P waves >3 mm (0.3 mV) in lead II; Woods, 1952). This is seen especially in older children. The electrocardiogram in the normal neonate shows right ventricular dominance, right-sided T waves (V4R and V_1) being upright at birth and inverted by the age of 1 week. The electrocardiogram in a neonate with tetralogy may, therefore, be normal for age. Failure of right-sided T waves to invert, however, is typically but not invariably found. Sinus rhythm is the rule, with a normal PR interval. The mean frontal QRS axis is between +90° and +150°. There is usually right ventricular hypertrophy, with dominant tall R waves in V4R and V, and a dominant S wave in V_6. Rarely, particularly in premature neonates, there may be dominant left-sided forces, as there are in a small proportion of adults (Burch et al, 1964). QRS duration is within normal limits prior to any intracardiac surgery, although complete right branch block frequently occurs postoperatively. When a superior mean frontal QRS axis is found, the additional presence of an atrioventricular septal defect should always be suspected. This would be virtually pathognomonic in a patient with Down's syndrome. Such an axis has also been reported, nonetheless, in patients with typical tetralogy (Feldt et al, 1966). A paucity of right ventricular forces may rarely be found when the right ventricle is small. This situation may reflect coexistent tricuspid stenosis (Kirklin and Karp, 1970) or a straddling tricuspid valve.

ECHOCARDIOGRAPHY

The echocardiographic features of tetralogy of Fallot are reliably demonstrated by cross-sectional techniques. Previous experience with the M-mode technique is now of historic interest (Caldwell et al, 1979). The suggestive, but not diagnostic, feature was overriding of the ventricular septum by the posterior (or at times apparently single) great artery (Gramiak and Shah, 1971). Although this feature distinguished patients with tetralogy from the normal, other conditions such as common arterial trunk gave a similar appearance. Differentiation could be made by demonstrating an anterior, often small, great artery (Chung et al, 1973). Diagnosis is now made directly by cross-sectional techniques.

Transthoracic cross-sectional echocardiography usually allows clear demonstration of all the intracardiac anatomy. As always, a sequential approach is used. The atrial arrangement is inferred from the location of the abdominal vessels, and the atrioventricular connections are demonstrated with apical four chamber views. Angulation upwards from a subcostal paracoronal view shows the narrowed subpulmonary outflow tract (Caldwell et al, 1979), with malalignment of the anteriorly displaced muscular outlet septum (Figure 46.19). Parasternal long-axis views demonstrate the aortic override (Figure 46.20). Biventricular connection is seen also in the four chamber view (Figure 46.21), the projection that will identify any additional muscular or inlet ventricular septal defects. A straddling or overriding tricuspid valve is seen in the four chamber view, as is the common atrioventricular junction in hearts with deficient atrioventricular septation (Figure 46.22). These views, together with a parasternal short-axis view, allow the margins of the ventricular septal defect to be identified. The defect is usually perimembranous but may have a muscular posteroinferior rim. The defect can also extend to become doubly committed and juxta-arterial when the outlet septum is very small or absent. When the pulmonary trunk is traced to its bifurcation, it is possible to determine the size of the pulmonary arteries (Figure 46.23) up to their first bifurcation, but not the more distal pattern of branching.

Views of the aortic arch show the branching pattern of the brachiocephalic arteries, a right brachiocephalic

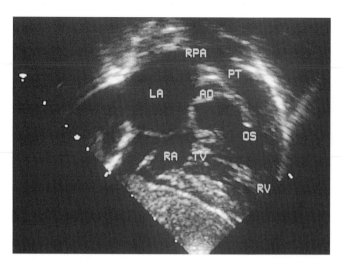

Figure 46.19. A cross-sectional echocardiogram in a subcostal paracoronal plane (equivalent to the right anterior oblique angiographic projection) demonstrates all the salient features of tetralogy. AO, overriding aorta; LA, left atrium; LPA, left pulmonary artery; OS, muscular outlet septum; PT, pulmonary trunk; RA, right atrium; RV, right ventricle; TV, tricuspid valve.

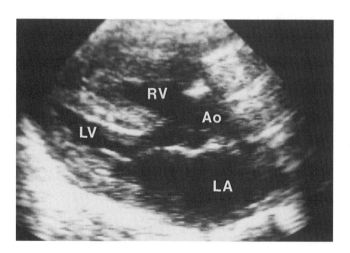

Figure 46.20. The parasternal long-axis section shows well the aortic valve (Ao) overriding the crest of the muscular ventricular septum. LA, left atrium; LV, left ventricle; RV, right ventricle.

(innominate) artery being found with a left aortic arch. When the first branching from the aorta itself divides into left carotid and subclavian arteries, then it can be inferred that the arch is right sided. These views will also show a persistent arterial duct, if present, while colour flow Doppler can confirm patency of previous palliative shunts and may show collateral arteries. As with the echocardiographic assessment of all anomalies, it is essential to confirm normal systemic and pulmonary venous connections. Anomalous pulmonary venous connections in particular, if present, must be identified (Redington et al, 1990). Associated anomalies, such as 'absence' of the pulmonary valve and dilation of the pulmonary trunk are readily identified (Figure 46.24)

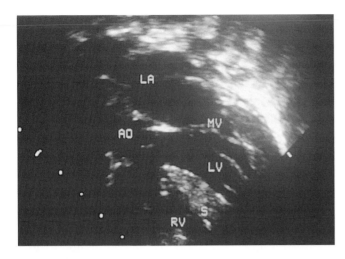

Figure 46.21. An angled four chamber section from the subcostal window also shows the biventricular connections of the overriding aorta (AO). MV, mitral valve; other abbreviations as in Figure 46.20.

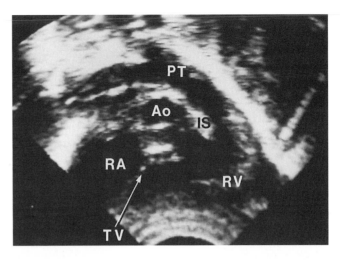

Figure 46.23. When the pulmonary trunk (PT) is traced beyond its bifurcation, seen here in the subcostal oblique section, it is possible to quantify the dimensions of the right and left pulmonary arteries. It is also possible to see these vessels in the short axis. Abbreviations as in Figures 46.19 and 46.22.

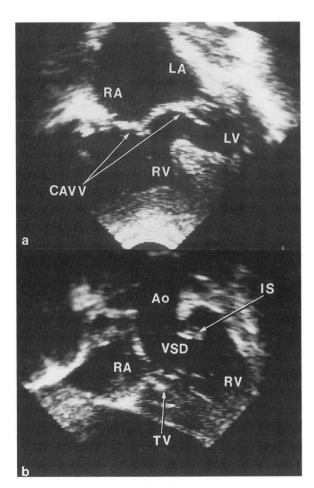

Figure 46.22. Examination of the atrioventricular junction with cross-sectional echocardiography from the subcostal window (a) reveals the presence of the bridging leaflets of a common atrioventricular valve (CAVV) when an atrioventricular septal defect (VSD) and common atrioventricular junction coexists with the typical morphology of tetralogy, revealed by scanning the outflow tracts (b). IS, muscular outlet septum; LV, left ventricle; other abbreviations as in Figure 46.19.

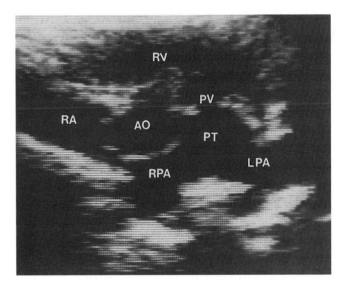

Figure 46.24. An echocardiogram in short axis shows the rudimentary nature of the leaflets of the pulmonary valve (PV) and dilatation of the right and left pulmonary arteries (RPA, LPA) in association with so-called 'absent' pulmonary valve. Other abbreviations as in Figure 46.19.

(Tenorio de Albuquerque et al, 1984). At the same time, it is possible to exclude anomalies with similar clinical features to tetralogy, such as double outlet right ventricle or complete transposition with ventricular septal defect and pulmonary stenosis. Indeed, cross-sectional echocardiography in skilled hands provides details of all the significant intracardiac morphological features of tetralogy of Fallot. In most patients, the origins of the right and left coronary arteries from the aorta can also be visualized, as can branching of the left artery into the circumflex and anterior descending arteries. Anomalous arteries can be identified crossing the subpulmonary infundibulum (Figure 46.25) (Sullivan, 1998).

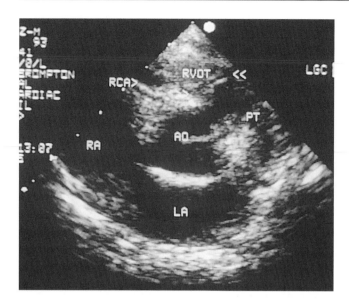

Figure 46.25. This short-axis echocardiogram shows an anomalous artery (arrowed) arising from the right coronary artery (RCA) and crossing the subpulmonary infundibulum (RVOT). Other abbreviations as in Figure 46.19.

CARDIAC CATHETERIZATION AND ANGIOGRAPHY

Prior to palliative surgery, sufficient information can be obtained from cross-sectional echocardiography to obviate the need for cardiac catheterization. In patients scheduled for total correction, cross-sectional echocardiography may also provide all the relevant clinical information; however in patients who have had prior palliation with a shunt, and in very young patients scheduled for correction, angiography still provides certain information not easily available from non-invasive techniques, such as the presence of peripheral pulmonary stenosis, systemic-to-pulmonary collaterals and the details of the pattern of branching of the coronary arteries.

Catheterization is performed percutaneously from the femoral vein and artery. The catheter is passed to the right atrium and right ventricle. From the right ventricle, the catheter can be passed via the ventricular septal defect to the aorta. Frequently a patent oval foramen or atrial septal defect will allow the venous catheter to be manoeuvred into the left atrium, permitting access to the pulmonary veins, and thence to the left ventricle. If the left ventricle was not entered across the oval foramen, the venous catheter can often be pulled back from the aorta and manipulated into this chamber through the ventricular septal defect. Alternatively, the left ventricle and right ventricles can be entered retrogradely. Whether or not attempts should be made to enter the pulmonary trunk is debatable, since this procedure can precipitate hypercyanotic attacks from infundibular shutdown. This can be prevented by giving propranolol (0.1 mg/kg) during or before catheterization. We do not make strenous efforts to enter the pulmonary trunk.

The saturations of oxygen in the various cardiac chambers depend on the severity of subpulmonary obstruction. When moderate to severe, a right-to-left shunt is usually detected in the aorta. Left ventricular blood, though frequently less than fully saturated, is then more highly saturated than aortic blood. At all ages, but especially in infants, right-to-left shunts are also detected at atrial level. Whereas pulmonary venous samples are fully saturated, there is some degree of left atrial desaturation. If subpulmonary obstruction is mild, a left-to-right shunt may be detected in the right ventricle. This is especially so in so-called 'acyanotic' patients. Systemic venous samples may be normal in such patients, although right-sided oxygen saturations may be reduced when there is cyanosis. Right and left atrial pressures are usually normal, but pressures will be equal in the body of the right ventricle and in the left ventricle. The subpulmonary infundibulum is often sequestrated as a discrete chamber. Systolic pressure is then between that measured in the pulmonary trunk and that in the body of the ventricle. The diastolic pressure in this infundibular chamber is also similar to, or marginally higher, than that in the body of the right ventricle. The pulmonary arterial pressure is typically lower than normal, with a small pulse pressure being found in these patients with moderate or severe infundibular stenosis. The pulmonary arterial pressure may be normal or slightly elevated when there is still a left-to-right shunt. Calculation of flows shows reduced pulmonary, and normal or increased systemic, blood flow, with a dominant right-to-left shunt. The degree of shunting, as well as the degree of aortic desaturation, depend on the severity of subpulmonary obstruction.

ANGIOCARDIOGRAPHY

Conventionally, angiograms should be performed in right ventricle, left ventricle and ascending aorta in order to delineate the anatomy fully. Whether a left ventriculogram is necessary after cross-sectional echocardiography has demonstrated the ventricular septal defect is not now certain. The introduction of axial angiography by Bargeron et al (1977) transformed angiographic assessment (Figure 46.26). These projections made it possible to demonstrate the entire pulmonary arterial tree from the supravalvar area up to and beyond its bifurcation (Elliott et al, 1977). If a left ventriculogram is performed, then the entire ventricular septum must be shown, both to demonstrate the subaortic ventricular septal defect and to confirm or exclude the presence of other defects. The size of both ventricles is demonstrated, although associated atrioventricular valvar abnormalities are better shown by cross-sectional echocardiography (Figure 46.22). Any other associated anomalies, such as anomalous systemic or pulmonary venous connections, or the presence of major systemic-to-pulmonary collateral arteries or an arterial duct, must be shown. So must the

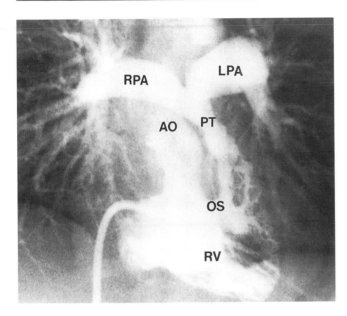

Figure 46.26. Right ventriculogram performed in right anterior oblique projection. The outlet (infundibular) septum (OS), profiled in cross-section, together with hypertrophied septoparietal trabeculations of the right ventricular free wall produce muscular subvalvar stenosis. The pulmonary trunk (PT) is seen, together with the size of the right and left pulmonary arteries (RPA, LPA, respectively). The aorta (AO) has been opacified by contrast passing through the ventricular septal defect. RV, right ventricle.

precise anatomy of any palliative shunts. Angiography will clearly demonstrate the dilated pulmonary arteries to be found when the pulmonary valvar leaflets are rudimentary (so-called 'absent valve'; Figure 46.27).

An aortogram is performed, first to exclude or demonstrate the presence of an arterial duct and/or major systemic-to-pulmonary collateral arteries and second to display the coronary arterial anatomy. In the neonate

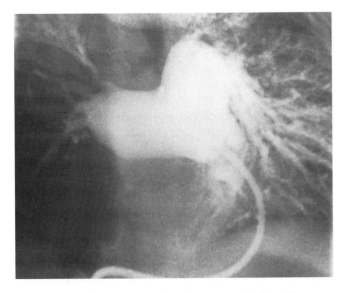

Figure 46.27. This injection in the pulmonary trunk shows the dilated pulmonary arteries in the setting of so-called absence of the leaflets of the pulmonary valve.

with severe infundibular stenosis, a duct (if present) will tend to have an abnormal course. Flow through it during fetal development will have been principally from the aorta to the pulmonary trunk rather than, as in normal fetuses, from the duct to the descending aorta (Rudolph et al, 1972; Miller et al, 1973).

The pattern of the coronary arteries can now be determined by cross-sectional echocardiography (Berry et al, 1988; Jureidini et al, 1989; Sullivan, 1998). Selective coronary angiography is not necessary to demonstrate the course of the major branches of right and left coronary arteries (Fellows et al, 1975), but the surgeon needs to be forewarned if a major vessel crosses in front of the subpulmonary infundibulum. This occurs in between 2 and 9% of patients with tetralogy of Fallot (White et al, 1972; Berry and McGoon, 1973). The most important variant is origin of the anterior descending artery from the right coronary artery (Longenecker et al, 1961). The only way to be certain whether or not such an abnormal vessel traverses the subpulmonary outlet is to obtain a root angiogram performed with a caudocranial and 30° left anterior oblique angulation (Carvalho et al, 1993). This so-called 'laid back' view was first introduced by Mandell et al (1990) to visualize the coronary arteries in complete transposition (see Chapter 48). It shows the aorta 'face on'. Its three sinuses are clearly seen, and there are no overlapping structures. The subpulmonary outflow tract in tetralogy is then anterior and to the left. The view is, therefore, analogous to the echocardiographic parasternal short-axis section taken at the level of the aortic valve. In these views, the main stem of the left coronary artery can be seen passing behind (beneath) the right ventricular outflow tract and dividing into its left anterior descending and circumflex branches. While this pattern of branching may be identified by cross-sectional echocardiography, and anomalous arteries identified crossing the subpulmonary infundibulum (Figure 46.25), there will be some patients where adequate imaging is difficult. Because of this, it is debatable whether angiography can completely be dispensed with. In our experience (Carvalho et al, 1993), false negatives can be avoided if angiography is used and identification of an anomalous anterior descending artery from the right coronary artery (Figure 46.28) is straightforward. False positives can be a problem, as the caudocranial view allows distinction between right and left and inferior and posterior but does not distinguish inferior and superior relationships (Carvalho et al, 1993). These problems can be resolved by obtaining simultaneous lateral projections of the aortic root injection (Li et al, 1998).

NATURAL HISTORY AND COMPLICATIONS

It is rare now, in developed countries, to encounter patients undergoing the natural history of tetralogy of

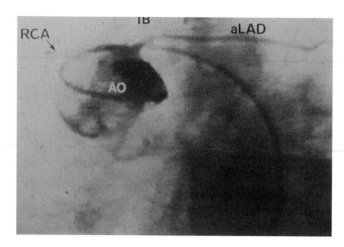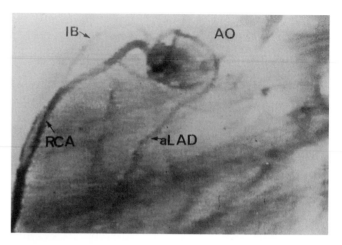

Figure 46.28. These angiograms taken after an injection in the aortic root are profiled in the 'laid back' view (left) and in lateral projection (right). The former shows an anomalous anterior interventricular artery (aLAD) arising from the right coronary aortic (AO) sinus and crossing the subpulmonary outflow tract. The lateral view discriminates between the anomalous artery and a prominent infundibular branch (IB) of the right coronary artery (RCA).

Fallot, as the defect will be repaired, or at least palliated, when symptoms occur. In poor countries, or those where cardiac surgery for children is not well developed, the situation is dramatically different. When the patient is not treated, subpulmonary obstruction, and hence depth of cyanosis, increases with time. Hypercyanotic crises become more frequent, more severe, more prolonged and may end in death. The effect of this progression upon the natural history was described in detail by Rygg et al (1971). Without surgical intervention, nine tenths of patients with tetralogy were dead by the age of 25 years (Figure 46.29). We now expect all patients undergoing total correction to survive, and any postoperative death is analysed in detail to determine what went wrong. This is a striking change in expectation and outcome.

As with many congenital cardiac anomalies with or without surgery, there is a risk of infective endocarditis both in the heart and at the site of systemic-to-pulmonary anastomoses. Without treatment, and following a palliative shunt, there is also a risk of cerebral abscess. This may occur in any cyanotic cardiac anomaly but is most common in tetralogy, especially after a Blalock–Taussig shunt. In Campbell's series (1958), cerebral abscess caused half the late deaths after this procedure, although these patients remained uncorrected for far longer than the present time. When an abscess develops, the causative organism is frequently, but not invariably, *Streptococcus viridans*. Clinical presentation is with drowsiness, altered consciousness, fever, headache and malaise. There may or may not be localizing neurological signs. As so-called 'pseudopapilloedema' has been described in patients with normal intracranial pressure but severe cyanotic heart disease, care must be taken in interpreting this sign. In this respect, Kohner et al (1967) showed that abnormal fundal appearances were more severe the higher the packed cell volume. Tortuous and dilated arterioles and venules are seen with increased vascularity of the funduses. When the haematocrit is above 65, frank papilloedema may be seen, even with normal intracranial pressure. Papilloedema alone, therefore, is not a reliable sign of cerebral abscess. If this diagnosis is suspected, blood cultures should be performed, although these are often negative. Emergency electroencephalography should be performed, which may demonstrate slow wave activity over the affected area, although again electroencephalographic abnormalities may be found simply with severe chronic cyanosis. Computed tomography or magnetic resonance imaging is the diagnostic technique of choice.

Pulmonary vascular obstructive disease is another late complication. This is related to sludging of red blood cells, stasis and intra-arterial thromboses (Rich, 1948). These pulmonary vascular complications are dealt with in more detail in Chapter 19. Massive macroscopic thrombosis has also been reported (Svane, 1977).

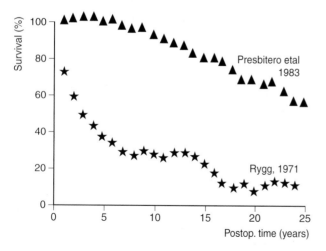

Figure 46.29. Data showing the prognosis for patients with tetralogy of Fallot without treatment (*; Rugg et al, 1971) and with palliation (▲; Presbitero et al, 1983).

MANAGEMENT

The asymptomatic child with tetralogy of Fallot requires surgical repair any time after the first 6 months of life, although some centres are now advocating even earlier correction (Reddy et al, 1995). Precise timing may depend on the experience of the particular unit involved, as will be discussed below. The medical management of a symptomatic child is devoted principally to preparation for surgery. This involves mostly treatment of hypercyanotic crises or spells, and occasionally treatment of polycythaemia. Medical treatment of heart failure in the atypical patient with a left-to-right shunt is as for heart failure complicating a large ventricular septal defect.

MEDICAL MANAGEMENT

MANAGEMENT OF HYPERCYANOTIC CRISES OR SPELLS

When called to a child undergoing a hypercyanotic crisis, the first actions should be to insert an intravenous line and administer oxygen by face mask. If the child is extremely restless, there is a place for morphine sulphate (0.1 mg/kg). This drug used to be the principal pharmacological agent used in management. It still has a part to play. Nonetheless, the drug of choice during an attack nowadays is a β-adrenergic blocking agent (Honey et al, 1964) such as propranolol (Cumming and Carr, 1966). The drug should be administered intravenously; 0.1 mg/kg is an adequate dose. Half of this should be given rapidly, and the remaining half more slowly over the next few minutes. It is uncommon for propranolol not to reverse infundibular spasm, providing that accompanying metabolic acidosis has been corrected. Arterial blood gases should be taken to check for this, and appropriate amounts of sodium bicarbonate given to correct any acidosis. Exceptionally, it will be necessary to construct an emergency systemic-to-pulmonary shunt. One hypercyanotic attack is, in our view, an indication for surgery. Beta blockade with propranolol may still be needed to tide a patient over in the few days or weeks before surgery can be arranged.

SURGICAL MANAGEMENT

The symptomatic infant or child requires surgery. Symptoms result principally from hypoxaemia, which can only adequately be relieved by surgical means. In the truly asymptomatic and acyanotic patient, operation may be delayed to 1 year of age, but in major centres no advantage is gained by further delay. The real decision in the symptomatic patient is whether to palliate or whether to attempt total correction. As surgical results have improved, preference for the latter course of action has increased.

It was Lillehei and his colleagues (1955) who first achieved successful repair using open intracardiac techniques. Then, in 1959, Kirklin et al reported an operative mortality of 28%, with four deaths in their last 25 patients (16%). Six years later, mortality had fallen to under 10% (Kirklin et al, 1965). By the 1970s, a mortality of under 5% was achieved in all children corrected under the age of 4 years (Pacifico et al, 1973). Consequently, by the early 1970s, total correction was being carried out in many centres with good results, but still the operative mortality was much higher in younger children (Puga et al, 1972; Chiariello et al, 1975). Primary repair in such young children had, however, been undertaken earlier with success (McMillan et al, 1965). Techniques for open heart surgery had so improved by the mid-1970s that primary repair in infancy came to be advocated as preferable to the protocols in which correction was carried out at a second operation following initial surgical palliation. Primary repair was championed by Barratt-Boyes and Neutze (1973) and Starr et al (1973), while favourable long-term results of this approach were reported by Muraoka et al (1973). By the late 1970s, primary correction was being performed with mortalities as low as 6% (Castaneda et al, 1977). This was the situation in the 1980s when we prepared the first edition of this book. What then is the position in the 2000s as we complete the second edition? Should all patients with tetralogy be subjected to primary repair whatever their age, or are there certain features that would make initial palliation, with secondary repair at a later date, a preferable approach? Before considering this question, we must deal first with the possible palliative procedures, and the major contemporaneous improvements in their evolution. We will also address the mechanics of open intracardiac repair of tetralogy, the procedure that, optimistically, is referred to as 'total correction'.

PALLIATIVE PROCEDURES

BLALOCK–TAUSSIG ANASTOMOSIS

In 1945, Blalock and Taussig noted that persistent patency of the arterial duct often prevented the onset of cyanosis in patients with tetralogy. From this, they developed the idea that it would be beneficial to use the subclavian artery to create an artificial duct. The procedure is traditionally performed on the side opposite to that of the aortic arch. On this side, the subclavian artery arises from the brachiocephalic (innominate) artery rather than directly from the aorta. Because of this, kinking is less likely to occur at its origin when it is turned down to become a shunt. Therefore, when the arch is right sided, a left-sided shunt is normally performed. Nowadays, modification of the classical shunt by placement of Gortex or Impra interposition grafts (McKay et al, 1980; Kay et al, 1983) has achieved such excellent results, with negligible mortality and adequate patency, that the modified shunt has become the procedure of choice. Following creation of such inter-position shunts in small infants, it is our policy to treat the patient with heparin in the initial postoperative period. We then use aspirin (acetylsalicylic acid) to decrease the adhesiveness of platelets for a further 3 months.

Nowadays, the shunt, be it classical or modified, will be required to have a relatively short period of function prior to correction, but longer-term results are excellent, as were the results of the classical shunt (Taussig et al, 1971). There was immediate symptomatic improvement and decrease in cyanosis in more than four fifths of patients, a feature that would be even higher at the present time. The fact that many of these older patients undergoing surgery between 1945 and 1951 were still alive over 30 years later, and sur-viving on their first shunt, was salutary. Indeed, these results bear comparison with modern outcomes of conduit surgery or the Fontan procedure. The Blalock–Taussig shunt, or its modification, therefore, is now generally accepted as the shunt of choice (Arciniegas et al, 1980; Kirklin et al, 1984). The classical or modified Blalock–Taussig shunt has no adverse influence on subsequent cor-rection (Chiariello et al, 1975; Daily et al, 1978; Arciniegas et al, 1980; Kirklin et al, 1984). Both procedures permit excellent growth of both pulmonary arteries (Guyton et al, 1983; Honda, 1993; Jahangiri et al, 1999), although not in all series (Laas et al, 1984).

WATERSTON ANASTOMOSIS

Intrapericardial anastomosis of the ascending aorta to the right pulmonary artery, as described by Waterston (1962), was considered by some surgeons (Alvarez Diaz et al, 1978; Azzolina et al, 1982) to be the shunt of choice in small infants. In this procedure, unlike the Blalock–Taussig shunt, the surgeon has carefully to judge the size of the anastomosis created between the posterior aspect of the ascending aorta and the anterior aspect of the right pulmonary artery. If the anastomosis is too small, severe hypoxaemia is a major problem in the immediate post-operative period. Too large an anastomosis produces plethora and pulmonary oedema, and may progress even-tually to pulmonary vascular disease. Problems described by Somerville et al (1975), such as inadequate size of the anastomosis, kinking of the right pulmonary artery and stenosis at the level of the anastomosis, were all avoided by care at surgery (Alvarez Diaz et al, 1978). Considerable surgical experience, nonetheless, was required to perform the procedure adequately, and to obtain optimal results. In contrast to the Blalock–Taussig shunt, some (Chiariello et al, 1975) but not all (Alvarez Diaz et al, 1978) showed a significant increase in mortality and morbidity related to closure of the shunt at the time of total correction.

POTT'S ANASTOMOSIS

Another systemic-to-pulmonary anastomosis was that described by Potts et al (1946). A communication is made between the descending aorta and left pulmonary artery. As with the Waterston shunt, there is a risk of making the anastomosis too big. Long-term follow-up showed a sig-nificant incidence of pulmonary vascular disease (Riker, 1963). There was also a considerable technical difficulty in closing the anastomosis at the time of total correction. The operation is used rarely, if ever, nowadays.

RELIEF OF SUBPULMONARY OBSTRUCTION AS A FIRST STAGE IN PALLIATION

It was Brock and Campbell (1950) who reported the results of a closed infundibulectomy via a transventricular approach to relieve subpulmonary obstruction. In present-ing the long-term result of this procedure, Brock (1974) reported a combined immediate and late mortality in 27% of 300 patients. The vast majority of those who survived surgery, however, made strikingly good progress. The pro-cedure results in symmetrical growth of the right and left pulmonary arteries. As emphasized more recently by Laas et al (1984), this may not occur after shunt procedures. This logical approach to palliation of tetralogy was also applied successfully in infants many years ago (Weinberg et al, 1962). Other groups achieved excellent results in early childhood (Flege and Ehrenhaft, 1967; Turski and Michalowski, 1968). These experiences were all achieved without use of cardiopulmonary bypass. This approach, however, is not applicable to neonates and smaller infants. It was logical, therefore, that 'open' infundibulectomy, using a patch to widen the subpulmonary outflow tract with cardiopulmonary bypass, should be advocated as palliation in early infancy in presence of diminutive pul-monary arteries (Gill et al, 1977; Tucker et al, 1979). The procedure was shown to cause growth, and not simply dis-tension, of the pulmonary arteries (Kirklin et al, 1977). It gives excellent relief of hypoxaemia with a low immediate mortality (Lane et al, 1983). But problems do occur. Some follow-up studies showed that many patients had multiple stenoses in the distal branches of the pulmonary arteries (Freedom et al, 1983). Further problems of narrowing of the pulmonary arteries at the distal insertion of the patch were encountered, especially when pericardium was used (Lane et al, 1983). Some centres continued to advocate infundibulectomy, nonetheless, as they found less peri-pheral stenoses in the pulmonary arteries than after shunts (Sebening et al, 1984). This was not our experience (Kay et al, 1983), nor that of many other units, who regard use of an Impra or Gortex interposition graft as the palliative procedure of choice (see above).

DEFINITIVE REPAIR

TECHNICAL CONSIDERATIONS

Intracardiac repair involves closing the ventricular septal defect and relieving subpulmonary obstruction. As with all open heart surgical procedures, it is necessary also to preserve the myocardium and to avoid damage to the conduction tissues. In children over 2 years, most surgeons use conventional cardiopulmonary bypass with cooling to either 28°C or to 20°C. Topical cold cardioplegic solutions may or may not be used. Varying periods of aortic cross-clamping are employed during intraventricular repair. Many centres use surface cooling followed by total circulatory arrest, with late bypass rewarming, for patients under 2 years of age (Barratt-Boyes et al, 1971). Others fibrillate the heart and use intermittent aortic cross-clamping. The right atrium is usually opened to close a patent oval foramen or atrial septal defect, and some now perform total repair via this portal (Edmunds et al, 1976; Binet et al, 1983). Most continue to use a ventriculotomy performed with a vertical incision in the outflow tract of the right ventricle. This is extended distally when a transannular patch is required. When this is not required, some surgeons prefer a transverse ventriculotomy. Alternatively, the right ventricle can be approached through the tricuspid valve (Edmunds et al, 1976). Others use a combined transventricular and transpulmonary approach (Karl and Sano, 1992).

The hypertrophied outlet septum, together with its parietal and septal extensions, are excised as indicated. Some surgeons make the decision as to whether a transannular patch is necessary from various measurements made on preoperative angiograms to determine the sizes of the pulmonary arteries relative to the aorta (Hawe et al, 1970; Blackstone et al, 1979; Tucker et al, 1979). The need for a patch can also be determined during the operation by using Hegar dilators to measure the narrowest part of the pulmonary outflow tract (Castaneda et al, 1977; Blackstone et al, 1979). Some degree of pulmonary incompetence is produced when transannular patching is used. A unicusp aortic homograft is inserted by some surgeons in an attempt to avoid this complication (Marchand, 1967; Radley-Smith and Yacoub, 1977; Monro 1978). The ventricular septal defect is repaired using a patch of knitted Dacron, Teflon or pericardium placed on its right ventricular aspect with either continuous or interrupted sutures.

It is essential, on discontinuing bypass, that the right ventricular pressure be lower than that in the left ventricle. It is no use permitting the patient to leave the operating theatre with suprasystemic right ventriculalr systolic pressures. Detailed angiographic studies should have demonstrated stenoses in the pulmonary arteries if present. Hypoplastic pulmonary arteries may still be the reason for residual high right ventricular pressures after adequate relief of subpulmonary obstruction even if pre- or intraoperative measurements were thought to exclude this possibility. Under these circumstances, the ventricular septal defect patch should be removed or fenestrated (Norwood et al, 1976).

Surgery should, ideally, result in normal right ventricular pressures, absence of a pressure gradient between the right ventricle and the pulmonary trunk and a competent pulmonary valve. Unfortunately, the nature of the subpulmonary obstruction rarely allows this ideal result (Pacifico et al, 1977). It is necessary, therefore, to choose the operation, or operations, that will give the closest result to the ideal with the lowest possible mortality and morbidity.

CHOICE OF OPERATIVE PROTOCOL

Symptomatic infants and/or children with tetralogy of Fallot require intervention to alleviate symptoms and to prevent neurological or other sequels of hypoxia. In the majority of patients, intervention will be surgical, although some advocate palliation by balloon dilation of the subpulmonary outflow tract (Sreeram et al, 1991). While this can be effective, damage to the ventriculo-arterial junction and pulmonary valvar leaflets is common, with tears not being confined to the valvar commissures (Battistessa et al, 1990). For this reason, and because the obstruction is predominantly subvalvar, the technique has a limited application. It can be considered if there are particular difficulties in undertaking a palliative shunt. We are unconvinced by the argument that increasing antegrade pulmonary blood flow via the outflow tract produces greater growth of the pulmonary arteries than does a well-constructed Blalock–Taussig shunt. Furthermore, after the latter, treatment with β-adrenergic blocking agents such as propranolol is unnecessary, whereas children palliated by balloon dilation of the subpulmonary infundibulum frequently continue to require pharmacological assistance to prevent infundibular shutdown. This not withstanding, one group have reported a reduction in the need for transanular patching at subsequent repair after early balloon dilation (Sluysmans et al, 1995).

Surgical repair of tetralogy of Fallot is now undertaken in virtually all patients, but what is not as yet resolved is whether total correction should be attempted in virtually all as a primary procedure or whether, in symptomatic neonates or young infants, it is preferable initially to construct a palliative shunt followed by correction in the second year of life.

In asymptomatic patients, corrective surgery should be deferred until after the first year of life, but there is no advantage to be gained by further deferment (Daily et al, 1978; Arciniegas et al, 1980). The same can be said for all those children presenting symptomatically above the age of 1 year and for some younger children presenting with good-sized pulmonary arteries. The key question is, 'When do the pulmonary arteries cease to be of good size?' Many of us have been considerably influenced by the experience of the University of Alabama in Birmingham, where the issue was treated in rigorous scientific fashion (Kirklin et al, 1983, 1984). The answer provided by this group is grounded in the concept of identification and neutralization of risk factors, with data derived from over 1000 patients undergoing surgery from 1967 onwards. We regard the principles of their approach as instructive, but, ultimately, each unit must use its own experience as the basis for determining the choice of operation. This is particularly the case in neonates or young infants, where the size of the pulmonary arteries may reflect low flow yet the vessels have the capacity to dilate if pulmonary blood flow increases, as occurs after corrective surgery.

Excluding the influence of pulmonary atresia, Kirklin et al (1984) identified nine factors that introduced a significant increment of risk. The first was the presence of diffusely small pulmonary arteries, the effect of which is to increase the postrepair ratio between the peak ventricular pressures. Their detrimental effect is neutralized by not attempting primary repair when the ratio of the combined diameter of the right and left pulmonary arteries (measured just before their first bifurcation) to that of the descending aorta is less than 1.5:1 (Blackstone et al, 1979). The second factor relates to abnormalities of the pulmonary arteries, such as anomalous origin of one artery or stenosis at its origin. These can all be alleviated by appropriate reconstructive procedures. Additional peripheral stenoses can now be dealt with by balloon dilation at later cardiac catheterization (Ring et al, 1985; Rothman et al, 1990), particularly using high-pressure balloons (Gentles et al, 1993). The third risk factor is a small pulmonary valvar orifice producing a high right ventricular pressure subsequent to repair if the obstruction is unrelieved. The necessary relief is provided by insertion of a transannular patch. Insertion of the patch, however, then becomes a fourth risk factor, though of less significance than a small 'annulus'. A transannular patch should not be used when the late postrepair peak ventricular pressure ratio after repair will be less than 0.7 without it. The first step in determining whether the patch is necessary is to measure the diameter of the subpulmonary outflow tract after infundibular resection. Use of prepared equations and nomograms then permits prediction of the immediate postoperative pressure ratio. This should be less than 0.85 about 30 minutes after repair, so that the final ratio will be less than 0.7. The second step is to verify that the right ventricular pressure 30 minutes after completion of repair without a patch is less than 0.85 of that in the left ventricle. If higher, a transannular patch should be inserted. Inherent in this approach is a reluctance to place a transannular patch, which may produce pulmonary incompetence. We will return to this point when considering long-term follow-up of corrected patients. A high postoperative peak pressure ratio is the fifth risk factor. This increases the risk of operative death if the patient survives and may lead to intolerance (Wessel et al, 1980a) and premature late death (Katz et al, 1982). The use of a valved conduit was the sixth factor identified in the Birmingham experience. This relates mostly to their inclusion of patients with pulmonary

atresia, since few would now place a conduit in patients with tetralogy. The exception to this may be when there is anomalous origin of the anterior descending artery from the right coronary artery. A transatrial–transpulmonary approach can also be used in this setting, thus avoiding the need for a conduit. Neutralization of the seventh risk factor, a previous Potts or Waterston shunt, is simple: avoid them. The next factor was a high haematocrit. Moderate elevation of the haematocrit does not alter the treatment. When the haematocrit is very high, a case can be made for constructing a shunt and wating 6 months, by which time the haematocrit will have fallen. The final risk factor is without question the most contentious, namely age at repair. Both old and young age appeared as incremental risks in the Birmingham analysis. Old age introduced risks for hospital death, poor postoperative exercise capacity (Wessel et al, 1980a) and impaired left ventricular function (Borow et al, 1980). Old age seemed to be more than 5 years. Ideally, repair should be accomplished before the age of 3 years. But how early should primary correction be recommended? In contrast to surgery for ventricular (Rizzoli et al, 1980) or atrioventricular septal defects (Studer et al, 1982), young age had still remained an incremental risk for repair of tetralogy in some series (Kirklin et al, 1983; Villani et al, 1983), but not all (Touati et al, 1990; Groh et al, 1991; Souza Uva et al, 1994; Hennein et al, 1995). In the past, some recommended construction of shunts for all patients less than 4 years of age (Arciniegas et al, 1980). Others argued for routine primary correction no matter how young the patient (Castaneda et al, 1977). The Birmingham group initially recommended primary repair down to the age at which the individual hospital risks of initial shunting and subsequent repair were thought to be less than those of primary repair (Kirklin et al, 1984). In their hands, this age had been about 6 months when a transannular patch was not needed, and 9 months when it was. We still have no argument with these recommendations. In contrast, those with excellent results in correcting young infants whatever their age, and for that matter whatever the size of their pulmonary arteries, still advocate primary repair at all ages. Therefore, Touati et al (1990) reported repair of 100 infants with symptomatic tetralogy undergoing surgery consecutively at under 1 year of age with only three deaths. Sousa Uva et al (1994) corrected 56 infants under 6 months, with 41 undergoing primary repair, and had only one death. Hennein et al (1995) gave details of 30 neonates, 11 with associated pulmonary atresia and five with non-confluent pulmonary arteries, with no deaths in hospital, but with some patients dying late. These exceptional surgical results show what can be achieved but raise important questions as to what, in the long term, is optimal. In these last series, 70%, 56% and 83% of the infants, respectively, required transannular patches. Of the series of Hennein et al (1995), five also had aortic homografts inserted between the right ventricle and the pulmonary arteries. Even the group from

Birmingham, Alabama have modified their views concerning pulmonary arterial size as a risk factor in infants, most of their earlier data having applied to older children. Thus, Groh et al (1991) reported a 'weak correlation, with considerable scatter' between the McGoon ratio and the ratio of ventricular pressure measured at the end of the operation in infancy. In a subsequent combined study with Boston Children's Hospital, 'size and configuration of the right and left pulmonary arteries had no demonstrable effect on survival, prevalence of transannular patching or post repair right ventricular–left ventricular pressure ratio' (Kirklin et al, 1992). Similar experience was reported by Reddy et al (1995). The most likely explanation for the apparently contradictory findings in the importance of pulmonary arterial size in infants and older children in influencing outcome of surgical correction is that 'small' arteries in infants may appear as such primarily because of low flow but yet remain able to be distended and to accommodate an increase in flow without appreciable increase in effective impedance. The structural composition of the central pulmonary arteries may also influence their capacity for subsequent growth, an inadequate proportion of elastin possibly being a hindrance to growth (Rosenberg et al, 1987).

When basing strategies for management exclusively on reported surgical series, it is important to be aware that surgeons only perform surgery on patients referred to them. Some degree of selection is inevitable. Therefore, the infants with truly minute pulmonary arteries may not be presented to a surgeon for correction, because of death before reaching hospital, because they are maintained on prostaglandins to allow a duct-dependent pulmonary circulation to permit pulmonary arterial growth or because they have had a palliative shunt elsewhere before they are considered for correction. Indeed, the Boston group recently reported their strategies for management of preoperative pulmonary valvar dilation, and transcatheter rehabilitation of pulmonary arteries, for tetralogy of Fallot with diminutive pulmonary arteries (Kreutzer et al, 1996).

Not all units, therefore, are so keen to pursue primary correction in small infants. A favourable outcome in correction of tetralogy of Fallot using a combined transatrial and transpulmonary approach beyond the neonatal period was reported by Karl and Sano (1992). They undertook correction in 366 patients, at a median age of 15.3 months, with two deaths in hospital and four occurring later. Actuarial survival was 97.5% at 4 years. Many of these patients had initially undergone construction of a shunt. The series also included patients with an anomalous coronary artery crossing the right ventricular outflow tract, and those with an atrioventricular septal defect.

One additional caveat, perhaps, is when an infant is having, or has on induction of anaesthesia, a hypercyanotic attack. Palliation rather than correction may then be prudent. Further problems are produced by associated lesions. If there is an atrioventricular septal defect, a second muscular inlet defect, or a straddling tricuspid valve, in our opinion it is imprudent to attempt immediate correction in infancy. Having diagnosed each of these lesions, we would initially palliate with an interposition shunt and undertake correction before the age of 5 years. With this approach, results for repair of tetralogy with atrioventricular septal defect have greatly improved (Gatzoulis et al, 1994). Comparable good results, nonetheless, are also reported by those who advocate primary correction (McElhinney et al, 1998).

So-called 'absence' of the pulmonary valve also produces complications, principally because of the dilated pulmonary arteries, coupled with incomplete development of the distal vascular bed. If the dilation extends far out into the pulmonary parenchyma, as happens in the most severely affected patients (Rabinovitch et al, 1982), surgery is unlikely to be of help no matter what procedure is performed. In the less severe cases, it is possible during correction of the intracardiac anomaly to reduce the size of the proximal pulmonary arteries, but concomitant bronchial distortion from compression cannot easily be relieved. Bronchomalacia can be expected, and hence obstruction to lung or airways may persist and complicate the postoperative course. Failure of development of the distal arterial bed may result in persistently high pulmonary arterial and right ventricular pressures despite adequate relief of subpulmonary obstruction. As previously indicated, this constitutes a major risk factor for correction that typically, but not necessarily, involves placement of a pulmonary homograft.

POSTOPERATIVE COURSE

In major centres nowadays, 95% or more of patients can be expected to survive corrective surgery, and the same percentages reach adult life. Indeed, two studies showed 98% of those surviving surgery to be alive following an observation period of over 20 years (Kirklin et al, 1981; Vogt et al, 1984). More recently, Murphy et al (1993) found an overall 86% actuarial survival among patients surviving 30 days after complete repair, compared with 96% in a control population. Further breakdown of this series showed survival rates after 30 years of 90%, 93% and 91% in patients operated on under 5 years, at 5–7 years and at 8–11 years, respectively. Patients who were 12 years or older at the time of operation had a survival rate of 76% compared with 93% in controls. As discussed, many centres now carry out surgery in infancy. The majority would certainly elect for surgery in the preschool period, usually before 3 years of age. It has also been shown that corrective surgery provides considerable benefits compared with the natural history even above the age of 40 years (Hu et al, 1985). Yet surgery is not without its complications. As Garson and McNamara (1981) commented, the striking relief of symptoms in all but a few patients tends to distract attention from haemo-dynamic, structural and psychological consequences or complications of the repair.

PHYSICAL RESPONSE TO CORRECTION

Following successful repair, almost all children rapidly 'catch up' in terms of height and weight. They grow faster than their peers (Page et al, 1978) and height and weight are normal 5 years after repair (Garson and McNamara, 1981). Murmurs frequently persist after operation, usually but not always related to (mild) residual subpulmonary obstruction or to acquired pulmonary incompetence (see below). The typical auscultatory findings on follow-up are a single second sound, an ejection systolic murmur in the second or third left intercostal space and a slightly delayed diastolic decrescendo murmur. If the pulmonary valve has been preserved, the second sound may be split; if subvalvar obstruction is completely relieved without a transannular patch, there may be no murmurs.

Presence of an ejection systolic murmur may complicate assessment of other problems, such as a residual ventricular septal defect, although cross-sectional echocardiography with Doppler studies easily allows quantification of residual intracardiac anomalies. Apart from a right aortic arch, when present, the chest radiograph may return to normal, but some will have a bulge over the upper left heart border as a consequence of patching the outflow tract. Cardiomegaly is observed in a proportion of those with complications (see below) but also persists in a small number of patients without any obvious cause (Garson and McNamara, 1981). When exercised, some will demonstrate normal values, although several studies have showed impaired exercise ability after complete repair (Strieder et al, 1975; Hirschfeld et al, 1978; Wessel et al, 1980a). The latter may reflect residual subpulmonary obstruction, residual ventricular septal defects or poor right ventricular function (Kinsley et al, 1974; Clayman et al, 1975). An increasing body of evidence points to the central importance of pulmonary incompetence, an inevitable consequence of a transannular patch, as a cause not only of impaired exercise tolerance but also of other late complications such as ventricular tachycardia or even sudden death (see below).

PSYCHOLOGICAL RESPONSE

Normal intelligence is to be anticipated following surgical repair (Garson et al, 1974; Castaneda and Rosenthal, 1977). There is no evidence of significant intellectual impairment in relation to the period of arterial oxygen desaturation prior to surgery. Some patients have been found to demonstrate persistent dependency, and this has been attributed to well-meaning but misguided parental overprotection (Garson et al, 1974). Some young adults may, therefore, need encouragement to be independent.

Once independence is attained, there need be no limit to achievement.

POSTOPERATIVE COMPLICATIONS

Problems can occur both in the immediate and late postoperative periods. Apart from the usual complications of cardiac surgery, such as bleeding, a low cardiac output may occur because of inadequate relief of subpulmonary obstruction or an obstructed or restrictive pulmonary vascular bed. A particular hazard is dehiscence of the patch in those patients where relief of subpulmonary obstruction is adequate. When this occurs, there will be a torrential left-to-right shunt with concomitant pulmonary oedema. This is because the thin-walled peripheral small pulmonary arteries cannot compensate and reduce the shunt by vasoconstriction. Paradoxically, if relief of subpulmonary obstruction is inadequate, patch dehiscence will not have such serious immediate consequences.

More recently, it has been appreciated that while most patients with a surgically adequate repair pass smoothly through the postoperative period, leaving the intensive care unit within 24 or 48 hours, a small proportion languish on inotropic support for many days before recovery. In the past, this had been attributed to prior treatment with β-blocking agents, but there is little evidence for this. In our experience, the majority of patients showing this phenomenom were not receiving β-blockers. Instead, echocardiographic Doppler studies in these patients show evidence of what has now been termed restrictive right ventricular physiology (Redington et al, 1992). There is antegrade diastolic flow in the pulmonary arteries coinciding with atrial systole throughout the respiratory cycle. As the pulmonary vascular resistance is low, atrial contraction causes flow to be transmitted through a poorly compliant right ventricle into the pulmonary arteries in such a way that, if pulmonary incompetence is present, its duration is shortened (Figure 46.30). Not only does atrial constriction cause antegrade diastolic flow in the pulmonary arteries, but retrograde flow can also be detected in the superior caval vein, again reflecting a poorly compliant right ventricle (Cullen, 1998). The mechanism of this phenomenon is not, at present, established. It does not appear to be related to age at operation but is more common on follow-up of patients in whom a transannular patch had been inserted (Norgard et al, 1996). Management consists of inotropic support with dopamine, and/or dobutamine, possibly with enoximone as a peripheral vasodilator. In severe cases, it may be necessary to cool the patient until ventricular function recovers.

In the late postoperative period, a residual ventricular septal defect and pulmonary incompetence, with or without impaired right ventricular function, are the most frequent unwelcome surgical sequels. A haemodynamically significant residual defect produces considerable

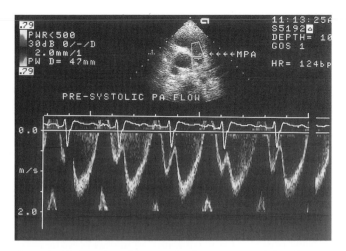

Figure 46.30. This Doppler trace of pulmonary arterial flow shows antegrade flow occurring in diastole coincident with atrial systole, thus shortening the duration of pulmonary regurgitation. This pattern is considered the hallmark of isolated right ventricular restriction. (Reproduced with kind permission of Dr Seamus Cullen and GMM Publishers, from 'The right heart in congenital heart disease' edited by Redington et al, 1998.)

morbidity and is by no means uncommon (Ruzyllo et al, 1974; Clayman et al, 1975; Poirier et al, 1977). It is also a potential cause of late death and, despite the not insignificant risk of reoperation, should probably be closed when recognized (Castaneda et al, 1974).

Pulmonary incompetence is found in between 60 and 90% of patients postoperatively. In the majority, it is well tolerated in the short and medium term, although occasionally it may exacerbate right-sided cardiac failure in the early postoperative period, thus prolonging recovery from surgery (Jones et al, 1973). Many groups, nonetheless, have produced optimistic results from medium-term follow-up (Bristow et al, 1970; Poirier al, 1977), especially if there is additional mild pulmonary stenosis (Hawe et al, 1972). Kaplan et al (1973), however, have reported that although pulmonary insufficiency is well-tolerated for the first few years it may result in a chronically dilated right ventricle and can lead to congestive heart failure. Pertinent to this is the study of Shimazaki et al (1984), who reviewed the natural history of isolated congenital pulmonary regurgitation. They showed that patients remain asymptomatic for up to 20 years, but thereafter freedom from symptoms declined rapidly with time. Symptoms included effort intolerance, right heart failure, arrhythmias and sudden death. Chronic pulmonary regurgitation may adversely affect exercise performance and right ventricular function. One of the difficulties hitherto has been lack of a technique to assess quantitatively the amount of pulmonary regurgitation. Qualitative assessment has suggested that impaired right ventricular function may be related to the degree of pulmonary regurgitation (Bove et al, 1983; Zakha et al, 1988), as may the degree of right ventricular dilation (Lange et al, 1982). Wessel et al (1980a) found a relation between the degree

of impairment of exercise and heart size on a chest radiograph. This led them to speculate that events of pulmonary regurgitation may correlate with decrease in exercise ability after operation. By using pressure–volume loops derived from simultaneous intraventricular pressure recordings during angiography, it has now become possible to quantify the pulmonary regurgitant fraction (Redington et al, 1988). Pulmonary regurgitation occurring during what should be right ventricular isovolumic relaxation is measured as the increase in right ventricular volume from the end of systole to opening of the tricuspid valve. Using this technique, exercise ability using a standard Bruce protocol has been combined with measurements of maximal consumption of oxygen and metabolic gas exchange using respiratory mass spectrometry (Carvalho et al, 1992). Maximal heart rate and total duration of exercise were less than in matched controls, and impairment of exercise capacity was shown to be directly related to the degree of pulmonary regurgitation. Similar findings had been reported by Rowe et al (1991), and by Norgard et al (1992), who used pulsed wave Doppler to classify pulmonary incompetence into mild, moderate or severe. The more severe categories were associated both with reduced exercise performance and with abnormalities such as reduced lung compliance. This group also reported a higher incidence of exercise-induced ventricular arrhythmias in patients with the most severe pulmonary regurgitation. Arrhythmias as found on 24-hour electrocardiographic tape recordings have also been detected in patients with severe pulmonary incompetence (Zahka et al, 1988), but there is no relationship between arrhythmias and residual subpulmonary obstruction.

Before dwelling in more detail on late conduction disturbances or arrhythmias and their relationship to haemodynamic disturbances, it is of note that, in the long term, the consequences of chronic pulmonary regurgitation may be modified by the diastolic properties of the right ventricle (Gatzoulis et al, 1995). Restrictive right ventricular physiology, found in some patients early after operation (Figure 46.30), is correlated with beneficial rather than adverse haemodynamic consequences when found on long-term follow-up. Exercise tolerance is enhanced, the heart does not enlarge despite pulmonary regurgitation and intraventricular conduction disturbances, as reflected by the QRS prolongation, may be less (Gatzoulis et al, 1995). In this respect, it should also be noted that the presence of peripheral pulmonary stenosis will increase the amount of pulmonary incompetence following surgery (Chaturvedi et al, 1997).

POSTOPERATIVE CONDUCTION DISTURBANCES AND ARRHYTHMIAS

Complete right bundle branch block is frequently produced following surgical correction of tetralogy (Zimmerman et al, 1958). There are three possible sites for damage to the right bundle. These are at the inferior border of the ventricular septal defect, where it could be damaged by sutures during insertion of a patch, within the moderator band, where it could be resected in the mistaken belief that this will relieve outflow tract obstruction, or distally, where the vertical ventriculotomy in the outflow tract may cut through the peripheral conduction fibres (Horowitz et al, 1979). Gelband et al (1971) produced convincing evidence from intraoperative bipolar electrode recordings that the ventriculotomy was responsible for a high proportion of cases. Further work then showed that the same pattern developed when the upper or middle third of the right ventricular free wall was incised. This suggested damage to a specific distal branch or branches of the right bundle rather than generalized interruption of distal conduction tissues (Krongrad et al, 1974). Postoperative intracardiac measurements of the time from initial ventricular polarization to depolarization at the right ventricular apex showed that, on rare occasions, isolated block could be caused by proximal damage (Sung et al, 1976).

Proximal damage to the conduction tissue is the more likely explanation when the electrocardiographic pattern of right bundle branch block is combined with a superior mean frontal QRS axis. This surface pattern can also result from damage at different sites (Steeg et al, 1975), which may explain the widely differing long-term prognoses observed in series of patients acquiring this postoperative electrocardiographic pattern. It occurs in between 8 and 20% of operated patients (Chesler et al, 1972; Downing et al, 1972; Wolff et al, 1972; Godman et al, 1974). When the damage is peripheral, the outlook is benign (Downing et al, 1972; Cairns et al, 1975; Steeg et al, 1975). Transient heart block was uncommon in the perioperative period of patients subsequently found to have a good prognosis, as was additional prolongation of the PR interval, the so-called 'trifascicular block pattern'. Conversely, some observed that the prognosis was less good when there was transient heart block (or a 'trifascicular block' pattern) after surgery (Moss et al, 1972; Wolff et al, 1972; Krongrad, 1978). They suggested that this combination pointed to central damage. Others have subsequently questioned this inference (Garson and McNamara, 1981). Godman et al (1974) have shown that a bad prognosis can, perhaps, be predicted instead by the presence of prolonged HV intervals on postoperative electrophysiological studies. Some abnormalities of atrioventricular conduction, therefore, are present in the majority of postoperative patients with tetralogy, but their precise prognostic significance is uncertain (Neches et al, 1977). What is not in doubt is that avoidance of conduction disturbances must be advantageous. By using as short a right ventriculotomy as possible, by limiting resection in the right ventricular outflow tract to the outlet septum and by not attacking the moderator band, the frequency of right bundle branch block can be significantly reduced (Hazan et al, 1980).

While heart block can be a cause of death at or soon after surgery and may cause some late sudden deaths, it is unlikely to account for the majority of deaths. Multiple ventricular premature beats may be a harbinger of more serious ventricular arrhythmias (James et al, 1975; Quattlebaum et al, 1976). Gillette et al (1977), indeed, concluded that ventricular arrhythmias, rather than conduction defects, were the likely basis for sudden death. The use of ambulatory monitoring, however, has greatly increased the detection of arrhythmias after surgery for congenital heart disease, or for that matter before surgery, bringing with it many dilemmas in management (Deanfield 1991).

Rhythm disturbances, such as frequent unifocal ventricular extrasysoles, more complex couplets, multifocal extrasystoles and even asymptomatic non-sustained ventricular tachycardia, were reported in two fifths or more of patients undergoing 24-hour monitoring on medium-term follow-up (Deanfield et al, 1980; Kavey et al, 1982). Attempts were made in these, and other, series to correlate arrhythmias with residual haemodynamic disorders, such as poorly relieved subpulmonary obstruction, but the results were conflicting. What has emerged is that frequency of arrhythmias correlates well with age at operation (Deanfield, 1991).

One possible explanation for this finding is the presence with older age of increasing amounts of fibrosis in the right but not the left ventricle (Jones et al, 1977; Deanfield et al, 1983; Hegerty et al, 1988). Not only age but more extensive surgery (Wessel et al, 1980b) and the extent of the ventriculotomy (Kobayashi et al, 1984) are associated with an increase in ventricular arrhythmias. Whether asymptomatic arrhythmias predict the risk of sudden death is a different matter. Sudden death occurs in about 6% of patients over the long term (Murphy et al, 1993), or 4.5 per 100 patients-years (Waien et al, 1992), but can it be predicted? As discussed previously, poor right ventricular systolic or diastolic function, residual subpulmonary obstruction or a residual ventricular septal defect have been associated with a poor prognosis, possibly owing to arrhythmias. The presence in asymptomatic patients of complex ventricular arrhythmias on 24-hour tape recordings, nonetheless, did not identify a group at risk (Cullen et al, 1994).

Perhaps the most important recent development in the ability to predict sudden death over the long term in patients with corrected tetralogy of Fallot comes from the work of Gatzoulis et al (1995). They have shown a relationship between QRS prolongation, right ventricular dilation, sustained ventricular arrhymias and late sudden death. In their study, prolongation of the QRS complex of 180 ms or more predicted with a 95% probability near-miss sudden death from sustained ventricular arrhymias. Conversely, no patient with sustained ventricular tachycardia dying suddenly had a duration less than 180 ms. Prolongation was associated with right ventricular dilation, often associated with pulmonary regurgitation, although this was not quantified in the study. When restrictive right ventricular physiology was identified on the late follow-up, duration of the QRS complex was always less than 180 ms. In these patients, the right ventricle has a limited end-diastolic volume; antegrade diastolic pulmonary flow owing to atrial systole limits the amount of pulmonary regurgitation. The myocardial structure that prevents right ventricular dilation even in the presence of pulmonary regurgitation is not known at present, but it appears to be protective in the long term against sudden death and sustained ventricular arrhythmias.

What emerges from these studies is that a mechano-electrical interaction in the right ventricle, namely ventricular dilation and stretch, may underly ventricular electrical instability. Such mechanisms have already been established for the left ventricle (Dean and Lab, 1989; Hansen et al, 1990). Of particular interest is that Waxman et al (1980) showed that a decrease in right ventricular volume, caused by a Valsalva manoeuvre, can terminate ventricular tachycardia in some patients. Electrophysiological studies (Kremers et al, 1988) have indicated a re-entry mechanism for sustained ventricular arrhythmias in this setting that requires areas of slow conduction. Further support to the notion that inhomogeneity in depolarization and repolarization may form the substrate for malignant ventricular arrhythmias late after repair of tetralogy of Fallot comes from the finding, in patients with QRS duration greater than 180 ms, that there are increased dispersions of the QT, QRS and JT intervals in those with, but not those without, episodes of ventricular tachycardia (Gatzoulis, 1997).

Fragmented electrograms indicative of localized areas of slowed conduction, however, have also been recorded from the inflow region (Kugler et al, 1983), the outflow tract (Donwar et al, 1992) and throughout the right ventricle in the absence of sustained ventricular tachycardia (Deanfield et al, 1985). It could be, therefore, that the mechanisms for non-sustained and sustained ventricular arrhythmias are different. This is an important consideration when we consider management of arrhythmias or conduction disorders on follow-up.

Treatment of arrhythmias and conduction disturbances at follow-up

The aims of treatment are relief of symptoms and prevention of sudden death. Non-sustained ventricular tachycardia is present in two fifths or more of asymptomatic patients on follow-up, but the incidence of late sudden death is low and cannot be predicted from analysis of 24-hour tape recordings. For this reason, we concur with the view that routine treatment of asymptomatic patients with non-sustained tachycardia is not currently indicated (Deanfield, 1991). Additional reasons for this conclusion are that non-sustained ventricular tachycardia may not be a marker for, nor have the same mechanism as, sustained tachycardia. Antiarrhythmic agents themselves may cause symptoms and can have a proarrhythmic action.

Atrial flutter causing symptoms requires treatment, and a class III agent such as amiodarone with or without digoxin may be effective. If ventricular function is well maintained, then sotalol, with both class III and β-blocking activity, is an alternative. Treatment of symptomatic ventricular arrhythmias is more difficult, and prevention is the best antidote. An early age of repair, a combined transatrial–transpulmonary approach to surgical correction or as small a right ventriculotomy as possible will all be expected to reduce risk, as will limiting the amounts of surgically induced pulmonary incompetence. With this in mind, reducing the need for transannular patching, even if this means submitting fewer young infants to primary correction, may also be advantageous. When sustained symptomatic tachycardia is present, or if an arrhythmia has induced an acute life-threatening event, antiarrhythmic agents such as amiodarone can be of benefit, but a more radical approach may be necessary. The importance of pulmonary incompetence in the long term has already been stressed. If this is present, then insertion of a pulmonary homograft may be indicated, both for haemodynamic reasons and to decrease right ventricular volume (Warner et al, 1993). This will then reduce the propensity to arrhythmias. The combination of even moderate pulmonary incompetence with duration of the QRS complex greater than 180 ms should also be considered as an indication for surgery, especially if there is additional downstream obstruction caused by peripheral pulmonary stenosis (Ibawi et al, 1987). Radiofrequency ablation also has a role when the site of origin of sustained tachycardia can be identified by electrophysiological studies.

REFERENCES

Alva C, Rigby M L, Ho S Y, Anderson R H 1998 Overriding and biventricular connection of aortic valves. Cardiology in the Young 8: 150–164

Alva C, Ho S Y, Lincoln C, Rigby M L, Wright A, Anderson R H 1999 The nature of the obstructive muscular bundles in double chambered right ventricle. Journal of Thoracic and Cardiovascular Surgery 117: 1180–1189

Alvarez Diaz F, Sanz E, Sanchez P A et al 1978 Fallot's tetralogy – palliation and repair with a previous shunt. In: Anderson R H, Shinebourne E A (eds) Paediatric cardiology 1977. Churchill Livingstone, Edinburgh, p 273–282

Anderson R H, Becker A E 1975 The surgical anatomy of Fallot's tetralogy. In: Longmore D B (ed.) The current status of cardiac surgery. MTP, Lancaster, UK, p. 49–61

Anderson R H, Becker A E, Van Mierop L H S 1977a What should we call the 'crista'? British Heart Journal 39: 856–859

Anderson R H, Monro J L, Ho S Y, Smith A, Deverall P B 1977b Les voies de conduction auriculo-ventriculaires dans le tetralogie de Fallot. Coeur 8: 793–807

Anderson R H, Allwork S P, Ho S Y, Lenox C C, Zuberbuhler J R 1981 Surgical anatomy of tetralogy of Fallot. Journal of Thoracic and Cardiovascular Surgery 81: 887–896

Ando M 1974 Subpulmonary ventricular septal defect with pulmonary stenosis. (Letter to Editor) Circulation 50: 412

Arciniegas E, Farooki Z Q, Hakimi M, Green E W 1980 Results of two-stage surgical treatment of tetralogy of Fallot. Journal of Thoracic and Cardiovascular Surgery 79: 876–883

Azzolina G, Russo P A, Maffei G, Marchese A 1982 Waterston anastomosis in two-stage correction of severe tetralogy of Fallot: ten years of experience. Annals of Thoracic Surgery 34: 413–421

Baker C, Brock R C, Campbell M, Suzman S 1949 Morbus caerulus; a study of 50 cases after the Blalock–Taussig operation. British Heart Journal 11: 170–198

Bargeron L M, Elliott L P, Soto B, Bream P R, Curry G C 1977 Axial cineangiography in congenital heart disease. Section I. Concept, technical and anatomic considerations. Circulation 56: 1075–1083

Barratt-Boyes B G, Neutze J M 1973 Primary repair of tetralogy of Fallot in infancy using profound cardiopulmonary bypass: a comparison with conventional two stage management. Annals of Surgery 178: 406–411

Barratt-Boyes B G, Simpson M, Neutze J M 1971 Intracardiac surgery in neonates and infants using deep hypothermia with surface cooling and limited cardiopulmonary bypass. Circulation 43: 1.25–30

Battistessa S A, Robles A, Jackson M, Miyamoto S, Arnold R, McKay R 1990 Operative findings after percutaneous pulmonary balloon dilatation of the right ventricular outflow tract in tetralogy of Fallot. British Heart Journal 64: 321–324

Becker A E 1992 Tetralogy of Fallot: from unifying pathology to variables. In: Yacoub M, Pepper J R (eds) Annals of cardiac surgery. Current Science, London, p. 81–91

Becker A E, Connor M, Anderson R H 1975 Tetralogy of Fallot: a morphometric and geometric study. American Journal of Cardiology 35: 402–412

Berry B E, McGoon D C 1973 Total correction for tetralogy of Fallot with anomalous coronary artery. Surgery 74: 894–898

Berry J M Jr, Einzig S, Krabill K A, Bass J L 1988 Evaluation of coronary artery anatomy in patients with tetralogy of Fallot by two-dimensional echocardiography. Circulation 78: 149–156

Bharati S, Kirklin J W, McAllister H A Jr, Lev M 1980 The surgical anatomy of common atrioventricular orifice associated with tetralogy of Fallot, double outlet right ventricle and complete regular transposition. Circulation 61: 1142–1149

Binet J-P, Patane L, Nottin R 1983 Correction of tetralogy of Fallot by combined transatrial and pulmonary approach. Modern Problems in Paediatrics 22: 152–156

Blackstone E H, Kirklin J W, Bertranou E G, Labrosse C J, Soto B, Bargeron L M Jr 1979 Preoperative prediction from cineangiograms of post-repair right ventricular pressure in tetralogy of Fallot. Journal of Thoracic and Cardiovascular Surgery 78: 542–552

Blalock A, Taussig H B 1945 The surgical treatment of malformations of the heart in which there is pulmonary stenosis or pulmonary atresia. Journal of the American Medical Association 128: 189–192

Borow K M, Green L H, Castaneda A R, Keane J K 1980 Left ventricular function after repair of tetralogy of Fallot and its relationship to age at surgery. Circulation 61: 1150–1158

Bove E L, Byrum C J, Thomas F D et al 1983 The influence of pulmonary insufficiency on ventricular function following repair of tetralogy of Fallot. Evaluation using radionuclide ventriculography. Journal of Thoracic and Cardiovascular Surgery 85: 691–696

Brinton W D, Campbell M 1953 Necropsies in some congenital diseases of the heart, mainly Fallot's tetralogy. British Heart Journal 15: 335–349

Bristow J D, Kloster F E, Lees M H, Menashe V D, Griswold H E, Starr A 1970 Serial cardiac catheterizations and exercise haemodynamics after correction of tetralogy of Fallot: average follow-up 13 months and 7 years after operation. Circulation 41: 1057–1066

Brock L 1974 Late results of palliative operation for Fallot's tetralogy. Journal of Thoracic and Cardiovascular Surgery 67: 511–518

Brock R C, Campbell M 1950 Infundibular resection or dilatation for infundibular stenoses. British Heart Journal 12: 403–424

Brotmacher L 1957 Oxygen administration in differential diagnosis in cyanotic patients. Guys Hospital Reports 106: 29–35

Brotmacher L, Campbell M 1958 Ventricular septal defect with pulmonary stenosis. British Heart Journal 20: 379–388

Burch G E, DePasquale N P, Phillips J H 1964 Tetralogy of Fallot associated with well developed left ventricular muscle mass and increased life span. American Journal of Medicine 36: 54–61

Burn J, Takao A, Wison D et al 1993 Conotruncal anomaly face syndrome is associated with a deletion within chromosome 22. Journal of Medical Genetics 30: 822–824

Cairns J A, Dobell A R C, Gibbons J E, Tessler I 1975 Prognosis of right bundle branch block and left anterior hemiblock after intracardiac repair of tetralogy of Fallot. American Heart Journal 90: 549–554

Caldwell R L, Weyman A G, Hurwitz R A, Girod D A, Feigenbaum H 1979 Right ventricular outflow tract assessment by cross-sectional echocardiography in tetralogy of Fallot. Circulation 59: 395–402

Campbell M 1958 Late results of operations for Fallot's tetralogy. British Medical Journal ii: 1175–1184

Campbell M, Deuchar D C 1961 Continuous murmurs in cyanotic congenital heart disease. British Heart Journal 23: 173–192

Campbell M, Gardner F E 1950 Radiological features of enlarged bronchial arteries. British Heart Journal 12: 183–200

Carvalho J S, Shinebourne E A, Busst C, Rigby M L 1992 Exercise capacity after complete repair of tetralogy of Fallot: deleterious effects of residual pulmonary regurgitation. British Heart Journal 67: 470–473

Carvalho J S, Silva C M, Rigby M L, Shinebourne E A 1993 Angiographic diagnosis of anomalous coronary artery in tetralogy of Fallot. British Heart Journal 70: 75–78

Castaneda A R, Rosenthal A 1977 Persistent abnormalities after repair of congenital heart defects. Ventricular septal defect and tetralogy of Fallot. Advances in Cardiology 20: 110–116

Castaneda A R, Sade R M, Lamberti J, Nicoloff D M 1974 Reoperation for residual defects after repair of tetralogy of Fallot. Surgery 76: 1010–1017

Castaneda A R, Freed M D, Williams R G, Norwood W I 1977 Repair of tetralogy of Fallot in infancy. Early and late results. Journal of Thoracic and Cardiovascular Surgery 74: 372–381

Celermajor J M, Varghese P J, Rowe R D 1969 Cardiovascular lesions in rubella embryopathy with special emphasis on pulmonary arterial disease. Israel Journal of Medical Sciences 5: 568–571

Chaturvedi R R, Kilner P J, White P A, Bishop A, Szwarc R, Redington A N 1997 Increased airway pressure and simulated branch pulmonary artery stenosis increase pulmonary regurgitation after repair of tetralogy of Fallot. Real-time analysis with a conductance catheter technique. Circulation 95: 643–649

Chesler E, Beck W, Schrire V 1972 Left anterior hemiblock and right bundle branch block before and after surgical repair of tetralogy of Fallot. American Heart Journal 84: 45–52

Chiariello L, Meyer J, Wukasch D C, Hallman G L, Cooley D A 1975 Intracardiac repair of tetralogy of Fallot. Five-year review of 403 patients. Journal of Thoracic and Cardiovascular Surgery 70: 529–535

Chung K J, Alexson C G, Manning J A, Gramiak R 1973 Echocardiography in truncus arteriosus: the value of pulmonic valve detection. Circulation 48: 281–286

Clayman J A, Ankeney J L, Liebman J 1975 Results of complete repair of tetralogy of Fallot in 156 consecutive patients. American Journal of Surgery 130: 601–607

Corvisart J N 1818 Essais sur les maladies et les lesions organiques du coeur et des gros vaisseaux, 3rd edn. Mequignon-Marvis, Paris

Cullen S 1998 The right ventricle in tetralogy of Fallot: the early postoperative period. In: Redington A N, Brawn W J, Deanfield J E, Anderson R H (eds) The right heart in congenital heart disease. GMM, London, p 81–84

Cullen S, Celermajer D S, Franklin R C G, Hallidie-Smith K A, Deanfield J E 1994 Prognostic significance of ventricular arrhythmia after repair of tetralogy of Fallot: a 12-year prospective study. Journal of the American College of Cardiology 23: 1151–1155

Cumming G R, Carr W 1966 Relief of dyspnoeic attacks in Fallot's tetralogy with propranolol. Lancet 1: 519–522

Czeizel A, Pornoi A, Péterffy E, Taral E 1982 Study of children of parents operated on for congenital cardiovascular malformations. British Heart Journal 47: 290–293

Daily P O, Stinson E B, Griepp R B, Shumway N E 1978 Tetralogy of Fallot. Choice of surgical procedure. Journal of Thoracic and Cardiovascular Surgery 75: 338–345

Dean J W, Lab M J 1989 Arrhythmia in heart failure: role of mechanically induced changes in electrophysiology. Lancet i: 1309–1311

Deanfield J E 1991 Late ventricular arrhythmias occurring after repair of tetralogy of Fallot: do they matter? International Journal of Cardiology. 30: 143–150

Deanfield J E, McKenna W J, Hallidie-Smith K A 1980 Detection of late arrhythmia and conduction disturbance after correction of tetralogy of Fallot. British Heart Journal 44: 248–253

Deanfield J E, Ho S Y, Anderson R H, McKenna W J, Allwork S P, Hallidie-Smith K A 1983 Late sudden death after repair of tetralogy of Fallot: a clinicopathologic study. Circulation 67: 626–631

Deanfield J E, McKenna W J, Presbitero P, England D, Graham G R, Hallidie-Smith K 1984 Ventricular arrhythmia in unrepaired and repaired tetralogy of Fallot. Relation to age, timing of repair, and haemodynamic status. British Heart Journal 52: 77–81

Deanfield J E, McKenna W J, Rowland E 1985 Local abnormalities of right ventricular depolarisation after repair of tetralogy of Fallot: a basis for ventricular arrhythmia. American Journal of Cardiology 55: 622–626

Dennis N R, Warren J 1981 Risks to the offspring of patients with some common congenital heart defects. Journal of Medical Genetics 18: 8–16

Dickinson D F, Wilkinson J L, Smith A, Hamilton D I, Anderson R H 1982 Variations in the morphology of the ventricular septal defect and disposition of the atrioventricular conduction tissues in tetralogy of Fallot. Thoracic and Cardiovascular Surgeon 5: 243–249

Digilio M C, Marino B, Grazioli S, Agostino D, Giannotti A, Dallapiccola B 1996 Comparison of occurrence of genetic syndromes in ventricular septal defect with pulmonary stenosis (classic tetralogy of Fallot) versus ventricular septal defect and major aortopulmonary collateral arteries. American Journal of Cardiology 77: 1375–1376

Donwar E, Harris L, Kimber S et al 1992 Ventricular tachycardia after surgical repair of tetralogy of Fallot: results of intraoperative mapping studies. Journal of the American College of Cardiology 20: 648–655

Downing J W, Kaplan S, Bore K E 1972 Post surgical left anterior hemiblock and right bundle branch block. British Heart Journal 34: 263–270

Edmunds L H, Saxena N C, Friedman S, Rashkind W J, Dodd P F 1976 Transatrial repair of tetralogy of Fallot. Surgery 80: 681–688

Edwards W E 1981 Double-outlet right ventricle and tetralogy of Fallot. Two distinct but not mutually exclusive entities. Journal of Thoracic and Cardiovascular Surgery 82: 418–422

Ehlers K H, Engle M A 1966 Familial congenital heart disease. I. Genetic and environmental factors. Circulation 34: 503–516

Elliott L P, Bargeron L M Jr, Bream P R, Soto B, Curry G C 1977 Atrial cineangiography in congenital heart disease. Section II. Specific lesions. Circulation 56: 1084–1093

Faggian G, Frescura C, Thiene G, Bortolotti U, Mazzucco A, Anderson R H 1983 Accessory tricuspid valve tissue causing obstruction of the ventricular septal defect in tetralogy of Fallot. British Heart Journal 49: 324–327

Fallot A 1888 Contribution a l'anatomie pathologique de la maladie bleue (cyanose cardiaque). Marseille Medicine 25: 77–403

Feldt R H, DuShane J W, Titus J L 1966 The anatomy of the atrioventricular conduction system in ventricular septal defect and tetralogy of Fallot: correlations with the electrocardiogram and vectorcardiogram. Circulation 34: 774–782

Fellows K E, Freed M D, Keane J F, Van Praagh R, Bernhard W, Castenada A C 1975 Results of routine preoperative coronary angiography in tetralogy of Fallot. Circulation 51: 561–566

Felge J B Jr, Ehrenhaft J L 1967 Transventricular pulmonary valvotomy and infundibular resection for tetralogy of Fallot. Diseases of the Chest 52: 727–731

Freedom R M, Olley P M 1976 Pulmonary arteriography in congenital heart disease. Catheterization and Cardiovascular Diagnosis 2: 309–312

Freedom R M, Pongiglione G, Williams W G, Trusler G A, Rowe R D 1983 Palliative right ventricular outflow tract construction for patients with pulmonary atresia, ventricular septal defect, and hypoplastic pulmonary arteries. Journal of Thoracic and Cardiovascular Surgery 86: 24–36

Garson A, McNamara D G 1981 Postoperative tetralogy of Fallot. In: Engle M A (ed.) Cardiovascular clinics, vol II: pediatric cardiovascular disease. Davis, Philadelphia, PA, p 407–429

Garson A Jr, Williams R B Jr, Reckless J 1974 Long-term follow-up of patients with tetralogy of Fallot: physical health and psychopathology. Journal of Pediatrics 85: 429–433

Gasul B M, Dillon R F, Urla V, Hait G 1957 Ventricular septal defects: their natural transformation into those with infundibular stenosis or into the cyanotic or noncyanotic types of tetralogy of Fallot. Journal of the American Medical Association 164: 847–853

Gatzoulis M A, Shore D, Yacoub M, Shinebourne E A 1994 Complete atrioventricular septal defect with tetralogy of Fallot: diagnosis and management. British Heart Journal 71: 579–583

Gatzoulis M A, Till J A, Somerville J, Redington A N 1995 Mechanoelectrical interaction in tetralogy of Fallot. QRS prolongation relates to right ventricular size and predicts malignant ventricular arrhythmias and sudden death. Circulation 15: 231–237

Gatzoulis M A, Till J A, Redington A N 1997 Depolarization– repolarization inhomogeneity after repair of tetralogy of Fallot. The substrate for malignant ventricular tachycardia? Circulation 95: 401–404

Gelband H, Waldo A L, Kaiser G A, Bowman F O Jr, Maim J R, Hoffman B F 1971 Etiology of right bundle- branch block in patients undergoing total correction of tetralogy of Fallot. Circulation 44: 1022–1033

Gentles T L, Lock J E, Perry S B 1993 High pressure balloon angioplasty for branch pulmonary artery stenosis: early experience. Journal of the American College of Cardiology 22: 867–872

Gibson S, Lewis K C 1952 Congenital heart disease following maternal rubella during pregnancy. American Journal of Diseases of Childhood 83: 317–319

Gill C C, Moodie D S, McGoon D C 1977 Staged surgical management of pulmonary atresia with diminutive pulmonary arteries. Journal of Thoracic and Cardiovascular Surgery 73: 436–442

Gillette P C, Yeoman M A, Mullins C E, McNamara D G 1977 Sudden death after repair of tetralogy of Fallot. Electrocardiographic and electrophysiologic abnormalities. Circulation 56: 566–571

Godman M J, Tham P, Kidd B S L 1974 Echocardiography in the evaluation of the cyanotic newborn infant. British Heart Journal 36: 154–166

Godman M J, Roberts N K, Izukawa T 1974 Late postoperative conduction disturbances after repair of ventricular septal defect and tetralogy of Fallot. Circulation 49: 214–221

Goldschmidt B 1974 Platelet function in children with congenital heart disease. Acta Paediatrica Scandinavica 61: 310–314

Goor D A, Lillehei C W 1975 The anatomy of the heart. Congenital malformations of the heart. Grune & Stratton, New York, p 1–37

Goor D A, Lillehei C W, Edwards J E 1971 Ventricular septal defects and pulmonic stenosis with and without dextroposition. Anatomic features and embryologic implications. Chest 60: 117–128

Gootman N L, Scarpelli E M, Rudolph A M 1963 Metabolic acidosis in children with severe cyanotic congenital heart disease. Pediatrics 31: 251–254

Gramiak R, Shah P M 1971 Cardiac ultrasonography and review of current applications. Radiologic Clinics of North America 9: 469–490

Griffin M L, Sullivan I D, Anderson R H, Macartney F J 1988 Doubly committed subarterial ventricular septal defect: new morphological criteria with echocardiographic and angiocardiographic correlation. British Heart Journal 59: 474–479

Groh M A, Meliones J N, Bove E L et al 1991 Repair of tetralogy of Fallot in infancy. Effect of pulmonary artery size on outcome. Circulation 84(suppl III): 206–212

Guntheroth W G, Morgan B C, Mullins G L 1965 Physiologic studies of paroxysmal hyperpnea in cyanotic congenital heart disease. Circulation 31: 70–76

Guntheroth W G, Morgan B C, Mullins G L, Baum D 1968 Venous return with knee–chest position and squatting in tetralogy of Fallot. American Heart Journal 75: 313–318

Guyton R A, Owens J E, Waumett J D, Dooley K J, Hatcher C R J, Williams W H 1983 The Blalock–Taussig shunt. Low risk, effective palliation, and pulmonary artery growth. Journal of Thoracic and Cardiovascular Surgery 85: 917–922

Hansen D E, Craig C S, Hodeghem L M 1990 Stretch-induced arrhythmias in isolated canine ventricle. Circulation 81: 1094–1105

Hastreiter A R, D'Cruz I A, Cantez T 1966 Right-sided aorta. British Heart Journal 28: 722–739

Hawe A, Rastelli G C, Ritter D G, Dushane J W, McGoon D C 1970 Management of right ventricular outflow tract in severe tetralogy of Fallot. Journal of Thoracic and Cardiovascular Surgery 60: 131–143

Hawe A, McGoon D C, Kincaid O W, Ritter D G 1972 Fate of the outflow tract in the tetralogy of Fallot. Annals of Thoracic Surgery 13: 137

Hazan E, Bical O, Bex J P, Dubuis C, Lecompte Y, De Riberolles C, Neveux J Y 1980 Is right bundle branch block avoidable in surgical correction of tetralogy of Fallot. Circulation 62: 852–854

Hegerty A, Anderson R H, Deanfield J E 1988 Myocardial fibrosis in tetralogy of Fallot: effect of surgery or part of the natural hisory? British Heart Journal 59: 123

Hennein H A, Mosca R S, Urcelay G, Crowley D C, Bove E L 1995 Intermediate results after complete repair of tetralogy of Fallot in neonates. Journal of Thoracic and Cardiovascular Surgery 109: 332–344

Higgins C B, Mulder D G 1972 Tetralogy of Fallot in the adult. American Journal of Cardiology 29: 837–846

Hirschfeld S, Tuboku-Metzger A J, Borkat G, Ankeney J, Clayman J, Liebman J 1978 Comparison of exercise and catheterization results following total surgical correction of tetralogy of Fallot. Journal of Thoracic and Cardiovascular Surgery 75: 446–451

Hoffman J I E, Rudolph A M, Nadas A S, Gross R E 1960a Pulmonic stenosis, ventricular septal defect and right ventricular pressure above systemic level. Circulation 22: 405–411

Hoffman J I E, Rudolph A M, Nadas A S, Paul M H 1960b Physiologic differentiation of pulmonic stenosis with and without an intact ventricular septum. Circulation 22: 385–404

Honda J 1993 Growth of the pulmonary arteries and morphological assessment after Blalock–Taussig shunt. Nippon Kyobu Geka Gakkai Zasshi 41: 569–577

Honey M, Chamberlain D A, Howard J 1964 The effect of beta-sympathetic blockade on arterial oxygen saturation in Fallot's tetralogy. Circulation 30: 501–510

Horowitz L N, Simson M B, Spear J F et al 1979 The mechanism of apparent right bundle branch block after transatrial repair of tetralogy of Fallot. Circulation 59: 1241–1252

Howell C E, Ho S Y, Anderson R H, Elliott M J 1990 Variations within the fibrous skeleton and ventricular outflow tracts in tetralogy of Fallot. Annals of Thoracic Surgery 50: 450–457

Hu D C K, Seward J B, Puga F J, Fuster V, Tajik A J 1985 Total correction of tetralogy of Fallot at age 40 years and older: long-term follow-up. Journal of the American Medical Association 5: 40–44

Hunter W 1784 Three cases of mal-conformation in the heart, Case II. Medical observations and inquiries by a Society of Physicians in London. 6: 291–303

Husson G, Otis A B 1957 Adaptive value of respiratory adjustments to shunt hypoxia and to altitude hypoxia. Journal of Clinical Investigation 36: 270–278

Ilbawi M N, Idriss F S, DeLeon S Y et al 1987 Factors that exaggerate the deleterious effects of pulmonary insufficiency on the right ventricle after tetralogy repair. Surgical implications. Journal of Thoracic and Cardiovascular Surgery 93: 36–44

Isaaz K, Cloez J L, MarÇon F, Worms A M, Pernod C 1986 Is the aorta truly dextroposed in tetralogy of Fallot? A two-dimensional echocardiographic answer. Circulation 73: 892–899

Jackson M, Connell M G, Smith A, Drury J, Anderson R H 1995 Common arterial trunk and pulmonary atresia: close developmental cousins? Results from a teratogen induced animal model. Cardiovascular Research 30: 992–1000

Jahangiri M, Lincoln C, Shinebourne E A 1999 Does the modified Blalock-Taussig shunt cause growth of the contralateral pulmonary artery? Annals of Thoracic Surgery 67: 1397–1399

James F W, Kaplan S, Chou T -C 1975 Unexpected cardiac arrest in patients after surgical correction of tetralogy of Fallot. Circulation 52: 691–695

Jones E L, Conti C R, Neill C A, Gott V L, Brawley R K, Haller J A Jr 1973 Long-term evaluation of tetralogy

patients with pulmonary valvular insufficiency resulting from outflow patch correction across the pulmonic annulus. Circulation 48(suppl III): 11–18

Jureidini S B, Appleton R S, Nouri S 1989 Detection of coronary artery abnormalities in tetralogy of Fallot by two-dimensional echocardiography. Journal of the American College of Cardiology 14: 960–967

Kaplan S, Helmsworth J A, McKinivan C E, Benzing G III, Schwartz D C, Schreiber J T 1973 The fate of reconstruction of the right ventricular outflow tract. Journal of Thoracic and Cardiovascular Surgery 66: 361–374

Karl T, Sano S 1992 Tetralogy of Fallot: favorable outcome of nonneonatal transatrial, transpulmonary repair. Annals of Thoracic Surgery 54: 903–907

Katz N M, Blackstone E H, Kirklin J W, Pacifico A D, Bargeron L M Jr 1982 Late survival and symptoms after repair of tetralogy of Fallot. Circulation 65: 403–410

Kay P H, Capuani A, Franks R, Lincoln C 1983 Experience with the modified Blalock-Taussig operation using polytetrafluoroethylene (Impra) grafts. British Heart Journal 49: 359–363

Kent J V 1953 The development of ribnotching after surgical intervention in congenital heart disease with a description of two cases. British Journal of Radiology 26: 346–351

Khoury G H, DuShane J W, Ongley P A 1965 The preoperative and postoperative vectorcardiogram in tetralogy of Fallot. Circulation 31: 85–94

King S B, Franch R H 1971 Production of increased right to left shunting by rapid heart rates in patients with tetralogy of Fallot. Circulation 44: 265–271

Kinsley R H, McGoon D C, Danielson G K, Wallace R B, Mair D D 1974 Pulmonary arterial hypertension after repair of tetralogy of Fallot. Journal of Thoracic and Cardiovascular Surgery 67: 110–120

Kirklin J W, Karp R B 1970 Tetralogy of Fallot from a surgical viewpoint. Saunders, Philadelphia, PA

Kirklin J W, Ellis F H, McGoon D C, Dushane J W, Swan H J C 1959 Surgical treatment for tetralogy of Fallot by open intracardiac repair. Journal of Thoracic and Cardiovascular Surgery 37: 22–46

Kirklin J W, Wallace R B, McGoon D C, DuShane J W 1965 Early and late results after intracardiac repair of tetralogy of Fallot: 5-year review of 337 patients. Annals of Surgery 162: 578–589

Kirklin J W, Blackstone E H, Pacifico A D 1977 The enlargement of small pulmonary arteries by preliminary palliative operations. Circulation 56: 612–617

Kirklin J W, Blackstone E H, Pacifico A D 1981 Natural and unnatural history of tetralogy of Fallot. In: Engle M A (ed.) Pediatric cardiovascular disease. Davis, Philadelphia, PA, p 442

Kirklin J W, Blackstone E H, Kirklin J K, Pacifico A D, Aramendi J, Bargeron L M Jr 1983 Surgical results and protocols in the spectrum of tetralogy of Fallot. Annals of Surgery 198: 251–261

Kirklin J W, Blackstone E H, Pacifico A D, Kirklin J K, Bargeron L M Jr 1984 Risk factors of early and late failure after repair of tetralogy of Fallot, and their neutralization. Thoracic and Cardiovascular Surgeon 32: 208–214

Kirklin J W, Blackstone E H, Jonas R A et al 1992 Morphologic and surgical determinants of outcome events after repair of tetralogy of Fallot and pulmonary stenosis. A two-institution study. Journal of Thoracic and Cardiovascular Surgery 103: 706–723

Kleinert S, Geva T 1993 Echocardiographic morphometry and geometry of the left ventricular outflow tract in fixed subaortic stenosis. Journal of the American College of Cardiology 22: 1501–1508

Kobayashi J, Hirose H, Nakano S, Masuda H, Shirakura R, Kawashima Y 1984 Ambulatory electrocardiographic study of the frequency and cause of ventricular arrhythmia after correction of tetralogy of Fallot. American Journal of Cardiology 54: 1310–1313

Kohner E M, Allen E M, Saunders K B, Emery V M, Pallis C 1967 Electroencephalogram and retinal vessels in congenital cyanotic heart disease before and after surgery. British Medical Journal 4: 207–210

Kontras S B, Bodenbender J G, Craenen J, Hosier D M 1970 Hyperviscosity in congenital heart disease. Journal of Pediatrics 76: 214–220

Kremers M S, Wells P J, Black W H, Solodyna M A 1988 Entrainment of ventricular tachycardia in postoperative tetralogy of Fallot. Pacing and Clinical Electrophysiology 11: 1310–1314

Kreutzer J, Perry S B, Jonas R A, Mayer J E, Castaneda A R, Lock J E 1996 Tetralogy of Fallot with diminutive pulmonary arteries: preoperative pulmonary valve dilation and transcatheter rehabilitation of pulmonary arteries. Journal of the American College of Cardiology 27: 1741–1747

Krongrad E 1978 Prognosis for patients with congenital heart disease and postoperative intraventricular conduction defects. Circulation 57: 867–870

Krongrad E, Heller S E, Bowman F O, Maim J R, Hoffman B F 1974 Further observations on the etiology of the right bundle branch block pattern following right ventriculotomy. Circulation 50: 1105–1113

Kugler J D, Pinsky W W, Cheatham J P, Hofshire P J, Mooring P K, Flemin W H 1983 Sustained ventricular tachycardia after repair of tetralogy of Fallot: new electrophysiologic findings. American Journal of Cardiology 51: 1137–1143

Kurosawa H, Imai Y, Becker A E 1988 Surgical anatomy of the atrioventricular conduction bundle in tetralogy of Fallot. New findings relevant to the position of the sutures. Journal of Thoracic and Cardiovascular Surgery 95: 586–591

Laas J, Engeser U, Meisner H et al 1984 Tetralogy of Fallot, development of the hypoplastic pulmonary arteries after palliation. Thoracic and Cardiovascular Surgeon 32: 133–138

Lane I, Treasure T, Leijala M, Shinebourne E, Lincoln C 1983 Diminutive pulmonary artery growth following right ventricular outflow tract enlargement. International Journal of Cardiology 3: 175–185

Lange P E, Onnasch D G, Bernhard A, Heintzen P H 1982 Left and right ventricular adaptation to right ventricular overload before and after surgical repair of tetralogy of Fallot. American Journal of Cardiology 50: 786–794

Lau K C, Calcaterra G, Miller G A H et al 1982 Aorto-pulmonary window. Journal of Cardiovascular Surgery 23: 21–27

Leatham A, Weitzman D 1957 Auscultatory and phonocardiographic signs of pulmonary stenosis. British Heart Journal 19: 303–317

Lev M 1959 The architecture of the conduction system in congenital heart disease. II. Tetralogy of Fallot. Archives of Pathology 67: 572–587

Lev M, Eckner F A O 1964 The pathologic anatomy of tetralogy of Fallot and its variants. Diseases of the Chest 45: 251–261

Li J, Soukias N D, Carvalho J S, Ho S Y 1998 Coronary arterial anatomy in tetralogy of Fallot: morphological and clinical correlations. Heart 80: 174–183

Lillehei C W, Cohen M, Warden H E et al 1955 Direct vision intracardial surgical correlation of the tetralogy of Fallot, pentalogy of Fallot, and pulmonary atresia defects: report of the first ten cases. Annals of Surgery 142: 418–443

Longenecker C G, Reemtsma K, Creech O Jr 1961 Anomalous coronary artery distribution associated with tetralogy of Fallot: a hazard in open cardiac repair. Journal of Thoracic and Cardiovascular Surgery 42: 258–262

Lund G W 1952 Growth study of children with the tetralogy of Fallot. Journal of Pediatrics 41: 572–577

Lurie P R 1953 Postural effects in tetralogy of Fallot. American Journal of Medicine 15: 297–306

Mandell V S, Lock J E, Mayer J E, Parness I A, Kulik T J 1990 The 'laid-back' angiogram: an improved angiographic view for demonstration of coronary arteries in transposition of the great arteries. American Journal of Cardiology 65: 1397–1383

Marchand P 1967 The use of a cusp-bearing homograft patch to the outflow tract and pulmonary artery in Fallot's tetralogy and pulmonary valvular stenosis. Thorax 22: 497–509

Marquis R M 1956 Longevity and the early history of the tetralogy of Fallot. British Medical Journal i: 819–822

Martin C E, Reddy P S, Leon D F, Shaver J A 1973 Genesis, frequency and diagnostic significance of ejection sound in adults with tetralogy of Fallot. British Heart Journal 35: 402–412

McElhinney D B, Reddy V M, Silverman N H, Brook M M, Hanely F L 1998 Atrioventricular septal defect with common valvar orifice and tetralogy of Fallot revisited: making a case for primary repair in infancy. Cardiology in the Young 8: 455–461

McKay R, de Leval M R, Rees P, Taylor J F N, Macartney F J, Stark J 1980 Postoperative angiographic assessment of modified Blalock–Taussing shunts using expanded polytetrafluoroethylene (Gore-Tex). Annals of Thoracic Surgery 30: 137–145

McMillan I K R, Johnson A M, Machell E S 1965 Total correction of tetralogy of Fallot in young children. British Medical Journal i: 348–350

Mehrizi A, Drash A 1962 Growth disturbance in congenital heart disease. Journal of Pediatrics 61: 418–429

Miller G A H, Restifo M, Shinebourne E A et al 1973 Pulmonary atresia with intact ventricular septum and critical pulmonary stenosis presenting in the first month of life. Investigations and surgical results. British Heart Journal 35: 9–16

Miller R A, Lev M, Paul M H 1962 Congenital absence of the pulmonary valve. The clinical syndrome of tetralogy of

Fallot with pulmonary regurgitation. Circulation
26: 266–278

Mitchell S C, Korones S B, Berendes H W 1971 Congenital
heart disease in 56 109 births. Incidence and natural
history. Circulation 43: 323–332

Momma K, Ando M, Takao A, Wu F-F 1990 Fetal
cardiovascular cross-sectional morphology of tetralogy of
Fallot in rats. Fetal Diagnostic Therapy 5: 196–204

Monro J L 1978 Surgery – necessity for outflow patch. In:
Anderson R H, Shinebourne E A (eds) Paediatric cardiology
1977. Churchill Livingstone, Edinburgh, p 295–303

Morgan B C, Guntheroth W G, Bloom R S, Fyler D C 1965
A clinical profile of paroxysmal hyperpnea in cyanotic
congenital heart disease. Circulation 31: 66–69

Moss A J, Klyman G, Emmanouilides G C 1972 Late onset
complete heart block. Newly recognized sequela of cardiac
surgery. American Journal of Cardiology 30: 884–887

Muraoka R, Yokota M, Matsuda K et al 1973 Long-term
hemodynamic evaluation of primary total correction of
tetralogy of Fallot during the first two years of life.
Archives of Japanese Chirurgerie 42: 315–324

Murphy J G, Gersh B J, Mair D D et al 1993 Long-term
outcome in patients undergoing surgical repair of
tetralogy of Fallot. New England Journal of Medicine
329: 593–599

Neches W H, Park S C, Mathews R A, Lenox C C, Marin-
Garcia J, Zuberbuhler J R 1977 Tetralogy of Fallot.
Postoperative electrophysiological studies. Circulation
56: 713–719

Neirotti R, Galindez E, Kreutzer G, Coronel A R, Pedrini M,
Becu L 1978 Tetralogy of Fallot with sub-pulmonary
ventricular septal defect. Annals of Thoracic Surgery
25: 51–56

Neufeld H N, McGoon D C, DuShane J W, Edwards J E 1960
Tetralogy of Fallot with anomalous tricuspid valve
simulating pulmonary stenosis with intact septum.
Circulation 22: 1083–1086

Nora J J, McGill C W, McNamara D G 1970 Empiric risks in
common and uncommon congenital heart lesions.
Tetralogy 3: 325–330

Norgard G, Gatzoulis M A, Moraes F et al 1996 Relationship
between the type of outflow tract repair and postoperative
right ventricular diastolic physiology in tetralogy of Fallot.
Implications for long-term outcome. Circulation
15: 3276–3280

Norwood W I, Rosenthal A, Castaneda A R 1976 Tetralogy
of Fallot with acquired pulmonary atresia and hypoplasia
of pulmonary arteries. Report of surgical management in
infancy. Journal of Thoracic and Cardiovascular Surgery
72: 454–457

O'Donnell T V, McIlroy M B 1962 The circulatory effects of
squatting. American Heart Journal 64: 347–356

Ongley P A, Rahimtoola S H, Kincaid O W, Kirklin J W 1966
Continuous murmurs in tetralogy of Fallot and pulmonary
atresia with ventricular septal defect. American Journal of
Cardiology 18: 821–826

Oppenheimer-Dekker A, Gittenberger-de Groot A C,
Bartelings M M, Wenink A C G, Moene R J, van der
Harten J J 1985 Abnormal architecture of the ventricles in
hearts with an overriding aortic valve and a
perimembranous ventricular septal defect ('Eisenmenger
VSD'). International Journal of Cardiology 9: 341–355

Pacifico A D, Bargeron L M Jr, Kirklin J W 1973 Primary
total correction of tetralogy of Fallot in children less than
four years of age. Circulation 48: 1085–1091

Pacifico A D, Kirklin J W, Blackstone E H 1977 Surgical
management of pulmonary stenosis in tetralogy of Fallot.
Journal of Thoracic and Cardiovascular Surgery
74: 382–395

Page R E, Deverall P B, Watson A, Scott O 1978 Height and
weight gain after total correction of Fallot's tetralogy.
British Heart Journal 40: 416–420

Patterson D F, Pyle R L, Van Mierop L, Melbin J, Olson M
1974 Hereditary defects of the conotruncal septum in
Keeshond dogs: pathological and genetic studies.
American Journal of Cardiology 34: 187–205

Peacock T B 1867 Malformations of the Human Heart.
Churchill, London, p 75

Pitt D B 1962 A family study of Fallot's tetrad. Australian
Annals of Medicine 11: 179–183

Poirier R A, McGoon D C, Wallace R B, Ritter D G, Moodie
D S, Wiltse C G 1977 Late results after repair of tetralogy
of Fallot. Journal of Thoracic and Cardiovascular Surgery
73: 900–908

Potts W J, Smith S, Gibson S 1946 Anastomosis of the aorta
to a pulmonary artery: certain types of congenital heart
disease. Journal of the American Medical Association
132: 629–631

Puga F J, DuShane J W, McGoon D C 1972 Treatment of
tetralogy of Fallot in children less than 4 years of age.
Journal of Thoracic and Cardiovascular Surgery
64: 247–253

Quattlebaum T G, Varghese P J, Neill C A, Donahoo J S
1976 Sudden death amongst post-operative patients with
tetralogy of Fallot. Circulation 54: 289–293

Rabinovitch M, Grady S, David I et al 1982 Compression of
intrapulmonary bronchi by abnormally branching
pulmonary arteries associated with absent pulmonary
valves. American Journal of Cardiology 50: 804–813

Radley-Smith R, Yacoub M 1977 Clinical and haemodynamic
results of primary total correction of Fallot's tetralogy in
the first two years of life. British Heart Journal 39: 353

Ramsay J M, Macartney F J, Haworth S G 1985 Tetralogy of
Fallot with major aortopulmonary collateral arteries.
British Heart Journal 53: 167–172

Reddy V M, Liddicoat J R, McElhinney D B, Brook M M,
Stanger P, Hanley F L 1995 Routine primary repair of
tetralogy of Fallot in neonates and infants less than
three months of age. Annals of Thoracic Surgery
60: S592–S596

Redington A N, Oldershaw P J, Shinebourne E A, Rigby M L
1988 A new technique for the assessment of pulmonary
regurgitation and its application to the assessment of right
ventricular function before and after repair of tetralogy of
Fallot. British Heart Journal 60: 57–65

Redington A N, Raine J, Shinebourne E A, Rigby M L 1990
Tetralogy of Fallot with anomalous pulmonary venous
connexion: a rare but clinically important association.
British Heart Journal 64: 325–328

Redington A N, Oldershaw P J, Shinebourne E A, Rigby M L
1992 A new technique for the assessment of pulmonary
regurgitation and its application to the assessment of right
ventricular function before and after repair of tetralogy of
Fallot. British Heart Journal 67: 470–473

Rich A R 1948 A hitherto unrecognized tendency to the development of widespread pulmonary vascular obstruction in patients with congenital pulmonary stenosis (tetralogy of Fallot). Bulletin of the Johns Hopkins Hospital 82: 389–401

Riker W L 1963 Intracardiac lesions from common congenital heart lesions. Surgical Clinics of North America 43: 133–145

Ring J C, Bass J L, Marvin W J et al 1985 Management of congenital stenosis of a branch pulmonary artery with balloon dilation angioplasty. Report of 52 procedures. Journal of Thoracic and Cardiovascular Surgery 90: 35–44

Rizzoli G, Blackstone E H, Kirklin J W, Pacifico A D, Bargeron L M Jr 1980 Incremental risk factors in hospital mortality rate after repair of ventricular septal defect. Journal of Thoracic and Cardiovascular Surgery 80: 494–505

Rosenberg H G, Williams W G, Trusler G A, Higa T, Rabinovitch M 1987 Structural composition of central pulmonary arteries. Growth potential after surgical shunts. Journal of Thoracic and Cardiovascular Surgery 94: 498–503

Rosenquist G C, Sweeney L J, Stemple D R, Christianson S D, Rowe R D 1973 Ventricular septal defect in tetralogy of Fallot. American Journal of Cardiology 31: 749–754

Rosenthal A, Nathan D G, Marty A T, Button L N, Miettenen O S, Nadas A S 1970 Acute haemodynamic effects of red cell volume reduction in polycythemia of cyanotic congenital heart disease. Circulation 42: 297–307

Rosenthal A, Button L N, Nathan D G, Miettenen O S, Nadas A S 1971 Blood volume changes in cyanotic congenital heart disease. American Journal of Cardiology 27: 162–167

Rothman A, Perry S B, Keane J F, Lock J E 1990 Early results and follow-up of balloon angioplasty for branch pulmonary artery stenosis. Journal of the American College of Cardiology 15: 1109–1117

Rowe R D, Vlad P, Keith J D 1955 Atypical tetralogy of Fallot. Noncyanotic form with increased lung vascularity: report of four cases. Circulation 12: 230–238

Rowe S A, Zahka K G, Manolio T A, Horneffer P J, Kidd L 1991 Lung function and pulmonary regurgitation limit exercise capacity in postoperative tetralogy of Fallot. Journal of the American College of Cardiology 17: 461–466

Rowland J W, Rosenthal A R, Castenada A R 1975 Double chamber right ventricle: experience with 17 cases. American Heart Journal 89: 455–462

Rudolph A M, Nadas A S, Borges W H 1953 Hematologic adjustments to cyanotic congenital heart disease. Pediatrics 11: 454–463

Rudolph A M, Heymann M A, Spitznas U 1972 Hemodynamic considerations in the development of narrowing of the aorta. American Journal of Cardiology 30: 514–525

Ruzyllo W, Nihill M R, Mullins C E, McNamara D G 1974 Hemodynamic evaluation of 221 patients after intracardiac repair of tetralogy of Fallot. American Journal of Cardiology 34: 565–576

Rygg I H, Olesen K, Boesen I 1971 The life history of tetralogy of Fallot. Danish Medical Bulletin 18: 2.25–30

Sebening F, Laas J, Meisner H, Struck E, Buhlmeyer K, Zwingers T 1984 The treatment of tetralogy of Fallot: early repair or palliation. Thoracic and Cardiovascular Surgeon 32: 201–207

Sharpey-Shafer E P 1956 Effects of squatting on the normal and failing circulation. British Medical Journal i: 1072–1074

Shimasaki Y, Blackstone E H, Kirklin J W 1984 The natural history of isolated congenital pulmonary valve incompetence: surgical implications. Thoracic and Cardiovascular Surgeon 32: 257–261

Shinebourne E A, Elseed A M 1974 Relation between fetal flow patterns, coarctation of the aorta and pulmonary blood flow. British Heart Journal 36: 492–498

Shinebourne E A, Anderson R H, Bowyer J J 1975 Variations in clinical presentation of Fallot's tetralogy. Angiographic and pathogenetic implications. British Heart Journal 37: 946–955

Sluysmans T, Neven B, Rubay J et al 1995 Early balloon dilatation of the pulmonary valve in infants with tetralogy of Fallot. Risks and benefits. Circulation 91: 1506–1511

Somerville J, Barbosa R, Ross D, Olsen E 1975 Problems with radical corrective surgery after ascending aorta to right pulmonary artery shunt (Waterston's anastomosis) for cyanotic congenital heart disease. British Heart Journal 37: 1105–1112

Sousa Uva M, Lacour-Gayet F, Komiya T et al 1994 Surgery for tetralogy of Fallot at less than six months of age. Journal of Thoracic and Cardiovascular Surgery 107: 1291–1300

Sreeram N, Saleem M, Jackson M et al 1991 Results of balloon pulmonary valvuloplasty as a palliative procedure in tetralogy of Fallot. Journal of the American College of Cardiology 18: 159–165

Starr A, Bonchek L I, Sunderland C O 1973 Total correction of tetralogy of Fallot in infancy. Journal of Thoracic and Cardiovascular Surgery 65: 45–57

Steeg C N, Krongrad E, Davachi F, Bowman F O Jr, Maim J R, Gersony W M 1975 Postoperative left anterior hemiblock and right bundle branch block following repair of tetralogy of Fallot. Clinical and etiologic considerations. Circulation 51: 1026–1029

Strieder D J, Aziz K, Zaver A G, Fellows K E 1975 Exercise tolerance after repair of tetralogy of Fallot. Annals of Thoracic Surgery 19: 397–405

Studer M, Blackstone E H, Kirklin J W et al 1982 Determinants of early and late results of repair of atrioventricular septal (canal) defects. Journal of Thoracic and Cardiovascular Surgery 84: 523–542

Sullivan I D 1998 Tetralogy of Fallot with pulmonary stenosis: imaging the abnormal anatomy. In: Redington A N, Brawn W J, Deanfield J E, Anderson R H (eds) The right heart in congenital heart disease. GMM, London, p 57–66

Sung R J, Tamer D M, Garcia O L, Castellanos A, Myerburg R J, Gelband H 1976 Analysis of surgically induced right bundle branch block pattern using intracardiac recording techniques. Circulation 54: 442–446

Svane S 1977 Primary thrombosis of pulmonary artery in child with tetralogy of Fallot. British Heart Journal 39: 815–819

Taussig H B 1947 Congenital malformations of the heart. The Commonwealth Fund, London

Taussig H B, Crocetti A, Eshaghpour E B 1971 Long-term observations on the Blalock–Taussig operation. I. Results of first operation. Johns Hopkins Medical Journal 129: 243–257

Tenorio de Albuquerque A, Rigby M L, Anderson R H, Lincoln C, Shinebourne E A 1984 The spectrum of atrioventricular discordance. A clinical study. British Heart Journal 51: 498–507

Titus J L, Daugherty G W, Edwards J E 1963 Anatomy of the atrioventricular conduction system in ventricular septal defect. Circulation 28: 72–81

Touati G D, Vouhé P R, Amodeo A et al 1990 Primary repair of tetralogy of Fallot in infancy. Journal of Thoracic and Cardiovascular Surgery 99: 396–402

Trainer A H, Morrison N, Dunlop A, Wilson N, Tolmie J 1996 Chromosome 22$_q$11 microdeletions in tetralogy of Fallot. Archives of Diseases in Childhood 74: 62–63

Tucker W Y, Turley K, Ullyot D J, Ebert P A 1979 Management of symptomatic tetralogy of Fallot in the first year of life. Journal of Thoracic and Cardiovascular Surgery 78: 494–501

Turski C, Michalowski J 1968 Brock's operation in treatment of tetralogy of Fallot's syndrome. Polish Medical Journal 7: 653–654

Van Mierop L H S, Wiglesworth F W 1963 Pathogenesis of transposition complexes. II Anomalies due to faulty transfer of the posterior great artery. American Journal of Cardiology 12: 226–232

Van Mierop L H S, Patterson D F, Schnarr W R 1977 Hereditary conotruncal septal defects in Keeshond dogs: embryologic studies. American Journal of Cardiology 40: 936–950

Van Praagh R 1968 What is the Taussig–Bing malformation? Circulation 38: 445–449

Van Praagh R, Corwin R D, Dahlguist E, Freedom R M, Matioli L, Nebesar R A 1970a Tetralogy of Fallot with severe left ventricular outflow tract obstruction due to anomalous attachment of the mitral valve to the ventricular septum. American Journal of Cardiology 26: 95–101

Van Praagh R, Van Praagh S, Nebesar R A, Muster A J, Sinha S N, Paul M H 1970b Tetralogy of Fallot: underdevelopment of the pulmonary infundibulum and its sequelae. American Journal of Cardiology 26: 25–33

Verel D 1961 Blood volume changes in cyanotic congenital heart disease and polycythemia rubra vera. Circulation 23: 749–753

Villani M, Gamba A, Tiraboschi R, Crupi G, Parenzan L 1983 Surgical treatment of tetralogy of Fallot. Recent experience using a prospective protocol. The Thoracic and Cardiovascular Surgeon 31: 151–155

Vogelpoel L, Schrire V 1955 The role of auscultation in the differentiation of Fallot's tetralogy from severe pulmonary stenosis with intact ventricular septum and right-to-left interatrial shunt. Circulation 11: 714–732

Vogelpoel L, Schrire V 1960 Auscultatory and phonocardiographic assessment of Fallot's tetralogy. Circulation 22: 73–89

Vogelpoel L, Schrire V, Nellen M, Goetz R H 1957 The differentiation of the tetralogy of Fallot from severe pulmonary stenosis with intact ventricular septum and right-to-left interatrial shunt. Angiology 8: 215–247

Vogelpoel L, Nellen M, Swanepoel A, Schrire V 1959 The use of amyl nitrite in the diagnosis of systolic murmurs. Lancet ii: 810–817

Vogelpoel L, Schrire V, Nellen M, Swanepoel A 1960 The use of phenylephrine in differentiation of Fallot's tetralogy from pulmonary stenosis with intact ventricular septum. American Heart Journal 59: 489–505

Vogt J, Wesselhoeft H, Luig H et al 1984 The preoperative and postoperative findings in 627 patients with tetralogy of Fallot. Thoracic and Cardiovascular Surgeon 32: 234–243

von Rokitansky C F 1875 Die Defects der Scheidewande des Herzens. Wilhelm Braumuller, Vienna, p 27–29

Waien S A, Liu P P, Ross B L, Williams W G, McLaughlin P R 1992 Serial follow-up of adults with repaired tetralogy of Fallot. Journal of the American College of Cardiology 20: 295–300

Warner K G, Anderson J E, Fulton D R, Payne D D, Geggel R L, Marx G R 1993 Restoration of the pulmonary valve reduces right ventricular volume overload after previous repair of tetralogy of Fallot. Annals of Thoracic Surgery 88: 189–197

Waterston D J 1962 Treatment of Fallot's tetralogy in children under 1 year of age. Rozhledy v Chirurgii 41: 181–183

Waxman M B, Wald R W, Finley J P, Bonet J F, Donwar E, Sharma A D 1980 Valsalva termination of ventricular tachycardia. Circulation 62: 843–851

Webber S A, Hatchwell E I, Barber J C K et al 1996 Importance of microdeletions of chromosomal region 22$_q$11 as a cause of selected malformations of the ventricular outflow tracts and aortic arch: a three-year prospective study. Journal of Pediatrics 129: 26–32

Weinberg M Jr, Bicoff J P, Buccheleres H G et al 1962 Pulmonary valvotomy and infundibulotomy in infants. Journal of Thoracic and Cardiovascular Surgery 44: 433–442

Wessel H U, Cunningham W J, Paul M H, Bastanier C K, Muster A J, Idriss F S 1980a Exercise performance in tetralogy of Fallot after intracardiac repair. Journal of Thoracic and Cardiovascular Surgery 80: 582–593

Wessel H U, Bastanier C K, Paul M H, Berry T E, Cole R B, Muster A J 1980b Prognostic significance of arrhythmia in tetralogy of Fallot after intracardiac repair. American Journal of Cardiology 46: 843–848

White R I Jr, French R S, Castaneda A, Amplatz K 1972 The nature and significance of anomalous coronary arteries in tetralogy of Fallot. American Journal of Roentgenology, Radium Therapy and Nuclear Medicine 114: 350–354

Whittemore R, Hobbins J C, Engle M A 1982 Pregnancy and its outcome in women with and without surgical treatment of congenital heart disease. American Journal of Cardiology 50: 641–651

Whittemore R, Wells J A, Castellsague X 1994 A second-generation study of 427 probands with congenital heart defects and their 837 children. Journal of the American Journal of Cardiology 23: 1459–1467

Wilcox B R, Ho S Y, Macartney F J, Becker A E, Gerlis L M, Anderson R H 1981 Surgical anatomy of double-outlet right ventricle with situs solitus and atrioventricular concordance. Journal of Thoracic and Cardiovascular Surgery 82: 405–417

Wolff G S, Rowland T W, Ellison R C 1972 Surgically induced right bundle branch block with left anterior hemiblock: an ominous sign in postoperative tetralogy of Fallot. Circulation 46: 587–594

Wood P 1958 Attacks of deeper cyanosis and loss of consciousness (syncope) in Fallot's tetralogy. British Heart Journal 20: 282–286

Woods A 1952 The electrocardiogram in the tetralogy of Fallot. British Heart Journal 14: 192–203

Young D, Elbl F 1971 Supraventricular tachycardia as cause of cyanotic syncopal attacks in tetralogy of Fallot. New England Journal of Medicine 284: 1359–1360

Zahka K G, Horneffer P J, Rowe S A et al 1988 Long-term valvular function after total repair of tetralogy of Fallot.

Relation to ventricular arrhythmias. Circulation 78(suppl III): 14

Zellers T M, Driscoll D J, Michels V V 1990 Prevalence of significant congenital heart defects in children of parents with Fallot's tetralogy. American Journal of Cardiology 65: 523–526

Zimmerman H A, de Oliviera J M, Nogueira C, Mendelsohn D, Kay E B 1958 The electrocardiogram in open heart surgery. Disturbances in the right ventricular conduction. Journal of Thoracic Surgery 36: 12–22

Zuberbuhler J R, Lenox C C, Neches W H, Park S C, Shaver J A 1975 Auscultatory spectrum of tetralogy of Fallot. Physiologic principles of heart sounds and murmurs. American Heart Association Monograph 46. American Heart Association, New York, p. 187

47

Tetralogy of Fallot with pulmonary atresia

E. J. Baker

INTRODUCTION

In this chapter we deal with one of the most complex, and difficult to treat of all congenital heart anomalies. In the first edition of this book, we called it 'pulmonary atresia with ventricular septal defect'. This name is still in widespread use, but here we have chosen to call it tetralogy of Fallot with pulmonary atresia. Why have we changed the name we use? It is a fact that all the patients to be discussed have pulmonary atresia with a ventricular septal defect. But so do many other patients who do not have this anomaly. For example, patients with complete transposition, corrected transposition, double inlet ventricle or atrioventricular valvar atresia can all have pulmonary atresia associated with a ventricular septal defect. Almost always, such patients have confluent pulmonary arteries fed by a patent arterial duct. They do not have the complexity of pulmonary arterial supply that is so characteristic of the anomaly to be discussed in this chapter. Patients with isomerism of the atrial appendages also frequently have pulmonary atresia with a ventricular septal defect as part of their complex intracardiac anatomy, but again almost always they have confluent pulmonary arteries fed by an arterial duct.

The particular complexity of the anomaly to be covered in this chapter, therefore, is that the pulmonary circulation is frequently, but not always, supplied by major systemic-to-pulmonary collateral arteries. Sometimes called major aortopulmonary collateral arteries, these vessels are often abbreviated to MAPCAs. As we will see, some patients do have confluent pulmonary arteries fed through an arterial duct. The unifying feature of these groups of patients is that the intracardiac anatomy is that of tetralogy of Fallot, or one of its variants, but with pulmonary atresia rather than pulmonary stenosis. This is why we have chosen to group the various forms of this anomaly together in this chapter under the title of tetralogy with pulmonary atresia.

PREVALENCE AND AETIOLOGY

Because there is no uniformity of how to classify the patients to be described, an exact incidence of tetralogy with pulmonary atresia is difficult to obtain. Tetralogy of Fallot, as a group, made up almost 4% of congenital heart defects in the series reported from Liverpool (Kenna et al, 1975). Up to one tenth of these will have had congenital pulmonary atresia rather than pulmonary stenosis. In many, the intracardiac anatomy indicates that an initially patent pulmonary outflow tract became atretic during fetal life. In others, particularly in those with systemic-to-pulmonary collateral arteries, the atresia was almost certainly part and parcel of the initial developmental abnormality (Jackson et al, 1996).

Tetralogy of Fallot with pulmonary atresia can occur as part of the velo-cardiofacial syndrome in association with facial and aural anomalies, cleft palate and developmental delay (Jedele et al, 1992). There is evidence that the more severe forms of tetralogy of Fallot, particularly those with pulmonary atresia, are often associated with chromosome 22q11 deletion (Momma et al, 1996; Chessa et al, 1998). Indeed, this chromosomal anomaly links velo-cardiofacial and Di George syndromes with ventricular septal defect, tetralogy of Fallot, common arterial trunk and interrupted aortic arch.

MORPHOLOGY AND MORPHOGENESIS

CLASSIFICATION

The term pulmonary atresia describes a complete obstruction, or absence of communication, between the cavities of the ventricular mass and the pulmonary arteries. As such it can, in the presence of tetralogy of Fallot or related lesions, result from an imperforate pulmonary

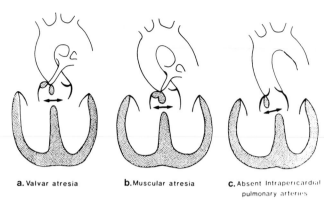

a. Valvar atresia   **b.** Muscular atresia   **c.** Absent intrapericardial pulmonary arteries

Figure 47.1. Diagram illustrating the arrangements of (a) an imperforate membrane, (b) a muscular subpulmonary infundibulum and (c) absence of the intrapericardial pulmonary arteries, which can produce pulmonary atresia in the setting of tetralogy of Fallot.

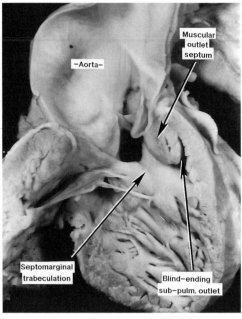

Figure 47.2. The typical pattern of extreme deviation of the outlet septum, which produces muscular pulmonary atresia in the setting of tetralogy. Note that, as in tetralogy, the outlet septum is inserted anterocephalad to the septomarginal trabeculation. Sub-pulm., subpulmonary.

valve. More usually, there is a muscular blockage of the ventriculo-pulmonary pathway, either at the entrance to the subpulmonary infundibulum or with the ventricular mass ending blindly at the distal extent of the muscular infundibulum. As an extension of this, the pulmonary trunk or even the intrapericardial pulmonary arteries may be absent (Figure 47.1).

Just as tetralogy of Fallot with pulmonary stenosis can be found with marked variability in intracardiac morphology, so can tetralogy with pulmonary atresia. Before discussing the crucial variations in pulmonary arterial anatomy, therefore, we will discuss the variations in morphology within the heart.

INTRACARDIAC STRUCTURE

Variations are to be found in the morphology of the ventricular outflow tracts, the morphology of the ventricular septal defect and the connection of the aorta to the ventricular mass. These features are, to a great extent, interrelated. To fulfil the basic diagnosis as tetralogy of Fallot, the aorta must be connected to the ventricles in posterior position relative to the atretic pulmonary trunk. In this position, the aortic orifice usually overrides the ventricular septum. The right ventricular outflow tract in most cases in then typical for tetralogy of Fallot, with the muscular outlet septum being displaced anteriorly and cephalad relative to the limbs of the septomarginal trabeculation (Figure 47.2). In a small number of cases, the muscular infundibulum is atretic at its mouth, and the pulmonary valve itself may then be patent. Alternatively, the subpulmonary infundibulum can be blind-ending at an imperforate pulmonary valve (Figure 47.3). In the most common pattern, nonetheless, the muscular outlet septum fuses directly with the parietal musculature of the right ventricle, obliterating the ventriculo-pulmonary junction. There is then a muscular wall between the cavities of the right ventricle and the pulmonary trunk.

Occasionally, the subpulmonary infundibulum is completely absent; as a result, the leaflets of the aortic valve are attached directly to the parietal ventricular wall (Figures 47.4a and 47.5b). This arrangement is reminiscent of common arterial trunk. In some cases, the aortic valve is in continuity with an imperforate pulmonary valve (Anderson et al, 1991). This arrangement is interpreted as tetralogy of Fallot with pulmonary atresia in the setting of a doubly committed and juxta-arterial ventricular septal defect (Figure 47.4b).

The ventricular septal defect itself is usually perimembranous (Figures 47.4b and 47.5a). It can also have a muscular posteroinferior rim when the posterior limb of the septomarginal trabeculation is fused with the ventriculo-infundibular fold (Figures 47.2, 47.4a and 47.5b). This muscular rim, when present, serves to protect the ventricular conduction tissues, separating them from the crest of the septum.

As discussed above, the defect can also extend to become doubly committed and juxta-arterial (Figure 47.4b). Such doubly committed defects can also be perimembranous or can have a muscular posteroinferior rim. Rarely, the ventricular septal defect may be restrictive, or even completely blocked, by tissue tags derived from the leaflets of the tricuspid valve (Fisher et al, 1980; Thiene and Anderson, 1983). The overall anatomy of the heart is then more like pulmonary atresia with intact ventricular septum, usually with a thick-walled right ventricle with a reduced cavity.

The precise connection of the aortic valve varies, as in tetralogy with pulmonary stenosis. In most instances, the

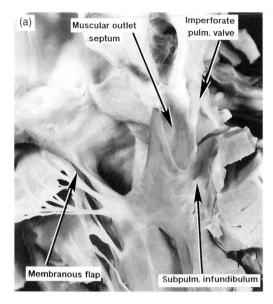

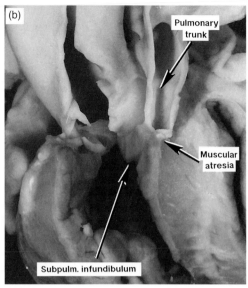

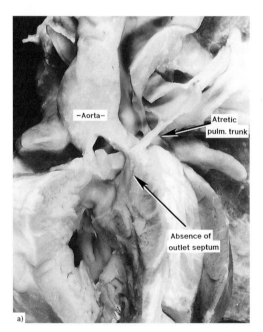

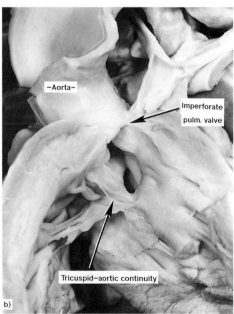

Figure 47.3. Pulmonary atresia in the setting of tetralogy of Fallot can be produced by an imperforate pulmonary (pulm.) valve (a) but, more usually, the subpulmonary (Sub pulm.) infundibulum shows evidence of muscular atresia (b).

Figure 47.4. (a) Rarely there is no evidence at all of a subpulmonary infundibulum, the aortic valve being attached directly to the parietal wall of the right ventricle. (b) In other cases, again very rarely, an imperforate pulmonary valve roofs a doubly committed and juxta-arterial defect. pulm, pulmonary.

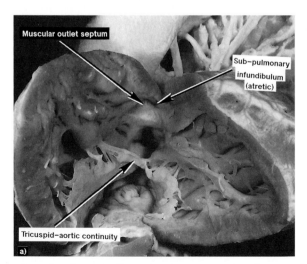

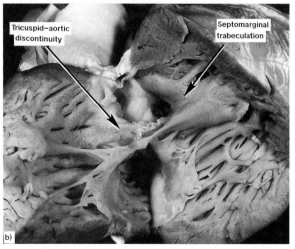

Figure 47.5. Tetralogy of Fallot with pulmonary atresia in hearts with (a) a perimembranous defect and (b) a muscular posteroinferior rim.

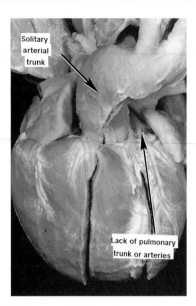

Figure 47.6. In this heart with discontinuous pulmonary arteries and a solitary trunk leaving the base of the heart, the left lung was initially supplied by an arterial duct and the right lung by systemic-to-collateral arteries (see Figure 47.16). In absence of the pulmonary trunk, the distinction cannot be made between the solitary vessel being an aorta or a common trunk. The arrangement is best described simply as a solitary arterial trunk.

valvar leaflets are connected largely within the left ventricle. With a perimembranous defect, the ventricular conduction axis is then exposed as it penetrates through the area of aortic–tricuspid valvar fibrous continuity. Hearts can also be found with predominant, or even total, commitment of the aorta to the right ventricle. If the pulmonary trunk is absent in such cases, then the arterial connection is still single outlet. When it is impossible to determine the origin of the pulmonary trunk, nonetheless, the solitary arterial trunk itself cannot be identified as aortic or common. It is described most accurately as a solitary arterial trunk (Figure 47.6) (Thiene and Anderson, 1983).

THE MORPHOLOGY OF THE INTRAPERICARDIAL PULMONARY ARTERIES——

When the pulmonary atresia is caused by an imperforate valve, the pulmonary trunk is present and patent down to the heart. But even in this setting, the trunk may supply only one pulmonary artery, the other either having no connection with the pulmonary trunk or else is completely absent. The pulmonary trunk, however, is often not completely patent. In extreme cases, it is recognizable only at postmortem as a fibrous strand running between the ventricular outflow tract and the pulmonary arterial confluence (Figure 47.4a), or joining to one or other of the pulmonary arteries. When the right and left pulmonary arteries are present, usually they are confluent. The confluence itself is usually tethered by either a patent or an atretic pulmonary trunk to the ventricular mass and

has the characteristic appearance of a flying seagull; however, it can vary markedly in size, usually dependent on its source of arterial supply (Figures 47.7 and 47.8).

The pulmonary arteries can also be non-confluent, but then one of them is usually attached to the remnant of the pulmonary trunk (Figure 47.9). Non-confluent pulmonary arteries can rarely be found in the absence of the pulmonary trunk. In this case, each artery is supplied either by one of bilateral arterial ducts or by systemic-to-pulmonary collateral arteries, or one arises from a duct and the other is fed by collateral arteries.

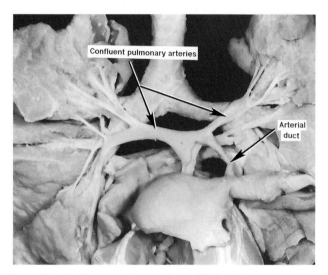

Figure 47.7. In this heart with tetralogy of Fallot with pulmonary atresia, there are confluent pulmonary arteries fed by an arterial duct.

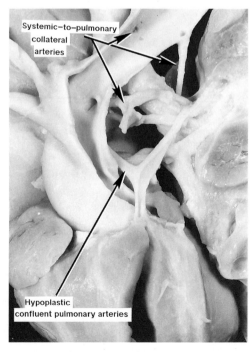

Figure 47.8. Compare this arrangement to the specimen shown in Figure 47.7. Here the pulmonary arterial confluence is fed through systemic-to-pulmonary collateral arteries.

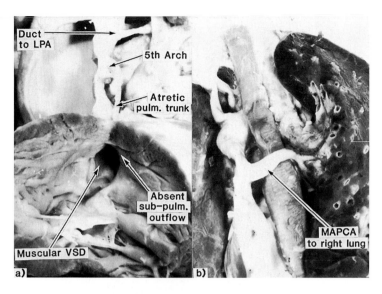

a)

b)

Figure 47.9. The blood supply to the right lung in this heart with discontinuous pulmonary arteries is through a fifth aortic arch. Note the atretic pulmonary (pulm.) trunk extending back to the heart and the absence of the subpulmonary infundibulum. The blood supply to the left pulmonary artery (LPA) is via an arterial duct. In addition (b) there is a major systemic to pulmonary collateral artery (MAPCA) supplying the right lung (multifocal supply). (Photographed and reproduced by kind permission of Dr M Kearney, University of Tromso, Norway.)

THE MORPHOLOGY OF PULMONARY ARTERIAL SUPPLY

The final common pathway of pulmonary supply is the capillaries supplying the air sacks of the lungs. These capillaries are connected to an intrapulmonary plexus of arteries that ramifies within the bronchopulmonary segments. Different parts of the plexus can be supplied with blood from different systemic sources (Figure 47.10). If all intrapulmonary arteries are connected to unobstructed and confluent pulmonary arteries, they supply all of both lungs, and pulmonary blood supply is said to be unifocal. When different parts of one lung are supplied from more than one source, the supply is said to be multifocal (Macartney et al, 1974).

UNIFOCAL PULMONARY BLOOD SUPPLY

When the pulmonary arterial supply is unifocal, it almost always comes from the arterial duct (Figure 47.10). Rarely, confluent pulmonary arteries feeding all of both lungs are supplied by only a single systemic-to-pulmonary collateral artery. In other rare cases, the confluent pulmonary arteries can be fed in unifocal fashion through an aortopulmonary window, via a fistula from the coronary arteries or through a fifth aortic arch (Figure 47.11).

MULTIFOCAL PULMONARY BLOOD SUPPLY

Of far more significance in the setting of tetralogy with pulmonary atresia is the arrangement of the pulmonary circulation where there is a multifocal supply. Hardly ever is this the result of an arterial duct coexisting with collateral arteries. Although once predicted to be embryologically impossible (Thiene et al, 1976), examples of a duct coexisting with systemic-to-pulmonary collateral arteries and supplying the same lung have now been

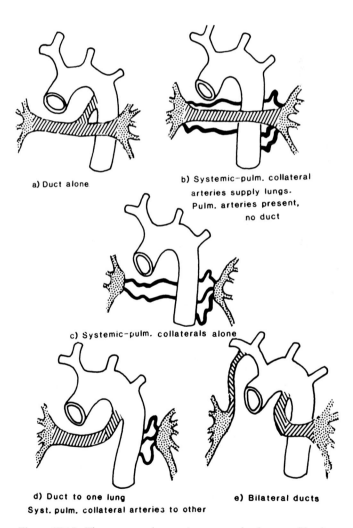

a) Duct alone

b) Systemic-pulm. collateral arteries supply lungs. Pulm. arteries present, no duct

c) Systemic-pulm. collaterals alone

d) Duct to one lung Syst. pulm. collateral arteries to other

e) Bilateral ducts

Figure 47.10. The more usual systemic sources of pulmonary blood supply in tetralogy of Fallot with pulmonary atresia are (a) an arterial duct alone, (b) systemic-to-pulmonary (pulm.) collateral arteries supplying one or both lungs with intrapericardial pulmonary arteries present but no duct, (c) systemic-pulmonary collaterals alone in the absence of intrapericardial pulmonary arteries, (d) an arterial duct to one lung and systemic-to-pulmonary (syst. pulm.) collateral arteries to the other, or (e) bilateral arterial ducts.

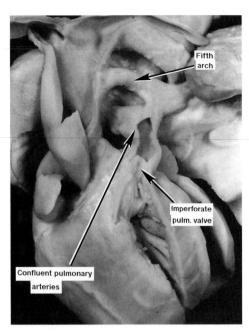

Figure 47.11. In this heart with tetralogy of Fallot and pulmonary atresia, unifocal supply to the confluent pulmonary (pulm.) arteries is from a fifth aortic arch.

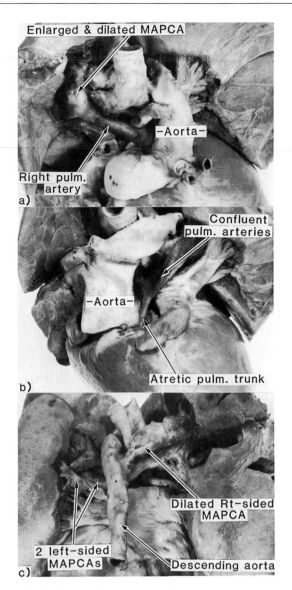

Figure 47.12. The multifocal supply in this patient is via systemic-to-pulmonary collateral arteries (MAPCA). (a) As is seen here, much of the blood is circulated through the intrapericardial pulmonary (pulm.) arteries. The union of a large right-sided collateral artery with the right pulmonary artery is seen. (b) Blood from this collateral artery is distributed via the central pulmonary arteries to the upper part of the left lung. (c) In addition, left-sided collateral arteries supply directly the lower part of the left lung, having no connection with the confluent intrapericardial pulmonary arteries. Note also the origin of the dilated right-sided (Rt-sided) collateral artery.

described (Macartney and Haworth, 1983), but such cases are exceedingly rare. In fact, it is a useful working rule that an arterial duct will not coexist in a lung that is also supplied by systemic-to-pulmonary collateral arteries.

But while systemic-to-pulmonary collateral arteries hardly ever coexist in the same lung with an arterial duct, they do usually coexist with confluent intrapericardial pulmonary arteries. In such circumstances, the confluent pulmonary arteries are hardly, if ever, connected to all of the bronchopulmonary segments of both lungs. Instead, it is the rule for different arteries to supply different segments of the two lungs. This arrangement constitutes the most common form of multifocal supply. The confluence of intrapericardial pulmonary arteries, itself fed by one or more major systemic-to-pulmonary collateral arteries, is connected to only part of the lungs, while the remainder of the pulmonary parenchyma is supplied directly by a variable number of major systemic-to-pulmonary collateral arteries. These individual arteries may directly feed individual intrapulmonary segments or groups of segments but can also communicate with the confluent intrapericardial arteries (Figure 47.12).

Another variety of multifocal supply is found when the pulmonary arteries are present but non-confluent. The different parts of the lungs may then be supplied by systemic-to-pulmonary collateral arteries, by a duct, by a coronary arterial fistula or aortopulmonary window or by a combination of these. Alternatively, the intrapulmonary arteries may not be supplied either by an arterial duct or by major systemic-to-pulmonary collateral arteries. Blood can then reach them only at precapillary level through acquired collateral arteries. These may enter the lungs either centrifugally through the bronchial arteries or centripetally via the intercostal or coronary arteries. These acquired collateral arteries can coexist with the other varieties of arterial supply.

MAJOR SYSTEMIC-TO-PULMONARY COLLATERAL ARTERIES

Major systemic-to-pulmonary collateral arteries are characteristic of tetralogy of Fallot with pulmonary atresia. The relationship between the collateral arteries and the

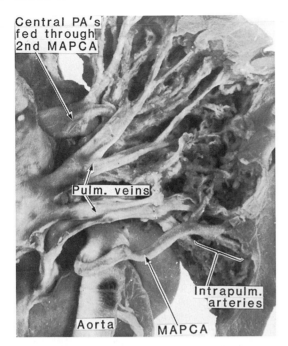

Figure 47.13. This is a dissection of the left lung of the patient illustrated in Figure 47.12. Note that the left-sided collateral artery (MAPCA) extends only from the aorta to the lung hilum. It supplies different segments of the lung compared to those perfused via the right-sided collateral artery (2nd MAPCA), which anastomoses with the confluent intrapericardial pulmonary arteries (PA's).

bronchial arteries has yet to be fully established. In most instances, the major collateral arteries have no independent course within the lung parenchyma, extending only from a systemic artery, usually the aorta, to the origin of the intrapulmonary arteries at or near the hilum (Figure 47.13). Arteries with this morphology are simple conduits. In certain circumstances, however, the collateral arteries extend into the lung and then branch in the pattern of a bronchial artery and supply the bronchial wall. A common embryological origin with the bronchial arteries cannot be excluded (de Ruiter et al, 1993).

The systemic-to-pulmonary collateral arteries, typically between two and six in number, usually arise from the anterior wall of the aorta opposite the origin of the intercostal arteries. Individual collateral arteries can take origin from the brachiocephalic arteries, or even from the coronary arteries. They frequently run a retro-oesophageal course. Usually they can be distinguished from a duct by their histological structure (Thiene et al, 1979). They can also be distinguished anatomically in most cases, since the arterial duct originates only from a given point within the aortic arch. Therefore, even when taking origin from a non-dominant aortic arch, the duct always originates more-or-less opposite the origin of a brachiocephalic or subclavian artery. It is this typical origin of a duct that helps to distinguish the rare fifth aortic arch (Figure 47.11), but to be sure of the existence of a fifth arch, it should coexist with the sixth arch (Gerlis et al, 1994).

CHARACTERISTIC PATTERNS OF PULMONARY BLOOD SUPPLY

If we try and simplify this complex situation, there are three major patterns of pulmonary arterial supply in tetralogy with pulmonary atresia (Figure 47.14). First, the most favourable arrangement is that in which the right and left pulmonary arteries are confluent and are supplied by an arterial duct. With this pattern, the

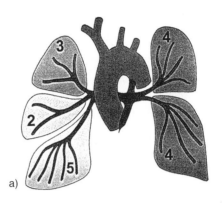

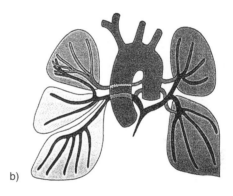

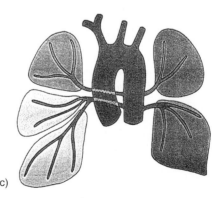

Figure 47.14. Three major patterns of pulmonary arterial supply are to be found in patients with tetralogy of Fallot and pulmonary atresia. (a) The first is for all bronchopulmonary segments to be supplied via confluent pulmonary arteries fed by the arterial duct. (b) In the second variant, supply of some segments is by systemic-to-pulmonary collateral arteries directly, while other segments are supplied by confluent intrapericardial pulmonary arteries themselves fed by the collateral arteries. (c) The third pattern is exclusive supply of all bronchpulmonary segments by multiple collateral arteries in the absence of confluent intrapericardial pulmonary arteries.

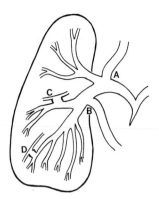

ANASTOMOSES

A. Extrapulmonary

B. Hilar

C. Lobar

D. Segmental

Figure 47.15. When the pulmonary artery supply is via systemic-to-pulmonary collateral arteries coexisting with confluent intrapericardial pulmonary arteries, the anastomosis with the pulmonary arteries can be extrapulmonary or at hilar, lobar or segmental levels.

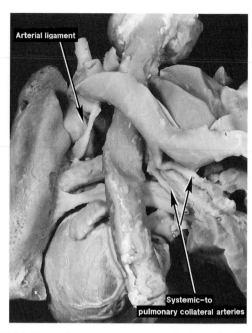

Figure 47.16. The pulmonary arterial supply is shown for the patient illustrated in Figure 47.6 with a solitary trunk. The left lung was initially fed by an arterial duct that had become ligamentous. The right lung is fed by multiple systemic-to-pulmonary collateral arteries.

pulmonary arteries themselves are usually distributed in normal fashion to all the bronchopulmonary segments. Such pulmonary arterial supply is unifocal.

In the second major pattern (Figure 47.14b), the intrapericardial pulmonary arteries are confluent but coexist with systemic-to-pulmonary collateral arteries. The distribution of the confluent pulmonary arteries itself is then variable, but the pulmonary arteries hardly ever supply all the bronchopulmonary segments and often supply only two thirds or less of the pulmonary parenchyma. Even then, the supply to the pulmonary arteries is via the collateral arteries, with anastomoses being possible at hilar, lobar or segmental levels (Figure 47.15). The confluent pulmonary arteries also vary markedly in size, reflecting the number of the bronchopulmonary segments they supply. In these cases, those parts of the lung not supplied by the intrapericardial pulmonary arteries are fed directly by systemic-to-pulmonary collateral arteries, with variation in the number of arteries present and the amount of lung supplied by each artery. In most cases, the peripheral supplies of central pulmonary arteries and the collateral arteries do not overlap, but in a proportion of segments two sets of arterial ramifications intermingle (Anderson et al, 1991; Ho et al, 1992).

The third typical pattern of arterial supply (Figure 47.14c) is complete absence of the central intrapericardial pulmonary arteries. In such circumstances, all the bronchopulmonary segments are supplied by multiple systemic-to-pulmonary collateral arteries.

In some instances, when the pulmonary arteries are non-confluent, one lung can have unifocal supply via an arterial duct, while the other lung has multifocal supply through a variable number of collateral arteries (Figure 47.16). In the presence of systemic-to-pulmonary collateral arteries, therefore, the key to diagnosis is to establish the course of each artery and to establish whether it runs directly into the lung or makes connections with intrapericardial and central pulmonary arteries.

EMBRYOLOGY

A great deal has been written about the morphogenesis of both the ventricular and pulmonary arterial features of tetralogy of Fallot with pulmonary atresia. Much of this has been derived from speculative embryological concepts and has not helped our understanding. From the stance of ventricular morphology, nonetheless, the anomaly is readily explained in terms of end-stage tetralogy of Fallot, with variation depending upon the specific morphology of the subarterial outlets. Some cases could be interpreted as representing common arterial trunk with absence of the intrapericardial pulmonary arteries. The arrangement in which a solitary trunk is connected to the ventricular mass in absence of central pulmonary arteries is a particular example (Figure 47.6). This anomaly was initially termed 'truncus arteriosus type IV' and was classified along with other variants of common arterial trunk (Collett and Edwards, 1949). On re-examination of these specimens, doubt was raised as to whether the central pulmonary arteries were indeed absent, or whether, instead, they were severely hypoplastic (Sotomora and Edwards, 1978). In this respect, Thiene and his colleagues (1976) described unequivocal examples of this anomaly in which not only were the intrapericardial pulmonary arteries absent but also no evidence was found within the right ventricle of the subpulmonary infundibulum. We have confirmed these observations (Crupi et al, 1977; Anderson et al, 1991). The argument of common trunk versus tetralogy then depends upon whether the absent pulmonary arteries,

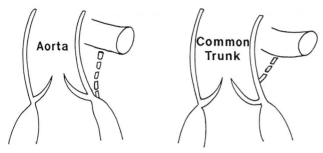

Figure 47.17. This diagram illustrates the conundrum in describing cases with absence of the pulmonary trunk (dotted line). Had the trunk been present, and connected to the ventricular mass (a) then the arterial trunk would be an aorta. However, if the pulmonary trunk was connected to the trunk itself (b) then the trunk would initially have been common. The best resolution is simply to describe, in this setting, a solitary arterial trunk (see Figures 47.6 and 47.16).

had they been present, would have taken origin from an arterial trunk or directly from the right ventricle (Figure 47.17). The argument is no longer hypothetical, since a heart has been described at postmortem in which the atretic pulmonary trunk arose from an arterial trunk – meaning that initially the trunk had indeed been a common structure (Schofield and Anderson, 1988). Furthermore, recent study of rats dosed with bisdiamine has shown that some fetuses develop classical tetralogy of Fallot, while others exhibit common arterial trunk with pulmonary atresia (Jackson et al, 1996). From the standpoint of anatomy, this conundrum is easily resolved simply by describing the ascending great artery found in absence of the pulmonary trunk as a solitary arterial trunk rather than an aorta (Thiene and Anderson, 1983). With regard to the overall morphogenesis of tetralogy of Fallot with pulmonary atresia, the anatomical prototypes can then be interpreted as developing in the setting of typical tetralogy, in the setting of tetralogy with doubly committed ventricular septal defects or, very rarely, in the setting of common arterial trunk.

Embryology has also been invoked to account for the typical patterns of pulmonary arterial supply (Thiene et al, 1981). Several observers had noted that, generally speaking, the lungs in tetralogy with pulmonary atresia are supplied either through the confluence of the pulmonary arteries fed by the arterial duct (derived from the embryological sixth aortic arch) or through systemic-to-pulmonary collateral arteries. Initially, the developing intrapulmonary arterial plexus is connected to the primitive intersegmental arteries, which, in turn, are connected to the aortic arch system, eventually via the fourth arch (Huntingdon, 1919). The concept advanced to explain the arrangement seen in the abnormal hearts is that when the intrapulmonary plexus eventually achieves its connection to the sixth arch it loses its connections with the fourth arch and the systemic arterial system. The systemic-to-pulmonary collateral arteries are then explained on the bais of persistence of the primitive intersegmental arteries, some of which also become bronchial

arteries. It is argued that these collateral arteries persist only in absence of the duct, which is the critical connection between the structures derived from the sixth arch and the aortic sack. This concept accounts adequately for the majority of cases and offers an excellent working hypothesis. It is undermined by those occasional instances when systemic-to-pulmonary collateral arteries coexist with the duct and both supply the intrapulmonary plexus in the same lung (Macartney and Haworth, 1983; Frescura et al, 1984).

Embryology, nonetheless, aids greatly in the understanding of the complexity of the pulmonary arterial supply in the majority of cases. In essence, the intrapulmonary arteries develop along with the lung. They are the final common pathway supplying arterial blood to the air sacs in the lungs. This common pathway can be supplied at the hilum, by the central intrapericardial pulmonary arteries fed through the arterial duct (sixth arch structures), by the rarer sources of unifocal supply or by systemic-to-pulmonary collateral arteries (primitive intersegmental arteries). These sources of supply can anastomose with different parts of the lungs in the same patient, although usually all the arteries in one lung are supplied either by the duct or by the systemic-to-pulmonary collateral arteries. The common pathway can subsequently be further enhanced by acquired collateral arteries, which reinforce the acinar supply at precapillary level.

PATHOPHYSIOLOGY

The ventricular septal defect is almost always large and non-restrictive. Rarely, the ventricular septal defect is small and obstructive. In a few reported cases (Fisher et al, 1980; Thiene and Anderson, 1983), the obstruction has been between the right ventricle and the aorta, making the right ventricular pressure suprasystemic. There is no reason why the obstruction should not also be between the left ventricle and the aorta.

There is complete mixing of pulmonary and systemic venous blood in the aorta (Macartney et al, 1973). Hence, distribution of blood to the body and lungs depends on the relative resistance offered by the two circulations. The systemic vascular resistance is no different from that in any other cyanotic condition. The complicated pattern of pulmonary arterial supply means that the pulmonary vascular resistance is both complex and variable.

PULMONARY VASCULAR RESISTANCE

The pulmonary vascular resistance results from obstruction at various sites between the aorta and the pulmonary capillaries (Figure 47.18). These are as follows.

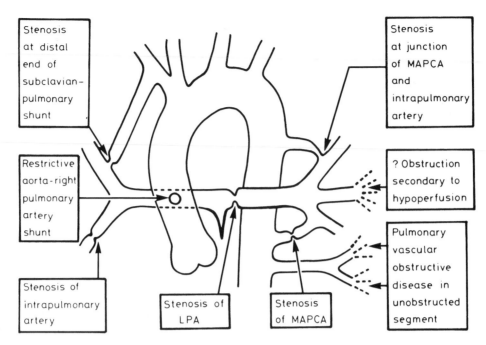

Figure 47.18. Possible sites of obstruction to pulmonary blood supply in pulmonary atresia with disease in ventricular septal defect. (Reproduced with permission from Anderson R H et al (eds) Paediatric cardiology 5. Churchill Livingstone, Edinburgh, 1983.)

OBSTRUCTION AT A DIRECT AORTOPULMONARY CONNECTION

It is rare for there to be a direct connection between the aorta and pulmonary arteries. Examples are an aortopulmonary window (Shore et al, 1983) and out-dated surgical anastomoses such as the Waterston and Potts shunts. The shunts should have been created with the objective of being obstructive. Another direct aortopulmonary connection that can be obstructed, albeit rarely, is a pulmonary artery arising anomalously from the ascending aorta.

OBSTRUCTION WITHIN AN AORTOPULMONARY CONDUIT

The connection between the aorta and pulmonary circulations more commonly is a vessel or surgical conduit between the aorta and either the central or intrapulmonary arteries (or the junction between the two). The same principles concerning haemodynamics apply to natural communications, such as a duct or major systemic-to-pulmonary collateral arteries, the rarer coronary-to-pulmonary arterial fistulas (Krongrad et al, 1972) or persistence of the fifth arch (Macartney et al, 1974), and to surgically created shunts or conduits inserted between the aorta or subclavian arteries and the pulmonary arteries. The difference in pressure between the aorta and the pulmonary arteries is not usually a gradual change in pressure over the whole length of the conduit or vessel. Instead, there is usually an abrupt drop at the pulmonary end (Macartney et al, 1974). This may be no more than a reflection of the Venturi effect, but

there may also be an anatomical obstruction at the pulmonary arterial end of the conduit (Figure 47.19a). This is particularly true in the case of surgical shunts created in early infancy. It is also true of a duct, which tends to become constricted at its pulmonary rather than its aortic end. Localized obstructions and pressure gradients also occur within major systemic-to-pulmonary collateral arteries (Figure 47.19a). In many cases, these obstructions can become more stenotic with time (Macartney et al, 1973; Reddy et al, 1995).

OBSTRUCTION WITHIN THE PULMONARY ARTERIES

If the central pulmonary arteries lie on the pathway of blood between the aorta and one lung, stenoses may be important, though their inaccessibility makes this difficult to prove (Figures 47.19–47.21) (McGoon et al, 1977; Macartney and Haworth, 1979). For example, in cases where the entire pulmonary blood flow is derived from a left duct (Figure 47.22), a stenosis of the central right pulmonary artery would be one factor limiting flow to the right lung. Pressure gradients may also occasionally be demonstrated in intrapulmonary arteries (Figure 47.23), whether or not these are connected to confluent intrapericardial pulmonary arteries.

OBSTRUCTION AT ARTERIOLAR LEVEL

Pulmonary vascular disease may develop in parts of the lungs. It can occur in pulmonary segments perfused at high pressure by unobstructed major systemic-to-pulmonary

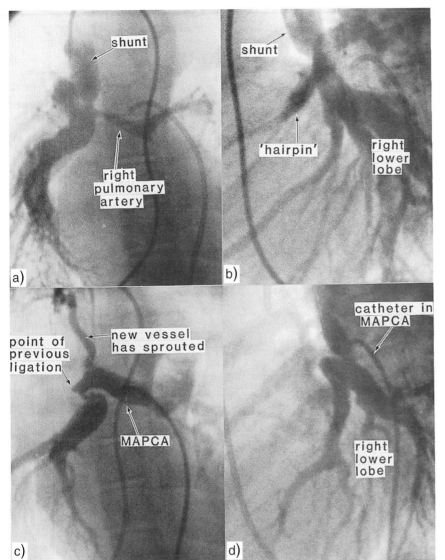

Figure 47.19. These frames, together with those from Figure 47.20 and 47.21 are all from the same patient, illustrating how a composite picture of total pulmonary blood supply is built up. (a) and (c) are frontal plane projections, while (b) and (d) are corresponding lateral projections. The new vessel in (c) was not present on a previous angiocardiogram. The segmental distribution of pulmonary blood supply, for example right lower lobe in (d), is inferred from summing the information in frontal and lateral projections. Note the obstruction at the end of the shunt in (a). The intrapericardial pulmonary arteries are seen as a 'hairpin' in the lateral projection.

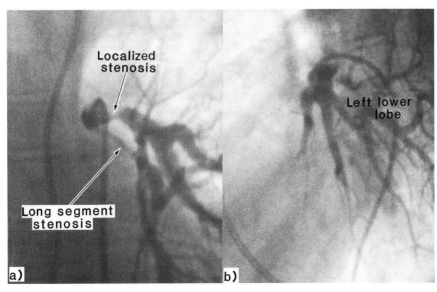

Figures 47.20. Selective injection in (a) frontal and (b) lateral projection in one systemic-to-pulmonary collateral artery in the patient illustrated also in Figures 47.19 and 47.21 (see legend to Figure 47.19). Note the obstruction in the collateral artery.

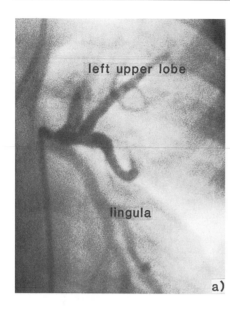

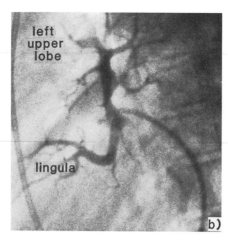

Figure 47.21. Selective injection shown in (a) frontal and (b) lateral projection into another may systemic-to-pulmonary collateral artery in the patient illustrated in Figures 47.19 and 47.20 (see legend to Figure 47.19).

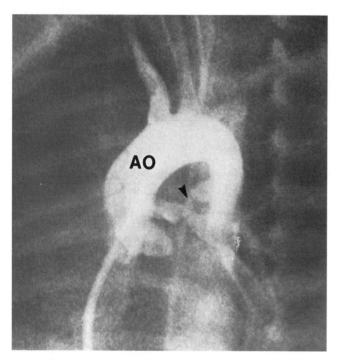

Figure 47.22. Ductal supply of confluent pulmonary arteries demonstrated by aortography. Note that the duct is narrowed at its pulmonary end (arrowed). AO, aorta.

collateral arteries (Jefferson et al, 1972; Thiene et al, 1979; Haworth and Macartney, 1980). Changes owing to hypoperfusion may also affect pulmonary vascular resistance. In particular, intimal proliferation in acquired collateral circulation appears to extend into the pulmonary arteries within the acinus, at least in experimental animals (Haworth et al, 1981). This is likely to raise pulmonary vascular resistance in affected segments.

The combination of all these obstructions is sufficient to reduce pulmonary blood flow below systemic levels in most patients, though in a few patients total pulmonary

blood flow may be markedly increased. Since pulmonary and systemic blood become completely mixed, systemic arterial hypoxaemia is most severe in patients with a low pulmonary and a high systemic flow. Total pulmonary resistance is, therefore, usually high (Macartney et al, 1974). But this, as outlined above, is the result of obstruction at a number of different levels. From the point of view of surgical repair, what matters is the resistance relative to the vessel to which the right ventricle is to be connected. Normally this is a central pulmonary artery.

When pulmonary blood supply is unifocal, all intrapulmonary arteries are connected to a single source of pressure (usually the pulmonary trunk or the confluence between right and left pulmonary arteries). Under these circumstances, pulmonary vascular resistance can be calculated, provided that mean arterial pressure at that point is known.

When pulmonary blood supply is multifocal, different intrapulmonary arteries are supplied from different sources. Since the different parts of the lung will then most probably be at different pressures, it is impossible to calculate the overall pulmonary vascular resistance. In fact, all the evidence indicates that regional pulmonary blood flow is extremely variable throughout the lungs. Hyperperfused and hypoperfused segments of lungs may be immediately adjacent to one another.

ACQUIRED COLLATERAL CIRCULATION TO THE LUNGS

Collateral arterial supply to the lungs may develop in any cyanotic heart condition. These collateral arteries, therefore, can develop in tetralogy with pulmonary atresia, but they are distinct from the major systemic-to-pulmonary collateral arteries that are typical of the condition. From the pathophysiological point of view, the most important distinction lies in the site of the anastomosis with the

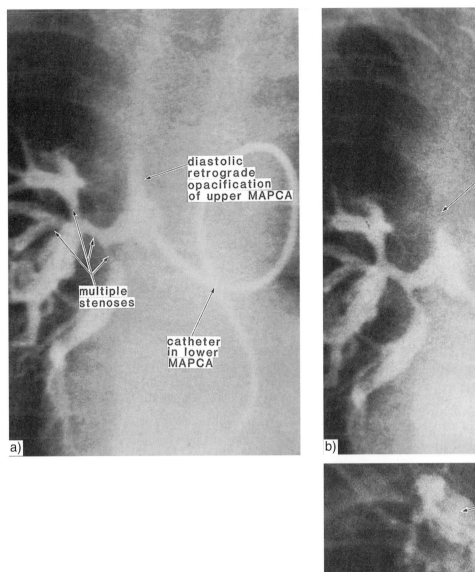

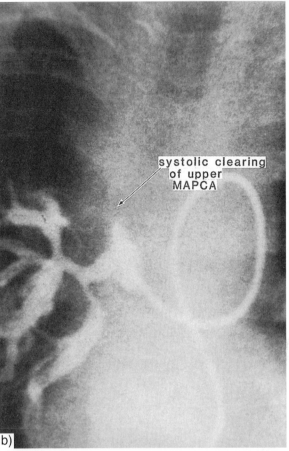

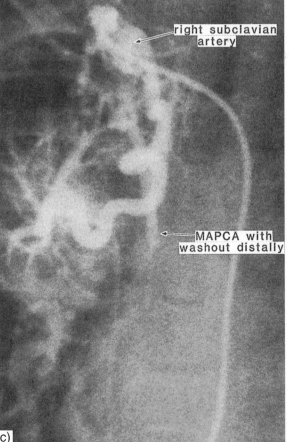

Figure 47.23. These selective injections into major aortopulmonary collateral arteries (a–c) all are viewed in the frontal projection and are from the same patient. They illustrate duplicate pulmonary blood supply, in that the right pulmonary artery is supplied by two different systemic-to-pulmonary collateral arteries (MAPCA).

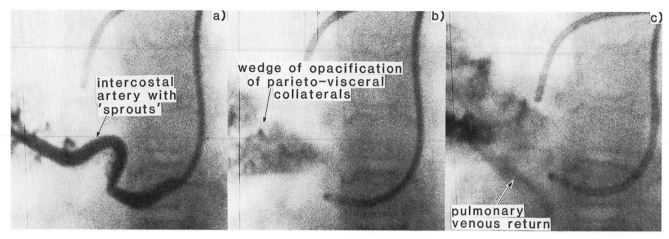

Figure 47.24. Selective injection into an intercostal artery in a patient with acquired pulmonary blood supply to the right lung. Successive panels (a through c) correspond to successive times during the injection and demonstrate the way in which the intercostal artery anastomoses through parieto-visceral collaterals with the pulmonary circulation, which then drain in normal fashion via the pulmonary veins.

pulmonary circulation. Acquired collaterals, with rare exceptions, join the pulmonary circulation at immediately precapillary level (Figure 47.24). Major systemic-to-pulmonary collateral arteries join at the hilum or at segmental level (Figures 47.19 and 47.20). Both types of collateral artery provide an effective pulmonary blood supply. Since acquired collateral circulation never produces heart failure, there must be a high resistance to blood flow between the aorta and the pulmonary arteries.

PRESENTATION

The clinical presentation of tetralogy with pulmonary atresia is almost entirely dependent on the amount of pulmonary blood flow. If the pulmonary blood supply depends on patency of a duct, then patients are liable to present as neonates with severe cyanosis when the duct narrows or closes. Major systemic-to-pulmonary collateral arteries, by comparison, form a relatively stable source of pulmonary blood supply. In these patients, therefore, the onset of clinically detectable cyanosis may be delayed well beyond the neonatal period. Indeed, of patients with major systemic-to-pulmonary collateral arteries, a small proportion have excessive pulmonary blood flow and present in heart failure (Miller et al, 1968).

Patients with pulmonary atresia usually present with the combination of cyanosis and exertional dyspnoea. Failure to thrive is often present. Many patients, however, have a balanced pulmonary blood flow with few if any symptoms and occasionally normal growth. Patients may initially present with non-cardiac clinical features of chromosome 22q11 deletion, such as feeding difficulties and developmental delay. Occasionally, they may present with evidence of immunodeficiency or hypocalcaemia as part of the picture of the Di George syndrome.

CLINICAL FINDINGS

Most, but by no means all, patients are clinically cyanosed from birth. In the minority with increased pulmonary blood flow, cyanosis may escape detection until the patient is a few months, or even years, old. Respiration is quiet unless pulmonary blood flow is excessive. Since there is run-off from the aorta, the peripheral pulses are equal and jerky in proportion to pulmonary blood flow. The jugular venous pressure is normal in height, though the A wave is dominant. The precordium feels characteristically quiet, since there are no thrills, and the degree of right ventricular hypertension is not usually sufficient to give a right ventricular lift. Only in infants with excessive pulmonary blood flow is the precordium active. It may be possible to feel both the ejection click and the second heart sound.

The first heart sound is followed by a loud aortic ejection click in all but young infants, this being related to the dilation of the aortic root. The second heart sound is invariably single. Blowing and continuous murmurs are almost always audible. They presumably originate from turbulence in the region of stenoses in the sites detailed above. For this reason, when the aortic arch is left sided, a murmur localized under the left clavicle is suggestive, but not diagnostic, of a persistent duct (Zutter and Somerville, 1971). A similar murmur on the right side would suggest a right duct. Widespread continuous murmurs are more characteristic of major systemic-to-pulmonary collateral arteries. There is no systolic ejection murmur such as would arise from infundibular stenosis. The continuous murmurs may obscure the early diastolic murmur or aortic regurgitation that often develops beyond the age of 8 years or so as a result of dilation of the aortic root or infective endocarditis (Capelli et al, 1982).

The continuous murmur may not be heard if pulmonary flow is too low to generate audible turbulence

(Macartney et al, 1972). This is the case in about half of severely cyanotic newborns with this condition (Miller et al, 1968). Such newborns are nearly always duct dependent. Severe pulmonary vascular obstructive disease in older children with unobstructed major systemic-to-pulmonary collateral arteries, however, may also prevent generation of a continuous murmur. We recall one barely cyanotic newborn with major collateral arteries and no murmurs where the absence of murmurs was presumably the result of unobstructed flow in the collateral arteries in association with a delayed fall in pulmonary vascular resistance, but this is exceptional and atypical. At least 95% of all children beyond the first month of life who have the combination of an aortic click, no systolic murmur, a single second heart sound, cyanosis and a continuous murmur will turn out to have tetralogy with pulmonary atresia. The remaining 5% of patients will have a common arterial trunk with stenosis of one or both pulmonary arteries, severe tetralogy of Fallot with major systemic-to-pulmonary collateral arteries (Ramsay et al, 1985) or pulmonary atresia with more complex ventricular morphology such as double inlet ventricle or discordant atrioventricular connections.

DIAGNOSIS

There is, in general, little difficulty with the diagnosis of tetralogy with pulmonary atresia. In older patients with surgical shunts, nonetheless, it may be impossible to distinguish between congenital and acquired pulmonary atresia. In all cases, other clinical features of the velocardiofacial and Di George syndromes should be looked for, and chromosomes should be analysed for the 22q11 deletion.

INVESTIGATIONS

CHEST RADIOGRAPHY

The so-called 'coeur-en-sabot' heart of tetralogy of Fallot is most often found when there is pulmonary atresia. This is because hypoplasia of the pulmonary trunk is usually more severe, the hollowness of the pulmonary bay is more pronounced and a right aortic arch is twice as common as in tetralogy with pulmonary stenosis. These findings occur in almost half of all patients with tetralogy and pulmonary atresia (Miller et al, 1968; Somerville, 1970). The lung markings are characteristically uneven in size and hence patchy, abnormal linear shadows indicating the position and course of collateral arteries. The unevenness exists because, in the presence of major systemic-to-pulmonary collateral arteries, some parts of the lung may be underperfused while others are overperfused. Furthermore, in older patients, particularly those who have had previous thoracotomies, the extensive acquired collateral circulation may produce rather granular lung fields.

ELECTROCARDIOGRAPHY

The electrocardiogram usually shows right atrial hypertrophy, and almost invariably right ventricular hypertrophy. This feature easily distinguishes the condition from newborns with pulmonary atresia with an intact ventricular septum, who usually have a conspicuous lack of right ventricular forces (Chapter 44). The mean frontal QRS axis is downward and to the right, usually between +100° and +180°.

ECHOCARDIOGRAPHY

The diagnosis of the intracardiac arrangement will be confirmed echocardiographically, but in most cases echocardiography will not be able to demonstrate all aspects of the complex pulmonary arterial supply.

The parasternal long-axis view shows a large aortic valve overriding the crest of the muscular ventricular septum. The atretic right ventricular outflow tract may be seen in short-axis parasternal cuts. Hypoplasia of the pulmonary trunk frequently permits the left lung to intrude between it and a precordial transducer, thus obscuring the pulmonary valve and trunk. This can be overcome by moving the transducer into a high precordial, or even suprasternal, position and obtaining a 'ductal cut' (Smallhorn et al, 1982b). This shows the left pulmonary artery, pulmonary trunk and right ventricular outflow tract in their long axis (Figure 47.25) (Smallhorn and Macartney, 1984). The same cut will image a left duct in the presence of a left aortic arch (Figure 47.26). From these, and subcostal cuts, the origin of the left and the proximal right pulmonary artery may be seen, as may their confluence when it is present.

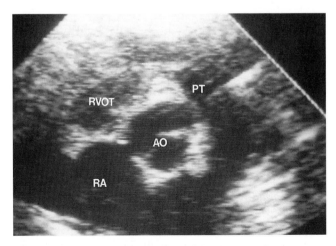

Figure 47.25. A high oblique parasternal short-axis cut demonstrating the atretic right ventricular outflow tract (RVOT). RA, right atrium; AO, aorta; PT, pulmonary trunk.

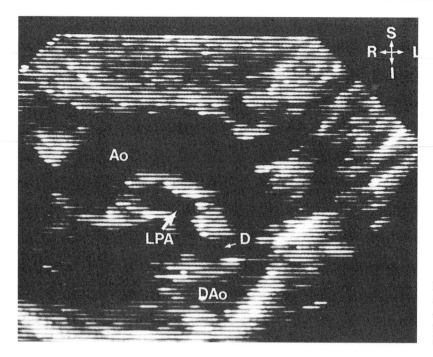

Figure 47.26. In this patient, a tortuous duct (D) supplies the left pulmonary artery (LPA), demonstrated by a suprasternal long-axis view of the aorta (Ao). DAo, descending aorta; I, inferior; L, left; R, right; S, superior.

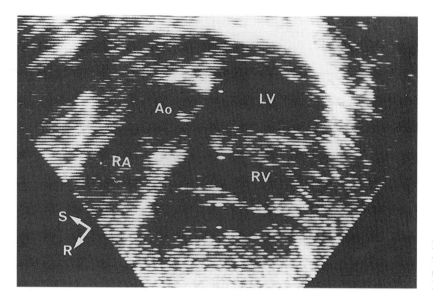

Figure 47.27. Subcostal long-axis section showing the aortic valve (Ao) overriding the ventricular septum. LV, left ventricle; R, right; RA, right atrium; RV, right ventricle; S, superior.

From the subcostal view, the overriding aorta can be seen when the transducer is depressed and angled anteriorly from the four chamber view (Figure 47.27). With clockwise rotation from this point, it is usually possible to demonstrate the blind-ending right ventricular infundibulum when present, and thereby rule out common arterial trunk in most cases (Figure 47.28) (Smallhorn et al, 1982a; Barron et al, 1983). Subcostal imaging can also demonstrate those rare cases in which the pulmonary arterial supply is derived through an aortopulmonary window (Figure 47.29).

Instances of an imperforate pulmonary valve can often only be differentiated from severe tetralogy by means of Doppler colour flow imaging. In both, the hypoplastic pulmonary trunk continues beyond the dense immobile echo immediately distal to the right ventricular outflow tract, which is either the imperforate or a severely stenotic pulmonary valve.

Suprasternal imaging of the right pulmonary artery is almost always possible when it is present, even if it is hypoplastic (Figure 47.30), though care must be taken not to confuse this structure with collateral arteries in the mediastinum (Figure 47.31). There is a good correlation between echocardiographic imaging and angiocardiographic size, though the echocardiographic 'lumen' is always slightly smaller than the true lumen (Huhta et al, 1982). Having found the right pulmonary artery, the operator should rotate the transducer while keeping it in view so as to demonstrate continuity with the left pulmonary artery. As continuity is most reproducibly assessed in a single cut, it is a good idea to move the transducer a little down from the suprasternal notch. The

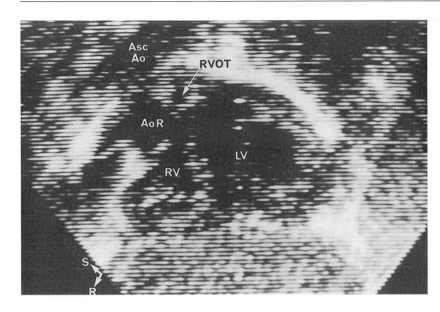

Figure 47.28. In this subcostal paracoronal cut, the very narrow right ventricular outflow tract (RVOT) is seen immediately to the left of the aortic root (AoR). Asc Ao, ascending aorta; other abbreviations as in Figure 47.27.

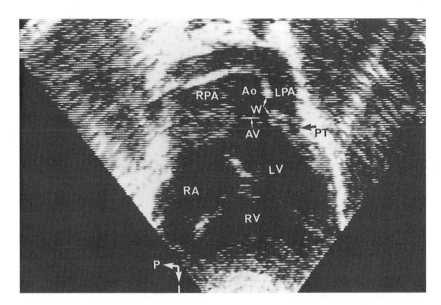

Figure 47.29. This subcostal oblique parasagittal section shows how the pulmonary arterial supply is derived via an aortopulmonary window (W). Note the short pulmonary trunk (PT), running back to an atretic valve. Ao, aorta; AV, aortic valve; I, inferior; LPA, left pulmonary artery; P, posterior; RPA, right pulmonary artery; other abbreviations as in Figure 47.27.

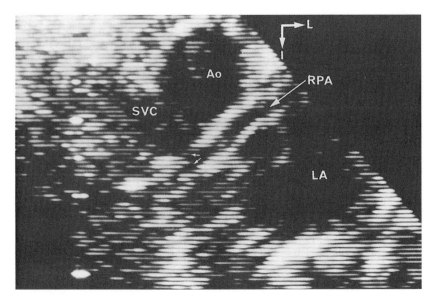

Figure 47.30. Suprasternal paracoronal picture of a hypoplastic right pulmonary artery (RPA), identified by its bifurcation (small white arrows). This is a suprasternal paracoronal section. Ao, aorta; I, inferior; L, left; LA, left atrium; SVC, superior caval vein.

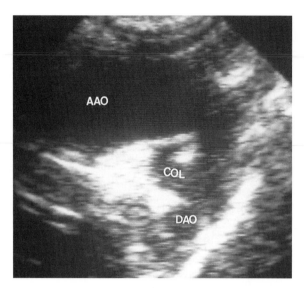

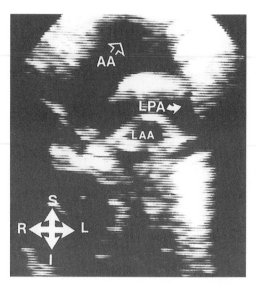

Figure 47.31. Suprasternal view of major systemic-to-pulmonary collateral artery (COL) originating from descending aorta (DAO); AAO, ascending aorta.

Figure 47.32. Origin of the left pulmonary artery (LPA) from the ascending aorta (AA) in a patient with tetralogy and pulmonary atresia. I, inferior; L, left; LAA, left atrial appendage; R, right; S, superior.

confluence will then appear as an inverted 'V'. As the transducer is rotated counterclockwise from suprasternally, a left aortic arch is normally seen. If this does not happen, the counter-clockwise rotation should be continued, for then it is likely that the bifurcation of a left brachiocephalic artery will be seen, indicating the presence of a right aortic arch. The region of the bifurcation should be scanned with colour Doppler imaging to search for an arterial duct. Then the transducer should be returned to its 'neutral' position imaging the right pulmonary artery and rotated clockwise. If there is indeed a right aortic arch, the round or elliptical section of the aorta seen above the right pulmonary artery will elongate as this rotation occurs, and the tight curve of a right arch will emerge. In the presence of a left arch, similar clockwise rotation will ultimately demonstrate the bifurcation of a right brachiocephalic artery, which should again be scrutinized for a duct.

Suprasternal views will also demonstrate anomalous origin of one pulmonary artery from the ascending aorta, the appearances usually being very similar to those of a common arterial trunk (Figure 47.32). The key to the differentiation between common trunk and tetralogy with pulmonary atresia in this situation is the presence of a blind right ventricular outflow tract and pulmonary trunk in those patients with tetralogy. If neither of these is seen, it can be impossible to distinguish echocardiographically between these two conditions in the presence of anomalous origin of one pulmonary artery (Smallhorn et al, 1982a). Colour Doppler usually allows the origins of major systemic-to-pulmonary collateral arteries to be established. The lungs themselves, however, obscure the intrapulmonary arteries; as a result, it is often not possible to establish the connections between the collateral arteries and the pulmonary arteries. As part of the echo-

cardiographic study, the function of the patent cardiac valves should be studied with colour Doppler. In particular, aortic regurgitation must be ruled out in adolescents or adults (Capelli et al, 1982).

RADIONUCLIDE IMAGING

Pulmonary perfusion imaging is of great value in demonstrating patterns of regional pulmonary perfusion in this anomaly. The perfusion images can only be interpreted once the anatomy of the pulmonary blood supply has been established by other means. They are of particular value in assessing the effect of surgical or interventional catheter procedures. Occasionally, administering radionuclide-labelled microspheres during catheterization can be of value in demonstrating the distribution of pulmonary perfusion from individual sources (Figure 47.33) (Baker et al, 1984).

MAGNETIC RESONANCE IMAGING

Magnetic resonance imaging (Figure 47.34) is excellent at demonstrating the anatomy of the central pulmonary arteries (Rees et al, 1987; Canter et al, 1989; Parsons et al, 1990). It can often demonstrate these arteries when other techniques, including angiography, have failed (Pagani et al, 1995). It can also show the presence and origin of major collateral arteries (Figure 47.35). For these reasons, if it is available, it should be used prior to angiography to help in planning invasive studies. Most magnetic resonance images are acquired over several minutes, and respiratory motion prevents imaging of the peripheral pulmonary perfusion. Recent faster imaging

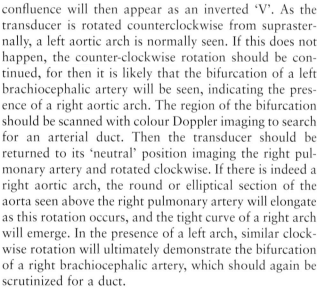

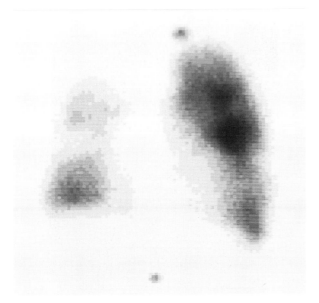

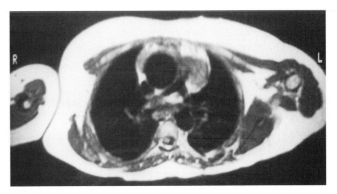

Figure 47.34. Hypoplastic confluent central pulmonary arteries in a patient with tetralogy with pulmonary atresia. In this transverse spin echo magnetic resonance image, the pulmonary arteries, approximately 2 mm in diameter, are seen dividing to the left and behind the ascending aorta.

Figure 47.33. A pulmonary perfusion image, seen in frontal projection, after technetium-99m-labelled microspheres have been injected into the central pulmonary arteries in a patient with tetralogy and pulmonary atresia. The distribution of perfusion to the lung parenchyma from the pulmonary arteries is clearly shown. There is good perfusion to the upper part of the left lung, but reduced perfusion to the lower half. The right lung has major defects in perfusion to the upper and middle zones. Major systemic to pulmonary collateral arteries supplied the lower part of the left lung and the majority of the right lung.

techniques are beginning to circumvent this problem, and magnetic resonance is likely to become more valuable in studying the distribution of pulmonary and collateral arteries (Figure 47.36).

CARDIAC CATHETERIZATION AND ANGIOGRAPHY

Complete investigation of the pulmonary arterial supply is essential in a patient with tetralogy and pulmonary atresia. It is best undertaken early in life, or as soon after presentation as possible. The cardiac anatomy is usually clearly shown by echocardiography. The source(s) of pulmonary perfusion, and the presence and size of central pulmonary arteries, should be established echocardiographically, by magnetic resonance or by angiography. The details of the distribution of pulmonary perfusion, nonetheless, can often only be ascertained by selective catheterization and angiography.

It is usually best to carry out upper descending aortography as the first stage of angiographic investigation. This will demonstrate patency of any normally positioned duct, as well as the majority of major systemic-to-pulmonary collateral arteries. A similar angiogram can be obtained if a balloon catheter is floated through the heart and aorta to lie in the lower descending thoracic aorta. During transitory occlusion of the aorta with the inflated balloon, contrast medium is injected through side holes proximal to the balloon. An isolated persistent duct is probably best left alone, as crossing such a duct with a catheter can lead to thrombosis.

Angiography in the aortic root is only necessary if non-invasive imaging has indicated that there is a more proximal source of pulmonary perfusion, such as a fistula between the coronary and pulmonary arteries, an aorto-pulmonary window, an anomalous origin of one pulmonary artery (Figure 47.37), a duct that arises from the brachiocephalic artery or major collateral arteries arising from the brachiocephalic arteries.

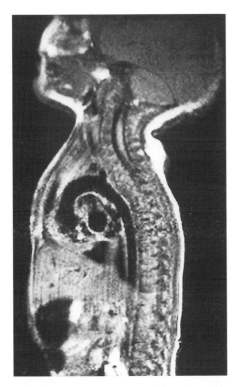

Figure 47.35. An oblique sagittal image of the aortic arch in an infant with tetralogy and pulmonary atresia. A major systemic-to-pulmonary collateral artery is seen arising from the descending aorta behind the left atrium.

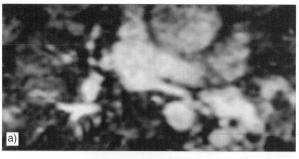

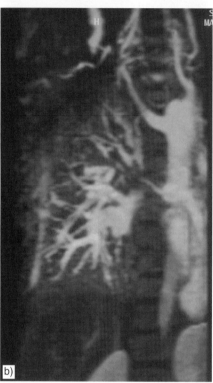

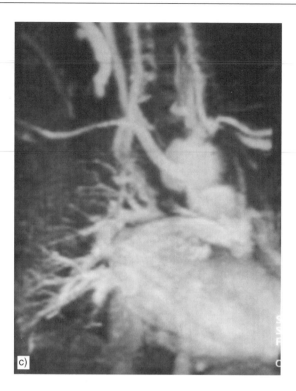

Figure 47.36. A contrast-enhanced (gadolinium) magnetic resonance angiogram of the aorta in tetralogy with pulmonary atresia. The whole series of images in this patient was acquired in 28 seconds while the patient held a breath. (a) A transverse slice through the descending aorta shows two collateral arteries arising together anteriorly from the aorta. (b) An oblique sagittal image from the same study reveals that one of the two collateral arteries seen in (a) supplies part of the right lung. (c) A separate sagittal image shows two further collateral arteries descending from the right subclavian artery to supply part of the right lung.

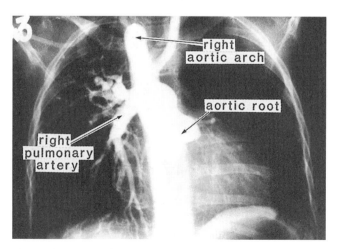

Figure 47.37. Anomalous origin of a right pulmonary artery from the ascending aorta in a patient with tetralogy with pulmonary atresia.

Posteroanterior and lateral projections (see Figures 47.19–47.21) with craniocaudal tilt are preferred. These are particularly helpful in showing small confluent pulmonary arteries since the craniocaudal angulation elongates the V-shaped confluence in the postoanterior projection. The craniocaudal tilt will also help separate the anterior pulmonary confluence from more posterior major systemic-to-pulmonary collateral arteries.

SELECTIVE CATHETERIZATION

Selective catheterization can be achieved for the major systemic-to-pulmonary collateral arteries, surgical shunts and central pulmonary arteries. It is best to enter the central intrapericardial pulmonary arteries whenever possible. This is particularly valuable when the pulmonary blood supply is unifocal, since pulmonary vascular resistance can then be determined. Catheters should always be passed as far distal into any collateral artery as is possible in order to detect pressure gradients.

Selective angiography needs to answer three questions. First, how does blood reach each part of the lungs? Second, are the central pulmonary arteries and the sources of pulmonary blood supply interconnected? Finally, are there any obstructions to the pulmonary blood flow?

Manipulation of catheters from a transvenous route through the heart into the aorta enables most of the necessary selective angiograms to be carried out. It is usually best, nonetheless, to use the retrograde arterial route. Though the approach from the axillary artery has much to commend it, percutaneous catheterization of the femoral artery is the most generally used technique.

Precurved catheters of cobra shape, with endholes so a guidewire can be used, are ideal for this. The long curve of the neck of the cobra keeps the tip pressed against the wall of the aorta and it is often difficult to avoid entering collateral arteries originating from the descending aorta. The tight curve at the tip is valuable for crossing surgical shunts. In the case of shunts between the subclavian and pulmonary arteries, the tip, once engaged in the shunt, then directs the guidewire down it.

If a central pulmonary artery can be entered, a pulmonary arteriogram is best taken in the right and left anterior oblique projections, since this permits assessment of which segments of the two lungs are connected to the central pulmonary arteries. The disadvantage of frontal and lateral projections in this case is the overlapping between the two lungs in the lateral projection.

Injection of contrast medium by hand is usually adequate for demonstration of smaller major systemic-to-pulmonary collateral arteries, but power injections are preferable for larger arteries. Otherwise, the large blood flow will excessively dilute the contrast medium.

During manipulation to enter major systemic-to-pulmonary collateral arteries originating from the descending aorta, intercostal arteries are frequently entered, particularly when they are enlarged as a result of supplying acquired collateral circulation to the lungs (see Figure 47.24). Entry to an intercostal artery may be suspected from the posterior course of the catheter from the aorta toward the paravertebral gutter, in contrast to the anterior course of major systemic-to-pulmonary collateral arteries toward the hilum. When contrast medium is injected, the patient may complain of pain in the muscles supplied by the intercostal artery, but no other harm appears to result.

Other varieties of preformed catheters may occasionally prove helpful, for example coronary arterial catheters when acquired or congenital pulmonary blood supply comes from the coronary arteries.

PULMONARY VENOUS WEDGE ANGIOGRAPHY

With good non-invasive imaging, and selective angiography of the major systemic-to-pulmonary collateral

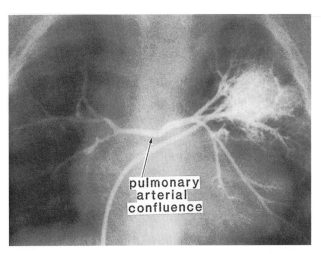

Figure 47.38. Pulmonary venous wedge injection, demonstrating pulmonary arterial confluence. (Original picture kindly supplied by Dr Robert Freedom, Hospital for Sick Children, Toronto, Canada.)

arteries, the anatomy of the pulmonary arteries should have been demonstrated. Only rarely will it be necessary to use pulmonary venous wedge angiography (Figure 47.38) (Nihill et al, 1978; Singh et al, 1978). The use of power injections is dangerous for this procedure (Alpert and Culham, 1979). We, therefore, recommend the technique suggested by Nihill and colleagues (1978). An end-hole catheter is wedged in a pulmonary vein and 0.5 ml/kg of contrast medium is then injected by hand, immediately followed by 1 ml/kg 5% dextrose. The effect of the first injection, if successful, is that contrast medium is forced retrogradely through the pulmonary capillaries and intrapulmonary arteries back to the hilum of the lung. The central pulmonary arteries and other intrapulmonary arteries may then opacify. Injection of dextrose continues this process while clearing away the 'blot' of contrast medium at the site of the injection.

A pulmonary venous wedge angiogram may fail to demonstrate central pulmonary arteries even when they are present. Either the pressure in the artery may be too high to permit contrast medium to be forced back to the hilum, or the vessel opacified may not be connected to the central pulmonary artery. Confident exclusion of the presence of central pulmonary arteries may, therefore, require pulmonary venous wedge angiography in multiple sites.

ANALYSIS OF ANGIOGRAPHY

Major systemic-to-pulmonary collateral arteries

The major systemic-to-pulmonary collateral arteries appear as large tortuous arteries, originating usually from the descending aorta (see Figures 47.19–47.21 and 47.23a,b), but occasionally from the brachiocephalic arteries (see Figure 47.23c) and, exceptionally, from coronary arteries. They anastomose with intrapulmonary arteries in the region of the hilum and are never connected to intercostal arteries. They accompany bronchuses but only rarely form a plexus around them. In essence, they are no different in appearance in the neonatal period from later life.

Arterial ducts

When a duct originates on the side opposite to the aortic arch, it is likely to arise close to the bifurcation of the brachiocephalic artery and pass to the intrapericardial pulmonary artery on that side, usually taking a straight course but sometimes 'wandering' (Figure 47.39). Rarely, the duct may originate from an anomalous retro-oesophageal subclavian artery arising as the last branch from the aorta (McKay et al, 1982). Exceptionally, bilateral ducts may be present.

Persistent fifth arch

A persistent fifth aortic arch would be expected to course from the distal ascending aorta proximal to the origin of the first brachiocephalic artery and extend to the pulmonary artery, as shown in Figure 47.11.

Intrapericardial pulmonary arteries

Central pulmonary arteries are most easily recognized when they are confluent, as they usually are. The confluent pulmonary arteries, together with the abbreviated pulmonary trunk, appear like a seagull in flight when seen in the frontal projection (Figure 47.40) (Somerville et al, 1978). This resemblance is heightened by craniocaudal tilt, this procedure elongating the pulmonary trunk. The confluent central pulmonary arteries appear in the lateral projection like a hairpin, extending anteriorly to the trachea (see Figure 47.19) (Fåller et al, 1981).

Where there is doubt as to the identity of an artery in the mediastinum, a particular problem when the central pulmonary arteries are not confluent, the fact that the pulmonary trunk is usually attached to the heart, if only by a fibrous cord, is helpful. Because of this, on a cine-angiogram viewed in motion, the intrapericardial

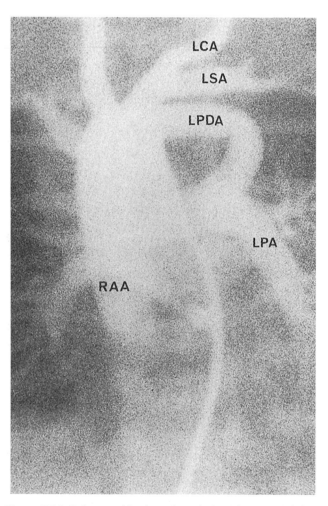

Figure 47.39. Pulmonary blood supply to the lungs by tortuous left duct (LPDA) in the presence of a right aortic arch (RAA). LCA, left carotid artery; LPA, left pulmonary artery; LSA, left subclavian artery.

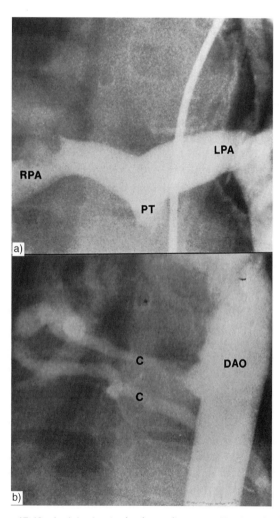

Figure 47.40. An injection in the descending aorta (Dao) is visualized in (a) frontal projection and (b) lateral projection. In (b) the injection is seen to fill two systemic-to-pulmonary collateral arteries (c). (a) With time, the contrast also opacifies the intrapericardial pulmonary arteries. The confluence of the right and left pulmonary arteries (RPA, LPA, respectively) from the atretic pulmonary trunk (PT) gives the appearance of a flying seagull.

pulmonary arteries are seen to move with the heart, whereas other mediastinal arteries move, if at all, with the lungs (Fåller et al, 1981).

Interconnections between major systemic-to-pulmonary collateral arteries, central pulmonary arteries and intrapulmonary arteries

The intraparenchymal pulmonary arteries in tetralogy with pulmonary atresia are essentially normal. In particular, with rare exceptions, their distribution is that of normal pulmonary arteries. Such abnormalities as exist are largely the result of the haemodynamic circumstances (Macartney and Haworth, 1979). Therefore, if they are hypoperfused at low pressure, they appear narrow, with deficient peripheral branching. By comparison, if they are hyperperfused and at high pressure, they appear large and tortuous, with increased background 'haze'. If pulmonary vascular obstructive disease supervenes, background 'haze' diminishes, but the arteries remain tortuous.

The abnormalities of the intrapulmonary arteries occur mainly at the hilum (Haworth and Macartney, 1980). Instead of fusing into a single hilar artery, as they normally do, they may remain separate. As a result, the pulmonary arterial supply to an entire lobe, segment or even part of a segment may be completely isolated from the remainder of the lung. The segmental or lobar arteries are connected proximally to a central pulmonary artery, to a major systemic-to-pulmonary collateral artery or to both (see Figures 47.19–47.21). The usual result is that pulmonary blood supply is compartmentalized, with each major collateral artery being the sole arterial blood supply to part of the lungs. Injection of contrast medium into that artery opacifies only that region of lung. Occasionally, on viewing a selective injection of contrast medium into a major collateral artery on a moving cineangiogram, wash-out of contrast medium may be seen as a result of non-opacified blood entering the intrapulmonary artery (see Figure 47.23). This is because more than one major systemic-to-pulmonary collateral artery is supplying the same region of lung, and hence there is a duplicate pulmonary arterial supply (Figure 47.41) (Fåller et al, 1981).

When a surgical shunt has been created to augment pulmonary arterial supply, and contrast medium is injected into the pulmonary artery by some route other than the shunt, wash-out of contrast medium is to be expected at the point of anastomosis of the shunt to the pulmonary artery.

By combining the information obtained from all the selective injections into major systemic-to-pulmonary collateral arteries, shunts and intrapericardial pulmonary arteries, it should be possible to state precisely the origin of blood supply to each pulmonary segment and, most importantly, how much of the parenchyma of each lung is connected to each pulmonary artery. In making this assessment, it is important to recognize duplicate supply when it exists. For example, if the left upper lobe is connected to a major systemic-to-pulmonary collateral artery

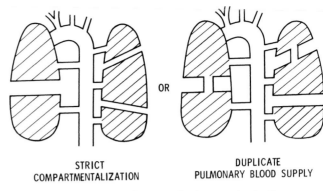

Figure 47.41. Diagram to illustrate what is meant by duplicate pulmonary blood supply in tetralogy with pulmonary atresia. (a) The more usual situation is strict compartmentalization, in which different regions of lung are supplied by a unique collateral. (b) In duplicate pulmonary blood supply, a given region of lung is supplied by more than one source.

and to the central left pulmonary artery, whereas the left lower lobe appears only to be connected to a major systemic-to-pulmonary collateral artery, a shunt into the central left pulmonary artery will, on the face of it, only increase blood supply to the left lower lobe. However, if careful inspection reveals wash-out from one lobe to the other, then it would increase blood supply to the entire left lung.

Obstructions within the entire system of pulmonary arterial supply

As has been described, obstructions and stenoses can occur at many levels in the pulmonary circulation. Haemodynamic pressure gradients are sometimes documented at sites where no angiocardiographic stenosis is seen (Macartney et al, 1973). Usually, obstructions are angiocardiographically obvious, as illustrated in Figure 47.20a. Craniocaudal tilt during injection into a central pulmonary artery increases the likelihood of detection of proximal stenosis of the central right or left pulmonary artery.

Acquired collateral arteries

Acquired collateral circulation is a rare finding in the first 3 months of life, but it develops over time, particularly after thoracotomies, when adhesion of the visceral and parietal pleural layers permits the development of centripetal collateral circulation from the chest wall to the lungs. Acquired collateral circulation appears on aortography as myriads of tiny vessels, which may originate from any artery in the thorax. Bronchial arteries are recognized by their relation to the trachea and bronchial tree, and the way in which they form a nutritive plexus in the bronchial walls. The result is that the bronchial tree 'lights up' in the course of the aortogram because of the contrast between the air in the lumen and the contrast medium in the walls.

More detailed analysis of acquired collateral circulation can be obtained by selective injection into intercostal, coronary or internal thoracic arteries. On injection into an intercostal artery, for example, a wedge of capillaries are first seen in the fused visceral and parietal pleuras, following which opacification occurs of the pulmonary veins and, occasionally, the pulmonary arteries (see Figure 47.24). Recognizable discrete anastomoses with intrapulmonary arteries in the region of the hilum are rare, in contrast with those formed by the major systemic-to-pulmonary collateral arteries.

NATURAL HISTORY

It is difficult to be sure of the natural history of tetralogy with pulmonary atresia, since before cardiac surgery was available the condition was frequently confused with either tetralogy of Fallot or common arterial trunk. Nevertheless, it is clear that the prognosis without treatment is extremely poor for patients with duct-dependent pulmonary blood supply. At the other end of the scale, patients with increased, but not excessive, pulmonary arterial supply can survive into the third and fourth decade of life without surgical treatment (Campbell and Deuchar, 1961; Stuckey et al, 1968). Systemic arterial oxygen saturation in these patients falls only slowly, if at all, with increasing age (Macartney et al, 1973). These two examples represent the two ends of the spectrum of prognosis. Overall, the majority of patients with tetralogy of Fallot and pulmonary atresia will not survive more than a few years without surgical treatment.

MANAGEMENT

MEDICAL MANAGEMENT

Neonates with duct-dependent pulmonary blood supply should be treated with parenteral prostaglandins E_1 or E_2 while waiting for surgical palliation. Treatment may be required to combat heart failure for patients with excessive pulmonary blood flow through major systemic-to-pulmonary collateral arteries.

DEFINITIVE REPAIR

When confluent pulmonary arteries are present, definitive repair consists of closing the ventricular septal defect and connecting the right ventricle to the pulmonary trunk or pulmonary arterial confluence. This was first reported in 1965 by Rastelli and colleagues, who used a valveless conduit. It was Ross who first established continuity using a valved conduit (Ross and Somerville, 1966). The long-term results using aortic or pulmonary homografts (Somerville and Ross, 1972) seem better, as obstruction

appears to be rare in this type of conduit. These are now the preferred surgical conduit. If possible, it is best to avoid the use of an extracardiac conduit (Kirklin et al, 1988). If there is continuity between the right ventricle and pulmonary trunk, correction can often be achieved with a patch reconstruction, similar to the technique for tetralogy with pulmonary stenosis.

Good results for radical correction in suitable patients were reported some time ago by Olin and colleagues (1976). Their overall mortality was about 14%. Just over half the patients required a valved conduit to restore right ventricular to pulmonary arterial continuity. The remainder had a patch reconstruction of the right ventricular outflow tract. Alfieri and colleagues (1978), and subsequently Kirklin et al (1988) and Blackstone et al (1988), then showed a strong positive correlation between the probability of hospital death and the ratio between the right and left ventricular systolic pressures after bypass. The risk of postoperative death rises steeply if the ratio of right ventricular to left ventricular pressures at the end of the repair is equal to or greater than unity. The causes of a high ratio are residual gradients in the right ventricular outflow, residual major systemic-to-pulmonary collateral arteries and hypoplasia and incompleteness of arborization of the intrapericardial pulmonary arteries. Definitive repair is possible if 15, out of the 20, bronchopulmonary segments are connected to confluent pulmonary arteries. Repair can also be achieved if 11 or more segments are connected to the central pulmonary arteries, but when the number is between 11 and 14, there is an increased risk of a high postoperative pressure ratio and an increased surgical mortality (Shimazaki et al, 1990; Kirklin and Barratt-Boyes, 1993). Other risk factors are related to the number of segments fed by the central pulmonary arteries. These are small size of the proximal right and left pulmonary arteries, non-confluent pulmonary arteries and a high number of systemic-to-pulmonary collateral arteries. There is also some evidence that very young age, or age greater than 8 years, adds to the risk of definitive repair (Kirklin and Barratt-Boyes, 1993).

The key to achieving satisfactory results is careful selection of patients: attempting repair only in patients who are predicted to have a low probability of severe postoperative right ventricular hypertension. More recent surgical reports have supported this view, with most authors favouring a staged approach to repair, patients unsuitable for primary repair having palliative procedures to encourage growth of hypoplastic pulmonary arteries: ligation of systemic-to-pulmonary collateral arteries or their anastomosis to the central pulmonary arteries (Iyer and Mee, 1991; Rome et al, 1993; Pagani et al, 1995; Yagihara et al, 1996).

An alternative approach has now been advocated by Reddy and colleagues (1995). They argue that systemic-to-pulmonary collateral arteries are not a reliable source of pulmonary blood. The flow may be too high, leading to pulmonary vascular disease, or the collateral artery may become progressively stenosed, leading to distal arterial hypoplasia. Either way, segments of lung may be lost to the pulmonary circulation. To counter this, they undertook complete repair in one procedure in 10 unselected patients aged from 1 month to 37 years. Complete unifocalization was achieved in all patients. This involved anastomosis of all the collateral arteries to the central pulmonary arteries or to the central conduit. The ventricular septal defect was left open in one patient. In the remainder, the ratio of right ventricular to left ventricular pressures at the end of the operation was between 0.29 and 0.75. There was one late death. Rome and colleagues (1993) compared the outcome of primary repair in 10 patients with hypoplastic pulmonary arteries with a staged approach in 30. Long-term survival after primary repair was poor, but about half of those who were treated by staged procedures eventually had a successful repair.

PALLIATIVE PROCEDURES

Palliative procedures may be needed to increase the pulmonary blood flow or, occasionally, to decrease the pulmonary blood flow. The long-term goal is definitive repair, so palliative procedures have a dual purpose, first to improve the management of the immediate clinical problem but also to make the patient suitable for definitive surgical repair. Preparation for definitive repair needs to address two problems: enlargement of hypoplastic central pulmonary arteries and unifocalization of pulmonary perfusion.

MANAGEMENT OF HYPOPLASTIC CENTRAL PULMONARY ARTERIES

Early intervention to increase the blood flow in diminutive central pulmonary arteries has long been advocated (Gill et al, 1977; Kirklin et al, 1977). There is good evidence that it can improve the eventual outcome (Iyer and Mee, 1991; Rome et al, 1993; Mee, 1996), even though the enlargement achieved may not affect uniformly the entire pulmonary arterial tree.

The choice is between a shunt and a reconstruction of the right ventricular outflow tract using a patch or conduit while leaving open the ventricular septal defect (Crupi et al, 1977; Gill et al, 1977; Lane et al, 1983). There is no clear consensus on which of these is preferred. There is evidence that early connection of the right ventricle to the pulmonary arteries promotes more pulmonary arterial growth than does a shunt (Piehler et al, 1980). Reconstruction of the right ventricular outflow also has the advantage of allowing direct access to the pulmonary arteries so that interventional procedures can be undertaken to address stenosis of the pulmonary arteries.

Since enlargement of the pulmonary arteries is not uniform, areas of pulmonary arterial stenosis may well remain following palliation. A combined surgical and interventional approach to the pulmonary arteries is now widely advocated. Balloon angioplasty, and the deployment of intravascular stents, are used after reconstruction of the right ventricular outflow tract to promote unobstructed flow to the maximum number of bronchopulmonary segments (Rome et al, 1993; Pagani et al, 1995).

One disadvantage of early reconstruction of the right ventricular outflow tract is that it needs cardiopulmonary bypass and carries a higher risk than does placement of a shunt. It is also recognized that patch reconstruction can lead to stenosis of the pulmonary arteries, especially the left, and that aneurysmal dilatation of the outflow patch can occur (Freedom et al, 1983). These considerations have led some surgeons to prefer a shunt as an initial procedure (Kirklin et al, 1988; Iyer and Mee, 1991). Peripheral shunts have fallen out of favour since they can lead to distortion of the pulmonary arteries. Central shunts, either constructed of Gore-Tex tube or by disconnecting the pulmonary trunk and anastomosing it end-to-side to the ascending aorta (Watterson et al, 1991), are now preferred.

UNIFOCALIZATION

There are two options for dealing with the major systemic-to-pulmonary collateral arteries. The first is to obliterate them either by surgical ligation or by embolization using coils and the second is surgical unifocalization. If there is a dual blood supply to pulmonary segments and this is combined with, or follows, a shunt or right ventricular outflow reconstruction, obliteration will encourage blood flow and hence growth and development of the central pulmonary arteries. If the collateral artery is the sole supply to an area of lung, ligation has been advocated in the hope that hypoplasia of that region of the lung will result, with compensatory hypertrophy of those regions connected to the central pulmonary arteries (Macartney et al, 1974). Necrosis of the region of lung supplied by the ligated collateral artery is unlikely but has been reported in exceptional cases (Olin et al, 1976; Alfieri et al, 1978). In practice, this approach has not been successful.

A better approach to collateral arteries that are the sole supply to parts of the lung is surgical unifocalization. The aim is to maximize the number of bronchopulmonary segments perfused from the central pulmonary arteries by connecting the collaterals to them. Technically this is not easy, as the collateral arteries are located posteriorly in the mediastinum while the pulmonary arteries are anterior. Early results were disappointing (Sullivan et al, 1988), but better results have now been achieved. Depending on the precise anatomy found, a number of techniques have been used, including direct and prosthetic anastomosis, division of a collateral artery with end-to-side anastomosis of its distal end to a pulmonary artery, and insertion of xenograft pericardial tubes (Iyer and Mee, 1991; Yagihara et al, 1996). Such operations rarely achieve unifocalization at a stroke, since it is often difficult to connect together all intrapulmonary arteries on one side, let alone both. The procedures can be carried out at the same time as a shunt or surgical relief of pulmonary arterial stenosis, but not in combination with reconstruction of the right ventricular outflow tract. Where the central pulmonary arteries are non-confluent, completely absent or are judged to be too hypoplastic to be amenable to the staging approach, an artificial pulmonary arterial confluence can be created using a prosthetic or xenograft pericardial tube graft. The confluence is connected to a shunt, and the collateral arteries unifocalized by connection to the confluence (Puga, 1991; Toyoda et al, 1996; Yagihara et al, 1996).

Coil embolization of collateral arteries can be used after definitive repair and when there is still a large left-to-right shunt through unligated collaterals. It is preferable to embolize collaterals before definitive repair is undertaken as part of a combined interventional and surgical strategy (Rome et al, 1993; Pagani et al, 1995).

Obstructions in major systemic-to-pulmonary collateral arteries can lead to a progressive reduction in overall pulmonary perfusion or to hypoperfusion of a significant part of the pulmonary parenchyma. There is little in the literature about balloon angioplasty and stenting of these obstructions, as a purely palliative measure, to improve systemic oxygenation or as a prelude to unifocalization. It may have a limited role in some circumstances, but some of these stenoses cannot be successfully dilated even with high-pressure balloons (Brown et al, 1998).

STRATEGIES FOR MANAGEMENT

In this complex and varied condition, generalizations about regions for treatment are unwise. Each patient requires detailed investigation, and an individual strategy for treatment must be devised by a team that has experience in managing this condition. Earlier in this chapter, we identified three characteristic patterns for pulmonary perfusion in this anomaly. These were confluent pulmonary arteries with a unifocal supply, confluent but hypoplastic central pulmonary arteries with major systemic-to-pulmonary collateral arteries and complete absence of the central pulmonary arteries with the pulmonary perfusion solely from major collateral arteries.

The first of these patterns is the easiest with which to deal. The pulmonary arteries are generally of a good size and are connected to all of the bronchopulmonary segments. The management is comparable to that for tetralogy of Fallot with pulmonary stenosis. Definitive repair can be carried out as a primary procedure (Di Donato et al, 1991), or a shunt is constructed in the neonatal period and definitive repair carried out in the first few years of life. The decision between the two will depend upon the size of the pulmonary arteries and the experience of the surgeon.

In patients with hypoplastic pulmonary arteries, it is essential to intervene early in life to encourage them to grow. This either involves reconstruction of the right ventricular outflow tract, with a patch or valveless conduit, or placement of a central aortopulmonary shunt. Major collateral arteries that form a dual supply to part of the lung with the central pulmonary arteries are ligated or embolized as part of the same procedure, or more commonly as a second staging procedure. Collateral arteries that form the sole supply to part of the lung are anastomosed to the central pulmonary arteries, ideally directly but if necessary using a prosthetic graft. The aim is to connect the central pulmonary arteries to as much of the pulmonary parenchyma as possible, and to achieve unobstructed blood flow within them. Balloon angioplasty, or stenting, of the pulmonary arteries may be necessary to deal with localized obstructions. Using this approach, approximately half of these patients will eventually have central pulmonary arteries of sufficient size and supplying sufficient of the lungs to make them suitable for definitive repair.

The third pattern is the most difficult to treat. Operations to create a central pulmonary confluence using grafts have been described (Puga, 1991; Toyoda et al, 1996; Yagihara et al, 1996). The long-term success of this approach, however, is not established. In patients with a stable and well-balanced pulmonary perfusion, many would advocate conservative management, with the eventual aim of offering them heart–lung transplantation (Kirklin and Barratt-Boyes, 1993; Bull et al, 1995).

RESULTS OF SURGERY

The majority of patients require multiple surgical interventions. Results of individual operations are, therefore, not as important as the results of the overall programme of treatment. These can be difficult to ascertain from published surgical series. What is clear is that the results of surgery for tetralogy with pulmonary atresia are much worse that those for tetralogy with pulmonary stenosis. The early mortality of definitive repair reported in published series varies between 4 and 15% (Kirklin et al, 1988; Iyer and Mee, 1991; Watterson et al, 1991; Rome et al, 1993; Pagani et al, 1995; Reddy et al, 1995; Yagihara et al, 1996). Many patients are never candidates for definitive repair despite palliative staging procedures. The proportion of patients that can be converted from being inoperable to operable by staging procedures is difficult to determine from the published series, but overall it seems to be little more than 50%. The staging procedures themselves carry a significant risk, with a reported mortality of at least 10% in most series. There does seem to be some evidence that the chances of achieving operability from staging operations are improved by starting early in life (Mee, 1996).

There is limited information about the long-term outcome for survivors of surgery. The most helpful and largest study is that of Kirklin and colleagues (1988). They found that there was a low, but constant, risk of dying in survivors of surgery. Survival was 82%, 69% and 58% at 1, 10 and 20 years, respectively. Taking into account the attrition rate before surgery, it is clear that the overall results of treatment for this condition are disappointing. In those patients with the most complex abnormalities of pulmonary perfusion, the choice between an aggressive surgical approach and conservative management remains finely balanced.

REFERENCES

Alfieri J, Blackstone E H, Kirklin J W, Pacifico A D, Bargeron L M Jr 1978 Surgical treatment in tetralogy of Fallot with pulmonary atresia. Journal of Thoracic and Cardiovascular Surgery 76: 321–335

Alpert B S, Culham J A G 1979 A severe complication of pulmonary vein angiography. British Heart Journal 41: 727–729

Anderson R H, Devine W A, Del Nido P 1991 The surgical anatomy of tetralogy of Fallot with pulmonary atresia rather than pulmonary stenosis. Journal of Cardiac Surgery 6: 41–58

Baker E J, Malamitsi J, Jones O D H, Maisey M N, Tynan M J 1984 Use of radionuclide labelled microspheres to show the distribution of the pulmonary perfusion with multifocal pulmonary blood supply. British Heart Journal 52: 72–76

Barron J V, Sahn D J, Attie F et al 1983 Two-dimensional echocardiographic study of right ventricular outflow and great artery anatomy in tetralogy with pulmonary atresia and in truncus arteriosus. American Heart Journal 105: 281–286

Blackstone E H, Shimazaki Y, Maehara T, Kirklin J W, Bargeron L M 1988 Prediction of severe obstruction to right ventricular outflow after repair of tetralogy of Fallot and pulmonary atresia. Journal of Thoracic Cardiovascular Surgery 96: 288–293

Brown S C, Eyskens B, Mertens L, Dumoulin M, Gewillig M 1998 Percutaneous treatment of stenosed major aortopulmonary collaterals with balloon dilatation and stenting: what can be achieved? Heart 79: 24–28

Bull K, Somerville J, Ty E, Spiegelhalter D 1995 Presentation and attrition in pulmonary atresia. Journal of the American College of Cardiology 25: 491–499

Campbell M, Deuchar D C 1961 Continuous murmurs in cyanotic congenital heart disease. British Heart Journal 23: 173–192

Canter C E, Guitierrez F R, Mirowitz S A, Martin T C, Hartmann A F Jr 1989 Evaluation of pulmonary arterial morphology in cyanotic congenital heart disease by magnetic resonance imaging. American Heart Journal 118: 347–354

Capelli H, Ross D, Somerville J 1982 Aortic regurgitation in tetrad of Fallot and pulmonary atresia. American Journal of Cardiology 49: 1979–1983

Chessa M, Butera G, Bonhoeffer P, et al 1998 Relation of genotype 22q11 deletion to phenotype of pulmonary vessels in tetralogy of Fallot and pulmonary atresia–ventricular septal defect. Heart 79: 186–190

Collett R W, Edwards J E 1949 Persistent truncus arteriosus: a classification according to anatomic types. Surgical Clinics of North America 29: 1245–1270

Crupi G, Macartney F J, Anderson R H 1977 Persistent truncus arteriosus. A study of 66 autopsy cases with special reference to definition and morphogenesis. American Journal of Cardiology 40: 569–578

Di Donato R M, Jonas R A, Lang P, Rome J J, Mayer J E, Castañeda A R 1991 Neonatal repair of tetralogy of Fallot with and without pulmonary atresia. Journal of Thoracic and Cardiovascular Surgery 101: 126–137

Fåller K, Haworth S G, Taylor J F N, Macartney F J 1981 Duplicate sources of pulmonary blood supply in pulmonary atresia with ventricular septal defect. British Heart Journal 46: 263–268

Fisher E A, Thanopoulos B D, Eckner F A O, Hastreiter A R, DuBrow I W 1980 Pulmonary atresia with obstructed ventricular septal defect. Pediatric Cardiology 1: 209–217

Freedom R M, Pongliglione G, Williams W G, Trusler G A, Rowe R D 1983 Palliative right ventricular outflow tract construction for patients with pulmonary atresia, ventricular septal defect, and hypoplastic pulmonary arteries. Journal of Thoracic and Cardiovascular Surgery 86: 24–36

Frescura C, Talenti E, Pellegrino P A, Mazzucco A, Faggian G, Thiene G 1984 Coexistence of ductal and systemic pulmonary arterial supply in pulmonary atresia with ventricular septal defect. American Journal of Cardiology 53: 348–349

Gerlis L M, Ho S Y, Anderson R H 1994 Maldevelopment of conotruncal and aortopulmonary septum with absent left central pulmonary artery: anatomical and clinical implications. (Letter) British Heart Journal 72: 210–211

Gill C C, Moodie D S, McGoon D C 1977 Staged surgical management of pulmonary atresia with diminutive pulmonary arteries. Journal of Thoracic and Cardiovascular Surgery 73: 436–442

Haworth S G, Macartney F J 1980 Growth and development of pulmonary circulation in pulmonary atresia with ventricular septal defect and major aortopulmonary collateral arteries. British Heart Journal 44: 14–24

Haworth S G, de Leval M, Macartney F J 1981 Hypoperfusion and hyperperfusion in the immature lung. Pulmonary arterial development following ligation of the left pulmonary artery in the newborn pig. Journal of Thoracic and Cardiovascular Surgery 82: 281–292

Ho S Y, Catani G, Seo J-W 1992 Arterial supply to the lungs in tetralogy of Fallot with pulmonary atresia or critical pulmonary stenosis. Cardiology of the Young 2: 65–72

Huhta J C, Piehler J M, Tajik A J et al 1982 Two dimensional echocardiographic detection and measurement of the right pulmonary artery in pulmonary atresia ventricular septal defect: angiographic and surgical correlation. American Journal of Cardiology 49: 1235–1240

Huntingdon G S 1919 The morphology of the pulmonary artery in the mammalia. Anatomical Record 17: 165–190

Iyer K S, Mee R B 1991 Staged repair of pulmonary atresia with ventricular septal defect and major systemic to pulmonary artery collaterals. Annals of Thoracic Surgery 51: 65–72

Jackson M, Connell M G, Smith A, Drury J, Anderson R H 1996 Common arterial trunk and pulmonary atresia: close developmental cousins? Results from a teratogen induced animal model. Cardiovascular Research 30: 992–1000

Jedele K B, Michels V V, Puja F J, Feldt R H 1992 Velo-cardiofacial syndrome associated with ventricular septal defect, pulmonary atresia, and hypoplastic pulmonary arteries. Pediatrics 89: 915–919

Jefferson K, Rees S, Somerville J 1972 Systemic arterial supply to the lungs in pulmonary atresia and its relation to pulmonary artery development. British Heart Journal 34: 418–427

Kenna A P, Smithells R W, Fielding D W 1975 Congenital heart disease in Liverpool: 1960–69. Quarterly Journal of Medicine 43: 2–44

Kirklin J W, Barratt-Boyes B G 1993 Cardiac Surgery. Churchill Livingstone, New York, p 942–973

Kirklin J W, Bargeron L M, Pacifico A D 1977 The enlargement of small pulmonary arteries by preliminary palliative operation. Circulation 56: 612–617

Kirklin J W, Blackstone E H, Shimazaki Y et al 1988 Survival, functional status, and reoperations after repair of tetralogy of Fallot with pulmonary atresia. Journal of Thoracic and Cardiovascular Surgery 96: 102–116

Krongrad E, Ritter D G, Hawe A, Kincaid O W, McGoon D C 1972 Pulmonary atresia or severe stenosis and coronary artery-to-pulmonary artery fistula. Circulation 46: 1005–1012

Lane I, Treasure T, Leijala M, Shinebourne E, Lincoln C 1983 Diminutive pulmonary artery growth following right ventricular outflow tract enlargement. International Journal of Cardiology 3: 175–185

Macartney F J, Haworth S G 1979 The pulmonary blood supply in pulmonary atresia with ventricular septal defect. In: Godman M J, Marquis R M (eds) Paediatric cardiology, vol 2 Heart disease in the newborn. Churchill Livingstone, Edinburgh, p 314–338

Macartney F J, Haworth S G 1983 Investigation of pulmonary atresia with ventricular septal defect. In: Anderson R H, Macartney F J, Shinebourne E A, Tynan M (eds) Paediatric Cardiology, vol 5. Churchill Livingstone, Edinburgh, p 111–125

Macartney F J, Deverall P B, Scott O 1972 Significance of continuous murmurs in cyanotic congenital heart disease, British Heart Journal 34: 205

Macartney F J, Deverall P, Scott O 1973 Haemodynamic characteristics of systemic arterial blood supply to the lungs. British Heart Journal 35: 28–37

Macartney F J, Scott O, Deverall P B 1974 Haemodynamic and anatomical characteristics of pulmonary blood supply in pulmonary atresia with ventricular septal defect–including a case of persistent fifth aortic arch. British Heart Journal 36: 1049–1060

McGoon M D, Fulton R E, Davis G D, Ritter D G, Neill C A, White R I 1977 Systemic collateral and pulmonary artery stenosis in patients with congenital pulmonary valve atresia and ventricular septal defect. Circulation 56: 473–479

McKay R, Stark J, de Leval M R 1982 Unusual vascular ring in infant with pulmonary atresia and ventricular septal defect. British Heart Journal 48: 180–183

Mee R B 1996 Presentation and attrition in complex pulmonary atresia, (Letter) Journal of the American College of Cardiology 28: 539–540

Miller W W, Nadas A S, Bernhard W F, Gross R E 1968 Congenital pulmonary atresia with ventricular septal defect. Review of the clinical course of fifty patients with assessment of the results of palliative surgery. American Journal of Cardiology 21: 673–680

Momma K, Kondo C, Matsuoka R. 1996 Tetralogy of Fallot with pulmonary atresia associated with chromosome 22q11 deletion. Journal of the American College of Cardiology 27: 198–202

Nihill M R, Mullins C E, McNamara D G 1978 Visualization of the pulmonary arteries in pseudotruncus by pulmonary vein wedge angiography. Circulation 58: 140–147

Olin C L, Ritter D G, McGoon D C, Wallace R B, Danielson G K 1976 Pulmonary atresia: surgical considerations and results in 103 patients undergoing definitive repair. Circulation 54(suppl III): 35–40

Pagani F D, Cheatham J P, Beekman R H, Lloyd T R, Mosca R S, Bove E L 1995 The management of tetralogy of Fallot with pulmonary atresia and diminutive pulmonary arteries. Journal of Thoracic and Cardiovascular Surgery 110: 1521–1532

Parsons J M, Baker E J, Hayes A et al 1990 Magnetic resonance imaging of the great arteries in infants. International Journal of Cardiology 28: 73–85

Piehler J M, Danielson G K, McGoon D C, Wallace R B, Fulton R E, Mair D D 1980 Management of pulmonary atresia with ventricular septal defect and hypoplastic pulmonary arteries by right ventricular outflow construction. Journal of Thoracic and Cardiovascular Surgery 80: 552–67

Puga F J 1991 Unifocalization for pulmonary atresia with ventricular septal defect. Annals of Thoracic Surgery 51: 8–9

Ramsay J M, Macartney F J, Haworth S G 1985 Tetralogy of Fallot with major aortopulmonary collateral arteries. British Heart Journal 53: 167–172

Rastelli G C, Ongley P A, Davis G D, Kirklin J W 1965 Surgical repair for pulmonary valve atresia with coronary–pulmonary artery fistula: report of a case. Mayo Clinic Proceedings 40: 521–527

Reddy V M, Liddicoat J R, Hanley F L 1995 Midline one-stage complete unifocalization and repair of pulmonary atresia with ventricular septal defect and major aortopulmonary collaterals. Journal of Thoracic and Cardiovascular Surgery 109: 832–844

Rees R S, Somerville J, Underwood S R et al 1987 Magnetic resonance imaging of the pulmonary arteries and their systemic connections in pulmonary atresia: comparison with angiographic and surgical findings. British Heart Journal 58: 621–626

Rome J J, Mayer J E, Castañeda A R, Lock J E 1993 Tetralogy of Fallot with pulmonary atresia. Rehabilitation of diminutive pulmonary arteries. Circulation 88: 1691–1698

Ross D N, Somerville J 1966 Correction of pulmonary atresia with a homograft aortic valve. Lancet ii: 1446–1447

Schofield D E, Anderson R H 1988 Common arterial trunk with pulmonary atresia. International Journal of Cardiology 20: 290–294

Shimazaki Y, Tokuan Y, Iio M et al 1990 Pulmonary artery pressure and resistance late after repair of tetralogy of Fallot and pulmonary atresia. Journal of Thoracic and Cardiovascular Surgery 100: 425

Shore D F, Ho S Y, Anderson R H, de Leval M, Lincoln C 1983 Aortopulmonary septal defect coexisting with ventricular septal defect and pulmonary atresia. Annals of Thoracic Surgery 35: 132–137

Singh S P, Rigby M L, Astley R 1978 Demonstration of pulmonary arteries by contrast injection into pulmonary vein. British Heart Journal 40: 55–57

Smallhorn J F, Macartney F J 1984 Suprasternal cross-sectional echocardiography in assessment of congenital heart disease. In: Hunter S, Hall R (eds) Echocardiography 2. Churchill Livingstone, Edinburgh, p 289–302

Smallhorn J F, Anderson R H, Macartney F J 1982a Two dimensional echocardiographic assessment of communications between ascending aorta and pulmonary trunk or individual pulmonary arteries. British Heart Journal 47: 563–572

Smallhorn J F, Huhta J C, Anderson R H, Macartney F J 1982b Suprasternal cross-sectional echocardiography in assessment of patent ductus arteriosus. British Heart Journal 48: 321–330

Somerville J 1970 Management of pulmonary atresia. British Heart Journal 32: 641–651

Somerville J, Ross D 1972 Long-term results of complete correction with homograft reconstruction in pulmonary outflow tract atresia. British Heart Journal 34: 29–36

Somerville J, Saravalli O, Ross D 1978 Complex pulmonary atresia with congenital systemic collaterals. Classification and management. Archives des Maladies du Coeur et des Vaisseaux 71: 322–328

Sotomora R F, Edwards J E 1978 Anatomic identification of so-called absent pulmonary artery. Circulation 57: 624–633

Stuckey D, Bowdler J D, Reye R D K 1968 Absent sixth aortic arch: a form of pulmonary atresia. British Heart Journal 30: 258–264

Sullivan I D, Wren C, Stark J, de Leval M R, Macartney F J, Deanfield J E 1988 Surgical unifocalization in pulmonary atresia and ventricular septal defect. Circulation 78 (suppl III): 5–13

Thiene G, Anderson R H 1983 Pulmonary atresia with ventricular septal defect. Anatomy. In: Anderson R H, Macartney F J, Shinebourne E A, Tynan M (eds) Paediatric cardiology, vol 5. Churchill Livingstone, Edinburgh, p 80–101

Thiene G, Bortolotti U, Gallucci V, Terribile V, Pellegrino P A 1976 Anatomical study of truncus arteriosus communis with embryological and surgical considerations. British Heart Journal 38: 1109–1123

Thiene G, Frescura C, Bini R M, Valente M, Gallucci V 1979 Histology of pulmonary arterial supply in pulmonary atresia with ventricular septal defect. Circulation 60: 1066–1074

Thiene G, Frescura C, Bortolotti U, del Maschio A, Valente M 1981 The systemic pulmonary circulation in pulmonary atresia with ventricular septal defect: concept of reciprocal development of the fourth and sixth aortic arches. American Heart Journal 101: 339–344

Toyoda Y, Yamaguchi M, Ohashi H et al 1996 Staged repair of tetralogy of Fallot and pulmonary atresia without central pulmonary arteries. Annals of Thoracic Surgery 61: 210–213

Watterson K G, Wilkinson J L, Karl T R, Mee R B 1991 Very small pulmonary arteries: central end-to-side shunt. Annals of Thoracic Surgery 52: 1132–1137

Yagihara T, Yamamoto F, Nishigaki K et al 1996 Unifocalization for pulmonary atresia with ventricular septal defect and major aortopulmonary collateral arteries. Journal of Thoracic and Cardiovascular Surgery 112: 392–402

Zutter W, Somerville J 1971 Continuous murmur in pulmonary atresia with reference to aortography. British Heart Journal 33: 905–909

48

Complete transposition

M. Tynan and R. H. Anderson

— INTRODUCTION —

The congenital malformation characterized by origin of the arterial trunks from morphologically inappropriate ventricles has probably been the source of as much confusion and controversy as any other single topic in paediatric cardiology. When Matthew Baillie gave the first case description (1797), he had no problems with nomenclature, simply describing the entity as a 'singular malformation' (Figure 48.1). His choice of terminology was echoed in the second case description by Mr Langstaff (1811), and this gentleman did not even give his readers the pleasure of knowing his initials! Since then, the entity, most usually described simply as 'transposition' has been defined in many different ways and has been used to describe many different types of

congenital cardiac malformations. Polemics have continued within the last decades, these being based for the most part on whether 'transposition' should be defined primarily on the way the ventricles support the arterial trunks (Van Praagh, 1971) or according to the relationship of the aorta relative to the pulmonary trunk (Van Mierop, 1971). Such disagreements are non-productive. If we distinguish between the features of the ventriculo-arterial connections on the one hand and relationships of the arterial trunks on the other, and we do not use the word transposition in isolation to describe either, we are able to circumvent all the controversies (Tynan and Anderson, 1979). There is little doubt, however, that in a clinical setting it is the manner of junctional union between the ventricles and arterial trunks which is paramount, since this feature determines the patterns of flow of blood through the heart. We use combinations of segmental connections, therefore, to define the various lesions that can be described in terms of transposition. Thus, we describe the topic of this chapter as complete transposition, defined as the combination of concordant atrioventricular and discordant ventriculo-arterial connections (Figure 48.2). This distinguishes this

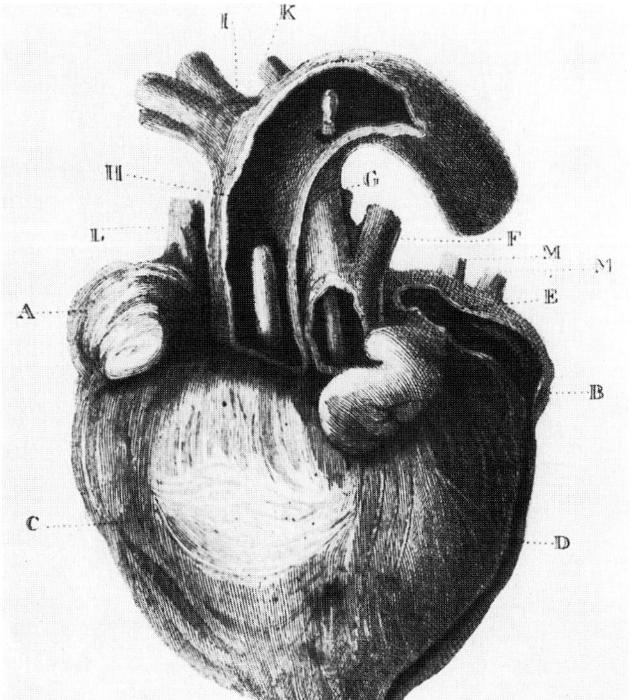

Figure 48.1. A reproduction of the original drawing by Matthew Baillie of the first case of complete transposition. Note the crow quill that has been inserted in the duct.

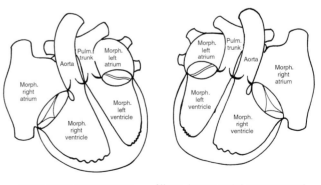

Usual atrial arrangement   **Mirror-image atrial arrangement**

COMPLETE TRANSPOSITION

Figure 48.2. The segmental combinations (concordant atrioventricular and discordant ventriculo-arterial connections) producing complete transposition. The diagrams are drawn with the most common arterial relationships, but these are variable (see text for discussion). Morph., morphological; Pulm., pulmonary.

particular group of patients with discordant ventriculo-arterial connections from those associated with discordant connections at the atrioventricular junction (congenitally corrected transposition; Chapter 49), those with isomeric atrial appendages (Chapter 31), with double inlet ventricle (Chapter 38) or with absent atrioventricular connections (Chapters 39 and 40). Relationships of the aorta relative to the pulmonary trunk are described separately as, when necessary, is the morphology of the ventricular outflow tracts.

——— HISTORICAL BACKGROUND ———

Before describing the morphology of complete transposition defined on the basis of concordant atrioventricular and discordant ventriculo-arterial connections, it is pertinent to give a brief review of the controversies underscoring the disagreements discussed above. It was John Farre (1814) who first used the term 'transposition' in the context of a cardiac malformation. He undoubtedly used it to describe origin of the great arterial trunks from morphologically inappropriate ventricles. Since then,

there have been vogues for defining transposition in terms of arterial relationships, or according to the morphology of the ventricular outflow tracts. Both Geipel (1903) and Monckeberg (1924) considered an aorta anterior to the pulmonary trunk to be the essence of transposition, irrespective of the ventriculo-arterial connections present. When the concept of transposition defined as an anterior aorta is combined with considerations of segmental connections at the atrioventricular and ventriculo-arterial junctions, it can be shown that there are eight basic types of transposition when each arterial trunk arises from its own ventricle (Figure 48.3). This concept for the eight variants of transposition was followed subsequently by Harris and Farber (1939) and by Cardell (1956). It underscores the use of the qualifiers 'congenitally corrected' as frequently applied to transposition. In Figure 48.3, some of the segmental combinations produce physiological correction of the circulatory patterns, with systemic venous blood reaching the lungs. Others produce anatomical correction, because the great arteries are connected to their morphologically appropriate ventricles despite the presence of an anterior aorta. Yet other combinations produce both anatomical and

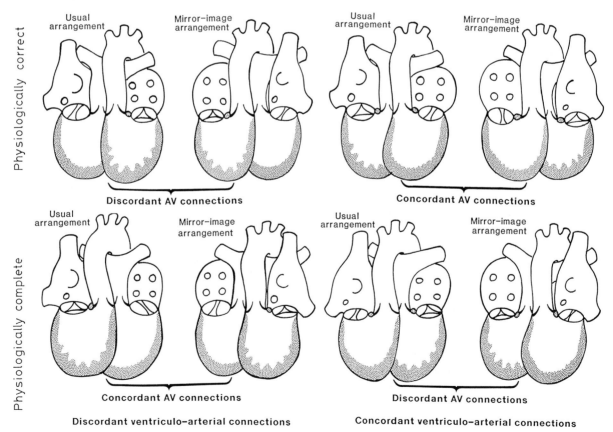

Figure 48.3. The combinations of atrial arrangement, atrioventricular (AV) connections and ventriculo-arterial connections that produce the eight prototypes initially considered to represent the different forms of 'transposition' when this entity was defined in terms of an anteriorly placed aorta. Note that some produce physiological transposition, whereas in others the circulatory pattern is 'corrected'. In two of the eight, there is both physiological and anatomical 'correction' of the position of the aorta.

physiological correction. This use of 'corrected' in an anatomical sense, however, being dependent upon the definition of transposition as an anterior aorta, produced considerable potential for confusion. It makes little sense in terms of patterns of flow through the heart to describe an anterior aorta arising from the left ventricle as representing transposition when the atrioventricular connections are concordant. Despite this, many continued to use this approach (Van Mierop, 1971; Angelini and Leachman, 1976). Over the same period, Grant (1962) had suggested that transposition would be better defined by the absence of fibrous continuity between the leaflets of the aortic and mitral valves, with the aortic having a muscular infundibulum and with fibrous continuity between the pulmonary and mitral valves. Van Praagh and Van Praagh (1966) also used a similar approach for a short period. Over recent years, there has been an increasing groundswell in favour of returning to the initial definition for transposition, namely the origin of the great arteries from morphologically inappropriate ventricles. The need for such a definition, in addition to removing the confusion of an anterior aorta arising from the left ventricle being considered as transposed, is further highlighted by the rare cases in which the arterial trunks are connected to morphologically inappropriate ventricles, but with the aorta in posterior position and with fibrous continuity between the leaflets of the aortic and mitral valves. This, of course, is the arrangement of arterial relationships and outflow tract morphology usually encountered in the normal heart (Van Praagh et al, 1971). Such abnormal hearts, with an aorta located posteriorly and rightward but arising from the morphologically right ventricle, cannot be described as transposition by those who insist upon an anterior position for the aorta as the essential criterion for definition. But, they produce haemodynamic and clinical findings identical to the combination usually considered by clinicians as producing transposition. Indeed, in clinical and anatomical terms, they are true examples of what we would call complete transposition. Faced with this dilemma, Van Praagh et al (1971) proposed that all previous definitions of transposition be abandoned, the word being reserved exclusively for description of discordant ventriculo-arterial connections. They proposed that the abnormal relationships encountered in hearts with connections other than transposition should be described as 'malposition'. Consequently, anatomically corrected transposition became anatomically corrected malposition, since the aorta in this segmental combination arose from its morphologically appropriate ventricle but in abnormal orientation compared with the pulmonary trunk. Malposition, however, was also used to describe the aortic position in other anomalies, such as double outlet right or left ventricle.

In response to this, the 'relationists' justifiably argued that, if they continued to define transposition as a relation, and if they found another term to describe those lesions with the great arteries connected to inappropriate ventricles with the aorta in posterior position, there was no reason why, in their system, they could not logically speak about 'double outlet right ventricle with transposition' (Angelini and Leachman, 1976).

Such a nomenclature based upon relations, without doubt, is internally consistent. It is inappropriate to insist that the users of an internally consistent system simply abandon it and adopt another system that may itself have deficiencies. This is particularly so when the strongest proponents of the approach based on segmental connections chose to qualify their own definition in terms of arterial relationships (Van Praagh et al, 1971). The resulting concept was, for a time, adopted so enthusiastically that the terms 'd-transposition' and 'l-transposition' frequently came to be used as though synonymous with complete and corrected transposition, respectively. Such usage is manifestly absurd. It is well known that the aortic valve is usually left-sided when complete transposition is found with mirror-imaged atrial arrangement (inversus). Furthermore, a proportion of patients with complete transposition and usual atrial arrangement have left-sided aorta (Carr et al, 1968). The same variability is found with congenitally corrected transposition, in which the majority have left-sided aortas but right-sided aorta is far from rare. The approach based on segmental alignments, therefore, unless used with extreme care, can be less logical and accurate than the 'relations' approach so denigrated by the advocates of d- and l-transposition (Van Praagh, 1971). Equally, the 'relations' approach, although internally consistent, is clumsy and unwieldy when used in a clinical setting (Angelini and Leachman, 1976).

The system that we prefer is a compromise. Although our approach is based primarily on segmental connections, we recognize the need to describe both arterial relationships and infundibular morphology; however, we use mutually exclusive terms for their description. In this way, we avoid the potentials for confusion to be found in all other systems of nomenclature.

PREVALENCE AND AETIOLOGY

Although a rare cardiac malformation, accounting for only 5–7% of all congenital cardiac malformations (MacMahon et al, 1953; Carlgren, 1969), complete transposition was responsible for up to 20% of cardiac deaths in infancy prior to the era of surgical correction (Hoffheinz et al, 1964). Boys are affected two to three times as frequently as girls (Liebman et al, 1969). No definite aetiological factors have been identified, but the condition is more frequent in infants of diabetic mothers (Liebman et al, 1969). Family studies have shown an association between complete transposition and tetralogy of Fallot (Fraser and Hunter, 1975).

—ANATOMY AND MORPHOGENESIS—

It is the basic combinations of concordant atrioventricular and discordant ventriculo-arterial connections that produce the entity we prefer to call complete transposition. This segmental combination can be complicated by the presence of a ventricular septal defect, an obstruction within the left ventricular outflow tract or both of these malformations. In the subsequent clinical sections, we will describe cases as being 'simple' when they have an intact interventricular septum and no obstruction of the left ventricular outflow tract, even if they are complicated by other lesions such as persistent patency of the arterial duct.

THE BASIC SEGMENTAL COMBINATIONS——

The essence of complete transposition is the presence of a morphologically right atrium joined to a morphologically right ventricle that gives rise to the aorta, together with a morphologically left atrium connected to a morphologically left ventricle that supports the pulmonary trunk (Figure 48.4). Such a combination of connections can occur with either usual (solitus) or mirror-imaged (inversus) atrial arrangements (Figure 48.2) but cannot exist when there is isomerism of the atrial appendages. Hearts with isomeric atrial appendages can, of course, have biventricular atrioventricular connections, right hand topology and discordant ventriculo-arterial connections. Such hearts are 'close-cousins' of complete transposition but are distinguished by the isomeric nature of the atrial segment and the abnormal venoatrial connections (see Chapter 31).

The internal anatomy of the atriums is basically normal, although most frequently the oval foramen is patent or there is a deficiency of the floor of the oval fossa. Even if the flap valve overlaps the rim of the oval fossa, it is flimsy and can be ruptured easily by balloon septostomy (Figure 48.5). In keeping with normal atrial anatomy, the sinus and atrioventricular nodes are in their anticipated position. There are no histologically specialized tracts of conduction tissue between the nodes (Figure 48.6). This is not to deny the importance of the prominent muscle bundles in the right atrium in conduction of the sinus impulse. These bundles, such as the terminal crest or the superior rim of the oval fossa, are, however, composed of ordinary working myocardium.

The arrangement of the central fibrous body, and the relations of the ventricular outflow tracts, are such that the ventricular morphology in complete transposition is not quite normal (Smith et al, 1986a,b). In well over half the cases in which the ventricular septum is intact, the ventricular outflow tracts run parallel to one another. Consequently, the entire ventricular septum is a straight structure, not showing the multiple curves so typical of the normal heart (Figure 48.7). Furthermore, the pulmonary valve is not wedged as deeply between the mitral and tricuspid valves as is the aortic valve in the normal heart (Figure 48.8). This, in turn, means that the area of off-setting of the leaflets of the atrioventricular valves is much less marked in complete transposition, as is the area occupied by the membranous septum. Indeed, in

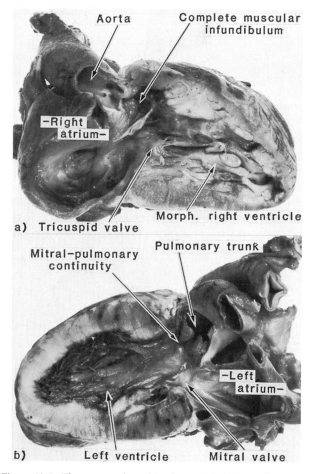

Figure 48.4. The segmental combinations producing complete transposition with intact ventricular septum as seen (a) from the right side and (b) from the left.

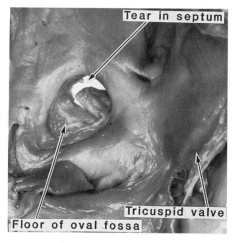

Figure 48.5. The oval fossa with its ruptured floor following balloon atrial septostomy.

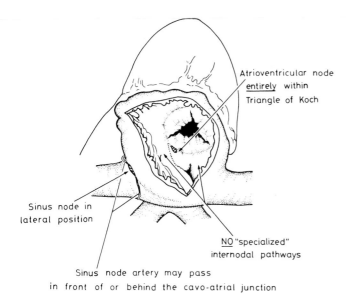

Figure 48.6. A drawing showing the disposition of the conduction tissues in complete transposition as they would be viewed by the surgeon at operation.

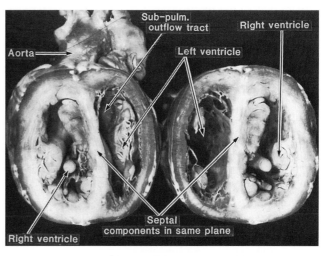

Figure 48.7. Because of the parallel arrangement of the ventricular outflow tracts, the ventricular septum has a basically straight configuration. Sub-pulm, subpulmonary.

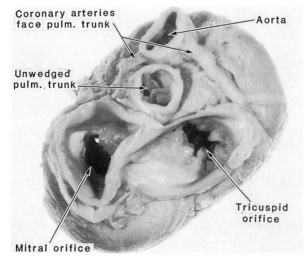

Figure 48.8. A dissection of the short axis of the heart viewed from its atrial aspect showing the unwedged position of the pulmonary (pulm.) trunk. Note also how the coronary arteries arise from the aortic sinuses, which are adjacent to, or 'face', the pulmonary trunk.

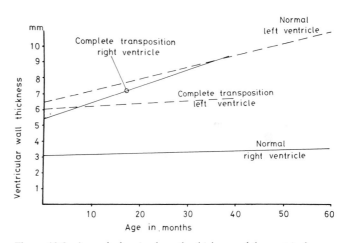

Figure 48.9. A graph showing how the thickness of the ventricular wall changes with increasing age in the normal heart and in complete transposition. (Adapted from the study of Dr Audrey Smith and colleagues (1981), Royal Liverpool Children's Hospital, Liverpool, UK, published with her kind permission.)

over half the hearts with intact septum, no membranous septum could be transilluminated (Smith et al, 1986b) and no fibrous partitions between the ventricles were found by histological studies (Oppenheimer-Dekker, 1978; Smith et al, 1986b). Another consequence of this abnormal arrangement is that the ratio of the dimensions of the inlet and outlet components of the ventricular mass in complete transposition are abnormal in favour of the outlet dimension, although not to the extent seen in atrioventricular septal defects (Chapter 36). From the standpoint of the thickness of the ventricular walls, at birth the morphologically left ventricular wall is marginally

thicker than that of the right ventricle. The right ventricular thickness then rapidly increases in the first 2 years of life, becoming much thicker than that of the left ventricle (Figure 48.9) (Bano-Rodrigo et al, 1980; Smith et al, 1982).

The most obvious external abnormality is the relationship of the aorta to the pulmonary trunk. In the majority of patients with an intact ventricular septum, the aortic root is to the right of the pulmonary trunk in hearts in the setting of usual atrial arrangement, and to the left in the mirror-imaged variant (Figure 48.10). This is by no means the rule, and patients are found with usual

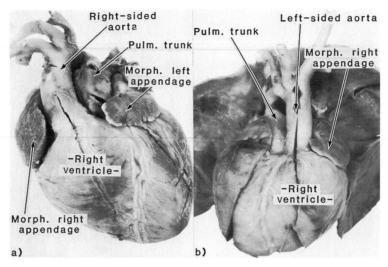

Figure 48.10. The usual position of the aorta relative to the pulmonary trunk as seen (a) in the patient with usual atrial arrangement and (b) in the heart with mirror-image arrangement.

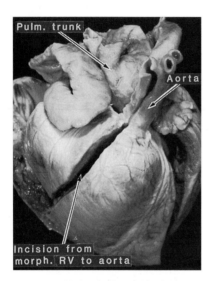

Figure 48.11. An unusual left-sided position of the aorta, together with spiralling of the great arteries, in a heart with usual atrial arrangement, concordant atrioventricular and discordant ventriculo-arterial connections. morph., morphological; Pulm., pulmonary; RV, right ventricle.

atrial arrangement and intact ventricular septum when the aorta is to the left (Figure 48.11). Indeed, in the angiographic study of Carr et al (1968), such an arrangement was found in one-fifth of the population examined. Very rarely, the aorta may be right sided and posterior when the ventricular septum is intact (Buchler et al, 1984).

Whenever the position of the aortic root is abnormal, the origins of the coronary arteries deviate from those found in the normal heart. The arteries, however, continue to arise from one or other, or both, of those aortic sinuses that face, or are adjacent to, the pulmonary trunk. This arrangement makes them particularly amenable to surgical transfer in the arterial switch procedure (Yacoub and Radley-Smith, 1978). The epicardial

course of the arteries arising from the facing sinuses is much less predictable. The various patterns have been well described by Rowlatt (1962), Elliott et al (1963) and Shaher and Puddu (1966). Attempts to account for the patterns in alpha-numeric fashion, however, led to truly formidable codifications that placed immense demands on the memory (Yamaguchi 1990; Amato and Galdieri, 1991; Kurosawa et al, 1991). It is much better to use a descriptive approach, accounting separately for the origins of the three major coronary arteries from the aortic sinuses, describing their course relative to the vascular pedicle and noting the arrangement of the artery supplying the sinus node (Anderson, 1991). As already stated, in our experience the coronary arteries in hearts with complete transposition have always arisen from one or both of the aortic sinuses which are adjacent to the pulmonary trunk. The position of these sinuses in space, however, can vary according to the relationship of the arterial trunks. It is not possible in an overall series, therefore, to describe their position in terms of right/left and anterior/posterior coordinates. Indeed, a system is required that is independent of spatial relationships. This can be achieved by considering the aortic sinuses as they would be visualized, figuratively speaking, by an observer standing in the non-adjacent aortic sinus and looking towards the pulmonary trunk. The sinuses supporting the coronary arteries are then located to the observer's right and left hands. That sinus to the observer's right hand is conventionally termed 'sinus 1', while that to the surgeon's left hand is called 'sinus 2' (Gittenberger-de Groot, 1986; Smith et al, 1986c). All patterns are then accounted for according to whether the right, circumflex and anterior interventricular arteries arise from sinus 1 or from sinus 2. The problem with this system is that, unless used regularly, it can be difficult to remember which sinus is which. Because of this, our own preference is to describe the sinuses simply as being right handed and left handed, as discussed above, being viewed from the aspect of the non-facing aortic sinus (Figure 48.12). But this concept is not without its own problems. This is because, in the most frequently encountered coronary arterial pattern encountered in complete transposition (Figure 48.13), the right coronary artery arises from the left hand facing sinus (# 2), and the main stem of the left coronary artery from the right hand aortic sinus (# 1). This offends many investigators, who would prefer to have the right coronary artery arising from the aortic sinus which can also be considered right handed. Such a viewpoint can be achieved if the surgeon places himself, figuratively speaking, in the pulmonary trunk and looks towards the aorta

(Amato and Galdieri, 1991; Amato et al, 1994). The whole purpose of the system is to account for departures from the 'norm' anticipated for complete transposition, since it is abnormalities in origins of the coronary arteries that are the major risk factors during the arterial switch procedure (see below). Because of this, and because of the need to have a system of description that accounts for all abnormalities and not just complete transposition, we prefer to retain our system of viewing the aortic sinuses from the non-adjacent aortic sinus (Figure 48.12) or resorting to the Leiden convention (Gittenberger-de Groot et al, 1983) and describing sinuses as # 1 and # 2, this having the inestimable advantage of being independent of spatial coordinates.

When considering the sinusal origin of the major coronary arteries, it is then necessary to note their radial, vertical and tangential origin relative to the sinuses themselves (Angelini and Leachman, 1976; Li et al, 2000). Most usually, the arteries arise within the sinus or at the level of the sinutubular junction, albeit usually eccentrically placed within the sinus (Figure 48.14). Significant problems can be created for the surgeon during the arterial switch procedure when the arteries take a high origin above the sinutubular junction, or if they have tangential origin through the aortic wall, crossing a commissure of the aortic valve (Figure 48.15). These arrangements are associated with an initial course of the artery running obliquely through the aortic wall, so-called intramural origin. With such intramural origin, the involved coronary artery tends to run between the walls of the aorta and those of the pulmonary trunk (Pasquini et al, 1993). In addition to sinusal origin, epicardial course is also important, in particular retropulmonary or anteroaortic position of any of the three major coronary arteries (Planché et al, 1988). It should then be remembered that

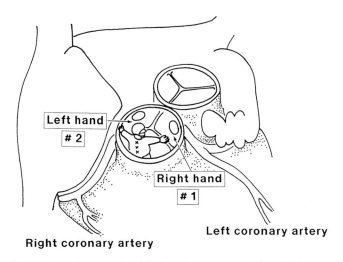

Figure 48.12. Irrespective of the location of the arterial trunks in space, the sinuses supporting the coronary arteries are always to the right hand and left hand of the observer 'standing' in the non-adjacent aortic sinus and looking towards the pulmonary trunk.

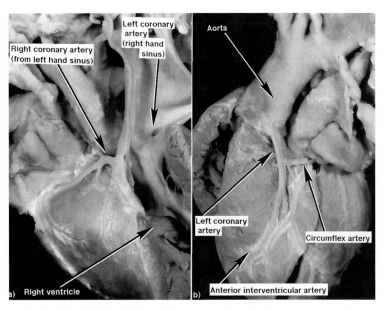

Figure 48.13. In this heart, the coronary arteries are arranged as in two thirds of examples of 'simple' complete transposition. The right coronary artery arises from the left hand facing sinus (# 2 in Figure 48.12) while the main stem of the left coronary artery, supplying the circumflex and anterior interventricular arteries, arises from the right hand facing sinus (# 1 in Figure 48.12).

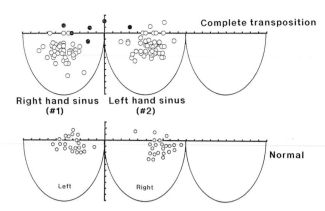

Figure 48.14. The arrangement of the coronary arteries within the aortic sinuses compared with a series of normal hearts. Black dots show the origins of arteries with an intramural segment.

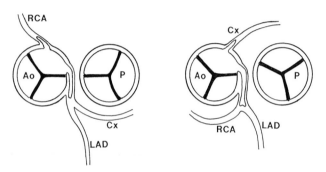

Figure 48.15. The aortic root (Ao) viewed from above. Note the intramural course of the left coronary artery, which has arisen from the left hand facing sinus (# 2 in Figure 48.12) and crossed the commissure, running between the arterial trunks to reach the interventricular groove. On the left, it gives rise to the circumflex (Cx) and interventricular (LAD) arteries. On the right, the right coronary artery (RCA), also arises from the main stem. The circumflex artery takes a retropulmonary (P) course. (After Gittenberger-de Groot et al 1986 Journal of Thoracic and Cardiovascular Surgery.)

the anterior interventricular artery can be duplicated. The artery to the sinus node is of further significance. It can arise from the initial course of either the right or the circumflex coronary arteries, or it can take a direct origin from one or other of the facing aortic sinuses. Its most important variation, however, is when it crosses the lateral margin of the right atrial appendage (Figure 48.16). In such lateral position, it is at surgical risk during a standard atriotomy (Barra Rossi et al, 1986).

When the ventricular septum is intact in complete transposition, the aorta almost always has a complete muscular infundibulum, while the leaflets of the pulmonary valve are in fibrous continuity with the mitral valve (see Figure 48.4). Variations in this infundibular morphology, for example the presence of bilaterally complete muscular infundibulums, are not seen nearly as frequently when the ventricular septum is intact as when there is a ventricular septal defect (see below). Other 'simple' malformations can coexist with complete trans-

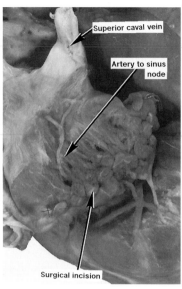

Figure 48.16. Lateral origin of the artery to the sinus node from the right coronary artery.

position and intact ventricular septum. Persistent patency of the arterial duct is particularly significant because it 'loads' the left ventricle, producing a thicker wall. This is advantageous should an arterial switch operation be contemplated for surgical correction. Other significant anomalies are infrequent but can occur. They include stenosis of the subaortic outflow tract, aortic coarctation (Milanesi et al, 1982; Waldman et al, 1984) or anomalous pulmonary venous connections (Shaher, 1973).

COMPLETE TRANSPOSITION WITH VENTRICULAR SEPTAL DEFECT

The most significant, and frequently occurring, associated lesion in complete transposition is a ventricular septal defect. As with isolated defects, these may be small, large or multiple, and they can be located within any part of the ventricular septum (Figure 48.17). The most characteristic defects are those that open beneath the ventricular outlets, with the muscular outlet septum being malaligned relative to the rest of the ventricular septum and located within the right ventricle (Figure 48.18). Such defects, which occupy a subpulmonary position, may have a muscular posteroinferior rim (Figure 48.18a) or may extend to become perimembranous (Figure 48.18b). Frequently, such defects are crossed by the tension apparatus of the tricuspid valve, which often inserts to a papillary muscle arising from the outlet septum. The superior and inferior margins, formed by the outlet and apical components of the muscular septum, diverge towards the parietal wall of the right ventricle; as a result, the gap between them increases anterosuperiorly. In consequence, the anterior margin of the defect is like the gap between a slightly open door (the outlet septum) and the doorframe (the

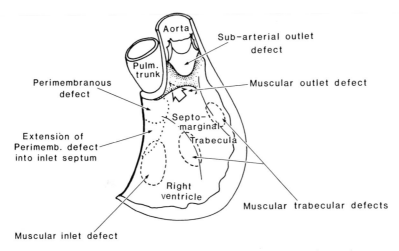

Figure 48.17. The different types of ventricular septal defect that may be found in association with complete transposition.

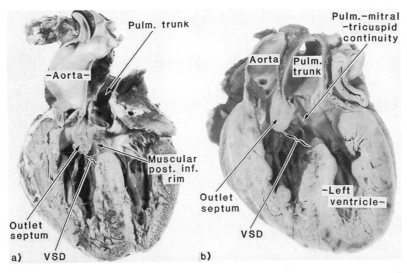

Figure 48.18. Subpulmonary outlet defects demonstrated by sectioning the heart in four chamber projection (a) with a muscular posteroinferior (post. inf.) rim and (b) extending to become perimembranous. Pulm., pulmonary; VSD, ventricular septal defect.

muscular ventricular septum). The outlet septum can also be malaligned into the left ventricle. This then narrows the left ventricular outflow tract, producing pulmonary stenosis (see below) in association with overriding and biventricular connection of the aortic valve (Figure 48.19). In the more common malalignment defects in which the outlet septum is positioned within the right ventricle, it is the pulmonary valve that overrides the septum. With ever greater degrees of overriding, and increasing connection of the leaflets of the pulmonary valve within the right ventricle, a spectrum of anomalies is seen culminating in double outlet right ventricle with subpulmonary ventricular septal defect. This whole series is often called the 'Taussig–Bing complex' (Bharati and Lev, 1976; Parr et al, 1983). It is our practice to divide the series at its midpoint. We then include only those with less than half the circumference of the overriding pulmonary valve connected within the right ventricle as examples of complete transposition (Stellin et al, 1987). Sometimes the distinction is

difficult, particularly when there is associated straddling of the mitral valve (see Chapter 41).

Equally significant from the surgical standpoint are those defects that extend to open to the inlet of the right ventricle. These are hidden beneath the septal leaflet of the tricuspid valve, complicating their surgical repair. When the defect extends to open into the right ventricular inlet, there is the potential for straddling and overriding of the tricuspid valve. In this setting, the muscular ventricular septum no longer extends to the crux, and the atrioventricular conduction axis takes origin from an anomalous posteroinferior atrioventricular node (see Fig. 41.33) (Milo et al, 1979).

Otherwise, in perimembranous and muscular outlet defects, the conduction tissue is carried on the left ventricular aspect of the septum, the posterocaudal rim of the defect being most vulnerable during surgical correction. As with isolated defects, the conduction axis is better protected when the posterior limb of the septomarginal

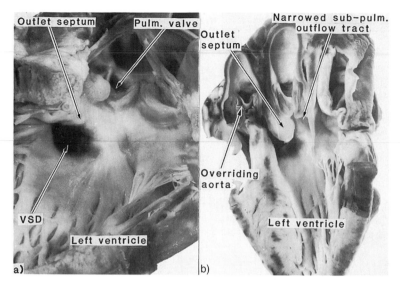

Figure 48.19. The outlet septum is deviated into the left ventricular outflow tract, producing subpulmonary (Sub-pulm.) obstruction in association with a ventricular septal defect (VSD) having a muscular posteroinferior rim. The heart is seen (a) as viewed from the left ventricle and (b) as in simulated long-axis section. Pulm., pulmonary.

trabeculation fuses with the ventriculo-infundibular fold (Figures 48.18a and 48.19). Should there be a muscular inlet defect, however, the conduction tissue axis is found in the anterocephalad position.

Other types of defect can be found, such as multiple muscular defects, solitary apical muscular defects or doubly committed defects roofed by the conjoined aortic and pulmonary valvar leaflets (Hoyer et al, 1992; Smith et al, 1994). They are less common. The doubly committed defect, when present, is of significance because it is usually associated with a left-sided aorta (Lincoln et al, 1976). This combination usually makes it an easy matter to patch the aorta to the left ventricle; however, coronary arterial anomalies are frequent (Houyel et al, 1995). When the aorta is left-sided, generally speaking the great arteries lie side by side; if there is a ventricular septal defect, the aorta may even lie posteriorly. The aorta is also occasionally found posteriorly and to the right in the presence of a ventricular septal defect. With this arrangement, there is usually aortic–mitral valvar continuity through the roof of the defect (Van Praagh et al, 1971; Wilkinson et al, 1975). Bilateral infundibulums are also seen more frequently in association with a defective ventricular septum, again most frequently when the arterial trunks are side by side. Other anomalies are also more frequent in association with ventricular septal defect, including juxtaposition of the atrial appendages, aortic stenosis and aortic coarctation (Milanesi et al, 1982).

COMPLETE TRANSPOSITION WITH OBSTRUCTION OF THE LEFT VENTRICULAR OUTFLOW TRACT

Any lesions that produce obstruction to the outflow tract of the morphologically left ventricle, and which in the normal heart produce aortic obstruction, will produce subpulmonary obstruction in the setting of complete transposition. Such lesions can be found at valvar or subvalvar level (Figure 48.20). Isolated valvar obstruction is rare (Shaher, 1973) and is more common in combination with subvalvar obstruction, which may be dynamic, fixed or both. Dynamic obstruction is produced by bulging of the ventricular septum. In its most severe form, this is reminiscent of hypertrophic obstructive cardiomyopathy in the heart with concordant ventriculo-arterial connections. When septal bulging itself is less severe, obstruction of the left ventricular outflow tract is frequently exacerbated by a fibrous ridge located on the septal bulge. This can progress to form a complete subvalvar shelf, the ridge

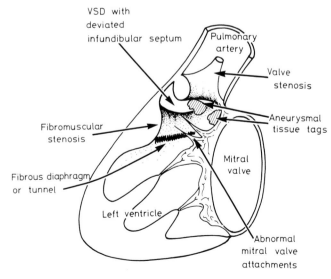

Figure 48.20. Different types of pulmonary stenosis found in combination with complete transposition and ventricular septal defect (VSD).

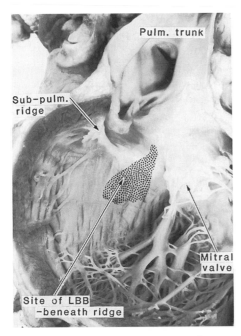

Figure 48.21. The fibrous ridge on the left ventricular aspect of the ventricular septum can progress to produce fixed subpulmonary (Subpulm.) stenosis. LBB, left bundle branch; Pulm., pulmonary.

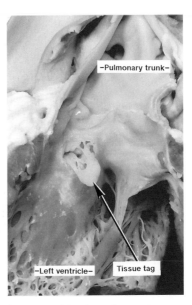

Figure 48.22. These tags arising from the membranous septum produce subpulmonary obstruction.

extending onto the facing surface of the mitral valvar leaflet (Figure 48.21). The extent of fibrous stenosis can also be more elongated, giving a tunnel lesion. The obstructive lesions associated with septal bulging are more prone to occur in hearts with a more directly anteroposterior relationship of the great arteries than when the arteries are side by side (Chiu et al, 1984). Other rarer forms of stenosis are produced by anomalous attachment of the tension apparatus of the mitral valve across the outflow tract or by aneurysms of fibrous tissue tags bulging into the outflow tract (Figure 48.22). All can exist with an intact ventricular septum or in association with a ventricular septal defect. When there is a septal defect, however, there is another most significant type of stenosis, namely a malalignment and deviation of the muscular outlet septum into the left ventricle that narrows the subpulmonary outflow tract in association with overriding of the aortic valve (Figure 48.19). Most of these fixed stenoses present major problems in surgical removal, either because of their own intrinsic morphology (for example a papillary muscle) or because of their proximity to vital structures, such as the left ventricular conduction tissues or the left coronary artery in the transverse sinus (Crupi et al, 1979). If removal is attempted, the safest area for resection is the area occupied by the muscular outlet septum, which can be reached without need for a ventriculotomy (Oelert and Borst, 1979; Wilcox et al, 1983).

MORPHOGENESIS

The morphogenesis of complete transposition is almost as contentious as the definition of transposition. In essence, there are two basic concepts. The first suggests that the anomaly is the consequence of malseptation of the arterial pole of the heart; as a result, the sixth aortic arches, destined to become the pulmonary arteries, are connected to the morphologically left ventricle, while the fourth aortic arches take their origin from the morphologically right ventricle. There have been various suggestions as to how this may occur. De la Cruz and da Rocha (1956) argued that it is because the ridges septating the arterial segment of the heart tube fuse in straight rather than in their normal spiral fashion. Van Mierop et al (1963) proposed a similar theory invoking abnormal development of the ridges. They contended that the abnormality is in the way the cushions in the ventricular outlet fuse with the ridges in the arterial segment, believing these two sets of cushions to be separate and discrete structures. A third possibility, suggested by Los (1976), was that the abnormal connections result from the aortopulmonary septum connecting with the septum in the outflow tract in reverse fashion.

The second theory puts the seat of maldevelopment not in the arterial trunks but in the ventricular outflow tracts. This hypothesis suggests that rather than the subaortic outflow portion of the right ventricle becoming connected to the left ventricle, as occurs in normal development, it is the subpulmonary outflow component, together with the pulmonary trunk, which is thus connected. This 'conal maldevelopment' concept was first proposed by Keith (1909). He invoked differential absorption of the infundibular structures as the causative mechanism. The concept was revitalized by Van Praagh under the guise of differential conal growth (Van Praagh et al, 1971). Evidence showing that abnormal formation of the infundibular regions is important in the genesis of complete transposition was subsequently marshalled by Goor and Edwards (1973) and Anderson et al (1974).

It now seems that, to explain all the known variants of complete transposition (including the arrangement in which the aorta arises posteriorly and to the right), it is necessary to invoke maldevelopment within both the outflow tracts and the arterial segment (Anderson, 1978; de la Cruz et al, 1981). One of the difficulties in adjudicating these various theories has been that complete transposition does not occur frequently in animals other than humans. It has, however, been induced by bombarding rat fetuses with neutrons (Okamoto et al, 1980). It has also been discovered in a mouse colony that had mirror-imaged bodily arrangement (situs inversus; Van Praagh et al, 1980) and is seen in mice dosed with teratogenic amounts of retinoic acid (Pexieder et al, 1995). A solitary chicken heart has now been found with complete transposition subsequent to experimental ablation of the cranial neural crest (Manner, 1998). The elucidation of the various theories will require more detailed studies of these experimental animal models, still as yet unavailable.

PATHOPHYSIOLOGY

The fundamental physiological derangement in complete transposition is that the systemic venous return is recirculated to the body via the right ventricle and aorta, while the pulmonary venous return is recirculated to the lungs via the left ventricle and pulmonary trunk (Figure 48.23). Thus, the pulmonary and systemic circulations are separate. This causes few, if any, problems in the fetus because the entire venous return, including that from the placenta, is normally distributed through the right atrium. Even in

the fetus, however, the discordant ventriculo-arterial connections will result in somewhat less-well-oxygenated blood going to the upper body than is normal. After birth, there is a major problem. Now the oxygenated pulmonary venous blood is unable to reach the systemic circuit, and the systemic venous return cannot reach the lungs for oxygenation. This results in severe systemic arterial desaturation. Fortunately, even in the absence of a pathological communication between the two circulations such as a ventricular septal defect, some mixing or cross-flow is possible through the arterial duct and the oval foramen. Persistence of the arterial duct allows blood to flow from the aorta to the pulmonary vascular bed, while the patent oval foramen allows bidirectional flow between the atrial chambers. Flow across the oval foramen is particularly important since, over a period of time, the total flow of blood from the pulmonary to the systemic circuit must equal the total flow from the systemic to the pulmonary circuit. With these naturally occurring communications, the bidirectional cross-flow between the two circulations, although small, is usually sufficient to support life for some days, or even weeks.

A less obvious, but important consequence of the separation of the two circulations is that the absolute flows in the systemic and pulmonary circuits may differ markedly from one another. In the normal circulation, the left and right ventricles are connected in series. Over a period of time, therefore, they must have similar outputs. The independence of the circuits in complete transposition absolves them of this limitation (Figure 48.23). Therefore, the flows in the pulmonary and systemic circulations usually differ. It has been suggested that the portion of systemic venous return recirculated to the body be called the

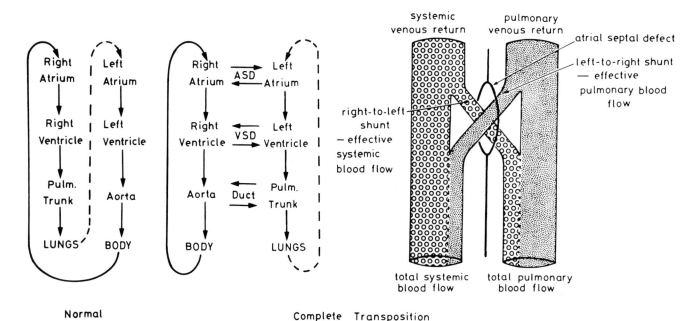

Figure 48.23. The pattern of circulation in the normal heart compared with that in complete transposition and the possibilities for cross-flows and their effect in complete transposition. ASD, atrial septal defect; VSD, ventricular septal defect.

'physiological right-to-left shunt'. The portion of pulmonary venous return recirculated to the lungs is then called the 'physiological left-to-right shunt' (Paul, 1983). Although this approach emphasizes the importance of the recirculation of the venous return in each circuit, it produces potential for confusion. We prefer to reserve the term 'shunt', when we use it at all, for the cross-flows through abnormal communications between the two circulations (Figure 48.23). In this context, the absolute flows in the two circuits, calculated from the consumption of oxygen and the arterio-venous difference in content of oxygen across the circuit, allows the calculation of resistances in the circuits. But this gives no information about adequacy of the communications between them. These cross-flows can be quantified by the calculation of the effective flows. The part of the systemic venous return that reaches the pulmonary vascular bed is the 'effective pulmonary flow' (Campbell et al, 1949). That proportion of the pulmonary venous return reaching the systemic vascular bed is the 'effective systemic flow'. These must be equal in magnitude. The effective pulmonary flow is easily calculated using the consumption of oxygen and the difference in content of oxygen between the systemic and the pulmonary venous blood. The effective systemic and pulmonary flows, and the adequacy of the bidirectional shunts, can, thus, be assessed from this one calculation.

DETERMINANTS OF SYSTEMIC ARTERIAL OXYGENATION

A prerequisite of life for the patient with complete transposition is that there be anatomical sites for intercirculatory shunting. These sites include the normally occurring oval foramen and, in the newborn, the arterial duct. There may be additional defects such as an atrial septal defect, a ventricular septal defect or pathological persistence of the duct. There is also evidence that systemic-to-pulmonary flow through the bronchial arteries may contribute to the total of intercirculatory shunts. As previously stated, when there are only the 'normal' sites for shunting, the magnitude of the cross-flows is small, and cyanosis is profound. The anatomical sites for cross-flows can, however, be of adequate size and not restrict intercirculatory mixing. Haemodynamic factors then determine the level of systemic arterial oxygenation and, hence, the degree of cyanosis. An increased ratio of pulmonary flow to systemic flow is associated with higher systemic arterial oxygen saturations than is a decreased ratio. With large unrestrictive communications at ventricular or great arterial level, resistance to pulmonary blood flow is the major limiting factor of systemic arterial oxygen content. Flow may be limited either by obstruction in the left ventricular outflow tract or by pulmonary vascular disease.

The site of the communication also has an effect. An unrestrictive ventricular septal defect is usually associated with a higher systemic arterial oxygen saturation than is an unrestrictive interatrial defect. This is almost certainly because of the greater flow of pulmonary blood generated in association with a ventricular septal defect. Even when only the atrial septum is deficient, the influence of the absolute flows is evident on the effective flows in the two circuits. The effect of bronchial collateral circulation on arterial oxygenation has not been determined. This is because no accurate quantification of this flow is available. Subjective assessment based on angiocardiography suggests that, even in infancy, this flow is significant but not large. The unknown magnitude of the bronchial collateral circulation remains a major source of inaccuracy in the estimation of absolute pulmonary blood flow (Paul, 1983).

The separation of the pulmonary and systemic circuits means that (even with the necessity for the left-to-right shunt to equal that from right-to-left), the absolute flows in the two circuits need not be equal. The absolute flows are determined by the individual characteristics for preload and afterload of the right and left ventricles. The left ventricle tends to become thin walled and more compliant than the right ventricle after the early weeks of infancy (Lev et al, 1961; Smith et al, 1982). This is reflected by the finding that left ventricular end-diastolic pressure is lower than that in the right ventricle (Aziz et al, 1979). The relative change in ventricular mural thickness reflects the fall in pulmonary vascular resistance occurring during this time. In a number of patients with complete transposition and only an atrial septal defect, the pulmonary flow exceeds that in the systemic circuit. In these patients, the higher pulmonary blood flow can be ascribed to the more compliant left ventricle ejecting against a lower pulmonary vascular resistance (afterload). A high ratio of pulmonary flow to systemic flow, however, is not always seen. In these circumstances, the explanation of low pulmonary flow is not certain. The role of the pressure–volume characteristics of the atriums, together with the pulmonary and systemic venous systems, in determining flow patterns is unknown, but they may play a part. Therefore, a high left atrial pressure, possibly resulting from a relatively low compliance, may reduce pulmonary flow by initiating reflex pulmonary arterial vasoconstriction. How the effective flows are maintained in balance is similarly speculative. In the simplest situation, with an intact ventricular septum and an interatrial communication, the patterns of flow are such that blood passes from the left to the right atrium when the atrioventricular valves are closed, and from the right to the left atrium when the atrioventricular valves are open (Carr, 1971). This suggests that the cross-flows are balanced, ar least in part, by the differences between left and right ventricular diastolic pressure–volume relationships. With a highly compliant left ventricle, the systemic-to-pulmonary shunt is promoted during ventricular diastole. By the same mechanism, a compliant left ventricle is conducive to high pulmonary blood flow. This, in turn, produces a high pulmonary venous return, which will promote the left-to-right atrial shunt. A poorly compliant left ventricle will have a limiting effect on the right-to-left shunt during diastole. By not promoting so high a pulmonary blood flow, it will also limit the left-to-right atrial shunt. The presence of a communication between the high-pressure components of the pulmonary and systemic circuits, either a ventricular septal defect or persistent patency of the arterial duct, will tend to promote a high absolute pulmonary blood flow. Timing within the cardiac cycle of the cross-flows between the two circuits in those with a ventricular septal defect is, as yet, less clearly understood than with an atrial septal defect. Another anatomical site for intercirculatory shunting is necessary when the arterial duct is patent. Unless the pulmonary vascular resistance is high, the flow through the duct will be largely from the systemic to the pulmonary circuit. Therefore, in general, the larger the communications between the two circulations, the higher will be the effective flow and, hence, the arterial oxygen saturation (Mair and Ritter, 1972).

CHANGES IN THE CIRCULATION AFTER BIRTH

Changes in the pulmonary vasculature with transition from fetal to extrauterine life are similar in complete transposition to those occurring in other forms of congenital heart disease (Tynan, 1971; Newfeld et al, 1979). The changes have been systematically observed only in patients palliated by creation of an atrial septal defect. The changes studied are those following initial palliation and may not be exactly the same as those occurring in the untreated infant. Any such differences, however, are of little practical importance, since the majority of unpalliated infants die. Those who survive with naturally occurring atrial septal defects usually have a low pulmonary vascular resistance. They are similar to the palliated infants. Observations in patients with intact ventricular septum show a fall in pulmonary arterial pressure from the high values in the first days of life to normal by the age of 2–3 months. The major changes occur over the early days and weeks. Although it might be expected that this fall in pulmonary vascular resistance would be accompanied by an age-related rise in pulmonary blood flow, this has not been established. One other feature is of note. At birth, it is unusual to detect a systolic pressure difference between the left ventricle and the pulmonary trunk. By the time the pressure in the pulmonary trunk has fallen to normal, however, a pressure difference of up to 20–30 mmHg has usually developed. This is a consequence of bulging of the ventricular septum towards the left ventricle. This occurs as the mass of the left ventricle, relative to the right, regresses because of its reduced afterload. Although these pressure gradients have an anatomical basis, they do not necessarily indicate the presence of progressive subvalvar pulmonary stenosis. The potential for this to occur is greater with a more anteroposterior relationship of the great arteries (Chiu et al, 1984).

THE CARDIAC EFFECTS OF COMPLETE TRANSPOSITION

Infants with inadequate intercirculatory communications suffer early cardiac decompensation. This is because of the combined effect of a high systemic blood flow in response to the profound systemic arterial hypoxaemia and the tendency to a high pulmonary blood flow. The changes are exacerbated by a metabolic acidosis occurring secondary to hypoxaemia. The presence of associated anomalies, such as aortic coarctation, will further promote early congestive cardiac failure. A sudden deterioration in the condition of the infant suggests closure of an anatomical communication between the two circuits: most probably closure of the arterial duct.

The presence of a ventricular septal defect may ameliorate the cyanosis. If this is unrestrictive, the interventricular communication will, of itself, lead to congestive cardiac failure when the pulmonary vascular resistance falls. The mechanism is similar to that seen in ventricular septal defect in the normally connected heart, although the onset is more rapid in complete transposition. Similarly, a high pulmonary blood flow, pulmonary venous congestion and congestive cardiac failure may be associated with persistent patency of the arterial duct.

The effect of obstruction of the left ventricular outflow tract, when not associated with a ventricular septal defect, is to increase the left ventricular afterload, reduce the pulmonary blood flow and, thus, cause more severe cyanosis (Tynan et al, 1969). Left ventricular hypertrophy will follow if the generated left ventricular pressures are high, in other words approaching or exceeding right ventricular pressures. Such degrees of severity are more likely to develop in the setting of progressive subpulmonary fibromuscular stenosis. When such obstruction is associated with an unrestrictive ventricular septal defect, the combination of a decreased pulmonary blood flow and the basic circulatory arrangement of complete transposition leads to early severe cyanosis. It is not associated with congestive cardiac failure and the patients tolerate the combination well. A minority with very severe systemic arterial hypoxaemia become ill early in life. They exhibit severe metabolic acidosis.

The long-term effects of the abnormal circulatory arrangement before or after surgical correction are, at present, unknown. Myocardial damage occurs in other situations where the morphologically right ventricle is operating against a high pressure and where cyanosis is present (Jones and Ferrans, 1977). There is no unanimity amongst those who have studied the function of the morphologically right ventricle after atrial redirection operations. Some have found it to perform less well than would a morphologically left ventricle under similar conditions (Graham et al, 1975; Hagler et al, 1978; Grahem, 1981), while others find both right and left ventricular performance to be well preserved in the majority of patients some 10 years after the Mustard operation (Hochreiter et al,

1994). A problem in interpreting these data is that we have no yardstick as to how the morphologically right ventricle should perform under these conditions. Nor do we know what these observations mean for the majority of patients who have undergone atrial surgery for 'correction' of complete transposition. Some encouragement may be taken from the fact that, although the pre-ejection period of the morphologically right ventricle may be prolonged, isovolumic contraction times are similar to those of the normal left ventricle (Fouron et al, 1980). Nonetheless, some individuals certainly do die from progressive right ventricular dysfunction (Brom, 1981) although systemic ventricular failure occurs in less than one-tenth of patients at 10 years of follow-up (Siebenmann et al, 1989). Systemic ventricular function appears to be best preserved in patients with an intact ventricular septum who have undergone an atrial switch during infancy (Siebenmann et al, 1989; Hochreiter et al, 1994). After the arterial switch operation, left ventricular mechanics have been reported to be normal and, in the intermediate term, have shown no time-related deterioration in those in whom the switch was the primary operation. When it was performed as a rapid two-stage strategy after left ventricular preparation, in contrast, indices of left ventricular performance were mildly depressed (Colan et al, 1995). Overall, although subtle impairment of ventricular performance has been detected after surgery, most patients can live a normal life, with the long-term expectancy being greater after the arterial switch.

At any event, in the intermediate term the majority of patients appear to have cardiac performance adequate to lead normal lives (Murphy et al, 1983). When considering the cardiac effects of complete transposition, account must also be taken of the competence of the morphologically tricuspid valve. Tricuspid regurgitation sufficiently severe to cause symptomatic and haemodynamic alterations does exist but is rare. The majority of severe cases probably occur following damage to the tricuspid valve or its tension apparatus either during surgical closure of ventricular septal defects or, more rarely, during balloon septostomy (Carrel et al, 1996). There is angiocardiographic evidence, however, that the tricuspid valve can be incompetent prior to any operative intervention (Tynan et al, 1972). The significance for long-term prognosis after atrial redirection operations is unclear. If there is doubt, then an early arterial switch operation with, if necessary, repair of the valve or its tension apparatus offers the best solution (Carrel et al, 1996).

THE PULMONARY EFFECTS OF COMPLETE TRANSPOSITION

Most of the effects of complete transposition upon the pulmonary vasculature relate to the magnitude of pulmonary blood flow and to the presence or absence of communications permitting flow at high pressure between the pulmonary and systemic circuits. One abnormality,

nonetheless, appears to be present even when pulmonary blood flow and pressure are not elevated – namely the preferential flow of blood to the right-sided lung (Muster et al, 1976). This preferential flow is thought to reflect the orientation of the outflow tract from the left ventricle. If not recognized as a normal finding in complete transposition, the differential pulmonary vascular markings seen in chest radiographs may be misinterpreted as representing an abnormality.

As already discussed, the high fetal levels of pulmonary resistance usually fall as expected in the first weeks of life. This is accompanied by the same anatomical changes as are seen in the normal lung (see Chapter 4). In the presence of communications permitting flows at high pressure between the circulations, such as an unrestrictive ventricular septal defect, it is common for the patient to develop pulmonary vascular disease. The majority of survivors with a large ventricular septal defect have developed the microscopic picture of severe pulmonary vascular disease by the age of 1 year (Ferencz, 1966; Wagenvoort et al, 1969; Newfeld et al, 1974; Rabinovitch et al, 1978). Severe changes have also been discovered during early infancy, suggesting that irreversible damage may be established within the first 6 months of life (Haworth, 1983). These findings are in keeping with experience that patients develop clinical and haemodynamic signs of irreversible pulmonary vascular disease as early as 6 months of age (Stark et al, 1969). The early development of pulmonary vascular disease can also occur with shunting across a large duct and, in a minority of cases, with only an atrial septal defect (Plauth et al, 1970; Lakier et al, 1975). The impression that pulmonary vascular disease develops very early is further supported by the finding that palliative procedures, such as banding of the pulmonary trunk, do not always prevent progression (Stark et al, 1969). It is also known that progression can occur after atrial redirection procedures (Mair et al, 1974; Rosengart et al, 1975).

EFFECTS ON GROWTH AND DEVELOPMENT

The presence of complete transposition has little effect on fetal development. Most patients are of normal size at birth, although Rosenthal (1996) has recently observed that affected newborns have smaller than normal cranial volumes relative to weight at birth. It is often thought that the patients are 'larger-for-dates', but this was not borne out by the studies of Liebman et al (1969) or Rosenthal (1996). Untreated survivors, and even those with adequate palliation, show evidence of retardation of growth during the second 6 months of life. This becomes progressively more obvious in older children who have not had definitive surgery. Retardation of motor skills is also evident by the end of the first year. As is the case in any form of cyanotic congenital heart disease, intellectual development may be limited. In the absence of a major cerebral complication, however, it is difficult to disentangle the physical from the psychosocial causes (Bentovim, 1983). Successful surgery certainly ameliorates the physical aspects of retardation. Its effect on intellectual development is as yet uncertain, but there does appear to be a possible relationship between intelligence and the timing of surgery, suggesting that delay in surgical correction may have a deleterious effect (Newburger et al, 1984).

CLINICAL FEATURES

PRESENTATION

The circulatory arrangement of complete transposition is such that all patients have significant degrees of arterial desaturation from birth. Cyanosis, therefore, is the presenting feature. It would seem that all patients should present in this way on the first day of life. Surprisingly, many do not. In our recent experience, a good proportion did present on the first day. Still, in a significant number of patients, no cardiac disease was suspected until after 1 week of life. Indeed, presentation in a few was delayed until after 1 month. Generally, it is those with intact ventricular septation who present within the first day or days of life. Those presenting later tend to have anatomical communications of sufficient size to permit maintenance of a relatively high arterial oxygen saturation. Such patients have large ventricular septal defects, persistent patency of the arterial duct or, more rarely, a large naturally occurring atrial septal defect. Other rare associated anomalies, such as totally anomalous pulmonary venous connection, may further delay recognition of the disease. Although there is always arterial systemic desaturation, it is often the onset of tachypnoea and dyspnoea caused by congestive heart failure that brings these infants to the attention of the paediatrician. As a result, there are two major modes of initial presentation. The first is cyanosis, which should be anticipated when the ventricular septum is intact. The second is congestive cardiac failure, which occurs when there is a significant shunt. The division between the two is not clear-cut. For instance, those patients with an intact ventricular septum in whom, for some reason, cyanosis is not recognized early can rapidly worsen and present with congestive cardiac failure. During the 1970s and 1980s, there was a significant change in the pattern of recognition of these patients. This was presumably the result of greater awareness of congenital heart defects by the neonatal paediatrician. In earlier standard textbooks, it was stated that most patients presented in the first week or month of life (Kidd, 1976). As indicated above, our recent experience is that many patients have reached the paediatric cardiologist by 12 hours of age. It has also long been known that those with severe cyanosis will develop a metabolic acidosis. Early recognition should obviate this development. Of patients recognized on the first day of life in our series, nonetheless, one fifth had significant metabolic acidosis and were collapsed on arrival in the cardiac centre.

Presentation may further be modified by the association of obstruction within the left ventricular outflow tract with deficient ventricular septation. With this combination, initial presentation is with cyanosis, as in those with an intact ventricular septum. Because of the pulmonary stenosis, the patients do not progress into congestive cardiac failure.

Fetal echocardiography has demonstrated the possibility of prenatal detection of congenital heart defects. The diagnosis of complete transposition can certainly be made in fetal life, and this has introduced a new mode of presentation (Allan et al, 1994). It cannot be suspected simply from screening the four chamber view (Sharland and Allan, 1992). Indeed, the diagnosis is quite difficult to make. The increase in numbers being detected during pregnancy testifies to the increase in awareness by those organizing programmes for fetal health in obstetric departments.

Most patients present with clinically detectable cyanosis. When congestive cardiac failure does supervene, all its signs and symptoms are present. On palpation, there will be a prominent right ventricular impulse. It is often possible to palpate both heart sounds because of the proximity of the aortic valve to the anterior chest wall. A systolic thrill may be felt when a ventricular septal defect is present. In patients who are not collapsed, the peripheral pulses are usually bounding and equal. Weak or impalpable femoral pulses, with normal or increased pulses in the arms, indicate the presence of associated aortic coarctation or interruption of the aortic arch. Coarctation can, however, in itself precipitate rapid deterioration in the clinical condition. Under these circumstances, all pulses may be weak. Hence, judgement of differences in the peripheral pulses is difficult. In this group, the possibility of coexisting obstruction in the aortic arch must be borne in mind when proceeding to more definitive investigations.

At auscultation, both heart sounds are loud. The second is usually perceived to be single, although careful auscultation usually reveals two components. Murmurs are not a prominent feature in those with an intact ventricular septum and no other abnormalities. There may be no murmurs or, at most, a mid-systolic ejection murmur may be heard. The presence of persistent patency of the arterial duct is occasionally associated with the typical continuous murmur, although this is far from the rule. The association with severe obstruction in the left ventricular outflow tract will produce a loud ejection systolic murmur heard at the upper left sternal edge and propagated into the lung fields. This will be present whether or not there is also a ventricular septal defect. When there is a ventricular septal defect without any obstruction within the left ventricular outflow tract, there will be a loud pan-systolic murmur at the lower left sternal edge. When pulmonary blood flow is high, an apical mid-diastolic murmur is heard. As with an isolated ventricular septal defect, the murmur may not be detected at birth. Its appearance depends on the anticipated fall in pulmonary vascular resistance from high fetal levels (see Chapter 4). Indeed, in some patients who retain a high pulmonary vascular resistance, the murmur may never become characteristic.

INVESTIGATIONS

LABORATORY FINDINGS

The crucial initial investigation in patients suspected of being cyanosed is the demonstration of systemic arterial hypoxaemia by analysis of arterial blood gases. In those without major intercirculatory mixing, the arterial content of oxygen is often in the range 15–25 mmHg (2–3 kPa). Although it will be higher when there are associated defects permitting mixing, it rarely exceeds 40–50 mmHg (5.5–7 kPa). In neither of these cases will the administration of 100% oxygen result in a rise of arterial oxygen above 180 mmHg (24 kPa). In general, there is little or no rise at all. The development of acidosis will also be reflected in the blood gas analysis. The more severely affected the patient, the lower will be the pH level. It is not uncommon to encounter values of 6.9–7.1 in a neonate with an intact ventricular septum. The arterial oxygen saturation is usually normal or low. The level of haemoglobin at birth is normal, but polycythaemia should be present with survival beyond 3 months of age, usually as a consequence of palliative treatment.

CHEST RADIOGRAPHY

The radiographic appearances reflect the haemodynamic disturbances present. At birth, the heart is of normal size and the lung fields are unremarkable (Counahan et al, 1973). Even at this age, the mediastinal shadow is narrow in almost one third of patients (Shaher, 1973). Although initially considered to be caused by the arterial relationships being more anteroposterior (Taussing, 1938), it is more likely that this impression represents lack of a prominent thymic shadow (Nogrady and Dunbar, 1969). After the first week of life, a narrow vascular pedicle is seen much more frequently (Schneeweiss et al, 1982). With the development of high pulmonary blood flow, or the onset of congestive cardiac failure, there is progressive cardiac enlargement and increase in the pulmonary vascular shadows. This progression does not occur in those patients with obstruction of the left ventricular outflow tract, particularly when associated with a ventricular septal defect. In this setting, the radiological picture is a normally sized heart with oligaemic lung fields. Such an appearance is, in many ways, similar to that of tetralogy. A right aortic arch is an uncommon finding. It is occasionally seen, and then usually in the presence of associated anomalies such as ventricular septal defect (Guerin et al, 1970; Mathew et al, 1974). The presence of a right arch should not, therefore, be taken as invalidating the diagnosis of complete transposition.

ELECTROCARDIOGRAPHY

The cardiac rhythm, as demonstrated by the standard electrocardiogram, is usually sinus in origin with no evidence of conduction abnormalities. Investigations of changes in the heart rhythm induced by operation, however, including 24-hour tape monitoring, have led to the discovery that conduction abnormalities are present as 'normal' findings in a significant number of patients with complete transposition prior to any definitive surgery (Southall et al, 1980). These abnormalities include Wenckebach block, two-to-one or complete sinuatrial block, atrial premature beats of less than 12 per hour or intermittent junctional escape rhythms. Such findings are also seen in patients without congenital heart disease (Southall, 1982). The P wave morphology of the standard electrocardiogram does not suggest atrial hypertrophy and the axis is normal in those with usual atrial arrangement with a left-sided heart. At birth, the mean frontal QRS axis is usually in the normal range (+90° to +120°). The usual right ventricular hypertrophy is evidenced by dominant R waves over the right chest leads and Rs morphology in the left chest leads. With passage of time, in patients with intact ventricular septum, there is absence of the expected normal evolution. Instead, right ventricular hypertrophy becomes more obvious, and the right axis deviation persists, as is the case with a large ventricular septal defect (Elliott et al, 1963). It might be expected that signs of left ventricular hypertrophy would be seen with obstruction in the left ventricular outflow tract or with pulmonary vascular disease, causing a high left ventricular pressure. The standard electrocardiogram rarely reveals this feature, although vectorcardiography has been suggested to be more valuable (Mair et al, 1970; Restieaux et al, 1972).

ECHOCARDIOGRAPHY

The echocardiographic diagnosis rests on the demonstration of the abnormal ventriculo-arterial connections. It cannot be inferred from the demonstration of an anterior right-sided aortic valve. This is because many patients with conditions other than complete transposition have this relationship, while the relationship is not present in a significant number of patients with complete transposition (Tynan and Anderson, 1979). Therefore, papers written concerning echocardiographic diagnosis that are based on this premise must be assessed cautiously. Historically, the diagnosis was inferred using M-mode techniques, the most reliable being contrast echocardiography evaluated from the suprasternal approach (Mortera et al, 1979). These

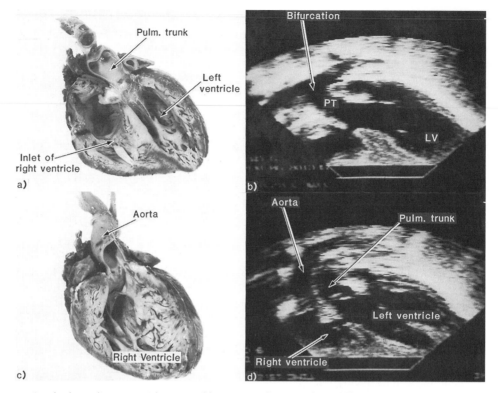

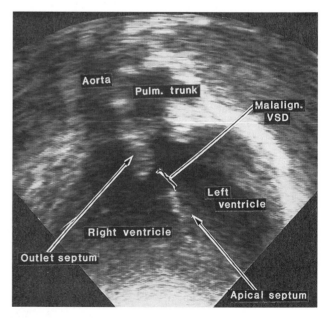

Figure 48.24. Cross-sectional echocardiograms, with comparable anatomical sections from different hearts, showing the discordant ventriculo-arterial connections that are the key to diagnosis. V, left ventricle, Pulm., pulmonary; PT, pulmonary trunk.

methods are no longer used. The echocardiographic diagnosis now rests on cross-sectional examination combined with colour Doppler. M-mode interrogation is reserved for measurements of size of chambers and ventricular function.

Cross-sectional echocardiography is the best diagnostic investigation. Both the concordant atrioventricular and the discordant ventriculo-arterial connections can be identified with certainty (Bierman and Williams, 1979). Once a usual or mirror-imaged atrial arrangement has been determined, then cross-sectional echocardiography in the four chamber planes will demonstrate concordant atrioventricular connections. Angulation of the transducer will enable the ventricles to be traced to their great arteries (Figure 48.24). The feature of particular value in demonstrating the discordant ventriculo-arterial connections is the branching pattern of the posterior arterial trunk arising from the left ventricle (Daskalopoulos et al, 1983). It is occasionally difficult to visualize the left ventricle, the pulmonary trunk and both its branches in a single subcostal cut, but the pulmonary trunk may be identified as such in the precordial long-axis cut by its abrupt posterior turn immediately above the valve. In the same cut, albeit with some angulation of the probe, the brachiocephalic artery may be seen to arise from the ascending aorta. These are definitive findings. The parallel arrangements of the great arteries found in the short axis is suggestive but can be seen with other ventriculo-arterial connections such as double outlet right ventricle. Suprasternal and high parasternal views will enable the aorta to be traced from the right ventricle to its

branches. Additional anomalies, such as the presence, size and site of a ventricular septal defect (Figure 48.25) or the position and nature of subpulmonary stenosis (Figure 48.26) can all be identified. Tension apparatus from the

Figure 48.25. A four chamber cross-sectional echocardiogram showing a subpulmonary ventricular septal defect (VSD) with malalignment (Malalign.) of the muscular outlet septum. Compare with Figure 48.18. Pulm., pulmonary. (Reproduced by kind permission of Prof. G. R. Sutherland.)

tricuspid valve inserting into the outlet septum can also be recognized (Huhta et al, 1982). This is important in planning surgical repair. Patency of the arterial duct is parti-

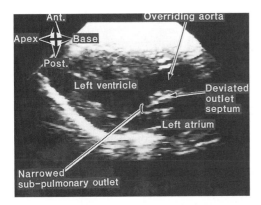

Figure 48.26. A long-axis parasternal cross-sectional echocardiogram showing subpulmonary stenosis owing to posterior (Post.) deviation of the outlet septum. Compare with Figures 48.19 and 48.32a. Ant, anterior.

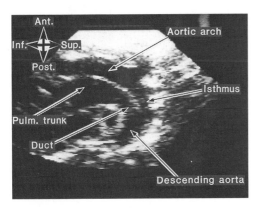

Figure 48.27. A parasagittal long-axis cross-sectional echocardiogram from the suprasternal notch showing the presence of an arterial duct in a patient with complete transposition. Ant., anterior, Inf., inferior; Post., posterior; Sup., superior.

cularly easy to demonstrate in complete transposition when assessed from the suprasternal approach (Figure 48.27) (Smallhorn et al, 1982). Detailed information concerning the symmetry of the pulmonary valve can be obtained, which may prove important in the long-term follow-up after the arterial switch operation (Kovalchin et al, 1994). Of particular importance is the assessment of the origins and proximal course of the coronary arteries (Elkins et al, 1994; Pasquini et al, 1994). Such interrogation is by no means foolproof, but it is now possible to identify the sinusal origin and epicardial course of the three major coronary arteries and to detect important anomalies such as high take-off (Figure 48.28) and origin adjacent to a commissure with intramural course of the proximal segment of the involved coronary artery (Figure 48.29).

Colour flow mapping makes the diagnosis easier and adds precision. The presence of additional lesions, such as

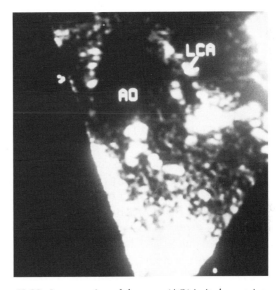

Figure 48.28. Interrogation of the aorta (AO) in its long axis reveals abnormally high take-off of one coronary artery. LCA, left coronary artery.

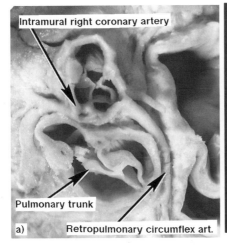

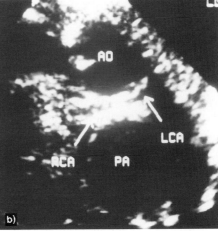

Figure 48.29. Interrogation in the short axis shows an intramural course of the proximal segment of a coronary artery. (a) Anatomical section; (b) echocardiograms. AO, aorta; art., artery; LCA and RCA, left and right coronary arteries, respectively; PA, pulmonary trunk.

patency of the arterial duct, aortic coarctation or obstruction of the left ventricular outflow tract, can readily be detected. The patterns of flow across the duct or a ventricular septal defect can be assessed. With the aid of such mapping, the continuous wave Doppler beam can be directed and, in the presence of tricuspid regurgitation, the right ventricular pressure can be assessed.

Both M-mode and cross-sectional echocardiography are of great value in the long-term follow-up of patients after definitive surgery, as will be discussed below.

NUCLEAR IMAGING

There is no doubt that a first-class nuclear angiogram can strongly suggest the presence of complete transposition by demonstrating early opacification of the aorta. Compared with the accuracy and convenience of cross-sectional echocardiography, however, such studies are of little value in initial diagnosis. The value of nuclear imaging is in the demonstration or exclusion of significant shunts after definitive surgery and in the long-term repetitive assessment of ventricular function and myocardial perfusion.

CARDIAC CATHETERIZATION

The course of the catheter reflects the anatomy, the aorta being entered from the right ventricle and the pulmonary trunk from the left ventricle. Entry to the pulmonary trunk from the right ventricle is often possible when there is an associated ventricular septal defect. The route to the pulmonary trunk is somewhat circuitous when the ventricular septum is intact, but entry can usually be made via the left atrium and left ventricle. Originally, this was performed using the coaxial flow-guided technique (Carr and Wells, 1966). Many workers now prefer to use a Swan–Ganz balloon catheter. Others have designed specially curved catheters (Macartney et al, 1975). It is usually possible to gain entry to the pulmonary trunk, nonetheless, using an appropriately curved Goodale Lubin catheter. This is done by bending the tip of the catheter into a J shape and immersing it in boiling water. The length of the J, and the radius of curvature chosen will depend upon the patient being investigated.

The haemodynamic findings vary with the age of the patient and the associated abnormalities. At all ages, the pulmonary arterial oxygen saturation is usually higher than that in the aorta. In the setting of complete transposition with intact ventricular septum, after the neonatal period, when the pulmonary vascular resistance has fallen, the pulmonary arterial pressure is usually normal. There is frequently a difference in systolic pressure between the left ventricle and the pulmonary arteries, which is usually of the order of 10–20 mmHg. The pressures in the right ventricle and aorta are normal for the

systemic circulation. An elevated pulmonary arterial pressure is seen in the presence of a large arterial duct or when there is an elevated pulmonary vascular resistance.

When there is an associated ventricular septal defect but no obstruction in the left ventricular outflow tract, the pulmonary arterial pressure will depend on the size of the defect and the pulmonary vascular resistance. The pressure may be normal when the defect is small. When the defect is nonrestrictive, the pulmonary arterial systolic pressure will be similar to that in the aorta. There is a spectrum of size and, therefore, of pulmonary arterial pressure, between these two extremes. With obstruction of the left ventricular outflow tract, there is also a spectrum of pressure gradients between the left ventricle and the pulmonary arteries. It is not possible on data derived from measurements of pressure alone to distinguish between the anatomical types of obstruction. When the ventricular septum is intact, a moderately elevated left ventricular pressure, with a gradient of 20–30 mmHg to the pulmonary trunk, is likely to result from dynamic subvalvar stenosis. Fixed anatomical stenosis, with or without a ventricular septal defect, is more likely to result in left ventricular pressures at or above those recorded in the right ventricle. The systolic pressure gradients will be concomitantly greater. The left atrial pressure in the majority of patients initially exceeds that measured in the right atrium. Early in the neonatal period, and after balloon septostomy or surgical septectomy, the mean pressures in the two atriums are similar even though their phasic wave forms may be different.

Oximetry allows the calculation of pulmonary and systemic blood flows. Using the effective pulmonary blood flow, the magnitude of the intercirculatory cross-flows can also be determined. These calculations are made in the usual fashion (see Chapter 17). To some extent, the site of these cross-flows can be detected by oximetry, but there is frequently evidence of bidirectional cross-flow at atrial level either through the oval foramen or an atrial septal defect, be it natural or iatrogenic. Furthermore, part of the pulmonary blood flow may be derived from bronchial collateral arteries. The extent to which this occurs in practice cannot be accurately measured. Consequently, the true oxygen content of blood in the pulmonary arteries is not known. This prevents precise measurement of the arterio-venous difference in content of oxygen across the pulmonary vascular bed, and hence calculation of pulmonary blood flow. This, in turn, makes unreliable the identification of the sites of shunting in the downstream cardiac segments. The pulmonary and systemic vascular resistances are calculated from the data concerning pressures and flow. This is best done using measured oxygen uptake. It is preferable in its absence to estimate the pulmonary vascular resistance using an assumed consumption of oxygen rather than relying on the ratio of pulmonary-to-systemic vascular resistances.

In the early days of life, when the pulmonary vascular resistance has not evolved fully from the high intrauterine levels, pressures in the pulmonary trunk and left ventricle will be high. The systolic pressure gradients from left ventricle to pulmonary arteries may not then be developed (Tynan, 1972). Consequently, findings at this time are not necessarily representative of the haemodynamics to be found later in infancy. Because of this, a complete haemodynamic study is not always necessary at the initial neonatal catheterization. This fact, together with the anatomical information obtained from cross-sectional echocardiography, means that the initial catheterization is in most centres the vehicle for balloon septostomy. The haemodynamic study can consequently be significantly abbreviated, or omitted entirely, at this initial catheterization. Indeed, cardiac catheterization is rarely needed today, since early diagnosis allows the arterial switch operation to be performed in the neonatal period. Such diagnosis is done on echocardiographic assessment alone, including nowadays identification of the coronary arteries. Complete characterization of the haemodynamic state is only necessary when patients present late and pulmonary vascular disease is suspected. Pulmonary vascular disease appears to be of more rapid onset and more florid in complete transposition than in other conditions. Those patients with a ventricular septal defect or an arterial duct are particularly at risk (Newfeld et al, 1974; see Chapters 37 and 52). The complete haemodynamic profile should, therefore, be established in such patients before surgery is performed.

ANGIOCARDIOGRAPHY

Just as a cardiac catheterization is rarely needed today, so angiocardiography is required infrequently. When it is performed, the discordant ventriculo-arterial connections can readily be demonstrated (Figure 48.30), as can associated defects. Where aortic coarctation is suspected, an

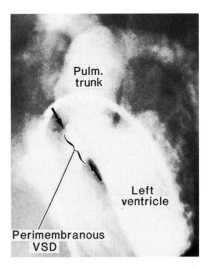

Figure 48.31. A long-axis left ventricular angiogram shows a perimembranous ventricular septal defect (VSD). (Reproduced by kind permission of Dr B. L. Soto, University of Alabama in Birmingham, USA.)

aortogram or right ventricular angiocardiogram may be indicated. This is best performed in the long-axis projection. Such angiocardiography or aortography will also demonstrate or exclude patency of the arterial duct or a ventricular septal defect. If left or right ventricular angiocardiograms are performed, then again the preferred projection is the long-axis one. These angiocardiograms will demonstrate the position of ventricular septal defects (Figure 48.31) and show whether they are single or multiple. Any anatomical obstruction within the left ventricular outflow tract can also be identified (Figure 48.32) (Shaher and Puddu, 1966; Tynan et al, 1969; Aziz et al, 1979; Sansa et al, 1979).

The role of coronary arteriography in the preoperative assessment of the newborn is even less clear. While the course and distribution of the coronary arteries can be demonstrated by angiography, particularly when using the 'laid-back' view, the important features can nowadays reliably be visualized echocardiographically. Most surgeons are happy to proceed to operation with this information. They then make their own evaluation in the operating theatre.

DIAGNOSIS

Complete transposition must be suspected in any cyanosed newborn, or in any infant who fails to show a normal increase in arterial oxygen saturation on breathing 100% oxygen. Clinical, ausculatory, electrocardiographic and chest radiological findings early in infancy may not differentiate this condition from other causes of cyanosis. A confident and accurate diagnosis depends on cross-sectional echocardiography. Although it is an exceedingly rare combination, it is in order to mention the combination of discordant atrioventricular and

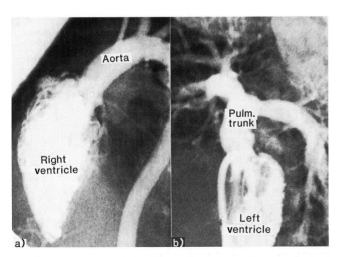

Figure 48.30. Angiocardiograms revealing discordant ventriculo-arterial connections in a patient with complete transposition. (Reproduced by kind permission of Dr B. L. Soto' University of Alabama in Birmingham, USA.)

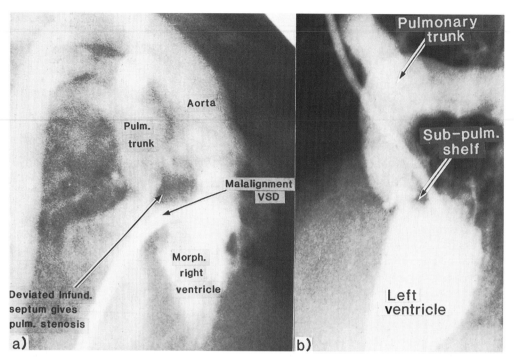

Figure 48.32. Subpulmonary stenosis caused by (a) posterior deviation of the muscular outlet septum in association with a ventricular septal defect (VSD) and (b) a fibrous shelf. Infund., infundibular; pulm., pulmonary; subpulm., subpulmonary. (Part (b) is reproduced by kind permission of Dr B. L. Soto, University of Alabama in Birmingham, USA.)

concordant ventriculo-arterial connections (Arciprete et al, 1985). This segmental arrangement produces haemodynamic findings identical to complete transposition. Distinction is important since, in presence of the discordant atrioventricular connections, there will be an abnormal disposition of the conduction tissues (see Chapter 49). It is also noteworthy that these rare cases are ideal for atrial redirection operations. This is because such procedures restore the morphologically left ventricle, supporting the aorta, to its appropriate systemic role.

COURSE AND PROGNOSIS

When untreated, complete transposition is a uniformly lethal lesion. In California from 1957 to 1964, nine tenths of patients with this lesion were dead by their first birthday (Liebman et al, 1969). This rate of death is supported by other studies (Boesen, 1963; Hoffheinz et al, 1964). The thorough study of Leibman and his colleagues (1969) showed that, at that time, the average life expectancy at birth was 0.65 years. If the patient survived until 1 week of age, this life expectancy rose to only 0.87 years. Comparable expectancy for life for patients reaching 1 month of age was 1.12 years; it was 3.92 years for those reaching 1 year. No patient in the series survived beyond the age of 22 years. The study also showed the minimal ameliorating effect of associated lesions. Even patients with the combination of ventricular septal defect and pulmonary stenosis had an average life expectancy of less than 5 years. While these data are not accurate figures of

the natural history, since they were collected during the evolving surgical era, they do indicate the bleak outlook for untreated patients. The major causes of death in untreated patients are anoxia and acidosis in the first week of life and congestive heart failure in the first month of life. Further causes of mortality and morbidity are thromboembolic phenomenons, particularly cerebrovascular accidents. Prior to the availability of palliative or corrective procedures, these were observed in about one tenth of patients (Tyler and Clark, 1957). The advent of balloon atrial septostomy and atrial redirection operations in infancy revolutionized the outlook. Analysis of the results of these measures for the years 1972–76 at the Hospital for Sick Children, Great Ormond Street, London showed a 5-year survival rate of 76.1% (Macartney et al, 1980). The outlook has been improved still further by the introduction of the arterial switch operation in the newborn period. When performed in babies up to 2 weeks of age, survival of 82% has already been reported at the age of 5 years (Kirklin et al, 1992). This must be anticipated to get better as diagnosis is made more rapidly and surgery continues to improve.

The early development of pulmonary vascular disease is now the most likely inhibitor of relatively normal life expectancy. This is exemplified by the lower survival rate of patients in whom banding of the pulmonary trunk was performed, at least in part to offset the development of pulmonary vascular disease (Macartney et al, 1980). The patient is certain to die prematurely if progressive pulmonary vascular disease does develop, even though the outlook may be somewhat better than the natural history if an operation such as a palliative Mustard procedure (Lindesmith et al, 1972), or palliative arterial switch (Pridjian et al, 1992), is performed (see below).

MANAGEMENT

SUPPORTIVE THERAPY AT PRESENTATION

There is no effective medical treatment for the physiological problem produced by the abnormal cardiac connections. Supportive measures should not, therefore, delay either the diagnosis or initial palliation by balloon atrial septostomy (see below). When metabolic acidosis is present, it should be corrected. Similarly, decongestive treatment should be started for those patients in heart failure. Prostaglandin E_2 (or E_1 in the USA) has a role in the initial treatment, as in other conditions such as pulmonary atresia with intact ventricular septum. Most paediatric cardiologists would advise that any severely hypoxic infant will benefit from this treatment and that it should be initiated prior to transfer to the cardiac centre (Bietzke and Suppan, 1983). Although oral administration of prostaglandin E_2 has been shown to be effective and to have a low rate of complications (Silove et al, 1981), this approach is now rarely used. Our own preference is for intravenous administration, with facilities for intubation and ventilation should apnoea develop.

BALLOON ATRIAL SEPTOSTOMY

Effective palliative treatment of complete transposition was introduced by Blalock and Hanlon (1950) with their surgical atrial septectomy. As the primary palliative procedure, however, this had a high mortality and morbidity (Deverall et al, 1969). The search for alternative methods of improving interatrial mixing led to the development of balloon atrial septostomy by Rashkind and Miller (1966). This has now become accepted as the initial palliative procedure and is performed as soon as the diagnosis is made. A balloon catheter is inserted and passed from right to left atrium through the oval foramen. It is then inflated with dilute contrast medium, starting initially with 2.5 ml; with a quick, short jerk, it is pulled into the right atrium. This procedure is then repeated, inflating the balloon to its maximum capacity. Up to eight passes may be necessary, although it is probably the first sharp jerk that tears rather than stretches the atrial septum (Figure 48.5). It is obviously of paramount importance that the balloon be inflated while free in the cavity of the left atrium. Serious damage, and even death, can result if the balloon is pulled back from any other location. Possibilities are from the right ventricle across the tricuspid valve, from the left ventricle across the mitral valve or from left to right ventricle through a ventricular septal defect. The procedure will be of no

value if the balloon is pulled from right atrial appendage to right atrium when there is left juxtaposition of the atrial appendages (Tyrrell and Moes, 1971). The left atrial location of the balloon prior to inflation is most easily ascertained by using cross-sectional echocardiography in the subcostal four chamber plane (Figure 48.33). This method not only allows accurate positioning of the balloon but also permits confirmation of septal rupture following the withdrawal. A further advantage of this technique (Allan et al, 1982) is that a single-lumen catheter can be used with absolute confidence. When the procedure is performed using X-ray screening alone, a double-lumen catheter is preferable, since it permits collection of data by measuring pressure and oximetry as well as injecting contrast medium to confirm the appropriate siting of the balloon. Many workers using single-lumen catheters perform the technique safely by passing the catheter into a pulmonary vein visualized outside the cardiac silhouette, thus confirming that the catheter has traversed the left

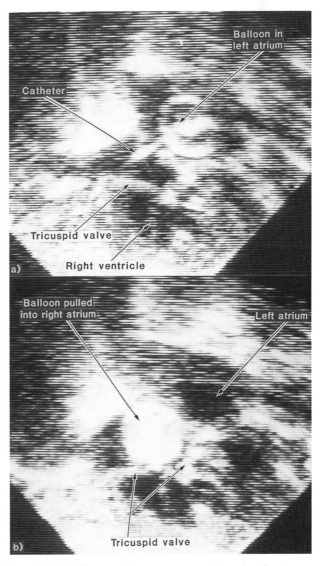

Figure 48.33. Balloon atrial septostomy as performed under cross-sectional echocardiographic control.

atrium. Slow withdrawal and inflation then extrudes the balloon from the pulmonary vein into the cavity of the left atrium, from whence the septostomy is performed as described. Even so, accurate positioning of the balloon, especially after initial septal rupture, is best and most easily demonstrated by cross-sectional echocardiography. Indeed, this is achieved with safety in the intensive care unit (Baker et al, 1984). If needs must, the technique can be accomplished via the umbilical vein, although this is not a recommended route (Abinader et al, 1970).

Balloon atrial septostomy, from its inception, produced a marked improvement in survival of infants with complete transposition. Early results showed an initial survival rate to 1 month of age of 80–85% with survival to 6 months of 70–75% (Tynan, 1971). With time, results improved; by 1981, survival to 6 months had reached 86% (Leanage et al, 1981). This improved survival probably reflects advances in intensive care, together with the willingness to perform early definitive surgery. The present practice of rapid septostomy with an abbreviated initial catheterization has contributed to this improvement. A successful septostomy results, in most patients, in a marked increase in arterial oxygen saturation. The biggest rise is found in those patients with an intact ventricular septum and a closed arterial duct. In a group of such patients, the mean oxygen saturation rose from 43 to 62%. In those with additional communications, the rise was from 56 to 67% (Tynan, 1972). These figures represent the measurements immediately before and after septostomy and do not indicate the long-term effects to be expected. In follow-up investigations in this group of patients as a whole, the mean arterial saturation fell to 59% (Tynan, 1972). Therefore, while in the best cases saturations of 60–70% may be seen, a successful septostomy in just as many may only result in an oxygen saturation of 50%. After a successful septostomy, the mean pressures in right and left atriums should be similar. Knowledge of interatrial pressure is important in assessing the adequacy of the defect when a subsequent investigation is indicated because of persistent systemic arterial hypoxaemia. In such cases, a left atrial pressure significantly in excess of the right is good evidence that the interatrial communication is of inadequate size. If performed in the first month of life, it is unlikely that balloon atrial septostomy will fail. The existence of an adequate atrial septal defect can be confirmed by subsequent cross-sectional echocardiography. In those rare patients who require creation of an atrial septal defect above 3 months of age, the balloon technique is unlikely to be effective. Should it be needed, surgical septectomy is the optimal treatment. Blade septostomy at catheterization is an alternative (Park et al, 1982).

SURGICAL PALLIATION

Two aspects of surgical palliation need to be considered. The first is the surgical creation of an atrial septal defect.

The second is the palliation designed to deal with associated cardiovascular malformations. Surgical atrial septectomy is now mainly of historical interest, since it is almost never indicated in patients with complete transposition, although it may on occasion be needed in more complex heart defects, such as those associated with mitral atresia. There were several methods of creating such a defect. The first, and most widely used, was introduced by Blalock and Hanlon (1950). It allowed creation of the defect without interruption of the systemic circulation. Nowadays, in the rare circumstances where it is needed, surgical septectomy would be achieved using cardiopulmonary bypass.

Palliation for associated abnormalities includes operations such as ligation of an arterial duct, or resection or arterioplasty for aortic coarctation. These should be performed at the time of the arterial switch operation. On rare occasions, it may be prudent to palliate an associated ventricular septal defect or defects by banding of the pulmonary trunk. Construction of a systemic-to-pulmonary arterial shunt may also be needed to allow time for growth when pulmonary stenosis occurs in the presence of a ventricular septal defect.

DEFINITIVE SURGICAL TREATMENT

The palliative procedures described above revolutionized the immediate prognosis for children born with complete transposition. They are, however, of extremely limited long-term value. More definitive surgical procedures are necessary to produce continued amelioration of the effects of the abnormal connections.

DEFINITIVE SURGERY: THE CONTEMPORARY APPROACH

There are several options now available for definitive surgery. For newborns having complete transposition with an intact ventricular septum, the arterial switch procedure should be performed within the first month of life, ideally within the first 2 weeks. An associated persistent arterial duct, or aortic coarctation, should be dealt with at the same time as the arterial switch is performed. Those having a ventricular septal defect, but in the absence of obstruction within the left ventricular outflow tract, should again undergo the arterial switch operation along with closure of the ventricular septal defect within the first month of life. If the infant does not present until later, surgery should be performed at the earliest opportunity. Should an infant with an intact ventricular septum present later than the first month of life with a low left ventricular pressure, there should be immediate banding of the pulmonary trunk followed by the arterial switch within 7 to 10 days. Should pulmonary vascular disease already have become irreversible in those with deficient ventricular septation, the arterial switch should be performed but the ventricular septal defect left open. In the setting of a ventricular septal defect combined with pulmonary stenosis, there are two options. The first is to close the ventricular septal defect so that the left ventricle is connected to the aorta and then to connect the right ventricle to the pulmonary arteries via a valved conduit. This procedure is known as the Rastelli operation. The second option is the procedure known as *reparation de l'etage ventriculaire* (REV; Lecompte et al, 1982). The concept is similar to that proposed by Rastelli, but the pulmonary trunk is connected to the right ventricle without the interposition of a conduit. The strategies nowadays employed for definitive surgery, therefore, all attempt, as near as is possible, to recreate concordant ventriculo-arterial connections. Earlier operations retained the discordant ventriculo-arterial connections, reversing the circulations at atrial level. These procedures, nonetheless, were so successful that there is a large population of patients who are long-term survivors of such atrial redirection. It is incumbent on us, therefore, to discuss also these operations in order to understand their strengths, weaknesses and complications.

AN HISTORICAL PERSPECTIVE: ATRIAL REDIRECTION PROCEDURES

Atrial redirection procedures corrected the haemodynamic abnormalities of complete transposition by redirecting the venous returns at atrial level. Originally suggested as a surgical option by Albert (1955), the first successful atrial redirection procedure was reported by Senning in 1959. During the 1960s, the operation devised by Mustard and his colleagues (1964) became the procedure to gain widespread approval. In the late 1970s and early 1980s, the Senning procedure experienced a major revival in a modified form and was used in many centres (Quaegebeur et al, 1977; Locatelli et al, 1978; Marx et al, 1983). Prior to the introduction of the arterial switch, it had become the most popular procedure for definitive correction of complete transposition with intact ventricular septum. We will review the salient points of these procedures in turn, before considering their overall complications.

The Mustard procedure

The atrioventricular connections were reversed in the Mustard procedure by removing the atrial septum and constructing an intra-atrial patch so that the superior and inferior caval venous channels were connected to the mitral valvar orifice, and the pulmonary veins to the tricuspid orifice (Figure 48.34). There were many modifications suggested for the design of the patch, and various materials were used in its construction. The most popular was the trouser-shaped patch devised by Brom (Quaegebeur and Brom, 1978), which was constructed either from pericardium or synthetic material. It was placed so that the legs of the trousers were attached round the caval venous orifices. The systemic venous return then ran down the legs to the mitral orifice. The waist of the trousers was attached to the parietal wall of the left atrium beyond the left pulmonary veins, and the pulmonary venous return ran across the crotch of the trousers to the tricuspid orifice (Figure 48.34). An alternative technique, using a Gore-Tex prosthesis, produced outstanding results in the hands of Oelert and his colleagues (1981). Irrespective of the precise technique or material used, and it was significant that the Toronto group continued to use a technique close to the original devised in that centre until they adopted the arterial switch procedure, the Mustard procedure provided excellent results throughout the world. At its zenith, most centres using the technique produced operative survival of 95% or better in patients born with an intact ventricular septum (Stark, 1981, 1984).

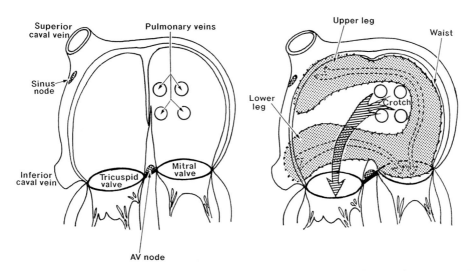

Figure 48.34. Diagram to show the effect of the Mustard operation. The pathways do not narrow down to the crossing points as shown in the right hand diagram, but it is difficult to demonstrate the full extent of the trouser-shaped patch in two dimensions. AV, atrioventricular.

The Senning procedure

The Senning procedure differed from the Mustard operation in that foreign material was used only as needed to make good the atrial septal deficiency. Venous redirection was accomplished by liberating a sleeve of right atrium between the superior and inferior caval venous orifices, interiorizing this within the left atrium so that the caval veins drained to the orifice of the mitral valve. The atrial wall was then reconstituted so that pulmonary venous return passed across what had originally been the epicardial surface of the intercaval right atrial sleeve, draining then to the tricuspid valve (Figure 48.35). As with the Mustard procedure, attempts were made to limit damage to the sinus node and its artery. Particular care was needed in the Senning procedure when the new pulmonary venous atrium was closed across the superior caval end of the right atrial sleeve, since this suture line could be taken close to the sinus node. If the sinus node and its artery were avoided, initial results showed that the modified Senning procedure could be accomplished with very low perioperative mortality, and with few problems of postoperative venous obstruction (Quaegebeur et al, 1977; Locatelli et al, 1978).

Problems persist, however, of late disturbances of rhythm and sudden death (Deanfield et al, 1983; Gewillig, 1998), and the question remains concerning right ventricular function (Bender et al, 1980). These complications are similar for both the Senning and the Mustard procedures. Although there was little or no objective evidence of its superiority, undoubtedly the Senning operation became the more popular of the two. Today, if an atrial redirection operation is deemed to be necessary, the choice between the two procedures is largely one of the personal preference of the surgeon (Marx et al, 1983).

Complications after atrial redirection procedures

Complications of the atrial redirection procedures were studied most extensively in survivors of the Mustard operation. Systemic and pulmonary venous obstruction proved to be a major problem (Clarkson et al, 1972; Champsaur et al, 1973; Stark et al, 1974). Early development of obstruction within the newly created caval venous channels produced high facial colour, facial oedema with engorged neck veins, sometimes accompanied by chylothorax, and hepatomegaly with or without ascites. This last complication was a frequent cause of reoperation in the early postoperative period. In the long term, severe superior and inferior caval venous obstruction can still be encountered in the absence of any signs or symptoms. The stenosis is usually produced at the junction between the patch and the left atrial tissues. Development of pulmonary venous obstruction is indicated by the onset of dyspnoea and signs of pulmonary oedema. Haemoptysis can occur in the long term. The stenotic area tends to be produced where the patch crosses the original site of the atrial septum. Once developed, the options for treatment include reoperation, but this is difficult and gives less than perfect results. Balloon dilation is another option and may relieve systemic or pulmonary venous stenosis. It tends to be of only temporary benefit in most patients. Implantation of stents is more reliable in the relief of systemic venous obstruction (MacLellan-Tobert et al, 1996; Brown et al, 1998) and can be accomplished even when the caval venous channel is totally obstructed (Abdulhamed et al, 1994). The role of stenting the pulmonary veins needs to be defined. The information presently available suggests that stents offer only temporary relief. Converting the patient directly to an arterial switch, subsequent to preparation of the left

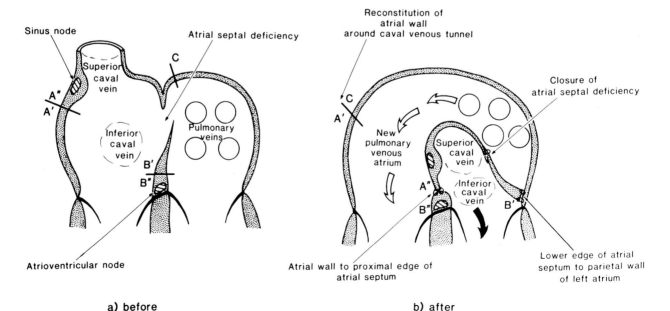

a) before   **b) after**

Figure 48.35. A diagrammatic representation of the Senning procedure. (a) The incisions made in the atrial walls and septum are shown. (b) The internalization of the systemic venous tributaries and reconstitution of the atrial wall (points A′ to C) can be seen.

ventricle, has more recently been suggested as a solution to the difficult problem of stenosis in the pulmonary venous pathway (de Jong et al, 1995).

A second major complication has been the development of serious postoperative atrial arrhythmias (El-Said et al, 1972; Isaacson et al, 1972; Clarkson et al, 1976; Saalouke et al, 1978). Analysis of these arrhythmias showed that, in most instances, they resulted from damage either to the sinus node or to its blood supply (Gillette et al, 1974, 1980). This was confirmed by subsequent anatomical studies (Edwards and Edwards, 1978; Bharati et al, 1979). Scrupulous avoidance of the area of the sinus node and its blood supply significantly reduced the incidence of arrhythmias (Ebert et al, 1974; Turley and Ebert, 1978; Ullal et al, 1979). Despite the most detailed attention to avoidance of these danger areas, including the artery to the sinus node (Barra Rossi et al, 1986), some patients continued to develop problems of rhythm after atrial redirection procedures (Janousek et al, 1994; Gelatt et al, 1997; Gewillig, 1998). In order to assess the incidence and significance of these problems accurately, it remains important to perform 24-hour recordings of the electrocardiogram. The detection of any arrhythmia is of concern in the light of the known incidence of sudden and unexpected death in postoperative patients (Deanfield et al, 1983). Even when the progressive loss of stable sinus rhythm is noted with time, however, no observations on standard or 24-hour electrocardiographic monitoring have so far identified those at risk for sudden death (Deanfield et al, 1988). Furthermore, electrophysiological studies of sinus nodal performance have been of little help in predicting those patients at high risk for serious arrhythmias. Consequently, there are no unequivocal criterions for prophylactic insertion of pacemakers in asymptomatic patients. It is generally accepted, nonetheless, that a pacemaker is indicated when 24-hour monitoring reveals long pauses of greater than 6 or more seconds, periods of severe bradycardia, or when a tachyarrhythmia requires drug therapy in the presence of episodes of profound bradycardia. Those arrhythmias that are associated with symptoms, such as syncope, should definitely be treated by insertion of a pacemaker.

A third major concern for patients after atrial redirection is the capability of the morphologically right ventricle to perform a systemic role over the long term. Various groups have identified abnormal right ventricular function in complete transposition, both before and after Mustard's operation (Graham et al, 1975; Hagler et al, 1978; Alpert et al, 1979; Arensman et al, 1983). It is still undecided if this depressed right ventricular function is related to the disease itself, to the surgery or to both. In the 100 patients of Oelert et al (1981) undergoing reinvestigation, impaired right ventricular function was found in only five. The follow-up of the patients initially reported by Ebert et al (1974) was also encouraging (O'Loughlin et al, 1983). More recent studies have shown preserved right ventricular function 10 years after surgery (Hochreiter et al, 1994), while reported instances of systemic right ventricular failure have been rare (Siebenmann, 1989). For the minority of patients with this complication, nonetheless, it is life threatening. It has been suggested that, for these patients, conversion to the arterial switch can be performed with reconstruction of the atrial septum. When the left ventricular pressure is high, this can be done directly. When the left ventricular pressure is low, the ventricle must be prepared by banding the pulmonary trunk (Cochrane et al, 1993). This strategy is not without risk but may be preferable to the alternative of heart transplantation (Uberfuhr et al, 1993). As Zuberbuhler (1983) commented, when summing-up the symposium published in the *American Journal of Cardiology*, 'My current attitude toward the Mustard operation is one of cautious optimism'. There is little evidence to warrant changing this prognosis. For patients with complete transposition and intact ventricular septum, therefore, the Mustard or Senning procedures were safe operations with excellent intermediate-term results. The long-term results are still being clarified, although a recent paper from New Zealand reported good survival after 28 years, with a 97% freedom from right ventricular failure (Wilson et al, 1998).

The results of atrial redirection procedures for patients with ventricular septal defect or left ventricular outflow tract obstruction were generally less good than when the ventricular septum was intact and there was no obstruction in the left ventricular outflow tract. In the best hands, the early results were still acceptable (Oelert et al, 1981), with survival rates in the region of 90%. When ventricular septal defects were associated with obstruction within the left ventricular outflow tract, most opted for the Rastelli procedure (see below), since it restored the left ventricle to the systemic role. In the past, however, some repaired this combination using the Mustard procedure, together with resection of the subpulmonary obstruction, albeit at a higher risk than for those with intact ventricular septum and no complications (Oelert et al, 1981). The Mustard procedure, combined with insertion of a conduit from the left ventricle to the pulmonary arteries, was also used with success for this combination (Crupi et al, 1979, 1985). Irrespective of the immediate results, there was generally an unacceptably high incidence of late complications. Particular problems were postoperative arrhythmias (Ullal et al, 1979) and tricuspid regurgitation (Tynan et al, 1972). The anatomy of the ventricular septal defect, which is frequently associated with malalignment of the muscular outlet septum and overriding of the pulmonary trunk, puts the tension apparatus of the tricuspid valve at risk in a large number of patients. If the tricuspid valve is damaged, this will increase the load on the morphologically right ventricle. Residual ventricular septal defects may also pose a haemodynamic problem. Overall, therefore, it was the poor results in those with ventricular septal defects that precipitated the move to arterial redirection.

THE ARTERIAL SWITCH OPERATION

Many investigators had considered and explored the possibility of correcting complete transposition by detaching the aorta and pulmonary trunk from their inappropriate ventricles and re-attaching them to their morphologically appropriate ventricles. Various ingenious manoeuvres were devised whereby the coronary arteries could then be relocated so as to receive their blood supply at systemic oxygen tension and pressure. These operations had proved uniformly fatal until Jatene reported the first success (Jatene et al, 1975). This caused considerable consternation when it was brought up in discussion at the second Henry Ford Symposium (1977). The surgical world was astounded. Jatene had successfully completed the procedure by translocating the coronary arteries to what had initially been the pulmonary trunk but which, after the arterial switch, was the base of the new aorta. Following this initial publication, others reported successful operations (Jatene et al, 1976, 1982; Ross et al, 1976; Yacoub et al, 1976). Four years later, in Amsterdam, Jatene presented a survey of the results for the arterial switch from 14 centres across the world. There were 54 deaths in 89 patients. The lowest mortality rate amongst those surveyed was 25%, and the highest was 100% (Jatene, 1981). Despite this, the arterial switch procedure retained its enthusiastic champions (Yacoub et al, 1982; Quaegebeur et al, 1986). Early versions of the operation had required a conduit to be placed between the 'new' pulmonary root and the pulmonary trunk. This had led to problems with obstruction in the newly created right ventricular outflow tract (Boyadjiev et al, 1990). To obviate the need to interpose such a conduit, an ingenious manoeuvre was described that liberated the posteriorly positioned bifurcation of the pulmonary trunk and threaded the aorta through it to gain access to the posterior arterial root (Lecompte et al, 1981). This manoeuvre then created sufficient length in

the pulmonary arteries for them to be anastomosed directly to the anterior arterial root. The 'French connection' is now almost invariably used. For the coronary arteries, they are detached from the initial aortic root together with a cuff of aortic wall, and the defects thus created are patched (Figure 48.36a). The coronary arteries are then reimplanted in the original pulmonary root, now the aortic arterial trunk (Figure 48.36b). The varied patterns of arterial supply in complete transposition have not prevented or compromised this transfer (Yacoub and Radley-Smith, 1978), although abnormal patterns proved to be risk factors (see below). Sometimes special procedures were required. Yacoub and Radley-Smith (1978) described the manoeuvre of turning a solitary coronary artery upside down during transfer. This option was further endorsed by Planché and his colleagues (1988). It was Brawn and Mee (1988), however, who pointed to the advantages gained from making a so-called 'trap door' incision hinged from a medial flap, and most surgeons now use this technique, or something similar. The most problematic cases, nonetheless, are the ones with an intramural course of a coronary artery (Gittenberger-de Groot et al, 1986). For many surgeons, identification of an intramural segment was considered justification for opting for an atrial redirection procedure (Day et al, 1992). The problem with this approach is that the intramural course remains after the atrial redirection, and such an arterial abnormality is known to be a risk for sudden death when found in the otherwise normally constructed heart (Mustafa et al, 1981). The innovative approach of Asou and colleagues (1994), permitting successful transfer of 12 examples of intramural arteries with varied anatomical patterns, seems much more preferable. Nowadays, therefore, it should prove possible to transfer all known patterns of origin of the coronary arteries. Indeed, it is fair to say that the surgical techniques have now become systematic (Brawn and Mee, 1988; Asou et al, 1994; Tamisier et al, 1997). Once

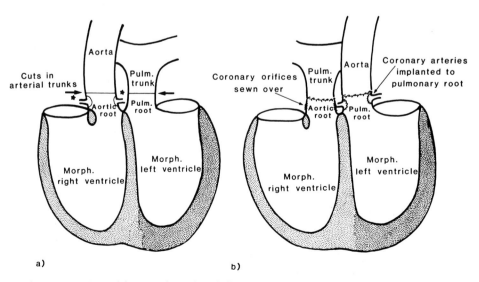

Figure 48.36. Diagrammatic representations of the arterial switch (a) before and (b) after the procedure. Morph., morphological; Pulm., pulmonary.

coronary arterial transfer is complete, the original aortic root is reconnected to the pulmonary trunk. Other ways to circumvent damage to the coronary arteries during relocation had been suggested (Aubert et al 1978) but have not been widely employed.

In the present era, in newborns with complete transposition and intact ventricular septum, and also in those with a ventricular septal defect, survival rates of greater than 90% are expected (Serraf et al, 1993; Wernovsky et al, 1995). Indeed, in the series reported by Asou et al (1994), including their 12 patients with intramural coronary arteries, overall survival was 96.7%. That the arterial switch is the treatment of choice has been reinforced by the demonstration in one institution of its superiority in the intermediate term over atrial redirection (Turley and Verrier, 1995). Questions do remain concerning its place in patients with organic subvalvar obstruction in the left ventricular outflow tract. Some patients may be suitable for the switch operation when the subvalvar stenosis can be resected in the presence of a normal pulmonary valve. When this is not the case, an alternative approach is needed, such as the Rastelli or REV operations (see below).

A further special circumstance is the patient with complete transposition and intact ventricular septum presenting later than the first month of life. In such patients, the left ventricular muscle mass may have involuted to such a degree that it is no longer able to support the systemic circulation. When this is the case, then the left ventricle has to be 'trained' to increase its mass. Banding the pulmonary trunk achieves this objective by increasing the left ventricular pressure, but it increases cyanosis. Therefore, in 1977, Yacoub and his colleagues suggested preparing the left ventricle with a combination of banding and placement of a shunt from a systemic to a pulmonary artery. These workers then waited several months before performing the arterial switch. More recently, it has been demonstrated that left ventricular hypertrophy occurs very rapidly; for example, left ventricular mass can double after a week in which the left ventricular pressure has been taken to 75% of systemic pressure by banding (Boutin et al, 1994). Nowadays, the interval between the preparatory procedure involving banding and shunting and the arterial switch has been reduced to 7 to 10 days, the so-called 'rapid two stage' approach (Jonas et al, 1989). This has the great advantage that the left ventricle, the function of which deteriorates after the preparatory banding, is no longer exposed to damage for longer than is absolutely necessary. An interesting new possibility for preparing the left ventricle is provided by raising the pulmonary arterial pressure by means of an indwelling balloon catheter introduced transvenously and inflated in the pulmonary trunk. This has been shown to induce right ventricular hypertrophy experimentally (Katayama et al, 1993) and has been used clinically in one patient (Bonhoeffer et al, 1992). The rapid two-stage arterial switch offers a good solution for patients presenting after the first month of life. Age is not the sole criterion for opting for two stages rather than primary arterial switch, since selected patients whose left ventricular pressures remain high (for example because of persistent patency of the arterial duct or dynamic obstruction of the left ventricular outflow tract) are suitable for primary repair. Most groups would perform the two-stage arterial switch if the patient was over 1 month of age, with a left ventricular pressure of less than 75% of systemic arterial pressure and a posterior left ventricular wall thickness less than 0.45 cm. Primary repair, nonetheless, has been achieved in infants up to 3 months of age in the presence of a relatively low left ventricular pressure (Davis et al, 1993).

As we have emphasized, pulmonary vascular disease develops rapidly in presence of a ventricular septal defect or an arterial duct sufficiently large to cause pulmonary hypertension. When vascular disease is established, the patients are no longer suitable candidates for corrective surgery. Providing the oxygen saturation in the pulmonary arteries is higher than that in the aorta, their condition can be ameliorated by redirecting the circulations but leaving open the ventricular septal defect or arterial duct. As a result of such rerouting, their systemic arterial oxygenation will be higher and their quality of life improved. Originally, this rerouting was achieved by atrial redirection (Lindesmith et al, 1972). Nowadays, a palliative arterial switch is employed (Pridjian et al, 1992).

The fate of the transplanted coronary arteries remains a cause of concern. The available data are somewhat conflicting. Defects in myocardial perfusion, as shown by radionuclide imaging, appear to be no more extensive or severe after the arterial switch operation than after other open heart procedures performed for congenital heart disease (Hayes et al, 1994). In contrast, occlusion or stenosis of coronary arteries revealed by coronary arteriography was found with some frequency in the patients studied by Bonnet et al (1996) from the cohort undergoing surgery in Paris. Disturbingly, many of the patients were asymptomatic. The problem in some of the patients could be traced to the technique used for surgical transfer of the coronary arteries, now discontinued in their centre. In many others, nonetheless, no cause could be identified. Late death has been associated with coronary stenosis (Tanel et al, 1995). Balloon coronary angioplasty has been used in the treatment of such coronary arterial stenosis after the switch (Hausdorf et al, 1995) and, by the time this book is published, stents will surely have been used.

Stenosis of the branches of the pulmonary arteries, often as a result of 'stretching' produced by the Lecompte procedure, is the second of the concerns. The true incidence of this complication is uncertain, but instances will be encountered in any centre performing this operation. Balloon angioplasty has been attempted for treatment, but most centres find it of little value. An exception is the Tokyo Womens' Medical College in Japan (Nakanishi et al, 1993). They report a 50% success rate and suggest that patients with an interval from operation of less than 3.5 years are most likely to have a successful outcome. Despite these data, most would recommend implantation of stents if relief is indicated.

The Rastelli procedure

The operation introduced by Rastelli et al (1969) specifically for those patients with a ventricular septal defect and obstruction in the subpulmonary outflow tract involves patching the ventricular septal defect to the right ventricular subaortic infundibulum. The pulmonary trunk is then ligated and divided, and an extracardiac conduit is placed between the right ventricle and the distal part of the divided pulmonary trunk (Figure 48.37). This operation, like the arterial switch procedure, has the advantage of restoring the left ventricle to its systemic role. For the procedure to be successful, the ventricular septal defect must be located so as to permit construction of a non-restrictive intracardiac tunnel extending to the subaortic infundibulum. This is usually possible in those patients with subpulmonary obstruction coexisting with a ventricular septal defect, since the outlet septum is deviated into the left ventricular outflow tract to produce the subpulmonary obstruction. The so-called malalignment defect is then ideally located to be connected surgically to the overriding aorta. In some patients, such a procedure may be compromised by tension apparatus of the tricuspid valve crossing the defect. Damage to these cords will then be of less significance than was the case after the Mustard procedure, since, postoperatively, the right ventricle will not be the systemic ventricle. If the outlet septum obstructs the intracardiac tunnel, it can safely be resected. The Rastelli procedure is less suitable for patients in whom pulmonary stenosis is associated with ventricular septal defects remote from the subaortic infundibulum, this arrangement precluding the construction of the required intraventricular tunnel.

In those patients suitable for the Rastelli operation, satisfactory results were reported up to the end of the 1970s (Marcelletti et al, 1976). The inevitable reoperation needed for replacement of the conduit, or closure of residual or recurrent ventricular septal defects, was usually achieved without mortality (McGoon et al, 1981). Subsequent to that time, there are various reports in textbooks of improved results (Stark and de Leval, 1994), but we have been unable to find any rigorous analysis of a large series of patients. The study reported by Vouhé and colleagues (1992) seems to be the most recent, but this questioned the place of the Rastelli procedure compared with 'reparation de l'etage ventriculaire' (the REV procedure; see below). Analysis of the patients undergoing surgery in Paris showed no difference between the two procedures in terms of risk factors or mortality, and the predicted survival in the latter part of the period of study was about 95%. The Rastelli procedure, therefore, now provides excellent results, but it does involve insertion of a prosthetic conduit. Ideally, it is performed between the ages of 4 and 6 years, when an adult-sized extracardiac conduit can be inserted. Even in these circumstances, late obstruction of the conduit by neointima with or without calcification is inevitable. Performance of the Rastelli carries with it the certainty that further operations will be needed during a normal life span.

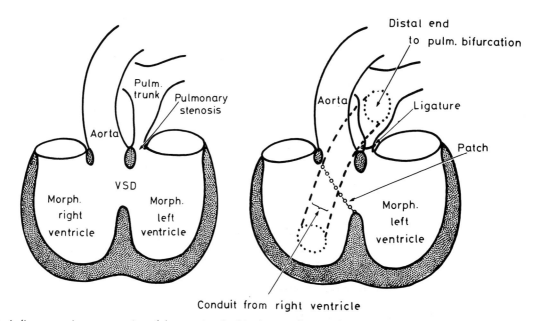

Figure 48.37. A diagrammatic representation of the steps involved in the Rastelli procedure. Morph., morphological; Pulm., pulmonary; VSD, ventricular septal defect.

The place for intraventricular repair for patients who have complete transposition with ventricular septal defect but no subpulmonary obstruction is not yet established. Patients do exist in which it would be possible to construct a tunnel between the ventricular septal defect and the subaortic infundibulum, but it is questionable if such patients could be tided over until the ideal age for insertion of a conduit in order to make the needed connection from the right ventricle to the pulmonary trunk. The anatomy in a very small number of patients may potentially permit construction of an intraventricular patch so that blood can be directed to the appropriate arterial trunks without having to insert an extracardiac conduit. Such an operation, mentioned briefly by Senning in 1959, had been performed in a solitary patient at the Mayo Clinic at the age of 2 years (McGoon, 1972). Subsequently, it became necessary to insert an extracardiac conduit for relief of acquired subpulmonary obstruction. Another patient in whom the procedure was attempted did not survive the operation. Since then, we are unaware of any significant experience with use of the so-called 'boomerang' patch (McGoon et al, 1981).

The REV procedure

The REV procedure consists of resection of the muscular outlet septum, suturing of an intraventricular baffle to direct blood from the left ventricle to the aorta and reconstruction of the pulmonary outflow tract by direct implantation of the posterior rim of the pulmonary arterial trunk to a right ventriculotomy, the anterior wall being completed by a patch. In most cases, the pulmonary bifurcation is translocated anterior to the ascending aorta (Figure 48.38). Following its original description (Lecompte et al, 1982), a larger series reporting good results in terms of both operative mortality and short-term clinical benefit was published by Rubay et al (1988). As already discussed, the results now obtained in Paris are in no way inferior to those achieved with the Rastelli operation (Vouhé et al, 1992). Choice between the procedures, therefore, will depend on the confidence of the surgeon; however, avoiding the need for a conduit must weigh in favour of the REV procedure.

The Damus–Stansel–Kaye procedure

The Damus–Stansel–Kaye operation, devised independently by its three eponymous originators, was designed to produce anatomical correction without the need to transplant the coronary arteries from the aortic to the pulmonary root (Figure 48.39). The pulmonary trunk is transected and its proximal end is attached in end-to-side fashion to the aorta. A conduit is then placed from the right ventricle to the distal end of the pulmonary trunk. A ventricular septal defect, if present, is closed. This permits the coronary arteries to be perfused retrogradely through the aortic root, which retains its connection to the ascending aorta, the left ventricular blood entering via the pulmonary root. Most experience with this procedure applied to patients with complete transposition came from the Mayo Clinic (Ceithaml et al, 1984). It was not widely adopted, although the concept is still used as a means of bypassing obstruction at the level of the ventricular septal defect in patients with univentricular atrioventricular connection.

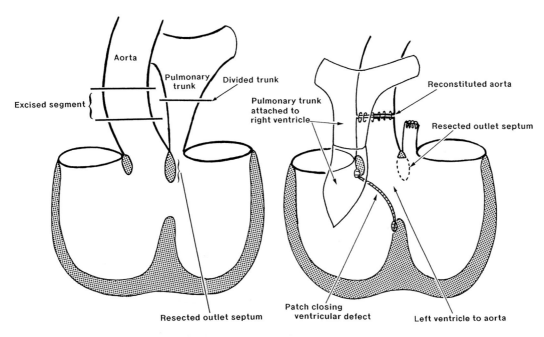

a) Initial morphology and preparatory procedures

b) Completed procedure

Figure 48.38. A diagrammatic representation of the REV (reparation de l'etage ventriculaire) procedure.

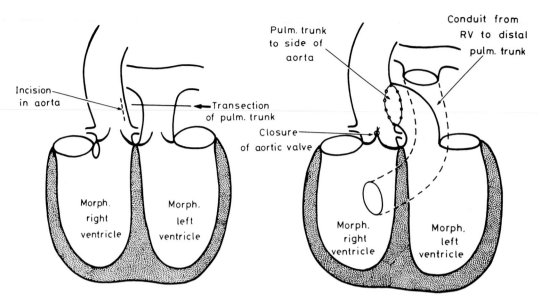

Figure 48.39. A diagrammatic representation of the steps involved in the Damus–Stansel–Kaye procedure.

REFERENCES

Abdulhamed J M, Yousef S A, Ali Khan M A, Mullins C 1994 Balloon dilatation of complete obstruction of the superior vena cava after Mustard operation for transposition of the great arteries. British Heart Journal 72: 482–485

Abinader E, Zeltzer M, Riss E 1970 Transumbilical atrial septostomy in the newborn. American Journal of Diseases of Childhood 119: 354–355

Albert H M 1955 Surgical correction of transposition of the great arteries. Surgical Forum 5: 75–77

Allan L D, Leanage R, Wainwright R, Joseph M C, Tynan M 1982 Balloon atrial septostomy under two dimensional echocardiographic control. British Heart Journal 47: 41–43

Allan L D, Sharland G K, Milburn A et al 1994 Prospective diagnosis of 1006 cases of congenital heart disease in the fetus. Journal of the American College of Cardiology 23: 1452–1458

Alpert B S, Bloom K R, Olley P M, Trusler G A, Williams C M, Rowe R D 1979 Echocardiographic evaluation of right ventricular function in complete transposition of the great arteries: angiographic correlates. American Journal of Cardiology 44: 270–275

Amato J J, Galdieri R J 1991 The arterial switch: surgical technique in respect to coronary artery patterns. In: D'Lessandro L C (ed.) Heart surgery 1991. Casa Editrice Scientifica Internazionale, Rome, p 237–248

Amato J J, Zelen J, Bushong J 1994 Coronary arterial patterns in complete transposition – classification in relation to the arterial switch procedure. Cardiology in the Young 4: 329–339

Anderson R H 1978 Another look at cardiac embryology. In: Yu P N, Goodwin J F (eds) Progress in cardiology, vol 7. Lea & Febiger, New York, p 1–53

Anderson R H 1991 Description of the origins and epicardial course of the coronary arteries in complete transposition. 1: 11–12

Anderson R H, Wilkinson J L, Arnold R, Becker A E, Lubkiewicz K 1974 Morphogenesis of bulboventricular malformations. II. Observations on malformed hearts. British Heart Journal 36: 948–970

Angelini P, Leachman R D 1976 Spectrum of double outlet right ventricle: an embryologic interpretation. Cardiovascular diseases. Bulletin of the Texas Heart Institute 3: 127–149

Arciprete P, Macartney F J, de Leval M, Stark J 1985 Mustard's operation for patients with ventriculo-arterial concordance: report of two cases and a cautionary tale. British Heart Journal 53: 443–450

Arensman F W, Radley-Smith R, Yacoub M H et al 1983 Catheter evaluation of left ventricular shape and function 1 or more years after anatomic correction of transposition of the great arteries. American Journal of Cardiology 52: 1079–1083

Asou T, Karl T R, Pawade A, Mee R B B 1994 Arterial switch: translocation of the intramural coronary artery. Annals of Thoracic Surgery 57: 461–465

Aubert J, Pannetier A, Couvelly J P, Unal D, Rouault F, Delarue A 1978 Transposition of the great arteries. New technique for anatomical correction: case report. British Heart Journal 40: 204–208

Aziz K U, Paul M H, Idriss F S, Wilson A D, Muster A J 1979 Clinical manifestations of dynamic left ventricular outflow tract stenosis in infants with d-transposition of the great arteries with intact ventricular septum. American Journal of Cardiology 44: 290–297

Baillie M 1797 The morbid anatomy of the most important parts of the human body, 2nd edn. Johnson & Nicol, London, p 38

Baker E J, Allan L D, Tynan M J, Jones O D H, Joseph M C, Deverall P B 1984 Balloon atrial septostomy in the neonatal intensive care unit. British Heart Journal 51: 377–378

Bano-Rodrigo A, Quero-Jimenez M, Moreno-Granado F, Gamallo-Amat G 1980 Wall thickness of ventricular chambers in transposition of the great arteries. Journal of Thoracic and Cardiovascular Surgery 79: 592–597

Barra Rossi M B, Ho S Y, Anderson R H, Rossi Filho R I, Lincoln C 1986 Coronary arteries in complete transposition–the significance of the sinus node artery. Annals of Thoracic Surgery 42: 573–577

Beitzke A, Suppan C H 1983 Use of prostaglandin E$_2$ in management of transposition of great arteries before balloon atrial septostomy. British Heart Journal 49: 341–344

Bender H W Jr, Graham T P, Boucek R J Jr, Walker W E, Boerth R G 1980 Comparative operative results of the Senning and Mustard procedures for transposition of the great arteries. Circulation 62: 1197–1203

Bentovim A 1983 Psychiatric and intellectual assessment. In: Anderson R H, Macartney F J, Shinebourne E A, Tynan M (eds) Paediatric cardiology, vol 3. Churchill Livingstone, Edinburgh, p 309–316

Bharati S, Lev M 1976 The conduction system in double outlet right ventricle with sub-pulmonic ventricular septal defect and related hearts (the Taussig–Bing group). Circulation 54: 459–466

Bharati S, Molthan M E, Veasy G, Lev M 1979 Conduction system in two cases of sudden death after the Mustard procedure. Journal of Thoracic and Cardiovascular Surgery 77: 101–108

Bierman F Z, Williams R G 1979 Prospective diagnosis of d-transposition of the great arteries in neonates by subxiphoid, two-dimensional echocardiography. Circulation 60: 1496–1502

Blalock A, Hanlon C R 1950 The surgical treatment of complete transposition of the aorta and pulmonary artery. Surgery 90: 1–15

Boesen I B 1963 Complete transposition of the great vessels: importance of septal defects and patent ductus arteriosus. Analysis of 132 patients dying before age 14. Circulation 28: 885–887

Bonhoeffer P, Carminati M, Parenzan L, Tynan M 1992 Non-surgical left ventricular preparation for arterial switch in transposition of the great arteries. Lancet 340: 549–550

Bonnet D, Bonhoeffer P, Piechaud J F et al 1996 Long-term fate of the coronary arteries after the arterial switch operation in newborns with transposition of the great arteries. Heart 76: 274–279

Boutin C, Jonas R A, Sanders S P, Wernovsky G, Mone S M, Colan S D 1994 Rapid two-stage arterial switch operation: acquisition of left ventricular mass after pulmonary artery banding in infants with transposition of the great arteries. Circulation 90: 1304–1309

Boyadjiev K, Ho S Y, Anderson R H, Lincoln C 1990 The potential for subpulmonary obstruction in complete transposition after the arterial switch procedure. An anatomic study. European Journal of Cardiothoracic Surgery 4: 214–218

Brawn W J, Mee R B B 1988 Early results for anatomic correction of transposition of the great arteries and for double-outlet right ventricle with subpulmonary ventricular septal defect. Journal of Thoracic and Cardiovascular Surgery 95: 230–238

Brom A G 1981 The Senning operation in the surgical treatment of complete transposition. In: Becker A E

Losekoot T G, Marcelletti C, Anderson R H (eds) Paediatric cardiology, vol 3. Churchill Livingstone, Edinburgh, p 211–217

Brown S C, Eyskens B, Mertens L, Stockx L, Dumoulin M, Gewillig M 1998 Self expandable stents for the relief of venous baffle obstruction after the Mustard operation. Heart 79: 230–233

Buchler J R, Bembom J C, Buchler R D 1984 Transposition of the great arteries with posterior aorta and subaortic conus: anatomical and surgical correlation. International Journal of Cardiology 5: 13–18

Campbell J A, Bing R J, Handelsman J C, Groswold H E, Hammond M 1949 Physiological studies in congenital heart disease. VIII. The physiological findings in two patients with complete transposition of the great vessels. Johns Hopkins Hospital Reports 84: 269–278

Cardell B S 1956 Corrected transposition of the great vessels. British Heart Journal 18: 186–192

Carlgren L E 1969 The incidence of congenital heart disease in Gothenberg. The third Edgar Mannheimer memorial lecture. Proceedings of the Association of European Paediatric Cardiologists 5: 2–8

Carr I 1971 Timing of bidirectional atrial shunts in transposition of the great arteries and atrial septal defect. Circulation 44 (suppl II): 70

Carr I, Wells B 1966 Coaxial flow-guided catheterization of the pulmonary artery in transposition of the great arteries. Lancet ii: 318–319

Carr I, Tynan M J, Aberdeen E, Bonham-Carter R E, Graham G, Waterston D J 1968 Predictive accuracy of the loop rule in 109 children with classical complete transposition of the great arteries. Circulation 38 (suppl VI): 52

Carrel T, Serraf A, Lacour-Gayet F et al 1996 Transposition of the great arteries complicated by tricuspid valve incompetence. Annals of Thoracic Surgery 61: 940–944

Ceithaml E L, Puga F J, Danielson G K, McGoon D C, Ritter D G 1984 Results of the Damus–Stansel–Kaye procedure of transposition of great arteries and for double outlet right ventricle with subpulmonary ventricular septal defect. Annals of Thoracic Surgery 38: 433–437

Champsaur G L, Sokol D M, Trusler G A, Mustard W T 1973 Repair of transposition of the great arteries in 123 paediatric patients: early and long-term results. Circulation 47: 1032–1041

Chiu I-S, Anderson R H, Macartney F J, de Leval M, Stark J 1984 Morphologic features of an intact ventricular septum susceptible to subpulmonary obstruction in complete transposition. American Journal of Cardiology 53: 1633–1638

Clarkson P M, Barratt-Boyes B G, Neutze J M, Lowe J B 1972 Results over a ten-year period of palliation followed by corrective surgery for complete transposition of the great arteries. Circulation 45: 1251–1258

Clarkson P M, Barratt-Boyes B G, Neutze J M 1976 Late dysrhythmias and disturbances of conduction following Mustard operation for complete transposition of the great arteries. Circulation 53: 519–524

Cochrane A D, Karl T R, Mee R B B 1993 Staged conversion to arterial switch for late failure of the systemic right ventricle. Annals of Thoracic Surgery 56: 854–861

Colan S D, Boutin C, Castaneda A R, Wernovsky G 1995 Status of the left ventricle after arterial switch operation for transposition of the great arteries. Hemodynamic and echocardiographic evaluation. Journal of Thoracic and Cardiovascular Surgery 109: 311–321

Counahan R, Simon G, Joseph M 1973 The plain chest radiograph in d-transposition of the great arteries in the first month of life. Pediatric Radiology 1: 217–223

Crupi G C, Anderson R H, Ho S Y, Lincoln C 1979 Complete transposition of the great arteries with intact ventricular septum and left ventricular outflow tract obstruction: surgical treatment and anatomical considerations. Journal of Thoracic and Cardiovascular Surgery 78: 730–738

Crupi G C, Pillai R, Parenzan L, Lincoln C 1985 Surgical treatment of sub-pulmonary obstruction in transposition of the great arteries by means of a left ventricular–pulmonary conduit. Late results and further considerations. Journal of Thoracic and Cardiovascular Surgery 89: 207–913

Daskalopoulos D A, Edwards W D, Driscoll D J, Seward J B, Tajik A J, Hagler D J 1983 Correlation of two-dimensional echocardiographic and autopsy findings in complete transposition of the great arteries. Journal of the American College of Cardiologists 2: 1151–1157

Davis A M, Wilkinson J L, Karl T R, Mee R B B 1993 Transposition of the great arteries with intact ventricular septum. Arteial switch repair in patients 21 days of age or older. Journal of Thoracic and Cardiovascular Surgery 106: 111–115

Day R W, Laks H, Drinkwater D C 1992 The influence of coronary anatomy on the arterial switch operation in neonates. Journal of Thoracic and Cardiovascular Surgery 104: 706–712

Deanfield J, Camm J, Macartney F et al 1983 Arrhythmia after interatrial repair of transposition: relation to sudden death. Circulation 68(Suppl III): 328

Deanfield J, Camm J, Macartney F et al 1988 Arrhythmia and late mortality after Mustard and Senning operation for transposition of the great arteries. Journal of Thoracic and Cardiovascular Surgery 96: 569–576

de Jong P L, Bogers A J, Witsenburg M, Bos E 1995 Arterial switch for pulmonary venous obstruction complicating Mustard procedure. Annals of Thoracic Surgery 59: 1005–1007

de la Cruz M V, da Rocha J P 1956 An ontogenetic theory for the explanation of congenital malformations involving the truncus and conus. American Heart Journal 51: 782–805

de la Cruz M V, Arteaga M, Espino-Vela J, Quero-Jimenez M, Anderson R H, Diaz G F 1981 Complete transposition of the great arteries: types and morphogenesis of ventriculoarterial discordance. American Heart Journal 102: 271–281

Deverall P B, Tynan M J, Carr I et al 1969 Palliative surgery in children with transposition of the great arteries. Journal of Thoracic and Cardiovascular Surgery 58: 721–729

Ebert P A, Gay W A Jr, Engle M A 1974 Correction of transposition of the great arteries. Relationship of the coronary sinus and postoperative arrhythmias. Annals of Surgery 180: 433–438

Edwards W D, Edwards J E 1978 Pathology of the sinus node in d-transposition following the Mustard operation. Journal of Thoracic and Cardiovascular Surgery 75: 213–218

Elkins R C, Knot-Craig C J, Ahn J H et al 1994 Ventricular function after the arterial switch operation for

transposition of the great arteries. Annals of Thoracic Surgery 57: 826–831

Elliott L P, Neufeld H N, Anderson R C, Adams P, Edwards J E 1963 Complete transposition of the great vessels. 1. An anatomic study of sixty cases. Circulation 27: 1105–1117

El-Said G, Rosenberg H S, Mullins C E, Hallman G L, Colley D A, McNamara D G 1972 Dysrhythmias after Mustard's operation for transposition of the great arteries. American Journal of Cardiology 30: 526–532

Farre J R 1814 Pathological research. In: Malformations of the heart. Longman, Hurst, Orm & Brown, London, p 1–46

Ferencz C 1966 Transposition of the great vessels: pathophysiologic considerations based upon a study of the lungs. Circulation 33: 232–241

Fouron J-C, Vallot F, Bourlon F, Lombaert M, Ducharme G, Davignon A 1980 Isovolumic contraction time of right ventricle in d-transposition of great arteries. British Heart Journal 44: 204–207

Fraser F C, Hunter A D W 1975 Etiologic relations among categories of congenital heart malformations. American Journal of Cardiology 36: 793–796

Geipel P 1903 Weitere Beitrage zum Situs Transversus und zur Lehre von den Transpositionen der grossen Gefasse des Herzens. Archiv für Kinderheilkunde 35: 112–161

Gelatt M, Hamilton R M, McCrindle B et al 1997 Arrhythmia and mortality after the Mustard procedure: a 30-year single-center experience. Journal of the American College of Cardiology 29: 194–201

Gewillig M 1998 The Mustard and Senning procedures: long-term follow-up of rhythm. In: Redington A N, Brawn W J, Deanfield J E, Anderson R H (eds) The right heart in congenital heart disease. G M M, London, p 197–201

Gillette P C, El-Said G M, Sivarajan N, Mullins C E, Williams R L, McNamara D G 1974 Electrophysiological abnormalities after Mustard's operation for transposition of the great arteries. British Heart Journal 36: 186–191

Gillette P C, Kugler J D, Garson A Jr, Gutgesell H P, Duff D F, McNamara D G 1980 Mechanisms of cardiac arrhythmias after the Mustard operation for transposition of the great arteries. American Journal of Cardiology 45: 1225–1230

Gittenberger-de Groot A C 1986 Elucidating coronary arterial anatomy or simplifying coronary arterial nomenclature. (Editorial note) International Journal of Cardiology 12: 305–308

Gittenberger-de Groot A C, Sauer U, Oppenheimer-Dekker A, Quaegbeur J 1983 Coronary arterial anatomy in transposition of the great arteries: a morphologic study. Pediatric Cardiology 4(suppl I): 15–24

Gittenberger-de Groot A C, Sauer U, Quaegbeur J 1986 Aortic intramural coronary artery in three hearts with transposition of the great arteries. Journal of Thoracic and Cardiovascular Surgery 91: 566–571

Goor D A, Edwards J E 1973 The spectrum of transposition of the great arteries, with special reference to developmental anatomy of the conus. Circulation 48: 406–415

Graham T P Jr 1981 Myocardial functional abnormalities in congenital heart disease–effects of cyanosis and abnormal loading conditions. In: Godman M J (ed.) Paediatric cardiology, vol 4. Churchill Livingstone, Edinburgh, p 102–116

Graham T P Jr, Atwood G F, Bouchek R J Jr, Boerth R C, Bender H W Jr 1975 Abnormalities of right ventricular function following Mustard's operation for transposition of the great arteries. Circulation 52: 678–684

Grant R P 1962 The morphogenesis of transposition of the great vessels. Circulation 26: 819–840

Guerin R, Soto B, Karp R B, Kirklin J W, Barcia A 1970 Transposition of the great arteries. Determination of the position of the great arteries in conventional chest roentgenograms. American Journal of Roentgenology, Radium Therapy and Nuclear Medicine 110: 747–756

Hagler D J, Ritter D G, Mair D D, Davis G D, McGoon D C 1978 Clinical, angiographic, hemodynamic assessment of late results after Mustard's operation. Circulation 57: 1214–1220

Harris J S, Farber S 1939 Transposition of the great cardiac vessels. Archives of Pathology and Laboratory Medicine 28: 427–502

Hausdorf G, Kampmann C, Schneider M 1995 Coronary angioplasty for coronary stenosis after the arterial switch procedure. American Journal of Cardiology 76: 612–613

Haworth S G 1983 Morphological changes and progression of pulmonary vascular disease. In: Anderson R H, Macartney F J, Shinebourne E A, Tynan M (eds) Paediatric cardiology, vol 5. Churchill Livingstone, Edinburgh, p 51–61

Hayes A M, Baker E J, Kakadeker A et al 1994 Influence of anatomic correction for transposition of the great arteries on myocardial perfusion: radionuclide imaging with technetium-99m 2-methoxy isobutyl isonitritle. Journal of the American College of Cardiology 24: 769–777

Hochreiter C, Snyder M S, Borer J S, Engle M A 1994 Right and left ventricular performance 10 years after Mustard repair of transposition of the great arteries. American Journal of Cardiology 74: 478–482

Hoffheinz H Z, Glaser E, Rodewald G 1964 Uber die Haufigheit angeborener im Hamburger Sektionsgut. Zentralblatt für Chirurgie 89: 326–340

Houyel L, Van Praagh R, Lacour-Gayet F et al 1995 Transposition of the great arteries (S,D,L): pathologic anatomy, diagnosis, and surgical management of a newly recognized complex. Journal of Thoracic and Cardiovascular Surgery 110: 613–624

Hoyer M H, Zuberbuhler J R, Anderson R H, del Nido P 1992 Morphology of ventricular septal defects in complete transposition. Surgical implications. Journal of Thoracic and Cardiovascular Surgery 194: 1203–1211

Huhta J C, Edwards W D, Danielson G K, Feldt R H 1982 Abnormalities of the tricuspid valve in complete transposition of the great arteries with ventricular septal defect. Journal of Thoracic and Cardiovascular Surgery 83: 569–576

Isaacson R, Titus J L, Meridith J, Feldt R H, McGoon D C 1972 Apparent interruption of atrial conduction pathways after surgical repair of transposition of the great arteries. American Journal of Cardiology 30: 533–535

Janousek J, Paul T, Luhmer I, Wilken M, Hruda J, Kallfelz H C 1994 Atrial baffle procedures for complete transposition of the great arteries: natural course of sinus node dysfunction and risk factors for dysrhythmias and sudden death. Zeitschrift für Kardiologie 83: 933–938

Jatene A D 1977 Report. In: Davila J C (ed.) 2nd Henry Ford international symposium on cardiac surgery. Appleton-Century-Crofts, New York, p 335

Jatene A D 1981 The switch operation for complete transposition. In: Becker A G, Losekoot T G, Marcelletti C, Anderson R H (eds) Paediatric cardiology, vol 3. Churchill Livingstone, Edinburgh, p 218–224

Jatene A D, Fontes V F, Paulista P P et al 1975 Successful anatomic correction of the great vessels. A preliminary report. Arquivos Brasilieros Cardiologia 28: 461–465

Jatene A D, Fontes V F, Paulista P P et al 1976 Anatomic correction of transposition of the great vessels. Journal of Thoracic and Cardiovascular Surgery 72: 364–370

Jatene A D, Fontes V F, Souza L C B, Paulista P P, Abdulmassih Neto C, Sousa J E M R 1982 Anatomic correction of transposition of the great arteries. Journal of Thoracic and Cardiovascular Surgery 83: 20–26

Jonas R A, Giglia T M, Sanders S P et al 1989 Rapid, two-stage arterial switch for transposition of the great arteries and intact ventricular septum beyond the neonatal period. Circulation 80(Suppl I): 203–208

Jones M, Ferrans V J 1977 Myocardial degeneration in congenital heart disease. American Journal of Cardiology 39: 1051–1063

Katayama H, Krzeski R, Frantz E G et al 1993 Induction of right ventricular hypertrophy with obstructing balloon catheter. Nonsurgical ventricular preparation for the arterial switch operation in simple transposition. Circulation 88(suppl I): 765–769

Keith A 1909 Hunterian lectures on malformations of the heart. Lancet ii: 433–435

Kidd B S L 1976 The fate of children with transposition of the great arteries following balloon atrial septostomy. In: Kidd B S L, Rowe R D (eds) The child and congenital heart disease after surgery. Futura, New York, p 153–164

Kirklin J W, Blackstone E H, Tchervenkov C I, Casteñeda A R 1992 Clinical outcomes after the arterial switch operation for transposition. Patient, support, procedural, and institutional risk factors. Congenital Heart Surgeons Society. Circulation 86: 1501–1515

Kovalchin J P, Allen H D, Cassidy S C, Lev M, Bharati S 1994 Pulmonary valve eccentricity in d-transposition of the arteries and implications for the arterial switch operation. American Journal of Cardiology 73: 186–190

Kurosawa H, Imai Y, Kawada M 1991 Coronary arterial anatomy in regard to the arterial switch procedure. Cardiology in the Young 1: 54–62

Lakier J B, Stanger P, Heymann M A, Hoffman J I E, Rudolph A M 1975 Early onset of pulmonary vascular obstruction in patients with aortopulmonary transposition and intact ventricular septum. Circulation 51: 875–880

Langstaff 1811 Case of a singular malformation of the heart. London Medical Review 4: 88

Leanage R, Agnetti A, Graham G, Taylor J, Macartney F J 1981 Factors influencing survival after balloon atrial septostomy for complete transposition of great arteries. British Heart Journal 45: 559–572

Lecompte Y, Zannini L, Hazan E et al 1981 Anatomic correction of transposition of the great arteries. New technique without use of a prosthetic conduit. Journal of Thoracic and Cardiovascular Surgery 82: 629–631

Lecompte Y, Neveux J Y, Leca F et al 1982 Reconstruction of the pulmonary outflow tract without prosthetic conduit. Journal of Thoracic and Cardiovascular Surgery 84: 727–733

Lev M, Rowlatt U F, Rimoldi H J A 1961 Pathologic methods for study of congenitally malformed hearts. Methods of electrocardiographic and physiologic correlation. Archives of Pathology 72: 493–511

Li J, Tulloh R M R, Cook A, Schneider M, Ho S Y, Anderson R H 2000 Coronary arterial origins in complete transposition. Heart in press

Liebman J, Cullum L, Belloc N 1969 Natural history of transposition of the great arteries: Anatomy, birth history and death characteristics. Circulation 40: 237–262

Lincoln C, Hasse J, Anderson R H, Shinebourne E A 1976 Surgical correction in complete levotransposition of the great arteries with an unusual subaortic ventricular septal defect. American Journal of Cardiology 38: 344–451

Lindesmith G G, Stiles Q R, Tucker B L, Gallaher M E, Stanton R E, Meyer B W 1972 The Mustard operation as a palliative procedure. Journal of Thoracic and Cardiovascular Surgery 63: 75–80

Locatelli G, Crupi G C, Villani M, Tiraboschi T, Vanini V, Parenzan L 1978 L'operazione di Senning nelle correzione della transposizione dei grossi vasi. Giornale Italiano di Cardiolgia 8: 299–308

Los J A 1976 Een eenvoigig ruimtelijk schema voor het classificeren van stoornissen in het scpteringproces van het menselijke hart naar morfogenetische criteria. Nederlandsch Tijdschrift Geneeskunde 120: 100–105

Macartney F J, Scott O, Deverall P B, Hepburn F 1975 New preformed catheter for entry into pulmonary artery in complete transposition of great arteries. British Heart Journal 37: 527–529

Macartney F J, Taylor J F N, Graham G R, de Leval M, Stark J 1980 The fate of survivors in cardiac surgery in infancy. Circulation 62: 80–91

MacLellan-Tolbert S G, Cetta F, Hagler D J 1996 Use of intravascular stents for superior vena caval obstruction after the Mustard operation. Mayo Clinic Proceedings 71: 1071–1076

MacMahon B, McKeown T, Record R G 1953 The incidence and life expectation of children with congenital heart disease. British Heart Journal 15: 121–129

Mair D D, Ritter D G 1972 Factors influencing intercirculatory mixing in patients with complete transposition of the great arteries. American Journal of Cardiology 30: 653–658

Mair D D, Macartney F J, Weidman W H, Ritter D G, Ongley P A, Smith R E 1970 The vectorcardiogram in complete transposition of the great arteries. Correlation with anatomic and haemodynamic findings and calculated left ventricular mass. Journal of Electrocardiology 3: 217–219

Mair D D, Danielson G K, Wallace R B, McGoon D C 1974 Long term follow up of Mustard operation survivors. Circulation 50 (suppl II): 46–53

Marcelletti C, Mair D D, McGoon D C, Wallace R B, Danielson G K 1976 The Rastelli operation for transposition of the great arteries. Journal of Thoracic and Cardiovascular Surgery 72: 427–434

Manner J 1998 The origin and course of the coronary vessels: embryological considerations. (Letter) Cardiology in the Young 8: 534–535

Marx G R, Hougen T J, Norwood W I, Fyler D G, Castañeda A R, Nadas A S 1983 Transposition of the great arteries with intact ventricular septum: results of Mustard and Senning operations in 123 consecutive patients. Journal of the American College of Cardiology 1: 476–483

Mathew R, Rosenthal A, Fellows K 1974 The significance of right aortic arch in d-transposition of the great arteries. American Heart Journal 87: 314–317

McGoon D C 1972 Intraventricular repair of transposition of the great arteries. Journal of Thoracic and Cardiovascular Surgery 64: 430–434

McGoon D C, Danielson G K, Wallace R B, Puga F J 1981 Surgical options for complicated complete transposition of great arteries. In: Becker A E, Losekoot T G, Marcelletti C, Anderson R H (eds) Paediatric cardiology, vol 3. Churchill Livingstone, Edinburgh, p 245–255

Milanesi O, Thiene G, Bini R M, Pellegrino P A 1982 Complete transposition of great arteries with coarctation of aorta. British Heart Journal 48: 566–571

Milo S, Ho S Y, Macartney F J et al 1979 Straddling and overriding atrioventricular valves: morphology and classification. American Journal of Cardiology 44: 1122–1134

Monckeberg J G 1924 Die Missbildungen des Herzens. In: Henke F, Lubarsch J (eds) Handbuch der speciellen pathologischen Anatomie und Histologie, vol 2. Springer, Berlin

Mortera C, Hunter S, Tynan M 1979 Contrast echocardiography and the suprasternal approach in infants and children. European Journal of Cardiology 9: 437–454

Murphy J H, Barlai-Kovach M, Mathews R A et al 1983 Rest and exercise right and left ventricular function late after the Mustard operation: Assessment by radionuclide ventriculography. American Journal of Cardiology 51: 1520–1525

Mustafa I, Gula G, Radley-Smith R, Durrer S, Yacoub M 1981 Anomalous origin of the left coronary artery from the anterior aortic sinus: a potential cause of sudden death. Journal of Thoracic and Cardiovascular Surgery 82: 297–300

Mustard W T, Keith J D, Trusler G A, Fowler R, Kidd L 1964 The surgical management of transposition of the great vessels. Journal of Thoracic and Cardiovascular Surgery 48: 953–958

Muster A J, Paul M H, van Grondelle A, Conway J J 1976 Asymmetrical distribution of pulmonary blood flow between the right and left lungs in d-transposition of the great arteries. American Journal of Cardiology 38: 352–361

Nakanishi T, Matsumoto Y, Seguchi M, Nakasawa M, Imai Y, Momma K 1993 Balloon angioplasty for postoperative pulmonary artery stenosis in transposition of the great arteries. Journal of the American College of Cardiology 22: 859–866

Newburger J W, Silbert A R, Buckley L P, Fyler D C 1984 Cognitive function and age at repair of transposition of the great arteries in children. New England Journal of Medicine 310: 1495–1499

Newfeld E A, Paul M H, Muster A J, Idriss F S 1974 Pulmonary vascular disease in complete transposition of the great arteries. A study of 200 cases. American Journal of Cardiology 34: 75–82

Newfeld E A, Paul M H, Muster A J, Idriss F S 1979 Pulmonary vascular disease in transposition of the great vessels and intact ventricular septum. Circulation 59: 525–530

Nogrady M B, Dunbar J S 1969 Complete transposition of the great vessels: re-evaluation of the so-called 'typical configuration' on plain films of the chest. Journal of the Canadian Association of Radiologists 20: 124–131

Oelert H, Borst H G 1979 Transmitral resection of subpulmonary stenosis in transposition of the great arteries. Thoracic and Cardiovascular Surgeon 27: 58–60

Oelert H, Schaps D, Luhmer I, Kalifelz H C, Borst H G 1981 Five years' experience with the Mustard operation. In: Becker A E, Losekoot T G, Marcelletti C, Anderson R H (eds) Paediatric Cardiology, vol 3. Churchill Livingstone, Edinburgh, p 200–210

Okamoto N, Satow Y, Hidaka N, Akimoto N 1980 Anomalous development of the conotruncus in neutron-irradiated rats. In: Van Praagh R, Takao A (eds) Etiology and morphogenesis of congenital heart disease. Futura, New York, p 195–214

O'Loughlin J E, Engle M A, Gay W A Jr, Klein A A, Ehlers K H, Levin A R 1983 Modified Mustard operation for simple and complex transposition of the great arteries –5–11 year follow-up. In: Engel M A, Perloff J K (eds) Congenital heart disease after surgery. Yorke Medical, New York, p 210–226

Oppenheimer-Dekker A 1978 Interventricular communications in transposition of the great arteries. In: Van Mierop L H S, Oppenheimer-Dekker A, Bruins C L D C H (eds) Embryology and tetratology of the heart and the great arteries. Boerhaave Series 13. Leiden University Press, the Hague, p 139–159

Park S C, Neches W H, Mullins C E et al 1982 Blade atrial septostomy: collaborative study. Circulation 66: 258–266

Parr G V S, Waldhausen J A, Bharati S, Lev M, Fripp R, Whitman V 1983 Coarctation in Taussing–Bing malformation of the heart. Surgical significance. Journal of Thoracic and Cardiovascular Surgery 86: 280–287

Pasquini L, Parness I A, Colan S D, Wernovsky G, Mayer J E, Sanders S P 1993 Diagnosis of intramural coronary artery in transposition of the great arteries using two-dimensional echocardiography Circulation 88: 1136–1141

Pasquini L, Sanders S P, Parness I A et al, 1994 Coronary echocardiography in 406 patients with d-loop transposition of the great arteries. Journal of the American College of Cardiology 34: 763–768

Paul M H 1983 Transposition of the great arteries. In: Adams F H, Emmanouilides G C (eds) Moss' heart disease in infants, children, and adolescents, 3rd edn. Williams & Wilkins, Baltimore, MD, p 296–332

Pexieder T, Blanc O, Pelouch V, Ostadalova I, Milerova M, Ostadal B 1995 Late fetal development of retinoic acid-induced transposition of the great arteries: morphology, physiology and biochemistry. In: Clark E B, Markwald R R, Takao A (eds) Developmental mechanisms of heart disease. Futura, Armonk, NY, p 297–307

Planché C, Bruniaux J, Lacour-Gayet F et al, 1988 Switch operation for transposition of the great arteries in neonates: a study of 120 patients. Journal of Thoracic and Cardiovascular Surgery 96: 354–363

Plauth W H Jr, Nadas A S, Bernhard W F, Fyler D C 1970 Changing hemodynamics in patients with transposition of the great arteries. Circulation 42: 131–142

Pridjian A K, Tacy T A, Teske D, Bove E L 1992 Palliative arterial repair for transposition, ventricular septal defect, and pulmonary vascular disease. Annals of Thoracic Surgery 54: 355–356

Quaegebeur J M, Brom A G 1978 The trouser-shaped baffle for use in the Mustard operation. Annals of Thoracic Surgery 25: 240–242

Quaegebeur J M, Rohmer J, Brom A G, Tinkelenberg J 1977 Revival of the Senning operation in the treatment of transposition of the great arteries. Thorax 32: 517–524

Quaegebeur J M, Rohmer J, OttenKamp J et al 1986 The arterial switch operation: an eight-year experience. Journal of Thoracic and Cardiovascular Surgery 92: 361–384

Rabinovitch M, Haworth S G, Castañeda A R, Nadas A S, Reid L M 1978 Lung biopsy in congenital heart disease: a morphometric approach to pulmonary vascular disease. Circulation 58: 1107–1121

Rashkind W J, Miller W W 1966 Creation of an atrial septal defect without thoracotomy. A palliative approach to complete transposition of great arteries. Journal of the American Medical Association 196: 991–992

Rastelli G C, Wallace R B, Ongley P A 1969 Complete repair of transposition of the great arteries with pulmonary stenosis. A review and report of a case corrected by using a new surgical technique. Circulation 39: 83–95

Restieaux N J, Ellison R C, Albers W H, Nadas A S 1972 The Frank electrocardiogram in complete transposition of the great arteries: its use in assessment of left ventricular pressure. American Heart Journal 83: 219–231

Rosengart R, Fishbein M, Emmanouilides G C 1975 Progressive pulmonary vascular disease after surgical correction (Mustard procedure) of transposition of the great arteries with intact ventricular septum. American Journal of Cardiology 35: 107–111

Rosenthal G L 1996 Patterns of prenatal growth among infants with cardiovascular malformations: possible fetal haemodynamic effects. American Journal of Epidemiology 143: 505–513

Ross D, Rickards A, Somerville J 1976 Transposition of the great arteries: logical anatomical arterial correction. British Medical Journal i: 1109–1111

Rowlatt U F 1962 Coronary artery distribution in complete transposition. Journal of the American Medical Association 179: 269–278

Rubay J, Lecompte Y, Batisse A et al 1988 Anatomic repair of anomalies of ventriculo-arterial connection (REV). Results of a new technique in cases associated with pulmonary outflow tract obstruction. European Journal of Cardiothoracic Surgery 2: 305–311

Saalouke M G, Rios G, Perry L W, Shapiro S R, Scott L P 1978 Electrophysiologic studies after Mustard's operation for d-transposition of the great vessels. American Journal of Cardiology 41: 1104–1109

Sansa M, Tonkin I, Bargeron L M Jr, Elliott L P 1979 Left ventricular outflow tract obstruction in transposition of the great arteries: an angiographic study of 74 cases. American Journal of Cardiology 44: 88–95

Schneeweiss A, Blieden L C, Shem-Tov A, Fiegal A, Neufeld H N 1982 Wide variety pedicle on thoracic roentgenogram in complete transposition of the great arteries. Clinical Cardiology 5: 75–77

Senning A 1959 Surgical correction of transposition of the great arteries. Surgery 45: 966–980

Serraf A, Lacour-Gayet F, Bruniaux J et al 1993 Anatomic correction of transposition of the great arteries in neonates. Journal of the American College of Cardiology 22: 193–200

Siebenmann R, von Segesser L, Schneider J, Senning A, Turina M 1989 Late failure of systemic ventricle after atrial correction for transposition of great arteries. European Journal of Cardiothoracic Surgery 3: 119–123

Shaher R M 1973 Complete transposition of the great arteries. Academic Press, New York, p 152–185

Shaher R M, Puddu G C 1966 Coronary arterial anatomy in complete transposition of the great arteries. American Journal of Cardiology 17: 355–361

Sharland G K, Allan L D 1992 Screening for congenital heart disease prenatally. Results of a 2 1/2 year study in the South East Thames Region. British Journal of Obstetrics and Gynaecology 99: 220–225

Silove E D, Coe J Y, Shill M F et al 1981 Oral prostaglandin E$_2$ in ductus-dependent pulmonary circulation. Circulation 63: 682–688

Smallhorn J F, Huhta J C, Anderson R H, Macartney F J 1982 Suprasternal cross-sectional echocardiography in assessment of patent ductus arteriosus. British Heart Journal 48: 321–330

Smith A, Wilkinson J L, Arnold R, Dickinson D F, Anderson R H 1982 Growth and development of ventricular walls in complete transposition of the great arteries with intact septum (simple transposition). American Journal of Cardiology 49: 362–368

Smith A, Wilkinson J L, Anderson R H, Arnold R, Dickinson D F 1986a Architecture of the ventricular mass and atrioventricular valves in complete transposition of the great arteries with intact septum compared with the normal heart. I. The left ventricle, mitral valve, and the interventricular septum. Pediatric Cardiology 6: 253–257

Smith A, Wilkinson J L, Anderson R H, Arnold R, Dickinson D F 1986b Architecture of the ventricular mass and atrioventricular valves in complete transposition with intact septum compared with the normal heart. II. The right ventricle and tricuspid valve. Pediatric Cardiology 6: 299–305

Smith A, Arnold R, Wilkinson J L, Hamilton D I, McKay R, Anderson R H 1986c An anatomical study of the patterns of the coronary arteries and sinus nodal artery in complete transposition. International Journal of Cardiology 12: 295–304

Smith A, Connel M G, Jackson M, Verbeek F J, Anderson R H 1994 Atrioventricular conduction system in hearts with muscular ventricular septal defects in the setting of complete transposition. Journal of Thoracic and Cardiolvascular Surgery 108: 9–16

Southall D P 1982 A new look at the normal range of heart rate and rhythm patterns in childhood. In: Anderson R H, Macartney F J, Shinebourne E A, Tynan M (eds) Paediatric cardiology, Churchill Livingstone, Edinburgh, p 3–21

Southall D P, Keeton B R, Leanage R et al 1980 Cardiac rhythm and conduction before and after Mustard's operation for complete transposition of the great arteries. British Heart Journal 43: 21–30

Stark J 1981 Complete transposition–surgeon's view. In: Becker A E, Losekoot T G, Marcelletti C, Anderson R H (eds) Paediatric cardiology, vol 3. Churchill Livingstone, Edinburgh, p 193–198

Stark J 1984 Transposition of the great arteries: which operation? Annals of Thoracic Surgery 38: 429–431

Stark J, de Leval M 1994 Surgery for congenital heart defects, 2nd edn. Saunders, Philadelphia, PA p 475

Stark J, Aberdeen E, Waterston D J, Bonham-Carter R E, Tynan M 1969 Pulmonary artery constriction (banding): a report of 146 cases. Surgery 65: 808–818

Stark J, Silove E D, Taylor J F N, Graham G R 1974 Obstruction to systemic venous return following the Mustard operation for transposition of the great arteries. Journal of Thoracic and Cardiovascular Surgery 68: 742–749

Stellin G, Zuberbuhler J R, Anderson R H, Slewers R D 1987 The surgical anatomy of the Taussig–Bing malformation. Journal of Thoracic and Cardiovascular Surgery 93: 560–569

Tamisier D, Ouaknine R, Pouard p et al 1997 Neonatal arterial switch operation: coronary artery patterns and coronary events. European Journal of Cardiothoracic Surgery 11: 810–817

Tanel R E, Wernovsky G, Landzberg M J, Perry S B, Burke R P 1995 Coronary artery abnormalities detected at cardiac catheterization following the arterial switch operation for transposition of the great arteries. American Journal of Cardiology. 76: 153–157

Taussig H B 1938 Complete transposition of the great vessels. American Heart Journal 16: 728–733

Turley K, Ebert P A 1978 Total correction of transposition of the great arteries. Conduction disturbances in infants younger than three months of age. Journal of Thoracic and Cardiovascular Surgery 76: 312–320

Turley K, Verrier E D 1995 Intermediate results from the period of the Congenital Heart Surgeon's Transposition Study: 1985 to 1989. Congenital Heart Surgeon's Society Database. Annals of Thoracic Surgery 60: 505–510

Tyler H R, Clark D B 1957 Cerebrovascular accidents in patients with congenital heart disease. American Medical Association Archives of Neurology and Psychiatry 77: 483–489

Tynan M J 1971 Survival of infants with transposition of great arteries after balloon atrial septostomy. Lancet i: 621–623

Tynan M J 1972 Transposition of the great arteries: changes in the circulation after birth. Circulation 46: 809–815

Tynan M J, Anderson R H 1979 Terminology of transposition of the great arteries. In: Godman M J, Marquis R M (eds) Paediatric cardiology, vol 2. Heart disease in the newborn. Churchill Livingstone, Edinburgh, p 341–349

Tynan M J, Carr I, Graham G, Bonham-Carter R E 1969 Subvalvular pulmonary obstruction complicating post-operative course of balloon atrial septostomy in transposition of the great arteries. Circulation 39(suppl I): 233–238

Tynan M J, Aberdeen E, Stark J 1972 Tricuspid incompetence after the Mustard operation for transposition of the great arteries. Circulation 45(suppl I): 111–115

Tyrrell M J, Moes C A F 1971 Congenital levoposition of the right atrial appendage: its relevance to balloon septostomy. American Journal of Diseases of Childhood 121: 508–510

Uberfuhr P, Reichenspurner H, Schmoeckel M et al 1993 Heart transplantation after Senning operation for transposition of the great arteries. Thoracic and Cardiovascular Surgeon 41: 369–371

Ullal R R, Anderson R H, Lincoln C 1979 Mustard's operation modified to avoid dysrhythmias and pulmonary and systemic venous obstruction. Journal of Thoracic and Cardiovascular Surgery 78: 431–439

Van Mierop L H S 1971 Transposition of the great arteries. Clarification or further confusion? [Editorial] American Journal of Cardiology 28: 735–738

Van Mierop L H S, Alley R D, Kausel H W, Stranahan A 1963 Pathogenesis of transposition complexes. 1. Embryology of the ventricles and great arteries. American Journal of Cardiology 12: 216–225

Van Praagh R 1971 Transposition of the great arteries. II. Transposition clarified. American Journal of Cardiology 28: 739–741

Van Praagh R, Van Praagh S 1966 Isolated ventricular inversion. A consideration of the morphogenesis, definition and diagnosis of nontransposed and transposed great arteries. American Journal of Cardiology 17: 395–406

Van Praagh R, Perez-Trevino C, Lopez-Cuellar M et al 1971 Transposition of the great arteries with posterior aorta, anterior pulmonary artery, subpulmonary conus and fibrous continuity between aortic and atrioventricular valves. American Journal of Cardiology 28: 621–631

Van praagh R, Layton W M, Van Praagh S 1980 The morphogenesis of normal and abnormal relationships between the great arteries and the ventricles: pathologic and experimental data. In: Van Praagh R, Takao A (eds) Etiology and morphogenesis of congenital heart disease. Futura, New York, p 271–316

Vouhé P R, Tamisier D, Leca F, Ouaknine R, Vernant F, Neveux J Y 1992 Transposition of the great arteries, ventricular septal defect and pulmonary outflow tract obstruction: Rasstelli or Lecompte procedure? Journal of Thoracic and Cardiovascular Surgery 103: 428–433

Wagenvoort C A, Nauta J, van der Schaar P J, Weeda H W H, Wagenvoort N 1969 The pulmonary vasculature in complete transposition of the great vessels. Judged from lung biopsies. Circulation 38: 746–754

Waldman J D, Schneeweiss A, Edwards W D, Lamberti J J, Shem-Tov A, Neufeld H N 1984 The obstructive subaortic conus. Circulation 70: 339–344

Wernovsky G, Wypij D, Jonas R A et al 1995 Postoperative course and hemodynamic profile after the arterial switch operation in neonates and infants. A comparison of low-flow cardiopulmonary bypass and circulatory arrest. Circulation 92: 2226–2235

Wilcox B R, Henry G W, Anderson R H 1983 The transmitral approach to left ventricular outflow tract obstruction. Annals of Thoracic Surgery 35: 288–293

Wilkinson J L, Arnold R, Anderson R H, Acerete F 1975 'Posterior' transposition reconsidered. British Heart Journal 37: 757–766

Wilson N J, Clarkson P M, Barratt-Boyes B G et al 1998 Long-term outcome after the Mustard repair for simple transposition of the great arteries. 28 year follow-up. Journal of the American College of Cardiology 32: 758–765

Yacoub M H, Radley-Smith R 1978 Anatomy of the coronary arteries in transposition of the great arteries and methods for their transfer in anatomical correction. Thorax 33: 418–424

Yacoub M H, Radley-Smith R, Ifilton C J 1976 Anatomical correction of complete transposition of the great arteries and ventricular septal defect in infancy. British Medical Journal i: 1112–1124

Yacoub M H, Radley-Smith R, Maclaurin R 1977 Two-stage operation for anatomical correction of transposition of the great arteries with intact interventricular septum. Lancet i: 1275–1278

Yacoub M H, Bernhard A, Radley-Smith R, Lange P, Sievers H, Heintzen P 1982 Supravalvular pulmonary stenosis after anatomic correction of transposition of the great arteries: causes and prevention. Circulation 66(suppl I): 193–197

Yacoub M H, Keck E, Radley-Smith R 1983 An evaluation of one and two stage anatomic correction of simple transposition of the great arteries. Circulation 68(suppl III): 48

Yamaguchi M 1990 Arterial switch operation. [Reply to the editor] Journal of Thoracic and Cardiovascular Surgery 100: 314

Zuberbuhler J R 1983 Symposium on results of the Mustard operation for complete transposition of the great arteries. Summary. American Journal of Cardiology 51: 1535–1536

49

Discordant atrioventricular connections and congenitally corrected transposition

R. M. Freedom*

INTRODUCTION

Discordant atrioventricular connections exist when the atrial chambers are connected to morphologically inappropriate ventricles. This segmental combination may occur in patients with either usual or mirror-imaged atrial arrangement (solitus or inversus). As described previously (Chapter 2), this junctional arrangement describes only part of the heart and cannot be considered an entity in itself. Discordant atrioventricular connections occur most frequently in combination with discordant ventriculo-arterial connections, the combination then usually being known as 'congenitally corrected transposition' (Figure 49.1). They can also be found with concordant ventriculo-arterial connections, with double outlet from either the morphologically right or left ventricle, or with single outlet of the heart (Losekoot, 1978; Freedom 1999).

The flow pathways in these various combinations are largely determined by the ventriculo-arterial connections, and by the additional anomalies present. On the basis of the principal pattern of flow of the saturated blood, two major groups can be distinguished. The first are those in which saturated blood tends to be conveyed into the aorta. This pattern exists in hearts with discordant ventriculo-arterial connections, in double outlet right ventricle with subpulmonary ventricular septal defect and in double outlet left ventricle with subaortic ventricular septal defect. The second group comprises those in which desaturated blood tends to be pumped into the aorta. This is produced by the much rarer combinations of concordant ventriculo-arterial connections, double outlet right ventricle with subaortic ventricular septal defect and double outlet left ventricle with subpulmonary

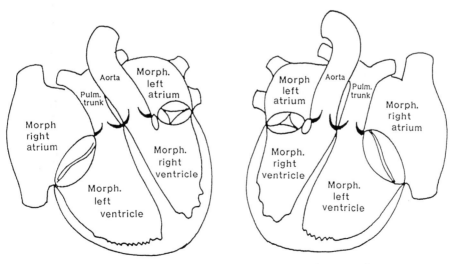

Usual atrial arrangement   **Mirror-imaged arrangement**

Figure 49.1. The segmental connections producing the entity best described as congenitally corrected transposition, being discordant at the atrioventricular and ventriculo-arterial junctions (double discordance), can exist in the usual or mirror-imaged arrangements, but not in patients with isometric atrial appendages. Morph, morphological; Pulm, pulmonary.

* The original chapter by T. G. Losekoot and A. E. Becker has been updated for the second edition.

ventricular septal defect. As emphasized, the first group is by far the largest. In hearts with a single outlet, the solitary arterial trunk will self-evidently receive mixed arterial and venous blood.

In all instances, however, the haemodynamic profile is moulded by the presence or absence of additional abnormalities. The most frequent ones are ventricular septal defects, pulmonary stenosis and atrioventricular valvar malformations. Of all these segmental combinations, congenitally corrected transposition is by far the most frequent and will receive the bulk of our attention.

CONGENITALLY CORRECTED TRANSPOSITION

DEFINITION

Congenitally corrected transposition is the arrangement in which discordant connections across the atrioventricular junctions are combined with discordant ventriculoarterial connections. This anomaly (Figure 49.1) can be encountered with usually arranged or mirror-imaged atrial chambers, but not in those with isomeric atrial appendages ('splenic syndromes' or visceral heterotaxy). Anomalies having only one atrioventricular connection are also excluded, as well as hearts with double inlet atrioventricular connection when the rudimentary right ventricle is left sided.

The greater majority of diagnosed patients have more or less severe complicating malformations. It is these associated lesions that have the greatest impact in the natural history. In those with pulmonary hypertension, there is also a marked tendency to develop pulmonary vascular obstructive disease. In addition to these intrinsic malformations, which can be considered part of the congenital anomaly, other complicating malformations can be acquired during life. These acquired changes most frequently involve the left atrioventricular valve and the conduction tissues. In postmortem material (Allwork et al, 1976), anomalies of the left atrioventricular valve are present in over nine tenths of patients. Haemodynamic changes are seen in only one third of these patients. During life, still further functional abnormalities can superimpose upon these structural changes, explaining why, in the older age group, the incidence of insufficiency of the left atrioventricular valve is high. This, perhaps, also accounts for the postoperative appearance of tricuspid insufficiency (Fox et al, 1976; Acar et al, 1998, Stümper and Braun, 1998; Freedom, 1999; Voskuil et al, 1999; Yeh et al, 1999). It is the unusual distribution of the conduction tissues that is probably responsible for the development and progression of conduction delay during life (see below). The acquisition of all these anomalies has significant influence on outcome. The prognosis for patients with initially uncomplicated conditions should, therefore, be guarded. This is the more so since, in con-

genitally corrected transposition, the morphologically right ventricle has to propagate the blood under high pressure in the high-resistance circulation, resulting in a pressure overload of this ventricle. This abnormal workload has considerable influence on the natural history in both isolated and complicated cases. The situation resembles severe isolated pulmonary stenosis, in which several studies have shown that life expectancy is significantly diminished (Nugent et al, 1977).

It is difficult, nonetheless, to evaluate precisely the influence of pressure overload on the morphologically right ventricle. Conclusive data are lacking. Occasionally, case reports have been published of patients with isolated congenitally corrected transposition, or with mild complicating malformations, who have reached older age. Patients have been described, however, who had isolated congenitally corrected transposition (or minor complicating malformations) and yet showed symptoms of severe circulatory insufficiency or died early (Losekoot et al, 1983). The question still remains unanswered as to whether the morphologically right ventricle, subjected to systemic workload for many years, will fail at an earlier age (Rotem and Hultgren, 1965). Recent experiences suggest that the morphologically right ventricle will fail sooner rather than later, affecting markedly the philosophy for surgical correction (see below), although conclusive proof of this deterioration has yet to be provided.

HISTORICAL BACKGROUND

It is now well over 100 years since the term corrected transposition was introduced by von Rokitansky (1875). He described two patients in whom, in his opinion, the abnormal relationship of the great arteries was corrected functionally by the position of the ventricular septum. Following his account, anatomical descriptions of specimens appeared regularly. It was the extensive clinical study from Anderson et al (1957) and the review of Schiebler et al (1961) that stimulated a greater clinical interest, this occurring concomitantly with the upsurge in sophisticated techniques for diagnosis and treatment. Surgical interventions in congenitally corrected transposition had always carried a high morbidity and mortality, but the improved knowledge of the anatomy of the conduction tissues (Anderson et al, 1973) produced more encouraging results (Fox et al, 1976; Danielson et al, 1978; de Leval et al, 1979; Marcelletti et al, 1980; Danielson, 1983). Even these successes, which followed intracardiac correction of the associated malformations, nonetheless, were much less than optimal (Connelly et al, 1996). As a result, there has been a trend towards the 'double switch' procedure (Ilbawi et al, 1990; Yamagishi et al, 1993). Even though this surgery is more complex, it has the inestimable advantage of restoring to the morphologically left ventricle its role in supporting the systemic circulation.

PREVALENCE

Surprisingly, the New England Regional Infant Cardiac Program identified only 16 infants with congenitally corrected transposition (Fyler et al, 1980). Neither the Baltimore–Washington Infant Study nor the Alberta Heritage studies provide data addressing the prevalence of doubly discordant connections (Ferencz et al, 1985; Grabitz and Joffres, 1988). The data subsequently provided by Fyler (1992) revealed that 89 patients with corrected transposition were seen at Boston Children's Hospital in the period 1972–1987. This accounted for 0.6% of those with congenital heart disease. Congenitally corrected transposition with mirror-imaged atrial chambers is rare. At the end of the 1980s, there were less than 100 well-documented cases (Attie et al, 1987).

The familial incidence of congenitally corrected transposition is very low. One publication mentions its occurrence in siblings (Shem-Tov et al, 1971), although there are occasional reports of siblings of children with congenitally corrected transposition having other cardiac anomalies (Losekoot et al, 1983). There are also a few observations in twins in which one had congenitally corrected transposition but the other child had either a normal heart (Schiebler et al, 1961; Keck et al, 1965; Bliddal, 1976a,b) or a different congenital cardiac malformation (Losekoot, 1967). Complicating non-cardiac anomalies have been described occasionally, and in great variety (Losekoot et al, 1983). The sex ratio in patients with usually arranged atrial chambers is about 1.6:1, with males predominating. The aetiology must be considered as multifactorial.

PHYSIOLOGY AND NATURAL HISTORY

The basic pattern for the circulation is normal, with the aorta in the pathway of the saturated blood and the pulmonary trunk in the pathway of the unsaturated blood (Figure 49.1). This pattern is usually influenced by complicating malformations present at birth or developing during life in the setting of congenital structural changes (Allwork et al, 1976). From a physiological point of view, there is another important aspect, which has already been emphasized. The morphologically right ventricle has to propagate blood into the aorta against a high resistance with a high systemic pressure. It is questionable if this ventricle is able to maintain such a high pressure for the full span of human life. Consequently, the natural history of congenitally corrected transposition is determined by the associated malformations, the acquired changes and the condition of the systemic ventricle. However, the notion of deterioration of the morphologically right ventricle is not yet proven. There are a number of reports of adults with congenitally corrected transposition surviving to the sixth, seventh and eighth decades of life, the patients coming to medical attention either for cardiac or non-cardiac reasons (Lieberson et al, 1969; Benchimol et al, 1971; Anderson and Becker, 1981; Lundstrom et al, 1990; Ikeda et al, 1992). The existence of such patients has been used to support the view that the morphologically right ventricle can function as the systemic right ventricle for many years. Evidence has also been presented, based on the radionuclide assessment of ventricular function, to support the notion of preservation of right ventricular integrity (Benson et al, 1986). A similar conclusion, based on different methodology, was reached by Dimas and colleagues (1989). Yet other data suggest that systemic ventricular ejection fraction does not increase from rest to exercise (Peterson et al, 1988), indicative of an abnormal exercise response. The issue, therefore, has not been completely resolved, although systolic function of the systemic morphologically right ventricle may be reasonably well preserved at rest. Relatively few data are available on morphologically right ventricular diastolic function.

Against this potentially encouraging information must be set the many studies, and increasing clinical experience, that point to the inability of the morphologically right ventricle to perform a systemic role, particularly in the face of a less than perfect atrioventricular valve. Very recent data, albeit from a small number of patients, have demonstrated ischaemic injury to the morphologically right ventricle in the absence of associated lesions (Hornung et al, 1998). Most patients, nonetheless, do have associated lesions. In this respect, Huhta and his colleagues (1985) analysed retrospectively the natural history of patients with congenitally corrected transposition seen at the Mayo Clinic. The only variable that correlated with decreased survival was insufficiency of the left atrioventricular valve. Survival was 70% at 5 years, and 64% at 10 years. Clearly this was an unusual series because mean age at diagnosis was 12.7 years, ranging from birth to 56 years. In a comparable study, Lundstrom and colleagues (1990) analysed patients from the United Kingdom managed over a 20-year period to 1988. The ages of survivors in their cohort ranged from 1 to 58 years, with a median of 20 years; all but 10 had additional cardiac difficulties. Of the patients, 26 had died by 1988, and 16 were considered unlikely to require surgery because of absent or trivial associated cardiac lesions. Patients who were very symptomatic from heart failure did not fare well. In addition, those young patients with severe tricuspid regurgitation and/or a failing morphologically right ventricle did poorly. McGrath and colleagues (1985) addressed death and other events after classical cardiac repair in 99 patients with discordant atrioventricular connections. The actuarial survival at 1 month, 1 year and 10 years was 86, 75 and 68%, respectively. These findings, combined with similar results reported by Connelly et al (1996), support strongly the trend towards surgical correction, when feasible, to restore the morphologically left ventricle to its systemic role (see below).

BASIC ANATOMY

The most common pattern is that with usual arrangement of the atrial chambers ('solitus'). As previously outlined, the segmental arrangement dictates that the right atrium connects to the morphologically left ventricle and the left atrium to the morphologically right ventricle (Figure 49.2a). The morphologically left ventricle, receiving desaturated blood, then empties into the pulmonary trunk (Figure 49.2b) and the morphologically right ventricle, receiving the pulmonary venous return, empties into the aorta (Figure 49.2c). The aorta usually arises from the right ventricle in anterior and leftward position relative to the pulmonary trunk (Figure 49.3). In a small proportion of hearts with usually arranged atriums and with the segmental arrangement of congenitally corrected transposition, the aorta is found in right-sided position (Allwork et al, 1976).

Irrespective of the arterial relationships, the discordant atrioventricular connections ensure that the right atrium empties into the morphologically left ventricle through a mitral valve, supported by typical paired papillary muscles located in posteromedial and anterolateral positions (Figure 49.4). The anterolateral papillary muscle group is particularly vulnerable during surgical ventriculotomy. The left atrium empties into the morphologically right ventricle through a morphologically tricuspid valve. When the septal structures are intact, the septal leaflet of this valve is attached at a lower level than the mitral valve (Figure 49.2a). The attachment of the tricuspid valve to the extensive membranous septum creates an interven-

tricular part, along with an atrioventricular portion between the left atrium and the right-sided morphologically left ventricle.

As a consequence of the discordant ventriculo-arterial connections, the pulmonary trunk is deeply wedged between the two atrioventricular valves (Figure 49.2b). The outflow of the morphologically left ventricle is thus hidden by the septal, or pulmonary, leaflet of the mitral valve (Figure 49.4). Indeed, the pulmonary valve is in fibrous continuity with this leaflet of the mitral valve. The anterior part of the left ventricular outflow forms a prominent recess, often nicely demonstrated on angled left ventricular angiograms. The outflow into the aorta shows the typical configuration of a morphologically right ventricle, with the leaflets of the aortic valve separated from those of the tricuspid valve by a complete muscular infundibulum (Figure 49.2c).

The two ventricles are often considered to be 'inverted', although in no way do they provide the mirror-image arrangement of the normal heart. This is largely because the outflow tracts are parallel to each other, rather than crossing (Figure 49.2). The ventricles, therefore, tend to be side by side, but other relationships do exist. Indeed, many hearts have either superoinferior relations from tilting or criss-cross relationships from rotation (Anderson, 1982).

The coronary arteries originate from the two aortic sinuses which are adjacent to the pulmonary trunk. Their precise position, relative to the heart, will vary according to the precise position of the aortic root. The epicardial distribution of these arteries, nonetheless, is

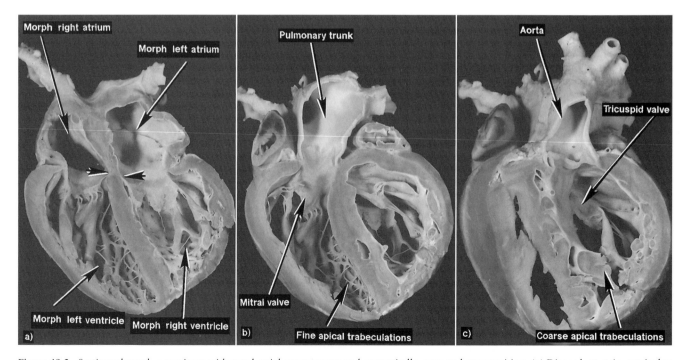

Figure 49.2. Sections through a specimen with usual atrial arrangement and congenitally corrected transposition. (a) Discordant atrioventricular connections (note the reversed off-setting of the hinges of the atrioventricular valves (arrowheads). (b) The pulmonary trunk arises from the morphologically (morph) left ventricle. (c) The aorta originates anteriorly and to the left from the morphologically right ventricle.

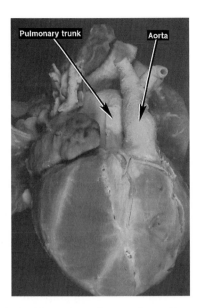

Figure 49.3. As in this specimen, the aorta is usually anterior and to the left in patients with congenitally corrected transposition in the setting of usual atrial arrangement.

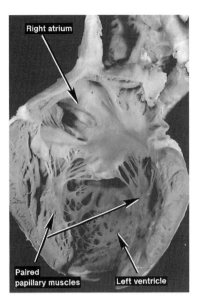

Figure 49.4. Paired papillary muscles support the tension apparatus of the mitral valve in the right-sided morphologically left ventricle in a typical heart with congenitally corrected transposition.

reasonably constant. The pattern is largely determined by the discordant atrioventricular junctional anatomy. Generally speaking, in persons with usual atrial arrangement, the coronary arteries are mirror imaged relative to the arrangement seen in the normal heart. Consequently, the right-sided coronary artery exhibits the pattern of a morphologically left coronary artery, with its short main stem dividing into anterior descending and circumflex branches (Figure 49.5). The circumflex artery encircles the mitral orifice, which is now right sided. The site of origin of the anterior descending coronary artery is a useful guide to the position of the ventricular septum. The left-sided coronary artery is a morphologically right coronary artery. It gives off infundibular and marginal branches while encircling the left-sided tricuspid orifice. Usually the posterior descending branch arises from this artery. These relationships are all mirror imaged when

there is mirror-imaged atrial arrangement (Figure 49.5b). A solitary coronary artery occurs as the most frequent anomaly (McKay et al, 1996; Uemura et al, 1996).

Because of the segmental arrangement of congenitally corrected transposition, there is gross malalignment between the interatrial septum and the inlet part of the ventricular septum (Becker and Anderson, 1978). In part, the gap between the two septums results from the wedged position of the left ventricular outflow tract incorporating the root of the pulmonary trunk (Figure 49.2b). The remainder of this gap, when the septal structures are intact, is filled by the extensive membranous septum. Not surprisingly, deficiency of this structure is common and produces a ventricular septal defect (see below).

The anatomy dictates that the regular atrioventricular node, located at the apex of the triangle of Koch in the base of the atrial septum, cannot give rise to a penetrating

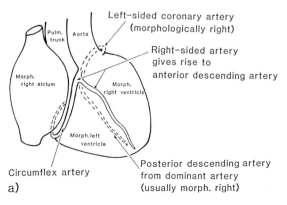

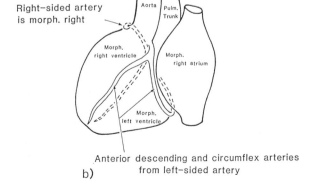

Figure 49.5. The arrangement of the coronary arteries in congenitally corrected transposition with (a) the usual atrial arrangement with left hand topology and (b) mirror-image atrial chambers with right hand topology. Note that the ventricles are arranged as expected for the normal heart when the atrial chambers are in mirror image.

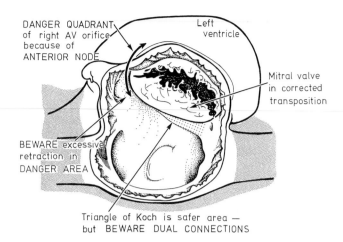

Figure 49.6. The salient surgical features of the abnormal disposition of the atrioventricular (AV) node in congenitally corrected transposition with usual atrial arrangement.

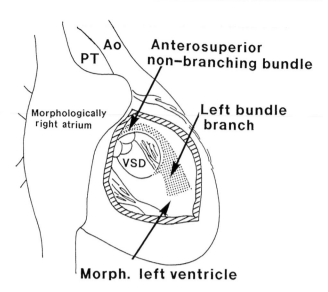

Figure 49.7. The unexpected relationship between the ventricular conduction tissues and a ventricular septal defect as viewed through a ventriculotomy in the right-sided morphologically left ventricle. Ao, aorta; Morph., morphological; PT, pulmonary trunk; VSD, ventricular septal defect.

atrioventricular conduction bundle. Hence, an anomalous second atrioventricular node is usually present. This additional node is located beneath the opening of the right atrial appendage (Figure 49.6). It is within the base of the right atrial parietal free wall, at the lateral margin of the area of pulmonary-to-mitral valvar fibrous continuity. It is this node that gives rise to the atrioventricular bundle, which penetrates through the fibrous trigone and comes to lie immediately underneath the pulmonary valvar leaflets. The extensive non-branching bundle then runs superficially underneath the right anterior facing leaflet of the pulmonary valve. It descends for some distance down the anterior septal surface of the subpulmonary left ventricular outflow tract before it branches. A cord-like right bundle branch extends leftwards to reach the morphologically right ventricular, whereas a fan-like left bundle branch cascades down the smooth left ventricular septal surface.

The precise anatomy of the bundle has far-reaching surgical significance in the presence of associated malformations. The close relationship between the non-branching bundle and the pulmonary valvar orifice is important in the presence of an obstructed left ventricular outflow tract. In patients with perimembranous ventricular septal defects, the bundle has a grossly abnormal position compared with the regular position of the conduction axis in hearts with ventricular septal defects in the setting of concordant atrioventricular connections (Chapter 3). When viewed through an anterior ventriculotomy, the bundle is to the right-hand side of the surgeon, rather than to the left-hand side as anticipated in a heart with normal junctional anatomy (Figure 49.7).

In hearts with less malalignment between the atrial and ventricular septums, the regular node may be positioned so as to enable it to make contact posteriorly with the ventricular septum. In such instances, both the regular and the anterior nodes may give rise to penetrating bundles, which can then both join with the branching

bundle. This produces a 'sling' of conducting tissues around the margin of a ventricular septal defect (if present). Such an arrangement was first described by Monckeberg (1913). The vulnerable position of the long non-branching bundle almost certainly explains why heart block remains a frequent complication after surgical closure of associated malformations. The block may sometimes be present at birth. More frequently, there is progressive acquired atrioventricular nodal dissociation, often culminating in complete heart block. This is usually caused by replacement of conduction fibres by fibrous tissue (Anderson et al, 1974).

In most patients encountered clinically, there will be associated malformations, of which three are so typical as to be considered almost part of the segmental combination. These are a ventricular septal defect, pulmonary stenosis and anomalies of the morphologically tricuspid valve (Van Praagh, 1970; Allwork et al, 1976). The morphology of each of these associated lesions can in itself be variable. Certain of the clinical features, however, are determined by the basic abnormal chamber connections. The clinical features of the basic lesion will be described first, followed by the morphology of the associated lesions and how these modify the clinical picture.

CLINICAL PRESENTATION

The clinical presentation is influenced by three factors: the architectural anomalies of the malformation itself, the position of the heart in the thoracic cavity and the complicating malformations present initially or developing subsequently.

As indicated, serious complicating malformations are frequent. Because of this, more than 70% of patients have symptoms in the first year of life (Kidd, 1978). Three groups may be recognized. First is the group with substantial left-to-right shunts who show failure to thrive, heart failure and murmurs at auscultation. In the second group, a right-to-left shunt is present, with reduction of pulmonary blood flow and cyanosis is the main finding. In the third group, the ventricular septum is intact. A murmur or an arrhythmia may then be the main symptom.

Presentation is not uncommon in the first days after birth and may reflect a significant disturbance of rhythm, such as congenital complete heart block, congestive heart failure owing to coarctation of the aorta, or functional or organic aortic atresia. Patients in this group with heart failure all have severe systemic atrioventricular valvar regurgitation. Early presentation may also reflect inadequate pulmonary blood flow, with either pulmonary atresia or very severe stenosis (Freedom et al, 1989; Freedom and Benson, 1992).

HISTORY

It is the complicating malformations that lead to all the well-known, but atypical, complaints. Specific symptoms for congenitally corrected transposition do not exist. Consequently, when complicating anomalies are mild or absent, the patient has no complaints at all.

PHYSICAL EXAMINATION

The findings at physical examination are again determined mainly by the complicating malformations. The well-known signs and symptoms of a large left-to-right shunt are present in about half of patients. Cyanosis and clubbing are seen regularly. Retarded growth may occur in the presence of large left-to-right shunts, severe insufficiency of the left atrioventricular valve or extreme cyanosis.

Some clues, nonetheless, may lead to the diagnosis of congenitally corrected transposition. The finding of the heart in a position unexpected for the atrial arrangement (for example a right-sided heart with usual arrangement or a left-sided heart in mirror-image arrangement) should always alert to the likelihood of congenitally corrected transposition (Anselmi et al, 1972; Liberthson et al, 1973; Squarcia et al, 1973). Another important finding may be a loud and unsplit second sound. This may sometimes even be palpable in the second left intercostal space, suggesting pulmonary hypertension. The sound originates from the aortic valve, with its loudness caused by the usual left-sided and anterior position of this structure. The pulmonary component of the second sound is often not audible because of its posterior position. The second sound, therefore, will often be single when there

is pulmonary stenosis (Caulfield et al, 1967; Perloff, 1978).

Two other symptoms may also draw attention to the existence of congenitally corrected transposition. They then suggest the presence of complicating malformations. First, a holosystolic murmur at the apex radiating to the axilla suggests insufficiency of the morphologically tricuspid valve. Second, a slow heart rate, especially in infants and young children, may be the first clue to the existence of high-degree atrioventricular block.

INVESTIGATIONS

ELECTROCARDIOGRAPHY

The electrocardiogram and vectorcardiogram are also influenced by several factors. The first is the anatomy of the heart itself, especially the disposition of the conduction tissue, the relationship of the two ventricles and the orientation of the ventricular septum. A second major feature is the position of the heart in the thoracic cavity. The third is the haemodynamic status.

In sinus rhythm with usual atrial arrangement, the atrial chambers are activated normally and the direction of the P waves does not differ from that seen in the normal subject (Figure 49.8). With mirror-image atrial arrangement, atrial activation is directed from left superior to right inferior, resulting in negative P waves in the leads I and aVL, and positive P waves in lead aVF (Figure 49.9) (Portillo et al, 1959; Van Praagh et al, 1965). The haemodynamic status will not influence the direction of the P waves but can express itself in the well-known changes in their configuration, duration and amplitude. These changes occur whatever the atrial arrangement. In the normal heart, ventricular activation starts in the septum and is directed from left to right and slightly anteriorly. This initial activation is responsible for septal Q waves in the left precordial leads, and absence of Q waves in the right precordial leads (Burchell et al, 1952; Durrer et al, 1965; Durrer, 1966). In congenitally corrected transposition with usual atrial arrangement, the ventricular bundle branches are arranged in mirror-image fashion. The initial activation of the ventricular septum, therefore, is from right to left in a more superior and anterior or posterior direction (Okamura et al, 1973; Ruttenberg, 1977). This results in Q waves in the right precordial leads, and absence of Q waves in the left precordial leads, the so-called 'reversal of the normal precordial Q waves pattern' (Figure 49.8) (Anderson et al, 1957). This pattern is present in up to three-quarters of patients with congenitally corrected transposition (Camier, 1967; Losekoot, 1967). Absence of Q waves over the left precordium is an even more constant finding. Besides the distribution of the Q waves, the morphology of the QRS complexes should also be taken into account when assessing the potential presence of a

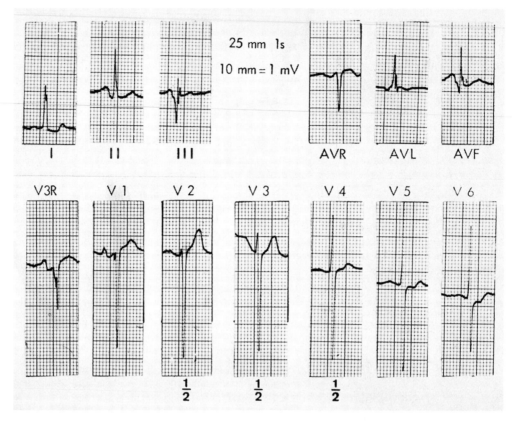

Figure 49.8. This electrocardiogram is from a boy aged 4 years, with usual atrial arrangement, a left-sided heart, moderate insufficiency of the left-sided atrioventricular valve, and mild pulmonary hypertension. Note the reversal of the pattern of the Q waves in the precordial leads, with positive T waves throughout these leads.

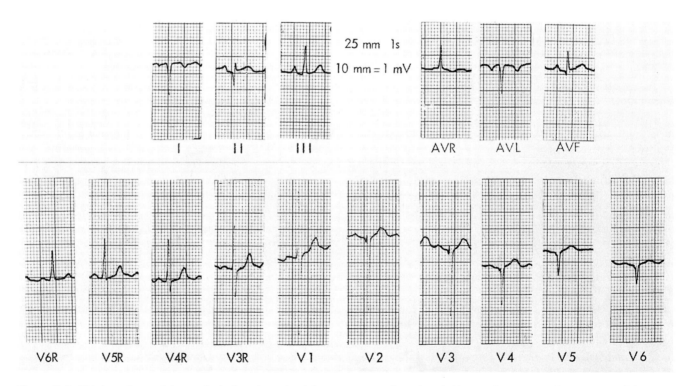

Figure 49.9. This boy, also aged 4 years, had mirror-imaged atrial arrangement and a right-sided heart. There is normal progression of the Q waves, and no evidence of ventricular hypertrophy.

reversed ventricular arrangement (de Carvalho Azevedo et al, 1958).

There are, of course, other reasons for discovering Q waves in the right precordial leads. Right ventricular hypertrophy is the most common cause. In congenitally corrected transposition, however, the Q wave is usually deep in relation to the R wave. This is not the case with right ventricular hypertrophy (Morgan et al, 1962). The initial septal activation in a left-superior direction is also responsible for the presence of a Q wave in the leads III and aVF, a phenomenon present in almost half of patients. The Q wave in lead III is nearly always deeper than one found in aVF (Figure 49.8). (Losekoot, 1967; Ruttenberg, 1977). This initial activation explains the almost constant absence of Q waves in lead I and aVL. In persons with mirror-imaged atrial arrangement, in contrast, the spatial arrangement of the ventricles is virtually normal. Because of this, the distribution of the Q waves is normal in the precordial as well as in the unipolar leads (Figure 49.9).

'Left-axis deviation' is often found in congenitally corrected transposition, particularly in uncomplicated disease or in the presence of overload of the left-sided ventricle (Burchell, 1962; Thibert et al, 1969). It seems justified to presume that this is the result of an early activation of the posterobasal parts of the left-sided morphologically right ventricle because of the abnormal anatomy of the conduction tissue. The abnormal initial activation of the ventricular septum, together with this left-axis deviation when present, produces a typical electrocardiogram with QS complexes in leads III and aVF and over the right precordium (Figure 49.8). In those with mirror imagery, the equivalent of the true left-axis deviation is not present, probably because of the more normal anatomy of the conduction tissue. Positive T waves are common in all precordial leads, being present in over 80% (Keck et al, 1965; Moffa et al, 1976; Losekoot et al, 1983).

The typical electrocardiographic pattern for uncomplicated cases can, therefore, be summarized as left-axis deviation, reversal of the precordial Q wave pattern and prominent Q waves in the leads III and aVF. Frequently there are QS complexes in the leads III and aVF and over the right precordium (Okamura et al, 1973; Victorica et al, 1973; Ruttenberg, 1977). This pattern may be greatly influenced by the haemodynamic status of the patient (Fernandez et al, 1970; Okamura et al, 1973; Victorica et al, 1973; Moffa et al, 1976; Losekoot et al, 1983). With only mild overload of the left-sided morphologically right ventricle, the electrocardiogram will not markedly change (Figure 49.8). In contrast, marked overload of the right-sided morphologically left ventricle will often lead to right-axis deviation, with QR complexes over the right precordium and deep S waves over the left precordium. In presence of biventricular hypertrophy, Q waves can be absent in all precordial leads, with large biphasic RS complexes in the mid-precordial leads.

The above discussions have all presumed the heart to occupy its usual position. When the heart is abnormally positioned, for example a right-sided heart in the patient with usual atrial arrangement, there are almost always severe intracardiac complications, with overload of the right-sided morphologically left ventricle. The morphologically left ventricle is usually displaced posteriorly. This results in the electrocardiogram showing right-axis deviation and RS waves in the precordial leads. Q waves over the right precordium are then a less constant finding. Impairment of atrioventricular conduction, particularly common in congenitally corrected transposition, will be discussed below.

Electrophysiological mapping during open heart surgery has been successfully accomplished in patients with both usual and mirror-imaged atrial arrangement (Kupersmith et al, 1974; Maloney et al, 1975; Waldo et al, 1975; Stewart et al, 1977; de Leval et al, 1979; Dick et al, 1979). In general, the findings during mapping were in agreement with the known anatomical disposition of the conduction tissues. Nowadays, therefore, mapping is never performed, except occasionally in presence of unusual complicating anomalies.

CHEST RADIOGRAPHY

The radiographic appearance of the heart, lung vascularity and vascular pedicle will be significantly influenced by the abnormal morphology of the heart and great vessels, the position of the heart in the thoracic cavity and the haemodynamic status. The frontal projection provides most relevant information. It almost always shows the position of the heart and the arrangement of the organs. The majority of patients with unexpected cardiac position will have either isomeric atrial appendages or discordant atrioventricular connections (Anselmi et al, 1972; Liberthson et al, 1973; Squarcia et al, 1973). In the absence of isomerism, atrial arrangement can accurately be predicted from the arrangement of the abdominal organs. The correlation with the thoracic organs is even more reliable, with the information derived from bronchial morphology also serving to indicate the presence of visceral symmetry (Van Mierop et al, 1970; Partridge et al, 1975; Macartney et al, 1978). Abnormal size and configuration of the atriums may be interpreted in the usual way. The plain chest radiograph, however, cannot give direct information about the atrioventricular connection nor about the relation of the two ventricles to each other. Dilation of one or both ventricles, caused either by complicating malformations or heart failure, is usually seen in the frontal film, but exposures in several projections may be necessary for full diagnosis. As complicating anomalies are common, the heart is enlarged in about four fifths of patients (Keck et al, 1965; Friedberg and Nadas, 1970).

Although the arrangement of the vascular pedicle gives no direct information about the ventriculo-arterial connections, it does give important information about the relationship of the two great arteries to each other. The most common relationship is side by side or oblique, with the aorta to the left and anterior (Barcia et al, 1967; Guerin et al, 1970). The ascending aorta is also to the left and anterior. Its left border then often becomes visible as a convex prominence at the left middle and upper border of the vascular pedicle, this being the expected location of the pulmonary trunk (Carey and Ruttenberg, 1964). This 'straight left heart border' may be pronounced in the presence of a dilated ascending aorta caused by a right-to-left shunt, or when the heart is right-sided (Figure 49.10). This sign may not be seen when the ascending aorta is small or when there is a more anteroposterior relation of the great arteries (Figure 49.11) (Carey and Ruttenberg, 1964; Edwards et al, 1965; du Bois et al, 1966). When viewed in lateral projection, the aorta can cause a shadow in the anterior mediastinum. The aortic arch is nearly always left sided with a sagittal course. Because of this, the aortic impression in the oesophagus is often faint or even absent (Anderson et al, 1957; Losekoot, 1978). In the presence of a right aortic arch, with a few exceptions, the prominence of the ascending aorta is absent (Losekoot et al, 1983).

The pulmonary trunk is displaced to a more postero-medial position and bears a close relationship with the oesophagus. This often results in a faint impression at the level of the tracheal carina (du Bois et al, 1966). Because

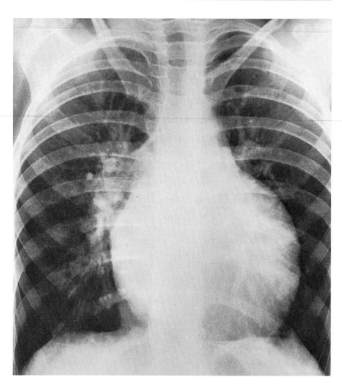

Figure 49.11. This chest radiograph is from a patient with usual atrial arrangement and left-sided heart in which there was insufficiency of the left atrioventricular valve and a ventricular septal defect. The aorta is small; consequently, the anticipated prominent left border of the vascular pedicle is lacking. Note the increased pulmonary vascular markings.

of the median position of the pulmonary trunk, the anticipated normal prominence of the pulmonary segment is missing. Even a dilated pulmonary trunk may be obscured, an obvious finding in pulmonary plethora. With extreme dilation, the shadow of the pulmonary trunk may be visible at the right border of the vascular pedicle, or at the left in those with mirror imagery (Watson, 1964; Losekoot et al, 1983).

The right and left branches of the pulmonary trunk are also displaced to the right. Because of this, the left branch is often projected in the cardiac shadow, resulting in an apparent difference in vascularization of the two lungs (Figure 49.11) (Thelen et al, 1969). The pulmonary vascularity depends on the complicating malformations present. Occasionally, the right hilum is displaced more cranially than the left and gives the impression of a waterfall (Ellis et al, 1962; Edwards et al, 1965; Guerin et al, 1970). As anticipated, all the features described for usual atrial arrangement are reversed in the setting of mirror-imaged arrangement.

ECHOCARDIOGRAPHY

The echocardiographic diagnosis of congenitally corrected transposition must be based on sequential segmental analysis. This necessitates use of the cross-sectional format. As the localization of the heart in the thoracic

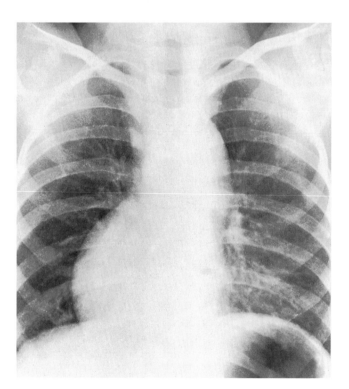

Figure 49.10. The typical chest radiograph as seen in frontal projection in a patient with usual atrial arrangement, a right-sided heart, a ventricular septal defect and pulmonary stenosis. Note the prominent ascending aorta at the left mediastinal border and the decreased pulmonary vascular markings.

cavity, along with the orientation of the ventricular septum, may be markedly abnormal, different transducer positions may be needed during the examination (Losekoot et al, 1983).

When the atriums are usually arranged, the atrial position can be inferred from the connection of the systemic veins to the morphologically right atrium and the pulmonary veins to the morphologically left atrium (Tajik et al, 1978). Finding abnormal venous connections should always alert the investigator to the possibility of isomerism of the atrial appendages. Once atrial arrangement has been determined, diagnosis of corrected transposition depends on the demonstration of the discordant atrioventricular connections. The ventricular morphology is identified on the basis of the morphology of the atrioventricular valves, the trabecular pattern of the ventricles and the infundibular morphology. Historically, when only M-mode techniques were available, one of the most striking features of corrected transposition was the fact that the images obtained were often confusing because of the abnormal relationship of the great arteries with the atrioventricular valves, and the abnormal spatial orientation of the ventricular septum. The first impression obtained was often that of a heart with a univentricular atrioventricular connection, or else an atrioventricular septal defect. Skilled investigators could demonstrate the presence of a septum, with atrioventricular valves to both sides of it (Meyer, 1977; Keutel and Hagenmuller, 1978; Losekoot et al, 1983). Such mental and manipulative gymnastics were rendered obsolete by the introduction of the cross-sectional formats, particularly when interrogation is possible from the oesophageal portal (Figure 49.12) (Hagler et al, 1981a; Foale et al, 1982; Sutherland et al, 1983). In the four chamber view,

the more apical insertion of the morphologically tricuspid valve, together with its direct cordal attachments to the ventricular septum, is found on the left side when the atriums are usually arranged, proving left-hand ventricular topology (Figure 49.13). The four chamber view also demonstrates that the atrioventricular component of the membranous septum is positioned between the outflow tract of the right-sided morphologically left ventricle and the left atrium (Losekoot et al, 1983). The parasternal long-axis view confirms that, in the left-sided ventricle, the atrioventricular valve is discontinuous from the anterior arterial valve and has multiple cords attaching it to the ventricular septum (Figure 49.14). Minor tilting of the transducer then makes it possible to traverse the septum and show that the right-sided atrioventricular valve is continuous with the posterior arterial valve. This information is almost diagnostic of corrected transposition (Losekoot et al, 1983). To demonstrate conclusively the ventriculo-arterial connections, nonetheless, it is necessary to trace the ventricular outflow tracts to the great arteries. This is readily achieved. The specific features of the aorta and pulmonary trunk are as in the normal heart. The four chamber section incorporating the arterial root or the long-axis views are usually sufficient for demonstration of the ventriculo-arterial connections. When the atriums are mirror imaged, the segmental morphology is approximately the mirror image of corrected transposition as described above. Knowledge of the basic anatomy should always permit accurate diagnosis with cross-sectional techniques once the presence of mirror-imaged atrial arrangement has been ascertained.

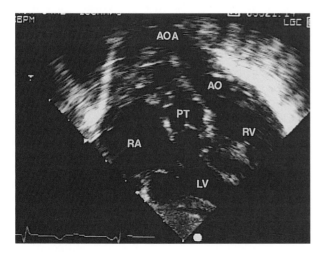

Figure 49.12. This cross-sectional image is obtained from the transgastric window in a patient with usual atrial arrangement and intact septal structures. All the salient features of the doubly discordant connections are readily seen. AO, aorta; AOA, aortic arch; PT, pulmonary trunk; RA, morphologically right atrium; LV, morphologically left ventricle; RV, morphologically right ventricle. The posterior left atrium is not seen.

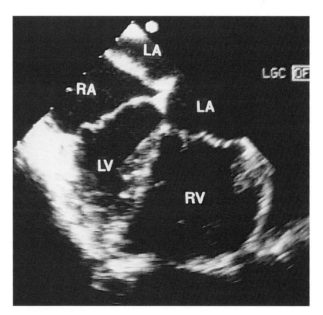

Figure 49.13. This view, again obtained from the transgastric window from a patient with intact septal structures, shows the reversed off-setting of the septal attachments of the atrioventricular valves. Note that the tricuspid valve is attached across the membranous septum, dividing into an atrioventricular component (between the right left atrium and left ventricle) and a much smaller interventricular component. LA, left atrium; other abbreviations as in Figure 49.12.

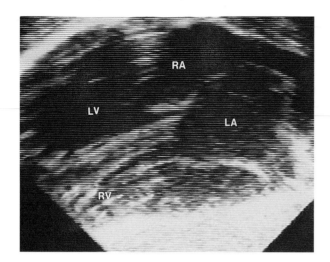

Figure 49.14. This transthoracic section in a patient with usual atrial arrangement and right-sided heart shows the multiple cords tethering the left-sided morphologically tricuspid valve to the ventricular septum. Abbreviations as in Figures 49.12 and 49.13.

The morphological details nowadays are seen with even greater clarity using transoesophageal and transgastric views (Figures 49.12 and 49.13). These also permit direct identification of the morphology of the atrial appendages, and hence unequivocal recognition of the discordant atrioventricular connections.

CATHETERIZATION

Catheterization became less important in the 1990s in determining the abnormal architecture of the heart but retains its role in establishing the haemodynamic status.

Venous catheterization demonstrates the atrial arrangement in nearly all patients and may help to distinguish isomeric atrial appendages because of the abnormal venoatrial connections. It gives no direct information about the ventricular morphology. By manipulating the catheter into the pulmonary trunk, its posteromedial position can be demonstrated clearly. The position of the aorta can also be established. In this way, an impression may be obtained about the relationship of the great arteries. Deduction of the connection between great vessels and ventricles, however, should be made with great care and reservation, especially in complicated cases with ventricular septal defect and/or other malformations.

ANGIOCARDIOGRAPHY

The angiocardiographic study of congenitally corrected transposition has also largely been made redundant by advances in echocardiography. When performed, interpretation progresses along the steps of segmental analysis. The morphologically right and left atrial chambers can be identified on the basis of the morphology of the appendages (Soto et al, 1978). The morphology of the atrial body and the connections with the venous system

add inferential information. The discordant atrioventricular connections in congenitally corrected transposition are best established by ventricular angiography. Occasionally, selective opacification of the atrium, with follow-through into the ventricles, is required for unequivocal identification, particularly in the presence of a criss-cross relationship between the ventricles (Symons et al, 1977; Freedom et al, 1978a).

Besides the classical anteroposterior and lateral views, axial projections are most helpful in demonstrating in detail the morphology of the ventricles and the presence of associated lesions (Bargeron et al, 1977; Losekoot et al, 1983). With usual atrial arrangement and left-sided heart (the arrangement found in over three fifths of patients with congenitally corrected transposition; Carey and Ruttenberg, 1964), the ventricles are positioned more or less side to side, with the ventricular septum in a sagittal plane. In the frontal plane, the right-sided morphologically left ventricle, usually located somewhat anteriorly and inferiorly, forms a triangular structure with the base directed superiorly and medially and the apex to the left and inferior (Figure 49.15a). The mitral valve forms a portion of the right and superior border. The left ventricular recess is projected over the outflow tract and is, therefore, poorly visualized.

The left-sided and morphologically right ventricle is located more superiorly and to the left. The shape is similar to that of a normally positioned right ventricle but with the long axis orientated inferiorly and to the left. The majority of the right border is formed by the tricuspid valve, which is separated from the arterial valve by the supraventricular crest (Figure 49.15b). The morphologically left ventricle is readily identified in the lateral projection on the basis of the prominent anterior recess (Figure 49.16). The inflow part of the ventricle is located in anteroinferior position, with the inflow tract superimposed over the trabecular zone. The outflow tract is situated posterosuperiorly. The arterial ventricle in lateral projection will be seen to have the typical features of the morphologically right ventricle. Posteriorly and inferiorly is seen the inflow portion, with the tricuspid valve viewed face on.

Anterosuperiorly is the infundibular component. The four chamber and elongated right anterior oblique views differ only marginally in appearance, but each may show certain details of the heart to better effect (Losekoot et al, 1983).

When the atriums are in usual position but the heart is right-sided in congenitally corrected transposition (an arrangement present in about one quarter of patients), the angiocardiographic anatomy is slightly different. The atrial septum is orientated anteriorly and somewhat to the right. The ventricles and the ventricular septum are also orientated to the right. The right-sided morphologically left ventricle now has an oval shape, and the 'tail' is absent in the anteroposterior view. In the situation with a right-sided heart and mirror-imaged atriums, the

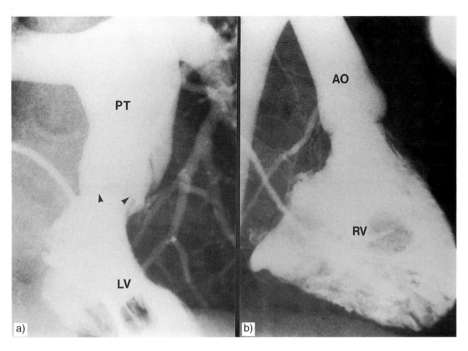

Figure 49.15. The classical angiographic appearances of (a) the morphologically left ventricle (LV) and the pulmonary trunk (PT) and (b) the morphologically right ventricle (RV) and aorta (AO) in a patient with usual atrial arrangement and intact septal structures. The arrowheads in (a) show the leaflets of the pulmonary valve in fibrous continuity with those of the mitral valve.

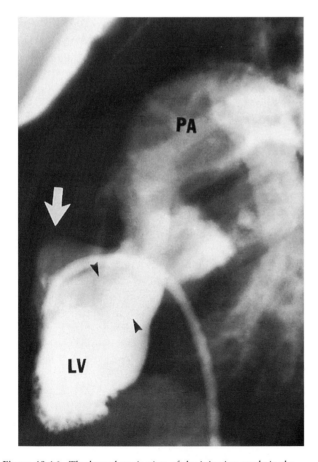

Figure 49.16. The lateral projection of the injection made in the morphologically left ventricle (LV) shows the typical anterior recess (arrowed) in front of the pulmonary trunk (PA). The black arrowheads show the mitral valvar orifice.

angiocardiographic appearances are the mirror image of the hearts with usual atrial arrangement and left-sided heart. The ventricular septum in these patients is orientated anteriorly, inferiorly and slightly to the right. As expected in patients with mirror-imaged atriums, the ventricles occupy the positions anticipated in the normal heart but with more side-by-side orientation and with parallel arterial trunks (Figure 49.17). In the posteriorly located left-sided morphologically left ventricle, the mitral valve is in left-superior and posterior position. The typical recess is again situated anterosuperiorly as viewed in the lateral projection (Attie et al, 1980; Losekoot et al, 1983).

As expected, angiocardiography clearly demonstrates the connections of the great arteries to the ventricles and their relationship to each other. With usual atrial arrangement, the aorta usually arises at the left border of the heart and the aortic arch is nearly always at the left (Figure 49.15). The aortic orifice is somewhat higher than that of the pulmonary trunk, which is situated in a posteromedial position with fibrous continuity between the leaflets of the pulmonary and mitral valves (Figure 49.16). The arrangements are reversed with mirror-imaged atrial arrangement (Figure 49.17).

Aortic root injections show the distribution of the coronary arteries. With usual atrial arrangement, the right-sided coronary artery, arising from the right-facing coronary sinus, is a morphologically left coronary artery. The artery arising from the left-facing sinus is a morphologically right coronary artery. In the mirror-imaged situation, the distribution of the coronary arteries is as found in the normal heart (Figure 49.5) (Schwartz and

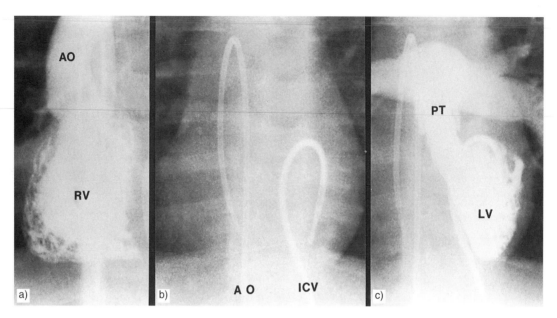

Figure 49.17. In this patient, the position of the arterial and venous catheters (b) show that there is mirror-imaged atrial arrangement, the catheter in the inferior caval vein (ICV) being to the left of the catheter in the aorta (AO). The ventricles occupy their anticipated position for the normal heart, with the aorta and morphologically right ventricle (RV) being right sided (a). The pulmonary trunk (PT) and morphologically left ventricle (LV) are left sided (c). Note the side-by-side ventricular relationships.

Wagner, 1974; Shea et al, 1979; Anderson and Becker, 1981).

THE BASIC LESION: UNCOMPLICATED CORRECTED TRANSPOSITION

Congenitally corrected transposition has been described without complicating anomalies, being identified at post-mortem or documented by the normal haemodynamic status at the time of observation. Study of the literature suggests that the incidence of uncomplicated corrected transposition is low, making up only about 1% of all cases (Losekoot, 1967; Ruttenberg, 1977; Kidd, 1978; Losekoot et al, 1983; Presbitero et al, 1995). However, structural anomalies are detected in a much higher incidence in anatomical studies than would be expected from clinical studies (Allwork et al, 1976). The possibility certainly exists that functional abnormalities that interfere significantly with the haemodynamic status may develop at a later age in response to these structural changes. The two most important anomalies developing during life are insufficiency of the left atrioventricular valve and high-degree atrioventricular block.

ASSOCIATED MALFORMATIONS

Amongst all persons with congenitally corrected transposition, the incidence of complicating malformations is sufficiently high to be considered the rule, albeit that a much higher incidence is detected in postmortem material than would be expected from clinical studies (Allwork

et al, 1976). Nearly all kinds of congenital cardiac malformation may be encountered, but three are so common that they are considered an integral part of the anomaly (Van Praagh, 1970). These are deficient ventricular septation, pulmonary stenosis and abnormalities of the left-sided atrioventricular valve. To these are usually added abnormalities of the conduction tissues. A fifth important feature is a positional anomaly of the heart (Losekoot, 1967; Kidd, 1978). The incidence of the remaining intracardiac malformations is more or less the same as in the normally structured heart.

It has been assumed that the incidence of intracardiac malformations is the same in those with mirror-imaged atriums as in those with usual atrial arrangement. It may be, however, that the incidence of ventricular septal defect is somewhat lower in the mirror-imaged situation, while that of pulmonary stenosis is slightly higher. More striking is the fact that well-documented cases of complete atrioventricular block are very rare in the mirror-imaged variant of congenitally corrected transposition (Losekoot et al, 1983). This is in keeping with the anatomical finding that the ventricular conduction axis takes origin more frequently from a regularly positioned atrioventricular node (Wilkinson et al, 1978; Dick et al, 1979).

VENTRICULAR SEPTAL DEFECT

Ventricular septal defect is the most common associated malformation. The incidence in clinical series is reported as 60–70% (Corone et al, 1966; Camier, 1967; Losekoot, 1967); postmortem series show an incidence of 78% (Allwork et al, 1976). As in hearts with concordant

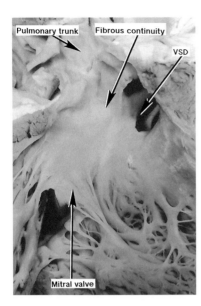

Figure 49.18. The typical ventricular septal defect (VSD) in congenitally corrected transposition is perimembranous and subpulmonary. Note the fibrous continuity between the leaflets of the pulmonary, mitral and tricuspid valves, which forms the posteroinferior margin of the defect.

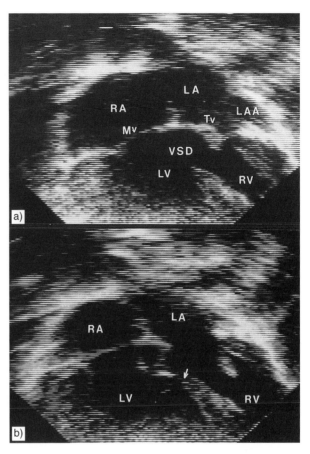

Figure 49.19. The transthoracic echocardiogram in four chamber section shows a perimembranous ventricular septal defect (VSD), but with lack of reversed off-setting (a) of the attachments of the mitral (Mv) and tricuspid (Tv) valves. Note the characteristic tubular shape of the left atrial appendage (LAA). (b) The attachment of a cord to the septum (arrowed) is evidence that this left-sided valve is morphologically tricuspid. Abbreviations as in Figures 49.12 and 49.13.

atrioventricular connections, the defects can be perimembranous, muscular or doubly committed and juxta-arterial.

The most common defect is perimembranous and, because of the discordant ventriculo-arterial connections, it is found in a subpulmonary position (Figure 49.18). Because of the deranged morphology of the atrioventricular junctions, the pulmonary outflow tract usually overrides the septum. The perimembranous defect extends posteriorly well towards the crux of the heart and erodes significantly the inlet part of the septum. The posterior edge of the defect is then formed by an extensive area of fibrous continuity between the leaflets of the pulmonary, mitral and tricuspid valves. The leaflets of the atrioventricular valves may, therefore, float through the defect, a characteristic often recognized on echocardiograms. The leaflets are also attached at the same level, removing the characteristic valvar off-setting (Figure 49.19). The roof of the defect is the pulmonary valve, and the anterior border is formed by the muscular septum. It should be reiterated that the conduction bundle will not be present in its anticipated position for a perimembranous defect with concordant atrioventricular connections, but instead will run along the upper and anterior border (Figure 49.20). In rare instances, the defect can be subpulmonary and muscular. The conduction bundle will still be anterosuperior. Muscular defects, however, may occur in any other part of the ventricular septum. If between the outlets, they may be above the bundle. Defects in juxta-arterial position, roofed by continuity between the leaflets of the aortic and pulmonary valves with absence of the septal component of the infundibulum (Figure 49.21), are particularly common in the Far East (Okamura and Konno, 1973).

The ventricular septal defect present in hearts with congenitally corrected transposition is usually large. It gives rise to an important shunt, with pulmonary hypertension and pulmonary vascular obstructive disease as the consequences. In most instances, however, ventricular septal defects occur in combination with other malformations, such as pulmonary stenosis and anomalies of the atrioventricular valves. The clinical picture does not differ from that in the normally structured heart. Even without pulmonary hypertension, the second heart sound may be accentuated because of the anterior position of the aortic valve.

The electrocardiogram reflects, to a great extent, the haemodynamic status. When the ventricular septal defect is small, it will not differ from the usual pattern seen in congenitally corrected transposition. Otherwise, the electrocardiogram should be interpreted according to the already discussed criterions of ventricular hypertrophy. Abnormal waves indicating dilation of one or both atriums are occasionally seen.

On the chest radiograph, the size of the heart reflects the haemodynamic changes with frequent dilation of the heart chambers and increase of vascular markings.

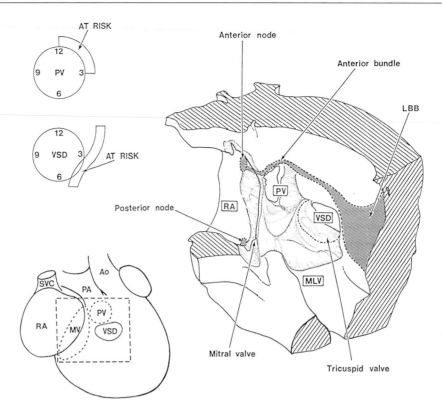

Figure 49.20. A diagram based on a reconstruction of the conduction system in a heart studied histologically emphasizes the anterosuperior location of the conduction bundle relative to the typical perimembranous ventricular septal defect (VSD). The insets show the areas at major surgical risk. Ao, aorta; LBB, left bundle branch; MLV, morphological left ventricle; MV, mitral valve; PA, pulmonary artery; PV, pulmonary valve; RA, right atrium; SVC, superior caval vein.

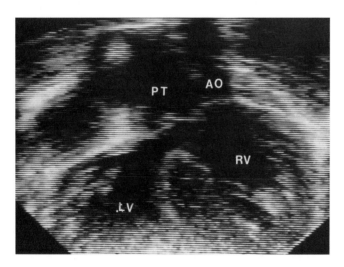

Figure 49.21. This transthoracic echocardiogram shows the fibrous continuity between the leaflets of the pulmonary (PT) and aortic (AO) valves, which identifies the ventricular septal defect as being doubly committed and juxta-arterial. Other abbreviations as in Figure 49.12.

Prominence of the pulmonary trunk is missing. In the presence of a large arterio-venous shunt, the convex prominence at the left side of the vascular pedicle is also absent (Figure 49.11). If the ventricular septal defect is combined with severe pulmonary stenosis and a veno-

arterial shunt, the prominence may be outspoken, especially when the heart itself is right sided.

Cross-sectional echocardiography in the four chamber and long-axis views demonstrates the site and morphology of a ventricular septal defect (Losekoot et al, 1983). When a perimembranous defect opens between the inlets, the valves are attached to the atrial septum at the same level (Figure 49.19) (Sutherland et al, 1983). Ventricular morphology is then distinguished on the basis of the attachments of the tendinous cords to the morphologically right ventricular aspect of the septum (Figure 49.19b).

Catheterization is invaluable for the evaluation of ventricular septal defects but has now been superceded by echocardiography for diagnosis. When performed the four chamber and elongated right oblique views may be necessary in addition to a frontal view to differentiate between perimembranous, doubly committed and muscular defects (Losekoot et al, 1983). Spontaneous closure of ventricular septal defects in congenitally corrected transposition has been described (Summerall et al, 1966; Allwork et al, 1976).

OBSTRUCTION TO THE OUTFLOW TRACT OF THE MORPHOLOGICALLY LEFT VENTRICLE

Excluding hearts with pulmonary atresia, stenosis occurs in approximately 30–50% of patients with usual atrial arrangement. It is isolated in less than one fifth of these. In approximately four fifths, the pulmonary stenosis is combined with a ventricular septal defect and, in about one third of these, abnormalities of the morphologically tricuspid valve are also found.

The anatomical nature of the stenosis varies. Valvar stenosis is usually accompanied by one or other variety of subpulmonary obstruction. The latter may take the form of muscular hypertrophy of the septum and the ventricular free wall, a fibrous diaphragm or an aneurysmal dilation of fibrous tissue derived from the interventricular component of the membranous septum (Figure 49.22). More rarely, tags may originate from either of the atrioventricular valves, or even from the leaflets of the pulmonary valve (Anderson et al, 1975). Subvalvar pulmonary obstructions, when present, are intimately related to the non-branching atrioventricular bundle.

When pulmonary stenosis is present, the clinical findings often suggest the appropriate diagnosis. A rough ejection-type murmur will be heard maximally in the second left intercostal space. Splitting of the second heart sound is an inconstant finding; sometimes the unsplit second sound can be accentuated, suggesting pulmonary hypertension. An early ejection click is only rarely heard. These findings are often altered by additional complicating malformations. Cyanosis is seen in about one sixth of the patients in whom pulmonary stenosis is combined with ventricular septal defect (Camier, 1967).

It is rare to see post-stenotic dilation of the pulmonary trunk on the chest radiograph. If the pulmonary trunk is present and severely dilated, it may be visible at the right border in the vascular pedicle in those with usual atrial arrangement, or at the left side in the mirror-

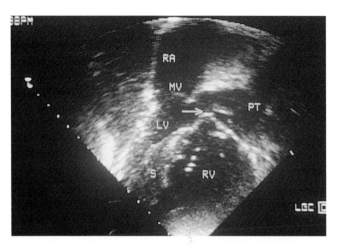

Figure 49.23. This transthoracic echocardiogram from the subcostal window in a patient with a right-sided heart shows marked narrowing of the subpulmonary outflow tract (arrowed) and post-stenotic dilatation of the pulmonary trunk (PT). S, septum; other abbreviations as in Figure 49.12.

imaged situation. The vascular markings of the lung are diminished.

The electrocardiogram correlates superficially with the severity of the diagnosis. Cross-sectional echocardiography is particularly helpful in defining the nature of the obstructive lesion. The four chamber view with the transducer in subcostal position gives the best information (Figure 49.23). Post-stenotic dilation of the pulmonary trunk is easily demonstrated when present.

Catheterization permits measurement of the pressure in the morphologically left ventricle, important information for assessing the severity of stenosis. Often it is difficult to advance the catheter into the pulmonary trunk. Should angiocardiography be considered necessary, the pulmonary trunk is clearly seen in the elongated right anterior oblique view, or in the four chamber view. Tags of accessory fibrous tissue in the morphologically left ventricular outflow tract are seen as filling defects in the outflow tract (Figure 49.24) or as bags full of contrast medium (Losekoot et al, 1983).

LESIONS OF THE MORPHOLOGICAL TRICUSPID VALVE

Lesions of the morphological tricuspid valve are almost an essential part of congenitally corrected transposition (Edwards, 1954; Schiebler et al, 1961). There is a marked discrepancy, however, between the incidence of such changes found at necropsy and those recognized during life. Postmortem material reveals anomalies of the tricuspid valve in almost nine tenths of cases, whereas only one in three patients have haemodynamic alterations owing to such abnormalities.

The most common underlying pathology is valvar dysplasia, with or without apical displacement of the septal and/or mural leaflets. Atrialization, with thinning and dilation of the ventricular inlet portion (as commonly

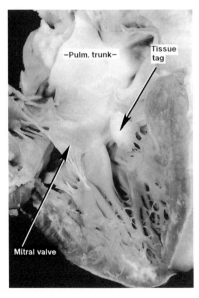

Figure 49.22. This view of the opened subpulmonary outflow tract from the morphologically left ventricle shows a tissue tag derived from the remnant of the interventricular component of the membranous septum. Pulm., pulmonary.

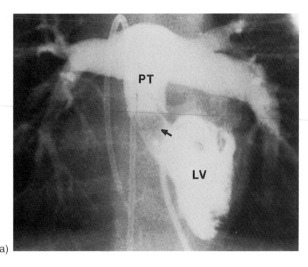
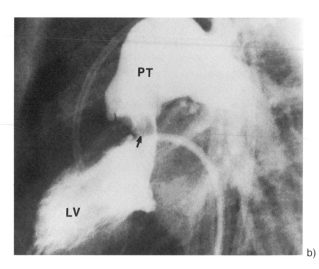

a)

b)

Figure 49.24. This angiogram taken following an injection in the morphologically left ventricle (LV) in a patient with mirror-imaged atrial chambers shows a subpulmonary tissue tag appearing as a filling defect in both frontal (a) and lateral (b) projections. PT, pulmonary trunk.

seen in Ebstein's malformation with concordant atrioventricular connections) is rare in hearts with congenitally corrected transposition (Figure 49.25). In about three quarters of patients, the tricuspid valvar anomalies are combined with a ventricular septal defect.

The clinical findings are those reflecting left atrioventricular valvar insufficiency. They do not differ importantly, therefore, from the findings of mitral regurgitation in the normal heart. The electrocardiogram will be normal for congenitally corrected transposition or may show the typical features of hypertrophy of the left-sided ventricle. 'Mitral' P waves are occasionally encountered.

In the frontal chest radiograph, the size of the heart depends upon the haemodynamic status. Prominence of the pulmonary segment is absent. The ascending aorta is small and, therefore, the convex bulge at the left of the mediastinum will be absent. There may be signs of pulmonary venous congestion.

Cross-sectional echocardiography demonstrates nicely the displacement of the valve septal leaflet, although it is often not possible to demonstrate dysplasia with certainty (Figure 49.26). The cross-sectional technique is also of great value in recognizing other valvar anomalies and in evaluating the function of an artificial valve.

Minimal anatomical changes of the left-sided valve may not be apparent angiocardiographically. False-positive interpretations are easily made (Losekoot et al, 1983). When Ebstein-like malformation is severe, nonetheless, it

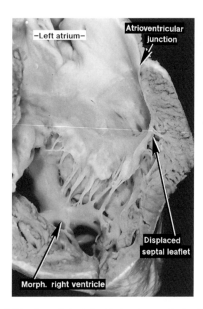

Figure 49.25. This view of the left-sided atrioventricular junction shows the typical appearances of Ebstein's malformation as seen in the setting of congenitally corrected transposition. The thinning of the inlet component as typically encountered when the atrioventricular connections are concordant is lacking in this heart. Morph., morphological.

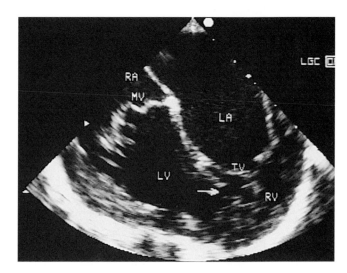

Figure 49.26. The transoesophageal echocardiogram shows the exaggerated off-setting of the hinge of the left-sided morphologically tricuspid valve (TV) that is typical of Ebstein's malformation as seen in congenitally corrected transposition. MV, mitral valve; other abbreviations as in Figures 49.12 and 49.13.

can be demonstrated angiocardiographically (Losekoot et al, 1983). Prolapse of the valve and the presence of abnormal tissue have also been demonstrated in angiocardiographic studies (Soto et al, 1978).

DELAY OR BLOCKING OF ATRIOVENTRICULAR CONDUCTION

Delay or blocking of atrioventricular conduction is a frequent complication of congenitally corrected transposition (Cardell, 1956). In most cases, the conduction delay is progressive during life. The incidence of the different degrees of block, therefore, varies with the age of the patients. First-degree atrioventricular block is seen in up to one third of patients (Camier, 1967; Losekoot, 1967). Second-degree atrioventricular block is much less frequent. About one tenth of patients may present with complete heart block.

Data presented by Fyler (1992) based on the experience from Boston Children's Hospital showed that 45% of their patients eventually developed complete heart block. This figure is somewhat higher than the 30% suggested by Mullins (1990). Because acquired heart block frequently occurs in the setting of associated cardiac anomalies, the bradycardia is not well tolerated, and a pacemaker may need to be inserted as a matter of urgency. It has been suggested that spontaneous complete heart block develops in about 2% of this population per year (Huhta et al, 1985).

In most cases of complete atrioventricular block, the QRS complexes are narrow. The ventricular rate differs from patient to patient. The genesis of these conduction anomalies is unclear but is almost certainly related to the abnormal anatomy of the conduction tissue (Walmsley, 1931). Fibrosis of the atrioventricular bundle and fibrosis at the junction with the anterior node are the most common pathological findings. Congenital anomalies may also be the cause for the conduction delay (Bharati et al, 1978). Electrophysiological studies have shown conduction delay in different levels of the specialized junctional area (Friedman et al, 1973; Wolff et al, 1973; Gillette et al, 1979).

There is a relatively high incidence of pre-excitation seen in patients with congenitally corrected transposition (Wellens et al, 1977; Losekoot et al, 1983). Types A and B have both been reported, with nearly the same incidence. Paroxysmal tachycardias have been present in some of the patients. When the Wolff–Parkinson–White syndrome is combined with Ebstein's malformation of the left atrioventricular valve, all patients have type-A pre-excitation. Other supraventricular disturbances of rhythm, typically atrial flutter, are also common in congenitally corrected transposition and are related to the haemodynamic status.

OTHER ASSOCIATED ANOMALIES

Any anomaly can coexist with congenitally corrected transposition. The incidence of other associated lesions is

high, but it is not clear whether their mutual relations differ from those found in the normally structured heart.

Abnormal relationships of the ventricles – so-called criss-cross heart or superoinferior ('upstairs–downstairs') ventricles – are found with some frequency. Nearly always other severe complicating cardiac malformations are then present, with ventricular septal defect, straddling valves and obstruction to pulmonary outflow being the most common. When these abnormal ventricular relationships are found with usual atrial arrangement, the aorta is usually situated to the right and anterior to the pulmonary trunk. This may give problems in diagnosis, particularly since other typical symptoms for corrected transposition may be absent. Angiocardiography, with contrast injections from both atriums and ventricles, gives diagnostic information (Freedom et al, 1978a; Losekoot et al, 1983), but the combination is readily diagnosed with cross-sectional echocardiography.

Straddling and overriding valves are particularly important, since the ventricle to which the overriding orifice should normally be connected is often underdeveloped (Freedom et al, 1978b). Straddling of the morphologically tricuspid valve is the more common (Figure 49.27). When such a valve straddles, the conduction tissue disposition is found in its anticipated position for corrected transposition (Milo et al, 1979). When it is the right-sided morphologically mitral valve that straddles (Figure 49.28), there may be significant departures from this norm (Becker et al, 1980; Gerlis et al, 1986). Diagnosis of a straddling atrioventricular valve creates diagnostic and surgical problems. The anomaly should always be considered when there is unexpected arterial desaturation or if there is underdevelopment of one ventricle. The definitive diagnosis is made by echocardiography, using either the transthoracic (Figure 49.29) or transoesophageal (Figure 49.30) portals. Angiocardiography can be diagnostic if performed by injection of contrast in the atrium

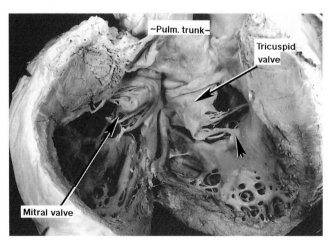

Figure 49.27. There is overriding of the orifice of the tricuspid valve in this heart with a perimembranous defect. The tension apparatus (arrowhead) just straddles the crest of the ventricular septum. Pulm., pulmonary.

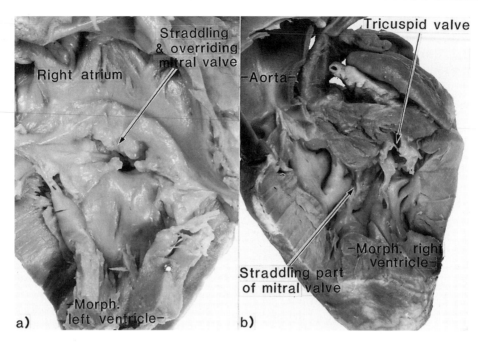

Figure 49.28. In this specimen, there is overriding and straddling of the morphologically (morph.) mitral valve, seen from the right-sided left ventricle (a) and from the left-sided morphologically right ventricle (b).

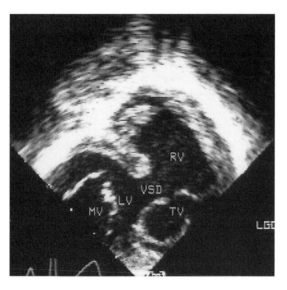

Figure 49.29. This transthoracic echocardiogram from a subcostal position shows straddling and overriding of the left-sided morphologically tricuspid valve (TV). Other abbreviations as in Figures 49.12 and 49.19.

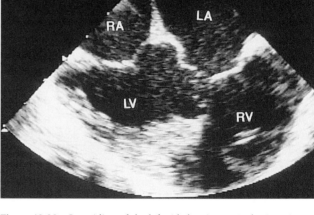

Figure 49.30. Overriding of the left-sided atrioventricular junction and straddling of the tension apparatus of the tricuspid valve is particularly clearly seen using the transoesophageal portal. Abbreviations as in Figures 49.12 and 49.13.

draining through the straddling valve. It may then be possible to demonstrate two separate contrast streams going to the ventricles (Becker et al, 1980). Dilution of the contrast media often masks this finding (Tandon et al, 1974; Freedom et al, 1978b). Injection of contrast in one or both ventricles with the camera angled for the left anterior or long-axis view (Bargeron et al, 1977) can be more conclusive (La Corte et al, 1976; Freedom et al, 1978b).

Atrial septal defect in the oval fossa is seen in about 12% of the clinical cases. Atrioventricular septal defects

also exist but are relatively rare (Attie et al, 1998). Patency of the arterial duct is also seen in about 12% of the clinical cases.

Aortic atresia is an uncommon association, but a number of instances with functional and anatomical atresia are described (Brenner et al, 1978; Craig et al, 1986; Freedom et al, 1989; Freedom, 1999). The unifying pathological feature is severe regurgitation of the systemic atrioventricular valve, producing a very abnormal and thinned morphologically right ventricle. The lungs, too, may exhibit some degree of hypoplasia (Deanfield et al, 1981; Matsukawa et al, 1985; Muster et al, 1985; Chan et al, 1989; Celermajer et al, 1991). Such patients may not be candidates for a classic Norwood-like approach unless the systemic atrioventricular valve is oversewn, as happened to one patient undergoing surgery in Toronto. Cardiac replacement is, perhaps, an alternative when the lungs are not disadvantaged.

Ventricular hypoplasia is seen most frequently in association with straddling valves (see above). Hypoplasia of the morphologically left ventricle can be seen in the setting of pulmonary atresia with intact (or nearly intact) ventricular septum (Steeg et al, 1971; Shimazu et al, 1981; Zahn et al, 1992). The left ventricle then resembles the situation more typically seen in hypoplastic left heart syndrome, with a patent aorta arising from the morphologically right ventricle.

Patients with significant ventricular hypoplasia, either morphologically right or left, or with major degrees of atrioventricular valvar straddling will rarely be suitable candidates for biventricular repair; rather, they will be placed on a Fontan protocol, as will those having pulmonary atresia with intact ventricular septum.

DIFFERENTIAL DIAGNOSIS

After careful non-invasive and invasive studies, it should now always be possible to make the proper diagnosis of congenitally corrected transposition and to identify all associated lesions. Some anomalies, nonetheless, may still give problems in differentiation. The lesions producing difficulty are those with discordant atrioventricular connections and other ventriculo-arterial connections, other anomalies with an anterior and left-sided ascending aorta in presence of usual atrial arrangement, or those with an anterior and right-sided aorta in the mirror-imaged situation.

In some hearts with a left-sided anterior aorta, the atrioventricular and ventriculo-arterial connections can both be concordant ('anatomically corrected malposition'). In these patients, as in congenitally corrected transposition, the basic circulation is normal. The combination is very rare and can be seen in persons with usually arranged, mirror-imaged or isomeric atrial chambers. There are nearly always bilateral infundibulums. In all reported cases there has been a ventricular septal defect, with subpulmonary outflow obstruction in three quarters. Left-sided juxtaposition of the atrial appendages was seen in half, the heart being right sided also in about half. Normal anatomy of the conduction tissue is to be expected. Careful interpretation of the electrocardiogram, echocardiogram and angiocardiogram, together with appropriate evaluation of the effect of complicating malformations on these findings, will lead to the correct diagnosis.

A left-sided anterior aorta is by no means a rare finding in complete transposition with usual atrial arrangement

(Carr et al, 1968; Otero Coto et al, 1978). The variation is easily recognizable echocardiographically, as well as by angiocardiography. More rarely, the aorta may be left sided and anterior in double outlet right ventricle with concordant atrioventricular connections and usual atrial arrangement. Nearly always there are bilateral infundibulums and a subaortic ventricular septal defect. Obstruction of the subpulmonary outflow tract and juxtaposition of the atrial appendages are very common (Otero Coto et al, 1978). Again electrocardiography, echocardiography and angiocardiography will demonstrate the pertinent aspects of the anomaly.

In the anomaly of double outlet left ventricle, itself rare, most patients have a right-sided aorta. A few patients with usual atrial arrangement and a left-sided aorta (and a right-sided aorta in the mirror-imaged situation) have been described (Sharratt et al, 1976; Urban, et al, 1977; Kinsley et al, 1979).

Isomeric atrial appendages with biventricular atrioventricular connections can closely resemble congenitally corrected transposition when the right-sided atrium is connected to the morphologically left ventricle, and the left-sided atrium to the morphologically right ventricle. This is particularly so when the ventriculo-arterial connections are also discordant. This combination can be found with either left or right isomerism (de Tommasi et al, 1981). The existence of isomerism may be suggested by an abnormal bronchial tree on the chest radiograph (Deanfield et al, 1980), an abnormal P wave (Blieden and Moller, 1973) or by the finding of abnormal pulmonary or systemic venous connections. In these anomalies, the conduction tissue arises from an anterior node or there is a sling between anterior and regular nodes (Dickinson et al, 1979).

Univentricular atrioventricular connection to a left ventricle with left-sided rudimentary right ventricle closely resembles congenitally corrected transposition when the ventriculo-arterial connections are also discordant. Reversal of the precordial Q wave pattern on the electrocardiogram is then the exception rather than the rule (Guller et al, 1975; Quero Jimenez et al, 1978). Furthermore, cross-sectional echocardiography demonstrates clearly that both atrioventricular junctions are committed to the dominant left ventricle. Angiocardiography confirms the combination of dominant left and rudimentary right ventricles (Chapter 38).

Univentricular atrioventricular connection to a dominant right ventricle is easy to distinguish from congenitally corrected transposition, even when the rudimentary morphologically left ventricle is right sided (Soto et al, 1979; Essed et al, 1980). Problems may arise when double inlet is associated with straddling of either the right (Becker et al, 1980) or the left atrioventricular valve (Otero Coto et al, 1981). Distinction can then largely be a matter of categorization, since it is well recognized that a spectrum exists from double inlet to congenitally corrected transposition (Losekoot et al, 1983).

SURGICAL TREATMENT

Since the segmental combinations in congenitally corrected transposition serve to correct the circulations, surgical correction of those associated malformations that initially have 'uncorrected' the malformation will restore normality, albeit that still the morphologically right ventricle will be called upon to pump the systemic circulation. Over the years, therefore, it was natural that surgeons should seek to provide correction by closing ventricular septal defects, relieving subpulmonary obstruction and repairing the morphologically tricuspid valve (El-Sayed et al, 1962; Bonfils-Roberts et al, 1974). In the very early days, significant problems were encountered because of the unexpected location of the atrioventricular conduction tissues, and surgically induced heart block was a well-recognized complication. Analysis of the results of surgery at the Mayo Clinic for the period from 1958 through 1979 showed that heart block was produced in 53% of patients who had, initially, been in sinus rhythm. Furthermore, in this undoubted centre of excellence, one quarter of the patients undergoing surgery died within 30 days of operation (Marcelletti et al, 1980). From the mid-1970s, however, surgeons had become aware of the precise location of the atrioventricular conduction axis and had devised means of avoiding the bundle during closure of ventricular septal defects (Danielson et al, 1978; de Leval et al, 1979) or relief of subpulmonary obstruction (Doty et al, 1983). Despite all these advances, results of 'classical' surgery remained disappointing. Important series were reported from acknowledged centres of excellence in the USA, Australia and the UK (McGrath et al, 1985; Sano et al, 1995; Szufladowicz et al, 1996). Although most patients had a satisfactory functional outcome, survival reported after 10 years was no more than 70–80% while the incidence of postoperative heart block remained disturbingly high, at 15–30%. Furthermore, correction of the associated malformations was frequently found to precipitate functional deterioration in the morphologically right ventricle and regurgitation across the tricuspid valve (Freedom, 1999; Voskuil et al, 1999; Yeh et al, 1999).

Because of these disappointing results, surgeons in several centres sought alternative means of repair that would not only correct the associated malformations but would also restore the morphologically left ventricle to its rightful role in pumping the systemic circulation. Placing the morphologically left ventricle beneath the aorta would provide anatomical as well as functional correction of the associated malformations. This can now be achieved by means of the so-called double switch procedure, combining atrial redirection with an arterial switch (Figure 49.31), or by tunnelling the left ventricle to the aorta through a large ventricular septal defect and combining this with redirection of flows at atrial level. To the best of our knowledge, it was Subirana and her

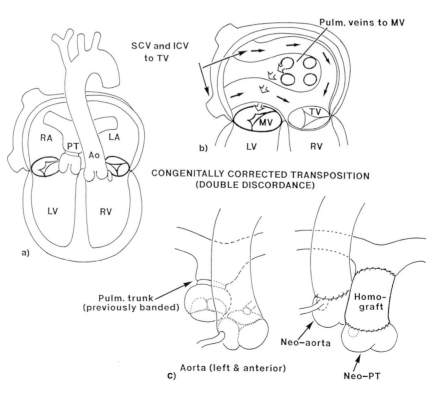

Figure 49.31. The steps involved in the so-called double switch procedure involve, first, banding of the pulmonary trunk (PT) unless associated lesions have already 'prepared' the left ventricle (a). An atrial redirection procedure (b) is then combined with an arterial switch (c). This then produces both physiological and anatomical correction. Ao, aorta; LA, left atrium; LV, left ventricle; MV, mitral valve; pulm., pulmonary; RA, right atrium; RV, right ventricle; SCV and ICV, superior and inferior caval veins; TV, tricuspid valve.

colleagues (1984) who first described such anatomical correction for a patient with discordant atrioventricular connections, although the patient, who also had double outlet right ventricle, died. Ilbawi and his associates (1990) then successfully restored the left ventricle to its systemic role in patients with either pulmonary atresia or pulmonary stenosis with a large interventricular communication, restoring continuity between the morphologically right ventricle and the pulmonary arteries by insertion of a conduit. Yamagishi and colleagues (1993) from Tokyo, and Yagihara and associates (1994) from Osaka, then showed that correction could also be achieved by means of the double switch procedures. For the double switch procedure to be successful it is also necessary that the morphologically left ventricle be capable of supporting the systemic circulation immediately at the conclusion of the operative procedures. This is not always the case. In those patients in whom it is judged that the left ventricle will not be appropriately 'prepared' therefore it is necessary to provide a period of training by banding the pulmonary trunk (Figure 49.31) (Mee, 1986; Stumper et al, 1995; Karl et al, 1997; Helvind et al, 1998).

Results of these procedures providing anatomical correction, with or without preliminary banding of the pulmonary trunk, have been very encouraging, but the surgical procedures required are extensive (Imai et al, 1994; Delius and Stark, 1996; Reddy et al, 1997; Imai, 1997; Acar et al, 1998, Stümper and Brawn, 1998; Bove, 1999; Sharma et al, 1999). Uemura and Yagihara (1998), describing their experience in Osaka, acknowledge that periods of nearly 4 hours for cardiopulmonary bypass, and almost 2.5 hours for aortic cross-clamping, are common place. Because of this, they emphasize the need for adequate myocardial protection, pointing out that retrograde cardioplegia is ineffective in protecting the morphologically left ventricle because the coronary sinus receives venous return from the morphologically right ventricle. Furthermore, not all patients with congenitally corrected transposition are suitable candidates for anatomical correction because of the compounding effects of some associated malformations (Alva et al, 1998). Analysis of the cohort of patients undergoing treatment at Hôpital Laennec, Paris, showed that certain groups did better than others after classical surgery (Vouhé and Sidi, 1998). In those with combined ventricular septal defect and subpulmonary obstruction, for example (this combination being a likely contraindication for anatomical correction), there was less risk of progressive deterioration in function of the morphologically right ventricle and the tricuspid valve. Despite this, the probability of late survival in this group after classical surgery was still disappointingly low, being 70% at 10 years.

Consequently, the potential benefits of placing the morphologically left ventricle in the systemic circuit subsequent to surgical repair are obvious. In a significant number of patients, this cannot be achieved because of severe anomalies of the mitral valve, relative hypoplasia of the morphologically left ventricle and either a small size or unusual position of the ventricular septal defect (Alva et al, 1998). These patients may profit from palliative procedures, including construction of a Fontan circulation or bilateral cavopulmonary connection, or may still be candidates for classical surgical procedures. When weighing the most appropriate surgical option, note must also be taken of the potential late drawbacks of anatomical correction, such as the need for revision of conduits, or the development of arrhythmias following atrial redirection procedures. The view of Brawn and his colleagues (1998) is that the more complex form of surgery needed to provide anatomical correction is justified in those patients who have primary failure of the morphologically right ventricle associated with problems of the tricuspid valve, and also in all those with pulmonary stenosis or atresia where the ventricular septal defect can safely be tunnelled to the aorta. They agree with Vouhé and Sidi (1998) that those patients with well-balanced systemic and pulmonary circulations, usually in the setting of a ventricular septal defect and moderate pulmonary stenosis, are best managed conservatively without surgical intervention until such time that they become symptomatic. The solution to these difficult decisions will become clearer when more information is available on the true ability of the morphologically right ventricle to support the systemic circulation over periods of greater than 40 years. This information will soon become available as the cohort of patients who underwent atrial redirection procedures for complete transposition live further into adult life (Chapter 48).

DISCORDANT ATRIOVENTRICULAR AND CONCORDANT VENTRICULO-ARTERIAL CONNECTIONS

As might be anticipated, the segmental combination of discordant connections across the atrioventricular junction with concordant ventriculo-arterial connections is found in patients with usual atrial arrangement (Figure 49.32) (Van Praagh and Van Praagh, 1966; Quero Jimenez and Raposo-Sonnenfeld, 1975) as well as in those with mirror-imaged atriums (Anderson et al, 1972; Clarkson et al, 1972; Leijala et al, 1981). Some of the reported cases, however, probably had isomeric atrial appendages and should be grouped accordingly. In most cases, the aorta is posterior and to the right of the pulmonary trunk. Because this arterial arrangement is seen in the otherwise normal heart, some describe the combination as isolated ventricular inversion. We do not find this particularly helpful, the more so since patients with this segmental combination have different positions of the great arteries (Espino-Vela et al, 1970). The important feature is that, clinically, the patients present with the

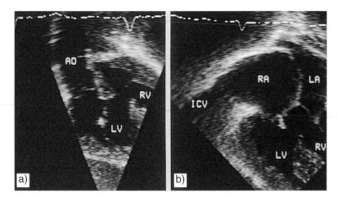

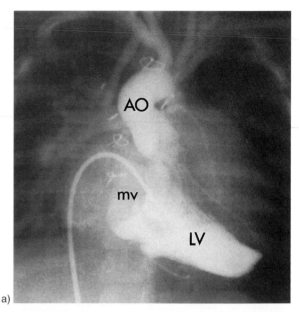

Figure 49.32. These cross-sectional echocardiograms show concordant ventriculo-arterial connections (a) in combination with discordant atrioventricular connections (b). This combination is ideal for atrial correction, restoring the left ventricle to its systemic role. Abbreviations as in Figure 49.31.

haemodynamics of complete transposition but the conduction tissues and electrocardiographic findings will be as for congenitally corrected transposition.

When this condition is not complicated by significant ventricular hypoplasia or abnormalities of the left atrioventricular valve, the affected patients are ideal candidates for surgical correction by simple atrial redirection (Leijala et al, 1981; Arciprete et al, 1985; Ranjit et al, 1991). This provides both anatomical and physiological correction of the circulations. For those with significant ventricular hypoplasia (Figure 49.33), long-term physiological palliation may be achieved by constructing a Fontan circulation.

DISCORDANT ATRIOVENTRICULAR CONNECTIONS WITH DOUBLE ─── OUTLET RIGHT VENTRICLE ───

Most patients in which discordant atrioventricular connections are combined with double outlet right ventricle have right-sided hearts and pulmonary stenosis: the so-called 'Mayo Clinic syndrome' (Kiser et al, 1968). Interestingly, it was in a heart such as this that Mönckeberg (1913) first described the unusual atrioventricular conduction system. This segmental combination can, of course, exist with the heart in any position within the chest. The ventricular septal defect is usually in subpulmonary position, but subaortic, doubly committed and noncommitted defects have all been described. All kinds of relation between the great arteries can also be present. In most cases, a Mönckeberg sling of conduction tissue is present, but solitary anterior connection of the penetrating bundle has also been found (de Leval et al, 1979). Any associated anomaly may be present when it is feasible for it to coexist. The clinical picture in patients who have an aorta that is anterior and left sided is identical in nearly all aspects to typically congenitally corrected transposition. The distinguishing feature, the

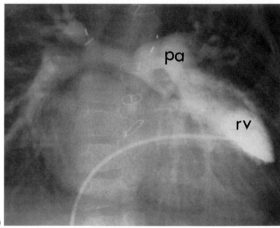

Figure 49.33. Angiograms from a patient with discordant atrioventricular but concordant ventriculo-arterial connections. The catheter shows the right-sided position of the inferior caval vein (a) and the connection to the morphologically left ventricle (LV) which gives rise to the aorta (AO). The left-sided morphologically right ventricle (rv) is grossly hypoplastic (b) and gives rise to the pulmonary trunk (pa).

origin of the pulmonary trunk from the left-sided morphologically right ventricle, can readily be demonstrated by echocardiography (Tabry et al, 1978; Hagler et al, 1981b; Battistessa and Soto, 1990). Angiography, nowadays, is rarely required.

DISCORDANT ATRIOVENTRICULAR CONNECTIONS AND DOUBLE OUTLET ─── LEFT VENTRICLE ───

The rarest ventriculo-arterial connection, that of double outlet left ventricle, can be found with all types of atrioventricular connection (Van Praagh and Weinberg, 1977). It seems likely that double outlet left ventricle with discordant atrioventricular connections can be found with various arterial relationships, and with the ventricular septal defect in different positions. This combination has been described with usual atrial arrangement and a left-sided aorta, and in mirror-imaged arrangement with a right-sided aorta (Brandt et al, 1976). The usual complicating lesions have been encountered, as seen in corrected transposition. Differentiation from discordant ventriculo-arterial connections is possible by cross-sectional echocardiography. It can also be demonstrated by angiography of high standard. Since the aorta is already taking origin from the morphologically left ventricle, these patients will be ideal candidates for anatomical correction, combining an atrial redirection procedure with placement of a conduit from the right ventricle to the pulmonary trunk.

DISCORDANT ATRIOVENTRICULAR CONNECTIONS WITH SINGLE OUTLET

There are three separate variants of discordant atrioventricular connection with a single outlet: common arterial trunk, single pulmonary trunk with aortic atresia and single aortic trunk with pulmonary atresia. Of these, the first two are extremely rare (Espino-Vela et al, 1970; Deanfield et al, 1981). With pulmonary atresia, however, there is usually a large ventricular septal defect in the subaortic position. This lends itself to tunnelling as part of anatomical correction. The conduction tissue is anterior to this defect, arising from an anterior atrioventricular node; consequently, extreme care is needed if enlargement of the defect is attempted as part of an anatomical correction (Brawn et al, 1998). Cases also exist of discordant atrioventricular connections with pulmonary atresia when the ventricular septum is intact (Steeg et al, 1971; Shimizu et al, 1981). Since, in these patients, the atretic pulmonary artery can usually be traced to the morphologically left ventricle, they are better classified as congenitally corrected transposition with pulmonary atresia. The arrangement of the left ventricle itself, however, is reminiscent of hypoplastic left heart syndrome.

In those with discordant atrioventricular connections, pulmonary atresia and ventricular septal defect, progressive cyanosis and tachypnoea are present from birth. At physical examination, the heart is not enlarged and the second sound is single. Murmurs are unimpressive but a continuous murmur may be heard in the second left intercostal space in the presence of a patent arterial duct. Prominence of the pulmonary trunk is lacking in the chest radiograph, with diminished pulmonary vascular markings. The bulge in the left contour of the vascular pedicle produced by the ascending aorta is outspoken when the heart is right sided. Signs of right ventricular hypertrophy may be absent on the electrocardiogram, and then the presence of a right precordial Q wave is of great diagnostic significance. The discordant atrioventricular connections, the connection of the aorta to the morphologically right ventricle and the ventricular septal defect can all readily be demonstrated echocardiographically, but it is difficult to trace the atretic pulmonary artery and its mode of connection to the heart. Angiocardiography will demonstrate the abnormal anatomy in detail. Almost always the pulmonary arterial supply is duct-dependent, but rare cases exist with supply through systemic-to-pulmonary collateral arteries. These patients will require investigation and treatment as for those having tetralogy of Fallot with pulmonary atresia. It must also be anticipated that even rarer forms of pulmonary arterial supply, such as patency of the fifth aortic arch or fistulous communications from the coronary arteries, will be encountered when patients with discordant atrioventricular connections have pulmonary atresia in association with a ventricular septal defect.

REFERENCES

Acar P, Sidi D, Bonnet D, Aggoun Y, Bonhoeffer P, Kachaner J 1998 Maintaining tricuspid valve competence in double discordance: a challenge for the paediatric cardiologist. Heart 80: 479–483

Allwork S P, Bentall H H, Becker A E et al 1976 Congenitally corrected transposition of the great arteries. Morphologic study of 32 cases. American Journal of Cardiology 38: 910–923

Alva C, Horowitz E, Ho S Y, Rigby M L, Anderson R H 1999 The feasibility of the double switch in the setting of discordant atrioventricular connections. Heart 81: 539–545

Anderson R C, Lillehei C W, Lester R G 1957 Corrected transposition of the great vessels of the heart. Pediatrics 20: 626–646

Anderson R H 1982 Criss-cross hearts revisited. Pediatric Cardiology 3: 305–313

Anderson R H, Becker A E 1981 Coronary arterial patterns: a guide to identification of congenital heart disease. In: Becker A E, Losekoot G, Marcelletti C, Anderson R H (eds) Paediatric cardiology, vol 3. Churchill Livingstone, Edinburgh, 251–262

Anderson R H, Arnold M B, Jones R S 1972 D-bulboventricular loop with L-transposition in situs inversus. Circulation 46: 193–199

Anderson R H, Arnold R, Wilkinson J L 1973 The conducting system in congenitally corrected transposition. Lancet i: 1286–1288

Anderson R H, Becker A E, Arnold R, Wilkinson J L 1974 The conducting tissues in congenitally corrected transposition. Circulation 50: 911–923

Anderson R H, Becker A E, Gerlis L M 1975 The pulmonary outflow tract in classical corrected transposition. Journal of Thoracic and Cardiovascular Surgery 65: 747–757

Anselmi G, Munoz S, Blanco P, Machado I, de la Cruz M V 1972 Systematization and clinical study of dextroversion, mirror-image dextrocardia and levoversion. British Heart Journal 34: 1085–1098

Arciprete P, Macartney F J, de Leval M, Stark J 1985 Mustard's operation for patients with ventriculo-arterial concordance: report of two cases and a cautionary tale. British Heart Journal 53: 443–450

Attie F, Soni J, Ovseyevitz J, Munoz-Castellanos L, Testelli M R, Buendia A 1980 Angiographic studies of atrioventricular discordance. Circulation 62: 407–415

Attie F, Cerda J, Richheimer R et al 1987 Congenitally corrected transposition with mirror-image atrial arrangement. International Journal of Cardiology 14: 169–175

Attie F, Iturralde P, Zabal C et al 1998 Congenitally corrected transposition with atrioventricular septal defect. Cardiology in the Young 8: 474–478

Bargeron L M, Elliott L P, Soto B, Bream P R, Curry G C 1977 Axial cineangiography in congenital heart disease. Section 1. Concept, technical and anatomical considerations. Circulation 56: 1075–1083

Barcia A, Kincaid O W, Davis G D, Kirklin J W, Ongley P A 1967 Transposition of the great arteries. An angiocardiographic study. American Journal of Roentgenology, Radiotherapy and Nuclear Medicine 100: 249–283

Battistessa S A, Soto B 1990 Double outlet right ventricle with discordant atrio-ventricular connexion: an angiographic analysis of 19 cases. International Journal of Cardiology 27: 253–260

Becker A E, Anderson R H 1978 The atrioventricular conduction tissues in congenitally corrected transposition. In: Van Mierop L H S, Oppenheimer-Dekker A, Bruins C L D C (eds) Embryology and teratology of the heart and the great arteries. Leiden University Press, Leiden, 79–87

Becker A E, Ho S Y, Caruso G, Milo S, Anderson R H 1980 Straddling right atrioventricular valves in atrioventricular discordance. Circulation 61: 1133–1141

Benchimol A, Tio S, Sundararajan V 1971 Congenital corrected transposition of the great vessels in a 58-year-old man. Chest 59: 634–638

Benson L N, Burns R, Schwaiger M et al 1986 Radionuclide angiographic assessment of ventricular function in isolated congenitally corrected transposition of the great arteries. American Journal of Cardiology 58: 319–324

Bharati S, McCue C, Tingelstad J B, Mantakas M, Shiel F, Lev M 1978 Lack of connection between the atria and the peripheral conduction system in a case of corrected transposition with congenital atrioventricular block. American Journal of Cardiology 42: 147–153

Bliddal J 1976a Congenitally corrected transposition: a detailed review of the world literature. Danish Medical Bulletin 23: 168–183

Bliddal J 1976b Four cases of congenitally corrected transposition with associated defects. Danish Medical Bulletin 23: 184–192

Blieden L C, Möller J H 1973 Analysis of the P-wave in congenital cardiac malformations associated with splenic anomalies. American Heart Journal 85: 439–444

Bonfils-Roberts E A, Guller B, McGoon D C, Danielson G K 1974 Corrected transposition, surgical treatment of associated anomalies. Annals of Thoracic Surgery 17: 200–209

Bove E L 1999 Congenitally corrected transposition of the great arteries: surgical options for biventricular repair. Progress in Pediatric Cardiology 10: 45–49

Brandt P W T, Calder A L, Barratt-Boyes B G, Neutze J M 1976 Double outlet left ventricle. Morphology, cineangiocardiographic diagnosis and surgical treatment. American Journal of Cardiology 38: 897–909

Brawn W J, Sethia B, de Giovanni J V, Wright J G C, Silove E D, Stumper O 1998 In: Redington A N, Brawn W J, Deanfield J E, Anderson R H (eds) The right heart in congenital heart disease. Greenwich Medical Media, London, 247–253

Brenner J I, Bharati S, Winn W C Jr, Lev M 1978 Absent tricuspid valve with aortic atresia in mixed levocardia (atria situs solitus, L-loop). A hitherto undescribed entity. Circulation 57: 836–840

Burchell H B 1962 Clinical value of left axis deviation in the electrocardiogram: a renaissance. Lancet 82: 51–56

Burchell H B, Essex H E, Pruitt D R 1952 Studies on the spread of excitation through the ventricular myocardium II. The ventricular septum. Circulation 6: 161–172

Camier P 1967 La transposition corrigée des gros vaisseaux. A propos de 14 observations. Thése, Lille

Cardell B S 1956 Corrected transposition of the great vessels. British Heart Journal 18: 186–192

Carey L S, Ruttenberg H D 1964 Roentgenographic features of common ventricle with inversion of the infundibulum. Corrected transposition with rudimentary left ventricle. American Journal of Roentgenology 92: 652–668

Carr I, Tynan M, Aberdeen E, Bonham-Carter R E, Graham G, Waterston D J 1968 Predictive accuracy of the 'loop rule' in 109 children with classical complete transposition of the great arteries. Circulation 38(suppl VI): 52

Caulfield W H, Bostock B, Perloff J K 1967 Corrected transposition of the great vessels with isolated pulmonic stenosis: the paradox of pulmonic stenosis with physical signs of pulmonary hypertension. American Journal of Cardiology 19: 285–289

Celermajer D S, Cullen S, Deanfield J E, Sullivan I D 1991 Congenitally corrected transposition and Ebstein's anomaly of the systemic atrioventricular valve: association with aortic arch obstruction. Journal of the American College of Cardiology 18: 1056–1058

Chan K C, da Costa P, Dickinson D F 1989 Functional aortic atresia in congenitally corrected transposition. International Journal of Cardiology 25: 237–239

Clarkson P M, Brandt P W T, Barratt-Boyes B G, Neutze J M 1972 'Isolated atrial inversion'. Visceral situs solitus, viscero-atrial discordance, discordant ventricular d-loop without transposition, dextrocardia: diagnosis and surgical correction. American Journal of Cardiology 29: 877–881

Connelly M S, Lui P P, Williams W G, Webb G D, Robertson P, McLaughlin P R 1996 Congenitally corrected transposition of the great arteries in adult: functional status and complications. Journal of the American College of Cardiology 27: 1238–1243

Corone P, Vernant P, Guerin F, Gaudeau S, Picat G 1966 Transposition corrigée, communication interventriculaire et rétécissement de l'artére pulmonaire (a propos de 8 observations). Archives des Maladies du Coeur 59: 1609–1639

Craig B G, Smallhorn J F, Rowe R D, Williams W G, Trusler G A, Freedom R M 1986 Severe obstruction to systemic blood flow in congenitally corrected transposition (discordant atrioventricular and ventriculo-arterial connexions): an analysis of 14 patients. International Journal of Cardiology 11: 209–217

Danielson G K 1983 Surgical treatment of atrioventricular discordance. In: Losekoot G, Anderson R H, Becker A E, Soto B, Danielson G K (eds) Congenitally corrected transposition. Churchill Livingstone, Edinburgh, 177–190

Danielson G K, McGoon D C, Wallace R B, Fiddler G I, Maloney J D 1978 Surgery for corrected transposition. In: Anderson R H, Shinebourne E A (eds) Paediatric cardiology, 1977. Churchill Livingstone, Edinburgh, 224–230

Deanfield J E, Leanage R, Stroobant J, Chrispin S R, Taylor J F N, Macartney F J 1980 Use of high kilovoltage filtered beam radiographs for detection of bronchial situs in infants and young children. British Heart Journal 44: 577–583

Deanfield J E, Anderson R H, Macartney F J 1981 A case of aortic atresia with 'corrected transposition of the great arteries'. Atrioventricular and ventriculo-arterial discordance. British Heart Journal 46: 683–686

de Carvalho Azevedo A, Ney Toledo A, Roubach R, Alves de Carvalho A, Zanolio W, Dohman H 1958 Corrected transposition of the great vessels: report on two clinical cases. Acta Cardiologica 13: 409–418

de Leval M R, Bastos P, Stark J, Taylor J F N, Macartney F J, Anderson R H 1979 Surgical technique to reduce the risks of heart block following closure of ventricular septal defect in atrioventricular discordance. Journal of Thoracic and Cardiovascular Surgery 78: 515–526

Delius R E, Stark J 1996 Combined Rastelli and atrial switch procedure: anatomic and physiologic correction of discordant atrioventricular connection associated with with ventricular septal defect and left ventricular outflow tract obstruction. European Journal of Cardiothoracic Surgery 10: 551–555

de Tommasi S M, Daliento L, Ho S Y, Macartney F J, Anderson R H 1981 Analysis of the atrioventricular junction, ventricular mass and ventriculo-arterial junction in 43 specimens with atrial isomerism. British Heart Journal 45: 236–247

Dick M II, Norwood W I, Chipman C, Castañeda A R 1979 Intraoperative recording of specialised atrioventricular conduction tissue electrograms in 47 patients. Circulation 59: 150–160

Dickinson D F, Wilkinson J L, Anderson K R, Smith A, Ho S Y, Anderson R H 1979 The cardiac conduction system in situs ambiguus. Circulation 59: 879–885

Dimas A P, Moodie D S, Sterba R 1989 Long-term function of the morphologic right ventricle in adult patients with corrected transposition of the great arteries. American Heart Journal 118: 526–530

Doty D B, Truesdell S C, Marvin W J J 1983 Techniques to avoid injury of the conduction tissue during the surgical treatment of corrected transposition. Circulation 68 (suppl II): 63–69

Du Bois R, Dupuis C, Remy J 1966 La transposition corrigée des gros vaisseaux; aspects radiographiques standard. Annales de Radiologie 9: 119–134

Durrer D 1966 The human heart: some aspects of its excitation. Transactions and Studies of the College of Physicians of Philadelphia 4th series 33: 159–170

Durrer D, Roos J P, Buller J 1965 The spread of excitation in canine and human heart. In: Taccardi B, Marchetti G (eds) Electrophysiology of the heart. Pergamon Press, Oxford, p 203

Edwards J E 1954 Differential diagnosis of mitral stenosis, a clinicopathologic review of simulating conditions. Laboratory Investigation 3: 89–115

Edwards J E, Carey L S, Neufeld H N, Lester R G 1965 Congenital heart disease. Correlation of pathologic anatomy and angiocardiography. Saunders, Philadelphia, PA, p 128

Ellis K, Morgan B C, Blumenthal S, Anderson D H 1962 Congenitally corrected transposition of the great vessels. Radiology 79, 35–50

El Sayed H, Cleland W P, Bentall H H, Melrose D G, Bishop M B, Morgan J 1962 Corrected transposition of the great arterial trunks: surgical treatment of the associated defects. Journal of Thoracic and Cardiovascular Surgery 44: 443–458

Espino-Vela J, de la Cruz M V, Munoz-Castellanos L, Plaza L, Attie F 1970 Ventricular inversion without transposition of the great vessels in situs inversus. British Heart Journal 32: 292–303

Essed C E, Ho S Y, Hunter S, Anderson R H 1980 Atrioventricular conduction system in univentricular heart of the right ventricular type with right-sided rudimentary chamber. Thorax 35: 123–127

Ferencz C, Rubin J D, McCarter R J et al 1985 Congenital heart disease: prevalence at livebirth. The Baltimore–Washington Infant Study. American Journal of Epidemiology 121: 31–36

Fernandez F, Laurichesse J, Siebat L, Lenégre J 1970 Electrocardiogram in corrected transposition of the great vessels of the bulbo-ventricular inversion type. British Heart Journal 32: 165–171

Foale R, Stefanini L, Rickards A, Somerville J 1982 Left and right ventricular morphology in complex congenital heart disease defined by two dimensional echocardiography. American Journal of Cardiology 49: 93–99

Fox L S, Kirklin J W, Pacifico A O, Waldo A L, Bargeron L M 1976 Intracardiac repair of cardiac malformations with atrioventricular discordance. Circulation 54: 123–127

Freedom R M 1999 Congenitally corrected transposition of the great arteries: definitions and pathologic anatomy. Progress in Pediatric Cardiology 10: 3–16

Freedom R M, Benson L N 1992 Congenitally corrected transposition of the great arteries. In: Freedom R M, Benson L N, Smallhorn J F (eds) Neonatal heart disease. Springer-Verlag, London, 523–542

Freedom R M, Culham G, Rowe R D 1978a The criss-cross heart and superoinferior ventricular heart, an angiocardiographic study. American Journal of Cardiology 42: 620–628

Freedom R M, Bini R, Dische R, Rowe R D 1978b The straddling mitral valve: morphological observations and clinical implications. European Journal of Cardiology 8: 27–50

Freedom R M, Benson L N, Smallhorn J F 1989 Congenitally corrected transposition of the great arteries. In: Moller J H, Neal W A (eds) Fetal, neonatal, and infant cardiac disease. Appleton and Lang, Norwalk CT, 550–570

Friedberg D Z, Nadas A S 1970 Clinical profile of patients with congenital corrected transposition of the great arteries. A study of 60 cases. New England Journal of Medicine 282: 1053–1059

Friedman H S, Lipski J, Pantazopoulos J, Genkins G, Donoso E 1973 Bundle of His electrocardiograms in congenital corrected transposition of the great arteries. A study of two adult cases. British Heart Journal 35: 1307–1314

Fyler D C 1992 Nadas' pediatric cardiology. Mosby-Year Book, Boston, MA, 701–708

Fyler D C, Buckley L P, Hellenbrand W E, Cohn H E 1980 Report of the New England Regional Infant Cardiac Program. Pediatrics 65(suppl): 375–461

Gerlis L M, Wilson N, Dickinson D F 1986 Abnormalities of the mitral valve in congenitally corrected transposition (discordant atrioventricular and ventriculoarterial connections). British Heart Journal 55: 475–479

Gillette P C, Busch U, Mullins C E, McNamara D G 1979 Electrophysiologic studies in patients with ventricular inversion and 'corrected transposition'. Circulation 60: 939–945

Grabitz R G, Joffres M R 1988 Congenital heart disease: incidence in the first year of life. The Alberta Heritage Pediatric Cardiology Program. American Journal of Epidemiology 128: 381–388

Guerin R, Soto B, Karp R B, Kirklin J W, Barcia A 1970 Transposition of the great arteries: determination of the position of the great arteries in conventional chest roentgenograms. American Journal of Roentgenology 110: 747–758

Guller B, Mair D D, Ritter D G, Smith R E 1975 Frank vectorcardiogram in common ventricle: correlation with anatomic findings. American Heart Journal 90: 290–294

Hagler D J, Tajik A J, Seward J B, Edwards W D, Mair D D, Ritter D G 1981a Atrioventricular and ventriculo-arterial discordance (corrected transposition of the great arteries). Wide angle two-dimensional echocardiographic assessment of ventricular morphology. Mayo Clinic Proceedings 56: 591–600

Hagler D J, Tajik A J, Seward J B, Mair D D, Ritter D G 1981b Double-outlet right ventricle: wide-angle two-dimensional echocardiographic observations. Circulation 63: 419–428

Helvind M H, McCarthy J F, Imamura M et al 1998 Ventriculo-arterial discordance: switching the morphologically left ventricle into the systemic circulation after 3 months of age. European Journal of Cardiothoracic Surgery 14: 173–178

Hornung T S, Bernard E J, Jaeggi E T, Howman-Giles R B, Celermajer D S, Hawker R E 1998 Myocardial perfusion defects and associated systemic ventricular dysfunction in congenitally corrected transposition of the great arteries. Heart 80: 322–326

Huhta J C, Danielson G K, Ritter D G, Ilstrup D M 1985 Survival in atrioventricular discordance. Pediatric Cardiology 6: 57–61

Ikeda U, Furuse M, Suzuki O, Kimura K, Sekiguchi H, Shimada K 1992 Long-term survival in aged patients with

corrected transposition of the great arteries. Chest 101: 1382–1385

Ilbawi M N, DeLeon S Y, Backer C L et al 1990 An alternative approach to the surgical management of physiologically corrected transposition with ventricular septal defect and pulmonary stenosis or atresia. Journal of Thoracic and Cardiovascular Surgery 100: 410–415

Imai Y 1997 Double-switch operation for congenitally corrected transposition of the great arteries. Advances in Cardiac Surgery 9: 65–86

Imai Y, Sawatari K, Hoshino S, Ishihara K, Nakazawa M, Momma K 1994 Ventricular function after anatomic repair in patients with atrioventricular discordance. Journal of Thoracic and Cardiovascular Surgery 107: 1272–1283

Karl T R, Weintraub R G, Brizard C P, Cochrane A D, Mee R B B 1997 Senning plus arterial switch for discordant (congenitally corrected) transposition. Annals of Thoracic Surgery 64: 495–502

Keck E W, Hauch H J, Lassrich M A et al 1965 Die Korrigierte Transposition der grossen Gefässe. Kardiologia 47: 158–206

Keutel J, Hagenmuller H 1978 Echocardiography in diagnosis of corrected transposition. In: Anderson R H, Shinebourne E A (eds) Paediatric cardiology, 1977. Churchill Livingstone, Edinburgh, 515–524

Kidd B S L 1978 Congenitally corrected transposition of the great arteries. In: Keith J D, Rowe R D, Vlad P (eds) Heart disease in infancy and childhood, 3rd edn. MacMillan, New York, 612–627

Kinsley R H, Levin S E, O'Donovan T G 1979 Transposition of the great arteries associated with a double left ventricular outflow tract. British Heart Journal 42: 483–486

Kiser J C, Ongley P A, Kirklin J W, Clarkson P M, McGoon D C 1968 Surgical treatment of dextrocardia with inversion of ventricles and double outlet right ventricle. Journal of Thoracic and Cardiovascular Surgery 55: 6–15

Kupersmith J, Krongrad E, Gersony W M, Bowman F O 1974 Electrophysiologic identification of the specialized conduction system in corrected transposition of the great arteries. Circulation 50: 795–800

La Corte M A, Fellows K E, Williams R G 1976 Overriding tricuspid valve: echocardiographic and angiocardiographic features. 8 cases of ventricular septal defect of atrioventricular canal type. American Journal of Cardiology 37: 911–919

Leijala M A, Lincoln C R, Shinebourne E A, Nellen M 1981 A rare congenital cardiac malformation with situs inversus and discordant atrioventricular and concordant ventriculo-arterial connections. diagnosis and surgical treatment. American Heart Journal 101: 355–356

Liberthson R R, Hastreiter A R, Sinha S N, Bharati S, Novaks M, Lev M 1973 Levocardia with visceral heterotaxy-isolated levocardia: pathologic anatomy and its clinical implications. American Heart Journal 85: 40–54

Lieberson A D, Schumacher R R, Chidress R H, Genouese P D 1969 Corrected transposition of the great vessels in a 73 year old man. Circulation 39: 96–100

Losekoot T G 1967 Gecorrigeerde transposities. Thesis. Scheltema en Holkema, Amsterdam

Losekoot T G 1978 Conditions with atrioventricular discordance: clinical investigations. In: Anderson R H,

Shinebourne E A (eds) Paediatric cardiology, 1977. Churchill Livingstone, Edinburgh, 198–206

Losekoot T G, Anderson R H, Becker A E, Danielson G K, Soto B 1983 Congenitally corrected transposition. Churchill Livingstone, Edinburgh

Lundstrom U, Bull C, Wyse R K H, Somerville J 1990 The natural and 'unnatural' history of congenitally corrected transposition. American Journal of Cardiology 65: 1222–1229

Macartney F J, Partridge J B, Shinebourne E A, Tynan M J, Anderson R H 1978 Identification of atrial situs. In: Anderson R H, Shinebourne E A (eds) Paediatric cardiology, 1977. Churchill Livingstone, Edinburgh, 16–26

Maloney J D, Ritter D G, McGoon D C, Danielson G K 1975 Identification of the conduction system in corrected transposition and common ventricle at operation. Mayo Clinic Proceedings 50: 387–394

Marcelletti C, Maloney J D, Ritter D G, Danielson G K, McGoon D C, Wallace R B 1980 Corrected transposition and ventricular septal defect: surgical experience. Annals of Surgery 191: 751–759

Matsukawa T, Yoshii S, Miyamura H, Eguchi S 1985 Aortic atresia with Ebstein's and Uhl's anomaly in corrected transposition of the great arteries: clinicopathologic findings. Japanese Circulation Journal 49: 325–328

McGrath L B, Kirklin J W, Blackstone E H, Pacifico A D, Kirklin J K, Bargeron L M Jr 1985 Death and other events after cardiac repair in discordant atrioventricular connection. Journal of Thoracic and Cardiovascular Surgery 90: 711–728

McKay R, Anderson R H, Smith A 1996 The coronary arteries in hearts with discordant atrioventricular connections. Journal of Thoracic and Cardiovascular Surgery 111: 988–997

Mee R B B 1986 Severe right ventricular failure after Mustard or Senning operations. Two stage repair: pulmonary artery banding and switch. Journal of Cardiovascular Surgery 92: 385–390

Meyer R A 1977 Pediatric Echocardiography. Lea & Febiger, Philadelphia, PA, 242–246

Milo S, Ho S Y, Macartney F J, Wilkinson J L et al 1979 Straddling and overriding atrioventricular valves: morphology and classification. American Journal of Cardiology 44: 1122–1134

Moffa P J, Transchesi J, Macruz R et al 1976 Corrected transposition of the great vessels: a vectorcardiographic study. Journal of Electrocardiology 9: 5–14

Mönckeberg J G 1913 Zür Entwicklungsgeschichte des Atrioventrikularsystems. Verhandlung der Deutschen Pathologischen Gesellschaft 16: 228–249

Morgan J, Pitman R, Goodwin J F 1962 Anomalies of the aorta and pulmonary arteries complicating ventricular septal defect. British Heart Journal 24: 279–292

Mullins C E 1990 Ventricular inversion. In: Garson A Jr, Bricker J T, McNamara D G (eds) The science and practice of pediatric cardiology. Lea & Febiger, Philadelphia, PA, 1233–1245

Muster A J, Idriss F S, Bharati S et al 1985 Functional aortic valve atresia in transposition of the great arteries. Journal of the American College of Cardiology 6: 630–634

Nugent E W, Freedom R M, Nora J J, Ellison R C, Rowe R D, Nadas A S 1977 Clinical course in pulmonary stenosis. Circulation 56(suppl I): 38–47

Okamura K, Konno S 1973 Two types of ventricular septal defect in corrected transposition of the great arteries: reference to surgical approaches. American Heart Journal 85: 483–490

Okamura K, Takao A, Hashimoto A, Hosoda S, Mimori K 1973 Electrocardiogram in corrected transposition of the great arteries with and without associated cardiac anomalies. Journal of Electrocardiology 6: 3–10

Otero Coto E, Quero Jimenez M, Cabrera A, Deverall P B, Caffarena J M 1978 Aortic levopositions without ventricular inversion. European Journal of Cardiology 8: 523–541

Otero Coto E, Calabro R, Marsico F, Lopez Arranz J S 1981 Right atrial outlet atresia with straddling left atrioventricular valve. A form of double outlet atrium. British Heart Journal 45: 317–324

Partridge J B, Scott O, Deverall P B, Macartney F J 1975 Visualization and measurement of the main bronchi by tomography as an objective indicator of thoracic situs in congenital heart disease. Circulation 51: 188–196

Perloff J K 1978 The clinical recognition of congenital heart disease. Saunders, Philadelphia, PA, 57–81

Peterson R J, Franch R H, Fajman W A, Jones R H 1988 Comparison of cardiac function in surgically corrected and congenitally corrected transposition of the great arteries. Journal of Thoracic and Cardiovascular Surgery 96: 227–236

Portillo B, Anselmi G, Sodi-Pallares D, Medrano G A 1959 Importance of the unipolar leads in the diagnosis of dextrocardias, levocardias, dextropositions and dextrorotations. American Heart Journal 57: 396–417

Presbitero P, Somerville J, Rabajoli F, Stone S, Conte M R 1995 Corrected transposition of the great arteries without associated defects in adult patients: clinical profile and follow-up. British Heart Journal 74: 57–59

Quero Jimenez M, Raposo-Sonnenfeld I 1975 Isolated ventricular inversion with situs solitus. British Heart Journal 37: 293–304

Quero Jimenez M, Rico Gomez F, Casanova Gomez M, Quero Jimenez C, Perez Martinez V 1978 The value of the electrocardiogram in the diagnosis of primitive ventricle. In: Anderson R H, Shinebourne E A (eds) Paediatric cardiology, 1977. Churchill Livingstone, Edinburgh, 339–344

Ranjit M S, Wilkinson J L, Mee R B B 1991 Discordant atrioventricular connexion with concordant ventriculo-arterial connexion (so-called 'isolated ventricular inversion') with usual atrial arrangement (situs solitus). International Journal of Cardiology 31: 114–117

Reddy V M, McElhinney D B, Silverman N H, Hanley F L 1997 The double switch procedure for anatomical repair of congenitally corrected transposition of the great arteries in infants and children. European Heart Journal 18: 1470–1477

Rotem C E, Hultgren H N 1965 Corrected transposition of the great vessels without associated defects. American Heart Journal 70: 305–318

Ruttenberg H D 1977 Corrected transposition (L-transposition) of the great arteries: splenic syndromes (asplenia, polysplenia). In: Moss A J, Adams F H, Emmanouilides G C (eds) Heart disease in infants, children and adolescents, 2nd edn. Williams & Wilkins, Baltimore MD, 338–354

Sano T, Risenfeld T, Karl T R, Wilkinson J L 1995 Intermediate-term outcome after intracardiac repair of associated cardiac defects in patients with atrioventricular and ventriculoarterial discordance. Circulation 92(suppl II): 272–278

Schiebler G L, Edwards J E, Burchell H B, DuShane J W, Ongley P A, Wood E H 1961 Congenital corrected transposition of the great vessels: a study of 35 cases. Pediatrics 27: 851–888

Schwartz H A, Wagner P I 1974 Corrected transposition of the great vessels in a 55-year-old woman; diagnosis by coronary angiography. Chest 66: 190–192

Sharma R, Bhan A, Juneja R, Kothari S S, Saxena A, Venugopal P 1999 Double switch for congenitally corrected transposition of the great arteries. European Journal of Cardiothoracic Surgery 15: 276–282

Sharratt G P, Sbokos C G, Johnson A M, Anderson R H, Monro J L 1976 Surgical 'correction' of solitus-concordant, double outlet left ventricle with L-malposition and tricuspid stenosis with hypoplastic right ventricle. Journal of Thoracic and Cardiovascular Surgery 71: 853–858

Shea P M, Lutz J F, Vieweg W V R, Corcoran F H, Van Praagh R, Hougen T J 1979 Selective coronary arteriography in congenitally corrected transposition of the great arteries. American Journal of Cardiology 44: 1201–1206

Shem-Tov A, Deutsch V, Yahini J H, Kraus Y, Neufeld H N 1971 Corrected transposition of the great arteries. A modified approach to the clinical diagnosis in 30 cases. American Journal of Cardiology 27: 99–113

Shimizu T, Ando M, Takao A 1981 Pulmonary atresia with intact ventricular septum and corrected transposition of the great arteries. British Heart Journal 45: 471–474

Soto B, Bargeron L M, Bream P R, Elliott L P 1978 Conditions with atrioventricular discordance–angiographic study. In: Anderson R H, Shinebourne E A (eds) Paediatric cardiology, 1977. Churchill Livingstone, Edinburgh, p 207–221

Soto B, Bertranou E G, Bream P R, Souza A, Bargeron L M 1979 Angiographic study of univentricular heart of right ventricular type. Circulation 60: 1325–1334

Squarcia U, Ritter D G, Kincaid O W 1973 Dextrocardia; angiocardiographic study and classification. American Journal of Cardiology 32: 965–977

Steeg C N, Ellis K, Bransilver B, Gersony W M 1971 Pulmonary atresia and intact ventricular septum complicating corrected transposition of the great vessels. American Heart Journal 82: 382–386

Stewart S, Manning J, Siegel L 1977 Automated identification of cardiac conduction tissue in L-TGA and Ebstein's anomaly. Annals of Thoracic Surgery 23: 215–220

Stümper O F, Brawn W J 1998 Anatomic repair of double-discordant hearts. Heart 80: 434–445

Stümper O F, Wright J G C, de Giovanni J V, Silove E D, Sethia B, Brawn W J 1995 Combined atrial and arterial switch procedure for congenital corrected transposition with ventricular septal defect. British Heart Journal 73: 479–482

Subirana M T, de Leval M, Somerville J 1984 Double outlet right ventricle with atrioventricular discordance. American Journal of Cardiology 54: 1385–1388

Summerall C P, Clowes G H A, Boone J A 1966 Aneurysm of ventricular septum defect with outflow obstruction of the venous ventricle in corrected transposition of great vessels. American Heart Journal 72: 525–529

Sutherland G R, Smallhorn J F, Anderson R H, Rigby M L, Hunter S 1983 Atrioventricular discordance. Cross sectional echocardiographic-morphological correlative study. British Heart Journal 50: 8–20

Symons J C, Shinebourne E A, Joseph M C, Lincoln C, Ho Y, Anderson R H 1977 Criss-cross heart with congenitally corrected transposition; report of a case with d-transposed aorta and ventricular pre-excitation. European Journal of Cardiology 5: 493–505

Szufladowicz M, Horath P, de Leval M, Elliot M, Wyse R, Stark J 1996 Intracardiac repair of lesion associated with atrioventricular discordance. European Journal of Cardiothoracic Surgery 10: 443–448

Tabry I F, McGoon D C, Danielson G K, Wallace R B, Davis Z, Maloney J D 1978 Surgical management of double-outlet right ventricle associated with atrioventricular discordance. Journal of Thoracic and Cardiovascular Surgery 76: 336–344

Tajik A J, Seward J B, Hagler D J, Mair D D, Lie J T 1978 Two-dimensional real-time ultrasonic imaging of the heart and great vessels: technique, image orientation, structure identification and validation. Mayo Clinic Proceedings 53: 271–303

Tandon R, Becker A E, Moller J H, Edwards J E 1974 Double inlet left ventricle: straddling tricuspid valve. British Heart Journal 36: 747–759

Thelen M, Thurn P, Schaede A, Behrenbeck D 1969 Die korrigierte Transposition der grossen Gefässe im Röntgenbild. Fortschritte Röntgenstrahle 110: 151–163

Thibert M, Jeune M, Simon G, Camus L, Nouaille J 1969 La transposition arterielle corrigée à propos de 41 observations. Archives du Maladies du Coeur 62: 1424–1428

Uemura H, Yagihara T 1998 Anatomic biventricular repair by intraventricular and intraarterial rerouting in patients with discordant atrioventricular connections. In: Redington A N, Brawn W J, Deanfield J E, Anderson R H (eds) The right heart in congenital heart disease. Greenwich Medical Media, London, p 237–242

Uemura H, Ho S Y, Anderson R H et al 1996 Surgical anatomy of the coronary circulation in hearts with discordant atrioventricular connections. European Journal of Cardiothoracic Surgery 10: 194–200

Urban A E, Anderson R H, Stark J 1977 Double outlet left ventricle associated with situs inversus and atrioventricular concordance. American Heart Journal 94: 91–95

Van Mierop L H S, Eisen S, Schiebler G L 1970 The radiographic appearance of the tracheobronchial tree as an indicator of visceral situs. American Journal of Cardiology 26: 432–435

Van Praagh R 1970 What is congenitally corrected transposition? New England Medical Journal 282: 1097–1098

Van Praagh R, Van Praagh S 1966 Isolated ventricular inversion. A consideration of morphogenesis, definition and diagnosis of non-transposed and transposed great arteries. American Journal of Cardiology 17: 395–406

Van Praagh R, Weinberg P M 1977 Double outlet left ventricle. In: Moss A J, Adams F J, Emmanouilides G C (eds) Heart disease in infants, children and adolescents. Williams & Wilkins, Baltimore, MD, p 367–380

Van Praagh R, Van Praagh S, Vlad P, Keith J D 1965 Diagnosis of the anatomic types of congenital dextrocardia. American Journal of Cardiology 13: 510–532

Victorica B E, Miller B L, Gessner I H 1973 Electrocardiogram and vectorcardiogram in ventricular inversion (corrected transposition). American Heart Journal 86: 733–744

Von Rokitansky C 1875 Die Defecte der Scheidewände des Herzens. Wilhelm Braumüller, Wien

Voskuil M, Hazenkamp M G, Kroft L J M et al 1999 Postsurgical course of patients with congenitally corrected transposition of the great arteries. American Journal of Cardiology 83: 558–562

Vouhé P R, Sidi D 1998 Congenitally corrected transposition: results of 'classical' surgery. In: Redington A N, Brawn W J, Deanfield J E, Anderson R H (eds) The right heart in congenital heart disease. Greenwich Medical Media, London, p 231–236

Waldo A L, Pacifico A D, Bargeron L M, James T N, Kirklin J W 1975 Electrophysiological delineation of the specialized A–V conduction system in patients with corrected transposition of the great vessels and ventricular septal defect. Circulation 52: 435–441

Walmsley T 1931 Transposition of the ventricles and the arterial stems. Journal of Anatomy 65: 528–540

Watson G H 1964 The diagnosis of corrected transposition of the great vessels. British Heart Journal 26: 770–777

Wellens H J J, Lubbers W J, Losekoot T G 1977 Preexcitation. In: Roberts N K, Gelband H (eds) Cardiac arrhythmias in the neonate, infant and child. Appleton-Century-Crofts, New York, p 231–263

Wilkinson J L, Smith A, Lincoln C, Anderson R H 1978 The conducting tissues in congenitally corrected transposition with situs inversus. British Heart Journal 40: 41–48

Wolff G S, Freed M D, Ellison R C 1973 Bundle of His recordings in congenital heart disease. British Heart Journal 35: 805–810

Yagihara T, Kishimoto H, Isobe F et al 1994 Double switch operation in cardiac anomalies with atrioventricular and ventriculoarterial discordance. Journal of Thoracic and Cardiovascular Surgery 107: 351–358

Yamagishi M, Imai Y, Hoshino H et al 1993 Anatomic correction of atrioventricular discordance. Journal of Thoracic and Cardiovascular Surgery 105: 1067–1076

Yeh T Jr, Connelly M S, Coles J G et al 1999 Atrioventricular discordance: results of repair in 127 patients. Journal of Thoracic and Cardiovascular Surgery 117: 1190–1203

Zahn E M, Smallhorn J F, Freedom R M 1992 Congenitally corrected transposition of the great arteries with hypoplasia of the morphologically left ventricle in the setting of situs inversus. International Journal of Cardiology 36: 9–12

50
═══ Double outlet ventricle ═══

J. L. Wilkinson

─────────────── INTRODUCTION ───────────────

The term double outlet ventricle refers to any cardiac anomaly in which both the aorta and pulmonary trunk are connected to the same ventricle. Since there are many examples in which one (or occasionally both) great arteries override a ventricular septal defect, it is necessary to frame the definition to allow for this contingency. An arterial trunk may be considered as being connected to a ventricle when more than half of its circumference, at the level of its arterial valve, is connected to that ventricle (Lev et al, 1972; Tynan et al, 1979). This is commonly referred to as the '50% rule'. In the individual case, the term double outlet ventricle may be applied accurately if the aorta and pulmonary trunk both arise *predominantly* from the same ventricle.

Double outlet ventricle is not a single anomaly, nor even a single group of malformations. Rather it represents a specific ventriculo-arterial connection (see Chapter 2) that may occur with each atrial arrangement, any atrioventricular connection and with all possible variations of ventricular morphology. Additionally, a host of associated defects may be found – some common and some rare. The clinical picture is as inconstant as the anatomical permutations and associations would suggest.

The malformations to be considered in this chapter are those in which the arteries are connected to one of two ventricles, each of which has an atrioventricular connection (in other words, those with *biventricular* atrioventricular connections). Excluded are those examples with double inlet or absent right or left atrioventricular connection.

─────────────── HISTORY ───────────────

The first example of double outlet right ventricle known to me was described in 1793 by Mr Abernethy of St Bartholomew's Hospital. In this case, the aorta arose entirely from the right ventricle and there was pulmonary stenosis: 'Both ventricles (the left by means of an opening in the upper part of the septum ventriculorum) projected their blood into the aorta'. This case was regarded by Farre (1814) as being in most respects similar anatomically, and in its clinical history, to a number of other cases that he documented and which were undoubtedly examples of what would now be termed tetralogy of Fallot, though he (Farre) draws attention particularly to the right ventricular origin of the aorta in Abernethy's case.

The term double outlet right ventricle appears to have been introduced by Witham (1957). Previous examples of hearts that would now be designated in this way were included in the collections of Peacock (1858), von Rokitansky (1875), Spitzer (1923) and Abbott (1936), generally under the terms partial transposition or complete dextroposition of the aorta (Abbott, 1936). Other early descriptions of the anomaly in its various forms

include those of Birmingham (1893) (in which the association with juxtaposition of the atrial appendages first appeared), Saphir and Lev (1941) (using the term tetralogy of Eisenmenger), Taussig and Bing (1949), Braun et al (1952) and Edwards et al (1952). Both Spitzer (1923) and Pernkopf (1926) included hearts with both great arteries arising from the right ventricle in their classifications of transposition.

It is not appropriate here to go into the tortuous semantic debate that continued through the 20th century, with regard to the use of the term transposition – particularly in relation to hearts with both great arteries arising from the right ventricle. The interested reader will find the more fundamental aspects of the debate well laid out by Van Mierop (1971), van Praagh (1971), Van Praagh et al (1971), Shinebourne et al (1976) and Tynan et al (1979).

RELATIONSHIP WITH TETRALOGY OF FALLOT ───

A debate that has also taxed anatomists, surgeons and cardiologists alike concerns the relationship between double outlet right ventricle and tetralogy of Fallot. The degree of aortic dextroposition seen in hearts with Fallot's tetralogy is extremely variable (Van Praagh et al, 1970; Goor et al, 1971). In a proportion of cases, the aorta may be connected predominantly to the right ventricle. In this setting, some workers have suggested that the presence of aortic–mitral continuity is an integral part of tetralogy of Fallot. If present, the heart should be categorized as tetralogy and if not as double outlet right ventricle (Stewart et al, 1979). Conversely, double outlet right ventricle has been said to be associated with mitral–aortic discontinuity in all cases (Baron, 1971), and the diagnosis has been considered contingent on this finding. Neufeld and colleagues (1961b), however, had previously included within the designation 'double outlet right ventricle with pulmonary stenosis' a patient with mitral–aortic continuity, and Lev et al (1972) subsequently established that the mitral–aortic relationship in double outlet right ventricle was extremely variable.

It becomes clear that double outlet right ventricle is a connection rather than a specific malformation and includes some examples that are morphologically similar to tetralogy of Fallot, others that resemble more closely complete transposition with ventricular septal defect, and others again that exhibit similarities to congenitally corrected transposition, or to yet other anomalies. Tetralogy of Fallot describes a well-known and familiar malformation with certain clearly defined morphological features: most notably 'infundibular stenosis or atresia, and a high ventricular septal defect' (Van Praagh et al, 1970). Some examples of this anomaly (with extreme overriding of the aorta) fall within the category of double outlet right ventricle (Edwards, 1981; Wilcox et al, 1981). Therefore, some specimens with the morphological features of tetralogy of Fallot may have the connection of double outlet right ventricle, the two designations not being mutually exclusive.

DOUBLE OUTLET LEFT VENTRICLE

Some early descriptions of double outlet left ventricle were examples of double outlet right ventricle with discordant atrioventricular connections (Fragoyannis and Kardalinos, 1962). Some morphologists and embryologists went on record as stating that 'double outlet from a morphologically left ventricle is an embryological impossibility' (Van Mierop and Wiglesworth, 1963). They considered that all described cases were probably examples of the former malformation. The first patient for whom the diagnosis was beyond doubt was published by Sakakibara et al (1967). Subsequently, numerous isolated cases have been described from both the pathological and the clinical viewpoint.

PREVALENCE

DOUBLE OUTLET RIGHT VENTRICLE

Double outlet right ventricle is a rare cardiac malformation, accounting for less than 1% of all congenital cardiac defects. It was found in 3% of a group of infants dying of congenital cardiac defects in the first month of life (Rowe and Mehrizi, 1968). It has been reported to be frequent in the trisomy 18 syndrome (Rogers et al, 1965). Although infrequent overall, nonetheless, it is sufficiently common for a number of authors to have accumulated large numbers of pathological, clinical or surgical cases (Lev et al, 1972; Sondheimer et al, 1977; Stewart et al, 1979; Wilcox et al, 1981). The more frequent variants of the anomaly are well documented and present a familiar enough problem to the paediatric cardiologist and surgeon.

DOUBLE OUTLET LEFT VENTRICLE

Double outlet left ventricle is a very much rarer malformation than double outlet right ventricle. Nevertheless, the total number of published cases is now substantial (Anderson et al, 1974d; Brandt et al, 1976; Van Praagh and Weinberg, 1977; Otero-Coto et al, 1981). Indeed, it may be more frequent than has previously been recognized. It probably accounts for less than 5% of all hearts with double outlet ventriculo-arterial and biventricular atrioventricular connections. This would correspond to an incidence of less than 1 in 200 000 births.

MORPHOLOGY AND CLASSIFICATION

The literature on double outlet right (and left) ventricle is extensive and includes descriptions of a bewildering variety of anatomical forms. In order to avoid confusion, it is essential that attention be focused separately on, first, the categorization and, second, the detail of the more common and more important malformations.

CATEGORIES

A logical, step-by-step, approach to the diagnosis and classification of double outlet right (and left) ventricle is essential. Analysis, in the clinical or pathological situation, must follow the same careful sequence that has been outlined earlier (Table 50.1). Atrial arrangement (and venous connections) must be ascertained, and the atrioventricular connections established with certainty. At the ventricular level, the anatomy of the connection between the ventricular mass and the great arteries is important, including their inter-relationships and the nature and severity of any

Table 50.1. Essential anatomical information required for analysis of hearts with double outlet ventricle

Atrial arrangement (situs)

Atrioventricular connections (type and mode)

Ventriculo-arterial connection (including information about arterial overriding)

Morphology and relations of ventricular septal defect(s)

Morphology of outflow tracts (especially obstructive lesions)

Relationships of arterial trunks

Associated defects (especially atrioventricular valves)

Table 50.2. Sites of ventricular septal defect in relation to arterial outlets in double outlet right ventricle with usual atrial arrangement and concordant atrioventricular connection

Site	Percentage[a]
Subaortic	52
Subpulmonary	24
Non-committed	14
Doubly committed	10

[a] Percentage of 84 specimens analysed.
Source: after Wilkinson et al (1981).

Table 50.3. Type of ventricular septal defect and relationship to arterial outlets in 84 specimens of double outlet right ventricle with usual atrial arrangement and concordant atrioventricular connections

Type of ventricular septal defect	Arterial outlet				Total
	Subaortic	Subpulmonary	Non-committed	Doubly committed	
Perimembranous	36	13	7	5	61
Muscular	9	9	5	4	27
Total	45	22	12	9	88

Source: after Wilkinson et al (1981).

obstructive problems. The size, site and morphology of the ventricular septal defect, which is categorized in a similar way to that used for isolated defects by Soto et al (1980), is also of great importance, particularly in reference to its relationship with the arterial outlets (Tables 50.2 and 50.3). Attention must also be paid to the integrity and function of the atrioventricular valves (especially the mitral valve) and to the presence of other associated cardiac defects, which are frequent (Table 50.4). It is neither practical nor desirable to use a rigid type of classification for the various forms of double outlet ventricle. In my view, the situation in each patient should be individually assessed for category, just as the medical and surgical management needs to be tailored to cater for the particular problems of the individual. Nonetheless, certain variants of double inlet right ventricle do occur frequently enough to merit separate discussion. These will be outlined below.

DOUBLE OUTLET RIGHT VENTRICLE

The more common variants of double outlet right ventricle (Figure 50.1a–c) (in approximate order of frequency) occur with:

- subaortic ventricular septal defect with the aorta to the right of the pulmonary trunk and with pulmonary stenosis (Fallot type)

Table 50.4. Associated defects in 84 specimens of double outlet right ventricle with usual atrial arrangement and concordant atrioventricular connections

Defect	Number	Percentage
Pulmonary stenosis	31	37
Atrial septal defect	19	23
Aortic coarctation	16	19
Mitral stenosis	7	8
Straddling mitral valve	6	7
Hypoplastic left ventricle	5	6
Aortic stenosis (valvar or subvalvar)	4	5
Restrictive ventricular septal defect	4	5
Juxtaposition of atrial appendages	4	5
Interrupted aortic arch	3	4
Complete atrioventricular septal defect	3	4
Hypoplastic right ventricle	2	2
Criss-cross atrioventricular connections	2	2
Imperforate mitral valve	1	1
Imperforate tricuspid valve	1	1
Parachute mitral valve	1	1
Cleft mitral valve	1	1
Cleft tricuspid valve	1	1
Totally anomalous pulmonary venous connection	1	1

Source: after Wilkinson et al (1981).

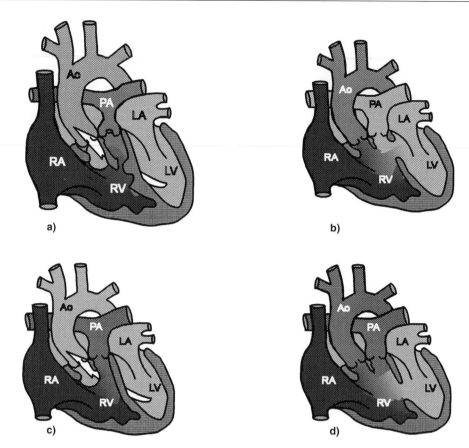

Figure 50.1. The more common variants of double outlet right ventricle. (a) Subaortic defect, pulmonary stenosis, aorta to right of pulmonary trunk, 'Fallot type'. (b) Subpulmonary defect (Taussig–Bing type). (c) Subaortic defect, aorta to right of pulmonary trunk, no pulmonary stenosis. (d) Non-committed ventricular septal defect. Darker shading indicates deoxygenated blood. Lighter shading indicates oxygenated blood. The white arrow indicates pathway of blood from the left ventricle to the aorta with subaortic ventricular septal defect. Ao, aorta; PA, pulmonary trunk; LV, left ventricle; RV, right ventricle; RA, right atrium; LA, left atrium.

- subpulmonary ventricular septal defect with the aorta to the right of the pulmonary trunk (Taussig–Bing type)
- subaortic ventricular septal defect with the aorta to the right of the pulmonary trunk in the absence of pulmonary stenosis.

Less common variants are given in Figure 50.1d and Figure 50.2a–d and include:

- non-committed ventricular septal defect with the aorta to the right of the pulmonary trunk
- doubly committed ventricular septal defect
- subaortic ventricular septal defect with the aorta to the left of the pulmonary trunk along with pulmonary stenosis
- double outlet right ventricle with usual atrial arrangement and discordant atrioventricular connections (aorta usually to the left of the pulmonary trunk)
- double outlet right ventricle with mirror-imaged atrial arrangement (any of the previously mentioned variations may occur)
- double outlet right ventricle with isomeric atrial appendages and, hence, ambiguous and

biventricular atrioventricular connections (not displayed in Figure 50.2).

ANATOMY OF THE COMMONER VARIANTS

Double outlet right ventricle with subaortic ventricular septal defect, aorta to right of pulmonary trunk and pulmonary stenosis (Fallot type)

In the 'classic' examples of this malformation (Figure 50.1a), the two great arteries are said to lie side by side (with the aorta to the right) with the arterial valves at approximately the same level. In many patients, however, the aorta lies slightly posterior to the pulmonary trunk in a relationship similar to that seen in typical tetralogy of Fallot. This pattern approximates more towards the normal arterial interrelationships. Frequently, there is a muscular infundibulum below each arterial valve, although fibrous continuity between the arterial and atrioventricular valves is found in a high proportion of patients (Wilcox et al, 1981; Wilkinson et al, 1981). The subpulmonary outflow tract shows stenosis, with or without hypoplasia of the infundibulum. Often the valve is additionally involved. The obstructive lesions are similar to those seen in Fallot's tetralogy. The ventricular septal defect is

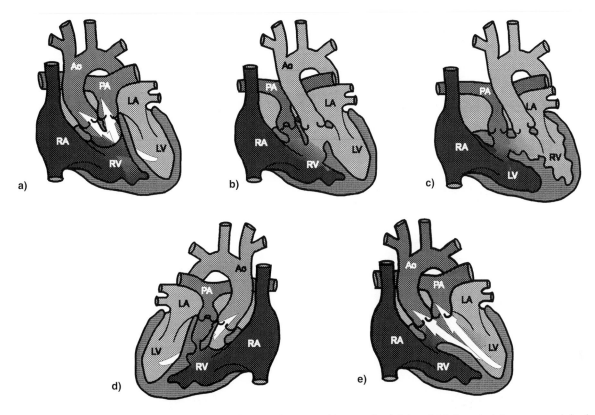

Figure 50.2. Other variants of double outlet right and left ventricle. (a) Doubly committed defect. (b) Subaortic defect, aorta to left of pulmonary trunk, pulmonary stenosis. (c) Double outlet right ventricle with discordant atrioventricular connections (usual atrial arrangement). (d) Double outlet right ventricle with mirror-imaged atrial arrangement (concordant atrioventricular connections). (e) Double outlet left ventricle with subaortic defect. Darker shading indicates de-oxygenated blood. Lighter shading indicates oxygenated blood. Arrows indicating passage of blood from the left ventricle to the aorta and pulmonary artery. Abbreviations as in Figure 50.1.

perimembranous in four fifths. It opens into the cavity of the right ventricle adjacent to the anteroseptal commissure of the tricuspid valve, to the right and posterior to the septal end of the outlet septum and below or into the subaortic infundibulum (Figure 50.3a). In approximately one fifth of patients the defect has a muscular posterior rim and is separated by this structure from the central fibrous body. This type of defect is similar to that seen in a proportion of those with tetralogy of Fallot (Dickinson et al, 1982). Its major significance clinically and surgically is the fact that the atrioventricular conduction axis is not related to the rim of the defect, being posterior to it, and hence is less vulnerable at operation. In those with more marked attenuation of the subaortic infundibulum (associated with mitral– aortic and/or tricuspid–aortic continuity), some aortic overriding is usual.

Important associated lesions include a restrictive ventricular septal defect, producing obstruction of the left ventricular outlet, and mitral stenosis (Figure 50.4c); the former occurs in up to one tenth of cases (Wilkinson et al, 1981).

Double outlet right ventricle with aorta to right and subpulmonary ventricular septal defect

The classical description by Taussig and Bing (1949) referred to a specimen in which the pulmonary trunk

(which was unobstructed) lay to the left of the aorta and above a large ventricular septal defect. Both great arteries had a muscular infundibulum. Although the pulmonary valve straddled the septal crest, the trunk arose predominantly from the right ventricle. The term Taussig–Bing anomaly has subsequently been used to refer to other malformations, such as complete transposition with subpulmonary septal defect and overriding (but posterior) pulmonary trunk (Beuren, 1960).

As has been well discussed by Van Mierop and Wiglesworth (1963) and by Van Praagh (1968), it could be argued that the term should be reserved for hearts in which the two great arteries are side by side (or nearly so) and in which there is a muscular subpulmonary infundibulum (Figure 50.1b). Nonetheless, it is important to acknowledge that double outlet right ventricle with subpulmonary defect may be associated with attenuation of the subpulmonary infundibulum, thus producing mitral–pulmonary continuity. The distinction in such cases between double outlet right ventricle and complete transposition with ventricular septal defect must depend on an assessment of the precise ventricular connection of the pulmonary trunk. An equally good case can be made, therefore, for using the term Taussig–Bing anomaly for this entire spectrum of hearts (Stellin et al, 1987). The ventricular septal defect is located anteriorly and, in two

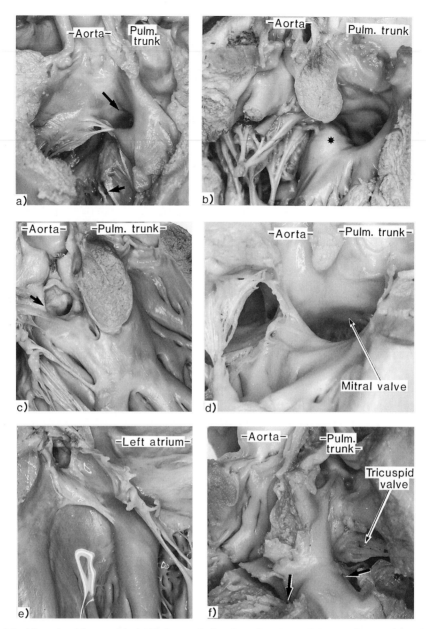

Figure 50.3. Morphology of double outlet right ventricle. (a) Right ventricular view of specimen showing subaortic defect (large arrow) in perimembranous site. Both great arteries have a muscular infundibulum. A second inlet muscular defect is indicated by the small arrow. (b) Right ventricular view of specimen with subpulmonary defect. Both great arteries have a muscular infundibulum. The posteroinferior rim of the defect (asterisk) is muscular. (c) Right ventricular view of specimen with restrictive subaortic defect but without pulmonary stenosis. The defect is perimembranous with a membranous septal remnant (arrow) in its rim. (d) Right ventricular view of specimen with doubly committed defect. The septal leaflet of the mitral valve is seen through the defect and is in continuity with both arterial valves (bilaterally deficient infundibulum). Both arterial valves override the defect, but each great artery arises predominantly (70%) from the right ventricle. The defect is perimembranous. (e) Left ventricular view in specimen with restrictive ventricular septal defect. (f) Right ventricular view of bizzare specimen with criss-cross concordant atrioventricular connections and left hand ventricular topology. Arrows indicate two defects. (Case included in Otero-Corto et al, 1979a.)

fifths of patients, has a muscular posterior rim separating it from the membranous septum (Figure 50.3b). In the remaining three fifths, however, the defect extends posteriorly and is perimembranous with a fibrous posterior margin (Wilkinson et al, 1981).

Double outlet right ventricle with subpulmonary defect is seldom associated with pulmonary stenosis. Aortic coarctation, in contrast, is a frequent association (8 out of 26 in the Toronto series; Sondheimer et al, 1977), often in association with straddling of the mitral valve. Mitral stenosis occurs (Lev and Bharati, 1973; Wilkinson et al, 1981). A restrictive subpulmonary defect producing left ventricular outlet obstruction is very infrequent.

Double outlet right ventricle with subaortic defect and no pulmonary stenosis (aorta to right of pulmonary trunk)

The malformation associated with a subaortic defect and no pulmonary stenosis (Figure 50.1c) is similar in many

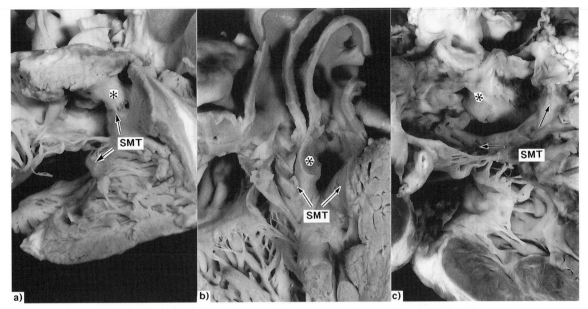

Figure 50.4. These specimens show how the position of the muscular outlet septum (asterisk) changes markedly even though the hole between the ventricles retains the same relationship to the septomarginal trabeculation (SMT) and right ventricle when both great arteries arise from that ventricle. The position of the muscular outlet septum determines whether the interventricular communication opens beneath the aorta (a), beneath the pulmonary trunk (b) or beneath both arterial trunks (when the outlet septum is absent) (c).

anatomical respects to the anomaly with pulmonary stenosis (see above). As in that situation, the arterial valves are usually side by side, or else the aortic valve is posterior and to the right of the pulmonary valve. The ventricular septal defect is usually perimembranous, though it may have a muscular posterior margin. A complete muscular infundibulum below the aortic valve is frequent, though aortic–tricuspid and/or aortic–mitral fibrous continuity may be present.

Aortic coarctation is frequently associated with this defect, as it is with the subpulmonary defect (see above). In the presence of aortic–mitral continuity, the aortic root usually overrides the septal crest. While the ventricular septal defect is often large in this group, restrictive defects may be seen (Figure 50.3c,e). This possibility should be borne in mind in the clinical situation (Lev and Bharati, 1973; Wilkinson et al, 1981).

Other anatomic variations

Even within the malformations already described, there is much individual anatomical variability. This applies to the site, size and detailed morphology of the ventricular septal defect (or defects), the relationships of the arterial outlets to one another and to the septal defect, and to the frequent presence of additional malformations (Tables 50.2–50.4 and Figure 50.5). With regard to the ventricular septal defect, it is noteworthy that both subaortic and subpulmonary defects are usually perimembranous, but defects with a muscular posteroinferior rim occur in a substantial minority (Table 50.3). Perimembranous defects may extend variably to open towards the inlet

and trabecular portions as well as opening into the outlet area of the right ventricle. Restrictive defects associated with left ventricular outlet obstruction are uncommon but are of great clinical and surgical importance (Serratto et al, 1967; Lavoie et al, 1971). Double or multiple defects occur occasionally.

Abnormalities of the atrioventricular valves occurred in one quarter of the 84 specimens described by Wilkinson et al in 1981. These included mitral stenosis (11% with subaortic defect) and straddling mitral valve (18% with subpulmonary defect). In addition, there were three hearts having an atrioventricular septal defect with common valve, two imperforate atrioventricular valves (one mitral and one tricuspid), and one each of parachute mitral valve, cleft mitral valve and cleft tricuspid valve (Table 50.4 and Figure 50.4a–c).

Obstruction to one of the arterial outlets occurs frequently (two thirds of the above series). The most common variety is infundibular and/or valvar pulmonary stenosis, with variable hypoplasia of the pulmonary arteries. This type of obstruction, usually similar to that seen in Fallot's tetralogy, was present in some three fifths of specimens with a subaortic defect but is infrequent in those with a subpulmonary defect. Obstruction of the systemic outlet is most often manifest by aortic coarctation, which occurred in one quarter of those with a subpulmonary defect and two fifths of those with a subaortic defect but without pulmonary stenosis. Interruption of the aortic arch occurred in an additional 14% with a subpulmonary defect, and subaortic and aortic stenosis also occur (Waldman et al, 1984). The total incidence of systemic outlet obstruction in those with a subpulmonary defect was nearly 50%.

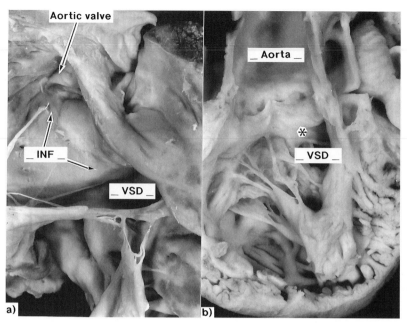

Figure 50.5. These two specimens show how the aorta can arise from the right ventricle with an extensive subaortic infundibulum (INF) (a) or with fibrous continuity between the aortic and mitral valves (b: asterisk). The aortic valve is closer to the roof of the interventricular communication (VSD) when the valvar leaflets are in fibrous continuity.

Other major associated malformations noted by Wilkinson et al (1981) included juxtaposition of the atrial appendages, totally anomalous pulmonary venous connection and criss-cross atrioventricular connections (see Figure 50.3). Wilcox et al (1981) have drawn attention to frequent variations in coronary arterial anatomy, which may be important surgically. Atrial septal defects within the oval fossa were present in almost one quarter of the specimens analysed by Wilkinson et al (1981).

LESS COMMON VARIANTS

Non-committed ventricular septal defect

In one tenth of cases, the sole ventricular septal defect is non-committed (Figure 50.1d). Such defects were perimembranous in site in most patients though unrelated to the arterial outlets. In only one was there an isolated muscular defect, this being in the inlet septum. Non-committed defects are important surgically (see below) and require careful delineation of the relationships of the defect to the arterial outlets and to other structures within the right ventricle – especially abnormal leaflet tissue derived from the tricuspid valve, which may interpose between the defect and the arterial outlets (Stellin et al, 1991). The majority (75%) have a bilateral muscular infundibulum, though in two patients (one with a common atrioventricular valve) there was pulmonary–tricuspid continuity.

Doubly committed ventricular septal defect

Just over one tenth of the 84 cases reported by Wilkinson et al (1981) had a doubly committed ventricular septal defect (Figure 50.2a), usually perimembranous in site and related to both arterial outlets (see Figure 50.3d). In about two fifths of specimens, the defect had a muscular posterior rim but in other respects was in a location similar to that in the perimembranous group. Three specimens had a bilaterally deficient infundibulum exhibiting both mitral–aortic and mitral–pulmonary continuity (Figure 50.3d). One additional patient had mitral–aortic continuity alone, while the remaining patients had bilaterally complete muscular outflow tracts.

In these small groups, there was wide variation in arterial interrelationships, in the presence and nature of associated defects and in the precise morphology of the septal defect. The associated defects included aortic co-arctation, pulmonary stenosis, straddling mitral valve, common atrioventricular valve, mitral stenosis, imperforate tricuspid valve, juxtaposition of the atrial appendages and subaortic stenosis.

CONSISTENT VARIATIONS IN MORPHOLOGY OF THE OVERALL GROUP

When previous accounts of the structure of the variants of double outlet are examined, the impression is often gained that when the ventricular septal defect is in subaortic rather than subpulmonary position it has moved relative to the muscular ventricular septum. To a certain extent, this must be the case, but when examined relative to the overall landmarks of the muscular ventricular septum, the location of the ventricular septal defect is remarkably constant (Capuani et al, 1995). Therefore, when the defect opens to the outlet of the right ventricle, be it subaortic subpulmonary or doubly committed, then always it is found between the limbs of the septomarginal trabeculation (septal band: Figure 50.4). The variation in morphology depends upon the connection of the muscular outlet septum relative to the septomarginal trabeculation. When the septal defect is subaortic (Figure 50.4a), then the muscular outlet septum is fused with the anterior limb of the trabeculation, as in tetralogy of Fallot. This fusion walls off the subpulmonary outlet from the ventricular septal defect. When the defect is in subpulmonary position in contrast, the muscular outlet septum is fused either to the posterior limb of the septomarginal trabeculation or to the ventriculo-infundibular fold (Figure 50.4b). This walls off the aorta from the septal defect and, almost always, produces a complete muscular subaortic infundibulum. The degree of 'squeeze' between the muscular outlet septum and the ventriculo-infundibular fold determines the extent of subaortic obstruction. The smaller the subaortic muscular area, the more likely it is that there will be aortic coarctation or interruption. The characteristics of the doubly committed defect (Figure 50.4c), also positioned between the limbs of the septomarginal trabeculation, is that almost always the muscular outlet septum and the adjacent portions of the subaortic and subpulmonary infundibulums are absent. This means that both arterial trunks tend to override the crest of the ventricular septum, producing an arrangement that some have likened to double outlet both ventricles (Brandt et al, 1976). It is noteworthy that absence of the outlet septum is a frequent (albeit not invariable) feature of double outlet right ventricle with doubly committed ventricular septal defect. It is, of course, also a characteristic feature of the so-called doubly committed subarterial ventricular septal defect

found with concordant ventriculo-arterial connections. The similarity of the terms (doubly committed defect with double outlet right ventricle and doubly committed ventricular septal defect), coupled with a comparable anatomical feature (absence of the muscular outlet septum), has led to some confusion. Trainees may perceive the two terms as being virtually synonymous. It is important to recognize that, despite some similarities (both semantic and anatomical) the conditions are, in most respects, very different. Most significantly, in double outlet right ventricle with doubly committed ventricular septal defect, the conjoined aortic and pulmonary valvar leaflets (or the remnant of the outlet septum, if present) are positioned above the cavity of the right ventricle. They do not form the superior rim of the septal defect, as is the case in the doubly committed subarterial defect seen with concordant ventriculo-arterial connections.

The interrelationships of the muscular structures around the septal defect condition other important anatomical features of double outlet. The size of the ventriculo-infundibular folds determines the extent of the subarterial infundibulums. When the folds are extensive, then long infundibulums are found supporting both arterial valves (Figure 50.5a). In contrast, when the fold is attenuated beneath each arterial valve, then there is atrioventricular-arterial valvar fibrous continuity (Figure 50.5b), but still with double outlet ventriculo-arterial connection. It is then the relationship between the posterior limb of the septomarginal trabeculation and the ventriculo-infundibular fold that determines whether the ventricular septal defect is perimembranous (Figure 50.6a) or has a muscular posteroinferior rim (Figure 50.6b). All of these anatomical

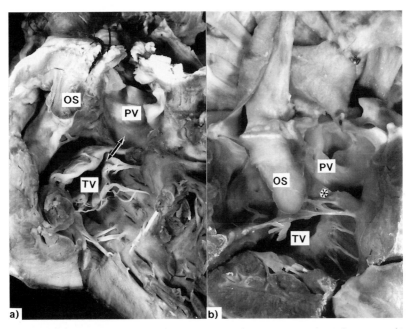

Figure 50.6. The crucial feature for the surgeon with regard to the interventricular communication is the nature of its posteroinferior rim. Both these specimens have subpulmonary defects. In the heart shown in (a), the defect is perimembranous because of the fibrous continuity between the leaflets of the tricuspid (TV) and pulmonary (PV) valves (arrowed). In the heart shown in (b), there is a muscular posteroinferior rim (asterisk), which protects the axis responsible for atrioventricular conduction. OS, muscular outlet septum.

details are readily demonstrated using cross-sectional echocardiography (Macartney et al, 1984).

MULTIPLE VENTRICULAR SEPTAL DEFECTS

In the series of Wilkinson et al (1981), 5 of the 84 cases had two ventricular septal defects. One had separate subaortic and subpulmonary defects. In the remaining four, there was an inlet muscular defect coexisting with a second subarterial defect (subaortic in two, subpulmonary in two) (see Figure 50.3a). Other than the presence of the second septal defect, these specimens showed similar features to others with subarterial defects.

DOUBLE OUTLET RIGHT VENTRICLE WITH INTACT VENTRICULAR SEPTUM

When the ventricular septum is intact, which can occur rarely in a patient with double outlet right ventricle, the left ventricle has no direct outlet. In such circumstances, the left ventricle is usually severely hypoplastic (Edwards et al, 1952; MacMahon and Lipa, 1964; Wilcox et al, 1981).

SUBAORTIC VENTRICULAR SEPTAL DEFECT WITH LEFT-SIDED AORTA AND PULMONARY STENOSIS

A subaortic ventricular septal defect with a left-sided aorta and with pulmonary stenosis (Figure 50.1c) was described by Paul et al in 1968 and termed by Van Praagh (1973) 'double outlet right ventricle with L-malposition'; it appears to be extremely uncommon. The septal defect in one of the cases reported by Lincoln et al (1975) was a perimembranous outlet defect, though in at least one other patient it appeared to have had a muscular posteroinferior rim (as appears also to have been the case in the specimen illustrated by Paul et al (1968). Pulmonary stenosis may be both valvar and subvalvar. The site of the septal defect makes these cases suitable for direct anatomical surgical correction, though relief of pulmonary stenosis may be difficult and an extracardiac conduit may be required. Associated defects, other than pulmonary stenosis, may include left juxtaposition of the atrial appendages (Lincoln et al, 1975; Van Praagh et al, 1975) and straddling mitral valve (see Figure 50.11, below).

DOUBLE OUTLET RIGHT VENTRICLE WITH DISCORDANT ATRIOVENTRICULAR CONNECTIONS

A double outlet right ventricle with discordant atrioventricular connections (Figure 50.2d; see also Figure 50.12d, below) has been described in association with both usual and mirror-imaged atrial arrangements. The largest reported set was a surgical series described by Tabry et al (1978). Most patients with usual atrial arrangement had

hearts placed in the right chest (dextrocardia), while those with mirror-imaged atriums had left-sided hearts (levocardia). Pulmonary stenosis was present in 16 of the 20 in the series. Subpulmonary defects were more frequent than subaortic defects (14 and 6, respectively). None was regarded as being non-committed or doubly committed. Valvar pulmonary atresia was noted in two. The relationships of the great arteries were very variable. The aorta lay to the left of the pulmonary trunk in 13, to the right in four and directly anterior in three. Common atrioventricular orifices have also been noted in association with the anomaly. This variant of double outlet right ventricle has much in common with congenitally corrected transposition, and is discussed further in Chapter 49.

DOUBLE OUTLET RIGHT VENTRICLE WITH MIRROR-IMAGED ATRIAL ARRANGEMENT AND ISOMERIC ATRIAL APPENDAGES

Mention of double outlet right ventricle with mirror-imaged atrial arrangement has already been made. While very few cases have been reported, it is likely that the same variability may be anticipated as has been described for double outlet right ventricle found with usual atrial arrangement (Stewart et al, 1976, 1979; Tabry et al, 1978).

Double outlet right ventricle in the presence of isomeric appendages occurs more commonly (Figure 50.2d). It has been stated that it is 'the rule in the asplenia syndrome' (Van Praagh and Vlad, 1978). This is not altogether borne out by the studies of Rose et al (1975) and de Tommasi et al (1981). In the latter study, however, double outlet right ventricle was found in one fifth (19% of right isomerism and 27% of left isomerism). In the syndromes of isomerism, it is well recognized that variability occurs at all levels of the heart (Chapter 31). This means that the complexity and multiplicity of the malformations seen in the presence of isomerism with double outlet right ventricle may be expected to be extreme. One combination in particular deserves mention: double outlet right ventricle with ambiguous and biventricular atrioventricular connections and a common atrioventricular orifice (Sridaromont et al, 1975). This may occur in both right isomerism and left isomerism, and with either right hand or left hand ventricular topologies.

DOUBLE OUTLET LEFT VENTRICLE

Because of the rarity of double outlet left ventricle (Figure 50.2e) few authors have reported a pathological, clinical or surgical series of any size from their own institution (see examples in Figure 50.6 and 50.14, below). Moreover, reviews of the subject and reports of individual cases have frequently included material relating to hearts with univentricular as well as biventricular atrioventricular connections (Van Praagh and Weinberg,

1977; Otero-Coto et al, 1979b, 1981). Otero-Coto and colleagues (1981) collected a total of 100 cases in their review of the literature, of which 81 had biventricular atrioventricular connections. The data from their analysis, and from that of Van Praagh and Weinberg (1977), form the basis for the following description.

Double outlet left ventricle most commonly occurs in hearts with usual atrial arrangement and concordant atrioventricular connections (89%). Discordant atrioventricular connections with usual atrial arrangement was noted in 5%, and mirror-imaged atrial chambers were present in the remaining 6% (with concordant atrioventricular connections in four out of five and discordant connections in the remaining one). Isomeric appendages were not found in any of the 81 with biventricular atrioventricular connections (though one case of right isomerism with double outlet from a left ventricle has been described with a univentricular atrioventricular connection).

Amongst the 72 with usual atrial arrangement and concordant atrioventricular connections, Otero-Coto et al (1981) described six major groups depending on the site of the ventricular septal defect, its relationship to the outlets and the arterial interrelations. Van Praagh and Weinberg (1977) did not clearly differentiate biventricular and univentricular atrioventricular connections. Their analysis included 13 distinct 'types', of which seven appear to relate to specimens with usual atrial arrangement and biventricular atrioventricular connections. It is clear from these studies that great variability exists even amongst those with usual atrial arrangement and concordant atrioventricular connections.

Apart from the unique specimen with intact ventricular septum described by Paul et al (1970), all the remaining hearts have had a ventricular septal defect. This has been subaortic in 68%, subpulmonary in 15% and doubly committed in 11%. Four (6%) had multiple defects. Arterial relationships are extremely variable. The aorta lay to the right of the pulmonary trunk, approximating to a normal relationship, in about one half of the hearts described by Otero-Coto et al (1981). In the remainder, it arose anteriorly or to the left of the pulmonary trunk. Infundibular morphology has also varied dramatically. Unfortunately, the incompleteness of documentation in some cases does not allow a clear picture to be drawn of the frequency of the different morphologies. A bilaterally deficient infundibulum is more frequently found with double outlet left ventricle than in any other situation. Nonetheless, it does not occur in the majority; the most common finding is a subpulmonary infundibulum with aortic–mitral continuity (Figure 50.6). A subaortic infundibulum with mitral–pulmonary continuity is also seen in a substantial number. Rarely, a bilateral infundibulum may be found. In other words, any possible infundibular morphology must be anticipated.

Associated abnormalities are the rule rather than the exception. Hearts with subaortic septal defects have a very high frequency of obstruction in the pulmonary outflow tract (present in more than 80%) (see Figure 50.12a,b, below). By contrast, those with a subpulmonary defect had a high incidence of systemic obstruction (usually coarctation), approximately half being so affected. These patients had a low incidence of pulmonary obstruction (10%).

The obstruction in the pulmonary outflow tract is frequently valvar (Bharati et al, 1978), but subvalvar obstruction is also a common finding (Otero-Coto et al, 1981). It is usually related to a stenotic and/or hypoplastic infundibulum, often with a displaced outlet septum. Systemic obstruction may take the form of aortic coarctation or interruption of the aortic arch, with or without subaortic stenosis (Otero-Coto et al, 1981). Anomalies of the atrioventricular valves occur in possibly one third of hearts and include hypoplasia, stenosis, straddling and Ebstein-like malformations. The tricuspid valve is more often abnormal than is the mitral valve. Hypoplasia of the right ventricle is also a frequent finding. Juxtaposition of the atrial appendages (on the left) has occurred in a few patients.

From the above description it may be seen that, as with double outlet right ventricle, extreme heterogeneity exists. It is doubtful whether it is justifiable to group or categorize the different specimens. Each 'type' is individually extremely rare and is subject to a host of associated defects and problems that may dominate the clinical picture and determine the surgical options.

In each case, the clinician must analyse the problem in the same logical sequence required for any complex defect. The anomaly must be investigated and categorized for each individual patient, systematically documenting it in terms of atrial arrangement, atrioventricular connection, morphology of septal defect and its relationship to the outlets, arterial relations, outlet obstruction, atrioventricular valvar abnormalities and other associated malformations.

CONDUCTION SYSTEM

The conduction system of hearts with double outlet right ventricle has been studied by several workers, though generally in small numbers of specimens and, in some cases, with rather bizarre and complex defects (Lev et al, 1964; Titus et al, 1964; Anderson et al, 1973; Lincoln et al, 1975; Bharati and Lev, 1976; Wilcox et al, 1981; Wilkinson et al, 1981). No studies have been reported in relation to double outlet left ventricle.

In double outlet right ventricle with usual atrial arrangement and concordant atrioventricular connections, the conduction system is related to the ventricular septal defect in a predictable way (Wilcox et al, 1981). When the defect is perimembranous (and regardless of its relation to the arterial outlets), the penetrating atrioventricular bundle runs onto the crest of the ventricular septum, usually with an extensive non-branching component, and usually branches close and to the left of the posteroinferior rim. This relationship to the septal defect is similar to that described in isolated ventricular septal defects (Milo et al, 1980) and in tetralogy of Fallot (Lev, 1959; Dickinson et al, 1982). As in those situations, some variability may be anticipated, with the branching component of the conduction axis being more-or-less vulnerable in the individual case. When the ventricular septal defect has a muscular posteroinferior rim, the conduction system is more distant from its margin and, hence, less vulnerable – apart from the right bundle branch (Wilcox et al, 1981). Again the situation is comparable with that seen in tetralogy of Fallot (Dickinson et al, 1982). Muscular defects in the inlet septum usually lie postero-inferior to the atrioventricular conduction axis, which may be related to their anterosuperior rim. In hearts with discordant atrioventricular connections, mirror-imaged atrial arrangement or isomeric atrial appendages, more complex anomalies of the conduction system may be anticipated. The possibility of the bundle relating to the anterosuperior rim of the defect should always be borne in mind (Anderson et al, 1973, 1974a; Tabry et al, 1978; Dickinson et al, 1979).

———— MORPHOGENESIS ————

During embryonic development, the normal heart passes through a phase during which both great arteries originate from the developing right ventricle. Indeed, this could be considered the default option. During horizons 16 and 17, the subaortic outflow tract becomes connected to the left ventricle. This process is associated with an effective leftward shift of the aorta, shortening of the sub-aortic infundibulum and attenuation of the ventriculo-infundibular fold in the area where it separates the leaflets of the developing mitral valve from those of the developing aortic valve. At the same time, the septum between the arterial outlets is realigned with the developing primary ventricular septum, and the primary inter-ventricular foramen is itself realigned to become the left ventricular outflow tract to the aorta (Goor et al, 1972; Anderson et al, 1974b). In order for this process to occur normally, it is necessary that certain earlier cardiac developmental processes have taken place in their correct sequence. These include formation of the ventricular loop and the development, in appropriate orientation, of the primordiums of the muscular ventricular and infundibulo-arterial septums. Errors in these, and other, phases of early cardiac development may profoundly affect subsequent morphogenesis involving the orientation and calibre of the outflow tracts and the ventriculo-arterial connections.

In hearts with double outlet right ventricle, the only universal feature is failure of complete incorporation of either of the arterial outflow tracts into the left ventricle. In many cases, an additional feature is the persistence of a muscular infundibulum in both subarterial outlets,

associated with lack of attenuation of the ventriculo-infundibular fold in the area between the atrioventricular and arterial valvar leaflets. In these cases, atrioventricular-arterial valvar fibrous continuity is not found. In addition, the muscular outlet septum remains an exclusively right ventricular structure, being malaligned, to a greater or lesser degree, relative to the trabecular muscular septum.

The fundamental cause of the embryological error or errors leading to double outlet right ventricle remains unclear. In the experimental situation, de la Cruz and her colleagues (Arteaga et al, 1982) have produced double outlet right ventricle in chick embryos by placing a loop around the infundibulum prior to its septation, thus preventing it from migrating and attenuating in the normal sequence. They concluded that double outlet right ventricle is basically an infundibular malformation. The relevance of these experimental data, however, to the naturally occurring malformation remains uncertain. In relation to the more bizarre variants of the anomaly (with abnormal atrial arrangement, discordant atrioventricular connections, abnormal arterial relationships, juxtaposition of the atrial appendages and so on), earlier and more severe errors in lateralization, loop formation and infundibulo-truncal spiralling must be implicated.

It has been established that, in their pathological features, many hearts with double outlet right ventricle are very similar to specimens of tetralogy of Fallot, while others bear a strong resemblance to complete transposition with ventricular septal defect. Lev et al (1972) proposed the presence of a pathological continuum from, on the one hand, tetralogy of Fallot to double outlet right ventricle with subaortic defect and, on the other hand, from the Taussig–Bing anomaly (double outlet right ventricle with subpulmonary defect) and to complete transposition with ventricular septal defect. Goor et al (1972) and Anderson et al (1974c) proposed that the different points of this spectrum could be related to different degrees of rotation (inversion) of the distal conus (infundibulum), coupled with varying failure of leftward migration and of absorption of the conoventricular flange (ventriculo-infundibular fold). In the rarer situation of double outlet right ventricle with left-sided aorta and subaortic defect, Goor and Edwards (1973) suggested that clockwise rather than counterclockwise inversion of the infundibulum had occurred. Lincoln et al (1975) raised the alternative possibility that malalignment of the aortopulmonary and muscular outlet (truncoconal) septum resulting in 'infundibulo-arterial discordance' might be an additional factor in this anomaly. All these workers took the view that these malformations were related to maldevelopment of the infundibulums. In this sense, they are in accord with the view of Arteaga et al (1982) based on the experimental work in chick embryos (see above).

In double outlet left ventricle, both outflow tracts are incorporated into the left ventricle. This is associated with exaggerated leftward shift of the arterial valves in relation to the ventricular septum. While this is sometimes associated with attenuation of the infundibular muscle below each arterial valve – producing a bilaterally deficient infundibulum – this is by no means the rule (Otero-Coto et al, 1981). In some hearts, one (or both) of the outflow tracts is a completely muscular structure. This appears to demonstrate that leftward shift of the arterial valves (relative to the ventricular septum) is not dependent on absorption and shortening (attentuation) of the infundibulum. It is notable that the muscular outlet septum is severely deficient in some cases of double outlet left ventricle and a doubly committed ventricular septal defect is related to both outlets (Figure 50.6). In such cases, it is tempting to hypothesize that the primordium of the outlet septum failed to form and became incorporated with the anterior part of the ventricular septum. Leftward shift of the aortic root towards its ultimate position in the left ventricular outlet might under these circumstances carry with it, to some degree, the abnormally mobile pulmonary root (which would not be 'fixed' to the right ventricle by the junction of muscular outlet and ventricular septums). Such a hypothesis, though attractive, could only explain a small proportion of cases of double outlet left ventricle (Ueda and Becker, 1986).

The apparent relationship between a rare variant of complete transposition with posterior aorta and subaortic ventricular septal defect (Van Praagh et al, 1971; Wilkinson et al, 1975) and double outlet left ventricle is also of some interest. In this malformation, the pulmonary trunk arises from the left ventricle and the aorta overrides the ventricular septum, arising predominantly from the right ventricle but with aortic–mitral valvar fibrous continuity. It is clear that the muscular outlet septum is grossly malaligned, with its leftward end being posteriorly orientated and the rightward part being anterior and incorporated with the muscular apical ventricular septum. The implication appears to be that, as a result of serious malalignment of the primordiums of the infundibular septum (but not of the great arteries themselves), the right (dextral) ridge fuses with the developing ventricular septum and walls off the pulmonary outflow tract from the right ventricle. Subsequent events include attenuation of the subaortic infundibulum and partial leftward shift (towards the 'normal' left ventricular outlet) of the aortic valve so that it overrides the septal defect. More marked leftward shift would clearly lead to double outlet left ventricle. As with most embryological theories, this concept still leaves unanswered the most important question: in this case, why should the muscular outlet septum be malaligned in the first place?

PATHOPHYSIOLOGY

The pathophysiology of double outlet ventricle is complex, being determined by the site of the ventricular septal defect in relation to the arterial outlets, the presence of pulmonary or systemic outlet obstruction, the pulmonary vascular resistance and by the presence of other associated cardiac defects.

The overall effect is largely determined by the level of pulmonary blood flow, the presence or absence of pulmonary hypertension and the effect of streaming. An additional important factor may be the presence of associated aortic coarctation, which, as well as producing an increase in systemic afterload, is liable to lead to hypoperfusion of the lower systemic segment after ductal closure, resulting in renal impairment and acute fluid retention. This usually leads to rapidly progressive cardiac failure in the newborn period.

PULMONARY BLOOD FLOW

Pulmonary flow is related to the presence and severity of pulmonary stenosis (valvar or subvalvar) and to the level of pulmonary resistance. Pulmonary arterial pressure and resistance are frequently normal or low in the presence of significant stenosis. Pulmonary flow is then also restricted, sometimes to markedly subnormal levels. Diminished pulmonary flow is inevitably associated with reduced arterial oxygen levels, though the degree of systemic hypoxia is also dependent on the effects of streaming. In the absence of pulmonary stenosis, the systolic pressure in the pulmonary trunk is usually equal to systemic pressure. Pulmonary flow is then dependent on the level of pulmonary vascular resistance. The behaviour of the pulmonary vasculature, in the presence of pulmonary hypertension, is similar to that observed in the presence of other congenital cardiac defects. In the early months of life, pulmonary resistance drops at a variable (though reduced) rate from the neonatal level. During this period, pulmonary blood flow increases progressively. Subsequently, sustained pulmonary hypertension leads to the development of obliterative pulmonary vascular disease (Heath and Edwards, 1958; Haworth et al, 1977) with rising pulmonary vascular resistance, until eventually pulmonary blood flow may fall to subnormal levels. Increased pulmonary blood flow tends to be associated with less severe systemic hypoxia, though, again, the effects of streaming are important in determining the arterial partial pressure of oxygen and oxygen saturation.

EFFECTS OF STREAMING

In the presence of a subaortic ventricular septal defect (with double outlet right ventricle), left ventricular blood tends to be directed predominantly to the aorta. This results physiologically in a situation resembling that seen with a simple ventricular septal defect (with concordant ventriculo-arterial connections). In the absence of pulmonary stenosis, little or no right-to-left shunting may be seen, aortic blood being almost fully saturated in many patients. When pulmonary stenosis coexists, some right-to-left shunting is almost always found and the extent of this (and of the associated systemic hypoxia) is related closely to the degree of obstruction. The physiology (as also the morphology) in this situation tends often to resemble closely that found in tetralogy of Fallot. In a minority of patients with a subaortic defect, these streaming effects are not seen, and in some the reverse may be the case, with lower oxygen saturation in the aorta than in the pulmonary trunk (Sridaromont et al, 1976, 1978).

When the septal defect is subpulmonary, the aorta is perfused preferentially with deoxygenated (systemic venous) blood. The physiology resembles that of complete transposition and, as in that condition, the degree of systemic hypoxia is dependent on the adequacy of 'mixing' between blood in the systemic and pulmonary circuits. As the double outlet situation tends to be associated with fairly good mixing in most cases, hypoxia may not be severe and the high pulmonary blood flow seen in most patients also militates against the development of severe hypoxia.

Non-committed and doubly committed ventricular septal defects result in variable streaming. In such cases, some degree of systemic hypoxia is almost invariable, and the main determinant of its severity is the degree of pulmonary stenosis.

INFLUENCE OF OTHER ASSOCIATED DEFECTS —

Mention has already been made of the serious effects that aortic coarctation may have on the pathophysiology. Many of the common associated defects may also affect the situation to a variable extent. Common atrioventricular orifice and straddling mitral valve probably reduce the 'streaming' effects that are otherwise often seen. Hypoplasia, stenosis or atresia of an atrioventricular valve may produce dramatic haemodynamic consequences, though mitral stenosis may produce surprisingly little effect if pulmonary blood flow is low owing to associated pulmonary stenosis. A restrictive ventricular septal defect produces pressure loading of the left ventricle, which consequently becomes hypertrophied (see Figure 50.4c); however, apart from elevated left ventricular pressure, the haemodynamics are usually not greatly affected unless the left ventricular outflow tract obstruction results in left atrial hypertension, with resulting pulmonary venous congestion etc.

CLINICAL FINDINGS

PRESENTATION

The clinical features of infants with double outlet ventriculo-arterial connection are extremely variable and may mimic those of many other defects.

Those with double outlet right ventricle, subaortic ventricular septal defect and pulmonary stenosis usually present a clinical picture that resembles that of tetralogy of Fallot. A systolic murmur is sometimes noted in the newborn period, but the onset of cyanosis may be delayed for several months.

Patients with double outlet right ventricle and subpulmonary ventricular septal defect, however, usually develop cyanosis in the newborn period, though the cyanosis may not be severe. Cardiac failure, developing later in the first month of life or subsequently, with tachypnoea, dyspnoea, failure to feed and thrive compounds the picture.

The appearance of severe cyanosis in the neonatal period is usually a reflection of the presence of severe pulmonary stenosis or atresia with very low pulmonary blood flow. Such a presentation is sometimes seen in those patients with a subaortic ventricular septal defect and pulmonary stenosis (Fallot type) but is also seen in more complex defects, especially those with isomerism.

Onset of symptoms of cardiac failure, but without cyanosis, at the end of the first month or in the second and third months of life is typical of those patients with a subaortic ventricular septal defect and no pulmonary stenosis. This clinical picture resembles that of a large isolated ventricular septal defect.

Early onset of cardiac failure is particularly a feature of those patients with an associated coarctation or interrupted aortic arch.

A small proportion of patients do not present in early infancy but are detected later in the first year of life, or rarely even later in childhood. While some such patients may have features similar to a late-presenting tetralogy of Fallot, others have evidence of severe pulmonary hypertension. They resemble more the child with a large ventricular septal defect, pulmonary hypertension and elevated pulmonary resistance who has survived without developing cardiac failure in infancy.

Data from the Hospital for Sick Children in Toronto showed that the majority of patients with double outlet right ventricle in all categories presented in the first 2 months of life, except for those with a subaortic ventricular septal defect and pulmonary stenosis, who usually presented later (Sondheimer et al, 1977).

The presenting features of double outlet left ventricle are similarly extremely variable. They do not permit distinction from double outlet right ventricle (or many other defects) on purely clinical grounds.

PHYSICAL SIGNS

The physical signs in double outlet ventricle vary with the clinical presentation and underlying pathology.

Manifestations of cardiac failure in early infancy, with or without cyanosis, are usually indicative of high pulmonary blood flow and pulmonary hypertension. When such features appear in the first week or two of life, they are usually associated with major or often multiple associated defects, such as aortic coarctation. Such infants usually have a hyperdynamic cardiac impulse with a parasternal systolic murmur of moderate amplitude, which often radiates fairly widely, particularly to the pulmonary area and the back. The second heart sound is usually loud, though this is often because of an aortic component, which, as in complete transposition, may be accentuated.

In the absence of cardiac failure, an ejection systolic murmur varying between grades 2/6 and 4/6 may be audible along the left sternal border and in the pulmonary area that radiates to the back. This is usually related to infundibular and/or valvar pulmonary stenosis. As in tetralogy of Fallot, the pulmonary component of the second sound is often inaudible. Cyanosis is variable and may not appear for several months.

An apical mid-diastolic murmur is occasionally heard and may reflect high pulmonary blood flow or associated mitral stenosis. A restrictive ventricular septal defect is associated with a harsh parasternal systolic murmur and a forceful apical impulse, on palpation, owing to left ventricular hypertrophy. The murmur from a restrictive defect may be masked if there is associated infundibular stenosis.

INVESTIGATIONS

ELECTROCARDIOGRAPHY

Early reports of the electrocardiogram in double outlet right ventricle (Neufeld et al, 1961a, 1962; Mirowski et al, 1963) suggested that certain features were of predictive diagnostic value. These included a superior frontal plane QRS axis with a counterclockwise vector loop in the presence of right ventricular hypertrophy. This pattern was said to be particularly frequent in those with a subaortic defect without pulmonary stenosis. Atrioventricular conduction delay, especially first-degree block, was found to be very common; intraventricular conduction disturbances, especially right bundle branch block, were also frequent. Some degree of left ventricular hypertrophy in the presence of severe right ventricular hypertrophy was also found in a high proportion of patients; right atrial hypertrophy was noted in 86% in the series of Mirowski et al (1963).

Krongrad and colleagues (1972) were unable to confirm that these electrocardiographic features were of any great diagnostic value. They found a superior QRS axis in 5 out of 12 patients without pulmonary stenosis, and also in 1 of 19 with pulmonary stenosis. The latter patient, and three of the former, had counterclockwise loops. Such electrocardiograms occur in a wide variety of other cardiac defects and are of little predictive value for this reason. In their patients, the other features were all found to be less frequent than previously suggested and were of no great predictive value either in the diagnosis of double outlet right ventricle or in the recognition of associated defects.

The most consistent electrocardiographic features in the more common types of double outlet right ventricle are the presence of right ventricular hypertrophy, right axis deviation (usually between +90° and +120°) and the presence of an rR', qR or rsR' pattern in right chest leads. QRS duration is normal in most patients. Right atrial hypertrophy is common, and bi-atrial or pure left atrial hypertrophy is seen in a minority of patients (Figure 50.7a).

The presence of left atrial hypertrophy or left ventricular hypertrophy has not been shown to correlate well with the haemodynamics (Krongrad et al, 1972). In two patients of our own, however, left atrial hypertrophy and diminished R waves in right chest leads were present in association with a restrictive ventricular septal defect and mitral valvar abnormalities (Figure 50.7b).

CHEST RADIOGRAPHY

Radiological features in double outlet right ventricle depend mainly on the associated malformations and are seldom of any diagnostic value. Atrial arrangement, as indicated by bronchial morphology on a penetrated or filter film, is normal ('usual') in most instances. Cardiac position is variable, though the substantial majority (approximately nine tenths) of patients with the more common types have left-sided hearts. A right aortic arch is seen in 25–30% of those with a subaortic ventricular septal defect and pulmonary stenosis (Sondheimer et al, 1977) and is occasionally present in other types.

Cardiomegaly of significant degree is, in general, associated with increased pulmonary blood flow. It is, therefore, an almost universal feature of instances with an unobstructed pulmonary outflow tract. Patients with pulmonary stenosis, however, frequently have little or no increase in cardiac diameter. Pulmonary oligaemia or plethora is again related to the presence or absence of significant pulmonary stenosis.

The cardiac contour may mimic tetralogy of Fallot, large ventricular septal defect or complete transposition with ventricular septal defect. No diagnostic characteristics are demonstrable. A straight right heart border is seen in some patients with left juxtaposition of the atrial appendages.

The site and size of the ventricular septal defect, and its relationship to the arterial outlets, has little influence on the radiological appearances on plain radiography.

ECHOCARDIOGRAPHY

M-mode echocardiography was used, in the early era of cardiac ultrasound, to assess mitral–arterial valvar discontinuity (Chesler et al, 1971). Since echocardiographic discontinuity can occur in a variety of situations,

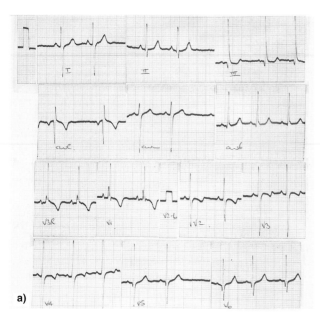

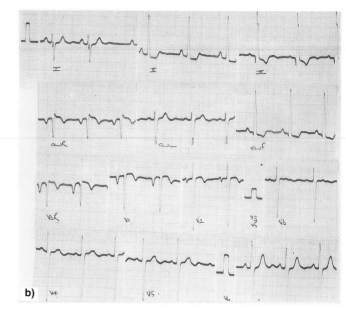

Figure 50.7. Electrocardiogram in double outlet right ventricle. (a) Typical pattern with axis + 100°, rR' in V₃R and V, and normal QRS duration. (b) Atypical record showing left atrial hypertrophy and diminished right ventricular potentials in patient with severe mitral stenosis and regurgitation and restrictive defect.

including left ventricular dilation (French and Popp, 1975; Feigenbaum, 1981), the inference that double outlet right ventricle might be present was frequently incorrect.

Cross-sectional echocardiography has a vitally important role in the comprehensive investigation of the patient with double outlet right ventricle. Not only may the diagnosis of double outlet be made with a high degree of certainty, but the relationship of the ventricular septal defect to the arterial outlets, the presence of arterial outlet narrowing or obstruction and the coexistence of important associated defects, especially those of the atrioventricular valves (such as common atrioventricular orifice or straddling mitral valve), may all be documented.

The diagnosis of double outlet right ventricle may be made in the long-axis view by demonstrating that both great arteries arise predominantly or entirely from the right ventricle, and that the only exit for the left ventricle is a ventricular septal defect (Figure 50.8) (Di Sessa et al, 1979; Hagler et al, 1981). Discontinuity between the septal leaflet of the mitral valve and the leaflets of the arterial valves may be seen when present but does not, in itself, establish the diagnosis as it may be present in other malformations. Moreover, mitral–arterial valvar continuity is characteristically present in tetralogy of Fallot, even when the aorta arises predominantly from the right ventricle. The degree of overriding of one or both great arteries over the ventricular septal defect can be assessed using a combination of long-axis, short-axis, apical and subcostal views. In most cases, the ventricular origin of each arterial trunk can be established with a high degree of accuracy, and true distinguished from spurious overriding. A combination of long-axis and serial short-axis views is helpful (Houston et al, 1977; Di Sessa

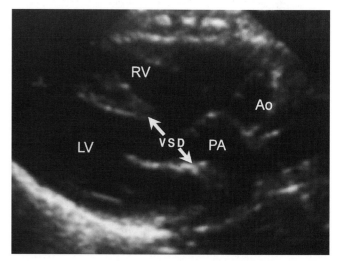

Figure 50.8. Cross-sectional echocardiogram, in parasternal long-axis cut, showing both great arteries originating from the right ventricle with a subpulmonary ventricular septal defect (VSD). Abbreviations as in Figure 50.1.

et al, 1979); and subcostal short- (Figures 50.9 and 50.10) and long-axis scans have been used extensively (Macartney et al, 1984). They are of particular value in assessing the relationship of the ventricular septal defect to the arterial outlets and in defining its superior margin.

Subcostal views are also helpful in analysing the relationships of the atrioventricular valves and their tension apparatus to the defect. Of particular importance in this respect, and particularly common, are abnormalities of insertion to the tricuspid valvar tension apparatus such that the pathway from the interventricular communication to one or both outflow tracts is impeded. This information

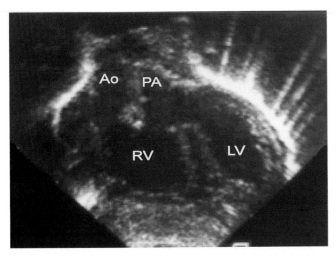

Figure 50.9. Cross-sectional echocardiogram, in subcostal short-axis cut, showing both great arteries originating from the right ventricle. The ventricular septal defect is again subpulmonary. Abbreviations as in Figure 50.1.

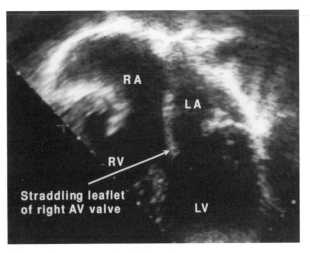

Figure 50.11. Cross-sectional echocardiogram, in apical four chamber view, demonstrating straddling of the tricuspid valve over the crest of the ventricular septal defect. AV, atrioventricular; other abbreviations as in Figure 50.1.

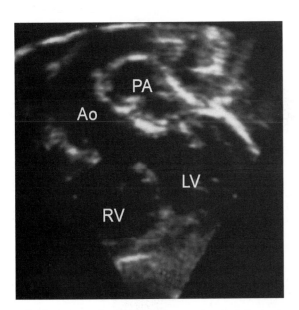

Figure 50.10. Cross-sectional echocardiogram, in apical short-axis view, showing a subaortic ventricular septal defect with the aorta arising entirely from the right ventricle. Abbreviations as in Figure 50.1.

may be of crucial importance to the surgeon. The views that give this information, however, may be misleading in assessing the extent of overriding of a great artery. This feature is probably better judged using parasternal long- and short-axis cuts.

The interrelationship of the great arteries and their relative sizes is usually readily demonstrable, as is the presence of valvar or subvalvar obstruction. Particular questions that are of surgical relevance and can be answered by cross-sectional echocardiography include the anatomy of the outlet septum, the anatomy of the roof of the ventricular septal defect, the relationships of atrio-ventricular valve tension apparatus to the septal defect, and the demonstration of which arterial outlet is most

closely adjacent to the defect (Macartney et al, 1984). In addition to these four features (which may be difficult to define by other means such as angiocardiography), echo-cardiography is of particular value in establishing the presence of major atrioventricular valvar abnormalities such as a common atrioventricular orifice or straddling of the mitral or tricuspid valve (Figure 50.11) across the septum (Hagler et al, 1981).

Other associated malformations, such as hypoplasia of the left or right ventricle, juxtaposition of the atrial appendages, aortic coarctation and interruption of the aortic arch may also be demonstrable echocardio-graphically.

The use of Doppler echocardiography is primarily of value in assessing obstructive lesions and atrioventricular valvar regurgitation. Colour flow mapping is especially helpful in the latter.

CARDIAC CATHETERIZATION AND ANGIOCARDIOGRAPHY

In catheterization of the patient with double outlet, the investigator must keep in mind two particular objectives. First, the intracardiac connections (especially the ventriculo-arterial connection) must be documented; second, all surgically important aspects of the malformation must be assessed.

In most cases, if appropriate preliminary investigations have been performed, the atrial arrangement, atrioventricular connections and ventriculo-arterial connection will all be known prior to catheterization. The bulk of the data required from cardiac catheterization, therefore, relate to the surgically important aspects of the defect.

In obtaining haemodynamic data, special attention must be paid to assessing any systolic pressure gradient between left and right ventricles (suggesting a restrictive septal defect) or any diastolic pressure gradient across the mitral valve. It is essential to gain access to the left side of the heart, either via the ventricular septal defect or at atrial level (by trans-septal puncture if necessary).

The relationship of the ventricular septal defect to the arterial outlets may, to some extent, be inferred by the behaviour of the catheter (such as easy passage of a retrograde aortic catheter to the left ventricle) or from an assessment of streaming. Haemodynamics resembling those of a large ventricular septal defect or of tetralogy of Fallot (in both of which aortic saturation exceeds that in the pulmonary trunk) suggest a subaortic ventricular septal defect. By contrast, a higher saturation in the pulmonary trunk than in the aorta is usually indicative of a subpulmonary defect.

Measurement of pulmonary arterial pressure, and calculation of the flow and resistance, is mandatory. The presence of pulmonary hypertension at systemic level, indicating absence of obstruction to the subpulmonary outlet, should always raise the suspicion of obstruction to the systemic outlet. A careful search should then be made for subaortic or aortic stenosis, and for aortic coarctation or interruption. The presence of pulmonary stenosis, by comparison, makes it unlikely that any obstruction to the systemic outlet will be present.

Angiocardiography should include selective left and right ventriculograms (Figure 50.12). The left ventriculogram should be carried out in a view designed to profile the ventricular septum (such as 45° left anterior oblique

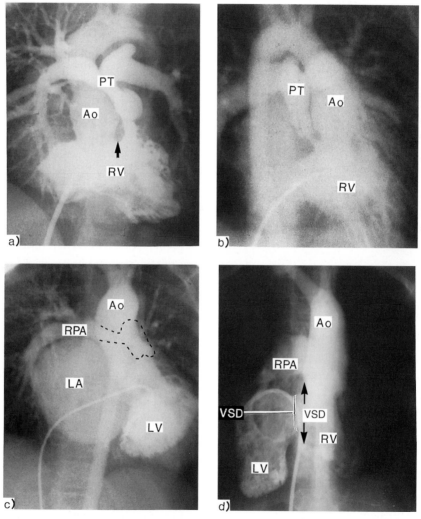

Figure 50.12. Angiography of double outlet right ventricle. (a) Anteroposterior view of right ventriculogram in Fallot-type double outlet right ventricle (RV). Contrast in the aorta (Ao) is less dense than that in the pulmonary trunk (PT) because of the passage of non-opacified blood from the left ventricle (LV) via the subaortic defect. The outlet septum (arrow) is seen in profile. The anatomy of the pulmonary stenosis (infundibular, valvar and supravalvar) is well demonstrated. (b) Anteroposterior view of right ventriculogram in a subaortic defect, left-sided aorta and pulmonary stenosis. Again the pulmonary obstruction is well defined, though the relationship of the outlets to the defect is not. (c) Anteroposterior view of left ventriculogram in a patient with mitral stenosis and regurgitation and restrictive defect. The left atrium (LA) is grossly dilated. The ventricular origin of the great arteries cannot be defined in this view. The aorta arose to the right and anterior to the pulmonary trunk (dotted) and only the right pulmonary artery (RPA) is well seen in this projection (same patient as in Figure 50.7b). (d) Anteroposterior projection of left ventriculogram in patient with usual atrial arrangement, discordant atrioventricular connections and double outlet right ventricle. The ventricular septal defect (VSD) is well profiled in this view, and the origin of the great arteries from the right ventricle and the mitral annulus are clearly demonstrated. The aorta in this case arose directly anterior to the pulmonary trunk.

inclination) with some craniocaudal tilt (20–30°). The precise orientation must be assessed individually and depends on the cardiac position and preliminary echocardiographic evidence. This view is intended to show the site and size of the ventricular septal defect (or defects) and its relationship to the arterial outlets (Figures 50.13–50.15). The presence of a common atrioventricular orifice, or overriding mitral valve, may also be demonstrated. The presence of mitral regurgitation may be assessed (Figure 50.12c) in the complementary plane (right anterior oblique) if biplane angiography is used.

Right ventriculography may be performed in a similar oblique projection, although frontal and lateral views may also be useful. This will normally demonstrate the relationship of the arterial outlets to one another and the presence and nature of obstructive lesions in either outflow tract (Figure 50.12a,b).

In patients with unobstructed pulmonary flow, a selective aortogram is often desirable (profiled in frontal and lateral projections) to demonstrate/confirm the presence of aortic coarctation (or interruption). Those with pulmonary stenosis may require selective pulmonary arteriography with 30° craniocaudal tilt (frontal projection) to define the anatomy of the pulmonary trunk and its bifurcation. In all cases, the investigator must bear in mind the high frequency of associated malformations and take whatever steps are necessary to define or exclude them. In cases where radical reconstruction of the pulmonary outflow tract (with or without a conduit) or an arterial switch operation is contemplated, it may be desirable to define the coronary arterial anatomy by aortography or by selective coronary arteriograms.

MAGNETIC RESONANCE IMAGING

Even with conventional angiography and echocardiography, the precise relationship of the great arteries to the ventricular septal defect may be difficult to determine. Recent work with magnetic resonance imaging suggests that this modality of investigation may provide useful additional information. The ability to generate cross-sectional images in almost any spatial plane may be of considerable assistance in clarifying the anatomy of these complex hearts (Parsons et al, 1991; Yoo et al, 1991).

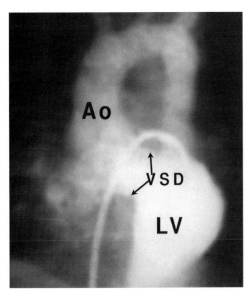

Figure 50.13. Left ventricular angiogram in four chamber projection showing subaortic ventricular septal defect (VSD). LV, left ventricle; Ao, aorta.

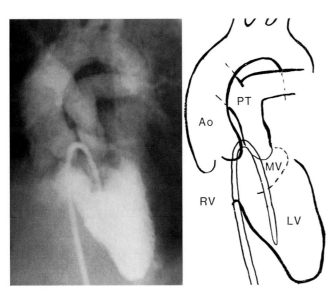

Figure 50.14. Four chamber view of left ventriculogram in patient with double outlet left ventricle, subaortic defect and pulmonary stenosis. The aorta (Ao) overrides the defect but arises predominantly from the left ventricle (LV). The pulmonary stenosis was mainly valvar (but is not well demonstrated). PT, pulmonary trunk; RV, right ventricle; MV, mitral valve.

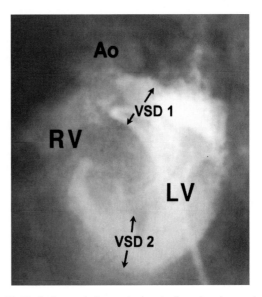

Figure 50.15. Left ventricular angiogram in four chamber projection showing multiple ventricular septal defects (VSD 1 and 2). The origin of the aorta (Ao) is seen faintly over the right ventricle (RV). LV, left ventricle.

DIFFERENTIAL DIAGNOSIS

As will be apparent from the foregoing description, the clinical picture, along with the radiographic and electro-cardiographic features, is very variable and non-specific. Double outlet may mimic many cardiac lesions. Those forms that do not include pulmonary stenosis may, when acyanotic, closely resemble a large isolated ventricular septal defect. In the presence of cyanosis, the picture may simulate that of complete transposition with a ventricular septal defect, or other cyanotic defects with high pulmonary flow. Coexisting coarctation may lead to the early development of cardiac failure, producing a clinical picture that resembles other variants of coarctation or hypoplastic left heart syndromes. The presence of pulmonary stenosis, by comparison, is more often associated with presentation at a later age and gives features similar to those of tetralogy of Fallot. In all cases, the differentiation depends on careful echocardiographic and angiographic delineation of the connections and relationship of the great arteries to the ventricles.

MANAGEMENT

Treatment of double outlet ventriculo-arterial connection is essentially surgical, including the palliative procedures that may be necessary after initial diagnosis. Other than for supportive measures, there is no place for medical treatment, although interventional catheterization may have a role in the treatment of complications of surgical palliation/repair.

SURGERY

The surgery of double outlet right ventricle has posed a great challenge to the ingenuity and skill of cardiac surgeons the world over. In the early years of cardiac surgery, the nature of the malformation was not always recognized preoperatively or intraoperatively. In this setting, closure of the ventricular septal defect without re-direction of left ventricular blood to the aorta led to some operative tragedies (Redo et al, 1963). Successful correction was first achieved by Kirklin in 1957 (Kirklin et al, 1964). Since that time, a large number of surgical reports have appeared (Kirklin et al, 1964; Kiser et al, 1968; Gomes et al, 1971; Danielson et al, 1972; Stewart et al, 1976; Harvey et al, 1977; Tabry et al, 1978; Stewart et al, 1979; Judson et al, 1983; Luber et al, 1983; Piccoli et al, 1983; Mazzucco et al, 1985; Aoki et al, 1994; Kleinert et al, 1997).

The surgical approach to the individual patient depends on the anatomical features present, and particularly on whether complicating additional abnormalities occur. In more complex cases, corrective surgery may not be feasible (Wilcox et al, 1981; Piccoli et al, 1983).

In those unsuitable patients, the use of a modified Fontan operation or other palliative procedures may be the preferred option. In the majority of patients, however, a biventricular repair is feasible.

In the early weeks of life, palliation may be required prior to subsequent correction. Patients with a subpulmonary ventricular septal defect, in whom the physiology resembles complete transposition, may benefit from balloon atrial septostomy. This is also worthwhile in those infants with severe left-sided obstructive lesions (such as mitral stenosis or atresia) to decompress the left atrium.

Infants with severe pulmonary hypertension and congestive failure may require palliation with banding of the pulmonary trunk if primary correction is likely to carry high risks (see below). Conversely, infants with restricted pulmonary blood flow owing to pulmonary stenosis may need construction of a systemic-to-pulmonary arterial shunt if primary correction is not considered either feasible or a satisfactory option at this age.

Those infants with aortic coarctation or interruption will usually require urgent surgical relief of the obstructive lesion in the newborn period, with or without simultaneous intracardiac repair. Banding of the pulmonary trunk may be considered desirable during the same procedure if early complete intracardiac repair is not possible.

Primary repair for those patients with a subaortic ventricular septal defect involves the placement of an intraventricular tunnel from the septal defect to the aorta (Kirklin et al, 1964). Subpulmonary or valvar pulmonary stenosis may be relieved by infundibulectomy, valvotomy or enlargement of the outflow tract with a gusset. An external conduit may be used where these methods are not appropriate.

In such patients, operative mortality is generally low in the modern era (Kirklin et al, 1986). Amongst 60 such patients (with 'non-complex' forms of double outlet right ventricle, with a subaortic ventricular septal defect) having biventricular repairs in Melbourne since 1978, there were two hospital deaths (3.33%; 70% confidence interval (CI) 0.9–7). Others have reported a generally favourable experience with this subgroup of patients (Judson et al, 1983; Luber et al, 1983; Piccoli et al, 1983; Mazzucco et al, 1985). Risks from total correction were considered to be significantly higher in younger age groups. This was not found to be the case in the recent analysis of Kirklin et al (1986). These concerns led some surgeons to prefer early palliation with banding of the pulmonary trunk or systemic-to-pulmonary arterial shunts (Judson et al, 1983). Other surgeons, however, report a low mortality except possibly in infants under 3 months of age. They recommend primary correction even in infancy (Piccoli et al, 1983). This has been the preferred approach in Melbourne and in Boston (Aoki et al, 1994; Kleinert et al, 1997). More complex anatomy in some hearts with a subaortic ventricular septal defect may complicate repair and increase the risks of operation. In the Melbourne experience, a range of such

Table 50.5. Surgery performed on patients with subaortic ventricular septal defects, in a cohort of 193 infants/children with double outlet right ventricle, having their initial palliation/repair between 1978 and 1993 at the Royal Children's Hospital, Melbourne

	Number	Hospital deaths
Biventricular repair: non-complex forms with additional lesion		
Pulmonary stenosis (other than Fallot's)	8	1
Tetralogy anatomy	37	1
Coarctation	1	0
No additional abnormality	14	0
Total	60	2 (3.33%)
Biventricular repair: complex forms with a complicating lesion		
Multiple VSDs (tetralogy type)	3	1
Multiple VSDs (not Fallot type)	4	0
Pulmonary atresia	2	0
Isomerism	3	0
Restrictive ventricular septal defect	3	0
Severe ascending aorta hypoplasia + coarctation (Konno)	1	1
Anomalous origin of one pulmonary artery	1	0
Pulmonary arterial sling	1	1
Aortopulmonary window	1	0
Exteriorized heart (ectopia cordis)	1	1
Total	20	4 (20%)
Other surgical procedures[a]		
Fontan (complex anatomy)	4	0
Palliation (band/shunt/coarctation repair)	6	3[b]

VSD, Ventricular septal defect.
[a] Patients undergoing other surgical procedures for coarctation (4), pulmonary atresia (1), hypoplastic left ventricle (2) and multiple VSD (3). Three patients awaited definitive surgery.
[b] Two died with severe hypoplasia of the left ventricle.

complicating features was encountered (Table 50.5). Among 20 such patients, hospital mortality after complete repair was 20%. This has led to our preference for adopting the Fontan procedure or construction of cavopulmonary shunts in these more complex patients, providing the haemodynamics are such that the patient is a suitable candidate for such procedures.

In patients with subpulmonary septal defects, surgical results in the past were less good. In selected patients, it proved possible to construct an intraventricular conduit from the left ventricle to the aorta (Patrick and McGoon, 1968; Kawashima et al, 1971, 1993). In most, however, it is necessary to close the defect so that left ventricular blood is directed to the pulmonary trunk. This then necessitates an additional arterial switch procedure, or an atrial redirection (Mustard or Senning operation). Atrial redirection in most cases was found to carry a high mortality (39%; Piccoli et al, 1983). For this reason, in the modern era, an arterial switch is preferable in almost all cases. It has been suggested that hearts in which the great arteries are in an anteroposterior relationship are particularly suitable for the repair incorporating an arterial switch, while those with side-by-side arterial relationships may be more suitable for intraventricular repair

(Yacoub and Radley Smith, 1984; Serraf et al, 1991). Others have employed arterial switch procedures in both situations (Kanter et al, 1986). Still other procedures have been attempted in some more complex cases. One such approach, the so called 'REV' (reparation a l'étage ventriculaire – repair at the ventricular level) procedure, involves sacrificing the pulmonary outflow tract in order to route an intraventricular baffle from the ventricular septal defect to the aorta. The pulmonary bifurcation is then brought in front of the ascending aorta using a Lecompte manoeuvre and is sutured directly to the upper edge of the ventriculotomy incision, using a pericardial patch or monocusp gusset to complete the attachment of the anterior wall of the new outflow tract to the pulmonary arteries (Lecompte et al, 1982; Borromee et al, 1988). This operation may be worth considering for patients with a subpulmonary septal defect with coexisting pulmonary stenosis, a combination that precludes an arterial switch repair. Another option in this situation is the use of a Rastelli-type repair incorporating insertion of an external valved conduit between the right ventricle and the pulmonary trunk (Vouhé et al, 1992).

The experience in Melbourne with subpulmonary defects is summarized in Table 50.6. The presence of

Table 50.6.　Surgery performed on patients with subpulmonary ventricular septal defects, in a cohort of 193 infants/children with double outlet right ventricle, having their initial palliation/repair between 1978 and 1993 at the Royal Children's Hospital, Melbourne

	Number	Hospital deaths
Biventricular repair: complicating lesion		
Multiple ventricular septal defects	6	2
Coarctation	9	0
Interrupted aortic arch	2	0
Pulmonary stenosis	1	0
Small right ventricle	1	0
No additional abnormality	20	1
Total	39	3 (7.7%)
Biventricular repair: surgical procedure		
Senning (palliative)	3	0
Senning + VSD (later converted to switch)	4	0
Senning + VSD repair	3	1
Primary arterial switch + VSD repair	27	2
REV procedure	1	0
Intraventricular baffle + conduit	1	0
Total	39	3 (7.7%)
Other surgical procedures		
Fontan (complex anatomy ± PS)	5	0
Palliation (coarctation/band/shunt)	5	2
Total	10	2 (20%)

PS, pulmonary shunt; REV, repair at the ventricular level; VSD, ventricular septal defect.

associated pulmonary stenosis may prejudice a satisfactory biventricular repair; in the absence of this complicating problem, however, almost all patients are suitable for an arterial switch procedure. The hospital mortality in 'non-complex' cases submitted to biventricular repair was 1/31 (3.2%; 70% CI 0.3–10), excluding patients with multiple ventricular septal defects. This is no different from that experienced in 'non-complex' cases with subaortic defects. Moreover, the presence of aortic coarctation or interruption did not impact on mortality at the time of repair – despite the fact that the arch was repaired at the same time as intracardiac repair in most patients. One infant with severe aortic coarctation died during attempted palliation (repair of aortic coarctation and atrial septectomy) early in the series. One patient with associated pulmonary stenosis and multiple ventricular septal defects underwent a Senning procedure, and was later converted to a Fontan, but died after the latter procedure. Three further children with subpulmonary ventricular septal defects were treated with Fontan operations, being considered unsuitable for biventricular repair, and all survived. A further five infants were palliated, being considered unsuitable for primary repair. One died late, of non-cardiac causes, and the others were awaiting definitive surgery at the time of audit.

Patients with doubly committed ventricular septal defects are usually suitable for intraventricular repair. The Melbourne series of 193 patients had only five with defects of this type, and all could be corrected in biventricular fashion using an intraventricular patch (Table 50.7). This type of defect was not identified as being a risk factor for death by Kirklin et al (1986) and is probably as favourable as a subaortic defect for biventricular repair.

Table 50.7.　Surgery performed on patients with doubly committed and non-committed ventricular septal defects, in a cohort of 193 infants/children with double outlet right ventricle, having their initial palliation/repair between 1978 and 1993 at the Royal Children's Hospital, Melbourne

Type of surgery	Number	Hospital deaths
Doubly committed VSD		
Intraventricular baffle	5	0
Non-committed VSD		
Intraventricular baffle	14	2
Arterial switch repair	4	0
Fontan procedure	9	0
Bidirectional cavopulmonary shunt	2	0
Palliation (band or shunt, etc.)	2	1
Total	31	3 (8.3%)

VSD, ventricular septal defect.

Non-committed defects, in contrast, may present a difficult problem. Selection of patients for biventricular repair or a Fontan or cavopulmonary shunt depends on careful assessment of the ventricular septal defect and its relationship to the arterial outlets, as well as any associated problems. Of 31 patients in the Melbourne experience, 18 were treated with either intraventricular baffles (14) or an arterial switch procedure (4). There were two hospital deaths. Fontan operations or bidirectional cavopulmonary shunts were performed in 11 patients with no mortality. The remaining two children had palliative treatment and one died (Table 50.7).

Other options include the use of a tubular internal conduit from the left ventricle to the aorta, accompanied by insertion of a valved external conduit from the right ventricle to the pulmonary trunk (Kirklin and Castaneda, 1977), or use of double external conduits (McGoon, 1976).

Additional risk factors identified in the surgery of double outlet right ventricle have included atrioventricular valvar abnormalities such as straddling or a common atrioventricular orifice (Luber et al, 1983). Patients with severe mitral or left ventricular hypoplasia, and those with superoinferior ventricles with an inlet septal defect, have been regarded as inoperable (Piccoli et al, 1983). This becomes less important if such patients are suitable for Fontan type surgery. Subpulmonary and non-committed defects were initially regarded as risk factors (Kirklin et al, 1986), but this has become less significant. The need for placement of a transannular patch or for an external valved conduit has also been regarded as a risk factor. Hence, the presence of pulmonary stenosis in itself may be an independent risk factor.

Multivariate analysis of the cohort of 193 Melbourne patients showed that the most significant anatomical features adversely affecting mortality were multiple defects ($p = 0.03$; odds ratio 3.86) and aortic coarctation ($p = 0.037$; odds ratio 3.75). The site of the ventricular septal defect did not have any significant effect on mortality in the series as a whole; neither did the presence of pulmonary stenosis, an atrioventricular septal defect with common atrioventricular junction or pulmonary atresia. Early age at the time of definitive surgery was associated with increased mortality, but only in the age group below 1 month ($p = 0.038$; odds ratio 7.79). Those patients operated on in the earlier years of the series (prior to 1985) were also at greater risk ($p = 0.011$; odds ratio 4.32). This effect was independent of the other identifiable variables. This is in keeping with the findings of Kirklin et al (1986) and others, namely that mortality has improved substantially since the mid-1980s. A report from Boston by Aoki and colleagues (1994) confirms the excellent results in those patients having a biventricular repair for various forms of double outlet right ventricle. Overall, early mortality was 11%. Risk factors identified as being of borderline significance, as in our series, included multiple ventricular septal defects and young age or low weight at repair. The last two were not independent variables in multifactorial analysis. No comparisons were made between those patients having biventricular repair and those being managed with Fontan or cavopulmonary shunt procedures. The subgroups of patients from the Melbourne series with multiple ventricular septal defects and with complete atrioventricular septal defects are summarized in Tables 50.8 and 50.9.

Apart from early mortality following surgery for double outlet right ventricle, late problems may also be significant. Late mortality has been reported as 21% by Judson et al (1983) amongst patients with a subaortic septal defect who underwent surgery. Most of these late deaths were related to arrhythmias. Continuing haemodynamic problems have included residual defects, subpulmonary stenosis and subaortic obstruction (which may be related to the intraventricular baffle). Reoperations were required for one of the above complications in 24% of 50 survivors of repair for double outlet right ventricle reported by Luber et al (1983). Aoki et al (1994) reported the need for reoperation in 19 of 62 survivors from their group of 73 patients, representing a reoperation rate amongst the surgical survivors of 31%. Indications for reoperation included 'subaortic'

Table 50.8. Surgery performed on patients with multiple ventricular septal defects, in a cohort of 193 infants/children with double outlet right ventricle, having their initial palliation/repair between 1978 and 1993 at the Royal Children's Hospital, Melbourne

Type of surgery	Number	Hospital deaths
Intraventricular baffle	8	2
Arterial switch repair	5	1
Senning operation	1	1
Fontan procedure	4	0
Bidirectional cavopulmonary shunt	1	0
Palliation (band)	4	1
Total	23	5 (22%)

Table 50.9. Surgery performed on patients with complete atrioventricular septal defect, in a cohort of 193 infants/children with double outlet right ventricle, having their initial palliation/repair between 1978 and 1993 at the Royal Children's Hospital, Melbourne

Type of surgery	Number	Hospital deaths
Intraventricular baffle	6	0
Fontan procedure	6	0
Bidirectional cavopulmonary shunt	4	0
Palliation (shunt)	2[a]	1
Total	18	1 (5.5%)

[a] One patient was awaiting further surgery.

obstruction (sometimes baffle related), residual defects, pulmonary stenosis and conduit obstruction. Actuarial freedom from reoperation was less than 50% at 8 years for patients with non-committed defects and for those with subpulmonary defects. By contrast, those with subaortic defects had a rate of freedom from reoperation better than 90% at 8 years. In the Melbourne series (Kleinert et al, 1997), the site of the ventricular septal defect was not a variable that influenced reoperation rate. Freedom from either death (operative or late) or reoperation was 65% at 10 years from the time of definitive operation for the entire cohort of 179 patients reaching 'repair' or Fontan/cavopulmonary shunt in that series.

Apart from these problems, quality of life following repair has, in most cases, been excellent, with 41 out of 42 survivors in the series reported by Judson et al (1983) being in New York Heart Association classes I or II.

ADDITIONAL PROBLEMS IN THE SURGERY OF DOUBLE OUTLET VENTRICLES

In hearts with a restrictive ventricular septal defect, intraventricular repair must be accompanied by surgical enlargement of the defect. Alternatively, an extracardiac conduit can be placed from left ventricle to aorta and the ventricular septal defect can then be closed. The presence of complicating intracardiac anomalies, such as mitral stenosis, straddling of an atrioventricular valve or a common atrioventricular orifice, may necessitate more extensive surgery involving valvar repair or replacement and so on (Pacifico et al, 1980).

Double outlet right ventricle with discordant atrioventricular connections is sometimes amenable to correction either by construction of an intraventricular tunnel to connect the morphologically left ventricle to the pulmonary trunk or by use of an external valved conduit inserted from the left ventricle to the pulmonary trunk combined with closure of the ventricular septal defect (Tabry et al, 1978). In the current era, use of the arterial switch procedure combined with a Senning or Mustard operation, or, in the presence of pulmonary stenosis, a Rastelli type repair, also coupled with a Senning or Mustard repair, has been employed with success (Yamagishi et al, 1993). Whether this is a better approach than to proceed towards a Fontan or bidirectional cavopulmonary shunt is debatable. Unfortunately, as with congenitally corrected transposition, there is a high incidence of heart block following surgical repair. This is almost certainly related to the abnormal disposition of the conduction system in hearts with discordant atrioventricular connections (Anderson et al, 1974a).

The Melbourne series contained only eight patients with discordant atrioventricular connections, one of whom was submitted to a biventricular repair. Four have had Fontan procedures, and one further child has been palliated with a bidirectional cavopulmonary shunt. The remaining two children had only had palliative proce-

dures at the time. One of these patients, with complex anatomy, had palliative treatment with an aortic valvotomy and implantation of a pacemaker; this patient died suddenly 2 years later. The other seven patients are all alive.

PROBABILITY OF LONG-TERM SURVIVAL

Actuarial probability of survival following biventricular repair was estimated by Aoki et al (1994) as being 81% at 8 years, which is similar to the experience in Melbourne: probability was 81% at 10 years (70% CI 62–92) (Figure 50.16). Overall probability of survival, from the time of initial surgery (palliative or corrective), in the entire cohort (193 patients) in Melbourne has been calculated as 76% at 13 years (70% CI 50–93) (Figure 50.17). It is noteworthy that those patients who were considered to be unsuitable for biventricular repair, and who were managed by a Fontan or cavopulmonary shunt procedure, have had a better record of survival in the short term, with a probability of 92% (70% CI 64–99) of survival at 6 years. Longer-term data is as yet

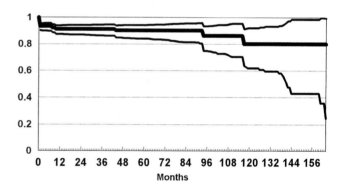

Figure 50.16. Actuarial survival probability for biventricular repair. Data (n = 143) from the Royal Children's Hospital, Melbourne series (1978–1993) analysed by the Kaplan–Meier method to give the probability (thick line) and the 70% confidence interval (thin lines).

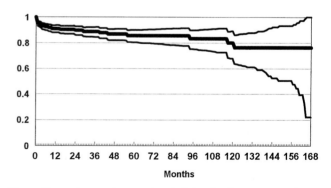

Figure 50.17. Actuarial survival probability for the entire Royal Children's Hospital, Melbourne series (1978–1993) from first surgery (n = 193). Data analysed by the Kaplan–Meier method to give the probability (thick line) and the 70% confidence interval (thin lines).

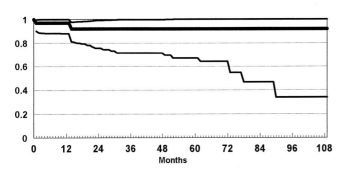

Figure 50.18. Actuarial survival probability for the Fontan procedure or a cavopulmonary shunt. Data (n = 32) from the Royal Children's Hospital, Melbourne series (1978–1993) analysed by the Kaplan–Meier method to give the probability (thick line) and the 70% confidence interval (thin lines).

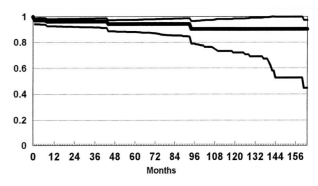

Figure 50.19. Actuarial survival probability for non-complex group after biventricular repair. Data (n = 108) from the Royal Children's Hospital, Melbourne series (1978–1993) analysed by the Kaplan–Meier method to give the probability (thick line) and the 70% confidence interval (thin lines).

unavailable for this cohort (Figure 50.18). Amongst the 193 children in the Melbourne series, it was possible to identify a subgroup of so-called complex cases (comprising patients with isomerism, a common atrioventricular valve, multiple ventricular septal defects, pulmonary atresia, discordant atrioventricular connections, hypoplasia of one ventricle or straddling/hypoplasia of one atrioventricular valve). Those within this group who were submitted to biventricular repairs had higher early mortality (23% CI 15–32) and a substantially lower probability of survival (77% CI 22–99 at 9.5 years) than the children with non-complex defects having biventricular repair (90% CI 72–98 at 10 years) (Figure 50.19). The difference in early survival was significant ($p = 0.03$) and has led to the conclusion that those who fall within the more complex category are likely to have a higher probability of early and medium-term survival if managed by a Fontan or a cavopulmonary shunt procedure.

REPAIR OF DOUBLE OUTLET LEFT VENTRICLE —

Surgical repair of double outlet left ventricle follows similar lines to that of double outlet right ventricle (Kerr et al, 1971; Pacifico et al, 1973). Those with pulmonary stenosis are usually best dealt with by insertion of an external valved conduit from the right ventricle to the pulmonary trunk. Placement of an intraventricular patch to direct right ventricular flow to the pulmonary trunk and left ventricular flow to the aorta may be possible in some cases.

Unfortunately, it appears that a high proportion of patients have significant right ventricular hypoplasia or other major complicating anomalies, making either of the above operations difficult or impossible. In such patients, a Fontan or cavopulmonary shunt procedure is likely to produce higher earlier and medium-term survival than an heroic attempt at biventricular repair (Sharratt et al, 1976; Otero-Coto et al, 1979a).

REFERENCES

Abbott M D 1936 Atlas of congenital cardiac disease. American Heart Association, New York, p 60

Abernethy J 1793 Surgical and physiological essays. James Evans, London, p 163

Anderson R H, Thapar M K, Arnold R, Jones R S 1973 Study of conducting tissue in a case of ventricular pre-excitation. British Heart Journal 35: 566–569

Anderson R H, Becker A E, Arnold R, Wilkinson J L 1974a The conducting tissues in congenitally corrected transposition. Circulation 50: 911–923

Anderson R H, Wilkinson J L, Arnold R, Lubkiewicz K 1974b Morphogenesis of bulboventricular malformations. I. Consideration of embryogenesis in the normal heart. British Heart Journal 36: 242–255

Anderson R H, Wilkinson J L, Arnold R, Becker A E, Lubkiewicz K 1974c Morphogenesis of bulboventricular malformations. II. Observations on malformed hearts. British Heart Journal 36: 948–970

Anderson R, Galbraith R, Gibson R, Miller G 1974d Double outlet left ventricle. British Heart Journal 36: 554–558

Aoki M, Forbess J M, Jonas R A, Mayer J E, Castañeda A R 1994 Result of biventricular repair for double-outlet right ventricle. Journal of Thoracic and Cardiovascular Surgery 107: 338–350

Arteaga M, de la Cruz M V, Sanchez C, Diaz G F 1982 Double outlet right ventricle: experimental morphogenesis in the chick embryo heart. Paediatric Cardiology 3: 219–227

Baron M G 1971 Radiologic notes in cardiology–angiographic differentiation between tetralogy of Fallot and double-outlet right ventricle. Relationship of the mitral and aortic valves. Circulation 43: 451–455

Beuren A 1960 Differential diagnosis of the Taussig–Bing heart from complete transposition of the great vessels with a posteriorly overriding pulmonary artery. Circulation 21: 1071–1087

Bharati S, Lev M 1976 The conduction system in double outlet right ventricle with subpulmonary ventricular septal defect and related hearts (the Taussig–Bing Group). Circulation 54: 459–467

Bharati S, Lev M, Stewart R, McAllister H A Jr, Kirklin J W 1978 The morphologic spectrum of double outlet left ventricle and its surgical significance. Circulation 58: 558–565

Birmingham A 1893 Extreme anomaly of the heart and great vessels. Journal of Anatomy and Physiology 27: 139–150

Borromee L, Lecompte Y, Batisse A et al 1988 Anatomic repair of anomalies of ventriculo-arterial connection associated with ventricular septal defect. II. Clinical results in 50 patients with pulmonary outflow tract obstruction. Journal of Thoracic and Cardiovascular Surgery 95: 96–102

Brandt P W T, Calder A L, Barratt-Boyes B G, Neutze J M 1976 Double outlet left ventricle, morphology, cineangiocardiographic diagnosis and surgical treatment. American Journal of Cardiology 38: 897–909

Braun K, de Vries A, Feingold D S, Ehrenfeld N E, Feldman J, Schorr S 1952 Complete dextroposition of the aorta, pulmonary stenosis, interventricular septal defect and patent foramen ovale. American Heart Journal 43: 773–780

Capuani A, Uemura H, Ho S Y, Anderson R H 1995 Anatomic spectrum of abnormal ventriculoarterial connections: surgical implications. Annals of Thoracic Surgery 59: 352–360

Chesler E, Joffe H S, Beck W, Schrire V 1971 Echocardiographic recognition of mitral–semilunar valve discontinuity: an aid to the diagnosis of origin of both great vessels from the right ventricle. Circulation 43: 725–732

Danielson G K, Ritter D G, Coleman H N III, Du Shane J W 1972 Successful repair of double-outlet right ventricle with transposition of the great arteries (aorta anterior and to the left) pulmonary stenosis, and subaortic ventricular septal defect. Journal of Thoracic and Cardiovascular Surgery 63: 741–746

De Tommasi S M, Daliento L, Ho S Y, Macartney F J, Anderson R H 1981 Analysis of atrioventricular junction, ventricular mass and ventriculo-arterial junction in 43 specimens with atrial isomerism. British Heart Journal 45: 236–247

Dickinson D F, Wilkinson J L, Anderson K R, Smith A, Ho S Y, Anderson R H 1979 The cardiac conduction system in situs ambiguous. Circulation 59: 879–885

Dickinson D F, Wilkinson J L, Smith A, Hamilton D I, Anderson R H 1982 Variations in the morphology of the ventricular septal defect and disposition of the atrioventricular conduction tissues in tetralogy of Fallot. The Thoracic and Cardiovascular Surgeon 5: 243–249

Di Sessa T G, Hagan A D, Pope C, Samtoy L, Friedman W F 1979 Two dimensional echocardiographic characteristics of double outlet right ventricle. American Journal of Cardiology 44: 1146–1154

Edwards J E, James J W, Du Shane J W 1952 Congenital malformations of the heart, origin of transposed great vessels from the right ventricle associated with atresia of the left ventricular outlet, double orifice of the mitral valve, and single coronary artery. Laboratory Investigations 1: 197–207

Edwards W D 1981 Double outlet right ventricle and tetralogy of Fallot. Two distinct but not mutually exclusive entities. Journal of Thoracic and Cardiovascular Surgery 82: 418–422

Farre J R 1814 Essay 1 on malformations of the human heart. Longman, Hurst, Orme and Brown, London, p 21

Feigenbaum H 1981 Echocardiography, 3rd Edn. Lea & Febiger, Philadelphia, PA, p 384

Fragoyannis S, Kardalinos A 1962 Transposition of the great vessels, both arising from the left ventricle (juxtaposition of the pulmonary artery), tricuspid atresia, atrial septal defect and ventricular septal defect. American Journal of Cardiology 10: 601–604

French J W, Popp R 1975 Variability of echocardiographic discontinuity in double outlet right ventricle and truncus arteriosus. Circulation 51: 848–854

Gomes M M R, Weidman W H, McGoon D C, Danielson G K 1971 Double-outlet right ventricle with pulmonic stenosis, surgical considerations and results of operation. Circulation 43: 889–894

Goor D A, Edwards J E 1973 The spectrum of transposition of the great arteries–with special reference to developmental anatomy of the conus. Circulation 48: 406–415

Goor D A, Lillehei C W, Edwards J E 1971 Ventricular septal defects and pulmonic stenosis with and without dextroposition. Chest 60: 117–128

Goor D A, Dische R, Lillehei C W 1972 The conotruncus. I. Its normal inversion and conus absorption. Circulation 46: 375–384

Hagler D J, Tajik A J, Seward J B, Mair D D, Ritter D G 1981 Double outlet right ventricle. Wide-angle two-dimensional echocardiographic observations. Circulation 63: 419–428

Harvey J C, Sondheimer H M, Williams W G, Olley P M, Trusler G A 1977 Repair of double outlet right ventricle. Journal of Thoracic and Cardiovascular Surgery 73: 611–615

Haworth S G, Sauer V, Buhlmeyer K, Reid L 1977 Development of the pulmonary circulation in ventricular septal defect: a quantitative structural study. American Journal of Cardiology 40: 781–788

Heath D, Edwards J E 1958 The pathology of hypertensive pulmonary vascular disease. Circulation 18: 533–547

Houston A B, Gregory N L, Coleman E N 1977 Two dimensional sector scanner echocardiography in cyanotic congenital heart disease. British Heart Journal 39: 1076–1081

Judson J P, Danielson G K, Puga F J, Mair D D, McGoon D C 1983 Double outlet right ventricle. Surgical Results 1970–1980. Journal of Thoracic and Cardiovascular Surgery 85: 32–40

Kanter K, Anderson R, Lincoln C, Firmin R, Rigby M 1986 Anatomic correction of double-outlet right ventricle with subpulmonary ventricular septal defect (the 'Taussig–Bing' anomaly). Annals of Thoracic Surgery 41: 287–292

Kawashima Y, Fugita T, Miyamoto T, Manabe H 1971 Intraventricular re-routing of blood for the correction of Taussig-Bing malformation. Journal of Thoracic and Cardiovascular Surgery 62: 825–829

Kawashima Y, Matsuda H, Yagihara T et al 1993 Intraventricular repair for Taussig–Bing anomaly. Journal of Thoracic and Cardiovascular Surgery 105: 591–596

Kerr A R, Barcia A, Bargeron L M, Kirklin J W 1971 Double outlet left ventricle with ventricular septal defect and pulmonary stenosis. Report of surgical repair. American Heart Journal 81: 688–693

Kirklin J K, Castañeda A R 1977 Surgical correction of double outlet right ventricle with non-committed ventricular septal defect. Journal of Thoracic and Cardiovascular Surgery 73: 399–403

Kirklin J W, Harp R A, McGoon D C 1964 Surgical treatment of origin of both vessels from right ventricle, including cases of pulmonary stenosis. Journal of Thoracic and Cardiovascular Surgery 48: 1024–1036

Kirklin J W, Pacifico A D, Blackstone E H, Kirklin J K, Bargeron L M Jr 1986 Current risks and protocols for operations for double outlet right ventricle. Journal of Thoracic and Cardiovascular Surgery 92: 913–930

Kiser J C, Ongley P A, Kirklin J W, Clarkson P M, McGoon D C 1968 Surgical treatment of dextrocardia with inversion of ventricles and double-outlet right ventricle. Journal of Thoracic and Cardiovascular Surgery 55: 6–15

Kleinert S, Sano T, Weintraub R G, Mee R B B, Karl T R, Wilkinson J L 1997 Anatomic features and surgical stratergies in double outlet right ventricle. Circulation 96: 1223–1239

Krongrad E, Ritter D G, Weidman W H, Du Shane J E 1972 Haemodynamic and anatomic correlation of electrocardiogram in double-outlet right ventricle. Circulation 46: 995–1004

Lavoie R, Sestier F, Gilbert G, Chameides L, Van Praagh R, Grondin P 1971 Double outlet right ventricle with left ventricular outflow tract obstruction due to a small ventricular septal defect. American Heart Journal 82: 290–299

Lecompte Y, Neveux J Y, Leca F et al 1982 Reconstruction of the pulmonary outflow tract without prosthetic conduit. Journal of Thoracic and Cardiovascular Surgery 84: 727–733

Lev M 1959 The architecture of the conduction system in congenital heart disease. II. Tetralogy of Fallot. Archives of Pathology 67: 572–587

Lev M, Bharati S 1973 Double outlet right ventricle – association with other cardiovascular anomalies. Archives of Pathology 95: 117–122

Lev M, Fell E H, Arcilla R, Weinberg M H 1964 Surgical injury to the conduction system in ventricular septal defect. American Journal of Cardiology 14: 464–476

Lev M, Bharati S, Meng C C L, Liberthson R R, Paul M H, Idriss F 1972 A concept of double outlet right ventricle. Journal of Thoracic and Cardiovascular Surgery 64: 271–281

Lincoln C, Anderson R H, Shinebourne E A, English T A H, Wilkinson J L 1975 Double outlet right ventricle with L malposition of the aorta. British Heart Journal 37: 453–463

Luber J M, Castañeda A R, Lang P, Norwood W I 1983 Repair of double outlet right ventricle: early and late results. Circulation 68(suppl II): 144–147

Macartney F J, Rigby M L, Anderson R H, Stark J, Silverman N H 1984 Double outlet right ventricle. Cross-sectional echocardiographic findings, their anatomical explanation, and surgical relevance. British Heart Journal 52: 164–177

MacMahon H E, Lipa M 1964 Double-outlet right ventricle with intact interventricular septum. Circulation 30: 745–748

Mazzucco A, Faggiona G, Stellin G, Bortolotte G, Livi U, Rizzoli G, Gallucci V, 1985 Surgical management of double-outlet right ventricle. Journal of Thoracic and Cardiovascular Surgery 90: 29–34

McGoon D C 1976 Left ventricular and biventricular extracardiac conduits. Journal of Thoracic and Cardiovascular Surgery 72: 7–14

Milo S, Ho S Y, Wilkinson J L, Anderson R H 1980 The surgical anatomy and atrioventricular conduction tissues of hearts with isolated ventricular septal defects. Journal of Thoracic and Cardiovascular Surgery 79: 244–255

Mirowski M, Mehrizi A, Taussig H B 1963 The electrocardiogram in patients with both great vessels arising from the right ventricle combined with pulmonary stenosis. Circulation 28: 1116–1127

Neufeld H N, Du Shane J W, Wood E H, Kirklin J W, Edwards J E 1961a Origin of both great vessels from the right ventricle. I. Without pulmonary stenosis. Circulation 23: 399–412

Neufeld H N, Du Shane J W, Edwards J E 1961b Origin of both great vessels from the right ventricle. II. With pulmonary stenosis. Circulation 23: 603–612

Neufeld H N, Lucas R V Jr, Lester R G, Adams P Jr, Anderson R C, Edwards J E 1962 Origin of both great vessels from the right ventricle without pulmonary stenosis. British Heart Journal 24: 393–408

Otero-Coto E, Wilkinson J L, Dickinson D F, Rufilanchas J J, Marquez J 1979a Gross distortion of atrioventricular and ventriculo-arterial relations associated with left juxta position of atrial appendages – bizarre form of atrioventricular criss-cross. British Heart Journal 41: 486–492

Otero-Coto E, Quero Jimenez M, Castañeda A R, Rufilanchas J J, Deverall P B 1979b Double outlet from chambers of left ventricular morphology. British Heart Journal 42: 15–21

Otero-Coto E, Quero Jimenez M, Anderson R H et al 1981 Double outlet left ventricle and univentricular heart of left ventricular type. In: Anderson R H, Shinebourne E A, Macartney F J, Tynan M (eds) Paediatric cardiology, Vol 5. Churchill Livingstone, Edinburgh

Pacifico A D, Kirklin J W, Bargeron L M, Soto B 1973 Surgical treatment of double-outlet left ventricle. Report of four cases. Circulation 48(suppl III): 19–23

Pacifico A D, Kirklin J W, Bargeron L M Jr 1980 Repair of complete atrioventricular canal associated with tetralogy of Fallot or double outlet right ventricle. Report of 10 cases. Annals of Thoracic Surgery 29: 351–356

Parsons J M, Baker E J, Anderson R H et al 1991 Double outlet right ventricle: morphologic demonstration using nuclear magnetic resonance imaging. Journal of the American College of Cardiology 18: 168–178

Patrick D L, McGoon D C 1968 Operation for double outlet right ventricle with transposition of the great arteries. Journal of Cardiovascular Surgery 19: 537–542

Paul M H, Van Praagh S, Van Praagh R 1968 Transposition of the great arteries. In: Watson H (ed) Pediatric cardiology. Lloyd Luke, London, p 583

Paul M H, Sinha S N, Muster A J, Cole R B, Van Praagh R 1970 Double outlet left ventricle. Report of an autopsy case with intact ventricular septum and consideration of its developmental implications. Circulation 41: 129–139

Peacock T B 1858 On malformations of the human heart. Churchill, London, p 36

Pernkopf E 1926 Der partielle situs inversus der Eingeweide beim Menschen. Zeitschrift für Anatomie und Entwicklungsgeschichte 79: 577–752

Piccoli G, Pacifico A D, Kirklin J W, Blackstone E H, Kirklin J K, Bargeron L M 1983 Changing results and concepts in the surgical treatment of double outlet right ventricle: Analysis of 137 operations in 126 patients. American Journal of Cardiology 52: 549–554

Redo S F, Engle M A, Holswade G R, Goldberg H P 1963 Operative correction of ventricular septal defect with origin of both great vessels from the right ventricle. Journal of Thoracic and Cardiovascular Surgery 45: 526–538

Rogers T R, Hagstrom J W C, Engle M A 1965 Origin of both great vessels from the right ventricle associated with the trisomy 18 syndrome. Circulation 32: 802–807

Rose V, Izukawa T, Moes C A F 1975 Syndromes of asplenia and polysplenia. A review of cardiac and non-cardiac malformations in 60 cases with special reference to diagnosis and prognosis. British Heart Journal 37: 840–852

Rowe R D, Mehrizi A 1968 The neonate with congenital heart disease: Vol V. Major problems in paediatrics. Saunders, Philadelphia, PA, p 204

Rowe R D, Freedom R M, Mehrizi A, Bloom K R 1981 The neonate with congenital heart disease, 2nd edn, Vol V. Major problems in clinical paediatrics. Saunders, Philadelphia, PA, p 313

Sakakibara S, Takao A, Arai T, Hashimoto A, Nogi M 1967 Both great vessels arising from the left ventricle (double outlet left ventricle) (origin of both vessels from the left ventricle). Bulletin of the Heart Institute of Japan 66–86

Saphir O, Lev M 1941 The tetralogy of Eisenmenger. American Heart Journal 21: 31–46

Serraf A, Lacour-Gayet F, Bruniaux J et al 1991 Anatomic repair of Taussig–Bing hearts. Circulation 84(suppl III): 200–205

Serratto M, Arevalo F, Goldman E J, Hastreiter A, Miller R A 1967 Obstructive ventricular septal defect in double outlet right ventricle. American Journal of Cardiology 19: 457–463

Sharratt G P, Slokos C G, Johnson A M, Anderson R H, Monro J L 1976 Surgical 'correction' of solitus-concordant double outlet left ventricle with 'L' malposition and tricuspid stenosis with hypoplastic right ventricle. Journal of Thoracic and Cardiovascular Surgery 71: 853–858

Shinebourne E A, Macartney F J, Anderson R H 1976 Sequential chamber localisation – logical approach to diagnosis in congenital heart disease. British Heart Journal 38: 327–340

Sondheimer H M, Freedom R M, Olley P M 1977 Double outlet right ventricle: clinical spectrum and prognosis. American Journal of Cardiology 39: 709–714

Soto B, Becker A E, Moulaert A J, Lie J T, Anderson R H 1980 Classification of ventricular septal defects. British Heart Journal 43: 332–343

Spitzer A 1923 Uber den bauplan des normalen und missbildeten Herzens. Virchows Archiv A. Pathological Anatomy and Histology 243: 81

Sridaromont S, Feldt R H, Ritter D G, Davis G D, Edwards J E 1975 Double outlet right ventricle associated with persistent common atrioventricular canal. Circulation 52: 933–942

Sridaromont S, Feldt R H, Ritter D G, Davis G D, Edwards J E 1976 Double outlet right ventricle, haemodynamic and anatomic correlations. American Journal of Cardiology 38: 85–94

Sridaromont S, Ritter D G, Feldt R H, Davis G D, McGoon D C, Edwards J E 1978 Double outlet right ventricle. Anatomic and angiographic correlations. Mayo Clinic Proceedings 53: 555

Stellin G, Zuberbuhler J R, Anderson R H, Slewers R D 1987 The surgical anatomy of the Taussig–Bing malformation. Journal of Thoracic and Cardiovascular Surgery 93: 560–569

Stellin G, Ho S Y, Anderson R H, Zuberbuhler J R, Siewers R D 1991 The surgical anatomy of double outlet right ventricle with concordant atrio-ventricular connection and noncommitted ventricular septal defect. Journal of Thoracic and Cardiovascular Surgery 102: 849–855

Stewart R W, Kirklin J W, Pacifico A D, Blackstone E H, Bargeron L M 1979 Repair of double outlet right ventricle. An analysis of 62 cases. Journal of Thoracic and Cardiovascular Surgery 78: 502–514

Stewart S, Farnham J D, Schreiner B, Manning J 1976 Complete correction of double outlet right ventricle with situs inversus. 1-loop, and 1-malposition (I.L.L.) with subaortic VSD and pulmonary stenosis. Journal of Thoracic and Cardiovascular Surgery 71: 129–133

Tabry I F, McGoon D C, Danielson G K, Wallace R B, Davis Z, Maloney J D 1978 Surgical management of double outlet right ventricle associated with atrio-ventricular discordance. Journal of Thoracic and Cardiovascular Surgery 76: 336–344

Taussig H B, Bing R J 1949 Complete transposition of the aorta and a levoposition of the pulmonary artery. American Heart Journal 37: 551–559

Titus J L, Neufeld H N, Edwards J E 1964 The atrioventricular conduction system in hearts with both great vessels originating from the right ventricle. American Heart Journal 67: 558–592

Tynan M J, Becker A E, Macartney F J, Quero-Jimenez M, Shinebourne E A, Anderson R H 1979 Nomenclature and classification of congenital heart disease. British Heart Journal 41: 544–553

Ueda M, Becker A E 1986 Double outlet right ventricle: an unusual variant with overriding of both great arteries, absent outlet septum and mitral to aortic to pulmonary valve continuity. International Journal of Cardiology 12: 155–164

Van Mierop L H S 1971 Transposition of the great arteries. I. Clarification or further confusion. American Journal of Cardiology 28: 735–738

Van Mierop L H S, Wiglesworth F W 1963 Pathogenesis of transposition complexes. II. Anomalies due to faulty transfer of the posterior great artery. American Journal of Cardiology 12: 226–232

Van Praagh R 1968 What is the Taussig Bing malformation? Circulation 38: 445–449

Van Praagh R 1971 Transposition of the great arteries. II. Transposition clarified. American Journal of Cardiology 28: 739–741

Van Praagh R 1973 Conotruncal malformations. In: Barratt-Boyes B G, Neutze J M, Harris E A (eds) Heart disease in infancy: diagnosis and surgical treatment. Churchill Livingstone, Edinburgh, p 141–188

Van Praagh R, Vlad P 1978 Dextrocardia, mesocardia and levocardia. In: Keith J D, Rowe R D, Vlad P (eds) Heart disease in infancy and childhood. Macmillan, New York, p 658

Van Praagh R, Weinberg M D 1977 Double outlet left ventricle. In: Moss A J, Adams F H, Emmanouilides M D (eds) Heart disease in infants, children and adolescents, 2nd edn. Williams & Wilkins, Baltimore, MD

Van Praagh R, Van Praagh S, Nebesar R A, Muster A J, Sinha S N, Paul M H 1970 Tetralogy of Fallot. Underdevelopment of the pulmonary infundibulum and its sequelae. American Journal of Cardiology 26: 25–33

Van Praagh R, Perez-Trevino C, Lopez-Cuellar M et al 1971 Transposition of the great arteries with posterior aorta, anterior pulmonary artery, subpulmonary conus and fibrous continuity between aortic and atrioventricular valves. American Journal of Cardiology 28: 621–631

Van Praagh R, Perez-Trevino C, Reynolds J L et al 1975 Double outlet right ventricle S D L with subaortic ventricular septal defect and pulmonary stenosis. American Journal of Cardiology 35: 42–53

Von Rokitansky C F 1875 Die Defecte der Scheidewande des Herzens. Braumuller, Vienna

Vouhé P R, Tamisier D, Leca F, Ouaknine R, Vernant F, Neveux J-Y 1992 Transposition of the great arteries, ventricular septal defect and pulmonary outflow tract obstruction: Rastelli or Lecompte procedure? Journal of Thoracic and Cardiovascular Surgery 103: 428

Waldman J D, Schneeweiss A, Edwards W D, Lamberti J J, Shem-Tov A, Neufeld H N 1984 The obstructive subaortic conus. Circulation 70: 339–344

Wilcox B R, Ho S Y, Macartney F J, Becker A E, Gerlis L M, Anderson R H 1981 Surgical anatomy of double outlet right ventricle with situs solitus and atrioventricular concordance. Journal of Thoracic and Cardiovascular Surgery 82: 405–417

Wilkinson J L, Arnold R, Anderson R H, Acerete F 1975 'Posterior' transposition reconsidered. British Heart Journal 37: 757–766

Wilkinson J L, Wilcox B R, Anderson R H 1981 The anatomy of double outlet right ventricle. In: Anderson R H, Macartney F J, Shinebourne E A, Tynan M (eds) Paediatric cardiology, Vol 5. Churchill Livingstone, Edinburgh, p 397–407

Witham A C 1957 Double outlet right ventricle. American Heart Journal 53: 928–939

Yacoub M H, Radley-Smith R 1984 Anatomic correction of the Taussig–Bing anomaly. Journal of Thoracic and Cardiovascular Surgery 88: 380–388

Yamagishi M, Imai Y, Hoshino S et al 1993 Anatomic correction of atrioventricular discordance. Journal of Thoracic and Cardiovascular Surgery 105: 1067–1076

Yoo S J, Lim T H, Park I S, Hong C V, Kim S H, Lee H J 1991 MR anatomy of ventricular septal defect in double outlet right ventricle with situs solitus and atrioventricular concordance. Radiology 181: 501–505

51

Common arterial trunk

R. H. Anderson and F. J. Macartney

── INTRODUCTION ──

The entity characterized by a common arterial trunk, exiting from the ventricular mass to supply directly the aortic, pulmonary and coronary arterial circulations, is an uncommon congenital malformation. Amongst populations of infants, its incidence was 1.4% in the New England Programme (Fyler et al, 1980), while it accounted for 2.1% of those who were symptomatic in the first year of life seen over a 10-year period at the Royal Brompton Hospital (Scott et al, 1984). With the advances in surgical repair achieved in the 1990s, most of these symptomatic infants should now survive to adult life. Consequently, the lesion can no longer be considered the province of the pathologist or the neonatologist. This is not to suggest that all problems have now been solved concerning its diagnosis and treatment. Those which remain will be the focus of this chapter.

── ANATOMY ──

Of all the congenital lesions that benefit from being described in straightforward fashion, common arterial trunk is the most obvious. When described in terms of truncus, or various expansions of this term that implicate persistence of an embryonic condition, it was always necessary to provide a definition of the lesion as it existed in the postnatal heart. Describing the entity as a common arterial trunk negates the need for further definition. A common trunk, of necessity, will exit from the base of the heart through a common arterial valve and will give rise directly to the systemic, pulmonary and coronary circulations (Figure 51.1) (Crupi et al, 1977). The situation can be complicated by absence, interruption or atresia of individual arteries within these circulations. The presence of the common trunk, nonetheless, distinguishes this entity from its close cousins in which a large patent trunk leaves the base of the heart in company with an atretic trunk, which can also be traced from its origin at the ventricular mass. The variant that still gives problems in terms of description is that in which there is complete absence of the intrapericardial pulmonary arteries. This entity (Figure 51.2) is best described as a solitary rather than a common trunk. This is because there is no way of knowing, had they been present, whether the intrapericardial pulmonary arteries would have originated from the arterial trunk or from the right ventricular outflow tract (Anderson and Thiene, 1989). In terms of clinical presentation and treatment, such patients with a solitary

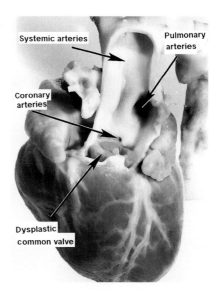

Figure 51.1. This specimen is dissected to show the typical features of a common arterial trunk, exiting from the ventricular mass through a common arterial valve and supplying directly the coronary, systemic and pulmonary circulations. Note the dysplastic nature of the truncal valve.

arterial trunk have more affinities with tetralogy and pulmonary atresia (see Chapter 47) than with common arterial trunk.

A common arterial trunk, as defined, represents one particular form of ventriculo-arterial connection. It must

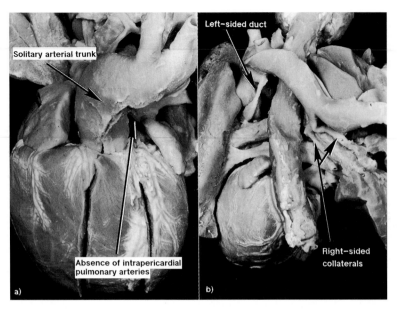

Figure 51.2. This heart (a) possesses a solitary arterial trunk in absence of any intrapericardial pulmonary arteries. The pulmonary supply (b) to the left lung was initially through a duct, while systemic-to-pulmonary collateral arteries supply the right lung. Had there been intrapericardial pulmonary arteries, it is impossible to say whether they would have arisen from the solitary trunk, making it a common trunk, or from the heart, making the solitary trunk an aorta. The most accurate description, therefore, is of solitary arterial trunk.

be anticipated to coexist, therefore, with all possible segmental combinations. In almost all instances, nonetheless, there will be usual atrial arrangement with concordant atrioventricular connections. Rare examples have been described in combination with discordant atrioventricular connections, or with absence of the right atrioventricular connection (tricuspid atresia: Scalia et al, 1984). While the atrioventricular junctions themselves are usually separate, and guarded by mitral and tricuspid valves, a common trunk can rarely be found in association with an atrioventricular septal defect and a common atrioventricular valve (Figure 51.3).

In the presence of the common trunk, almost always the truncal valve is connected in both ventricles, with the orifice overriding the ventricular septal crest but with its leaflets in fibrous continuity with the mitral valve in the left ventricle (Figure 51.4). Such a biventricular connection necessitates the presence of a subarterial interventricular communication. This ventricular septal defect is generally large. Its floor is the crest of the ventricular septum, reinforced on the right ventricular aspect by the limbs of the septomarginal trabeculation. The defect is roofed by the leaflets of the truncal valve (Anderson and Wilcox, 1993), with the cone of space thus subtended

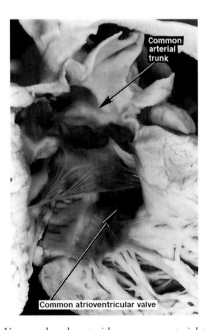

Figure 51.3. Very rarely, a heart with a common arterial trunk can also have a common atrioventricular junction guarded by a common valve in association with deficient atrioventricular septation. Note the extreme bridging of the superior leaflet, and the fibrous continuity with the truncal valve.

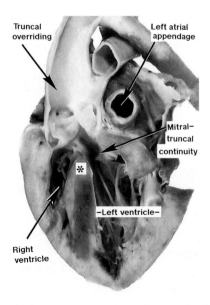

Figure 51.4. This long-axis section shows the truncal valve overriding the crest of the muscular ventricular septum (asterisk), with the valvar leaflets supported in both ventricles but, typically as shown, in fibrous continuity with the anterior leaflet of the mitral valve.

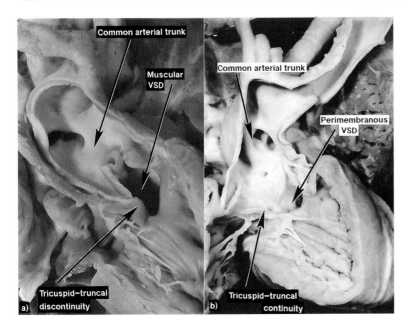

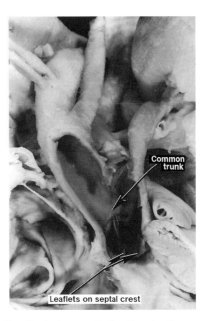

Figure 51.5. The presence (a) or absence (b) of a muscular rim along the posteroinferior margin of the ventricular septal defect (VSD) determines whether or not the defect is considered to be perimembranous. This has important connotations concerning the vulnerability of the conduction axis during surgical correction.

Figure 51.6. Usually, during ventricular diastole, the truncal valvar leaflets close at a distance from the crest of the ventricular septum. Occasionally, as shown here, the leaflets can coapt on the septal crest, meaning that ventricular shunting can occur only during systole.

having right and left ventricular margins. It is usually the right ventricular margin that is considered to represent the ventricular septal defect. In the majority of cases, fusion of the inferior limb of the septomarginal trabeculation with the ventriculo-infundibular fold along this right ventricular margin produces muscular discontinuity between the leaflets of the tricuspid and the truncal valves (Figure 51.5a) (Crupi et al, 1977). When this fusion fails to occur, there is continuity between the tricuspid and truncal valvar leaflets, making the ventricular septal defect perimembranous (Figure 51.5b). The presence or absence of the muscular bar in the posteroinferior margin is important for the surgeon because, when present, it protects the specialized axis responsible for atrioventricular conduction (Anderson and Wilcox, 1993). There is usually a large distance between the coapting leaflets and the crest of the septum during ventricular diastole when the truncal valvar leaflets are closed. In some instances, however, this space may be reduced, producing restriction during diastole. Alternatively, the leaflets may close directly on the septal crest (Figure 51.6). This latter arrangement has been described as 'intact ventricular septum' (Carr et al, 1979). This is somewhat misleading because, even in this arrangement, a septal deficiency is seen when the truncal valve opens during ventricular systole. It is possible to find hearts where the ventricular septum is truly intact, albeit very rarely. This occurs when the common trunk arises exclusively from the right ventricle (Alves and Ferrari, 1987). The ventricular septal defect, when present, can also be restrictive when the common trunk takes an exclusive origin from one or other ventricle. Such a restrictive ventricular septal defect (Rosenquist et al, 1976) is more likely to produce problems when the trunk arises exclusively from the right ventricle (Figure 51.7).

The truncal valve itself has three leaflets in approximately two thirds of patients. In most of the remaining patients, either two or four leaflets are seen guarding the common arterial orifice, though on rare occasions valves with five or more leaflets have been reported (Collett and Edwards, 1949; Van Praagh and Van Praagh, 1965; Calder et al, 1976; Crupi et al, 1977). As already stated, the truncal valvar leaflets are almost always in fibrous continuity with the anterior leaflet of the mitral valve (Figure 51.2), but there can be a completely muscular subtruncal infundibulum, particularly when the common trunk arises exclusively from the right ventricle (Figure 51.7). Insufficiency of the truncal valve is not uncommon and can be caused by thickened and dysplastic leaflets

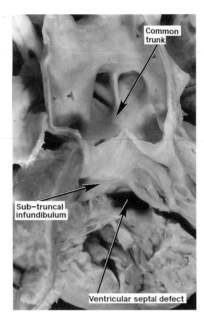

Figure 51.7. Although usually the truncal valve overides the ventricular septal crest (as shown in Figure 51.2), occasionally the trunk can arise exclusively from one or other ventricle, here from the right ventricle. Note the completely muscular subtruncal infundibulum and the potentially restrictive ventricular septal defect.

(Figure 51.1), or by prolapse of unsupported leaflets as a result of annular dilation (Becker et al, 1971; Gelband et al, 1972). Truncal valvar stenosis is relatively uncommon; when present, it is usually associated with dysplastic valvar tissue (Ledbetter et al, 1976; Patel et al, 1978).

The greatest variability in patients with common trunk is found in the pattern of its branching. Presence of a right-sided aortic arch, with mirror-imaged branching of the brachiocephalic arteries, is associated more often with common trunk, occurring in up to one third of patients, than with any other congenital cardiac malformation (Van Praagh and Van Praagh, 1965; Calder et al, 1976; Crupi

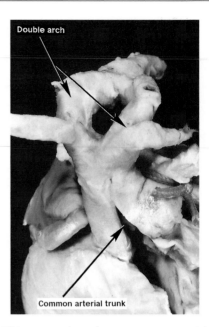

Figure 51.8. This rare specimen shows a common arterial trunk with a double aortic arch.

et al, 1977). Very rarely, a double aortic arch may be present (Figure 51.8). Hypoplasia of the aortic arch, with or without coarctation, is a particularly important associated finding (Figure 51.9a) (Bharati et al, 1974; Crupi et al, 1977). Interruption of the aortic arch (Figure 51.9b) is chosen as a major feature for categorization in the alpha-numeric system favoured by Van Praagh and Van Praagh (1965). In postmortem series (Van Praagh and Van Praagh, 1965; Calder et al, 1976; Crupi et al, 1977), such interruption is found in up to one fifth of specimens. When the arch is interrupted, an arterial duct feeds the descending thoracic aorta and part of the brachiocephalic circulation, the precise proportion depending on the site of interruption. As with other forms of interruption (see Chapter 56), retro-oesophageal origin of the right

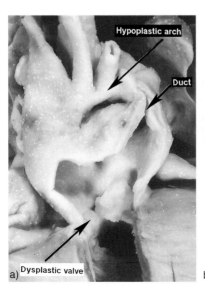

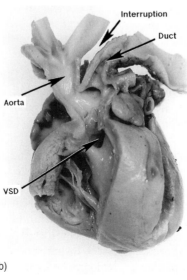

Figure 51.9. These specimens show obstruction to flow through the systemic pathways, with coarctation (b) and interruption between the left common carotid and subclavian arteries (a). In both instances, the duct feeds the descending aorta, either in part or in its entirety. VSD, ventricular septal defect.

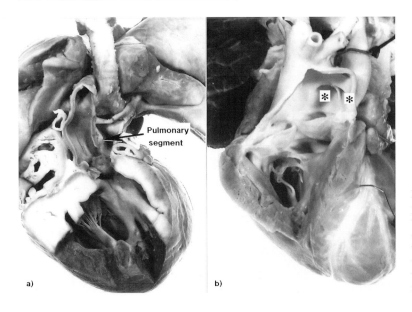

Pulmonary segment

a) b)

Figure 51.10. The most common pattern of origin of the pulmonary arteries from the common trunk is either through a short confluent segment, known as type I (a) or directly from the leftward and posterior margin of the trunk, type II (b). The asterisks indicate the openings of the pulmonary arteries. In a good proportion of patients with this condition, nonetheless, the situation is intermediate between these patterns.

subclavian artery is frequently seen. Apart from those hearts with severe coarctation or interruption, or in which the pulmonary arteries are discontinuous and one is fed through a patent duct, it is rare to find ductal patency coexisting with common arterial trunk, although it does exist (Gerlis et al, 1990).

While the state of the aortic arch is possibly most significant clinically, by tradition it has been the arrangement of origin of the pulmonary arteries that is most frequently used for numeric classification (Collett and Edwards, 1949). The pulmonary arteries arise most commonly from the left posterolateral aspect of the common trunk, taking origin a short distance above the truncal valve. When the arteries arise in this typical location, there can be a short confluent arterial segment (so-called type I: Figure 51.10a), or the right and left arteries can take separate origin from the trunk (so-called type II: Figure 51.10b). In most instances, however, the morphology is intermediate, and this pattern is sometimes described in jocular fashion as 'type 1½'. Other patterns of origin can be found, such as origin from each side of the common trunk, often at some distance from the truncal valve (type III: Figure 51.11), distal origin from the underside of the common segment (Rubay et al, 1987), or origin from within a truncal sinus (Figure 51.12). It is also possible to find examples in which only one pulmonary artery arises from the common trunk, the other being supplied initially through a duct that became ligamentous. This can then present as 'unilateral absence' of one pulmonary artery, but almost always the 'absent' artery is identified within the hilum of the lung. In this setting, the discontinuous pulmonary artery initially fed by the duct is most frequently on the same side as the aortic arch. This is in contrast to the finding in tetralogy of Fallot with 'absent' pulmonary artery, in which the absent, or discontinuous, artery is more frequently on the side opposite the aortic arch. In some circumstances, when the pulmonary arteries arise separately from the

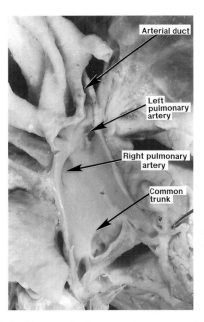

Arterial duct

Left pulmonary artery

Right pulmonary artery

Common trunk

Figure 51.11. In this example, the two pulmonary arteries arise from either side of the common trunk but at a considerable distance from the truncal valve (type III). Note that the aortic arch is interrupted, with the descending aorta supplied through the arterial duct.

trunk, the right artery is positioned to the left at its origin relative to the left pulmonary artery. The two arteries then spiral as they extend to the pulmonary hilums. This entity is called crossed pulmonary arteries (Becker et al, 1970).

This chapter will not deal with so-called pseudotruncus arteriosus, which is a form of tetralogy of Fallot but with pulmonary atresia rather than stenosis (see Chapter 47). Nor will we consider so-called hemitruncus, a term often used to describe the situation in which one pulmonary artery arises from the ascending aorta when the other takes origin from the right ventricle. Of necessity, such hearts have two arterial valves. They cannot, therefore, be examples of common arterial trunk.

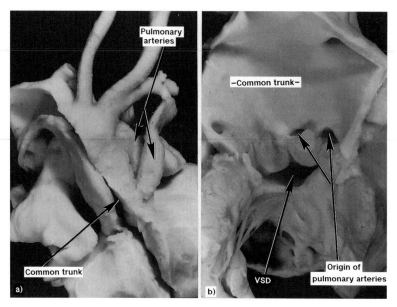

Figure 51.12. In contrast to the specimen shown in Figure 51.11, in this heart the pulmonary arteries arise remarkably close to the pulmonary valve, indeed, within the truncal arterial sinus. The specimen is shown externally (a) and internally (b). VSD, ventricular septal defect.

Anomalies of the origin and distribution of the coronary arteries are frequent (Shrivastava and Edwards, 1977; Anderson et al, 1978; Suzuki et al, 1989). Knowledge of these variations, and of the location of the conduction tissue, is important when planning surgical repair. The sinus node and the atrioventricular node are normal in location and structure. The atrioventricular bundle courses to the left of the central fibrous body, and the left bundle branch originates along the left ventricular septal endocardium (Thiene et al, 1976). The right bundle branch travels within the myocardium of the ventricular septal crest, attaining a subendocardial course at the level of the moderator band. In those hearts in which musculature interposes between the truncal and tricuspid valves, the membranous septum is intact behind the muscular rim and the atrioventricular conduction tissues are somewhat distant from the rim of the defect. In patients in which the ventricular septal defect is perimembranous, in contrast, the conduction tissue passes along the left aspect of the posteroinferior rim of the defect. It is then at greater surgical risk.

The most common associated cardiovascular anomalies have already been mentioned, including right aortic arch, interrupted aortic arch, patency of the arterial duct, discontinuity of one pulmonary artery, coronary arterial anomalies and incompetent truncal valve. A defect within the oval fossa has been noted in up to one fifth of patients, persistence of the left superior caval vein draining to the coronary sinus in up to one tenth and an aberrant subclavian artery in between one tenth and one twentieth (Van Praagh and Van Praagh, 1965; Bharati et al, 1974; Marcelletti et al, 1977). Partially anomalous pulmonary venous connection has also been reported (Mair et al, 1974).

—AETIOLOGY AND MORPHOGENESIS—

There is increasing evidence that at least some cases of common arterial trunk result from a genetic defect. The evidence comes from interpretation of morphology, experiments in animals, studies on the role of cells migrating from the neural crest in the development of the outlet components of the heart and the arterial trunks, and the discovery of deletions in chromosome 22q11 in patients with so-called conotruncal defects.

The morphology of common arterial trunk supports very strongly the notion that, during development, there has been failure of septation of the ventricular outlets and the proximal arterial segment of the heart tube. It has also been suggested that the entity represents failure of formation of the subpulmonary conus, with the common arterial trunk in essence representing the aorta (Van Praagh and Van Praagh, 1965). There is little evidence to support this latter notion, and much to contradict it. Specimens with common arterial trunk show no evidence of a blind-ending subpulmonary outflow tract, such as is seen in tetralogy with pulmonary atresia. It is this latter entity that provides the paradigm for underdevelopment of the subpulmonary outflow tract. In such hearts with tetralogy and pulmonary atresia, four fifths of specimens have perimembranous ventricular septal defects; by comparison, in the setting of common arterial trunk, four fifths of hearts have a muscular posteroinferior rim to the ventricular septal defect. Additionally, if the arterial root truly represented the aorta, then coronary arteries would be anticipated to arise in patterns comparable to those seen in the normal heart. This is rarely the case in the setting of common arterial trunk, where the origins and course of the coronary arteries are frequently bizarre (Crupi et al, 1977; Suzuki et al, 1989).

There is then much additional evidence from developmental studies to support the notion that common trunk exists because of failure of septation of the developing outflow tracts. In an elegant study using Keeshond dogs, Van Mierop and colleagues (1978) showed that the cushions which normally divided the outflow segment of the heart failed to fuse in the setting of common arterial trunk. This concept of failure of septation of the ventricular outlets was endorsed by Bartelings and colleagues (1991). They showed the importance of fusion of the aortopulmonary septum (which divided the proximal part of the arterial segment) with the ridges or cushions dividing the outlet component of the heart itself. When the cushions themselves failed to fuse, then there was no scaffold for union with the septum dividing the arterial segment. Significantly, this aortopulmonary septum grows down towards the heart, originating within the aortic sack. In normal development, it is populated by cells migrating from the neural crest. Much recent work, extending the original studies of Le Lievre and Le Douarin (1975) and Kirby and colleagues (1983), has shown that the septal structures do not develop properly in the face of inadequate migration from the neural crest. One of the resulting malformations is common arterial trunk. But common trunk is not the only lesion to be produced when there is abnormal migration of cells from the neural crest. Kirby and colleagues (1983) demonstrated their findings by removing surgically the occipital neural crest prior to migration of cells. When Besson and his associates (1986) removed smaller parts of the crest, they produced embryos with ventricular septal defect and double outlet right ventricle rather than common arterial trunk. Similar effects are seen when the populations of cells migrating from the crest are perturbed by treatment of the developing embryos with bis-diamine. Although some of the abnormal embryos have common arterial trunk, others have tetralogy of Fallot with or without pulmonary atresia, or doubly committed and juxta-arterial ventricular septal defects (Momma et al, 1991; Jackson et al, 1995). This, in turn, is in keeping with the results of selective inbreeding of the Keeshond dogs, which Van Mierop and colleagues (1978) used in their developmental study. Using the same colony of animals, Patterson and colleagues (1993) observed a similar spectrum of malformations to that obtained either by surgical removal of the neural crest or by dosing with bis-diamine: many animals had common arterial trunk, but others had ventricular septal defects or tetralogy of Fallot. Significantly, the pattern of inheritance was consistent with a defect at a single autosomal locus. The genetic basis for such malformations is further supported by observations made in the homozygous mutant Splotch mouse, which has common arterial trunk arising exclusively from the right ventricle (Franz, 1989; Conway et al, 1997). These embryos also show reduction or absence of the dorsal root ganglions, further derivatives of the neural crest. The Splotch mutation itself is known to be

the consequence of deletion of 32 base pairs from the homeodomain of the gene *pax3* (Epstein et al, 1991).

Common arterial trunk has also now been produced when there is deficiency of *sox4*, a gene which normally populates the endocardial cushions of the developing outflow tracts (Schilham et al, 1996). Some of the afflicted embryos in these experiments, however, had doubly committed ventricular septal defects rather than common arterial trunk (Ya et al, 1998). This is of particular interest, since the morphology of the outflow tracts is almost identical in those with common arterial trunk and those with doubly committed defects, apart from the finding of separate aortic and pulmonary valvar orifices in the latter. All of this is pertinent to findings in humans with microdeletions of chromosome 22q11.

It was in 1981 that de la Chapelle and colleagues first reported a family with a chromosomal translocation resulting in partial trisomy for chromosome 20 and partial monosomy for chromosome 22. The four afflicted patients all had DiGeorge syndrome, and one had common arterial trunk. Another translocation resulting in common arterial trunk in combination with DiGeorge syndrome was then reported by Lupski and colleagues (1991). These initial reports led to searching for microdeletions in the 22q11 region, first by high resolution banding (Wilson et al 1992), and then by fluorescent in situ hybridization (Carey et al, 1992). These investigations revealed that a majority of patients with DiGeorge syndrome have 22q11 deletions (Wilson et al, 1992; Driscoll et al, 1993). The gene itself is being hotly pursued (Halford et al, 1993; Lindsay et al, 1993). Meanwhile, Wilson and colleagues (1993) have proposed that DiGeorge syndrome is best considered as the severe end of a clinical spectrum, now frequently called CATCH 22: reflecting cardiac defects, abnormal facies, thymic hypoplasia, cleft palate and hypocalcaemia produced by deletions of 22q11. Nearly one third of patients with non-syndromic defects involving the ventricular outflow tracts, and three quarters of those with common arterial trunk, have been shown to have microdeletions in this DiGeorge critical region (Goldmuntz et al, 1993). An association between common arterial trunk, and other anomalies of the outflow tracts, and CHARGE syndrome (coloboma, heart disease, choanal atresia, retardation (mental and physical) genital hypoplasia and ear anomalies) has long been recognized. The anomalies of the outflow tracts found with CHARGE syndrome are much the same as in DiGeorge syndrome, except that tetralogy of Fallot and double outlet right ventricle predominate in the former, whereas, in the latter, common arterial trunk and interruption of the aortic arch proximal to the left subclavian artery are more common (Lin et al, 1987).

Consequently, it is likely that chromosomal damage leads to deletions of 22q11, which, in some way, interfere with the migration of neural crest cells and thereby cause damage to the third and fourth pharyngeal pouches. We have come a long way since Freedom and colleagues

(1972) drew the attention of paediatric cardiologists to the association between anomalies of these pharyngeal pouches and congenital cardiac malformations.

It should not be thought, however, that all is now resolved. One fifth of patients with terminal deletions of the long arm of chromosome 7 have been reported to have cardiac anomalies (Tiller et al, 1988). There is one such case with common arterial trunk diagnosed before and after birth by echocardiography, but not by post-mortem or angiocardiography (Finley et al, 1993). Anomalies of the outflow tracts encountered in the Baltimore–Washington Infant Study showed no recurrences from 109 parents or siblings (Ferencz et al, 1985). This is in keeping with the findings of Nora and Nora (1978), who suggested a lower than usual recurrence rate of 1% for common arterial trunk. It may well be notable, nonetheless, that common arterial trunk and double outlet right ventricle were significant in offspring of mothers with diabetes mellitus (Ferencz et al, 1990).

There are other pertinent family studies. Pierpont et al (1988) elected to look at the relatives of patients with either common arterial trunk or interrupted aortic arch. In common arterial trunk with no other aortic malformations, the recurrence rate in siblings was 1.6%, corresponding to one sibling pair. When common arterial trunk was associated with additional problems of the aortic arch, the recurrence rate in siblings was 13.6%, corresponding to six siblings. Four of these had malformations involving the outflow tracts, including one with interruption of the aortic arch distal to the left carotid artery. There were no recurrences of interruption distal to the left subclavian artery, but when the interruption was distal to the left common carotid artery, there were two with recurrences (2.5%), one with complete transposition and one with persistence of the arterial duct.

Rein and colleagues (1990) reported two siblings with a diagnosis at open heart surgery of common arterial trunk. They were the only children of consanguineous parents. The mother then produced two more children, one with common arterial trunk and the other with tetralogy, pulmonary atresia and systemic-to-pulmonary collateral arteries (Rein and Sheffer, 1994). A first cousin of the four affected sisters had an atrioventricular septal defect with severe pulmonary stenosis. Another first cousin, once removed, had complete transposition. This kindred suggests autosomal recessive inheritance but is not conclusive. If it were, this would be a very important observation that would change our understanding of the aetiology of congenital heart disease. There are four other reliably documented reports of common arterial trunk in siblings (Goodyear, 1961; Shapiro et al, 1981; Pierpont et al, 1988; Ferry et al, 1994). Furthermore, Brunson and colleagues (1978) and le Marec and colleagues (1989) each reported a set of three siblings with common arterial trunk. Two sets of twins concordant for common arterial trunk have been described, one being monochorionic and diamniotic, presumably monozygotic (Benešová & Šikl, 1954) and the other dizygotic (Lang et al, 1991).

Patients with common arterial trunk, therefore, continue to be a fertile population is which to study the genetic background of congenital cardiac malformations.

PATHOPHYSIOLOGY

Most patients with a common arterial trunk will present during the first year of life, the majority now being seen as neonates. The reasons for such an early presentation in most cases are the excessive pulmonary blood flow and the low systemic arterial diastolic pressure. Both of these may, in turn, compromise coronary arterial flow. These features reflect the more rapid fall in pulmonary vascular resistance compared with normal, an event that seems to be characteristic of the lesion. The reason for this early fall is, to the best of our knowledge, undetermined. Early presentation is even more frequent when there are associated anomalies of the common truncal valve, or other associated lesions such as interruption of the aortic arch. The other major physiological consequence of the anatomical lesion is the opportunity it provides for common mixing. This occurs primarily within the common trunk; as a result, the ensuing cyanosis is mild. There is also, nonetheless, a large interventricular communication in nearly all cases. Because the common trunk also has a biventricular connection in most patients, this communication is of lesser physiological significance.

The higher pulmonary blood flow will, of course, result in an increased return to the left atrium, producing raised left atrial pressure and left ventricular volume overload. This will then contribute to the tachypnoea that, together with signs of cardiac failure, is typical of the early presentation. Because of the confluent defect between the ventricles and the arterial trunks, there will be equalization of pressures at both ventricular and arterial levels. This is another characteristic pathophysiological feature.

These regular features can then be modified markedly by associated malformations. Truncal valvar insufficiency, for example, leads to varying degrees of right or left ventricular volume overload, the extent depending on the site of the incompetent valvar segments. Truncal valvar stenosis results in ventricular pressure overload. Incompetence or stenosis will exacerbate the congestive cardiac failure. These valvar lesions will also produce, relatively rapidly, marked ventricular hypertrophy, which will be seen on the echocardiogram. The other significant associated lesion is interruption of the aortic arch, which, of necessity, leads to a duct-dependent circulation. Progressive narrowing or closure of the duct will lead to even earlier cardiac failure. This progresses to cardiogenic shock and metabolic acidosis, usually within the first week of life. The effect of the rare combination of a

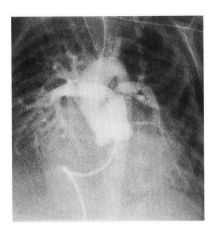

Figure 51.13. This angiogram made in the common trunk, and viewed in frontal projection, shows stenosis at the origin of the right and left pulmonary arteries.

restrictive interventricular communication and high pulmonary blood flow is to produce obstruction of the left ventricular outflow tract and concomitant left ventricular hypertrophy.

In some cases, the pulmonary vascular resistance fails to fall so precipitously. Pulmonary blood flow in these patients then tends to be in balance with the systemic flow. Under these circumstances, there is no congestive cardiac failure but rather more intense cyanosis. Decreasing pulmonary flows beyond infancy may be the consequence of progressive pulmonary vascular disease.

The other reason for more intense cyanosis, particularly in infancy, but also in older children, is the presence of stenosis at the origins of the pulmonary arteries (Figure 51.13). This will produce a decrease in pulmonary arterial pressures, less pulmonary flow and a greatly decreased chance of developing cardiac failure. This is at the cost of still further decreased systemic arterial saturation.

CLINICAL FINDINGS

The typical patient with common arterial trunk will present during the neonatal period, or in early infancy, with mild central cyanosis, a hyperactive precordium and signs of increasing congestive cardiac failure. There will be difficulties in feeding, failure to thrive, often extreme tachypnoea and hepatic enlargement. A wide pulse pressure, with bounding pulses, is to be anticipated. Obvious cyanosis is a feature of either raised pulmonary vascular resistance or pulmonary stenosis. Once cardiac failure is established, the chest may bulge in consequence of the cardiomegaly.

At auscultation, the first heart sound is usually normal, while the second sound is accentuated. It might be anticipated that the second sound would always be single in the presence of a common arterial valve. This is not the case. In approximately one half of infants, there is close

splitting of the second sound, documented by phonocardiography as well as by auscultation (Victorica et al, 1968). Possible explanations for this finding are asynchronous closure of the valvar leaflets or production of a duplicate sound by vibrations within the arterial trunk. In most infants, there will also be a loud systolic ejection click, heard best at the apex, which coincides with the opening of the truncal valve. A systolic murmur is almost always heard but can be of varying intensity and duration. Other findings often include an ejection systolic murmur of grade II or III heard maximally at the mid-to-upper left sternal border, or a harsh pansystolic murmur of grade III or IV heard maximally at the lower left sternal border. Less common murmurs include the apical mid-diastolic one, which results from flow, and an early diastolic murmur heard maximally along the left sternal edge, indicating truncal valvar insufficiency. Rarely, the murmur may be continuous and heard not only over the precordium but also the back. This is indicative of pulmonary stenosis. Surprisingly, in perhaps one tenth of patients, no murmur is heard at all at the time of presentation. This indicates an absence of turbulence within the ventricles or their outflow tracts.

INVESTIGATIONS

ELECTROCARDIOGRAPHY

Normal sinus rhythm is the rule, and conduction through the heart is similarly normal. The QRS axis as seen in the frontal plane is extremely variable and non-specific but is almost always directed inferiorly. The distribution of ventricular forces is also variable, reflecting the variability encountered in ventricular hypertrophy. According to the data cited in Keith et al (1978), the majority of patients showed evidence of combined ventricular hypertrophy, with those having isolated right ventricular hypertrophy forming the second largest group. It was infrequent in the series at Toronto to find either evidence of isolated left ventricular hypertrophy or a normal pattern. There are, therefore, no specific electrocardiographic features for patients with common arterial trunk, except perhaps that inversion of the T waves is seen with frequency in the left precordial leads, probably reflecting the impaired coronary arterial diastolic flow.

RADIOLOGIC FEATURES

The chest radiograph shows significant cardiomegaly, together with an increase in pulmonary vascular markings (Figure 51.14). The aortic arch is right sided in approximately one third of patients. This finding, in association with increased pulmonary vascularity, is strongly suggestive of common trunk. It may be possible to see an unusually high origin of the left pulmonary artery with

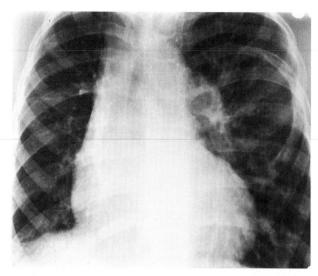

Figure 51.14. The chest radiograph typically shows cardiomegaly and increased pulmonary vascular markings. Note the high origin of the left pulmonary artery.

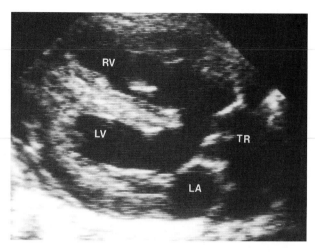

Figure 51.15. The long-axis echocardiogram from the parasternal window shows the common truncal valve (TR) overriding the crest of the muscular ventricular septum. LA, left atrium; LV, left ventricle; RV, right ventricle.

no intervening confluent pulmonary arterial segment (Figure 51.14). Although the truncal root itself is dilated, the arterial pedicle tends to appear narrow simply because of its commonality. When pulmonary blood flow is decreased, the heart is less enlarged and the pulmonary vascular markings are closer to normal. Pronounced discrepancy between the vascular markings on the two sides suggests unilateral atresia (or absence) of one pulmonary artery. As with the electrocardiogram, there are no specific findings, but the association of right arch and plethora is highly suggestive of the diagnosis.

CROSS-SECTIONAL AND DOPPLER ECHOCARDIOGRAPHY

It is now possible, in most instances, to evaluate neonates and infants with common arterial trunk with such precision that only cross-sectional echocardiography is required prior to corrective surgery. The goals of echocardiography are to define the ventricular origin and pattern of branching of the common arterial trunk, to determine the morphology and any functional abnormalities of the truncal valve, to exclude any stenosis at the origins of the pulmonary arteries, to distinguish a perimembranous ventricular septal defect from one with a muscular posteroinferior rim, to exclude any abnormalities of the aorta and to define all other associated lesions. In the majority of patients, transthoracic echocardiography provides all the diagnostic information. It is unusual, therefore, for transoesophageal studies to be needed. Only for older patients, or following palliative surgery, is it possible that cardiac catheterization and angiography may be required.

The parasternal long-axis section of the left ventricle will usually show the common arterial trunk overriding the ventricular septum, with its valve forming the superior border of the ventricular septal defect (Figure 51.15). This feature, of course, is lacking when the trunk has a univentricular origin (Figure 51.16). If the pulmonary arteries have a confluent segment, it will be seen arising posteriorly from the common trunk in this section (Figure 51.17). The leaflets of the truncal valve are frequently dysplastic (Figure 51.18) and, occasionally, can prolapse, causing the ventricular septal defect to be restrictive. Indeed, as shown morphologically (Figure 51.6), the leaflets may occasionally coapt directly on the crest of the ventricular septum. Colour flow Doppler will demonstrate flow to the aorta from both the right and left ventricle and will document any truncal valvar insufficiency, which can be predominantly or exclusively to either the right or the left ventricle. When the valve is stenotic, there is limited excursion of the leaflets. Turbulent flow distal to the truncal valve will then be evident on colour flow or continuous wave interrogation (Figure 51.19). The parasternal long-axis sections will demonstrate the expected fibrous continuity between the leaflets of the truncal valve and the truncal leaflet of the mitral valve, the degree of dilation of the left ventricle and the extent of biventricular hypertrophy. The ventricular septal defect, if restrictive, will be diagnosed in this section. Continuous wave Doppler will then record a pressure drop across the defect, which may either be from left to right or right to left, depending upon the ventricular origin of the common trunk.

The parasternal short-axis section taken just above the level of the truncal valve demonstrates the pulmonary arteries as they arise from the common trunk. In the so-called type I variant of common trunk, a short pulmonary arterial segment arises from the left lateral aspect of the common trunk and then divides into right and left pulmonary arteries (Figure 51.17). Stenosis at the origin of the right or left pulmonary arteries, or pulmonary

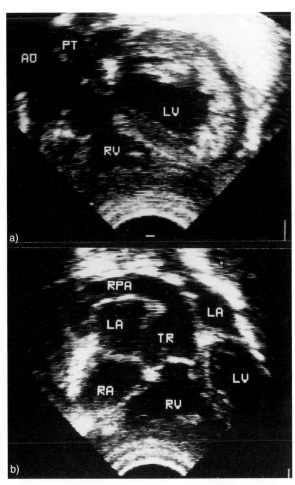

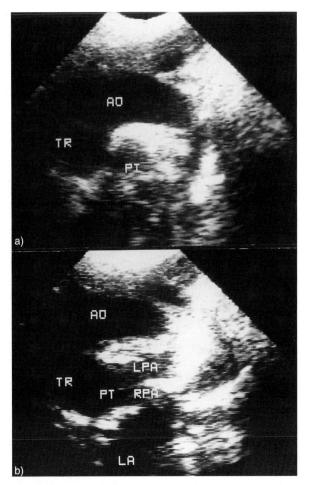

Figure 51.16. These echocardiograms were obtained from the subcostal window. (a) The common trunk divides into aorta (AO) and pulmonary trunk (PT) and arises exclusively from the right ventricle (RV), with the left ventricle (LV) exiting to the trunk through the ventricular septal defect. (b) The univentricular origin of the trunk is clearly seen. RPA, right pulmonary artery; RA, right atrium; other abbreviations as in Figure 51.15.

Figure 51.17. Parasternal long-axis sections show that a confluent arterial segment (PT) arises from the common trunk (TR) (a) before dividing (b) to become the right and left pulmonary arteries (RPA, LPA, respectively). Abbreviations as in Figures 51.15 and 51.16.

arterial hypoplasia, will be evident in this section. In the so-called type II pattern, the right and left pulmonary arteries arise from the posterior wall of the common trunk through separate but adjacent orifices. In practice, it is often difficult to distinguish these patterns, even in postmortem specimens. In contrast, the type III variant is easily distinguished, the right and left pulmonary arteries arising from the common trunk via two widely separated orifices. Other rarer origins of the pulmonary arteries must be anticipated, including atresia or even absence of one pulmonary artery. The parasternal short-axis section will also identify the number of truncal valvar leaflets (Figure 51.18). Discontinuity between the tricuspid and truncal valvar leaflets will be seen in this cut when there is a muscular posteroinferior rim to the ventricular septal defect, expected in four fifths of patients.

The apical and parasternal four chamber sections also demonstrate the large subarterial ventricular septal defect and the overriding of the truncal valve. Colour flow

Doppler will usually demonstrate biventricular shunting across the defect. Any truncal valvar insufficiency will be evident in this section, while duplex scanning with continuous wave Doppler documents any systolic gradient should the truncal valve be stenotic. The diastolic pressure drop between the common trunk and the ventricular mass can be demonstrated when there is valvar insufficiency. The drop in pressure identified across a stenotic truncal valve, however, will exaggerate the severity of stenosis. This is because the high pulmonary blood flow gives rise to a large left ventricular output. Gradients of up to 60 mmHg as estimated with Doppler, therefore, will become insignificant after corrective surgery. Although the parasternal long- and short-axis sections will demonstrate the pulmonary arteries arising posteriorly from the common trunk, the subcostal long-axis sections are unique in their ability to display most of the morphological features of common arterial trunk. The subcostal paracoronal sections demonstrate the ventricular septal

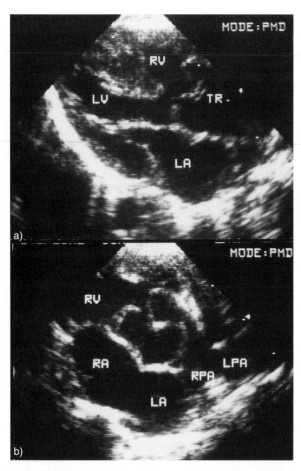

Figure 51.18. These long- (a) and short-axis (b) sections taken from the parasternal window show a dysplastic truncal valve (TR) with three leaflets. During diastole, the leaflet prolapses close to the crest of the ventricular septum. Abbreviations as in Figures 51.15 and 51.16.

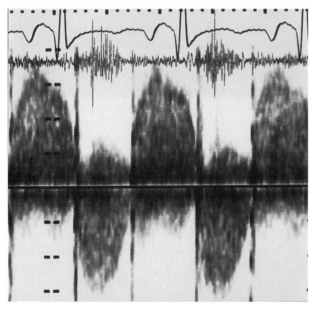

Figure 51.19. Doppler interrogation shows regurgitant and turbulent flow across a stenotic truncal valve.

defect, the nature of its posteroinferior rim, the overriding of the common trunk and the origin of both the ascending aorta and the pulmonary arteries (Figure 51.20). The right oblique section identifies the entirety of the proximal right pulmonary artery, whereas leftward rotation can be used to demonstrate the features of the left pulmonary artery. These sections also permit identification of any stenosis at the origins of the left and right pulmonary arteries and will reveal rare findings such as 'crossed' origins of the pulmonary arteries (Becker et al, 1970). Duplex scanning can be used to measure the pressure drop across any identified stenoses. Characteristically, continuous wave Doppler identifies both systolic and diastolic flow immediately distal to the site of stenosis. Suprasternal sections can also be used to identify the origin of the pulmonary arteries from the common trunk. These cuts, in addition, will demonstrate the presence of interruption of the aortic arch, the side of the aortic arch and additional anomalies such as an arterial duct or aortic coarctation. Retrograde diastolic flow is observed quite frequently in the aortic arch, reflecting the low diastolic pressure in the pulmonary arteries.

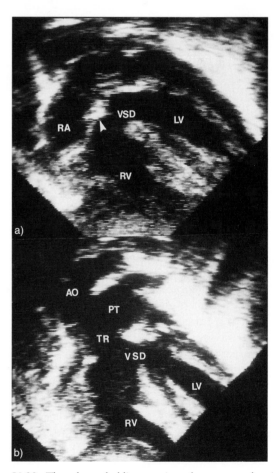

Figure 51.20. The subcostal oblique sections show a muscular rim (arrowed) of the ventricular septal defect (VSD) between the leaflets of the truncal and tricuspid valves (a) and the division of the trunk (TR) into its aortic (AO) and pulmonary (PT) components (b). Abbreviations as in Figure 51.15.

It is not unusual for interruption of the aortic arch to be associated with common arterial trunk (Figure 51.21), often in combination with significant dysplasia of the truncal valvar leaflets producing insufficiency and/or stenosis. Almost always the ascending aorta is relatively hypoplastic, being smaller than the proximal pulmonary arteries. The interruption can occur at any of the classical sites. At the time of echocardiographic investigation, most neonates will already be receiving prostaglandins intravenously; consequently, the arterial duct will be relatively large. The high left parasternal echocardiographic section demonstrates the duct (Figure 37.21b), and colour flow will then usually demonstrate bidirectional flow. Pulsed Doppler reveals that systolic flow is from the pulmonary arteries to the descending aorta; however, there is reversal of flow during diastole, providing the pulmonary vascular resistance is low. The suprasternal parasagittal sections (Figure 51.21a) reveal the site of the aortic interruption relative to the origin of the brachiocephalic, left common carotid and left subclavian arteries.

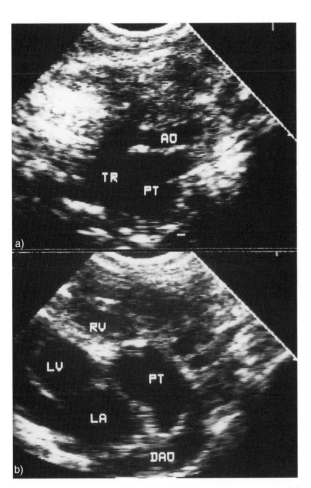

Figure 51.21. The suprasternal section (a) shows interruption of the aortic arch, with the characteristic V at the termination of the aorta (AO). The parasternal section (b) shows the descending aorta (DAO) taking origin from the pulmonary segment of the trunk (PT) via an arterial duct. Abbreviations as in Figures 51.15 and 51.16.

CARDIAC CATHETERIZATION AND ANGIOCARDIOGRAPHY

It is possible nowadays to refer patients with typical non-invasive findings directly for corrective surgery (Stark et al, 1983; Ebert et al, 1984; Bove et al, 1989, 1993; Hanley et al, 1993). Should there be any doubt about any aspect of the presentation, however, cardiac catheterization should be performed, particularly if there is any suggestion of pulmonary vascular obstructive disease. If pulmonary vascular disease is to be properly evaluated, pulmonary venous saturations of oxygen cannot be assumed because pulmonary oedema or chest infection can result in pulmonary venous desaturation. Nor can it be assumed that either the pressure or the saturation of oxygen is the same in the two pulmonary arteries, or is the same in one of them and the aorta. In most cases, there is streaming of blood preferentially from right ventricle to pulmonary arteries, and from the left ventricle to the aorta (Mair et al, 1974; Calder et al, 1976). Furthermore, there may be obstruction at the point of origin of pulmonary arteries from the aorta (Figure 51.14) or in one pulmonary artery. Such differences in pressure between the aorta and the pulmonary arteries were found in almost half of the patients studied by Calder et al (1976). Therefore, if catheterization is to be performed, ideally separate catheters should be placed in each pulmonary artery, a systemic artery, the superior caval vein and at least one pulmonary vein. Consumption of oxygen should be measured while the catheter in the superior caval vein is withdrawn to the inferior caval vein to obtain a second measurement of systemic venous oxygen. Then, with further manipulation, more pulmonary venous saturation values should be obtained. The effect of administration of 100% oxygen or pulmonary vasodilators should be measured. Entry to the pulmonary arteries is achieved most readily by retrograde arterial catheterization, looping the catheter in the truncal root so that it can then pass upwards into the pulmonary arteries. Any differences in systolic pressure should be noted across the truncal valve. These were reported to occur in one third of the patients investigated by Calder et al (1976) and varied from 10 to 60 mmHg. Criterions for distinguishing such differences in pressure owing to truncal stenosis from those caused by excessive flow are, in most cases, not yet available. Any difference noted in neonates in systolic pressure across the arterial duct (Calder et al, 1976) is an important indication for administration of prostagladin.

Selective angiocardiography should consist, first, of injecting contrast medium into the truncal root, filming in frontal and lateral projections. Elongated right anterior oblique views show well the aortopulmonary septum (Ceballos et al, 1983). Rapid injections are necessary to avoid excessive dilution of the contrast medium by the torrential flow. Such an injection should demonstrate the anterior tilt of the truncal root (Calder et al, 1976), the

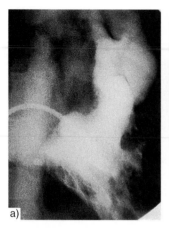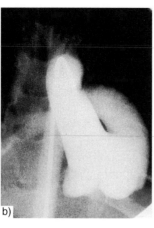

a) b)

Figure 51.22. These angiograms show a ventricular injection (a) filling the common trunk and an injection in the truncal root (b) revealing the right pulmonary artery, which has a direct origin from the trunk, but is discontinuous from the pulmonary artery.

origin of one or both pulmonary arteries from the ascending trunk, the degree of truncal regurgitation (found in two thirds of patients by Hallermann and colleagues (1969)) and, in some cases, a jet of non-opacified blood traversing the truncal valve (Patel et al, 1978). Exceptionally, the pulmonary arteries may be seen arising from the underside of the aortic arch (Rubay et al, 1987) or from other unusual sites, such as one of the truncal sinuses (Figure 51.7). It may still be difficult after angiography to be sure that the diagnosis is not aortopulmonary window, but this distinction should already have been made echocardiographically. An injection in the truncal root will usually demonstrate any interruption of the aortic arch. The injection in the truncal root should also reveal any unilateral 'absence' of one pulmonary artery (Figure 51.22). This malformation was found in almost one tenth of the series of Calder and colleagues (1976) and in one sixth of the surgical series reported by Mair and colleagues (1974). If suspected, then a further descending aortogram, and selective injection(s) into collateral arteries, or even pulmonary venous wedge injections on the side of the 'absent' pulmonary artery, should clarify whether the artery really is absent or whether it originally derived its blood supply from an arterial duct (van der Horst and Gotsman, 1974). Abnormalities of the origins of the coronary arteries have been identified as a risk factor in one large surgical series of infants (Hanley et al, 1993). Although it was suggested that such abnormalities should be identified by coronary arteriography, or by echocardiography prior to surgery (Hanley et al, 1993), there is no evidence as yet that such findings have reduced surgical mortality.

———— DIFFERENTIAL DIAGNOSIS ————

Subsequent to clinical examination, and study of the chest radiograph and an electrocardiogram, the main dif-

ferential diagnosis is ventricular septal defect or patency of the arterial duct. Patients with common arterial trunk tend to present earlier than either of these. The presence of cyanosis would favour common trunk but is rare. Jerky pulses militate against ventricular septal defect but do not help in differentiation from patent arterial duct. The electrocardiogram is of little value, and neither is the chest radiograph, although the presence of a right aortic arch favours common trunk. Aortopulmonary window must also be considered but is extremely rare. Double outlet right ventricle without pulmonary stenosis usually has the mild cyanosis but not the jerky pulses.

With cross-sectional echocardiography, the most likely problem is failure adequately to demonstrate the absence of the right ventricular outflow tract and its arterial valve. Tetralogy of Fallot, because it is common, is the most likely source of difficulty. Aortopulmonary window looks like common trunk if attention is directed only to the great arteries, but the problem disappears once the separate nature of the pulmonary valve is identified. Anomalous origin of one pulmonary artery from the ascending aorta can cause problems if the great arteries alone are imaged but, again, the dilemma is resolved by demonstration of separate origin of the pulmonary valve and trunk. Problems in differentation do arise for those hearts in which a true common trunk is associated with either a duct or systemic-to-pulmonary collateral arteries feeding one lung. Once again, careful examination of the right ventricular outflow tract, and search for a long tortuous arterial duct, should resolve the dilemma (Smallhorn et al, 1982). All these problems concerned with evaluation of the right ventricular outflow tract are equally applicable to angiocardiography should this investigation now be performed.

———— COURSE AND PROGNOSIS ————

The Central Bohemian study (Šamánek et al, 1988) has provided the most reliable indicator of prognosis for infants. This is because all patients dying below the age of 15 years in Central Bohemia between 1952 and 1979 had a compulsory postmortem, which was performed or supervised by one pathologist. Prior to 1979, only shunts, bandings and ductal ligations were performed. Of the infants born with common arterial trunk, over nine tenths died in the first year and half of the few survivors died in the second year. Looking at the first year, two thirds died in the first month, and nearly one third of those surviving died in the second month. In the face of this unbiased study, it becomes easier to interpret those studies that were obviously biased by treatment (Marcelletti et al, 1976). Isolated reports tell us that long-term survival is possible without treatment in rare patients with common arterial trunk, and who currently holds the world record for survival, but tell us almost nothing else. Survival until identification at postmortem has been reported at the ages of 36 years (Carr et al, 1935) and 38 years (Hicken et al, 1966). The median age at death in a series of patients coming to attention largely through postmortem, in contrast, was no more than 5 weeks (Calder et al, 1976). If one pulmonary artery was absent, the median age at death was 5 months. Truncal valvar insufficiency has an additional marked deleterious effect on survival in young infants (Gelband et al, 1972). Di Donato and colleagues (1985), however, found that the group of patients with minimal truncal insufficiency was significantly younger than the group with severe insufficiency. All patients with severe insufficiency were aged over 5 years. This, nonetheless, is based on a surgical series in which those neonates or infants with severe valvar insufficiency almost certainly never survived to reach the centre for management.

MANAGEMENT

MEDICAL TREATMENT

Sick infants require maximal medical treatment and correction of metabolic acidosis. If there is interruption of the aortic arch, prostaglandin E will be necessary to maintain patency of the duct. Even if the patient appears to be responding well to medical treatment, early surgery should be planned. Ebert and colleagues (1984) described six infants dying during maximal medical treatment, even though five of them had shown dramatic immediate improvement. This, coupled with recent results, shows that there is no reason for delaying surgical repair.

SURGICAL TREATMENT

Until recently, surgical treatment had commenced by banding the pulmonary arteries, either at the level of a confluent pulmonary arterial segment or separately for the right and left arteries. The rationale behind banding (Heilbrunn et al, 1964; Smith et al, 1964) is that it will reduce volume overload on the left ventricle and prevent pulmonary arterial hypertension distal to the band. Banding, however, cannot be expected to work as well as it does in ventricular septal defect. This is because cyanosis and truncal regurgitation, if present, must increase from the moment the surgeon begins to constrict the band. By contrast, in ventricular septal defect, the surgeon can apply the band much tighter because the aortic valve is usually competent. Furthermore, in patients with a ventricular septal defect, as the band is constricted, pulmonary arterial flow and pressure can be diminished without producing a right-to-left shunt. Therefore, although strict criterions were developed to optimize banding for common arterial trunk (Poirier et al, 1975), results of correction subsequent to banding have proven to be less good than the current results of

immediate correction. Most centres nowadays, therefore, opt directly for definitive repair during the neonatal period.

DEFINITIVE REPAIR

The first successful 'complete' repair of common arterial trunk, using a valved conduit to restore continuity from the right ventricle to the pulmonary arteries, was achieved at the Mayo Clinic in September 1967 (McGoon et al, 1968). It was the culmination of extensive research in dogs (Rastelli et al, 1967) using freeze-dried and irradiated homografts. Ross and Somerville (1966) had previously used a conduit incorporating a homograft valve preserved with antibiotics to repair tetralogy of Fallot with pulmonary atresia. Furthermore, in 1974, Behrendt and colleagues reported that a patient was doing well 11 years after repair of common arterial trunk using a simple tube graft to join right ventricle and pulmonary trunk. It is, nonetheless, with the Mayo Clinic that early success is associated, and subsequent to that with the group at San Francisco (Ebert et al, 1976).

The operation begins with dissecting both pulmonary arteries down to their branching points in the hilums of both lungs. The aorta is fully mobilized, particularly if it is intended to transect the common trunk in order to detach the pulmonary arteries when there is no pulmonary trunk (Griepp et al, 1977). The surgery is performed under hypothermic cardiopulmonary bypass. The degree of truncal incompetence is carefully assessed, because this is difficult to predict from preoperative investigation (de Leval et al, 1974), except perhaps from colour flow mapping. Significant regurgitation interferes with myocardial protection, irrespective of whether that is carried out by intermittent cross-clamping or cardioplegia. It may be necessary to inject cardioplegic solution into the coronary arteries or coronary sinus as a counter measure. If the regurgitation is severe, or if there is severe and dysplastic truncal stenosis, there is no alternative to replacing the truncal valve (Di Donato et al, 1985). The pulmonary arteries are detached from the common trunk, taking care to avoid any coronary arterial origins. The defect in the aorta is closed by direct suture. If there is no pulmonary trunk, access is improved by transecting the ascending component of the common trunk. The separate pulmonary arteries are excised with the interposed portion of trunk as a single button, and the ascending aorta is reconstructed as an end-to-end anastomosis. The ventricular septal defect is then closed with a patch in such a way as to connect the remaining aortic component of the trunk with the left ventricle. Continuity between the pulmonary arteries and the right ventricle can often be established with the aorta cross-clamped while the patient is being rewarmed. With adequate mobilization of the pulmonary arteries, it should be possible to anastomose the homograft directly onto the right ventriculotomy without any prosthetic interposition. Use of a valveless conduit (Spicer et al, 1984) made sense at the time, but a valved conduit is to be preferred since a competent pulmonary valve is desirable in the postoperative period, particularly when there are pulmonary hypertensive crises.

Continuity between the right ventricle and pulmonary arteries can also be achieved without use of a conduit. This operation, popularized by Barbero-Marcial and his colleagues (1990), was initially performed in a single patient by Reid and his associates (1986). The Brazilian series as initially reported involved seven infants aged 2–9 months. There was one hospital death and no late deaths. The monocusps seemed to close well, as judged echocardiographically, but were regurgitant. This novel approach was then used by Losay and colleagues (1991) in six patients, with two early deaths and one late death. A more recent experience was described by Nakae and colleagues (1996) from Kanagawa, Japan, but again with unduly high initial mortality. As Hanley (1996) pointed out when commenting on the Japanese experience, despite these valiant attempts to avoid conduits, the gold standard for surgical repair remains insertion of a valved allograft, preferably of pulmonary origin. Only in the absence of such allografts should the initial procedure be to avoid the use of a conduit. Successful surgical correction can also be achieved when the aortic arch is interrupted. The original successful repair, described by Gomes and McGoon (1971), and repeated by Davis and colleagues (1985), left the duct in place to supply blood to the descending aorta. This, of course, can only be done after the age of a year or so, when there is no chance of ductal closure. In younger patients, the duct and all ductal tissue must be excised. The entire thoracic aorta, the pulmonary arteries, the head and neck vessels and the duct must then be thoroughly mobilized, otherwise it will be impossible to join the ascending to the descending aorta. Successful repairs in the setting of interruption were usually confined to solitary patients (Schumacher et al, 1986; Fujiwara et al, 1988; Scott et al, 1988) until a remarkable series was reported from Melbourne with no early or late deaths (Sano et al, 1990). This is now achieved in other centres of excellence.

In terms of overall surgical approach, analysis of risk factors in the early days had shown that young age was the most potent cause of early death. This was the incentive towards postponing operation, if necessary by banding (Poirier et al, 1975). Such protocols were able to improve the rate of survival after definitive repair in a given centre, but only at the cost of worse overall survival in the population as a whole. The most important factor in selecting such older patients for surgical repair was the pulmonary vascular resistance. Excluding complicated cases and patients with unilateral absence of a pulmonary artery, surgical mortality in this era for patients with a resistance below 8 units/m^2 was 10%. For those with pulmonary vascular resistance of 8–12 units/m^2, the mortality was 33%. All patients with a pulmonary vascular

resistance of greater than 12 units/m^2 died (Mair et al, 1974). Apart from age, pulmonary vascular resistance and year of operation, no other risk factors were found in the analysis carried out at the Mayo Clinic based on their first 92 patients (Marcelletti et al, 1977). Earlier, severe truncal insufficiency had also been found to be a risk factor (Mair et al, 1974). In the subsequent experience at the Mayo Clinic, reported in 1985 by Di Donato and colleagues, actuarial freedom from reoperation was 85.5% at 5 years and 52.9% at 10 years. All these patients had undergone two-stage repair. In this respect, by using data from the literature on survival with and without surgery of various types, Stark and his associates were able to show that, of 100 patients considered at birth, only nine would survive with a policy of definitive repair at age 5, 30 would survive with initial banding followed by repair at 5 years, but 58 would survive with immediate repair in infancy and subsequent replacement of the conduit. Consequently, although the contribution of the Mayo Clinic to the surgery of common arterial trunk cannot be overestimated, it became clear that the patients referred to the surgeons at Mayo Clinic represented only a tiny subset of the overall population of patients with common arterial trunk, namely that subset selected for survival. To make any impact on the entire group of patients with common arterial trunk, it was essential to accomplish definitive repair in infants.

Already in the mid-1970s, 8 years after the first repair reported at Mayo Clinic, reports had started to appear of such definitive repair during infancy. These began with success in solitary patients (Singh et al, 1975; Sullivan et al, 1976) but soon extended to reports of series. In 1976, Ebert and colleagues reported survival of four of five infants undergoing repair of common arterial trunk at less than 6 months of age. They used either a 12 mm Hancock prosthesis or an aortic allograft to establish continuity with the pulmonary arteries, siting the valve as close to the pulmonary anastomosis as possible to avoid compression by the sternum.

This seminal paper was, in due course, followed by description of a remarkable series of 100 patients, all undergoing definitive repair within the first 6 months of life (Ebert et al, 1984). Amongst these patients, there were 11 early and three late deaths. Of the 86 infants surviving over 2 years, 55 had already returned for replacement of the conduit. None died. Similar results, in a smaller series, had been reported by Sharma and colleagues (1985). Still better results, albeit in smaller series, have been reported by Bove and colleagues (1993) and by Hanley et al (1993). Multivariate analysis of the latter experience, from Boston Children's Hospital, demonstrated four risk factors: severe truncal regurgitation, interrupted aortic arch, age at repair greater than 100 days and anomalous origin of the coronary arteries. In the 33 patients without these risk factors, there were no deaths. In the 30 with at least one risk factor, hospital survival was only 63%. Age as a risk factor, therefore, has now been reversed in comparison with the earlier experience from Mayo Clinic. In part, this reflects the general advances in technique, understanding and postoperative care. It also relates to the lower incidence of pulmonary hypertensive crises in younger infants, who, therefore, require less ventilatory support after the operation.

One factor that might limit success after operative repair is the fate of the valved conduit, which almost always is used as part of the operative procedure. Even in the early days, it was clear that there was a problem of medial calcification in the wall of the aortic homograft then employed (Rastelli et al, 1967). One way of avoiding this complication was to use pulmonary rather than aortic homografts. These were first tried in dogs (Seki et al, 1970) but were relatively little used initially in patients. Another much more popular method was to use the Hancock prosthesis: a tube of Dacron containing a porcine aortic valve preserved in glutaraldehyde (Bowman et al, 1973). This conduit had the great advantage of being freely available to those who could afford it. Even in the experience of the Mayo Clinic when patients were repaired in childhood (Di Donato et al, 1985), about one quarter of patients required replacement of the conduit. Now that repair is usually undertaken during the neonatal period, replacement of the conduit becomes almost inevitable simply because of growth. In recent analysis of the patients undergoing surgery in San Francisco (Rajasinghe et al, 1997), two thirds of those repaired during infancy over a 20-year period had required replacement of their conduits. The only factor significantly associated with a shorter time to replacement was a smaller size of the conduit first inserted. This inevitable replacement of conduits was, of course, the stimulus to attempt repair without need for such a device (Reid et al, 1986; Barbero-Macial et al, 1990). As already discussed, the increased mortality and morbidity of the reconstructive procedures means that use of the conduit remains the 'gold standard', even during infancy (Hanley, 1996). Replacement of the conduit can be achieved with very little morbidity and no mortality.

It is, nonetheless, important to recognize obstruction of the conduit when it occurs. This is suspected on clinical grounds when a loud, rough, ejection systolic murmur develops at the left sternal edge, usually accompanied by a thrill and a lift. A prominent a wave is seen in the jugular venous pulse, reflecting an elevated right ventricular end-diastolic pressure. As obstruction develops, so does tricuspid regurgitation, which gives a cv wave in the jugular venous pulse. Regurgitation through the conduit is suggested by a loud diastolic murmur commencing with the sound of closure of the valve within the conduit. Doppler estimation of the pressure difference across the conduit is a valuable means of monitoring progress. Arrhythmias, occasionally life threatening, may accompany obstruction. When the conduit is replaced, the arrhythmia usually goes away (Moodie et al, 1976). Replacement of the conduit necessitates care with the midline sternotomy to avoid uncontrolled entry (Merin and McGoon, 1973). If demonstration of the relationship between sternum and conduit is deemed helpful, the best method is magnetic resonance imaging. In most series, the risk of replacement so far has been zero (Moodie et al, 1976; Ebert et al, 1984; Bove et al, 1993; Heinemann et al, 1993; Slavik et al, 1994).

It does now seem that the use of a fresh, antibiotic-sterilized homograft gives the best results over the long term (Moore et al, 1976), though this has never been demonstrated in any controlled way. Slavik and colleagues (1994), nonetheless, reported a remarkable follow-up of a series of infants repaired in the first year of life using such an antibiotic-sterilized aortic homograft. Only two patients required replacement of the conduit; in one of these, the aim of the operation had been to replace the truncal valve, but the conduit was replaced electively at the same time. In the 14 patients retaining the original homograft, the median of the residual peak gradient across the right ventricular outflow tract was 15 mmHg (range 10–40 mmHg) as assessed by Doppler velocimetry. In contrast, a report from Boston Children's Hospital (Heinemann et al, 1993) revealed two risk factors for obstruction of the conduit. These were choice of an aortic rather than a pulmonary homograft, and a gradient obtained on the first postoperative day when pulling back from the pulmonary arteries to the right ventricle. The size of the conduit itself was not a risk factor. In this series, the actuarial survival at 2 years without stenosis of the conduit was 75% for aortic homografts, while no patients had developed obstruction of a pulmonary homograft. It is possible to relieve obstruction by balloon dilation, using a balloon equal in diameter to the conduit (Murdoch et al, 1991). Better results are obtained following insertion of stents (Hosking et al, 1992; Hayes et al, 1997); however, with the inevitability of eventual replacement, surgery seems the best option.

The long-term results of surgical repair are now outstanding considering that less than one tenth of a cohort of 100 patients would be alive after 5 years without surgical correction of any kind (as shown by Stark et al (1978)). As we have discussed, to achieve optimal results it is necessary to undertake repair during infancy. Results are now available for the 20-year period subsequent to the initial repair of infants with common arterial trunk achieved in San Francisco in 1975 (Rajasinghe et al, 1997). The medium age at repair for the 165 patients corrected in this period was 3.5 years, and four fifths underwent surgery in the first year of life. Previous banding had been performed in 15 patients. Actuarial survival amongst the survivors of the initial repair was 83% at 15 years. As emphasized, replacement or revision of the conduit is almost inevitable but can be achieved with no mortality and little morbidity. Truncal valvar insufficiency still remains a problem. Freedom from replacement of the truncal valve amongst those without preoperative insufficiency was 95% at 10 years, but significantly lower, at 63%, in those who had a regurgitant valve prior to repair. The problem of the regurgitant truncal valve has been assessed in detail by McElhinney and colleagues (1998), using the same cohort of patients from the University of California at San Francisco. Despite improving prospects for the overall subset of patients with truncal valvar insufficiency, the results in those patients with severe regurgitation continue to be poor even in this centre of excellence. This, however, is a very small group amongst the overall cohort of patients with common arterial trunk. For the greater majority, the outlook of surgical repair undertaken in infancy is excellent, even for those with the added complication of interruption of the aortic arch.

REFERENCES

Alves P M, Ferrari A H 1987 Common arterial trunk arising exclusively from the right ventricle with hypoplastic left ventricle and intact ventricular septum. International Journal of Cardiology 16: 99–102

Anderson K R, McGoon D C, Lie J T 1978 Surgical significance of the coronary arterial anatomy in truncus arteriosus communis. American Journal of Cardiology 41: 76–81

Anderson R H, Thiene G 1989 Categorization and description of hearts with common arterial trunk. European Journal of Cardiothoracic Surgery 3: 481–487

Anderson R H, Wilcox B R 1993 Surgical anatomy of ventricular septal defects associated with overriding valvar orifices. Journal of Cardiac Surgery 8: 130–142

Barbero-Marcial M, Riso A, Atik E, Jatene A 1990 A technique for correction of truncus arteriosus types I and II without extracardiac conduits. Journal of Thoracic and Cardiovascular Surgery 99: 364–369

Bartelings M M, Gittenberger-de Groot A C 1991 Morphogenetic considerations on congenital malformations of the outflow tract. Part 1: common arterial trunk and tetralogy of Fallot. International Journal of Cardiology 32: 213–230

Becker A E, Becker M J, Edwards J E 1970 Malposition of pulmonary arteries (crossed pulmonary arteries) in persistent truncus arteriosus. American Journal of Roentgenology Radium Therapy and Nuclear Medicine 110: 509–514

Becker A E, Becker M J, Edwards J E 1971 Pathology of the semilunar valve in persistent truncus arteriosus. Journal of Thoracic and Cardiovascular Surgery 62: 16–26

Behrendt D M, Kirsch M M, Stern A, Sigmann J, Perry B, Sloan H B 1974 The surgical therapy for pulmonary artery – right ventricular discontinuity. Annals of Thoracic Surgery 18: 122–137

Benešová D, Šikl H 1954 A rare concordant malformation in monochoriate twins: persistent common arterial trunk. Journal of Pathology and Bacteriology 47: 367–371

Besson W T III, Kirby M L, Van Mierop L H S, Teabeaut J R II 1986 Effects of the size of lesions of the cardiac neural crest at various embryonic ages on incidence and type of cardiac defects. Circulation 73: 360–364

Bharati S, McAllister H A, Rosenquist G C, Miller R A, Tatooles C J, Lev M 1974 The surgical anatomy of truncus arteriosus communis. Journal of Thoracic and Cardiovascular Surgery 67: 501–510

Bove E L, Beekman R H, Snider R et al 1989 Repair of truncus arteriosus in the neonate and young infant. Annals of Thoracic Surgery 47: 499–506

Bove E L, Lupinetti F M, Pridjian A K et al 1993 Results of a policy of primary repair of truncus arteriosus in the neonate. Journal of Thoracic and Cardiovascular Surgery 105: 1057–1066

Bowman F O, Hancock W D, Malm J R 1973 A valve-containing dacron prosthesis. Archives of Surgery 107: 724–728

Brunson S C, Nudel D B, Gootman N, Aftalion B 1978 Truncus arteriosus in a family. American Heart Journal 96: 419–420

Calder L, Van Praagh R, Van Praagh S et al 1976 Truncus arteriosus communis. American Heart Journal 92: 23–38

Carey A H, Kelly D, Halford S et al 1992 Molecular genetic study of the frequency of monosomy 22q11 in DiGeorge syndrome. American Journal of Human Genetics 51: 964–970

Carr F B, Goodale R H, Rockwell A E P 1935 Persistent truncus arteriosus in a man aged thirty-six years. Archives of Pathology 19: 833–837

Carr I, Bharati S, Kusnoor V S, Lev M 1979 Truncus arteriosus communis with intact ventricular septum. British Heart Journal 42: 97–102

Ceballos R, Soto B, Kirklin J W, Bargeron L M 1983 Truncus arteriosus: an anatomical–angiographic study. British Heart Journal 49: 589–599

Collett R W, Edwards J E 1949 Persistent truncus arteriosus; a classification according to anatomic types. Surgical Clinics of North America 29: 1245–1269

Conway S J, Henderson D J, Kirby M L, Anderson R H, Copp A J 1997 Development of a lethal congenital heart defect in the splotch (Pax3) mutant mouse. Cardiovascular Research 36: 163–173

Crupi G, Macartney F J, Anderson R H 1977 Persistent truncus arteriosus. A study of 66 autopsy cases with special reference to definition and morphogenesis. American Journal of Cardiology 40: 569–578

Davis J T, Ehrlich R, Blakemore W S, Lev M, Bharati S 1985 Truncus arteriosus with interrupted aortic arch: report of a successful surgical repair. Annals of Thoracic Surgery 39: 82–85

de la Chapelle A, Herva R, Koivisto M, Aula P 1981 A deletion in chromosome 22 can cause diGeorge syndrome. Human Genetics 57: 253–256

de la Cruz M V, Cayre R, Angelini P, Noriega-Ramos N, Sadowinski S 1990 Coronary arteries in truncus arteriosus. American Journal of Cardiology 66: 1482–1486

de Leval M R, McGoon D C, Wallace R B, Danielson G K, Mair D D 1974 Management of truncal valvular regurgitation. Annals of Surgery 180: 427–432

Di Donato R M, Fyfe D A, Puga F J et al 1985 Fifteen year experience with surgical repair of truncus arteriosus. Journal of Thoracic and Cardiovascular Surgery 89: 414–422

Driscoll D A, Salvin J, Sellinger B et al 1993 Prevalence of 22q11 microdeletions in DiGeorge and velocardiofacial syndromes: implications for genetic counselling and prenatal diagnosis. Journal of Medical Genetics 30: 813–817

Ebert P A, Robinson S J, Stanger P, Engle M A 1976 Pulmonary artery conduits in infants younger than six months of age. Journal of Thoracic and Cardiovascular Surgery 72: 351–356

Ebert P A, Turley K, Stanger P, Hoffman J I E, Heymann M A, Rudolph A M 1984 Surgical treatment of truncus arteriosus in the first 6 months of life. Annals of Surgery 200: 451–456

Epstein D J, Vekemans M, Gros P (1991) Splotch (sp²ᴴ), a mutation affecting development of the mouse neural tube, shows a deletion within the paired homeodomain of pax-3. Cell 67: 767–774

Ferencz C, Rubin J D, McCarter R J et al 1985 Congenital heart disease: prevalence at live birth. The Baltimore–Washington Infant Study. American Journal of Epidemiology 121: 31–36

Ferencz C, Rubin J D, McCarter R J, Clark E B 1990 Maternal diabetes and cardiovascular malformations: predominance of double outlet right ventricle and truncus arteriosus. Teratology 41: 319–326

Ferry P, Massias C, Salzard C, Anguill C, Olleac A, Quentin M 1994 Récurrence de tronc artériel commun. A propos d'un cas de diagnostic anténatal. Journal de Gynécologie Obstétrique, et Biologie de la Réproduction 23: 696–700

Finley B E, Sequin J H, Bennett T L et al 1993 Terminal deletion of 7q presenting in utero with a truncus arteriosus and nonimmune hydrops. American Journal of Medical Genetics 47: 221–222

Franz 1989 Persistent truncus arteriosus in the Splotch mutant mouse. Anatomy and Embryology 180: 457–464

Freedom R M, Rose F S, Nadas A S 1972 Congenital cardiovascular disease and anomalies of the third and fourth pharyngeal pouch. Circulation 46: 165–172

Fujiwara K, Yokota Y, Okamoto F et al 1988 Successful surgical repair of truncus arteriosus with interrupted aortic arch in infancy by an anterior approach. Annals of Thoracic Surgery 45: 441–444

Fyler D C, Buckley L P, Hellebrand W E, Cohn H E 1980 Report of the New England Regional Infant Cardiac Program. Pediatrics 65 (suppl): 376–461

Gelband H, van Meter S, Gersony W M 1972 Truncal valve abnormalities in infants with persistent truncus arteriosus. Circulation 45: 397–403

Gerlis L M, Ho S Y, Smith A, Anderson R H 1990 The site of origin of nonconfluent pulmonary arteries from a common arterial trunk or from the ascending aorta: its morphological significance. American Journal of Cardiovascular Pathology 3: 115–120

Goldmuntz E, Driscoll D, Budarf M L et al 1993 Microdeletions of chromosomal region 22q11 in patients with congenital conotruncal cardiac defects. Journal of Medical Genetics 30: 807–812

Gomes M M R, McGoon D C 1971 Truncus arteriosus with interruption of the aortic arch: report of a case successfully repaired. Mayo Clinic Proceedings 46: 40–43

Goodyear J E 1961 Persistent truncus arteriousus in two siblings. British Heart Journal 23: 194–196

Griepp R B, Stinson E B, Shumway N E 1977 Surgical correction of types II and III truncus arteriosus. Journal of Thoracic and Cardiovascular Surgery 73: 345–352

Halford S, Wadey R, Roberts C et al 1993 Isolation of a putative transcriptional regulator from the region of 22q11 deleted in DiGeorge syndrome, Shprintzen syndrome and familial congenital heart disease. Human Molecular Genetics 2: 2099–2107

Hallerman F J, Kincaid O W, Tsakiris A G, Ritter D G, Titus J L 1969 Persistent truncus arteriosus: a radiographic and angiocardiographic study. American Journal of Roentgenology 107: 827–834

Hanley F L 1996 Invited commentary. Annals of Thoracic Surgery 62: 129

Hanley F L, Heinemann M K, Jonas R A et al 1993 Repair of truncus arteriosus in the neonate. Journal of Thoracic and Cardiovascular Surgery 105: 1047–1056

Hayes A M, Nykanen D G, Smallhorn J S et al 1997 Use of balloon expandable stents in the palliative relief of obstructed right heart conduit obstruction. Cardiology of the Young 7: 423–433

Heilbrunn A, Kittle C F, Diehl A M 1964 Pulmonary arterial banding in the treatment of truncus arteriosus. Circulation Supplement, Cardiovascular Surgery 29: 102–107

Heinemann M K, Hanley F L, Fenton K N, Jonas R A, Mayer J E, Castañeda A R 1993 Fate of small homograft conduits after early repair of truncus arteriosus. Annals of Thoracic Surgery 55: 1409–1412

Hicken P, Evans D, Heath D 1966 Persistent truncus arteriosus with survival to the age of 38 years. British Heart Journal 28: 284–286

Hosking M C, Benson L N, Nakanishi T, Burrows P E, Williams W G, Freedom R M 1992 Intravascular stent prothesis for right ventricular outflow obstruction. Journal of the American College of Cardiology 20: 371–380

Jackson M, Connell M G, Smith A, Drury J, Anderson R H 1995 Common arterial trunk and pulmonary atresia: close developmental cousins? Results from a teratogen induced animal model. Cardiovascular Research 30: 992–1000

Keith J D, Rowe R D, Vlad P 1978 Heart Disease in infancy and childhood. MacMillan, New York, p 464

Kirby M L, Gale T F, Stewart D E 1983 Neural crest cells contribute to normal aorticopulmonary septation. Science 220: 1059–1061

Lang M J, Aughton D J, Riggs T W, Milad M P, Biesecker L G 1991 Dizygotic twins concordant for truncus arteriosus. Clinical Genetics 39: 75–79

Ledbetter M K, Tandon R, Titus J L, Edwards J E 1976 Stenotic semilunar valve in persistent truncus arteriosus. Chest 69: 182–187

Le Lievre C S, Le Douarin N M 1975 Mesenchymal derivatives of the neural crest: analysis of chimaeric quail and chick embryos. Journal of Embryological and Experimental Morphology 34: 125–154

le Marec B, Odent S, Almange C, Journel H, Roussey M, Defawe G 1989 Truncus arteriosus: an autosomal disease? Journal de Genetique Humaine 37: 225–230

Lin A E, Chin A Y, Devine W, Park S C, Zackai E 1987 The pattern of cardiovascular malformation in the CHARGE association. American Journal of Disease in Childhood 141: 1010–1013

Lindsay E A, Halford S, Wadey R, Scambler P J, Baldini A 1993 Molecular cytogenic characterization of the DiGeorge syndrome region using flourescence in situ hybridization. Genomics 17: 403–407

Losay J, Planché C, Lacour-Gayet F, Touchot A, Bruniaux J 1991 Immediate and mid-term results of complete repair of truncus arteriosus during the first year of life. Archives des Maladies de Cour et Vaisseaux 84: 691–695

Lupski J R, Langston C, Friedman R, Ledbetter D H, Greenberg F 1991 DiGeorge anomaly associated with a de novo Y: 22 translocation resulting in monosomy del(22)(q11.2). American Journal of Medical Genetics 40: 196–198

Mair D D, Ritter D G, Davis G D, Wallace R B, Danielson G K, McGoon D C 1974 Selection of patients with truncus arteriosus for surgical correction. Anatomic and hemodynamic considerations. Circulation 49: 144–151

Marcelletti C, McGoon D C, Mair D D 1976 The natural history of truncus arteriosus. Circulation 54: 108–111

Marcelletti C, McGoon D C, Danielson G K, Wallace R B, Mair D D 1977 Early and late results of surgical repair of truncus arteriosus. Circulation 55: 636–641

McElhinney D, Reddy V M, Rajasinghe H A, Mora B N, Silverman N H, Hanley F J 1998 Trends in the management of truncal valve insufficiency. Annals of Thoracic Surgery. 65: 517–524

McGoon D C, Rastelli G C, Ongley P A 1968 An operation for the correction of truncus arteriosus. Journal of the American Medical Association 205: 59–63

McGoon D C, Rastelli G C, Wallace R B 1970 Discontinuity between right ventricle and pulmonary artery. Surgical Treatment. Annals of Surgery 172: 680–689

Merin G, McGoon D C 1973 Reoperation after insertion of aortic homograft as a right ventricular outflow tract. Annals of Thoracic Surgery 16: 122–126

Momma K, Ando M, Takao A, Miyagawa-Tomita S 1991 Fetal cardiovascular morphology of truncus arteriosus with or without truncal valve insufficiency in the rat. Circulation 83: 2094–2100

Moodie D S, Mair D D, Fulton R F, Wallace R B, Danielson G K, McGoon D C 1976 Aortic homograft obstruction. Journal of Thoracic and Cardiovascular Surgery 72: 553–561

Moore C H, Martelli V, Ross D N 1976 Reconstruction of right ventricular outflow tract with a valved conduit in 75 cases of congenital heart disease. Journal of Thoracic and Cardiovascular Surgery 71: 11–18

Murdoch I A, Parsons J M, Dos Anjos R, Qureshi S A 1991 Balloon dilatation of a stenosed aortic homograft following repair of the common arterial trunk. Pediatric Cardiology 12: 175–176

Nakae S, Kasahara S, Kuroyama N et al 1996 Correction of truncus arteriosus with autologous arterial flap in neonates and small infants. Annals of Thoracic Surgery 62: 123–128

Nora J J, Nora A H 1978 The evolution of specific and environmental counselling in congenital heart disease. Circulation 57: 205–213

Patel R G, Freedom R M, Bloom K R, Rowe R D 1978 Truncal or aortic valve stenosis in functionally single arterial trunk. American Journal of Cardiology 42: 800–809

Patterson D F, Pexieder T, Schnarr W R, Navratil T, Alaili R 1993 A single major-gene defect underlying cardiac conotruncal malformations interferes with myocardial growth during embryonic development: studies in the CTD line of Keeshond dogs. American Journal of Human Genetics 52: 388–397

Pierpont M E M, Gobel J C, Moller J H, Edwards J E 1988 Cardiac malformations in relatives of children with truncus arteriosus or interruption of the aortic arch. American Journal of Cardiology 61: 423–427

Poirier R A, Berman M A, Stansel H C Jr 1975 Current status of the surgical treatment of truncus arteriosus. Journal of Thoracic and Cardiovascular Surgery 69: 169–182

Rajasinghe H A, McElhinney D B, Reddy V M, Mora B N, Hanley F L 1997 Long-term follow-up of truncus arteriosus repaired in infancy: a twenty-year experience. Journal of Thoracic and Cardiovascular Surgery 113: 869–878

Rastelli G C, Titus J L, McGoon D C 1967 Homograft of ascending aorta and aortic valve as a right ventricular outflow. Archives of Surgery 95: 698–708

Reid K G, Godman M J, Burns J E 1986 Truncus arteriosus: successful surgical correction without the use of a valved conduit. British Heart Journal 56: 388–390

Rein A J J T, Sheffer R 1994 Genetics of cono-truncal abnormalities: further evidence of autosomal recessive inheritance. American Journal of Medical Genetics 50: 302–303

Rein A J J T, Dollberg S, Gale R 1990 Genetics of conotruncal malformations: review of the literature and report of a consanguinous kindred with various conotruncal malformations. American Journal of Medical Genetics 36: 353–355

Rosenquist G C, Bharati S, McAllister H A, Lev M 1976 Truncus arteriosus communis: truncal valve anomalies associated with small conal or truncal septal defects. American Journal of Cardiology 37: 410–412

Ross D N, Somerville J 1966 Correction of pulmonary atresia with a homograft aortic valve. Lancet ii: 1446–1447

Rubay J E, Macartney F J, Anderson R H 1987 A rare variant of common arterial trunk. British Heart Journal 57: 202–204

Šamánek M, Benešová D, Goetzová J 1988 Distribution of age at death in children with congenital heart disease who died before the age of 15. British Heart Journal 59: 581–585

Sano S, Brawn W J, Mee R B B 1990 Repair of truncus arteriosus and interrupted aortic arch. Journal of Cardiac Surgery 5: 157–162

Scalia D, Russo P, Anderson R H et al 1984 The surgical anatomy of hearts with no direct communication between the right atrium and the ventricular mass – so-called tricuspid atresia. Journal of Thoracic and Cardiovascular Surgery 87: 743–755

Schilham M W, Oosterwegel M A, Moerer P et al 1996 Defects in cardiac outflow tract formation and pro-B-lymphocyte expansion in mice lacking Sox-4. Nature 320: 711–714

Schumacher G, Schreiber R, Meisner H, Lorenz H P, Sebening F, Bühlmeyer K 1986 Interrupted aortic arch. Natural history and operative results. Pediatric Cardiology 7: 89–93

Scott D J, Rigby M L, Miller G A H, Shinebourne E A 1984 The presentation of symptomatic heart disease in infancy based on 10 years' experience (1973–1982) – implications for the provision of services. British Heart Journal 52: 248–257

Scott W A, Rocchini A P, Bove E L et al 1988 Repair of interrupted aortic arch in infancy. Journal of Thoracic and Cardiovascular Surgery 96: 564–568

Seki S, Rastelli G C, McGoon D C, Titus J L 1970 Replacement of the pulmonary artery with a pulmonary arterial homograft. Journal of Thoracic and Cardiovascular Surgery 60: 853–858

Shapiro S R, Ruckman R N, Kapur S et al 1981 Single ventricle with truncus arteriosus in siblings. American Heart Journal 102: 456–459

Sharma A K, Brawn W J, Mee R B B 1985 Truncus arteriosus. Surgical approach. Journal of Thoracic and Cardiovascular Surgery 90: 45–49

Shrivastava S, Edwards J E 1977 Coronary arterial origin in persistent truncus arteriosus. Circulation 55: 551–554

Singh A, de Leval M, Stark J 1975 Total correction of type I truncus arteriosus in a 6-month-old infant. British Heart Journal 37: 1314–1316

Slavik Z, Keeton B R, Salmon A P, Sutherland G R, Fong L V, Monro J L 1994 Persistent truncus arteriosus operated during infancy: long-term follow-up. Pediatric Cardiology 15: 112–115

Smallhorn J F, Anderson R H, Macartney F J 1982 Two dimensional echocardiographic assessment of communications between ascending aorta and pulmonary trunk or individual pulmonary arteries. British Heart Journal 47: 563–572

Smith G W, Thompson W M, Dammann J F, Muller W H 1964 Use of the pulmonary artery banding procedure in treating type II truncus arteriosus. Circulation Supplement, Cardiovascular Surgery 29: 108–113

Spicer R L, Behrendt D, Crowley D C et al 1984 Repair of truncus arteriosus in neonates with the use of a valveless conduit. Circulation 70(suppl I): 26–29

Stark J, Gandhi D, de Leval M, Macartney F, Taylor J F N 1978 Surgical treatment of persistent truncus arteriosus in the first year of life. British Heart Journal 40: 1280–1287

Stark J, Smallhorn J, Huhta J, de Leval M, Macartney F J, Rees P G, Taylor J F 1983 Surgery for congenital heart defects diagnosed by cross-sectional echocardiography. Circulation 68(suppl II): 129–138

Sullivan H, Sulayman R, Replogle R, Arcilla R A 1976 Surgical correction of truncus arteriosus in infancy. American Journal of Cardiology 38: 113–116

Suzuki A, Ho S Y, Anderson R H, Deanfield J E 1989 Coronary arterial and sinusal anatomy in hearts with a common arterial trunk. Annals of Thoracic Surgery 48: 792–797

Thiene G, Bortolotti U, Gallucci V, Terribile V, Pellegrino P A 1976 Anatomic study of truncus arteriosus communis with embryological and surgical considerations. British Heart Journal 38: 1109–1123

Tiller G E, Watson M S, Duncan L M, Dowton S B 1988 Congenital heart defect in a patient with deletion of chromosome 7q. American Journal of Medical Genetics 29: 283–287

van der Horst R L, Gotsman M S 1974 Type 3c truncus arteriosus. Case report with clinical and surgical implications. British Heart Journal 36: 1046–1048

Van Mierop L H S, Patterson D F, Schnarr W R 1978 Pathogenesis of persistent truncus arteriosus in light of observations made in a dog embryo with the anomaly. American Journal of Cardiology 41: 755–762

Van Praagh R, Van Praagh S 1965 The anatomy of common aortico-pulmonary trunk (truncus arteriosus communis) and its embryologic implications. American Journal of Cardiology 16: 406–426

Victorica B E, Krovetz L J, Elliot L P et al 1968 Persistent truncus arteriosus in infancy. American Heart Journal 77: 13–25

Wilson D I, Cross I E, Goodship J A et al 1992 A prospective cytogenetic study of 36 cases of DiGeorge syndrome. American Journal of Human Genetics 51: 957–963

Wilson D I, Burn J, Scambler P, Godship J 1993 DiGeorge syndrome: part of CATCH 22. Journal of Medical Genetics 30: 852–856

Ya J, van den Hoff M J, de Boer P A et al 1998 Normal development of the outflow tract in the rat. Circulation Research 82: 464–472

52

The arterial duct: its persistence and its patency

L. N. Benson and K. N. Cowan

All these arrangements are marvellous, without any question. But we have to consider that it exceeds all expectations how soon the occlusion of all these openings takes place.

(Galen, 129–200 AD)

INTRODUCTION

When Siegal (1962) re-examined Galen's original Greek text, as published by Kuehn (1821–1833), he pointed out that Galen was familiar with many aspects of the fetal circulation even though he did not realize that blood circulated. He understood that fetal blood was aerated in the placenta, and that blood was diverted away from the liver by a short vessel connecting the portal to the inferior caval vein. Galen also knew that blood crossed the oval foramen to bypass the right ventricle and reach the left heart directly. He realized, nonetheless, that some blood still entered the right ventricle and pulmonary trunk, from whence it was shunted into the aorta through a special fetal channel, thereby bypassing the lungs. The quotation at the head of the chapter, taken from Siegal's paper, clearly indicates Galen's understanding of the dramatic readjustment of the circulation at birth.

Botallo described postnatal patency of the oval foramen. By a series of misinterpretations, and careless translations, his name became, quite unjustifiably, attached to the arterial duct (Franklin, 1941). Fabrizi d'Acquapendente, in his *De formate foetu*, provided detailed descriptions of fetal anatomy in humans and other mammals. William Harvey, who was a pupil of Fabrizi in Padova for 2 years, synthesized previous anatomical descriptions in his own writings, but his genius resided in proposing the concept of active circulation of the blood. He stressed the large size of the arterial duct and the fact that blood flowed from right to left through it during fetal life (1628). Harvey was incorrect only in his belief that flow of blood to the lungs was completely lacking in the fetus. Highmore (1651), a friend of Harvey, described closure of the oval foramen and arterial duct as occurring with the onset of respiration. He believed that the arterial duct collapsed as a consequence of blood being diverted to the lungs. Several ingenious theories to explain closure of the duct have been reviewed by Dawes (1982), all being based on postmortem appearances, and all invoking mechanical factors. Strassman (1894) revived an older suggestion of Aranzi (1564). He proposed that the tongue of tissue lying between the duct and the anterior wall of the aortic isthmus functioned as a flap-like valve to close the vessel. It is now generally accepted, however, that no such valve exists. It was Virchow (1856) who first suggested that closure of the arterial duct results from contraction of its mural smooth muscle, while Gerard (1900) introduced the concept of two-stage closure, in which functional constriction is followed by anatomical obliteration. When Huggett (1927) exteriorized a fetal goat and maintained it in stable condition with the placental circulation intact, he brought further studies of the duct into the realm of the physiologist rather than the anatomist. His experimental technique led to the first systematic investigation of how the duct constricts at birth. This eventually led to our understanding of the role of oxygen in effecting functional closure by muscular contraction. These studies will be discussed later in the chapter.

In 1907, in an address to the Philadelphia Academy of Surgery, John Munro first suggested surgical ligation of a patent arterial duct. Thirty-one years later, Graybiel et al (1938) reported the first attempt to perform this operation in a 22-year-old woman with bacterial endocarditis. Unfortunately, although the patient survived the surgery, she died a few days later from complications of the infection. As a result, it was Robert Gross of Boston who performed the first successful ligation of a patent duct in a 7-year-old child with intractable heart failure (Gross and Hubbard, 1939). He thereby introduced an amazing era of progress in the surgery of congenital malformations of the heart. No historical review of the arterial duct, however brief, would be complete without recognizing Gibson's exquisite description of the murmur that typifies its persistence (1898).

NOMENCLATURE

From time to time, authors have argued that the terms 'patent' or 'persistent' are redundancies that should be avoided when describing the arterial duct. In our view, this oversimplifies the situation, and both terms remain useful. Persistence implies that the duct is present after the time of its expected closure and, therefore, distinguishes a pathological from a physiological state. The term patent remains useful in the perinatal period, especially in the premature infant in whom patency can be used to signify a duct that is functionally open, as opposed to one that is functionally closed but retains the potential to reopen.

EMBRYOLOGY AND PATHOGENESIS

During early fetal development, six arterial arches link the aortic sack with the paired dorsal aortas, although all six arches are never present simultaneously. This symmetrical arrangement is transformed to the configuration seen in postnatal life, as some arterial segments disappear and others realign (Congdon, 1922). The normal duct develops from the dorsal portion of the left sixth arch. From their inception, the sixth arches, which are first identifiable at the 5 mm crown–rump stage and become canalized by the 7 mm stage, are associated with the developing lung buds. These buds are initially supplied by a plexus of capillaries that develops from the aortic sack and later connects to the dorsal aorta. The sixth arches develop from the resulting vascular connections between the aortic sack and the dorsal aorta. When the developing arterial segment is divided to form the aorta and the pulmonary trunk, the sixth arches remain continuous with the latter. On the right side, the ventral portion of the sixth arch ultimately becomes the proximal portion of the right pulmonary artery, while the dorsal portion regresses. On the left side, the ventral portion is absorbed into the pulmonary trunk and the dorsal segment becomes the arterial duct.

Developmental anomalies of the aortic arch may be associated with an abnormally situated duct, either patent or represented by a ligament. In such cases, the duct may form part of a vascular ring (Stewart et al, 1964). A right aortic arch, in the greater majority of patients, tends to be associated with intracardiac anomalies (Stewart et al, 1964). These cause blood to be ejected towards the right rather than the left of the primitive arterial arches. One quarter to one third of patients with tetralogy of Fallot have such right-sided aortic arches, usually with mirror-imaged branching, along with a left-sided arterial duct or ligament arising from the

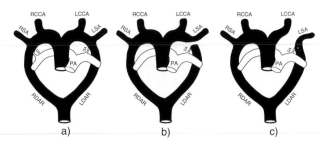

Figure 52.1. The formation of a right aortic arch with mirror-imaged branching, a retro-oesophageal arterial duct and aberrant left subclavian artery: (a) the hypothetical double arch pattern (Edwards, 1948); (b) a retro-oesophageal duct, and (c) an aberrant left subclavian artery (Edwards, 1953). RCCA, right carotid artery; LCCA, left carotid artery; DA, arterial duct; PA, pulmonary artery; LSA, left subclavian artery; RSA, right subclavian artery; RDAR, right dorsal aortic arch; LDAR, left dorsal aortic root.

brachiocephalic trunk. The duct may then connect the left pulmonary artery either to the subclavian portion of the brachiocephalic (innominate) artery or to the upper descending aorta by a remnant of the left dorsal aorta. In the latter, there is a complete vascular ring (Figure 52.1) (Edwards, 1953). A right-sided duct can also be found with a right-sided ascending and descending arch (Akiyama et al, 1992). Such a right-sided duct, or ligament, occurs much less frequently with a right arch and mirror-imaged branching, but it is also associated with the presence of intracardiac anomalies, especially tetralogy of Fallot.

A right aortic arch with an aberrent left subclavian artery and a left duct is the most common form of a complete vascular ring, and this probably arises as an independent developmental error. It is less frequently associated with intracardiac anomalies (Figure 52.2) (Stewart et al, 1964). Numerous reports exist of this anomaly both in children and adults (Stewart et al, 1964). A very rare ductal anomaly also associated with a vascular ring is the so-called ductal sling (Binet et al, 1978), where the duct connects a left descending aorta to the right pulmonary artery, passing between the trachea and oesophagus. A right aortic arch with an aberrent left subclavian artery and a right-sided duct is exceedingly rare but does occur (Gross and Newhauser, 1951; Sones and Effler, 1951–1952).

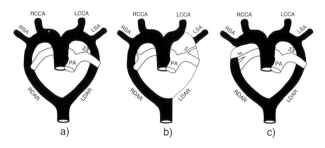

Figure 52.2 Arrangement of different types of double aortic arch. (a) The double aortic arch (Edwards, 1948), with a left duct. (b) Sites of atresia in the left arch (dotted line). (c) Sites of atresia in the right arch. Abbreviations as in Figure 52.1.

In the most common form of double aortic arch, both arches are patent, usually with the right being larger than the left, while the upper part of the descending aorta is also to the left. In these cases, the duct is also on the left and connects the left pulmonary artery to the aorta. Double aortic arch, in which both limbs are patent with either a right duct or bilateral ducts, has not been reported, although the arrangement with bilateral ducts has been induced experimentally in rats deficient for vitamin A (Wilson and Warkany, 1950). Atresia may also occur between the left duct and descending aorta, the left subclavian artery and the duct, or between the left common carotid and subclavian arteries (Figure 52.2) (Shulford et al, 1972). If the atresia is between the left subclavian artery and the duct, or between the left common carotid and subclavian arteries, the duct passes between the left pulmonary artery and the caudal end of the left dorsal aortic root (descending aortic diverticulum). An atretic right arch is exceedingly rare (Figure 52.2). In at least two reported cases, the atresia involved segments of the subclavian artery and a right duct (Ergin et al, 1981; Burrows et al, 1986).

A right duct associated with a normally branching left aortic arch has also been observed. Similarly, the combination of a left aortic arch, right descending aorta and left duct has been described (Airan et al, 1989; Sanchez Torres and Roldan Conesa, 1989). There is no ring when the duct connects the right pulmonary artery to the base of the brachiocephalic artery. If the connection is to the descending aorta by means of a partially persistent right aortic arch, however, then it produces a complete vascular ring.

Bilateral arterial ducts, although rare, have been reported and are associated with intracardiac anomalies (Freedom et al, 1984; Formigari et al, 1992). Kelsey et al (1953) reported a patient who also had a right-sided heart, ventricular septal defects and pulmonary atresia with a patent right duct and a left ligament. The aortic arch was left sided and branched normally. Bilateral ducts with a right aortic arch and a right-sided descending aorta, or isolation of the left subclavian artery, have also been described (Barger et al, 1956; Nair et al, 1992), as has the same combination with the additional anomaly of absence of the proximal left pulmonary artery (Steinberg et al, 1964).

Persistent right, left or bilateral ducts may replace the proximal pulmonary artery (Figure 52.3). The origin of one pulmonary artery from a duct on the same side is not uncommon (Freedom et al, 1992), particularly in the setting of tetralogy with pulmonary atresia (Thiene et al, 1981; Frescura et al, 1984). Bilateral ductal origins for the pulmonary arteries are rare (Murray et al, 1970; Berry et al, 1974; Todd et al, 1976; Freedom et al, 1984).

Absence of the arterial duct was first described as a postmortem finding in 1671, being seen in a grossly malformed infant with an extrathoracic heart and tetralogy of Fallot (see Steno, 1948). Emmanouilides et al (1976)

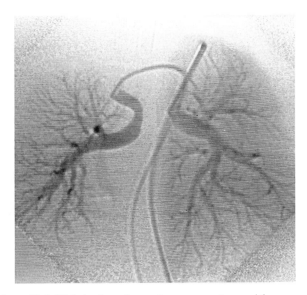

Figure 52.3 Digital subtraction angiogram, superimposed from two different injections, showing ductal origins of both pulmonary arteries. No central pulmonary arteries were present.

reported on four neonates with the syndrome of tetralogy of Fallot, absent pulmonary valve and absent duct; they were able to find seven other reports of this combination of anomalies (Figure 52.4). They postulated that absence of the duct early in fetal life might contribute to the massive dilation of the pulmonary arteries that typifies this syndrome. In the presence of high fetal pulmonary vascular resistance, and increased right ventricular stroke volume secondary to pulmonary regurgitation, the pulmonary arteries become progressively distended because the normal outlet through the duct for most of the right ventricular output is lacking (Emmanouilides et al, 1976; Fischer et al, 1984, Ettedgui et al, 1990). Lack of such marked aneurysmal dilation in those patients with absence of the leaflets of the pulmonary valve and intact ventricular septum in whom the duct is patent tends to support their hypothesis (Freedom et al, 1979; Lau et al, 1990). Isolated examples with a patent duct and dilated arteries, nonetheless, have been reported (Mainwaring et al, 1993).

The duct is also absent in approximately three quarters of patients with a common arterial trunk. Absence of significant flow through the duct in the presence of a larger aortopulmonary connection permits the duct to disappear early in fetal life. In more complex varieties of common arterial trunk, however, such as those with so-called 'absence' of one pulmonary artery, the pulmonary artery itself may originate from a duct. Similarly, in those patients with an associated interruption or atresia of the aortic arch, patency of the duct is essential to maintain systemic perfusion (Freedom et al, 1992; Rossiter et al, 1978).

A number of teratogens that may influence the development of the duct have been identified, including rubella, alcohol, amphetamines and the anticonvulsant

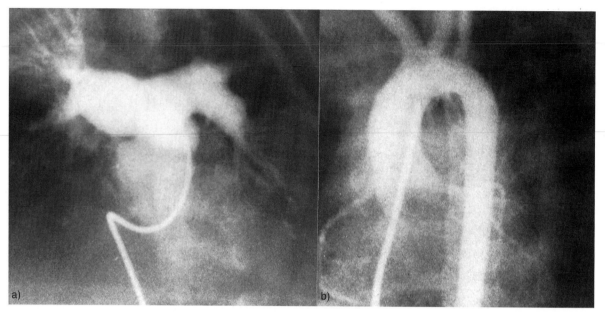

Figure 52.4 Angiogram performed in a neonate with tetralogy of Fallot and rudimentary formation of the leaflets of the pulmonary valve. (a) The massively dilated pulmonary arteries can be seen. (b) The aortogram reveals absence of the duct.

hydantoin (Nora and Nora, 1978). The most sensitive period during which the duct is susceptible to teratogens is from 18 to 60 days of gestation. Absence of the duct has been induced experimentally in chick embryos by the administration of β-adenoceptor agonists. Associated malformations, including anomalies of the aortic arch, ventricular septal defect, overriding aorta or double outlet right ventricle, aortopulmonary window or common arterial trunk, were also induced. Frequencies of malformations were related to the β-stimulating potency of the drug used, and frequency was reduced by pretreatment with blocking agents, especially β-1 blockers. Caffeine and theophylline both potentiated the frequency of malformations, as did cocaine. These findings led Gilbert et al (1977) to propose a mechanism of cardiovascular teratogenesis mediated by cyclic adenosine 3′,5′-monophosphate (cyclic AMP).

ANATOMY

The fetal arterial duct is a short and wide vessel of variable length. It connects the pulmonary arteries to the lesser curve of the arch of the aorta at the point of transition from arch to descending aorta, joining just distal and opposite to the origin of the left subclavian artery. In the fetus, the duct appears very much as the direct continuation of the pulmonary trunk, while the left and right pulmonary arteries are seen as considerably smaller branches from the trunk.

The duct is related posteriorly to the left main bronchus, while anteriorly it is crossed by the vagus nerve. This gives off the left recurrent laryngeal nerve, which encircles the duct before ascending behind the aortic arch into the neck. The pulmonary arterial end of the vessel is covered by a reflection of the pericardium.

Langer (1857) is credited with being the first to recognize that the histological features of the duct differ from those of the adjacent pulmonary artery and aorta. Normal structure of the unconstricted vessel is difficult to study. Most reports relate to tissues that have either undergone partial or complete constriction or to those that have been subjected to mechanical handling and fixation. Many studies fail, however, to distinguish between structural changes resulting from functional constriction and those leading to anatomical obliteration. There is general agreement that the duct is a muscular artery endowed with an intima, media and adventitia. Microscopically, it differs from the adjacent pulmonary trunk and aorta. While the media of the aorta is composed mainly of circumferentially arranged elastic fibers, the media of the duct consists largely of spirally arranged smooth muscle cells directed clockwise and counterclockwise and has an increased content of hyaluronic acid. The intimal layers are thicker than the adjoining vessels and contain increased amounts of mucoid substance (Fay and Cooke, 1972; Gittenberger-de-Groot et al, 1980, 1985). The tissues of the duct in the newborn are rather loosely arranged, with a well-defined internal elastic lamina that may be single or focally duplicated, with small interruptions encountered regularly. The outer two thirds of the lamellas of the aorta and pulmonary arteries merge into the adventitia of the duct without forming an external elastic layer, whereas the inner third passes into the internal elastic lamella. The internal elastic laminas of the great vessels disappear during gestation by splitting into the elastic lamellas. Scattered throughout the media are concentrically arranged layers of elastic tissue, with sparse elastic fibrils running irregularly between them. In longitudinal sections, the elastic fibres of the aorta and pulmonary artery are seen to condense into a coarse elastic band at the orifice of the duct (Jager and Wollenman, 1942). This description of the elastic tissue was confirmed by Holmes (1958). In contrast, Danesino et al (1955) stated that there was no 'true elastic network', and Desligneres and Larroche (1970) described only 'very rare, frail and fragmented' elastic fibres. Electron microscopic studies, nonetheless, confirmed the presence of fine branching strands of microfibril-coated elastin between the layers of smooth muscle cells (Silver et al, 1981)

The arrangement of the smooth muscle cells within the medial layer of the duct has been the subject of numerous light microscopic studies. Graper (1927) described an inner longitudinal layer of muscle fibres, and an outer circular layer interspersed with longitudinal running bundles. Melka (1926) reported a similar arrangement but with a more clearly defined outer longitudinal layer. In contrast, von Hayek (1936) considered the muscle to run in spirals. Silver et al (1981) re-examined this question, finding a predominantly circular arrangement, especially in the outer media. Longitudinally orientated smooth muscle seen in the inner media is sometimes aggregated into one or more columns. This feature of the newborn is not found in stillborn infants. No collagen is seen in the media by light microscopy, but abundant material that strains positively for acid mucopolysaccharides is observed between the muscle and elastic laminas. By electron microscopy, however, it is possible to detect fine collagen fibrils lying between adjacent lamellas of smooth muscle cells and elastin. This is especially so in full-term specimens. At the junctional zones between the duct and the adjacent vessels, the ductal smooth muscle inserts between the endings of the elastic–collagen lamellas of the great arteries. During the second half of gestation, the smooth muscle cells show decreasing evidence of secretory activity, and increasing maturation of their contractile elements.

Vessels cannot close by isolated contraction of circularly arranged muscle (Roach, 1973). Coincident shortening of the less abundant longitudinally arranged muscle fibres is, therefore, critical to effective closure. This shortening probably depends on active attachment of the muscle to the collagen framework of the great vessels in the junctional zones.

The innervation of the duct was examined by Boyd (1941), using light microscopy in fetal newborn and adult ligamental specimens from rabbits and other species. He observed both thick neural fibres, with well marked medullary sheaths, and fine fibres of sympathetic origin. Subsequent studies have confirmed the presence of fine non-myelinated fibres (Holmes, 1958; Boreus et al, 1969; Silver et al, 1981). Histochemical studies have shown adrenergic fibres to be fairly abundant, especially in the adventitia and outer media. Cholinergic fibres are

extremely sparse or totally absent (Aronson et al, 1970). Allan (1955) dissected 15 full-term infants and found that the nerve supply to the duct was predominantly from the inferior cervical sympathetic cardiac nerve. The duct possesses vessels in its walls that may have a role in fuelling contraction at birth (Desligneres and Laroche, 1970; Silver et al, 1981b). Some degree of hyperaemia of these vessels is common in newborn infants.

The appearance of the intima during fetal life is controversial. Many authors have described eccentrically placed intimal cushions or mounds composed of smooth muscle and elastic tissue, the formation of which preceeds normal ductal closure after birth. Beneath these mounds, the internal elastic lamina is often fragmented and split (Figure 52.5) (Melka, 1926; Costa, 1930; Swenson, 1939; Jager and Wollerman, 1942; Danesino et al, 1955; Bakker, 1962; Silver et al, 1981). These mounds are observed early in fetal development. They become progressively thicker and more extensive towards term. Danesino and associates (1955) found them to be most abundant in the mid-portion of the inferior curve of the vessel, attributing them to constriction and shortening of the duct. Electron microscopical studies in rat fetuses towards the end of their gestation revealed striking differences between the contiguous great arteries and the duct (Jones et al, 1969). These observers described striking endothelial projections into the lumen, with large vacuoles in the subendothelial spaces. This formation of subendothelial oedema is the first stage in development of the internal cushions, which is initiated by the separation of the endothelial cells from the internal elastic

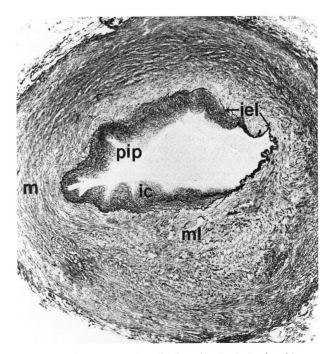

Figure 52.5 Transverse section of a duct showing intimal cushions (ic), postnatal intimal proliferation (pip), media (m) containing no elastic lamallas, mucoid lakes (ml), and a fragmented internal elastic lamina (iel) (van Gieson stain).

lamina, with changes in the components of the extra-cellullar matrix (de Reeder et al, 1989a). This development may herald the sloughing and necrosis of the centrally placed endothelial cells seen in the closed duct. Medial smooth muscle extended through the internal elastic lamina into the protrusions, while many of the medial smooth muscle cells had markedly distended cisterns within the endoplasmic reticulum, suggesting active synthesis of protein. Jones and colleagues (1969) concluded that ductal closure, at least in the rat, is an active morphological process beginning well before birth, thereby supporting several previous similar proposals. Mato and colleagues (1970) studied radioautograms and proposed that migration of medial cells towards the lumen was more important than intimal proliferation as a prelude to closure. This hypothesis was supported by Toda et al (1980), who also attributed prenatal intimal thickening to migration of smooth muscle cells through the internal elastic lamina.

Do the intimal cushions really develop during normal fetal maturation, or do they only occur in a duct that has undergone partial constriction or collapse? Considering the high flow of blood through the fetal duct, it is difficult to conceive that prominent protrusions of intima into the lumen could exist without inducing turbulent flow and a bruit. No such bruit can be heard in the undisturbed duct of the fetal lamb at term. In all the studies in which intimal cushions are described, the structure has been subjected to one or more perturbations, such as relatively slow fixation, mechanical stimulation or cessation of circulation with loss of intraluminal distending pressure. Hornblad and his associates (1969a) challenged the existence of intimal cushions as prenatal structures. In preliminary studies, they showed that storage, mechanical manipulation and fixation in formalin can all induce artefactual changes. Using rapid freezing techniques with either liquid nitrogen or isopentane, the rate of closure of the duct in the rat was found to be temperature dependent. Independent of the degree of closure, the lumen remained round, was without deformation and showed no evidence of formation of mounds. Wall thickness increased, while the internal elastic lamina became corrugated, especially in the mid-portion of the vessels. A decrease in the lumen was associated with accumulation of endothelial cells within the lumen. No mitoses were seen. Hornblad and his associates concluded that closure was aided by passive central displacement of endothelial and inner medial cells but that, in the rat, no part of the media was prenatally prepared for this process. They found significant variation between species in rates of closure and morphology (Hornblad and Larsson, 1967a,b). Closure was most rapid in the guinea pig and rabbit, and more gradual in the rat, pig and lamb (Hornblad, 1969b; Hornblad et al, 1969). In the latter two species, although considerable contraction occurred during the first 30 minutes after delivery, the lumen was not occluded until 8 hours postnatally. Morphological

differences related to the ratio of diameters of the wall thickness and the lumen. Further observations on fetal tissues from various species persuaded Hornblad and colleagues that neither antenatal proliferation of the intima nor migration of medial muscle were important in normal closure of the duct.

Bakker (1962) fixed human fetal ducts with intraluminal formalin at distending pressures comparable to fetal blood pressure. He described the duct as having a wide round lumen in which the intimal cushions can be seen only with 'some difficulty' as 'level thickenings embedded in the rest of the wall with a concave lumen side'. He regarded the cushions as a normal reparative reaction to distending forces during fetal existence.

At birth, the vessel constricts. The intimal thickenings, or cushions, become irregular ridges protruding into the lumen, running mainly lengthwise. By their extrusion, they exert traction on the media causing disorganization and formation of mucoid lakes (Figure 52.6) located mainly on the border between cushions and media.

Anatomical obliteration follows functional closure (Gerard, 1900). The process begins with necrosis of the inner wall caused by anoxia, followed by the formation of dense fibrous tissue. This cytolytic necrosis is characterized by loss of nucleuses, absence of cellular infiltration and persistence of an unaltered elastic skeleton within the wall. Nutrition to the intima and inner media is maintained by diffusion from the lumen and by the still functioning vessels in the wall. The lumen is progressively obliterated by a process of luminal fibrosis, probably representing organization of mural or occlusive thrombus. Eventually, the duct becomes converted into a fibrous strand, the arterial ligament, which may become calcified.

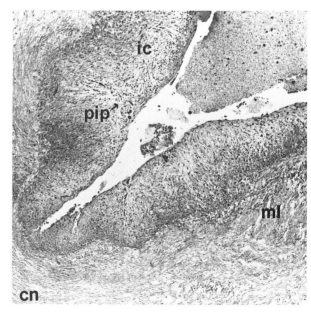

Figure 52.6 Transverse section of the constricted duct. Note the mucoid lakes. cn, connective tissue; other abbreviations as in Figure 52.5.

Anatomical obliteration may take several weeks to complete. About two thirds of ducts are obliterated by 2 weeks (Christie 1930), and almost all by 1 year.

— PHYSIOLOGICAL CONSIDERATIONS—

PATENCY OF THE DUCT DURING FETAL LIFE AND FUNCTIONAL CLOSURE

Ingenious theories concerning closure of the duct abound in the 19th century literature. They have been admirably reviewed by Sciacca and Condorelli (1960). It is now clear that functional closure results from muscular contraction of the wall. How this comes about will be considered in this section. First, we will discuss patency during fetal life.

Although patency was long considered a passive process (Coceani, 1994), there is now considerable evidence to suggest that ductal patency during fetal life is actively maintained by a continuous production of prostaglandin E_2 within the vessel wall (Mathew, 1998). This is, perhaps, augmented by the action of circulating prostanoids (Olley and Coceani, 1981). Prostaglandin E_2 is one of a family of fatty acids synthesized in mammalian tissues from arachidonic acid (Samuelson, 1978). This synthesis, and that of the other prostaglandins, requires the incorporation of molecular oxygen into arachidonic acid. This is then released by various forms of stimulation from the phospholipid of cell membranes. The release of arachidonic acid is inhibited by corticosteroids, but, once it has occurred, it is rapidly transformed by several biosynthetic pathways to form a remarkable array of biologically active compounds. Best known of these pathways is that which depends on cyclooxygenase enzymes; this produces the stable compounds prostaglandin I_2 (prostacyclin) and thromboxane. This pathway is blocked by aspirin, indomethacin (indometacin) and other non-steroidal anti-inflammatory agents, which thus prevent the formation of all the above named products.

The importance of active vasodilation was first shown by Coceani and Olley (1973), who identified the ability of prostaglandins E_1 and E_2 to dilate lamb duct in isolated preparations (Smith, 1998; Mathew, 1998). Since that time, additional work has supported a predominant role for a variety of prostaglandins as ductal vasodilators in several species (Cassin, 1987), including humans (Heymann and Rudolph, 1973; Noah, 1978). In particular, prostaglandin E_2 exhibits the most potent effects (Coceani et al, 1975; Clyman et al, 1978). It appears to be the main prostaglandin regulating ductal tone (Coceani et al, 1978). Prostaglandin E_2 binds to a receptor subtype, prostanoid E_4, that is coupled to a G-protein (Pierce et al, 1995), as characterized in rabbit duct (Smith et al, 1994). This induces a rise in cyclic AMP (Walsh and Mentzer, 1987) through association of the G-protein with adenylyl cyclase (Nishigaki et al, 1995). The mechanism of action was suggested by the studies of Crichton and co-workers (1997), in which the intrinsically high sensitivity of the contractile proteins of the ductal smooth muscle to calcium ions (mediating sustained vasoconstriction) was reduced by a cyclic AMP-dependent pathway initiated by prostaglandin E_2 binding to its prostanoid receptor (Crichton et al, 1997). In addition, the duct may respond in a fashion similar to other tissues, in which elevated cyclic AMP reduces release of calcium from intracellular stores (Karaki et al, 1997). As the contractile apparatus of the smooth muscle is stimulated by calcium ions (Alberts et al, 1994), this mechanism may function to inhibit the contractile processes, thereby maintaining ductal patency in the fetus. Indeed, the importance of prostaglandins to the maintenance of ductal patency has been confirmed using indomethacin, which inhibits production of prostaglandin E_2.

In additional studies, the role of the vasodilator nitric oxide in maintaining ductal patency has also been investigated. Walsh and colleagues (1988) were able to show that oxygen-induced ductal closure was markedly attenuated by donors of nitric oxide, either nitroprusside or glyceryl trinitrate (nitroglycerin). This effect was shown to be mediated through a rise in intracellular concentrations of cyclic nucleotides (Walsh and Mentzer, 1987) and could be correlated with the regulation of calcium-dependent contraction, similar to the situation with prostaglandin E_2. Application of nitric oxide, both in vitro (Coceani et al, 1994a) and in vivo (Fox et al, 1996), induced ductal contraction associated with a reduction in cyclic 3′,5′-guanosine monophosphate (cyclic GMP) (Coceani et al, 1996). This contractile response was not entirely abolished by denudation of the ductal endothelium, implying the involvement of additional sources of nitric oxide (Coceani et al, 1994a). Subsequent descriptive studies of the fetal ductal wall during late gestation have identified local sites of production that are richly immunoreactive to antibodies against endothelial nitric oxide synthetase. These are found along the endothelium (Fox et al, 1996), and within the vessels supplying the wall. Specific reactivity for inducible nitric oxide synthase is also seen in the luminal endothelium (Clyman et al, 1998). More recent studies have also implicated ductal smooth muscle cells, immunoreactive for nitric oxide synthetase, in the production of nitric oxide. Despite this supportive evidence, Fox et al (1996) have reported that inhibition of nitric oxide synthases by Nω-nitro-L-arginine induces a very modest contraction of the duct in fetal lambs compared with that observed with indomethacin, when ductal flow was decreased while resistance increased. Consequently, the role of nitric oxide in maintaining ductal patency is likely accessory to the more profound effect on ductal tone exerted by prostaglandin E_2. This was further supported by the finding in indomethacin-treated, and endothelium-denuded, rabbit ducts that the maximal effect of sodium nitroprusside was only a small part of the maximal relaxation caused by prostaglandin E_2 (Smith and McGrath, 1993). This indicates that nitric oxide, on its own, cannot overcome the vasoconstriction caused by indomethacin.

Enzymes capable of producing other gaseous biological messengers have been localized by Coceani and colleagues (1994a) to ductal endothelial and smooth muscle cells. Following characterization of carbon monoxide as a potent vasodilatory substance (Coceani, 1993), this group has characterized the expression of haem oxygenase-1, the inducible form of the carbon monoxide synthesizing enzyme, in lamb ductal endothelial cells. Both the type 1 and type 2 constitutive forms of haem oxygenase were identified in ductal smooth muscle cells (Coceani et al, 1997). The dilation induced by carbon monoxide is mediated either through stimulation of cyclic GMP or through effects on membrane potassium channels (Werkstrom et al, 1997). Contraction of the duct by a haem oxygenase inhibitor, zinc protoporphyrin IX, in contrast, occurred only under restricted conditions (Coceani et al, 1997). Taken together, these data indicate that, while numerous dilatory agents may interact in concert to counteract vasoconstriction (probably through regulation of intracellular stores of calcium and responsiveness of the contractile apparatus to these ions), the greatest consistent influence on ductal patency is exerted by prostaglandins, in particular prostaglandin E_2. Other prostaglandins, including prostaglandin I_2, similarly relax the duct, but much less strongly and with a higher threshold for their action.

Blockade of synthesis of prostaglandin by inhibition of cyclooxygenase close to term constricts the fetal duct, both experimentally and during life (Sharpe et al, 1974; Olley et al, 1975; Heymann and Rudolph, 1976; Clyman, 1980, 1987; Coceani and Olley, 1980). The degree of indomethacin-induced constriction under hypoxic conditions equals that produced by oxygen in control tissues. This constricting effect is more marked in tissues from immature animals. It is fully reversed by treatment with prostaglandin E_2 or E_1 (Heymann and Rudolph, 1976; Coceani et al, 1979), indicating that the prostaglandins play an active role in maintaining ductal patency during fetal life. Both indomethacin and ibuprofen, when given in therapeutic doses to near-term pregnant ewes, constrict the fetal duct. Although the constriction varies in degree, it is as marked in some cases as that observed in the untreated newborn lamb. It results in virtual complete closure of the duct.

The exact sites of production of prostaglandin are unclear (Clyman, 1980; Coceani and Olley, 1980; Clyman and Heymann, 1981; de Reeder, 1989b), but both prostaglandin E_2 and prostaglandin I_2 are formed intramurally (de Reeder, 1989b). Although prostaglandins are detectable in very low concentrations in the plasma of adults, there is little evidence that they act as circulating hormones, because they are rapidly catabolized in the lung. In the fetus, however, high circulating concentra-

tions are present, partly because of the reduced pulmonary blood flow and partly because of their placental production. At birth, concentrations are reduced when the placental source is removed and flow of blood to the lungs allows for increased catabolism. Ductal patency or closure appears to be a balance between the constricting effects of oxygen (see below) and, perhaps, other vasoactive constricting and relaxing substances (Clyman, 1987).

Present evidence suggests that increased oxygen tension, loss of dilatory prostaglandins and activity of contractive prostaglandins together contribute to induce constriction of the duct in the neonate (Smith, 1998). A fall in the levels of both locally released prostaglandin (E_2 and E_1) and circulating prostaglandins (E_2), which are believed to be synthesized mainly in the placenta (Thorburn, 1992; Clyman, 1987), may thus contribute to vasoconstriction of the duct in the neonate. Clyman et al (1980) have demonstrated that circulating levels of prostaglandin E_2 decrease tenfold by 1 hour, and 20-fold by 3 hours, after birth in the newborn lamb. Furthermore, treatment of humans, as well as experimental animals, with prostaglandins alone prevents postnatal closure of the duct (Olley et al, 1976; Host et al, 1988; Jarkovska et al, 1992). Consequently, loss of the vasodilatory effect of prostaglandin is probably central to constriction of the duct in the neonate, although the major factor stimulating contraction appears to be a consequence of increased arterial tension of oxygen. The duct experiences this shortly after delivery as a result of the flow of highly oxygenated blood from the aorta following reversal of the shunt (Smith, 1998).

Increases in oxygen tension stimulate an antagonistic, vasoconstrictive prostaglandin pathway. Studies by Smith and McGrath (1995) have documented the presence of both dilator and contractile receptors to prostaglandin in the duct. Inhibition of prostaglandin I_2 synthase by elevated oxygen tension (Needleman et al, 1981), promotes the formation of prostaglandin H_2. As prostaglandin H_2 is a precursor of prostaglandin E_2, this may account for reports showing increased production of prostaglandin E_2 by the isolated lamb duct in response to oxygen (Coceani et al, 1986). In this context, however, modulation of the function of the vasodilatory prostaglandin receptor by stimulation of vasoconstrictive receptors may potentiate the constrictive response by promoting interaction of prostaglandin E_2 with its normally unligated contractile receptor (Smith and McGrath, 1995). Indeed, Coceani and colleagues (1975) have documented an insensitivity of ductal tissue to dilation by prostaglandin E_2 at the physiological tensions of oxygen observed in the neonate, suggesting a dilatory receptor. Therefore, a shift in the balance of usage of receptors to prostaglandin has been proposed as a mechanism of amplification that would increase ductal vasoconstriction after birth in response to increased tensions of oxygen (Smith and McGrath, 1991).

In addition to this contractile pathway involving prostaglandin, vasoconstriction is induced in response to increased oxygen saturation of oxygen through release of the potent vasoconstrictor endothelin-1 from ductal endothelial and smooth muscle cells. This is mediated by cytochrome P450 (Fay, 1971; Coceani et al, 1992). Cyanide inhibited the contraction of the duct induced by oxygen, and this demonstrated a link in the balance between oxygen and exposure to carbon monoxide to modulation of the activity of membrane-bound cytochrome P450 (Coceani et al, 1988a,b). In response to oxygen, this cytochrome is selectively expressed in the duct. It regulates production of endothelin-1 through a putative monooxygenase intermediate (Coceani et al, 1994b). Production and secretion of endothelin-1 by both ductal endothelium and smooth muscle cells alike (Coceani and Kelsey, 1991) is controlled by the rate-limiting cytochrome oxygen sensor. This potently induces vasoconstriction of the duct (Coceani et al, 1989) following ligation of a population of endothelin subtype A receptors (Coceani et al, 1992). Endothelin A receptor signalling involves phospholipase C and mediates both a rapid transient and subsequently sustained rise in intracellular release of calcium ions (Miyauchi and Masaki, 1999). Consequently, relaxation of isolated ductal tissue from fetal lambs and guinea pigs close to term is induced by independent administration of carbon monoxide, an inhibitor of cytochrome P450 (1-aminobenztriazole), an antagonist for the cytochrome P450 endothelin A receptor (phosphoramidon), an inhibitor of endothelin-converting enzyme (BQ-123) or an antagonist for the endothelin A receptor (Coceani et al, 1988b, 1992, 1996).

It appears that ductal patency during fetal life is maintained by inhibition of intracellular release of calcium and by insensitivity of the contractile proteins of smooth muscle cells to calcium ions. The cyclic monophosphate secondary messengers mediating this response are induced by circulating and local prostaglandins, together with nitric oxide and carbon monoxide. The relaxed state of the duct is rapidly reversed at birth by loss of placental derived prostaglandins and a rise in oxygen tension. This inhibits prostaglandin synthases and induces the contractile prostaglandin receptors. The subsequent drop in cyclic AMP levels increases the sensitivity of ductal smooth muscle cells to calcium and enhances vasoconstriction through cytosolic calcium released by endothelin-1.

Prostaglandin $F_{2\alpha}$ is unique among the prostaglandins in contracting the lamb duct when administered in high doses. Starling and Elliot (1974) reported a contractile effect of prostaglandin $F_{2\alpha}$ on the isolated duct of the calf, and they proposed that it might be the elusive 'oxygen messenger'. In their experiments, not only did prostaglandin $F_{2\alpha}$ contract the vessel, but the contraction increased in intensity when the content of oxygen was increased. It abated after treatment with an antagonist of prostaglandin or a blocker of its synthesis. The findings

of Coceani and Olley (1973) suggested, however, that this hypothesis was incorrect, or at least that it did not apply to other species. Although prostaglandin $F_{2\alpha}$ does constrict the duct in the lamb, this action only occurs at doses that are several orders of magnitude greater than those at which prostaglandin E_2 exerts its relaxant effect. Moreover, the action does not correlate with oxygen tension of the medium, and the oxygen-induced contraction is not reduced by pretreatment with agents that block synthesis. In fact, the action is often enhanced. The contractile response to prostaglandin $F_{2\alpha}$, therefore, is pharmacological rather than physiological.

Thromboxane A_2, a related derivative of the cyclooxygenase pathway, has also been proposed as the chemical mediator of ductal constriction (Friedman, 1978). There is little to support this view. Neither thromboxane A_2 nor its more stable metabolite thromboxane B_2 have any experimental effect on the duct. Thromboxane A_2 does not appear to be produced in the duct.

More recently, other products of the lipoxygenase-controlled biosynthetic pathways of arachidonic acid have been screened. They, also, have been shown to have little effect on muscular tone in the duct of the lamb.

At present, the hypothesis that ductal patency depends on a continuous production of prostaglandin E_2 within the walls of vessels is secure (Olley and Coceani, 1987; Coceani and Olley, 1988). This role has now been exploited clinically, as will be discussed later in the chapter.

THE MECHANISM OF FUNCTIONAL CLOSURE OF THE DUCT

Functional closure of the duct depends on abrupt contraction of its muscular wall. Systematic study of this dramatic event was first undertaken by Kennedy and Clark (1941, 1942), and by Barcroft and colleagues (1946). It was Kennedy and Clark who first suggested that closure was initiated by the increased content of oxygen in the circulating blood after the first breath. During fetal life, the duct is exposed to the intraluminal oxygen contained in pulmonary arterial blood, which has a tension of around 18 mmHg, and to the oxygen of blood that perfuses the vessels of the ductal wall. Additional vessels originating from the descending aorta just below the insertion of the duct, and from the left coronary artery, have also been described as supplying the wall. The tension of oxygen in the blood in these vessels would be somewhat higher, but the maximum would not exceed 28 mmHg. Normally, arterial tension of oxygen increases rapidly after the first breath, to above 50 mmHg (Kennedy and Clark, 1942).

Barcroft et al (1938) originally believed that closure was neurogenic. Using guinea pigs, they showed that a wide variety of stimulation induced ductal constriction. The work of Barclay and associates (1939) deserves special mention, because they used the then novel diagnostic tool of angiography. In fetal sheep close to term, using serial radiographs, they demonstrated ductal closure shortly after delivery. Kennedy and Clark (1941, 1942) also studied ductal closure in guinea pigs. They observed that closure occurred within 10 minutes of either normal breathing or artificial inflation of the lungs with air, even after all nervous input to the vessel was obliterated. Expansion of the lungs with nitrogen failed to induce closure, but injection of oxygen into a vein without inflation of the lungs did. Kennedy and Clark concluded that oxygen was the primary stimulus to ductal constriction and that it acted independently of nervous input. Record and McKeown (1953a, 1955) exposed newborn guinea pigs to inspired air with a reduced content of oxygen for 24 hours. At postmortem, they found the duct to be more visibly patent than in control animals.

Closure of the duct was then studied in exteriorized lamb fetuses. The actions of various types of stimulation on the vessel could be measured by direct observation (Born et al, 1956). Ventilation of the lamb with oxygen, so that systemic saturation rose to 90% or more, caused the duct to constrict. This response could not be prevented by bilateral sympathectomy, vagotomy or even complete disruption of the brain and spinal cord. Cross-perfusion experiments using a second lamb further supported the concept of a direct action of oxygen on the duct. In the same series of experiments, constriction of the duct was observed in response to asphyxia, and to infusions of adrenaline (epinephrine) and noradrenaline (norepinephrine). Further support for the Kennedy–Clark hypothesis was provided by the experiments of Assali et al (1963), and by those of Zapol and colleagues (1971). Although, by the mid-1950s, the importance of oxygen as the trigger to ductal closure was firmly established, there was little information concerning its mechanism of action.

Kovalcik (1963) studied isolated spiral strips of the duct of lambs, or rings of the guinea pig duct, in an organ bath. During equilibrium at extremely low tensions of oxygen, the tissues slowly contracted over a period of 2 to 3 hours before stabilizing. Oxygen induced large and sustained contractions that developed within 5 minutes of exposure. Repeated exposure to oxygen abolished this reaction, although responsiveness to certain drugs was maintained. No difference in behaviour was found between tissues from premature lambs and those born at term. The findings in the guinea pig were the same. In the presence of oxygen, both acetylcholine and noradrenaline contracted the duct, with the action of acetylcholine being more marked. In the absence of oxygen, the effect of both agents was much reduced. Histamine had no effect, and bradykinin was contractile. The action of noradrenaline was blocked by dibenamine and that of acetylcholine by atropine, although the response to oxygen was preserved. From these experiments, Kovalcik concluded that oxygen acts directly on the arterial duct. He speculated that this responsiveness to oxygen represented an especially well-developed example of a general biological phenomenon in which vascular smooth muscle tone is dependent upon the tension of oxygen. He further proposed that oxygen acts by releasing an endogenous hormone from receptive cells, or by accelerating a rate-limiting enzyme.

From studies on ducts from guinea pig mounted in an organ bath so that both the luminal and exterior surfaces could be exposed to solutions of differing oxygen tension, Fay (1971) found that responsiveness of the duct to oxygen was more sensitive than appeared from Kovalcik's experiments. Fay showed that the postnatal rise in tension from 25 to 80 mmHg was sufficient to initiate and maintain ductal closure against arterial pressures of up to 100 mmHg. Furthermore, the action of oxygen was independent of neural involvement. There was no evidence favouring site-specific oxygen receptors. He obtained evidence of a stimulatory action of oxygen on cytochrome a_3, resulting in accelerated synthesis of high energy phosphates. In later work, Fay et al (1977) demonstrated a steep gradient in tensions of oxygen within ductal tissue, such that the core tension could be sufficiently low to limit activity of the respiratory chain. He suggested that changes in the electrical activity of the surface membranes might be involved in the response to oxygen. There is some evidence to indicate that oxygen induces a conductance change in the sarcolemma of the smooth muscle cell, which results in depolarization coupled to contraction (Roulet and Coburn, 1981). In the same experiments, evidence was also obtained that favoured a mechanism of contraction which was independent of membrane potentials.

While Kovalcik (1963) observed no difference in sensitivity to oxygen between the immature and mature tissue, McMurphy and Boreus (1971) found definite age-dependent differences. Ducts from legally aborted mid-term fetuses proved sensitive to acetylcholine, and somewhat less so to histamine. They did not respond to oxygen. The investigators suggested that sensitivity to oxygen is a late development in the duct. This concept was further explored by McMurphy et al (1972) in isolated ducts obtained from fetal lambs ranging in age from 90 to 150 days. With increasing maturity of the duct, they again found lack of responsiveness of immature tissues and a progressively lower threshold for oxygen.

REMODELLING OF THE ARTERIAL DUCT ——

Ductal closure becomes permanent following completion of a phase of remodelling that begins in the last third of gestation and continues into neonatal life. The duct differs from both the aorta and the pulmonary trunk in terms of the orientation of its smooth muscle cells and the deposition of extracellular matrix. Rather than the circumferential orientation of smooth muscle cells observed in the other vessels, ductal smooth muscle cells are arranged in cylindrical layers that spiral in opposing directions (Brook and Heymann, 1995). These layers, which tend to be thicker than in the other vessels, underline a relatively thick intima that contains excess mucoid substance. Pre-emptive changes in the orientation of the smooth muscle cells, and the content and structure of the extracellular matrix, are observed during late gestation (Gittenberger-de-Groot et al, 1980). These alterations, which parallel those characterized in many occlusive vascular diseases (Ross, 1986; Rabinovitch, 1998), involve the formation of vascular lesions known in the duct as 'intimal cushions'. Unlike in pathogenesis, the observed vascular changes in the duct appear to be driven and orchestrated by a developmental programme (Rabinovitch, 1996). Morphological studies of the formation of cushions in humans and in animal models revealed a variety of features, which included fragmentation of elastic laminas, subendothelial accumulation of glycosaminoglycans and apparent proliferation of smooth muscle cells with migration into the subendothelium (Yoder, 1978; Gittenberger-de-Groot et al, 1980; Silver et al, 1981; Rabinovitch, 1996). These changes, which have been divided into four developmental stages by Gittenberger-de-Groot et al (1980), commence at both ends of the duct at approximately 5 months of gestation (Hammerman, 1995). In the first stage, this duct is characterized by a continuous circumferential internal elastic lamina upon which rests the basement membrane and an endothelial monolayer. The media is layered by longitudinally oriented smooth muscle cells and surrounded by adventitia, thus resembling a normal muscular systemic artery. Progression through the second and third stages involves increased intimal thickening related to accumulation of smooth muscle cells and expansion of the subendothelial space. In the fourth and final stage of ductal development, contact and fusion of the cushions promotes luminal accumulation of loose fibrous matrix, which anatomically closes the conduit. A variable rate of progression accounts for preterm and term infants exhibiting ductal maturation ranging through the second to the fourth stages (Gittenberger-de-Groot et al, 1980). In addition, infants presenting with a clinically patent duct that persists beyond the first week of life, a concept explored later in detail, have led to an additional classification by Gittenberger-de-Groot et al (1980). Based on structural morphology, these vessels still have a subendothelial elastic lamina bordering the lumen and are often identical to the normal first stage. It is unclear whether this represents the original elastic lamina or an additional lamina deposited on top of the first (Gittenberger-de-Groot, 1977).

The earliest changes, detected by descriptive studies, are associated with modifications of the extracellular matrix (Gittenberger-de-Groot et al, 1985; Rabinovitch et al, 1988). In particular, de Reeder et al (1988) examined ducts from normal neonatal beagles, as well as a strain of dogs in which an uncharacterized genetic defect leads to a persistently patent arterial duct. As part of the early events mediating intimal thickening in normal dogs, endothelial cells were observed to detach. An increase in hyaluronan and chondroitin sulphate did not occur in the line of beagles with patent ducts, and there was a reduction in the amount of additional extracellular matrix proteins, specifically fibronectin and collagen type III. The extracellular matrix components laminin and collagen type I were also lost from within the basal lamina (de Reeder et al, 1989a). These features are consistent with other models; in fetal lambs impairment of elastin assembly, together with high levels of monomeric tropoelastin, is added to the extensive remodelling of the extracellular matrix occurring within the duct (Zhu et al, 1993). This pre-emptive remodelling suggests roles for a modified extracellular matrix in mediating proliferation, migration and/or differentiation of ductal cells.

Consistent with the concept that remodelling of the extracellular matrix correlates with, and may promote, changes in cellular function, ultrastructural reports by Yoder et al (1978) in rabbit duct during late gestation documented the appearance of mitotic smooth muscle cells, as well as migratory smooth muscle cells as based on their altered radial orientation. Many of these migratory cells were protruding through breaks within the internal elastic lamina, suggesting an important role for proliferation and migration in formation of the cushions (Hinek and Rabinovitch, 1993). Zhou and colleagues (1998) used cell culture to characterize further the unique activities of ductal smooth muscle cells as suggested by their morphological development. The central 'orchestrator' of these changes appears to be transforming growth factor-β (TGF-β). A 'developmentally programmed' enhancement of translational efficiency of the messenger RNA results in abundant secretion by ductal endothelial cells (Zhou et al, 1998) and regulates increased production of hyaluronan (Boudreau and Rabinovitch, 1991; Boudreau et al, 1992). Sequestration of the growth factor with neutralizing antibodies arrests accumulation of hyaluronan. This temporal induction of synthesis is attenuated as a result of destabilization of its message following completion of formation of the cushions, and correspondingly, synthesis of hyaluronan declines. Very recently, the growth factor has also been shown to suppress apoptosis of the smooth muscle cells, thus contributing to modulation of the smooth muscle cell phenotype by enabling survival and proliferation on a remodelled matrix (Inishi et al, 1998). The mechanism related to activation of this programme remains unknown, although it may be related to activation by retinoic acid, as the expression of the promoter for this molecule temporally parallels that of TGF-β (Rabinovitch, 1996).

Further characterization and comparison of the biochemical nature of these smooth muscle cells relative to those of the surrounding vessels indicated a rise in the glycosaminoglycan chondroitin sulphate in response to endothelially derived factors, probably TGF-β (Boudreau and Rabinovitch, 1991). This glycosaminoglycan contributes to remodelling by dissociating elastin-binding proteins from the surfaces of the ductal smooth muscle cells (Hinek et al, 1991). Elastin-binding proteins, together with additional complex components, are proposed to mediate the assembly of elastin fibres on the surface of the cells (Hinek et al, 1988). In addition, unlike smooth muscle cells from the aorta or pulmonary arteries, cultured ductal smooth muscle cells produce a truncated form of tropoelastin (Hinek et al, 1993). This product lacks the carboxy-terminus, suggesting that impaired movement out of solution may result from an inability to align and cross-link on the microfibrillar scaffolding provided by elastin. Truncated elastin causally arises in these cells because of their deficiency of the elastin-binding protein, as this protein normally acts as a 'protective' companion (Hinek et al, 1991). Since elastin-binding protein shares the elastin-binding motif of serine elastases (Hinek et al, 1993), it prevents these enzymes from attaching to the newly synthesized tropoelastin during intracellular trafficking (Hinek and Rabinovitch, 1994). Subsequently, the degradation of tropoelastin in the absence of elastin-binding protein results in a truncated product. Moreover, following transfection of the elastin-binding protein, increased expression in the ductal smooth muscle cells results in a phenotypic modulation from the migratory to the quiescent contractile characteristics of normal vascular smooth muscle cells. These findings correlate with observations pertaining to, and accounting for, the abnormal assembly of elastic laminas in the duct.

As smooth muscle cells are positively chemotactic for peptides derived from elastin (Mecham et al, 1984; Senior et al, 1984), these soluble tropoelastin peptides can promote chemotaxis of ductal smooth muscle cells into the subendothelium during ductal thickening. Furthermore, with reduction in expression of elastin-binding proteins, these smooth muscle cells show enhanced motility through assembled elastin membranes (Hinek et al, 1992). Indeed, induction of migration by aortic smooth muscle cells on elastin requires treatment with chondroitin sulphate, and 'shedding' of their elastin-binding proteins. Therefore, loss of elastin-binding protein permits the migration of ductal smooth muscle cells through the elastin laminas by preventing immobolizing adhesion to elastin. Recent evidence, however, suggests that elastin peptides also stimulate synthesis of fibronectin.

The phenotype of the migratory ductal smooth muscle cell is also enhanced by temporal increases in the production of both fibronectin and hyaluronan, while changes in the synthesis of other extracellular matrix proteins, such as laminin and collagen type IV, were unremarkable (Boudreau et al, 1991; Boudreau and Rabinovitch, 1991). This temporal induction occurs at the end of the second third of gestation in fetal lambs. Hyaluronan is an extraordinarily large, negatively charged glycosaminoglycan that associates with osmot-

ically active cations, therefore, and is heavily hydrated. This provides expansion of the connective tissue space, which is permissive to cell migration. Cells, however, can directly migrate on hyaluronan through expression of the cell surface hyaluronan-binding protein, the receptor for hyaluronan-mediated motility (Turley and Torrance, 1985; Turley et al, 1991). In this regard, hyaluronan-supplemented collagen gels had enhanced migration of ductal smooth muscle cells that was blocked by antibodies to motility receptors (Boudreau et al, 1991). Consistent with studies in transformed cells (Hall et al, 1994), this enhanced motility was shown to be co-dependent on increased incorporating of fibronectin into the matrix, being arrested by soluble integrin peptides and functional blocking antibodies. It also involved the formation and rapid turnover of focal adhesion contacts (Boudreau et al, 1991). The observed directional migration from the media, through the elastin lamina and into the subendothelium, is probably related to the formation of a gradient of fibronectin between these vascular compartments produced by the combined deposition of fibronectin by endothelial and smooth muscle cells. In addition, the elongated migratory ductal smooth muscle cells accumulate the motility receptors preferentially on their leading edge (Boudreau et al, 1991). This, therefore, may act to polarize the cell towards the hyaluronan-rich basement membrane synthesized by the endothelial cells.

Synthesis of fibronectin, which is critical for migration of the smooth muscle cells and, thus, ductal closure, is regulated by the efficiency of translation of messenger RNA. Zhou et al (1997) have shown that translation of this message is controlled, at least in part, by an AU-rich element in the 3′-untranslated region. Production of nitric oxide, as a result of increased neuronal and endothelial expression of nitric oxide synthetases, specifically in the arterial duct compared with the aorta increases expression and phosphorylation of the binding protein light chain-3 microtubules. The phosphorylated light chain-3 binds to the AU-rich elements of the fibronectin message. This enhances sorting and localization of the fibronectin message onto the rough endoplasmic reticulum for translation and, hence, increases synthesis of fibronectin (Zhou and Rabinovitch, 1998). Therefore, apart from its minor contribution to ductal patency, the primary role of nitric oxide in the duct appears to be the temporal increase of expression of fibronectin, which is translated into enhanced directional migration of the ductal smooth muscle cells.

While the pathways involved in the selective upregulation of expression of nitric oxide synthetase, and production of nitric oxide in the duct, remain unclear, recent observations have suggested two potential mechanisms. As previously indicated, ductal smooth muscle cells increase their synthesis of fibronectin in response to soluble elastin peptides. This pathway may be mechanistically linked through effects on release of nitric oxide following stimulation by elastin peptide. Alternatively, a very recent report indicates that TGF-β stimulates transport and metabolism of L-arginine in vascular smooth muscle cells (Durante et al, 1998). As L-arginine is the precursor of nitric oxide, TGF-β may be involved in regulating ductal dynamics by enhancing and/or promoting the effects of nitric oxide. Consequently, as TGF-β mediates loss of elastin-binding protein, and this promotes elastin peptide biosynthesis, TGF-β continues to be implicated as the master orchestrator of the formation of the intimal cushions within the duct.

While considerable research remains to be done, these processes describe a specific and temporal sequence of developmentally programmed events within the duct that initiate and mediate the remodelling phase of ductal closure, associated with formation of the intimal cushions. Together, the intimal cushions and muscular constriction at birth probably trigger pathways that culminate in permanent anatomical closure of the arterial duct. This transition ultimately depends on fibrotic changes, potentially mediated through loss of flow and the resultant ischaemia. This involves destruction of the endothelial cells, apoptosis and necrosis of smooth muscle cells and extensive alterations in, and loss of, extracellular matrix (Clyman, 1987; Slomp et al, 1992).

STEROIDS AND THE ARTERIAL DUCT

Glucocorticoids inhibit the release of arachidonic acid from cell membranes. This probably occurs via binding to a specific glucocorticoid receptor. This initiates a series of events that cause synthesis of a specific modulating protein (Russo-Marie and Duval, 1980). Reduced availability of arachidonic acid, the precursor for prostaglandin E_2, might be anticipated to induce ductal constriction in the fetus. Momma et al (1981) induced fetal ductal contraction by injecting glucocorticoids into rats at the 21st day of pregnancy. The fetuses were studied using the rapid whole-body freezing technique described by Hornblad (1969a). For all glucocorticoids tested, constriction began in the first hour after injection and was maximal between 1 and 4 hours after hydrocortisone, at 2 hours after prednisolone, and at 4 hours after betamethasone. Mild but significant ductal constriction persisted at 24 hours after each glucocorticoid. Injection of massive doses of each glucocorticoid resulted in complete constriction, the relative potency being roughly 1, 2 and 20 for hydrocortisone, prednisolone and betamethasone, respectively. A definite effect on the duct was observed with 0.2 mg/kg betamethasone. Momma et al (1981) also observed a more marked effect on premature than on mature fetuses. This finding accords with other data indicating that the prostaglandin system is aged dependent, being more active in the immature fetus.

Hydrocortisone also decreases the sensitivity of the duct to prostaglandin E_2. Rings of lamb duct from fetuses treated with hydrocortisone show a significantly larger oxygen-induced contraction than do age-matched controls. Baseline tensions developed in an environment of low oxygen were similar. Indomethacin induced a further contraction in both pretreated tissues. Consequently, the overall tension developed in the two groups was not significantly different. These findings are certainly consistent with the concept that endogenous prostaglandins maintain patency of the duct during fetal life by reducing its ability to contract in response to oxygen. Hydrocortisone, by reducing the availability of the precursor of prostaglandin E_2 and, therefore, of prostaglandin E_2, increases the sensitivity to oxygen. This raises the possibility that endogenous corticoids, which normally increase in the plasma towards term, may be important in priming the duct for normal closure (Clyman et al, 1981a).

Support for this view derives from another observation by Clyman and colleagues (1981b). They studied premature infants born to women given betamethasone prior to labour to reduce the incidence of respiratory distress syndrome. Among infants delivered more than 24 hours after treatment, the overall incidence of ductal patency was significantly lower compared with unmatched controls. This trend was apparent irrespective of weight and was independent of the duration of rupture of the membranes. In a blinded placebo-controlled study, however, antenatal treatment with betamethasone was shown to have had no constrictive effect (Eronen et al, 1993). Similar observations were noted when betamethasone and indomethacin were given in the fetal rat (Momma and Takao, 1989), with a marked increase in ductal constriction when administered together. No increase in indomethacin-induced constriction was found when betamethasone was given 24 hours prior to indomethacin. These observations need further confirmation in other properly designed prospective studies. Nonetheless, they certainly fit well with current concepts concerning the control of fetal ductal tone.

BRADYKININ AND THE ARTERIAL DUCT

Bradykinin is a vasoactive nonapeptide released from its inactive precursor kininogen by a serine protease, kallikrein. Kovalcik (1963) found that bradykinin constricts the duct of both the lamb and the guinea pig when the tension of oxygen exceeds 5.3 kPa. This action was confirmed in fetal sheep (McMurphy et al, 1972). The peptide is also a potent vasoconstrictor of human and lamb umbilical vessels in an environment of greater tension of oxygen. It has minimal effects, however, at concentrations that resemble those of the fetus. Bradykinin, furthermore, is a potent pulmonary vasodilator in both fetal and newborn lambs (Campbell et al, 1968). Melmon and associates (1968) proposed that bradykinin might mediate the circulatory transition from fetal to adult states. Support for this novel hypothesis came from their own experiments, which showed, first, that concentrations of bradykinin in human cord blood were some sixfold greater than adult levels and, second, that arterial blood from the cord contained both kallikrein and kininogen. Plasma kallikrein was activated, with subsequent production of kinin, both by exposure to neonatal granulocytes or by a decrease in temperature from 37° to 27°C. This drop in temperature is comparable to that which occurs in blood from the umbilical artery at birth. Unfortunately for their theory, some infants included in their study showed no increase in blood kinin levels but had normal neonatal transitions, with normal closure of the duct. Expansion of the fetal lamb lungs with oxygen apparently activates kininogen and releases bradykinin, most probably from the lungs. Mechanical expansion alone has no effect (Heymann et al, 1969). These findings can be related to more recent knowledge linking the bradykinin system to the prostaglandin cascade. Kinins induce formation and release of prostaglandin from both bovine umbilical arteries and veins (Terragano et al, 1977). Human umbilical vessels synthesize two or three times more prostaglandins than other vascular tissues. While production of prostaglandin I_2 predominates in all other fetal vessels, however, the umbilical artery produces predominantly prostaglandin E_2 and the umbilical vein produces prostaglandin $F_{2\alpha}$. Both of these agents constrict the vessels from which they are produced.

Present knowledge would suggest that bradykinin is unlikely to be involved in physiological closure of the duct. Its stimulatory action is on phospholipase activity. It is, therefore, more likely to induce formation of prostaglandin I_2 within the duct. This relaxes rather than constricts the smooth muscle.

To summarize, oxygen is the trigger that initiates contraction, but other factors may reduce or counteract its effect on the smooth muscle of the duct (Figure 52.7).

THE IMPORTANCE OF THE DUCT IN THE FETAL CIRCULATION

The arrangement of the fetal circulation, with the ventricles working in parallel, permits fetal needs to be met most efficiently (Figure 52.8). Early in the first trimester, the fetal duct is sufficiently developed to carry most of the right ventricular output, which accounts for about two thirds of the total combined ventricular outputs. The relative sizes of the great vessels and duct are dependent on the magnitude of this flow and significantly influence the form of many cardiovascular malformations (Heymann and Rudolph, 1972; Rudolph et al, 1972). In the normally developing heart, the duct meets the aorta proximally at an acute angle of less than 45 degrees, while the distal angle is obtuse, at around 130 degrees (Cassels, 1973). This is in contrast to the situation in the setting of many congenital cardiac malformations (see below). Most of the output from the right ventricle traverses the

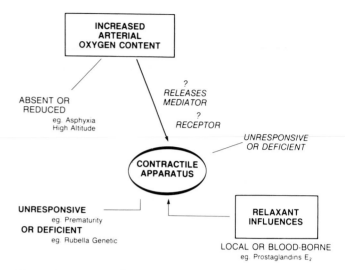

Figure 52.7 Factors influencing the contractile apparatus of the duct. The existence of a chemical mediator, and/or a specific receptor for the effect of oxygen, is still speculative.

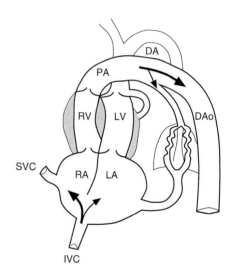

Figure 52.8 Fetal cardiac circulation. The majority of systemic venous return, particularly from the inferior caval vein (IVC), is directed through the right ventricle (RV), and through the duct (DA) to the descending aorta (DAo). LA, left atrium; LV, left ventricle; PA, pulmonary trunk; RA, right atrium; SVC, superior caval vein.

duct, accounting for approximately three fifths of the combined flow (Heymann and Rudolph, 1975), and provides eight to nine tenths of the flow to the descending aorta (that is, the majority of placental flow). Only about one tenth of the output of the right ventricle in the fetal lamb is directed to the lungs (Heymann and Rudolph, 1975). Consequently, the arterial duct diverts blood from the high-resistance pulmonary circulation to the descending aorta and the low-resistance placenta. Unlike the adult circulation, in which blood always traverses the heart twice in any one total circulation, the fetal circulation minimizes 'double pumping' to the small volume of pulmonary venous return. The demands on the fetal myocardium for work are thereby reduced to a minimum. This is perhaps fortunate in view of its limited capabilities (Friedman, 1973).

Although some workers have reported a small pressure gradient across the fetal duct, with the pulmonary arterial pressure being slightly greater than that of the aorta, this is probably an artefact of acutely exteriorized animals. Friedman (1978) was unable in chronically instrumented lambs to induce further relaxation of the vessel with prostaglandins. Under physiological conditions, pulmonary arterial and aortic pressures are equal.

Whether the duct regulates the distribution of right ventricular output in the fetus is unknown. It is conceiv-able that the fetal lungs have significant metabolic functions. In this case, the ability to alter the amount of blood directed to the lungs would be advantageous.

THE ROLE OF THE DUCT IN THE PATHOPHYSIOLOGY OF CONGENITAL CARDIAC MALFORMATIONS

The behaviour of the duct in the immediate postnatal period may be crucial when the heart is congenitally malformed (Figure 52.9). When either the pulmonary or the systemic circulation is entirely supplied through the duct,

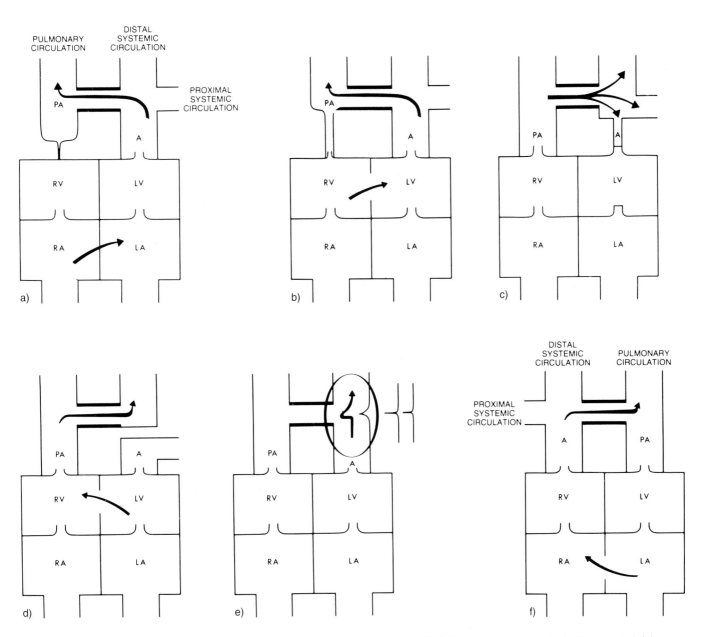

Figure 52.9 Role of the duct in various congenital malformations. (a) Pulmonary atresia. (b) Critical pulmonary stenosis. (c) Hypoplastic left heart. (d) Interrupted aortic arch. (e) Aortic coarctation. (f) Complete transposition. Flow through the duct (heavy lines) maintains or significantly contributes to pulmonary blood flow (a,b), systemic blood flow (c,d), bypasses a coarctation, which becomes apparent when the duct closes (e) or contributes to mixing between the two parallel circulations (f). A, aorta; PA, pulmonary artery; other abbreviations as in Figure 52.8.

survival itself depends on the behaviour of the duct. The duct that closes despite an obligatory need to remain patent has been aptly named 'the suicidal duct'.

Flow of blood to the lungs may be entirely duct dependent. This situation is epitomized by pulmonary atresia with an intact ventricular septum, and by tetralogy of Fallot with pulmonary atresia but no systemic-to-pulmonary collateral arteries. In these settings, the duct tends to be long and narrow, appearing as a downwardly directed branch of the distal aortic arch; as a result, the proximal angle is much less acute, and often obtuse (Calder et al, 1984). The distal angle, in contrast, is often acute (Rudolph et al, 1972). When this is not the case, it can be inferred that the development of pulmonary atresia occurred in late gestation (Santos et al, 1980). In other situations, such as pulmonary stenosis, some flow may reach the lungs through the normal channels, but the duct is essential for adequate flow. Major obstruction to normal flow of blood to the lungs may also coexist in other complex malformations, such as tricuspid atresia. Arterial oxygen saturation in all these settings depends on the volume of pulmonary blood flow, which needs to be sufficient to provide adequate oxygenated blood to mix with systemic venous return in the left heart. Although these patients never experience a normal postnatal rise in arterial tension of oxygen, closure of the duct usually occurs. Frequently it is delayed for 24 to 48 hours, or longer (Marino et al, 1992). It is not known what is the stimulus for closure despite the presence of coexisting hypoxaemia in these circumstances. As constriction occurs, pulmonary blood flow progressively diminishes. This causes a progressive fall in tension and saturation of arterial oxygen. Deprived of adequate supplies of oxygen, the tissues switch to anaerobic metabolism. This, in turn, results in metabolic acidosis, which further depresses cardiac function and causes pulmonary vasoconstriction. Without medical and/or surgical intervention, this sequence of events can only end in death. Pharmacological manipulation to prevent ductal closure prior to surgical creation of an aortopulmonary shunt has met with great success and is discussed later in this chapter.

Systemic blood flow may also be partially or entirely dependent on the duct. In patients with aortic atresia as part of the hypoplastic left heart syndrome, no blood can reach the systemic circulation except through the duct. In this instance, the distal angle of ductal insertion to the descending aorta is closer to normal, although the proximal angle is less acute and the duct is shorter and broader (Calder et al, 1984). Flow occurs retrogradely via the aortic isthmus to supply the head and neck vessels, including the ascending aorta and the coronary circulation. Partial dependence of the systemic circulation exists when there is interruption of the aortic arch. In these patients with duct-dependent systemic blood flow, heart failure rather than hypoxia predominates. The failure becomes rapidly more severe as the duct constricts, as it usually does within the first 24 hours of life. When the systemic circulation is totally dependent upon the duct, a 'shock-like' clinical picture develops, with poorly palpable peripheral pulses. Decreased coronary arterial perfusion compromises cardiac function. Decreased renal perfusion leads to renal insufficiency and a poor response to anti-failure therapy. Reopening of the duct by infusion of prostaglandin will reverse this trend and perhaps permit time for palliative surgical procedures (Heymann et al, 1979; Freed et al, 1981).

The duct also plays an important role in patients with aortic coarctation (Figure 52.9e) (Heymann et al, 1979; Freed et al, 1981). While the duct remains open, its aortic end can act as a bypass for flow from the aortic isthmus to the descending aorta. When it closes, the full significance of the coarctation becomes apparent. Perfusion of the lower half of the systemic circulation is then reduced, the femoral pulses become weak or absent, and output of urine decreases. With infusion of prostaglandin to reopen the duct, systemic perfusion can be improved, with reversal of acidosis and improved renal function. Moreover, when a ventricular septal defect is associated with the coarctation, left-to-right shunting tends to increase, causing pulmonary oedema and left heart failure. When the duct remains partially patent, flow is normally directed from the aorta to the pulmonary trunk. This adds further to the already increased pulmonary blood flow if pulmonary resistance is low.

Patients with complete transposition, especially when the ventricular septum is intact, depend on adequate mixing between the two parallel systemic and pulmonary circulations. Much of this mixing takes place at the atrial level, especially after balloon septostomy or atrial septectomy. Its amount is then determined by the relative compliances of the two ventricles. Patency of the duct can contribute favourably to mixing in complete transposition. Left-to-right flow of desaturated blood from the aorta to the pulmonary trunk via the duct is balanced by increased left-to-right flow of fully saturated blood from left atrium to right atrium. The net effect is to increase arterial oxygen saturation, and this can acutely stabilize the infant until medical or surgical intervention can safely be accomplished (Benson et al, 1979). This advantageous result is offset by an increased likelihood of pulmonary oedema with heart failure, and an increased risk of pulmonary vascular disease, if the atrial septum is restrictive.

The duct may also act as a safety valve for patients with severe pulmonary vascular obstruction or with pulmonary arterial stenosis beyond the duct. By facilitating run-off from the pulmonary circulation, it may prevent right ventricular failure, but at the cost of differential cyanosis. Maternal intake of inhibitors of prostaglandin during pregnancy should be avoided, particularly when duct-dependent cardiac malformations are uncovered by fetal echocardiography (Menahem, 1991; Saenger et al, 1992).

INTRAUTERINE DUCTAL CLOSURE

The duct can close in early gestation. Intimal cushions, the substrate for functional and anatomical closure, have been noted as early as the fourth month of gestation. Several drugs are known to influence intrauterine ductal constriction and closure, particularly the inhibitors of prostaglandin (Momma and Takeuchi, 1983; Niebyl, 1992; Schoenfield, 1992; Moise, 1993; van den Veyver, 1993). These can result in fetal heart failure and intra-uterine death (Harlass et al, 1989; Menahem, 1991; Mohen et al, 1992; Eronen, 1993). Transient neonatal tricuspid regurgitation and persistent fetal circulation have also been postulated to be the result of premature ductal closure (Berry et al, 1983; Harker, 1981). Fetal echocardiography, combined with Doppler studies of flow, can reveal restriction in ductal flow and could be of some benefit during administration of such drugs to the mother, if required. Technical difficulties in reliably imaging the duct, nonetheless, limit their clinical utility. The fetus with duct-dependent blood flow should not be exposed to such agents (Saenger et al, 1992; Menahem, 1991).

POSTNATAL DUCTAL CLOSURE

Functional ductal closure is normally initiated by constriction of the spiral medial muscle layer, with shortening and thickening of the duct, disruption of the intima and formation of intimal cushions (Gittenberger-de-Groot et al, 1980). A secondary process of migration of smooth muscle into the subintimal layers, haemorrhage and necrosis, endothelial disruption and, finally, fibrosis obliterates the lumen and forms the arterial ligament. Although closure was originally thought to be functionally complete within the first postnatal day (Moss et al, 1963), careful auscultation reveals a murmur in many infants in the first hours of life (Burnard, 1959; Braudo and Rowe, 1961; Moss et al, 1963). The murmur is very soft in intensity, crescendo systolic or continuous, and has a decrescendo diastolic component. It may be evident only during inspiration during auscultation at the second to third intercostal space. The pulmonary component of the second heart sound is normal when pulmonary arterial pressures are normal, and it can occasionally be heard to split (Brando and Rowe, 1961). With further ductal constriction, only the systolic component is audible, which usually disappears by the second or third day. Chest radiography and electro-cardiography are normal. Early haemodynamic studies (Moss et al, 1963) demonstrated small left-to-right shunts with normal pulmonary arterial pressures. Echographic evaluation using conventional and Doppler colour flow, combined with high-resolution imaging, has documented ductal shunting up to 72 hours after birth in healthy babies born at term (Gentile et al, 1981;

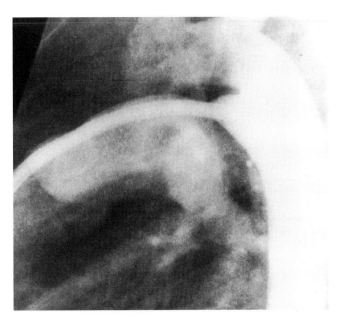

Figure 52.10 A lateral angiogram showing the typical conical duct in a patient about to undergo ductal occlusion.

Daniels et al, 1982; Huhta et al, 1984; Liao et al, 1988; Lim et al, 1992; Silverman, 1993), and even longer in preterm infants (Milne et al, 1989; Reller et al, 1989). Intimal cushions have been seen echocardiographically as echodense protrusions in the ductal lumen and are a first sign of impending ductal closure. Lack of formation of these mounds have been associated with prolonged rates of patency (Hiraishi et al, 1987a). The initial constriction occurs at the pulmonary arterial end and extends towards the aorta, giving a typical conical shape (Figure 52.10). This conical aortic end, the ampulla, may persist for many weeks, or occasionally years, after closure. In some, there may be a diverticulum originating from the proximal left pulmonary artery, from which the arterial ligament also arises (Figure 52.11). The duct is completely closed by 8 weeks of age in nine tenths of infants without additional cardiovascular anomalies (Christie, 1930).

THE PERSISTENT ARTERIAL DUCT

Persistence of the duct implies an abnormal state in which patency continues beyond the time at which normal closure should occur. Functional closure in full-term infants occurs within 10 to 15 hours of birth. Anatomical closure may not be complete for up to 3 months. On this basis, true persistence of the duct has been defined as continued patency in infants older than 3 months (Cassels, 1973). This definition should be applied only to infants born at term. Patency of the duct associated with prematurity is an entirely separate problem, and this will be discussed in a subsequent section.

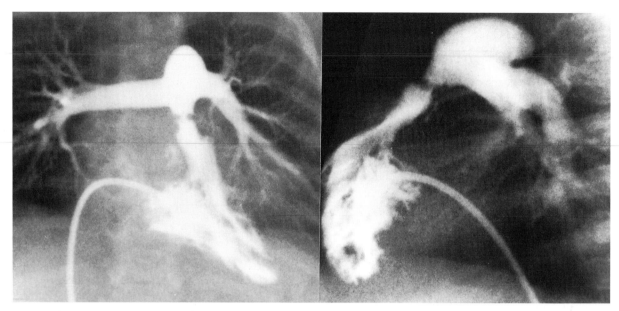

Figure 52.11 Pulmonary arterial angiograms from a patient with Fallot's tetralogy and a persistent ductal diverticulum, originating near the mouth of the left pulmonary artery. The aortic end of the duct had closed.

AETIOLOGY

Theoretically, the duct may persist for one or more of several reasons. Normal constriction may fail because of structural or biochemical abnormalities, which may be genetic or environmental in origin. Alternatively, the contractile 'apparatus' may be completely normal, but the stimulus to contraction, such as oxygen, may be lacking. Relaxant agents could also prevent closure, even when the duct is normal and the usual stimulus is present.

Persistence of the duct is associated with chromosomal aberrations, with asphyxia at birth, with birth at high altitude and with congenital rubella. In some cases, particularly in the preterm infant, the duct may reopen after functional closure owing to reduced arterial oxygen tension or increased concentration of prostaglandins, as occurs in asphyxial states or pulmonary disease, such as aspiration of meconium (Clyman et al, 1980). In the majority of cases, however, no cause is identifiable. These are considered to stem from interactions between multiple genetic and environmental influences.

Undamaged tissue from well-documented examples of a persistently patent duct is seldom available for study. Nonetheless, a few observations have been made. These are always open to the objection that the observed changes result from, rather than cause, the persistence. Gittenberger-de-Groot (1977) reported the presence of an unfragmented wavy subendothelial elastic lamina in some, but not all, persistently patent ducts, combined with an increase in elastic tissue in the media. Intimal cushions were rather sparse. She was unable to correlate the quantity of elastic material with the duration of patency, or with the presence or absence of associated cardiac defects. The abnormal elastic tissue was regarded

as being a primary prenatal abnormality. Bakker (1962) had applied the term 'aortification' to the increase in elastic tissue he observed in persistent ducts.

The studies of Patterson and Buchanan (Patterson et al, 1971; Patterson, 1980) are worthy of description at some length. Poodles, and some other species of pure-bred dogs, suffer a high incidence of persistent patency of the duct. As in humans, this is more common in females. In the normal animal, the smooth muscle is evenly distributed within the duct. The internal elastic lamina is not unduly prominent, and there are no prenatal intimal mounds. The vessel closes during the first 24 hours of life, with degenerative changes often being present by the third day, and always by the seventh. Conversion to a ligament is completed by 2 months. By contrast, the wall thickness in affected dogs is asymmetric. The segment of duct adjacent to the aorta is thinner than the opposing wall. It resembles the aorta in possessing alternating layers of elastic and collagen tissue. This unusual extension of elastic tissue into the ductal wall is associated with a corresponding decrease in smooth muscle, and the duct is shorter. Identical changes can be seen in fetuses of bitches belonging to families predisposed to persistent patency. This suggests that the defective structure is a cause rather than a result of persistence. When the degree of structural abnormality was graded, the mean grade for each litter correlated in a linear fashion with the gene dosage for persistent patency. Therefore, in this species at least, underdevelopment of smooth muscle appears to explain persistence of the duct. This underdevelopment could be genetically determined or the result of environmental insults (Buchanan, 1978). Tissues from normal dog fetuses, and from fetuses receiving various known proportions of their genes from dogs with persistent ducts, were studied experimentally (Knight et al, 1973). Ducts from the offspring of the dogs with ductal patency tended to be more widely patent under hypoxic conditions, and they showed a lesser response to oxygen, acetylcholine and noradrenaline. The abnormal findings were more marked as the degree of relationship increased to dogs having naturally persistent ducts. The families of dogs with congenitally persistent ducts provide further evidence in support of a role for intimal cushions in anatomical closure. In these dogs, lack of formation of intimal cushions was associated with relatively normal elastin architecture and failure to expand the subendothelium. In contrast to the normal ducts, the absence of subendothelial changes were reflected in a failure to increase hyaluronan, chondroitin sulphate and fibronectin production, together with a quiescent morphology of the smooth muscle cells (Gittenberger-de-Groot et al, 1985; de Reeder et al, 1988). This atypical extension of elastin throughout the wall was associated with decreased smooth muscle cells and morphological expansion of this vessel. The precocious luminal extension of proliferating vascular smooth muscle cells in knock-out mice without elastin production (Li et al, 1998) suggests a role for intact elastin scaffolding in mediating arrest of growth and differentiation of the smooth muscle cells. The distribution of vascular elastin observed in the dogs with persistently patent ducts may be responsible for the untimely differentiation and quiescence of the ductal smooth muscle cells. While the defect resulting in this phenotype is unknown, failure to disassemble the elastin matrix may prevent the formation of the intimal cushions and lead to a persistently patent duct.

Zetterquist (1972) made a thorough study of the families of 435 patients undergoing surgical closure of persistent ducts in Sweden. Females predominated in a ratio of 3 to 1. He found an incidence of $2.5 \pm 0.7\%$ among 484 children of these patients. This figure is almost identical to that found for the siblings of the original patients ($2.3 \pm 0.6\%$), thereby excluding simple recessive inheritance. Nora (1968) reported a somewhat higher risk to the offspring of 4.3%, given one affected parent. This incidence is some 45 times greater than the risk for the general population. It accords extremely well with the predicted incidence in first-degree relatives according to the multifactorial hypothesis. In this hypothesis, the incidence is obtained from the square root of the general incidence. For persistent duct, this is 0.057, or 2.4% (Edwards, 1960). Rarely, several generations may be affected, suggesting a dominant pattern of inheritance (Wei al, 1984; Martin et al, 1986; Lee et al, 1991; Rogers et al, 1992; Davidson, 1993; Schwartz et al, 1993). Neither Zetterquist nor Nora found any increased risk for defects other than persistent duct in the offspring of patients who had a persistent duct.

The risk to further children in sibships where two children have already been affected is probably in the order of 10%. It undoubtedly increases for each affected sibling. Sibships of up to five with persistently patent duct have been observed (Burnell and Stern, 1971).

Twin studies support the multifactorial hypothesis (Nora, 1968). Despite the extremely small sizes of the samples, Nora was able to collect eight cases involving monozygotic twins, of which four were concordant. This compared with only one of five dizygotic twins. Concordance for the specific cardiac defect was also found to be high in the study by Anderson (1977).

Persistent ductal patency may be a feature of several syndromes associated with well-defined chromosomal abnormalities. It is commonly present in the various trisomies, either in isolation or, more often, combined with other malformations. The defect is especially common in the +14q syndrome, with over half having congenital cardiac malformations. The XXY syndrome is also often associated with persistence of the duct.

Maternal rubella was first linked to persistent ductal patency by Gregg (1941). It is also associated with other lesions, especially pulmonary arterial stenosis. Histological examination of ducts from patients with rubella syndrome showed them to have a thinner wall, with absence of both an internal elastic lamina and intimal proliferation. They, therefore, resemble a very immature duct (Gittenberger-de-Groot et al, 1978). The amount of smooth muscle was also reduced (Campbell, 1961). Persistence of the duct also occurred as part of the thalidomide syndrome (Keck et al, 1972), while deficiency of copper in rats has resulted in high rates of ductal patency (Alliende-Gonzales et al, 1991). Some differences in ductal ultrastructure have also been demonstrated in patients with cyanotic cardiac malformations, compared with acyanotic lesions, and may partly explain the prolonged patency of the duct in some of these children.

Persistence of the duct is more likely to be found in infants born at high altitude (Alzamora-Castro et al, 1960). According to Penaloza et al (1964), the incidence of ductal persistence in schoolchildren born at sea level in Peru (0.05%) was similar to that in North American children. There was a progressive rise to 0.72% in the incidence among Peruvian children born at altitudes in excess of 3.5 km. At 5 km, the partial pressure of oxygen is decreased, suggesting that hypoxia may be a factor. These findings, however, were not confirmed in studies in Denver and Leadville, Colorado in the United States of America. This raises the question of whether other genetic or environmental factors explain the Peruvian findings (Vogel et al, 1964).

Record and McKeown (1953b) similarly studied aetiological factors. The ratio of incidence in females and males was over 2:1. They found that, for males, persistence was more common in first-born compared with later-born children. In girls, the defect was unrelated to order of birth but was related to maternal age under 25 years. A history of fetal asphyxia was present in two fifths, while rubella accounted for only three cases in their study. These findings were substantially confirmed by Polani and Campbell (1960), except that maternal age and birth rank were not significant factors in their study. In both investigations, there appeared to be a seasonal incidence in girls. Thus, there was a sharp increase in births of affected girls during the summer, which then persisted during the remainder of the year. This seasonal incidence in girls was unrelated to the incidence of rubella. In a study in New England, births of children with the defect showed a distinct seasonal increase during October through January. The first trimester of gestation for these children coincided with the peak seasonal incidence of rubella in the later winter and early spring (Rutstein et al, 1952). These authors concluded that rubella probably accounted for the seasonal excess, since births were otherwise uniformly distributed through the year. Seasonal incidence of births in either females or males was not present in the large cohort studied by Zetterquist (1972), and neither was asphyxia at birth a factor.

Most examples of the truly persistent duct, therefore, represent the influence of multifactorial inheritance. Rubella is clearly a causative factor in some cases, and it probably accounts for early reports of seasonal variations in incidence. Birth at high altitude resulting in ductal persistence represents lack of the usual stimulus to closure. Birth asphyxia is more likely to delay closure than to prevent it. Occasional cases are associated with specific genetic defects. Persistent patency is more common in females, except in those where it is caused by rubella, in which case the ratio of genders is almost equal (Krovetz and Warden, 1962).

INCIDENCE

Several attempts have been made to estimate the incidence of the persistent duct seen in isolation, but all studies published thus far contain potential sources of error. This is particularly evident when cases caused by prematurity or maternal rubella are included. Anderson (1954) estimated the incidence to lie between 1 in 2500 and 1 in 5000 births. In this study, isolated patency of the duct accounted for 12% of all congenital cardiac malformations. The most extensive study of a relatively homogeneous population is that by Carlgren (1959). He charted the incidence of congenital heart disease in children born in the Swedish city of Gothenburg during the period 1941–1950. He found an overall incidence for all malformations of 6.4 per 1000. Persistent patency of the duct was the third most common lesion identified, accounting for 35 patients out of 58 105 livebirths. Of these patients, five were probably the consequence of maternal infection with rubella. Another seven patients died in the first month of life, suggesting that prematurity may have been a factor. Therefore, the number of patients with true persistent patency of unknown cause was probably about 24, or 0.04% of the overall series of livebirths. Data from 12 North American centres was collected on 55 044 livebirths. Again there were 35 patients found with isolated persistent patency, giving an incidence of 0.06% (Mitchell et al, 1971). As with Carlgren's study, some of these were probably associated with prematurity or rubella, suggesting good agreement with the findings from the Swedish population.

Not surprisingly, since the constrictive effects of oxygen and the dilatory effects of prostaglandins are related to gestational age, there is an extremely high incidence of ductal patency in infants born at low body weight (Reller et al, 1990; Gonzalez and Ventura-Junca, 1991; Mouzinho et al, 1991). Almost half of infants weighing less than 1750 g at birth, and up to four-fifths of those weighing less than 1200 g, have clinical evidence of patency of the duct (Auld, 1966; Danilowicz et al, 1966; Siassi et al, 1969; Girling et al, 1971; Kitterman et al, 1972; Clarkson, 1974; Baylen et al, 1975; Lee, 1975; Ellison et al, 1983; Clyman, 1984). With the advent of therapy with surfactant to reduce pulmonary arterial pressures and improve pulmonary mechanics, many more preterm infants are now encountered with ductal patency (Fujiwara et al, 1980; Clyman et al, 1982; Heldt et al, 1989; Shimada et al, 1989; Kinsella et al, 1991; Reller et al, 1991). The overall incidence in infants born prematurely is 8 per 1000 livebirths.

PATHOPHYSIOLOGY

Isolated persistent patency results in shunting of blood from one side of the circulation to the other. The volume depends on the length and internal diameter of the duct, and on the systemic and pulmonary vascular resistances. As pulmonary resistance is usually much lower than systemic, the flow is from the aorta to the pulmonary trunk. Hence, flow to the lungs is increased and may result in left atrial and left ventricular overload, these two chambers being enlarged in the presence of a significant shunt. If the duct is widely patent, flow depends entirely on the ratio of resistances. Right ventricular failure may occur in the presence of a large duct with pulmonary hypertension or pulmonary oedema, and an elevated left atrial pressure. Right-to-left shunting may also occur through a stretched incompetent oval foramen because of left atrial hypertension (Rudolph et al, 1958). In lesser degrees of heart failure, left-to-right shunting can also be seen. Pulmonary arterial systolic pressure will normally equal systemic pressure. In most patients, the duct is partially constricted, and the degree of constriction is the major factor limiting flow. Under these conditions, pulmonary arterial pressure is normal or only mildly elevated. It is exceeded by the systemic pressure both in systole and diastole, thereby permitting shunting throughout the cardiac cycle. Symptomatology and clinical findings are largely determined by the magnitude of the shunt.

CLINICAL FEATURES

Most patients are asymptomatic. The malformation is recognized concomitant with detection of the characteristic murmur. Occasionally, there may be a history of prematurity, asphyxia during birth or maternal rubella. Patients with large shunts may fail to thrive, experiencing difficulty with feeding during infancy and frequently suffering recurrent infections of the upper respiratory tract. Occasionally, congestive heart failure develops.

PHYSICAL EXAMINATION

Growth is retarded in about one third of patients. They are acyanotic in the absence of complicating factors. All the peripheral pulses are easily palpable, with a rapid upstroke and decay. The pressure of the pulse is widened, with lowering of the diastolic component. Arterial pulsation in the neck may be prominent in those with large shunts. Examination of the precordium reveals an active cardiac impulse, with the forceful cardiac apex displaced to the left. When the shunt is small, the only abnormal finding may be the murmur. The continuous, or 'machinery', murmur of the uncomplicated persistent duct is best heard in the left infraclavicular area, although it is occasionally maximal at the third left interspace. Gibson's (1898) description of the murmur, deservedly, has been widely quoted: 'the murmur begins after the commencement of the first sound, it persists through the second sound and dies away gradually during the long pause. The murmur is rough and thrilling. It begins softly and increases in intensity so as to reach its acme, just about, or immediately after, the second sound, and from that point gradually wanes, until its termination. The second sound can be heard to be loud and clanging.' The murmur is caused by turbulent flow through the duct itself.

Additional murmurs may be present because of increased flow across the aortic valve, producing an ejection systolic sound, and across the mitral valve, giving a diastolic murmur with loud onset. The systolic component of the continuous murmur may be transmitted into the neck, and it may be associated with a thrill in the second left intercostal space. With small shunts, the murmur may be quite soft; it can be augmented by administering a systemic vasoconstrictor (Crevasse and Logue, 1959). It may also increase in intensity during inspiration as a result of the fall in pulmonary vascular resistance. Recent echocardiographic studies using colour flow Doppler have further identified the presence of small ductal communications in the absence of any typical murmur of patency, this degree of shunting giving uncharacteristic soft vibratory systolic murmurs (Salazar et al, 1990; Houston et al, 1991). These observations may have a significant impact on estimates of the incidence of ductal patency and the risk of endocarditis.

Systolic ejection sounds are common in patients with large shunts (Hubbard and Neis, 1969). Most are of pulmonary arterial origin, but occasionally both pulmonary and aortic sounds are present, in which case the pulmonary sound usually precedes that from the aorta. Such distinctions are difficult to make clinically but have been observed using simultaneous phonocardiographic and catheterization studies.

The second heart sound is difficult to analyse clinically, but phonocardiography suggests that it is usually paradoxically split when there is a large shunt (Neill and Mounsey, 1958). Rudolph et al (1964) showed experimentally that, in the presence of aortopulmonary shunting, late opening and early closure of the pulmonary valve results in marked shortening of right ventricular systole.

Many patients with loud continuous murmurs also have multiple 'clanging' sounds. These are relatively localized to the pulmonary area and are most frequent in the second half of systole, corresponding to the period of peak flow within the duct. Neill and Mounsey (1958) attributed these sounds to the turbulence caused by the 'head on' collision of directionally opposed flow from the duct and the right ventricle, and they named them 'eddy sounds'. To this point, we have considered the auscultatory findings only for an uncomplicated persistent duct in a child. It should be remembered that these features may differ in infancy or be altered by the development of complications.

INVESTIGATIONS

ELECTROCARDIOGRAM

Patients with isolated persistency of the duct usually have some electrocardiographic evidence of left ventricular hypertrophy, with dominant R waves in all standard leads. Tall peaked T waves may be observed in aVF and the left precordial leads, reflecting volume overload of the left ventricle. Except in infancy, inversion of the T waves, or depression of the ST segment, is most unusual in patients with an isolated duct. Left atrial hypertrophy may be identified by prolongation of the P wave. Occasionally, the electrocardiogram may show combined ventricular hypertrophy, or it can be entirely normal should the duct be small. The electrical axis is usually normal (Ash and Fischer, 1955). Estimates of the distribution of abnormalities have been made by several authors but are of limited value because of the selected case material on which the figures are based. Deviation of the electrical axis to the right with right atrial and/or right ventricular hypertrophy suggests the presence of additional defects or of pulmonary hypertension. The electrocardiographic changes are less predictable in infants and clinically less helpful (Marcano and Goldberg, 1969). In older children, ligation of the duct is usually followed by fairly rapid regression of the electrocardiographic abnormalities, with return to normality (Watson and Keith, 1962).

Prolongation of the PR interval, which disappears or decreases after surgery, has been observed in about one fifth of those affected (Mirowski et al, 1962). Atrial fibrillation may develop in adult life (Cosh, 1957). In patients with persistent patency resulting from rubella, the electrical axis may be superior and directed to the left or right (Halloran et al, 1966).

Complications will modify the electrocardiogram. When the shunt is large enough to equalize the systemic and pulmonary arterial pressures, biventricular hypertrophy is likely to develop. With the onset of pulmonary vascular disease, the predominant findings will be those of right ventricular hypertrophy.

CHEST RADIOGRAPHY

The chest film may be normal in patients with a small shunt. Cardiomegaly is present in those where flow to the lungs is close to twice systemic flow or greater. Increased pulmonary vascular markings are then seen, with an obvious bulge of the pulmonary trunk at the left mid-border of the cardiac silhouette. The aorta is also prominent. Both it and the pulmonary trunk tend to enlarge with age (Cosh, 1957). Enlargement of the left atrium is usually present and reflects increased pulmonary venous return owing to the left-to-right shunt. Increased pulmonary vascularity may be more marked on the right, as is often seen with other left-to-right shunts (Figure 52.12) (Garfunkel and Kirkpatrick, 1963; Whitley et al, 1963). During the era of fluoroscopy, it was possible to see obvious pulsations in both the aorta and pulmonary trunk, with a characteristic see-saw motion between the left ventricle and pulmonary trunk. This technique is no longer recommended. If necessary, left atrial enlargement can be confirmed by a barium swallow in the right anterior oblique view. The duct may calcify, although this complication is more common when the vessel is closed rather than patent. The aortic end of the duct, the ductal ampulla, may be seen on the chest radiograph, and it can be demonstrated angiographically during the first week of life. It occasionally persists as an aortic diverticulum (Berdon et al, 1965). These findings may be modified, especially if pulmonary vascular disease develops.

ECHOCARDIOGRAPHY

Persistent patency beyond the neonatal period is readily diagnosed from the characteristic clinical features. Cross-sectional or M-mode echocardiography may help to exclude other structural cardiac malformations. The duct can be imaged throughout its length using a high left parasternal view (Smallhorn et al, 1982; Vick et al, 1985). This view allows accurate evaluation of ductal size (Sahn and Allen, 1978). It also shows the presence of tissue within the lumen, indicating imminent closure (Hiraishi et al, 1987a). In preterm infants, imaging may be difficult owing to a poor echographic window because of emphysematous lungs from high ventilatory pressures. A subxiphoid view can then be used. Characteristic dias-

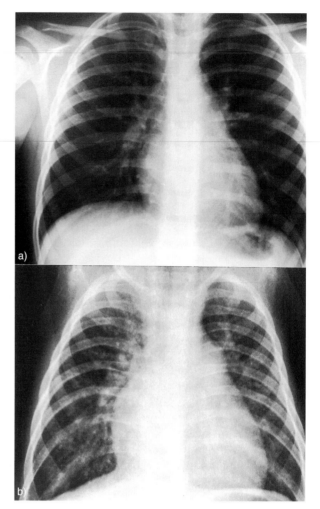

Figure 52.12 Two chest radiographs from patients with a small duct. (a) Note the minimally increased pulmonary vascularity. (b) A younger child with a large ductal communication. There is increased pulmonary vascularity and cardiomegaly.

tolic flow in the pulmonary trunk identified by Doppler interrogation increases the confidence of diagnosing ductal shunting (Huhta et al, 1984).

Flow through the duct can be quantified by analysis of Doppler tracings of diastolic flow in the left pulmonary artery (Hiraishi et al, 1987b) or the descending aorta (Serwell et al, 1982; Drayton and Skidmore, 1987), but it is difficult. Colour flow Doppler techniques, however, have been more useful in revealing ductal patency. This is, at present, the most sensitive method for detecting and semiquantifying ductal flow (Stephenson et al, 1980; Liao et al, 1988; Reller et al, 1989). Evaluation of patterns of flow in the duct can provide a window to assess pulmonary haemodynamics in babies with structurally normal or abnormal hearts (Shiraishi et al, 1989). Qualitatively, the presence of bidirectional, or pure right-to-left, shunting has been found highly specific for elevated pulmonary arterial pressures (Stevenson et al, 1979; Musewe et al, 1987). Additionally, using colour flow mapping, measurements of velocity can be used to estimate pulmonary arterial pressures (Figure 52.13) (Houston et al, 1989;

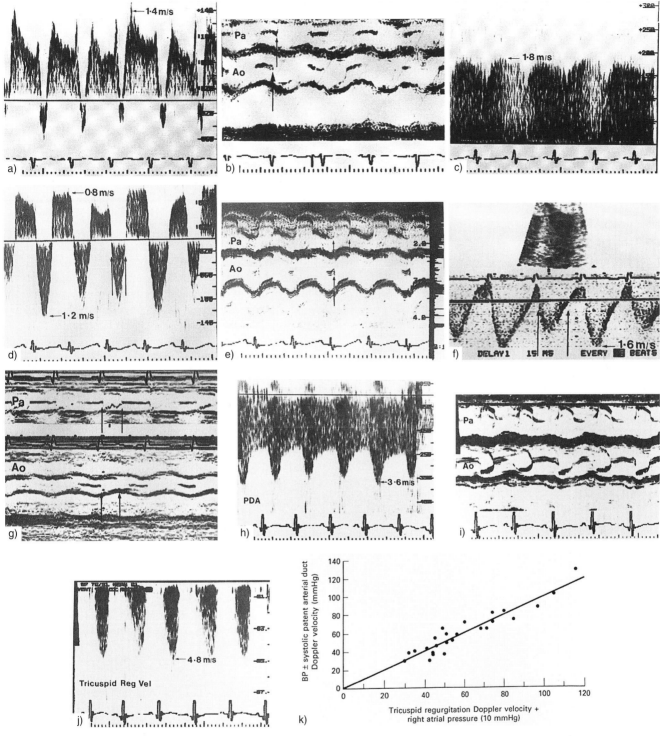

Figure 52.13 Evaluation of pulmonary arterial systolic pressures from profiles of ductal velocity. A patient with transient tachypnoea.
(a) Bidirectional shunting can be seen on the first day of life. Note the brief right-to-left flow (below the horizontal zero flow line). (b) The M-mode tracings taken on the first day. These can be used to determine the duration of systole from the images obtained in the aortic (Ao) and pulmonary trunk (Pa). Arrows show opening of valves. (c) the Doppler trace from the same patient at 48 hours of age. Ductal flow is now entirely left-to-right, consistent with lower pulmonary arterial pressures (d–g) An infant (1 day of age) with persistent pulmonary hypertension. (d) Patterns of ductal flow are significantly different to those in the previous patient, with a longer duration of right-to-left flow. (e) The M-mode trace shows the nearly simultaneous opening of the arterial valves. The duration of right-to-left shunting (between arrows) is as long or longer than the duration of systole, suggesting systemic or suprasystemic pulmonary arterial pressures. (f) The Doppler trace from the same patient, on day 2 of life, shows nearly pure right-to-left shunting. (h–j) An infant showing pure right-to-left shunting. (h) The Doppler trace. (i) The M-mode trace shows the motion of the arterial valvar leaflets. (j) The Doppler display was obtained from the tricuspid valve (tricuspid regurgitation) in the same patient, confirming the suprasystemic pulmonary arterial pressures (95 versus 55 mmHg). (k) A linear regression analysis compares ductal Doppler-derived pulmonary arterial systolic pressure with that obtained by adding right atrial pressure to the velocity of tricuspid regurgitation. (Modified from Musewe et al, 1990 with permission.)

Aziz and Tasneen, 1990; Musewe et al, 1990; Ge et al, 1993a,b). Furthermore, ultrasonic studies, by providing an assessment of left atrial and left ventricular enlargement, may give some idea of the magnitude of the shunt. Echocardiography is probably most valuable in the diagnosis of ductal patency in the premature infant. It will be discussed further in that section.

CARDIAC CATHETERIZATION AND ANGIOGRAPHY

Most cardiologists would not consider catheterization a necessary diagnostic procedure for patients with typical clinical findings of persistent ductal patency. If it is undertaken, it is usually possible to probe the duct from the pulmonary trunk and to pass a catheter through the vessel and down the aorta. When the catheter apparently crosses a duct but then turns in a headward direction, the alert investigator should consider the presence of an aortopulmonary window. The size of the shunt may be difficult to quantify by oximetry because it is difficult to obtain a truly representative sample distal to the site of shunting. Pulmonary arterial pressure is usually normal or slightly elevated. The duct can be visualized by selective aortography with injection of contrast media in the last part of the aortic arch (Figure 52.14).

Other imaging modalities are available to confirm the presence of ductal patency. Radionuclide scanning can be used to detect the presence of shunting, but anatomical localization is lacking. Magnetic resonance imaging provides anatomical detail (Higgins et al, 1990) and is particularly useful in the setting of complex anomalies (Friese et al, 1992). With velocity encoding of cinemagnetic resonance signals, patterns of shunting can be detected (Chien et al, 1991; Brenner et al, 1992). In general, however, the

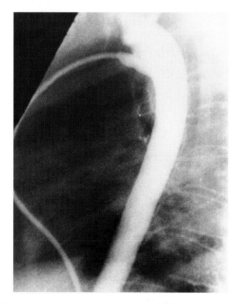

Figure 52.14 A descending aortogram, outlining a long and narrow duct, obtained by cannulating the pulmonary end of the duct from the right heart.

simpler technique of cross-sectional echocardiography with colour flow Doppler provides sufficient anatomical and haemodynamic detail to define the anatomy and its variations and to indicate proper management.

DIAGNOSTIC PROBLEMS

Other causes of a continuous murmur may create confusion. The venous hum (Potain, 1867) often causes difficulty for the inexperienced auscultator. This noise, which can be loud, is usually best heard in the supraclavicular fossas. While audible bilaterally, it is usually louder on the right. A venous hum, when loud, may be transmitted below the clavicle. Here, it may be misdiagnosed as being from a patent duct. This error can be avoided by exerting pressure over the root of the neck, turning the head to the side, or lying the child down. These manoeuvres readily obliterate the venous hum, while having no effect on the murmur generated by ductal flow.

An aortopulmonary window rarely can cause a continuous murmur similar to that of persistent ductal patency. More typically, however, the communication is large and does not cause a continuous murmur. Even with careful aortography, nonetheless, this condition may be misdiagnosed. The true situation may then be appreciated only at thoracotomy. Echocardiography should now help to avoid this error.

Major aortopulmonary collateral arteries, pulmonary arterio-venous fistulas and collateral arteries associated with coarctation all cause continuous murmurs. These seldom cause diagnostic problems because of the general clinical picture and the location of the murmur. Other causes of continuous murmurs heard in the chest include ruptured sinus of Valsalva, peripheral pulmonary arterial stenosis, common arterial trunk, coronary artery fistulas, the supracardiac form of totally anomalous pulmonary venous connection, mitral atresia, surgically created systemic-to-pulmonary arterial shunts and, rarely, anomalous origin of the left coronary artery from the pulmonary trunk. Prolapse of an aortic valvar leaflet into a ventricular septal defect may also simulate persistent patency of the duct (Bonham-Carter and Walker, 1955). Most, if not all, of these potential pitfalls can be avoided by careful clinical evaluation and good echocardiography.

MANAGEMENT

Once the diagnosis of uncomplicated persistent patency of the arterial duct is established, elimination of the shunt should be recommended by surgical ligation or catheter occlusion, even when the shunt is small. The justification for closure of small communications resides in the prevention of infective endocarditis, coupled with an extremely low procedural morbidity and mortality.

In the occasional patient who develops congestive heart failure, excluding those patients to be discussed below in the context of prematurity, drugs should be administered to combat the failure, but only until intervention can conveniently be arranged.

SURGICAL INTERVENTION

The first successful ligation of a persistent arterial duct, achieved in a 7-year-old girl by Robert Gross in 1939, has already been mentioned. The duct is usually approached through a left posterolateral incision, using the third interspace in infants, and the fourth space in children over 1 year. Uncommonly, the duct is on the right side, especially in the presence of a right aortic arch. It must then be approached from the right. The duct may be ligated or divided. The relative merits of each procedure continue to be hotly debated by surgeons. Excellent results have been reported using both procedures.

Ligation using two heavy silk ligatures, plus an umbilical tape ligature, is simple and safe (Trusler, 1979). Transfixation, as proposed by Blalock, does not appear necessary. Using this technique, the incidence of recanalization is about 1% (Bickford, 1960; Trusler, 1979; Daniels et al, 1984). Jones (1965), however, reported 12 instances of recurrent or residual ductal flow amongst 61 patients in whom the duct had been ligated using heavy tape. Clinically detectable shunts after surgical intervention have ranged from 0.4% to 3.1% (Panagopoulos et al, 1971; Trippestad and Efskind, 1971). Recent echo Doppler studies, however, have detected flow in clinically silent ducts, suggesting the incidence of residual flow to be higher (Musewe et al, 1989; Sorensen et al, 1991). Large ducts, exceeding 7–10 mm diameter, or those associated with pulmonary hypertension should be divided. Recurrent ducts, short wide vessels or those with spontaneous or infected aneurysms should also be divided, using an approach through the left chest. Controlled hypotension may help to control bleeding in patients with pulmonary hypertension or friable ducts (Groves et al, 1954).

By 1939, Gross was able to publish details of ductal ligation in 14 patients varying in age from 3 to 24 years, with two having endarteritis caused by infection with *Streptococcus viridans*. There were no deaths, and no significant complications, in his early series, but he advocated division rather than ligation. Further reports of more extensive experience followed (Holman et al, 1953; Bickford, 1960; Jones, 1965). Jones (1965), reporting on a large experience extending over 25 years, had only 1 of 431 patients dying with an uncomplicated duct, giving a rate of mortality of 0.2%. A figure of 0.5% was reported by Panagopoulos et al (1971).

Once the safety of the operation was established in older children and adults, it was natural for surgeons to attempt closure in infancy (Ghani and Hashim, 1989). Mustard (1951) reported successful ligation in four infants. Many surgeons then demonstrated the ease with which the duct can be ligated even in premature infants (Wagner et al, 1984). In most units, surgical ligation is reserved for those premature infants who have failed an adequate course of indomethacin, or when there are contraindications to its administration (see below). Some have advocated prophylactic ductal ligation, although the only demonstrated advantage of such a prophylactic approach has been a reduction in the incidence of necrotizing enterocolitis in babies weighing less than 1000 g (Cassady et al, 1979). The need for accurate anatomical definition prior to intervention in the premature infant was underscored by Fleming et al (1983).

Ligation or division of the duct is usually associated with an immediate rise in systemic arterial pressure. This may be sustained for several days before subsiding to normal levels (Taylor et al, 1950). Pulmonary arterial pressure, if elevated and in the absence of pulmonary vascular disease, falls to normal. The continuous murmur disappears and the size of the heart is reduced. Left atrial and left ventricular enlargement, as judged by echocardiography (Ash and Fischer, 1955), also diminish.

Complications are uncommon. Injury to the recurrent laryngeal nerve injury can occur occasionally and is usually temporary (Jones, 1965; Fan et al, 1989), although it can be permanent. Rarely, a false aneurysm may develop, prompting urgent surgical re-operation after ligation (Ross et al, 1961; Powell, 1963; Payne and Jordan, 1968) or division (Crafoord, 1947, Hallman and Cooley, 1964; Egami et al, 1992). Damage to the phrenic nerve has also been reported, occurring most frequently in the premature infant (Berger et al, 1960; Fan et al, 1989). Chylothorax can also occur. Inadvertent ligation of the distal left pulmonary artery occurs infrequently. This is a hazard when the duct is large and the recurrent laryngeal nerve has an unusual course (Pontius et al, 1981). Ligation of the descending aorta can occur, especially when the duct is approached from a median sternotomy. Signs of aortic coarctation may also be unmasked after ductal ligation (Elseed et al, 1974). This is a constant hazard in the premature infant. Abnormal findings after ductal ligation, such as decreased femoral pulses or declining urinary output, should prompt rapid re-evaluation.

Thoracoscopic closure without thoracotomy is a recent innovation. Laborde et al (1993) first reported use of the video-assisted endoscopic technique in 38 patients with a mean age of 23.3 months, and mean weight of 9.5 kg (22 lb). Clinical evidence of successful closure was found in all, although two attempts were necessary in two patients. Damage to the recurrent laryngeal nerve occurred in one, while four suffered pneumothorax. Increasing experience with the procedure has reduced the incidence of complications. Continued experience has shown this approach to shorten hospital stay and to provide a cost-effective, safe and rapid technique compared with open thoracotomy. Damage to the recurrent laryngeal nerve, and residual shunts, can occur (Rothenberg et al, 1995;

Das et al, 1997; Laborde et al, 1997; Tsuboi et al, 1997; Hines et al, 1998). Recently, a transaxillary muscle-sparing thoracotomy has been developed for the neonate and infant. This provides excellent exposure for ductal division, produces less postoperative pain and achieves an acceptable cosmetic result (Kyoku et al, 1989; Karwande and Rowles, 1992; Cetta et al, 1997; Kennedy et al, 1998).

CLOSURE IN THE CATHETERIZATION LABORATORY

Porstmann (1967, 1968, 1971, 1974), on the basis of his experience with over 100 patients, has long advocated closure using a percutaneous technique through the femoral artery. In this techniques, closure is accomplished using an Ivalon plug. A prerequisite for this approach is that the lumen of the duct must be conical in shape, and it must be smaller than the lumen of the femoral artery. The technique is complicated, requiring placement of a large sheath in the femoral artery. A loop is then constructed from the femoral artery through the duct and to the femoral vein. Because of this, the technique has not been found suitable for infants and small children. Other devices, such as polyvinyl alcohol umbrellas with steel wires, umbrella-sponge plugs, or polymers with a memory for their shape, have been used to close artificial ducts created in dogs from either the arterial or venous circulations (Mills and King, 1976; Leslie et al, 1977; Echigo et al, 1990). A detachable silicone double balloon has been described by Warnecke et al (1984) but has not had extensive clinical trials. Magal and colleagues (1989) described a device consisting of a small nylon sack that could be filled with segments of guidewire and fixed with a distal flexible crossbar. Rao et al (1993) described a successful modification of a single disc device originally designed for closure of atrial communications. Rashkind and Cuaso, as long ago as 1979, proposed using a device consisting of a stainless steel grappling hook filled with a cone of foam. The prosthesis was introduced in a collapsed state and then expanded when released from the tip of the catheter. Since that initial clinical application, and with improvements in the design of the equipment, experience from a multicentre clinical trial (Rashkind et al, 1987) has defined the setting for successful occlusion in the catheterization laboratory and has led to its use as an effective alternative to surgery. Still more recently, spring coils, originally designed for peripheral vascular embolization, have been used to achieve closure (Lloyd et al, 1993).

The Rashkind ductal occluder

Closure can be accomplished using the Rashkind ductal occluder from either venous or arterial entry (Rashkind et al, 1987). The use of a long sheath placed across the duct from the venous circulation, as decribed by Bash and Mullins (1984), has now become the technique of choice (Figure 52.15). Closure in this fashion is achievable in infants and young children. It is not, however,

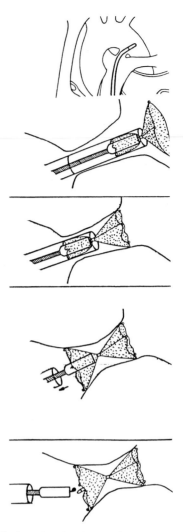

Figure 52.15 The long-sheath technique for delivery of the occluder system through the right heart for ductal occlusion using the Rashkind device.

possible to close ducts larger than 8 or 9 mm in diameter, nor to achieve closure in premature infants. The occluder consists of two open-pore discs made of medical grade polyurethane foam mounted on opposing spring assemblies with three arms resembling opposing umbrellas (Figure 52.16). When released, the arms spring perpendicular to the shaft of the catheter and self-seal. The device is available with diameters of 12 and 17 mm, the larger device being made with four arms per disc, but with the same spring and mechanism for attachment to the catheter.

As with surgical management, the clinical diagnosis should be confirmed non-invasively prior to catheterization by colour flow Doppler echocardiography, with particular emphasis placed on the presence of associated lesions that could complicate the procedure, such as azygos continuation of the inferior caval vein, presence of an additional lesion that requires surgical intervention or the presence of pulmonary vascular disease. Special attention should also be directed to the transverse arch

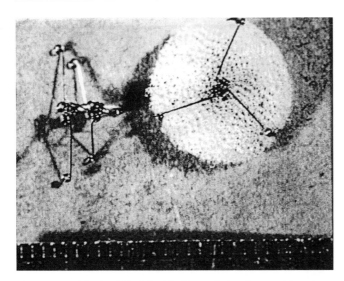

Figure 52.16 The Rashkind double-disc occluder shown with and without the foam on the occluding arms.

and isthmic region to exclude unsuspected coarctation. The procedure is ideally suited for patients weighing 10 kg (23 lb) or more. It should not be performed in smaller infants because of the risk of compromising the left pulmonary artery (Musewe et al, 1989; Ottenkamp et al, 1992). There is considerable variation in procedural details as practised amongst centres, such as the use of coincident arterial cannulation, the number and type of angiogram and so on. The majority of procedures, however, can be performed in an out-patient setting, with discharge the afternoon of study (Benson et al, 1988; Wessel et al, 1988).

A number of clinical series have been published involving hundreds of patients (Rashkind et al, 1987; Benson et al, 1988; Dyck et al, 1988; Wessel et al, 1988; Latson et al, 1989; Ballerini et al, 1990; Rey et al, 1990; Rohmer et al, 1990; Hosking et al, 1991; Ali Khan et al, 1992; Anonymous, 1992; Ng et al, 1992; Galal et al, 1993; Verin et al, 1993a; Wilson et al, 1993). Successful implantation can be accomplished in almost all, with elimination of clinical signs of left-to-right shunting. Within the first 48 hours, ductal murmurs can still be heard in a few patients despite correct placement, although a number may have residual shunts without murmurs. Evidence of shunting is often provided by Doppler interrogation over the superior aspect of the device (Plate 52.1) (Dyck et al, 1988; Musewe et al, 1989).

Complications are few. Acute bacterial endarteritis has occured after implantation when appropriate prophylactic medication was not applied (Dyck et al, 1988; Latson et al, 1989). Embolization to both systemic and pulmonary circulations has been encountered, with several patients requiring surgical referral. Retrieval has also been accomplished in both situations using snares, baskets or grasping forceps (Rashkind et al, 1987; Latson et al, 1989).

Pulsed and colour flow Doppler techniques have been used to evaluate the rates of occlusion (Musewe et al, 1989; Hosking et al, 1991; Ali Khan et al, 1992; Anonymous, 1992; Huggon et al, 1993). In one study (Hosking et al, 1991), just over one third had Doppler evidence of shunting detected 1 year after the procedure, falling to one fifth at 2 years and less than one tenth at 40 months (Figure 52.17). Similar observations have been reported by others (Latson et al, 1991; Anonymous, 1992; Huggon et al, 1993). A number of patients have undergone repeat procedures, with successful placement of a second device (Hosking et al, 1989; Huggon et al, 1993; Moore, 1995). In a few patients, there is evidence of increased flow at the origin of the left pulmonary artery subsequent to implantation, presumably as a result of turbulence or encroachment of the device into the mouth of the left pulmonary artery. There was an increased incidence of this finding when the Rashkind device was placed in children under 10 kg in weight (Fadley et al, 1993). A few patients have also experienced haemolysis after placement of the device, with coexistent residual shunting (Ladusans et al, 1989; Grifka et al, 1992; Hayes et al, 1992).

Closure using the transfemoral plug

The Porstmann plug is inserted using a catheter placed from the femoral artery and threaded across the duct into the right heart (Figure 52.18). Either the catheter itself, or an exchange guidewire, is snared from the vein on the opposite side and exteriorized, forming an arterio-venous loop through the duct. The Ivalon plug is introduced through a tubular applicator and threaded over the track wire. The lower age for closure using this device is between 3 and 4 years (Porstmann et al, 1971; Sato et al, 1975). The success of the technique depends on the ratio of the lumen of the femoral artery to that of the duct, allowing an appropriately sized plug to be placed retrogradely (Qian, 1992).

Several hundred cases of persistently patent duct have undergone occlusion in this fashion. In 109 cases commented upon by Porstmann (1974), no mortality and only minor morbidity were noted. The method was unsuccessful in eight patients, in five because the duct was too large and the plug slipped into the pulmonary artery. Since the plug was still attached to the guidewire, it could be manoeuvred into the femoral vein and removed by venectomy. In the remaining three patients the plug could not be fixed because of the rigidity or small size of the duct. It was permitted to embolize to the aortic bifurcation and removed by arteriotomy.

Disadvantages of the Porstmann technique include, first, arterial entry, with need for arterial exposure under certain circumstances, and possible arterial damage; second, the requirement for a transductal arterio-venous loop, necessitating venectomy should be device have to be retrieved; and, third, the limitation on age for closure.

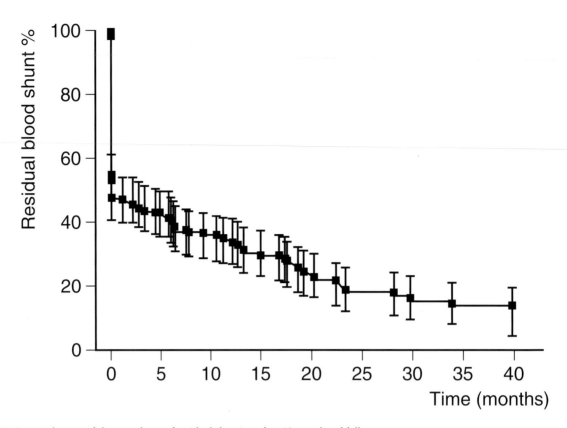

Figure 52.17 Actuarial curve of the prevalence of residual shunting after 40 months of follow-up.

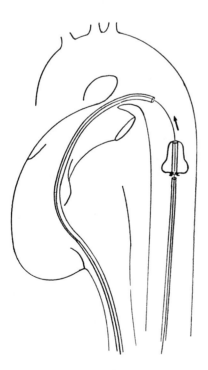

Figure 52.18 Schematic representation of Porstmann's technique for occlusion of the duct.

Advantages, however, include a secured delivery system that avoids free embolization with placement and little or no residual or recurrent shunting (Wang, 1991). Despite the early clinical trials and success of this approach, it remains technically complex. Except for a few centres, it has not achieved large clinical application (Kitamura et al, 1976; Schrader et al, 1993, 1994).

A similar conical polyurethane plug, the Botalloccluder, requires only transvenous delivery but suffers from the requirement of a large bore catheter (Saveliev et al, 1992; Verin et al, 1993b). Using a Nitinol wire framework, Amplatz has now designed a ductal plug delivered through a long transvenous sheath technique using small catheters. This system is uniquely suited for the small child with a large duct, measuring 4 mm or greater, where coil implantation may be unstable. Early clinical applications have been encouraging (Masura et al, 1998). The device will certainly find a place in the armamentarium of transcatheter occluders (Figure 52.19).

Closure using spring coils

Using spring coils designed for embolization of peripheral vessels, Cambier et al (1992) reported successful occlusion of ducts smaller than 2.5 mm in diameter. Lloyd

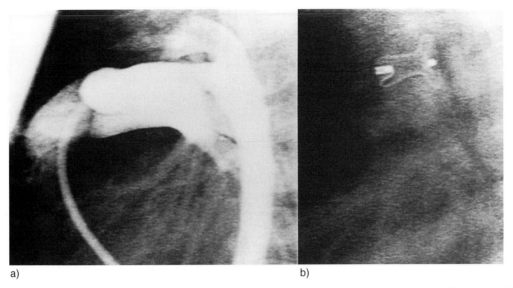

a)   b)

Figure 52.19 A large arterial duct with left-to-right shunting. (a) A lateral projection of an aortogram showing the large arterial duct. (b) The wire mesh of the Amplatzer device in the duct.

et al (1993), and Moore (1994a), then applied the procedure to a larger number of patients, commenting that the approach was simple, not technically demanding and could safely be performed in an outpatient setting. In particular, the requirement for only small catheters for delivery makes this approach attractive even in the small infant or child. The duct may be cannulated from either a venous or arterial approach, or both for simultaneous implantations (Figure 52.20). This technique has now been used worldwide, because of the availability of the implant, its low cost (Prieto et al, 1998) and high rates of occlusion: 95% or better in long-term follow-up of more than 6 months (Weber et al, 1996; Nishimoto et al, 1997; Rothman et al, 1997; Dalvi et al, 1998; Ino et al, 1998; Goyal et al, 1999). Occlusion using spring coils compares well with results achieved using the double umbrella implant, in terms of rates of occlusion (Galal et al, 1996; Zeevi et al, 1996), and has been used successfully for closure of residual surgical shunts (Podnar and Masura, 1999) or after attempted occlusion using the double umbrella (Moore et al, 1994b, 1995; Hijazi et al, 1995; de Moor et al, 1996). While comparatively fewer procedures have been performed in the adult (Ing et al, 1996), similar rates of occlusion are possible. As with other techniques for transcatheter ductal occlusion, recannulation has been noted, albeit rarely (Nishimoto et al, 1997; Goyal et al, 1999). Coils have also been used to close larger ducts, wider than 4 mm diameter, although heavier gauge wire (0.052 inch (0.13 cm) in contrast to 0.038 inch (0.095 cm)) (Owada et al, 1997) or multiple implants (Hijazi et al, 1996) are often required. Improvements in the technique of delivery, using detachable control mechanisms (Tometzki et al, 1996; Arora et al, 1997; Podnar and Masura, 1997; Bermudez-Canete

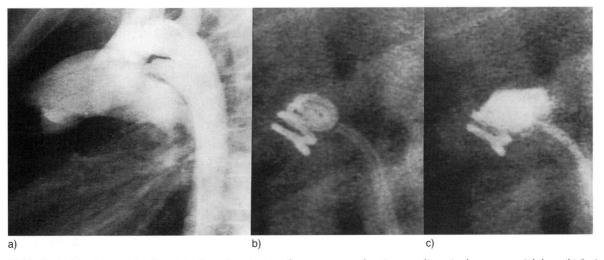

a)   b)   c)

Figure 52.20 Occlusion of an arterial duct. (a) A lateral projection of an aortogram showing a medium-sized patent arterial duct. (b) Spring coils can be seen astride the duct. (c) A contrast injection confirming occlusion of the ductal flow by implantation of the coil.

et al, 1998; Oho et al, 1998; Uzun et al, 1998; Johnston et al, 1999), a snare (Sommer et al, 1994; Ing and Bierman, 1995; Ing and Sommer, 1999), modified delivery catheters (Kuhn and Latson, 1995), forceps (Hays et al, 1996) or balloon occlusion (Bendjis and Moore, 1997; Dalvi et al, 1998) have further simplified the procedure. Whether these modifications will lead to improved rates of occlusion or lessen complications is not known as yet. Complications reported so far have been few and are limited primarily to embolization of the device to the pulmonary arteries, from which it can often be retrieved using a snare. More rarely, there may be left pulmonary arterial stenosis (Dalvi et al, 1998) or haemolysis through a partially occluded shunt (Ono et al, 1998; Uzun et al, 1999).

NATURAL HISTORY

Like most congenital cardiac malformations, completely reliable information concerning the natural history of untreated patients with a persistently patent duct is non-existent. The data available stem from the short period of time that elapsed between the condition being diagnosed with any frequency and to its being relieved by operation. Campbell (1968) attempted an overview of the natural history, based on his own extensive clinical experience and on the literature. Inevitably, such calculations tend to overemphasize the number of patients who experience events, be they favourable or adverse. They perhaps underestimate the number of patients with an asymptomatic and undetected duct.

SPONTANEOUS CLOSURE

By definition, a persistent duct is one that remains open beyond 3 months in an infant born at fullterm. Delayed closure in premature infants, or that occurring within the first 3 months, is, therefore, excluded from consideration in this section. Campbell analysed four series of patients in which 11 examples of spontaneous closure occurred over 1842 patient-years, giving a rate of 0.6% per annum. Several of the examples, however, were based on quite tenuous clinical impressions. In none was catheterization performed before and after the event. The figure calculated by Campbell is almost certainly an overestimate. He did not suggest that surgery should be delayed, except, perhaps, in patients with small shunts and signs that the duct was already closing. Few cardiologists would now agree even with these exceptions.

EFFECT ON LIFE EXPECTANCY

By combining four series, consisting mainly of 'unselected' schoolchildren with persistent duct, Campbell deduced a mortality rate of 0.42% per annum during the first two decades. Thereafter, he calculated mortality

rates per year as 1–1.5% in the third decade, 2–2.5% in the fourth and 4% for each subsequent year. These calculations indicate that one third of patients with a persistent duct die by the age of 40, in contrast to less than one twentieth of the normal population. Many of the figures are based on data obtained in the era before antibiotics were available. As infective endocarditis is a major cause of death, the impact of antibiotics must also be taken into account.

These figures agree fairly well with age at death as reported in necropsy series. Abbott (1936), for example, found the mean age at death, having excluded those who died in infancy, to be 30 years. In another series, the mean age was 36.5 years (Keys and Shapiro, 1943). Despite this agreement, the fact remains that calculations from postmortem series, and from clinical series, are extrapolations from rather small numbers. They undoubtedly exaggerate the adverse aspects of the natural history.

COMPLICATIONS

The important complications of persistent patency of the duct include congestive heart failure, infective endarteritis, pulmonary vascular disease, aneurysmal formation, thromboembolism and calcification.

CONGESTIVE HEART FAILURE

Congestive heart failure resulting from an isolated persistent duct either develops in infancy or during adult life. Infective endarteritis may rarely precipitate heart failure during childhood. Heart failure in infancy usually has its onset before the age of 3 months. Occasionally, its presence may not be recognized until after that time. A delayed normal fall in pulmonary vascular resistance may cause the left-to-right flow to increase progressively. The clinical picture is initially that of left heart failure, with tachypnoea and pulmonary oedema. Ultimately, signs of right-heart failure appear with hepatomegaly. Although initially there may be a good response to digoxin and diuretics, this is seldom maintained. Closure is advisable. These infants born at term do not respond to indomethacin when over 3 months of age. The occasional occurrence of sudden death in infants treated medically further encourages a policy of early intervention (Keith et al, 1978).

Amongst adults, there used to be a group with cardiomegaly and features of left ventricular overload and strain. Such patients must now be rare in countries with well-developed systems of health care, as it is unlikely their lesion will have escaped detection. Congestive heart failure may also occur as a terminal event in patients in whom severe pulmonary vascular disease complicates a persistently patent duct. If so, transcatheter closure appears to be the treatment of choice (Bonhoeffer et al, 1993).

INFECTIVE ENDARTERITIS

Infective endarteritis in a patient with an uncomplicated persistent duct is uncommon in childhood and appears to be prevented by successful surgery. In the era preceding antibiotics and surgical treatment, it was a major cause of death. It accounted for almost half of all deaths in several pooled postmortem series (Abbott, 1936; Bullock et al, 1939; Keys and Shapiro, 1943). Campbell (1968) calculated an infection rate of between 0.45 and 1.0% per annum based on the figures of Cosh (1957) for patients after the first decade. Infection occasionally follows surgery, when it is probably secondary to infected sutures. The first line of treatment should be with antibiotics, following the recommendations as established by the American Heart Association, with surgery being delayed until sterilization is completed. Occasionally, this proves impossible, in which case surgery should be performed under continuing antibiotic therapy (Stejskal and Stark, 1992). Vegetations are usually found at the pulmonary arterial end of the duct. They may give rise to recurrent pulmonary embolization, with the clinical picture suggesting 'recurrent pneumonia'. Infection may cause some examples of ductal aneurysms, especially those occurring postoperatively (Rangel-Abundis et al, 1991). A single case of endarteritis on a clinically silent and non-hypertensive duct has been reported. This has implications for treatment in such situations (Balzer et al, 1993).

PULMONARY HYPERTENSION AND THE PERSISTENT DUCT

Although the pulmonary arterial pressure is usually normal, or only slightly elevated, in patients with persistently patent ducts, occasionally it is raised sufficiently to modify the physical findings. Pulmonary hypertension develops either because of a torrential left-to-right shunt or as the consequence of raised pulmonary vascular resistance. The latter may be caused by vasoconstriction or by structural changes within the pulmonary vascular bed. The implications of pulmonary hypertension secondary to an increased flow, as opposed to that caused by increased resistance, are markedly different. The two situations should be clearly differentiated.

When the duct is widely patent, and pulmonary vascular resistance is low, pulmonary arterial systolic equals systemic systolic pressure. Flow of blood to the lungs is then several times greater than that in the systemic circuit. The pulmonary arterial diastolic pressure may equal or be slightly lower than that in the aorta. These patients usually experience severe congestive heart failure, with failure to thrive and recurrent respiratory infections. Their electrocardiogram shows combined ventricular hypertrophy, while the chest radiograph reveals cardiomegaly with marked pulmonary plethora. The echocardiogram will reveal enlargement of the left

heart chambers. Such patients respond poorly to medical therapy. The correct management is to eliminate the shunt. Successful ligation, or occlusion, usually restores pulmonary arterial pressure to normal. There appears to be little risk of subsequent pulmonary vascular changes in this group of patients.

Some individuals respond to pulmonary venous distension, and to the left atrial enlargement that occurs secondary to high pulmonary blood flow because of reflex pulmonary vasoconstriction. They thereby partially protect themselves against the full effects of an unrestricted ductal shunt. If studied haemodynamically, these patients will be found to have a moderate left-to-right shunt. Pressure in the pulmonary circulation is at systemic levels, with or without a high pulmonary capillary wedge pressure. Pulmonary arterial pressure usually falls with administration of oxygen, or in response to pulmonary vasodilators. Successful elimination of the shunt usually restores pulmonary arterial pressure to normal.

Fixed and high pulmonary vascular resistance may result from progressive structural changes in patients who originally have large left-to-right shunts and normal pulmonary vessels. Alternatively, it may exist from birth. Civen and Edwards (1951) have suggested that patients in the latter category represent a form of persistence of the fetal pulmonary circulation. As yet, there is poor understanding of the factors that initiate and maintain the progressive pulmonary vascular damage which may occur with any large left-to-right shunt. They include the shearing forces of high flow and the high pressures exerted on the intima, perhaps associated with changes in the pulmonary handling of vasoactive agents and mitogens.

It is instructive to follow the clinical changes that accompany the onward rise in pulmonary vascular resistance. The pulmonary diastolic pressure reaches systemic levels in advance of the systolic pressure. The first alteration is, therefore, a decrease in diastolic flow across the duct. As flow diminishes, so the diastolic component of the continuous murmur becomes attenuated. Eventually, it disappears. At this stage the patient has a pan-systolic murmur. With a further increase in resistance, systolic pressures begin to equalize. Systolic flow diminishes, the systolic murmur shortens and, eventually, it also disappears. Concurrent with these changes, the second sound becomes closely split, or even single. There is accentuation of the pulmonary component. The clinical findings become those of severe pulmonary hypertension, with marked right ventricular hypertrophy and a loud, usually palpable, second pulmonary sound. A pulmonary ejection click is almost always audible. The second sound is loud and difficult to split. A high-pitched early diastolic murmur, the Graham Steel murmur, indicating pulmonary regurgitation may be added to these sounds, as may a pan-systolic murmur of tricuspid regurgitation when right heart failure supervenes.

Equalization of pressures with balanced resistances also brings reversal of the direction of flow through the duct. The magnitude of this flow then increases concomitant with the rise in pulmonary vascular resistance. In some patients, it is possible to recognize differential cyanosis, the blue discoloration being confined to the lower body; there is clubbing of the toes but not the fingers.

Unless there is differential cyanosis, it is not possible to recognize a duct clinically in patients with severe pulmonary hypertension and high pulmonary vascular resistance. Its diagnosis will depend on cardiac catheterization and angiography, or cross-sectional echocardiography and colour flow Doppler studies.

Until heart failure develops, the chest radiograph shows at most mild cardiomegaly, with marked prominence of the pulmonary arterial segment (Figure 52.12). Right-axis deviation, right atrial hypertrophy and right ventricular enlargement are usually evident in the electrocardiogram. In some patients, however, a picture of combined, or even left, ventricular hypertrophy may still be seen.

It is impossible to calculate accurately the risk of progressive pulmonary vascular disease in patients with a large persistent duct. Surgical treatment has been available almost as long as clinical recognition. The information in terms of natural history necessary to answer the question is not available, nor would such a study now be feasible. Campbell (1968) does not address this problem in his calculations. There are several reports in the literature, nonetheless, concerning this complication (Whitaker et al, 1955; Ellis et al, 1956; Wallgren, 1962). These are based on selected groups of patients. They overemphasize the frequency of the problem. Nor do they all distinguish adequately between pulmonary hypertension with high flow and true pulmonary vascular disease. The presence of pulmonary hypertension secondary to structural changes within the pulmonary vasculature increases the surgical risk, especially once there is right-to-left shunting. Ellis et al (1956) reported mortality in more than half of a small group of such patients. The complication should be largely avoided by early recognition and treatment of the hypertensive duct. In the occasional patient who escapes early detection, pulmonary arterial wedge angiography, with or without lung biopsy, may be useful in determining the extent of pulmonary vascular changes, and their potential for reversal.

ANEURYSM OF THE DUCT

True aneurysm of the duct is rare. It manifests in two distinct forms. The first is present at or shortly after birth (Heikkinen et al, 1974; Lund et al, 1992); this is the spontaneous aneurysm of infancy (Figure 52.21). The second form presents in childhood or later life. Cruickshank and Marquis (1958) reviewed the early cases reported in the literature. Rutishauser et al (1977) were able subsequently to cite 60 cases reported in infancy. Ductal closure usually begins at the pulmonary

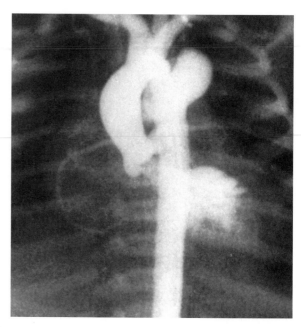

Figure 52.21 Anteroposterior retrograde aortogram defining a ductal aneurysm. Note the associated moderate aortic insufficiency.

arterial end of the vessel. If closure of the aortic end fails to occur, it becomes, in effect, an aortic diverticulum under systemic pressure. While formation of such a diverticulum is not uncommon, it is less clear why this occasionally progresses to aneurysmal formation. Structural abnormalities are possibly present in the aortic, but not the pulmonary, end of the duct. Sepsis may be involved in the pathogenesis of some cases in infancy. A diverticulum arising from the pulmonary trunk is also not uncommon.

The type found in infancy is much more common. It is usually asymptomatic and may not be uncovered until postmortem for death from other causes (Das and Chesterman, 1956). It presents as a tumour-like left-sided mediastinal mass (Rutishauser et al, 1977). Of the cases occurring in infancy and analysed by Cruickshank and Marquis (1958), death occurred by rupture in one and by embolism in a further tenth. Dissection and infection may also occur. Regression can occur, presumably owing to thrombosis and organization, but progressive enlargement, or the onset of hoarseness because of damage to the recurrent laryngeal nerve, is an indication for surgical excision (Heikkinen et al, 1974). In view of the frequency of life-threatening complications, angiographic confirmation and prompt surgical removal are advisable. Rupture, with survival owing to prompt surgery, has also been described (Ferlic et al, 1975), as has presentation with pulmonary arterial obstruction (Fripp et al, 1985).

Aneurysm of the duct is even more uncommon in adults. The duct may be patent at both ends, but it is usually closed at the pulmonary arterial end (Graham, 1940; Tutassaura et al, 1969; Ueno et al, 1990). Possible pathogenic mechanisms include arrested closure, with persistence of an aortic diverticulum; delayed spontaneous closure of the pulmonary arterial end of a persistent duct; infective arteritis; and external trauma in a patient with a persistent duct (Rangel-Abundis et al, 1991). Aneurysm of the duct should be considered in the differential diagnosis of adult with unexplained mediastinal masses seen on chest radiography. The diagnosis can be confirmed by aortography, and perhaps by computed tomography (Cohen et al, 1981). Like the pattern seen in infancy, the high incidence of rupture and embolization and the effects of pressure suggest that surgical excision is advisable.

Surgical ligation may itself be followed by aneurysmal formation (Kerwin and Jaffe, 1959; Ross et al, 1961), almost always associated with recanalization. In the experience of Ross et al (1961), infection was present in two thirds of the patients, predating surgery in two cases. In patients with staphylococcal arteritis, the infection originated with surgery and persisted because of contaminated sutures. The aneurysm was successfully excised or closed in all.

THROMBOEMBOLISM

Thrombosis of the duct was first described as a source of neonatal embolus by Rauchfuss (1859). Several cases, mostly fatal, have been described (Stout and Koehl, 1970; Dworsky et al, 1980). Early diagnosis may provide an opportunity for successful intervention, which may include thrombectomy, heparin and resection of infarcted tissue.

PATENCY OF THE ARTERIAL DUCT IN THE PREMATURE INFANT

Since the 1970s, there has been a marked increase in premature delivery in many, but not all, developed countries. While the reasons for this are obscure, the increase has been met by the development of neonatal intensive care units and, more recently, units for pregnancies considered to be at high risk. The art and science of caring for the extremely premature infant have developed to the point where survival of infants weighing no more than 500 g is not uncommon.

PATHOPHYSIOLOGY

There are several factors that tend to prevent closure of the arterial duct in the immature infant. Both the sensitivity to oxygen and the action of prostaglandin are age dependent (Clyman, 1990). On one hand, the tension output per unit of muscle in response to oxygen increases towards term, while the threshold for onset of contraction decreases. On the other hand, the relaxant mechanism of prostaglandin is more active in the immature duct (Coceani et al, 1979; Clyman, 1980). Levels of

circulating relaxant prostaglandins are also higher in the premature infant than in the infant at term, in part because of the immaturity of catabolic mechanisms in the lungs. Other factors, such as strategies for fluid balance (Stevenson, 1977; Bell et al, 1980), the type and duration of ventilatory support, drug therapy, phototherapy, blood transfusions and diuretics, undoubtedly account for the wide variations in incidence of problematic patients reported from different institutions (Clyman, 1984; Furzan et al, 1985; Rosenfeld et al, 1986).

The thickness of the well-muscularized fetal vessels responsible for pulmonary vascular resistance changes very little during the last trimester of gestation. Because the number of vessels increases rapidly, total pulmonary vascular resistance falls during this period. The vessels of the immature lung also constrict less for a given stimulus than at term. Constrictive stimuluses include hypoxia, acidaemia and, possibly, circulating vasoactive peptides and prostaglandins. There is also evidence that there is increased leakage of water from the vessels in the immature lungs. This decreases pulmonary compliance and may occur even when left atrial pressure is normal (Bland and McMillan, 1977). These factors render the immature infant especially liable to develop left-to-right shunting when the duct remains patent. Systemic vasoconstriction, so often a feature of the sick premature infant, may further encourage the shunt. Increased pulmonary blood flow may also exacerbate the respiratory distress syndrome (Jacob et al, 1980).

The immature infant is further handicapped by its reduced cardiac reserve. The immature, as opposed to mature, myocardium contains relatively more water and connective tissue. The immature ventricles are hence less distensible. Increased volume overload secondary to a left-to-right shunt produces an inordinate rise in left ventricular end-diastolic pressure, and a concomitant rise in pulmonary venous pressure. Experimental (Clyman, 1987) and human (Ellison et al, 1983) studies, however, suggest the newborn heart may be capable of significant response to a volume load, achieved by increasing stroke volume with no consequences to perfusion (Linder et al, 1990). Sympathetic innervation is also incomplete. With a large left-to-right shunt through the duct, systemic diastolic pressure falls. This compromises the flow through the coronary arteries, which, combined with a shortened diastole because of tachycardia and raised ventricular end-diastolic pressures, predisposes to subendocardial ischaemia. Systemic hypoxia secondary to pulmonary problems, combined with a reduced capacity to carry and deliver oxygen because of the presence of the fetal form of haemoglobin and concurrent anaemia, may further impair myocardial function. Ischaemic changes in the electrocardiogram are frequent in the sick premature infant. Other important circulations, such as those of the gut, kidneys and brain, may be compromised by the haemodynamic changes, related in part to the diastolic run-off from the aorta into the pulmonary arteries

(Clyman, 1987; Gleason et al, 1988; Bomelburg and Jorch, 1989; Alpan et al, 1990; Wong et al, 1990). The duct may be an aetiological factor in necrotizing entero-colitis (Kitterman, 1975) and cerebral haemorrhage (Perlman et al, 1981; Bejar et al, 1982).

Because of its potentially catastrophic effects, cerebral haemorrhage as a complication of patent duct has been the subject of several studies. External Doppler tech-niques have been used to study the velocity of cerebral flow in premature infants (Perlman et al, 1981; Martin et al, 1982). Perlman et al (1981) suggested that fluctua-tions in such velocities during opening and closing of the duct create the necessary conditions for subependymal haemorrhage. Lipman et al (1982) proposed that bleed-ing is triggered by a 'surge' in diastolic flow and arterial pressure after closure of the duct in the absence of autoregulation of cerebral blood flow. Bejar et al (1982) observed significant increases in the size of pre-existing haemorrhages when the duct was surgically ligated during the first 96 hours of life. The precise role of the duct in the pathogenesis of cerebral haemorrhage remains uncertain, although the association between the two con-ditions seems well established (Dykes et al, 1980; Ichihashi et al, 1990; Shortland et al, 1990).

CLINICAL FEATURES

The clinical picture of patency of the duct in the prema-ture infant depends on the size of the left-to-right shunt, on the maturity of the heart and lungs to adjust to the increased volume load, and on the presence of other pathology, which may obscure the more typical findings. As many premature infants have respiratory distress syn-drome, the stage of this illness and the use of surfactant will also modify the clinical expression of ductal shunt-ing by influencing pulmonary vascular resistance. The presence of a significant duct can often be difficult to rec-ognize even by experienced clinicians. Echocardiography is of great value. Three fairly distinct patterns of clinical presentation may be observed (Heymann and Hoffman, 1978); these occur in the absence or presence of pulmo-nary disease and in infants recovering from pulmonary disease.

ABSENCE OF PULMONARY DISEASE

Patients with patency of the duct who do not have pul-monary disease generally have birthweights exceeding 1500 g. Smaller infants may be encountered, nonetheless, whose mothers may have received steroids or who have themselves received surfactant. Sometimes a systolic murmur is detected in the first week of life. This becomes louder and longer as pulmonary vascular resistance falls, and eventually it spills into early diastole. The murmur is best heard in the second and third left interspaces. It is associated with accentuation of pulmonary closure, with

the typical continuous murmur as heard in older children usually not being present. If the shunt becomes large, the precordium becomes hyperactive, the pulse pressure wide and the peripheral pulses bounding. An apical third sound may also occur associated with a diastolic flow murmur. If the left ventricle fails, tachycardia and tachypnoea develop, and moist sounds can be heard in the chest. Apnoea and bradycardia may complicate severe left ventricular failure. Hepatomegaly may only develop late. Most infants in this group do not develop massive shunts and can be managed by simple medical means. The duct closes spontaneously in the majority at an age approximating to fullterm. These older infants tend to respond less well to indomethacin than more immature infants (Peckham et al, 1984).

INFANTS RECOVERING FROM LUNG DISEASE

Left-to-right ductal shunting may develop in infants recovering from respiratory distress syndrome. Usually they weigh between 1000 and 1500 g. Most probably the duct is patent from birth, and left-to-right shunting only develops during recovery when pulmonary vascular resistance falls. At this same time, increased administra-tion of fluids may further aggravate the loading effects of the left-to-right shunt on left ventricular function. Many of these infants are still maintained on mechanical venti-lators or continuous positive airway pressure when shunting first develops. Because of this, the initial systolic murmur may be difficult to detect. Often the clinical find-ings are quite labile. If the shunt increases, the murmur becomes more obvious. As in those with lung disease, it may eventually spill into diastole. Other signs of a large shunt may be present, including bounding pulses, a hyperdynamic precordium and tachycardia. This group of patients tends to be more immature and to develop left ventricular failure with relatively smaller shunts. Ventilatory status may deteriorate so that higher con-centrations of oxygen and increased pressure or rate settings are required to counter a deteriorating status of the blood gases. Apnoeic episodes and bradycardia are common.

INFANTS WITH LUNG DISEASE

Infants with patency of the duct and lung disease tend to be the most immature infants, with birthweights below 1000 g. Usually they are dependent upon a ventilator. The development of a left-to-right ductal shunt in these patients is associated with increasing requirement for ventilator support and deterioration of the status of the blood gases. Murmurs may be difficult to hear, and occa-sionally a very large duct may be silent (Thibeault et al, 1975; McGraph et al, 1978). Signs of a large left-to-right shunt may occur, but left ventricular failure is often difficult to differentiate from signs resulting from pulmonary disease or sepsis.

INVESTIGATIONS

Neither the electrocardiogram nor the chest radiograph are particularly helpful in making the diagnosis of a significant duct in premature infants. The electrocardiogram may show left ventricular hypertrophy in the group without lung disease, especially if the shunt is substantial and has been present for some time. In the other two groups, right ventricular predominance is more usual. As mentioned, ischaemic changes may also be present. The chest radiograph may show cardiomegaly with increased pulmonary blood flow. Often the heart is not obviously enlarged, and pulmonary changes owing to flow or failure are difficult to differentiate from those caused by primary pulmonary problems.

ECHOCARDIOGRAPHY

Persistent patency of the duct after the neonatal period is readily diagnosed by its characteristic clinical features. Ligation is normally advised, even when the shunt is small. Cross-sectional echocardiography and Doppler flow studies are invaluable in ruling out other structural malformations prior to surgery. In premature infants, however, especially those with respiratory distress syndrome, the recognition of significant shunting across a patent duct can be extremely difficult. Indeed, patients with severe ventilator-dependent respiratory distress syndrome may have a large ductal shunt, which may be entirely silent owing to lack of turbulent flow within the vessel (Thibeault et al, 1975; McGraph et al, 1978). Cardiomegaly may also be absent, especially in infants who are fluid restricted.

Hirata and colleagues (1969) reported a good correlation between M-mode echocardiographic and angiographic measurements of left atrial volume. Left atrial diameter also correlates well with the magnitude of left-to-right shunts through a ventricular septal defect (Carter and Bowmen, 1973). In the light of these observations, Silverman et al (1974) evaluated the use of M-mode echocardiography to recognize ductal shunting in premature infants. In the absence of age-related normals for such patients, they measured the ratio of the dimensions of the left atrium and the aortic root. A value of 1.0 for this ratio in normal full-term infants had been found by Hagan et al (1973). Using a slightly modified technique, Silverman et al (1974) found that this ratio was increased in patients with a patent duct compared with controls. The ratio fell after surgical ligation of the duct. Measurements of left ventricular end-diastolic dimension, shortening fraction and systolic time intervals were added to those of the ratio of the left atrium to the aortic root in an effort to improve specificity and sensitivity (Baylen et al, 1977; Hirschklau et al, 1978). Although echocardiographic evidence of patency using these criterions often precedes clinical recognition of a left-to-right shunt, it is also clear that many important ducts will be missed, especially in fluid-restricted infants (Hirschklau et al, 1978; Sahn and Allen, 1978; Voldez-Cruz and Dudell, 1981). This type of echocardiographic evaluation became widely adopted in critically ill infants with pulmonary disease but has now been superseded by cross-sectional echocardiography combined with Doppler assessment of flow. Further refinements in echocardiographic diagnosis of ductal patency can be anticipated with high-resolution imaging. The full length of the duct can be imaged, along with other arch structures, using the suprasternal approach. Definition may be further improved in the premature infant by the use of high frequency 7 MHz probes (Figure 52.22).

MANAGEMENT

Because many ducts will eventually close in premature infants, there has been an understandable reluctance to advise aggressive intervention as soon as a significant left-to-right shunt is recognized. The presence of a ductal shunt, however, has been implicated in the pathogenesis of bronchopulmonary dysplasia, and as a factor in the

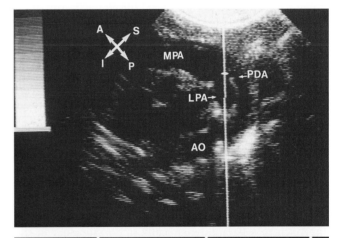

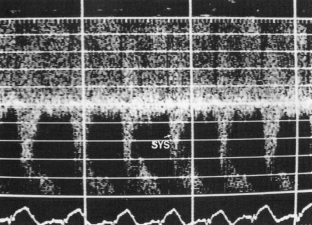

Figure 52.22 Cross-sectional echocardiographic image of the duct (PDA). The lower panel shows a Doppler recording from its pulmonary end with flow during systole (SYS). LPA, left pulmonary artery; MPA, pulmonary trunk; AO, aorta.

duration of ventilator support. This increased risk of chronic lung disease has led many to advocate early and effective treatment. Early experience with surgical ligation demonstrated that congestive heart failure could quickly be controlled, although mortality and morbidity from the respiratory distress syndrome remained high. With further surgical experience, mortality directly resulting from the operation has been reduced to less than 1%. Some centres have advocated, and successfully performed, surgery in the nursery, thereby avoiding the hazards of transport to and from the operating room.

Once the role of E-type prostaglandins in maintaining ductal patency during fetal life was established, pharmacologically induced closure using indomethacin was soon reported in the premature infant (Sharpe, 1975; Friedman et al, 1976; Heymann et al, 1976). Rates of success varying between 18 and 89% were reported in a number of subsequent uncontrolled clinical trials in which various doses of oral indomethacin were used. Vert and colleagues (1980) showed that the plasma half-life of indomethacin correlates inversely with postnatal age. This, and the fact that the bioavailability of oral indomethacin varies quite considerably, probably account for many of the reported differences. Transient renal insufficiency and mild gastrointestinal bleeding are the main side effects.

Despite its widespread usage, questions remain concerning proper dosage, duration of treatment and optimal timing of administration. Several studies involving large numbers of infants were performed (Cotton et al, 1978; Gersony et al, 1983) to address some of these issues; these have been summarized by Clyman (1987). Although the effectiveness of indomethacin in prompting ductal closure depends on both dosage and the timing of administration (Brash et al, 1981; Yeh et al, 1989; Gal et al, 1990), the major determinants of success are gestational and postnatal age.

There is, as yet, no consensus regarding the optimal approach to a haemodynamically important duct in the premature infant. The trend is to earlier closure, by medical or surgical means (Figure 52.23) (Musewe and Olley, 1992). In infants weighing less than 1000 g, without evidence of cardiac compromise, the administration of indomethacin has been associated with improved outcomes (Mahoney, 1982, 1985; Cotton et al, 1991). This was in contrast to those infants weighing more than 1000 g, where outcomes were unaltered. As only one third of such infants with low birthweight become symptomatic, this approach would result in the needless administration of indomethacin to some babies. Once the problem is recognized, however, intake of fluid should be restricted, and frusemide (furosemide) given in a dose of 1 mg/kg. Digoxin is of dubious benefit in this situation. If the shunt remains large after 24 hours, indomethacin should be given, preferably intravenously although nasogastric administration can be successful. Extreme prematurity, very low birthweight and advanced

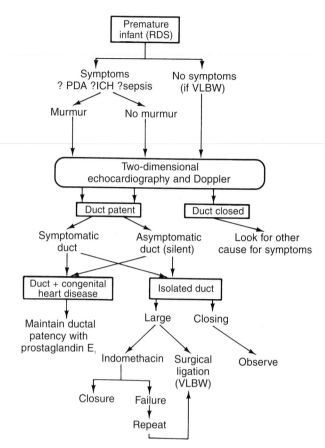

Figure 52.23 Flow diagram for the management of the premature infant with respiratory distress syndrome and a suspected patent duct. ICH, intracranial haemorrhage; PDA, patent arterial duct; VLBW, very low birthweight. (From Musewe N N, Olley P M 1992 Patent ductus arteriosus. In: Neonatal Heart Disease, Freedom R M, Benson L N, Smallhorn J F (eds), Springer-Verlag, London p 598, with permission.)

conceptional or postnatal age are all factors that reduce the chances of successful closure using indomethacin. Renal and/or hepatic insufficiency, serious hyperbilirubinaemia or problems with coagulation are contraindications to its use.

Dosage is largely selected on an empirical basis. The initial dose is 0.2 mg/kg, while subsequent doses depend on age at time of initial treatment. The subsequent two doses are 0.1 mg/kg in those less than 48 hours of age, 0.2 mg/kg in those aged 2–7 days and 0.25 mg/kg in those older than 7 days. Prolonged treatment with indomethacin has also been attempted to prevent recurrence, and with good effect (Hammerman and Aramburo, 1990; Rennie and Cooke, 1991). The rate of re-opening is highest in the very premature, occurring in one third at weights less than 1000 g and in less than one tenth of those weighing 1500 g (Mellander et al, 1984; Clyman et al, 1985). If there is no response to indomethacin, surgical ligation should be considered.

Indomethacin-induced closure of the duct is followed by immediate and progressive clinical improvement, with a decrease in requirements for oxygen and in mean airway inflation pressure during mechanical ventilation (Jacob et al, 1980). Lung compliance has been shown to improve both after surgical ligation and closure with indomethacin (Naulty et al, 1978; Yeh et al, 1981). Duration of ventilation, length of hospitalization and the costs of medical care are also reduced by early treatment (Cotton et al, 1978; Merritt et al, 1979; Gersony et al, 1983). Such studies have not been able to demonstrate any substantial difference in the outcome of infants treated either surgically or medically. They did observe a generally favourable neurological developmental, visual, audiological and renal outcome of infants given indomethacin. Reversal of indomethacin-induced ductal closure by administration of prostaglandin, in the presence of ductal-dependent cardiac malformations, has been possible (Strauss et al, 1982).

Surgical ligation of the persistent duct in premature infants was first reported by Powell (1963) and de Cancq (1963). Overall mortality remains high but is more often related to continuing respiratory distress, intracranial haemorrhage or coagulopathy (Brandt et al, 1981; Massone et al, 1990; Matsuo et al, 1991) rather than the surgery itself. As with therapy with indomethacin, surgery has been associated with a decreased need for ventilatory support and reduced hospital stay (Cotton et al, 1978; Coster et al, 1989), particularly in infants weighing less than 1500 g (Ring-Mrozik et al, 1991; Canarelli et al, 1993). Surgery can be safely carried out in the neonatal intensive care unit to avoid the stress of transportation to the operating theatre (Hoffman et al, 1991; Kewitz et al, 1991).

Many questions remain unanswered concerning the true impact of a large left-to-right ductal shunt on the course and outcome of prematurity and respiratory distress syndrome. In a large multicentred trial, one third of patients with a significant duct had spontaneous closure, while indomethacin induced closure in seven tenths of patients treated. There was no difference in the rate of closure if indomethacin was given immediately on diagnosis or after 48 hours of intensive medical therapy. Mortality rates were identical in patients treated with indomethacin early, with indomethacin given late or with surgery, being about 13% overall in each group (Nadas, 1982).

USE OF PROSTAGLANDINS TO — MAINTAIN PATENCY OF THE DUCT —

The critical role of the duct during the newborn period in the pathophysiology of many congenital heart malformations has been discussed earlier in the chapter. The demonstration that E-type prostaglandins maintain ductal patency during fetal life suggested the clinical use of prostaglandin E_1 or E_2 in newborns with heart disease. Successful maintenance of the duct was first reported in patients with duct-dependent pulmonary blood flow,

Table 52.1. Indications for therapy with prostaglandins E_1 (or E_2) in newborn

	Defects
Clear benefit	
Duct-dependent pulmonary blood flow	Pulmonary atresia, critical pulmonary stenosis, severe tetralogy
Duct-dependent systemic blood flow	Interruption of the aortic arch, hypoplastic left heart syndrome, aortic coarctation
Duct-dependent mixing	Complete transposition, provided there is adequate communication at atrial level
Possible benefit	
Tricuspid valve lesions	Ebstein's anomaly, isolated tricuspid incompetence
Duct-dependent systemic blood flow	Critical aortic stenosis

such as occurs in pulmonary atresia with or without a ventricular septal defect (Elliott et al, 1975; Olley et al, 1976; Saji et al, 1991). Favourable responses were subsequently observed in other lesions (Table 52.1).

Prostaglandin E_1 is infused intravenously in a starting dose of 0.05–0.1 mg/min per kg body weight. This can often be further reduced to 0.01–0.02 mg/min per kg after an initial effect, thus reducing side effects. Intra-arterial administration does not appear to have any therapeutic advantages and may cause potent systemic vasodilatation associated with local oedema. Furthermore, potential complications from the arterial line are likely to be more serious. Arterial tension of oxygen usually rises within minutes of starting treatment in patients with duct-dependent pulmonary blood flow.

The response is remarkably uniform. It is usually possible to increase arterial oxygen saturation to around 80%. Infants under 4 days of age, and those with the lowest tensions of oxygen prior to infusion, tend to show the most dramatic increases. Those with birthweights exceeding 4 kg (9 lb) tend to respond less well (Freed et al, 1981). The improved oxygenation provides 'a period of grace', during which metabolic acidosis can be reversed and palliative surgery organized on a semielective basis. Treatment with prostaglandin E_1 generally needs to be maintained for only 1 or 2 days. Under special circumstances, such as low birthweight, prolonged administration appears to be safe, and tolerance does not develop (Lewis and Lurie, 1978).

Prostaglandin E_1 is also valuable in the emergency care of infants with duct-dependent systemic blood flow, such as those with aortic coarctation, interruption of the aortic arch and hypoplastic left heart syndrome. In patients with interruption of the aortic arch, the pressure in the descending aorta increases markedly, and differences in pressure across the duct are reduced or abolished. Patients with aortic coarctation show a trend to equalize the blood pressures in the upper and lower limbs. In both lesions, previously suppressed urinary output usually increases. The partially constricted duct relaxes more slowly than in those patients with cyanotic malformations. The infusion should be continued for 2–3 hours before concluding that a response is unlikely. Clinical improvement can be anticipated in about four fifths of acyanotic patients.

Failure to respond may be a consequence of previous complete closure of the duct, congenital absence or intrauterine closure of the vessel or extreme hypoplasia of the pulmonary arteries, which will of themselves limit pulmonary blood flow despite adequate dilation of the duct.

Reported side effects of prostaglandin include fever, bradycardia, hypotension, apnoeic spells, cutaneous flushing and seizure-like activity. Apnoeic spells occur in about one tenth of treated infants. They are more common in those under 2 kg (4.5 lb) and are probably dependent on dose. Assisted ventilation should be available when prostaglandin E_1 therapy is initiated.

Pulmonary arterial smooth muscle may also be reduced by infusion of prostaglandin E_1. This effect may be associated with the formation of localized aneurysmal dilatations (Haworth et al, 1980). This latter finding has not yet been confirmed. Long-term treatment with prostaglandins may induce cortical hyperostosis in the long bones. This effect seems to be completely reversible when therapy is discontinued.

Oral prostaglandin E_2 has been used to maintain ductal patency over several weeks or months (Coe and Silove, 1979). While successful in raising the tension of oxygen, oral therapy carries the disadvantage of frequent administration, uncertain absorption and potential vascular damage (Schlesinger et al, 1989; Baji et al, 1991). Even after prolonged systemic or oral therapy, in the majority (but not all), the duct retains its ability to constrict when administration is discontinued.

The impact of prostaglandin E_1 on the mortality and morbidity of serious congenital heart malformations in the newborn period is difficult to measure because of the many concurrent improvements in surgical technique and postoperative management. It seems probable that it has been a significant factor in the improved outlook for these children. The only group of patients in which its effect may be adverse are those with pulmonary venous obstruction. In these, administration of prostaglandin may precipitate pulmonary oedema and cause a marked deterioration in condition (Freedom et al, 1978).

INFILTRATION OF FORMALIN, BALLOON DILATION AND IMPLANTATION OF STENTS

Rudolph et al (1975) described a technique of subadventitial formalin infiltration of the wall of the duct designed to maintain long-term patency of the vessel in patients with duct-dependent cardiac malformations in whom surgery was either inadequate or not feasible. Satisfactory results were reported when formalin infiltration was combined with valvotomy or infundibuloplasty (Melo et al, 1980). When used alone, the technique seemed less successful (Hatem et al, 1980). Deanfield and colleagues (1981), however, found that infiltration of formalin did not ensure ductal patency even for a short time. They abandoned the technique in favour of infusion of prostaglandin E_1. Furthermore, Seibert et al (1981) reported two patients who developed delayed damage to the function of the left recurrent laryngeal nerve after infiltration of formalin. In view of the alternatives, therefore, there is little now to recommend this procedure.

Percutaneous balloon dilation has also been proposed as a method to maintain ductal patency (Corwin et al, 1981; Suarez de Lezo et al, 1985; Lund et al, 1989; Walsh et al, 1992, 1993). Temporary patency can be achieved, but abrupt closure, thrombosis or rupture can occur, making this a less reliable means of assuring patency. Except for special instances, this technique has not been pursued clinically.

To provide a mechanical scaffold for the ductal wall, resistant to the constrictive forces of ductal closure, Coe and Olley (1991) proposed the implantation of endovascular stents. This approach, using either self- or balloon-expandable stents, has had limited clinical application. The implantation in anatomically uncomplicated ducts, such as in pulmonary atresia, critical pulmonary stenosis or the hypoplastic left heart syndrome (Figure 52.24), has been encouraging (Gibbs et al, 1993; Ruiz et al, 1993). The application in more complex situations, such as occurs in tetralogy with pulmonary atresia, however, can be technically difficult (Gibbs et al, 1992). The role of stents in the management of these infants has yet to be defined.

BIOENGINEERING OF THE ARTERIAL DUCT FOR THERAPEUTIC GAIN

Novel methodology for maintaining ductal patency into the postnatal period to sustain life and allow surgical intervention of duct-dependent cardiac malformations is emerging. Very recently, Mason et al (1999) described the maintenance of ductal patency through surgical transfection of fetal lambs. By targeting the ductal smooth muscle cells with an expression vector encoding a 'decoy' of the fibronectin message, it proved possible to sequester the protein, thereby preventing upregulation of fibronectin and arresting intimal cushions. This approach both emphasizes the importance of fibronectin to the process of ductal closure and identifies a new therapeutic modality and target. While fetal surgery is probably not feasible in the clinical setting, an alternative approach,

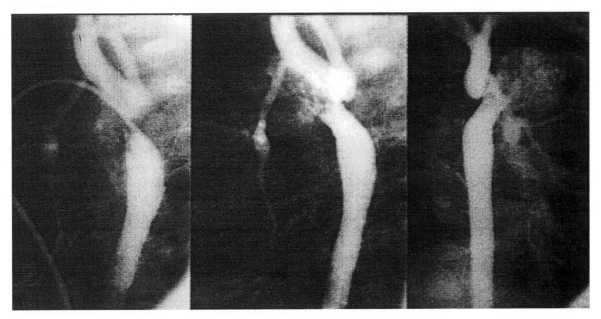

Figure 52.24 A patient with hypoplastic left heart syndrome awaiting cardiac transplantation. The duct became stenotic and unresponsive to prostaglandin. Here, a pulmonary arterial angiogram depicts a stent placed transvenously across the duct to relieve the stenosis.

such as that employed by Rajotte et al (1998) and Arap et al (1998), targeting chemotherapeutic agents given by systemic infusion to different vascular beds by unique peptide 'zipcodes', may offer bright therapeutic avenues.

These studies identifying and characterizing the cellular and molecular mechanisms involved in ductal patency and closure have tremendously advanced our understanding of this developmentally programmed fetal vessel. The impact of these advances extends beyond the scope of ductal remodelling, as they have provided insight into the pathogenesis of occlusive vascular diseases, processes which utilize similar pathways. This work has also provided the basis for further advances to develop safe therapeutic measures by which to maintain ductal patency for patients with cyanotic congenital heart disease, ultimately translating into improved care and clinical outcome.

SUMMARY

At first sight, there seem to be few questions remaining about the arterial duct. The reality is quite different. There is still much to learn about its structure and innervation. What is the process that links oxygen to contraction of its smooth muscle, and to closure of the lumen? What are the factors that determine true persistence of the vessel? What is the true significance of the duct in prematurity? What are the factors that cause significant left-to-right shunts to develop? How is this problem best managed? Can mechanical devices, or perhaps more specific pharmacological agents, substitute for surgical closure or maintain patency? And what will be the role of the molecular mechanisms discussed above? Further study of the arterial duct both in the laboratory and by careful clinical observation should continue to be rewarding.

REFERENCES

Abbott M 1936 Atlas of congenital heart disease. American Heart Association, New York

Airan B, Bhan A, Rao I M 1989 The combination of a left aortic arch, a right-sided descending thoracic aorta with a left-sided arterial duct. International Journal of Cardiology 24: 107–109

Akiyama K, Hasegawa T, Kitamura S et al 1992 Right-sided patent ductus arteriosus with a right aortic arch and right descending aorta. Japanese Journal of Thoracic Surgery 45: 442–445

Alberts B, Bray D, Lewis J, Raff M, Roberts K, Watson J D 1994 In: Robertson and Adams (eds) Molecular biology of the cell. Garland, New York

Ali Khan M A, Al Yousef S, Mullins C E, Sawyer W 1992 Experience with 205 procedures of transcatheter closure of the ductus areteriosus with special reference to residual shunts and longterm followup. Journal of Thoracic and Cardiovascular Surgery 104: 1721–1727

Allan F D 1955 The innervation of the human ductus arteriosus. Anatomical Record 122: 611–631

Alliende-Gonzales F, Villa Elizage I, Antillon Klussmann F 1991 Copper deficiency and persistence of the ductus arteriosus. Developmental Pharmacology and Therapeutics 17: 172–179

Alpan G, Mauray F, Clyman R I 1990 The effects of the patent ductus arteriosus on diaphragmatic blood flow and function. Pediatric Research 28: 437–445

Alzamora-Castro V, Battilana G, Abugattas R, Sialer S 1960 Patent ductus arteriosus and high altitude. American Journal of Cardiology 5: 761–763

Anderson R C 1954 Causative factors underlying congenital heart malformations. I, patent ductus arteriosus. Pediatrics 14: 143–151

Anderson R C 1977 Congenital cardiac malformations in 109 sets of twins and triplets. American Journal of Cardiology 39: 1045–1050

Anonymous 1992 Transcatheter occlusion of persistent arterial duct, Report of the European Registry. Lancet 340: 1062–1066

Aranzi G C 1564 De humano foetus libellus. Bononiae, Rubrius. In: Aronson S, Gennser G, Owman C H, Sjoberg N O 1970 Innervation and contractile response of the human ductus arteriosus. European Journal of Pharmacology 11: 178–186

Arap W, Pasqualini R, Ruoslahti E 1998 Chemotherapy targeted to tumor vasculature. Current Opinions in Oncology 10: 560–565

Aronson S, Gennser G, Owman C H, Sjoberg N O 1970 Innervation and contractile response of the human ductus arteriosus. European Journal of Pharmacology 11: 178–186

Arora R, Verma P K, Trehan V, Passey R, Nigam M, Kalra G S 1997 Transcatheter coil occlusion of persistent ductus arteriosus using detachable steel coils: short-term results. Indian Heart Journal 49: 60–64

Ash R, Fischer D 1955 Manifestations and results of treatment of patent ductus arteriosus in infancy and childhood. An analysis of 138 cases. Pediatrics 16: 695–703

Assali N S, Morris J A, Smith R W, Manson W A 1963 Studies on ductus arteriosus circulation. Circulation Research 13: 478–489

Auld P A M 1966 Delayed closure of the ductus arteriosus. Journal of Pediatrics 69: 61–66

Aziz K, Tasneem H 1990 Evaluation of pulmonary arterial pressure by Doppler color flow mapping in patients with a ductus arteriosus. British Heart Journal 63: 295–299

Bakker P M 1962 Morfogenese en involutie van de ductus arteriosus. Thesis, Leiden

Ballerini L, Mullins C E, Cifarelli A et al 1990 Non-surgical closure of patent ductus arteriosus in children with the Rashkind double disk occluder. Gionale Italian Di Cardiologia 20: 805–809

Balzer D T, Spray T L, McMufflin D, Cottingham W, Canter C E 1993 Endarteritis associated with a clinically silent patent ductus arteriosus. American Heart Journal 125: 1192–1193

Barclay A E, Barcroft J, Barron D H, Franklin K J 1939 A radiographic demonstration of the circulation through the heart in the adult and in the fetus, and the identification of the ductus arteriosus. British Journal of Radiology 12: 505–517

Barcroft J 1946 Researches on prenatal life. Blackwell, Oxford

Barcroft J, Kennedy J A, Mason M F 1938 The relation of the vagus nerve to the ductus arteriosus of the guinea pig. Journal of Physiology 92: 1P

Barger J D, Bregman E H, Edwards J E 1956 Bilateral ductus arteriosus with right aortic arch and right-sided descending aorta. American Journal of Roentgenology, Radium Therapy and Nuclear Medicine 76: 758–761

Bash G E, Mullins C E 1984 Insertion of patent ductus occluder by transvenous approach: a new technique. Circulation 70(suppl II): 285

Baylen B G, Meyer R A, Kaplan S, Ringenburg W E, Korfhagen J 1975 The critically ill premature infant with patent ductus arteriosus and pulmonary disease: an echocardiographic assessment. Journal of Pediatrics 86: 423–432

Baylen B G, Mayer R A, Korfhagen J, Benzing G, Bubb M E, Kaplan S 1977 Left ventricular performance in the critically ill premature infant with patent ductus arteriosus and pulmonary disease. Circulation 55: 182–188

Bejar R, Merritt T A, Coen R W 1982 Pulsatility index, patent ductus arteriosus and brain damage. Pediatrics 69: 818–822

Bell E F, Warburton D, Stonestreet B S, O W 1980 Effect of fluid administration on the development of symptomatic patent ductus arteriosus and congestive heart failure in premature infants. New England Journal of Medicine 302: 598–604

Benson L N, Patel R, Olley P M, Coceani F, Rowe R D 1979 Prostaglandin E$_1$ in the management of d-transposition of the great arteries. American Journal of Cardiology 44: 691–699

Benson L N, Dyck J, Hecht B 1988 Technique for closure of the small patent ductus arteriosus using the Rashkind occluder. Catheterization and Cardiovascular Diagnosis 14: 82–84

Berdjis F, Moore J W 1997 Balloon occlusion delivery technique for closure of patent ductus arteriosus. American Heart Journal 133: 601–604

Berdon W E, Baker D H, James L S 1965 The ductus bump. American Journal of Radiology 95: 91–98

Berger M, Ferguson C, Hendry J 1960 Paralysis of the left diaphragm, left vocal cord and aneurysm of the ductus arteriosus in a 7-week-old infant. Journal of Paediatrics 56: 800–802

Bermudez-Canete R, Santoro G, Bialkowsky J et al 1998 Patent ductus arteriosus occlusion using detachable coils. American Journal of Cardiology 82: 1547–1559

Berry B E, McGoon D C, Ritter D G, Davis G D 1974 Absence of anatomic origin from heart of pulmonary arterial supply: clinical application of classification. Journal of Thoracic and Cardiovascular Surgery 68: 119–125

Berry T E, Muster A J, Paul 1983 Transient neonatal tricuspid regurgitation: possible relation with premature closure of the ductus arteriosus. Journal of the American College of Cardiology 2: 1178–1182

Bickford B J 1960 Surgical aspects of patent ductus arteriosus. Archives of Disease in Childhood 35: 92–96

Binet J P, Conso J F, Losay J 1978 Ductus arteriosus sling: report of a newly recognized anomaly and its surgical correction. Thorax 33: 72–75

Bland R D, McMillan D D 1977 Lung fluid dynamics in awake newborn lambs. Journal of Clinical Investigation 60: 1107–1115

Bomelburg T, Jorch G 1989 Abnormal blood flow patterns in renal arteriosus of small preterm infants with patent ductus arteriosus detected by Doppler ultrasonography. European Journal of Pediatrics 148: 660–664

Bonham-Carter R E, Walker C H M 1955 Continuous murmurs without patent ductus arteriosus. Lancet i: 272–276

Bonhoeffer P, Borglii A, Onorato E, Carminati M 1993 Transfemoral closure of patent ductus arteriosus in adult patients. International Journal of Cardiology 39: 181–186

Boreus L O, Malmfors T, McMurphy D M, Olson L 1969 Demonstration of adrenergic receptor function and innervation in the ductus arteriosus of the human fetus. Acta Physiologica Scandinavica 77: 316–321

Born G V R, Dawes G S, Mott J C, Rennick B R 1956 The constriction of the ductus arteriosus caused by oxygen and asphyxia in newborn lambs. Journal of Physiology 132: 304–342

Boyd J D 1941 The nerve supply of the mammalian ductus arteriosus. Journal of Anatomy 75: 457–468

Brandt B, Marvin W J, Ehrenhaft J L, Heintz S, Doty D B 1981 Ligation of patent ductus arteriosus in premature infants. Annals of Thoracic Surgery 32: 167–170

Brash A R, Hickey D E, Graham T P, Stahlman M T, Oates J A, Cotton R B, 1981 Pharmokinetics of indomthacin in the neonate: the relationship of plasma levels to response of the ductus arteriosus. New England Journal of Medicine 303: 67–72

Braudo M, Rowe R D 1961 Ausculatation of the heart: early neonatal period. American Journal of Diseases of Childhood 101: 575–586

Brenner L D, Caputo G R, Mostbeck G 1992 Quantitation of left to right atrial shunts with velocity-encoded cine nuclear magnetic imaging. Journal of the American College of Cardiology 20: 1246–1250

Brook M M, Heymann M A 1995 Patent ductus arteriosus. In: Allen H and Gutgesell H (eds) Emmanouilides, Riemenschneider, Moss and Adams: heart disease in infants, children, and adolescents: including the fetus and young adult. Williams & Wilkins, Baltimore, MD, pp. 746–764

Boudreau N, Rabinovitch M 1991 Developmentally regulated changes in extracellular matrix in endothelial and smooth muscle cells in the ductus arteriosus may be related to intimal proliferation. Laboratory Investigation 64: 187–199

Boudreau N, Turley E, Rabinovitch M 1991 Fibronectin, hyaluronan, and a hyaluronan binding protein contribute to increased ductus arteriosus smooth muscle cell migration. Developmental Biology 143: 235–247

Boudreau N, Clausell N, Boyle J, Rabinovitch M 1992 Transforming growth factor-beta regulates increased ductus arteriosus endothelial glycosaminoglycan synthesis and a post-transcriptional mechanism controls increased smooth muscle fibronectin, features associated with intimal proliferation. Laboratory Investigation 67: 350–359

Buchanan J W 1978 Morphology of the abnormal ductus arteriosus in dogs. In: Heymann M A, Rudolph A M (eds) The ductus arteriosus: proceedings of the seventy-fifth Ross conference on pediatric research. Columbus, OH, Ross Laboratories, p 9–15

Bullock L T, Jones J C, Dolley F S 1939 The diagnosis and effects of ligation of the patent ductus arteriosus. Journal of Pediatrics 15: 786–801

Burnard E D 1959 A murmur that may arise from the ductus arteriosus in the human baby. Proceedings of the Royal Society of Medicine 52: 77–78

Burnell R H, Stern L M 1971 Five instances of persistent ductus arteriosus in one sibship. Clinical Pediatrics 10: 541–542

Burrows P E, Moes C A F, Freedom R M 1986 Doule aortic arch with atretic right dorsal segment. Pediatic Cardiology 6: 331–334

Calder A L, Kirker J A, Netuze J M, Starling M B 1984 Pathology of the ductus arteriosus treated with prostaglandin: comparisons with untreated cases. Pediatric Cardiology 5: 85–89

Cambier P A, Kirby W C, Wortham D C, Moore J W 1992 Percutaneous closure of the small (less than 2.5 mm) patent ductus arteriosus using coil embolization. American Journal of Cardiology 69: 815–816

Campbell A G M, Dawes G S, Fishman A P, Hyman A I, Perks A M 1968 The release of a bradykinin-like pulmonary vasodilator substance in foetal and newborn lambs. Journal of Physiology 195: 83–96

Campbell M 1961 Place of maternal rubella in the aetiology of congenital heart disease. British Medical Journal 1: 691–696

Campbell M 1968 Natural history of persistent ductus arteriosus. British Heart Journal 30: 4–13

Canarelli J P, Poulain H, Clamadieu C, Ricard J, Maingourd Y, Quintard J M 1993 Ligation of the patent ductus arteriosus in premature infants – indications and procedures. European Journal of Pediatric Surgery 3: 3–5

Carlgren L E 1959 The incidence of congenital heart disease in children born in Gothenburg 1941–1950. British Heart Journal 21: 40–50

Carter W H, Bowman R 1973 Estimation of shunt flow in isolated ventricular septal defect by echocardiogram. Circulation 48(suppl IV): 64

Cassady G, Crouse D T, Kirklin J W, Raddle I C, Soldin J C 1979 A randomized controlled trial of very early prophylactic ligation of the ductus arteriosus in babies who weighed 1000 grams or less at birth. New England Journal of Medicine 320: 1511–1516

Cassels D E 1973 The ductus arteriosus. Thomas, Springfield

Cassin S 1987 Role of prostaglandins, thromboxanes and leukotrienes in the control of the pulmonary circulation in the fetus and the newborn. Seminars in Perinatology 11: 53

Cetta F, Deleon S Y, Roughneen P T et al 1997 Cost-effectiveness of transaxillary muscle-sparing same-day operative closure of patent ductus arteriosus. American Journal of Cardiology 79: 1281–1282

Chien C T, Lin C S, Hsu Y H, Lin M C, Chen K S, Wu D J 1991 Potential of hemodynamic abnormalities in patent ductus arteriosus by cine magnetic resonance imaging. American Heart Journal 122: 1065–1073

Christie A 1930 Normal closing time of the foramen ovale and the ductus arteriosus. An anatomic and statistical study. American Journal of Diseases in Children 40: 323–326

Civen W H, Edwards J E 1951 The postnatal structural changes in the intrapulmonary arteries and arterioles. Archives of Pathology 51: 192–200

Clarkson P M, Orgil A A 1974 Continuous murmurs in infants of low birth weight. Journal of Pediatrics 84: 208–211

Clyman R L 1980 Ontogeny of the ductus arteriosus response to prostaglandins and inhibitors of their synthesis. Seminars in Perinatology 4: 115–124

Clyman R L 1984 The role of the patent ductus arteriosus in respiratory distress syndrome. Seminars in Perinatology 8: 293–299

Clyman R L 1987 Ductus arteriosus: current theories of prenatal and postnatal regulation. Seminars in Perinatology 11: 64–71

Clyman R L 1990 Developmental physiology of the ductus arteriosus. In: Long W (ed.) Fetal and Neonatal Cardiology. W B Saunders, Philadelphia, PA, p 64–75

Clyman R L, Heymann M A 1981 Pharmacology of the ductus arteriosus. Pediatric Clinics of North America 28: 77–93

Clyman R I, Mauray F, Roman C, Rudolph A M 1978 PGE$_2$ is a more potent vasodilator of the lamb ductus arteriosus than is either PGI$_2$ or 6-keto PGF$_{1\alpha}$. Prostaglandins 16: 259–264

Clyman R L, Brett C, Murray F 1980 Circulating prostaglandin E$_1$ concentrations and incidence of patent ductus arteriosus in preterm infants with respiratory distress syndrome. Pediatrics 66: 725–729

Clyman R L, Mauray F, Roman C, Rudolph A M, Heymann M A 1981a Glucocorticoids alter the sensitivity of the lamb ductus arteriosus to prostaglandin E$_2$. Journal of Pediatrics 98: 126–128

Clyman R L, Ballard P L, Sniderman S et al 1981b Prenatal administration of betamethasone for prevention of patent ductus arteriosus. Journal of Pediatrics 98: 123–126

Clyman R I, Jobe A, Heymann M A 1982 Increased shunt through the patent ductus arteriosus after surfactant replacement therapy. Journal of Pediatrics 100: 101–107

Clyman R I, Campbell D, Heymann M A, Mauray F 1985 Persistent responsiveness of the neonatal ductus in immature lambs a possible cause for reopening of patent ductus arteriosus after indomethacin–induced closure. Circulation 71: 141–145

Clyman R I, Walsh N, Black S M, Riemer R K, Mauray F, Chen Y Q 1998 Regulation of ductus arteriosus patency by nitric oxide in fetal lambs: the role of gestation, oxygen tension, and vasa vasorum. Pediatric Research 43: 633–644

Coceani F 1993 Carbon monoxide and dilation of blood vessels. Science 260: 739

Coceani F 1994 Control of the ductus arteriosus – a new function for cytochrome P450, endothelin and nitric oxide. Biochemistry and Pharmacology 48: 1315–1318

Coceani F, Kelsey L 1991 Endothelin-1 release from lamb ductus arteriosus: relevance to postnatal closure of the vessel. Canadian Journal of Physiology and Pharmacology 69: 218–221

Coceani F, Olley P M 1973 The response of the ductus arteriosus to prostaglandins. Canadian Journal of Physiology and Pharmacology 51: 220–225

Coceani F, Olley P M 1980 Role of prostaglandins, prostacyclin, and thromboxanes in the control of prenatal patency and postnatal closure of the ductus arteriosus. Seminars in Perinatology 4: 109–113

Coceani F, Olley P M 1988 The control of cardiovascular shunts in the fetal and neonatal period. Canadian Journal of Physiology and Pharmacology 66: 1129–1134

Coceani F, Olley P M, Bodach E 1975 Lamb ductus arteriosus: effect of prostaglandin synthesis inhibitors on the muscle tone and the response to prostaglandin E$_2$. Prostaglandins 9: 299–308

Coceani F, Bodach E, White E, Bishai I, Olley P M 1978 Prostaglandin I$_2$ is less relaxant than prostaglandin E$_2$ on the lamb ductus arteriosus. Prostaglandins 15: 551–556

Coceani F, White E, Bodach E, Olley P M 1979 Age-dependent changes in the response of the ductus arteriosus to oxygen and ibuprofen. Canadian Journal of Physiology and Pharmacology 57: 825–831

Coceani F, Huhtanen D, Hamilton N C, Bishai I, Olley P M 1986 Involvement of intramural prostaglandin E$_2$ in prenatal patency of the lamb ductus arteriosus. Canadian Journal of Physiology and Pharmacology 4: 737–744

Coceani F, Breen C A, Lees J G, Falck J R, Olley P M 1988a Further evidence implicating a cytochrome P-450-mediated reaction in the contractile tension of the lamb ductus arteriosus. Circulation Research 62: 471–477

Coceani F, Hamilton N C, Labuc J, Olley P M 1988b Cytochrome P450-linked monooxygenase: involvement in the lamb ductus arteriosus. American Journal of Physiology 254: H640–H643

Coceani F, Armstrong C, Kelsey L 1989 Endothelin is a potent constrictor of the lamb ductus arteriosus. Canadian Journal of Physiology and Pharmacology 67: 902–904

Coceani F, Kelsey L, Seidlitz E 1992 Evidence for an effector role of endothelin in closure of the ductus arteriosus at birth. Canadian Journal of Physiology and Pharmacology 70: 1061–1064

Coceani F, Kelsey L, Seidlitz E 1994a Occurrence of endothelium-derived relaxing factor–nitric oxide in the lamb ductus arteriosus. Canadian Journal of Physiology and Pharmacology 72: 82–88

Coceani F, Kelsey L, Ackerley C, Rabinovitch M, Gelboin H 1994b Cytochrome P450 during ontogenic development: occurrence in the ductus arteriosus and other tissues. Canadian Journal of Physiology and Pharmacology 72: 217–226

Coceani F, Kelsey L, Seidlitz E, Korzekwa K 1996 Inhibition of the contraction of the ductus arteriosus to oxygen by 1-aminobenzotriazole, a mechanism-based inactivator of cytochrome P450. British Journal of Pharmacology 117: 1586–1592

Coceani F, Kelsey L, Seidlitz E et al 1997 Carbon monoxide formation in the ductus arteriosus in the lamb: implications for the regulation of muscle tone. British Journal of Pharmacology 120: 599–608

Coe J Y, Olley P M 1991 A novel method to maintain ductus arteriosus patency. Journal of the American College of Cardiology 18: 837–841

Coe J Y, Silove E D 1979 Oral prostaglandin E$_2$ in pulmonary atresia. Lancet i: 1297–1298

Cohen B A, Efremidis S C, Dan S J, Robinson B, Rabinowitz J G 1981 Aneurysm of the ductus arteriosus in an adult. Journal of Computer Assisted Tomography 5: 421–423

Congdon E D 1922 Transformation of the aortic-arch system during the development of the human embryo. Contributions to Embryology 14: 47–110

Corwin R D, Singh A K, Karlson K E 1981 Balloon dilation of ductus arteriosus in a newborn with interrupted aortic arch and ventricular septal defect. American Heart Journal 102: 446–447

Cosh J A 1957 Patent ductus arteriosus. A follow-up study of 73 cases. British Heart Journal 19: 13–22

Costa A 1930 La minuta struttura e le trasformazioni involutive del dotto arterioso di Botallo nelia specie umana. Cuore e Circolazione 14: 546–568

Coster D D, Gorton M E, Grooters R K, Thieman K C, Schneider R F, Soltanzadeh H 1989 Surgical closure of the patent ductus arteriosus in the neonatal intensive care unit. Annals of Thoracic Surgery 48: 386–389

Cotton R B, Stahlman M T, Bender H W, Graham T P, Cutterden W Z, Kovar I 1978 Randomized trial of early closure of symptomatic patent ductus arteriosus in small preterm infants. Journal of Pediatrics 93: 647–651

Cotton R B, Haywood J L, FitzGerald G A 1991 Symptomatic patent ductus arteriosus following prophylactic indomethacin. A clinical and biochemical appraisal. Biology of the Neonate 60: 273–282

Crafoord G 1947 Discussion of paper by Gross R E: Complete division for the patent ductus arteriosus. Journal of Thoracic Surgery 16: 314

Crevasse L E, Logue R B 1959 Atypical patent ductus. The use of a vasopressor agent as a diagnostic aid. Circulation 19: 332–337

Crichton C A, Smith G C, Smith G L 1997 Alpha toxin permeabilised rabbit fetal ductus arteriosus is more sensitive to Ca²⁺ than aorta or main pulmonary artery. Cardiovascular Research 33: 223–229

Cruickshank B, Marquis R M 1958 Spontaneous aneurysm of the ductus arteriosus. American Journal of Medicine 25: 140–149

Dalvi B, Nabar A, Goyal V, Naik A, Kulkarni H, Ramakanthan R 1998 Transcatheter closure of patent ductus arteriosus in children weighing <10 kg with Gianturco coils using the balloon occlusion technique. Catheterization and Cardiovascular Diagnosis 44: 303–308

Danesino V L, Reynolds S R M, Rehman I H 1955 Comparative histological structure of the human ductus arteriosus according to topography, age, and degree of constriction. Anatomical Record 121: 801–829

Daniels O, Hopman J C W, Steolinger G B A, Burch H J, Peer P G M 1982 Doppler flow characteristics in the main pulmonary artery and the LA/AO ratio before and after ductal closure in healthy newborns. Pediatic Cardiology 3: 99–104

Daniels S R, Reller M D, Kaplan S 1984 Recurrence of patency of the ductus arteriosus after surgical ligation in premature infants. Pediatrics 73: 56–58

Danilowicz D, Rudolph A M, Hoffman J I E 1966 Delayed closure of the ductus arteriosus in premature infants. Pediatrics 37: 74–78

Das J B, Chesterman J T 1956 Aneurysms of the patent ductus arteriosus. Thorax 11: 295

Das M B, Kapoor L, Moulick A et al 1997 Video-assisted thoracoscopic surgery for closure of patent ductus arteriosus in children. Indian Heart Journal 49: 300–302

Davidson H R 1993 A large family with patent ductus arteriosus and unusual face. Journal of Medical Genetics 30: 503–505

Dawes G 1982 Physiological changes in the circulation after birth. In: Fishman A F, Richards D W (eds) Circulation of the blood, men and ideas. American Physiological Society, Bethesda, MD, pp. 743–816

Dawes G S, Mott J C, Widdicombe J G 1955 The patency of the ductus arteriosus in newborn lambs and its physiological consequences. Journal of Physiology 128: 361–383

Deanfield J E, Rees P G, Bull C M et al 1981 Formalin infiltration of ductus arteriosus in cyanotic congenital heart disease. British Heart Journal 45: 573–576

de Cancq H E Jr 1963 Repair of patent ductus arteriosus in a 1417 g infant. American Journal of Diseases of Children 106: 402–404

de Moor M, Al Fadley F, Galal O 1996 Closure of residual leak after umbrella occlusion of the patent arterial duct, using Gianturco coils. International Journal of Cardiology 56: 5–9

de Reeder E G, Girard N, Poelmann R E, Van M J, Patterson D F, Gittenberger-de-Groot A C 1988 Hyaluronic acid accumulation and endothelial cell detachment in intimal thickening of the vessel wall. The normal and genetically defective ductus arteriosus. American Journal of Pathology 132: 574–585

de Reeder E G, Poelmann R E, van Munsteren J C, Patterson D F, Gittenberger-de Groot A C 1989a Ultrastructural and immunohistochemical changes of the extracellular matrix during intimal cushion formation in the ductus arteriosus of the dog. Atherosclerosis 79: 29–40

de Reeder E G, Gittenberger-de Groot A C, van Munsteren J C, Poelmann R E, Patterson D F, Keirse M J 1989b Distribution of prostacyclin synthase, 6-keto-prostaglandin F₁ alpha, and 15-hydroxy-prostaglandin dehydrogenase in the normal and persistent ductus arteriosus of the dog. American Journal of Pathology 135: 881–887

Desligneres S, Larroche J C 1970 Ductus arteriosus. I. Anatomical and histological study of its development during the second half of gestation and its closure after birth. II. Histological study of a few cases of patent ductus arteriosus in infancy. Biology of the Neonate 16: 278–296

Drayton M R, Skidmore R 1987 Ductus arteriosus blood flow during first 48 hours of life. Archives of Disease in Childhood 62: 1030–1034

Durante W, Liao L, Peyton K J, Schafer A I 1998 Transforming growth factor-β₁ stimulates ʟ-arginine transport and metabolism in vascular smooth muscle cells. Circulation 98(suppl I): 183

Dworsky M, Kohaut E, Jander H P, Ceballos R 1980 Neonatal embolism due to thrombosis of the ductus arteriosus. Radiology 134: 645–646

Dyck J D, Benson L N, Smallhorn J F, McLaughlin P, Freedom P M, Rowe R D 1988 Catheter occlusion of the persistently patent ductus arteriosus: initial experience and early followup. American Journal of Cardiology 62: 1089–1092

Dykes F, Lazzara A, Ahmann P, Blumenstein B, Schwartz J, Brann A W 1980 Intraventricular hemorrhage: a prospective in evaluation of etiopathogenesis. Pediatrics 66: 42–49

Echigo S, Matsuda T, Kamiya T et al 1990 Development of a new transvenous patent ductus arteriosus occluder technique using a shape memory polmer. ASAIO Transactions 36: M195–M198

Edwards J E 1953 Malformations of the aortic arch system manefested as 'vascular rings'. Laboratory Investigation 2: 56–75

Edwards J H 1960 The simulation of mendelism. Acta Genetica 10: 63–70

Egami J, Tada Y, Takagi A, Sato O, Idezuki Y 1992 False aneurysm as a late complication of division of a patent ductus arteriosus. Annals of Thoracic Surgery 53: 901–902

Elliott R B, Starling M B, Neutze J M 1975 Medical manipulation of the ductus arteriosus. Lancet i: 140–142

Ellis F H Jr, Kirklin J W, Callaghan J A, Wood E H 1956 Patent ductus arteriosus with pulmonary hypertension. Journal of Thoracic Surgery 31: 268–282

Ellison R C, Peckman G H, Lang P 1983 Evaluation of the preterm infant for patent ductus arteriosus. Pediatrics 71: 364–372

Elseed A M, Shiebourne E A, Paneth M 1974 Management of juxtaductal coarctation after surgical ligation of persistent ductus arteriosus. British Heart Journal 36: 687–692

Emmanouilides G C, Thanopoulos B, Siassi B, Fishbein M 1976 'Agenesis' of ductus arteriosus associated with the syndrome of tetralogy of Fallot and absent pulmonary valve. American Journal of Cardiology 37: 403–409

Ergin M A, Jayaram N, LaCorte M 1981 Left aortic arch and right descending aorta: diagnostic and therapeutic implications of a rare type of vascular ring. Annals of Thoracic Surgery 31: 82–85

Eronen M 1993 The hemodynamic effects of antenatal indomethacin and a beta-sympathomimetic agent on the fetus and the newborn: a randomized study. Pediatric Research 33: 615–619

Eronen M, Kari A, Pesonen E, Hallman M 1993 The effect of antenatal dexamethasone administration on the fetal neonatal ductus arteriosus. A randomized double-blind study. American Journal of Diseases of Children 147: 187–192

Ettedgui J A, Sharland G K, Chita S K, Cook A, Fagg N, Allan L D 1990 Absent pulmonary valve syndrome with ventricular septal defect: role of the arterial duct. American Journal of Cardiology 15: 233–234

Fadley F, Al Halees Z, Galal O, Kumar N, Wilson N 1993 Left pulmonary artery stenosis after transcatheter occlusion of the persistent arterial duct. Lancet 341: 559–560

Fan L L, Campbell D N, Clarke D R, Washington R L, Fix E J, White C W 1989 Paralyzed left vocal cord associated with ligation of patent ductus arteriosus. Journal of Thoracic and Cardiovascular Surgery 98: 611–613

Fay F S 1971 Guinea pig ductus arteriosus. I: Cellular and metabolic basis for oxygen sensitivity. American Journal of Physiology 221: 470–479

Fay F S, Cooke P H 1972 Guinea pig ductus arteriosus. II: Irreversible closure after birth. American Journal of Physiology 222: 841–849

Fay F S, Nair P, Whalen W J 1977 Mechanism of oxygen-induced contraction of the ductus arteriosus. In: Reivich M, Coburn R F, Lahiri S, Chance B (eds) Tissue hypoxia and ischaemia. Plenum Press, New York, p 123–134

Ferlic R M, Jofschire P J, Mooring P K 1975 Ruptured ductus arteriosus aneurysm in an infant. Report of a survivor. Annals of Thoracic Surgery 20: 456–468

Fischer D R, Neches W H, Beerman L B 1984 Tetralogy of Fallot with absent pulmonary valve: analysis of 17 patients. American Journal of Cardiology 53: 1433–1437

Fleming W H, Sarafian L B, Kugler J D, Nelson R M, Jr 1983 Ligation of patent ductus arteriosus in premature infants: importance of accurate anatomic definition. Pediatrics 71: 373–375

Formigari R, Vairo U, de Zorzi A, Santoro G, Marino B 1992 Prevalence of bilateral patent ductus arteriosus in patients with pulmonic valve atresia and asplenia syndrome. American Journal of Cardiology 70: 1219–1220

Fox J J, Ziegler J W, Ivy D D, Halbower A C, Kinsella P, Abman S H 1996 Role of nitric oxide and cGMP system in regulation of ductus arteriosus tone in ovine fetus. American Journal of Physiology 270: H2638–H2645

Franklin K J 1941 Ductus venosus (Arantii) and ductus arteriosus (Botalli). Bulletin of the History of Medicine 9: 580–584

Freed M D, Heymann M A, Lewis A B, Roehl S L, Kensey R C 1981 Prostaglandin E$_1$ in infants with ductus dependent congenital heart disease. Circulation 64: 899–905

Freedom R M, Olley P M, Coceani F, Rowe R D 1978 The prostaglandin challenge. Test to unmask obstructed total anomalous pulmonary venous connections in asplenia syndrome. British Heart Journal 40: 91–94

Freedom R M, Patel R G, Bloom K R 1979 Congenital absence of the pulmonary valve, associated imperforate membrane type of tricuspid atresia, right ventricular tensor apparatus and intact ventricular septum: a curious developmental complex. European Journal of Cardiology 10: 171–196

Freedom R M, Moes C A F, Pelech A 1984 Bilateral ductus arteriosus (or remnant): an analysis of 27 patients. American Journal of Cardiology 53: 884–889

Freedom R M, Smallhorn J F, Burrows P E 1992 Pulmonary atresia and ventricular septal defect. In: Freedom R M, Benson L N, Smallhorn J F (eds) Neonatal heart disease. Springer-Verlag London p 229–256

Frescura C, Talenti E, Pellegrino P A, Mazzucco A, Faggian G, Thiene G 1984 Coexistence of ductal and systemic pulmonary arterial supply in pulmonary atresia with ventricular septal defect. American Journal of Cardiology 53: 884–889

Friedman W F 1973 The intrinsic physiologic properties of the developing heart. In: Friedman W F, Leshc M, Sonnenblick E M (eds) Neonatal heart disease. Grune & Stratton, New York, p 21–49

Friedman W F 1978 Studies of the response of the ductus arteriosus. In: Heymann M A, Rudolph A M (eds) The ductus arteriosus. Proceedings of the seventy-fifth Ross conference on pediatric research. Columbus, OH, p 35–43

Friedman W F, Hirschlkau M J, Printz M P, Pitlick P T, Kirkpatrick S E 1976 Pharmacologic closure of patent ductus arteriosus in premature infant. New England Journal of Medicine 295: 526–529

Friese K K, Dulce M C, Higgins C B 1992 Airway obstruction by right aortic arch with right-sided patent ductus arteriosus: demonstration by MRI. Journal of Computer Assisted Tomography 16: 888–892

Fripp R P, Whitman V, Walhausen J A, Boal D K 1985 Ductus arteriosus aneurysm presenting as pulmonary artery obstruction: diagnosis and management. Journal of the American College of Cardiology 6: 234–236

Fujiwara T, Maeta H, Morita T, Watanabe V, Chida S, Abe T 1980 Artificial surfactant therapy in hyaline membrane disease. Lancet i: 55–59

Furzan J A, Reisch J, Tyson J E, Laird P, Rosenfeld C R 1985 Incidence and risk factors for symptomatic patent ductus arteriosus among newborn very-low birth weight infants. Early Development 12: 39–48

Gal P, Ransom J L, Schall S, Weaver R L, Bird A, Brown Y 1990 Indomethacin for patent ductus arteriosus closure. Application of serum concentrations and pharmacodynamics to improve response. Journal of Perinatology 10: 20–26

Galal O, Schmaltz A A, Fadely F, Fawzy M E, Wilson N, Mimish L 1993 Transcatheter obliteration of patent ductus arteriosus in young adults with the Rashkind occluder. Zeitschrift für Kardiologie 82: 432–435

Galal O, de Moor M, al-Fadley F, Hijazi Z M 1996 Transcatheter closure of the patent ductus arteriosus: comparison between the Rashkind occluder device and the anterograde Gianturco coils technique. American Heart Journal 131: 368–373

Galen C 1821–1833 Medicorum graecorium opera quae exstant. Kuehn C G (ed) Lipsiae

Garfunkel J M, Kirkpatrick J A 1963 Decreased vascularity of the left lung and unequal aeration of the lungs as a manifestation of patent ductus arteriosus. American Journal of Radiology 89: 1012–1016

Ge Z M, Zhang Y, Fan D S, Kang W, Hatle L, Duran C 1993a Simultaneous measurement of pulmonary artery diastolic pressure by Doppler echocardiography and catheterization in patients with patent ductus arteriosus. American Heart Journal 125: 263–266

Ge Z M, Zhang Y, Fan D S, Fan J X, Ji X P, Zhao Y X, Hatle L 1993b Reliability and accuracy of measurement of transductal gradient by Doppler ultrasound. International Journal of Cardiology 40: 35–43

Gentile R, Stevenson G, Dooley T, Franklin D, Kawabori I, Pearlman A 1981 Pulsed Doppler echocardiography determination of time of ductus closure in normal newborn infants. Journal of Pediatrics 98: 443–448

Gerard G 1900 De l'obliteration du canal arterial, les theories et les faits. Journal of Anatomy 36: 323–357

Gersony W M, Peckham G J, Ellison R C, Miettinen O S, Nadas A S 1983 Effects of indomethacin on premature infants with patent ductus arteriosus: results of a national collaborative study. Journal of Pediatrics 102: 895–860

Ghani S A, Hashim R 1989 Surgical management of patent ductus arteriosus. A review of 413 cases. Journal of the Royal College of Surgeons of Edinburgh 34: 33–36

Gibbs J L, Rothman M T, Rees M R, Parsons J M, Blackburn M E, Ruiz C E 1992 Stenting the arterial duct: a new approach to palliation for pulmonary atresia. British Heart Journal 67: 240–245

Gibbs J L, Wren C, Watterson K G, Hunter S, Hamilton J R L 1993 Stenting the arterial duct combined with banding of the pulmonary arteries and atrial septostomy or septectomy: a new approach to palliation for the hypoplastic left heart syndrome. British Heart Journal 69: 551–553

Gibson G A 1898 Diseases of the heart and aorta. Edinburgh, Pentland, p 61, 303, 310–312

Gilbert E F, Bruyere H J J Jr, Ishikawa S, Cheung M O, Hodach R J 1977 The effect of practalol and butoxamine on aortic arch malformation in beta adrenoreceptor stimulated chick embryos. Teratology 15: 317–324

Girling D J, Hallidie-Smith K A 1971 Persistent ductus arteriosus in ill and premature babies. Archives of Disease in Children 46: 177–181

Gittenberger-de-Groot A C 1977 Persistent ductus arteriosus: most probably a primary congenital malformation. British Heart Journal 39: 610–618

Gittenberger-de-Groot A C, Moulaert A J, Harinck E, Becker A E 1978 Histopathology of the ductus arteriosus after prostaglandin E_1 administration in ductus-dependent cardiac anomalies. British Heart Journal 40: 215–220

Gittenberger-de-Groot A C, van Ertbruggan I, Moulaert A J, Harinck E 1980 The ductus arteriosus in the preterm infant: histologic and clinical observations. Journal of Pediatrics 96: 88–93

Gittenberger-de-Groot A C, Strengers J L, Mentink M 1985 Histologic studies on normal and persistent ductus arteriosus in the dog. Journal of the American College of Cardiology 6: 394–404

Gleason C A, Clyman R I, Heymann M A, Mauray E, Leake R, Roman C 1988 Indomethacin and patent ductus arteriosus: effects on renal function on preterm lambs. American Journal of Physiology 254: F38–F44

Gonzalez A, Ventura-Junca P 1991 Incidence of clinically apparent ductus arteriosus in premature infants less than 2000 g. Revista Chilena de Pediatria 62: 354–358

Goyal V S, Fulwani M C, Ramakantan R, Kulkarni H L, Dalvi B V 1999 Follow-up after coil closure of patent ductus arteriosus. American Journal of Cardiology 83: 463–466

Graham E A 1940 Aneurysm of the ductus arteriosus, with a consideration of its importance to the thoracic surgeon. Archives of Surgery 41: 324

Graper L 1927 Die anatomischen Veranderungen kurz nach der Gebert III. Ductus Botalli. Zeitschrift für Anatomie und Entwicklungsgeschichte 61: 312–329

Graybiel A, Strieder J W, Boyer N H 1938 An attempt to obliterate the patent ductus arteriosus in a patient with bacterial endocarditis. American Heart Journal 15: 621–624

Gregg N M 1941 Congenital cataract following german measles in the mother. Transactions of the Ophthalmalogical Society of Australia 3: 35–46

Grifka R G, O'Laughlin M P, Mullins C E 1992 Late transcatheter removal of a Rashkind PDA occlusion device for persistent hemolysis using a modified transeptal sheath. Catheterization and Cardiovascular Diagnosis 25: 140–143

Gross R E 1939 Complete surgical division of the patent ductus arteriosus. A report of fourteen successful cases. Surgery, Gynaecology and Obstetrics 36–43

Gross R E, Hubbard J P 1939 Surgical ligation of a patent ductus arteriosus. A report of first successful case. Journal of the American Medical Association 112: 729–731

Gross R E, Neuhauser E D 1951 Compression of the trachea or esophagus by vascular anomalies: surgical therapy in 40 cases. Pediatrics 7: 69–88

Groves L K, Etter D B, Sones F M 1954 Controlled hypotension in the surgical treatment of certain cases of patent ductus arteriosus. Cleveland Clinic Quarterly 21: 169–175

Hagan A D, Deely W J, Sahn D J, Friedman W F 1973 Echocardiographic criteria for normal newborn infants. Circulation 48: 1221–1226

Hall C L, Wang C, Lange L A, Turley E A 1994 Hyaluronan and the hyaluronan receptor RHAMM promote focal adhesion turnover and transient tyrosine kinase activity. Journal of Cell Biology 126: 575–588

Hallman A L, Cooley D A 1964 False aortic aneurysm following division and suture of a patent ductus arteriosus. Successful excision with hypothermia. Journal of Cardiovascular Surgery 5: 23–27

Halloran K H, Sanyal S K, Gardner T H 1966 Superiorly orientated electrocardiographic axis in infants with the rubella syndrome. American Heart Journal 72: 600–606

Hammerman C 1995 Patent ductus arteriosus. Clinical relevance of prostaglandins and prostaglandin inhibitors in PDA pathophysiology and treatment. Clinics in Perinatology 22: 457–479

Hammerman C, Aramburo M J 1990 Prolonged indomethacin therapy for the prevention of recurrences of patent ductus arteriosus. Journal of Pediatrics 117: 771–776

Harker J C 1981 Effects of indomethacin on fetal rat lungs: a possible cause of persistent fetal circulation. Journal of Perinatology 12: 41–47

Harlass F E, Duff P, Brady K, Read J 1989 Hydrops fetalis and premature closure of the ductus arteriosus: a review. Obstetrics and Gynecology 44: 541–543

Harvey W 1628 Exercitatio anatomica de motu cordis et sanguinis in animalibus. Francofurti, Fitzeri

Hatem J, Sade R M, Upshur J K, Hohn A R 1980 Maintaining patency of the ductus arteriosus for palliation of cyanotic congenital cardiac malformation. The use of prostaglandin E$_1$ and formaldehyde infiltration of the ductal wall. Annals of Surgery 192: 124–128

Haworth S G, Sauer U, Buhimeyer K 1980 Effect of prostaglandin E$_1$ on pulmonary circulation in pulmonary atresia. A quantitative morphometric study. British Heart Journal 43: 306–314

Hayes A M, Redington A N, Rigby M L 1992 Severe haemolysis after transcatheter duct occlusion: a non-surgical remedy. British Heart Journal 67: 321–322

Hays M D, Hoyer M H, Glasow P F 1996 New forceps delivery technique for coil occlusion of patent ductus arteriosus. American Journal Cardiology 77: 209–211

Heikkinen E S, Simila S, Laitinen J, Larmi T 1974 Infantile aneurysm of the ductus arteriosus. Acta Paediatrica Scandinavica 63: 241

Heldt G P, Pesonen E, Merritt T A, Elias W, Sahn D J 1989 Closure of the ductus arteriosus and mechanics of breathing in preterm infants after surfactant replacement therapy. Pediatric Research 25: 305–310

Heymann M A, Hoffman J I 1978 Problem of patent ductus arteriosus in premature infants. Pediatrician 7: 3–17

Heymann M A, Rudolph A M 1972 The effects of congenital heart disease on the fetal and neonatal circulation. Progress in Cardiovascular Diseases 15: 115–143

Heymann M A, Rudolph A M 1973 Ductus arteriosus dilatation by prostaglandin E$_1$ in infants with pulmonary atresia. Pediatrics 59: 325–329

Heymann M A, Rudolph A M 1975 Control of the ductus arteriosus. Physiological Reviews 55: 62–68

Heymann M A, Rudolph A M 1976 Effects of acetylsalicylic acid on the ductus arteriosus and circulation in fetal lambs in utero. Circulation Research 38: 418–422

Heymann M A, Rudolph A M, Nies A S, Melmon K L 1969 Bradykinin production associated with oxygenation of the fetal lamb. Circulation Research 25: 521–534

Heymann M A, Rudolph A M, Silverman N H 1976 Closure of the ductus arteriosus in premature infants by inhibition of prostaglandin synthesis. New England Journal of Medicine 295: 530–533

Heymann M A, Berman W, Jr, Rudolph A M, Whitman V 1979 Dilation of the ductus arteriosus by prostaglandin E$_1$ in aortic arch anomalies. Circulation 59: 169–173

Higgins C B, Silverman N H, Kersting-Sommerhoff B A, Schmidt K 1990 Patent ductus arteriosus. In: Congenital heart disease: echographic and magnetic resonance imaging. Raven Press, New York, p 128

Highmore N 1651 Corporis humani disquisitio anatomica. Hagae-Comitis, Ex Officina Sammuelis Brown, Bibliopolae Anglici

Hijazi Z M, Geggel R L 1996 Transcatheter closure of large patent ductus arteriosus (> or = 4 mm) with multiple Gianturco coils: immediate and mid-term results. Heart 76: 536–540

Hijazi Z M, Geggel R L, al-Fadley F 1995 Transcatheter closure of residual patent ductus arteriosus shunting after the Rashkind occulder device using single or multiple Gianturco coils. Catheter and Cardiovascular Diagnosis 36: 255–258

Hinek A, Rabinovitch M 1993 The ductus arteriosus migratory smooth muscle cell phenotype processes tropoelastin to a 52-kDa product associated with impaired assembly of elastic laminae. Journal of Biological Chemistry 268: 1405–1413

Hinek A, Rabinovitch M 1994 67-kD elastin-binding protein is a protective 'companion' of extracellular insoluble elastin and intracellular tropoelastin. Journal of Cell Biology 126: 563–574

Hinek A, Wrenn D S, Mecham R P, Barondes S H 1988 The elastin receptor: a galactoside-binding protein. Science 239: 1539–1541

Hinek A, Mecham R P, Keeley F, Rabinovitch M 1991 Impaired elastin fiber assembly related to reduced 67-kD elastin-binding protein in fetal lamb ductus arteriosus and in cultured aortic smooth muscle cells treated with chondroitin sulfate. Journal of Clinical Investigation 88: 2083–2094

Hinek A, Boyle J, Rabinovitch M 1992 Vascular smooth muscle cell detachment from elastin and migration through elastic laminae is promoted by chondroitin sulfate-induced 'shedding' of the 67-kDa cell surface elastin binding protein. Experimental Cell Research 203: 344–353

Hinek A, Rabinovitch M, Keeley F, Okamura O Y, Callahan J 1993 The 67-kD elastin/laminin-binding protein is related to an enzymatically inactive, alternatively spliced form of beta-galactosidase. Journal of Clinical Investigation 91: 1198–1205

Hines M H, Bensky A S, Hammon J W Jr, Pennington D G 1998 Video-assisted thoracoscopic ligation of patent ductus arteriosus: safe and outpatient. Annals of Thoracic Surgery 66: 853–858

Hiraishi S, Misawa H, Onguchi K 1987a Two-dimensional Doppler echocardiographic assessment of closure of the ductus arteriosus in normal newborn infants. Journal of Pediatrics 111: 755–760

Hiraishi S, Horiguchi Y, Misawa H, Kadoi N, Fujino N, Yashiro K 1987b Noninvasive Doppler echocardiographic evaluation of shunt flow dynamics of the ductus arteriosus. Circulation 75: 1146–1153

Hirata T, Wolfe S B, Popp R L, Helmen C H, Feigenbaum H 1969 Estimation of left atrial size using ultrasound. American Heart Journal 78: 43–52

Hirschklau M J, Kirkpatrick S E, Higgins C G, Friedman W F 1978 Echocardiographic diagnosis: Pitfalls in premature infant with a large patent ductus arteriosus. Journal of Pediatrics 92: 474–477

Hoffmann M, Greve H, Kortmann C 1991 Surgical closure of persistent ductus arteriosus in small premature infants in an incubator. Klinische Padiatrie 203: 20–23

Holman E, Gerbode F, Purdy A 1953 The patent ductus. A review of seventy-five cases with surgical treatment including an aneurysm of the ductus and one of the pulmonary artery. Journal of Thoracic Surgery 25: 111–142

Holmes R L 1958 Some features of the ductus arteriosus. Journal of Anatomy 92: 304–309

Hornblad P Y 1969a Experimental studies on closure of the ductus arteriosus utilizing whole-body freezing. Acta Paediatrica Scandinavica (Suppl) 190: 1–21

Hornblad P Y 1969b Embryological observation of the ductus arteriosus in the guinea pig, rabbit, rat and mouse. Studies on closure of the ductus arteriosus. IV. Acta Physiologica Scandinavica 76: 49–57

Hornblad P Y, Larsson K S 1967a Studies on closure of the ductus arteriosus II. Closure rate in the rat and its relation to environmental temperature. Cardiologia 51: 242–252

Hornblad P Y, Larsson K S 1967b Studies on closure of the ductus arteriosus III. Species differences in closure rate and morphology. Cardiologia 51: 262–282

Hornblad P Y, Larsson K S, Marsk L 1969 Studies on closure of the ductus arteriosus VII. Closure rate and morphology of the ductus arteriosus in the lamb. Cardiologia 54: 336–342

Hosking M C K, Benson L N, Musewe N, Freedom R M 1989 Reocclusion for persistent shunting after catheter placement of the Rashkind patent ductus arteriosus occluder. Canadian Journal of Cardiology 5: 340–342

Hosking M C K, Benson L N, Musewe N, Dyck J D, Freedom R M 1991 Transcatheter occlusion of the persistent patent ductus arteriosus: forty month follow-up and prevalence of residual shunting. Circulation 84: 2312–2317

Host A, Halken S, Kamper J, Lillquist K 1988 Prostaglandin E₁ treatment in ductus dependent congenital cardiac malformation. A review of the treatment of 34 neonates. Dan Medical Bulletin 35: 81–84

Houston A B, Lim M K, Doig W B et al 1989 Doppler flow characteristics in the assessment of pulmonary artery pressure in ductus arteriosus. British Heart Journal 62: 284–290

Houston A B, Gnanapragasam J P, Lim M K, Doig W B, Coleman E N 1991 Doppler ultrasound and the silent ductus arteriosus. British Heart Journal 65: 97–99

Hubbard T F, Neis D D 1969 The sounds at the base of the heart in cases of patent ductus arteriosus. American Heart Journal 59: 807–815

Huggett A St G 1927 Foetal blood-gas tensions and gas transfusion through the placenta of the foetal goat. Journal of Physiology 62: 373–384

Huggon I C, Tabatabaei A H, Qureshi S A, Bakker E J, Tynan M, 1993 Use of a second Rashkind arterial duct occluder for persistent flow after implantation of the first device. British Heart Journal 69: 544–550

Huhta J C, Cohen M, Gutgesell H P 1984 Patency of the ductus arteriosus in normal neonates: two dimensional echocardiography versus Doppler assessment. Journal of the American College of Cardiology 4: 561–564

Ichihashi K, Shiraishi H, Endou H, Kuramatsu T, Yano S, Yanagisawa M 1990 Cerebral and abdominal arterial hemodynamics in preterm infants with patentductus arteriosus. Acta Paediatrica Japonica: Overseas Edition 32: 349–356

Ing F F, Bierman F Z 1995 Percutaneous transcatheter coil occlusion of the patent ductus arteriosus aided by the nitinol snare: further observations. Cardiovascular Interventional Radiology 18: 222–226

Ing F F, Sommer R J 1999 The snare-assisted technique for transcatheter coil occlusion of moderate to large patent ductus arteriosus: immediate and intermediate results. Journal of the American College of Cardiology 33: 1710–1718

Ing F F, Mullins C E, Rose M, Shapir Y, Bierman F Z 1996 Transcatheter closure of the patent ductus arteriosus in adults using the Gianturco coil. Clinical Cardiology 19: 875–879

Inishi Y, Bai H-Z, Pollman M J, Gibbons G H 1998 Transforming growth factor-beta 1 inhibits human vascular smooth muscle cell apoptosis via mitogen-activated protein kinase pathway. Circulation 98 (suppl I): 598

Ino T, Nishimoto K, Okubo M et al 1998 Spring coil retraction in coil occlusion of persistent ductus arteriosus. Heart 80: 327–329

Jacob J, Gluck L, Disessa T et al 1980 The contribution of PDA in the neonate with severe RDS. Journal of Pediatrics 96: 79–87

Jager B V, Wollenman O J 1942 An anatomical study of the closure of the ductus arteriosus. American Journal of Pathology 18: 595–613

Jarkovska D, Janatova T, Hruda J, Ostadal B, Samanek M 1992 Effect of prostaglandin E₂ on the ductus arteriosus in the newborn rat. An ultrastructural study. Physiology Research 41: 323–30

Johnston T A, Stern H J, O'Laughlin M P 1999 Transcatheter occlusion of the patent ductus arteriosus: use of the retrievable coil device. Catheter and Cardiovascular Interventions 46: 434–437

Jones J C 1965 Twenty-five years experience with the surgery of patent ductus arteriosus. Journal of Thoracic and Cardiovascular Surgery 50: 149–165

Jones M, Barrow M V, Wheat M W 1969 An ultrastructural evaluation of the closure of the ductus arteriosus in rats. Surgery 66: 891–898

Karaki H, Ozaki H, Hori M et al 1997 Calcium movements distribution and functions in smooth muscle. Pharmacology Reviews 49: 157–230

Karwande S V, Rowles J R 1992 Simplified muscle-sparing thoracotomy for patent ductus arteriosus ligation in neonates. Annals of Thoracic Surgery 54: 164–165

Keck E W, Roloff D, Markworth P 1972 Cardiovascular findings in children with the thalidomide dysmelia syndrome. Proceedings of the Association of European Pediatric Cardiology

Keith J D, Rowe R D, Vlad P 1978 Heart disease in infancy and childhood. MacMillan, New York

Kelsey J R Jr, Gilmore C E, Edwards J E 1953 Bilateral ductus arteriosus representing persistence of each sixth aortic arch. Archives of Pathology 55: 154–161

Kennedy A P Jr, Snyder C L, Ashcraft K W, Manning P B 1998 Comparison of muscle-sparing thoracotomy and thoracoscopic ligation for the treatment of patent ductus arteriosus. Journal Pediatric Surgery 33: 259–261

Kennedy J A, Clark S L 1941 Observations on the ductus arteriosus of the guinea pig in relation to its method of closure. Anatomical Record 79: 349–371

Kennedy J A, Clark S L 1942 Observations on the physiological reactions of the ductus arteriosus. American Journal of Physiology 136: 140–147

Kerwin A J, Jaffe F A 1959 Postoperative aneurysm of the ductus arteriosus with fatal rupture of a mycotic aneurysm of a branch of the pulmonary artery. American Journal of Cardiology 3: 397–403

Kewitz G, Garde K, Lusebrink R et al 1991 Surgical ligation of patent ductus arteriosus on the intensive care unit in small premature infants. Monatsschrift Kinderheilkunde 139: 39–43

Keys A, Shapiro M J 1943 Patency of the ductus arteriosus in adults. American Heart Journal 25: 158–186

Kinsella J P, Gerstmann D R, Gong A K, Taylor A F, deLemos R A 1991 Ductal shunting and effective systemic blood flow following single dose surfactan treatment in the premature baboon with hyaline membrane disease. Biology of the Neonate 60: 283–291

Kitamura S, Sato K, Naito Y et al 1976 Plug closure of patent ductus arteriosus by transfemoral catheter method. Chest 70: 631–635

Kitterman J 1975 Effects of intestinal ischemia. In: Moore T (ed) Necrotizing enterocolitis in the newborn infant. Report of the sixty-eighth Ross conference on pediatric research. Ross Laboratories, Columbus, OH, p 38–40

Kitterman J A, Edmunds L H Jr, Gregory G A, Heymann M A, Tooley W H, Rudolph A M 1972 Patent ductus arteriosus in premature infants: incidence, relation to pulmonary disease, and management. New England Journal of Medicine 287: 473–477

Knight D H, Patterson D F, Melbin J 1973 Constriction of the fetal ductus arteriosus induced by oxygen acetylcholine and norepinephrine in normal dogs and those genetically predisposed to persistent patency. Circulation 47: 127–132

Kovalcik V 1963 The response of the isolated ductus arteriosus to oxygen and anoxia. Journal of Physiology 169: 185–197

Krovetz L J, Warden H E 1962 Patent ductus arteriosus. An analysis of 515 surgically proved cases. Diseases of the Chest 42: 241–250

Kuhn M A, Latson L A 1995 Transcatheter embolization coil closure of patent ductus arteriosus – modified delivery for enhanced control during coil positioning. Catheter and Cardiovascular Diagnosis 36: 288–290

Kyoku I, Yokota M, Kitano M et al 1989 Axillary vertical incision thoracotomy sparing pectoralis major muscle and latissimus dorsi muscle: an approach for patent ductus arteriosus. Kyobu Geka 42: 371–373

Laborde F, Noirhomme F, Karam J, Batisse A, Bourel F, Saint Maurice O 1993 A new video-assisted thoracoscopic surgical technique for interruption of patent ductus arteriosus in infants and children. Journal of Thoracic and Cardiovascular Surgery 105: 278–280

Laborde F, Folliguet T A, Etienne P Y, Carbognani D, Batisse A, Petrie J 1997 Video-thoracoscopic surgical interruption of patent ductus arteriosus. Routine experience in 332 pediatric cases. European Journal of Cardiothoracic Surgery 11: 1052–1055

Ladusans E J, Murduch I, Franciosi J 1989 Severe haemolysis after percutaneous closure of a ductus arteriosus (arterial duct). British Heart Journal 61: 548–550

Langer C 1857 Zür anatomie der fotalen kreislaufsorgane. Zeitschrift Gesellschaft Wien Arzte 13: 328–338

Latson L A 1991 Residual shunts after transcatheter closure of patent ductus arteriosus. A major concern or benign 'techno-malady'? Circulation 84: 2591–2593

Latson L A, Hofschire P J, Kugler J D, Cheatham J P, Gumbiner C H, Danford D A 1989 Transcatheter closure of patent ductus arteriosus in pediatric patients. Journal of Pediatrics 115: 549–553

Lau K C, Cheung H H, Mok C K 1990 Congenital absence of the pulmonary valve, intact interventricular septum, and patent ductus arteriosus: management in a newborn infant. American Heart Journal 120: 711–714

Lee C C, Wu Y C, Lin F C 1991 Familial patent ductus arteriosus. Report of a family. Chang Keng I Hsueh-Chang Gung Medical Journal 14: 50–53

Lee M H 1975 Patent ductus arteriosus in premature infants; a diagnostic and therapeutic dilemma. [Commentary] Journal of Pediatrics 86: 132–134

Leslie J, Lindsay W, Amplatz K 1977 Nonsurgical closure of patent ductus arteriosus: an experimental study. Investigational Radiology 12: 142–145

Lewis A B, Lurie P R 1978 Prolonged PGE, infusion in an infant with cyanotic congenital heart disease. Pediatrics 61: 534–536

Li D Y, Brooke B, Davis E C et al 1998 Elastin is an essential determinant of arterial morphogenesis. Nature 393: 276–280

Liao P K, Su W S, Hung J S 1988 Doppler echocardiographic flow characteristics of isolated patent ductus arteriosus: better delineation by Doppler color flow mapping. Journal of the American College of Cardiology 12: 1285–1291

Lim M K, Hanretty K, Lilley S, Murtagh E P 1992 Intermediate ductal patency in healthy newborn infants: demonstration by color Doppler flow mapping. Archives of Disease in Childhood 67: 1217–1218

Linder W, Seidel M, Versmold H T, Dohlemann C, Riegel K P 1990 Stroke volume and left ventricular output in premature infants with patent ductus arteriosus. Pediatric Research 27: 278–281

Lipman B, Serwer G A, Brazy J E 1982 Abnormal cerebral hemodynamics in preterm infants with patent ductus arteriosus. Pediatrics 69: 778–781

Lloyd T R, Fedderly R, Mendelson A M, Sandhu S, Beekman R H 1993 Transcatheter occlusion of patent ductus with Gianturco coils. Circulation 88: 1412–1420

Lund G, Rysavy J, Cragg A 1989 Long-term patency of the ductus arteriosus after balloon dilatation: an experimental study. Circulation 69: 772–774

Lund J T, Hansen D, Brocks V, Jensen M B, Jacobson J R 1992 Aneurysm of the ductus arteriosus in the neonate: three case reports with a review of the literature. Pediatric Cardiology 13: 222–226

Magal C, Wright K C, Dupart G Jr, Wallace S, Gianturco C 1989 A new device for transcatheter closure of the patent ductus arteriosus: a feasibility study in dogs. Investigational Radiology 24: 272–276

Mahoney L, Carnero V, Brett C, Heymann M A, Clyman R I 1982 Prophylactic indomethacin therapy for patent ductus arteriosus in very low birthweight infants. New England Journal of Medicine 306: 506–508

Mahoney L, Caldwell R L, Girod D A 1985 Indomethacin therapy on the first day of life with very low birthweight. Journal of Pediatrics 106: 801–803

Mainwaring R D, Lamberti J J, Spicer R L 1993 Management of absent pulmonary valve syndrome with patent ductus arteriosus. Journal of Cardiac Surgery 8: 148–155

Marcano B, Goldberg S J 1969 Patent ductus arteriosus: a correlation of electrocardiographic and physiologic information. American Journal of Diseases in Children 117: 194–197

Marino B, Guccione P, Carotti A, De Zorzi A, Di Donato R, Marcelleti C 1992 Ductus arteriosus in pulmonary artesia with and without ventricular septal defect. Anatomic and functional differences. Scandinavian Journal of Thoracic and Cardiovascular Surgery 26: 93–96

Martin C G, Snider A R, Katz S M, Peabody J C, Brady J P 1982 Abnormal cerebral blood flow patterns in preterm infants with large patent ductus arteriosus. Journal of Pediatrics 101: 587–593

Martin R P, Banner N R, Radley-Smith R 1986 Familial persistent ductus arteriosus. Archives of Disease in Childhood 61: 906–907

Mason C A, Bigras J L, O'Blenes S B et al 1999 Gene transfer in utero biologically engineers a patent ductus arteriosus in lambs by arresting fibronectin-dependent neointimal formation. Nature Medicine 5: 176–182

Massone M L, Soliani M, Puccio V et al 1990 The relationship between ligation of the ductus arteriosus and intracranial hemorrhage in preterm infants. Minerva Anesiesiologica 56: 179–183

Masura J, Walsh K P, Thanopoulous B et al 1998 Catheter closure of moderate- to large-sized patent ductus arteriosus using the new Amplatzer duct occluder: immediate and short-term results. Journal of the American College of Cardiology 31: 878–882

Mathew R 1998 Development of the pulmonary circulation: metabolic aspects. In: Polin and Fox (eds) Fetal and neonatal physiology. Saunders, Philadelphia, PA, p 924–929

Mato M, Aikawa E, Uchiyama Y 1970 Radioautographic study on the obliteration of the ductus arteriosus Botalli. Virchows Archiv Abteilung A. Pathologische Anatomie 349: 10–20

Matsuo K, Baba H, Kusaba E, Yamaguchi H, Masumoto T, Yoshinaga M 1991 Surgical treatment of patent ductus arteriosus in extremely premature infants. Kyobu Geka [Japanese Journal of Thoracic Surgery] 44: 445–446

McGraph R L, McGuinness G A, Way G L, Wolfe R R, Nora J J, Simmons M A 1978 The silent ductus arteriosus. Journal of Pediatrics 93: 110–113

McMurphy D M, Boreus L O 1971 Studies on the pharmacology of the perfused human fetal ductus

arteriosus. American Journal of Obstetrics and Gynaecology 109: 937–942

McMurphy D M, Heymann M A, Rudolph A M, Melmon K L 1972 Developmental changes in constriction of the ductus arteriosus: responses to oxygen and vasoactive agents in the isolated ductus arteriosus of the fetal lamb. Pediatric Research 6: 231–238

Mecham R P, Griffin G L, Madaras J G, Senior R M 1984 Appearance of chemotactic responsiveness to elastin peptides by developing fetal bovine ligament fibroblasts parallels the onset of elastin production. Journal of Cell Biology 98: 1813–1816

Melka J 1926 Beitrag zur kemtuis der morphologic und obliteration des ductus arteriosus Botalli. Anatomischer Anzeiger 61: 348–356

Mellander M, Leheup B, Lindstrum D P 1984 Recurrence of symptomatic patent ductus arteriosus in extreme premature infants treated with indomethacin. Journal of Pediatrics 105: 138–141

Melmon K L, Cline M J, Hughes T, Nies A S 1968 Kinins: possible mediators of neonatal circulatory changes in man. Journal of Clinical Investigation 1295–1302

Melo J, Norwood W, Freed M, Castañeda A 1980 Formalin infiltration of patent ductus arteriosus. In: Proceedings of the World congress of pediatric cardiology. CIBA, London, p 60

Menahem S 1991 Administration of prostaglandin inhibitors to the mother; the potential risk to the fetus and neonate with duct-dependent circulation. Reproduction, Fertility and Development 3: 489–494

Merritt T A, White C L, Jacob J et al 1979 Patent ductus arteriosus treated with ligation or indomethacin: a follow-up study. Journal of Pediatrics 95: 588–594

Mills M L, King T D 1976 Nonoperative closure of left-to-right shunts. Journal of Thoracic and Cardiovascular Surgery 72: 371–378

Milne M J, Sung R Y T, Fok T F, Crozier I G 1989 Doppler echocardiographic assessment of shunting via the ductus arteriosus in newborn infants. American Journal of Cardiology 64: 102–105

Mirowski M, Arevelo F, Medrano G A, Cisneros F A 1962 Conduction disturbances in patent ductus arteriosus. A study of 200 cases before and after surgery with determination of the P–R index. Circulation 15: 807–813

Mitchell S C, Korones S B, Berendes H W 1971 Congenital heart disease in 56 109 births. Incidence and natural history. Circulation 43: 323–332

Miyauchi T, Masaki T 1999 Pathophysiology of endothelin in the cardiovascular system. Annual Review of Physiology 61: 391–415

Mohan D, Newnham J P, D'Orsogna L 1992 Indomethacin for the treatment of polyhydramnios: a case of constriction of the ductus arteriosus. Australian New Zealand Journal of Obstetrics and Gynecology 32: 243–246

Moise K J Jr, 1993 Effects of advanced gestational age on the frequency of fetal ductal constriction in association with maternal indomethacin use. American Journal of Obstetrics and Gynecology 168: 1350–1353

Momma K, Takao A 1989 Increased constriction of the ductus arteriosus with combined administration of indomethacin and betamethasone in fetal rats. Pediatric Research 25: 69–75

Momma K, Takeuchi H 1983 Constriction of fetal ductus arteriosus by non-steroidal anti-inflammatory drugs: study of additional 34 drugs. Prostaglandins 26: 631–643

Momma K, Nishihara S, Ota Y 1981 Constriction of the fetal ductus arteriosus by glucocorticoid hormones. Pediatric Research 15: 19–21

Moore J W 1995 Repeat use of occluding spring coils to close residual patent ductus arteriosus. Catheter and Cardiovascular Diagnosis 35: 172–175

Moore J W, George L, Kirkpatrick S E et al 1994a Percutaneous closure of the small patent ductus arteriosus using occluding spring coils. Journal American College of Cardiology 23: 759–765

Moore J W, George L, Kirkpatrick S E 1994b Closure of residual patent ductus arteriosus with occluding spring coil after implant of a Rashkind occluder. American Heart Journal 127: 943–945

Moss A J, Emmanouilides G, Duffie E R, Jr 1963 Closure of the ductus arteriosus in the newborn infant. Pediatrics 32: 25–30

Mouzinho A I, Rosenfeld C R, Risser R 1991 Symptomatic patent ductus arteriosus in very-low-birth-weight infants: 1987–1989. Early Human Development 27: 65–77

Munro J C 1907 Ligation of the ductus arteriosus. Annals of Surgery 46: 335–338

Murray C A, Korns M E, Amplatz K, Edwards J E 1970 Bilateral origin of the pulmonary artery from the homolateral ductus arteriosus. Chest 57: 310–317

Musewe N N, Olley P M 1992 Patent ductus arteriosus. In: Freedom R M, Benson, L N, Smallhorn J F (eds) Neonatal heart disease. Springer-Verlag, London, p 598

Musewe N N, Smallhorn J F, Benson L N, Burrows P E, Freedom R M 1987 Validation of ductul-derived pulmonary artery pressure in patients with ductus arteriosus under different hemodynamic states. Circulation 76: 1081–1091

Musewe N N, Benson L N, Smallhorn J F, Freedom R M 1989 Two-dimensional echocardiographic and color flow Doppler evaluation of ductal occlusion with the Rashkind prosthesis. Circulation 80: 1706–1710

Musewe N N, Poppe D, Smallhorn J F 1990 Doppler echocardiographic measurement of pulmonary artery pressure from ductal Doppler velocities in the newborn. Journal of the American College of Cardiology 15: 446–456

Mustard W T 1951 Suture ligation of the patent ductus arteriosus in infancy. Canadian Medical Association Journal 64: 243–244

Nadas A F 1982 The Mannheimer lecture. Pediatric Cardiology 3: 71–76

Nair S K, Subramanyam R, Venkitachalam C G, Valiathan M S 1992 Right aortic arch with isolation of the left subclavian artery and bilateral patent ductus arteriosus. A case report. Journal of Cardiovascular Surgery 33: 242–244

Needleman P, Holmberg S, Mandelbaum B 1981 Ductus arteriosus closure may result from suppression of prostacyclin synthetase by an intrinsic hydroperoxy fatty acid. Prostaglandins 22: 675–682

Neill C, Mounsey P 1958 Auscultation in patent ductus arteriosus with a description of two fistulae simulating patent ductus. British Heart Journal 20: 61–75

Ng M P, Wong K Y, Tan A, Ong K K 1992 Non-surgical closure of patent ductus arteriosus with the Rashkind PDA occluder system. Journal of the Singapore Paediatric Society 34: 185–190

Niebyl J R 1992 Drug therapy during pregnancy. Current Opinion in Obstretics and Gynecology 4: 43–47

Nishigaki N, Negishi M, Honda A et al 1995 Identification of prostaglandin E receptor 'EP2' cloned from mastocytoma cells as EP4 subtype. FEBS Letters 364: 339–341

Nishimoto K, Ino T, Ohkubo M, Akimoto K, Yabuta K 1997 Mid-term follow-up results of coil embolization for patent ductus arteriosus. Journal of Cardiology 30: 131–136

Noah M L 1978 Use of prostaglandin E_1 for maintaining the patency of the ductus arteriosus. Advances in Prostaglandin and Thromboxane Research 4: 355–362

Nora J J 1968 Multifactorial inheritance hypothesis for the etiology of congenital heart diseases: the genetic–environmental interaction. Circulation 38: 604–617

Nora J J, Nora A H 1978 The evolution of specific genetic and environmental counselling in congenital heart disease. Circulation 57: 205–213

Oho S, Ishizawa A, Koike K et al 1998 Transcatheter occlusion of patent ductus arteriosus with a new detachable coil system (DuctOcclud): a multicenter clinical trial. Japanese Circulation Journal 62: 489–493

Olley P M, Coceani F 1981 Prostaglandins and the ductus arteriosus. Annual Review of Medicine 32: 375–385

Olley P M, Coceani F 1987 Lipid mediators in the control of the ductus arteriosus. American Review of Respiratory Diseases 136: 218–219

Olley P M, Bodach E, Heaton J, Coceani F 1975 Further evidence implicating E-type prostaglands in the patency of the lamb ductus arteriosus. European Journal of Pharmacology 34: 247–250

Olley P M, Coceani F, Bodach E 1976 E-type prostaglandins. A new emergency therapy for certain cyanotic congenital heart malformations. Circulation 53: 728–731

Ono M, Furuse A, Kotsuka Y, Yagyu K, Isoda T 1998 Persistent hemolysis after coil occlusion of a patent ductus arteriosus in a patient with aortic regurgitation. Japanese Heart Journal 39: 243–246

Ottenkamp J, Hess J, Talsma M D, Buis-Liem T N 1992 Protrusion of the device: a complication of catheter occlusion of patent ductus arteriosus. British Heart Journal 68: 301–303

Owada C Y, Teitel D F, Moore P 1997 Evaluation of Gianturco coils for closure of large (≥ 3.5 mm) patent ductus arteriosus. Journal of the American College of Cardiology 30: 1856–1862

Panagopoulos P H G, Tatooles C J, Aberdeen E, Waterston D J, Bonham-Carter R E 1971 Patent ductus arteriosus in infants and children. A review of 936 operations (1946–1969). Thorax 26: 137–144

Patterson D F 1980 Genetic aspects of cardiovascular development in dogs. In: Van Praagh R, Takao A (eds) Etiology and morphogenesis of congenital heart disease. Futura, New York, p 1–19

Patterson D F, Pyle P L, Buchanan J W, Trautvetter E, Abt D A 1971 Hereditary patent ductus arteriosus and its sequelae in the dog. Circulation Research 29: 1–13

Payne R F, Jordan S C 1968 Postoperative aneurysms following ligation of the patent ductus arteriosus. British Journal of Radiology 42: 858–861

Peckham G J, Miettinen O S, Ellison R C et al 1984 Clinical course to 1 year of age in premature infants with patent ductus arteriosus. Results of a multicenter randomized trial of indomethacin. Journal of Pediatrics 105: 285–290

Penaloza D, Arias-Stella J, Sime F, Recavarren S, Marticorena E 1964 The heart and pulmonary circulation in children at high altitudes. Pediatrics 34: 568–582

Perlman J M, Hill A, Volpe J J 1981 The effect of patent ductus arteriosus on flow velocity in the anterior cerebral arteries: ductal steal in the premature newborn infant. Journal of Pediatrics 99: 767–771

Pierce K L, Gil D W, Woodward D F, Regan J W 1995 Cloning of human prostanoid receptors. Trends in Pharmacologic Science 16: 253–256

Podnar T, Masura J 1997 Percutaneous closure of patent ductus arteriosus using special screwing detachable coils. Catheter and Cardiovascular Diagnosis 41: 386–391

Podnar T, Masura J 1999 Transcatheter occlusion of residual patent ductus arteriosus after surgical ligation. Pediatric Cardiology 20: 126–130

Polani P E, Campbell M 1960 Factors in the causation of persistent ductus arteriosus. Annals of Human Genetics 24: 343–357

Pontius R G, Danielson G K, Noonan J A, Judson J P 1981 Illusions leading to surgical closure of the distal left pulmonary artery instead of the ductus arteriosus. Journal of Thoracic and Cardiovascular Surgery 82: 107–113

Porstmann W, Wierny L, Warnke H 1967 Der Verschluss des Ductus arteriosus persistens ohne Thorakotomie (vor 1 a ufige Mitterlung). Thoraxchicurgie 15: 199–203

Porstmann W, Wierny L, Warnke H 1968 Der Vershluss des Ductus arteriosus persistens ohne Thorakotomie (zweite Mitterlung). Fortschritte Rontgenstrade 109: 133–148

Porstmann W, Wierny L, Warnke H, Gerstberger G, Romaniuk P A 1971 Catheter closure of patent ductus arteriosus. Radiology Clinics of North America 9: 203–218

Porstmann W, Hieronymi K, Wierny L, Warnke H 1974 Nonsurgical closure of oversized patent ductus arteriosus with pulmonary hypertension. Report of a case. Circulation 50: 346–381

Potain S C 1867 Des mauvements et des bruits qui se passent dans les veines jugulaires. Bulletin et Memoires de la Societe de Medecine de Paris 4: 3

Powell M L 1963 Patent ductus arteriosus in premature infants. Medical Journal of Australia 2: 58–63

Prieto L R, de Camillo D M, Konrad D J, Scalet-Longworth L, Latson L A 1998 Comparison of cost and clinical outcome between transcatheter coil occlusion and surgical closure of isolated patent ductus arteriosus. Pediatrics 101: 1020–1024

Qian J 1992 Catheter closure of patent ductus arteriosus without thoracotomy. Chung-Hua Hsin Hsueh Kuan Ping Tsa Chih 20: 167–168

Rabinovitch M 1996 Cell–extracellular matrix interactions in the ductus arteriosus and perinatal pulmonary circulation. Seminars in Perinatology 20: 531–541

Rabinovitch M 1998 Diseases of the pulmonary vasculature. In: Topol E J (ed.) Lippincott-Raven, Philadelphia, PA, p 3001–3029

Rabinovitch M, Beharry S, Bothwell T, Jackowski G 1988 Qualitative and quantitative differences in protein synthesis comparing fetal lamb ductus arteriosus endothelium and smooth muscle with cells from adjacent vascular sites. Developmental Biology 130: 250–258

Rajotte D, Arap W, Hagedorn M, Koivunen E, Pasqualini R, Ruoslahti E 1998 Molecular heterogeneity of the vascular endothelium revealed by in vivo phage display. Journal of Clinical Investigation 102: 430–437

Rangel-Abundis A, Badui E, Verdin R, Escobar C V, Enciso R, Valdespino A 1991 Spontaneous aneurysm of the patent ductus arteriosus with endarteritis. A case report. Archives del Instituto de Cardiologia de Mexico 61: 59–64

Rao P S, Sideris E B, Haddad J et al 1993 Transcatheter occlusion of patent ductus arteriosus with adjustable buttoned device. Initial clinical experience. Circulation 88: 1119–1126

Rashkind W J, Cuaso C C 1979 Transcatheter closure of patent ductus arteriosus: successful use in a 3.5 kilogram infant. Pediatric Cardiology 1: 3–7

Rashkind W J, Mullins C E, Hellenbrand W E, Tait M A 1987 Nonsurgical closure of the patent ductus arteriosus: clinical application of the Rashkind PDA Occluder System. Circulation 75: 583–592

Rauchfuss C 1859 Ueber thrombose des ductus arteriosus Botalli. Virchows Archiv A. Pathology Anatomy and Histology 17: 376–397

Record R G, McKeown T 1953a Anatomical closure of the ductus arteriosus in the guinea pig. Clinical Science 14: 213–217

Record R G, McKeown T 1953b Observations relating to the aetiology of patent ductus arteriosus. British Heart Journal 15: 376–386

Record R G, McKeown T 1955 The effect of reduced atmospheric pressure on closure of the ductus arteriosus in the guinea pig. Clinical Science 16: 225–228

Reller M D, Ziegler M L, Rice M J, Solin R C, McDonald R W 1989 Duration of ductal shunting in healthy preterm infants: an echographic color flow Doppler study. Journal of Pediatrics 112: 441–446

Reller M D, Colasurdo M A, Rice M J, McDonald R W 1990 The timing spontaneous closure of the ductus arteriosus in infants with respiratory distress syndrome. American Journal of Cardiology 1: 75–78

Reller M D, Buffkin D C, Colasurdo M A, Rice M J, McDonald R W 1991 Ductal patency in neonates with respiratory distress syndrome. A randomized surfactant trial. American Journal of Diseases of Children 145: 1017–1020

Rennie J M, Cooke R W 1991 Prolonged low dose indomethacin for persistent ductus arteriosus of prematurity. Archives of Disease in Childhood 66: 55–58

Rey C, Piechaud, J F, Bourlon F 1990 Endoluminal closure of ductus arteriosus. A cooperative study. Archives des Maladies du Coeur et des Vaisseaux 83: 615–619

Ring-Mrozik E, Hecker W C, Huterer C, Hofmann D 1991 Indication and results of thoracic surgical procedures in premature infants. Progress in Pediatric Surgery 27: 244–250

Roach M R 1973 A biophysical look at the relationship of structure and function in the umbilical artery: In: Fetal and neonatal physiology. Proceedings of the Joseph Barcroft centenary symposium. Cambridge University Press, Cambridge, p 141

Rogers J C, Begleiter M L, Harris D J 1992 Patent ductus arteriosus in four generations of a family. [letter] Journal of Medical Genetics 29: 758

Rohmer J, Hess J, Talsma M D 1990 Closure of the persistent ductus arteriosus (Botalli) using a catheter procedure; the initial 50 patients treated in the Netherlands. Nederlands Tijdschrift voor Geneeskunde 134: 2347–2351

Rosenfeld W, Sadhev S, Brunot V, Jhaveri R, Zabaleta I, Evans H E 1986 Phototherapy effects on the incidence of patent ductus arteriosus in premature infants: prevention with chest shielding. Pediatrics 78: 10–14

Ross R 1986 The pathogenesis of atherosclerosis–an update. New England Journal of Medicine 314: 488–500

Ross R S, Feder F P, Spencer F C 1961 Aneurysms of the previously legated patent ductus arteriosus. Circulation 23: 350–357

Rothenberg S S, Chang J H, Toews W H, Washington R L 1995 Thoracoscopic closure of patent ductus arteriosus: a less traumatic and more cost-effective technique. Journal of Pediatric Surgery 30: 1057–1060

Rothman A, Lucas V W, Sklansky M S, Cocalis M W, Kashani I A 1997 Percutaneous coil occlusion of patent ductus arteriosus. Journal of Pediatrics 130: 447–454

Roulet M J, Coburn R F 1981 Oxygen-induced contraction in the guinea pig neonatal ductus arteriosus. Circulation Research 49: 997–1002

Rudolph A M, Mayer F E, Nadas A S, Gross R E 1958 Patent ductus arteriosus: a clinical and hemodynamic study of patients in the first year of life. Pediatrics 22: 892–904

Rudolph A M, Scarpelli E M, Golinko R J, Gootman N L 1964 Hemodynamic basis for clinical manifestations of patent ductus arteriosus. American Heart Journal 68: 447–458

Rudolph A M, Heymann M A, Spitznas V 1972 Hemodynamic considerations in the development of narrowing of the aorta. American Journal of Cardiology 30: 514–525

Rudolph A M, Heymann M A, Fishman N, Lakier J B 1975 Formalin infiltration of the ductus arteriosus. New England Journal of Medicine 292: 1263–1268

Ruiz C E, Zhang H P, Larsen R L 1993 The role of interventional cardiology in pediatric heart transplantation. Journal of Heart and Lung Transplantation 12: S164–S167

Russo-Marie F, Duval D 1980 Mechanism of action of glucocorticoids on prostaglandin secretion. In: Ramwell P (ed.) Prostaglandin synthetase inhibitors: new clinical applications. Alan R. Liss, New York, p 13–29

Rutishauser M, Ronen G, Wyler F 1977 Aneurysm of the nonpatent ductus arteriosus in the newborn. Acta Pediatrica Scandinavica 66: 649–651

Rutstein D D, Nickerson R J, Heald F P 1952 Seasonal incidence of patent ductus arteriosus and maternal rubella. American Journal of Diseases in Children 84: 199–213

Saenger J S, Mayer D C, D'Angelo L J, Manci E A 1992 Ductus-dependent fetal cardiac defects contraindicate indomethacin tocolysis. Journal of Perinatology 12: 41–47

Sahn D J, Allen H D 1978 Real-time cross-sectional echocardiographic imaging and measurement of the patent ductus arteriosus in infants and children. Circulation 58: 343–354

Saji T, Matsuura H, Hoshino K, Yamamoto S, Ishikita T, Matsuo N 1991 Oral prostaglandin E$_1$ derivative (OP-1206) in an infant with double outlet right ventricle and pulmonary stenosis. Effect on ductus-dependent pulmonary circulation. Japanese Heart Journal 32: 735–740

Salazar J, Olivan P, Ibarra F et al 1990 Silent uncomplicated patent ductus arteriosus in children. Diagnosis with echo-Doppler. Servicio de Espanola De Cardiologia 43: 410–412

Samuelsson B, Goldyne M, Granstrom E, Hamberg M, Hammarstrom S, Maimstein C 1978 Prostaglandins and thromboxanes. Annual Review of Biochemistry 997–1029

Sanchez Torres G, Roldan Conesa D 1989 Left aortic arch without a circumflex segment and a right descending aorta: a hypothetical case a real example. Archivos del Institution de Cardiologia de Mexico 59: 125–131

Santos M A, Moll J N, Drummond C, Aranjo W B, Romano N, Reiss N B 1980 Development of the ductus arteriosus in right ventricular outflow tract obstruction. Circulation 62: 818–822

Sato K, Fujino M, Kozuka T et al 1975 Transfemoral plug closure of patent ductus arteriosus. Circulation 51: 337–341

Saveliev V S, Prokubovski V I, Kolody S M, Saveliev S V, Verin V E 1992 Patent ductus arteriosus: transcatheter closure with a transvenous technique. Radiology 184: 341–344

Schlesinger Y, Schimmel M S, Eidelman A I, Glaser Y 1989 Oral prostaglandin E$_2$ for the management of ductus dependent congenital heart disease. Is there a role for home therapy? Acta Paediatrica Scandinavica 78: 635–636

Schoenfeld A 1992 NSAID's: maternal and fetal considerations. American Journal of Reproduction and Immunology 28: 141–147

Schrader R, Kadel C, Cielinski G, Bussmann W D, Kaltenbach M 1993 Non-thoracotomy closure of persistent ductus arteriosus beyond 60 years. American Journal of Cardiology 72: 1319–1321

Schrader R, Hofstetter R, Fassbender D et al 1999 Transvenous closure of patent ductus arteriosus with Ivalon plugs. Multicenter experience with a new technique. Investigative Radiology 34: 65–70

Schwartz J, Rabinovitz H, Leibovitz H et al 1993 Patent ductus arteriosus involving three generations – a case history. Angiology 44: 751–753

Sciacca A, Condorelli M 1960 Involution of the ductus arteriosus. A morphological and experimental study, with a critical review of the literature. Bibliothera Cardiologica [Supplement to Cardiologics] Karger, Basle

Seibert R W, Seibert J J, Norton J B, Williams D 1981 Recurrent laryngeal nerve damage following formalin infiltration of ductus arteriosus. Laryngoscope 91: 392–393

Senior R M, Griffin G L, Mecham R P, Wrenn D S, Prasad K U, Urry D W 1984 Val–Gly–Val–Ala–Pro–Gly, a repeating peptide in elastin, is chemotactic for fibroblasts and monocytes. Journal of Cell Biology 99: 870–874

Serwer G A, Armstrong B E, Anderson P A W 1982 Continuous wave Doppler ultrasonographic quantitation of patent ductus arteriosus flow. Journal of Pediatrics 100: 297–300

Sharpe G L 1975 Indomethacin and closure of the ductus arteriosus. [Letter] Lancet i: 693

Sharpe G L, Thalme B, Larsson K S 1974 Studies on closure of the ductus arteriosus. XI Ductal closure in utero by a prostaglandin synthesis inhibitor. Prostaglandins 8: 363–368

Shimada S, Raju T N, Bhat R, Maeta H, Viyasagar D 1989 Treatment of patent ductus arteriosus after exogenous surfactant in baboons with hyaline membrane disease. Pediatric Research 26: 565–569

Shiraishi H, Endo H, Ichihashi K et al 1989 Bidirectional ductal shunts in the early neonatal period: evaluation by Doppler color flow imaging. Journal of Cardiology 19: 541–550

Shortland D B, Gibson N A, Levene M I, Archer L N, Evans D H, Shaw D E 1990 Patent ductus arteriosus and cerebral circulation in preterm infants. Developmental Medicine and Child Neurology 32: 386–393

Shulford W H, Sybers R G, Weens H S 1972 The angiographic features of double aortic arch. American Journal of Roentgenography 116: 125–140

Siassi B, Emmanouilides G C, Cleveland R J, Hirose F 1969 Patent ductus arteriosus complicating prolonged assisted ventilation in respiratory distress syndrome. Journal of Pediatrics 74: 11–19

Siegal R E 1962 Galen's experiments and observations on pulmonary blood flow and respiration. American Journal of Cardiology 10: 738–745

Silver M M, Freedom R M, Silver M D, Olley P M 1981 The morphology of the human newborn ductus arteriosus: a reappraisal of its structure and closure with special reference to prostaglandin E_1 therapy. Human Pathology 12: 1123–1136

Silverman N H 1993 Patent ductus arteriosus. In: Pediatric echocardiograpy. Williams & Wilkins, Baltimore, MD, p 167–177

Silverman N H, Lewis A B, Heymann M A, Rudolph A M 1974 Echocardiographic assessment of ductus arteriosus shunt in premature infants. Circulation 50: 821–825

Slomp J, van M J, Poelmann R E, Bogers A J, Gittenberger-de-Groot A C 1992 Formation of intimal cushions in the ductus arteriosus as a model for vascular intimal thickening. An immunohistochemical study of changes in extracellular matrix components. Atherosclerosis 93: 25–39

Smallhorn J F, Huhta J C, Anderson R H, Macartney F J 1982 Suprasternal cross-sectional echocardiography in assessment of patent ductus arteriosus. British Heart Journal 48: 321–330

Smith G C 1998 The pharmacology of the ductus arteriosus. Pharmacology Reviews 50: 35–58

Smith G C, McGrath J C 1991 Prostaglandin E_2 and fetal oxygen tension synergistically inhibit response of isolated fetal rabbit ductus arteriosus to norepinephrine. Journal of Cardiovascular Pharmacology 17: 861–866

Smith G C, McGrath J C 1993 Characterisation of the effect of oxygen tension on response of fetal rabbit ductus arteriosus to vasodilators. Cardiovascular Research 27: 2205–2211

Smith G C, McGrath J C 1995 Contractile effects of prostanoids on fetal rabbit ductus arteriosus. Journal of Cardiovascular Pharmacology 25: 113–118

Smith G C, Coleman R A, McGrath J C 1994 Characterization of dilator prostanoid receptors in the fetal rabbit ductus arteriosus. Journal Pharmacology and Experimental Therapeutics 271: 390–6

Sommer R, Gutierrez A, Lai W W, Parness I A 1994 Use of preformed nitinol snare to improve transcatheter coil delivery in occlusion of patent ductus arteriosus. American Journal of Cardiology 74: 836–839

Sones F M Jr, Effler D B 1951–1952 Diagnosis and treatment of aortic rings. Cleveland Clinic Quarterly 18–19: 310–320

Sorensen K E, Kristensen B O, Hansen O K 1991 Frequency of occurence of residual ductal flow after surgical ligation by color-flow mapping. American Journal of Cardiology 67: 653–654

Starling M B, Elliott R B 1974 The effects of prostaglandins, prostaglandin inhibitors, and oxygen on the closure of the ductus arteriosus, pulmonary arteries and umbilical vessels in vitro. Prostaglandins 8: 187–203

Steinberg I, Miscall L, Goldberg H P 1964 Congenital absence of left pulmonary artery with patent ductus arteriosi. Journal of the American Medical Association 190: 394–396

Stejskal L, Stark J 1992 Surgical treatment of persistent ductus arteriosus complicated by bacterial endocarditis. European Journal of Cardiothoracic Surgery 6: 272–273

Steno N 1948 Reprinted with historical note: an unusually early description of the so-called tetralogy of Fallot. Mayo Clinic Proceedings 23: 316–320

Stevenson J G 1977 Fluid administration in the association of patent ductus arteriosus complicating respiratory distress syndrome. Journal of Paediatrics 90: 257–261

Stevenson J G, Kawabori I, Guntheroth W G 1979 Noninvasive detection of pulmonary hypertension in patent ductus arteriosus by pulsed Doppler echocardiography. Circulation 60: 355–359

Stevenson J G, Kawabori I, Guntheroth W G 1980 Pulsed Doppler echocardiographic diagnosis of patent ductus arteriosus: sensitivity, specificity, limitations and technical features. Catheterization and Cardiovascular Diagnosis 6: 255–263

Stewart J R, Kincaid O W, Edwards J E 1964 An atlas of vascular rings and related malformations of the aortic arch system. Thomas, Springfield, IL

Stout C, Koehl G 1970 Aortic embolism in a newborn infant. American Journal of Diseases in Children 120: 74–76

Strassman P 1894 Anatomische und physiologische untersuchingen uber den blutkreislauf bein neugebornen. Archiv für Gynakologie 45: 393–445

Strauss A, Mondanlou H D, Gyepes M, Wittner R 1982 Congenital heart disease and respiratory distress syndrome: reversal of indomethacin closure of patent ductus arteriosus by prostaglandin therapy in a preterm infant. American Journal of Diseases of Childhood 136: 934–936

Swenson A 1939 Beitrag zur kenuntris von dem histologischeu bau und dem postembryonolen verschlub des ductus arteriosus. Botalli Zeitschrift Mikroanat Forschung 46: 275–298

Taylor B E, Pollack A A, Burchell H B, Clagen O T, Wood E H 1950 Studies of the pulmonary and systemic arterial pressure in cases of patent ductus arteriosus with special reference to the effects of surgical closure. Journal of Clinical Investigation 29: 745–753

Terragano N A, Terragano A, McGill J C, Rodriguez D J 1977 Synthesis of prostaglandin by the ductus arteriosus of the bovine fetus. Prostaglandins 14: 721–727

Thibeault D W, Emmanouilides G C, Nelson R J, Lachman R S, Rosenbart R M, Oh W 1975 Patent ductus arteriosus complicating the respiratory distress syndrome in preterm infants. Journal of Pediatrics 86: 120–126

Thiene G, Frescura C, Bortolotti U, Del Maschio A, Valente M 1981 The systemic pulmonary circulation in pulmonary atresia with ventricular septal defect: concept of reciprocal development of the fourth and sixth aortic arches. American Heart Journal 101: 339–344

Thorburn G D 1992 The placenta, PGE$_2$ and parturition. Early Human Development 29: 63–73

Toda T, Tsuda N, Takagi T, Nishimori I, Leszczynski D, Kummerow F 1980 Ultrastructure of the developing human ductus arteriosus. Journal of Anatomy 131: 25–37

Todd E P, Lindsay W G, Edwards J E 1976 Bilateral ductus origin of the pulmonary arteries. Systemic pulmonary arterial anatomosis as first stage in planned total correction. Circulation 54: 834–836

Tometzki A J, Arnold R, Peart I et al 1996 Transcatheter occlusion of the patent ductus arteriosus with Cook detachable coils. Heart 76: 531–535

Trippestad A, Efskind L 1971 Patent ductus arteriosus. Surgical treatment of 686 patients. Scandinavian Journal of Thoracic Cardiovascular Surgery 6: 38–43

Trusler G A 1979 Surgery for patent ductus arteriosus – 1979. In: Tucker B W, Lindesmith G G (eds) Congenital heart disease. Grune & Stratton, New York, p 39–45

Tsuboi H, Ikeda N, Minami Y et al 1997 A video-assisted thoracoscopic surgical technique for interruption of patent ductus arteriosus. Surgery Today 27: 439–442

Turley E A, Torrance J 1985 Localization of hyaluronate and hyaluronate-binding protein on motile and non-motile fibroblasts. Experimental Cell Research 161: 17–28

Turley E A, Austen L, Vandeligt K, Clary C 1991 Hyaluronan and a cell-associated hyaluronan binding protein regulate the locomotion of ras-transformed cells. Journal of Cell Biology 112: 1041–1047

Tutassaura H, Goldman B, Moes C A F, Mustard W T 1969 Spontaneous aneurysm of the ductus arteriosus in childhood. Thoracic and Cardiovascular Surgery 57: 180–182

Ueno Y, Shinozaki T, Shimamoto M, Ohkubo K, Ueda M, Akiyama F 1990 Aneurysm of the diverticulum of the ductus arteriosus in the adult. Journal of the Japanese Association for Thoracic Surgery 83: 1356–1361

Uzun O, Dickinson D, Parsons J, Gibbs J L 1998 Residual and recurrent shunts after implantation of Cook detachable duct occlusion coils. Heart 79: 220–222

Uzun O, Veldtman G R, Dickinson D F, Parsons J M, Blackburn M E, Gibbs J L 1999 Haemolysis following implantation of duct occlusion coils. Heart 81: 160–161

Valdez-Cruz L M, Dudell G G 1981 Specificity and accuracy of echocardiographic and clinical criteria for diagnosis of patent ductus arteriosus in fluid-restricted infants. Journal of Pediatrics 298–305

van den Veyver I R 1993 The effect of gestational age and fetal indomethacin levels on the incidence of constriction of the fetal ductus arteriosus. Obstetrics and Gynecology 82: 500–503

Verin V E, Friedli B, Oberhansli I, Urban P, Meier B 1993a Closure of patent ductus arteriosus using interventional catheterization. Schweizerische Medizinische Wochenschrift 123: 530–532

Verin V E, Saveliev S V, Kolody S M, Prokubovski V I 1993b Results of transcatheter closure of the patent ductus arteriosus with the Botallo occluder. Journal of the American College of Cardiology 22: 1509–1514

Vert P, Bianchetti G, Morchal F, Monin P, Morselli P L 1980 Effectiveness and pharmacokinetics of indomethacin in premature newborns with patent ductus arteriosus. European Journal of Clinical Pharmacology 18: 83–88

Vick G W, III, Huhta J C, Gutgesell H P 1985 Assessment of the ductus arteriosus in preterm infants utilizing suprasternal two-dimensional/Doppler echocardiography. Journal of the American College of Cardiology 5: 973–977

Virchow R 1856 Die thrombosen der neugeboren. In: Gesamnelte abhandlunger zur wissenschafthchen medicin. Maidinger Frankfurt, p 591

Vogel J H K, Pryor R, Blount G S 1964 The cardiovascular system in children from high altitude. Journal of Pediatrics 64: 315–322

Hayek H V 1936 Der funktionelle bau der nabelarterien und des ductus Botaii. Zeitschrift für Anatomie und Entweicklungsgeschichte 105: 15–24

Wagner H R, Ellison R C, Zierler S 1984 Surgical closure of patent ductus arteriosus in 268 preterm infants. Journal of Thoracic Cardiovascular Surgery 87: 870–875

Wallgren E I 1962 Pulmonary and renal circulation in children with patent ductus arteriosus. Acta Paediatrica (Suppl.) 51: 138

Walsh K P, Sreeram N, Franks R, Arnold R 1992 Balloon dilatation of the arterial duct in congenital heart disease. Lancet 339: 331–332

Walsh K P, Abrams S E, Arnold R 1993 Arterial duct angioplasty as an adjunct to dilatation of the valve for critical pulmonary stenosis. British Heart Journal 69: 260–262

Walsh R S, Mentzer R J 1987 Role of cyclic nucleotides in relaxation of fetal lamb ductus arteriosus. Surgery 102: 313–318

Walsh R S, Ely S W, Mentzer R J 1988 Response of lamb ductus arteriosus to nitroglycerin and nitroprusside. Journal Surgical Research 44: 8–13

Wang Y 1991 Transfemoral plug closure in 45 cases of patent ductus arteriosus. Chung-Hua Hsin Hsueh Kuan Ping Tsa Chih 19: 18–20

Warnecke I, Frank J, Hohle R, Lemm W, Bucherl E S 1984 Transvenous double-balloon occlusion of the persistent ductus arteriosus: an experimental study. Pediatric Cardiology 5: 79–84

Watson D G, Keith J D 1962 The Q wave in lead V$_6$ in heart disease of infancy and childhood with special reference to diastolic loading. American Heart Journal 63: 629–635

Weber H S, Cyran S E, Gleason M M, White M G, Baylen B G 1996 Transcatheter vascular occlusion of the small patent ductus arteriosus: an alternative method. Pediatric Cardiology 17: 181–183

Wei J, Chang Y, Ko G, Sheih S 1984 Familial patent ductus arteriosus. American Journal of Cardiology 54: 235–236

Werkstrom V, Ny L, Persson K, Andersson K E 1997 Carbon monoxide-induced relaxation and distribution of haem oxygenase isoenzymes in the pig urethra and lower oesophagogastric junction. British Journal of Pharmacology 120: 312–318

Wessel D L, Keane J F, Parness I, Lock J E 1988 Outpatient closure of the patent ductus arteriosus. Circulation 77: 1068–1071

Whitaker W, Heath D, Brown J W 1955 Patent ductus arteriosus with pulmonary hypertension. British Heart Journal 17: 121–137

Whitley J E, Rudhe U, Herzenberg H 1963 Decreased left lung vascularity in congenital left-to-right shunts. Acta Radiologics: Diagnosis 1: 1125–1131

Wilson J G, Warkany J 1950 Cardiac and aortic arch anomalies in offsprings of vitamin A deficient rats correlated with similar human anomalies. Pediatrics 5: 708–725

Wilson N J, Neutze, J M, Mawson J B, Calder A L 1993 Transcatheter closure of patent ductus arteriosus in children and adults. New Zealand Medical Journal 26: 299–301

Wong S N, Lo R N, Hui P W 1990 Abnormal renal and splanchnic arterial Doppler pattern in premature babies with symtomatic patent ductus arteriosus. Journal of Ultrasound in Medicine 9: 125–130

Yeh T F, Thalji A, Luken L, Lilien L, Carr I, Pildes R S 1981 Improved lung compliance following indomethacin therapy in premature infants with persistent ductus arteriosus. Chest 80: 698–700

Yeh T F, Achanti B, Patel H, Pildes R S 1989 Indomethacin therapy in premature infants with patent ductus arteriosus – determination of therapeutic plasma levels. Developmental Pharmacology and Therapeutics 12: 169–178

Yoder M J, Baumann F G, Grover J N, Brick I, Imparato A M 1978 A morphological study of early cellular changes in the closure of the rabbit ductus arteriosus. Anatomical Record 192: 19–39

Zapol W M, Kolobow T, Doppman J, Pierce J E 1971 Response of the ductus arteriosus and pulmonary blood flow to blood oxygen tension in immersed lamb fetuses perfused through an artificial placenta. Journal of Thoracic and Cardiovascular Surgery 61: 891–903

Zeevi B, Berant M, Bar-Mor G, Blieden L C 1996 Percutaneous closure of small patent ductus arteriosus: comparison of Rashkind double-umbrella device and occluding spring coils. Catheter and Cardiovascular Diagnosis 39: 44–48

Zetterquist P 1972 A clinical and genetic study of congenital heart defects. The Institute for Medical Genetics, University of Uppsala, Sweden

Zhu L, Dagher E, Johnson D J et al 1993 A developmentally regulated program restricting insolubilization of elastin and formation of laminae in the fetal lamb ductus arteriosus. Laboratory Investigation 68: 321–331

Zhou B, Rabinovitch M 1998 Microtubule involvement in translational regulation of fibronectin expression by light chain 3 of microtubule-associated protein 1 in vascular smooth muscle cells. Circulation Research 83: 481–489

Zhou B, Boudreau N, Coulber C, Hammarback J, Rabinovitch M 1997 Microtubule-associated protein 1 light chain 3 is a fibronectin mRNA-binding protein linked to mRNA translation in lamb vascular smooth muscle cells. Journal of Clinical Investigation 100: 3070–3082

Zhou B, Coulber C, Rabinovitch M 1998 Tissue-specific and developmental regulation of transforming growth factor-beta 1 expression in fetal lamb ductus arteriosus endothelial cells. Pediatric Research 44: 865–872

53

═══ Pulmonary stenosis ═══

M. Tynan and R. H. Anderson

In this chapter we will consider the malformations characterized by obstruction (at some level) to flow of blood from the right ventricle into the pulmonary circulation. Most frequently, the obstruction is at the level of the pulmonary valve. Less frequently, it is at infundibular level, within the trabecular component of the right ventricle or within the pulmonary arterial pathways. Lesions at any of these levels can occur as part of more complex malformations such as tetralogy of Fallot (Chapter 46) or complete transposition (Chapter 48). The more complex variants will be discussed in the appropriate chapters. In this section, we are concerned with those patients in whom the pulmonary obstruction is the primary lesion. There is no ideal term to describe this situation. The lesion is certainly not 'isolated' because, as we shall see, it has profound influences on other parts of the heart. Equally, pulmonary stenosis with an intact septum is less than an ideal description, since small muscular defects in the apical trabecular part of the ventricular septum produce little change in the clinical picture. We will exclude from consideration, however, those cases in which pulmonary stenosis co-exists with a perimembranous ventricular septal defect, whatever its size. In this respect we are following the lead of Rowe (1978a), who, for much the same reasons as we have listed, concluded that the most appropriate term was 'pulmonary stenosis with normal aortic root' (a term introduced by Abrahams and Wood, 1951).

─── INCIDENCE AND AETIOLOGY ───

Although the lesion was initially considered rare (Abbott, 1936), increasing clinical experience has shown that pulmonary stenosis can account for a tenth or more of congenital cardiac malformations. Abrahams and Wood (1951) found an incidence of 11.6% amongst 689 patients, while Campbell (1954) reported 113 examples (10%) in a survey of 1130 cases. The corresponding figure in the extensive case material of the Hospital for Sick Children, Toronto was 9.9%. There is no difference in the incidence between the sexes, but a surprising difference is noted in the seasonal pattern of birth. Campbell (1962) first noted this when he observed that most affected males were born between the months of July and September. The maximal period for females was between January and March. He commented that his figures were too small to be significant, but in a much larger series studied in Ontario, Rose and her colleagues (1972) confirmed peaks for males born in the autumn and females born in the spring.

From the standpoint of aetiology, there is considerable evidence pointing to a genetic basis for the occurrence of the lesion in its various forms. Thus, although McKeown et al (1953) found no familial trait in their study, subsequent investigators found strong evidence supporting familial influence. Lamy et al (1957) found two subjects with pulmonary stenosis among four siblings of patients with pulmonary stenosis, a recurrence rate of 4%. Campbell (1962) found six occurrences of congenital heart disease in 282 siblings of 125 patients, giving, in his series, a recurrence rate of 2.1%. The figure found by Fabricius (1959) was 4%. These are all significantly higher than would be expected by chance. Furthermore, Campbell (1962), combining his series with that of Lamy et al (1957), found an incidence of 2% of consanguinity amongst the parents. The rate in the general population of the United Kingdom at that time was 0.4%. Nora and Spangler (1972) also found an increased incidence of the same lesion amongst siblings of patients with pulmonary stenosis. Added to these studies, there are several examples of numerous members of the same family having pulmonary stenosis. Outstanding in this respect are the remarkable families reported by Fournier and his colleagues (1963) and by Koroxendis et al (1966). In the latter example, the last child, also affected, had been born of a different father from the others. Two of the earlier children also had deaf mutism and hypertelorism. The conclusion was drawn that the constellation of lesions was caused by a point mutation, the deafness being a variably expressed part of the syndrome. In the family reported by Fournier and his colleagues (1963), four of five sisters had pulmonary stenosis together with the nephrotic syndrome. A less convincing family history was reported by Klinge and Baekgaard Laursen (1975), since their index patient had only mild pulmonary stenosis in the setting of an atrioventricular septal defect with left ventricular dominance. The finding on the paternal side of the family, however, of a relative with valvar pulmonary stenosis, together with a bifoliate pulmonary valve in a paternal cousin, suggested a sex-influenced monogenic pattern of inheritance. Klinge and Baekgaard Laursen (1975) also pointed to the fact that pulmonary stenosis was well-recognized as being part of several inherited syndromes, such as trisomy 18, Marchesani's syndrome and the cardiofacial syndrome. The last, described first by Linde et al (1973), is recognized to be closely related to the Ullrich–Noonan syndrome (Noonan and Ehmke, 1963), in which there is known familial occurrence of a dysplastic pulmonary valve.

In contrast to the genetic background of pulmonary valvar stenosis, specific causative agents have been identified for pulmonary arterial stenosis. For example, infection with rubella virus is well established as producing this lesion (Rowe, 1963; Emmanouilides et al, 1964; Campbell, 1965). Peripheral pulmonary arterial stenosis coexisting with supravalvar aortic stenosis is known to be part of the syndrome associated with infantile hypercalcaemia (the so-called 'William's syndrome': Beuren et al, 1964; Jue et al, 1965). Even with arterial stenosis, however, genetic factors cannot be excluded, since familial occurrences were reported by Gay et al (1963), McCue et al (1965) and Roberts and Moes (1973).

ANATOMY AND PATHOGENESIS

PULMONARY VALVAR STENOSIS

Stenosis at valvar level is by far the most common lesion producing pulmonary stenosis. An understanding of the mechanisms responsible for stenosis needs to be founded on an appropriate appreciation of normal valvar anatomy. The pulmonary valve consists, in essence, of three leaflets supported in semilunar fashion within the sinuses of the pulmonary trunk. The most distal attachment of the hingepoints of each leaflet is to the sinutubular junction (the discrete ring marking the transition from the clover-like sinuses to the tubular trunk), while the most proximal attachment of each leaflet is to the muscular infundibulum of the right ventricle (Figure 53.1). This means that each semilunar hingepoint, marking the haemodynamic ventriculo-arterial junction, crosses twice the circular anatomical junction to be found between the muscular infundibulum and the fibroelastic wall of the pulmonary trunk. As a consequence of this arrangement, crescents of muscular infundibulum are incorporated at the base of each pulmonary sinus, while three tapering triangles of fibrous pulmonary truncal wall extend beyond the anatomical ventriculo-arterial junction as parts of the

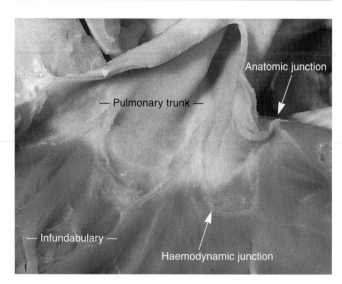

Figure 53.1. This normal pulmonary valve has been opened by an incision through the front of the right ventricular outflow tract, and the leaflets have been removed from their semilunar attachments. Note that the attachments incorporate triangles of arterial wall in the ventricular outflow tract, and crescents of infundibular musculature in the valvar sinuses (both cross-hatched). See also Figure 53.2. (Photographed by kind permission of Dr J. R. Zuberbuhler, University of Pittsburgh, USA.)

ventricular outflow tract, reaching to the level of the sinutubular junction (Figure 53.2). When the pulmonary valve is normally structured, the free edge of each leaflet is appreciably longer than the mathematical chord of the sinus that supports it, this arrangement permitting the three leaflets to fit snugly together to close the valvar orifice. When the overall arrangement of the valve is examined (Figure 53.3, left hand panel), it becomes evident that there is no such thing as a collagenous 'annulus' supporting the leaflets in circular fashion. It is the semilunar nature of their suspension that permits competent closure and unobstructed opening, with the zones of apposition between the adjacent leaflets extending in triradiate fashion from the centroid of the valvar orifice

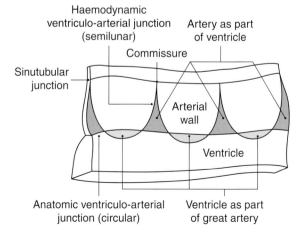

Figure 53.2. Diagrammatic representation of the morphology shown in Figure 65.1.

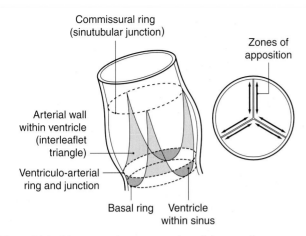

Figure 53.3. Diagrammatic representation of the overall arrangement of the pulmonary valve (left hand panel) together with the mode of apposition of the valvar leaflets when viewed from above during ventricular diastole (right hand panel).

to the sinutubular junction at its periphery (Figure 53.3, right hand panel).

When we consider the mechanics of valvar stenosis in the light of this anatomo-functional arrangement, it becomes evident that the abnormality most obviously narrowing the orifice will be fusion of adjacent leaflets along their zones of apposition – the so-called commissures. This is precisely what is seen in the typical form of pulmonary valvar stenosis. Each zone of apposition shows evidence of peripheral fusion, usually to comparable degree, so that the orifice of the valve is narrowed to produce a central opening (Figure 53.4). The more the fusion extends towards the centre of the valve, the narrower will be the central opening, and the more severe will be the valvar stenosis. Therefore, in relatively minor forms of stenosis, the opening in the valve has a triangular configuration (Figure 53.4). In the most severe forms, which produce the typical critical stenosis seen in neonates, the leaflets fuse along their zones of apposition almost to the valvar centroid, leaving a pin-prick opening. In this so-called domed stenosis (Figure 53.5), the central cupola tends to be smooth, with evidence of the fused zones of apposition seen to varying degrees as peripheral raphes. In some instances, four such raphes are seen, suggesting that the valve itself initially had four leaflets (Selzer et al, 1949). Quadrifoliate pulmonary valves are by no means unusual, being discovered once in each 250 postmortems by Becker (1972). The chance findings at postmortem, however, were benign lesions. It is also unusual in our experience to find commissural fusion producing pulmonary stenosis in the setting of a bifoliate valve. Although Rowe (1978a) described 20% of the postmortem material with pulmonary stenosis at Toronto as having bicuspid valves, we found only two such hearts in the comparable material in the files of Children's Hospital of Pittsburgh (Figure 53.6) and have no such case in the records of the Royal Brompton Hospital, London.

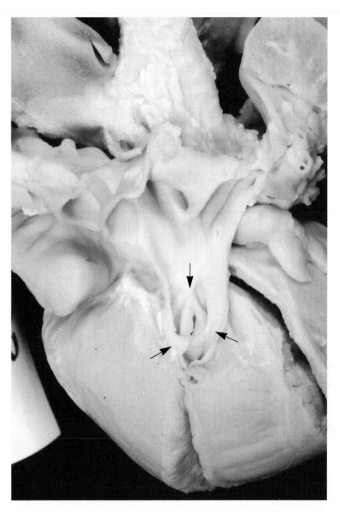

Figure 53.4. This stenotic pulmonary valve with three leaflets is displayed by removing the anterior wall of the pulmonary trunk. Note the fusion of the peripheral ends of the zones of apposition between adjacent leaflets (arrowed). (Photographed by kind permission of Dr J. R. Zuberbuhler, University of Pittsburgh, USA.)

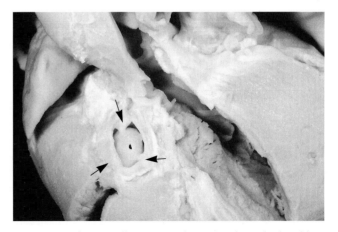

Figure 53.5. This critically stenotic pulmonary valve is displayed by removing the entirety of the pulmonary trunk. The zones of apposition are fused uniformly to the centre of the valve, producing typically dome-shaped stenosis. The arrows show the peripheral attachments to the sinutubular junction, demonstrating the initially trifoliate nature of the valve. (Photographed by kind permission of Dr J. R. Zuberbuhler, University of Pittsburgh, USA.)

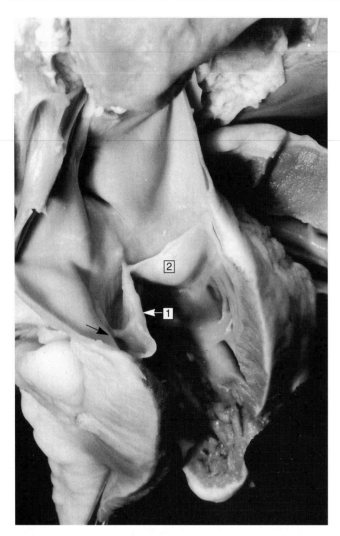

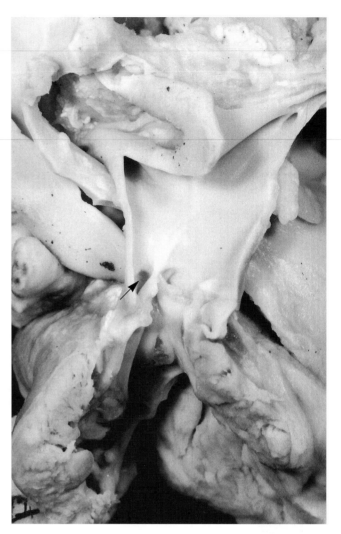

Figure 53.6. This minimally stenotic pulmonary valve, from the collection of the Children's Hospital of Pittsburgh, has only two leaflets (1,2), with a raphe seen in one of the leaflets (arrowed). (Photographed by kind permission of Dr J. R. Zuberbuhler, University of Pittsburgh, USA.)

Figure 53.7. In this stenotic valve, there is minimal fusion of the leaflets. Instead, it is dysplasia of the leaflets and pinching in at the sinutubular junction (arrowed) that produces the stenosis. (Photographed by kind permission of Dr J. R. Zuberbuhler, University of Pittsburgh, USA.)

The typical lesion producing pulmonary valvar stenosis, therefore, is uniform fusion of the peripheral zones of apposition of a trifoliate valve, leaving a central aperture. Usually this arrangement is associated with some degree of thickening at the union of the zones of apposition with the sinutubular junction, the arrangement being described surgically as 'tethering'. An accentuation of such tethering can produce marked narrowing at the sinutubular junction, giving an hourglass appearance that is often described as 'supravalvar'. In reality, the sinutubular junction is an integral part of the valvar complex. Such pinching-in can also be found at the sinutubular junction in the absence of fusion of adjacent leaflets. This produces two different types of valvar stenosis, which probably reflect different manifestations of dysplasia of the valvar leaflets. It was Koretzky et al (1969) who first focused attention on the so-called 'dysplastic' variant, in which the leaflets themselves are markedly thickened and mucoid (Figure 53.7). The

thickening of the leaflets themselves is sufficient to produce some obstruction of the valvar orifice, but clinical experience indicates that such thickened leaflets usually coexist with a narrowed sinutubular junction. Most of the patients with Ullrich– Noonan syndrome have this type of stenosis (Rodriguez-Fernandez et al, 1972). There is then still a third type of valvar stenosis where the major narrowing is at the sinutubular junction, with poststenotic dilation of the pulmonary trunk excacerbating the hourglass appearance (Figure 53.8). First described by Milo et al (1988) on the basis of surgical observations, the major feature is a shortening of the free-edge of the dysplastic leaflets in addition to the sinutubular constriction. This produces an arrangement whereby each sinus takes on the appearance of a bottle with a narrow neck. A similar arrangement can be found in so-called supravalvar aortic stenosis, where again the major area of narrowing is found at the pinched-in sinutubular junction (see Chapter 54).

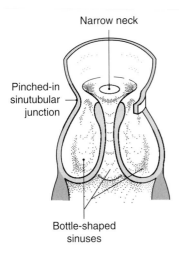

Narrow neck

Pinched-in
sinutubular
junction

Bottle-shaped
sinuses

Figure 53.8. Diagrammatic representation of the variant of valvar pulmonary stenosis emphasized by Milo et al (1988). The bottle-shaped sinuses, with narrow necks, result from pinching-in of the sinutubular junction.

Although pulmonary valvar stenosis may be considered a simple lesion, it is rare for the lesion to be totally isolated. Almost always there is hypertrophy of the right ventricular wall. In the neonate with critical valvar stenosis, such hypertrophy may be severe, with accompanying fibrosis of the endocardium and thickening of the tricuspid valvar tension apparatus. The ventricle then resembles the less severely affected right ventricles seen in pulmonary atresia with intact septum (Figure 53.9). It is often possible to find areas of subendocardial right ventricular infarction in the absence of coronary arterial disease (Franciosi and Blanc, 1968). Rowe (1978a) argued (on clinical evidence) that such right ventricular ischaemia was probably more common than previously realized. Harinck and his colleagues (1977) found left ventricular myocardial hypertrophy in over half the cases they studied with pulmonary stenosis, while Becu et al (1976) described extensive areas of disarray in the myocardial and arterial walls in hearts from patients aged 6 days to 9 years. This all points to the disease being more generalized than would be expected from a simple valvar lesion producing direct haemodynamic effects. When the right ventricular wall is hypertrophied, the size of the ventricular cavity is usually relatively reduced. Apart from this relative reduction, there is a further group of patients with true diminution in cavity size as a consequence of overgrowth and obliteration of the trabecular component. This finding is more typically seen in pulmonary atresia with intact septum (Chapter 44). First described with pulmonary stenosis by Finlay (1879), more recent accounts of this combination were given by Williams et al (1963) and Freed et al (1973).

In a good proportion of cases with pulmonary valvar stenosis of whatever type, there is an associated deficiency of the atrial septum. Rowe (1978a) observed that three quarters of his postmortem specimens had either a probe patent septum or else a defect within the oval fossa. Such defects were more commonly seen in those who had only moderate stenosis. The combination of pulmonary stenosis, atrial septal defect and right ventricular hypertrophy is referred to by French investigators as the 'trilogy of Fallot' (Souliè et al, 1951). This recalls Fallot's original description (1888), when he identified such a combination as an alternative cause of 'le maladie bleu' and distinguished it from the tetralogy. While having good historical pedigree, there now seems little justification for retaining the term. Tetralogy is now identified from the specific morphology of the right ventricular outflow tract, a feature that is not present in cases referred to as 'trilogy'. Retention of this latter term seems to create an unnecessary potential for confusion.

Although Campbell (1954) observed marked cardiac cirrhosis in adults dying with pulmonary stenosis, such hepatic changes are unlikely to be encountered now. Rowe (1978a), however, reported early fibrotic changes in the liver of two of his patients dying at age 6 and 7 years, respectively.

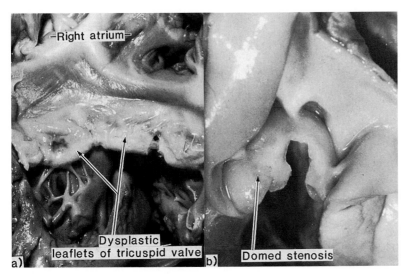

Right atrium

Dysplastic
leaflets of tricuspid valve

a)

Domed stenosis

b)

Figure 53.9. The right ventricle is thickened and the tricuspid valve dysplastic (a) in a patient with severe stenosis and (b) child dying in infancy. Reproduced by kind permission of Dr Leon M. Gerlis, Imperial College School of Medicine at National Heart and Lung Institute, London, UK.)

INFUNDIBULAR STENOSIS

Pure narrowing of the muscular subpulmonary infundibulum in the setting of an intact ventricular septum (or with an apical ventricular septal defect) is rare. Although reported with an incidence of up to 10% in older series (Abrahams and Wood, 1951; Brock, 1961), more recent experience has shown it to be much less common. Zaret and Conti (1973) found only three cases among their 228 patients. Of the cases seen at the Hospital for Sick Children, Toronto during the 23 years prior to publication of their book, only 2.7% had this type of stenosis (Rowe, 1978a). It is probable that many of the cases described as having isolated infundibular stenosis have previously also had a ventricular septal defect that closed spontaneously (Brock, 1961; Gamble and Nadas, 1965; Zaret and Conti, 1973).

COMBINED VALVAR AND INFUNDIBULAR STENOSIS

Hypertrophy of the subpulmonary infundibulum occurs along with hypertrophy of the rest of the right ventricle in response to valvar stenosis. This reduces the infundibular diameter, and endocardial fibroelastosis may be seen along with the hypertrophy. Fixed stenosis of the infundibulum coexisting with valvar stenosis is exceedingly rare (Rowe, 1978a). The reactive stenosis, however, is an important component to be noted when judging the results of balloon valvoplasty (see below), since time is needed for its regression.

OTHER TYPES OF STENOSIS OCCURRING WITHIN THE RIGHT VENTRICLE

Other types of stenosis within the right ventricle are also very rare, but they must be considered as possible causes of pulmonary stenosis. Hypertrophy of the body of the septomarginal trabeculation (which in its severest form produces the typical 'two-chambered right ventricle') is usually found with a ventricular septal defect (Alva et al, 1999). It can exist with an intact septum (Restivo et al, 1984). In other patients, the valve of the embryonic venous sinus (sinus venosus) can persist and become so expanded and aneurysmal that it can pass through the tricuspid valve and obstruct the pulmonary outflow tract (the 'spinnaker syndrome': Jones and Niles, 1968). A similar case has been described in which it was a huge aneurysm of the membranous septum that produced subpulmonary stenosis (Bonvicini et al, 1982). More rarely, tumours can cause subvalvar right ventricular obstruction (Simcha et al, 1971), as may aneurysm of the right coronary sinus of the aorta (Edwards and Burchell, 1957). Hypertrophic cardiomyopathy can also afflict the right ventricle, particularly in the setting of lentiginosis, although left ventricular obstruction usually dominates.

PULMONARY ARTERIAL STENOSIS

Stenoses of the pulmonary arterial tree are frequent in association with complex malformations such as tetralogy of Fallot or complete transposition. They can also complicate more simple lesions such as pulmonary valvar stenosis or ventricular septal defect. Stenoses in the pulmonary arteries can also occur in isolation, and in various parts of the pulmonary arterial tree. These lesions have been classified in detail by Smith (1958) and by Franch and Gay (1963). These systems were simplified by Rowe (1978a). Thus, the stenosis may be localized and central (within the pulmonary trunk or right and left pulmonary arteries), localized and peripheral (at the branch points of major intrapulmonary arteries) or more extensive (existing as a hypoplastic arterial segment commencing either at the end of the right or left main pulmonary artery or a major intrapulmonary branch point). The arterial stenoses, when peripheral, may be unilateral. As Rowe (1978b) indicated, there is a paucity of post-mortem descriptions of these cases. We have yet to encounter such a specimen. Rowe (1978b) summarized the reported cases, opining that an anomaly of medial elastic tissue together with intimal proliferations could be the cause. It is likely that the disease process will not be limited to the pulmonary arteries but will involve also the systemic vessels (Rowe, 1972). In this respect, it is noteworthy that the pulmonary arteries are also involved in the so-called 'Macaroni' syndrome, a condition that primarily narrows the ascending aorta.

PATHOGENESIS

Dome-shaped pulmonary stenosis has now been shown to develop as an acquired condition during intrauterine life (Allan et al, 1994). The degree of severity seen at birth depends upon the extent of the process during gestation. Peripheral pulmonary arterial stenoses may be caused by congenital rubella, and they are seen in recognizable syndromes of malformation such as William's and Alagille's syndromes (Alagille et al, 1975). Stenosis, or even acquired atresia, of one of the main branches of the pulmonary trunk may follow the construction of a modified Blalock–Taussig shunt (Waldman et al, 1996; Godart et al, 1997). This is probably the most common cause of stenosis of a major pulmonary arterial branch.

PATHOPHYSIOLOGY

The haemodynamic consequences depend on the severity of the stenosis. When severe, the right ventricular systolic pressure may exceed that in the left ventricle. With valvar pulmonary stenosis, the elevated pressure is present right up to the undersurface of the pulmonary valvar leaflets. With infundibular or apical obstruction, high pressures are encountered proximal to the obstruction. Lower, or even normal, pressures are then found in the downstream portion of the ventricle. In contrast, with supravalvar or peripheral stenoses, the high pressure is encountered not only in the ventricle but also in the pulmonary trunk. When stenoses occur at more than one level, then more than one systolic pressure gradient will be present. Right ventricular hypertension is always present. Its severity depends on the severity of the obstruction.

Reactive right ventricular hypertrophy will occur, again depending on the severity of the obstruction. Marked right ventricular hypertrophy is associated with elevation of the end-diastolic pressure, which, in turn, leads to hypertension and hypertrophy of the right atrium. In the presence of patency of the atrial septum (either an atrial septal defect or a patent oval foramen), such right atrial hypertension can produce a right-to-left atrial shunt with consequent cyanosis. Similar haemodynamics are seen when there is underdevelopment of the right ventricle, even when the pulmonary stenosis is only moderately severe (Williams et al, 1963). Pulmonary stenosis in the neonate may be of such severity that the pulmonary circulation is adequately perfused only while the arterial duct remains patent. The cardiac effects of pulmonary stenosis are limited in the majority of patients to the right heart chambers, but exceptions do occur. Obstruction of the left ventricular outflow tract caused by septal hypertrophy is seen in severe disease.

When hypertrophic cardiomyopathy is severe, both left and right ventricular outflow tracts may be obstructed. Enlargement of the left ventricular cavity, and mild degrees of left ventricular muscular hypertrophy, are seen when an associated ventricular septal defect or persistent arterial duct produces a left-to-right shunt. Indeed, as discussed above, Harinck et al (1977) found morphological evidence of left ventricular hypertrophy in half the patients they studied. It is difficult to account for these changes on haemodynamic grounds, but they are rarely clinically manifest.

As a result of severe pulmonary stenosis (and in the presence of severe right ventricular hypertrophy), myocardial infarction may occur in the right ventricle (Franciosi and Blanc, 1968). Typically this is subendocardial, but extensive septal and free wall infarction has been observed (Dimond and Lin, 1954). The hypertrophy and increased left ventricular fibrosis observed by Harinck et al (1977), taken together with the much more extensive myocardial and arterial wall changes reported by Becu et al (1976), suggests that pulmonary stenosis is rarely an 'isolated' lesion. Instead, it may be part of a much more widespread cardiopathy. Increase in the bronchial arterial collateral circulation has been observed (Thomas, 1964). This is probably an adaptive process,

since these arteries appear to be normal in both size and number in the younger patients.

PRESENTATION AND CLINICAL FEATURES

The majority of patients are asymptomatic during childhood, regardless of the severity of the stenosis. The possibility of a cardiac malformation is usually uncovered by the discovery of a cardiac murmur. Growth is usually normal. An exception to this is pulmonary stenosis in the setting of the Ullrich–Noonan syndrome. Growth is then retarded and the children have a typical facies and build. It is also observed that many children, other than those with the Ullrich–Noonan syndrome, have a facial appearance typical of pulmonary stenosis. This 'moon face' (Wood, 1962) is neither invariable nor pathognomonic. Symptoms, when they occur, are usually associated with severe stenosis. Patients with mild to moderately severe stenosis remain asymptomatic throughout their lives. Even with severe stenosis, the onset of symptoms is usually delayed for some years, even into adult life. Cyanosis occurs when severe stenosis is associated with an atrial septal defect or, in some instances, a patent oval foramen. Cyanosis is also frequent in infants with critical stenosis. The mode of presentation in these may then be indistinguishable from pulmonary atresia with intact septum. Cyanosis may also be seen in a small proportion of older children (Campbell, 1954). Central cyanosis is not seen when there is no anatomical site for a right-to-left shunt. Peripheral cyanosis still occurs (Campbell, 1954). Other symptoms include diminished exercise tolerance and dyspnoea on exertion, particularly in those with cyanosis. Unlike tetralogy (Chapter 46), squatting is very rarely seen. Syncope may occur as a consequence of the inability to increase the cardiac output, or because of arrhythmias. Chest pain of an ischaemic nature is not infrequent in older patients, but it may occur even in young children. Dyspnoea, syncope and chest pain are all of sinister import and (together with the cyanosis) indicate the need for urgent surgery.

The most obvious physical sign in valvar and subvalvar stenosis is an ejection systolic murmur heard maximally at the left sternal edge in the second intercostal space. In all but the mildest disease, a thrill is felt at the same site. Although the murmur is the most obvious physical sign, systematic examination reveals others. Central cyanosis is rare in older children and adults. When present it is usually mild and may be seen on exertion. The jugular venous pulse is usually normal in the setting of mild or moderate stenosis. When stenosis is severe, a prominent A wave is evident (particularly in older children and adults). The cardiac impulse is of right ventricular type, associated with a tapering apex beat (Abrahams and Wood, 1951). The thrill is localized to the pulmonary area and, unlike the murmur (see below), is never propagated to the neck. The first heart sound is normal. In all but the mildest cases, the second sound is widely split. Unlike the splitting found with an atrial septal defect, there is normal respiratory variation in the setting of pulmonary stenosis. The wide splitting results from delayed closure of the pulmonary valve. This delay is probably not caused by prolonged right ventricular systole but by increased capacitance in the pulmonary vascular bed. Because of this, the pulmonary valve remains open after right ventricular pressure has fallen to levels that usually would have induced closure (Shaver et al, 1975; Zuberbuhler, 1981). The delay in pulmonary closure in these circumstances has led to a further addition to our jargon: namely, pulmonary 'hangout'. In older patients with severe stenosis, there may be a right ventricular fourth heart sound (Vogelpoel and Schrire, 1960). In valvar pulmonary stenosis, an ejection click (sometimes difficult to separate from the first heart sound) precedes the murmur in all but the severe cases. Such an ejection sound is not heard in the subvalvar or supravalvar types of stenosis.

The murmur itself is long and ejection in type. Although maximal in the second left interspace, it is sometimes heard as low as the fourth space in infundibular or apical stenosis. When stenosis is mild, the murmur may not occupy the whole of systole but peaks in mid-systole. In more severe stenosis, the murmur peaks later and occupies the whole of systole. In the severest forms, it may pass beyond the aortic component of the second heart sound. An ejection click is a further indication of the severity of the condition when the stenosis is valvar. Its timing varies with the respiratory cycle (Hultgren et al, 1969; Weyman et al, 1974). The presence of an audible click means that, during systole, atrial contraction has opened the pulmonary valve only a little way at most. Therefore, the onset of rapid ejection from ventricular systole quickly opens the valve to its fullest extent. At this point, the valve is suddenly limited in its motion at the free edge. It then 'domes', the entire valvar mechanism stops moving suddenly and, like a gybing sail, it emits a cracking sound. Atrial systole always tends to open the pulmonary valve before the onset of ventricular systole. In mild cases of pulmonary stenosis with little right ventricular hypertrophy and no detectable right atrial hypertrophy, however, right atrial pressure is never sufficient to move the pulmonary valve even close to its 'domed' position. Ventricular systole then produces sufficient motion to give the ejection click. In moderately severe stenosis, increased venous return during inspiration increases atrial systolic pressures sufficiently to open the pulmonary valve almost completely, with consequent loss of the ejection click. Hence, the click is audible only in expiration. In severe stenosis (when right atrial hypertrophy is evident), atrial systolic pressures are sufficient to open the valve almost to its 'domed' position in all phases of the respiratory cycle. An ejection click is then never heard.

Supravalvar stenosis (if limited to the pulmonary trunk) will have similar physical signs to the other forms, except that an ejection click is not heard. The second sound is frequently entirely normal (Perloff and Lebauer, 1969). The ejection systolic murmur is usually clearly heard in the axilla and in the back. Indeed, it may be loudest there. The murmur may continue to obscure even the pulmonary component of the second heart sound (Perloff and Lebauer, 1969). It is rarely continuous when the stenosis is limited to the pulmonary trunk or to the origin of the right or left main branches (D'Cruz et al, 1964). Multiple peripheral pulmonary arterial stenoses present different physical signs. In these subjects, the pulmonary component of the second heart sound is accentuated. It may be as loud as in patients with severe pulmonary vascular disease. In addition, the murmur extends further into diastole and is frequently continuous. Such a murmur is best heard over the back.

In patients with supravalvar pulmonary stenosis, the clinical features of one of the systemic diseases associated with this anomaly may be obvious. They should certainly be sought. The typical facies of William's syndrome are readily recognized. The auditory, ocular and mental stigmata of congenital rubella, or jaundice in Alagille's syndrome, may dominate the picture. When this type of pulmonary stenosis is suspected, careful examination and investigation must be made to exclude the frequently associated left-sided obstructive disease.

Tricuspid regurgitation may complicate the picture in any type of severe pulmonary stenosis. Hepatic pulsations may then be felt and, particularly in older children or adults, a prominent V wave will be seen in the jugular venous pulse. A systolic murmur may also be heard in the fourth and fifth intercostal spaces at the left sternal edge.

INVESTIGATIONS

Blood chemistry and haemotological investigations are normal in the majority of patients. Polycythaemia will be found when cyanosis has been present for some time. The serum calcium may be elevated in William's syndrome but is frequently normal, particularly in older children. The obstructive nature of the jaundice found in Alagille's syndrome will be demonstrated by appropriate laboratory investigations.

CHEST RADIOGRAPHY

In the mildest disease, the cardiac contour may be normal. The classical abnormal features are a heart of normal size, with prominence of the pulmonary knob and dilatation of the left pulmonary artery (Figure 53.10) (Gay and Franch, 1960). These features are seen with all grades of severity in valvar stenosis. Enlargement of the pulmonary knob is rarely, if ever, seen in infundibular, apical or supravalvar stenosis. In all forms, however, right ventricular

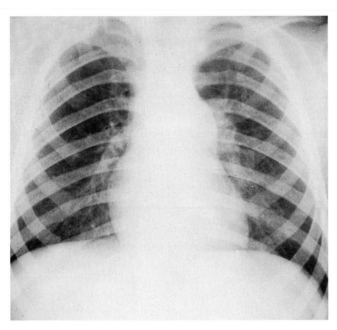

Figure 53.10. A typical frontal chest radiograph showing prominence of the pulmonary knob and dilation of the left pulmonary artery.

enlargement may be detectable on the lateral chest film. Cardiac enlargement becomes evident with the advent of tricuspid regurgitation or congestive cardiac failure. On close examination, the lung vascularity is usually found to be normal, although a superficial examination may suggest diminished markings. Pulmonary oligaemia is only present when there is a right-to-left shunt via an interatrial communication or a ventricular septal defect. There are no specific features of subvalvar or supravalvar stenosis.

ELECTROCARDIOGRAPHY

It has been known for many years that the electrocardiogram reflects the severity of the stenosis (Abrahams and Wood, 1951; Marquis, 1951; Soulié et al, 1951; Campbell and Brock, 1955; Bassingthwaighte et al, 1963). The electrocardiogram, however, provides no information concerning the site of the stenosis. There are no features that distinguish subvalvar from valvar from supravalvar stenosis.

A normal tracing is usually found in mild stenosis. Even with moderately severe obstruction, there may be discernible right atrial or ventricular hypertrophy (Levine and Blumenthal, 1965). In moderately severe stenosis, the QRS axis tends to be between +90 and +130 degrees. In the transition from mild to moderately severe stenosis, evidence of conduction delay in the right ventricle, together with an RSR pattern (Ellison and Restieaux, 1972), suggests a milder degree of stenosis than does an exclusive R wave complex in V_1 (Ellison and Miettinen, 1974). The R to S ratio in the right chest leads is frequently 4:1, but R waves rarely measure more than 20 mm, and never more than 28 mm.

Severe stenosis is never associated with a normal tracing. The P waves frequently show right atrial hypertrophy. The mean frontal QRS axis is between +110 and +150 degrees. The R:S ratio is inverted in the left as well as the right chest leads. The R waves in V_1 are in excess of 28–30 mm in two thirds of cases, while a QR complex is seen in approximately one half. The tall R waves may extend across the anterior chest leads to V_4 or V_5, and rarely to V_6. The T waves almost always are inscribed in the opposite direction to the dominant deflection in the QRS complexes. Rare abnormalities include complete right bundle branch block. In some, particularly those with Ullrich–Noonan syndrome, the QRS axis is directed superiorly.

The electrocardiogram in some individuals shows increasing right ventricular hypertrophy with increasing age. It is not clear whether this results from increasing severity of the stenosis, or from increasing hypertrophy as a time-related response to a stable degree of stenosis. A further age-related problem is the superimposition of mild-to-moderate degrees of right ventricular hypertrophy on the normally evolving electrocardiogram during infancy and early childhood. A failure of evolution to the normal left ventricular dominance may be the only electrocardiographic evidence of mild-to-moderate stenosis in the early years of life.

ECHOCARDIOGRAPHY

Both cross-sectional and M-mode techniques may appear normal in the presence of mild stenosis. If the valve is thickened and doming, these abnormal features of the leaflets should be detected on cross-sectional examination (Figure 53.11). When the valve is dysplastic, thickening and immobility of its leaflets will be seen, together with narrowing of the sinutubular junction (Musewe et al, 1987). In mild-to-moderate valvar stenosis, an accentuation of the A dip on

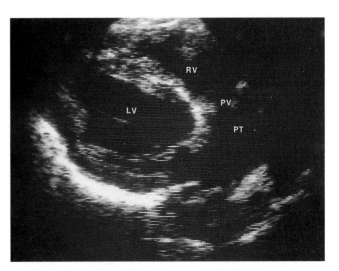

Figure 53.11. A subcostal short-axis section showing thickening of a stenotic pulmonary valve (PV). Note the post-stenotic dilation of the pulmonary trunk (PT). RV, right ventricle; LV, left ventricle.

the M-mode tracing of the pulmonary valve has been reported (Weyman et al, 1974). This is an inconsistent finding. Right ventricular hypertrophy, if severe, will be detected by both methods, as will dilation of the cavity of the right ventricle. Apical or infundibular stenosis can be seen in the subcostal views. Similarly, stenosis of the pulmonary trunk (and even stenosis of the right and left pulmonary arteries at their origin) can be demonstrated. The cross-sectional echocardiogram is accurate at identifying the site of stenosis, but is of limited value in isolation in assessing severity. Peripheral pulmonary stenoses, however, require angiocardiography or magnetic resonance imaging for their demonstration. Imaging techniques can thus provide useful information concerning the anatomy of pulmonary stenosis, but the non-invasive assessment of severity requires a different approach. Attempts have been made to predict the right ventricular pressure from the electrocardiogram, or from a combination of clinical features and the electrocardiogram (Ellison et al, 1977). Although significant correlations can be produced, there is such a wide scatter that the more elaborate methods are hardly worth the effort. It is important to recognize, nonetheless, that, if the right ventricular pressure exceeds 80 mmHg, there is never a normal electrocardiogram after the early weeks of life. An R wave in V_1 of more than 30 mm indicates a right ventricular pressure in excess of 100 mmHg. Perhaps the simplest guide has been proposed by Rudolph (1974). When there is a pure R wave in V_4R or V_1 between the ages of 2 and 20 years, the height of the R wave in millimetres multiplied by 5 gives an estimate of the right ventricular pressure. The advent of Doppler echocardiography has provided a more direct non-invasive method of assessing the severity of valvar stenosis (Chapter 13). Providing the jet of highest velocity (V_{max}) is accurately identified, the transvalvar gradient is given by the formula $V_{max}^2 \times 4$. This technique, now available in most specialized centres, and applicable to valvar stenosis, augments rather than supplants the electrocardiogram.

MAGNETIC RESONANCE IMAGING

Spin echo images can define most types of pulmonary stenosis, but it is rarely necessary to resort to magnetic resonance imaging save in the case of stenosis of the pulmonary arterial branches. Here, resonance imaging is superior to echocardiography, since the first- and second generation branches can usually be seen. When there are multiple peripheral narrowings of the branches, then angiography is necessary.

CARDIAC CATHETERIZATION

The typical finding in all variants but supravalvar stenosis is an elevation of right ventricular pressure in the presence of normal pulmonary arterial pressures. When supravalvar stenosis is present, the right ventricular and proximal pulmonary arterial pressures are elevated. A pressure drop is only encountered when the catheter is manipulated peripherally across the site of the stenosis or stenoses.

Withdrawal traces show the level of the stenosis. In supravalvar stenosis, the pulmonary arterial systolic pressure rises before the pulmonary valve is crossed. When valvar stenosis is present, an abrupt gradient is seen, with the systolic pressure rising to high levels and the diastolic pressure falling to that found in the ventricle. With subvalvar stenosis, a fall of diastolic pressure to ventricular levels is noted before the systolic pressure rises to high proximal right ventricular pressures. In valvar stenosis, a fall of pressure is seen as the catheter passes through the valvar orifice. This fall occurs in peak systole and results from the Bernouilli effect occurring in the high-velocity flow through the valvar orifice. This must not be misinterpreted as reduced ventricular diastolic pressure, which would indicate subvalvar stenosis. Pressure gradients may be encountered at more than one level. In this setting, it is difficult to assess the severity of all but the most proximal stenosis. It may be impossible when there is peripheral stenosis to manoeuvre the catheter sufficiently into the periphery to enter a zone of low pressure. Furthermore, in the newborn, it is important not to confuse the normal 5–10 mmHg systolic pressure gradient across the bifurcation of the pulmonary trunk with peripheral pulmonary stenosis.

The degree of right ventricular hypertension is the main indicator of severity. Mild stenosis exists when the systolic pressure proximal to it is below 60 mmHg. With moderate stenosis, this pressure may be up to 100 mmHg. Above this level, the stenosis is considered severe. Other haemodynamic findings in severe stenosis include elevation of right ventricular end-diastolic and right atrial A wave pressures. A high V wave in the right atrium indicates tricuspid regurgitation. A right-to-left shunt at atrial or ventricular level should be sought in all cyanosed patients. A left-to-right shunt may occasionally be encountered in the presence of an atrial or ventricular septal defect. Catheterization of the left heart is indicated in all patients with supravalvar stenosis, together with those in whom subvalvar stenosis may be a component of hypertrophic cardiomyopathy.

ANGIOCARDIOGRAPHY

Right ventricular angiography in right anterior oblique projection will demonstrate obstruction within the apical trabecular component ('two-chambered right ventricle' – Figure 53.12). The best all-purpose projection for evaluation of the pulmonary outflow tract and pulmonary arteries, nonetheless, is an anteroposterior one with 45 degree head-up tilt. When taken together with the lateral projection (Figure 53.13), a good view is obtained of all the

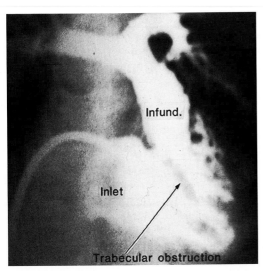

Figure 53.12. A right ventricular angiogram reveals the presence of an obstructive shelf within the apical trabecular component ('two-chambered right ventricle'). Infund, infundibulum.

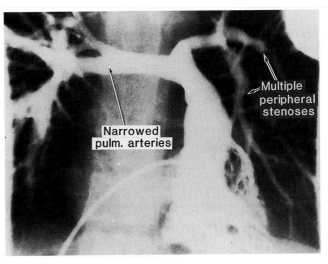

Figure 53.14. A four-chamber projection of the pulmonary arteries in a patient with William's syndrome showing hypoplasia of the bifurcation of the pulmonary trunk and multiple peripheral stenoses (pulm., pulmonary).

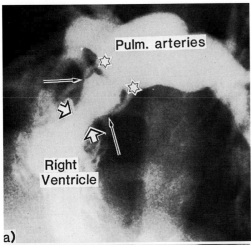

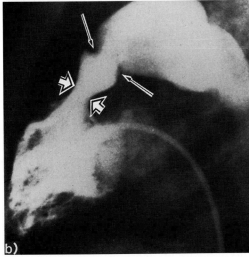

Figure 53.13. Pulmonary (pulm.) valvar stenosis is seen in the anteroposterior projection with head-up tilt (a) and lateral projection (b) following a right ventricular injection. Note the site of origin of the domed leaflets (long arrows), the narrowed orifice (stars) and the secondary infundibular narrowing (open arrows). It is the orifice that is the key point in balloon dilation (see Figure 53.16).

important structures. In this way, it is possible to distinguish 'domed' stenosis from a dysplastic valve (Jeffrey et al, 1987). It is also possible to recognize the hourglass variant with bottle-shaped sinuses (Milo et al, 1988). With regard to balloon valvoplasty, the lateral projection is the best for measurement of the diameter of the root of the pulmonary trunk. On occasion, a four-chamber axial oblique projection may be preferred in order to visualize the pulmonary arterial bifurcation. This also shows advantage to peripheral stenoses when these are present (Figure 53.14). Left-sided angiocardiograms are indicated when there is a ventricular septal defect, or when there is left-sided obstruction. The long-axis oblique projection is the most useful.

DIAGNOSIS

The differentiation of mild pulmonary stenosis from an atrial septal defect may present initial difficulty in the small child. The murmurs and the electrocardiogram are often similar. The normal respiratory variation of the second heart sound, together with an ejection click, will indicate the diagnosis of pulmonary stenosis. In cyanosed patients, the obvious differential is from tetralogy. In infancy this usually requires cross-sectional echocardiography. When squatting is present in toddlers and young children, however, it suggests tetralogy rather than isolated pulmonary stenosis.

Pulmonary stenosis associated with an atrial septal defect and a left-to-right shunt must be distinguished from an atrial septal defect with a dynamic pressure gradient across the right ventricular outflow tract. This depends on the demonstration by echocardiography, angiography (or both) of an anatomically abnormal pulmonary valve or obstruction within the right ventricular outflow tract.

Pulmonary stenosis may be mimicked by conditions associated with a murmur but in which the heart is structurally normal. Idiopathic dilation of the pulmonary trunk is, perhaps, the most difficult to exclude, since the murmur may be accompanied by a systolic click and, radiologically, the pulmonary knob is prominent. The pulmonary second sound is usually accentuated, however, and rarely does the electrocardiogram or the echocardiogram suggest right ventricular hypertrophy or an abnormal pulmonary valve. Murmurs associated with 'pectus excavatum' may suggest right ventricular hypertrophy or an abnormal pulmonary valve. The skeletal abnormality may give rise to the false impression of a prominent pulmonary knob on the frontal projection of the chest radiograph. But there is rarely any abnormality of the heart sounds, while the electrocardiogram and echocardiogram show a normal heart.

Obstruction to right ventricular outflow may be seen in generalized systemic diseases such as glycogen storage disease. Carcinoid disease is also associated with pulmonary stenosis, but this is rarely seen in children. Neurofibromas and rhabdomyomas have been incriminated, as have isolated cardiac tumours such as right ventricular myxomas (Rosenquist et al, 1970; Simcha et al, 1971). Echocardiography is of great assistance in identifying the cause of right ventricular outflow obstruction when tumours are involved. With modern investigative techniques, the diagnosis of the site, type and severity of pulmonary stenosis can be made with certainty.

COURSE AND PROGNOSIS

The morbidity and mortality of pulmonary stenosis depend, in general, on the severity of the obstruction to right ventricular outflow. Patients with mild-to-moderate stenosis, with right ventricular pressures of less than 60 mmHg, live normal lives with no symptoms. Apart from the risk of bacterial endocarditis, they do not die prematurely. Severely affected subjects, with right ventricular pressure in excess of systemic arterial pressures, are at risk of premature death. Such deaths are scattered throughout childhood and early adult life (Abbott, 1936). The highest death rate is amongst those most severely affected who present with symptoms in the first year of life (Rowe, 1978a). Those infants with congestive cardiac failure (Levine and Blumenthal, 1965) or paroxysmal dyspnoeic episodes are particularly at risk. Complicating features (such as hypoplasia of the right ventricle) must play a part in many such patients. So must the fact that many infants not only have heart failure but are also cyanosed, with all the risks that that entails. Assessment of the severity of stenosis is particularly difficult in infants and young children. This is because heart failure occurs in the first 2 years of life, with right ventricular pressures of less than 80 mmHg. These levels of right ventricular pressure are lower than those found in older children in heart failure (Nugent et al, 1977). Cyanosis also occurs in infancy with manometrically less severe stenosis than it is associated with in later life. If the right ventricular pressure is hardly elevated at all, then an alternative cause of cyanosis must be sought (for example, Ebstein's malformation).

The fact that pulmonary stenosis is not in all cases a static disease complicates the assessment of its severity. Data on changes with time are available from patients treated medically as part of the United States Natural History Study (Nugent et al, 1977). Cardiac catheterization separated by 4–8 years showed that, although the measured systolic gradient from right ventricle to pulmonary arteries remained stable in the majority, there was a significant increase in 14%, and a decrease in a further 14%. In only three patients did an initial gradient of less than 40 mmHg increase to one greater than 60 mmHg. In a further four patients, the initial gradient of 60–90 mmHg increased to over 130 mmHg. A significant number, however, showed increases in the gradient from 40–60 mmHg to over 70 mmHg. It is, therefore unlikely that a patient with mild stenosis will progress to severe stenosis. With moderate stenosis, such progression occurs in perhaps one tenth. The most dramatic increases in gradient were seen in those whose initial investigation was performed under the age of 2 years, although serious progression was seen in some patients up to 12 years of age. Unless the stenosis is manometrically mild at the first examination, therefore, predictions concerning the eventual outcome must be made with reservations in subjects under the age of 12 years. Predictions based on initial studies are likely to be extremely unreliable in those under 2 years of age.

There is little detailed information concerning the prognosis for pulmonary arterial stenosis. Deaths may occur in infancy, but many affected children certainly live into adolescence. The condition is rarely recognized in adult life, however, suggesting that deaths occur in later childhood, adolescence and early adult life.

MANAGEMENT

The initial role of the paediatric cardiologist is to assess the severity of obstruction, including careful charting of its progression. The decision must then be made as to when the gradient across the outflow tract is sufficiently severe to warrant mechanical relief. Since balloon valvoplasty (Kan et al, 1982) now provides a means of effecting this relief during cardiac catheterization, the contribution of surgery must also be carefully evaluated. As discussed above, changes in severity are not uncommon under the age of 12 years, so careful follow-up of all patients is necessary. Decisions regarding the timing of cardiac catheterization, or repeat catheterization, must be made on the results of non-invasive studies. The onset of symptoms (such as hypoxic spells and angina, signs of congestive cardiac failure or radiological evidence of cardiomegaly) means that medical management has continued for too long. Increasing right ventricular hypertrophy on the electrocardiogram or echocardiogram suggests that a particular patient has entered the severe category, and that relief should not be delayed. Regular monitoring of the velocity of blood flow across the stenosis using Doppler techniques is mandatory. This is best ascertained by continuous wave techniques (Chapter 13), the location of the maximum velocity of the jet through the stenotic valve having been ascertained by colour flow mapping. The electrocardiogram should also be monitored regularly (if less frequently).

Medical treatment is indicated as a temporary measure in those in congestive cardiac failure. Similarly, E-type prostaglandins will improve the condition of those neonates who present with cyanosis and associated patency of the arterial duct. Their use is indicated as part of resuscitation and preparation for catheterization and/or surgery. It is not necessary to have a precise anatomical diagnosis to start such therapy. We recommend that they be given in the referring hospital to any cyanosed newborn in whom congenital heart disease is suspected. The only indication for indefinite medical management is inoperability. This is confined to supravalvar stenosis with multiple peripheral stenoses. Only supportive measures can be offered with confidence in these patients, although the role of balloon angioplasty is now being explored.

Infective endocarditis is a rare complication of pulmonary stenosis (Gersony and Hayes, 1977), but all paediatric cardiologists have encountered cases even after surgical relief. Routine prophylaxis is, therefore, indicated throughout life in all patients, irrespective of the site or severity of stenosis.

BALLOON VALVOPLASTY

The use of balloon valvoplasty is a direct progression from the use of balloons to dilate obstructive lesions in peripheral and coronary arteries. Its role in valvar pulmonary stenosis was pioneered by Kan and her colleagues (1982) at the Johns Hopkins Hospital, Baltimore, and for peripheral stenoses by Lock et al (1983) in Minneapolis.

The technique for valvoplasty consists of introducing an angioplasty catheter over a guidewire into the pulmonary valvar orifice (Figure 53.15). The balloon is rapidly inflated (Figure 53.16) and deflated under radiological control. This cycle is best performed three times, although it is the first inflation that appears to achieve the result. Inflation is performed to the maximum recommended pressure of the chosen balloon. Since all currently available balloons have a taper at each end, the balloon should be placed so that its midpoint occupies the valvar orifice (this point having been determined on

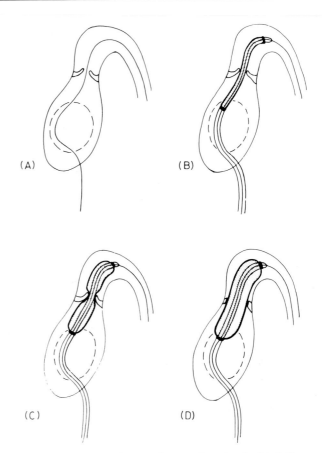

Figure 53.15. Diagram showing the procedures involved in balloon valvoplasty. (Reproduced by kind permission of Dr D. A. Girod, University of Indiana, Indianapolis, USA.)

a previous angiogram; see Figure 53.13). It is also on the basis of this angiogram that the size of the balloon is selected. This should be equal to, or 10–20% greater than, the diameter of the pulmonary trunk at the origin of the proximal hingepoints of the valvar leaflets (see Figure 53.13). Following dilation, the balloon catheter is exchanged over the guidewire for a Goodale–Lubin catheter. The guidewire is then removed, and a postprocedural withdrawal pressure tracing is performed. It is considered best practice not to attempt to cross again an angioplastied segment once the guidewire is removed. This is occasionally unavoidable when dilation has not produced an acceptable result.

In adults, where the root of the pulmonary trunk is large, it is occasionally necessary to perform the dilation with two balloons simultaneously. The combined diameter of the balloons should be approximately 20% larger than that of the optimal balloon, if it were available.

Arterial pressure is monitored throughout the procedure, as is the electrocardiogram.

Adverse haemodynamic and arrhythmic events have, in our experience and that of others, usually proved to be transient (Rocchini et al, 1984; Tynan et al, 1985). In order to minimize any adverse effects, we administer atropine and oxygen prior to the procedure, which is performed with an effectively anaesthetized patient (using

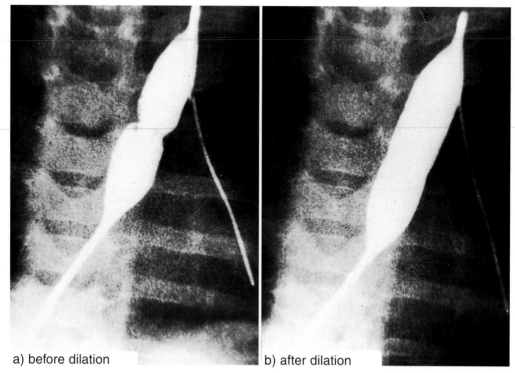

a) before dilation   b) after dilation

Figure 53.16. Balloon valvoplasty (a) The balloons in position having been placed across a stenotic pulmonary valve (note minimal indentation at site of ruptured valve). (b) Full inflation of the balloon removes the indentation.

ketamine for this purpose). Although serious complications of balloon pulmonary valvoplasty are rare, it is recommended that the procedure only be performed by experienced staff working in a well-equipped centre for paediatric cardiology. Backup of a surgical team is essential. This team should be as enthusiastic for the procedure as the physicians who performed it.

Short- and intermediate-term results have shown that balloon valvoplasty is the initial treatment of choice for isolated valvar pulmonary stenosis (Kan et al, 1982; Lababidi and Wu, 1983; Rocchini et al, 1984; Tynan et al, 1985; O'Connor et al 1992; Witsenburg, 1993). It has not been our practice to perform the procedure in those patients who have associated lesions that would require subsequent surgical treatment. An exception is the neonate with pulmonary stenosis and a right-to-left atrial shunt. Here, we would perform a balloon valvoplasty as the initial treatment. Deaths following valvoplasty are rare. A report from the United Kingdom (Hubner et al, 1992) detailed 3 deaths in 258 patients undergoing the procedure during 1990. Mortality after valvoplasty is concentrated in those needing the procedure during the first months of life. In patients older than this, complications are also infrequent and usually transient (First report of VACA registry: Stanger et al, 1990). Occasionally, following a technically adequate valvoplasty, a pressure gradient may be observed at subvalvar level, and this in the absence of structural subvalvar stenosis. This 'infundibular reaction' resolves with time, but some have given beta blockers with apparent good effect. It appears to us that this 'reaction' is less frequent when ketamine is used for anaesthesia. Today,

success rates in achieving valvoplasty are high, and relief of the obstruction is the rule (Witsenburg, 1993). Reasons for failure may be technical, namely the use of too small a balloon, or they may be anatomical, usually because of either severe dysplasia of the valve or a small pulmonary root (McCrindle, 1994). Despite the possibility of failure in the presence of a dysplastic valve, we would still perform the procedure because the degree of dysplasia that negates success has not been systematized. Children over a month or two of age undergoing the procedure are discharged from hospital routinely as they would be for any other catheterization (in our units, the next day). On follow-up so far, there has been no evidence of significant pulmonary regurgitation.

The haemodynamic indications for balloon valvoplasty are as unclear as those for surgical intervention (see below). Inevitably, the ease and safety of the procedure have led to its use in patients with only mild stenosis. In these patients, it is difficult to assess efficacy. We, therefore, only perform the procedure when the right ventricular pressure exceeds 55–60 mmHg.

Balloon pulmonary valvoplasty in the newborn infant presents particular challenges. These infants are frequently ill, often cyanosed and frequently receiving prostaglandins to maintain patency of the arterial duct. In contrast to older children, there is a 5.6% chance of not being able to achieve the dilation (Colli et al, 1995; Tabatabaei et al, 1996). The use of guidewires designed primarily for coronary arteries, and the introduction of low profile balloons, means that this problem is less frequently encountered now. The procedure is greatly facilitated if the guidewire can be manipulated from the pulmonary trunk through the arterial duct into the descending aorta. The balloon can then be manoeuvred into the valve on the stiff part of the wire. In addition to the procedure being technically more demanding in this age group, complications are more frequent, including right ventricular perforation and femoral venous tears. The outcome may be adversely influenced by the small size of the right ventricle and pulmonary root (Fedderly et al, 1995), but there is some evidence of increase in size of these structures following successful valvoplasty (Tabatabaei et al, 1996). Despite all these problems, survival after balloon pulmonary valvoplasty in the newborn is now in excess of 80%, with rates for reintervention in the region of 20%. These results compare well with those of surgery in the newborn (Hanley et al, 1993).

SURGICAL MANAGEMENT

Balloon valvoplasty (Figure 53.17) has now superseded surgery as the initial treatment of pulmonary valvar stenosis. Nowadays, the only indication for operation is failure of a technically adequate balloon dilation. Most frequently, this occurs because of dysplasia of the valvar leaflets, and relief of this stenosis requires either a transjunctional patch or 'debulking' of the valve. There are, however, still many survivors of surgery, so knowledge of this approach is of more than historical importance. There

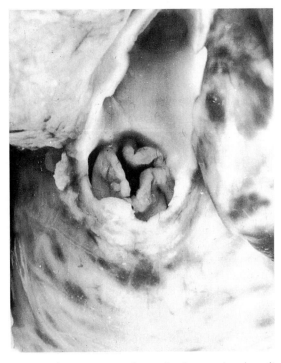

Figure 53.17. The appearance of a previously stenotic valve relieved by balloon angioplasty. The stenotic leaflets have been split cleanly along the commissures and the valve does not appear to be regurgitant. The patient died from a cause unrelated to the valvoplasty (multiple hepatic arteriovenous fistulas).

was no unanimity concerning the level of right ventricular systolic pressure at which surgery was indicated. The preoperative pressure gradients in the patients treated surgically in the United States Natural History Study (Nugent et al, 1977) ranged from less than 25 mmHg (albeit in only 1% of those undergoing surgery) to greater than 80 mmHg. Of the 304 patients undergoing surgery, 28% had systolic pressure gradients of 50–70 mmHg. The pressure gradients in this last group represent right ventricular pressures in the range 70–110 mmHg. There is little doubt that all centres would recommend surgery when the resting right ventricular pressure is greater than 100 mmHg. A pressure of 75 mmHg would be the cut-off point for many. Few would operate if the right ventricular pressure was less than 60 mmHg.

The surgical techniques included closed pulmonary valvotomy (Brock, 1948). This is rarely indicated save in the critically ill neonate. Good results have been obtained, nonetheless, even in this group of patients (Milo et al, 1980). Good results have also been reported in this age group when a transarterial approach has been used together with inflow occlusion at normothermia (Litwin et al, 1973). The limitations of this approach include the inability to correct associated defects, the difficulty of dealing with dysplastic valves (especially those with small valvar dimensions), the limited time it provides for the surgical procedure and the limited exposure for resection of any associated subvalvar stenosis. It is probable that these techniques were in many cases only palliative (Nugent et al, 1977), since subsequent revision was often necessary.

Open pulmonary valvotomy on cardiopulmonary bypass is now the surgical method of choice in the majority of patients in the majority of centres. Using this approach, the 'domed' valve can be incised and mobilized and redundant leaflet tissue excised. Subvalvar stenosis can also be dealt with when present. Patency of the atrial septum (be it a true atrial septal defect or an oval foramen) should be closed if present. Dysplastic valves may require excision (Watkins et al, 1977). If associated with a narrow ventriculo-arterial junction, they may be dealt with by insertion of a transvalvar patch (Vancini et al, 1980).

A rare form of subvalvar stenosis occurs when redundant tissue from the tricuspid valve obstructs both a ventricular septal defect and the pulmonary outflow tract. This can be readily removed using cardiopulmonary bypass.

Results of surgery for pulmonary valvar stenosis are extremely good. Postoperative deaths are almost entirely limited to emergency operations in infants (Nugent et al, 1977; Hanley et al, 1993). Mortality rates below 3% have long been achieved (Tandon et al, 1965). Similar results should be attained in the subvalvar variant of stenosis.

PROGRESS AFTER VALVOPLASTY OR SURGERY

The United States Natural History Study (Nugent et al, 1977) provides the most comprehensive long-term follow-up of patients who have undergone surgery. In this cohort of 234 patients catheterized before and after surgery, 81% had postoperative pressure gradients of 25 mmHg or less. Only 4% had gradients of greater than 50 mmHg. Of these 10 patients, six were under 2 years of age at surgery and only one had undergone surgery using cardiopulmonary bypass. Therefore, these surgical failures can, in part, be attributed to the age at surgery and, in part, to the surgical technique. Prior to surgery, 69% of the overall group were judged to be in poor condition. On long-term follow-up, only 3% were still considered 'poor', while 61% were judged to be 'excellent'. When analysed by ages at operation, those under 2 years of age appeared to fare less well than the older children. Only 37% of the younger children were deemed 'excellent' at follow-up. Since 92% were graded poor prior to surgery, these less favourable results are a reflection of the more severe disease encountered in the youngest patients. They are not a rational reason for delay in treatment, be it by surgery or balloon valvoplasty. Including all the categories of pre- and postoperative condition ('excellent', 'good', 'fair' and 'poor'), nearly nine tenths of the patients had improved as a consequence of surgery. Therefore, surgery has, in the past, provided good results in valvar pulmonary stenosis. Similarly, surgical relief of subvalvar stenosis provides excellent results.

The data accumulated during the 1990s indicate that balloon valvoplasty, when performed properly, provides long-term relief to valvar pulmonary stenosis. In children over 1 month of age, there is little evidence of increase in severity with the passage of time. When the immediate pressure gradient is low after the procedure, later follow-up rarely shows a clinically significant increase (Witsenburg et al, 1993; McCrindle, 1994). There is some evidence to suggest that pulmonary regurgitation is less severe after balloon dilation than after surgery (O'Connor et al, 1992). Therefore, balloon valvoplasty appears to impart at least as good a long-term haemodynamic state as does surgery. Even in the most problematic group, the newborns, the results in terms of survival and the need for reintervention are comparable between the two approaches (Hanley et al, 1993; Tabatabaei et al, 1996).

TREATMENT OF STENOSIS OF THE PULMONARY ARTERY AND ITS BRANCHES

The treatment of stenosis of the pulmonary arterial branches is dependent on the sites and number of the stenoses. Localized proximal narrowing of the pulmonary trunk and its bifurcation can be relieved by surgical patch arterioplasty (McGoon and Kincaid, 1964). This is rarely undertaken as a procedure in its own right but is usually part of a more extensive operation, such as the repair of the tetralogy. Patch arterioplasty gives good initial relief, but recurrence of the stenosis is not uncommon. Long tubular narrowing, or discrete stenosis of more peripheral generations of the pulmonary arteries, are not accessible to surgical relief. Treatment of recurrent or isolated stenoses of the major pulmonary arterial branches, along with more peripheral stenoses, is now the province of the interventionist. Historically, balloon angioplasty was the first treatment undertaken, and good immediate results were reported in about half the patients (Hosking et al, 1992; Worms et al, 1992). Long-term results, in contrast, were disappointing (Hosking et al, 1992), so the technique was modified by the use of high-pressure balloons (Gentles et al, 1993). Again, early results were encouraging, but recurrence has proved to be frequent. Overall, good prolonged relief was obtained in less than one third when balloon angioplasty was used. The procedure itself is not devoid of risk, rupture of the pulmonary artery being the most obvious, since the balloon must be inflated to several times the diameter of the stenosed segment. One reason for immediate failure to dilate the artery is the fibroelastic nature of many primary stenoses; consequently despite prolonged inflation of the balloon, deflation results in elastic recoil of the vessel to its original calibre. Failure can also occur because it is impossible to dilate the artery with a balloon alone. This circumstance may be encountered with stenoses occurring subsequent to surgery, such as those following construction of systemic-to-pulmonary arterial shunts. Reasons for initial success but late restenosis are not apparent. The relatively poor success rate, and unpredictability, of balloon dilation, together with the risk of complications, have led many to abandon this technique in favour of implantation of stents. There are a multitude of stents available, but most experience in the treatment of stenosis of the pulmonary artery has been with the Palmaz–Schatz stent. This is a steel stent that is mounted on an angioplasty balloon, usually of the high-pressure type, and expanded to the desired diameter by inflation of the balloon. The advantages of the use of stents are that overdilation of the artery is not necessary. Also, there is no elastic recoil of the stent. Furthermore, since the stent can be redilated with growth of the patient, there is no need to overexpand at the time of implantation (Ing et al, 1995). Initial, and subsequent, results have shown good immediate and intermediate term relief (O'Laughlin et al, 1993; Ing et al, 1995). There is a tendence to build up 'neo-intima' within the stent, resulting in some decrease in lumen over time, but this can be relieved by redilation of the stent. Because of this build up of neo-intima, the long-term fate of stented arteries is uncertain.

At the present time, this approach offers the best treatment of stenosis of the pulmonary arterial branches. Stenosis of the first- and second-generation branches can certainly be successfully treated by implantation of stents, but, as yet, the possibilities for dealing with more peripheral branches are still developing.

The indications for treating stenosis of the pulmonary arterial branches include elevation of the proximal pulmonary arterial pressure. This is usually seen when both pulmonary arteries are affected. The exact level of pressure has not been systematized. It depends to some extent on the lesion. Most workers would not implant stents if the proximal pressure was below 60 mmHg but, in the case of the Alagille syndrome, some surgeons will not perform a liver transplant if the right ventricular pressure is above 40 mmHg. When the stenosis or stenoses are unilateral, then a gross asymmetry of lung perfusion is an indication. The lesions must be accessible to implantation. This is rarely the case when multiple stenosis are present, as in Williams syndrome.

REFERENCES

Abbott M E 1936 Atlas of congenital heart disease. The American Heart Association, New York

Abrahams D G, Wood P 1951 Pulmonary stenosis with normal aortic root. British Heart Journal 13: 519–548

Alagille D, Odievre M, Gautier M, Dommergues J P 1975 Hepatic ductular hypoplasia associated with characteristic facies, vertebral malformations, retarded physical, mental and sexual development, and cardiac murmur. Journal of Pediatrics 86: 63–71

Allan L D, Sharland G, Cook A 1994 Color atlas of fetal cardiology. Times-Mirror, London, p 100

Alva C, Ho S Y, Lincoln C R, Wright A, Anderson R H 1999 The nature of the obstructive muscular bundles in double chambered right ventricle. Journal of Thoracic and Cardiovascular Surgery 117: 1180–1189

Bassingthwaighte J B, Parkin T W, DuShane J W, Wood E H, Burchell H B 1963 The electrocardiographic and hemodynamic findings in pulmonary stenosis with intact ventricular septum. Circulation 28: 893–905

Becker A E 1972 Quadricuspid pulmonary valve. Anatomical observations in 20 hearts. Acta Morphologica Neerlando-Scandinavica 10: 299–309

Becu L, Somerville J, Gallo A 1976 Isolated pulmonary valve stenosis as part of more widespread cardiovascular disease. British Heart Journal 38: 472–482

Beuren A J, Schultze C, Eberle P, Harmjanz D, Apitz J 1964 The syndrome of supravalvular aortic stenosis, peripheral pulmonary stenosis, mental retardation and similar facial appearance. American Journal of Cardiology 13: 471–483

Bonvicini M, Piovaccari G, Picchio F M 1982 Severe subpulmonary obstruction caused by an aneurysmal tissue tag complicating an infundibular perimembranous ventricular septal defect. British Heart Journal 48: 189–191

Brock RC 1948 Pulmonary valvulotomy for the relief of congenital pulmonary stenosis. British Medical Journal i: 1121–1126

Brock R 1961 The surgical treatment of pulmonary stenosis. British Heart Journal 23: 337–356

Campbell M 1954 Simple pulmonary stenosis. Pulmonary stenosis with closed ventricular septum. British Heart Journal 16: 273–300

Campbell M 1962 Factors in the aetiology of pulmonary stenosis. British Heart Journal 24: 625–632

Campbell M, Brock R C 1955 The results of valvotomy forsimple pulmonary stenosis. British Heart Journal 17: 229–246

Campbell P E 1965 Vascular abnormalities following maternal rubella. British Heart Journal 27: 134–138

Colli A M, Perry S B, Lock J E, Keene J F 1995 Dilation of critical pulmonary stenosis in the first month of life. Catheterization and Cardiovascular Diagnosis 34: 23–28

D'Cruz I A, Arcilla R A, Agustsson M H 1964 Dilatation of the pulmonary trunk in stenosis of the pulmonary valve and of the pulmonary arteries in children. American Heart Journal 68: 612–620

Dimond E G, Lin T K 1954 The clinical picture of pulmonary stenosis (without ventricular septal defect). Annals of Internal Medicine 40: 1108–1124

Edwards J E, Burchell H B 1957 The pathological anatomy of deficiencies between the aortic root and the heart, including aortic root sinus aneurysms. Thorax 12: 128–139

Ellison R C, Miettinen O S 1974 Interpretation of RSR in pulmonic stenosis. American Heart Journal 88: 7–10

Ellison R C, Restieaux N J 1972 Vectorcardiogram in congenital heart disease. A method for estimating severity. Saunders, Philadelphia

Ellison R C, Freedom R M, Keane J F, Nugent E W, Rowe R D, Miettinen O S 1977 Indirect assessment of severity in pulmonary stenosis. Circulation 56(suppl I): 114–119

Emmanouilides G C, Linde L M, Crittenden I H 1964 Pulmonary artery stenosis associated with ductus arteriosus following maternal rubella. Circulation 29: 514–522

Fabricius J 1959 Isolated pulmonary stenosis. Munksgaard, Copenhagen

Fallot A 1888 Contribution a l'anatomie pathologique de la maladie bleue (cyanose cardiague). Marseille Medicine 25: 77–403

Finlay D W 1879 Malformation of the heart: stenosis of the pulmonary valve, with dilatation of the pulmonary artery and hypertrophy of the right ventricle: patency of the foremen ovale, with a cribriform opening in the septum of the auricies (ductus arteriosus closed). Transactions of the Pathological Society of London 30: 262–265

Fournier A, Paget M, Pauli A, Devin P 1963 Syndromes nephrotiques familiaux. Syndrome nephrotique associe a une cardiopathie congenitale chez quatre soeurs. Pediatrie 18: 677–685

Franch R H, Gay B B Jr 1963 Congenital stenosis of the pulmonary artery branches. A classification, with postmortem findings in two cases. American Journal of Medicine 35: 512–529

Franciosi R A, Blanc W A 1968 Myocardial infarcts in infants and children. 1. A necropsy study in congenital heart disease. Journal of Pediatrics 73: 309–319

Freed M D, Rosenthal A, Bernhard W F, Litwin S B, Nadas A S 1973 Critical pulmonary stenosis with a diminutive right ventricle in neonates. Circulation 48: 875–881

Gabriele O F, Scatliff J H 1970 Pulmonary valve calcification. American Heart Journal 80: 299–302

Gamble W J, Nadas A S 1965 Severe pulmonic stenosis with intact ventricular septum and right aortic arch. Circulation 32: 114–119

Gay B B Jr, Franch R H 1960 Pulsation in the pulmonary arteries as observed with roentgenoscopic image amplification. Observation in patients with isolated pulmonary valvular stenosis. American Journal of Roentgenology 83: 335–344

Gay B B, Franch R H, Shuford W H, Rogers J V 1963 Roentgenologic features of simple and multiple coarctations of the pulmonary artery and branches. American Journal of Roentgenology 90: 599–613

Gersony W M, Hayes C J 1977 Bacterial endocarditis in patients with pulmonary stenosis, aortic stenosis or ventricular septal defect. Circulation 56(suppl I): 1184–1187

Godart F, Qureshi S A, Simcha A et al 1997 Patency of and development of stenoses in modified Blalock–Taussig shunts constructed using expanded polyterafluoroethylene. Cardiology in the Young 9: 153–159

Hanley F L, Sade R M, Freedom R M and the Congenital Heart Surgeons Society 1993 Outcomes in critically ill neonates with pulmonary stenosis and intact ventricular septum: a multiinstitutional study. Journal of the American College of Cardiology 22: 183–192

Harinck E, Becker A E, Gittenberger-de-Groot A C, Oppenheimer-Dekker A, Versprille A 1977 The left ventricle in congenital isolated pulmonary valve stenosis. A morphological study. British Heart Journal 39: 429–435

Hosking M C, Thomaidis C, Hamilton R, Burrows P E, Freedom R M, Benson L N 1992 Clinical impact of balloon angioplasty for branch pulmonary arterial stenosis. American Journal of Cardiology 69: 1467–1470

Hubner P J B on behalf of the British Cardiovascular Intervention Society 1992 Cardiac interventional procedure in the United Kingdom during 1990. British Heart Journal 68: 434–436

Hultgren H N, Reeve R, Cohn K, McLeod R 1969 The ejection click of valvular pulmonic stenosis. Circulation 40: 631–640

Jeffrey R F, Moller J H, Amplatz K 1972 The dysplastic pulmonary valve: a new roentgenographic entity. With the discussion of the anatomy and radiology of other types of valvular pulmonary stenosis. American Journal of Roentgenology, Radium Therapy and Nuclear Medicine 114: 322–329

Ing F F, Grifka R G, Nihill M R, Mullins C E 1995 Repeat dilation of intravascular stents in congenital heart defects. Circulation 92: 893–897

Jones R N, Niles N R 1968 Spinnaker formation of the sinus venosus valve. Circulation 38: 468–473

Jue K L, Noren G R, Anderson R C 1965 The syndrome of idiopathic hypercalcemia of infancy with associated congenital heart disease. Journal of Pediatrics 67: 1130–1140

Kan J S, White R I Jr, Mitchell S E, Gardner T J 1982 Percutaneous balloon valvuloplasty: a new method for treating congenital pulmonary-valve stenosis. New England Journal of Medicine 307: 540–542

Klinge T, Baekgaard Laursen H 1975 Familial pulmonary stenosis with underdeveloped or normal right ventricle. British Heart Journal 37: 60–64

Koretzky E D, Moller J H, Korns M E, Schwartz C J, Edwards J E 1969 Congenital pulmonary stenosis resulting from dysplasia of valve. Circulation 40: 43–53

Koroxenedis G T, Webb N C, Moschos C B, Lehan P H 1966 Congenital heart disease, deaf mutation and associated somatic malformations occurring in several members of one family. American Journal of Medicine 40: 149–153

Lababidi Z, Wu J R 1983 Percutaneous balloon pulmonary valvuloplasty. American Journal of Cardiology 52: 560–562

Lamy M, De Grouchy J, Schweisguth O 1957 Genetic and non-genetic factors in the aetiology of congenital heart disease: a study of 1188 cases. American Journal of Human Genetics 9: 17–41

Levine O R, Blumenthal S 1965 Pulmonic stenosis. Circulation 32(suppl III): 33–41

Linde L M, Turner S W, Sparkes R S 1973 Pulmonary valvular dysplasia. A cardiofacial syndrome. British Heart Journal 35: 301–304

Litwin S B, Williams W H, Freed M D, Bernhard W F 1973 Critical pulmonary stenosis in infants: a surgical emergency. Surgery 74: 880–886

Lock J E, Castaneda-Zuniga W R, Fuhrman B P, Bass J L 1983 Balloon dilation angioplasty of hypoplastic and stenotic pulmonary arteries. Circulation 67: 962–967

Marquis R M 1951 Unipolar electrocardiography in pulmonary stenosis. British Heart Journal 12: 265–276

McCrindle B W for the VACA Registry Investigators 1994 Independent predictors of long-term results after balloon pulmonary valvoplasty. Circulation 89: 1751–1759

McCue C M, Robertson L W, Lester P G, Mauck HP Jr 1965 Pulmonary artery coarctations: a report of 20 cases with review of 319 cases from the literature. Journal of Pediatrics 67: 222–238

McGoon D C, Kincaid O W 1964 Stenosis of branches of the pulmonary artery: surgical repair. Medical Clinics of North America 48: 1083–1088

McKeown T, MacMahon B, Parsons C G 1953 The familial incidence of congenital malformation of the heart. British Heart Journal 15: 273–277

Milo S, Yellin A, Smolinsky A, Blieden L C, Neufeld H N, Goor DA 1980 Closed pulmonary valvotomy in infants under six months of age: report of 14 consecutive cases without mortality. Thorax 35: 814–818

Milo S, Fiegl A, Shem-Tov A, Neufeld H N, Goor D A 1988 Hour-glass deformity of the pulmonary valve: a third type of pulmonary valve stenosis. British Heart Journal 60: 128–133

Noonan J A, Ehmke D A 1963 Associated noncardiac malformations in children with congenital heart disease. Journal of Pediatrics 63: 468–470

Nora J J, Spangler R D 1972 Risks and counseling in cardiovascular malformations. Birth Defects Original Article Series 8: 154–159

Nugent E W, Freedom R M, Nora J J, Ellison R C, Rowe R D, Nadas AS 1977 Clinical course in pulmonary stenosis. Circulation 56(suppl I): 38–47

O'Connor B K, Beekman R H, Lindauer A, Rocchini A 1992 Intermediate term outcome after pulmonary balloon valvoplasty: comparison with a matched surgical control group. Journal of the American College of Cardiology 20: 169–173

O'Laughlin M P, Slack M C, Grifka R G, Perry S B, Lock J E, Mullins C E 1993 Paediatric cardiovascular medicine: implantation and intermediate-term follow-up of stents in congenital heart disease. Circulation 88: 605–614

Perloff J K, Lebauer E J 1969 Auscultatory and phonocardiographic manifestations of isolated stenosis of the pulmonary artery and its branches. British Heart Journal 31: 314–321

Restivo A, Cameron A H, Anderson R H, Allwork S P 1984 Divided right ventricle: a review of its anatomical varieties. Pediatric Cardiology 5: 197–204

Roberts N, Moes C A F 1973 Supravalular pulmonary stenosis. Journal of Pediatrics 82: 838–844

Rocchini A P, Kveselis D A, Crowley D, Dick M, Rosenthal A 1984 Percutaneous balloon valvuloplasty for treatment of congenital pulmonary valvular stenosis in children. Journal of the American College of Cardiology 3: 1005–1012

Rodriguez-Fernandez H L, Char F, Kelly D T, Rowe R D 1972 The dysplastic pulmonic valve and the Noonan syndrome. Circulation 46(suppl II): 98

Rose V, Hewitt D, Milner J 1972 Seasonal influences on the risk of cardiac malformations. Nature of the problem and some results from a study of 10 007 cases. International Journal of Epidemiology 1: 235–244

Rosenquist G C, Krovetz L J, Haller J A Jr, Simon A L, Bannayan G A 1970 Acquired right ventricular outflow obstruction in a child with neurofibromatosis. American Heart Journal 79: 103–108

Rowe R D 1963 Maternal rubella and pulmonary artery stenoses. Report of eleven cases. Pediatrics 32: 180–185

Rowe R D 1972 Stenosis of conducting arteries in infants and children. Birth Defects Original Article Series 8: 69–73

Rowe R D 1978a Pulmonary stenosis with normal aortic root. In: Keith J D, Rowe R D, Vlad P (eds) Heart disease in infancy and childhood, 3rd edn. Macmillan, New York, p 761–788

Rowe R D 1978b Pulmonary arterial stenosis. In: Keith J D, Rowe R D, Vlad P (eds) Heart disease in infancy and childhood, 3rd edn. Macmillan, New York, p 789–801

Rudolph A M 1974 Congenital diseases of the heart. Year Book Medical, Chicago

Selzer A, Carnes W H, Noble C A, Higgins W H, Holmes R C 1949 Syndrome of pulmonary stenosis with patent foremen ovale. American Journal of Medicine 6: 3–23

Shaver J A, O'Toole J D, Curtiss E I, Thompson M E, Reddy P S, Leon D F 1975 Second heart sound: the role of altered greater and lesser circulation. Physiologic principles of heart sounds and murmurs. American Heart Association Monograph No 46. American Heart Association, New York, p 58–73

Simcha A, Wells B G, Tynan M J, Waterston D J 1971 Primary cardiac tumours in infancy and childhood. Archives of Diseases in Childhood 46: 508–514

Smith W G 1958 Pulmonary hypertension and a continuous murmur due to multiple peripheral stenoses of the pulmonary arteries. Thorax 13: 194–200

Stanger P, Cassidy S C, Girod D A, Kan J S, Lababidi Z, Shapiro S R. 1990 Balloon pulmonary valvuloplasty: results of the Valvuloplasty and Angioplasty of Congenital Anomalies Registry. American Journal of Cardiology 65: 775–783

Souliè P, Joly F, Carlotti J, Sicot J-R 1951 Etude comparde de l'himodynamique dans les tetralogies et dans les trilogies de Fallot. Archives des Maladies du Coeur et des Vaisseaux 44: 577–601

Tabatabai H, Boutin C, Nykanan D G, Freedom R M, Benson L N 1996 Morphologic and haemodynamic consequences after percutaneous balloon valvotomy for neonatal pulmonary stenosis: medium-term follow-up. Journal of the American College of Cardiology 27: 473–478

Tandon R, Nadas A S, Gross R E 1965 Results of open heart surgery in patients with pulmonic stenosis and intact ventricular septum. Circulation 31: 190–201

Thomas M A 1964 Pulmonary vascular changes in pulmonary stenosis with and without ventricular septal defect. British Heart Journal 26: 655–661

Tynan M, Baker E J, Rohmer J et al 1985 Percutaneous balloon pulmonary valvuloplasty. British Heart Journal 53: 520–524

Vancini M, Roberts K D, Silove E D, Singh S P 1980 Surgical treatment of congenital pulmonary stenosis due to dysplastic leaflets and small valve annulus. Journal of Thoracic and Cardiovascular Surgery 79: 464–468

Vogelpoel L, Schrire V 1960 Auscultatory and phonocardiographic assessment of pulmonary stenosis with intact ventricular septum. Circulation 22: 55–72

Waldman J D, Karp R B, Gittenberger-de Groot A C, Agarwala B, Glagov S 1996 Spontaneous acquisition of discontinuous pulmonary arteries. Annals of Thoracic Surgery 62: 161–168

Watkins L J, Donahoo J S, Harrington D, Haller J A Jr, Neill C A 1977 Surgical management of congenital pulmonary valve dysplasia. Annals of Thoracic Surgery 24: 498–506

Weyman A E, Dillon JC, Feigenbaum H, Chang S 1974 Echocardiographic patterns of pulmonary valve motion in valvular pulmonary stenosis. American Journal of Cardiology 34: 644–651

Williams J C P, Barratt-Boyes B G, Lowe J B 1963 Underdeveloped right ventricle and pulmonary stenosis. American Journal of Cardiology 11: 458–468

Witsenburg M, Talsma M, Rohmer J, Hess J 1993 Balloon valvoplasty for valvular pulmonary stenosis in children over 6 months of age: initial results and long-term follow-up. European Heart Journal 14: 1657–1660

Wood P 1962 Diseases of the heart and circulation, 2nd edn. Eyre & Spottiswood, London, p 441

Worms A M, Marcon F, Chehab G, Michalski H 1992 Angioplastic percutanée de stenoses de branch arterielles pulmonaires. Etude cooperative. Archives des Maladies du Coeur er des Vaisseaux 85: 527–531

Zaret B L, Conti R C 1973 Infundibular pulmonic stenosis with intact ventricular septum in the adult. Johns Hopkins Medical Journal 132: 50–60

Zuberbuhler J R 1981 Clinical diagnosis in pediatric cardiology. Churchill Livingstone, Edinburgh, p 64–70

54

Congenital anomalies of the aortic valve and left ventricular outflow tract

S. Hunter

INTRODUCTION

Obstruction to the left ventricular outflow of the heart may be above the aortic valve, at the valve or in the subvalvar region. Valvar or subvalvar stenosis may be associated with other congenital defects such as pulmonary valvar stenosis, an arterial duct, anomalies of the mitral valve and, less commonly, defects of the interatrial septum. Shone's syndrome (Shone et al, 1963) is an example of diffuse left heart abnormality with subvalvar aortic stenosis, a parachute mitral valve and sometimes coarctation of the aorta.

Congenital aortic stenosis accounts for 5% of all cardiac abnormalities (Jordan and Scott, 1973). If all bicuspid aortic valves are included, then this may be the most common congenital abnormality (Roberts, 1970a,b). It is difficult to know the true incidence, however, as congenitally abnormal aortic valves may not be recognized in childhood.

Within the whole group, 75% have valvar stenosis, 23% discrete subaortic stenosis, and 1–2% supravalvar obstruction. The three forms may occur separately or together, and each may be associated with aortic regurgitation. Dominant aortic regurgitation irrespective of cause is discussed later in the chapter.

Hypertrophic obstructive cardiomyopathy must be differentiated from 'fixed' subvalvar stenosis. Left ventricular hypertrophy is associated with all three lesions and is usually concentric, although asymmetric septal hypertrophy can be found in association with all forms of 'fixed' obstruction from discrete subvalvar ledges to coarctation of the aorta. This septal anomaly may physiologically and morphologically mimic hypertrophic obstructive cardiomyopathy. An abnormal arrangement with disarray of septal myocardial fibres has been described in this situation (Somerville, 1981).

AORTIC VALVAR STENOSIS

Valvar stenosis is the most common obstruction in the left ventricular outflow tract. When isolated, it is usually congenital; the presence of a mitral lesion may suggest a rheumatic origin. In developed countries today, however, rheumatic fever is rare and congenital mitral abnormalities may be found with aortic stenosis, although they are more frequently associated with discrete subvalvar obstruction. Aortic stenosis has also been described in association with mitral stenosis as part of the congenital rubella syndrome (Rowe, 1973).

MORPHOLOGY

To understand the mechanisms of obstruction in the left ventricular outflow tract, it is necessary to understand the normal arrangement. This is not always easy, particularly as most accounts are based on the idea of an aortic 'annulus'. While there are rings within the normal aortic root, none of them support the leaflets of the aortic valve, which are hinged within the root in semilunar fashion (Figure 54.1). The outflow tract represents an interlocking of the aortic valvar sinuses and the supporting ventricular structures, with marked variation of the location of the haemodynamic as opposed to the anatomical ventriculo-arterial junctions. This is a slightly difficult concept; consequently, it is helpful to describe these junctions very precisely. The anatomical ventriculo-arterial junction is the line at which the fibroelastic walls of the aortic sinuses are supported by the base of the left ventricle. When the root is opened out in a pathological specimen, this line can be seen to form a complete ring, the anterosuperior parts of which are supported by the musculature of the ventricular septum and the parietal left ventricular wall. The posteroinferior parts are attached to the anterior or aortic leaflet of the mitral valve and the

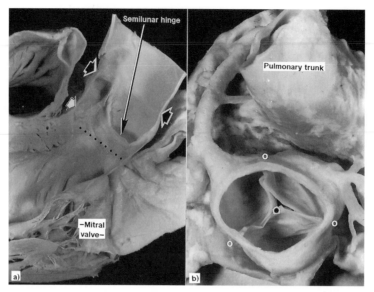

Figure 54.1. These preparations of the normal heart show (a) the simulated long-axis section of the aortic root and (b) the valve seen from the aortic aspect having transected the aorta. The long-axis section shows the semilunar haemodynamic junction, the sinutubular junction (closed arrows), and the anatomical junction seen anteriorly (closed arrow). The short-axis cut shows how the zones of apposition between the leaflets (commissures) extend from the sinutubular junction to the centre of the valvar orifice. The dotted line in (a) joins the basal extent of the attachments of the leaflets.

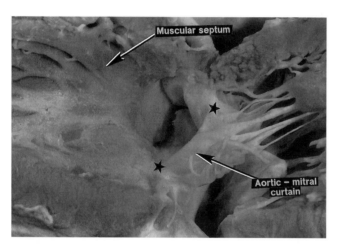

Figure 54.2. The outflow tract of the left ventricle is viewed from beneath. The aortic-mitral curtain (between stars) spans the ventricular roof. Note that the aortic valvar leaflets are attached in part to muscle and in part to fibrous structures.

membranous ventricular septum (Figure 54.2). In contrast, the haemodynamic junction is marked by the semilunar lines of attachment of the aortic valvar leaflets (Figure 54.1). These semilunar hinges cross the ring at six points; as a result, three crescents of ventricular tissue (partly muscular and partly fibrous) are incorporated into the bases of the three aortic sinuses of Valsalva, while three fibrous triangles are incorporated within the ventricular outflow tract (Sutton et al, 1995) (Figure 54.3). The triangles extend down as far as the most distal attachment of the leaflets. These attachments, the so-called commissures, are at the level of a second discrete ring, namely the sinutubular junction. This important structure, which is clearly seen in cross-sections of the root (Figure 54.1),

marks the junction between the expanded aortic sinuses and the tubular aorta. It is part of the aortic root; therefore, it is somewhat illogical to describe such stenosis at this level as supravalvar, though this is the traditional way. It is perhaps also illogical to consider only the peripheral attachment of the valvar leaflets to this ring as the commissures. Literally, a commissure is a line of apposition, and the lines of apposition between the normal valvar leaflets extend from the centre to the periphery of the valve. It is important that all parts of these junctions open without hindrance if the valve is to function properly (Figure 54.1b).

There is another ring within the outflow tract that can be constructed by joining together the most basal parts of the three semilunar leaflets. This is, however, an abstract concept, whereas the sinutubular junction and the anatomic ventriculo-arterial junctions are true annular structures. The line of attachment of the leaflets when considered in its entirety looks like a crown rather than a circle (Figure 54.3). Annulus does not seem the most obvious word to describe such a structure. The semilunar configuration of the leaflets and their suspension within the root are also important when measurements are being made of the outflow from the left ventricle. Diagrams are often taken to illustrate the concept of measurement showing lines being drawn between adjacent low points of attachment (Figure 54.4). These diagrams obviously depend on poetic licence, since such sections would never cut the full diameter of the root.

All this anatomy is important when considering the structure of stenosis of the outflow tract. It should be noted that the larger part of supravalvar stenosis is found at the level of the sinutubular junction, and it is also true that many examples of obstruction involve all three levels.

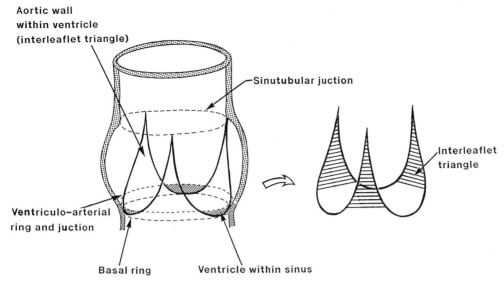

Figure 54.3. The aortic root is built up on the basis of a crown like configuration, with the semilunar hinges of the leaflets crossing the annular ventriculo-arterial junction. Note also the presence of a basal ring, and another ring at the sinutubular junction. The extension of the leaflets to the sinutubular junction produces the interleaflet triangles.

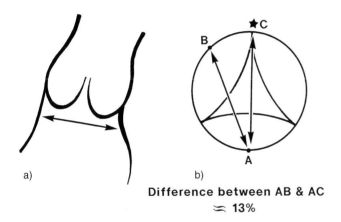

Figure 54.4. Diagrams are often drawn to show measurements of the aortic outflow taken at the base of the semilunar hinges (a). If such measurements were truly at the nadir of attachment with the ventricle (b), the section would be a cord of the outflow tract (BA) rather than a full diameter (CA).

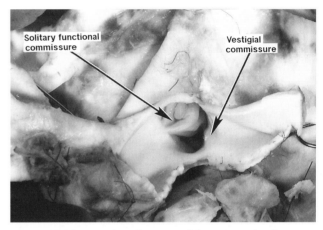

Figure 54.5. The typical configuration of the 'unicuspid and unicommissural' valve as seen from the aortic aspect. Compare with Figure 54.6.

VALVAR STENOSIS

Stenosis of the leaflets of the aortic valve is traditionally grouped as unicuspid, bicuspid or tricuspid. It is interesting also to note the number of sinuses present and the nature of the support of the valvar leaflets. In the presence of what appears to be a unicuspid aortic valve (Figure 54.5), examination from underneath (Figure 54.6) may show a solitary slit-like opening within the valvar curtain, but reveal three interleaflet triangles beneath the leaflets, even if two of them are vestigial (McKay et al, 1992). Some valves previously diagnosed as bicuspid have been shown to be formed on a trisinuate prototype (Leung et al, 1991). Unicuspid or unicommissural valves in infancy and early childhood often end up in the autopsy room. The keyhole opening within the

valvar curtain represents the only properly developed commissure (Figure 54.5). This is usually between the left and non-coronary aortic leaflets so that it points towards the mitral valve. The other leaflets are abnormally attached in annular fashion to the anterior ventricular wall and the commissures between the potential leaflets are vestigial (Figure 54.6). It is difficult to see how such valves are ever amenable to balloon dilation or open surgical valvotomy. They occur frequently in postmortem collections, probably because they are associated with small fibroelastotic left ventricles fulfilling many of the anatomic criteria for inclusion within the hypoplastic left heart syndrome (Chapter 45).

The bicuspid aortic valve (Figure 54.7) is often described in association with critical aortic stenosis but is also found in asymptomatic individuals. The valvar

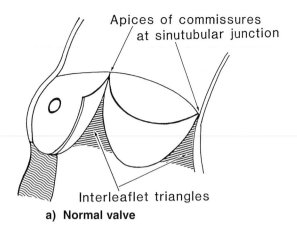

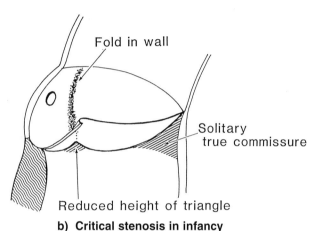

a) Normal valve

- Apices of commissures at sinutubular junction
- Interleaflet triangles

b) Critical stenosis in infancy

- Fold in wall
- Solitary true commissure
- Reduced height of triangle

Figure 54.6. When the 'unicuspid' arrangement seen in critical stenosis in infancy (b) is compared with the normal valve (a), vestigial commissures are found within the unicuspid leaflet, showing that it is formed on a trisinuate prototype and that the leaflet truly has an annular hinge. (Copyright Paediatrics, NHLI.)

leaflets are of markedly dissimilar size (Edwards, 1965), one being formed by fusion of what was potentially two leaflets. Examination of a large number of aortic valves with two leaflets (Angelini et al, 1989) has shown that most abnormal valves have three sinuses, with the conjoined leaflet representing either fusion of the two coronary leaflets, or fusion of the right and non-coronary leaflets (Figure 54.8). From time to time, truly bisinuate valves are encountered, or at least trisinuate valves without evidence of a raphe between the presumed conjoined leaflets. Stenosis, when it occurs, is the result of fusion of the ends of the zone of apposition between the two leaflets. Such fusion is more likely to be subject to disruption by balloon intervention. Bicuspid aortic valves produce problems when they become incompetent, or if they provide a nidus for endocarditis, but this is more likely to occur in adult life and is rarely seen in childhood.

A stenotic aortic valve with three leaflets can produce problems in early life or be the seat of senile aortic calcification (Vollebergh and Becker, 1976). Grossly dysplastic and lumpy valves occur in 10% of cases of congenital aortic valvar stenosis. They are found much more frequently in infancy. This finding is rare in older children and adolescents unless they have undergone previous surgery.

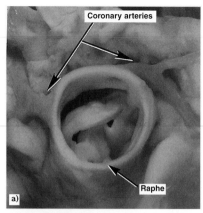

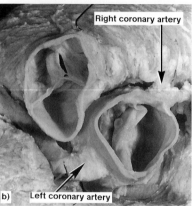

Figure 54.7. The two valves shown are both bileaflet. (a) The anterior leaflet represents both the usual 'coronary' leaflets but is smaller than the non-coronary leaflet. (b) The conjoined leaflet is supported in right and non-coronary sinuses.

Calcification of the aortic valve develops from the third decade in all patients with mildly stenotic or bicuspid valves. It may start as early as the second decade, particularly if the valves are lumpy and myxomatous. Patients often present in later life with severe calcific aortic stenosis in what was an unobstructed mildly stenosed valve. It is more common in males than females. Patients with familial hypocholesterolaemia, progeria and rickets develop calcification earlier even if the aortic valve is only mildly abnormal. Bicuspid aortic valves with minimal stenosis usually do not develop calcific stenosis until the sixth or seventh decade, but moderate or severe stenosis in childhood will lead to quite heavy calcification in the third and fourth decades. Isolated calcific valvar stenosis is always caused by a congenital abnormality of the aortic valve.

Aortic valvar stenosis is three times more common in males. Families with a greater than usual incidence of bicuspid aortic valve have been described (Emmanuel et al, 1978) with or without stenosis. Stenosis of valves with three leaflets, in contrast appears not to have such a familial tendency.

CLINICAL FINDINGS

Valvar stenosis can usually be differentiated from other types of aortic obstruction by the clinical signs

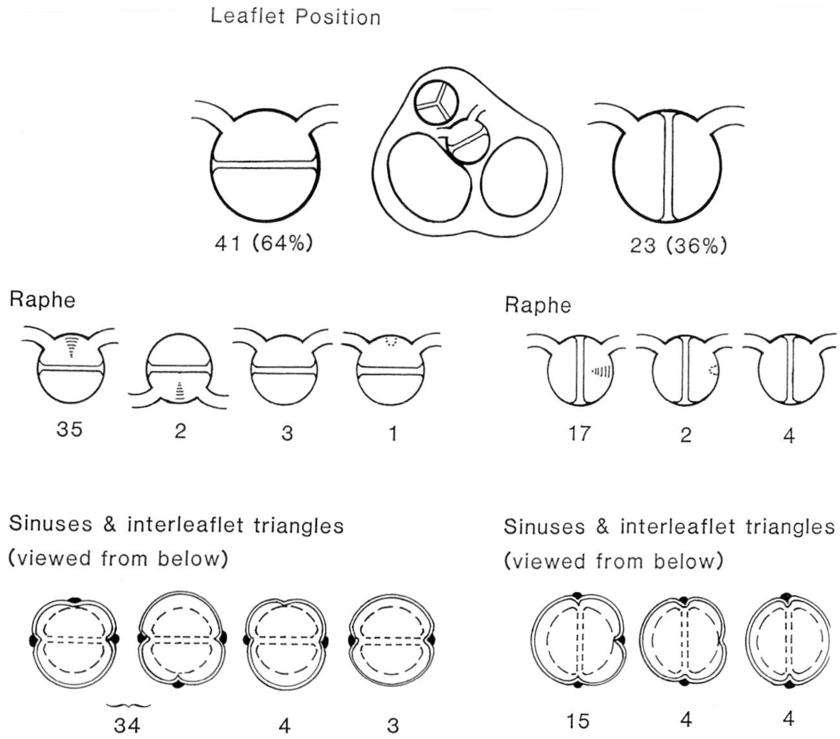

Leaflet Position

41 (64%)   23 (36%)

Raphe   Raphe

35   2   3   1   17   2   4

Sinuses & interleaflet triangles
(viewed from below)

Sinuses & interleaflet triangles
(viewed from below)

34   4   3   15   4   4

Figure 54.8. Although largely of academic interest, analysis of a large series of bicuspid valves by Angelini and her colleagues (1989) showed that most were formed on the basis of a trisinuate and initially trifoliate prototype.

Table 54.1. Clinical signs that differentiate the type of left ventricular outflow obstruction

Sign	Valvar[a]	Subvalvar	Supravalvar
Pulse			
Different in each arm	±	–	± (if stenoses)
Character	Sharp, normal or small	Normal or sharp	Sharp
Click	+	–	–
Maximal site of systolic murmur	Left or right sternal edge	Left sternal edge	Right sternal edge
Early diastolic murmur	±	+	Rare
Poststenotic dilation of ascending aorta	+	±	–

[a] The common pliant domed form. When the valve is thick and lumpy, the signs resemble subvalvar stenosis and the ascending aorta is not usually dilated.

(Table 54.1). Isolated congenital aortic valvar stenosis has several modes of presentation in childhood and young adult life:

- critical aortic valvar stenosis in infancy
- bicuspid valves but no sign of obstruction
- domed aortic valve presenting in childhood with mild, moderate or severe stenosis.

The more severe forms of valvar stenosis may be associated with excessive hypertrophy of the muscular ventricular septum, producing an additional dynamic mid-ventricular obstruction. There is then a further group of patients with critical valvar stenosis who have hypoplastic aortic roots and excessive septal hypertrophy. These frequently have tunnel obstruction, and fixed subaortic stenosis may also be present.

CRITICAL AORTIC VALVAR STENOSIS IN INFANCY

Aortic stenosis is a common cause of heart failure in infancy. It may be diagnosed before birth, and is a recognized cause of intrauterine morbidity and mortality. When aortic stenosis is diagnosed in fetal life, the outlook is uniformly poor and the pregnancy is frequently terminated. Critical aortic stenosis presents commonly in the neonatal period with severe heart failure, dyspnoea, poor peripheral circulation and low cardiac output. The aortic valve is thick, poorly formed and frequently unicuspid, with a small eccentric opening. The aortic root and valvar orifice are small. The appearance of the left ventricle is very variable. The cavity may be small, immobile and lined with endocardofibroelastic tissue (Figure 54.9).

This is a bad prognostic sign, and such hearts differ only minimally from the milder end of the hypoplastic left heart syndrome (Chapter 45). In other infants, the left ventricle may be enlarged and immobile, with poor systolic function and mitral regurgitation resulting either from ventricular dilation or infarction of papillary muscles from coronary arterial insufficiency (Figure 54.10). The left atrium is dilated, often with hypertrophic walls. Histologically, the left ventricular myocardium is fibrotic and, hypertrophic, with evidence of subendocardial ischaemia and even calcium deposits; this suggests that myocardial damage has been present for some time, even before birth. A third, and rarer, ventricular finding is gross concentric hypertrophy with a small left ventricular cavity, similar to that seen in hypertrophic cardiomyopathy.

After birth, patency of the arterial duct may help the child with critical aortic stenosis to maintain the haemodynamic status quo. Age at presentation may depend, therefore, not only on the severity of the stenosis, but also on the time of ductal closure. The pulses are often of small volume. There is an aortic systolic ejection murmur and an apical third heart sound.

The murmur at the aortic area may be soft if left ventricular function is poor. Ejection clicks are uncommon as the valve is usually thick and immobile. Chest radiographs show cardiomegaly, left atrial enlargement, and prominent pulmonary veins. The electrocardiogram may initially show little evidence of hypertrophy but, as the weeks pass, left ventricular hypertrophy develops, often with mitralization of the P wave and with conduction defects associated with myocardial fibrosis. Sometimes the initial traces reveal diffuse T wave inversion and ST flattening, suggesting myocardial hypoxic changes. The diagnosis is reliably and easily made using cross-sectional echocardiography (Figure 54.11). The aortic valve is usually thickened and is frequently domed. The varying appearances of the left ventricle have already been described. Doppler ultrasound is used to identify the severity of stenosis and the presence of mitral regurgitation. Peak velocity of flow in the ascending aorta is increased, sometimes to over 4 m/s. In the presence of impaired left ventricular function, the peak velocity may be reduced to less than 3 m/s, although the flow in the ascending aorta is obviously turbulent. After successful intervention, either by surgery or balloon valvotomy, the ascending aortic velocity may increase, indicating an improvement in left ventricular systolic function.

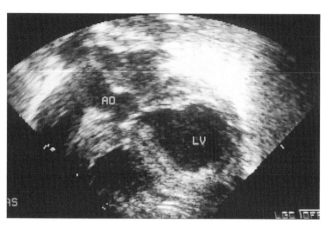

Figure 54.9. Echocardiogram showing critical aortic valvar (AO) stenosis with severe concentric left ventricular (LV) hypertrophy and small cavity.

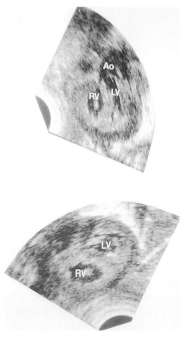

Figure 54.10. Critical aortic valvar (AO) stenosis in a neonate with dilated poorly contracting left ventricle (LV). RV, right ventricle.

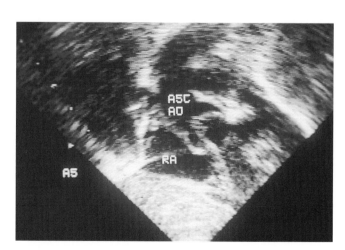

Figure 54.11. Long-axis subcostal echocardiographic view of domed aortic valve with eccentric orifice. RA, right atrium; AS, aortic stenosis; ASC, ascending aorta.

MANAGEMENT OF CLINICAL AORTIC VALVAR STENOSIS IN INFANCY

Medical treatment is at best a stop-gap measure in these sick infants. In the past, standard treatment was open valvotomy (Messina et al, 1984), although closed valvotomy (Duncan et al, 1986) was also advocated. More recent reports suggest that the results from balloon valvotomy are as good as surgery (Sullivan et al, 1988; Mosca et al, 1995). It appears that the critical factors predicting outcome are the systolic function and the morphology of the left ventricle and the valve (Zeevi et al, 1989). When the left ventricle is small and dysfunctional, neither surgical nor balloon valvotomy give good results; both have high risks. When the left ventricle is bigger, bulkier and has reasonable systolic function, then the results from either form of treatment are satisfactory. The choice depends on local expertise and preference. If the left ventricle is very small, and the circulation is duct-dependent, surgical management is undertaken using the Norwood techniques, as described for hypoplastic left heart (Chapter 45).

BICUSPID AORTIC VALVE WITH MILD AORTIC VALVAR STENOSIS

Children with such a bicuspid aortic valve are asymptomatic. They present with murmurs at routine examination, or occasionally with infective endocarditis. It is important to make the correct diagnosis in childhood to establish appropriate and lifelong protection against endocarditis, to offer parental reassurance, and to ensure that unnecessary restrictions on activities are avoided. Bicuspid aortic valves may be associated with ventricular septal defects, atrial septal defects, arterial ducts, coarctation of the aorta and pulmonary valvar stenosis.

The carotid and brachial pulses, blood pressure and apex beat are normal. An ejection click is heard after the first heart sound at the left sternal edge. It is easily heard towards the apex and increases on expiration. The click may be the only sign of a bicuspid aortic valve, but it commonly precedes a short ejection systolic murmur. An early diastolic murmur of mild aortic regurgitation may follow aortic valvar closure. The femoral pulses should be checked because of the common association with aortic coarctation. Blood pressure and the electrocardiogram are normal. The radiograph may show poststenotic dilation, but the heart size is usually normal. When the valve calcifies in adult life, this is visible on the lateral chest radiograph.

Cross-sectional echocardiography in the parasternal short-axis view reveals the morphology of the valve (Figure 54.12). The valve, if truly bicuspid, may have a vertical or horizontal line of opening. More commonly, the valve is functionally bicuspid with three leaflets of unequal size (Figure 54.13). Most truly bicuspid aortic

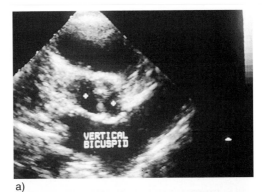

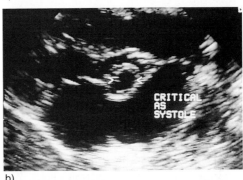

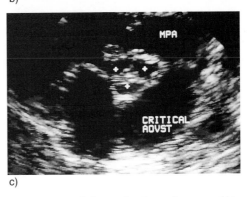

Figure 54.12. Parasternal short-axis echocardiograms of bicuspid aortic valves. (a) With vertical commissure; (b) with horizontal commissure between arrowheads. (c) with raphe on superior leaflet (between upper plus signs). MPA, main pulmonary artery.

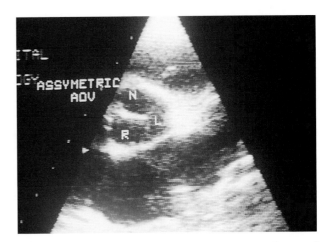

Figure 54.13 Parasternal short-axis echocardiogram showing functionally biscupid aortic valve with three leaflets, two of which are fused. N, non-coronary sinus; R, L, right and left coronary sinuses.

valves are trivially regurgitant on Doppler examination, even when a diastolic murmur is not audible. Bicuspid valves are usually associated with normal ascending aortic Doppler velocity. Associated mild aortic valvar stenosis produces turbulent flow in the ascending aorta, with a peak velocity up to 3 m/s measured from the suprasternal notch or the second right intercostal space.

Dilation of the aortic root is commonly found with bicuspid aortic valve, even in the absence of significant stenosis or regurgitation (Hahn et al, 1992). These authors postulate that the bicuspid aortic valve and aortic dilation may reflect a common developmental abnormality. Other studies have previously suggested a connection between bicuspid aortic valve, cystic medial necrosis of the aortic wall and dissection of the aorta (McKusick, 1972; Edwards et al, 1978). What the link between these two anomalies might be is not clear, since overwhelmingly the great majority of patients with bicuspid aortic valvar stenosis or aortic regurgitation do not suffer gross dilation of the root or dissection. A prospective study is needed to clarify this.

Differential diagnosis includes pulmonary valvar stenosis and other causes of ejection clicks. Pulmonary valvar stenosis normally has a murmur and click maximal at the pulmonary area and not conducted into the carotid arteries. In small children, nonetheless, the murmur of pulmonary stenosis may be conducted into the carotid arteries and the echocardiogram is needed to differentiate. Many normal young women have mitral valvar prolapse that is associated with a click and sometimes a mid systolic murmur at the apex. This click occurs significantly later in systole and alters with change in position.

A patient with a perimembranous ventricular septal defect undergoing spontaneous closure as a result of formation of an aneurysm may present with a click in mid-systole at the left sternal edge. The click arises from the aneurysm billowing into the defect.

Patients with trivial aortic valvar stenosis or a bicuspid aortic valve should be allowed to lead a normal active life but will require antibiotic prophylaxis against infective endocarditis.

DOMED PLIANT VALVE WITH MODERATE OR SEVERE AORTIC STENOSIS

Most patients with a domed pliant valve present at routine examination with loud murmurs and a carotid thrill. Symptoms are rare, although syncope, angina and dyspnoea on exertion have been described with severe stenosis. Heart failure is rare in childhood but is occasionally seen in adolescents or young adults. Although sudden death is more common in aortic stenosis than in other forms of congenital heart disease (Lambert et al, 1974), the risk is small. It was no more than 2% in a series of 300 cases described by Peckham et al (1964).

The danger of sudden death is confined to those with severe stenosis. The exact cause of sudden death is uncertain, but ventricular arrhythmias following myocardial ischaemia may be the underlying problem.

Although syncope may occur after extreme effort with mild or moderate obstruction, it is usually only found with severe stenosis. It results from inability of the left ventricle to increase its output appropriately with exercise (Braunwald et al, 1963). Fatigue is often mentioned but is difficult to assess and frequently relates to parental anxiety. Most young people, even with quite significant congenital aortic stenosis, appear energetic and asymptomatic.

The physical signs depend upon the severity of the stenosis and the valvar pathology. The character of the peripheral pulses is normal in moderate stenosis, and the resting heart rate is usually slow. With even greater severity, the upstrokes of the right brachial and carotid pulses are sharp. They differ from the left carotid and brachial pulses, which tend to be smaller and slightly anacrotic (Figure 54.14). These differences in the pulse are explained by the initial rapid ejection of blood, which conducts a pulse wave primarily up the brachiocephalic artery. With greater severity of stenosis all the pulses are small. Carotid and suprasternal systolic thrills are common, and the apex beat is localized and thrusting without significant lateral displacement. On auscultation, a click is heard followed by a long ejection systolic murmur with maximum intensity late in systole. The click is best heard at the apex away from the maximum intensity of the murmur (Figure 54.15). In very severe stenosis, the aortic component of the second heart sound is delayed and the sound becomes single or appears reversed on expiration. Soft aortic early-diastolic murmurs are uncommon with a pliable valve, while lumpy valves tend not to have an ejection click and more frequently have early diastolic murmurs.

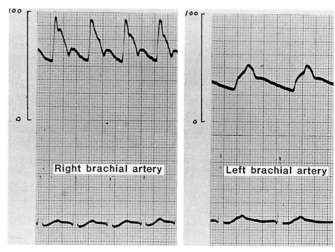

Figure 54.14. Brachial arterial pulses from a 12-year-old boy with domed aortic valve.

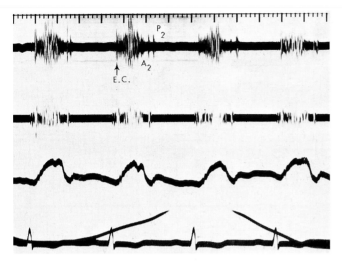

Figure 54.15. An ejection click (E.C.) preceding an ejection systolic murmur recorded at the apex and pulmonary area in a patient with domed and pliable stenotic aortic valve.

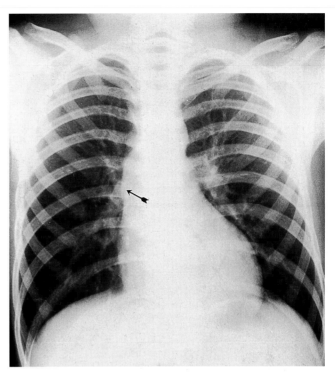

Figure 54.16. Chest radiograph from a patient with critical aortic valvar stenosis requiring aortic valvotomy. It shows post-stenotic dilation of the ascending aorta (arrow).

The electrocardiogram shows variable degrees of left ventricular hypertrophy depending on the degree of severity. Left ventricular voltage increases, with upright T waves, which, as time passes, many invert with associated ST depression. This shows first of all in leads II, III and AVE, appearing some considerable time before the ST–T changes occur in the left chest leads. The presence of Q waves in the left ventricular leads is uncommon in congenital aortic stenosis and may suggest associated lesions. The electrical axis is usually normal. Forms of left bundle branch block are unusual and frequently suggest myocardial pathological changes secondary to aortic stenosis.

Exercise testing may be useful in the follow-up and assessment of children with moderate stenosis. It used to be said that ST depression of greater than 1 mm indicated a gradient of more than 50 mmHg, but James et al (1981) reported significant ST changes with gradients of 30 mmHg or less. In general, the ST–T wave changes during exercise do appear to be related to the severity of stenosis and symptoms such as chest pain, breathlessness or syncope.

If the systolic blood pressure falls or fails to rise normally with exercise, this indicates severe stenosis (Riopel et al, 1977). Even with severe stenosis, however, ventricular function is generally normal in children (Orsmond et al, 1980).

Even with quite severe stenosis, the chest radiograph need not show cardiac enlargement. A rounded outline of the apex can be seen as a result of left ventricular hypertrophy and poststenotic dilation of the ascending aorta is frequently present (Figure 54.16). Aortic dilation is often absent in patients with dysplastic lumpy aortic valves, where the ascending aorta is small or even hypoplastic. Left atrial enlargement seen on the radiograph is an indication of very severe stenosis and left ventricular abnormality. Calcium deposits are not usually present in children or adolescents except after endocarditis. Cross-sectional echocardiography demonstrates very variable morphology. Although doming is commonly seen in parasternal long-axis sections (Figure 54.17), it is less obvious in truly bicuspid valves, which often appear to prolapse slightly in diastole. As mentioned above, the most common arrangement is a functionally bicuspid valve with three asymmetric leaflets. The degree of obstruction obviously bears a close relationship to the reduction in the area of the valvar orifice. Direct measurement by planimetry from the cross-sectional echocardiogram is difficult because of the eccentric nature of the orifice and the thickened leaflets; the inherent error is unacceptably great. The continuity equation offers a theoretically satisfying method for measuring valvar area using echocardiography and Doppler (Skjaerpe et al, 1985). Stroke volume in the left ventricular outflow tract (LVOT) is the same as that across the aortic valvar orifice. Consequently, the area of the valvar orifice can be calculated from:

$$\text{Aortic valve area} = \frac{\text{Area of LVOT} \times \text{systolic velocity integral in LVOT}}{\text{Systolic velocity integral at aortic valve}}$$

Although its protagonists stress the usefulness of this method, it has inherent practical problems and is not of proven clinical value.

The major source of error in using the continuity theorum lies in the difficulty in measuring accurately the

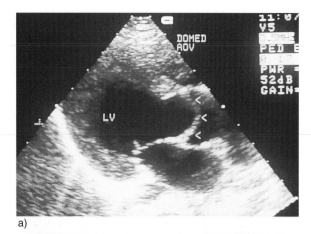

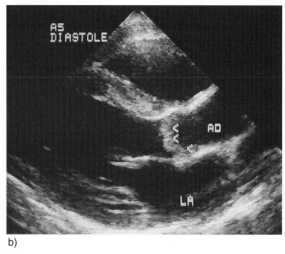

Figure 54.17. Long-axis parasternal views of domed aortic valve (arrow) in systole (a) and diastole (b). LA, left atrium; LV, left ventricle; AO, aorta.

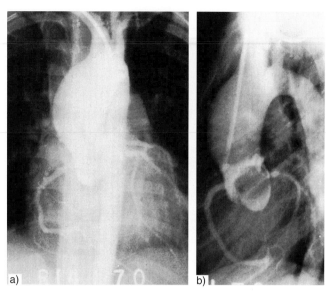

Figure 54.18. An aortogram, seen in frontal (a) and lateral (b) projections, showing a domed aortic valve with jet of blood passing through the contrast-filled aorta.

left ventricular outflow tract (Figure 54.4). Doppler ultrasound seems to provide a workable method for assessing severity of stenosis. The peak velocity in the ascending aorta beyond the valve is easily and reproducibly measured using continuous wave Doppler. This peak velocity may then be used to infer the instantaneous pressure difference across the aortic valve. Peak instantaneous pressure difference occurs earlier and is greater than the 'peak to peak' pressure difference, which is the usual measurement at catheterization. The Bernoulli equation in its modified form gives a fair estimate of pressure difference and, therefore, severity of stenosis. In mild stenosis, in mixed stenosis and regurgitation, and where there are multiple or lengthy areas of stenosis, it becomes less predictable and reliable. For clinical purposes, it probably makes most sense to forget the Bernoulli equation (binomial distribution) and to use the peak velocity of flow in the ascending aorta as an index of stenosis. A simple rule of thumb is that mild stenosis produces a velocity in the ascending aorta of 3 m/s or less. Moderate stenosis exists when the velocity is 3–4.5 m/s, and anything over 4.5 m/s is indicative of severe obstruction.

Most patients with aortic valvar stenosis do not nowadays require diagnostic cardiac catheterization if the clinical, electrocardiographic and echocardiographic features are in agreement. Catheterization is undertaken only when doubt exists about the level of obstruction, when clinical echocardiographic or electrocardiographic features are at variance, or if other lesions coexist. Left-heart catheterization is usually sufficient and should include crossing the valve with an end-hole catheter to demonstrate the level of obstruction correctly. There appears to be no need now for the inotropic provocation tests in vogue in the past at cardiac catheterization.

An aortogram in the frontal and left lateral view should be performed to elucidate the valvar morphology. If there is an associated left ventricular gradient or dysfunction, a left ventriculogram may also be indicated (Figures 54.18 and 54.19).

AORTIC VALVAR STENOSIS ASSOCIATED WITH THICKENED AND MYXOMATOUS LEAFLETS ——

Aortic valvar stenosis associated with thickened and myxomatous leaflets (Figure 54.20) occurs mainly in infancy and is rare in later childhood. The symptoms occur as in other forms of obstruction within the left ventricular outflow tract. The valve does not dome and is less mobile, giving an appearance on echocardiogram or angiogram of a flat thick plate-like structure with a rather small ascending aorta (Figure 54.19). There is often a wasted appearance above the attachments of the leaflets and the valve root is often small. Asymmetric septal hypertrophy and a cardiomyopathic appearance to the left ventricle is not uncommon. It is important to recognize this variant because surgical treatment is

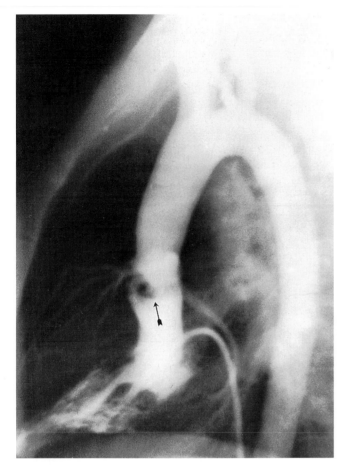

Figure 54.19. A left ventriculogram, in lateral projection, showing a thick, lumpy aortic valve that does not dome (arrow). Note the small ascending aorta. The left ventricle shows septal bulging with unusually large papillary muscles and an appearance of midventricular obstruction.

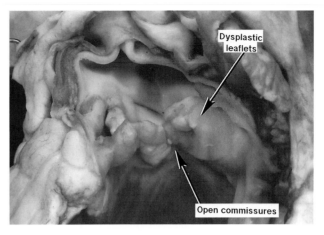

Figure 54.20. The typical 'rubbery' valve without commissural fusion frequently seen in children with trifoliate valvar stenosis.

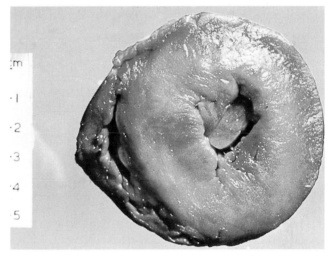

Figure 54.21. A cross-section of the left ventricle from a 15-year-old boy, showing massive hypertrophy. His heart would not function after bypass for open aortic valvotomy.

difficult and often has a poor haemodynamic result (Somerville and Ross, 1971). Late survivors present a formidable problem for re-operation and it is frequently not possible to relieve the gradient.

MANAGEMENT OF PATIENTS WITH SIGNIFICANT AORTIC VALVAR STENOSIS ——————BEYOND INFANCY——————

The patient with congenital aortic valvar stenosis needs lifelong medical supervision. Even with bicuspid or mildly stenotic valves, early advice about the prevention of bacterial endocarditis is vital, and careful dental care must be provided at all times. The incidence of bacterial endocarditis is less than 1%, or 2.7 episodes per 1000 patient-years (Hossack et al, 1980). Mouth organisms are not the only source of infection, however, and all sources must be looked for and prevented.

Once the diagnosis of aortic valvar stenosis is made in a child severity must be assessed. Management has three basic aims. First, to prevent sudden death, second, to prevent permanent damage and fibrosis secondary to ventricular hypertrophy (Figure 54.21), and third, to relieve symptomatology. This last aim is necessary frequently in infancy but rarely in childhood.

Although sudden death is rare, it is probably wise to restrict patients from competitive or excessive sporting activities. Regular severe exercise may increase the stimulus to hypertrophy and resultant potential subendocardial ischaemia.

The electrocardiograph and the echocardiograph together allow the cardiologist to assess changes in the severity of stenosis. Frequently, moderate stenosis progresses in later childhood and adolescence, when the ascending aortic Doppler velocities rise and ST and T wave changes invert in the left ventricular leads of the electrocardiogram (Figure 54.22). Children with moderate aortic stenosis should be reviewed on an annual outpatient basis until around puberty, when the interval should be shortened to six months.

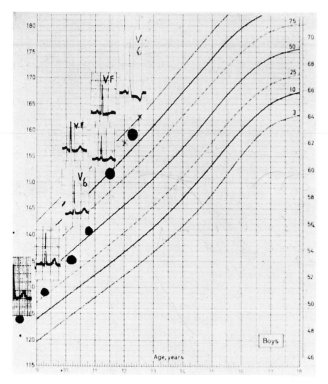

Figure 54.22. The electrocardiogram (lead V6) plotted against the growth chart from a boy followed from age 6 to 13 years with simple aortic valvar stenosis. Note the rapid deterioration in electrocardiographic findings at the pubertal growth spurt.

The indications for surgical intervention have been summarized as follows.

- Moderate aortic valvar stenosis with ST–T wave changes in the left ventricular leads at rest
- No symptoms but electrocardiographic changes or an altered response to exercise in serial tests
- A resting peak-to-peak systolic pressure difference greater than 60 mmHg in the absence of ST–T wave changes at catheterization
- Symptoms related to aortic stenosis with signs of at least moderate valvar obstruction.

Open surgical valvotomy has been the treatment of choice for many years. Mortality is low: usually less than 2% (Sandor et al, 1980). The incidence of residual stenosis or regurgitation, however, is not inconsiderable although infrequently remarked upon in surgical reviews. Long-term surgical reports suggest that survival immediately following operation is excellent. Long-term outlook is much less trouble-free, with a cumulative mortality of 16% reported at 15 years (Hossack et al, 1980). Johnson et al (1984) further suggested that there was only a 56% chance actuarially of being free of re-operation at 10 years. Hsieh et al (1986) applied actuarial analysis to young people and children following surgical valvotomy. The probability of survival fell from 94% at 5 years to 77% at 22 years. Of the patients in the study, 36% required re-operation, with a 12% surgical mortality. Of

25 re-operations in this series, 20 were for valvar replacement because of regurgitation or residual stenosis. These features highlight the fact that aortic stenosis is not a benign condition in childhood, and that open surgical valvotomy is at best a palliative procedure.

Balloon valvotomy of the aortic valve, as described by Labadidi et al (1984) and Sullivan et al (1989), may now be reasonably considered as the initial treatment of choice. It is at least as safe as open valvotomy and probably has a lower incidence of regurgitation and residual stenosis. In theory, balloon valvotomy should postpone surgery for a number of years. The indications for intervention are the same as for surgery. Since the advent of balloon valvotomy in our department, open surgical valvotomy has certainly become a rare occurrence.

The ease and efficacy of balloon valvotomy, and the advantage to the patient of no immediate surgery, suggests that, in the future, we may wish to intervene earlier or when the pressure difference is smaller. For instance, if a pressure difference of 50 mmHg could be reduced to 20 mmHg, restriction of physical activity might reasonably be relaxed to allow relatively normal activities. Nonetheless, the new technique does fail from time to time, and open valvotomy remains a safe alternative. As the incidence of calcification increases from the third decade onwards, the efficacy of balloon valvoplasty diminishes. While balloon valvotomy will postpone surgery, it is important to realise that any young person who requires intervention for aortic valvar stenosis will inevitably require replacement of the valve at some time in the future (Presbitero and Somerville, 1982).

Replacement of the aortic valve in children and young people has always been problematical. Aortic homografts, and other tissue valves, are haemodynamically excellent but liable to early deterioration, necessitating replacement. Synthetic valves, particularly the bileaflet valves, are mechanically reliable and very durable but condemn the patient to anticoagulation treatment for the rest of their lives. This may limit their options for career and employment; for girls, it makes pregnancy difficult and inconvenient.

A number of centres are now returning to the procedure first described by Ross in 1967 (Gerosa, 1991). In this operation, the original aortic valve and root are completely excised, and the pulmonary root is inserted into the aortic position. The coronary arteries are re-implanted into the pulmonary autograft (Somerville and Ross, 1982). The continuity of the right ventricular outflow tract is restored using a pulmonary homograft. The advantages of this procedure to the child and young adult are that the autograft grows and the patient does not need anticoagulation therapy. The pulmonary homograft will require replacement with time and growth, but this is a lesser procedure, with lesser risks to the patient.

SUBVALVAR STENOSIS

A variety of lesions can obstruct the subaortic outflow tract, with or without a coexisting ventricular septal defect. When there is an interventricular communication, then posterior deviation of the muscular outlet septum is usually the most important lesion (al Marsafawy et al, 1995). This is considered in Chapter 56. Obstruction can also be produced by hypertrophy of the ventricular septum, as seen in hypertrophic cardiomyopathy (Chapter 59), by anomalous tissue tags derived from the membranous septum or the leaflets of the atrioventricular valves or by anomalous attachment of the tension apparatus of the left atrioventricular valve (McElhinney et al, 1998). The last two are more likely to be found when there is also a ventricular septal defect, or in the setting of common atrioventricular junction and deficient atrioventricular septation. When the ventricular septum is intact, the most significant lesion is the so-called subvalvar ridge (Figure 54.23). This lesion has been described in many ways and has been the subject of multiple investigations. Although often termed 'membranous', almost always the lesion is a firm fibrous shelf that encircles the outflow tract in diaphragmatic fashion (Somerville, 1985) (Figure 54.23a). The ridge often extends to be attached to the aortic valvar leaflets themselves (Figure 54.23b) and overlies the left bundle branch as it crosses the ventricular septum. A discrete plan of cleavage almost always exists, nonetheless, between the shelf and the musculature. Because of this, it can readily be stripped away by surgery. Since the lesion is acquired, there is always the likelihood of recurrence. The toughness of the lesion makes it unlikely that balloon dilation would be effective, but this has certainly been attempted and reputedly with some success. The shelf tends to be a discrete structure, although its position can vary with regard to its proximity to the valvar leaflets. If extensive, it can produce so-called 'tunnel' stenosis. In florid cases, there is a marked abnormality in the alignment between the plane of the aortic root and the ventricular septum. This has been promoted as a potential cause of the malformation (Gewillig et al, 1992). Subaortic ridges are not congenital (Figure 54.24). They are acquired as a result of some haemodynamic abnormality and are not usually found before the age of 9 months (Kitchiner et al, 1994).

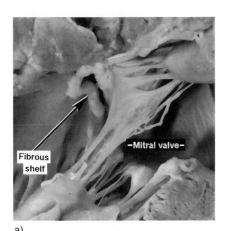

a)

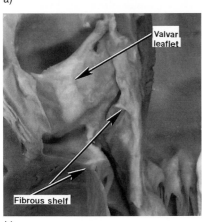

b)

Figure 54.23. The typical pattern of the diaphragmatic form of subvalvar aortic stenosis, seen intact (a) and in long-axis section (b).

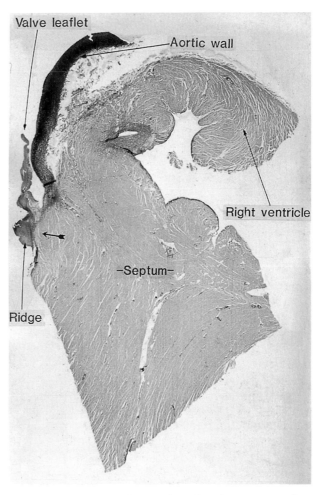

Figure 54.24. A histological section from the subaortic region of a 14-month-old child who died from heart failure and pneumonia with a large duct. The arrow points to a non-obstructive ridge beneath the aortic valvar leaflet. This might be the forerunner of fixed subaortic obstruction. (Given by the late Dr L. Becu.)

CLINICAL FEATURES

Symptoms are uncommon with this subvalvar stenosis, even when the narrowing is severe; however, occasionally syncope and giddiness occur. If undiagnosed and presenting in middle life, congestive heart failure, dyspnoea and syncope have been described.

The physical signs are similar to aortic valvar stenosis with a carotid thrill, a left ventricular apex and an aortic ejection systolic murmur maximal at the left sternal edge and conducted to the carotid arteries. The pulses are generally symmetrical, sometimes with a sharp upstroke depending on the degree of dynamic muscular obstruction. There is no ejection click. The aortic second sound is audible and, in most patients as the years go by, is followed by an early diastolic murmur. Chest radiograph is often normal, although enlargement of left ventricle and left atrium may be present. There is sometimes post-stenotic dilation of the ascending aorta.

The electrocardiogram, as might be expected, shows varying degrees of left ventricular hypertrophy, normally without a Q wave. Upright T waves are preserved even with quite severe obstruction. The electrical axis is normal except in older patients with myocardial damage.

Echocardiography with Doppler ultrasound is the quickest and best way of making the diagnosis and differentiating the common from the rarer forms. Cross-sectional examination in the parasternal long axis shows the characteristic ridge in the outflow tract (Figure 54.25). The full extent of the crescent may be difficult to assess from this approach. In older children or young adults, transoesophageal echo demonstrates this lesion more fully and is probably a better way to identify associated lesions of the mitral and aortic valves. M-mode echo allows identification of the degree of left ventricular hypertrophy, the presence of septal hypertrophy and characteristic mid-systolic vibration of the aortic leaflets during ejection (Figure 54.26). Doppler ultrasound is used to assess the extent of aortic regurgitation and the degree of obstruction within the left ventricular outflow tract. As in aortic valvar stenosis, peak ascending aortic velocities are the most reliable indicator of severity, although significant aortic regurgitation and long segment obstruction may invalidate the Bernoulli equation, as already described. Catheterization may be needed to identify the severity of the obstruction. Angiography should include an aortogram profiled in left anterior oblique projection (Figure 54.27), and a left ventriculogram profiled in frontal and lateral or left anterior oblique views (Figures 54.28–54.30). In about 20% of patients, the angiogram will show clearly a linear diaphragm within the left ventricular outflow tract, but it is rather more common to see a broader shadow (Figure 54.30).

Because of the progressive nature of the disorder, and the presence of a regurgitant aortic valve, surgery is indicated even when the narrowing is thought to be only mild or moderate (Somerville et al, 1980). The risks are similar to surgery for valvar stenosis.

Clinical management should be the same as for valvar stenosis, with serial echocardiography and electrocardiography providing the mainstay of follow-up.

Recurrence of the fixed obstruction may be a problem in as many as one third of patients. This may be the result of incomplete initial relief of obstruction or it may reflect residual myocardial hypertrophy. Patients sometimes develop a tunnel obstruction, which may necessitate total replacement of the root and valve to relieve the narrowing. Those who undergo surgery under the age of 8 years of age seem to have a good long-term result without recurrence and with no cardiomyopathic appearances (McKay and Ross, 1982). The conduction tissues are vulnerable at operation, and this is particularly so in patients with associated ventricular septal defects.

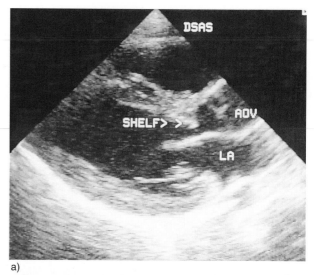

a)

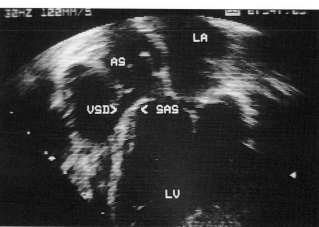

b)

Figure 54.25. Fixed subaortic stenosis. (a) Long-axis parasternal view (b) four chambered apical view with subaortic shelf and ventricular septal defect (VSD). AOV; aortic valve; LA, left atrium; DSAS, discrete subaortic stenosis; AS, aortic stenosis; SAS, subaortic stenosis; LV, left ventricle.

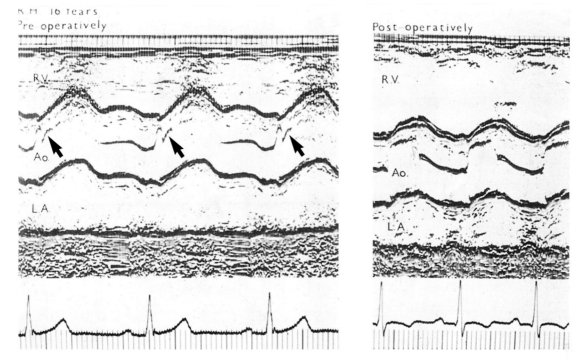

Figure 54.26. An M-mode echocardiogram from a patient with fixed subaortic stenosis. Before operation it shows premature closure of the aortic valve (arrow) with shuddering as it opens. This has disappeared in the postoperative record on the right.

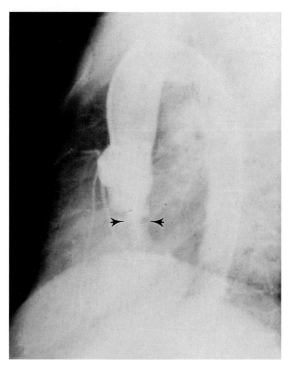

Figure 54.27. Subaortic shelf outlined (arrows) by aortic regurgitation following an aortogram in a patient with severe fixed subaortic stenosis.

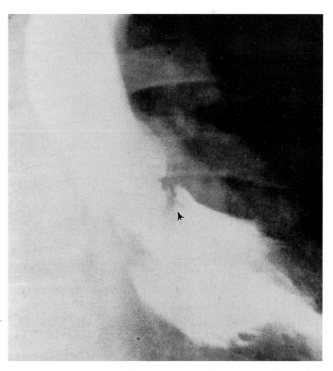

Figure 54.28. A ventricular angiogram, in frontal projection, showing unusually well-developed and easily seen fixed subaortic stenosis (arrow). It is this appearance that gives rise to the term 'membrane'.

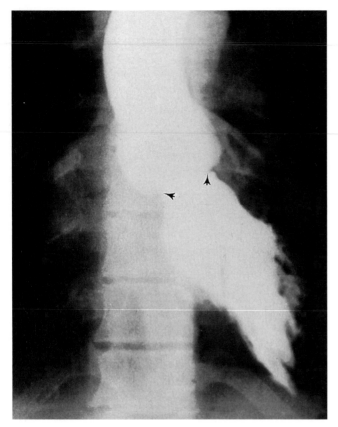

Figure 54.29. A left ventriculogram, frontal projection, showing notching under aortic valve. Frequently, this is the only sign of fixed subaortic stenosis. The patient did well after resection of a full subaortic ring.

——SUPRAVALVAR AORTIC STENOSIS——

Supravalvar stenosis accounts for only 1–2% of aortic stenosis seen in childhood. The condition may be familial or may be associated with disorders of calcium metabolism. It was first described in association with a characteristic facial appearance by Williams et al (1961). The original description also included failure to thrive, gastrointestinal upset, and mental retardation. Black and Bonham Carter (1963) then described infantile hypercalcaemia, and noted that the patients had characteristic facial features when the hypercalcaemia was associated with signs of aortic stenosis. They recognized that the face described by Williams et al (1961) was also seen in infantile idiopathic hypercalcaemia (Figure 54.31), thus establishing a link between disturbance of calcium metabolism and supra-aortic stenosis. It is now accepted, however, that supravalvar aortic stenosis may occur in William's syndrome but also occurs in normal children without any history of metabolic abnormality.

Supravalvar aortic obstruction is probably not present at birth, although the aorta is often small and thick-walled. Obstruction appears later for reasons that are unclear. It may be associated with other congenital abnormalities such as coarctation, pulmonary valvar

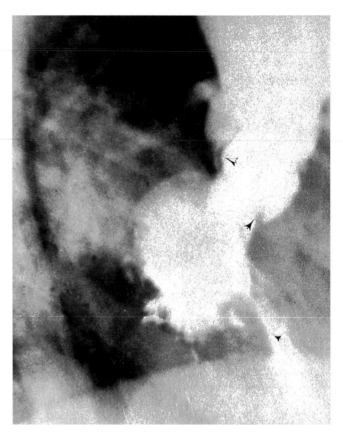

Figure 54.30. Lateral angiocardiogram from a patient with fixed subaortic stenosis. A small notch is seen as a filling defect from the bulging ventricular septum (upper arrow). Intense irregular muscular hypertrophy causes mid-ventricular obstruction (lower arrow). This has the angiocardiographic appearance of hypertrophic cardiomyopathy. The aortic valve is mildly stenosed and doming (uppermost open arrow).

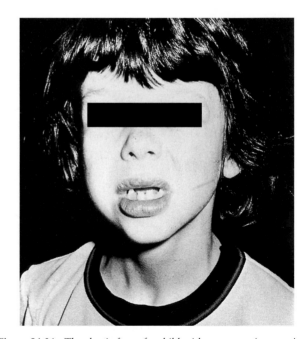

Figure 54.31. The classic face of a child with supra-aortic stenosis and infantile hypercalcaemia. Note the prominent orbital ridges and jaw, with the thick lips, large ridged teeth and slight strabismus. The features are neither pixie-like nor elfin.

stenosis, pulmonary arterial stenosis or atrial septal defect. Children with several anomalies like this do not, as a rule, have the characteristic facies. The aetiology is unknown, although the loss of the long arm of chromosome 4 was implicated in one patient (Jefferson et al, 1986).

The stenosis lies above the aortic sinuses and the coronary orifices at the sinutubular junction (Plate 54.1). The aortic sinuses are enlarged and bulge laterally. The aortic leaflets are often slightly thickened, and the coronary arteries, which take origin below the obstruction, are dilated, thick walled and ectatic. The coronary arterial thickening is mainly medial; later in life, premature coronary atherosclerosis is described. The nature of the aortic narrowing is variable (Stamm et al, 1997). The most common form is the 'hour glass' variety with dilation of the distal aorta (Figure 54.32). There are also diffuse or tubular varieties, and, very rarely, a diaphragmatic or localized form (Figure 54.32a,c). The ascending aorta is grossly abnormal irrespective of type, with a thickened wall and disorganization of the media (Peterson et al, 1965). The intima is scarred with fibrosis, and there are pits large enough to be seen on aortography. The narrowing and scarring are not exclusive to the aorta and may be found in the iliac arteries and in the abdominal and renal vessels. Stenosis of the origin of the carotid and subclavian arteries, and less frequently the renal and mesenteric arteries, occurs in up to half the patients. The pulmonary circulation is also affected. In 20% of patients, there are multiple pulmonary arterial stenoses. These are mostly peripheral, being seen where the major vessels enter the lung. Consequently, supravalvar aortic stenosis in most, but not all, patients is part of a more widespread abnormality of the cardiovascular system involving the major conducting arteries. Histological findings away from the site of the obstruction in the aorta show irregular thickening and branching of medial elastic fibres: an appearance that has been called a 'mosaic' by Edwards (1965) and 'higgledy-piggledy' arteriopathy by Becu et al (1976).

Supravalvar aortic stenosis and its attendant lesions may be the result of an early, perhaps intrauterine, disturbance with distortion of the normal development of the walls of the major conducting arteries. At points of vulnerability, such as the major divisions and the supraaortic area, more major damage occurs, resulting in a scar. The resultant disproportionate growth of the abnormal aorta leads to a stenotic area. It is unclear why the supravalvar aortic area is so vulnerable, but the pathology of the aorta and the tendency to multiple lesions does support the hypothesis that a diffuse cardiovascular disease is present that is not eradicated by successful surgery.

CLINICAL FEATURES

Infants with supravalvar aortic stenosis may fail to thrive and suffer vomiting, constipation and delayed development. All of these are probably related to disturbed calcium metabolism. Cardiovascular symptoms are rare. When present, they are those of aortic obstruction and ventricular dysfunction. Dyspnoea and angina only occur much later, and syncope is extremely rare. Peripheral arterial stenosis may be associated with hypertension. Bacterial endocarditis is described on the aortic valve, and antibiotic prophylaxis is mandatory.

The characteristic appearance of William's syndrome (Figure 54.31), when present, is easily identified. The prominent ridged teeth, jaw, heavy brows and the amiable temperament are very characteristic. Patients

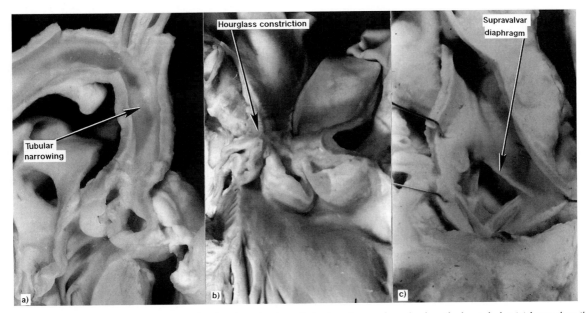

Figure 54.32. 'Supravalvar' aortic stenosis most often involves the sinutubular junction, and can be described as tubular (a) hour-glass (b) and diaphragmatic (c).

having supravalvar aortic stenosis with a positive family history, nonetheless, usually have normal appearance and normal intelligence. There is then no history of failure to thrive in infancy.

If supravalvar aortic stenosis is present, all pulses may be full but the right carotid and brachial pulses are sharper and fuller than the rest. This is attributed to the Coanda effect, where the jet stream hugs the aortic wall and selectively streams into the brachiocephalic artery. When the supravalvar obstruction is very severe, small pulses will be present throughout.

Carotid, suprasternal, and right upper parasternal thrills are usual. The apex beat is localized and of left ventricular type. There is a systolic ejection murmur maximal at the right sternal edge and conducted to the carotid arteries. The closure of the aortic valvar leaflets is usually normal, and is rarely delayed or reduced. There is no ejection click, but there is frequently an aortic diastolic murmur. In the presence of pulmonary arterial stenosis, long systolic murmurs are heard widely over the lungs posteriorly. Pulmonary valvar closure may be quite loud if the stenosis is severe enough to increase pulmonary arterial pressure. Bruits are heard in the loins in the presence of renal arterial stenosis. Systemic hypertension is not infrequent in this condition. It may be the result of renal arterial stenosis, or may occur without stenosis, presumably as a result of diffuse arterial pathology. Even if the blood pressure is normal, or only mildly elevated at rest, it may show a grossly abnormal response to exercise.

The electrocardiogram is the same as in other forms of obstruction within the left ventricular outflow tract. T wave changes occur late. In the presence of pulmonary arterial stenosis, right axis deviation and right ventricular hypertrophy may be seen.

Chest radiographs sometimes show slight dilation of the ascending aorta, but the lung fields are normal and the pulmonary trunk is prominent in the presence of severe pulmonary arterial stenosis. Severe left ventricular hypertrophy and dysfunction will lead to enlargement of the left atrium, and sometimes the left ventricle.

Cross-sectional echocardiography is helpful, but visualization of the narrowing in the aorta is often difficult from the parasternal view (Plate 54.1). The enlarged coronary arterial orifices from the aortic sinuses are easily seen in the short-axis views. The aortic valvar leaflets may be thickened but move normally. The ventricular septum often bulges into the outflow tract, and the papillary muscles are usually large. Doppler examination of the ascending aorta reveals a pattern of high-velocity and turbulent flow. High velocities are frequently recorded in the ascending aorta when quite small gradients are measured invasively. According to Levine et al (1989), this is the result of the phenomenon of pressure recovery. Doppler estimates of pressure drop more accurately identify the inherent haemodynamic anomaly than the invasive measurement of peak-to-peak gradients. Aortography is the

most important part of the investigation, demonstrating the site and extent of the narrowing and the origins of the coronary arteries (Figure 54.33). Ideally, an injection should be carried out in the abdominal aorta to identify renal arterial abnormalities. Aortography frequently shows diffuse abnormalities in the ascending aorta, with pitting irregularity and hypoplasia. Left ventricular angiography shows irregular hypertrophy, with a small cavity and an intrusive septum (Figure 54.34).

Surgical treatment is usually advised in patients when peak-to-peak gradients are measured in excess of

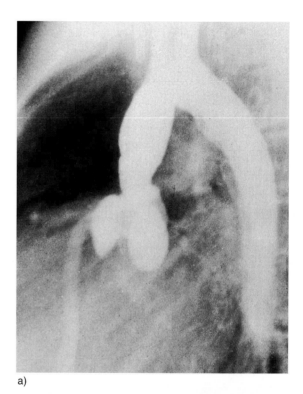

a)

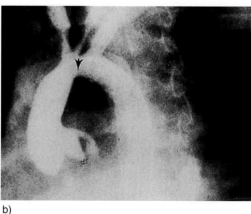

b)

Figure 54.33. Aortogram from a patient with supra-aortic stenosis. (a) Recording taken when the child was 9 years old, prior to surgery. Pitting of the ascending aorta can be seen, depicting diffuse abnormality away from the site of the supra-aortic obstruction. (b) The same patient aged 18 years (9 years after relief of supra-aortic stenosis) has developed an obstruction in the aortic arch (arrow). There are narrowings at the origins of the bracheocephalic and left carotid arteries.

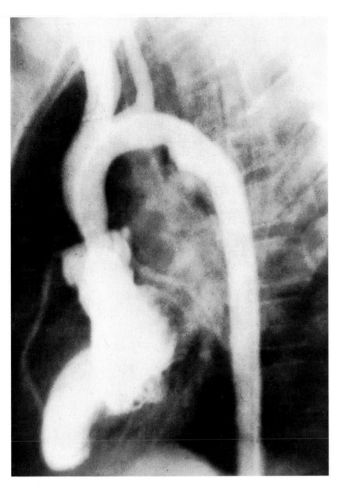

Figure 54.34. A left ventricular angiogram from a patient with supra-aortic stenosis showing marked septal hypertrophy. There is bulging into the outflow tract and irregular hypertrophy of the muscle and papillary muscle on the inferior border of the left ventricle.

60 mmHg at cardiac catheterization to relieve outflow obstruction, and to preserve the left ventricle. Usually a gusset is inserted into the aorta just above the valve. Myectomy is occasionally needed if the subvalvar region is very hypertrophied. Although the majority of patients will benefit, there are some in whom tunnel obstruction exists. These cannot be relieved by a gusset and require replacement of the root. Surgical mortality is low unless there is serious myocardial damage and dysfunction. Following surgery, mild aortic regurgitation is common and there is often systemic hypertension. Surgery on patients in the first decade of life is usually very successful but recurrence is described, sometimes more distally in the aortic arch. The diffuse arterial changes will persist; consequently long-term supervision as for other cardiovascular disorders is important.

——— AORTIC REGURGITATION ———

Aortic regurgitation presenting as an isolated lesion in childhood is very uncommon. Aortic regurgitation may, however, result from congenital abnormalities, acquired primary heart disease or a combination of acquired pathology on a congenital disorder. Any of the stenotic lesions may develop regurgitation, either as a result of endocarditis or because the lesion itself interferes with aortic valvar function as in fixed subaortic stenosis.

CLINICAL FEATURES ———

Symptoms occur late in aortic regurgitation unless the lesion develops acutely. Symptoms from chronic regurgitation result from left ventricular dysfunction, with effort dyspnoea, pulmonary oedema and sometimes heart failure. Angina is very unusual but may occur with acquired lesions and aortic root or coronary orifice involvement (Table 54.2).

The pulse pressure reflects the degree of aortic regurgitation except in the presence of heart failure. The carotid arterial pulsations are usually easily visible in severe regurgitation. The patient's head may nod in time with systole; this is de Musset's sign. It commemorates a Frenchman who suffered from syphilitic aortitis and aortic valvar disease.

There are systolic and diastolic murmurs at the left sternal edge, an overactive enlarged left ventricle, a mid-diastolic murmur at the apex (the Austin–Flint murmur), and a loud sound of aortic valvar closure. The diastolic murmur is usually loudest at the right sternal edge and may even accompany a thrill in lesions where the aortic root is grossly dilated. Rupture of an aortic leaflet produces aortic regurgitation with a very characteristic mewing or seagull murmur. Since the peripheral pulse reflects the severity of regurgitation, it may be anything from normal through jerky to collapsing. In very severe cases of regurgitation, even the retinal arteries show increased pulsation.

The electrocardiographic changes depend on severity and duration of regurgitation. Voltages in the left ventricular leads increase, with deep S waves in V1 and R waves in I, AVL, V5 and V6. T waves usually remain tall and upright until left ventricular dysfunction has

Table 54.2. Aetiology of aortic regurgitation

Aortic valvar abnormality: bicuspid, unicuspid or quadricuspid
Aorta to left ventricle tunnel
Ventricular septal defect and aortic regurgitation (Chapter 37)
Fistula from left coronary artery to left ventricle (Chapter 60)
Rheumatic fever
Endocarditis
Prolapsing chondritis
Wegener's granuloma
Ruptured aneurysm sinus of Valsalva
Viral arteritis
Postoperative occurrence following surgery to the left
  ventricular outflow tract

occurred, when ST depression and inversion is present. Unless there is aortic root disease involving the coronary arterial orifices, Q waves from cavity dilation precede the tall R waves in the left ventricular lead. Once regurgitation is severe and long established, P mitrale is sometimes seen on the electrocardiogram.

The chest radiograph shows cardiomegaly with left atrial dilation and prominence of the ascending aorta and aortic knuckle. The mildest lesions are associated with a normal chest radiograph.

Cross-sectional echocardiography and Doppler ultrasound confirm the diagnosis and often give the clinician further information about the degree of severity. Parasternal long-axis views show a large, vigorously contracting left ventricle, moderate left ventricular hypertrophy, and often a morphologically normal aortic valve. Prolapse of an aortic leaflet associated with deficient septation or following endocarditis is well demonstrated on this view (Figure 54.35). Similar appearances are also seen from the apical long-axis view. Colour flow mapping readily identifies the area at which regurgitation occurs, often localizing it very accurately to one or other leaflet. Although one may guess at the degree of regurgitation by how far the colour in the jet spreads down into the left ventricular cavity, this is not a reliable index and cannot be quantified accurately (Plate 54.2). There is no completely satisfactory ultrasonic method for measuring regurgitation, although echo Doppler volumetric assessments of regurgitant fraction have been employed. The methodology here is fraught with inaccuracy, and it is almost certainly not worth the trouble. Left ventricular size at end diastole is still the best indicator of the degree of left ventricular volume overload, and should be measured on a regular basis to try to determine the optimal timing for reparative surgery or valvar replacement.

AORTIC–LEFT VENTRICULAR TUNNEL

Although described as a tunnel (implying that it has length and two openings) this lesion is more correctly described as a defect (Serino et al, 1983). The defect lies between the right aortic sinus and its leaflet, it is separate from the right coronary arterial orifice (Ho et al, 1998) (Figure 54.36). Free reflux occurs from the aorta to the left ventricle, producing aneurysmal dilation of the right aortic sinus, dilation of the left ventricle, and widening of the ascending aorta. In time, the whole aortic root becomes dilated with secondary valvar regurgitation. The lesion may be associated with aortic valvar stenosis or abnormalities of the origins of the coronary arteries. This diagnosis should be considered in any child who presents with severe aortic regurgitation in infancy or in the newborn period.

An aortic–left ventricular tunnel can produce heart failure in the infant, but more often the patient presents with well compensated and impressive aortic regurgitation and dilation and hypertrophy of the left ventricle. The physical signs suggest severe aortic regurgitation, with loud aortic valvar closure and a systolic thrill at the left and right sternal edges. The dilated ascending aorta may be palpable on the right side of the chest. On the chest radiograph, the dilated right aortic sinus may protrude on to the left heart border and the aorta is enlarged (Figure 54.37). Diagnosis can be made by cross-sectional echocardiography, but angiocardiography is usually carried out, and shows the characteristic distortion of the right aortic sinus (Figure 54.38). In the older child, it is easy to confuse rupture of the sinus of Valsalva with the tunnel abnormality. Surgical repair is carried out as soon as the diagnosis is made in the hope of preventing valvar regurgitation. Usually, however, the regurgitation persists despite closure, and replacement of the aortic valve may be necessary.

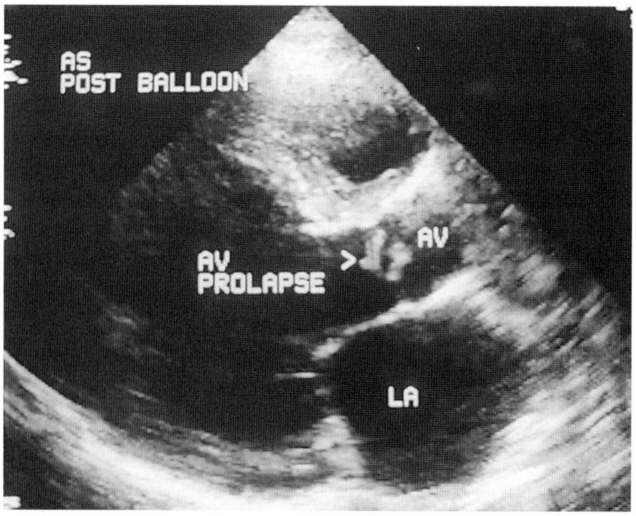

Figure 54.35. Aortic valvar (AV) prolapse in parasternal long-axis view. AS, aortic stenosis; LA left atrium; RV, right ventricle.

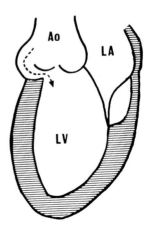

Figure 54.36. Diagram illustrating the morphology of the aorto-left ventricular defect, formerly presumed to be a 'tunnel'. Ao, aorta; LA, left atrium; LV, left ventricle.

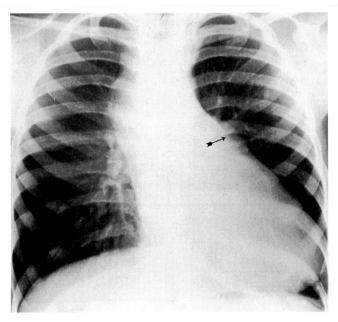

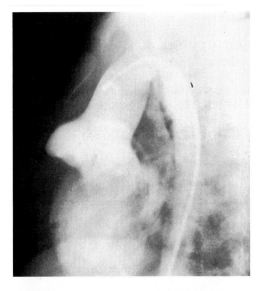

Figure 54.37. Chest radiograph of 6-year-old patient with aorto-left ventricular defect showing a dilated right aortic sinus on the left cardiac border (arrow). The ascending aorta is also dilated as a result of chronic aortic regurgitation. The left ventricle is large.

OTHER CAUSES OF AORTIC REGURGITATION —

Patients with congenital floppiness of a bicuspid or multicusp valve may present with aortic regurgitation. Echocardiography makes the diagnosis quickly and easily. Acquired aortic regurgitation may be caused by relapsing chondritis. This is an autoimmune problem presenting in childhood or adolescence as a long-standing illness with cycles of fever and illness. The acute regurgitation in this condition results from avulsion of the leaflet. Rheumatic aortic regurgitation can be the lone lesion in a young patient with a history of rheumatic fever, although additional involvement of the mitral valve is much more common. This condition is discussed in detail in Chapter 43.

In almost all forms of isolated aortic regurgitation in childhood that is severe enough to cause a haemodynamic abnormality, replacement of the aortic valve is the treatment of choice. The surgical options are discussed earlier in this chapter, and include the Ross procedure or insertion of a mechanical valve.

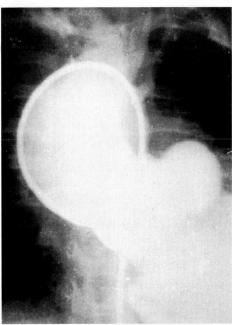

Figure 54.38. Aortograms from two patients with aorto-left ventricular defect. The frontal projection in one patient shows huge dilation of the aortic sinus, which protrudes on the bottom cardiac border. The lateral view is from the other patient. Both had severe aortic regurgitation.

REFERENCES

Al Marsafawy H M F, Ho S Y, Redington A N, Anderson R H 1995 The relationship of the outlet septum in the aortic outflow tracts in hearts with interruption of the aortic arch. Journal of the Thoracic and Cardiovascular Surgery 109: 1225–1236

Angelini A, Ho S Y, Anderson R H et al 1989 The morphology of the normal aortic valve as compared with the aortic valve having two leaflets. Journal of Thoracic and Cardiovascular Surgery 98(3): 362–367

Becu L, Somerville J, Galio A 1976 'Isolated' pulmonary valve stenosis as a part of more widespread cardiovascular disease. British Heart Journal 38: 472–482

Black J A, Bonham Carter R E 1963 Association between aortic stenosis and facies of severe infantile hypercalcaemia. Lancet ii: 745–749

Braunwald G, Goldblatt A, Aygen M M, Rockoff S D, Morrow A G 1963 Congenital aortic stenosis, I. Clinical and haemodynamic findings in 100 patients. Circulation 27: 426–432

Duncan K, Sullivan I, Robinson P, Horvath P, de Leval M, Stark J 1986 Transventricular aortic valvotomy for critical aortic stenosis in infants. Journal of Thoracic and Cardiovascular Surgery 93: 546–550

Emmanuel R, Withers R, O'Brien K, Ross P, Feizi O 1978 Congenitally bicuspid aortic valves. Clinicogenetic study of 41 families. British Heart Journal 40: 1402–1407

Edwards J E 1965 Pathology of left ventricular outflow tract obstruction. Circulation 31: 586–599

Edwards W D, Leaf D S, Edwards J E 1978 Dissecting aneurysm associated with congenital bicuspid aortic valve. Circulation 57: 1022–1025

Gerosa G, McKay R, Ross D N 1991 Replacement of the aortic valve or root with a pulmonary autograft in children. Annals of Thoracic Surgery 51: 424–429

Gewilling M, Daenen W, Dumoulin M, vans der Hauwaert T 1992 Rheologic genesis of discrete subvalvular aortic stenosis: A Doppler echocardiographic study. Annals of Thoracic Surgery 19(4): 818–824

Hahn R T, Roman M J, Mogtader A H, Devereux R B 1992 Association of aortic dilatation with regurgitant, stenotic and functionally normal bicuspid aortic valves. Journal of the American College of Cardiology 19(2): 283–288

Ho S Y, Muriago M, Cook A C, Thieme G, Anderson R H 1998 Surgical anatomy of aorto-left ventricular tunnel. Annals of Thoracic Surgery 65: 509–514

Hossack K F, Neutze J M, Lowe J B, Barratt-Boyes B G 1980 Congenital valvar aortic stenosis. Natural history and assessment for operation. British Heart Journal 43: 561–573

Hsiech K, Keane J F, Nadas A S, Bernhard W F, Castaneda A R 1986 Long term follow-up of valvotomy before 1968 for congenital aortic stenosis. American Journal of Cardiology 58: 338–341

James F W 1981 Exercise testing in normal individuals and patients with cardiovascular disease. Cardiovascular Clinics 11(2): 227–246

Jefferson R D, Burn J, Gaunt K L, Hunter S, Davison E V 1986 A terminal deletion of the long arm of chromosome 4 [46, XX, del (4) q33] in an infant with phenotypic features of William's syndrome. Journal of Medical Genetics 23: 474–477

Johnson R G, Williams G R, Razook J D, Thompson W M, Lane M M, Elkins R C 1984 Re-operation in congenital aortic stenosis. Annals of Thoracic Surgery 40(2): 156–162

Jordan S C, Scott O 1973 Heart disease in paediatrics. Butterworth, London

Kitchiner D, Jackson M, Malaiya N, Walse K, Arnold R, Smith A 1994 Morphology of left ventricular outflow tract structures in patients with subaortic stenosis and a ventricular septal defect. British Heart Journal 72(3): 251–260

Labadidi Z, Wu J, Walls J T 1984 Percutaneous aortic valvuloplasty: results in 23 patients. American Journal of Cardiology 53: 194–197

Lambert E C, Menon V A, Wagner H R, Vlad P 1974 Sudden unexpected death from cardiovascular disease in children. A cooperative international study. American Journal of Cardiology 34: 89–94

Leung M P, McKay R, Smith A, Anderson R H, Arnold R 1991 Critical aortic stenosis in early infancy. Anatomic

and echocardiographic substrates of successful open valvotomy. Journal of Thoracic and Cardiovascular Surgery 101(3): 526–535

Levine R A, Jimoh A, Cape E G, McMillan S, Yoganshan A P, Weyman A E 1989 Pressure recovery distal to a stenosis: potential cause of gradient 'over estimation' by Doppler echocardiography. Journal of the American College of Cardiology 13(3): 706–715

McElhinney D B, Reddy V M, Silverman N H, Hanley F L 1998 Accessory and anomalous atrioventricular valvar tissue causing outflow tract obstruction; surgical implications of a heterogeneous and complex problem. Journal of the American College of Cardiology 32: 1741–1748

McKay R, Ross D 1982 Technique for the relief of discrete subaortic stenosis. Journal of Thoracic and Cardiovascular Surgery 84: 917–920

McKay R, Smith A, Leung M P, Arnold R, Anderson R H 1992 Morphology of the ventriculoaortic junction in critical aortic stenosis. Implications for haemodynamic function and clinical management. Journal of Thoracic and Cardiovascular Surgery 104(2): 434–442

McKusick V A 1972 Association of congenital bicuspid aortic valve and Erdheim's cystic medial necrosis. Lancet 1: 1026–1027

Messina L M, Turley K, Stanger P, Hoffman J I E, Ebert P A 1984 Successful aortic valvotomy for severe congenital valvular aortic stenosis in the newborn infant. Journal of Thoracic and Cardiovascular Surgery 88: 92–96

Mosca R S, Iannettoni M D, Schwartz S M et al 1995 Critical aortic stenosis in the neonates. Journal of Thoracic and Cardiovascular Surgery 109(1): 147–154

Orsmond G S, Bessinger F B, Müller J H 1980 Rest and exercise haemodynamics in children before and after aortic valvotomy. American Heart Journal 29: 76–86

Peckham G B, Keith J O, Eyans J R 1964 Congenital aortic stenosis – some observations on the natural history and clinical assessment. Canadian Medical Association Journal 91: 639–643

Peterson T A, Todd D B, Edwards J E 1965 Supraventricular aortic stenosis. Journal of Thoracic and Cardiovascular Surgery 50: 734–741

Presbitero P, Somerville J, Revel-Chion R, Ross D 1982 Open aortic valvotomy for congenital aortic stenosis. Late results. British Heart Journal 47: 26–34

Riopel D A, Taylor A B, Hohn A R 1977 Blood pressure response to treadmill exercise in children with aortic stenosis. In: 46th annual meeting of the American Academy of Paediatrics, New York

Roberts W C 1970a The congenitally bicuspid aortic valve in clinically isolated aortic stenosis. An autopsy study of 162 patients over 15 years of age. Circulation 42: 91–97

Roberts W C 1970b The congenitally bicuspid aortic valve: a study of 85 autopsy cases. American Journal of Cardiology 26: 72–83

Rowe R D 1973 Cardiovascular disease in the rubella syndrome. Cardiovascular Clinics 5: 61–80

Sandor G G S, Olley P M, Trusler G A, Williams W G, Row R D, Morch J E 1980 Long term follow up patients after valvotomy for congenital valvular aortic stenosis in children. Journal of Thoracic and Cardiovascular Surgery 80: 171–178

Serino W, Andrade J, Ross D, de Leval M, Somerville J 1983 Aorto-left ventricular communication after closure. Late post operative problems. British Heart Journal 49: 501–506

Shone J D, Sellers R D, Anderson R C, Adams P Jr, Lillehei C W, Edwards J E 1963 The developmental complex of 'parachute mitral valve', supravalvar ring of left atrium, subaortic stenosis and coarctation of the aorta. American Journal of Cardiology 11: 714–725

Skjaerpe T, Hegrenaes L, Hatle L 1985 Non-invasive estimation of valve area in patients with aortic stenosis by Doppler ultrasound and two dimensional echocardiography. Circulation 72: 810–818

Somerville J 1981 Congenital cardiovascular disease or congenital heart disease – a time for change in concepts? In: Becker A E, Loosekoot T G, Marcelletti C, Anderson R H (eds) Paediatric cardiology. Churchill Livingstone, Edinburgh, vol. 3, p 324–345

Somerville J 1985 Fixed subaortic stenosis – a frequently misunderstood lesion. [Editorial note] International Journal of Cardiology 8: 145–148

Somerville J, Ross D 1971 Congenital aortic stenosis – an unusual form. Consideration of surgical management. British Heart Journal 33: 552–558

Somerville J, Ross D 1982 Homograft replacement of aortic root with re-implantation of coronary arteries. Results after one to five yars. British Heart Journal 47: 473–482

Somerville J, Stone S, Ross O 1980 Fate of patients with fixed subaortic stenosis after surgical removal. British Heart Journal 43: 429–647

Stamm C, Li J, Ho S Y, Redington A N, Anderson R H 1997 The aortic root in supravalvular stenosis: the potential surgical relevance of morphologic findings. Journal of Thoracic and Cardiovascular Surgery 114: 16–24

Sullivan I D, Wren C, Bain H H et al 1989 Balloon aortic valvotomy for congenital aortic stenosis in childhood. British Heart Journal 61: 186–191

Sutton J P III, Ho S Y, Anderson R H 1995 The forgotten interleaflet triangles: a review of the surgical anatomy of the aortic valve. Annals of Thoracic Surgery 59: 419–427

Vollebergh F E, Becker A E 1977 Minor congenital variations of cusp size in tricuspid aortic valves. Possible link with isolated aortic stenosis. British Heart Journal 39: 1006–1011

Williams J C P, Barratt-Boyes B G, Lowe J B 1961 Supravalvular aortic stenosis. Circulation 24: 1311–1318

Zeevi B, Keane J F, Castaneda A R, Perry S B, Lock J E 1989 Neonatal critical valvar aortic stenosis. Circulation 80: 831–839

55

Anomalies of the coronary arteries

N. H. Silverman and P. R. Lurie

This chapter will deal with coronary anomalies in hearts in which the overall structure is normal. The special coronary arterial circulations found with major cardiac anomalies will be dealt with in the corresponding chapters. These defects are rare, occurring in 0.3 to 1.3% of one autopsy series (Alexander and Griffith, 1956), but it is extremely difficult to estimate prevalence, as it depends upon recognition. The milder anomalies escape notice both during life and at postmortem.

MORPHOLOGY

Normal coronary arterial anatomy may be summarized as described by James (1961) (Figure 55.1). Two arterial orifices are placed relatively centrally in the right and left sinuses of Valsalva. The right coronary artery arises from the right sinus of Valsalva. Having entered the atrioventricular groove, it sends an infundibular branch anteriorly and then courses backward and inferiorly, terminating in the majority of hearts in the posterior interventricular groove. In approximately 50% of people, there is a separate origin of the infundibular branch (Schlesinger et al, 1949; Baroldi and Scomazzoni, 1967). The main stem of the left coronary artery arises from the left sinus of Valsalva and emerges perpendicularly for a few millimeters. It then bifurcates into an anterior descending branch (which traverses the anterior inter-

ventricular groove) and a circumflex branch, which courses around the left atrioventricular groove and may terminate in the posterior interventricular groove. In only 1% of people are there separate origins of the left circumflex and anterior descending coronary arteries from the left sinus (Schlesinger et al, 1949; Baroldi and Scomazzoni, 1967; Ogden and Goodyer, 1970; Vlodaver et al, 1975; Dicicco et al, 1982; Roberts, 1986).

When both right and left coronary arteries supply a branch to the posterior interventricular groove, the system is said to be 'balanced'. In the right-dominant system, which occurs in 90% of normals, the right coronary supplies one large or two smaller branches to this groove with no contribution from the left. In the left-dominant system, the converse is true. All three alternatives are normal variations (Figure 55.1).

The three principal arteries all give off branches superiorly to the atriums and inferiorly to the ventricles. The major branches remain superficial and visible through the epicardium until they terminate in broom-like arborizations that penetrate the myocardium. Over the left ventricle, these penetrating arteries proceed perpendicularly through the wall, being occluded by ventricular contraction; consequently, the left ventricular myocardium is perfused during diastole (Gregg and Fisher, 1963).

There may be anomalies in the locations, numbers and patency of the coronary orifices, and in the course of the proximal portions of the coronary arteries (Ogden, 1970). More distally, anomalies include a totally or partially intramural course and fistulous communication from a coronary artery to a coronary vein, to myocardial sinusoids, or to a cardiac chamber.

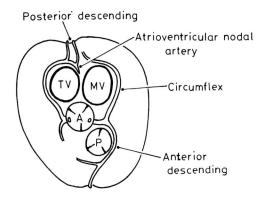

Figure 55.1. The normal coronary arteries are shown looking at the heart from above and in front, with the atriums removed. In this instance, with both arteries to the posterior interventricular grove taking origin from the right coronary artery, the system is right dominant. TV, tricuspid valve; MV, mitral valve; A, aorta; P, pulmonary trunk.

MORPHOGENESIS

The morphogenesis of these anomalies is easily related to what is known of early embryonic development. When myocardial cells are first observed to contract, there is no defined coronary circulation. The cells are loosely assembled and bathed in the blood, which they pump. The walls of the heart only gradually condense, with normal persistence of sinusoids within the walls connecting with the ventricular cavities. According to Hackensellner (1956), the coronary arteries themselves appear as buds from both the aorta and pulmonary trunk in the seventh week of life shortly after partition of the truncus. Subsequent workers have been unable to confirm the origin of buds from the pulmonary trunk, while questions also have arisen concerning the outgrowth of buds from the aorta. More recent evidence suggests that the arteries develop from a network of capillaries that appears in the epicardium, and that this system then sends major branches into the aortic sinuses Bogers et al, 1988). Various combinations in this system of faulty persistence, failure to develop or atrophy after appearance are sufficient to explain the more proximal arterial anomalies. Anastomoses of the coronary arterial branches with ingrowing veins and the primitive sinusoidal spaces explain the various types of fistulous communication.

INVESTIGATION

Abnormalities of the coronary arteries can be investigated by means of electrocardiography, nuclear isotope techniques, magnetic resonance imaging, fast scanning computed tomography, echocardiography and angiography from the aortic root and coronary arterial system itself.

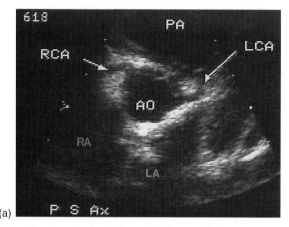 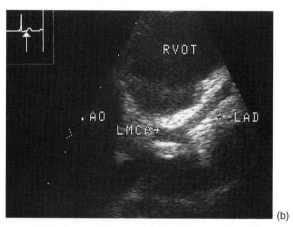

Figure 55.2. The normal echocardiographic images of the coronary arteries can usually be seen from the parasternal long-axis view. (a) A parasternal short-axis view of the aortic root (AO) shows the origins of the right (RCA) and left (LCA) coronary arteries. The left coronary artery runs posterior to the pulmonary trunk (PA). Posteriorly lie the right atrium (RA) and left atrium (LA). (b) A magnified view of the main stem of the left coronary artery (LMCA) dividing into the left anterior descending aorta (LAD) and the circumflex coronary arteries. RVOT, right ventricular outflow tract.

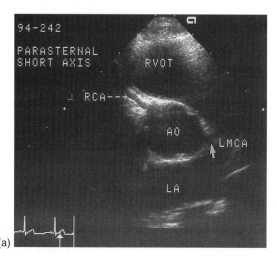 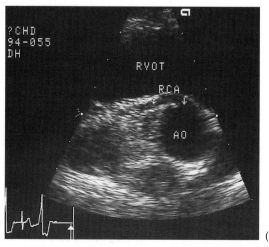

Figure 55.3. (a) This parasternal short-axis view of the coronary arteries focuses on the right coronary artery arising from the right sinus of Valsalva. The main stem of the left coronary artery (LMCA, arrow) is also seen to arise from the left sinus. The right ventricular outflow tract lies anteriorly. (b) A magnified, slightly cranially obtained view of the right coronary artery as it enters the right atrioventricular groove. Abbreviations as in Figure 55.2.

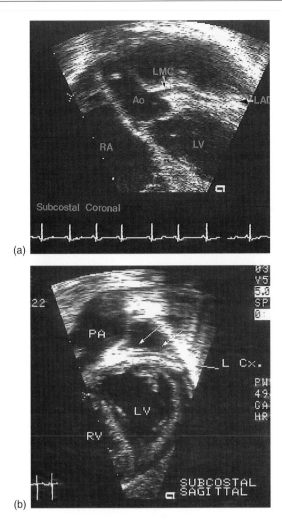

(a)

(b)

Figure 55.4. Subcostal views of the proximal left coronary arterial system in normal children. (a) A magnified subcostal coronal view of the heart. The left ventricle (LV), aortic root (Ao), and right atrium (RA) are identified. The main stem of the left coronary artery (LMC) can be seen to arise from the aortic root and to continue on the surface of the heart as the left anterior descending coronary artery (LAD). (b) The subcostal sagittal view of the left circumflex (L Cx.) coronary artery as it courses in the atrioventricular groove. PA, pulmonary trunk; RV, right ventricle.

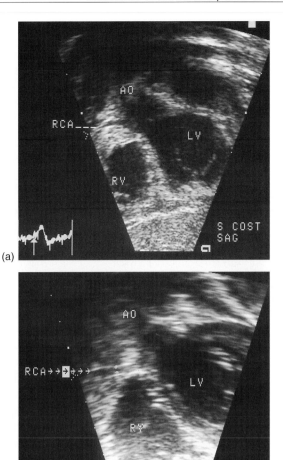

(a)

(b)

Figure 55.5. Subcostal views of the proximal right coronary arterial system in normal children. (a) An oblique subcostal sagittal view shows the origin and proximal course of the right coronary artery arising from the aortic root. (b) A magnified view of the more distal course of the right coronary artery as it runs in the atrioventricular groove above the right ventricle. Abbreviations as in Figure 55.2.

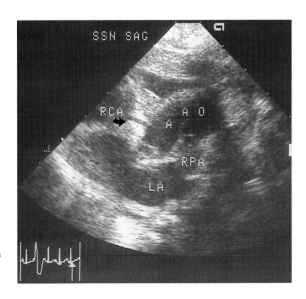

Figure 55.6. A suprasternal sagittal view demonstrates the right coronary artery (RCA) arising from the aorta and running anteriorly (arrow). The right pulmonary artery (RPA) running in cross-section can be seen in the crux of the arch, and the left atrium (LA) can be seen posteriorly.

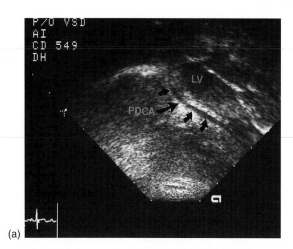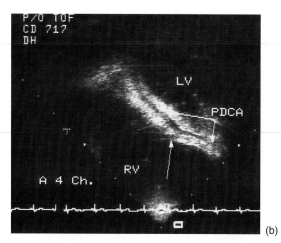

(a) (b)

Figure 55.7. Apical views of the posterior descending coronary artery. (a) A subcostal coronal view near the crux of the heart. The scan plane has passed superiorly from the diaphragm, and the posterior descending coronary artery (PDCA) comes into view on the ventricular surface. (b) The posterior portion of the left ventricle is seen superiorly. The posterior descending coronary artery can also be seen from the apical view (arrows) as the scan plane is directed posteriorly from the apical four chamber view. The left (LV) and right (RV) ventricles can be seen to straddle the artery. A single arrow points toward a right ventricular branch of this vessel.

Echocardiographic imaging of the coronary system has improved greatly since the first edition of this volume appeared. It is now possible to evaluate coronary arterial morphology with considerable accuracy, particularly the proximal segments of the coronary arteries (Figures 55.2–55.7; Plate 55.1).

ORIGIN OF THE LEFT CORONARY ARTERY FROM THE PULMONARY TRUNK

INCIDENCE

A left coronary artery originating from the pulmonary trunk occurs in 1:250 to 1:400 of all cases of congenital heart disease. The male:female incidence is 2.3:1 (Neufeld and Schneeweis, 1983).

PATHOPHYSIOLOGY

HAEMODYNAMICS RELATED TO MORPHOLOGY

In the fetus, the heart develops quite normally. After birth, as long as the pulmonary arterial pressure remains at or near systemic levels, the left ventricular myocardium supplied by the anomalous artery remains well perfused. The avidity of myocardium for oxygen is such that normal perfusion with blood of mixed-venous oxygen content presents no problem. As pressure in the pulmonary trunk falls postnatally, perfusion of the left ventricle begins to suffer because the period during which pressure in the coronary artery exceeds intramural left ventricular pressure becomes shorter. This circulatory handicap reduces left ventricular function, raising left

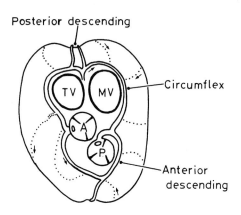

Figure 55.8. Origin of the left coronary artery from the pulmonary trunk. Small arrows indicate direction of collateral circulation from branches of the right coronary artery to those of the left. Dotted lines indicate enlarged collateral connections. Abbreviations as in Figure 55.1.

ventricular end-diastolic pressure and leading to pulmonary vasoconstriction, thus slowing the postnatal reduction of pulmonary arterial pressure and mitigating the handicap in perfusion. At the same time, the ischemic myocardium is being perfused increasingly by a developing set of collateral connections from the right coronary artery, which arises normally (Figure 55.8). Ideally, a superb set of perfectly distributed collateral arteries could be developed before the pulmonary arterial pressure had fallen sufficiently to result in significant ischaemic damage to the left ventricle. In less than ideal circumstances, the collateral connections may develop but are poorly distributed; consequently some portions of the left ventricle may be well perfused while others become ischaemic. In another pattern of abnormal distribution of the collateral arteries, there are large interconnections proximal to the branches supplying contracting myocardium that act as left-to-right (aortopulmonary) arterial shunts, requiring extra work from the left ventricle while deviating blood supply from its myocardium. This malformation presents a picture postnatally that may vary enormously from patient to patient, and also from time to time in a given patient (Wesselhoeft et al, 1968; Perry and Scott, 1970; Askenazi and Nadas, 1975). The end result is best evaluated in terms of time of onset of clinically observable myocardial ischaemia. At one extreme, this may never occur, while, at the other, disastrous damage to the myocardium occurs in the first weeks of infancy.

HAEMODYNAMIC RESPONSE

Anatomically, the right coronary artery at its origin enlarges, while the left tends to be small and thin walled, resembling a vein. The collateral circulation between the right and left systems may be diffusely large and well distributed and, as a result, the left ventricle is well perfused and the heart retains normal form and function. When the collateral connections are poorly developed or so distributed as to form a fistula between right coronary artery and pulmonary trunk, the left ventricle becomes ischaemic, dilated, infarcted and fibrosed. Often the fibrosis extends into the papillary muscles and the mitral valve itself (Foster et al, 1964). Mitral valvar competence may be compromised by these changes as well as by dilatation caused by ischaemia, resulting in stretching of the annulus. The right ventricle, and parts of the left, which are perfused by the right coronary artery, continue to contract well. The left atrium tends to enlarge and there is passive congestion of the lungs.

CLINICAL FINDINGS

PRESENTATION

The infant with myocardial ischaemia tends to have both the classic symptoms and signs of congestive heart failure and exhibits a very special type of anginal attack, which is recognized in infancy (Bland et al, 1933). Brought on usually by the stress of feeding or defecation, these are episodes in which the infant suddenly appears to be in severe distress, grunting or crying in short gasps, and is dyspnoeic, grey and sweaty. The child who has escaped myocardial ischaemia in infancy may present rather innocuously on a routine examination with an unexplained heart murmur, mild cardiomegaly or an abnormal electrocardiogram. Myocardial ischaemia may first present in adolescence or young adult life when, under the stress of maximally motivated exertion, either anginal pain or arrhythmia may occur. The latter may produce sudden unexplained death or near-miss death. The patient also may present with progressive mitral regurgitation, which may or may not be accompanied by electrocardiographic signs of ischaemia.

PHYSICAL SIGNS

The sick infant may have the general appearance of a baby in chronic congestive heart failure, may have the episodes described above, or may have both. The heart is usually large and is overactive parasternally, with an apex that may be hypo- or even dyskinetic. The first heart sound may be loud, normal or faint, with the second heart sound being loud, and third and fourth heart sounds often present. An apical holosystolic murmur of mitral regurgitation may be heard, and there may be an apical diastolic rumble.

The older child with adequate collateral circulation may have completely normal cardiac findings. Sometimes a continuous murmur is heard, leading to consideration of the diagnosis of a small patent arterial duct. Such a child may also have apical murmurs in systole and diastole owing to mild degrees of mitral valvar damage.

INVESTIGATIONS

ELECTROCARDIOGRAPHY

The sick infant with ischaemia and infarction in the portions of left ventricular myocardium supplied by the left coronary artery has sinus tachycardia. Rarely there may be premature ventricular contractions or ventricular tachycardia, pathological Q waves and abnormalities of the QRS and ST–T segments, compatible with anterior, anteroseptal or anterolateral infarction (Wesselhoeft et al, 1968). Electrocardiographic changes may be progressive as infarcts evolve. While the electrocardiogram is not likely to be normal, it may not show the classic findings for ischaemia or infarction; therefore, there are occasions in this disease when the electrocardiogram is not diagnostic. The vector cardiogram typically shows a counterclockwise loop in the horizontal plane. Again, this is far from invariable. The older child who has survived without symptoms may very well have a normal electrocardiogram.

RADIOLOGICAL FINDINGS

In the sick infant, the heart is in the normal position but is generally enlarged, with left atrial enlargement and pulmonary venous engorgement. In the older child, a normal chest radiograph may be expected.

ECHOCARDIOGRAPHIC FINDINGS

In the sick infant, echocardiography demonstrates left ventricular enlargement and depressed ventricular contractions. Mitral regurgitation is almost invariably present, and brightness of the endocardium is frequently observed, often associated with endocardial fibroelastosis (Silverman, 1993).

Previously, the echocardiographic findings were not specific in any patient (Fisher et al, 1981). In particular, the transverse sinus of the pericardium had been confused with a normal left coronary artery (Robinson et al, 1984). The advent of high-resolution scanning, and greater understanding of this phenomenon, have clarified the problems produced by imaging of the transverse coronary sinus through errors in lateral resolution of ultrasound (Robinson et al, 1984; Schmidt et al, 1988).

Definitive imaging of abnormal origin of the left coronary artery from the pulmonary trunk can now be achieved. As the artery enters the pulmonary trunk posteriorly, the cut to demonstrate this is required in the sagittal plane image (Figure 55.9 and Plate 55.2) (Martin et al, 1986; Sanders et al, 1989).

NUCLEAR IMAGING

Thallium-201 scintigraphy can yield a 'cold' area in the affected portion of the left ventricle (Finley et al, 1978; Rabinovitch et al, 1979); however, the same effect has been seen in some patients with cardiomyopathy (Gutgesell et al, 1980). The significance of gallium scanning in myocardial and coronary arterial disease requires further evaluation.

CARDIAC CATHETERIZATION

The physiological study using cardiac catheterization is performed to measure cardiac output, left ventricular end-diastolic pressure and pulmonary arterial pressure. The objective of angiocardiography is to establish the integrity and the source of the coronary arteries. In a very sick infant, the less done the better within the limits of adequate diagnosis. An aortic root injection may be sufficient to show clearly the early filling of the right coronary artery and the delayed passage via collateral vessels into the left coronary distribution and, finally, the pulmonary trunk. If the pulmonary trunk never clearly opacifies, it is desirable next to inject the pulmonary trunk, looking very carefully for small, usually diastolic, phasic filling of the left main stem and its circumflex and anterior descending branches. The finding of coronary arterial filling from the pulmonary trunk should rule out ligation of the main stem of the left coronary artery at its origin as a form of treatment for the patient (Figure 55.10).

Should adequate injections of both the aortic root and the pulmonary trunk still leave no clue as to the origin of the left coronary artery, one may consider selective injection of the right coronary artery, as recommended by Formanek et al (1980). If filming is available only in a single plane, a left anterior oblique projection gives optimal discrimination between the right and left coronary arterial beds. Though it may superimpose the origin of the right coronary artery on the origin of the left, if the aortic root is empty while the contrast is still reaching the pulmonary trunk, one injection will provide all the necessary data. With biplane filming, one can choose combinations of either posteroanterior plus lateral or right plus left anterior obliques, usually with equally good result.

In the sick infant, one is most concerned with the close resemblance of such patients to those with congestive cardiomyopathy (Ruttenberg et al, 1964). We now believe that any patient considered to have unexplained congestive cardiomyopathy should have high-quality cross-sectional echocardiographic imaging, with Doppler colour flow interrogation of the left coronary arterial system. In this manner, it is possible to exclude a large number of patients suspected of having anomalous arterial origin from the pulmonary trunk. If any doubt about the diagnosis remains, the patient should be given the benefit of cineangiography.

Much less likely statistically, but even more easily confused, is stenosis or atresia of the aortic origin of the left coronary artery. In such patients, the left coronary arterial branches are also filled from collateral connections with branches of the right coronary artery. No contrast, however, will enter the pulmonary trunk. Usually, it is not possible to find any contrast reaching the left coronary artery either from the aortic root or from the enlarged right coronary artery. It will at least be clear from aortography that such a patient does not have cardiomyopathy and does require an attempt at improving vascularization of the left ventricle.

COURSE AND PROGNOSIS

Some patients will stabilize and improve spontaneously as collateral circulation improves. The overall outlook for the group left untreated, however, is poor. Death may occur suddenly, owing to arrhythmia or to cardiogenic shock from further infarction. In the review of Wesselhoeft and colleagues (1968), 88% of the infants with angina and/or failure died. Prompt recognition and surgical treatment is the aim. Progressive mitral regurgitation is another course of disease progression. Close examination of coronary arteries is mandatory in all children with mitral regurgitation.

MANAGEMENT

Unless the patient is symptomatic, no treatment is likely to be called for as no diagnosis will usually have been made.

MEDICAL MANAGEMENT

In the ideal situation, when the diagnosis is suspected clinically, and catheterization studies are to be done to confirm the diagnosis as a preliminary to early surgery, low cardiac output and congestive heart failure preferably should be managed with carefully titrated dopamine or dobutamine given intravenously. An agent that adjustabli reduces afterload (such as nitroprusside or glyceryl trinitrate (nitroglycerin)) may be given by infusion, provided blood pressure is adequate. Digoxin is

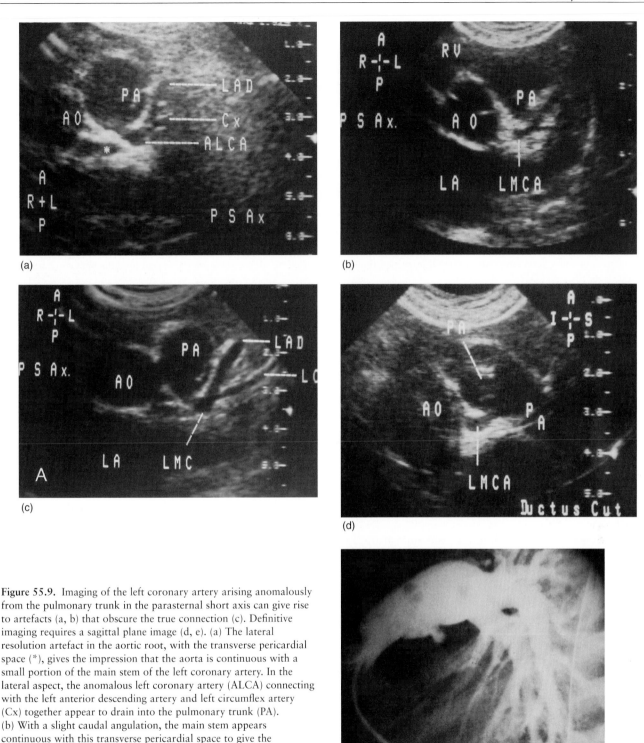

(a)

(b)

(c)

(d)

(e)

Figure 55.9. Imaging of the left coronary artery arising anomalously from the pulmonary trunk in the parasternal short axis can give rise to artefacts (a, b) that obscure the true connection (c). Definitive imaging requires a sagittal plane image (d, e). (a) The lateral resolution artefact in the aortic root, with the transverse pericardial space (*), gives the impression that the aorta is continuous with a small portion of the main stem of the left coronary artery. In the lateral aspect, the anomalous left coronary artery (ALCA) connecting with the left anterior descending artery and left circumflex artery (Cx) together appear to drain into the pulmonary trunk (PA). (b) With a slight caudal angulation, the main stem appears continuous with this transverse pericardial space to give the artefactual appearance directed toward the aortic root. (c) The main stem of the left coronary artery (LMC) is seen to originate from the pulmonary trunk. By connecting the transverse pericardial space with the artery and the aortic root, this makes it possible to misconstrue a continuity between the aorta, the transverse pericardial space, and the main stem of the left coronary artery. (d) A so-called sagittal cut demonstrates the main stem of the left coronary artery (LMCA) draining into the pulmonary trunk. This example was taken just prior to angiography (e) and demonstrates the double lines of the echo from the catheter within the pulmonary trunk. The aortic root can be seen to lie immediately below and adjacent to the pulmonary root. We have termed this a 'ductal cut' because it is a truly sagittally oriented image. (e) A catheter is placed through the right ventricular outflow tract and into the pulmonary trunk and a pulmonary artery angiogram is carried out. At the time of this still frame, the proximal origin of the anomalous left coronary artery could be seen as a bulge coming off the posterior and inferior aspect of the pulmonary trunk. A, anterior; P, posterior; L, left; R, right; other abbreviations as in Figure 55.2. (Published with permission of the *Journal of the American College of Cardiology*, from (Schmidt et al, 1988.))

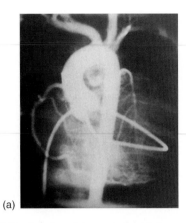
(a)

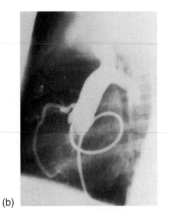
(b)

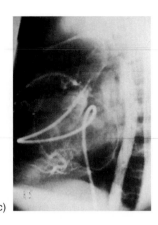
(c)

Figure 55.10. A series of cineangiographic images from the patient shown in Plate 55.2. (a) The posteroanterior projection, showing the left coronary artery entering into the pulmonary trunk. (b) Lateral projection shows the right coronary artery filling from the aorta, and no filling of the left coronary artery. (c) A later frame in lateral projection shows the filling of the left coronary arterial system from the right coronary artery.

to be avoided, because it promotes arrhythmias in the postoperative period when the ischaemic myocardium is reperfused (Kaplinsky et al, 1981). The diagnosis often is not considered initially, however, and most of these patients are given digoxin. Substitution of an inotropic catecholamine for digoxin should be made as soon as possible. Pain, anxiety and air-hunger should be treated with morphine in order to diminish myocardial requirements for oxygen.

SURGICAL MANAGEMENT

The diagnosis of this condition is the indication for operation. The specific aim is to preserve as much myocardium as possible (Castañeda et al, 1994). In the small subset where the cardiac function is profoundly depressed, heart transplantation may be a more desirable option. Modern surgical techniques make it possible to support the circulation further by means of devices that assist the left ventricle or provide extracorporeal membrane oxygenation.

The aim of surgery is to re-establish prograde perfusion of the left coronary arterial system with aortic blood. To these ends, the experience gained in transplanting coronary arteries with the arterial switch procedure for complete transposition has made this approach the most popular. It also provides the best option for surgery. When technical considerations make this operation difficult, such as when the orifice of the artery is in an unfavourable position, the transpulmonary baffle described by Takeuchi et al (1979) can be performed. Bypass grafting using the carotid and internal mammary arteries, or saphenous venous grafts, is now performed much less frequently. The procedure of ligating the left coronary artery has, quite correctly, been all but abandoned. As indicated, when the ischaemia has become global and irreversible, the option of a cardiac transplant is an alternative therapy.

OTHER ANOMALIES AND VARIATIONS —OF ORIGIN AND COURSE—

Most of the anomalies covered in this section are of little clinical importance in childhood. They may become important in adolescence and early adult life, when extremes of physical exertion may cause significant intolerance of malfunction previously well tolerated. They may also be significant in middle age, when the additional effects of atherosclerotic changes have become clinically manifest. Anomalies then may be discovered in the performance or interpretation of selective coronary arteriography. The malformations are also being recognized increasingly, albeit still very rarely, in the investigation of syncopal episodes or 'near-miss' sudden death.

STENOSIS OR ATRESIA OF THE MAIN STEM OF THE LEFT CORONARY ARTERY

Stenosis of the main stem of the left coronary artery is an exception to the above statement, as it may be lethal in infancy and may be treatable. The origin, and sometimes a short length of the artery, either fail to canalize or involute (Figure 55.11). Much as when the left coronary artery arises from the pulmonary trunk, the circulation on the left side depends upon collateral blood flow from the branches of the right coronary artery. Byrum et al (1980) reviewed this rare problem, probably less than one tenth as common as origin of the left coronary artery from the pulmonary trunk. The severity of symptoms, signs and laboratory findings is related inversely to the size and distribution of the collateral vessels. Some patients have survived without symptoms for many years (Fortuin and Roberts, 1971). Infants who present with evidence of myocardial ischaemia are urgently in need of diagnosis and treatment. Results obtained by catheterization in these infants may easily be confused with those

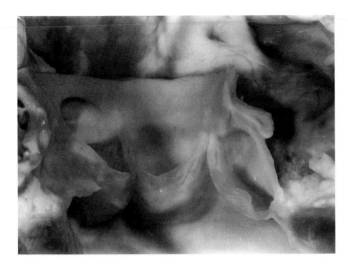

Figure 55.11. This specimen, from a child who died suddenly, shows atresia of the main stem of the left coronary artery. (Reproduced by kind permission of Dr J R. Zuberbuhler, Children's Hospital of Pittsburgh, PA.)

occurring with origin of the left coronary artery from the pulmonary trunk. On aortography, the large right coronary artery will be seen to fill the distribution of the left coronary artery via multiple connections from collateral branches. No contrast material will be seen entering the pulmonary trunk. There may be a wisp of filling of the left coronary artery from the aorta. There will certainly be no filling of the left coronary circuit from the pulmonary trunk on pulmonary arteriography. Cross-sectional echocardiography will demonstrate the left coronary artery in its normal location, but it will be diminutive or atretic for a few millimetres. In contrast with the more encouraging outlook today for the infant with anomalous left coronary artery from the pulmonary trunk, this lesion has never been treated successfully in early infancy. If the symptoms in a given patient are life threatening, an attempt at some sort of canalization, dilation or bypass graft seems warranted.

OTHER ABNORMALITIES OF ARTERIAL ORIGIN

The orifice of the artery may be ovoid instead of round. They may be located eccentrically in the sinus of Valsalva or just above or totally remote from the sinus. In this regard, it should be noted that a significant proportion of the normal population, up to 20%, have the coronary arteries arising at or above the level of the sinutubular junction (Muriago et al, 1997). A coronary artery may originate from an artery other than the aorta, such as an intercostal or internal thoracic artery. A 12-year-old girl who died suddenly with no previous cardiac history was observed by us at postmortem to have a left coronary artery arising from the internal thoracic (mammary) artery. The artery then passed between, and was apparently compressed by, the aorta and the pulmonary trunk.

Two orifices within a single sinus usually occur along with anomalous proximal arterial segments.

ANOMALIES OF THE PROXIMAL SEGMENTS

A very common normal variation in the proximal segments is a second small orifice in the right sinus of Valsalva that gives rise directly to the infundibular (conus) artery (Figure 55.12). Instead of originating from the left main coronary artery, the circumflex artery may arise as a branch of the right coronary artery (Figure 55.13), or from a separate orifice in the right aortic sinus. It may pass between the front of the aorta and the free-standing subpulmonary infundibulum in such a way as to be compressed between them in systole. Partial intramural course of such arteries through the wall of the aortic sinus has been shown to be significant as a cause of sudden death in juveniles (Corrado et al, 1992).

Another anomalous origin of the left circumflex artery occurs when it is a first branch from the right coronary artery that winds around behind the aorta to the left atrioventricular groove and then travels normally (Figure 55.14).

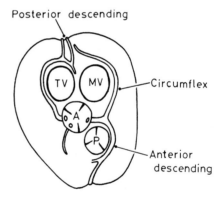

Figure 55.12. Origin of the infundibular (conus) artery from an accessory orifice in the right sinus of Valsalva. Abbreviations as in Figure 55.1.

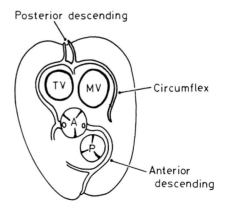

Figure 55.13. The circumflex artery arising as a terminal extension of the right coronary artery. Abbreviations as in Figure 55.1.

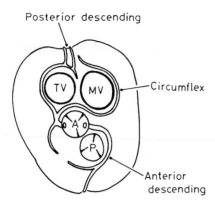

Figure 55.14. The circumflex artery arising as a first branch of the right coronary artery. Abbreviations as in Figure 55.1.

Single coronary arteries, whether arising from the right (Figure 55.15) or the left (Figure 55.16) sinus of Valsalva, are large vessels that pass completely around the heart, giving off all the usual normal branches (Sharbaugh and White, 1974). A single coronary artery has no pathological implications except when atherosclerosis occurs; or when it takes an anomalous course resulting in compression (see below). There may or may not be an atrophic relic of the opposite artery. It differs from stenosis or

atresia of the orifice in that the flow to the side without the orifice is directly through the large single coronary artery with normal branches, as opposed to collateral flow through branches of the arterial bed with the normal artery to branches of the bed with the deficient orifice.

ABERRANT COURSE

Cheitlin and colleagues (1974) have pointed out the pathological significance of a single coronary artery (Figure 55.17) or of both coronary arteries (Figure 55.18) arising from the right sinus of Valsalva when the branch or artery that supplies the left coronary distribution courses leftward between the aorta and pulmonary artery and, can, therefore, be compressed. They showed a striking incidence of sudden unexplained death in adolescents and young adults, and a strong relation of death to heavy exertion. Maron et al (1980) studied 29 hearts of competitive athletes dying during play, aged 13–30 years, and found the left coronary artery arising from the right sinus of Valsalva and coursing leftward in this way in three of them. As indicated, Corrado et al (1992) have further

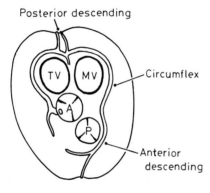

Figure 55.15. A single coronary artery arising from the right sinus of Valsalva. Abbreviations as in Figure 55.1.

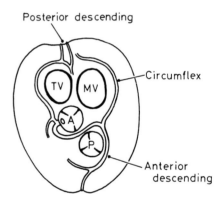

Figure 55.17. A single coronary artery arising from the right sinus of Valsalva with the left branch coursing between the aorta and pulmonary trunk (or right ventricular outflow tract); as a result, can be compressed. Abbreviations as in Figure 55.1.

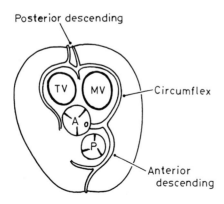

Figure 55.16. A single coronary artery arising from the left sinus of Valsalva. An atrophic relic from the right sinus is also represented. Abbreviations as in Figure 55.1.

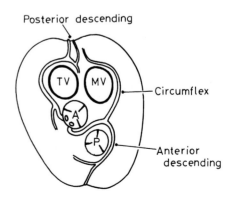

Figure 55.18. Both coronary arteries arising from separate orifices in the right sinus of Valsalva, with the left coronary artery coursing between the aorta and pulmonary trunk and subject to compression. Abbreviations as in Figure 55.1.

emphasized the significance of an intramural course complicating this anomaly.

This lesion has been defined by echocardiography. The most important finding relates to the detection of the left artery having its intramural, or almost intramural, course. Doppler colour flow confirms the direction of the flow within the coronary artery (Plate 55.3).

In contrast, when a single coronary arises from the left sinus of Valsalva (Figure 55.19) or both coronary arteries arise from separate orifices in that sinus (Figure 55.20), with the right coronary artery coursing between aorta and subpulmonary infundibulum, compression can occur but sudden death usually does not, probably because of the low perfusion pressure required for the right ventricle (Liberthson et al, 1979a; Benge et al, 1980).

Both coronary arteries arising from the pulmonary trunk constitute a rare situation. It is compatible with life only if associated with pulmonary hypertension (Roberts, 1962). Small accessory coronary arteries from the pulmonary trunk may uneventfully supply a part of the right ventricle. If they are larger, they tend to form connections

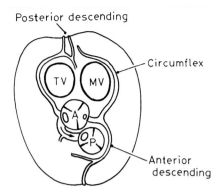

Figure 55.21. This diagram illustrates a large accessory coronary artery arising from the pulmonary trunk, which has anastomosed with the infundibular branch of the right coronary artery, resulting in fistulous left-to-right shunt. It equally well illustrates a short, direct rapidly flowing fistula from the coronary artery to the pulmonary trunk (the difference is semantic only). Abbreviations as in Figure 55.1.

with branches of normal origin, resulting in fistulous flow from aorta to pulmonary trunk (Figure 55.21).

When the right coronary artery originates from the pulmonary trunk, there is no ischaemia because the supply to the right ventricle is under low pressure (Tingelstad et al, 1972). Without ischaemia, there is no stimulus to form collateral anastomoses with branches of the left coronary artery, and thus there is no great tendency to establish fistulous flow.

MYOCARDIAL BRIDGES

Rather than running on the surface of the heart, part of any of the epicardial coronary arteries can dip into the muscle, creating a bridge of muscle running over the coronary artery. This occurs most frequently in the proximal half of the left coronary artery. Most are not significant, but occasionally longer and thicker bridges can cause ischaemia (Geiringer, 1951; von Pólacek, 1961; Angelini et al, 1983; Visscher et al, 1983).

CORONARY ARTERY FISTULA

The most distal malformations in the coronary arterial tree are communications between branches of the coronary arteries and another large vessel or cardiac chamber (McNamara and Gross, 1969; Rittenhouse et al, 1975; Liberthson et al, 1979b). The source is most often the right coronary artery, with the left being much less frequently involved, and both coronary arteries less frequently still. The 'sink' may be in any one or several of the following: the superior caval vein, the coronary sinus, the right atrium, the right ventricle, the pulmonary trunk, a pulmonary vein, the left atrium or the left ventricle. Embryologically, these fistulas seem to represent persistent junctions of primordial epicardial vessel with intramyocardial sinusoidal circulation. They vary from

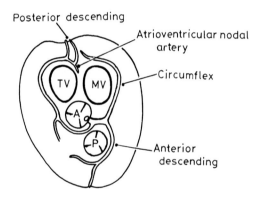

Figure 55.19. A single coronary artery arising from the left sinus of Valsalva, with the right branch coursing between the aorta and the pulmonary trunk and subject to compression. Abbreviation as in Figure 55.1.

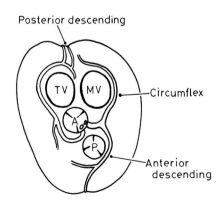

Figure 55.20. Both coronary arteries arising from separate orifices in the left sinus of Valsalva, with the right coronary artery coursing between the aorta and the pulmonary trunk and subject to compression. Abbreviations as in Figure 55.1.

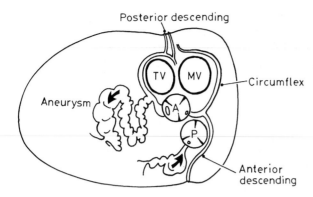

Figure 55.22. This diagram illustrates a complex, circuitous slowly flowing fistula running from a coronary artery to the pulmonary trunk, a large portion of which is an aneurysm that may contain clot and may be, in part, calcified. Abbreviations as in Figure 55.1.

simple direct connections of a coronary artery with the lumen of a chamber or large vessel (Figure 55.21) to complex, worm-like aneurysmal cavities in which blood may stagnate, clot and calcify (Figure 55.22). They are as varied pathophysiologically as they are anatomically. In the simple direct connections with large communicating orifices, there may be appreciable shunts. The increased volume loading begins with the aorta and left ventricle in all cases, and, depending upon where the fistula drains, is reflected farther back into left atrium, pulmonary vascular bed, right ventricle, right atrium or caval veins. The largest shunts tend to be in those that connect to the right side of the heart rather than the left. This is probably because of the greater period of systolic narrowing when the orifice of communication is into the left ventricle as well as because of the lesser pressure gradient between aorta and left ventricle. Even in those communications ending in the right side of the heart and contributing to pulmonary blood flow, rarely is the ratio between pulmonary and systemic flows greater than 3:1.

Some fistulas have been found to be large in the newborn. Further postnatal enlargement does occur. The aneurysmal sections of the fistula, in particular, may gradually dilate over time. It striking cardiac enlargement is noted, it is more likely to be caused by a dilated complex fistula on the surface of the heart than by functional enlargement of the heart from volume overload. Dilation of a complex fistula tends to occur slowly, stretching the pericardium and compressing softer cardiac structures, potentially producing arrhythmias and obstructing veins entering the right or left side of the heart.

Other effects and complications include fistulous 'steal' from the neighbouring myocardium, with ischaemia, atherosclerotic changes at points of stress, thrombosis and embolization, rupture and infective endocarditis.

Over half of patients are clinically asymptomatic with normal exercise tolerance, despite their moderate volume overloads. Symptoms of congestive heart failure may occur, especially when the anomaly presents in infancy.

Other symptoms include exercise intolerance with dyspnoea and angina, and occasionally arrhythmia.

The presenting physical finding that brings many such patients to the cardiologist is a continuous murmur over the heart. This may resemble that from an arterial duct, except that it is often heard maximally in unusual locations, and may peak in diastole rather than during systolic ejection.

Electrocardiographically, there is no characteristic finding. Radiologically, the heart may be normal in size and shape and moderately enlarged; it may be overactive when there is a short, rapidly flowing fistula. It may be very large but not overactive when there is a huge cavernous slow-flowing fistula. The cross-sectional echocardiogram, especially with Doppler colour flow imaging, has permitted the display of the site of entry of these fistulas (Reeder et al, 1980; Miyatake et al, 1984; Cooper et al, 1985; Ludomirsky et al, 1987; Lloyd et al, 1988; Sanders et al, 1989; Velvis et al, 1989).

Echocardiographic awareness of coronary arterial abnormalities has been heightened by recognition of the aneurysms associated with the mucocutaneous lymph-node syndrome. The use of Doppler colour flow, accompanied by imaging, now allows the recognition of the site of origin, course and site of entry of the fistula.

Pulsed and continuous wave Doppler ultrasound confirm the nature of the disturbed flow at the site of entry in most patients, particularly when guided by the colour flow map. Coil embolization now can be monitored directly with transoesophageal echocardiography (Nguyen et al, 1989; Doorey et al, 1991). Arterial contrast echocardiography can be used in the cardiac catheterization laboratory by placing the contrast directly into the aortic root and detecting the origin, course and site of drainage (Figures 55.23 and 55.24; Plates 55.4 and 55.5).

Treatment of coronary artery fistulas nowadays is increasingly the province of the interventional catheterizer. Transoesophageal echocardiography plays an important role in monitoring the success of this procedure (Plate 55.5).

CORONARY–PULMONARY FISTULAS

Doppler colour flow also detects fistulas from the coronary arteries to the pulmonary trunk or its branches. The major differential diagnoses are anomalous coronary arteries and patency of the arterial ductus. Colour flow mapping and imaging define the site of drainage. These fistulas are usually asymptomatic and lack the other ancillary and associated features described for anomalous coronary arteries.

Ventricular size and function are normal, but the proximal coronary arteries are abnormal. In addition, because of the low velocity of flow, the Doppler controls must be adjusted carefully in order to identify the area of disturbance of flow. We have found high-frequency transducers,

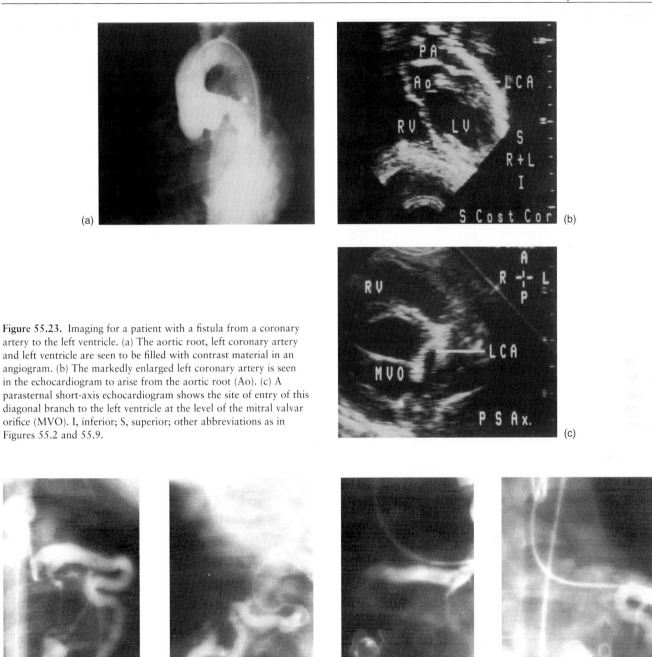

Figure 55.23. Imaging for a patient with a fistula from a coronary artery to the left ventricle. (a) The aortic root, left coronary artery and left ventricle are seen to be filled with contrast material in an angiogram. (b) The markedly enlarged left coronary artery is seen in the echocardiogram to arise from the aortic root (Ao). (c) A parasternal short-axis echocardiogram shows the site of entry of this diagonal branch to the left ventricle at the level of the mitral valvar orifice (MVO). I, inferior; S, superior; other abbreviations as in Figures 55.2 and 55.9.

Figure 55.24. Angiographic findings in a fistula from the left coronary artery to the right ventricle. (a) Filling of the aorta is shown with the left coronary artery, and its fistulous course of entry into the right ventricle. (b) The same findings as in (a) shown in lateral projection. (c, d) Complete obstruction of the fistula after embolization.

together with lowering of the Nyquist limit, paramount in defining these lesions, which reportedly have been recognized by angiography and missed by echocardiography (Lloyd et al, 1988). The disturbances in flow may be quite limited and difficult to locate, and careful scanning of the pulmonary trunk, particularly the anterior aspect, is necessary. With this approach, and using high-resolution equipment, we have been able to define the lesion (Plate 55.6).

Cardiac catheterization with aortography provides the definitive diagnosis. Selective coronary arteriography, by separating the overlapping coronary arterial trees, is even more helpful. In the event that the laboratory does not have the equipment or expertise for selective injections, a deliberate injection into the right sinus of Valsalva can provide virtually selective filling of the right coronary artery.

The differential diagnosis of duct-like murmurs is given in Chapter 51. Angiographically, there may be confusion with ruptured sinus of Valsalva. Careful analysis in more than one plane usually provides a correct interpretation.

Not much is known about the course of these lesions without surgery, because surgical treatment was available during the years in which accurate diagnosis was feasible. The mortality has been low since the earliest period of surgical treatment, and the tendency has been practically universal to proceed with surgery on these rare patients in order to prevent complications. Jaffe et al (1973) did observe a small group of patients prospectively, and noted that most of them changed very little, with some tendency to resolve spontaneously by thrombosis. The other side of the coin is represented by patients who have come to attention because of infective endocarditis, aggravated atherosclerotic complications or thrombotic complications. Inevitably, coil embolization, where this can be performed, will supplant surgical treatment in managing this lesion.

Once a decision is made to proceed to surgery, the plan is usually to attempt closure of the point at which the fistula enters the heart without interrupting the continuity of the coronary artery beyond the fistula. This may be accomplished while the heart is beating, but a pump oxygenator must at least be kept on standby in case entry into a cardiac chamber or bypass coronary arterial grafting becomes necessary. A small percentage of patients submitted to surgery have postoperative infarction or ischaemia downstream from the ligation. This is an especially disturbing complication when a fistula from the right coronary artery to the atrium or superior caval vein is ligated and the atrioventricular nodal artery is interrupted. Because of the ability to treat coronary arterial fistula by coil embolization through a transcoronary catheter, it is inappropriate to use surgery before trying this method of resolution.

In this discussion, nothing has been said of the fistulous communications seen in patients with pulmonary or aortic atresia with intact ventricular septum. These are discussed in the appropriate chapters on those major anomalies (Chapters 43 and 53).

DISEASE STATES

ARTERIOPATHIES OF INFANCY INVOLVING THE CORONARY ARTERIES

Infantile arterial calcification is the usual term for an idiopathic disease that, in most cases, causes death in the first 6 months of life. The disease probably begins in fetal life (Traisman et al, 1956; Weens and Marin, 1956). It involves the coronary arteries, as well as retinal, carotid,

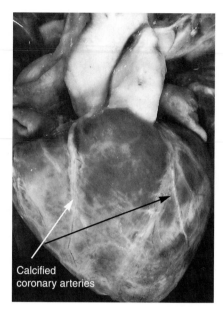

Calcified coronary arteries

Figure 55.25. These coronary arteries are calcified as a result of occlusive infantile arteriopathy.

renal and other medium-sized arteries. It is not clear whether it is a single pathological process or several that overlap with a similar end result (Robertson, 1960; Macartney et al, 1976). Even in the same patient, intimal fibrous proliferation dominates in some sections of muscular arteries, while in others, fragmentation of the internal elastic lamina with deposition of calcium is the striking finding (Figure 55.25). There may be more generalized interruption in elastic arteries, with patchy discontinuity of the elastic lamellae of the media. Williams (quoted McKusick, 1960 in material positive for periodic acid–Schiff reaction defects polysaccharides, mucins, glycoproteins) found preceding the deposition of calcium and suggested that the disease is an anomaly of mucopolysaccharide metabolism rather than of calcium metabolism. Because in some severe cases there is very little calcification, Witzleben (1970) offered the more general term 'occlusive infantile arteriopathy'.

The diagnosis has been made during life by palpation of arteries, from radiographs of soft tissues showing calcification, and with ophthalmoscopy. Cardiac symptoms are of angina or myocardial infarction with arrhythmia and congestive failure. The involvement is progressive and widespread, and no effective treatment has been found.

MUCOCUTANEOUS LYMPH NODE SYNDROME (KAWASAKI DISEASE)

Kawasaki disease has attained great importance in paediatric cardiology, both in Japan (where it was first described) and throughout the world (Kawasaki et al, 1974). While there may be myocarditis and pericarditis

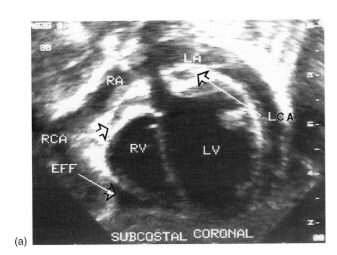

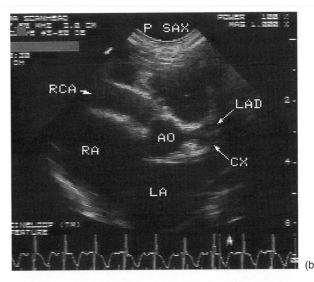

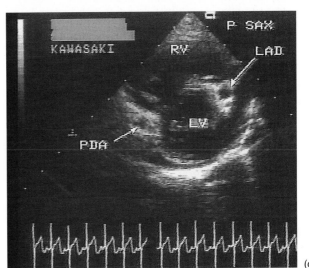

Figure 55.26. (a) Enlargement of the left and right coronary arteries occurs in the recovery phase of the Kawasaki syndrome. A moderate pericardial effusion (EFF) is present. (b) This parasternal short-axis view shows a giant fusiform aneurysm of the right coronary artery, 8 mm in diameter. The left coronary artery is also enlarged, and the enlargement continues into the origins of the left anterior descending and circumflex coronary (CX) arteries. (c) This frame was taken at a later date in the same patient. It shows the interrogation of the coronary arteries in a more distal site. Here the delimiting left anterior descending and posterior descending (PDA) coronary arteries can be seen on the surfaces of the front and back of the heart as they run on the ventricular septal junctions with the ventricles. Abbreviations as in Figure 55.2.

in its early phase, the great danger is coronary arteritis with aneurysmal formation, a complication that ensues in about 10% of patients. An extensive description of this disease and its diagnosis may be found in Chapter 61. Here we emphasize the importance of echocardiographic recognition, which allows imaging of major sections of the coronary arteries and definition of the length and extent of aneurysms. The technique also can be used to chart the size of aneurysms over time. Angiography best defines the presence of stenoses and the state of the microcirculation, but if the disease is found to be mild and the extent of the aneurysm is small, this invasive technique may not be necessary (Figure 55.26 and Plate 55.7).

INFANTILE POLYARTERITIS NODOSA

Infantile polyarteritis nodosa is an extremely rare disease, usually diagnosed at postmortem, in infants dying with

febrile illness (Munro-Faure, 1959; Roberts and Fetterman, 1963; Crouch and Diehl, 1973). Pathologically, the arteritic lesions, including those of the coronary arteries, are indistinguishable from those of Kawasaki disease (Landing and Larson, 1977). The clinical features are not nearly as pathognomonic as those of Kawasaki disease; consequently, the clinician is unaware of the potential underlying pathology. One might suspect the disease in an infant with an acute or subacute febrile illness, possibly associated with rash, but with none of the other hallmarks of Kawasaki disease, if there were cardiomegaly and/or ischaemic changes in the electrocardiogram. Such a presentation might suggest an acute viral myocarditis, but the finding of aneurysms on crosssectional echocardiography could enable the diagnosis to be made during life. Chamberlain and Perry (1971) were led to the diagnosis by palpation of brachial arterial aneurysms. Once diagnosed, the treatment would be acetylsalicylic acid as in Kawasaki disease.

REFERENCES

Alexander R W, Griffith G C 1956 Anomalies of the coronary arteries and their clinical significance. Circulation 14: 800–805

Angelini P, Trivellato M, Donis J, Leachman R D 1983 Myocardial bridges: a review. Progress in Cardiovascular Diseases 26: 75–88

Askenazi J, Nadas A S 1975 Anomalous left coronary artery originating from the pulmonary artery. Report on 15 cases. Circulation 51: 976–987

Baroldi G, Scomazzoni G 1967 Coronary circulation in the normal and the pathologic heart, Vol? ed? Office of the Surgeon General, Washington, DC

Benge W, Martins J B, Funk D C 1980 Morbidity associated with anomalous origin of the right coronary artery from the left sinus of Valsalva. American Heart Journal 99: 96–100

Bland E F, White P D, Garland J 1933 Congenital anomalies of the coronary arteries. American Heart Journal 8: 787–797

Bogers A J J C, Gittenberger-de Groot A C, Dubbledam J A, Huysmans H A 1988 The inadequacy of existing theories on development of the proximal coronary arteries and their connexions with the arterial trunks. International Journal of Cardiology 20: 117–123

Byrum C J, Blackman M S, Schneider B, Sondheimer H M, Kavey R E 1980 Congenital atresia of the left coronary ostium and hypoplasia of the left main coronary artery. American Heart Journal 99: 354–358

Castañeda A R, Jonas R A, Mayer J E, Hanley F L 1994 Cardiac surgery of the neonate and infant. Saunders, Philadelphia

Chamberlain J L III, Perry L W 1971 Infantile periarteritis nodosa with coronary and brachial aneurysms: a case diagnosed during life. Journal of Pediatrics 78: 1039–1042

Cheitlin M D, de Castro C M, McAllister H A 1974 Sudden death as a complication of anomalous left coronary origin from the anterior sinus of Valsalva, A not-so-minor congenital anomaly. Circulation 50: 780–787

Cooper M J, Bernstein D, Silverman N H 1985 Recognition of left coronary artery fistula to the left and right ventricles by contrast echocardiography. Journla of the American College of Cardiology 6: 923–926

Corrado D, Thiene G, Cocco P, Frescura C 1992 Non-atherosclerotic coronary artery disease and sudden death in the young. British Heart Journal 68: 601–607

Crouch J A, Diehl A M 1973 Cardiac complications. Periarteritis nodosa of infancy. Journal of the Kansas Medical Society 74: 78–81

Dicicco B S, McManus B M, Waller B F, Roberts W C 1982 Separate aortic ostium of the left anterior descending and left circumflex coronary arteries from the left aortic sinus of Valsalva (absent left main coronary artery). American Heart Journal 104: 153–154

Doorey A J, Sullivan K L, Levin D C 1991 Successful percutaneous closure of a complex coronary-to-pulmonary artery fistula using a detachable balloon: benefits of intra-procedural physiologic and angiographic assessment. Catheterization and Cardiovascular Diagnosis 23: 23–27

Finley J P, Howman-Giles R, Gilday D L, Olley P M, Rowe R D 1978 Thallium-201 myocardial imaging in anomalous left coronary artery arising from the pulmonary artery. Applications before and after medical and surgical treatment. American Journal of Cardiology 42: 675–680

Fisher E A, Sepehri B, Lendrum B, Luken J, Levitsky S, Barron S 1981 Two-dimensional echocardiographic visualization of the left coronary artery in anomalous origin of the left coronary artery from the pulmonary artery: pre-and post-operative studies. Circulation 63: 698–704

Formanek A, Nath P H, Zollikofer C, Moller J H 1980 Selective coronary arteriography in children. Circulation 61: 84–95

Fortuin N J, Roberts W C 1971 Congenital atresia of the left main coronary artery. American Journal of Medicine 50: 385–389

Foster H R Jr, Hagstrom J W C, Ehlers K H, Engle M A 1964 Mitral insufficiency due to anomalous origin of the left coronary artery from the pulmonary artery. Pediatrics 34: 649–654

Geiringer E 1951 The mural coronary artery. American Heart Journal 41: 359–364

Gregg D E, Fisher L C 1963 Blood supply to the heart. In: Handbook of physiology, Section 2, vol ed. American Physiological Society, Washington, DC, p 26–35

Gutgesell H P, Pinsky W W, DePuey E G 1980 Thallium-201 myocardial perfusion imaging in infants and children. Value in distinguishing anomalous left coronary artery from congestive cardiomyopathy. Circulation 61: 596–599

Hackensellner H A 1956 Aksessorische Kransgeffäsanlagen der Arteria pulmonalis unter 63 meschlichen Embryonenserien mit einer grössten Lange von 12 bis 36 mm. Mikroscopischanat Forschung 62: 153–163

Jaffe R B, Glancy D L, Epstein S E, Brown B G, Morrow A G 1973 Coronary arterial–right heart fistulae. Long-term observations in seven patients. Circulation 47: 133–143

James T N 1961 Anatomy of the coronary arteries. Hoeber, New York

Kaplinsky E, Ogawa S, Michelson E L, Dreifus L S 1981 Instantaneous and delayed ventricular arrhythmias after reperfusion of acutely ischemic myocardium: evidence for multiple mechanisms. Circulation 63: 333–340

Kawasaki T, Kosaki F, Okawa S, Shigematsu I, Yanagawa H 1974 A new infantile acute febrile mucocutaneous lymph node syndrome (MLNS) prevailing in Japan. Pediatrics 54: 271–276

Landing B H, Larson E J 1977 Are infantile periarteritis nodosa with coronary artery involvement and fatal mucocutaneous lymph node syndrome the same? Comparison of 20 patients from North America with patients from Hawaii and Japan. Pediatrics 59: 651–662

Liberthson R R, Dinsmore R E, Fallon J T 1979a Aberrant coronary artery origin from the aorta. Report of 18 patients, review of literature and delineation of natural history and management. Circulation 59: 748–754

Liberthson R R, Sagar K, Berkoben J P, Weintraub R M, Levine F H 1979b Congenital coronary arteriovenous fistula: report of 13 patients, review of the literature and delineation of management. Circulation 59: 849–854

Lloyd T R, Mahoney L T, Marvin W J, Knoebel D 1988 Identification of coronary artery to right ventricular fistulae by color flow mapping. Echocardiography 5: 115–120

Ludomirsky A, Danford D A, Glasow P F, Blumenschein S D, Murphy D J, Huhta J C 1987 Evaluation of coronary artery: fistula by color flow Doppler echocardiography. Echocardiography 4: 383–385

Macartney F J, Bain H H, Ionescu M I, Deverall P B, Scott O 1976 Angiocardiographic/pathologic correlations in congenital mitral valve anomalies. European Journal of Cardiology 4: 191–211

Maron B J, Roberts W C, McAllister H A, Rosing D R, Epstein S E 1980 Sudden death in young athletes. Circulation 62: 218–229

Martin G R, Cooper M J, Silverman N H, Soifer S J 1986 Contrast echocardiography in the diagnosis of anomalous left coronary artery arising from the pulmonary artery. Pediatric Cardiology 6: 203–205

McKusick V A 1960 Heritable disorders of connective tissue, 2nd edn. Mosby, St Louis, MO

McNamara J J, Gross R E 1969 Congenital coronary artery fistula. Surgery 65: 59–69

Miyatake K, Okamoto M, Kinoshita N, Fusejima K, Sakakibara H, Nimura Y 1984 Doppler echocardiographic features of coronary arteriovenous fistula. British Heart Journal 51: 508–518

Munro-Faure H 1959 Necrotizing arteritis of the coronary vessels in infancy: case report and review of the literature. Pediatrics 25: 914–926

Muriago M, Sheppard M N, Ho S Y, Anderson R H 1997 The location of the coronary arterial orifices in the normal heart. Clinical Anatomy 10: 297–302

Neufeld H N, Schneeweiss A (eds) 1983 Coronary artery disease in infants and children. Lea & Febiger, Philadelphia, PA, p 1

Nguyen K, Myler R K, Hieshima G, Ashraf M, Stertzer H S 1989 Treatment of coronary artery stenosis and coronary arteriovenous fistula by interventional cardiology techniques. Catheterization and Cardiovascular Diagnosis 18: 240–243

Ogden J A 1970 Congenital anomalies of the coronary arteries. American Journal of Cardiology 25: 474–479

Ogden J A, Goodyer A V 1970 Patterns of distribution of the single coronary artery. Yale Journal of Biology and Medicine 43: 11–21

Perry L W, Scott L P 1970 Anomalous left coronary artery from pulmonary artery: report of 11 cases; review of indications for and results of surgery. Circulation 41: 1043–1052

Rabinovitch M, Rowland T W, Castañeda A R, Treves S 1979 Thallium 201 scintigraphy in patients with anomalous origin of the left coronary artery from the main pulmonary artery. Journal of Pediatrics 94: 244–247

Reeder G S, Tajik A J, Smith H C 1980 Visualization of coronary artery fistula by two-dimensional echocardiography. Mayo Clinic Proceedings 55: 185–189

Rittenhouse E A, Doty D B, Ehrenhaft J L 1975 Congenital coronary artery–cardiac chamber fistula. Review of operative management. Annals of Thoracic Surgery 20: 468–485

Roberts F B, Fetterman G H 1963 Polyarteritis nodosa in infancy. Journal of Pediatrics 63: 519–525

Roberts W C 1962 Anomalous origin of both coronary arteries of the newborn. American Journal of Cardiology 10: 595–601

Roberts W C 1986 Major anomalies of coronary arterial origin seen in adulthood. American Heart Journal 111: 941–963

Robertson J H 1960 Significance of intimal thickening in the arteries of the newborn. Archives of Diseases in Childhood 35: 588–594

Robinson P J, Sullivan I D, Rumpeng V, Anderson R H, Macartney F J 1984 Anomalous origin of the left coronary artery from the pulmonary trunk: potential for false negative diagnosis with cross-sectional echocardiography. British Heart Journal 52: 272–277

Ruttenberg H D, Jue K L, Elliott L P, Anderson R C, Edwards J E 1964 Cardiac myopathy, probably of congenital origin: a case simulating anomalous origin of the left coronary artery from the pulmonary trunk. Circulation 29: 768–771

Sanders S P, Parness I A, Colan S D 1989 Recognition of abnormal connections of coronary arteries with the use of Doppler color flow mapping. Journal of the American College of Cardiology 13: 922–926

Schlesinger M J, Zoll P M, Wessler S 1949 The conus artery: a third coronary artery. American Heart Journal 38: 823–836

Schmidt K G, Cooper M J, Silverman N H, Stanger P 1988 Pulmonary artery origin of the left coronary artery: diagnosis by two-dimensional echocardiography, pulsed Doppler ultrasound and color flow mapping. Journal of the American College of Cardiology 11: 396–402

Sharbaugh A H, White R S 1974 Single coronary artery. Analysis of the anatomic variation, clinical importance, and report of five cases. Journal of the American Medical Association 230: 243–246

Silverman N H 1993 Pediatric echocardiography, ed. Williams & Wilkins, Baltimore, MD, p 628

Takeuchi S, Imamura H, Katsumoto K et al 1979 New surgical method for repair of anomalous left coronary artery from pulmonary artery. Journal of Thoracic and Cardiovascular Surgery 78: 7–11

Tingelstad J B, Lower R R, Eldredge W J 1972 Anomalous origin of the right coronary artery from the main pulmonary artery. American Journal of Cardiology 30: 670–673

Traisman H S, Limperis N M, Traisman A S 1956 Myocardial infarction due to calcification of the arteries in an infant. American Journal of Diseases of Children 91: 34–42

Velvis H, Schmidt K G, Silverman N H, Turley K 1989 Diagnosis of coronary artery fistula by two-dimensional echocardiography, pulsed Doppler ultrasound and color flow imaging. Journal of the American College of Cardiology 14: 968–976

Visscher D W, Miles B L, Waller B F 1983 Tunneled ('bridged') left anterior descending coronary artery in a newborn without clinical or morphologic evidence of myocardial ischemia. Catheterization and Cardiovascular Diagnosis 9: 493–496

Vlodaver Z, Neufeld H N, Edwards J E 1975 Coronary arterial variations in the normal heart and in congenital heart disease. Academic Press, New York

von Pólacek P 1961 Relation of myocardial bridges and loops on the coronary arteries to coronary occlusion. American Heart Journal 61: 44–52

Weens H S, Marin C A 1956 Infantile arteriosclerosis. Radiology 67: 168–176

Wesselhoeft H, Fawcett J S, Johnson A L 1968 Anomalous origin of the left coronary artery from the pulmonary trunk. Its clinical spectrum, pathology, and pathophysiology, based on a review of 140 cases with seven further cases. Circulation 38: 403–425

Witzleben C L 1970 Idiopathic infantile arterial calcification – a misnomer? American Journal of Cardiology 26: 305–309

56

Aortic coarctation and interrupted aortic arch

J. Brierley and A. N. Redington

INTRODUCTION

Coarctation derives from the Latin term *coartatio*, which translated literally means a drawing together. Aortic coarctation, therefore, indicates a narrowing at some point along the course of the aorta. When used in the context of congenital heart disease, coarctation refers to an area of narrowing of the thoracic aorta in the region of the insertion of the arterial duct, with or without additional abnormalities of the aortic arch. The more proximal obstructive lesions of the aorta, those directly above the left ventricular outflow tract, are conventionally considered along with lesions of the aortic valve. Those distal to the thoracic aorta, together with acquired lesions, are beyond the remit of this chapter.

Interruption of the aortic arch is a condition in which there is complete anatomical discontinuity between two adjacent segments of the aortic arch. It can be considered as the extreme end of the spectrum of obstruction of the aorta.

AORTIC COARCTATION

The first description of aortic coarctation is generally attributed to Johann Freidrich Meckel, the famous Prussian anatomist who presented the case of an 18-year-old female to the Royal Academy of Sciences of Berlin in 1750. At postmortem, she was found to have an aorta that was 'so narrow that its diameter was smaller by half than that of the pulmonary artery, which it should have exceeded or at least have equalled in calibre'.

A more recognizable description of the entity we now recognize as coarctation was published in Desault's *Journal de Chirurgie* in 1791, the title being *Considerable Stenosis of the Thoracic Aorta Observed at the Hotel-Dieu of Paris*. M. Paris, Prosector of the Amphitheatre at the Hotel-Dieu described the postmortem of 'a very emaciated woman about 50 years old'. An injection of equal parts resin and tallow, dyed with lampblack, was introduced into the beginning of the aorta. 'The material penetrated so easily that a great deal more than is usually possible might have been injected.' As well as recognizing that the thoracic arteries were thicker and more tortuous than the normal, Paris went on to give the following description. 'The part of the aorta which is beyond the arch, between the ligamentum arteriosum and the first inferior intercostal, was so greatly narrowed that it had at most the thickness of a goosequill. Hence in taking apart its walls, which had not decreased in this place, there remained only a small lumen. The part of the vessel which was above the constriction was slightly dilated; the distal part was of normal calibre. The most careful dissection did not reveal either in the aorta or in its vicinity any cause to which this extraordinary condition could be attributed.'

PREVALENCE AND AETIOLOGY

Aortic coarctation accounts for 6–8% of livebirths with congenital heart disease (Mitchell et al, 1971; Šamanak et al, 1989; Bower and Ramsey, 1994). An even higher incidence is found in stillborn infants (Hoffman, 1995) while, in another study, aortic coarctation was identified at postmortem in 17% of neonates dying from congenital heart disease (Izakuwa et al, 1979). The overall incidence is in the region of 1 in 12 000. Campbell and Polani (1961) reported a ratio of males to females of 1.74:1. Noting that the ratio was the same in each decade of life, they concluded that the increased prevalence in males was not a consequence of increased female mortality. The New England Regional Infant Cardiac Program (Fyler et al, 1980), which also included interrupted aortic arch, put the ratio at only 1.27 males to each famale.

Coarctation is generally said to show multifactorial inheritance, although genetic factors are clearly important in certain groups. For example, in a large Danish series of patients with Turner's syndrome, aortic coarctation was found in one tenth (Gotzche et al, 1994). Interestingly, the incidence is lower in patients with Turner mosaicism, or those with structural anomalies of the X chromosome. Turner's syndrome is characterized by abnormalities of lymphatic drainage, and it is possible that this provides a clue to the aetiology of the associated coarctation. Those with the XO genotype are more likely to have classical neck webbing compared with the other genotypes. In a recent report, Greally et al (1996) described a 1-month-old infant presenting with an aortic coarctation who was found to have mosaic trisomy of chromosome 16 on analysis of peripheral blood and in structurally affected tissues, including the aorta. Inheritance as an autosomal dominant trait was reported by Beekman and Robinow in 1985, while monozygotic twins have been encountered with coarctation (Sehested, 1982). It is also of interest that cells migrating from the neural crest are known to populate the aortic arches, the finding of coarctation in an infant has prompted Momma (1998) to query an association with 22q11 deletion.

Seasonal incidence is seen, with a paucity of males born between April and August (Miettinen et al, 1970), but no exogenous aetiological agent has yet been identified. A recent study in Finland, although only involving a small cohort, failed to implicate any direct teratogens in the aetiology of coarctation (Tikkanen and Heinonen, 1993). Nonetheless, the overall recurrence rate given a sibling with any congenital heart defect is increased by many orders of magnitude, being calculated at about 2% (Park, 1996).

MORPHOLOGY

The lesions to be considered in this chapter all occur in proximity to the junction of the aortic arch and the arterial duct. This ductal–aortic junction is clearly of fundamental importance to their evolution and morphology, although isolated coarctation has been described, rarely, proximal to the subclavian arteries (d'Abreu et al, 1961) and, more frequently, in the descending thoracic aorta (Konai et al, 1955). Aortic coarctation cannot, however, be considered to be a uniform entity. Instead, it represents a spectrum of lesions, generally encompassing variable degrees of tubular hypoplasia along with additionally stenotic areas within the aortic arch. These variants are more common in neonates and infants, whereas more discrete coarctation in association with arterial collateral vessels and degenerative aortic changes is more likely in those presenting at later age. The extreme end of the variety seen during infancy is interruption of the aortic arch (see below). In terms of definitions, tubular hypoplasia describes a uniform narrowing of part of the arch, whereas discrete coarctation is usually produced by a localized shelf-like lesion, often with a degree of proximal tapering of the aortic arch towards the lesion. Often

the two are grouped together; for precise clinical evaluation, however, it is necessary to differentiate between the two.

DISCRETE COARCTATION

Discrete coarctation is much commoner than tubular hypoplasia, and has been the subject of manifold classifications. In his classical article, Bonnet (1903) divided coarctation into an infant type, occurring proximal to the aortoductal junction with patency of the arterial duct, and an adult type, tending to occur distally to the point of insertion of the arterial ligament and associated with the development of collateral vessels. This distinction was simplistic. Many further attempts at classification followed (Evans, 1933; Bramwell, 1947; Johnson et al 1951; Clagget et al, 1954). Although more anatomical in their description, these classifications continued to include ductal patency and the presence of associated intracardiac defects within their definitions.

The approaches were made more systematic by Edwards (1968), who provided an account that described precisely the site of coarctation, no matter whether the arterial duct is patent, closed or ligamentous, and irrespective of the presence of additional anomalies. This remains our favoured method of description.

A convention, describing the site of coarctation as juxtaductal (Rudolph et al, 1972), is unhelpful in that, since the majority of coarctation lesions are in proximity to the arterial duct, the term adds little to descriptive anatomy. If it indicates an obstruction exactly opposite the site of the ductal insertion, then such lesions do exist, but they are relatively rare (Becker et al, 1970). In our opinion, the terms preductal, paraductal (Bruins, 1974; Elzenga and Gittenberger-de Groot, 1985) and postductal provide a much more precise description of the location of these lesions (Figure 56.1).

Preductal lesions

The most common site for discrete coarctation is between the left subclavian artery and the aortoductal junction. If the duct is open, there is usually a degree of isthmal hypoplasia, with the isthmus tapering down towards the junction with the duct, which takes the form of a discrete waist, often with some infolding of the aortic wall (Figure 56.2). In the majority of cases, this is associated with a shelf-like extension of ductal tissue (Figure 56.3) which completely encircles the lumen of the isthmus, being in continuity with the muscular ductal wall (Wielangar and Dankmeijer, 1968; Ho and Anderson, 1979; Gittenberger-de Groot, 1981). It is the ductal shelf that produces the greater obstruction to flow and, therefore, physiologically is the most important factor in coarctation. The waisting of the aortic wall and the ductal shelf usually coexist but can occur in isolation (Pellegrino et al, 1985). There was, initially, a marked discrepancy concerning these findings.

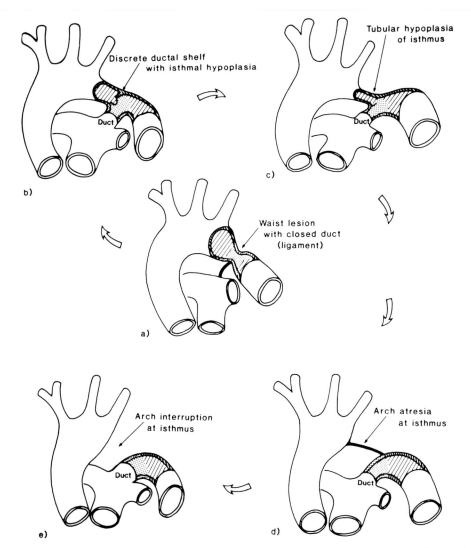

Figure 56.1 The hypothetical sequence of anomalies leading from discrete waist-like coarctation (a), through the discrete shelf lesion (b), to tubular hypoplasia (c), to atresia at the isthmus (d) and, finally, to interruption between the left subclavian artery and the descending aorta (e). The duct is shown as a patent structure in (b) to (e).

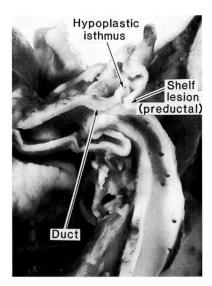

Figure 56.2 In this specimen, the duct is still open, and the coarctation lesion is formed by a discrete ductal shelf combined with marked hypoplasia of the aortic isthmus.

Several investigators reported an inability to find ductal tissue in the shelf (Edwards, 1968; Hutchins, 1971). Elzenga and Gitenberger de Groot (1983) provided an explanation for this failure when they showed that the shelf had the capacity to 'migrate' with increasing age, eventually to be replaced by fibrous tissue.

In normal adult life, the isthmus is proportionately much larger than in infancy. This differential growth of the components of the thoracic aorta probably accounts for the apparent cranial migration of aortic insertion of the duct, with relative caudal migration of the ductal shelf. In earlier life, this usually lies proximal relative to the site of ductal insertion (Figures 56.2 and 56.3).

In later life, it was often possible to see histological changes distal to the site of coarctation. These were caused by the high velocity jet through the site of coarctation impacting on the aortic wall, the intimal proliferation and thinning of the elastic component of the wall thus produced predisposing to infective endocarditis, aneurysmal formation and even acute aortic dissection. Such changes

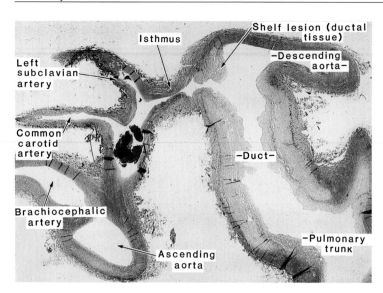

Figure 56.3 This histological section shows the structure of the isthmus, duct and descending aorta in a heart from a patient with discrete coarctation. The stenotic shelf is clearly formed of pale-staining ductal tissue.

are now of historical interest since, as we will see, virtually all cases are recognized and repaired in infancy.

Inspection of gross pathological specimens, nonetheless, shows that the major pattern of flow in neonatal hearts is from the duct to the descending aorta, with the isthmus inserting end-to-side into the junction of the arterial duct with the descending aorta (Figure 56.4). Whether this is cause or effect is discussed lucidly by Rosenberg (1973). Protagonists of the concept that decreased isthmal flow during fetal life causes coarctation, emphasize the frequent coexistence of preductal coarctation with intracardiac lesions' which tend to channel flow to the pulmonary artery in preference to the ascending aorta (Rudolph et al, 1972; Shinebourne et al, 1976). These associate anomalies, nonetheless, are not a universal pre-

requisite for the formation of coarctation, which may occur in the setting of an otherwise apparently normal heart. Furthermore, there have been occasional reports of preductal coarctation occurring more proximally, for example between the left common carotid and left subclavian arteries (Clagget et al, 1954; Poulias et al, 1984). As we have already stated, discrete lesions have been found even proximal to both subclavian arteries (d'Abreau et al, 1961), and the flow hypothesis fails to explain the morphogenesis of postductal lesions. This is not to deny the importance of differential flow, but it is more likely that this simply exaggerates the effect of the ductal sling (Hoffman, 1988).

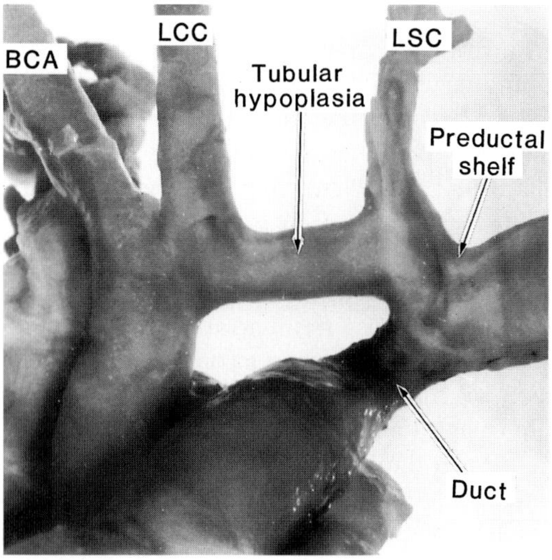

Paraductal lesions

Paraductal coarctation occurs directly opposite the mouth of the duct at its insertion to the aorta. Becker (1970) found eight cases of paraductal coarctation in his study of 71 patients. Elzenga and Gittenberger de Groot (1985) demonstrated that coarctation in this site occurs much more frequently in association with aortic atresia and a hypoplastic left ventricle (Figure 56.5).

Postductal lesions

Postductal lesions occur distal to the aortic origin of the arterial duct. In the series described by Becker (1970), there were nine examples, with five occurring with a closed duct. The realization that immediate surgery was required in infants with this type of coarctation predated the era of pharmacological manipulation of the duct. The most important consequence of this variant today is the lack of improvement of such critically ill infants despite maintenance of ductal patency with prostaglandin. Indeed, recognition of postductal coarctation represents one of the few remaining indications for urgent surgery, day or night. Fortunately, there is a characteristic pattern to the Doppler recording in the aortic arch and arterial

Figure 56.4 This specimen has been dissected along the aortic arch. It shows a discrete lesion in preductal position, together with tubular hypoplasia of the segment of aortic arch between the left common carotid (LCC) and left subclavian (LSC) arteries, and a short hypoplastic isthmus. BCA, brachiocephalic artery.

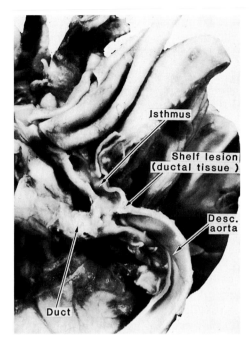

Figure 56.5 This specimen, sectioned along the isthmus and descending (desc.) aorta, shows how the discrete stenotic shelf is composed of ductal tissue that encircles the mouth of the isthmus. The lesion itself is in paraductal position.

duct that helps to establish the diagnosis. There is a continuous left-to-right shunt at the level of the arterial duct, with a pan-diastolic gradient and prolonged pressure half-time (Cullen and Redington, 1993). Such postductal coarctation is the norm in adults, although occurring postligamental rather than postductal. As discussed above, it is likely that the site of the coarctation seen in older patients results from differential growth of the components of the thoracic aorta, such that an initially preductal lesion becomes postligamental with the passage of time.

Anomalies of the subclavian arteries

Although rare, anomalies of the subclavian arteries are important both clinically and surgically. The most common, albeit much more frequently associated with interruption of the aortic arch, is origin of the right subclavian artery from the aorta distal to the site of ductal insertion. The anomalous artery then pursues a retro-oesophageal course, often arising from the expanded segment of aorta called the diverticulum of Kommerrell. Clinically, this can form the substrate for vascular ring (see Chapter 57). It may account for an uncharacteristically weak pulse in the right arm, along with failure to detect a difference in blood pressure between the right brachial artery and lower body.

The left subclavian artery can arise paraductally. In this setting, the isthmus itself is exceedingly short or non-existent. The mouth of the subclavian artery can then be incorporated in the ductal sling and has a tendency to be stenosed at its origin.

Collateral circulation

Although rarely present in infants (Matthew et al, 1972), collateral circulation gradually develops throughout childhood in those with subcritical coarctation. Such collateral arteries bypass the obstruction and augment perfusion to the lower body. The most common pattern involves a large 'arterial aberrans' from the right subclavian artery supplying the aorta below the coarctation, together with various branches of the left subclavian artery, including the thyrocervical trunk, the left intercostal arteries via the left internal thoracic artery (leading to rib notching) and the anterior spinal artery through the left vertebral artery (Edwards et al, 1948). One particular vessel in this circulation has achieved recognition as 'Abbot's artery'. This is an anomalous vessel arising from the posterior aspect of the isthmus and passing medially behind the carotid artery and transverse arch (Lerberg, 1981).

Associated anomalies

The presence of associated cardiovascular lesions was one of the criterions commonly used to differentiate coarctation found in infancy from those presenting, often in isolation, in later childhood and adulthood. While such a classification is flawed in absolute terms, the general relationship is a real one. Shinebourne et al (1976) demonstrated an inverse relationship between age at presentation and frequency of associated lesions, with 85% of those presenting as neonates having a significant associated lesion, compared with only 50% of those first seen at from 1 month to 1 year of age.

Patency of the arterial duct and anomalies of the subclavian arteries have already been alluded to, while tubular hypoplasia will be addressed below. In fact, the presence of aortic coarctation, hypoplasia of the isthmus, patent arterial duct, and the presence of an interatrial communication or patency of the oval foramen, is so common as to be referred to sometimes as part of a coarctation complex in neonates.

The typical associated anomalies are dominated by the appearance of lesions that tend preferentially to potentiate flow to the pulmonary rather then systemic arterial pathway. Such lesions lead to reduced flow through the aortic isthmus in fetal life.

There are two main mechanisms by which this occurs. The first is through a defect that allows left-to-right flow at either ventricular or great arterial level. The most common of these lesions is a ventricular septal defect. When found in the presence of coarctation, the ventricular septal defect can be similar to the archetypal pattern seen in hearts with interruption of the aortic arch, namely a septal defect associated with posterior deviation of the muscular outlet septum (Figure 56.6). More frequently, however, the defects are perimembranous and associated with posteroinferior overriding of the aortic valve (Figure 57.7). Such defects produced no obstruction to flow of

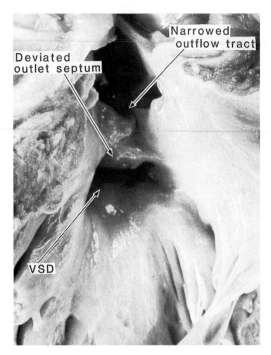

Figure 56.6 This view of the subaortic outflow tract, from a specimen with aortic coarctation, shows posterior deviation of the muscular outlet septum narrowing the outflow tract. VSD, ventricular septal defect.

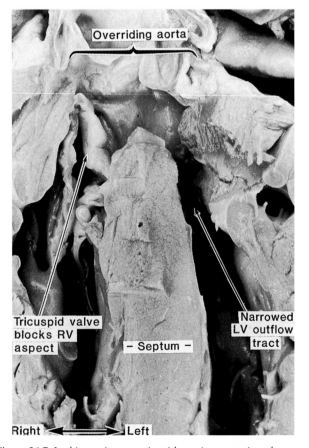

Figure 56.7 In this specimen, again with aortic coarctation, the aortic root overrides the crest of the muscular ventricular septum. The outflow from the left ventricle (LV) is narrowed by muscular bundles, while the entrance to the aortic root from the right ventricle (RV) is narrowed by tissue tags derived from the tricuspid valve.

blood to the pulmonary arteries, but the right ventricular aspect of the defects are usually obstructed by tissue tags derived from tricuspid valve, giving the impression that the overall arrangement could reduce aortic blood flow (Anderson et al, 1983).

The second mechanism provides overt obstruction to the outflow from the left ventricle both pre- and postnatally. Lesions falling into this second category include aortic atresia, valvar and subvalvar aortic stenosis and bicuspid aortic valve (Moulaert and Oppenheimer-Dekker, 1976). Congenital lesions of the mitral valve are also typically associated with coarctation, and decreased flow through the left ventricular inlet will also lead to decreased flow across the isthmus. Similarly, supravalvar mitral shelf, stenosing left atrial ring and divided left atrium may all present with aortic coarctation (Rosenquist, 1974; Ruckman et al, 1978). The combination of several of these lesions carries a particularly poor prognosis and overlaps with the hypoplastic left heart syndrome. This combination involves co-existence of parachute mitral valve, supravalvar left atrial ring, subaortic stenosis and aortic coarctation as described by Shone and his colleagues in 1963. Recent review of a series of such patients with Shone's syndrome showed that, despite initial good results following surgical repair of the coarctation, mortality from later repair of the mitral valve was significant, and the morbidity in the survivors was substantial (Bolling et al, 1990).

Bicuspid aortic valve, although usually haemodynamically insignificant in early postnatal life, is very commonly seen in patients with aortic coarctation. In later life, this predisposes to calcific stenosis, regurgitation and infective endocarditis. Its frequency has varied greatly in different reported series, ranging from a high of 85% in the review of Edwards (1968) to the more conservative estimates of 23% in the cases studied by Abbott (1928), 25% of the series of Benkwitz and Hunter (1937), and 27% in the investigation of Tawes et al (1969a). Reifenstein and colleagues (1947) discovered bicuspid aortic valves in 43% of patients then referred to as 'adult' coarctation. In the series reported by Becker et al (1970), two fifths of those dying with coarctation under 6 months of age had a bicuspid aortic valve, in contrast to two thirds of those surviving longer. All these figures, however, were derived from post-mortem series. The true incidence would best be described using echocardiography in life.

The morphology of the bicuspid aortic valve associated with coarctation, nonetheless, has been shown to be significantly different from that occurring as an isolated lesion (Folger et al, 1984). The valve found with coarctation had two equally sized leaflets, whereas that seen in isolation usually had leaflets of unequal size. Irrespective of that, there is a known association between bicuspid aortic valve and weakness in the aortic wall, this accounting for the long-term incidence of dilation of the aortic root and subsequent dissection in those with bicuspid valves (Edwards et al, 1978; Lindsay et al, 1988). Whether this produces problems in the long-term follow-up of patients with coarctation has still to be established.

As might be anticipated, coarctation also occurs when the aortic arch is right sided. Anomalous origin of the left subclavian artery, and other abnormalities in branching patterns, is then frequently encountered (Grossman and Jacoby, 1969; Honey et al, 1975). Coarctation can also be found in the setting of a double aortic arch (Beekman et al, 1986).

Secondary pathology

Secondary pathology can be divided into local effects, effects on the myocardium and distant effects, the last in general caused by hypertension. The local changes tend to be characteristic. In older children and adults, fibrous intimal thickening is superimposed on the site of coarctation. The thickened layer is composed of concentric layers of collagen, with varying degrees of elastin and smooth muscle cells. The characteristic depletion and disarray of elastic tissue seen with cystic medial necrosis has also been observed (Isner et al, 1987). Distally, the coarctation protrudes into the aortic lumen in a nipple-like manner, probably as a result of the pressure exerted from above. The intimal proliferation, together with superimposed thrombus, can lead to near or actual obliteration of the lumen (Clagett et al, 1954). In such instances, all distal perfusion becomes dependent on the collateral circulation. The distal aortic wall often shows poststenotic dilation and is somewhat thinner than normal. The abdominal aorta may, however, be somewhat hypoplastic owing to diminished flow. The combination of these local changes accounts for the occasional development of aortic dissection in patients with advanced disease without treatment.

Pregnancy imposes an increased haemodynamic strain on the aortic wall owing to the physiological changes that occur, particularly in the last trimester and peripartum. Aortic dissection, and even rupture, are described in patients with uncorrected coarctation, perhaps initially misdiagnosed as pre-eclampsia (Kinney et al, 1945; Mandel et al, 1954). Such complications have also followed apparently successful repair (Wray et al, 1975). Whether earlier surgical intervention decreases the occurrence of the changes in the aortic wall is unknown. Close monitoring and meticulous control of blood pressure is, nonetheless, mandatory in all pregnant patients known to have coarctation.

The direct effect on the myocardium of obstruction to left ventricular ejection depends on the rapidity of the onset as well as the degree of increase in afterload, the left ventricle having numerous compensatory mechanisms. In the neonate undergoing rapid decompensation with ductal closure, left ventricular systolic and diastolic dysfunction rapidly lead to congestive heart failure. Diastolic flow in the coronary arteries decreases as left ventricular wall stress increases. This leads to ischaemia, especially of the subendocardium. The resultant decrease in cardiac output causes, and then perpetuates, a metabolic acidosis, which further depresses left ventricular contractility. In part, in infancy, this is a consequence of the inability of the myocardium to mount the usual adaptive responses to increased impedance to outflow. These will be discussed below under pathophysiology. Unless intervention is performed, death can be rapid. Of those who survive the initial insult, some develop marked subendocardial fibrosis (Cheitlin et al, 1980). If the onset of obstruction is less abrupt, compensatory adaptations can occur, primarily in the form of left ventricular hypertrophy. Ischaemic heart disease eventually occurs in many even in the absence of proximal coronary arterial occlusion (Tawes et al, 1969b).

Distant complications include the well recognized and classic 'berry' or saccular aneurysm of the circle of Willis. All the organs in the upper body can, nonetheless, sustain pathology secondary to hypertension. These changes are not entirely ameliorated by the initial relief of obstruction. This will be discussed at greater length below.

TUBULAR HYPOPLASIA

Tubular hypoplasia describes a uniformly narrow segment of the aortic arch. It frequently coexists with discrete coarctation in infants but must be considered separately. Tubular hypoplasia is also distinct from the gradual tapering of the isthmus characteristically seen with discrete coarctation. Histologically, the wall of an affected segment is normal, in contrast to the ductal and fibrous nature of discrete coarctation. The lesion is not usually clinically obstructive when found in isolation.

The most frequently affected sites of tubular hypoplasia are between the isthmus and the segment between the common carotid and left subclavian arteries (Figure 56.8). Rarely, the segment between the brachiocephalic and common carotid arteries is affected. There is a large variability in the size of the aortic arch in normal neonates; consequently, any attempt to define hypoplasia on pure numerical grounds is invalid.

Moulaert et al (1976) attempted to quantify the degree of hypoplasia by comparing the diameter of the affected segment with that of the distal ascending aorta, hypoplasia being defined as a proximal arch less than 60%, a distal arch less than 50% and an isthmus less than 40%. Both Morrow et al (1986) and Vouhe et al (1988) have subsequently suggested that comparisons are better made in relation to the descending aorta, since the ascending aorta can be smaller than expected in some of these patients. The descending aorta is also easier to measure echocardiographically.

MORPHOGENESIS

Three main abberations in embryological development have been proposed to explain abnormalities of the aortic

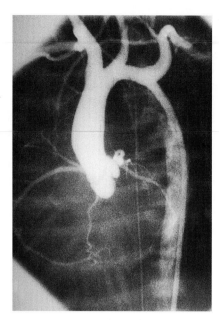

Figure 56.8 This angiogram is from a neonate and shows severe tubular hypoplasia of the isthmus.

arch. The first, abnormal embryogenesis of the vessels of the arch, and the second, abnormal development of the arterial duct, are closely interlinked. The third implicates changes in the ratio of flow between the pulmonary and systemic arterial pathways. We will consider the hypotheses in isolation for clarity.

In the usual situation, that with a left arch, it is the left fourth branchial arch that becomes the definitive aortic arch. The arterial duct then derives from the connection of the sixth brachial arch to the dorsal aorta. The left subclavian artery, in contrast, forms from the seventh segmental artery. This must undergo a cephalad migration through differential growth before assuming a position proximal to the aortic isthmus. In its migration, it must cross many structures. Derangements in this process were claimed by Clagett et al (1954) to be of importance in the pathogenesis of coarctation, but these views have not received widespread support.

The hypothesis implicating the arterial duct was based on findings of ductal tissue extending as a shelf into the lumen of the aorta at the site of the aortic insertion of the duct, thus forming a 'sling' of tissue around the entire circumference of the aorta at that site. Such ectopic ductal tissue had initially been described by Skoda as long ago as 1855, but his observations were doubted by those who were unable to find ductal tissue in the coarctation shelf (see above). Unequivocal evidence of the ductal sling, nonetheless, was provided by Wielanga and Dankmeijer (1968) and their findings were confirmed by Ho and Anderson (1979) and Gittenberger de Groot (1981). Hence, theories first advanced in the 19th century that coarctation was a malformation that only became apparent postnatally, after ductal closure, still hold some relevance today.

The third proposal is that the patterns of flow of blood in the fetal circulation influence embryogenesis. Rudolph et al (1972) postulated that it was a reduction in the volume of blood passing through the ascending aorta in fetal life that led postnatally to the development of coarctation. Such a hypothesis is strongly supported by the common association of coarctation with other obstructive lesions in the left side of the heart, along with those malformations that result in decreased flow in the fetal ascending aorta.

It had been widely assumed that, as only 10 to 20% of the combined fetal ventricular outputs passed through the aortic isthmus, there would be little in the way of adverse haemodynamic effects of coarctation in fetal life. It has now been shown, however, that infants born at full term with coarctation have an increased incidence of cranial abnormalities (van Houten et al, 1996). This is presumably the consequence of reduced flow in the ascending aorta leading to decreased cerebral perfusion. Similar abnormalities have also been found in children with isolated ventricular septal defects, perhaps giving further credence to the 'flow' theory. The secondary haemodynamic effects are also underscored by the relatively consistent finding of enlarged right-sided compared with left-sided structures in the fetal echocardiograms of those with coarctation. Indeed, the enlargement of the pulmonary trunk and its valve, and increased right-to-left ventricular ratios when compared with normal infants, have been proposed as diagnostic of the disease in fetal life (Sharland et al, 1994).

No single hypothesis can explain the morphogenesis of all coarctation lesions. It is more likely that there is interplay between the various mechanisms. It is highly likely that decreased flow to the aorta in some way influences the distribution of ductal tissue in the distal aortic arch (Hoffman, 1988). These basic mechanisms certainly help in the understanding of clinical presentation, early management and even successful treatment of coarctation lesions, to be described below.

PRESENTATION AND CLINICAL SYMPTOMATOLOGY

INFANTS AND NEONATES

Presentation

Most infants present with varying degrees of heart failure in infancy. When seen immediately, this is manifested by collapse, or later by poor feeding, sweating, breathlessness and failure to thrive. The group that survives infancy without symptoms will be discussed subsequently. The onset of cardiac failure is commonly within the first 3 months of life, but a significant number present within the first week of life. These patients uniformly will have critical narrowing of the aorta. They present when the supplementary effect of blood flow through the duct from the right ventricle to the descending aorta is interrupted. At this stage, they present acutely with shock, renal failure and necrotizing enterocolitis. Often described as having a duct-dependent systemic circulation, it is only the flow to the lower body that is initially limited. The secondary effects of acidosis on the myocardium, nonetheless, may lead to a global reduction in cardiac output. The coarctation itself may only be recognized as the infant is resuscitated.

The management of these infants has been revolutionized with the emergence, in the 1970s, of treatment with prostaglandin E$_1$ to maintain ductal patency. This will be discussed below.

Physical findings

These infants will be tachypnoeic, with intercostal recession. Those with markedly low cardiac output will often show profound skin mottling, slow capillary refill and peripheral cyanosis. Central cyanosis will only occur in the presence of an associated cyanotic congenital heart lesion, or when there is persistence of the fetal circulation. The presence of palpable femoral pulses in the first day or two of life does not exclude the diagnosis of coarctation, since flow of blood to the lower body may be maintained antegradely through the patent arterial duct. By the time the infant presents with symptoms, nonetheless, the femoral pulses are usually impalpable, or at least considerably weaker when compared with the brachial pulses. Occasionally, the infant is so shocked that no pulses are palpable; with resuscitation, the pulses in the right arm should return. The precordium is often active, unless myocardial function is depressed. On auscultation, there is usually a summation gallop rhythm. There is often a systolic murmur found along the left sternal edge, from the site of coarctation, and this may also be audible posteriorly. The continuous murmur classically ascribed to coarctation is unusual in infancy. Associated murmurs from other lesions, such as the arterial duct, may also be heard. An ejection click indicates an associated bicuspid aortic valve. Hepatomegaly and pulmonary crepitations are common, indicating heart failure.

Measurement of blood pressure in all four limbs reveals a gradient between the upper and lower limbs irrespective of whether the flush or Doppler method is used. The latter technique is preferable (Elseed et al, 1973). It should be remembered that differences in pressure of up to 20 mmHg may be revealed by Doppler interrogation in the normal neonate, presumably owing to the isthmal narrowing that is normal at this stage (de Swiet and Shinebourne, 1977). It is sometimes necessary to measure blood pressures serially if the diagnosis remains unclear. Indeed, in the presence of a marked run-off between the right subclavian and the iliac arteries as occurs with a large arterial duct or a cerebral arteriovenous malformation, for example, it may be possible to detect a large difference between systolic blood pressures measured in the arms and legs and yet the femoral pulses will remain easily palpable. Therefore, it is the combination of weak or absent femoral pulses together with a gradient in pressure between the limbs that is virtually pathognomonic of aortic coarctation. Paradoxically, the diagnosis of coarctation can be made more difficult by the administration of prostaglandin. Although greatly improving the physical condition, the manoeuvre leads to the pressure difference between the arms and legs becoming significantly diminished. All of these points may be important when facilities for cross-sectional echocardiography are lacking but are less important now that this is rarely the case.

OLDER CHILDREN AND ADULTS

Presentation

A large number of patients with coarctation pass through infancy without difficulty, either because initially the coarctation was not severe enough to become critical following closure of the arterial duct or because of the rapid development of a collateral circulation. The diagnosis in these children, or indeed adults, usually follows a routine medical examination. Only at this late event is there discovery of a heart murmur, absence or weakness of the femoral pulses, or systemic hypertension. When pressed, such patients will occasionally admit to a history of headaches, nosebleeds, cold feet, or calf pain on exercise (Tawes et al, 1969c). At the extreme, these patients may present with the end stages of hypertensive disease, such as subarachnoid haemorrhage or hypertensive retinopathy. Alternatively, they may be discovered during investigation for coronary arterial disease in later life.

Physical findings

The physical findings in older patients usually rest upon the appreciation of diminished or delayed femoral pulses compared with the right brachial or radial pulse. The femoral pulse is normally fractionally earlier than the radial, with a similar character, waveform and volume. Any departure from this norm requires further investigation.

In a recent study comparing the ability of primary care physicians in North America to detect coarctation during two decades, 1980–1990 and 1970–1980, Ing et al (1996) disappointingly noted that 'despite current recommendations to screen for coarctation with four extremity blood pressures, pediatricians had not improved their ability to diagnose this condition or make early appropriate referrals'. In the United Kingdom, there is also a tendency to rely only on the palpation of radial and femoral pulses to exclude coarctation. Yet, as the above study showed, this finding is unreliable compared with measurement of blood pressures in all four limbs.

The jugular venous pressure is normal, and hepatic enlargement is unusual. On palpation of the precordium, the apex is often displaced and heaving in nature as a result of left ventricular hypertrophy. On auscultation, the first and second heart sounds are usually normal but may be accompanied by an apical fourth heart sound if the left ventricle is becoming non-compliant.

The classical continuous murmur of coarctation is best heard in the left infraclavicular fossa and radiates to the back over the left scapula. It generally peaks late in systole and continues into early diastole, corresponding with the diastolic tail seen on Doppler echocardiography. Flow through significant collateral arteries from the ascending to descending aorta can also generate continuous murmurs. Physiologically, these collateral arteries can restore flow of blood to the lower body to normal. They then pemit palpable femoral pulses, albeit usually reduced and delayed. This is important because, if a well-developed collateral circulation is present, the aorta can be cross-clamped with impunity during operative repair, with little risk of damage to the spinal cord.

At this age, the physical findings of associated abnormalities, such as an ejection click with bicuspid aortic valve or a murmur owing to a small ventricular septal defect, will be typical of those lesions. A search for disease caused by hypertension is often unrewarding in childhood, although fundoscopic changes with a unique 'corkscrew' appearance to the retinal arteries has been described. These changes are different from the usual hypertensive change (Tabandeh, 1996).

INVESTIGATIONS

CHEST RADIOGRAPHY

The most frequent abnormalities seen in infants are cardiomegaly and increased pulmonary vascular mark-ings. Distinguishing between pulmonary venous congestion and excessive pulmonary flow may be difficult. In older children, the heart size is often normal, but if cardiomegaly is present it is usually caused by left ventricular enlargement. There are two pathognomonic signs that can be seen on the plain chest radiograph in older children. The first is rib notching, which usually is not seen until 4 years of age, although appearance in the first year has been described (Martelle and Moss, 1962). By adulthood, around three quarters of untreated patients have rib notching. It is most commonly seen posteriorly in the lower borders of the fourth to eighth ribs, around one third of the way from the spine to the lateral chest wall (Figure 56.9). This is the point where the intercostal artery crosses the rib. The notching in coarctation is classically bilateral. It must be distinguished from the unilateral notching seen after a classical Blalock–Taussig shunt, although unilateral notching can also occur with coarctation when a subclavian artery arises distal to the site of obstruction. The other cardinal radiological sign is known as the 'figure three' sign (Figure 56.9b). This appears to the left of the mediastinum and is caused by pre- and poststenotic dilation of the aorta.

ELECTROCARDIOGRAPHY

The majority of young infants presenting with coarctation will have normal right ventricular dominance, with extreme right-axis deviation. Later, left ventricular hypertrophy supervenes. There are early electrocardiographic signs of left ventricular dominance and strain in some infants. This has been linked to subendocardial ischaemia (Shinebourne et al, 1976) or coexisting aortic stenosis. Other changes are related to coexistent pathology.

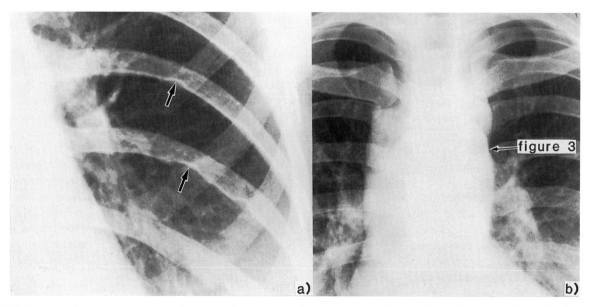

Figure 56.9 Evidence of coarctation is seen in the chest radiograph, with these pictures showing (a) rib notching (arrowed) and (b) the so-called 'figure 3' sign.

MAGNETIC RESONANCE IMAGING

Although echocardiography is a superior modality for the diagnosis of congenital heart disease in infants and young children and magnetic resonance imaging is limited in smaller children because of the need for sedation or anaesthesia, it has recently been shown that magnetic resonance imaging combined with phase velocity mapping can be used as a complete diagnostic tool in obtaining both morphological and physiological information in coarctation (Oshinski et al, 1996). In addition, resonance imaging is an excellent tool in the assessment of post-operative repair. This will be discussed below.

ECHOCARDIOGRAPHY

Echocardiography has become the diagnostic method of choice in infancy. The best view to image the aortic arch is the superior paracoronal section. This is obtained from the suprasternal notch and allows visualization of the entire aortic arch (Figure 56.10). In those with coarcta-

tion there is most commonly a short narrowed segment just distal to the left subclavian artery caused by the obstructive shelf projecting into the aorta posteriorly. More rarely, there is a longer segment of narrowing involving the isthmus (Figure 56.11). It must be remembered that the apparent anterior shelf often seen on the anterior wall of the aorta is not a part of the coarctation but the overlapping point of entry of the duct (Smallhorn et al, 1982b).

It is important, especially in infants, to assess the size of the transverse aortic arch. It can often be hypoplastic (Figure 56.12) or stenotic and can result in residual obstruction after distal repair. In the absence of an arterial duct, the haemodynamic severity of coarctation can

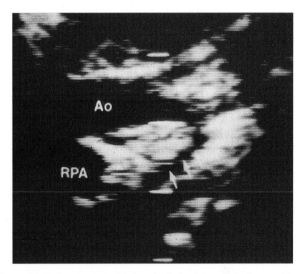

Figure 56.11 Long segment isthmal tubular hypoplasia (arrows) in suprasternal paracoronal section (see Figure 56.8 for angiographic correlation). Ao, aorta; RPA, right pulmonary artery.

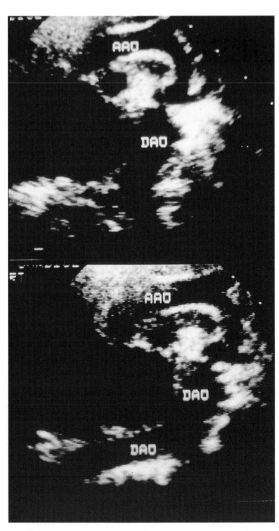

Figure 56.10 Suprasternal echocardiographic sections of severe discrete coarctation in a neonate. AAO, ascending aorta; DAO, descending aorta.

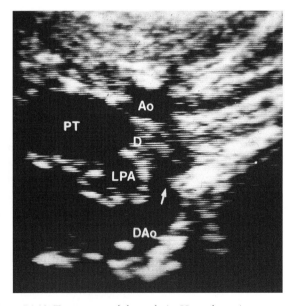

Figure 56.12 Transverse arch hypoplasia. Here, the entire transverse arch is tortuous and small, with relative sparing of the isthmus (arrow). Ao, aorta; DAo, descending aorta; d, duct; LPA, left pulmonary artery; PT pulmonary trunk.

readily be assessed by Doppler echocardiography. The spectral recording shows an extension of antegrade flow, and a persisting gradient into diastole, the so-called diastolic tail. There is rarely any doubt to its significance, but if uncertainty does exist, the spectral recording can be analysed further (Carvalho et al, 1990) according to the peak velocity and the half-time of diastolic velocity decay. This predicts accurately the severity of anatomical coarctation (Figure 56.13).

In isolated coarctation, the peak instantaneous pressure drop across the obstruction can be calculated from the peak velocity of the jet by using the simplified Bernoulli equation. In the presence of a significant associated obstructive lesion in the left heart, it is necessary to quantify the peak velocity of the jet proximal to the site of coarctation. This can often be significantly raised and, if not taken into account by using the expanded Bernoulli equation ($P = 4[V_{22} - V_{12}]$), there can be a significant overestimation of the gradient (Snider et al, 1997).

The remaining examination must be focused on the potential associated malformations, with care taken to assess the mitral and aortic valves accurately. Left ventricular wall thickness should be measured and an M-mode assessment of left ventricular shortening fraction should be made. It must always be remembered that, in the presence of coarctation severe enough to cause low cardiac output, the severity of associated obstructive lesions in the left heart can be underestimated. All of these observations must be modified in the presence of an arterial duct. When large, any gradient across the site of coarctation will be obviated, and the pattern of flow altered. Under these circumstances, much more reliance is placed upon adequate imaging of the stenotic area. In experienced hands, the diagnosis of coarctation using echo Doppler can be made with 95% sensitivity and 99% specificity (Huhta et al, 1984).

FETAL ECHOCARDIOGRAPHY

There are significant advantages to making the diagnosis of congenital heart defects during fetal life, especially those lesions that can be deemed duct dependent, as intervention electively with prostaglandin can prevent shock and acidosis. The difficulties in prenatal diagnosis of coarctation were well described by Sharland et al (1994). They found that, although a certain combination of features was strongly suggestive of abnormalities in the aortic arch, there was a significant rate of false-positive diagnosis, particularly in late pregnancy. These findings were confirmed by Brown et al (1997). They looked at the predictive value and sensitivity of one parameter, discrepancy in ventricular size, in the fetal diagnosis of coarctation. There was a moderate sensitivity at 62% but a mediocre positive predictive value. They also commented on the high rate of false-positive diagnosis beyond 34 weeks of gestation. Therefore, although severe coarctation is associated with relative hypoplasia of left heart structures compared with the right, which is visible in early pregnancy, this can be a feature of the normal fetus later in pregnancy. Milder forms of coarctation are compatible with an entirely normal fetal echocardiogram, especially in the last trimester.

CARDIAC CATHETERIZATION AND ANGIOGRAPHY

In most cases, sufficient information can be obtained from clinical and non-invasive examination to decide on an appropriate plan for management. Cardiac catheterization is of limited value in delineating further the anatomy in the neonate, and it is associated with significant morbidity. It is rarely necessary for the assessment of associated anomalies. Indeed, even if significant mitral obstruction, mitral regurgitation or aortic stenosis is

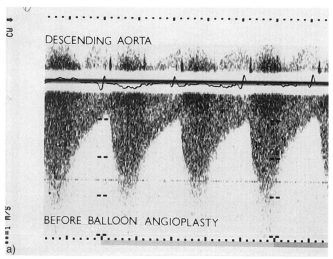

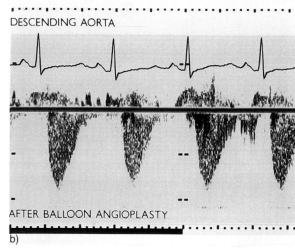

Figure 56.13 Typical spectral Doppler recordings from a patient with severe aortic coarctation before (a) and after (b) balloon angioplasty. The peak velocity is 3 m/s but more importantly there is a prolonged diastolic tail, which is abolished immediately after balloon angioplasty.

present, the baby is often better assessed after repair of the coarctation, when cardiac output, the effects of the arterial duct, and other abnormalities of ventricular performance, have resolved.

One potential indication for invasive assessment, nonetheless, is for intervention. Ever since Singer and colleagues (1982) first described primary balloon angioplasty of coarctation, controversy has existed as to its role in the management of coarctation in patients of all ages. This will be discussed in detail below.

COURSE AND PROGNOSIS

Campbell (1970) quoted a mean age of death of 31 years for those with coarctation surviving the first year without an operation, three quarters being dead by the age of 46 years. His information was derived from clinical records and postmortem studies. Although infants dying in the first year were excluded, he suggested that those presenting with congestive heart failure might have had a survival rate at 1 year as low as 16%, this figure taking no account of associated lesions. In older patients, the cause of death was often related to systemic hypertension, the two most common findings being congestive cardiac failure (25.5%) and aortic dissection or rupture (21%). Bacterial endocarditis was also common (18%). An additional significant group (11.5%) died as a result of ruptured berry or saccular aneurysms causing intracranial bleeding. These congenital lesions are more common in those with coarctation (Hodes et al, 1959). Hypertension secondary to coarctation is not, however, thought to be the only pathogenic factor. Abnormalities of the vessel wall are important, certainly in intracerebral catastrophes, but also with the other causes of death such as aortic dissection or rupture. Cystic medial necrosis and new structural abnormalities are seen in areas remote from the coarcted segment itself and may be unrelated to the type and age at surgery.

The mortality from bacterial endocarditis has fallen markedly in recent years through improved diagnostic techniques, especially cross-sectional echocardiography, and aggressive early treatment with antibiotics. When found, the site of endocarditis is often in the aorta, distal to the coarctation site, or on an associated bicuspid aortic valve. It is recommended, nonetheless, that children with coarctation receive prophylactic antibiotics against endocarditis, even after definitive surgical repair, during dental, colonic and genitourinary procedures.

MANAGEMENT

STABILIZATION OF NEONATES AND INFANTS

The management of those presenting with coarctation in infancy was revolutionized in the early 1980s by the ability to maintain, and restore pharmacologically, the patency of the arterial duct. In the majority of infants with preductal coarctation who present with heart failure, shock and deteriorating renal function, the ability to perfuse the lower body, albeit with systemic venous blood, will reverse the physiological insult as long as ductal patency and flow is maintained.

Prostaglandin E_1 was first demonstrated to maintain ductal patency under both aerobic and anaerobic conditions by Coceani and Olley in 1973. It was not until around a decade later, nonetheless, that it started to be applied clinically to patients with obstructive lesions such as coarctation (Leoni et al, 1984). Prostaglandin E_1 is given initially at a dose of 0.05–0.1 µg/min per kg body weight. This can be increased to 0.4 µg/min per kg if required, although lower initial doses have been shown to be equally therapeutic and less likely to cause apnoea (Kramer et al, 1995). Freed et al (1981) showed that the maximal response occurred between 15 minutes and 4 hours. Occasional improvement has been documented in infants as old as 5 weeks, but treatment is generally less impressive in older neonates and in those whose ducts are closed at presentation (Lewis et al, 1978; Freed et al, 1981). Side effects can occur, most commonly decreased respiratory drive leading to apnoea, occasionally requiring ventilation. There can also be hypotension with cutaneous vasodilation, jitteriness (which can lead to seizures), fever, susceptibility to infections, diarrhoea and, more rarely, coagulopathy (British National Formulary, 1997). For the neonate, management depends on timing of diagnosis. If the diagnosis has been made, or is strongly suspected, antenatally, then there is little to be lost from starting prostaglandin E_1 at birth. Certain centres advocate antenatal transfer and delivery in or close to the cardiac centre. If a neonate is found to have weak or absent femoral pulses and remains well, it is justifiable to arrange transfer to a tertiary centre, having commenced prostaglandin E_1 to avoid the catastrophe of an acute closure of the duct during transfer.

In any infant becoming shocked within the first few weeks of life, and in whom lower limb pulses are absent, it should be mandatory to start prostaglandin along with the normal resuscitatory manoeuvres while expert assistance is sought. Ventilation with positive pressure will reduce systemic consumption of oxygen and may directly ameliorate cardiac failure. During ventilation, manoeuvres to increase pulmonary vascular resistance, and hence reduce the ratio of pulmonary to systemic blood flow, will lead to increased right-to-left flow through the arterial duct, thus improving perfusion of the lower body. The management is similar to that in the pre- and postoperative infant with hypoplastic left heart syndrome (see Chapter 45). This will include minimizing the fraction of inspired oxygen, maintaining arterial partial pressure of carbon dioxide at 6 kPa or more, and the judicious use of volume and ionotropes. As the group from Paris recently demonstrated, the outcome in these children with multiorgan failure is much more favourable if time is taken medically to stabilize them before carrying out definitive intervention (Lupoglazoff et al, 1995).

In a proportion of infants, the infusion of prostaglandin E_1 produces no effect. Definitive treatment then becomes urgent. Cullen et al (1993) described four such infants and demonstrated postductal coarctation characterized by left-to-right flow through the duct along with a stenotic Doppler profile in the descending aorta. These infants required immediate definitive treatment because maintaining ductal patency failed to improve systemic blood flow.

DEFINITIVE TREATMENT

As with any therapeutic manoeuvre, it would be preferable if evidence-based medicine had provided a technique that was clearly superior in terms of immediate and long-term relief of coarctation, had minimal side effects and was cost effective. Hanley (1996), discussing balloon dilation of congenital coarctation, makes two important points on this subject. First, the pursuit of 'a single ideal form of therapy for all forms of coarctation' is almost certainly misguided, as the obstructive lesions show great variability in their morphology, even before ductal patency and associated intracardiac lesions are considered. Second, studies spanning a period of 50 years, during which both general surgical techniques and medical resuscitation have improved greatly and prostaglandin has been introduced, cannot be compared as the studies have different groups of patients from different periods treated with different techniques.

The fact that the various surgical repairs have all had their vociferous proponents at various stages, and that most of the debate has been adversarial in nature, has not led towards a resolution of the question of optimal treatment. And when the debate is further complicated by the issue of balloon dilation for 'native' coarctation, then Hanley's call for prospective, randomized studies involving a large number of subjects seems imperative to implement.

NON-ELECTIVE SURGICAL REPAIR

The majority of duct-dependent infants can be medically stabilized and will benefit from an interlude before definitive treatment while metabolic derangements are corrected. These infants, nonetheless, will need relief of their aortic obstruction within 1 or 2 days of presentation. There have been reports that minimally symptomatic infants with isolated coarctation can be managed medically for a period of time (Fyler et al, 1980; Hesslein et al, 1983). In the majority of tertiary centres nowadays, any symptomatic infant is repaired surgically with little delay. There is considerable debate about the procedure of choice, and whether one- or two-stage treatment of associated defects should be performed. A large part of

the debate regarding the best method of repair centres on the high incidence of recoarctation, although this is clouded by the fact that some groups cite residual gradients from arm to leg, others consider blood pressures in the arms, and yet others measure the difference in the pressure between upper and lower limbs exposed by exercise. The matter is then further complicated by the confusion of whether many cases of 'recoarctation' are residual coarctation. The need for precision in terminology was elucidated by Waldman et al (1983). They recognized four patterns of gradients between the arms and legs after initial surgery. These were, first, complete and permanent abolition. Second was initial abolition followed by late recurrence. The third option was initial residual obstruction followed by late resolution, and, finally, persistent residual obstruction. Furthermore, the common practice of defining rates of recoarctation as the percentage of patients undergoing surgery who are known to have recoarctation at the time of reporting is almost worthless. As with any other late operative complication, this percentage is heavily dependent on the period over which progress has been monitored. Actuarial rates of recoarctation must be given (Macartney et al, 1980; Williams et al, 1980). In this chapter we will not try to compare the techniques (see below), rather we will describe them along with their intrinsic potential advantages and disadvantages. As stated, no comparative review can be definitive. Even if it were, it would be ignored by the protagonists of alternative approaches!

MANAGEMENT OF ASSOCIATED LESIONS IN INFANCY

If the arterial duct is patent, it should be ligated if surgery is performed. There has been extensive debate regarding the best approach to associated ventricular septal defects in neonates and infants with coarctation. The coarctation can be repaired and an expectant policy can be adopted, whereby failure to wean from the ventilator or failure to thrive are indications for reoperation to close the defect or, much more rarely nowadays, to band the pulmonary trunk. Although argued against by some, this strategy does have the advantage of allowing improvement in ventricular performance, pulmonary oedema and general condition of the infant. It may even buy time for spontaneous closure of small defects. An increasingly popular option, particularly in the presence of a large defect, is one-staged repair. This involves closing the defect together with repair of coarctation via a midline sternotomy. The main disadvantage here used to be the high mortality, up to 30% in some series. More recently, following the general trend, the mortality for one-staged repair has diminished markedly (Park et al, 1992). The final, and least fashionable, option is repair of the coarctation and concomitant banding of the pulmonary trunk. This option is particularly valid in the presence of multiple ventricular septal defects, or for those that are judged inaccessible. It is rarely recommended for the management of single large defects. A method of reliably assessing which defects will close spontaneously would be beneficial. Brouwer and colleagues (1996), addressing this issue, found that the presence of a left-to-right shunt prior to repair of the coarctation, and extension of the defect into the right ventricular inlet or outlet, were the two significant risk factors for eventual surgical closure of the defect. It is also necessary to address the problems of more complicated associated defects, such as complete transposition, double outlet right ventricle, tricuspid atresia or double inlet ventricle, at the time of repair of coarctation. These lesions are discussed elsewhere in this book.

In those infants at the extreme end of the spectrum with multiple obstructive lesions in the left heart, so-called Shone's anomaly, the outlook is generally considered to be poor. A recent experience shows some benefit from aggressive reconstructive surgery with early attention paid to the mitral valve (Brauner et al, 1997). Although there remains a significant early mortality (16%), the late functional outcome was favourable compared with more conservative approaches (Bolling et al, 1990).

ELECTIVE REPAIR

In those who are asymptomatic, there is an added area of contention, namely the optimal age to repair the coarctation. Again, there has been much debate as to the nature of the intervention. There are three main factors to consider. First, it is known that the overall operative mortality is greatest in those under 1 year of age, although this has improved greatly in recent years through a combination of improved medical management and better surgical techniques. Second, the likelihood of recoarctation is related not only to the type of repair but also to the timing of repair, being more common in those undergoing surgery under 1 year of age. Brouwer et al (1994), while acknowledging the importance of weight at operation, showed that recoarctation in patients undergoing resection and end-to-end anastomoses was dependent on age. In those having surgery as neonates, one third were affected; in contrast, 15% of those operated on between 1 and 18 months, and only 3% of older children, were affected. The last major factor to consider was also addressed by Brouwer and colleagues (1994), namely the effect of age at operation on the incidence of late hypertension. This occurred in 10% after neonatal and early repair, but increased mortality in children over the age of 5 years. Maron and colleagues (1973) had already demonstrated that patients undergoing repair of coarctation in their late teens had an excessively high mortality from cardiovascular causes in later life. One of these was persistent hypertension. Their study made it clear that there was an age beyond which

operative repair may not change the natural history of the disease. In the rather selected group they studied, life expectancy was no better than for untreated coarctation. This justifiably changed the prevailing opinion. These findings were subsequently confirmed by Lawrie and colleagues (1981), who also showed that residual hypertension was a poor prognostic factor. Others have since shown that hypertension can occur late after repair (Clarkson et al, 1983), while Naton and Olley (1976) found a much higher incidence of permanent hypertension not caused by recoarctation in patients undergoing surgery above 4 years of age. Shinebourne and colleagues (1976) made similar observations, but the 'break-point' in their cohort was 1 year of age. Their recommendation at that time was for elective repair during the second 6 months of life, thereby neatly steering a course between the Scylla of recoarctation and the Charybdis of permanent hypertension. At this point, everything seemed quite clear. Subsequently, however, scattered reports have appeared of permanent hypertension occurring in patients undergoing repair of coarctation in infancy, or even the neonatal period (Patel et al, 1977; Herrmann et al, 1978; Shinebourne et al, 1979). To keep this problem in perspective, it should be noted that Williams et al (1980) found no patient with permanent hypertension without recoarctation among 118 survivors of repair of coarctation in infancy. It does seem, however, that there may be a few patients in whom permanent hypertension will ensue irrespective of the age of repair. To some extent, all of this discussion has become irrelevant to contemporary management. 'Elective' surgery is performed in most centres at, or shortly after, presentation at any age. This discussion does serve as a reminder of the potential long-term implications for the disease, no matter when, or how, it is repaired.

HISTORY AND TECHNIQUES OF REPAIR APPROACHES

RESECTION AND END-TO-END REPAIR

It was Blalock and Park (1944) who performed the first experimental repair of coarctation in the mid 1940s, using either the turned-down left subclavian artery or the carotid artery to bypass the induced stenosis (Blalock and Park, 1944). Gross and Hufnagel (1945), at the Childrens' Hospital in Boston, had also performed studies in animal models of coarctation in which they had demonstrated that aortic cross-clamping, followed by resection with end-to-end anastomosis, was feasible. The first surgical repair of congenital coarctation was reported in 1945 by Crafoord and Nylin of Sabbatsberg hospital, Stockholm. Crafoord, the chief surgeon, had been discussing the feasibility of repair for some time when two patients (a 12-year-old schoolboy and a 27-year-old farmer) presented to his institution with isolated coarctation. Considering the poor prognosis of both, and after discussion with Nylin, the chief physician, it was decided that attempted repair was justified. Both underwent lateral thoracotomy with aortic cross-clamping just proximal and distal to the coarctation. The coarctation was resected, and end-to-end anastomosis of the adjacent aortic segments was performed. To this day, this remains the standard surgical procedure in older patients with discrete narrowing.

INTERPOSITION GRAFTS

Although the first report (Calodney and Carson, 1950) ended in failure, Gross (1951) introduced the interposition of an aortic homograft across the coarcted segment. For a time, this was considered the treatment of choice for infants with coarctation. Thus, Kirklin et al (1952) successfully repaired coarctation in this fashion in a 10-week-old infant, and Mustard and colleagues (1955) reported successful neonatal repair. A similar approach, but using prosthetic conduits, was introduced later (Morris et al, 1960). This remained useful in older patients with aneurysms, in those with complex anatomy, or for those in which approximation of the cut ends could not be accomplished during attempted end-to-end anastomoses (Edie et al, 1975). Its disadvantages include use of prosthetic material, and hence increased risk of infection, lack of potential for growth and obviously the need for two anastomoses.

PATCH AORTOPLASTY

Because of early poor results of end-to-end anastomosis, with recoarctation reported in up to 60% (Hartmann et al, 1970; Sade et al, 1979; Williams et al, 1980), different mechanisms of repair were sought. Vosschulte (1961) had already introduced 'isthmuloplasty' in 1957, and from this developed the technique of patch aortoplasty. An elliptical patch of dacron, or polytetrafluoroethylene, was placed over the site of coarctation opposite the site of ductal insertion.

Patch angioplasty was claimed to reduce rates of recoarctation (Sade et al, 1978). Differences in pressure between arms and legs induced by exercise were shown by two independent groups to be less after patch angioplasty than after resection followed by end-to-end anastomosis (Connor and Baker, 1981; Smith et al, 1984). The very high frequency of true aneurysms (Figure 56.14) developing late and opposite the site of repair, nonetheless, has led many centres to use this technique only if no alternative is available. The pathogenesis of aneurysms is not fully elucidated. It has been suggested that excessive resection of the ductal shelf weakens the aortic media (DeSanto et al, 1987). Others have implicated deviations in haemodynamic patterns caused by differing tensile strength between the prosthetic patch and the posterior aortic wall (Rheuban et al, 1986) and intensification of

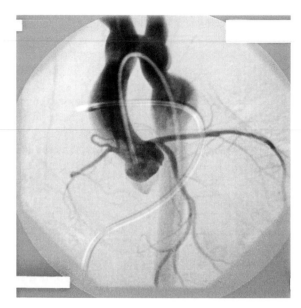

Figure 56.14 Postoperative ascending aortogram showing obvious aneurysmal dilatation of the aorta at the site of previous patch aortoplasty.

the pulse wave at the native wall. A more recent study using polytetrafluoroethylene for the patch, but without resection of ductal tissue, promises improved results (Backer et al, 1995), but, generally, this technique has been consigned to the history books.

SUBCLAVIAN FLAP REPAIR

Waldhausen and Narhwold (1966) introduced the subclavian flap aortoplasty also in an attempt to decrease the very high incidence of recoarctation that complicated its contemporary alternatives. The subclavian artery is mobilized through a standard left thoracotomy and ligated at its first branch, attempting to preserve the thyrocervical trunk and the internal thoracic artery in order to improve perfusion to the left arm (Moulton et al, 1984). A longitudinal incision is made across the coarctation from the subclavian artery to the area of poststenotic dilation. The proximal stump of the subclavian artery is then opened anteriorly, turned down over the incision and anastomosed. The vertebral artery is ligated to prevent any subsequent subclavian steal leading to cerebral ischaemia.

The advantages of the technique include the use of exclusively native material, with consequent decreased risk of infection and improved potential for growth (Moulton et al, 1984), no circumferential anastomosis and less extensive dissection compared with the end-to-end repair. Furthermore, this repair is held to leave less tension on the suture lines in comparison with end-to-end-repair. Obviously, the major disadvantage is the loss of the main arterial supply to the left arm. Indeed, deleterious effects on growth of the arm have been reported. These range from mild discrepancy in limb length, similar to that following a Blalock–Taussig shunt, to rare reports of gangrene (Geiss et al, 1980; Todd et al, 1983; van Son et al, 1989). Aneurysms have also been described (Martin et al, 1988) but are less common than after patch aortoplasty. Early studies, suggesting a much lower incidence of recoarctation compared with other repairs, led to the technique being advocated as the treatment of choice in infancy (Campbell et al, 1984; Penkoske et al, 1984). More recent studies have refuted these claims (Cobanoglu et al, 1985; Beekman et al, 1986; von Son et al, 1989; Rubay et al, 1992).

Variations on the original method have been described. Waldhausen, the original proponent (Waldhausen and Narhwold, 1966), together with Hart et al (1983), described a 'reversed' technique for coarctations occurring proximal to the left subclavian artery. This variant has now been used for those with significant associated tubular hypoplasia. Attempts have also been made to address the loss of the subclavian artery, using techniques involving reimplantation (de Mendonca et al, 1985; Meier et al, 1986) or by using the internal thoracic artery to preserve the arterial supply to the arm (Fournier et al, 1985). Further variants have been described to deal with rare anatomical variants, such as anomalous origin of the right subclavian artery, involvement of coarctation in the left subclavian artery and hypoplasia of the arch (Campbell et al, 1982; Odell and Spilkin, 1984).

EXTENDED END-TO-END REPAIR

The occurrence of recoarctation in the experience of some centres using subclavian flap repair, particularly in very young infants, led Lansman and colleagues (1986) to modify the classic resection and end-to-end operation, introducing the extended end-to-end repair. Many now use this technique, or one of its modifications, electively, especially if there is associated tubular hypoplasia of the transverse arch or isthmus. Whether tubular hypoplasia needs to be so specifically addressed is itself a contentious point. Proponents of the subclavian flap repair argue that, in most patients, subsequent growth of the arch is sufficient once the obstruction has been relieved. Some evidence (Siewers et al, 1991) certainly suggests that the hypoplastic arch does have significant potential for growth after repair. The main precepts underscoring the more radical resections are, first, that it is the retention of ductal tissue in the lumen of the main conduit to the lower body that fosters the development of an obstructing shelf and thereby leads to recoarctation. This concept was explored by Jonas (1991). Second, correction must address hypoplasia of the isthmus and distal arch. The initial modification consisted of a similar approach to that used in the classic end-to-end procedure, but the first cross-clamp was applied proximal to the left subclavian artery. Patency of the common carotid artery is closely monitored. The distal clamp is placed clear of the coarctation, and the entire obstructive segment is excised. The proximal anastomotic site is the longitudinally cut underside of the aortic arch, the distal end being the obliquely cut descending aorta. Zannini et al (1985) and Elliot (1987) further modified the technique specifically to address hypoplasia of the transverse arch. Their dissection is much more extensive, including the arteries to the head and neck and the descending aorta down to the diaphragm. The proximal clamp is applied across the left subclavian, left common carotid and part of the brachiocephalic artery, the tip being well down the left wall of the ascending aorta. Although this latter technique has led to an apparent reduction in recoarctation (Elliot 1987), questions must be posed concerning the very high rates of recoarctation that the advocates of the newer technique seem to produce with more conservative approaches. Indeed, a consensus operation is unlikely ever to be achieved, simply because of individual surgical experience, technique and results.

BALLOON ANGIOPLASTY

Although an accepted form of treatment for recurrent coarctation after surgical repair (see later), percutaneous balloon angioplasty of native coarctation as a primary intervention remains highly controversial. Originally adopted because of the significant morbidity and mortality associated with operative repair of recoarctation, its extension to include native coarctation has been contentious.

Sos and colleagues (1979) demonstrated that percutaneous balloon dilation of native coarctation was feasible by dilating a lesion during a neonatal postmortem. Animal studies followed (Casteñada-Zuniga et al, 1982; Lock et al, 1982). Once Singer et al (1982) reported the first clinical dilation in a 7-week-old child shortly following surgical repair, primary balloon intervention was soon attempted (Finley et al, 1983; Lock et al, 1983; Sperling et al, 1983).

Most reports describe retrograde arterial placement of the balloon via femoral or umbilical arterial catheter (Attia et al, 1988; Rao et al, 1992). Antegrade venous placement, via a patent oval fossa, the left ventricle and ascending aorta, has been advocated by some (Rao et al, 1988; Lo et al, 1989). Choice of the appropriate size of balloon has been the subject of much discussion, with various comparisons made to the size of the aortic isthmus, the coarcted site, the poststenotic area and the aorta at the level of the diaphragm. Suffice to say, no consensus exists, but few would choose a balloon larger than any part of the aorta in which the balloon is to be inflated but which is not part of the discrete narrowing. Hence, many consider it unwise to dilate areas of associated tubular hypoplasia. Angiography should always be repeated after dilation to assess the degree of overt damage to the arterial wall. Importantly, most interventionists who perform the procedure advocate never crossing the recently dilated site with catheter tips or guidewires. This is because of the very real risks of aortic dissection and even rupture (Finlay et al, 1983). Following dilation, it is probably wise to monitor the patient in the intensive care or high-dependency unit. One death has been reported 6 hours after uncomplicated dilation of recoarctation that was caused by ventricular fibrillation (Kan et al, 1983).

Initial results with balloon dilation of native coarctation were disappointing (Lock et al, 1983). Of particular concern was the occasional incidence of aneurysms developing at the site of dilation (Cooper et al, 1987; Brandt et al, 1987). Our own early institutional experience in neonates (Redington et al, 1990) compared unfavourably with contemporary surgical results (Figure 56.15). Because of this, we abandoned balloon dilation of native coarctation. We remain unconvinced by the subsequent literature in neonates and infants. Rates of recoarctation of 83% for the former, and 40% for the latter, with complications involving the femoral artery in 20% and 10%, respectively, have been quoted by the most ardent proponents of angioplasty for native coarctation (Rao et al, 1996). We consider this unacceptable in the face of continually improving surgical results, and this is supported by prospective randomized studies (Shaddy et al, 1993). The data are less clear cut in older children, and the lower incidence of certain surgical complications, such as para-

plegia and postoperative hypertension must be borne in mind (see complications).

As Lock demonstrated, however, successful balloon angioplasty requires tearing of the intimal and medial walls of the aorta (Lock et al, 1982), a finding confirmed by Ho et al (1988). Sohn and colleagues (1994) demonstrated, using intravascular ultrasound, that there is a high incidence of aortic dissection following balloon dilation of either native or residual coarctation (Figure 56.16). Even though the majority of these tears remain clinically unimportant, dissection requiring surgical intervention is reported (Erbel et al, 1990; Fawzy et al, 1992; Beitzke et al, 1997). With such a relatively unsighted technique, the most frequent local problems are, unsurprisingly, residual coarctation and the aforementioned development of aneurysms. The other serious complication occurs at the site of vascular access. It is worth noting that balloon dilation is not entirely free from neurological sequels, particularly if associated with anomalies in cerebral vasculature (Benson et al, 1986).

Yetman et al (1997) recently showed that when a recurrent coarctation is successfully dilated, the likelihood of remaining free from reintervention 12 years later was over 70%. Hypoplasia of the transverse arch was the primary predictor for the need to reintervene. Generally, the results of balloon valvoplasty for recurrent coarctation are considered more successful, with lower incidences of aneurysmal formation (Hess et al, 1986; Hijazi et al, 1991), perhaps because of the surrounding scar tissue. Of recent interest, however, are the results of the investigations of the Valvuloplasty and Angioplasty of

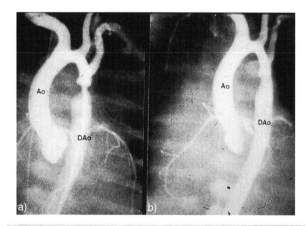

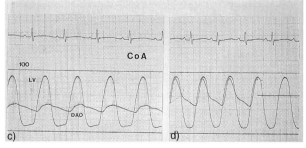

Figure 56.15 Balloon dilation for aortic coarctation. Ascending aortic angiograms from a neonate before (a) and after (b) balloon dilation. The Doppler tracing shows the initial gradient across the narrowed aorta (a) and confirms the excellent early haemodynamic result, showing abolition of the initial gradient. Severe recoarctation occurred within 4 weeks. CoA, aortic coarctation; DAo, descending aorta; LV, left ventricle.

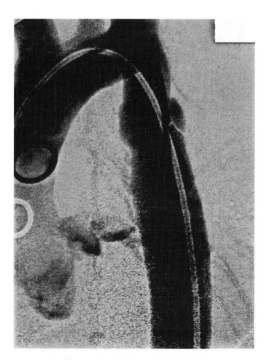

Figure 56.16 Ascending aortic angiogram immediately after balloon dilation of severe aortic coarctation. There is early aneurysmal formation, with an obvious intimal flap posteriorly.

Congenital Anomalies Registry. They recently reviewed the previous 12 years of angioplasty for coarctation from their 25 centres. The results of acute angioplasty of native coarctation were marginally superior to those for recurrent coarctation (McCrindle et al, 1996).

Whether the advantages of avoiding conventional surgery, and its attendant morbidity, are outweighed by these disadvantages is the nub of the ongoing debate. To some extent, the answer must depend on the institutional results for the surgical alternative.

COMPLICATIONS

Repair of coarctation is a life-saving procedure, most obviously when performed in early infancy for an isolated lesion (Macartney et al, 1980; Williams et al, 1980). There are, however, significant complications. All the complications of a lateral thoracotomy or dissection of tissue can occur, along with the problems of cardiopulmonary bypass should associated defects be repaired. It is more appropriate here to consider only those complications specific to the repair itself.

EARLY COMPLICATIONS

The most catastrophic early complication is bleeding. Any procedure involving arterial anastomosis can be associated with leakage from the suture lines, and any continued blood loss from chest drains or worsening haemodynamics, perhaps indicating loss into the mediastinum, must result in immediate surgical exploration. Ideally, any associated coagulopathy must first be corrected. The phenomenon of paradoxical hypertension occurring after coarctectomy (see below) can put undue pressure on the suture lines, hence hypertension must be aggressively controlled in the immediate postoperative period. Those with Turner's syndrome are known to be at especial risk, perhaps because of their abnormal connective tissue (Brandt et al, 1984).

Neurological complications are occasionally seen. Damage to local structures can result in transient paralysis of the vocal cords, Horner's syndrome or diaphragmatic paralysis. The last of these can be especially troublesome in younger patients, who occasionally require diaphragmatic plication, or even long-term ventilation. Damage to the thoracic duct can result in persistent chylous effusions.

Perhaps the most feared complication of elective repair is injury to the spinal cord. Brewer (1972) showed that poor collaterals around the coarctation at the time of repair predisposed to later paraplegia, as did poor distal perfusion. Most authors suggest pharmacological intervention when the distal arch pressure falls below 50 mmHg (Moreno et al, 1980; Watterson et al, 1990). Although Brewer (1972) showed no particular correlation to the length of cross-clamping, it seems prudent to minimize this. Other attempts to protect the spinal cord have included measuring somatosensory potentials (Pollock et al, 1986) and drainage of cerebrospinal fluid (McCullough et al, 1988). If there is a limited collateral supply, and the distal aortic pressure drops, many centres utilize a temporary 'jump graft' (Luosto et al, 1980; Foster, 1984). Occasionally, more central damage can result from aortic cross-clamping and, as mentioned earlier, subclavian steal from the circle of Willis can result if the vertebral artery is left open during subclavian flap aortoplasty.

There are two distinct periods of paradoxical hypertension following repair of aortic coarctation. The first occurs almost immediately and is almost certainly caused by a major outpouring from the carotid and aortic baroreceptors, which respond to reduced stretch caused by, for them, relative hypotension. The finding of increased levels of noradrenaline subsequent to repair in these patients supports this theory (Goodall and Sealy, 1969), although the fact that pressure has been shown to remain elevated for up to 6 months (Benedict et al, 1978) somewhat confuses the matter, as the first period tends to abate after 24–72 hours.

The second period occurs later, around the second or third postoperative day and has often been referred to as post-coarctectomy syndrome. It was initially believed to be caused by acute mesenteric arteritis associated with relative hypertension. Subsequently, it has been shown potentially to affect all the vessels distal to the site of repair. Sealy (1990) postulated that this second period of hypertension could be analogous to the arteritis seen with malignant hypertension in that the vessels below the coarctation site, used to lower perfusion pressures, are suddenly exposed to much higher pressures after repair and respond with intense arterial vasospasm sufficient to cause endothelial ischaemia. The role of the renin–angiotensin system in the two responses has been extensively studied, yet no unifying theory exists. Studies have shown that plasma levels of renin are normal prior to surgery (Amsterdam et al, 1969; Strong et al, 1970; Alpert et al, 1979). Following surgery, perhaps paradoxically, the levels increase (Parker et al, 1982). It further complicates matters that diverse pharmacological manipulations all abate the second period, namely depletion of adrenergic transmitters by reserpine, β-blockade, smooth muscle relaxation and inhibition of angiotensin-converting enzyme. Preoperative β-blockade has been shown, in a randomized unblinded trial, to reduce postoperative systolic and diastolic blood pressure and to lower the activity of renin in the plasma, without affecting the usual rise in postoperative plasma noradrenaline concentration, suggesting a major role for the sympathetic nervous system (Gidding et al, 1985). Interestingly, there does not seem to be a clear relationship between transient postoperative and long-term hypertension (Rocchini et al, 1976; Stansel et al, 1977).

LATE COMPLICATIONS

The problem of defining recoarctation has already been discussed, together with some idea as to its aetiology (Merrill et al, 1994). Symptomatic individuals need re-intervention, but criterions regarding the degree of hypertension in the arm, and noninvasively measured gradients across the site of repair, are unreliable. In younger children, clinical examination and Doppler echocardiographic assessment can be relied upon (see earlier) but this may not be the case in older patients. Many centres now use magnetic resonance imaging to assess recoarctation in these older children and adults. The multi-image planes that are obtained (Greenberg et al, 1997) offer unparalleled anatomical views of sites of repair and are particularly useful in assessing the development of aneurysmal change. More recently, magnetic resonance phase velocity mapping has been used to provide accurate estimates of the severity of stenosis and pressure gradients in coarctation (Mohiaddin et al, 1993; Kilner et al, 1996; Oshinski et al, 1996). Truly diagnostic cardiac catheterization is now rarely required.

Since Maron and colleagues (1973) highlighted an optimal time for elective repair of coarctation, there have been many studies showing abnormal physiological responses, even in those repaired in infancy. Initially, most concern focused on the prevalence of hypertension. Cardiovascular complications were presumed secondary to this, with long-term studies showing a reduced life expectancy after 'successful' repair in late childhood (Presbitero et al, 1987; Cohen et al, 1989). Furthermore, although studies suggest normal exercise capacity and cardiovascular function in those undergoing surgery below school age (Balderston et al, 1992), as these children age there is a tendency for abnormal physiological responses to exercise testing to develop, notably hypertension in the arms and detectable gradients between the pre- and postcoarctation vascular beds. Hypertension in the arms is seen even in the absence of other evidence of recoarctation at rest (Simsolo et al, 1988; Heger et al, 1997). Simsolo and colleagues (1988) postulated that preoperative hypertension may induce irreversible changes in the arterial wall along with long-term baroreceptor dysfunction. This was confirmed by Gardiner and colleagues (1994), who demonstrated abnormal endothelial responses in the precoarctation vascular bed in adults after 'successful' surgical repair in childhood. Guenthard and Wyler (1995) later demonstrated that the hypertensive response to exercise was not related to anatomical narrowing, but to an interaction between an enhanced sympathetic nervous system and structural and functional abnormalities of the precoarctation vessels (Guenthard et al, 1996). It has also been shown that these children have abnormal left ventricular mass and diastolic dysfunction (Moskowitz al, 1990; Leandro et al, 1992). Some consider postoperative hypertension to be secondary to occult gradients manifested during exercise, which have resulted in a persistent hyperdynamic and hypercontractile left ventricle (Kimball et al, 1994). It is likely that further research in these children will result in the elucidation of a more complex interaction between the physiology of the precoarctation vascular bed and hypertension. It remains to be seen whether more rigid 'prophylactic' antihypertensive medication in those found to have asymptomatic gradients on exercise will be efficacious in decreasing long-term cardiovascular complications.

These patients, however, should not avoid exercise. At the Bethesda conference, the recommendations were that participation in sports be permitted 6 months after intervention for those who had a gradient of less than 20 mmHg between the limbs at rest, and a normal systolic pressure on exercise. In those with aortic dilation, wall thinning or aneurysmal formation, participation should be restricted to low-impact sports (Graham et al, 1994).

——— INTERRUPTED AORTIC ARCH ———

Interruption of the aortic arch defines a condition in which there is complete anatomical discontinuity between two adjacent segments of the aortic arch (Figure 56.17). In the rare cases that show anatomical continuity, via a solid cord (Figure 56.18), the term arch atresia is better used. Both conditions, nonetheless, show physiological discontinuity and can be considered the extreme end of the spectrum of obstruction of the aortic arch.

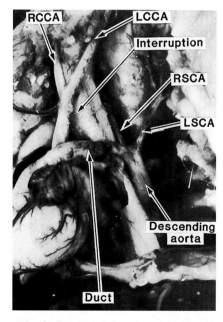

Figure 56.17 This fetal specimen shows interruption of the aortic arch between the left common carotid artery (LCCA) and the left subclavian artery (LSCA), with retro-oesophageal origin of the right subclavian artery (RSCA). RCCA, right common carotid artery.

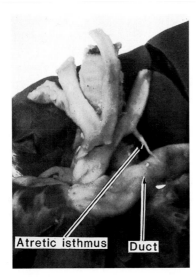

Figure 56.18 In this specimen, a fibrous strand is present at the site of the isthmus, which is, therefore, atretic.

It was Celoria and Patton (1959) who described the commonly used classification as types A, B and C. Interruption distal to the left subclavian artery (type A) was the first described in 1778 by Stiedele in Vienna. The more common variety, type B, interruption between the left common carotid and left subclavian artery, was described some 40 years later (Siedel, 1818), while the least frequent, type C, interruption between the brachiocephalic and left common carotid arteries, was not seen until 1948 (Weisman and Kesten, 1948) (Figure 56.19). As with most congenital heart disease, a rigorous description of the anatomy as seen is often more accurate than eponymous or alphanumeric divisions. In the interests of brevity, we will use this time-honoured classification throughout the subsequent discussions in this chapter.

INCIDENCE AND AETIOLOGY

Van Praagh (1971) found an overall incidence of interrupted aortic arch of 1% in congenital heart defects, with a distribution of 40% type A, 55% type B and a mere 5% as type C. Sell et al (1988) found a higher incidence of type B (69%), whereas the Congenital Heart Surgeons Society found type B to represent 73% of its 250 cases. The total incidence of interruption of the aortic arch in the New England Regional Infant Cardiac Program was 19 per million livebirths, representing 1.3% of critical congenital heart disease (Fyler et al, 1980). It accounted for 8.6% of deaths in the first month of life in postmortem material at the Royal Brompton Hospital, London (Hegerty et al, 1985). Interruption as an isolated lesion is rare (Dische et al, 1975). The combination of congenital absence of the aortic isthmus, patency of the arterial duct and ventricular septal defect was such a usual triad that Everts-Suarez and Carson (1959) deemed it a trilogy. The multi-institutional study of the Congenital Heart Surgeons Society showed a coexisting ventricular septal defect in 72% of 97 cases with interruption encountered between 1987 and 1990 (Jonas et al, 1994). The sex incidence is equal (Van Praagh et al, 1971).

The high incidence of chromosome 22q11 deletion, the Di George syndrome or Catch 22 sequence in those with type B interruption gives an indication as to the genesis of this condition. Van Mierop and Kutsche (1986) showed that as many as one third of those with Di George phenotype had type B interruption, and, conversely, that 68% of those with type B interruption had Di George syndrome. This suggests that the two entities are both caused by abnormal migration of tissue from the neural crest. A more recent study of cytogenetic

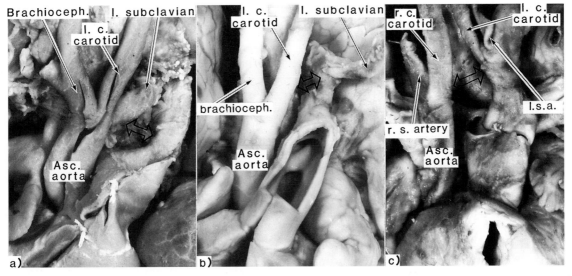

Figure 56.19 These three specimens show interruption (double-headed arrow) at the isthmus (a), between the left common (l.c.) carotid artery and the left (l) subclavian artery (b), and between the right common (r.c.) and the left common carotid arteries (c). Asc., ascending; brachioceph, brachiocephalic artery; l.s.a., left subclavian artery; VSD, ventricular septal defect; r. s., right subclavian.

abnormalities in congenital heart disease found a lower incidence of 44% of those with type B interruption having the microdeletion of chromosome 22 (Johnson et al, 1997). Occurrence in siblings is described (Buch et al, 1980) and, in one family, two siblings and their half sibling were affected (Gobel et al, 1993).

MORPHOLOGY

A full description of the anatomy must include the morphology of the abnormal aortic arch and the structure of the associated intracardiac defects. The aortic arch is, by definition, discontinuous. This is the end of an anatomical spectrum passing from aortic coarctation and tubular hypoplasia, through arch atresia to interruption of the aortic arch. Although this concept is intuitively valid, the different genetic and cardiovascular associations suggest that, at least in some subgroups, interrupted aortic arch is a distinct anatomical entity.

The associated lesions are of great importance in the aetiology, clinical course and prognosis. As already discussed, although interruption can occur in isolation, this is exceptional (Dische et al, 1975; Milo et al, 1982). The most frequently observed lesions are the classic combination of a 'posterior malalignment' ventricular septal defect and patency of the arterial duct. The former is better described as a perimembraneous or muscular outlet defect with posterior deviation of the outlet septum into the subaortic area, the deviation leading to subaortic obstruction (Figure 56.20). This defect was first described by Becu et al (1955), and its importance further emphasized by Van Praagh et al (1971). Indeed, it was originally thought that the 'posterior malalignment' was inevitably associated with overriding of the pulmonary trunk with respect to the ventricular septum. This concept is now known to be erroneous (al-Marsafawy et al, 1995), overriding of the pulmonary trunk being only rarely encountered, and then usually where the defect is doubly committed (Figure 56.21). As Freedom and colleagues (1977) demonstrated, other types of ventricular septal defect can occur, but these are much less frequently seen than the malalignment variant.

Interruption can be one of the components of the Shone complex of multiple obstructive lesions in the left heart, yet hypoplasia of the left ventricle and mitral valve is uncommon. The size of the left ventricular outflow tract and ascending aorta is crucial to management and will be discussed below. Abnormal ventriculo-arterial connections are also described, including discordant ones, double outlet right ventricle (occasionally with the Taussig–Bing malformation) (Liddicoat et al, 1994), aortopulmonary window with intact septum (Figure 56.22) (Moes and Freedom, 1980; Ho et al, 1983) and congenitally corrected transposition (Cottrell et al, 1981).

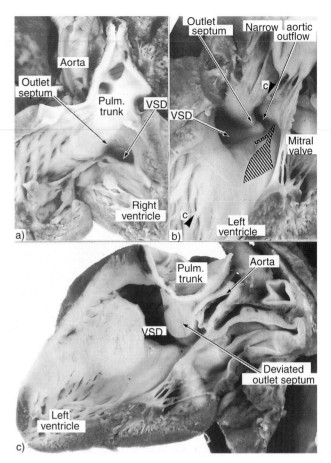

Figure 56.20 This panel shows the typical arrangement seen within the heart in association with ventricular septal defect (VSD) and interruption of the aortic arch. (a) Posterior deviation of the outlet septum through the ventricular septal defect can be seen from the right ventricle. (b) The left ventricular aspect reveals the narrowed subaortic outlet. (c) The long-axis sectional equivalent shows the marked disproportion between the size of the pulmonary (pulm.) trunk and the aorta.

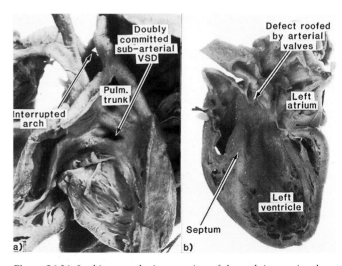

Figure 56.21 In this example, interruption of the arch is associated with a doubly committed and subarterial ventricular septal defect (VSD), seen from the right ventricle (a) and in sectional format (b). Pulm., pulmonary.

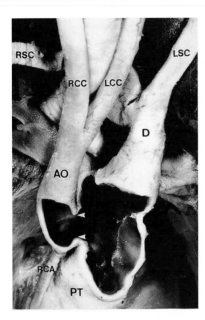

Figure 56.22 Interruption between the left common carotid (LCC) and left subclavian (LSC) artery in this case is associated with an aortopulmonary window (arrowheads). There was also aortic valvar atresia. AO, aorta; D, duct; PT, pulmonary trunk; RCA, right carotid artery; RCC, right common carotid; RSC right subclavian artery.

PATHOPHYSIOLOGY

In the most common situation, where interruption is associated with a patent arterial duct and ventricular septal defect, the infant will initially be well because the pulmonary vascular resistance is high and blood will, therefore, pass through the arterial duct to the systemic circulation. One of two events will precipitate collapse in these infants. First, ductal closure will lead to a critical reduction in lower body perfusion and rapid development of acidosis and shock. Second, a falling pulmonary vascular resistance in the presence of a widely patent duct will lead to preferential flow of blood to the pulmonary circulation to the detriment of the systemic circulation. More slowly progressive, but potentially equally important, tissue acidosis leading to collapse may also occur.

In those with the rarer variant of interruption occurring in isolation, there must be a collateral circulation, usually via the head and neck vessels.

CLINICAL PRESENTATION AND SYMPTOMATOLOGY

As with other obstructive lesions in the left heart that are duct dependent, interrupted aortic arch tends to present with heart failure of acute onset simultaneous with closure of the arterial duct within the first few days of life. Four fifths are admitted to a specialist hospital within 2 weeks (Espulgas, 1979). The signs of heart failure are non-specific, being similar to those discussed previously for aortic coarctation.

The most specific sign in clinical diagnosis is palpation of differential upper body pulses. Most often the femoral pulses, together with both or one arm pulse or one carotid pulse, are weak. If only the femoral pulses are weak, the differentiation of type A interruption from coarctation is impossible. Indeed, even when one or both arm pulses is absent, the diagnosis may still be that of coarctation with anomalous origin of the subclavian artery distal to the narrow segment (Subramanian, 1972). Classically, weak left arm and femoral pulses in the presence of normal right arm and carotid pulses occur with interruption between the left common carotid and left subclavian arteries (type B). If the left carotid pulse is also weak, interruption may be present between the common carotid arteries (type C). Interestingly, in the presence of type B interruption with origin of both subclavian arteries distal to the interruption, pulses may be impalpable in all limbs, while both carotid arteries remain palpable. Hence, if palpation of the neck vessels is not performed, an incorrect diagnosis of aortic atresia could be made (Sharratt et al, 1979).

Difference in pulses, however, is not a static entity. Ductal reopening, either occurring spontaneously or with prostaglandin therapy, can change the clinical picture. Because of this, many of the earlier reviews of the subject did not mention inequality of pulses as a feature of interruption (Roberts et al, 1962; McNamara and Rosenberg, 1968; Nadas and Fyler, 1972; Collins-Nakai et al, 1976).

Auscultation is usually unhelpful. Often a gallop rhythm is present, and the heart sounds are usually easily audible, the second being closely split. An ejection click may indicate the presence of associated bicuspid aortic valve, but this is non-specific. If a murmur is present, it is often pan- or mid-systolic and of low intensity, indicating the non-restrictive nature of the ventricular septal defect.

INVESTIGATIONS

CHEST RADIOGRAPHY

The heart is usually left sided with normal abdominal and bronchial arrangement. Cardiomegaly, particularly enlargement of the left atrium, is present in 90% of neonates (Neye-Bock and Fellows, 1980). Increased pulmonary vascular markings with pulmonary oedema are also the norm. In the rare patients who survive infancy untreated, Jaffe (1975) found more specific signs, including absence of the aortic knob (52%), midline trachea (33%), absent aortic impression on barium swallow (29%) and termination of the descending aorta at the level of the pulmonary trunk (14%). He also described rib notching on the side of the subclavian arteries arising from the ascending aorta in the presence of a restrictive or closed arterial duct.

A narrow mediastinum may suggest absence of the thymus gland, a feature of the Di George sequence.

ELECTROCARDIOGRAPHY

There are no specific electrocardiographic features to aid diagnosis. Again strongly influenced by associated abnormalities, the tracings may show any combination of ventricular hypertrophy, right, left or both, or they may be normal. Occasionally, a prolonged QT interval may be seen secondary to the hypocalcaemia of Di George syndrome.

ECHOCARDIOGRAPHY

In those with Di George syndrome, absence of the thymic window means that echocardiographic imaging is more difficult. The examination must focus on the intracardiac anatomy as well as on the aortic arch. From subcostal views, it is evident that there is a marked discrepancy between the sizes of the great arteries. The suprasternal view allows further delineation of a relatively small ascending aortic arch following an obviously straight course and leading to at least one arch branch, and a much larger pulmonary trunk leading, via an arterial duct, to the proximal end of a much larger descending aorta (Smallhorn et al, 1982a). A complete description of the aorta, the site of interruption and the anatomy of the great vessels should now be possible in almost all neonates (Figures 56.23 and 56.24.) The borders of the classical ventricular septal defect, described above, are further assessed from the parasternal long axis, as is the degree of subaortic obstruction and other parameters predictive of obstruction of the left ventricular outflow tract subsequent to surgical repair (Geva et al, 1993). Particular care is needed to exclude an aberrant right subclavian artery or right duct in the setting of a left arch.

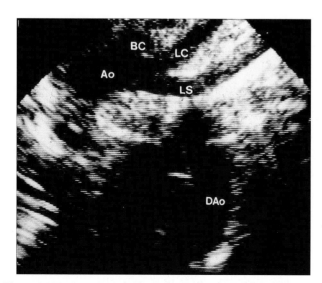

Figure 56.23. Suprasternal echocardiographic section showing typical appearances of interruption of the aortic arch distal to the left subclavian artery. Ao, aorta; BC, brachiocephalic artery; DAO, descending aorta; LC, left carotid artery; LS, left subclavian artery.

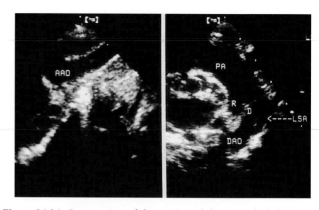

Figure 56.24. Interruption of the aortic arch between the left carotid artery and left subclavian artery (LSA), the latter arising from the descending aorta (DAO), opposite the arterial duct (D). AAO, ascending aorta; PA, pulmonary trunk.

CARDIAC CATHETERIZATION

Cardiac catheterization is rarely necessary at presentation as the anatomy of the aortic arch and associated lesions is demonstrable on echocardiographic assessment. Cardiac catheterization in an unstable infant also carries a significant risk.

If catheterization is undertaken, the infant must be stabilized (see below). Then, via the minimum number of approaches, it is important to access all four cardiac chambers and both great arteries.

Generally, an antegrade venous approach allows access to all four chambers, to the left atrium via the oval foramen, to the pulmonary trunk and thence to the arterial duct and descending aorta, and, via the ventricular septal defect, to the ascending aorta.

In much rarer cases, such as those with aortic atresia, access may need to be gained from the arm (Norwood and Stellin, 1981), and angiography will then define the anatomy of the arch and associated anomalies.

Haemodynamic investigations will demonstrate right-to-left shunting at atrial and ventricular levels in the usual cases across the stretched oval foramen and the ventricular septal defect, secondary to the systemic pressures in the right side of the heart.

Ascending aortography

An injection into the ascending aorta demonstrates in 60% the classic V sign of the brachiocephalic and left common carotid arteries (Figure 56.25) viewed in the frontal projection (Neye-Bock and Fellows, 1980). Occasionally, the V more resembles a U or W if all three arteries take origin proximal to the interruption. The appearance is still characteristic in that the aortic arch continues smoothly into its most distal branch proximal to the interruption regardless of whether this is the brachiocephalic, left common carotid, or subclavian artery. If the aortic arch continues beyond its last branch and appears to taper down to apparent complete obstruction,

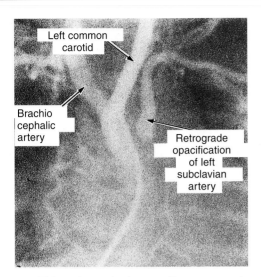

Figure 56.25. This angiogram in the ascending aorta reveals interruption of the arch between the left common carotid artery and the left subclavian artery, the latter filled retrogradely.

the diagnosis is either aortic atresia or severe coarctation with distal wash-in from the arterial duct and not interruption (Morera et al, 1983).

Origin of subclavian arteries distal to the interruption is suggested by retrograde filling from the carotid artery, in a form of 'subclavian steal', from the vertebral artery on the same side. A subclavian artery proximal to the interruption can occasionally provide supply distal to it via the intercostal arteries (Jaffe, 1976; Neye-Bock and Fellows, 1980). Subclavian steal can also result in retrograde opacification of an isolated subclavian artery originating from the pulmonary trunk via a duct. Such an artery will also be opacified by injection into the pulmonary artery (Jaffe, 1976).

Sometimes, the differentiation between coarctation and interruption distal to the right subclavian artery requires retrograde arterial catheterization to the descending aorta, with balloon occlusion angiography, which should demonstrate an aortic isthmus in the former (Figure 56.26). In the rare hearts with an aorto-pulmonary window, ascending aortography will demonstrate filling of the pulmonary trunk (Moes and Freedom, 1980; Fisher et al, 1974). Right ventricular angiography may be necessary in such patients to confirm the presence of two arterial valves and rule out a common arterial trunk.

Left ventriculography

The ventricular septal defect is best seen with caudo-cranial tilt in the left anterior oblique position. The lateral long-axis view profiles the defect and demonstrates the subaortic stenosis caused by the displaced outlet septum (Figure 56.27).

COURSE AND PROGNOSIS

The natural history is poor. Without surgery, three quarters die in the first month of life, the majority in the first 10 days. Less than one tenth survive without correction beyond the first year of life if there is coexisting ductal patency (Roberts et al, 1962; Van Praagh et al, 1971; Freedom et al, 1977).

With the evolution of prostaglandin therapy and surgical intervention over the past decades, the impact of the associated cardiac and extracardiac defects has become of greater relevance, although little long-term follow up is available.

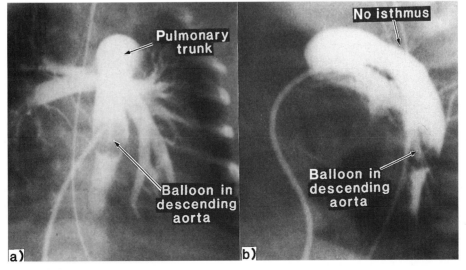

Figure 56.26. This injection is made in the descending aorta with a ballon catheter blown up to block the arch. The contrast shows continuity from the pulmonary trunk through the duct, but no evidence of the isthmus caused by interruption of the aortic arch. The injection is shown in frontal (a) and lateral (b) projections.

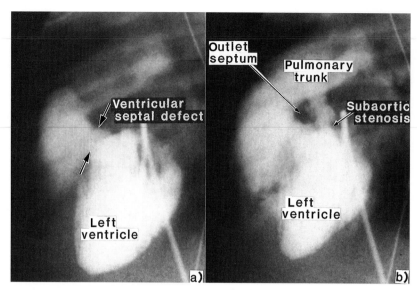

Figure 56.27. These angiograms taken in sequence in lateral projection following an injection in the left ventricle show a ventricular septal defect (a) associated with posterior deviation of the muscular outlet septum (b), with consequent subaortic stenosis. There was interruption of the aortic arch. Compare with Figure 56.20.

MANAGEMENT

MEDICAL MANAGEMENT

As in the majority of obstructive lesions of the left heart, the management of interruption was revolutionized by the ability to manipulate pharmacologically the closing arterial duct. The stabilization of the infant is the same as that discussed for neonates with duct-dependent coarctation, from which interruption must be distinguished. With the usual anatomy, arterial lines in the right radial and umbilical arteries allow accurate assessment of both the ascending aortic and the duct-dependent perfusion.

Chromosomes should be assessed, and the specific deletion in chromosome 22 looked for using fluorescent in situ hybridization. It is important to be vigilant to the possibility of hypocalcaemia and to anticipate it before clinical sequels, such as convulsions, develop. Infusions of calcium are useful in the acute phase. Subsequently, the management is identical to that of isolated hypoparathyroidism, involving oral supplementation of calcium and administration of vitamin D. Documentation of decreased levels of parathormone in the setting of a low normal calcium are diagnostically important before embarking on treatment, which should ideally be conducted with advice from a paediatric endocrinologist. Abnormalities in T cell function can occur, and it is important for assays of T cell number and function to be performed. In the acute phase, it is important that infants with interruption should be presumed to have T cell defects. Blood transfusion (including bypass) should only be performed with irradiated blood to avoid the possibility of transfused lymphocytes and causing graft-versus-host disease. Later, the susceptibility to infection may lead to the need for rotational antibiotics or other immune manipulation.

Other later problems in those with chromosome 22 deletions are developmental delay and feeding problems, both of which need a significant amount of medical input after repair.

SURGICAL MANAGEMENT

History and evolution

The first repair of an interruption was performed in a 3-year-old female by Samson in 1955 (Merrill et al, 1957). It entailed the direct end-to-end anastomosis of a short segment interruption using the divided arterial duct. As this first operation was performed before the advent of open heart surgery, the associated ventricular septal defects could not be addressed at the time but were closed some 4 years later.

There followed a period of progressive intervention, a successful technique similar to subclavian flap repair of coarctation with banding of the pulmonary trunk being reported by Sirak et al (1968). Other palliative procedures followed, such as interposition of a Dacron graft between the pulmonary trunk and the descending aorta (Litwin et al, 1972). The first one-stage repair was reported in 1972 by Barratt-Boyes and his colleagues in a neonate with interruption distal to the left subclavian artery, a ventricular septal defect and totally anomalous pulmonary venous connections. The repair using direct anastomosis occurred 5 years later (Trusler and Izakuwa, 1975).

Following the introduction of prostaglandin, the ability to operate on a metabolically stable neonate enabled improved surgical techniques to be developed. As in the case with coarctation, there has been much debate concerning the optimal surgical management, notably whether a one- or two-staged procedure should be performed. Initially, two-staged repair allowed shorter and less-invasive initial procedures in unstable neonates (Irwin et al, 1991). However, as preoperative resuscitation, techniques for cardiopulmonary bypass and postoperative intensive care have improved, the trend worldwide has been to use one-stage repairs (Vouhe et al, 1990; Jonas et al, 1994; Tlaskal et al, 1997).

A further area of contention involves the method of restoring continuity in the arch, either direct end-to-end anastomosis or interposition of a Dacron graft. The problems of rapid outgrowth of artificial grafts, and later anatomical distortion secondary to induced fibrotic reaction, mean that the latter option is less favourable.

Our own preference in those with interruption and associated anomalies is for one-stage repair with direct end-to-side anastomosis of the distal segment to the ascending aorta, along with standard repair of the ventricular septal defect. This concurs with current practice in most centres (Sell et al, 1988; Menahem et al, 1992; Serraf et al, 1996).

In those unsuitable for biventricular repair, a Fontan-type procedure must be considered. In this instance, definitive surgery for associated anomalies is not undertaken.

The degree of subaortic obstruction is critical in those whose interruption is associated with the other classical components of the hypoplastic left heart spectrum (Ho et al, 1983). If the diagnosis is the latter, then operative intervention will be dominated by that malformation, and a Norwood operation must be performed. There are, however, cases in which, although the left ventricle is of good size, there is a significantly small subaortic diameter. Generally if this is less than 3 mm, standard repair is contraindicated. Certain centres have then advocated Norwood procedures (Jacobs et al, 1995; Rychik et al, 1991). Alternatively, the left ventricle outflow can be baffled via the ventricular septal defect to the pulmonary trunk, which is in turn divided, its distal end being anastamosed to the right ventricle with a homograft and its proximal end anastomosed to the ascending aorta in a form of Damus–Kaye–Stansel procedure (Yasui et al, 1987). Many prefer to perform anatomical correction, with resection of the subaortic stenosis if at all possible (Ilbawi et al, 1988; Bove et al, 1993).

Preoperative stabilization must be meticulously maintained during transport to the operating theatre. Particular care must be taken to avoid hyperventilation and hyperoxaemia, as discussed under management of duct-dependent coarctation.

Technique

Once stability is ensured, access is via a midline sternotomy. Thymic tissue, absent in chromosome 22 deletion, is noted and, if present, largely removed to facilitate dissection. The pericardium is opened, and a piece harvested if closure of the atrial septum is envisaged. Cannulas are inserted initially into the ascending aorta and right atrium. If the arterial duct is patent, cannulation of the pulmonary trunk is crucial to optimize coronary and cerebral perfusion during cooling.

Immediately on instituting cardiopulmonary bypass, both pulmonary arteries are snared to preferentialize flow through the arterial duct to the lower body. While the patient is cooling, the branches of the aorta and the arterial duct are extensively dissected and the common carotid arteries snared. On reaching a nasopharyngeal temperature below 20°C, bypass is stopped. The aortic cross-clamp is applied and cardioplegia solution delivered. Only now can the prostaglandin be stopped. The carotid arterial snares are tightened and the cannulas and cross-clamp removed.

The arterial duct is ligated, the aorta opened and any obvious ductal tissue in the aortic lumen excised. Any anomalous subclavian arteries are ligated. The distal aortic segment is fully mobilized and a small C-clamp is applied to it and approximated to the left posterolateral aspect of the ascending aorta. This end-to-side anastomosis is sutured with polypropylene sutures. It is vital that this is achieved under no tension. Other defects are then addressed, including inspection of the atrial septum, the intactness of which is crucial. Vigorous de-airing drill is performed and the aortic cannula re-inserted for warming. Lines vital for postoperative management are now inserted, namely left atrial and pulmonary arterial lines.

COMPLICATIONS

EARLY COMPLICATIONS

On completion of surgery, anastomotic gradients should be rigorously excluded before closure. Once stable, the infant is transferred to intensive care.

Initially, as discussed under coarctation, bleeding is the most potentially dangerous problem, especially in the area of the anastomosis. Any worsening haemodynamics in the face of increased chest drainage in the absence of coagulopathy should prompt surgical exploration. Any deviation from a routine postoperative recovery once other problems are excluded, notably infection, respiratory complications or factors resultant from intraoperative perfusion, should lead to a rigorous reassessment of the haemodynamics. Echocardiography or cardiac catheterization must be performed to look for additional atrial or ventricular septal defects, residual subaortic obstruction. If any are discovered, urgent surgical intervention must be performed.

The majority of complications discussed for coarctation can occur in addition to the complications of intracardiac surgery and cardiopulmonary bypass.

LATE COMPLICATIONS

All those who have artificial grafts inserted as neonates will require graft replacement eventually. In those undergoing direct anastomosis, significant gradients occur, but it has been known for some time that balloon dilation can successfully be used to relieve such gradients across the site of repair (Saul et al, 1987; Bove et al, 1993; Bogers et al, 1997).

Left ventricular outflow tract obstruction, if not significant perioperatively, can become worse over the supervening years and require surgical intervention (Jonas et al, 1989; Bogers et al, 1997). Geva and colleagues (1993) showed that the size of the left ventricular outflow tract preoperatively, the type of interruption and the presence of an aberrant right subclavian artery were all predictive of postoperative obstruction. They postulated that these factors influence the volume of flow of blood across the left ventricular outflow tract leading to its obstruction. Knowledge of these factors should enable preoperative identification of infants who may require surgical relief of subaortic stenosis.

OUTCOME

The outcome of repair of interrupted aortic arch is, to a large degree, dependent on the preoperative state of the infant. A recent review has confirmed that preoperative condition is the greatest predictor of late neurological outcome in these children (Schreiber et al, 1997). It had been shown earlier that preoperative renal function, intracerebral haemorrhages, number of cardioplegic injections and age at operation were important determinants of outcome (Seraff et al, 1996). The overall survival is dominated by the associated lesions but should approach 70% at 5 years (Seraff et al, 1996; Bogers et al, 1997; Tlaskal et al, 1997).

--- REFERENCES ---

Abbott M E 1928 coarctation of the aorta of the adult type. II. Statistical study and historical retrospect of 200 recorded cases, with autopsy, of stenosis or obliteration of the descending arch in subjects above the age of two years. American Heart Journal 3: 392–421

Alpert B S, Bain H, Balfe J W, Kidd B S L, Olley P N 1979 Role of renin–angiotensin–aldosterone system in hypertensive children with coarctation of the aorta. American Journal of Cardiology 43: 823–834

al-Marsafawy H M, Ho S Y, Redington A N, Anderson R H 1995 The relationship of the outlet septum to the aortic outflow tract in hearts with interruption of the aortic arch. Journal of Thoracic and Cardiovascular Surgery 109: 1225–1236

Amsterdam E A, Albers W H, Christlieb A R, Morgan C L, Nadas A S, Hickler R B 1969 Plasma renin activity in children with coarctation of the aorta. American Journal of Cardiology 23: 396–399

Anderson R H, Lenox C C, Zuberbuhler J R 1983 Morphology of ventricular septal defect associated with coarctation of the aorta. British Heart Journal 50: 176–181

Attia I M, Lababidi Z A 1988 Transumbilical balloon coarctation angioplasty. American Heart Journal 116: 1623–1624

Backer C L, Paape K, Zales V R, Weigel T J, Mavroudis C 1995 Coarctation of the aorta. Repair with polytetrafluoroethylene patch aortoplasty. Circulation 92(Suppl II): 132–136

Balderston S M, Daberkow E, Clarke D R, Wolfe R R 1992 Maximal voluntary exercise variables in children with postoperative coarctation of the aorta. Journal of American College of Cardiology 19: 154–158

Barratt-Boyes B G, Nicholls T T, Brandt P W, Neutze J M 1972 Aortic arch interruption associated with patent ductus arteriosus, ventricular septal defect, and total anomalous pulmonary venous connection. Total correction in an 8-day-old infant by means of profound hypothermia and limited cardiopulmonary bypass. Journal of Thoracic and Cardiovascular Surgery 63: 367–373

Becker A, Becker M, Edwards J 1970 Anomalies associated with coarctation of aorta: particular reference to infancy. Circulation 41: 1067–1075

Becu L M, Tauxe W N, DuShane J W, Edwards J E 1955 A complex of congenital cardiac anomalies: ventricular septal defect, biventricular origin of the pulmonary trunk and subaortic stenosis. American Heart Journal 50: 901–911

Beekman R H, Robinow M 1985 Coarctation of the aorta inherited as an autosomal dominant trait. American Journal of Cardiology 56: 818–819

Beekman R H, Rocchini A P, Behrendt D M et al 1986 Long-term outcome after repair of coarctation in infancy: subclavian angioplasty does not reduce the need for reoperation. Journal of American College of Cardiology 8: 1406–1411

Beitzke A, Stein J I, Gamillscheg A, Rigler B 1997 Dissection of the descending aorta after balloon angioplasty of native coarctation. Pediatric Cardiology 18: 222–225

Benedict C R, Grahams-Smith D G, Fisher A 1978 Changes in plasma catecholamines and dopamine beta-hydroxylase after corrective surgery for coarctation of the aorta. Circulation 57: 598–602

Benkwitz K B, Hunter W C 1937 Combined infantile and adult coarctation of aorta with coincident occlusion of vena cava superior: report of a case. American Journal of Pathology 13: 289–310

Benson L N, Freedom R M, Wilson G J, Halliday W C 1986 Cerebral complications following balloon angioplasty of coarctation of the aorta. Cardiovascular Intervention and Radiology 9: 184–186

Blalock A, Park E A 1944 The surgical treatment of experimental coarctation of the aorta. Annals of Surgery 119: 445–452

Bolling S F, Iannettoni M D, Dick M II, Rosenthal A, Bove E L 1990 Shone's anomaly: operative results and late outcome. Annals of Thoracic Surgery 49: 887–893

Bogers A J, Contant C M, Hokken R B, Cromme-Dijkhuis A H 1997 Repair of aortic arch interruption by direct anastomosis. European Journal of Cardiothoracic Surgery 11: 100–104

Bonnet L M 1903 Sur la lesion dite sténose congénitale de l'aorte dans le region de l'isthme. Reune Medicale 23: 108, 255, 335 (cited by Edwards J E 1953 Laboratory Investigations 2: 56–75)

Bove E L, Minich L L, Pridjian A K et al 1993 The management of severe subaortic stenosis, ventricular septal defect, and aortic arch obstruction in the neonate. Journal of Thoracic and Cardiovascular Surgery 105: 289–295 [discussion 295–296]

Bower C, Ramsay J M 1994 Congenital heart disease: a 10 year cohort. Journal of Paediatric Child Health 30: 414–418

Bramwell C 1947 Coarctation of the aorta: clinical feature. British Heart Journal 9: 100–124

Brandt B, Heinz S F, Rose E F et al 1984 Repair of coarctation of the aorta in children with Turner's syndrome. Pediatric Cardiology 5: 175

Brandt B III, Marvin W J Jr, Rose E F, Mahoney L T 1987 Surgical treatment of coarctation of the aorta after balloon angioplasty. Journal of Thoracic and Cardiovascular Surgery 94: 715–719

Brauner R A, Laks H, Drinkwater D C Jr, Scholl F, McCaffery S 1997 Multiple left heart obstructions (Shone's anomaly) with mitral valve involvement: long-term surgical outcome. Annals of Thoracic Surgery 64: 721–729

Brewer L A, Fosberg R G, Mulder G A et al 1972 Spinal cord complications following surgery for coarctation of the aorta. Journal of Thoracic and Cardiovascular Surgery 64: 368

Brouwer R M, Erasmus M E, Ebels T, Eijgelaar A 1994 Influence of age on survival, late hypertension, and recoarctation in elective aortic coarctation repair. Including long-term results after elective aortic coarctation repair with a follow-up from 25 to 44 years. Journal of Thoracic and Cardiovascular Surgery 108: 525–531

Brouwer R M, Cromme-Dijkhuis A H, Erasmus M E et al 1996 Decision making for the surgical management of aortic coarctation associated with ventricular septal defect. Journal of Thoracic and Cardiovascular Surgery 111: 168–175

Brown D L, Durfee S M, Hornberger L K 1997 Ventricular discrepancy as a sonographic sign of coarctation of the fetal aorta: how reliable is it? Journal of Ultrasound Medicine 16: 95–99

Bruins C L D C 1974 De arterial pool van het hart. Thesis, Leiden.

Buch J, Wennevold A, Efsen F, Andersen G E 1980 Interrupted aortic arch in two siblings. Acta Paediatrica Scandinavica 69: 783–785

Calodney M M, Carson M J 1950 Coarctation of the aorta in early infancy. Journal of Pediatrics 37: 46–52

Campbell D B, Waldhausen J A, Pierce W S et al 1984 Should elective repair of coarctation be done in infancy? Journal of Thoracic and Cardiovascular Surgery 88: 929

Campbell D N, Paton B C, Wiggins J W, Wolfe R R, Clarke D R 1982 Infant coarctation of the aorta. Alternatives to subclavian flap repair. Pediatric Cardiology 3: 139–142

Campbell M 1970 Natural history of coarctation of the aorta. British Heart Journal 32: 633–640

Campbell M, Polani P E 1961 The aetiology of coarctation of the aorta. Lancet i: 463–468

Carvalho J S, Redington A N, Shinebourne E A, Rigby M L, Gibson D 1990 Continuous wave Doppler echocardiography and coarctation of the aorta: gradients and flow patterns in the assessment of severity. British Heart Journal 64: 133–137

Castañeda-Zuniga W R, Lock J E, Vlodaver Z et al 1982 Transluminal dilatation of coarctation of the abdominal aorta. An experimental study in dogs. Radiology 143: 693–697

Celoria G C, Patton R B 1959 Congenital absence of the aortic arch. American Heart Journal 56: 407–426

Cheitlin M D, Robinowitz M, McAllister H, Hoffman J I, Bharati S, Lev M 1980 The distribution of fibrosis in the left ventricle in congenital aortic stenosis and coarctation of the aorta. Circulation 62: 823–830

Clagett D T, Kirklin J W, Edwards J E 1954 Anatomic variations and pathological changes in coarctation of the aorta. A study of 124 cases. Surgical Gynecology and Obstetrics 98: 103–114

Clarkson P M, Nicholson M R, Barratt-Boyes B G, Neutze J M, Whitlock R M 1983 Results after repair of coarctation of the aorta beyond infancy: a 10 to 28 year follow-up with particular reference to late systemic hypertension. American Journal of Cardiology 51: 1481–1488

Cobanoglu A, Teply J F, Grunkemeier G L, Sunderland C O, Starr A 1985 Coarctation of the aorta in patients younger than three months. A critique of the subclavian flap operation. Journal of Thoracic and Cardiovascular Surgery 89: 128–135

Coceani F, Olley P M 1973 The response of the ductus arteriosus to prostaglandins. Canadian Journal of Physiology and Pharmacology 51: 220–225

Cohen M, Fuster V, Steele P M, Driscoll D, McGoon D C 1989 Coarctation of the aorta. Long-term follow-up and prediction of outcome after surgical correction. Circulation 80: 840–845

Collins-Nakai R L, Dick M, Parisi-Buckley L, Fyler D C, Castañeda A R 1976 Interrupted aortic arch in infancy. Journal of Pediatrics 88: 959–962

Connor T M, Baker W P 1981 A comparison of coarctation resection and patch angioplasty using postexercise blood pressure measurements. Circulation 64: 567–572

Cooper R S, Ritter S B, Rothe W B, Chen C K, Griepp R, Golinko R J 1987 Angioplasty for coarctation of the aorta: long-term results. Circulation 75: 600–604

Cottrell A J, Holden M P, Hunter S 1981 Interrupted aortic arch type A associated with congenitally corrected transposition of great arteries and ventricular septal defect. British Heart Journal 46: 671–674

Crafoord C, Nylin G 1945 Congenital coarctation of the aorta and its surgical treatment. Journal of Thoracic Surgery 14: 347–362

Cullen S, Redington A N 1993 Doppler-detected aortic coarctation with PDA. American Heart Journal 126: 1493–1494

d'Abreu A L, Aldridge A G V, Astley R, Jones M A C 1961 Coarctation of the aorta proximal to both subclavian arteries producing reversible papilloedema. British Journal of Surgery 48: 525–527

de Mendonca J T, Carvalho M R, Costa R K, Franco Filho E 1985 Coarctation of the aorta: a new surgical technique. Journal of Thoracic and Cardiovascular Surgery 90: 445–447

DeSanto A, Bills R G, King H, Waller B, Brown J W 1987 Pathogenesis of aneurysm formation opposite prosthetic patches used for coarctation repair. An experimental study. Journal of Thoracic and Cardiovascular Surgery 94: 720–723

de Swiet M, Shinebourne E A 1977 Blood pressure in infancy. American Heart Journal 94: 399–401

Dische M R, Tsai M, Baltaxe H A 1975 Solitary interruption of the arch of the aorta. Clinicopathologic review of eight cases. American Journal of Cardiology 35: 271–277

Edie R N, Janani J, Attai L A, Malm J R, Robinson G 1975 Bypass grafts for recurrent or complex coarctations of the aorta. Annals of Thoracic Surgery 20: 558–566

Edwards J E 1968 Aortic arch system. In: Gould S E (ed.) Pathology of the heart and blood vessels, 3rd edn. Charles C Thomas, Springfield, IL, p 416–454

Edwards J E, Christensen N A, Clagett O T, McDonald J R 1948 Pathologic considerations in coarctation of the aorta. Proceedings of the Staff Meetings of the Mayo Clinic 23: 324–332

Edwards W D, Leaf D S, Edwards J E 1978 Dissecting aortic aneurysm associated with congenital bicuspid aortic valve. Circulation 57: 1022–1025

Elliot M J 1987 Coarctation of the aorta with arch hypoplasia: improvements on a new technique. Annals of Thoracic Surgery 44: 321–323

Elseed A M, Shinebourne E A, Joseph M C 1973 Assessment of techniques for measurement of blood pressure in infants and children. Archives of Disease in Childhood 48: 932–936

Elzenga N J, Gittenberger-de Groot A C 1983 Localised coarctation of the aorta. An age dependent spectrum. British Heart Journal 119: 317–323

Elzenga N J, Gittenberger-de Groot A C 1985 Coarctation and related aortic arch anomalies in hypoplastic left heart syndrome. International Journal of Cardiology 8: 379–393

Erbel R, Bednarczyk I, Pop T et al 1990 Detection of dissection of the aortic intima and media after angioplasty of coarctation of the aorta. An angiographic, computer tomographic, and echocardiographic comparative study. Circulation 81: 805–814

Esplugas E 1979 Interruption of the aorta – anatomical, clinical and angiocardiographic observations. In: Godman M J, Marquis R M (eds) Paediatric cardiology 2, Heart disease in the newborn. Churchill Livingstone, Edinburgh, p 187–195

Evans W 1933 Congenital stenosis (coarctation), atresia and interruption of the aortic arch: a study of 28 cases. Quarterly Journal of Medicine 2: 1–32

Everts-Suarez E A, Carson C P 1959 The triad of congenital absence of aortic arch (isthmus aortas), patent ductus arteriosus and ventricular septal defect – a trilogy. Annals of Surgery 150: 153–159

Fawzy M E, Dunn B, Galal O et al 1992 Balloon coarctation angioplasty in adolescents and adults: early and intermediate results. American Heart Journal 124: 167–171

Finley J P, Beaulieu R G, Nanton M A, Roy D L 1983 Balloon catheter dilatation of coarctation of the aorta in young infants. British Heart Journal 50: 411–415

Fisher E A, DuBrow I W, Hastreiter A R 1974 Aortopulmonary septal defect and interrupted aortic arch: a diagnostic challenge. American Journal of Cardiology 34: 356–359

Folger G, Stein P 1984 Bicuspid aortic valve morphology when associated with coarctation of the aorta. Catheterization and Cardiovascular Diagnosis 10: 17–25

Foster E D 1984 Reoperation for aortic coarctation. Annals of Thoracic Surgery 38: 81–89

Fournier A, Chartrand C, Guerin R, Davignon A, Stanley P 1985 Use of the internal mammary artery for preservation of circulation to the left arm after subclavian flap aortoplasty in correction of coarctation in children. Journal of Thoracic and Cardiovascular Surgery 90: 926–928

Freed M D, Heymann M A, Lewis A B, Roehl S L, Kensey R C 1981 Prostaglandin E$_1$ infants with ductus arteriosus-dependent congenital heart disease. Circulation 64: 899–905

Freedom R M, Bain H H, Esplugas E, Dische R, Rowe R D 1977 Ventricular septal defect in interruption of aortic arch. American Journal of Cardiology 39: 572–582

Fyler D C, Buckley D C, Hellenbrand W C, Cohn H E 1980 Report of the New England Regional Infant Cardiac Program. Pediatrics 65: 375–461

Gardiner H M, Celermajer D S, Sorensen K E et al 1994 Arterial reactivity is significantly impaired in normotensive young adults after successful repair of aortic coarctation in childhood. Circulation 89: 1745–1750

Geiss D, Williams W G, Lindsay W K, Rowe R D 1980 Upper extremity gangrene: a complication of subclavian artery division. Annal of Thoracic Surgery 30: 487–489

Geva T, Hornberger L K, Sanders S P, Jonas R A, Ott D A, Colan S D 1993 Echocardiographic predictors of left ventricular outflow tract obstruction after repair of interrupted aortic arch. Journal of American College of Cardiology 22: 1953–1960

Gittenberger-de Groot A C 1981 Structural variation of the ductus arteriosus in congenital heart disease and in persistent fetal circulation. In: Godman M J (ed.) Paediatric cardiology, Vol 4. Churchill Livingstone, Edinburgh, p. 56–63

Gidding S S, Rocchini A P, Beekman R et al 1985 Therapeutic effect of propranolol on paradoxical hypertension after repair of coarctation of the aorta. New England Journal of Medicine 312: 1224–1228

Gobel J W, Pierpont M E, Moller J H, Singh A, Edwards J E 1993 Familial interruption of the aortic arch. Pediatric Cardiology 14: 110–115

Goodall M C, Sealy W C 1969 Increased sympathetic nerve activity following resection of coarctation of the thoracic aorta. Circulation 39: 345–351

Gotzsche C O, Krag-Olsen B, Nielsen J, Sorensen K E, Kristensen B O 1994 Prevalence of cardiovascular malformations and association with karyotypes in Turner's syndrome. Archives of Disease in Childhood 71: 433–436

Graham T P, Bricker T, James F W, Strong W B 1994 26th Bethesda Conference: recommendations for determining eligibility for competition in athletes with cardiovascular abnormalities. 6–7 January, 1994. Journal of American College of Cardiology 24: 845–899

Greally J M, Neiswanger K, Cummins J H et al 1996 A molecular anatomical analysis of mosaic trisomy 16. Human Genetics 98: 86–90

Greenberg S B, Marks L A, Eshaghpour E E 1997 Evaluation of magnetic resonance imaging in coarctation of the aorta: the importance of multiple imaging planes Pediatric Cardiology 18: 345–349

Gross R E 1951 Treatment of certain aortic coarctations by homologous grafts. Annals of Surgery 134: 753–768

Gross R M, Hufnagel C A 1945 Coarctation of the aorta. Experimental studies regarding its surgical correction. New England Journal of Medicine 233: 287–293

Grossman L M, Jacoby W J Jr 1969 Right aortic arch and coarctation of the aorta. Diseases of the Chest 56: 158–160

Guenthard J, Wyler F 1995 Exercise-induced hypertension in the arms due to impaired arterial reactivity after successful coarctation resection. American Journal of Cardiology 75: 814–817

Guenthard J, Zumsteg U, Wyler F 1996 Arm–leg pressure gradients on late follow-up after coarctation repair. Possible causes and implications. European Heart Journal 17: 1572–1575

Hanley F L 1996 The various therapeutic approaches to aortic coarctation: is it fair to compare? Journal of American College of Cardiology 27: 471–472

Hart J C, Waldhausen J A 1983 Reversed subclavian flap angioplasty for arch coarctation of the aorta. Annals of Thoracic Surgery 36: 715–717

Hartmann A F Jr, Goldring D, Hernandez A et al 1970 Recurrent coarctation of the aorta after successful repair in infancy. American Journal of Cardiology 25: 405–410

Heger M, Gabriel H, Koller-Strametz J et al 1997 Aortic coarctation – long-term follow-up in adults. Zeitschrift für Kardiologie 86(1): 50–55.

Hegerty A S, Anderson R H, Ho S Y 1985 Congenital heart malformations in the first year of life – a necropsy study. British Heart Journal 54: 583–592

Herrmann V M, Laks H, Fagan L, Terschluse D, William V L 1978 Repair of aortic coarctation in the first year of life. Annals of Thoracic Surgery 25: 57–63

Hess J, Mooyaart E L, Busch H J, Bergstra A, Landsman M L 1986 Percutaneous transluminal balloon angioplasty in restenosis of coarctation of the aorta. British Heart Journal 55: 459–461

Hesslein P S, Giitgesell H P, McNamara D G 1983 Prognosis of symptomatic coarctation of the aorta in infancy. American Journal of Cardiology 51: 299–303

Hijazi Z M, Fahey J T, Kleinman C S, Hellenbrand W E 1991 Balloon angioplasty for recurrent coarctation of aorta. Immediate and long-term results. Circulation 84: 1150–1156

Ho S Y, Anderson R H 1979 Coarctation, tubular hypoplasia, and the ductus arteriosus. Histological study of 35 specimens. British Heart Journal 41: 268–274

Ho S Y, Wilcox B R, Anderson R H, Lincoln J C R 1983 Interrupted aortic arch – anatomical features of significance. Thoracic and Cardiovascular Surgeon 31: 199–205

Ho S Y, Somerville J, Yip W C, Anderson R H 1988 Transluminal balloon dilation of resected coarcted segments of thoracic aorta: histological study and clinical implications. International Journal of Cardiology 19: 99–105

Hodes H L, Steinfeld L, Blumenthal S 1959 Congenital cerebral aneurysms and coarctation of the aorta. Archives of Pediatrics 76: 28–43

Hoffman J I E 1995 Incidence of congenital heart disease: II. Prenatal incidence. Pediatric Cardiology 16: 155–165

Hoffman J I E, Heyman M A, Rudolph A M 1988 Coarctation of the aorta: significance of aortic flow. In: Anderson R H, Neches W H, Park S C, Zuberbuhler J R (eds) Perspectives in Pediatric Cardiology, Volume 1. Mount Kisco, New York: Futura Publishing Co. Inc., pp 347–351

Honey M, Lincoln J C, Osborne M P, de Bono D P 1975 Coarctation of aorta with right aortic arch. Report of surgical correction in 2 cases: one with associated anomalous origin of left circumflex coronary artery from the right pulmonary artery. British Heart Journal 37: 937–945

Huhta J C, Gutlesell H P, Latson L A, Huffities F D 1984 Two-dimensional echocardiographic assessment of the aorta in infants and children with congenital heart disease. Circulation 70: 417–424

Hutchins G M 1971 Coarctation of the aorta explained as a branch-point of the ductus arteriosus. American Journal of Pathology 63: 203–214

Ilbawi M N, Idriss F S, de Leon S Y, Muster A J, Benson D W Jr, Paul M H 1988 Surgical management of patients with interrupted aortic arch and severe subaortic stenosis. Annals of Thoracic Surgery 45: 174–180

Ing F F, Starc T J, Griffiths W M 1996 Early diagnosis of coarctation of the aorta in children: a continuing dilemma. Pediatrics 98: 378–382

Irwin E D, Braunlin E A, Foker J E 1991 Staged repair of interrupted aortic arch and ventricular septal defect in infancy. Annals of Thoracic Surgery 52: 632–636

Isner J M, Donaldson R F, Fulton D, Bhan I, Payne D D, Cleveland R J 1987 Cystic medial necrosis in coarctation of the aorta: a potential factor contributing to adverse consequences observed after percutaneous balloon angioplasty of coarctation sites. Circulation 75: 689–695

Izakuwa T, Mullholland H C, Rowe R D 1979 Structural heart disease in the newborn. Archives of Diseases in Childhood 54: 281–285

Jacobs M L, Rychik J, Murphy J D, Nicolson S C, Steven J M, Norwood W I 1995 Results of Norwood's operation for lesions other than hypoplastic left heart syndrome. Journal of Thoracic and Cardiovascular Surgery 110: 1555–1561 [discussion 1561–1562]

Jaffe R B 1975 Complete interruption of the aortic arch. 1. Characteristic radiographic findings in 21 patients. Circulation 52: 714–721

Jaffe R B 1976 Complete interruption of the aortic arch. 2. Characteristic angiographic features with emphasis on collateral circulation to the descending aorta. Circulation 53: 161–168

Johnson A L, Frencz C, Wiglesworth F W, McRae D L 1951 Coarctation of the aorta complicated by patency of the ductus (physiologic considerations in the classification of coarctation of the aorta). Circulation 4: 242–250

Johnson M C, Hing A, Wood M K, Watson M S 1997 Chromosome abnormalities in congenital heart disease. American Journal of Medical Genetics 70: 292–298

Jonas R A 1991 Coarctation: do we need to resect ductal tissue? Annals of Thoracic Surgery 52: 604–607

Jonas R A, Sell J E, Van Praagh R et al 1989 Left ventricular outflow obstruction associated with interrupted aortic arch and ventricular septal defect. In: Crupi C, Parenzan L,

Anderson R H (eds). Perspectives in Pediatric Cardiology Volume 2. Pediatric Cardiac Surgery part 1. Mount Kisco, New York: Futura Publishing Company Inc. pp 61–65

Jonas R A, Quaegebeur J M, Kirklin J W, Blackstone E H, Daicoff G 1994 Outcomes in patients with interrupted aortic arch and ventricular septal defect. A multiinstitutional study. Congenital Heart Surgeons Society. Journal of Thoracic and Cardiovascular Surgery 107: 1099–1109 [discussion 1109–1113]

Kan J S, White R I Jr, Mitchell S E, Farmlett E J, Donahoo J S, Gardner T J 1983 Treatment of restenosis of coarctation by percutaneous transluminal angioplasty. Circulation 68: 1087–1094

Kilner P J, Shinohara T, Sampson C et al 1996 Repaired aortic coarctation in adults – magnetic resonance imaging with velocity mapping shows distortion of anatomy and flow. Cardiology of the Young 6: 20–27

Kimball T R, Reynolds J M, Mays W A, Khoury P, Claytor R P, Daniels S R 1994 Persistent hyperdynamic cardiovascular state at rest and during exercise in children after successful repair of coarctation of the aorta. Journal of American College of Cardiology 24: 194–200

Kinney T D, Sylvester R E, Levine S A 1945 Coarctation and acute dissection of the aorta associated with pregnancy. American Journal of Medical Science 210: 725–732

Kirklin J W, Burchell H B, Pugh G B et al 1952 Surgical treatment of coarctation of the aortic in a ten week old infant. Report of case. Circulation 6: 411–414

Konai N R, Chaudhurg D C R, Basu A 1955 A case of coarctation of aorta in an unusual site. American Heart Journal 49: 275–280

Kramer H H, Sommer M, Rammos S, Krogmann O 1995 Evaluation of low dose prostaglandin E1 treatment for ductus dependent congenital heart disease. European Journal of Pediatrics 154: 700–707

Lansman S, Shapiro A J, Schiller M S et al 1986 Extended aortic arch anastomosis for repair of coarctation in infancy. Circulation 74(Suppl I): 37–41

Lawrie G M, DeBakey M E, Morris G C Jr, Crawford E S, Wagner W F, Glaeser D H 1981 Late repair of coarctation of the descending thoracic aorta in 190 patients. Results up to 30 years after operation. Archives of Surgery 116: 1557–1560

Leandro J, Smallhorn J F, Benson L et al 1992 Ambulatory blood pressure monitoring and left ventricular mass and function after successful surgical repair of coarctation of the aorta. Journal of American College of Cardiology 20: 197–204

Leoni F, Huhta J C, Douglas J et al 1984 Effect of prostaglandin on early surgical mortality in obstructive lesions of the systemic circulation. British Heart Journal 52: 654–659

Lerberg D B 1981 Abbott's artery. Annals of Thoracic Surgery 33: 415–416

Lewis A B, Takahashi M, Lurie P R 1978 Administration of prostaglandin E$_1$ in neonates with critical congenital cardiac defects. Journal of Pediatrics 93: 481–485

Liddicoat J R, Reddy V M, Hanley F L 1994 New approach to great-vessel reconstruction in transposition complexes with interrupted aortic arch. Annals of Thoracic Surgery 58: 1146–1150

Lindsay J Jr 1988 Coarctation of the aorta, bicuspid aortic valve and abnormal ascending aortic wall. American Journal of Cardiology 61: 182–184

Litwin S B, Van Praagh R, Bernhard W F 1972 A palliative operation for certain infants with aortic arch interruption. Annals of Thoracic Surgery 14: 369–375

Lo R N, Leung M P, Yau K K, Cheung D L 1989 Transvenous antegrade balloon angioplasty for recoarctation of the aorta in an infant. American Heart Journal 117: 1157–1159

Lock J E, Niemi T, Burke B A, Einzig S, Castañeda-Zuniga W R 1982 Transcutaneous angioplasty of experimental aortic coarctation. Circulation 66: 1280–1286

Lock J E, Bass J L, Amplatz K, Fuhrman B P, Castañeda-Zuniga W 1983 Balloon dilation angioplasty of aortic coarctations in infants and children. Circulation 68: 109–116

Luosto R, Kyllonen K E, Merikallio E 1980 Surgical treatment of coarctation of the aorta with minimal collateral circulation. Scandinavian Journal of Thoracic and Cardiovascular Surgery 14: 217–220

Lupoglazoff J M, Hubert P, Labenne M, Sidi D, Kachaner J 1995 Therapeutic strategy in newborn infants with multivisceral failure caused by interruption or hypoplasia of the aortic arch. Archives des Maladies du Coeur et des Vaisseaux 88: 725–730

Macartney F J, Taylor J F, Graham G R, De Level M, Stark J 1980 The fate of survivors of cardiac surgery in infancy. Circulation 62: 80–91

Mandel B J, Evans E W, Walford R L 1954 Dissecting aortic aneurysm during pregnancy. New England Journal of Medicine 251: 1059–1061

Maron B J, Humphries J O, Rowe R D, Mellits E D 1973 Prognosis of surgically corrected coarctation of the aorta. A 20-year postoperative appraisal. Circulation 47: 119–126

Martelle R R, Moss A J 1962 Fifty-three cases of coarctation of the aorta. American Journal of Diseases of Children 103: 556–563

Martin M M, Beekman R H, Rocchini A P, Crowley D C, Rosenthal A 1988 Aortic aneurysms after subclavian angioplasty repair of coarctation of the aorta. American Journal of Cardiology 61: 951–953

Matthew R, Simon G, Joseph M 1972 Collateral circulation in coarctation of the aorta in infancy and childhood. Archives of Diseases in Childhood 47: 950–953

McCrindle B W, Jones T K, Morrow W R et al 1996 Acute results of balloon angioplasty of native coarctation versus recurrent aortic obstruction are equivalent. Valvuloplasty and Angioplasty of Congenital Anomalies (VACA) Registry Investigators. American Journal of Cardiology 28: 1810–1817

McCullough J L, Hollier L H, Nugent M 1988 Paraplegia after thoracic aortic occlusion: influence of cerebrospinal fluid drainage. Journal of Vascular Surgery 7: 153

McNamara D G, Rosenberg H S 1968 Interruption of the aortic arch. In: Watson H (ed.) Paediatric cardiology. Lloyd-Luke, London, p 224–232

Meier M A, Lucchese F A, Jazbik W, Nesralla I A, Mendonca J T 1986 A new technique for repair of aortic coarctation. Subclavian flap aortoplasty with preservation of arterial blood flow to the left arm. Journal of Thoracic and Cardiovascular Surgery 92: 1005–1012

Menahem S, Rahayoe A U, Brawn W J, Mee R B 1992 Interrupted aortic arch in infancy: a 10-year experience. Pediatric Cardiology 13: 214–221

Merrill D L, Webster C A, Samson P C 1957 Congenital absence of the aortic isthmus. Journal of Thoracic Surgery 33: 311

Merrill W H, Hoff S J, Stewart J R, Elkins C C, Graham T P Jr, Bender H W Jr 1994 Operative risk factors and durability of repair of coarctation of the aorta in the neonate. Annals of Thoracic Surgery 58: 399–402

Miettinen O S, Reiner M L, Nadas A S 1970 Seasonal incidence of coarctation of the aorta. British Heart Journal 32: 103–107

Milo S, Massini C, Goor D A 1982 Isolated atresia of the aortic arch in a 65 year old man. Surgical treatment and review of published reports. British Heart Journal 47: 294–297

Mitchell S C, Korones S B, Berendes H W 1971 Congenital heart disease in 56 109 births: incidence and natural history. Circulation 43: 323–332

Moes C A F, Freedom R M 1980. Aortic arch interruption with truncus arteriosus or aorticopulmonary septal defect. American Journal of Roentgenology 135: 1011–1016

Mohiaddin R H, Kilner P J, Rees S, Longmore D B 1993 Magnetic resonance volume flow and jet velocity mapping in aortic coarctation. Journal of American College of Cardiology 22: 1515–1521

Momma K 1998 Right aortic arch with coarctation proximal to the right subclavian artery and Kommerell's diverticulum. Cardiology of the Young 8: 413–414

Moreno N N, de Campo T, Kaiser G A et al 1980 Technical and pharmacological management of distal hypotension during repair of coarctation of aorta. Journal of Thoracic and Cardiovascular Surgery 80: 182

Morera J A, Celano V, Roland J M A et al 1983 A rare form of isolated interrupted aortic arch: the value of two-dimensional echocardiography in the precatheterization evaluation. Pediatric Cardiology 4: 289–292

Morris G C, Cooley D A, DeBakey M E, Crawford E S 1960 Coarctation of the aorta with particular emphasis upon improved techniques of surgical repair. Journal of Thoracic Surgery 40: 705–712

Morrow W R, Huhta J C, Murphy D J Jr, McNamara D G 1986 Quantitative morphology of the aortic arch in neonatal coarctation. Journal of American College of Cardiology 8: 616–620

Moskowitz W B, Schieken R M, Mosteller M, Bossano R 1990 Altered systolic and diastolic function in children after 'successful' repair of coarctation of the aorta. American Heart Journal 120: 103–109

Moulaert A J, Bruins C C, Oppenheimer-Dekker A 1976 Anomalies of the aortic arch and ventricular septal defects. Circulation 53: 1011–1015

Moulaert A J, Oppenheimer-Dekker A 1976 Anterolateral muscle bundle of the left ventricle, bulboventricular flange and subaortic stenosis. American Journal of Cardiology 37: 78–81

Moulton A L, Brenner J I, Roberts G et al 1984 Subclavian flap repair of coarctation of the aorta in neonates. Realization of growth potential? Journal of Thoracic and Cardiovascular Surgery 87: 220–235

Mustard W T, Rowe R D, Keith J D, Sirek A 1955 Coarctation of the aorta with special reference to the first year of life. Annals of Surgery 141: 429–435

Nadas A S, Fyler D C 1972 Interrupted aortic arch. In: Pediatric cardiology, 3rd edn. Saunders, Philadelphia, PA, p 507–508

Nanton M A, Olley P M 1976 Residual hypertension after coarctation in children. American Journal of Cardiology 37: 769–772

Neye-Bock S, Fellows K E 1980 Aortic arch interruption in infancy: radio- and angiographic features. American Journal of Roentgenology 135: 1005–1010

Norwood W I, Stellin G J 1981 Aortic atresia with interrupted aortic arch. Reparative operation. Journal of Thoracic and Cardiovascular Surgery 81: 239–244

Odell J A, Spilkin S 1984 Anomalous right subclavian artery and coarctation of the aorta. Surgical implications and the use of the right subclavian artery as a flap. British Heart Journal 51: 666–669

Oshinski J N, Parks W J, Markou C P et al 1996 Improved measurement of pressure gradients in aortic coarctation by magnetic resonance imaging. Journal of American College of Cardiology 28: 1818–1826

Park J K, Dell R B, Ellis K, Gersony W M 1992 Surgical management of the infant with coarctation of the aorta and ventricular–septal defect. Journal of American College of Cardiology 20: 177–180

Park M K 1996 The pediatric cardiology handbook. Mosby Year Book, Mosby, New York

Parker F B Jr, Streeten D H P, Farrell B, Blackman M S, Sondheimer H M, Anderson G H Jr 1982 Preoperative and postoperative renin levels in coarctation of the aorta. Circulation 66: 513–514

Patel R, Singh S P, Abrams L, Roberts K D 1977 Coarctation of the aorta with special reference to infants. Long-term results of operation in 126 cases. British Heart Journal 39: 1246–1253

Pellegrino A, Deverall P B, Anderson R H et al 1985 Aortic coarctation in the first three months of life. An anatomopathological study with respect to treatment. Journal of Thoracic and Cardiovascular Surgery 89: 121–127

Penkoske P A, Williams W G, Olley P M et al 1984 Subclavian arterioplasty. Repair of coarctation of the aorta in the first year of life. Journal of Thoracic and Cardiovascular Surgery 87: 894–900

Pollock J C, Jamieson M P, McWilliam R 1986 Somatosensory evoked potentials in the detection of spinal cord ischaemia in aortic coarctation repair. Annals of Thoracic Surgery 42: 251

Poulias G E, Polemis L, Skoutas B, Doundoulakis N, Papaioannou K 1984 Coarctation of the aorta of unusual morphology. Journal of Cardiovascular Surgery 25: 211–215

Presbitero P, Demarie D, Villani M et al 1987 Long term results (15–30 years) of surgical repair of aortic coarctation. British Heart Journal 57: 462–467

Rao P S, Solymar L 1988 Transductal balloon angioplasty for coarctation of aorta in the neonate. American Heart Journal 116: 1558–1562

Rao P S, Wilson A D, Brazy J 1992 Transumbilical balloon coarctation angioplasty in neonates with critical aortic coarctation. American Heart Journal 124: 1622–1624

Rao P S, Galal O, Smith P A, Wilson A D 1996 Five- to nine-year follow-up results of balloon angioplasty of native aortic coarctation in infants and children. Journal of American College of Cardiology 27: 462–470

Redington A N, Booth P, Shore D F, Rigby M L 1990 Primary balloon dilatation of coarctation of the aorta in neonates. British Heart Journal 64: 277–281

Reifenstein G H, Levine S A, Gross R E 1947 Coarctation of the aorta: a review of 104 autopsied cases of the 'adult type', 2 years of age or older. American Heart Journal 33: 146–168

Rheuban K S, Gutgesell H P, Carpenter M A et al 1986 Aortic aneurysm after patch angioplasty for aortic isthmic coarctation in childhood. American Journal of Cardiology 58: 178–180

Roberts W C, Morrow A G, Braunwald E 1962 Complete interruption of the aortic arch. Circulation 26: 39–59

Rocchini A P, Rosenthal A, Barger A C, Castaneda A R, Nadas A S 1976 Pathogenesis of paradoxical hypertension after coarctation repair. Circulation 54: 382–387

Rosenberg 1973 Coarctation of the aorta: morphology and pathogenic considerations. Perspectives in Pediatric Pathology 1: 339–368

Rosenquist G C 1974 Congenital mitral valve disease associated with coarctation of the aorta. Circulation 49: 985–989

Rubay J E, Sluysmans T, Alexandrescu V et al 1992 Surgical repair of coarctation of the aorta in infants under one year of age. Long-term results in 146 patients comparing subclavian flap angioplasty and modified end-to-end anastomosis. Journal of Cardiovascular Surgery (Torino) 33: 216–222

Ruckman R N, Van Pragh 1978 Anatomic types of congenital mitral stenosis: report of 49 autopsy cases with consideration of diagnosis and surgical implications. American Journal of Cardiology 42: 592–601

Rudolph A M, Heymann M A, Spitznas U 1972 Hemodynamic considerations in the development of narrowing of the aorta. American Journal of Cardiology 30: 514–525

Rychik J, Murdison K A, Chin A J, Norwood W I 1991 Surgical management of severe aortic outflow obstruction in lesions other than the hypoplastic left heart syndrome: use of a pulmonary artery to aorta anastomosis. Journal of American College of Cardiology 18: 809–816

Sade R M, Taylor A B, Chariker E P 1978 Aortoplasty compared with resection for coarctation of the aorta in young children. Annals of Thoracic Surgery 28: 346–353

Sade R M, Taylor A B, Chariker E P 1979 Aortoplasty compared with resection for coarctation of the aorta in young children. Annals of Thoracic Surgery 28: 346–353

Šamanak M, Slavik Z, Zborilova B, Hrobonova V, Voriskova M, Skovranek J 1989 Prevalence, treatment and outcome of heart disease in live-born children: a prospective analysis of 91 823 live-born children. Pediatric Cardiology 10: 205–211

Saul J P, Keane J F, Fellows K E, Lock J E 1987 Balloon dilation angioplasty of postoperative aortic obstructions. American Journal of Cardiology 59: 943–948

Schreiber C, Mazzitelli D, Haehnel J C, Lorenz H P, Meisner H 1997 The interrupted aortic arch: an overview after 20 years of surgical treatment. European Journal of Cardiothoracic Surgery 12: 466–469

Sealy W C 1990 Paradoxical hypertension after repair of coarctation of the aorta: a review of its causes. Annals of Thoracic Surgery 50: 323–329

Sehested J 1982 Coarctation of the aorta in monozygotic twins. British Heart Journal 47: 619–620

Seidel J F 1818 Index Musei Anatomici Kiliensis. CF Mohr, Kiel, 61

Sell J E, Jonas R A, Mayer J E, Blackstone E H, Kirklin J W, Castañeda A R 1988 The results of a surgical program for interrupted aortic arch. Journal of Thoracic and Cardiovascular Surgery 96: 864–877

Serraf A, Lacour-Gayet F, Robotin M, Bruniaux J, Sousa-Uva M, Roussin R, Planche C 1996 Repair of interrupted aortic arch: a ten-year experience. Journal of Thoracic and Cardiovascular Surgery 112: 1150–1160

Shaddy R E, Boucek M M, Sturtevant J E et al 1993 Comparison of angioplasty and surgery for unoperated coarctation of the aorta. Circulation 87: 793–799

Sharland G K, Chan K Y, Allan L D 1994 Coarctation of the aorta: difficulties in prenatal diagnosis. British Heart Journal 71: 70–75

Sharratt G P, Leanage R, Monro J O, Shinebourne E A 1979 Aortic arch interruption presenting with absence of all limb pulses. Archives of Disease in Childhood 54: 49–53

Shinebourne E A, Tam A S, Elseed A M, Paneth M, Lennox S C, Cleland W P 1976 Coarctation of the aorta in infancy and childhood. British Heart Journal 38: 375–380

Shinebourne E A, Hart S, de Swiet M 1979 Management of symptomatic coarctation of the aorta in infancy: subsequent blood pressure compared with a normal population. In: Godman M J, Marquis R M (eds) Paediatric cardiology, Vol 2. Heart disease in the newborn. Churchill Livingstone, Edinburgh, p 243–256

Shone J D, Sellers R D, Anderson R C et al 1963 The development complex of 'parachute mitral valve', supravalve ring of left atrium, subaortic stenosis and coarctation of the aorta. American Journal of Cardiology 11: 714–725

Siewers R D, Ettedgui J, Pahl E, Tallman T, del Nido P J 1991 Coarctation and hypoplasia of the aortic arch: will the arch grow? Annals of Thoracic Surgery 52: 608–613

Simsolo R, Grunfeld B, Gimenez M et al 1988 Long-term systemic hypertension in children after successful repair of coarctation of the aorta. American Heart Journal 115: 1268–1273

Singer M I, Rowen M, Dorsey T J 1982 Transluminal aortic balloon angioplasty for coarctation of the aorta in the newborn. American Heart Journal 103: 131–132

Sirak H D, Ressallat M, Hosier D M, de Lorimier A A 1968 A new operation for repairing aortic arch atresia in infancy. Report of three cases. Circulation 37 (suppl II): 43–50

Skoda J 1855 Protokoll der Sections – Sitzung far Physiologie und Pathologic. Wbl Zeitschrift Gls Aerzte Wien 1: 720

Smallhorn J F, Anderson R H, Macartney F J 1982a Cross-sectional echocardiographic recognition of interruption of aortic arch between left carotid and subclavian arteries. British Heart Journal 48: 229–235

Smallhorn J F, Anderson R H, Macartney F J 1982b Two dimensional echocardiographic assessment of communications between ascending aorta and pulmonary trunk or individual pulmonary arteries. British Heart Journal 47: 563–572

Smith R T Jr, Made R M, Riopel D A, Taylor A B, Crawford F A Jr, Hohn A R 1984 Stress testing for comparison of synthetic patch aortoplasty with resection and end to end anastomosis for repair of coarctation in childhood. Journal of the American College of Cardiology 4: 765–770

Sinder A, Serwer G, Ritter S 1997 Echocardiography in pediatric heart disease. Mosby-Year Book, Mosby, New York

Sohn S, Rothman A, Shiota T et al 1994 Acute and follow-up intravascular ultrasound findings after balloon dilation of coarctation of the aorta. Circulation 90: 340–347

Sos T, Sniderman K W, Rettek-Sos B, Strupp A, Alonso D R 1979 Percutaneous transluminal dilatation of coarctation of thoracic aorta post mortem. Lancet ii: 970–971

Sperling D R, Iorsey T J, Rowen M, Gazzaniga A B 1983 Percutaneous, transluminal angioplasty of congenital coarctation of the aorta. American Journal of Cardiology 51: 562–564

Stansel H C Jr, Tabry I F, Poirier R A, Berman M A, Hellenbrand W E 1977 One hundred consecutive coarctation resections followed from one to thirteen years. Journal of Pediatric Surgery 12: 279–286

Steidele R J. Samml Chir Med Beiob 1778 Vienna 2: 114

Strong W B, Botti R E, Silbert D R, Liebman J 1970 Peripheral and renal vein plasma renin activity in coarctation of the aorta. Pediatrics 45: 254–259

Subramanian R 1972 Coarctation or interruption of aorta proximal to origin of most subclavian arteries. Report of three cases presenting in infancy. British Heart Journal 34: 1225–1226

Tabandeh H 1996 Retinal vascular abnormalities in aortic coarctation. Eye 10: 525–527

Tawes R L, Aberdeen E, Waterston D J, Bonham Carter R E 1969a Coarctation of the aorta in infants and children. A review of 333 operative cases, including 179 infants. Circulation 39(suppl I): 173–184

Tawes R L Jr, Berry C L, Aberdeen E, Graham G R 1969b Myocardial ischemia in infants. Its role in three common congenital cardiac anomalies. Annals of Thoracic Surgery 8: 383–390

Tawes R, Berry C, Aberdeen E 1969c Congenital bicuspid aortic valves associated with coarctation of the aorta in children. British Heart Journal 31: 127–128

Tikkanen J, Heinonen O P 1993 Risk factors for coarctation of the aorta. Teratology 47: 565–572

Tlaskal T, Chaloupecky V, Marek J et al 1997 Primary repair of interrupted aortic arch and associated heart lesions in newborns. Cardiovascular Surgery (Torino) 38: 113–118

Todd P J, Dangerfield P H, Hamilton D I, Wilkinson J L 1983 Late effects on the left upper limb of subclavian flap aortoplasty. Journal of Thoracic and Cardiovascular Surgery 85: 678–681

Trusler G A, Izukawa T 1975 Interrupted aortic arch and ventricular septal defect. Direct repair through a median sternotomy incision in a 13-day-old infant. Journal of Thoracic and Cardiovascular Surgery 69: 126–131

van Houten J P, Rothman A, Bejar R 1996 High incidence of cranial ultrasound abnormalities in full-term infants with congenital heart disease. American Journal of Perinatology 13: 47–53

Van Mierop L H, Kutsche L M 1986 Cardiovascular anomalies in DiGeorge syndrome and importance of neural crest as a possible pathogenetic factor. American Journal of Cardiology 58: 133–137

Van Praagh R, Bernhard W F, Rosenthal A, Parisi L F, Fyler D C 1971 Interrupted aortic arch: surgical treatment. American Journal of Cardiology 27: 200–211

van Son J A, Daniels O, Vincent J G, van Lier H J, Lacquet L K 1989 Appraisal of resection and end-to-end anastomosis for repair of coarctation of the aorta in infancy: preference for resection. Annals of Thoracic Surgery 48: 496–502

Vorsschulte K 1961 Surgical correction of the aorta by an 'isthmus plastic' operation. Thorax 16: 338–342

Vouhe P R, Trinquet F, Lecompte Y et al 1988 Aortic coarctation with hypoplastic aortic arch. Results of extended end-to-end aortic arch anastomosis. Journal of Thoracic and Cardiovascular Surgery 96: 557–563

Vouhe P R, Mace L, Vernant F et al 1990 Primary definitive repair of interrupted aortic arch with ventricular septal defect. European Journal of Cardiothoracic Surgery 4: 365–370

Waldhausen J A, Nahrwold D L 1966 Repair of coarctation of the aorta with a subclavian flap. Journal of Thoracic and Cardiovascular Surgery 51: 532–533

Waldman J D, Lamberti J J, Goodman A H et al 1983 Coarctation in the first year of life. Patterns of postoperative effect. Journal of Thoracic and Cardiovascular Surgery 86: 9–17

Watterson K G, Dhasmana J P, Higgins J W, Wisheart J D 1990 Distal aortic pressure during coarctation operation. Annals of Thoracic Surgery 49: 987–990

Weisman D, Kesten H D 1948 Absence of transverse aortic arch with defects of cardiac septums. Report of a case simulating acute abdominal disease of a newborn infant. American Journal of Diseases in Childhood 76: 326

Wielenga G, Dankmeijer J 1968 Coarctation of the aorta. Journal of Pathology and Bacteriology 95: 265–274

Williams W G, Shindo G, Trusler G A, Dische M R, Olley P M 1980 Results of repair of coarctation of the aorta during infancy. Journal of Thoracic and Cardiovascular Surgery 79: 603–608

Wray T M, Page D L, Glick A, Smith R F 1975 Aortic dissection fifteen years after surgical repair of aortic coarctation. Johns Hopkins Medical Journal 136: 51–53

Yasui H, Kado H, Nakano E et al 1987 Primary repair of interrupted aortic arch and severe aortic stenosis in neonates. Journal of Thoracic and Cardiovascular Surgery 93: 539–545

Yetman A T, Nykanen D, McCrindle B W et al 1997 Balloon angioplasty of recurrent coarctation: A 12 year review. Journal of American College of Cardiology 30: 811–816

Zannini L, Lecompte Y, Galli R et al 1985 Aortic coarctation with hypoplasia of the arch: description of a new surgical technic. Giornale Italiano di Cardiologia 15: 1045–1048

57

— Vascular ring and pulmonary sling —

S. C. Park and J. R. Zuberbuhler

INTRODUCTION

The trachea and bronchuses are closely related anatomically to the aorta and its brachiocephalic branches and to the pulmonary arteries. Certain anomalies of these arteries may cause obstruction to the airways. The term 'vascular ring' has been used somewhat loosely to describe a variety of such vascular abnormalities that can cause tracheal or oesophageal compression. It should probably be limited to malformations in which there is encirclement of the trachea and oesophagus by vascular structures. Not all vascular rings defined in this way necessarily result in compromise of the airways nor produce symptomatic oesophageal compression. Conversely, there are vascular anomalies that do not form a true ring and yet may produce highly significant obstruction of the airways. This chapter reviews a variety of vascular abnormalities that may compromise the lumen of either the airways or the oesophagus.

INCIDENCE

Although minor variations in the morphology of the aortic arch morphology are relatively common, symptomatic abnormalities are rare. According to Gasul et al (1966), the prevalence of vascular rings was 0.7% in 1943 patients with congenital heart disease. Vascular rings occurred in 21 of 1606 (1.3%) heart specimens with congenital cardiac malformations in the Heart Museum at the Children's Hospital of Pittsburgh.

CLASSIFICATION AND MORPHOLOGY

A review of the embryological development of the aortic arch is helpful in understanding the genesis of certain vascular abnormalities. In an early stage of development, the aortic arches are paired structures connecting ventral and dorsal aortas (Figure 57.1a). The proximal portions of the ventral aortas take origin from the aortic sack with the paired dorsal aortas uniting to form the descending aorta. Between the ventral and dorsal aortas, six paired brachial arches develop, giving the basic so-called 'Rathke arrangement' (Figure 57.1b). The fifth arches regress entirely. The first and second arches almost disappear, persisting only as small arteries in the head. Large components of the primitive paired dorsal aortas between the third and fourth arches also regress bilaterally. At the same time, the aortic sack divides to form the ascending aorta and the pulmonary trunk. The third arches, and the dorsal aortas cephalad to the fourth arches, become the right and left internal carotid arteries, while the ventral aortas cephalad to these arches become the external carotid arteries. The fourth arch forms the aortic arch proper (Figure 57.1c), and the sixth arches form the arterial duct (ductus arteriosus) and the proximal pulmonary arteries. The seventh cervical members of the series of parietal intersegmental arteries migrate in a cephalad direction and become the subclavian arteries (Figure 57.1d).

It is unlikely that the Rathke concept of the bilateral system of archs ever exists in its entirety at one given point of development. Extrapolating from this concept, however, Edwards (1984, 1953) hypothesized the existence of a primitive double aortic arch system with a duct, a common carotid and a subclavian artery arising independently from each arch (Figure 57.1d). Most aortic arch anomalies are assumed to be the result either of regression of a part of this system that normally persists, or persistent patency of a component that normally regresses. Figure 57.2 illustrates the possible morphological abnormalities resulting from interruption at various sites.

1559

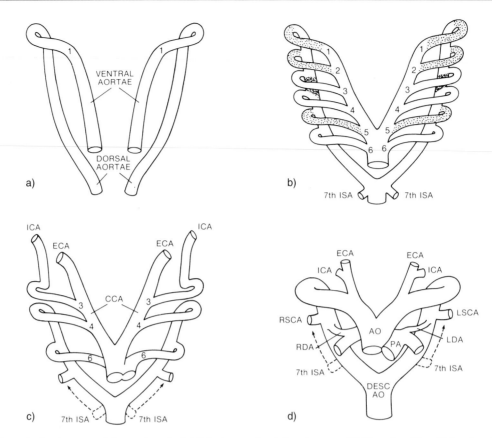

Figure 57.1. Embryonic development of the aortic arch. (a) Paired ventral and dorsal aortas. (b) Six pairs of brachial arches develop between the dorsal and ventral aortas; the first, second and fifth arches subsequently regress, as shown by shaded areas. (c) The common carotid arteries (CCA) consist of remnants of the ventral aorta between the third and fourth arches; the external carotid arteries (ECA) are the continuation of the ventral aortas. The third arches become internal carotid arteries (ICA). (d) The sixth arches form both arterial ducts (LDA, left duct; RDA, right duct) and the proximal right and left pulmonary arteries. The seventh intersegmental arteries (ISA) migrate in the cephalic direction and become the subclavian arteries (RSCA, right; LSCA, left). Eventually a primitive double aortic arch system is formed with bilateral ducts.

ANOMALIES RESULTING FROM INTERRUPTION

INTERRUPTION DISTAL TO THE DUCT

When the interuption occurs distally in the right-sided arch (position 1 in Figure 57.2, centre), the result is a normal left-sided aortic arch and a left-sided duct with a right brachiocephalic (innominate) artery (Figure 57.2, R-1). When the interruption is on the left side of the arch, there is a right-sided aortic arch with mirror-imaged branching of the head and arm vessels, including a left-sided brachiocephalic (innominate) artery. This latter arrangement is frequently associated with serious cyanotic congenital heart disease, most commonly with tetralogy of Fallot with pulmonary stenosis or atresia, common arterial trunk, and a left-sided heart with mirror-imaged visceral arrangement (situs inversus). On reviewing 105 heart specimens with right aortic arch in the Heart Museum of the Children's Hospital of Pittsburgh, the arterial duct or its ligament was left-sided in 55%, right-sided in 28%, bilateral in 3% and absent in 14% (Figure 57.2, L-1). It should be noted that when a left-sided duct arises from the base of the brachiocephalic (innominate) artery and connects to the left pulmonary artery a vascular ring does not result (Figure 57.2, L-1). Similarly, a right-sided duct with a normal left arch does not form a ring (Figure 57.2, R-1).

INTERRUPTION BETWEEN THE DUCT AND THE SUBCLAVIAN ARTERY

When the left arch is interrupted between the duct and the subclavian artery (position 2 in Figure 57.2, centre), the duct originates from a diverticular remnant of the left dorsal aorta, the so-called 'diverticulum of Kommerell' (Kommerell, 1936; Shannon, 1961; Blake and Manion, 1962). It passes retro-oesophageally, connects with the left pulmonary artery and forms a vascular ring (Figure 57.2, L-2) (Grollman et al, 1967; Wychulis et al, 1971). Theoretically, a right-sided duct arising from a diverticulum of Kommerell with left arch is possible (Figure 57.2, R-2) but, to our knowledge, has not been reported.

INTERRUPTION BETWEEN THE SUBCLAVIAN AND COMMON CAROTID ARTERIES

Interruption between the subclavian and common carotid arteries (position 3 in Figure 57.2, centre) results in a

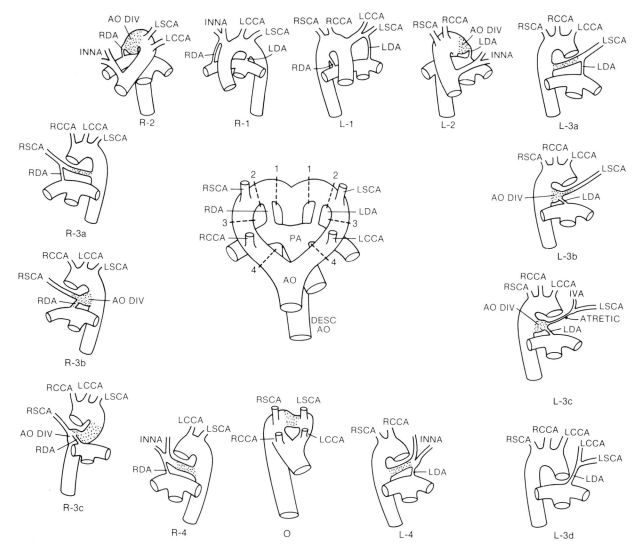

Figure 57.2. Possible aortic arch anomalies depending on the site of interruption (dotted lines) in the primitive double aortic arch system (centre diagram). The letter code under each figure indicates the sidedness of the aortic arch and site of the aortic arch. The dotted areas are retro-oesophageal components. AO, aorta; Desc, descending; Div, diverticulum; INNA, brachiocephalic (innominate) artery; LCCA, left common carotid artery; LDA, left-sided duct; LSCA, left subclavian artery; RCCA, right common carotid artery; RDA, right-sided duct; RSCA, right subclavian artery; VA, vertebral artery.

contralateral aortic arch with anomalous distal origin of the subclavian artery on the side of the interruption and lack of a brachiocephalic (innominate) artery. The carotid artery is the first vessel to arise from the arch. If the arterial duct arises from the affected subclavian artery, a loose vascular ring results (Figure 57.2, R-3a, L-3a) (Felson and Palayew, 1963; Stewart et al, 1964). When the arch is right-sided and the anomalous subclavian artery is left-sided, the arch is to the right of the trachea, the aberrant subclavian artery is posterior, the duct is to the left and the pulmonary trunk is anterior. The loose 'ring' is not continuous, since the right pulmonary artery and right arch are not physically connected. But the vascular structures are interlocked, and there is complete encirclement of the trachea. If the duct originates from a diverticulum of Kommerell rather than from the subclavian artery

(Figure 57.2, R-3b, L-3b), the resultant ring is much tighter (Stewart et al, 1964).

An aberrant subclavian artery with bilateral ducts causes a true vascular ring but is exceedingly rare (Stewart et al, 1964). The mirror-image dvariant does occur, with the aberrant subclavian artery being right-sided in association with a left arch and a right descending aorta (Figure 57.2, R-3c) (Paul, 1948; Park et al, 1976).

INTERRUPTION DISTAL TO THE DUCT COMBINED WITH INTERRUPTION BETWEEN THE CAROTID AND SUBCLAVIAN ARTERIES

Interruption of the aortic arch at positions 1 and 3 in Figure 57.2 (centre) causes 'isolation' of the subclavian artery from the aorta. The subclavian artery is connected to the pulmonary artery by a duct (Figure 57.2, L-3d), and a vascular ring does not result (Stewart et al, 1964; Shuford et al, 1970). The isolated subclavian artery is supplied retrogradely with blood from the vertebral artery and may cause a subclavian steal syndrome (Shuford et al, 1970; Victorica et al, 1970; Rodriguez et al, 1975). When, with this arrangement, the left duct arises from an aortic diverticulum, a tight vascular ring does result (Figure 46.2, L-3c).

INTERRUPTION PROXIMAL TO THE COMMON CAROTID ARTERY

Interruption proximal to the common carotid artery (position 4 in Figure 57.2, centre) results in distal and retro-oesophageal origin of the brachiocephalic (innominate) artery (Figure 57.2, R-4, L-4) (Grollman et al, 1968). If there is an associated duct or ligament arising from the affected artery, there will be a complete ring, but it is loose and does not cause symptoms.

NO INTERRUPTION

Lack of interruption of either the right or left aortic arch results in a double aortic arch (Figure 57.2, O).

ANOMALIES CAUSING A VASCULAR RING ———

DOUBLE AORTIC ARCH (NO INTERRUPTION)

The anomaly most likely to cause a symptomatic vascular ring is persistence of both right and left fourth arches. Most commonly both arches are patent, the right being larger than the left, and there is a left duct and a left descending aorta (Tables 57.1 and 57.2). Occasionally, there is anatomical continuity but luminal atresia of one arch. Atresia has only been reported in the left arch, either between the left common carotid artery and the left subclavian artery, or distal to the left subclavian artery. Theoretically, the duct could be on the left or right or it could be bilateral; however, only a left-sided duct has been reported to date (Moës, 1978).

Table 57.1. Size of aortic arch in patients with double aortic arch

Side of descending aorta	Size of aortic arch(%)		
	Right > left	Right = left	Left > right
Left 71%	72	8	20
Right 29%	75	11	14
Overall	73	9	18

Based on 139 cases from data of Ekström and Sandblom (1951) and Théodoridès (1960); reviewed by Klinkhamer (1969).

Table 57.2. Patency and site of atresia in double aortic arch with left arch smaller than right

Side of descending aorta	Patency (%)		Site of atresia (%)	
	Patent	Atretic	Distal to left subclavian artery	Between left subclavian and left carotid arteries
Left	85	15	86	14
Right	76	24	67	33
Overall	83	17	77	23

Based on 139 cases from data of Ekström and Sandblom (1951) and Théodoridès (1960); reviewed by Klinkhamer (1969).

Approximately one-fifth of patients with double aortic arches also have some form of congenital heart disease. Associated anomalies include tetralogy of Fallot, ventricular septal defect, coarctation of the aorta, patency of the arterial duct, complete transposition and common arterial trunk (Romanos et al, 1957; Stewart et al, 1964; Lincoln et al, 1969; Zdebska et al, 1977).

RIGHT AORTIC ARCH WITH LEFT DUCT

With a right aortic arch and a left duct (interruption at position 2 in Figure 57.2, centre) there may be a mirror-imaged arrangement of the arteries to the head and arms (a left brachiocephalic (innominate), right common carotid and right subclavian artery, in order of their origin). The left duct then extends from a diverticulum of Kommerell to the left pulmonary artery (Figure 57.2, L-2), passing retro-oesophageally and forming a tight vascular ring. This anomaly is exceedingly rare (Wychulis et al, 1971; Shuford and Sybes, 1974). Bennett et al (1984) reported a patient with a right aortic arch with mirror-imaged arrangement of the arteries to the head and arms and a right-sided descending aorta, which gave rise to a blind-ending diverticulum of Kommerell. A partially patent duct connected the diverticulum and the left pulmonary artery, forming a vascular ring. The duct causes a significant compression of the left main bronchus, producing respiratory distress and hyperinflation of the left lung.

ABERRANT SUBCLAVIAN ARTERY WITH AN IPSILATERAL DUCT

A left aortic arch with an aberrant right subclavian artery (interruption at position 3 in Figure 57.2, centre) is a common aortic arch anomaly, occurring in 0.5% of the population (Klinkhamer, 1969). This malformation almost never produces dysphagia or respiratory symptoms, since the duct or ligament is usually left-sided and there is, therefore, no vascular ring. Rarely, an aberrant right subclavian artery passes between the oesophagus

Table 57.3.   Right aortic arch and associated aberrant left subclavian artery

Primary anomaly	Incidence	
	Right aortic arch	Associated aberrant left subclavian artery
Pulmonary atresia with ventricular septal defect	18/65 (28%)	0
Common arterial trunk	12/46 (26%)	1 (8%)
Tetralogy of Fallot	74/366 (20%)	3 (4%)
Ventricular septal defect	26/216 (12%)	7 (27%)
Double inlet left ventricle	10/85 (12%)	0
Tricuspid atresia	3/438 (7%)	0
Complete transposition	6/136 (4%)	1 (17%)
Atrial septal defect	4/191 (2%)	1 (25%)
Miscellaneous	11	–
None	16	13 (81%)
Total	*180*	*26 (14%)*

Data from 180 cases at the Children's Hospital of Pittsburgh.

and the trachea rather than behind the oesophagus (Holzapfel, 1899). Bayford (1794) reported a case of an adult with this anomaly who had dysphagia.

A right arch with an aberrant left subclavian artery is also common. Hastreiter et al (1966) reported an incidence of 0.1%. Of 180 patients diagnosed as having right aortic arch at the Children's Hospital of Pittsburgh, 26 (14%) had an aberrant left subclavian artery. Half of these 26 patients had various congenital cardiac anomalies including tetralogy of Fallot, ventricular septal defect, atrial septal defect, common arterial trunk and complete transposition (Table 57.3).

A vascular ring is formed when the anomalous subclavian artery arises distally and there is a duct on the same side. If the duct arises from the subclavian artery itself (Figure 57.2, L-3a, R-3a), the ring is usually loose and symptoms are rare. If the duct arises from an aortic diverticulum (Figure 57.2, L-3b, L-3c), the ring will be tight. This has been reported only with a left-sided duct (Antia and Ottensen, 1966; Victorica et al, 1970).

LEFT AORTIC ARCH, RIGHT DESCENDING AORTA AND RIGHT DUCT

A left arch with a retro-oesophageal right descending aorta and right duct (interruption at position 3 on the right aortic arch in Figure 57.2 centre; Figure 57.3), produces marked posterior indentation of the oesophagus but rarely causes symptoms. A left arch with a retro-oesophageal right descending aorta and aberrant right subclavian artery, in contrast, may cause compression of the right main bronchus if there is a right-sided duct that connects the aortic diverticulum and the right pulmonary artery (Figures 57.2 (R-3c) and 57.4). Compromise of the

airways (Schlamowitz et al, 1962; Park et al, 1976) and dysphagia (Edwards, 1948; Sterz, 1961) have been reported. This anomaly is rare and only 12 cases had been discovered by Park et al in 1976.

ABERRANT BRACHIOCEPHALIC (INNOMINATE) ARTERY WITH AN IPSILATERAL DUCT

An aberrant brachiocephalic (innominate) artery with a duct on the same side (interruption at position 4 in Figure 57.2, centre) forms a loose ring and usually causes no clinical symptoms (Figure 57.2, L-4, R-4). Theoretically, an aberrant brachiocephalic (innominate) artery could exist with either a right or a left aortic arch, but only the left variety has been reported and this is itself very rare (Grollman et al, 1968). Only two patients with a right aortic arch and aberrant brachiocephalic (innominate) artery have been documented angiocardiographically at the Children's Hospital of Pittsburgh (Figure 57.5). One had a ventricular septal defect, while the other had valvar and peripheral pulmonary stenosis. Neither had clinical signs nor symptoms of airway or oesophageal compromise.

CLINICAL FINDINGS

The clinical manifestations of abnormalities of the aortic arches vary primarily with the severity of encroachment by the abnormal vessel on the trachea, bronchus or oesophagus. Some anomalies (an aberrant subclavian artery, for instance) rarely cause symptoms. Others (such as double aortic arch) almost always produce significant obstruction. The most prominent clinical manifestations

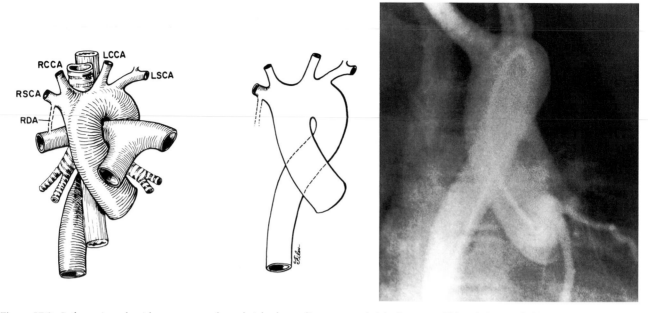

Figure 57.3. Left aortic arch with a retro-oesophageal right descending aorta and right ligament. Abbreviations as in Figure 57.2.

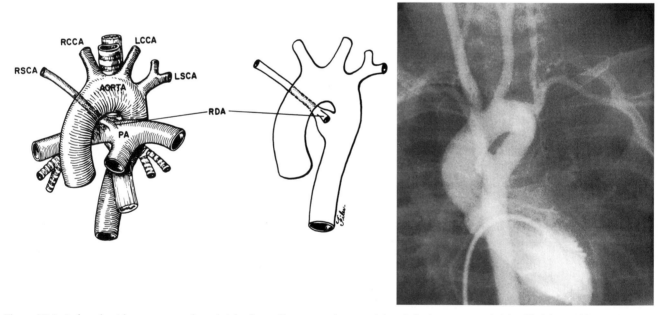

Figure 57.4. Left arch with a retro-oesophageal right descending aorta, aberrant right subclavian artery and right-sided duct. Abbreviations as in Figure 57.2.

include stridor, wheezing and cough. The characteristic stridor is inspiratory, but it may be both inspiratory and expiratory. Although respiratory symptoms are usually mild and rarely recognized in the newborn period, they often become apparent during the first few months of life. Patients with a double aortic arch tend to have symptoms at an earlier age than do patients with other types of vascular ring. Even with double aortic arch, the onset of symptoms can be insidious and there may be no obvious stridor during the first few months of life. There may be a history of recurrent respiratory infections requiring

medical attention, and some patients have been referred for an evaluation of an 'allergic problem' such as asthma. Even with the most severe form of a vascular ring, airway symptoms can vary considerably and may disappear during sleep or quiet play. Symptoms are often exacerbated by exertion or crying, and upper respiratory tract infection also aggravates the airway compromise. Although patients with a double aortic arch are usually symptomatic in early infancy, they can rarely have no symptoms, with the anomaly being found only as an incidental finding at cardiac catheterization or at postmortem.

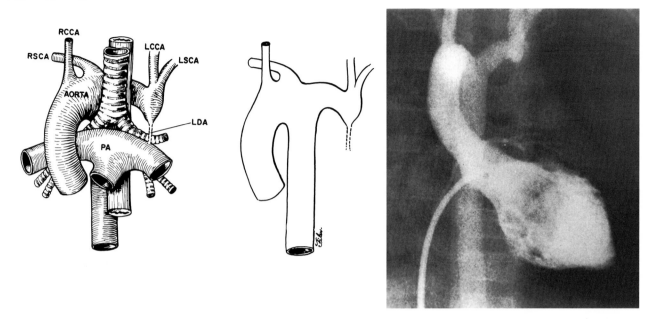

Figure 57.5. Right aortic arch with an aberrant brachiocephalic (innominate) artery.

Patients with a right aortic arch, an aberrant left sub-clavian artery and a left-sided retro-oesophageal duct (Figure 57.2, L-3b) may present early, but symptoms tend to be less severe than in those with a double aortic arch.

Dysphagia is quite rare in children with a retro-oesophageal vessel. The majority of patients with vascular abnormalities gain weight and develop adequately, but those with frequent pulmonary infections and/or difficulties with feeding may fail to thrive and have poor physical development.

— DIAGNOSIS AND INVESTIGATION —

Some vascular rings cause no clinical symptoms and are noted incidently at postmortem or during cardiac catheterization. Others are symptomatic. Although there are a number of causes of chronic stridor in infancy and childhood, the possibility of a vascular abnormality should always be considered in any patient with signs and symptoms of airway obstruction. In review of a large number of children with stridor, 4–8% were found to have a vascular ring or some other vascular anomaly (Kahn et al, 1977; Holinger, 1980).

Since most patients with recurrent or persistent respiratory problems have already had chest radiographs, a careful review of these films may be helpful. The single most valuable non-invasive study is a series of radiographs taken with barium in the oesophagus. The sidedness of the arch is usually readily apparent, and retro-oesophageal arteries are marked by a posterior oesophageal indent-ation. A double aortic arch may be suggested by bilateral indentations, usually at slightly different levels, in addition to a large posterior indentation (Figures 57.6 and 57.7).

In some cases, a barium swallow under fluoroscopy adds additional information, particularly when dysphagia or aspiration are also present.

Some investigators (Nikaidoh et al, 1972; Arciniegas et al, 1978; Lam et al, 1978) suggest that angiography is unnecessary or less useful than barium oesophagraphy for diagnosis. It should be stressed, however, that different anomalies may produce similar findings on the barium-filled oesophagram (Figures 57.6–57.8). A precise anatomical diagnosis cannot then be made without angiography or other diagnostic procedures such as echo-cardiography or magnetic resonance imaging. Tonkin et al (1980) have advocated simultaneous angiographic and barium oesophagraphic studies during cardiac catheterization to evaluate the anatomical relationship between the blood vessels and oesophagus. We have found that leaving a small radiopaque tube, such as a feeding tube or a Swan–Ganz catheter, in the oesophagus during the study is equally helpful in determining spatial relationships. If a Swan–Ganz catheter is used, the balloon can be inflated with contrast material and slowly withdrawn from the stomach to the oropharynx to evaluate the site and severity of the oesophageal constriction. A cinefluoroscopic record of this catheter withdrawal is made for correlation with cineangiograms.

Certain vascular structures (such as an atretic segment of an aortic arch or an arterial ligament) cannot be visualized by angiography. Tenting or distortion of the arteries to the head and arms, or the presence of a large aortic diverticulum of Kommerell, may suggest their presence (Figure 57.9). Biplane angiography in multiple views using selective injections of contrast material in the artery suspected of producing compromise is the most precise way of defining the anatomy. Since an aortic vascular ring

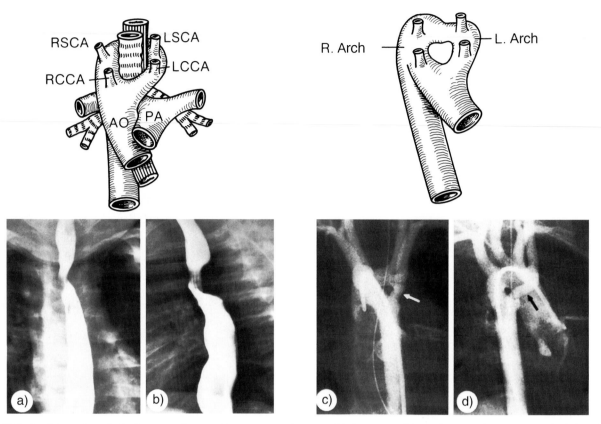

Figure 57.6. Double aortic arch. Barium oesophagrams in anteroposterior (a) and left anterior oblique (b) views demonstrate right, left and posterior indentations. Selective aortograms in anteroposterior (c) and right anterior oblique (d) views demonstrate a typical double aortic arch with the left arch (arrows) smaller than the right. The radiopaque line is a Swan–Ganz catheter in the oesophagus.

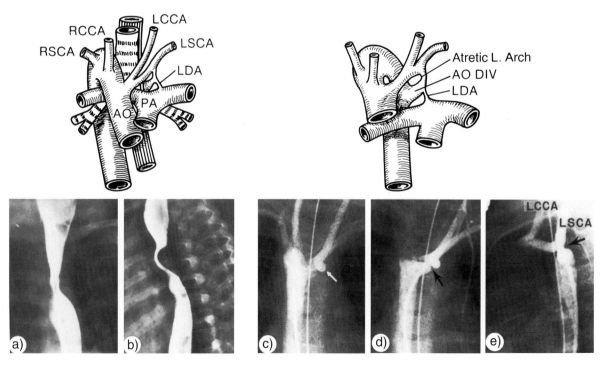

Figure 57.7. Double aortic arch with near-atresia of the left arch (probe patent only). Barium oesophagrams in the anteroposterior (a) and left anterior oblique (b) views are similar to that of a double aortic arch (Figure 57.3). Selective aortogram in the anteroposterior view (c) simulates a right aortic arch with mirror-imaged head and arm arteries, the left-sided brachiocephalic (innominate) artery being the first branch. The arrow indicates an unusual projection from the brachiocephalic (innominate) artery. A communication between the diverticulum of Kommerell and the left innominate artery is shown in (d) and (e) (arrows), confirming the double aortic arch.

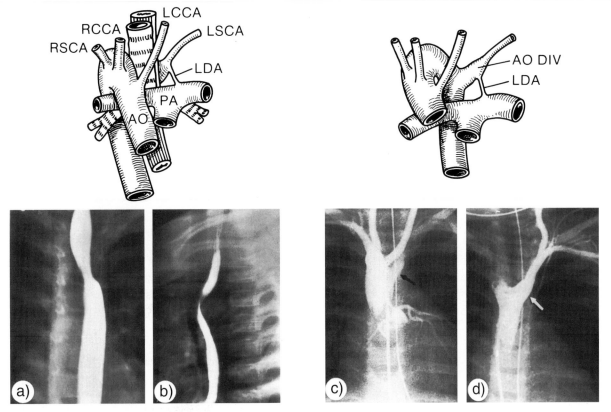

Figure 57.8. Right aortic arch with an aberrant left subclavian artery and left duct. Barium oesophagrams in the anteroposterior (a) and left anterior oblique (b) views demonstrate oesophageal indentations similar to those seen in double aortic arch (Figures 57.3 and 57.4). Aortogram in the anteroposterior view (c) shows an aberrant left subclavian artery (arrow). Selective injection of contrast material in the aberrant vessel shows dilatation of the origin of the artery, which represents a remnant of the embryonic left arch (d).

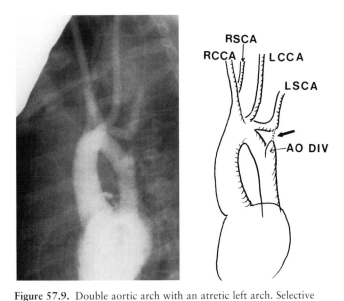

Figure 57.9. Double aortic arch with an atretic left arch. Selective left ventriculogram in the left anterior oblique view shows an aortic diverticulum (AO DIV) and tenting of the origin of the left subclavian artery (LSCA), suggesting the presence of ligamentous atretic left arch (arrow) (confirmed at surgery). Abbreviations as in Figure 57.2.

and pulmonary sling (distal origin of the left pulmonary artery) may coexist (Ahlstrom et al, 1973), pulmonary

arteriography should be performed routinely if there is unilateral atelectasis or hyperinflation of the lung.

Cross-sectional echocardiography sometimes provides accurate diagnostic imaging of anomalies such as double aortic arch by visualization of both aortic arches (Figure 57.10). Colour flow mapping enhances the visualization of the anomaly and confirms patency of the vessel or aortic arch. When two aortic arches are present, even if one is atretic, there is separate branching of the common carotid and subclavian arteries instead of common branching as seen with a brachiocephalic artery. Such separate branching should suggest the presence of a double arch. Identifying the dominant arch is important from the surgical point of view. In recent years, surgical intervention has been performed on the basis of echocardiographic study without further angiographic study or magnetic resonance imaging. Only when non-invasive imaging does not provide adequate diagnostic information is a selective angiographic study mandatory. Bronchoscopy may exacerbate symptoms in a patient with a compromised airway and should be undertaken only under special circumstances. Tracheobronchography should be discouraged in view of the high morbidity of this study in patients with a compromised airway.

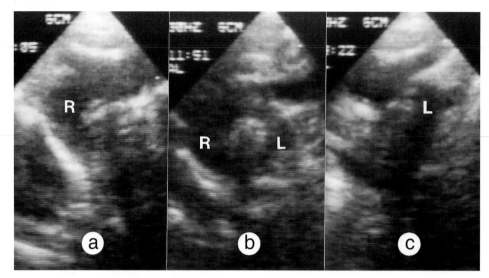

Figure 57.10. Cross-sectional echocardiograms of a double aortic arch from the suprasternal view. The right oblique view (a) shows a dominant right arch (R) while the left oblique view (c) shows a smaller left arch (L). The coronal oblique view (b) demonstrates simultaneous visualization of both right and left arches.

MANAGEMENT

The simple existence of a vascular ring is not an indication for surgical intervention. Godtfredsen et al (1977) reported spontaneous improvement of respiratory symptoms in patients with vascular rings in a long-term follow-up study (median 7 years) and suggested conservative medical management of these patients. It is generally accepted, however, that surgical intervention should be undertaken whenever there is significant compromise to the airways. Unnecessary delay may cause irreversible tracheobronchial damage, leading to chronic compromise of the airways even after surgical repair of the anomalous arch.

A double aortic arch usually requires surgery in early infancy. The smaller of the two arches (or the atretic arch) should be divided. In most cases of double aortic arch, the left arch is the smaller one (or is atretic). It can be approached from a left anterolateral thoracotomy. Patients with a right aortic arch, aberrant left subclavian artery and left duct may rarely have significant dysphagia or respiratory symptoms. Division of the duct usually relieves the obstruction of the airways, but division of the aberrant subclavian artery is necessary very rarely to alleviate dysphagia.

The reported operative mortality in patients with a double aortic arch has ranged from 6 to 30% (Arciniegas et al, 1978; Moës et al, 1978). Operative complications in the past included development of chylothorax, aortaoesophageal fistulae (Arciniegas et al, 1978) and paralysis of the vocal cords as a result of damage to the recurrent laryngeal nerve (Nikaidoh et al, 1972). More recent experience in large series (Checa et al, 1983; Roesler et al, 1983) has shown that the ring can be surgically divided without mortality. The postoperative course after relief of

a vascular ring is variable. Although symptomatic improvement may occur shortly after surgery, persistent respiratory symptoms are not unusual, since distortion of the tracheobronchial tree persists following surgery. Severe associated tracheomalacia may rarely require a direct surgical approach to the trachea. Inoue et al (1973) reported a high incidence of facial and nasopharyngeal abnormalities in patients with a vascular ring. Postoperative residual respiratory problems may be related to pre-existing anomalies of the airways. Although respiratory symptoms may persist for a variable period of time after surgical repair, the ultimate prognosis is generally good.

COMPRESSION OF THE TRACHEA BY THE BRACHIOCEPHALIC (INNOMINATE) ARTERY

Gross and Neuhauser in 1948 were the first to report respiratory problems associated with an anomalous brachiocephalic (innominate) artery, and they described a surgical procedure for its correction. The largest experience with this lesion has been reported from the Hospital for Sick Children in Toronto (MacDonald and Fearon, 1971; Moës et al, 1975). Despite earlier scepticism concerning the existence of this entity, it has gradually become more widely recognized as a cause of compromised airways. The underlying problem is thought to be an unusually distal origin of the brachiocephalic (innominate) artery that causes it to pass from left to right in front of the trachea. Although the artery may pass anterior to the trachea in asymptomatic individuals, it usually has a more posterior origin in patients with compromised airways. The length of the artery has also been thought to be an important contributing factor in producing tracheal compression (Moës, 1978). In some patients with this condition, the left common carotid artery also arises directly from a common brachiocephalic trunk. Since this occurs in one-tenth of the general population (Edwards, 1960), it should not be implicated as a sole cause of tracheal compression. Resonance imaging studies in patients with endoscopically suspected tracheal compression by the brachiocephalic artery suggest that the symptoms may result from an intrinsic deficiency of tracheal cartilage rather than an anatomical abnormality of the mediastinum or its vasculature (Fletcher and Cohn, 1989). Further investigation and confirmation of this observation is needed.

INCIDENCE

The true incidence of compression of the trachea by an anomalous brachiocephalic (innominate) artery is difficult to determine. There is considerable disparity in the frequency of diagnosis from institution to institution. The male:female ratio is approximately 3:1 (Moës et al, 1975).

CLINICAL FINDINGS

The clinical manifestations depend on the severity of encroachment of the trachea by the anomalous artery. The most common sign is stridor, either inspiratory or biphasic. Other respiratory problems include wheezing, cough and recurrent pneumonia. The most severe manifestation of this anomaly is reflex apnoea, which may lead to sudden death. In a review of 60 patients undergoing surgery, Moës et al (1975) reported that 84% had stridor, 38% experienced reflex apnoea and 33% had recurrent pulmonary infections. The onset of symptoms varied from birth to 30 months of age, with a mean of 4 months. Patients may become symptomatic as late as 8 years of age (Ardito et al, 1980). Despite respiratory symptoms, patients with this condition seldom have feeding difficulties and their physical growth is usually well maintained.

Moës et al (1975) and Ardito et al (1980) reported that some patients with this anomaly have coexisting abnormalities of the airways, such as subglottic stenosis, tracheo-oesophageal fistula, laryngomalacia and asthma. The contribution of the anomalous brachiocephalic (innominate) artery to the problem with the airways is then difficult to assess.

DIAGNOSTIC PROCEDURES

Chest radiographs may provide important diagnostic information (Ericsson and Soderlund, 1969; Berdon and Baker, 1972). In particular, the lateral view shows anterior indentation of the trachea in around one half of the patients (Moës et al, 1975; Ardito et al, 1980). The barium oesophagram is normal (Figure 57.11).

Tracheobronchoscopy should delineate the exact location and the severity of obstruction. The classical bronchoscopic finding is an oblique anterior pulsatile compression extending from the left inferiorly to right superiorly (Figure 57.11). The compressed segment is short and is located 1–2 cm above the carina. Fearon and Shortreed (1963) reported that the right radial or temporal arterial pulse could be obliterated or diminished when the pulsatile bulge on the anterior wall of the trachea was compressed with the tip of the bronchoscope. The degree of compression may be assessed by bronchoscopy, although Ardito et al (1980) noted poor correlation between the bronchoscopically estimated degree of tracheal obstruction and the severity of clinical symptoms. The need for angiographic study of this abnormality has been questioned. Some investigators (Moës et al, 1975) have felt that it is unnecessary. Although angiographic study has not been routinely performed in our institution, a selective angiographic study is sometimes helpful in delineating the anatomical derangement and in ruling out associated malformations. An aortogram shows the brachiocephalic (innominate) artery originating to the left of the midline; however, since the arteries to the head and arms overlap in the lateral view, it is often difficult to determine whether the artery compresses the trachea. Selective injection of contrast into the proximal portion of the artery itself is helpful when viewed in the anteroposterior, lateral and right and left oblique projections. Overpenetrated lateral and left anterior oblique views often demonstrate the anatomical relationship between the trachea and the abnormal artery and may also determine the severity of the tracheal compression. Tracheobronchographic study is generally not recommended.

MANAGEMENT

Management of compression of the trachea by the brachiocephalic artery varied from institution to institution. MacDonald and Fearon (1971) managed about one sixth of their 285 patients surgically, while Ardito et al (1980) reported surgical intervention in one third of their 78 patients. Mildly symptomatic patients are usually managed medically. But there is agreement that patients with reflex apnoea should undergo surgery without delay. The operation consists of suspension of the anomalous brachiocephalic (innominate) artery to the under-surface of the sternum (Mustard et al, 1969). Recently, Hawkins et al (1992) advocated a new surgical technique of reimplantation of the artery more proximally on the ascending aorta to the right of the trachea. Long-term results of this technique remain to be observed. Management of patients with moderate respiratory symptoms should be

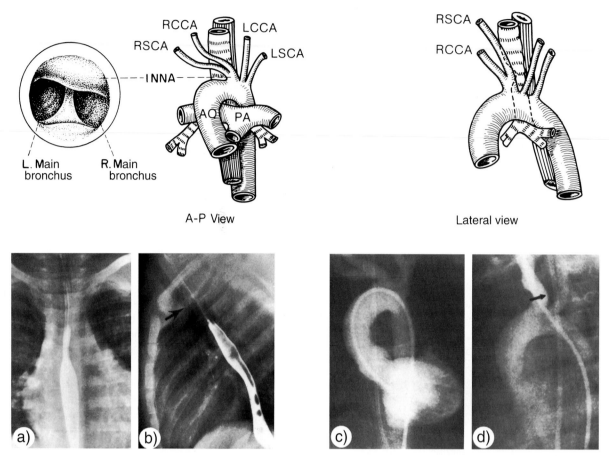

Figure 57.11. Compression of the trachea by an anomalous brachiocephalic (innominate) artery. An endoscopic view shows anterior compression of the trachea just above the carina, running obliquely from left inferiorly to right superiorly. The barium oesophagram in anteroposterior (a) and lateral (b) views is normal. However, anterior compression of the trachea is seen in the lateral view (b) (arrow). Selective left ventriculography in the anteroposterior view (c) shows distal take-off of the anomalous brachiocephalic (innominate) artery. The left anterior oblique view of the selective arteriogram (d) demonstrates its relatively posterior origin and also reveals compression of the anterior aspect of the trachea.

tailored to the individual and depends upon the frequency and severity of respiratory symptoms and the degree of tracheal compression, as determined endoscopically and/or angiographically. There have been no operative deaths reported in major series. Most patients have had either complete relief of symptoms or improvement following surgery (Moës et al, 1975). Persistent respiratory symptoms following operation may result from inadequate operative relief of the tracheal compression or, more frequently, from associated intrinsic airway problems.

DISTAL ORIGIN OF THE LEFT PULMONARY ARTERY —(PULMONARY SLING)—

In pulmonary sling, the left pulmonary artery originates from the right pulmonary artery. It then passes over the right mainstem bronchus and courses posterior to the trachea to reach the hilum of the left lung (Figure 57.12). It has many appellations, including 'distal origin of the left pulmonary artery', 'anomalous left pulmonary artery', 'aberrant left pulmonary artery', 'vascular sling', 'pulmonary sling', 'pulmonary arterial sling' and 'pulmonary arterial ring'. The earliest report of this condition was by Glaevecke and Doehle in 1897, but the first surgical correction was not attempted until 1954 (Potts et al, 1954).

The embryological basis of the distal origin of the left pulmonary artery is unknown, but it has been postulated that there is faulty development of the left sixth aortic arch, with the right pulmonary artery (derived from the right sixth arch) vascularizing the undivided primitive lung. With maturation and separation of the primitive lung buds, there is then enlargement of a branch of the right pulmonary artery which leads to the left lung and which becomes the definitive left pulmonary artery. Associated cardiovascular malformations occur in about one quarter of patients. They include ventricular septal defect, atrial septal defect, patency of the arterial duct, coarctation of the aorta, tetralogy of Fallot with right aortic arch, double inlet left ventricle, persistent left superior caval vein and common arterial trunk with an interrupted aortic arch. Rarely, an accessory left pulmonary artery may supply the left upper lobe (Figure

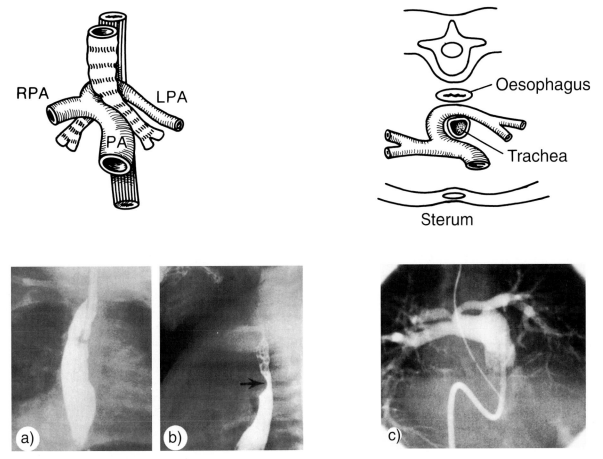

Figure 57.12. Pulmonary vascular sling. Barium oesophagram in the anteroposterior view (a) is normal. A marked anterior indentation (arrow) is seen in the lateral view (b). Selective pulmonary arteriogram in the anteroposterior view in the sitting position (c) demonstrates the anomalous origin of the left pulmonary artery from the right pulmonary artery.

57.13a). Of 68 postmortem examinations of pulmonary vascular sling, 51% had associated tracheobronchial abnormalities such as hypoplasia of the distal trachea (38% with complete cartilaginous rings and 13% without normal cartilaginous rings), stenosis of the left main bronchus (5%) and direct origin of the right epi-arterial bronchus from the trachea (12%) (Figure 57.13b) (Gikonyo et al, 1989). The so-called 'bronchus suis' (Figure 57.13b) is an anomalous right upper bronchus branching from the trachea. The portion of the trachea distal to the origin of such a right upper bronchus is usually hypoplastic.

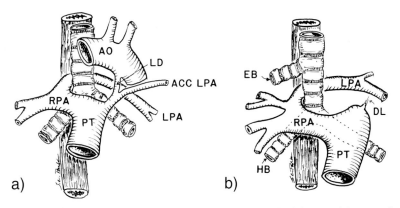

Figure 57.13. Atypical pulmonary vascular sling. (a) An accessory artery (ACC LPA) to the left upper lobe arises from the pulmonary trunk and is connected to the left arterial duct (LD). (b) Association with an abnormal branching of the trachea, 'bronchus suis'. The right upper lobe bronchus arises independently as an epiarterial bronchus (EB) proximal to the usual hyparterial right bronchus (HB). DL, ductal ligament; LPA, left pulmonary artery; PT, pulmonary trunk; RPA, right pulmonary artery. (Illustrations modified from Gikonyo et al, 1989.)

INCIDENCE

This anomaly is rare, with 130 cases being collected by Gikonyo et al by 1989.

CLINICAL MANIFESTATIONS

The anomalous left pulmonary artery almost always compresses the proximal portion of the right main bronchus and the distal end of the trachea. The dominant clinical manifestations are respiratory, including stridor, wheezing and cough. Stridor is often expiratory, in contrast to the usual inspiratory stridor of aortic vascular rings, but can be either inspiratory or biphasic. Signs of obstruction to the airways may begin in the neonatal period (Clarkson et al, 1967; Corbett and Washington, 1971), may be severe and may lead to death in the first few months of life. Rarely, patients with this anomaly have minimal or no respiratory symptoms and are identified incidently during cardiac catheterization for other forms of congenital heart defects or at work-up for a gastrointestinal disorder (Rudhe and Zetterqvist, 1959; Murphy et al, 1964; Lenox et al, 1979).

DIAGNOSIS

Since patients with pulmonary sling may die early in life, it is important to consider distal origin of the left pulmonary artery in any infant with signs of obstruction to the airways. The chest radiograph may demonstrate a variety of findings, depending on the degree of obstruction of the right main stem bronchus and lower portion of the trachea. Hyperinflation of the right lung with mediastinal shift to the left is common. If obstruction to the right main bronchus is severe, the right lung may be atelectactic. Barium-filled oesophagraphy is a useful non-invasive study. The characteristic findings were described by Wittenborg et al (1956) and Capitanio et al (1971). In the lateral view, the aberrant vessel produces an anterior indentation on the oesophagus and a posterior indentation on the trachea at the level of the carina. The anterior oesophageal indentation is not pathognomonic of this anomaly since it can also occur with the rare form of aberrant right subclavian artery that passes between the oesophagus and trachea (Bayford, 1794; Holzapfel, 1899). It can also be produced by an intrinsic mass in the oesophagus.

Another even rarer condition, the so-called 'ductal sling', may give a similar oesophagraphic finding as well as identical clinical manifestation. In this malformation, the anomalous arterial duct connects the right pulmonary artery and the left descending aorta, passing over the right main bronchus and between the trachea and the oesophagus (Binet et al, 1978). Despite these other possibilities, an anterior oesophageal indentation most likely indicates distal origin of the left pulmonary artery.

A definitive diagnosis may be made by selective pulmonary arteriography, which demonstrates the origin of the left pulmonary artery from the right pulmonary artery and its passage between the trachea and oesophagus. The anomalous origin of the left pulmonary artery usually overlaps the right pulmonary artery on a conventional anteroposterior view, and a sitting-up view with 45 degree elevation provides better visualization (Figure 57.12c). Cross-sectional echocardiography may visualize the anomalous origin of the left pulmonary branch from the right pulmonary artery (Figure 57.14a). Colour flow mapping enhances the visualization of the anomalous vessel (Figure 57.14b). Magnetic resonance imaging can demonstrate the lesion clearly (Figure 57.14c). Therefore, unless an associated abnormality or intracardiac defect is suspected, routine cardiac catheterization and angiographic study are unnecessary prior to surgical intervention. Since there is a high incidence of associated serious abnormalities of the airways, routine endoscopic examination is mandatory. If necessary, resonance imaging should be performed to rule out and/or to determine the extent of any abnormalities involving the airways (Azarow et al, 1992).

MANAGEMENT

Early recognition of pulmonary sling is important if management is to be successful. Symptomatic patients with this anomaly should undergo surgical intervention without delay. The surgical procedure most often used consists of removing the left pulmonary artery from the right pulmonary artery using cardiopulmonary bypass, and then reimplanting it into the pulmonary trunk anterior to the trachea. A branch from the anomalous left pulmonary artery to the right upper lobe may be identified on the preoperative angiogram or at operation. If so, it should be sacrificed so that the entire left pulmonary artery can be mobilized.

Some investigators have reported a high operative mortality and a high incidence of occlusion of the left pulmonary artery following operation (Sade et al, 1975; Lenox et al, 1979; Baker et al, 1992). Phelan and Venables (1978) have even suggested conservative medical management. Dunn et al (1979), however, reported successful reimplantation of the left pulmonary artery into the pulmonary trunk in four patients whose ages ranged from 5 to 54 months. The operation was performed without cardiopulmonary bypass by utilizing microsurgical techniques and heparinization. All patients were proven postoperatively to have patency of the left pulmonary artery by ventilation perfusion scanning. Most centres now prefer an approach through a median sternotomy combined with extracorporeal circulatory support. Tracheal stenosis and bronchial abnormalities are common, so morbidity and mortality remain significant. Associated problems with the airways may require

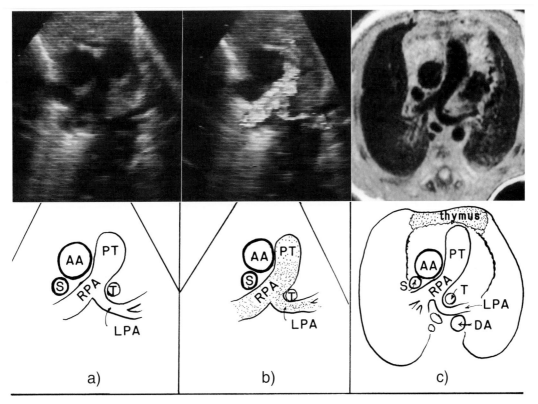

Figure 57.14. Pulmonary vascular sling. Suprasternal short-axis echocardiographic views (a,b) demonstrate the anomalous origin of the left pulmonary artery (LPA) from the right pulmonary artery (RPA). Flow mapping enhances the visualization of the vessel (b). Resonance imaging (c) provides superior diagnostic information. AA, ascending aorta; DA, descending aorta; PT, pulmonary trunk; S, superior caval vein; T, trachea.

correction at the time of the surgery to the arteries. Various techniques have been utilized for repairing tracheal stenosis. Hickey and Wood (1987) resected the distal third of the trachea. Jonas et al (1989) translocated the left pulmonary artery anterior to the trachea before tracheal reanastomosis, thus obviating the need for vascular division or anastomosis. Idriss et al (1984) used a pericardial patch tracheoplasty with good results. More recently, Yamaguchi et al (1990) advocated a tracheoplasty technique using a piece of cartilage.

There is usually prompt symptomatic improvement following operation, but some patients have persistent respiratory symptoms owing to pre-existing tracheobronchial stenosis or hypoplasia of the distal trachea. Others obtain symptomatic relief after the operation despite complete obstruction of the left pulmonary artery, presumably as a result of thrombosis at the site of the anastomosis between the left pulmonary artery and the pulmonary trunk. Postoperative patency of the left pulmonary artery should always be checked, either by echocardiography or ventilation perfusion scan. Reoperation may be successful in establishing continuity between the pulmonary trunk and the left pulmonary artery.

REFERENCES

Ahlstrom H, Lundstrom N, Mortensson W 1973 Occurrence of two vascular rings in the same infant. Acta Paediatrica Scandinavica 62: 201–204

Antia E U, Ottesen O E 1966 Collateral circulation in subclavian stenosis or atresia: Angiographic demonstration of retrograde vertebral–subclavian flow in two cases with right aortic arch. American Journal of Cardiology 18: 599–604

Arciniegas E, Hakimi M, Hertzler J H, Farooki Z Q, Green E W 1978 Surgical management of congenital vascular rings. Journal of Thoracic and Cardiovascular Surgery 77: 724–727

Ardito J M, Ossoff R H, Tucker G F, DeLeon S Y 1980 Innominate artery compression of the trachea in infants with reflex apnea. Annals of Otology, Rhinology and Laryngology 89: 401–405

Azarow K S, Pearl R H, Hoffman M A, Zucher R, Edwards F H, Cohen A J 1992 Vascular Ring: does magnetic resonance imaging replace angiography? Annals of Thoracic Surgery 53: 882–885

Baker C L, Idriss F S, Holinger L D, Mavroudis C 1992 Pulmonary artery sling: results of surgical repair in infancy. Journal of Thoracic and Cardiovascular Surgery 103: 683–691

Bayford D 1794 An account of a singular case of obstructed deglutition. Memoirs of the Medical Society of London 2: 271

Bennett E V, Grover F L, Trinkle J K 1984 Right aortic arch causing left bronchus obstruction. Texas Heart Institute Journal 11: 204–207

Berdon W E, Baker D H 1972 Vascular anomalies and the infant lung: rings, slings and other things. Seminars in Roentgenology 7: 39–64

Binet J P, Conso J F, Losay J et al 1978 Ductus arteriosus sling: report of a newly recognised anomaly and its surgical correction. Thorax 33: 72–75

Blake H A, Manion W C 1962 Thoracic arterial arch anomalies. Circulation 26: 251–265

Capitanio M A, Ramos R, Kirkpatrick J A 1971 Pulmonary sling, roentgen observations. American Journal of Roentgenology, Radium Therapy and Nuclear Medicine 112: 28–34

Checa S L, Santalla A, Villagra F et al 1983 Vascular rings: Surgical experience. Revista Espanola de Cardiologia 36: 55–59

Clarkson P M, Ritter D G, Rahimtoola S H, Hallermann F J, McGoon D C 1967 Aberrant left pulmonary artery. American Journal of Diseases of Children 113: 373–377

Corbett D P, Washington J E 1971 Respiratory obstruction in the newborn and excess pulmonary fluid. American Journal of Roentgenology, Radium Therapy, and Nuclear Medicine 112: 18–22

Dunn J M, Gordon I, Chrispin A R, de Leval M R, Stark J 1979 Early and late results of surgical correction of pulmonary artery sling. Annals of Thoracic Surgery 28: 230–238

Edwards J E 1948 Retro-esophageal segment of the left aortic arch, right ligamentum arteriosum and right descending aorta causing a congenital vascular ring about the trachea and esophagus. Proceedings of the Staff Meetings of the Mayo Clinic 23: 108–116

Edwards J E 1953 Malformations of the aortic arch system manifested as 'vascular rings'. Laboratory Investigation 2: 56–75

Edwards J E 1960 Congenital malformations of the heart and great vessels. In: Gould S E (ed.) Pathology of the heart, 2nd edn. Thomas, Springfield, NJ p 438–480

Ekström G, Sandblom P 1951 Double aortic arch. Acta Chirurgica Scandinavica 102: 183–202

Ericsson N O, Soderlund S 1969 Compression of the trachea by an anomalous innominate artery. Journal of Pediatric Surgery 4: 424–431

Fearon B, Shortreed R 1963 Tracheobronchial compression by congenital cardiovascular anomalies in children: Syndrome of apnea. Annals of Otology, Rhinology and Larynogology 72: 949–969

Felson B, Palayew M J 1963 The two types of right aortic arch. Radiology 81: 745–759

Fletcher B D, Cohn R C 1989 Tracheal compression and the innominate artery: MR evaluation in infants. Radiology 170: 103–107

Gasul B M, Arcilla R A, Lev M 1966 Heart disease in children: diagnosis and treatment. Lippincott, Philadelphia, PA, p 2

Gikonyo B M, Jue K L, Edwards J E 1989 Pulmonary vascular sling: report of seven cases and review of the literature. Pediatric Cardiology 10: 81–89

Glaevecke L, Doehle 1897 Uber eine seltene angeborene Anomalie der Pulmonalarterie. Munchener Medizinische Wochenschrift 44: 950

Godtfredsen J, Wennevold A, Efsen F, Lauridsen P 1977 Natural history of vascular ring with clinical manifestations. Scandinavian Journal of Thoracic Cardiovascular Surgery 11: 75–77

Grollman J H, Paris C H, Hamilton L E 1967 Congenital diverticula of the aortic arch. New England Journal of Medicine 276: 1178–1182

Grollman J H, Bedynek J L, Henderson H S, Hall R J 1968 Right aortic arch with an aberrant retroesophageal innominate artery: angiographic diagnosis. Radiology 90: 782–783

Gross R E, Neuhauser E B D 1948 Compression of the trachea by an anomalous innominate artery: an operation for its relief. American Journal of Diseases of Children 75: 570–574

Hastreiter A R, D'Cruz I A, Cantez T 1966 Right-sided aorta: part I. Occurrence of right aortic arch in various types of congenital heart disease. British Heart Journal 28: 722–739

Hawkins J A, Bailey W W, Clark S M, Ivey I D 1992 Innominate artery compression of the trachea: treatment by reimplantation of the innominate artery. Journal of Thoracic and Cardiovascular Surgery 103: 678–682

Hickey M St J, Wood A E 1987 Pulmonary artery sling with tracheal stenosis: one stage repair. Annals of Thoracic Surgery 44: 416–417

Holinger C D 1980 The etiology of stridor in the neonate, infant and child. Annals of Otology, Rhinology and Laryngology 89: 397–400

Holzapfel G 1899 Ungewohnlicher Unsprung und Verlauf der Arteria Subclavia Dextra. Anatomische Hefts 12: 369–523

Idriss F S, DeLeon S Y, Ilbawi M N, Gerson C R, Tucker G F, Holinger L D 1984 Tracheoplasty with pericardial patch for extensive tracheal stenosis in infants and children. Journal of Thoracic and Cardiovascular Surgery 88: 527–535

Inoue T, Shohtsu A, Kawada K, Takeuchi S, Sohma Y 1973 Late results following surgery for vascular ring in infancy, with special reference to associated extracardiac anomalies. Journal of Cardiovascular Surgery 14: 404–407

Jonas R A, Spevak P J, McGill T, Castaneda A R 1989 Pulmonary artery sling: primary repair by tracheal resection in infancy. Journal of Thoracic and Cardiovascular Surgery 97: 548–550

Kahn A, Baran D, Spehl M, Dab L, Blum D 1977 Congenital stridor in infancy. Clinical lesions derived from a survey of 31 instances. Clinical Pediatrics 16: 19–26

Klinkhamer A C 1969 Esophagography in anomalies of the aortic arch system. Williams & Wilkins, Baltimore, MD, p 16–30, 64–65

Kommerell B 1936 Verlagerung des Osophagus durch eine abnorm verlaufende Arteria subclavia dextra (Arteria lusoria). Fortschritte auf dem Gebiete der Roentgenstrahlen und der Nuklearmedizin 54: 590–595

Lam C R, Kabbani S, Arciniegas E 1978 Symptomatic anomalies of the aortic arch. Surgery, Gynecology and Obstetrics 147: 673–681

Lenox C C, Crisler C, Zuberbuhler J R et al 1979 Anomalous left pulmonary artery. Journal of Thoracic and Cardiovascular Surgery 77: 748–752

Lincoln J C, Deverall P B, Stark J, Aberdeen E, Waterston D J 1969 Vascular anomalies compressing the oesophagus and trachea. Thorax 24: 295–306

MacDonald R E, Fearon B 1971 Innominate artery compression syndrome in children. Annals of Otology, Rhinology and Laryngology 80: 535–540

Moës C A F 1978 Vascular rings and anomalies of the aortic arch. In: Keith J D, Rowe R D, Vlad P (eds) Heart disease in infancy and childhood, 3rd edn. Macmillan, New York, p 856–881

Moës C A F, Izukawa T, Trusler G A 1975 Innominate artery compression of the trachea. Archives of Otolaryngology 101: 733–738

Murphy D R, Dunbar F S, MacEwen D W, Sanchez F R, Perey D Y E 1964 Tracheobronchial compression due to a vascular sling. Surgery, Gynecology and Obstetrics 118: 572–578

Mustard W T, Baylies C E, Fearon B, Pelton D, Trusler G A 1969 Tracheal compression by the innominate artery in children. Annals of Thoracic Surgery 8: 312–319

Nikaidoh H, Riker W L, Idriss F S 1972 Surgical management of 'vascular rings'. Archives of Surgery 105: 327–333

Park S C, Siewers R D, Neches W H, Lenox C C, Zuberbuhler J R 1976 Left aortic arch with right descending aorta and right ligamentum arteriosum. Journal of Thoracic and Cardiovascular Surgery 71: 779–784

Paul R N 1948 A new anomaly of the aorta: left aortic arch with right descending aorta. Journal of Pediatrics 32: 19–29

Phelan P D, Venables A W 1978 Management of pulmonary artery sling (anomalous left pulmonary artery arising from right pulmonary artery): a conservative approach. Thorax 33: 67–71

Potts W J, Holinger P H, Rosenblum A H 1954 Anomalous left pulmonary artery causing obstruction to right main bronchus: report of a case. Journal of the American Medical Association 155: 1409–1411

Rodriguez L, Izukawa T, Moës C A F, Trusler G A, Williams W G 1975 Surgical implications of right aortic arch with isolation of left subclavian artery. British Heart Journal 37: 931–936

Roesler M, de Leval M, Chrispin A, Stark J 1983 Surgical management of vascular ring. Annals of Surgery 197: 139–146

Romanos A N, Bruins C L, Brom A D 1957 Rare anomaly of the aortic arch combined with coarctation of the aorta. Diseases of the Chest 31: 540–547

Rudhe U, Zetterquist P 1959 Aberrant left pulmonary artery. Acta Chirurgica Scandinavica Supplement 245: 331–335

Sade R M, Rosenthal A, Fellows K, Castaneda A R 1975 Pulmonary artery sling. Journal of Thoracic and Cardiovascular Surgery 69: 333–346

Schlamowitz S T, DiGiorgi S, Gensini G G 1962 Left aortic arch and right descending aorta. American Journal of Cardiology 10: 132–137

Shannon J M 1961 Aberrant right subclavian artery with Kommerell's diverticulum: report of a case. Journal of Thoracic and Cardiovascular Surgery 41: 408–411

Shuford W H, Sybers R G 1974 The aortic arch and its malformations. Thomas, Springfield, NJ, p 4–9, 51

Shuford W H, Sybers R G, Schlant R C 1970 Right aortic arch with isolation of the left subclavian artery. American Journal of Roentgenology, Radium Therapy and Nuclear Medicine 109: 75–83

Sterz H 1961 Dysphagie durch eine seltene Anomalie der Aorta thoracalis: Arcus Aortae sinistir circumflexus und Dextroposition der Aorta desendens. Wiener Zeitschrift für Innere Medizin und Ihre Grenzgebiete 42: 420–424

Stewart J R, Kincaid O W, Edwards J E 1964 An atlas of vascular rings and related malformations of the aortic arch system. Thomas, Springfield, NJ, p 8–13, 124, 219

Theodoridès T H 1960 Contributions a l'etude du double arch aortique complet. Thesis, Utrecht (Quoted by Klinkhamer A C, 1969)

Tonkin I L, Elliott L P, Bargeron L M 1980 Concomitant axial cineangiography and barium esophagography in the evaluation of vascular rings. Radiology 135: 69–76

Victorica B E, Van Mierop L H S, Elliott L P 1970 Right aortic arch associated with contralateral congenital subclavian steal syndrome. American Journal of Roentgenology, Radium Therapy and Nuclear Medicine 108: 582–590

Wittenborg M H, Tantiwongse T, Rosenberg B F 1956 Anomalous course of left pulmonary artery with respiratory obstruction. Radiology 67: 339–345

Wychulis A R, Kincaid O W, Weidman W H, Danielson G K 1971 Congenital vascular ring: surgical considerations and results of operation. Mayo Clinic Proceedings 46: 182–188

Yamaguchi M, Oshima Y, Hosokawa Y et al 1990 Concomitant repair of congenital tracheal stenosis and complex cardiac anomaly in small children. Journal of Thoracic and Cardiovascular Surgery 100: 181–187

Zdebska E, Smolska I, Markowa M, Miezynski W 1977 Early diagnosis and surgical treatment of children with congenital vascular rings and accompanying heart lesions. Journal of Pediatric Surgery 12: 121–124

58

Abnormal positions and relationships of the heart

R. H. Anderson

---------------------------- INTRODUCTION ----------------------------

An abnormally positioned heart is not usually in itself a malformation of utmost significance. The exceptions are the extreme examples of exteriorization of the heart (ectopia cordis) or junction of hearts in the setting of conjoined twins. A heart unusually positioned within the chest, an abnormal orientation of the cardiac apex or the finding of unexpected relationships of structures within the heart, nonetheless, can all lead to considerable diagnostic problems and potential confusion in description. We have outlined our philosophy and approach to these situations in Chapter 2. Those who have not studied this chapter in detail should, perhaps, return for refreshment concerning our 'ground rules'. In this chapter, we will synthesize our concepts in the setting of abnormally positioned hearts and unexpected intracardiac relationships. Thus, we will discuss the major problems produced by an extrathoracic position of the heart, or ectopia cordis, in its various degrees, and follow this with a brief account of congenital absence of the pericardium. We will summarize the cardiac problems encountered in the setting of conjoined twins. We will then provide a simple formula for coping with location of the heart in an unexpected part of the thoracic cavity, or the orientation of its apex in a disharmonious fashion. We will account for the problems produced by, and the anomalies associated with, juxtaposition of the atrial appendages, before concluding with a discussion of the arrangements now usually described as 'criss-cross hearts' and 'supero-inferior ventricles'.

---------------- EXTERIORIZATION OF THE HEART (ECTOPIA CORDIS) ----------------

Although it is often maintained that Neil Stensen's famous case of tetralogy was also the first reported case of an extrathoracic heart (Van Praagh et al, 1983), Rashkind has argued that such malformations were almost certainly recognized long before 1671. In Rashkind's opinion, they were recorded in the writings of the ancient Babylonians (Rashkind, 1982), although there is some dispute concerning the precise translation of the tablet involved. Be that as it may, a heart positioned in part or completely out of the thorax remains a very rare and, with relatively few exceptions, a uniformly fatal condition. The lesion is usually termed 'ectopia', but Kanagasuntheram and Verzin (1962) have pointed to the deficiency in such description. The Greek word *ektopos* simply means 'away from a place'. As such, a heart found in the right chest of an otherwise normal person is ectopic. Despite this semantic failing, which represents yet another example of deficient use of a 'classical' term and supports the use of the vernacular, ectopia is used universally to account for a heart located in part or completely outside the thoracic cavity.

The known cases of an extrathoracic heart were extensively reviewed by Byron (1948). Scott (1955) noted the description of 10 further cases, including his own. Kanagasuntheram and Verzin (1962) discovered an additional six cases not included by Byron in his catalogue of 142 examples. In addition, they encounted 33 cases reported between Byron's study and their own. In terms of categorization, it was Townsend (1845) who originally divided extrathoracic hearts according to their location, identifying cervical, thoracic and abdominal groups. Subsequently, it was suggested that the combined thoraco-abdominal position made up a further distinct pattern. Kanagasuntheram and Verzin (1962) then added a combined thoracocervical group to this list. Cases encountered and described since the catalogue of Kanagasuntheram and Verzin (1962) continue to fall within these groupings.

When the heart is found in the neck, the sternum is usually intact. According to Kanagasuntheram and Verzin (1962), this arrangement reflects a retention of the normal initial site of cardiac development. Byron reported four examples, commenting on their exceedingly poor prognosis. Van Praagh and his colleagues (1983) dismissed the type, arguing that it is found only in malformed fetuses. They are in error in this respect. Byron reported how one infant with a cervical heart lived a few hours, while Laliberte's patient (1918) survived to adult life. This example, however, would probably be better placed in the thoracocervical group. Van Praagh et al (1983) further sought to distinguish between a cleft to the sternum and an extrathoracic heart. This seems to be unnecessarily divisive, since a heart within the neck is certainly not within the thorax irrespective of whether the sternum is cleft or not. Irrespective of such niceties, the cervical type is by far the rarest group. There is also a question mark over the abdominal group. Van Praagh and his colleagues (1983) argue that most of the reported cases, with 38 catalogued in Byron's series, had part of the heart retained within the chest. They would group these as combined abdominothoracic, finding only one example, that of Deschamps (1806) in which the heart was exclusively within the abdomen. The greater majority of cases, therefore, either protrude from the chest or else extend through a diaphragmatic defect. They then occupy a midline deficiency of the body wall, lying partly in the chest and partly within the abdomen. In the cases exteriorized from the chest, the hearts are usually covered by neither skin nor pericardium. This was certainly the situation in the cases of Byron (1948) and Kanagasuntheram and Verzin (1962). In both of these, the myocardium of the heart was exposed, covered only by the serous pericardium. As Byron observed, during treatment of his patients it was necessary continually to moisten the cardiac surface. Various means had been employed in previous cases to provide this moisture. Martinez (1747) covered the exposed heart with a contraption made of pliable osiers and linen that was anointed with wine and melted butter. Scott (1955) reports that Goode (1904) covered the heart in his patient with a pasteboard cone and used oil for the anointing agent, while others used saline sponges. Irrespective of the method employed, most patients survived for only a matter of hours or days. The difference in those cases grouped as being abdominothoracic is that the extrathoracic heart is better covered by the body wall, having at least a covering of skin or membrane. It is this group of patients that have been placed together as a syndrome unified by five anomalies, namely a midline deficiency of the abdominal wall, a defect of the lower part of the sternum, a deficiency of the pericardial sack, a deficiency of the diaphragm and an intracardiac congenital lesion (Cantrell et al, 1958). Not all patients with extrathoracic hearts extending into the abdomen have all of these features. Indeed, a small number of patients have been described in which the malpositioned heart was, in itself, anatomically normal (Toyama, 1972). As the scholarly review of Toyoma showed, the cases can themselves be grouped according to the number of Cantrell's five features that are present. This is probably of more pedagogic than practical importance. Treatment of the abdominothoracic type is probably more hopeful than the patients with exclusively thoracic exteriorization. This is more so when only a small part of the heart is exteriorized, as in a case we saw with only a long ventricular diverticulum extending through the deficiency

of the body wall (Figure 58.1). Even in this patient, however, when the cavities of both ventricles extended into the diverticulum in the presence of a perimembranous ventricular septal defect, surgery proved unsuccessful. In another patient seen personally, the heart was much more malformed and was exteriorized together with the liver into a large midline defect (Figure 58.2). The heart itself exhibited tricuspid atresia (Figure 58.3). This patient was diagnosed during fetal life by echocardiography (Figure 58.4) and did not come to term.

Very few patients have survived reparative surgery, although several persons with abdominal hearts who did not undergo surgery survived into adult life. An example is the old soldier observed by Deschamps and reported by Breschet (1826). He fought through several campaigns and died of suppurative nephritis of the right kidney. But there have been surgical successes. One instance of an extrathoracic heart extending into the abdomen was corrected at surgery by Brock in 1950 and reported by Scott (1955). The heart was entirely covered by skin. A diverticulum of the left ventricle was the only intracardiac defect. Two similar successful operations were recorded by Major (1953). A case of an extrathoracic heart exteriorized on the chest wall was successfully repaired by Saxena and his team at the Children's Hospital of Philadelphia (reported by Van Praagh et al, 1983). The postoperative course was exceedingly stormy and, even by 1981, the child still had a tracheostomy, although described by then as a 'cute kid'. Although Jones et al (1979) have advocated immediate surgery for all patients diagnosed with an extrathoracic heart, the problems to be encountered, not least being the small size of the deficient thoracic cavity, the excessive length of the venous and arterial connections to the extrathoracic heart, and the

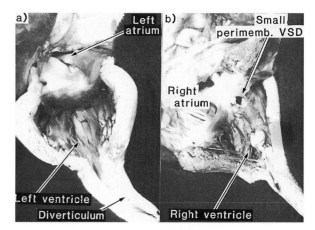

Figure 58.1. A congenital diverticulum of the ventricles in a case of abdominothoracic exteriorization of the heart. The diverticulum extended through the deficiency of the sternum into an omphalocoele. The cavities of both ventricles extended into the diverticulum and there was a perimembranous ventricular septal defect (perimemb. VSD). The five anomalous features of Cantrell's syndrome were present. Although surgical repair of the deficiencies of the body wall was attempted, it was unsuccessful. (Reproduced by kind permission of Dr N. Fagg, Guy's Hospital, London, UK.)

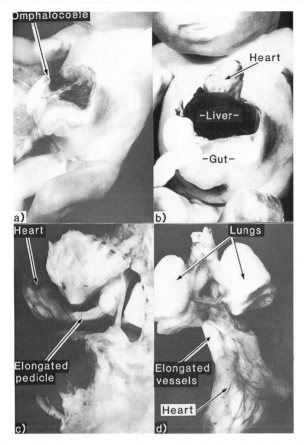

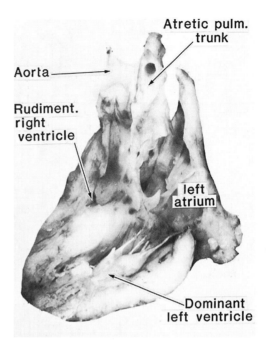

Figure 58.2. A more extensive thoracoabdominal exteriorization of the heart diagnosed by fetal echocardiography (see Figure 58.4). The heart extends from the thorax into a large omphalocoele and is covered by membrane of the umbilical cord (a and b). Note the extensive arterial and venous pedicles extending from the heart into the thorax (c and d). (Reproduced by kind permission of Dr N. Fagg, Guy's Hospital, London, UK.)

Figure 58.3. A long-axis section of the heart described in Figure 58.2. There is a dominant left ventricle and rudimentary (rudiment.) right ventricle with the aorta overriding the ventricular septal defect in the setting of pulmonary (pulm.) atresia. There was also absence of the right atrioventricular connection (tricuspid atresia).

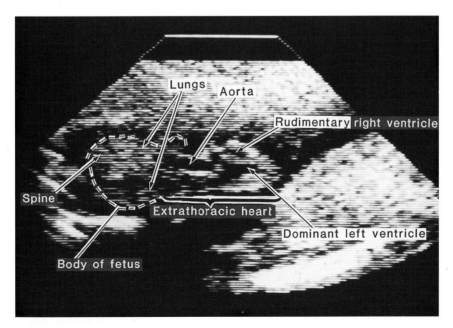

Figure 58.4. A cross-sectional echocardiogram taken during fetal life showing the exteriorized heart illustrated in Figures 58.2 and 58.3. The dominant left and rudimentary right ventricles are clearly seen in addition to the long arterial pedicle. (Reproduced by kind permission of Prof L. D. Allan, Guy's Hospital, London, UK.)

frequent coexistence of a large omphalocoele, suggest that the success rate of such heroic surgery will be depressingly small. The difficulty, and rarity of opportunity, for successful corrections is bone out by the collected experience of Amato and his colleagues (1995, 2000), albeit that Morales and associates (2000) reported four successful cases encountered over a period of six years.

CONGENITAL DEFICIENCY OF THE PERICARDIUM

An integral part of the various forms of extrathoracic heart is a gross deficiency of the fibrous pericardial sack. A deficiency of this firm bag can also be found when the heart is in its anticipated intrathoracic position. According to Van Praagh and his colleagues (1983), the anomaly was first observed by Columbus in 1559. Since then, about 150 cases have been described. It is, therefore, exceedingly rare. Only three examples were discovered amongst the 1716 hearts in the Boston collection (Van Praagh et al, 1983). We have knowingly observed only a single case at postmortem, this being a chance finding in a 68-year-old patient (Becker and Anderson, 1981). Cases can, therefore, be entirely asymptomatic.

Alternatively, such patients may have chest pain that can resemble angina (Wallace et al, 1971). When associated with other anomalies, such as diaphragmatic hernia or lesions of the heart, it is the associated malformations that dominate the clinical picture. The biggest intrinsic problems occur with relatively localized left-sided deficiencies of the pericardium. Either the ventricles or the left atrial appendage can become herniated through a small opening with strangulation and, in extreme cases, death (Sunderland and Wright-Smith, 1944; Robin et al, 1975). Limited deficiency of the fibrous sack on the right side can result in herniation of the lung into the pericardial cavity with subsequent obstruction of the superior caval vein (Moene et al, 1973).

The diagnosis is often made, or at least suggested, from the chest radiograph (Ellis et al, 1959). A large left-sided deficiency permits the entire heart to shift leftwards with production of three rather than two knuckles on the left heart border as seen on the chest radiograph. When the defect is small and there is herniation of the left appendage, the heart is normally positioned but the malpositioned auricle produces an exaggerated bulge in the region of the pulmonary knob. Angiocardiography can confirm herniation of the appendage if it is suspected, and, presumably, the anomalous position should be located by cross-sectional echocardiography. Only the small defects require surgical treatment, although large deficiencies may not be entirely benign. This is because the pericardial sack functions as the heart's 'seat belt'. It has been noted that the heart is more prone to traumatic injury when the pericardium is deficient (Reginato et al, 1980). Surgical treatment of small defects is done either by enlargement of the defect, then incurring the small risk of losing the 'seat belt' effect, or else by closure using a flap of mediastinal pleura.

CONJOINED TWINS

A malformation in the process of monozygotic twinning, which usually produces separate but identical individuals by cleavage of the single fertilized egg, can result in the twins becoming incompletely divided. This produces the rare examples of conjoined twins that, for centuries, have fascinated both medical and lay persons. The incidence is calculated at approximately 1 conjunction per 50 000 births (Morrison, 1963). The fanciful accounts of monsters and prodigies provided by Ambrose Pare (cited by Guttmacher and Nichols, 1967) are not that far removed from reality. The possibilities and sites for conjunction are legion. Accordingly, the categories provided for classification are formidable (Guttmacher and Nichols, 1967). The famous Siamese twins Eng and Chang, who survived into old age, were joined only at the abdomen, sharing no more than a common cord of liver substance. Twins with cardiac involvement are all joined at the chest, although not necessarily with common cardiac chambers. Indeed, those with separate hearts in a common thoracic cavity have the best chance of survival. Even when the hearts themselves are quite separate, there can be extensive intermingling of the circulations between the twins (Figure 58.5). The problems of such circulatory mixing were encountered clinically by Joffe and his colleagues (1977). We have had the opportunity to study three sets of joined twins which exemplify the even greater problems underscoring attempted treatment when the hearts themselves are joined.

In one case, the twins faced each other and were joined at the thorax and abdomen with a common rib-cage, with a sternum at each side common to both twins (Figure 58.6). The right side of one twin faced the left side of the other, and each had its organs arranged in usual fashion. There were separate lungs but a common liver. Each twin possessed a spleen in its own left side. The hearts were joined at ventricular and atrial level, even though each heart had two atriums and two ventricles. The latter were unconnected even though set in a common ventricular mass. The interconnections of the great veins, however, were complex in the extreme and would have precluded any attempt at surgical separation.

One of the other sets of twins we studied was joined at atrial level in a fascinating fashion. The hearts were joined in the fashion of leaves of a book rather than 'face-to-face' (Gerlis et al, 1993). Within this arrangement, the twins shared a midline morphologically right atrium; consequently, while the one twin had usual atrial arrangement, the other exhibited isomerism of the right atrial appendages (Figure 58.7). In keeping with the right isomerism, the right-sided twin also had lungs and bronchuses bilaterally of right morphology, and there was no spleen in its

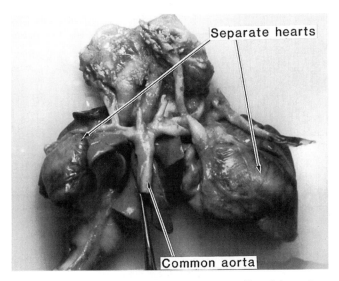

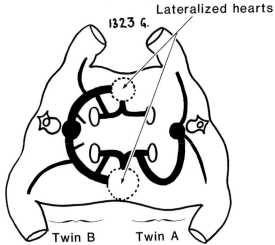

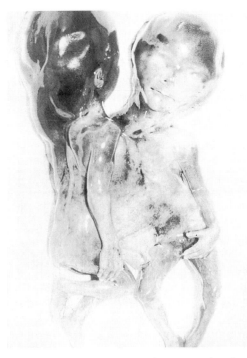

Figure 58.6. The overall arrangement of twins joined at the chest and abdomen. Dissection revealed presence of lateralized sternums shared by both twins together with a common liver. Each twin had its own spleen on the left side. The hearts were joined at atrial and ventricular levels.

Figure 58.5. Intermingling of the circulation in two sets of conjoined twins studied by Dr Leon Gerlis. The upper panel shows separate hearts giving rise to separate aortas, which then fuse to form a common descending arterial trunk. The lower panel is a diagrammatic representation of the complex intermingling of the pulmonary and systemic arterial pathways in a different set of twins with the rare occurrence of lateralized and separate hearts. (Reproduced by kind permission of Dr Leon M. Gerlis.)

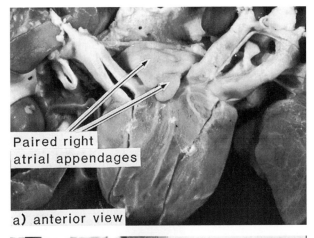

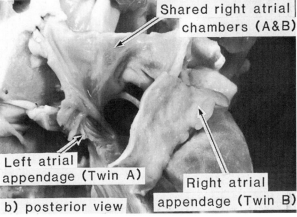

Figure 58.7. The atrial chambers from a set of joined twins sharing a common atrium. The shared chamber provides a right atrium to each twin, so that the left-hand twin (conventionally termed 'twin A') has the usual atrial arrangement while the right-hand twin (twin B) has isomerism of the right atrial appendages. Twin B also exhibited right pulmonary isomerism and had absence of the spleen.

abdominal cavity (Rossi et al, 1987). Several other examples of conjoined twins have been recorded where the one twin had usual arrangement of its organs and the other had right isomerism. We are aware of at least eight occurrences (Morrill, 1919; Mudaliar, 1930; Williams, 1944; Singer and Rosenberg, 1967; Beischer and Fortune, 1968; Edwards et al, 1977; Ursell and Wigger, 1983). Always it is the right-sided twin (usually labelled 'twin B') that is afflicted by the isomerism. Similar findings have been recorded in fishes (Morrill, 1919). Recent work in chick embryos (Levin et al, 1996) has served to provide the concept of 'cross-talk' between the conjoined embryos as the basis for failure of lateralization. The left-sided twin is hypothesized to synthesize an inhibitor of the gene *sonic hedgehog*, activin being proposed as the inhibitor. It is then suggested that diffusion of the inhibitor to the right-sided twin prevents the induction of *nodal*, this latter gene being considered necessary for the formation of morphologically left structures (see also Chapter 31; Anderson et al, 1998).

Ursell and Wigger (1983) have suggested that fusion of the twins in 'bookleaf' fashion rather than face-to-face is suggestive of isomerism in the right-sided twin. In the set of twins we studied in which the right-sided twin had isomerism, and in all those reported previously, the cardiac malformations were severe in both twins. They would have precluded success for either had surgical separation been attempted. Indeed, successful surgery is remarkably rare in cases of twins conjoined at the chest (Simpson et al, 1970).

Diagnosis of conjunction is not now likely to be a problem. Intrauterine cross-sectional ultrasonography is now likely to reveal the diagnosis in the majority of cases.

Although analysis will be difficult, an assessment can be made of the degree of cardiac involvement (Figure 58.8). If surgical separation is to be attempted, a full investigation will be needed. It had been suggested that palpation of pulses or electrocardiography might point to union or separation of the hearts, particularly at the vital ventricular level (Leachman et al, 1967; Simpson et al, 1970). These findings, however, are not always reliable (Izukawa et al, 1978). Angiocardiography (Patel et al, 1977; Izukawa et al, 1978) and echocardiography should always be performed, although interpretation of the images may be difficult. As indicated, even in potentially suitable cases, survivors of attempted separation are rare (De Angelis et al, 1970; Simpson et al, 1970).

MALPOSITION OF THE HEART

Normally the heart is located in the mediastinum with one third of its bulk to the right and two thirds to the left of the midline. With this arrangement, the apex usually points inferiorly and to the left. This combined pattern is traditionally described as 'levocardia'. The heart can be deviated from this position, or its apex can point in an unexpected direction, for several reasons. A pneumothorax of the right lung will produce a rightward shift of the thoracic contents and result in the heart becoming right-sided. Space-occupying lesions of the thoracic cavity can push the heart in rightward direction. Alternatively, the heart can be right-sided because of a congenital malformation of the thorax or its contents. This in itself is not necessarily an abnormality. For

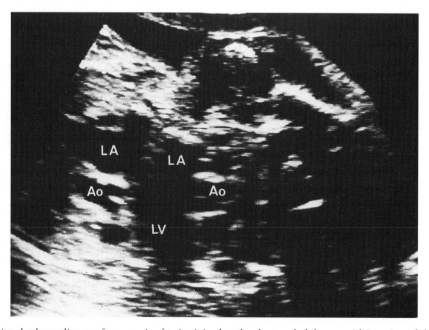

Figure 58.8. A cross-sectional echocardiogram from a pair of twins joined at the chest and abdomen with junction of the hearts and major intermingling of the circulations. This shows two left atrial chambers (LA) connecting to a left ventricle (LV) common to both twins, which gives rise to two aortas (Ao). The echocardiographic diagnoses were subsequently confirmed at postmortem following an unsuccessful attempt surgically to separate the twins. (Reproduced by kind permission of Prof. Lindsey D. Allen.)

example, otherwise normal individuals with completely mirror-imaged arrangement of the organs will 'normally' have a right-sided heart.

When assessing the significance of a right-sided heart, therefore, or a heart with its apex pointing to the right, it is necessary to take account of these various features. Several questions should be asked. What is the overall arrangement of the organs? Is there an abnormality of the lungs or the thoracic contents? If present, is it of congenital or acquired aetiology? Is the heart itself abnormally structured, or are its chambers grotesquely enlarged? Only when these questions have been posed, and answered, can the significance of a malpositioned heart be fully appreciated (Figures 58.9 and 58.10). Attempts to compress all this information into short phrases or single words have led to complex and confusing usage of the terms 'dextrocardia' and 'levocardia', particularly when combined with adjectives such as 'isolated', 'pivotal' or 'mixed' (see Wilkinson and Acerete (1973) for review). For these reasons, we choose not to use these cryptic conventions. Instead, we opt for a purely descriptive approach.

When describing a malpositioned heart, we account first for its overall location. This can be simply accomplished by describing it as left-sided, central (midline) or right-sided. Thereafter, it is necessary to account for the orientation of its apex. This also can be left-sided, central or right-sided. All locations can simply be categorized in terms of these two variables: position of the heart and orientation of its apex. It is then necessary to place this information in the context of the overall arrangement of the thoracic and abdominal organs, and the presence of acquired or congenital disease of the heart and/or lungs, as described above. If, for example, the heart is described

as lying mostly in the right chest, and with its apex orientated to the left, there can be little room for misunderstanding this arrangement irrespective of the precise nature of the malposition.

In this context, recognition of an unusually located heart should no longer be regarded as a diagnosis in its own right. Finding a right-sided heart, for example, gives no clue as to what is happening inside the organ. The heart itself may be entirely normal. The abnormal cardiac location, therefore, is simply described as the first step of subsequent full sequential segmental analysis (see Chapter 2). A right-sided heart, or a left-sided heart in the person with mirror imagery, is, however, associated with certain well-recognized lesions, or combinations of lesions. The heart is typically right-sided in association with hypoplasia of the right lung in the Scimitar syndrome and its variants (Chapter 33; Neill et al, 1960). The heart is also right-sided in well over a third of individuals who have an isomeric arrangement of their organs (Chapter 31). The single lesion most associated with a right-sided heart, or left-sided heart with mirror-imaged arrangement, is discordant atrioventricular connections (Chapter 49). At best, these are clues to the final diagnosis. The variety of lesions that can exist in

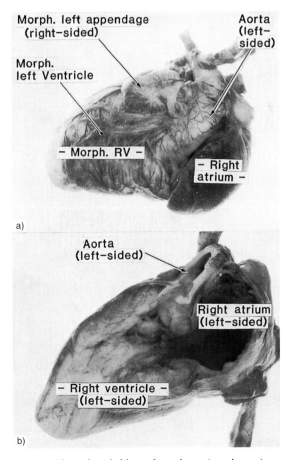

Figure 58.10. The right-sided heart from the patient shown in Figure 58.9 exhibits mirror-imaged atrial arrangement (a), together with the segmental combination of complete transposition, again in the mirror-imaged pattern (b).

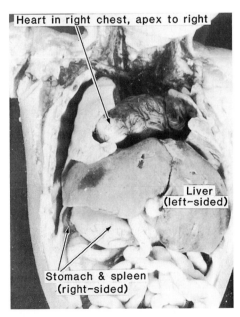

Figure 58.9. The abdominothoracic organs in a fetus with a right-sided heart. There is completely mirror-imaged arrangement of all the organs.

malpositioned hearts is protean (Van Praagh et al, 1964; Lev et al, 1968; Squarcia et al, 1973; Calcaterra et al, 1979; Huhta et al, 1982). The abnormal position of the heart in itself, nonetheless, has a fundamental effect on the electrocardiogram. This is discussed fully in Chapter 12.

JUXTAPOSITION OF THE ATRIAL APPENDAGES

Although not necessarily representing malposition of the heart itself, but often occurring in the setting of a malpositioned heart, juxtaposition of the atrial appendages is a potentially confusing feature of a congenitally malformed heart. The two appendages in the normally constructed heart lie one to each side of the arterial pedicle. It is, of course, the morphological nature of each appendage that determines the arrangement of the atrial chambers (see Chapter 2). Juxtaposition of the appendages occurs when both the appendages arc to the same side of the arterial pedicle. The presence of juxtaposition, however, in no

way interferes with recognition of the structure of each juxtaposed appendage on the basis of the extent of the pectinate muscles. Consequently, juxtaposition can occur in the person with usual atrial arrangement (Figure 58.11a,b) in the individual with mirror-imaged arrangement (Figure 58.11d) or in the presence of isomeric appendages (Figure 58.11c).

Juxtaposition in the presence of usual atrial arrangement occurs most frequently when the right appendage is deviated leftward through the transverse sinus so that it lies beneath the left appendage (Figure 58.12). This is conventionally called 'left juxtaposition'. It tends to be associated with relatively complex anatomical lesions. Noteworthy associated malformations are tricuspid atresia, hypoplasia of the right ventricle and abnormal ventriculo-arterial connections (Melhuish and Van Praagh, 1968; Freedom and Harrington, 1974; Allwork et al, 1977). Sometimes the juxtaposition is only partial, with a small pouch of right appendage continuing to protrude in rightward direction (Figure 58.13a). The effect of the juxtaposition is to distort the internal morphology of the atrial septum. On opening the relatively small atrial

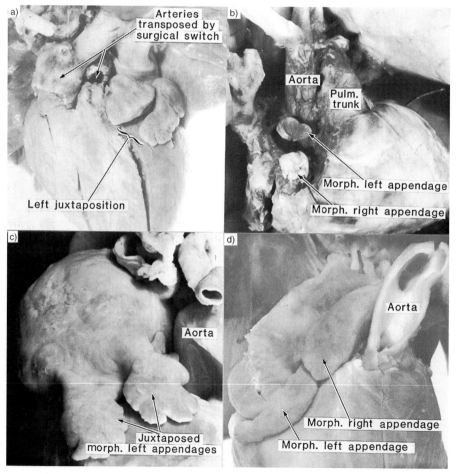

Figure 58.11. Juxtaposition of the atrial appendages occurs in two basic patterns. (a) Left-sided juxtaposition in a person with usual atrial arrangement. (b) Right-sided juxtaposition, again with usual atrial arrangement. The two other examples of right-sided juxtaposition are shown with (c) left isomerism and (d) mirror-imaged atrial arrangement, respectively. Note that, in each case, the morphology of the appendage can be readily recognized despite the presence of juxtaposition. Morph., morphological; Pulm., pulmonary.

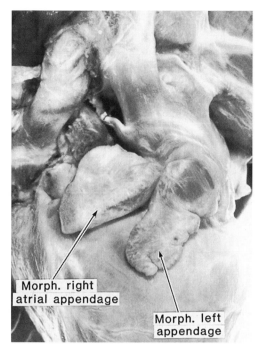

Figure 58.12. In left-sided juxtaposition, the right atrial appendage comes to lie medial to and slightly beneath the left appendage. This is in contrast to right-sided juxtaposition (see Figure 58.11b), where the morphologically (Morph.) left appendage is above the right appendage.

when complete. The terminal groove is orientated in horizontal rather than vertical fashion, and the sinus node itself is deviated towards the atrioventricular junction.

Much more rarely with usual atrial arrangement, the appendages can be juxtaposed to the right of the arterial pedicle. It is then the left appendage that occupies the transverse sinus and comes to lie superiorly to the right appendage (Figure 58.11). Right is much rarer than left juxtaposition when there is usual atrial arrangement. In some cases, right juxtaposition is found in virtually normal hearts when the only associated lesion may be an atrial septal defect (Becker and Becker, 1970). In other instances, it may accompany exceedingly complex lesions (Anderson et al, 1976). In the person with mirror-imaged arrangement, right-sided juxtaposition (Figure 58.11d) is the expected variant. It is associated with the same constellation of lesions as is left-sided juxtaposition in the individual with usual atrial arrangement. Juxtaposition can be either right-sided (Figure 58.11c) or left-sided in the presence of isomerism. The associated lesions are then dictated by the isomeric arrangement (see Chapter 31).

Plain chest radiography in left juxtaposition usually shows a straight right heart border because the right atrial appendage is not in its usual place. The diagnosis is made more readily from cross-sectional echocardiography (Chin et al, 1983; Rice et al, 1983), provided that the possibility of its existence is entertained. Subcostal sections (Figure 58.14), approximating to the standard four chamber view, demonstrate continuity on either side of the arterial pedicle between the body of the right atrium and its appendage. Precordial short-axis sections (Figure 58.15) demonstrate the neck of the appendage within the transverse sinus separating the left atrium from the posterior great artery. During cardiac catheterization, if the diagnosis has not already been made by echocardiography, the first pointer to the diagnosis is sampling systemic

surface, which is obvious to the surgeon, the orifice of the juxtaposed appendage occupies the anticipated site of the oval fossa (Figure 58.13b). The fossa itself is more slit-like and is deviated posteroinferiorly. The distortion and reduced volume of the right atrium can be potential problems in the Mustard and Senning procedures. Another consequence of the juxtaposition is to distort the landmarks to the sinus node (Ho et al, 1979). This is less marked with partial juxtaposition but more obvious

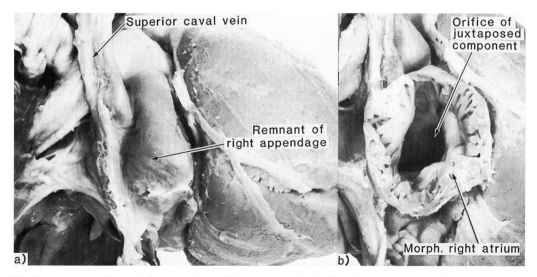

Figure 58.13. This illustrates partial left-sided juxtaposition of the morphologically (Morph.) right appendage in the setting of tricuspid atresia. (a) A small pouch remains in the anticipated site of the right appendage. (b) Opening the atrium shows the orifice of the juxtaposed auricle at the anticipated site of the oval fossa. Note also the absent right atrioventricular connection.

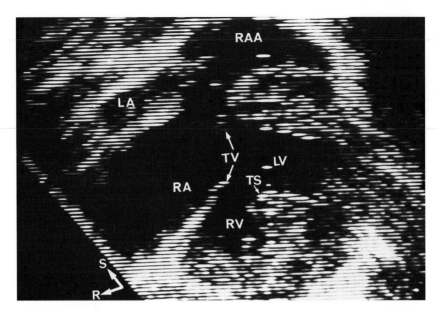

Figure 58.14. Subcostal echocardiograms approximating to a standard four chamber view showing the left-sided right atrial appendage (RAA) in continuity with the normally located atrium (RA) in a case of left juxtaposition of the atrial appendages. LA, left atrium; TV, tricuspid valve; TS, trabecular part of the ventricular septum; RV, right ventricle; LV, left ventricle.

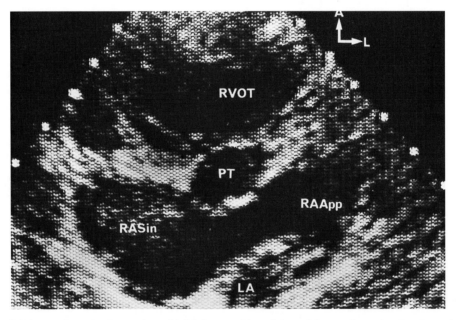

Figure 58.15. A precordial short-axis section in a patient with left juxtaposition of the atrial appendages showing the neck of the appendage within the transverse sinus and separating the left atrium (LA) from the posterior great artery (PT). RAsin, body (sinus) of right atrium; RAApp, appendage; RVOT, right ventricular outflow tract.

venous blood from the left side of the heart in a low pressure zone. Selective injection of contrast medium into the appendage will establish the diagnosis.

CRISS-CROSS HEARTS AND SUPERO-INFERIOR VENTRICLES

The last group of hearts to be considered are those where the relationship of the cardiac chambers or great arteries is not as expected for the given segmental connections. The significance of these malformations has diminished markedly since it has been appreciated that segmental connections cannot, and should not, be inferred from abnormal relationships of cardiac structures. The abnormal relationships in themselves, however, can still be a confusing feature.

The essence of the criss-cross heart is rotation of the ventricular mass around its long axis (Anderson et al, 1974; Anderson, 1982). This can occur with any known

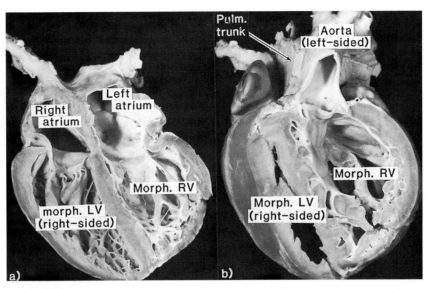

Figure 58.16. The anticipated relationships of the ventricles and great arteries in a patient with congenitally corrected transposition (discordant atrioventricular and ventriculo-arterial connections in the setting of usual atrial arrangement). The morphologically (morph.) left ventricle (LV) is right-sided (a) while the aorta (b) is left-sided. RV, right ventricle; Pulm., pulmonary.

combination of connections of the cardiac segments. It results in the ventricles and great arteries achieving unexpected relationships. For example, in the patient with congenitally corrected transposition in the setting of usual atrial arrangement, the morphologically left ventricle is expected to be a right-sided structure, while the aortic valve most frequently is located anteriorly and to the left (Figure 58.16). The ventricular mass in the presence of a criss-cross malformation is rotated such that the morphologically left ventricle achieves a left-sided position, while the aortic valve becomes anterior and right-sided

(Figures 58.17 and 58.18). In the presence of usual atrial arrangement, a right-sided and anterior aorta arising from a right-sided morphologically right ventricle is more typically found with the segmental combinations of complete transposition (Chapter 48). When, in the presence of such a criss-cross heart with congenitally corrected transposition, a catheter traversing the right atrium passes through a ventricular septal defect and opacifies the morphologically right ventricle and aorta despite the discordant atrioventricular connections, the potential for misdiagnosis and incorrect treatment is considerable (Symons et al,

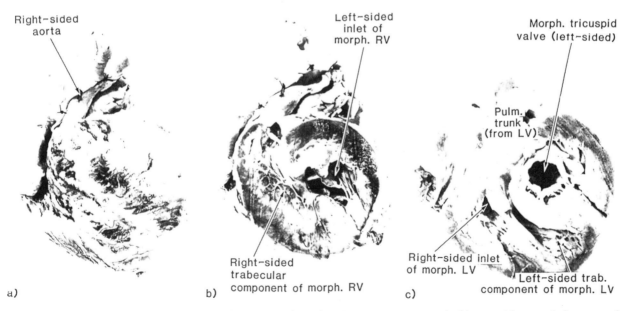

Figure 58.17. Rotation of the ventricles around their long axis produces the criss-cross arrangement, in this case with congenitally corrected transposition. Despite the discordant connections at both atrioventricular and ventriculo-arterial junctions, the aorta is right sided to the outflow and apical parts of the morphologically (morph.) left ventricle (LV), which are left sided. The heart is sectioned in four chamber plane and three progressively deeper slices (a–c) are shown. RV, right ventricle; trab, trabecular.

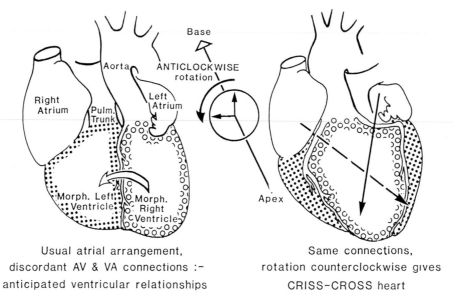

Figure 58.18. Diagram illustrating the rotation along the long axis of the ventricular mass that produces a criss-cross arrangement in the setting of congenitally corrected transposition. Morph., morphological; AV, atrioventricular; VA, ventriculo-arterial.

1977). The criss-cross arrangement in the setting of congenitally corrected transposition, therefore, gives the arterial and ventricular relationships anticipated for complete transposition. In similar fashion, criss-crossing and rotation can occur with the connections of the segments that produce complete transposition, and then the spurious impression is provided of congenitally corrected transposition (Figure 58.19).

It has been stated that the criss-cross arrangement is an illusion (Van Praagh et al, 1983). This depends upon what is considered to be illusory. As described above, the potential for misdiagnosis provided by the ventricular rotation is real. Equally, there is nothing illusory about the crossing of the ventricular inlets, nor the unusual

positions of the apical ventricular components. Once the investigator is aware of the possibility, both the abnormal relationships and the true segmental connections are readily demonstrated both by cross-sectional echocardiography (van Mill et al, 1982; Robinson et al, 1985; Figure 58.20) and by angiocardiography (Figure 58.21; Robinson et al, 1985). The key is first to analyse the connections between the cardiac segments, and then the relations of the ventricles and arterial trunks. The secret is not to be surprised when the relationships observed are not as anticipated for the demonstrated segmental connections (Anderson, 1982).

In the examples cited and illustrated above, which can be encountered with any combination of atrioventricular

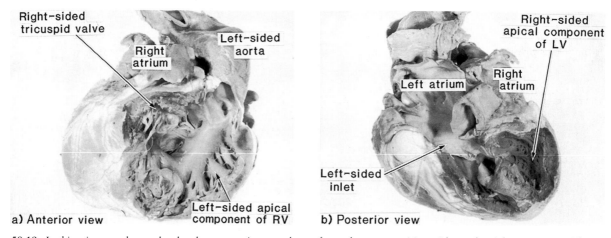

Figure 58.19. In this criss-cross heart, the chamber connections are those of complete transposition with usual atrial arrangement. The morphologically right ventricle (RV) and aorta, however, are left sided (a) relative to the morphologically left ventricle (LV) and the pulmonary trunk. In keeping with the concordant atrioventricular connections, however, there is right hand topology of the ventricular mass (compare with Figure 58.22). (b) The posterior aspect illustrates the right-sided position of the apical trabecular component of the morphologically left ventricle.

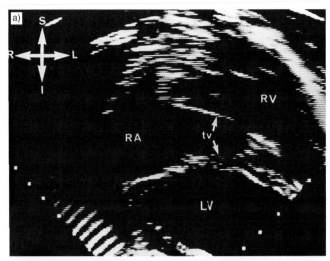

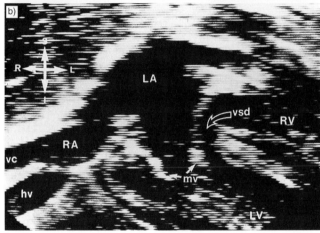

Figure 58.20. Echocardiograms illustrating a criss-cross arrangement in a patient with concordant atrioventricular and discordant ventriculo-arterial connections (complete transposition). (a) The right atrium (RA) connected via a tricuspid valve (tv) with the right ventricle (RV), which is unequivocally left sided. (b) The left atrium (LA) connected to the right-sided morphologically left ventricle (LV) through a mitral valve (mv). vsd, ventricular septal defect; hv, hepatic vein; vc, inferior caval vein.

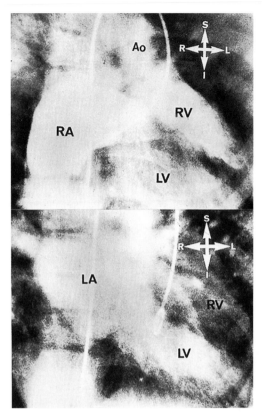

Figure 58.21. Angiocardiograms (from the patient illustrated in Figure 58.20) illustrating the typical connections and relationships of complete transposition complicated by the criss-cross anatomy. The upper panel shows the right atrium (RA) connected to the left-sided right ventricle (RV), which supports the aorta (Ao) in left-sided position. The lower panel shows the left atrium (LA) connected to the right-sided left ventricle (LV), which gives rise to the pulmonary trunk.

and ventriculo-arterial connections, the ventricular topology in each heart was as anticipated for the atrioventricular connections. Thus, in the patient with congenitally corrected transposition (see Figure 58.17), although the morphologically left ventricle was left-sided despite the discordant atrioventricular connections in the setting of usual atrial arrangement, the morphologically right ventricle accepted only the palmar surface of the observer's left hand with its thumb (figuratively speaking) in the tricuspid valve (left hand ventricular topology; see Chapter 2). This is because the criss-cross arrangement in the example cited was the simple result of rotation of the ventricular mass along its long axis (see Figure 58.18). Such rotation does not disturb the left hand ventricular topology ('l-loop'), which is characteristic of discordant atrioventricular connections in the patient with usual atrial arrangement. Similarly, in the patients with

usual atrial arrangement and complete transposition (Figures 58.19–58.21), there was right-handed ventricular topology, as expected for the concordant atrioventricular connections, despite the morphologically right ventricle being left-sided. Indeed, when Van Praagh and his colleagues (1964) first formulated their segmental approach to diagnosis, they used the terms 'concordance' and 'discordance' specifically to describe the harmony that almost always exists between the arrangements of the cardiac segments, irrespective of their precise connections and relationships. As far as they were concerned, the coexistence of usual atrial arrangement and a ventricular 'd-loop' (right hand topology), or of a mirror-image atrial arrangement and ventricular 'l-loop' (left hand topology), was concordant irrespective of how the atriums were connected to the ventricles. Similarly, irrespective of connections between atriums and ventricles, discordance was considered to represent the coexistence of either usual atrial arrangement and left hand ventricular topology (l-loop), or else mirror-imaged atrial arrangement and right-hand topology (d-loop). It was potentially confusing, therefore, when initially we chose to describe the connections between the atriums and ventricles in terms of atrioventricular 'concordance' and 'discordance'

(Shinebourne et al, 1976). At first, the potential for confusion was not too obvious. This was because, almost without exception, those patients with concordant atrioventricular connections also exhibited concordance between the anticipated arrangement of atrial chambers and the ventricular topology, namely usual atrial arrangement with right hand topology, and mirror-imaged arrangement with left hand topology. Similarly, almost without exception, all patients with discordant atrioventricular connections showed the expected discordance between the segments, in other words usual arrangement with left hand topology, and mirror-imaged arrangement with right hand topology. More recently, however, rare cases have been discovered that emphasize the need to distinguish separately the connections between the segments from their topological arrangement. This, in turn, dictates the need for us precisely to use 'discordant' and 'concordant' in their adjectival context as modifiers of the connections, that is to state specifically the presence of discordant or concordant atrioventricular connections. We should not have used them as nouns to describe the connections when Van Praagh and his colleagues (1964) had previously used them in this way to describe segmental harmony or disharmony. The particular cases that emphasized the need to distinguish these different usages were described by Weinberg and his colleagues at the First World Congress of Paediatric Cardiology in London in 1980. As far as we know, they have been published only in abstract form. We ourselves, however, had previously seen one similar case at postmortem (Otero Coto et al, 1979) and have now encountered two further cases (Anderson et al, 1987). The reason for describing these cases here, and for the lengthy preamble leading to their description, is that they make up a much rarer form of criss-cross heart. This rare variant cannot be explained simply on the basis of the rotation of the ventricular mass.

In the examples we studied at postmortem, the atrial chambers were arranged in usual fashion. The right atrium connected to the morphologically right ventricle, which was left sided relative to the left ventricle, the latter being connected to the left atrium (Figure 58.22). In this respect, therefore, the heart was similar to the one shown in Figure 58.19. Despite the concordant atrioventricular connections, however, there was left hand ventricular topology (Figure 58.23). According to the convention of Van Praagh and his colleagues (1964), this combination, of usual atrial arrangement and ventricular l-loop produces atrioventricular discordance. In addition, there was double outlet from the morphologically right ventricle, straddling of the left atrioventricular valve and left-sided juxtaposition of the atrial appendages. In the example studied clinically, there was again the usual atrial arrangement. In this case, however, the right atrium connected to a left-sided morphologically left ventricle, which gave rise to the pulmonary trunk. The left atrium connected to the right-sided morphologically right ventricle, which supported the aorta. The heart, therefore, had the segmental

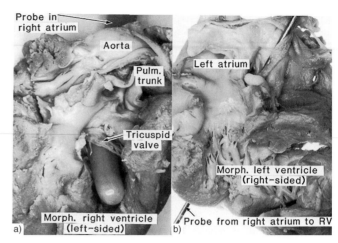

Figure 58.22. An unusual form of criss-cross heart where the ventricular topology is not as expected for the atrioventricular connection. (a) A probe is placed through the right atrium, which connects to the morphologically (Morph.) right ventricle (RV) (concordant atrioventricular connections). (b) The left atrium connects with the right-sided morphologically left ventricle. The probe is through the right atrioventricular connection. Pulm., pulmonary. (Reproduced by kind permission of Dr J. L. Wilkinson and A. Smith, University of Liverpool, UK.)

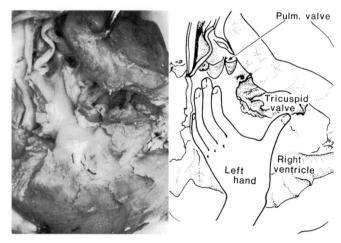

Figure 58.23. Finding the right ventricle in left-sided position occurs in any criss-cross heart (see Figure 58.19). What is particularly unusual in this case, however, is that the ventricular mass has a left-hand topological pattern. The septal surface of the right ventricle accepts (figuratively) only the palmar surface of the observer's left hand placed with its thumb in the inlet and its fingers in the outlets. Pulm., pulmonary. (Reproduced by kind permission of Drs J. L. Wilkinson and A. Smith, University of Liverpool, UK.)

connections producing congenitally corrected transposition. But, in this case, despite the discordant atrioventricular connections, the ventricular topology was right-handed. This combination, usual atrial arrangement and ventricular d-loop, should be described as atrioventricular concordance according to the convention of Van Praagh et al (1964). The patient had straddling of the right atrioventricular valve and right-sided juxtaposition of the atrial appendages. Juxtaposition of the atrial appendages, and straddling atrioventricular valves, were also features of the cases described by Weinberg and his colleagues (1980). The existence of the usual types of crisscross heart emphasized the need to describe the connections of the cardiac segments and the relationships of the ventricles and arterial trunks separately. These rarer, and much more complex, cases emphasize the need on occasions also to specify the topology of the cardiac segments when they differ from the anticipated arrangement. Provided that all these features are recognized, and accounted for separately, there should be little room for confusion or misunderstanding, irrespective of the specific words used for their description. The term criss-cross itself, however, describes a particular relationship of the ventricular inlets. It does not describe the complete heart. Full sequential segmental description is needed for that purpose.

In comparison with the potential problems encountered with criss-cross hearts, few should be posed by ventricles that are arranged in supero-inferior, or upstairs–downstairs, fashion. This abnormal relationship simply reflects a tilting of the ventricular mass along its long axis (Anderson, 1982). Supero-inferior ventricles are usually described in the setting of discordant atrioventricular connections, where it is the rule for the ventricles to be arranged in side-by-side fashion (see Figure 58.16). Tilting of the ventricular mass to either side then produces a stacking effect of the ventricles one on top of the other (Figure 58.24). Like the criss-cross pattern, supero-inferior ventricles are often seen in the presence of straddling and/or overriding atrioventricular valves (Freedom et al, 1978; Van Praagh et al, 1980). As was also the case with the criss-cross arrangement, 'upstairs–downstairs', or supero-

inferior, describes not the complete heart, but only a particular ventricular relationship. Sequential segmental description is mandatory for full categorization of the hearts thus described.

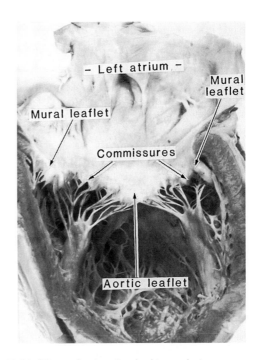

Figure 58.24. The mechanisms involved in producing a supero-inferior arrangement of the ventricle in the setting of congenitally corrected transposition. MLV and MRV, morphologically left and right ventricles, respectively; Pulm., pulmonary.

REFERENCES

Allwork S P, Urban A E, Anderson R H 1977 Left juxtaposition of the auricles with I-position of the aorta. Report of six cases. British Heart Journal 39: 299–308

Amato J J, Zelen J, Talwalker N G 1995 Single-stage repair of thoracic ectopia cordis. Annals of Thoracic Surgery 59: 518–520

Amato J J, Douglas W I, Desai V, Burke S 2000 Ectopia cordis. Chest Surgical Clinics of North America 10: 297–316

Anderson R H 1982 Criss-cross hearts revisited. Pediatric Cardiology 3: 305–313

Anderson R H, Shinebourne E A, Gerlis L M 1974 Criss-cross atrioventricular relationships producing paradoxical atrioventricular concordance or discordance. Their significance to nomenclature of congenital heart disease. Circulation 50: 176–180

Anderson R H, Smith A, Wilkinson J L 1976 Right juxtaposition of the auricular appendages. European Journal of Cardiology 4: 495–503

Anderson R H, Smith A, Wilkinson J L 1987 Disharmony between atrioventricular connexions and segmental combinations–unusual variants of 'criss-cross' hearts. Journal of the American College of Cardiology 10: 1274–1277

Anderson R H, Webb S, Brown N A 1998 Defective lateralisation in children with congenitally malformed hearts. Cardiology in the Young 8: 512–531

Becker A E, Anderson R H 1981 Pathology of congenital heart disease. Butterworths, London, p 413–415

Becker A E, Becker M J 1970 Juxtaposition of atrial appendages associated with normally oriented ventricles and great arteries. Circulation 41: 685–688

Beischer N A, Fortune D W 1963 Double monsters. Obstetrics and Gynecology 32: 158–170

Breschet G 1826 Memoirs sur l'ectopie de appareil de la circulation et particuherement sur celle du coeur. Repertoires general d'anatomie et de physiologie pathologiques et de Clinique chirurgie chirurgicale (Paris) 2: 1–39

Byron F X 1948 Ectopia cordis. Report of a case with attempted correction. Journal of Thoracic Surgery 17: 717–722

Calcaterra G, Anderson R H, Lau K C, Shinebourne E A 1979 Dextrocardia–value of segmental analysis in its categorization. British Heart Journal 42: 497–507

Cantrell J R, Haller J A, Ravitch M M 1958 A syndrome of congenital defects involving the abdominal wall sternum, diaphragm, pericardium and heart. Surgery, Gynecology and Obstetrics 107: 602–614

Chin A J, Bierman F Z, Williams R G, Sanders S P, Lang P 1983 Two-dimensional echocardiographic appearance of complete left-sided juxtaposition of the atrial appendages. American Journal of Cardiology 52: 346–348

De Angelis R R, Dursi J F, Ibach J R 1970 Successful separation of xiphagus conjoined twins. Annals of Surgery 172: 302–305

Deschamps 1806 Observation sur un deplacement remarquable du coeur; par M. Cullerier, medecin a Laval. Journal General de Medecine, de Chirugie et de Pharmacie 26: 275–279

Edwards W D, Hagel D R, Thompson J, Whorton C M, Edwards J E 1977 Conjoined thoraeopagus twins. Circulation 56: 491–497

Ellis K, Leeds N E, Himmelstein A 1959 Congenital deficiences in the parietal pericardium. A review with 2 new cases including successful diagnosis by plain roentgenography. American Journal of Roentgenology 82: 125–137

Freedom R M, Harrington D P 1974 Anatomically corrected malposition of the great arteries. Report of 2 cases, one with congenital asplenia; frequent association with juxtaposition of atrial appendages. British Heart Journal 36: 207–215

Freedom R M, Culham G, Rowe R D 1978 The criss-cross and supero-inferior ventricular heart: an angiocardiographic study. American Journal of Cardiology 42: 620–628

Gerlis L M, Seo J-W, Ho S Y, Chi J G 1993 Morphology of the cardiovascular system in conjoined twins: spatial and sequential segmental arrangements in 36 cases. Teratology 47: 91–108

Goode J G 1904 Cited by Scott G W 1955 Virginia M (semi-monthly) 13: 555

Guttmacher A F, Nichols B L 1967. Tetralogy of conjoined twins. Birth Defects Original Article Series 3: 3–9

Ho S Y, Monro J L, Anderson R H 1979 Disposition of the sinus node in left-sided juxtaposition of the atrial appendage. British Heart Journal 41: 129–132

Huhta J C, Hagler D J, Seward J B, Tank A J, Julsrud P R, Ritter D G 1982 Two-dimensional echocardiographic assessment of dextrocardia: a segmental approach. American Journal of Cardiology 50: 1351–1360

Izukawa T, Langford Kidd B S, Moes C A F et al 1978 Assessment of the cardiovascular system in conjoined thoracopagus twins. American Journal of Diseases of Childhood 132: 19–24

Joffe H S, Rose A, Gersh B J, Beck W 1977 Figure-of-eight circulation in thoracopagus conjoined twins with a shared heart. European Journal of Cardiology 6: 157–166

Jones A F, McGrath R S, Edwards S M, Lilly J R 1979 Immediate operation for ectopia cordis. Annals of Thoracic Surgery 28: 484–486

Kanagasuntheram R, Verzin J A 1962 Ectopia cordis in man. Thorax 17: 159–167

Laliberte J H 1918 Line ectopie cardiaque. Bulletin Medicale de Quebec 20: 241–243

Leachman R D, Latson J R, Kohler C M, McNamara D G 1967 Cardiovascular evaluation of conjoined twins. Birth Defects Original Article Series 3: 52–65

Lev M, Liberthson R R, Eckner F A O, Arcilla R A 1968 Pathologic anatomy of dextrocardia and its clinical implications. Circulation 37: 979–999

Levin M, Roberts D J, Holmes L B, Tabin C 1996 Laterality defects in conjoined twins. Nature 384: 321

Major J W 1953 Thoracoabdominal ectopia cordis: report of case successfully treated by surgery. Journal of Thoracic Surgery 26: 306–317

Martinez M 1747 De corde in monstroso infanulo, ubi obiter, et noviter de motu cordis et sanguinis. In: Haller A (ed) Disputations anatomical selectre. Vandenhoeck, Gottingen, vol. 2, p 973–1001

Melhuish B P P, Van Praagh R 1968 Juxtaposition of the atrial appendages. A sign of severe cyanotic congenital heart disease. British Heart Journal 30: 269–284

Moene R J, Dekker A, van der Harten H J 1973 Congenital rightsided pericardial defect with herniation of part of the lung into the pericardial cavity. American Journal of Cardiology 31: 519–522

Morales M J, Patel S G, Duff J A, Villareal Rl, Simpson JW 2000 Ectopia cordis and other midline defects. Annals of Thoracic Surgery 70: 111–114

Morrill C V 1919 Symmetry reversal and mirror imaging in monstrous trout and a comparison with similar conditions in human double monsters. Anatomical Record 16: 265–291

Morrison J E 1963 Foetal and neonatal pathology, 2nd edn. Butterworths, London

Mudaliar A L 1930 Double monsters—a study of their circulatory system and some other anatomical abnormalities—and the complications in labour. Journal of Obstetrics and Gynaecology 37: 753–768

Neill C A, Ferencz C, Sabiston D C, Sheldon H 1960 The familial occurrence of hypoplastic right lung with systemic arterial supply and venous drainage 'scimitar syndrome'. Johns Hopkins Medical Journal 107: 1–21

Otero Coto E, Wilkinson J L, Dickinson D F, Rufilanchas J J, Marquez J 1979 Gross distortion of atrioventricular and ventriculoarterial relations associated with left juxtaposition of atrial appendages—bizarre form of atrioventricular criss-cross. British Heart Journal 41: 486–492

Patel R, Fox K, Dawson J, Taylor J F N, Graham G R 1977 Cardiovascular anomalies in thoracopagus twins and importance of preoperative evaluation. British Heart Journal 39: 1254–1258

Rashkind W J 1982 Congenital heart disease. Benchmark papers in human physiology. Hutchinson Ross, Stroudsberg, PA, vol. 16, p 91

Reginato E, Riccardi M, Verunelli F, Eufrate S 1980 Post-traumatic mitral regurgitation and ventricular septal defect in absence of left pericardium. Thoracic and Cardiovascular Surgeon 28: 213–217

Rice M J, Seward J B, Hagler D J, Edwards W D, Julsrud P R, Tajik A J 1983 Left juxtaposed atrial appendages: diagnostic two dimensional echocardiographic features. Journal of the American College of Cardiology 1: 1330–1336

Robin E, Ganguly S N, Fowler M S 1975 Strangulation of the left arterial appendage through a congenital partial pericardial defect. Chest 67: 354–355

Robinson P J, Kumpeng V, Macartney F J 1985 Cross sectional echocardiographic and angiocardiographic correlation in criss-cross hearts. British Heart Journal 54: 61–67

Rossi M B, Burn J L, Ho S Y, Thiene G, Devine W A, Anderson R H 1987 Conjoined twins and right atrial isomerism. British Heart Journal 58: 518–524

Scott G W 1955 Ectopia cordis. Report of a case successfully treated by operation. Guys Hospital Reports 104: 55–66

Shinebourne E A, Macartney F J, Anderson R H 1976 Sequential chamber localization–logical approach to diagnosis in congenital heart disease. British Heart Journal 38: 327–340

Simpson J S, Mustard W T, Moes C A F, Izukawa T 1970 Emergency separation of thoracopagus (twins conjoined at thorax) in the newborn period: importance of careful preoperative cardiac evaluation. Pediatric Surgery 67: 697–702

Singer D B, Rosenberg H S 1967 Pathologic studies of thoracopagus conjoined twins. Birth Defects Original Article Series 3: 97–105

Squarcia U, Ritter D G, Kincaid O W 1973 Dextrocardia, angiographic study and classification. American Journal of Cardiology 32: 965–977

Sunderland S, Wright-Smith R J 1944 Congenital pericardial defects. British Heart Journal 6: 167–175

Symons J C, Shinebourne E A, Joseph M C, Lincoln C, Ho Y, Anderson R H 1977 Criss-cross heart with congenitally corrected transposition: report of a case with d-transposed aorta and ventricular preexcitation. European Journal of Cardiology 5: 493–505

Townsend R 1845 In: Tweedie A (ed.) Cyclopaedia of practical medicine. Lea & Blanchard, Philadelphia, PA, vol. 2, p 387–391

Toyama W M 1972 Combined congenital defects of the anterior abdominal wall, sternum, diaphragm, pericardium and heart. A case report and review of the syndrome. Pediatrics 50: 788–792

Ursell P C, Wigger H J 1983 Asplenia syndrome in conjoined twins: a case report. Teratology 27: 301–304

van Mill G, Moulaert A, Harinck E, Wenink A, Oppenheimer-Dekker A 1982 Subcostal two-dimensional echocardiographic recognition of a criss-cross heart with discordant ventriculo-arterial connection. Pediatric Cardiology 3: 319–323

Van Praagh R, Van Praagh S, Vlad P, Keith J D 1964 Anatomic types of congenital dextrocardia. Diagnostic and embryologic implications. American Journal of Cardiology 13: 510–531

Van Praagh S, LaCorte M, Fellows K E et al 1980 Superoinferior ventricles: anatomic and angiographic findings in ten postmortem cases. In: Van Praagh R, Takao A (eds) Etiology and morphogenesis of congenital heart disease. Futura, New York, p 317–378

Van Praagh R, Weinberg P M, Matsuoka R, Van Praagh S 1983 Malpositions of the heart. In: Adams F H, Emmanoulides G C (eds) Moss' heart disease in infants, children and adolescents. Williams & Wilkins, Baltimore, MD, p 422–458

Wallace H W, Shen D, Baum S, Blakemore W S, Zinsser H F 1971 Angina pectoris associated with a pericardial defect. Journal of Thoracic and Cardiovascular Surgery 61: 461–465

Weinberg P M, Van Praagh R, Wagner H R, Cuaso C C 1980 New form of criss-cross atrioventricular relation: an expanded view of the meaning of d and l-loops. World Congress of Paediatric Cardiology 1980, London (Abstract 319)

Wilkinson J L, Acerete F 1973 Terminological pitfalls in congenital heart disease. Reappraisal of some confusing terms, with an account of a simplified system of basic nomenclature. British Heart Journal 35: 1166–1177

Williams M H L 1944 Thoracopagus tribranchius dipus. Medical Journal of Australia 2: 275–278

59

Cardiomyopathies

J. S. Carvalho

INTRODUCTION

Cardiomyopathies have previously been defined as primary disorder of the myocardium without a known cause (WHO/ISFC, 1980). This definition excluded conditions such as systemic disorders that might involve the myocardium as part of the disease process, previously known as 'specific heart muscle disease'. This splitting of the diseases of the myocardium into two separate compartments has generated much debate. In clinical practice, however, conditions known to involve the cardiac muscle, such as metabolic disorders, have continued to be described as a secondary form of cardiomyopathy. To some extent, this reflected our inability, particularly in childhood, to recognize the aetiological factor at presentation. This, in turn, at least from a clinical standpoint, reflected the multiplicity of aetiological factors that, via different pathways, lead to a similar response of the myocardium.

Greater understanding of aetiological and pathogenetic factors affecting the myocardium has now led to new definitions and classifications. According to the most recent revision proposed by the World Health Organization (WHO/ISFC, 1996), 'cardiomyopathy' is now defined as any disease of the myocardium associated with cardiac dysfunction. Classification is now based primarily on the dominant pathophysiology and takes into account, if possible, both aetiology and pathogenesis (Table 59.1). Currently, there are four recognized types:

'dilated', 'hypertrophic', 'restrictive' and 'arrhythmogenic right ventricular'. Those cases that do not fulfil the criterions for any of these categories are described as 'unclassified cardiomyopathies'. Those forms that have a known association with cardiac or systemic disorders are additionally recognized and described as 'specific cardiomyopathies', acknowledging the association, for example, as in 'metabolic cardiomyopathy'. Within the new classification, it is now accepted that dilated cardiomyopathy, for example, can have different aetiologies, such as genetic, viral or ischaemic.

This chapter addresses the dilated, hypertrophic and restrictive cardiomyopathies as encountered in children. Myocarditis, or inflammation of the myocardium, is a common basis for dilated cardiomyopathy. It will be discussed together with dilated cardiomyopathy, since the two entities have many clinical similarities, and differentiation between them in a clinical context may not be so straightforward. Specific points of relevance to better understanding of myocarditis will be given separately. Endocardial fibroelastosis, an unclassified cardiomyopathy, is also considered in this chapter, as it usually presents as a dilated cardiomyopathy. Arrhythmogenic right ventricular cardiomyopathy will be dealt with in Chapter 26, while specific cardiomyopathies are reviewed in Chapter 67.

DILATED CARDIOMYOPATHY AND MYOCARDITIS

Dilated cardiomyopathy is characterized by enlargement of a ventricular cavity, most commonly the left, associated with impairment of systolic function. Abnormalities of diastolic function are also recognized. Within this new definition, it is recognized that the entity can be caused by a known agent, such as alcohol. When associated with cardiovascular disease, nonetheless, the extent of myocardial dysfunction must be beyond what is expected

from the severity of the condition alone. An abnormality that could cause similar findings but also could explain the degree of impaired function, such as an anomalous origin of the left coronary artery from the pulmonary trunk, should not, therefore, be considered a cardiomyopathy. Myocarditis is defined simply as inflammation of the myocardium (Roper, 1987). This is also the end-point of myocardial involvement by a variety of agents, such as

Incorporating modifications from the original chapters by T. G. Losekoot and A. E. Becker in the first edition.

Table 59.1 Classification of cardiomyopathies

Characteristics	Aetiology/association
Dilated cardiomyopathy Dilatation and impaired contraction of left and/or right ventricle	Idiopathic Familial/genetic Viral and/or immune Alcoholic/toxic Associated with cardiovascular disease but disproportional myocardial dysfunction

Hypertrophic cardiomyopathy
  Left and/or right ventricular hypertrophy
  Usually normal or decreased ventricular volume
	Familial disease with autosomal dominant pattern of inheritance and incomplete penetrance, resulting from mutations in genes for sarcomeric contractile proteins

Restrictive cardiomyopathy
  Restrictive filling and reduced diastolic volume of left and/or right ventricle
  Normal or near normal systolic function and wall thickness
	Idiopathic
	Associated with amyloidosis
	Associated with endomyocardial disease with or without hypereosinophilia

Arrhythmogenic right ventricular cardiomyopathy
  Fibrofatty replacement of right and/or left ventricular myocardium (local, then global involvement)
  Some left ventricular involvement with septal sparing
	Familial disease is common with autosomal dominant pattern of inheritance and incomplete penetrance
	Recessive form described

Unclassified cardiomyopathies	Fibroelastosis Non-compacted myocardium Systolic dysfunction with minimal dilation Mitochondrial dysfunction
Specific cardiomyopathies Associated with specific cardiac disorder, but degree of myocardial involvement not explained by cardiovascular disease, or associated with systemic disorders	Ischaemic Valvar Hypertensive Inflammatory (myocarditis): autoimmune, infectious, idiopathic Metabolic: endocrine (e.g. diabetes, thyrotoxicosis), storage diseases and infiltrations (e.g. glycogen), deficiency (e.g. selenium, anaemia), amyloid General system disease: connective tissue disorders, infiltrations and granulomas (sarcoidosis, leukaemia), muscular dystrophies (e.g. Duchenne), neuromuscular disorders (e.g. Friedriech's ataxia, Noonan syndrome) Sensitivity and toxic reactions (e.g. anthracyclines, irradiation, alcohol) Peripartal

an infectious, toxic or autoimmune process that could lead to myocardial inflammation, albeit that infection with an enterovirus is most common. Based on histology, a group of cardiac pathologists set out criterions for the diagnosis of myocarditis and its differentiation from dilated cardiomyopathy. These have become known as the Dallas criterions (Aretz, 1987). Within this system, myocarditis can only be diagnosed in the presence of myocytic necrosis or degeneration associated with an increase in number of T lymphocytes. In dilated cardiomyopathy, in contrast, myocytic hypertrophy and fibrosis are the main findings. This distinction is not always

easy to make. As was pointed out by Davies and McKenna (1994), 'in dilated cardiomyopathy there can be anything from no increase in T-lymphocytes to a large increase'. Formal counting of T-lymphocytes, furthermore, suffers from 'ill defined quantification methods'.

Despite these distinctions, both myocarditis and dilated cardiomyopathy can present in a similar way and can have similar clinical, echocardiographic and angiographic findings. This makes it difficult, if not impossible, to differentiate between the two entities. In a number of cases, the history is suggestive of an illness of recent onset, possibly preceded by a viral infection, thus permitting a presumptive diagnosis of myocarditis. However, a recent respiratory or gastrointestinal illness might well precipitate symptoms in a patient with dilated cardiomyopathy who had previously been asymptomatic (Taliercio et al, 1985; Schmaltz et al, 1987). Attempts to isolate an aetiological agent, and, therefore, to distinguish directly between the two entities, are often unsuccessful. Definitive diagnosis according to the Dallas consensus can be achieved only on a histological basis. At least in theory, therefore, endomyocardial biopsy should be the most reliable way of diagnosing myocarditis. But there are manifold difficulties with this technique imposed by interobserver variability in interpreting endomyocardial biopsies (Davies and Ward, 1992). These difficulties are aggravated by limitations that are inherent to the technique itself, such as those related to analysing only a small sample of the myocardium (Aretz, 1987). For all these reasons, it is now advantageous to think of the two entities as part of one clinical spectrum, an interpretation now acknowledged by the latest classification of the World Health Organization (WHO/ISFC, 1996).

PREVALENCE AND EPIDEMIOLOGY

From a population-based study reported from the Mayo Clinic over the period from 1975 to 1984 (Codd et al, 1989), dilated cardiomyopathy represented 36.5 per 100 000 cases in all age groups. In infancy, the estimated prevalence of all types of cardiomyopathy from the Baltimore–Washington epidemiologic study was 1 in 10 000 livebirths (Ferencz and Neill, 1992). As a prenatal diagnosis, dilated cardiomyopathy accounted for 5 out of 1158 fetal scans (0.4%) carried out over 10 years, and it accounted for 5% of all fetal cardiac abnormalities in the Vancouver series. During the same period of time in Vancouver, a further two stillborns, and 10 neonates seen in the first week of life, were diagnosed as having dilated cardiomyopathy, including endocardial fibroelastosis and myocarditis (Webber et al, 1993).

Most series, however, are hospital based. True prevalence in the general population, therefore, is difficult to ascertain. Furthermore, there are differences regarding the criterions used for inclusion or exclusion with regard to cases of endocardial fibroelastosis and myocarditis, and possibly for other types of secondary cardiomyopathy, which may remain undiagnosed. Dilated cardiomyopathy, when used in a broad sense to include endocardial fibroelastosis and myocarditis, represented less than 3% of children admitted to hospital with cardiac disease in Boston (Greenwood et al, 1976; Colan et al, 1992) over a period spanning more than 40 years. It accounted for 2–3% of neonates seen at the Toronto Hospital for Sick Children over a period of more than 25 years (Rowe et al, 1981a; Benson 1992).

Children with dilated cardiomyopathy usually present in the first 2 years of life (Greenwood et al, 1976;

Pongpanigh and Iasraprasart, 1985; Taliercio et al, 1985; Schmaltz et al, 1987), with about half seen in the first year (Greenwood et al, 1976). Both sexes are similarly affected (Stein et al, 1964; Greenwood et al, 1976; Pongpanigh and Iasraprasart, 1985; Taliercio et al, 1985; Griffin et al 1988; Chen et al 1990). In one study, having excluded myocarditis and endocardial fibroelastosis, a ratio of two females to one male was reported (Schmaltz et al, 1987). At the Royal Brompton Hospital, we have encountered 40 new cases of dilated cardiomyopathy in the echocardiographic records over a 10-year period from 1983. Patients subsequently shown to have myocarditis or endocardial fibroelastosis were included. Approximately three quarters of the patients had been seen since 1988. Our incidence was similar between the sexes, with approximately half presenting in the first year of life.

MYOCARDITIS

For similar reasons to those discussed above, it is impossible to obtain epidemiological data in the general population. Mild cases will almost certainly resolve spontaneously without the condition becoming recognized. In those who come to medical attention, clinical diagnosis overlaps with idiopathic dilated cardiomyopathy. Histological confirmation is not feasible in all patients and has its own limitations, as discussed above. With all these caveats in mind, myocarditis represented 0.3% of all children seen in the Texas Children's Hospital from 1954 to 1977 and accounted for just over 1% of postmortem cases (Friedman, 1995). Liu (1992) estimated that 0.1 per 1000 people each year will have myocarditis and stressed the vulnerability of populations with altered immunological states, for example children, young adults and pregnant women. Individual susceptibility to myocarditis is likely to represent a genetic predisposition to the disease. At an experimental level, variability of expression has been shown in different strains of mice (Huber and Lodge, 1986; Chow et al, 1991).

NATURAL HISTORY

From the experience of Greenwood and colleagues (1976) with primary myocardial disorders seen in 171 children prior to 1974, it was shown that approximately one third died, one third improved and one third remained with a cardiac abnormality. The population described at that time was mixed and possibly included other types of heart disease. Over one third of all patients reviewed were diagnosed as having non-obstructive cardiomyopathy on clinical grounds alone, since cross-sectional echocardiography was not then available. Nevertheless, although there is still uncertainty as far as the prognosis of individual patients is concerned, it is clear that, in any population studied, some recover, some continue with dilated cardiomyopathy and some die (Pongpanigh and Iasraprasart, 1985; Taliercio et al, 1985; Schmaltz et al, 1987; Griffin et al, 1988; Burch et al, 1994; Matitiau et al, 1994). Some patients, presumably considered unlikely to survive with conventional therapy alone, undergo cardiac transplantation, thus modifying the natural history.

An analysis of survival of adults with dilated cardiomyopathy (including some with high alcohol intake and others with rheumatic carditis) seen between 1960 and 1973 showed survivals at 1 and 5 years of 70% and 40%, respectively (Fuster et al, 1981). Even in a more selected group of idiopathic cases, a survival rate of 56% has been reported at 5 years (Romeo et al, 1989). A changing and improving mortality has been documented in recent years (Di Lenarda et al, 1995), partly through the introduction of new therapeutic agents such as inhibitors of angiotensin-converting enzyme (ACE inhibitors). Life tables have been published for cases encountered in childhood. Our own group of 40 newly diagnosed children seen over a period of 10 years at the Royal Bromptom Hospital includes all those initially diagnosed as having dilated cardiomyopathy, even if their subsequent course has shown some to have either myocarditis or endocardial fibroelastosis. The Kaplan–Meyer survival table (Figure 59.1) shows a 72% survival at 1 year and 61% at 5 years. The absolute numbers of survivors, however, become progressively smaller. The most striking feature, common to all series, is the much higher attrition rate during the first year following presentation compared with subsequent years. Then, despite a continuing risk of premature death, risk of death falls progressively. Taliercio and colleagues (1985) suggested that age at presentation appeared as a possible risk factor for death, but it did not achieve statistical significance. Subsequently, Griffin and colleagues (1988) showed a striking difference in survival if patients were grouped according to age at diagnosis. Those diagnosed prior to the age of 2 years had a survival rate at 5 years of 60%, compared with 20% in patients diagnosed when older than 2 years. When analysed in combination, these two series had an alarming mortality on follow-up, amount-

ing to 96% for the older children, and 30% for the younger ones (Taliercio, 1988). This finding is by no means universal. Other series showed age not to influence outcome (Schmaltz et al, 1987; Chen et al, 1990; Lewis and Chabot, 1991; Wiles et al, 1991). These inconsistencies in establishing the true relevance of age as a prognostic sign must represent not only difficulties in defining age of the start of the disease but also the impossibility of positively making a precise diagnosis of myocarditis or endocardial fibroelastosis. The latter point is reflected in the heterogeneity of patients studied in each series. Parameters such as family history, shortening fraction (Chen et al, 1990), ejection fraction (Agaki et al, 1991), persistent cardiomegaly (Pongpanigh and Iasraprasart, 1985; Griffin et al, 1988), left ventricular end-diastolic pressure (Lewis and Chabot, 1991; Burch et al, 1994) and arrhythmias (Griffin et al, 1988; Lewis and Chabot, 1991) have been suggested to correlate with outcome. Their predictive prognostic value, however, again varies significantly among different series.

Among a series of indexes derived from M-mode echocardiograms taken at the time of presentation for our children seen at Royal Brompton Hospital, the ratio of the thickness of the posterior wall of the left ventricle, to the left ventricular dimension at end-diastole were shown to be higher (> 0.17; median 0.19) in those who survived and whose left ventricular function improved compared with those who died or required transplantation (≤ 0.16, median 0.13) (Carvalho et al, 1996). We speculate that the reason for a better prognosis in the group with a higher ratio is that the potential for recovery will be greater if the left ventricular mass is relatively preserved.

AETIOLOGY AND PATHOGENESIS

Most cases of dilated cardiomyopathy remain idiopathic but, in a few examples, it is possible to establish a cause and effect relationship for specific agents. These conditions are now recognized as 'specific cardiomyopathies', such as anthracycline and metabolic cardiomyopathies. They are dealt with in greater detail in Chapter 67. In the so-called 'idiopathic group', factors such as genetic origin, altered immune response and viral infections have been implicated.

IMMUNOLOGICAL HYPOTHESIS

Various studies have shown some association between dilated cardiomyopathy and immunological defects, as well as the presence of autoantibodies directed towards cardiac tissue. The immunological problems include defects in natural killer cells in suppressor lymphocyte activity (Fowles et al, 1979; Anderson et al, 1982; Gerli et al, 1986), and in cytotoxic T cell responses (Wong et al, 1977). Cardiac autoantibodies have been shown to

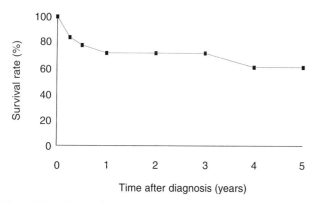

Figure 59.1. Actuarial survival for patients (*n* = 40) with dilated cardiomyopathy seen at the Royal Brompton Hospital, London.

occur more frequently in patients with dilated cardiomyopathy than in those with other forms of heart disease, or in normal controls (Caforio et al, 1990; Latif et al, 1993). The presence of autoantibodies, however, does not appear to differentiate between familial and non-familial cases (Michels et al, 1994). These findings might point to an immune component to the pathogenesis of dilated cardiomyopathy, but there is no definitive aetiological link. There is also some evidence to suggest that the immune response might be, to some extent, genetically determined (Anderson et al, 1984; Bender 1991; Carlquist et al, 1991).

FAMILIAL CARDIOMYOPATHY AND GENETIC BASIS

The occurrence of familial cases of dilated cardiomyopathy might have been underestimated in the past. A study of first-degree relatives of patients with the disease has shown familial incidence in 20% (Michels et al, 1992). Furthermore, analysis of the pedigree of affected families has shown that the inheritance can be autosomal dominant, recessive or X-linked (Moller et al, 1979; Michels et al, 1985; Berko and Swift 1987; Goldbaltt et al, 1987; Mestroni et al, 1995). As far as the molecular basis for dilated cardiomyopathy is concerned, the genes affected are little known. Defects in the gene for dystrophin, known to be abnormal in Becker and Duchenne variants of muscular dystrophy, have been demonstrated in families with X-linked dilated cardiomyopathy (Muntoni et al, 1993; Towbin et al, 1993; Milasin et al, 1996; Muntoni et al, 1997). However, they have also been encountered in patients with sporadic disease (Oldfors et al, 1994; Muntoni et al, 1997). Abnormalities at chromosome 1q32 have also been linked to a family with dilated cardiomyopathy (Durand et al, 1995), and deletions of chromosome 1p-1q were associated with an autosomal pattern of inheritance in another family with abnormalities of atrioventricular conduction and dilated cardiomyopathy (Michels, 1993). A further subgroup of familial cases might be associated with mutations of mitochondrial DNA (Suomalainen et al, 1992).

THE CONTROVERSIAL INTERACTION: VIRAL MYOCARDITIS AND CHRONIC DILATED CARDIOMYOPATHY

Inflammation of the myocardium may be caused by an infection, most commonly viral, or it may result from a non-infectious response of the myocardium. Various organisms may cause myocardial inflammation. The myocardial response to these agents may be a direct consequence of the organism itself, its toxins or an autoimmune response to the infection.

Clinical and serological studies have suggested that a number of cases of dilated cardiomyopathy are caused by persistent viral infection following viral myocarditis.

Although no virus has been isolated from the myocardium of patients with dilated cardiomyopathy, prospective follow-up of patients with acute myocarditis support this possible link between the two entities. In order to test this hypothesis further, molecular biological techniques have been employed to try to detect enteroviral genome directly in myocardial tissue obtained from endomyocardial biopsies, or from hearts explanted at the time of transplantation. Results appear conflicting. Bowles and colleagues (1986, 1989) have demonstrated the presence of Coxsackievirus B RNA sequences not only in about half the cases of myocarditis and dilated cardiomyopathy with histological evidence of inflammation but also in nearly a quarter of cases with end-stage disease. Similar results could not be reproduced by Cochrane and colleagues (1991), who failed to demonstrate enteroviral sequences in 40 samples obtained at transplantation using comparable hybridization techniques. Studies using in situ hybridization have also detected enteroviruses in samples from dilated cardiomyopathy more commonly than in samples from normals (Kandolf and Hofschneider, 1989). With amplification of genes by the polymerase chain reaction, providing more sensitive and specific tests, one study suggested a link between viral infection and dilated cardiomyopathy in a small number of patients, with no link found in controls (Jin et al, 1990). Others, in contrast, showed a similar prevalence of enterovirus in the myocardium of patients with dilated cardiomyopathy and in controls (Keeling et al, 1992; Muir et al, 1993). Still others did not show enteroviral sequences either in controls or hearts showing dilated cardiomyopathy (Grasso et al, 1992; Liljeqvist et al, 1993). The evidence for a role of enteroviruses in the pathogenesis of dilated cardiomyopathy, therefore, remains unclear.

PATHOLOGY

Characteristically, there is dilation of all four cardiac chambers, but the left ventricular dilation is obvious (Figure 59.2). The dilation of the chambers may mimic mural hypertrophy. The gross aspect of the myocardium itself is unremarkable, but there are usually secondary changes of fibroelastosis, which may be diffuse or patchy. Intracavity thrombosis is common. The histopathological features are non-specific. Biopsies will reveal myocytic hypertrophy with varying degrees of interstitial fibrosis. It is often possible to see scant inflammatory cells and lymphocytes, making it difficult, if not impossible, always to distinguish between cardiomyopathy and viral myocarditis, as discussed above.

PATHOPHYSIOLOGY

Whatever the cause of dilated cardiomyopathy, there is impaired contractile function of the myocardial cells. The

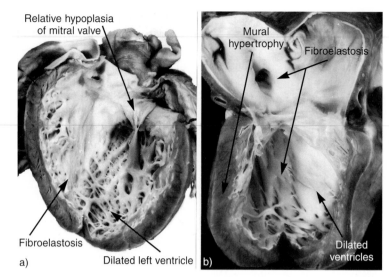

Relative hypoplasia
of mitral valve

Mural
hypertrophy

Fibroelastosis

Fibroelastosis

Dilated left ventricle

Dilated
ventricles

a)

b)

Figure 59.2. These hearts both show the features of dilated cardiomyopathy. (a) The dilated nature of the ventricle is obvious, giving the impression that the mitral valve is small, although it is of normal size. (b) There is also hypertrophy of the left ventricular wall, and the degree of dilation is not as marked. There was a coincidental association with aortic coarctation in this case.

left ventricular cavity is dilated, with increased end-systolic and end-diastolic volumes, and a decreased shortening fraction. Maintenance of cardiac output is, to a certain extent, a result of the Frank–Starling mechanism by which ventricular dilation leads to an increased stroke volume, with consequent increased wall tension and myocardial consumption of oxygen. Sympathetic stimulation, with a secondary tachycardia, also contributes to the maintenance of cardiac output, especially in the very young child. Within physiological limits, these mechanisms compensate for abnormal function and, consequently, cardiac failure may not be overt. Extending the limits of the initial compensatory mechanisms, however, leads to a decrease in both stroke volume and cardiac output. Reduced flow of blood to the kidneys stimulates the renin–angiotensin mechanism, with retention of sodium and water, thus aggravating the increase in ventricular diastolic pressures and promoting pulmonary and systemic venous congestion.

CLINICAL FEATURES

Clinical presentation of patients with dilated cardiomyopathy is usually related to heart failure. Decreased exercise tolerance, with breathlessness on exertion or feeding, is common. Pallor, irritability and failure to thrive may also occur. Older children may have a history of nocturnal cough and orthopnoea. Intercurrent infections, frequently of the upper respiratory tract, increase myocardial demands and worsen symptoms. Diagnosis of bronchitis or asthma is not uncommon before a diagnosis is made of heart disease. Some children may present extremely ill, with severe heart failure and frank pulmonary oedema. In others, the presentation can be related to the presence of arrhythmias. Under these cir-

cumstances, it is important to exclude abnormalities of rhythm as the primary cause of myocardial dysfunction.

Physical examination usually reveals an unwell child, with tachypnoea and tachycardia. Occasionally, the presenting symptom has been abdominal pain caused by acute distension of the liver. Pulses are frequently weak, and the point of maximal cardiac impulse is often displaced downward and laterally. A third heart sound is common. The pulmonary component of the second heart sound may be increased, depending on the pulmonary vascular resistance. Murmurs of atrioventricular valvar regurgitation, most commonly mitral, may or may not be present, even in the presence of valvar insufficiency.

INVESTIGATIONS

ELECTROCARDIOGRAPHY

The electrocardiogram frequently shows sinus tachycardia and non-specific abnormalities of repolarization. Left ventricular hypertrophy is seen in a significant proportion of patients (Taliercio et al, 1985). Progressive electrocardiographic changes, such as prolongation of the PR interval and QRS duration, are also reported (Wilensky et al, 1988). Some patients exhibit a left bundle branch block pattern. Arrhythmias of both atrial and ventricular origin are most commonly detected on Holter monitoring but do not seem to predict outcome (Friedman et al, 1991).

CHEST RADIOGRAPHY

The chest radiograph (Figure 59.3) essentially shows cardiomegaly of varying degrees and pulmonary venous congestion, with frank pulmonary oedema in some cases. Elevation of the left main bronchus can occur as a result

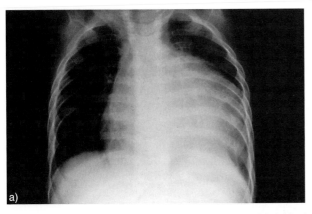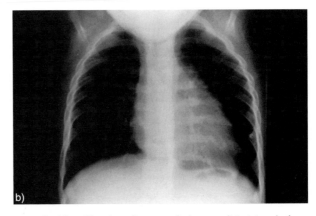

Figure 59.3. Chest radiographs obtained from a 6-month-old child who presented with a dilated cardiomyopathy/myocarditis (a) and after 6 weeks following treatment for failure (b). Note the gross cardiomegaly at presentation, with normalization of the heart size on follow-up.

of left atrial enlargement, and its compression can lead to pulmonary collapse.

ECHOCARDIOGRAPHY

Echocardiography (Figure 59.4) is certainly the most useful investigation, not only to document ventricular dilatation and function but also to rule out possible aetiological factors that may require specific treatment. By its non-invasive nature, it allows serial measurements to be made, these being essential in the short- and long-term follow-up. All cardiac chambers can be enlarged, especially the left-sided ones. M-mode recordings allow assessment of ventricular dimensions and function as well as wall thickness (Figure 59.5). Pulsed and colour Doppler studies will define atrioventricular, and sometimes arterial, valvar regurgitation. When the tricuspid or

pulmonary valves are insufficient, it is possible to infer pulmonary arterial systolic and diastolic pressures.

CARDIAC CATHETERIZATION AND ANGIOGRAPHY

Cardiac catheterization and angiography is seldom, if ever, necessary to make the diagnosis of dilated cardiomyopathy. One of the reasons for performing cardiac catheterization is to rule out anomalies of the coronary arteries, but in most instances this can be achieved by echocardiography alone. Other indications relate to measurement of pulmonary vascular resistance in the assessment for possible transplantation, or to perform endomyocardial biopsy. The pressure tracing in the left ventricle is typically abnormal owing to a slower rate of rise and fall of pressure. This produces a triangular

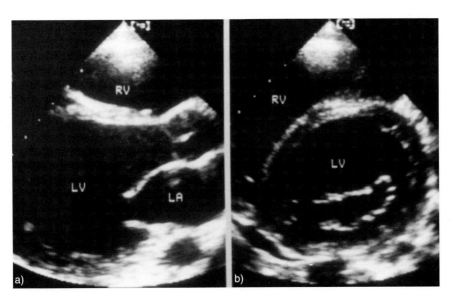

Figure 59.4. Long-axis (a) and short-axis (b) left ventricular cross-sectional images obtained from a child with dilated cardiomyopathy. Images were taken at end-diastole and illustrate the enlarged ventricular cavity. RV–right ventricle; LV–left ventricle; LA–left atrium.

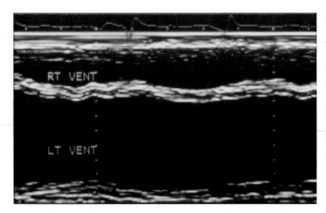

Figure 59.5. M-mode echocardiographic recording obtained from the same child as in Figure 59.4. Note the increase in both end-diastolic and end-systolic dimensions of the left ventricle, with a corresponding shortening fraction of 8%. RT–right ; LT–left; VENT–ventricle.

appearance, associated with elevation of both end-diastolic and minimal diastolic pressures (Grossman 1986).

MAGNETIC RESONANCE IMAGING

Other investigations include magnetic resonance imaging and nuclear studies. Both are usually unnecessary, since information on anatomy, ventricular function and wall motion are provided most commonly by echocardiography. Myocardial uptake of gallium-67 (O'Connell et al, 1981, 1984) and indium-111-labelled antimyosin antibody (Dec et al, 1990) have been used for cardiac imaging to detect myocarditis. The technique may yet play a role in identifying patients with myocardial inflammation.

CLINICAL MANAGEMENT

Conventional treatment of patients with dilated cardiomyopathy and heart failure includes use of digoxin and diuretics. For patients who are very sick, in severe heart failure and with pulmonary oedema, further cardiovascular support might be necessary, including positive pressure ventilation and the use of intravenous inotropic agents and systemic vasodilators. Adequate sedation, and sometimes muscular paralysis, are deemed necessary in an attempt to minimize consumption of oxygen and achieve a stable haemodynamic status.

VASODILATORS

Administration of agents that decrease afterload reduces cardiac workload and improves cardiac output in patients with impaired myocardial function (Beekman et al, 1984; Agostini et al, 1986). Intravenous hydralazine, when given to infants in the cardiac laboratory, was shown to increase cardiac index by increasing both stroke volume and heart rate, and to decrease pulmonary capillary wedge pressure. When used orally, hydralazine

was again associated with sustained clinical improvement (Artman et al, 1987). Prospective trials in adults with congestive heart failure have shown that the use of inhibitors of angiotensin-converting enzyme improves survival (Consensus Trial Study Group, 1987), a factor that has contributed to the observed improvement since the late 1980s in the survival of patients with dilated cardiomyopathy (Di Lenarda et al, 1995). One study showed greater improvement of ventricular function and lower mortality in a group of children treated with hydralazine compared with a non-treated group (Rao, 1995). Lewis and Chabott (1993) have also shown improved survival during the first year in patients treated with inhibitors of angiotension-converting enzyme, and a trend to better survival during the second year.

ANTICOAGULANTS

Intracavity thrombus, and embolic episodes, have been documented in both adults (Fuster et al, 1981) and children with dilated cardiomyopathy. Thrombus is more commonly found at postmortem, being seen in nearly half the cases in one series (Agaki et al, 1991), than in patients who underwent echocardiography (Taliercio et al, 1985). In the latter group, reported embolization varied between 8 and 17% (Stein et al, 1964; Taliercio et al, 1985; Schmaltz et al, 1987; Agaki et al, 1991). Pulmonary embolism and infarction occurred in about one sixth of children awaiting transplantation. Echocardiography failed to demonstrate thrombus in two thirds of all cases followed up (Hsu et al, 1991). It is reasonable, nonetheless, to consider anticoagulation or use of antiplatelet therapy in those children who remain with a dilated and poorly contractile ventricle, in particular if thrombus has been documented. Difficulties in controlling anticoagulation, coupled with the potential hazards of therapy, do influence its widespread use.

IMMUNOSUPPRESSION

Immunosuppression may play a role in treating patients with myocarditis and dilated cardiomyopathy, but there has been no definitive evidence that steroids, or other immunosuppressive agents such as azathioprine and cyclosporin A (cyclosporine), influence the outcome in either adults or children. The fact that active and persistent myocarditis does not appear to be a common cause of dilated cardiomyopathy in children (Lewis et al, 1985), and the risks of long-term administration of steroids in the young, do not support chronic use of steroids. In acute cases, one is often tempted to use immunosuppression in the hope that immune mechanisms will be halted, with consequent recovery of myocardial function. Reports of improvement of biopsy-proven myocarditis in adults and children who received immunosuppression often are uncontrolled (Fitchett et al, 1984; Chan et al, 1991). The significance of 'improvement', therefore, is questionable. In a compilation of published clinical trials of immunosuppression, Liu and colleagues (1992) showed the overall efficacy of steroids to be 64%, with spontaneous clinical improvement in 48%. A randomized controlled trial of prednisone in adults with dilated cardiomyopathy, nonetheless, failed to demonstrate any improvement of ejection fraction after 6 months of follow-up (Parrilo et al, 1989). The large American randomized trial was designed to see if immunosuppression improved prognosis in patients with biopsy-documented myocarditis. Over 100 patients had been randomized to treatment from an initial population of 2000 by 1992 (Davies and Ward, 1992; Liu, 1992). Improvement of ventricular function at 1 year, and mortality rates at 1 and 2 years, were similar in the groups with and without treatment. Immunosuppression, therefore, has not yet been proven to alter outcome. So far, its use to treat patients with myocarditis diagnosed either clinically or by biopsy has no scientific justification.

MODULATION OF IMMUNE STATE

Reports based on viral-induced myocarditis in animals suggested that other means of modulating the immune system rather than by immunosuppression might have a role in treatment. Use of synthetic immunostimulants, prior to or just after viral innoculation, permitted better survival and inhibited myocardial viral replication in treated mice, possibly by activating mechanisms of host defence (Yukihito et al, 1992). Mice infected with coxsackie-virus B3, and treated with T cell monoclonal antibody, showed reduced histological evidence of myocarditis and reduced mortality (Kishimoto and Abelman, 1989). Polyclonal immunoglobulin, used to prevent myocarditis as well as to treat mice with myocarditis, also reduced necrosis and inflammation (Weller et al, 1992). The mechanisms for this protection remain speculative, but probably involve providing antibodies against viruses or altering the immune response. The latter could be achieved by blocking the ability of the immune system to respond to an antigen, or by providing antibodies against autoantibodies (Nydegger, 1984).

In a report from the Boston Children's Hospital, polyclonal immunoglobulin was used to treat consecutive children admitted with presumed acute myocarditis. Results were compared with a retrospective control group. These data suggested that the treated children were more likely to recover ventricular function and had a tendency for better survival over the first year following presentation (Drucker et al, 1994). This preliminary report will prompt further studies to assess the clinical utility of immunoglobulin and its impact on long-term outcome.

ENDOMYOCARDIAL BIOPSY

Endomyocardial biopsy was introduced as early as 1962 (Sakakibara and Konno, 1962), but has been used in children only from the late 1970s (Lurie et al, 1978; Yukihito et al, 1992). It is a relatively safe procedure, and in most instances, can be performed without adverse complications (Schmaltz et al, 1982; Rios et al, 1984; Bhargava et al, 1987; Shaddy and Bullock, 1993). It is, nevertheless, invasive, and serious complications have been reported, including right ventricular perforation (Yoshizato et al, 1990) and death (Leatherbury et al, 1988; Webber et al, 1994). Risks and benefits, therefore, have to be weighed on an individual basis. One of the main reasons for performing biopsy in children with suspected dilated cardiomyopathy is the potential for diagnosing or refuting the presence of active myocarditis, with the possible implications regarding management. There is poor correlation, nonetheless, between the clinical and histological diagnosis of myocarditis and evidence of inflammation in samples obtained from children with dilated cardiomyopathy (Lewis et al, 1985; Leatherbury et al, 1988; Yoshizato et al, 1990; Webber et al, 1994). This could be related to a sampling error of the biopsy technique, or to overdiagnosis of myocarditis on clinical grounds. The question 'should patients with biopsy-proven myocarditis be treated with immunosuppressive therapy?' remains controversial. There is still lack of evidence to prove that such treatment is beneficial. Reports of its utility, as well as its lack of utility, are often non-randomized and non-controlled (Mason et al, 1980; Chan et al, 1991). The randomized trial organized by the National Institute of Health failed to demonstrate beneficial effects of immunosuppression either on outcome or on ventricular function (Davies and Ward, 1992; Liu, 1992). At present, therefore, there is no evidence to support the use of endomyocardial biopsy as a diagnostic clinical tool in patients with either dilated cardiomyopathy or suspected myocarditis. At the Royal Brompton Hospital, we do not routinely perform endomyocardial biopsy in this group of children. This approach, however, does not and should not preclude performing biopsies in a properly controlled trial, or in selected cases where further specific information is sought (Davies and Ward, 1992).

——ENDOCARDIAL FIBROELASTOSIS——

The diagnosis of endocardial fibroelastosis is a histological one. There is thickening of the endocardium by collagen and elastic tissue. It can occur in association with cardiac malformations, especially left-sided obstructive lesions such as aortic stenosis and atresia, and it can also occur in the presence of an anomalous coronary artery arising from the pulmonary trunk. When it is not associated with any structural cardiac abnormality, the endocardial fibroelastosis is considered primary. It is this primary form of the condition that can present clinically as a cardiomyopathy, although the diagnosis of endocardial fibroelastosis itself can be confirmed only by histological analysis. Under the most recent classification of cardiomyopathies by the

World Health Organization (WHO/ISFC, 1996), endocardial fibroelastosis has been 'unclassified'. In other words, the condition does not fit readily into any of the four main categories of cardiomyopathies. From the clinical standpoint, however, primary endocardial fibroelastosis is better grouped under dilated cardiomyopathy, from which it is often indistinguishable, especially if there is no involvement of other organs.

Edwards (1954) classified the primary form of endocardial fibroelastosis as occurring in 'dilated' and 'contracted' forms based upon the size of the left ventricle. During fetal development, however, a dilated left ventricle has been shown to be the initial stage of the contracted form (Carceller et al, 1990). When contracted, the left ventricle has characteristically hypertrophied walls, with a small cavity, and the left atrium is grossly enlarged (Farrell and Skinner, 1992). The contracted form simulates mitral stenosis in the neonate and ultimately leads to right-sided failure (Maron, 1983). It is, however, seldom encountered (Hashimoto et al, 1988; Farrell and Skinner, 1992). The dilated form is characterized by enlargement of the left ventricular cavity. It is by far the commoner of the two types, but it is still rare.

PREVALENCE, EPIDEMIOLOGY AND NATURAL HISTORY

One of the difficulties in establishing the occurrence of endocardial fibroelastosis, as well as its clinical course, is that its diagnosis is dependent on histological analysis. False-positive and false-negative clinical diagnoses, therefore, are bound to occur. Primary endocardial fibroelastosis is, nonetheless, an extremely rare condition. Mitchell et al (1966) found 7 among the 41 078 livebirths they had followed over the first year of life: an incidence of 0.17 per 1000. These authors, together with Keith and his colleagues (1978), estimated the incidence of primary endocardial fibrosis to be 1–2% of all cases of congenital heart disease. Among postmortems performed on neonates and children, the incidence of primary endocardial fibroelastosis varies from 0.3 to 1.4% (Fischer, 1962; Sobaniec-Zotowska et al, 1991). In those with cardiac malformations, endocardial fibroelastosis is found in 4 to 7% (Lambert and Vlad, 1958; Fontana and Edwards, 1962; Forfar et al, 1964).

The condition may occur sporadically, although a familial incidence is reported in both humans and animals (Chen et al, 1971; Westwood et al, 1975; Paasch and Zook, 1980). Accumulated experience supports an autosomal recessive mode of transmission although X-linked cases are also known (Barth et al, 1983, 1996; D'Adamo et al, 1997). Presentation is usually in the first year of life (Ino et al, 1988) and frequently mimics that of dilated cardiomyopathy. Over two thirds present with respiratory distress (Ino et al, 1988). Data on natural history of the disease is inevitably based on cases diagnosed mainly on clinical grounds, although some might have had histological confirmation of the diagnosis. Even if the study of these populations does not reflect the true natural history of endocardial fibroelastosis, it probably represents the spectrum commonly seen in clinical practice. The information provided, therefore, is somehow helpful for counselling. Ino and colleagues (1988) reported actuarial survival rates of 83% at 1 year, and 77% at 4 years. Over 70% of patients presenting in the first 2 years of life are said to be cured over a mean period of follow-up of nearly 9 years (Jarrar et al, 1994); these results being attributed to prolonged treatment with digitalis.

Endocardial fibroelastosis usually presents in infancy, but it has occasionally been reported both in the contracted (Hashimoto et al, 1988) and dilated forms (Mandel and Bruner, 1995) in adults with pulmonary hypertension. At times, its first clinical manifestation is that of sudden death in infancy or childhood. Its occurrence in the developing fetus has also been documented (Carceller et al, 1990; Newbould et al, 1991; Revel et al, 1994; Agnoletti et al, 1995). Endocardial fibroelastosis, with or without cardiac malformation, is recognized to be associated with hydrops (Newbould et al, 1991), even occurring subsequent to resolution of the condition (Carvalho and Markiewicz, 1997). Newbould and colleagues (1991) found that nearly one third of those with hydrops had endocardial fibroelastosis at postmortem. The endocardial changes had been present from fetal life in all cases, since the population included both stillborns and neonates who died in the first day of life.

AETIOLOGY AND PATHOGENESIS

The aetiology and pathogenesis of the endocardial changes in endocardial fibroelastosis remain unclear. The pathology gives no clear indication of the underlying mechanisms. The endocardium apparently shows a productive response, although the causative factors remain obscure. It seems likely that the classical examples of endocardial fibroelastosis, dominated by the dense layers of collagen and elastic tissue, represent an end-stage of several pathways. This is in keeping with the concept that primary endocardial fibroelastosis constitutes a heterogeneous group of diseases but is not a disease in itself (Lurie, 1988). Primary endocardial fibroelastosis has been reported in association with a variety of conditions. Viral-induced myocarditis has been implicated in its pathogenesis (Hutchins and Vie, 1972; Factor, 1978), including mumps virus (Noren et al, 1963; Gersony et al, 1966) and parvovirus (Levin, 1980). More recently, with the advent of molecular studies by polymerase chain reaction, there has been an increased awareness for the role of viruses, especially that for mumps, in the pathogenesis. Myocardial samples from postmortems of those with endocardial fibroelastosis have been shown to be positive for mumps virus RNA in over 70% of cases, compared with none in the control group, with nearly 30% positive for adenovirus (Ni et al, 1997). Storage disorders are also well recognized in association with endocardial fibroelastosis (Dincsoy et al, 1965; Westwood, 1977; Miller and Partridge, 1983; Schulz et al, 1987; Stephan et al, 1989) and, at times, involvement of the heart can be the first clinical manifestation of the disease. Other metabolic defects include carnitine deficiency (Tripp et al, 1981; Bennett et al, 1996) and respiratory chain abnormalities (Ruesch et al, 1996). Clinical cases involving multiple organs have been recognized, in particular the so-called cardioskeletal syndromes (Marles and Chudley, 1990; Ades et al, 1993; Orstavik et al, 1993; Devi et al, 1995; Bleyl et al, 1997). Morphological abnormalities of the mitochondria have been documented in some instances. Sobaniec-Zotowska and colleagues (1991) pointed out that, in postmortem series from the first year of life, nearly 30% of cases found to have endocardial fibroelastosis coexisted with skeletal and respiratory tract defects. The so-called Barth syndrome is an X-linked disease that is characterized by dilated cardiomyopathy and/or endocardial fibroelastosis, neutropenia, short stature and skeletal myopathy. It has been mapped to region Xq28 (Ades et al, 1993).

Other families with an X-linked mode of inheritance and cardiac and skeletal muscular involvement have been mapped to the same region of chromosome X (Bleyl et al, 1997; D'Adamo et al, 1997). Other associated factors that might play a role in the pathogenesis include hypoxia (Johnson, 1952), lymphatic obstruction (Kline et al, 1964) and raised intramyocardial tension (Hutchins et al, 1981) It has also been reported in a neonate who was the recipient fetus in the syndrome of twin-to-twin transfusion (Zosmer et al, 1994), again supporting the theory that the histological changes observed in endocardial fibroelastosis may represent a response to different insults, including haemodynamic disturbances, that may have occurred early in fetal life.

PATHOLOGY

The principal abnormality in endocardial fibroelastosis is the thickened endocardium. Gross inspection will show a typical porcelain-like appearance of the inner side of the affected chamber (Figure 59.6a). Usually the left ventricle is involved, but occasionally other heart chambers may also be affected (Bjorkhem et al, 1981). The

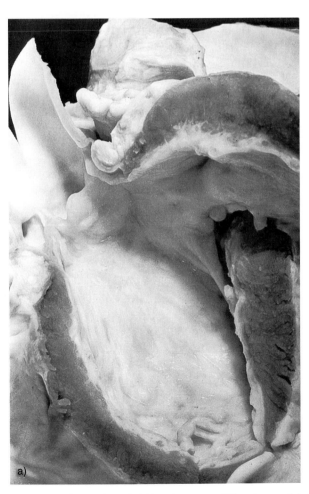
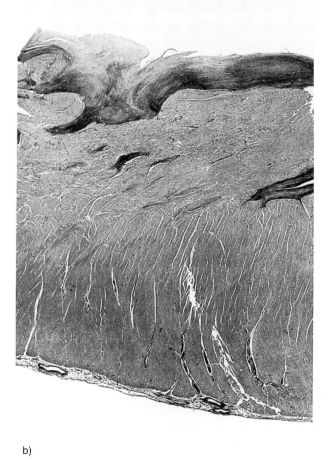

a) b)

Figure 59.6. Primary endocardial fibroelastosis. (a) There is porcelain-like thickening of the endocardium of the left ventricle. (b) Histology shows the fibroelastic thickening.

ventricular walls show distinct hypertrophy. The abnormal endocardium is composed of layers of collagen and elastic fibres intermixed with numerous spindle-shaped fibroblast-like cells (Figure 59.6b). The collagen and elastic components usually dominate the picture, but occasionally hearts can be encountered where the cellular aspect is more apparent. The adjacent myocardial wall is usually unremarkable, except for ischaemic changes that occur in the zone bordering the endocardial fibroelastosis. Slit-like 'sinusoids' are commonly encountered. Usually these channels are also lined by endocardial fibroelastosis that extends from the ventricular cavity. Otherwise, the myocardium is normal. In some instances, particularly in the 'dilated' form, the mitral valve may show a rolled free edge as an expression of long-lasting insufficiency. This abnormality is generally considered to be secondary to the fibroelastosis.

PATHOPHYSIOLOGY

The pathophysiological characteristics of endocardial fibroelastosis are similar to that described in dilated cardiomyopathy. Cardiac output and stroke volume may initially be normal (Graham et al, 1968; McLoughlin et al, 1968). The left ventricular cavity is dilated, as is the left atrium. Mitral insufficiency may ensure and accentuate the dilation of the left atrium, with subsequent increase in pulmonary arterial and right ventricular pressure.

In the rare 'contracted' variant, the mitral valvar orifice is usually small. The dominating feature in these patients is that of obstruction at the left ventricular inlet. As a consequence, the left atrial pressures are high from the very start, often with a diastolic gradient across the mitral valve. The pulmonary arterial pressure is elevated and may reach systemic levels. Heart failure occurs early in life and is usually rapidly progressive (Chandar et al, 1990).

CLINICAL FEATURES

Presentation of endocardial fibroelastosis is usually in infancy, and its clinical course is similar to that of infants with dilated cardiomyopathy or acute myocarditis. It is difficult to make the differential clinical diagnosis among these conditions if, by definition, confirmation of acute myocarditis and endocardial fibroelastosis is dependent on histological findings. If there is history of confirmed endocardial fibroelastosis in another member of the family, it is reasonable to assume the same clinical diagnosis (Benson, 1992). Clinical onset is often abrupt, with rapidly progressive deterioration. Initial symptomatology is related to left heart failure and, hence, is dominated by respiratory problems. Difficult breathing with recession is common, along with poor feeding and lethargy. Respiratory complications may further contribute to

relapses, with subsequent cardiac failure. A more fulminating course is occasionally seen in neonates. Indeed, even sudden death in a healthy infant may be the first and only manifestation. A more chronic course is occasionally observed, with an initial good response to medical treatment followed by relapses, mainly after infection of the respiratory tract.

On examination, findings are again similar to an infant with dilated cardiomyopathy or myocarditis. Grunting, pallor, peripheral cyanosis and shock may be observed. Gallop rhythm is frequent. The pulmonary component of the second heart sound may be accentuated. Signs of mitral insufficiency develop in half the patients (Moller et al, 1964).

INVESTIGATIONS

ELECTROCARDIOGRAPHY

The electrocardiogram usually shows sinus rhythm. Ventricular hypertrophy is seen in most patients, with high voltages in the left precordial leads. The configuration of the T waves may vary, as may the ST segments. The typical 'strain pattern', with asymmetrical inverted T waves and depression of the ST segments is often present. Rowe and co-workers (1987), and Benson (1992), pointed out that, in patients with a histological diagnosis of endocardial fibroelastosis, four-fifths had tracings suggestive of left ventricular hypertrophy with strain, whereas none of those with myocarditis or dilated cardiomyopathy without endocardial fibroelastosis showed similar patterns. Occasionally, the T waves show a symmetrical inversion or have a flat, biphasic or positive configuration (Figure 59.7) (Hastreiter and Fisher, 1977).

Combined left and right ventricular hypertrophy is seen in patients who have a long protracted course of left ventricular failure and pulmonary hypertension (Sellers et al, 1964; Hastreiter and Fisher, 1977). Pure right ventricular hypertrophy may be encountered in the first weeks of life, mainly in the presence of acute cardiac failure. In the contracted type, right ventricular hypertrophy may also be present with low or normal left ventricular potentials, and with left or combined atrial hypertrophy. Low voltage tracings are seen occasionally and may be encountered both in the initial and terminal stages of cardiac failure (Hastreiter and Fisher, 1977). A pattern suggestive of myocardial infarction may be seen in some patients. This phenomenon nearly always points to extensive myocardial fibrosis or necrosis. Dilation of the left atrium is a regular finding. Right atrial dilation is seen mostly in far advanced disease.

ECHOCARDIOGRAPHY

The echocardiographic findings are, in general, similar to those seen in myocarditis and dilated cardiomyopathy.

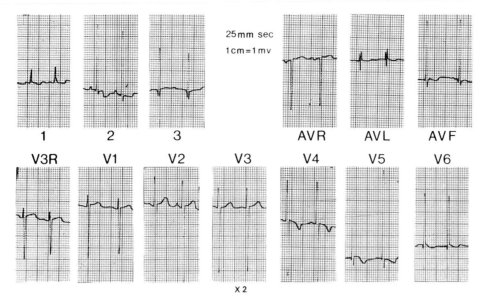

Figure 59.7. This electrocardiogram is from a 3-month-old infant with postmortem-proven endocardial fibroelastosis. There are signs of left ventricular hypertrophy with flat or negative T waves in leads I, II, aVF, V_5 and V_6.

The fibroelastosis of the endocardium may result in a multitude of dense echoes, which are highly suggestive of the diagnosis (Rowe et al, 1981b). We have also observed children for whom there was either a presumptive diagnosis of endocardial fibroelastosis because of a sibling dying with the condition or a postmortem diagnosis of endocardial fibroelastosis and in whom the echocardiogram failed to demonstrate such hyperechogenicity (Figure 59.8). In the 'contracted' form, the thick layer of endocardial fibroelastosis may almost completely fill the cavity of the left ventricle (Feigenbaum, 1981b).

CARDIAC CATHETERIZATION

As with dilated cardiomyopathy, cardiac catheterization may offer additional information if measurement of pulmonary vascular resistance is deemed necessary in the assessment for transplantation, or it may be needed to perform endomyocardial biopsy.

TREATMENT

There is no specific treatment for the condition, which in many instances is not recognized until a postmortem is performed. The therapeutic regimen will be as described above for dilated cardiomyopathy.

— HYPERTROPHIC CARDIOMYOPATHY —

The first case of hypertrophic cardiomyopathy is generally considered to have been described by Schminke in 1907 (Braunwald et al, 1964). Already in the 19th century, however, there were reports in the German and

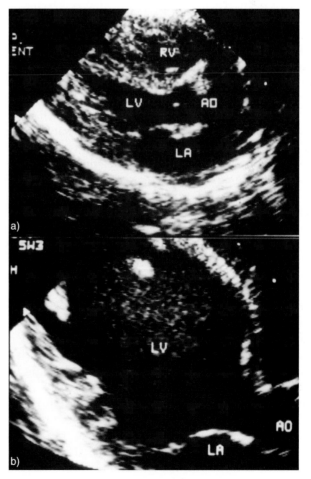

Figure 59.8. Long-axis echocardiographic views of the left ventricle obtained from an infant with a family history of endocardial fibroelastosis that was also shown at postmortem. (a) The left ventricular cavity size was normal at the age of 2 weeks, when the neonate was asymptomatic. (b) At the age of 4.5 months, there was gross left ventricular dilation with poor contractile function. Abbreviations as Fig. 59.4. AO–aorta.

French literature of specimens with the gross aspect of what we now recognize as hypertrophic cardiomyopathy (cited by Meerschwam, 1968; Ten Cate, 1978). It was the publications of Brock (1957, 1959), Teare (1958) and Bercu et al (1958), nonetheless, that focused on the clinical and pathological aspects of this disease and that set the scene for an era of waxing interest in hypertrophic cardiomyopathy. From the historical point of view, it is of interest that Bernheim, in 1910, described a syndrome of right heart failure in patients with left ventricular hypertrophy of diverse origin. The impediment to right heart function was thought to be bulging of the hypertrophied ventricular septum into the right ventricular cavity. It is likely, in retrospect, that some of his cases would also now be classified as hypertrophic cardiomyopathy.

Over recent years, our knowledge has evolved enormously, mainly through advances in molecular genetics and in understanding pathophysiological mechanisms, as well as our awareness of the great variability in its expression. Hypertrophic cardiomyopathy is now recognized as a genetic cardiac disease with an autosomal dominant pattern of inheritance, but with variable penetrance and expression (Maron et al, 1984; Greaves et al, 1987), albeit that sporadic cases occur (Watkins et al, 1992b). There is genetic heterogeneity, with more than one gene being associated with the clinical condition. There is also great phenotypic variability, not only among unrelated families, but also within the same family (Ciro et al, 1983).

Hypertrophic cardiomyopathy is a disease characterized by unexplained ventricular hypertrophy, which can affect the right or left ventricles. It is often asymmetrical (Henry et al, 1973a), usually involving the mid and upper parts of the interventricular septum. The site and extent of the hypertrophied segment may not be restricted to the septum; it may occur at other sites, including the right ventricular free wall, or even be present in a diffuse manner. Hypertrophy may also affect predominantly the apex (Klues et al, 1995). Asymmetric septal thickening, moreover, should be distinguished from disproportionate septal thickening, which may accompany a variety of other disease processes, with acquired myocardial hypertrophy as the common denominator (Maron et al, 1979). In childhood, in particular, the hypertrophy may involve the right ventricle (Barr et al, 1973), or both ventricles in combination, with marked obstruction of the right ventricular outflow tract being common in infancy (Maron and Roberts, 1981a; Maron et al, 1982b). Of further relevance to the paediatrician are closely related conditions such as Noonan syndrome (Ehlers et al, 1972; Burch et al, 1992) and Friedreich's ataxia (Perloff, 1980; Alboliras et al, 1986). The condition is also well recognized in infants of diabetic mothers (Gutgesell et al, 1980).

Extensive myocardial disarray is an important microscopic feature of hypertrophic cardiomyopathy (Teare, 1958; Maron and Roberts, 1979; St John Sutton et al, 1980; Maron and Roberts, 1981a). This particular histological texture in isolation, nonetheless, is far from pathognomonic (for reviews see Becker and Caruso (1982) and Bulkley et al (1983). Likewise, systolic anterior motion of the mitral valvar apparatus is often considered an important feature of the disease but, again, in itself is non-diagnostic.

PREVALENCE AND NATURAL HISTORY

Hypertrophic cardiomyopathy usually does not express itself clinically prior to adolescence (Maron and Roberts, 1981a), although the disease does occur at all ages, including childhood and infancy. Indeed, hypertrophic cardiomyopathy has occasionally been encountered in stillborns.

Its prevalence, as defined by unexplained ventricular hypertrophy, usually encountered on echocardiography, is estimated to be 1 in 500 (Savage et al, 1983; Hada et al, 1987; Maron et al, 1995). In some families with hypertrophic cardiomyopathy, if molecular genetic studies are taken into account, up to one fifth of adults are thought to carry the gene that causes the disease, even though they do not fulfil standard echocardiographic criterions (McKenna et al, 1997). Diagnosis may be at any time from infancy to old age (Cannan et al, 1995), but the condition is relatively rare in childhood. Morbidity and mortality, however, are greater at younger ages. Quoted annual mortality rates of 3–6% for children (Fiddler et al, 1978; Maron et al, 1978; McKenna and Deanfield, 1984; Romeo et al, 1990) are higher than those for the adult population (2–4%) (McKenna and Camm, 1989). This produces a 5-year actuarial survival up to 80% (Romeo et al, 1990). The clinical course is extremely variable. Patients may remain stable for many years, although premature death is common. McKenna and Deanfield (1984) reviewed a group of children who presented at a mean age of 9 years, reporting death in just over half, with a mean follow-up period of 9 years. In another study of children seen below the age of 14 years, death occurred in about one quarter during a mean follow-up time of 9 years. Most deaths occurred during physical exercise, and a decreased ejection fraction and history of syncope at presentation were independent negative predictors of survival (Romeo et al, 1990). Apart from age, other clinical characteristics can be considered risk factors for sudden death in children, such as adverse family history and syncopal episodes (McKenna et al, 1981a; McKenna and Deanfield, 1984). Hardarson et al (1973) and Goodwin (1982) consider the occurrence of symptoms in prognosis and early mortality. They have stated that it is moderate-to-marked septal hypertrophy associated with distinct abnormal electrocardiographic changes, together with a family history of multiple premature deaths, that identifies the young patient with an increased risk of sudden death. Others have not been able to confirm this opinion (Maron and Roberts, 1981a).

Ventricular tachycardia on a 24-hour electrocardiogram appears to identify a subgroup of adults at increased risk of sudden death (McKenna et al, 1981a), but the role of arrhythmias in precipitating sudden death in childhood is less clear. Arrhythmias were rare in infants and children with hypertrophic cardiomyopathy, although periods of non-sustained ventricular tachycardia were found in one fifth of adolescents in the study of McKenna and colleagues (1988a). Furthermore, the absence of arrhythmias during 24-hour monitoring does not indicate a low risk of sudden death. Premature death occurs more frequently in some families than others. It is possible that marked and diffuse left ventricular hypertrophy confers a predisposition to early death in minimally symptomatic or asymptomatic patients (Spirito and Maron, 1990). Concomitant right ventricular hypertrophy also appears to be associated with more severe disease (McKenna et al, 1988b). The prognostic value of these features in childhood remains unknown, as no large long-term follow-up is available. Other symptoms, such as exertional dyspnoea, fatigue and chest pain, do not predict sudden death.

Most series reported thus far, however, are hospital based. They are, therefore, biased towards referral of those with more severe and symptomatic disease. Two recent studies that are population based and that included patients from infancy to adulthood have reported a more benign outlook (Cannan et al, 1995; Cecchi et al, 1995). The annual risk of cardiac death and sudden death was low in both studies, although a group of patients who experienced atrial fibrillation had a worse clinical course (Cecchi et al, 1995). Atrial fibrillation is known to be poorly tolerated by patients with hypertrophic cardiomyopathy (Glancy et al, 1970; Stafford et al, 1986). Its presence, in general, is taken as a bad prognostic sign. The actuarial survival rate at 15 years of 76% for those patients who developed atrial fibrillation, compared with 97% for patients in sinus rhythm (Cecchi et al, 1995), is in contrast with the data of Robinson and colleagues (1990), who showed similar survival at 5 years for patients with arrhythmia and those who remained in sinus rhythm. None of their patients under the age of 21 years, with or without atrial fibrillation, died within the period of study.

In infancy, however, progressive heart failure is a more common mode of death. Historically, marked cardiac failure in the first year of life has been associated with unfavourable prognosis (Maron and Roberts, 1981b; Maron et al, 1982b). In the early 1980s, Maron and colleagues (1982b) reported that most infants with this condition who experienced heart failure died in their first year of life. It is worth noting, nonetheless, that most infants who died had been treated with digitalis! Subsequently, Schaffer and colleagues (1983) from Toronto reported their experience for children seen under the age of 2 years. Only one sixth presented with heart failure, with a much more favorable clinical course attributed to early treatment. Half the patients received

propranolol. More recently, a regional follow-up study of infants (Skinner et al, 1997) has shown that mortality is less than previously reported. The reasons are not entirely clear, but recognition and inclusion of those with less-severe disease as a consequence of echocardiographic diagnosis, as well as introduction of alternative forms of treatment, probably play an important role in modifying natural history.

AETIOLOGY AND PATHOGENESIS

The classical description by Teare in 1958 identified the familial nature of the condition by recognizing two siblings who died with asymmetrical hypertrophy. Subsequently, reports of two generations of the same family demonstrated the likely autosomal dominant pattern of inheritance (Hollman et al, 1960). Techniques of molecular biology have now identified the location of the abnormal gene for β-myosin heavy chain on chromosome 14q1 in a large family studied by Jarcho and colleagues (1989). This was the gene responsible for the disease in the original family described by Teare (Watkins et al, 1992a). A further locus for familial hypertrophic cardiomyopathy has been mapped to the regions of the genes coding for heavy chain myosins on chromosome 14 (Solomon et al, 1990). It has increasingly become clear, however, that there is marked genetic heterogeneity. Five separate genes are currently known to produce hypertrophic cardiomyopathy (Geisterfer-Lowrance et al, 1990; Carrier et al, 1993; Thierfelder et al, 1994; MacRae et al, 1995; Watkins et al, 1995). Four of these are known genes and code for different proteins that are related to the myofibril: β-cardiac myosin heavy chain on chromosome 14, α-tropomyosin on chromosome 15, cardiac troponin T on chromosome 1, and myosin-binding protein C on chromosome 11. An unknown gene on chromosome 7 is linked not only with the cardiomyopathy but also with pre-excitation (Burn et al, 1997).

In most cases, both in children and in adults, the condition behaves as an autosomal dominant disorder. Affected individuals, therefore, are heterozygous. There is incomplete penetrance, however, and the disease may not be fully expressed in affected persons despite their carriage of the gene (Maron et al, 1984; Greaves et al, 1987).

Watkins and colleagues (1992b) showed that new mutations of myosin heavy chain can account for some sporadic cases, which, in turn, can be transmitted to offspring. It remains possible, however, that some cases are sporadic and non-genetic. A more complete appraisal of the underlying genetics is given in Chapter 7.

In considering pathogenesis of hypertrophic cardiomyopathy, it is important to be aware of its definition as unexplained myocardial hypertrophy, and the clinical context within which this hypertrophy is usually recognized. Certain diseases are known to mimic hypertrophic cardiomyopathy on echocardiography. They may or may not share some of the pathogenetic mechanisms of the true familial condition.

PATHOLOGY

The disease is characterized by excessive hypertrophy of the myocardium, often asymmetric in nature, with a preference for the ventricular septum and the adjacent anterior free wall (Figure 59.9). In most cases, gross inspection will reveal a markedly narrowed left ventricular outflow tract (Figure 59.9). The endocardium of the septal surface overlying the zone of septal hypertrophy is usually slightly thickened, from fibrosis, and is often shaped as an imprint of the facing aortic leaflet of the mitral valve. In other cases, the hypertrophy can be more diffuse in nature, affecting the greater part of the left ventricular musculature (Figure 59.10). In rare instances, the disease may affect only the left ventricular apex or the right ventricular free wall.

The cut surface of the thickened wall may reveal an abnormal texture of the myocardial fibres (Figure 59.11). In other instances, particularly in the very young, gross inspection may not display any characteristic change other than hypertrophy. Microscopical examination usually reveals disorganization of the myocardial fibres. Small and broad bundles of fibres form an intricate lacework, often with an abundance of perpendicular junctions of individual cells (Figure 59.12). The extent of this unusual architecture may vary but, in 'classical' cases, it is extensive, involving the full thickness of the septum or the affected ventricular free wall. Fibrosis may accompany the myocardial disorganization, and thickening of the walls of intramural coronary arteries can occur. It is as yet speculative whether the abnormalities in fibral arrangement of the myocardial fibres are responsible for the

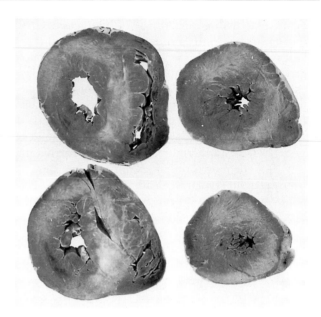

Figure 59.10. Cross-sections of the ventricles in the setting of hypertrophic cardiomyopathy shows extensive hypertrophy which, at the base of the heart, is localized preferentially in the ventricular septum and anterior free wall. Towards the apex, it becomes circumferential in distribution.

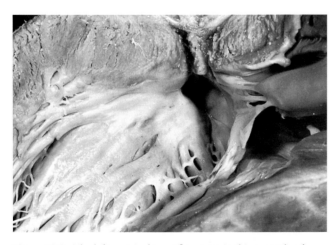

Figure 59.9. The left ventricular outflow tract in this example of hypertrophic cardiomyopathy shows extensive bulging of the ventricular septum and thickening of the adjacent anterior free wall. The endocardium of the left ventricular septal surface is thickened, shaped as an imprint of the aortic leaflet of the mitral valve.

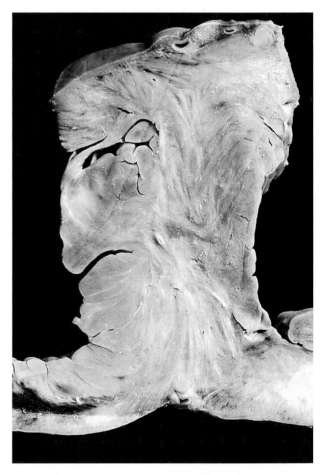

Figure 59.11. This transverse cut through the ventricular septum in a heart with hypertrophic cardiomyopathy shows marked septal thickening and an unusual disarray of the myocardial fibres.

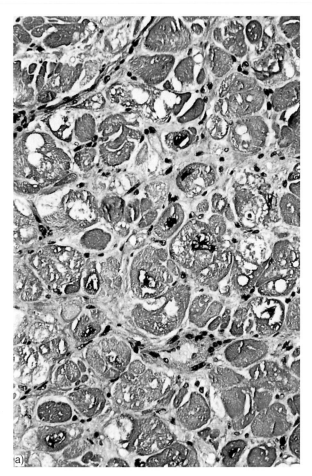 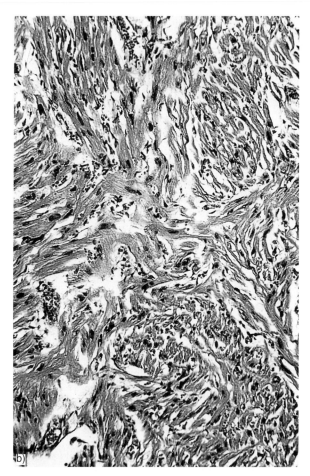

Figure 59.12. The histology picture of hypertrophic cardiomyopathy is characteristic. (a) Immense hypertrophy of the myocytes can be seen with bizarre nucle uses and some (mostly artefactual) vacuolization. There is a slight increase in interstitial fibrous tissue (haematoxylin–eosin, ×320). (b) In addition, there is disorganization of the myocardial cells (haematoxylin–eosin, ×210).

abnormal myocardial compliance encountered in hypertrophic cardiomyopathy (see below). The marked variability in degree and extent of the changes, however, could explain the wide spectrum of clinical signs and symptoms.

PATHOPHYSIOLOGY

Ventricular hypertrophy is the characteristic finding despite the great genotypic and phenotypic variability. The pathophysiological consequences of the myocardial abnormality, nonetheless, are variable; hence, the clinical signs and symptoms are varied. The dominant pathophysiological abnormality is impairment of relaxation. This abnormality of diastolic function can result in elevation of the left ventricular end-diastolic pressure, with resulting pulmonary congestion and dyspnoea. This is the most common symptom in hypertrophic cardiomyopathy, particularly when the condition presents in early infancy. Similar elevations of atrial pressures occur in the right side of the heart when the right ventricle is also affected by the myocardial hypertrophy. Several studies have shown that the diastolic abnormalities are exceed-

ingly complex (Sutton et al, 1978; Hanrath et al, 1980b) and may vary from one patient to another, as well as from one moment to the other in the same patient (Goodwin, 1982). Probably of less importance than the diastolic abnormalities producing 'inflow obstruction' is the presence of obstruction of the outflow tract, which occurs in some patients. This underscores the obstructive versus non-obstructive forms. The obstruction to either outflow tract has a dynamic characteristic. In the left ventricle, the hypertrophied ventricular septum typically bulges towards, and potentially narrows, the subaortic outflow tract. The distal portions of the mitral valvar apparatus are seen to move anteriorly across the outflow tract during ventricular contraction, making contact with the ventricular septum in mid-systole, a finding known as 'systolic anterior motion' (Glasgow et al, 1980). This latter feature is probably a secondary phenomenon consequent to the altered haemodynamic forces occurring during systole (Pollick et al, 1982).

The dynamic nature of this obstruction remains one of the most accepted explanations for the altered haemodynamics in the obstructive form of hypertrophic cardiomyopathy. It also explains how physical signs may vary with different clinical manoeuvres and influences the choice of drugs when medical therapy is contemplated. On the one hand, in general, the gradient will rise with an increase in ventricular contractility, a decrease in intraventricular volume and a decrease in afterload. On the other hand, the obstruction will diminish with a decrease in ventricular contractility, an increase in ventricular volume and an increase in the peripheral arterial resistance. As a consequence, the haemodynamic findings in these patients with obstruction of ventricular outflow may vary from one instance to the next, and the pressure gradient may change spontaneously, even during a single study. This aspect is often considered unique for hypertrophic cardiomyopathy.

It is evident that all manoeuvres and pharmacological agents that affect ventricular volume, myocardial contractility or afterload will influence also the pressure gradient and, hence, may be of diagnostic or therapeutic value. The dynamic nature of the obstruction can sometimes be demonstrated following a premature beat. As a consequence of the prolonged diastolic filling phase, the contractility of the ventricular myocardium will increase. In normal individuals, or in patients with a fixed aortic stenosis, the postextrasystolic contraction will result in a higher pressure in the left ventricle, and a larger pulse pressure in the systemic circulation. In patients with hypertrophic cardiomyopathy, however, the increase in contractility will result in a concomitant increase in the obstruction, which, thus, leads to a rise in left ventricular pressure but a decrease of the arterial pulse pressure (Brockenbrough et al, 1961). Heart failure may ensue in the terminal phase of the disease, accompanied by ventricular dilation and disappearance of the outflow obstruction (Epstein and Maron, 1982).

The increased contractility of the myocardium in hypertrophic cardiomyopathy leads to a rapid rise in left ventricular pressure at the beginning of systole. Directly after opening of the aortic valve, there is unimpeded, early ejection at high velocity, with a supranormal ejection fraction. The obstruction then develops during contraction; probably most of the forward flow occurs in the presence of the pressure gradient (Ross et al, 1966).

Mitral insufficiency is a common finding and often accompanies obstruction of the left ventricular outflow tract. The insufficiency is mainly caused by dyssynergic traction on both valvar leaflets. On occasion, it may have a greater and more deleterious haemodynamic effect than the outflow obstruction itself.

Since its introduction by Brock (1957), the mechanism of a dynamic impediment to mid-systolic outflow, as discussed above, has remained the most widely accepted explanation for the abnormal haemodynamics in obstructive hypertrophic cardiomyopathy. Others believe that left ventricular ejection in the 'obstructive' type is not impeded at all in systole, and that true obstruction does not exist, despite the fact that systolic pressure gradients can be recorded (Criley et al, 1965; Goodwin,

1980, 1982; Murgo et al, 1980, 1983). In their opinion, the ejection in 'obstructive' hypertrophic cardiomyopathy is characterized by hyperdynamic flow into the aorta, with 90% of left ventricular stroke volume ejected in the first half of the systole, and little or no flow occurring in late systole, this pattern having been demonstrated in several studies (Hernandez et al, 1964; Pierce et al, 1964; Criley et al, 1965; Murgo et al, 1983). How they explain the mechanisms by which the pressure gradients are generated remains unclear, but one suggestion is 'trapping' of the catheter, or alternatively the virtual elimination of any appreciable ventricular cavity during systole (Criley et al, 1965; Goodwin, 1980, 1982; Murgo et al, 1980, 1983).

CLINICAL FEATURES

In general, there is no correlation between the severity of the disease and the symptomatology. Children often lack symptoms; not infrequently, the disease is detected because of the presence of a murmur, often thought to be innocent or an arrhythmia. As a rule, hypertrophic cardiomyopathy does not interfere with the physical development of the patient except in its most severe forms. Those affected may remain asymptomatic for a long period; eventually, however, they almost always develop complaints.

Tiredness, poor exercise tolerance, exertional dyspnoea and palpitations may occur, but chest pain is rare. As in adults, sudden death can be the mode of presentation in childhood. Of those diagnosed in infancy, about one third will be seen because of a heart murmur. Over half are in heart failure (Skinner et al, 1997), manifested by tachypnoea and failure to thrive because of obstruction to left ventricular inflow. Although there may be gradients across both ventricular outflow tracts, this is not usually the reason for presentation in infancy. Other infants will present with cyanosis caused by right-to-left interatrial shunting associated with high right-sided pressures.

The most important signs are a 'jerky' arterial pulse, a palpable double apical impulse resulting from the left atrial 'kick', a late-onset systolic ejection murmur at the left sternal border or the apex and a fourth heart sound (Goodwin, 1982). These findings are all understandable on the basis of the haemodynamic disturbances. They may differ, however, from one patient to the other, as well as from one moment to the next in one and the same patient. A variety of physical findings can, therefore, be expected.

The increased left ventricular contractility, together with the explosive ejection in the initial phase of systole, may result in a sharp rise in the arterial pulse (Braunwald et al, 1964; Wellens et al, 1977; Goodwin, 1980). In patients with outflow obstruction, a sudden decrease in cardiac output in the mid-systolic phase may lead to a double-peaked arterial pulse. This particular characteristic of the pulse is difficult to identify by palpation only, but non-invasive tracings of the carotid arterial pressure curve, as well as intra-arterial pressure recordings, will unequivocally show these features. A rapid upstroke to a sharp early peak, the percussion wave, is followed by a steep downstroke, after which a lower late systolic positive wave, the tidal wave, is inscribed (Figure 59.13) (Brachfeld and Gorlin, 1961; Benchimol et al, 1963; Braunwald et al, 1964).

The blood pressure is usually within normal limits, but occasionally the pulse pressure is raised. Physical examination occasionally reveals cardiac enlargement, but precordial bulging is rare. On inspection or palpation of the heart, a left ventricular heave can be found, caused by left ventricular hypertrophy. A double apical impulse can often be recorded. The first one is caused by the 'atrial kick'. The second is caused by the left ventricular contraction (Figure 59.14) (Braunwald et al, 1960; Wigle, 1962; Cohen et al, 1964). The double impulse is typically found in the more severe forms of hypertrophic cardiomyopathy with subaortic stenosis.

The apex cardiogram (Figure 59.14) allows expression of the amplitude of the A wave as a percentage of the height of the main wave. The elevated 'A wave ratio' correlates roughly with the diminished ventricular diastolic compliance (Braunwald et al, 1964; Meerschwam, 1968), although the systolic plateau of the apex cardiogram is unreliable in this respect.

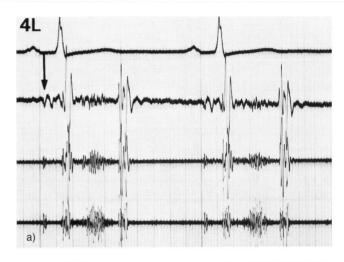

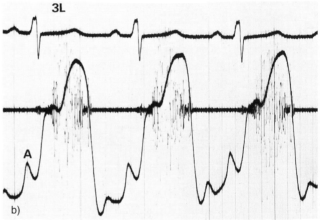

Figure 59.14. Phonocardiograms in patients with inflow obstruction. (a) This phonocardiogram in hypertrophic cardiomyopathy with inflow obstruction is taken in the fourth left intercostal space; tracings are the same as in Figure 59.13a. There is a high-frequency and late-systolic murmur. A fourth heart sound (arrow) is registered, even in the high-frequency tracing. (b) The apexcardiogram in another patient with inflow obstruction shows a clear atrial 'kick'. Note the high frequency and late onset of the systolic murmur. There was also reversed splitting of the second heart sound.

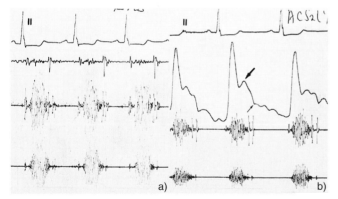

Figure 59.13. Phonocardiograms in hypertrophic cardiomyopathy. (a) This phonocardiogram is taken in the 4th left intercostal space. The traces shown are, from top to bottom: lead II of the electrocardiogram, low-frequency, mid-frequency and high-frequency tracings of the phonocardiogram. Note the late-onset and high-frequency character of the systolic murmur. The second sound is constantly split. (b) A carotid arterial tracing and phonocardiogram were also taken in the second left intercostic space. The traces shown are, from top to bottom: lead II of the electrocardiogram, carotid arterial tracing, mid-frequency and high-frequency tracings of the phonocardiogram. The carotid arterial tracing shows a rapid upstroke leading to a rather small peak (the percussion wave). It is followed by a lower, late-systolic peak (the tidal wave; large arrow). The second component of the second sound is, in time, related to the incisura (small arrow) and must, therefore, be the aortic component. Note that the pulmonary component of the second sound precedes the aortic component, demonstrating reversed splitting.

A precordial systolic thrill may be palpable. It is almost always a sign of outflow obstruction, although it does not permit any further classification as to the severity of the narrowing. The first heart sound is normal, and an early systolic ejection click is rare. Systolic murmurs are almost always present, but they may pass unnoticed in patients without mitral insufficiency or outflow obstruction (Maron and Roberts, 1981a). In patients with outflow obstruction, a grade 2–4/6 ejection type systolic murmur is almost always present. The late onset of the murmur relative to the first heart sound is most likely a result of the development of obstruction during ventricular contraction (Figures 59.13 and 59.14). The murmur has a coarse character and is loudest at the lower left sternal border or just inside the apex (Braunwald et al, 1964; Wigle, 1964). The intensity of the murmur, however, may change, intensifying during a Valsalva manoeuvre, which leads to a decrease in left ventricular volume, and also in the postpremature beat, which leads to an increase of the gradient. An increase in venous return, such as occurs with squatting or postural changes, has the opposite effect. Diminishing the afterload of the heart with amyl nitrite or a similar drug results in an increase in the loudness of the murmur, whereas an increase in afterload, for instance by phenylephrine, decreases the intensity of the murmur (Nellen et al, 1971). A holosystolic, high-frequency murmur may be heard at the apex of the heart in the presence of mitral insufficiency, which radiates to the axilla. The second heart sound is unsplit or narrowly split in most cases (Maron and Roberts, 1981a).

Paradoxical splitting of the second heart sound, caused by lengthening of the left ventricular ejection time, is a regular phenomenon, particularly in patients with marked obstruction of the left ventricular outflow tract (Braunwald et al, 1964; Cohen et al, 1964; Wigle, 1964). This feature is best detected by phonocardiography (Figure 59.13b). Absence of paradoxical splitting does not exclude the presence of haemodynamically important left ventricular outflow obstruction.

A third heart sound, or a mid-diastolic murmur, is also a frequent finding. It is interpreted as a sign of either inflow obstruction or increased flow over the atrio-ventricular valve, as occurs in patients with mitral insufficiency (Braunwald et al, 1964; Wigle, 1964; Meerschwam, 1968).

A fourth heart sound is of even greater significance, since it reflects diminished diastolic ventricular compliance. A high-frequency fourth heart sound on the phonocardiogram nearly always indicates the existence of an elevated left ventricular end-diastolic pressure (Figure 59.14a) (Wigle, 1964).

INVESTIGATIONS

ELECTROCARDIOGRAPHY

The electrocardiogram is usually abnormal, but findings are non-specific. Right ventricular hypertrophy is seen in approximately 50% of infants (Maron and Roberts, 1981b; Maron et al, 1982b), while older children show more left ventricular hypertrophy, abnormal Q waves and ST–T wave changes (Maron and Roberts, 1981b).

The P waves are usually broad and notched in the limb leads, and biphasic with a broad negative component in V_1. These anomalies are mostly caused by a delay of conduction in the left atrium, often accompanied by atrial dilatation. Signs of right atrial or biatrial dilatation occur occasionally. Hence, abnormal P waves are a common feature in more advanced disease, particularly in those in whom the major problem is inflow obstruction or atrio-ventricular valvar insufficiency (Frank and Braunwald, 1968; Bahl and Massie, 1972).

An abnormal long PQ interval, in other words first-degree atrioventricular block, occurs in a very small pro-

portion of patients with hypertrophic cardiomyopathy. The conduction delay has been attributed to myocardial fibrosis. Higher degrees of deficient atrioventricular conduction have been described but appear to be exceedingly rare. In incidental cases, hypertrophic cardiomyopathy is associated with signs and symptoms of ventricular pre-excitation (Bahl and Massie, 1972; Wellens et al, 1977). A variety of abnormalities are seen in the QRS complexes. Signs of left ventricular hypertrophy are the most common, with the highest incidence being encountered in patients in whom the obstructive form prevails (Figure 59.15) (Wigle 1962; Frank and Braunwald, 1968; Bahl and Massie, 1972; Maron and Roberts, 1981a). Signs of right ventricular hypertrophy are encountered in a relatively high proportion of those presenting in infancy, obstruction of the right ventricular outflow tract being

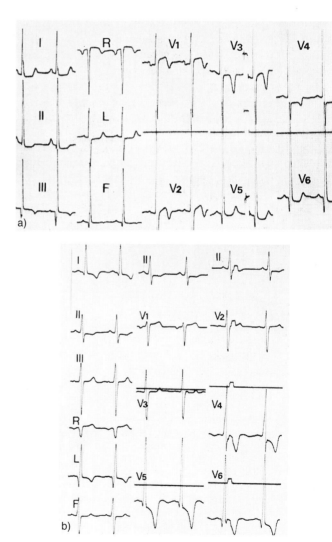

Figure 59.15. These electrocardiograms are from a boy with hypertrophic cardiomyopathy taken at the ages of 7 years (a) and 12 years (b). There are signs of left ventricular hypertrophy with abnormal ST–T segments. There is significant progression over the intervening period, with deep negative T waves in leads I, aVL, V_4–V_6 in the later electrocardiogram, in which all leads are taken at half sensitivity.

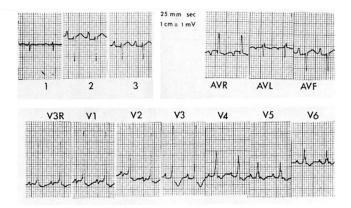

Figure 59.16. This electrocardiogram is from a 14-day-old infant with hypertrophic cardiomyopathy and right ventricular outflow obstruction. There is evidence of slight right atrial dilation and severe right ventricular hypertrophy.

much more common in these young patients (Figure 59.16). Patterns mimicking myocardial infarction can occur, typified by abnormal Q waves (particularly in leads I and AVL and in the left precordial leads), together with abnormal ST segments and T waves. These abnormalities are caused by hypertrophy of the ventricular septum and myocardial fibrosis (Bahl and Massie, 1972). Septal hypertrophy may first be noticed because of the combined occurrence of deep Q waves and normal R waves over the left precordium. In time, these changes may subside and the typical, albeit otherwise non-diagnostic, pattern of left ventricular hypertrophy may develop (Braudo et al, 1964; Bloom, 1978).

Intraventricular conduction defects, left bundle branch block in particular, are common features in advanced cases. The change is considered secondary to myocardial fibrosis. Septal fibrosis may cause a change in direction of early depolarization, resulting in the absence of Q waves in the leads I, aVL, V_5 and V_6. Left-axis deviation, with a mean QRS axis between $-30°$ and $-90°$, is seen regularly; it is caused by myocardial fibrosis, which results in a conduction block in the anterior ramifications of the left branch (Frank and Braunwald, 1968; Bahl and Massie, 1972). Abnormalities of the ST segment and T waves occur in almost every patient, usually as a consequence of left ventricular hypertrophy or an intraventricular conduction delay. Inversion of T waves in the right and mid-precordial leads has been described and probably relates to septal hypertrophy (Braudo et al, 1964).

All types of arrhythmia have been described. The two most important ones are atrial fibrillation and ventricular extrasystoles. Atrial fibrillation develops mainly in advanced disease and is generally considered an ominous sign. Ventricular extrasystoles, particularly when multiple and multifocal, may lead to ventricular tachycardia and, hence, may predispose to ventricular fibrillation. Ventricular arrhythmias found during 24-hour electro-cardiographic monitoring are rare in children, in contrast

to the situation reported in adults (McKenna et al, 1988a).

It has been reported that the presence of low-amplitude signals late in the QRS complex and early ST segment in signal-averaged electrocardiograms have a 77% positive predictive value in detecting patients with history of cardiac arrest or who have had episodes of non-sustained ventricular tachycardia (Cripps et al, 1990). As this type of arrhythmia is infrequent in childhood, its use as a possible tool in identifying children at risk of dying unexpectedly is limited.

CHEST RADIOGRAPHY

The chest radiograph will usually reveal a heart of almost normal size, with a cardiothoracic ratio of less than 60% and a non-characteristic cardiac silhouette. Cardiomegaly is seen in virtually all infants, but in only a quarter of older children (Maron and Roberts, 1981b). Left ventricular enlargement, when observed, does not correlate with the severity of the disease. In an occasional patient, the frontal projection may disclose a bulge at the left heart border, albeit in itself non-diagnostic (Wigle, 1964; Meerschwam, 1968). Atrial dilation, when marked, may be observed. Isolated right ventricular enlargement is exceedingly rare. Unless heart failure has developed, vascular markings of the lungs are usually normal.

ECHOCARDIOGRAPHY

Since asymmetric septal hypertrophy is a common anatomical feature in both obstructive and non-obstructive disease, the echographic demonstration of a thickened ventricular septum disproportionate to the thickness of the posterior wall of the left ventricle is a key feature. A ratio of 1.3:1 or more between the septal thickness and that of the left ventricular posterior wall has generally been considered to be diagnostic, and this has been the main M-mode echocardiographic finding used to diagnose hypertrophic cardiomyopathy (Figure 59.17) (Henry et al, 1973b). It is, however, a non-specific marker (Menapace et al, 1977; Gibson et al, 1979). Hypertrophy of the septo-marginal trabeculation may mimick septal thickening and, thus, may lead to an erroneous diagnosis of hypertrophic cardiomyopathy. Furthermore, a ratio of over 1.3:1 is seen relatively often in normal neonates and is certainly found in children with congenital cardiac malformations (Maron et al, 1979, 1982b). The abnormal ratios of the septum to the free wall frequently encountered in normal children gradually disappear by 2 years of age, concomitant with greater thickening of the left ventricle, and this criterion is worthless in young children. Small errors in absolute measurement also become greater with the use of a ratio (Maron and Roberts, 1981b). It is better to use absolute values for septal and free wall thickness and compare them with normal values.

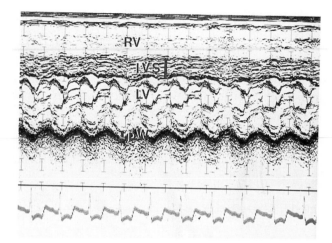

Figure 59.17. M-mode echocardiogram in a girl with hypertrophic cardiomyopathy. There is thickening of the ventricular septum (IVS, 16 mm) and of the left ventricular posterior wall (pW, 6 mm). The ratio is 2.7:1. In the left ventricular cavity (LV), the leaflets of the mitral valve show systolic anterior motion of the aortic leaflet. There is markedly reduced motion of the ventricular septum. RV, right ventricle.

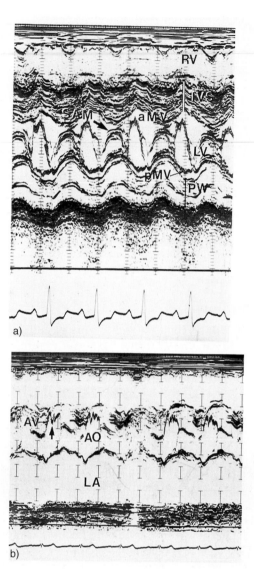

Figure 59.18. M-mode echocardiograms in a child with hypertrophic cardiomyopathy. (a) A view taken through the mitral valve shows the aortic leaflet of the mitral valve (aMV) moving anteriorly in the beginning of systole and remaining in close contact with the left side of the ventricular septum (IVS), the so-called 'systolic anterior motion' (SAM). In this view the asymmetric septal hypertrophy is not clearly demonstrated. (b) In the M-mode echocardiogram through the aorta (AO) and left atrium (LA), the aortic leaflets (AV) show partial mid-systolic closure (large arrow) and a coarse flutter. LV, left ventricle; pMV, mural valvar leaflet; PW, posterior wall left ventricle; RV, right ventricle.

Other M-mode features, such as systolic anterior movement of the mitral valve and mid-systolic closure of the aortic valve, often assumed to be associated with gradients across the left ventricular outflow tract (Doi et al, 1980; Wong et al, 1980), are also non-specific for hypertrophic cardiomyopathy. Systolic anterior motion of the aortic leaflet of the mitral valve is a common feature. It is best recorded with the M-mode technique. The abnormal anterior motion starts in first third of the systolic interval. The leaflet remains in an anterior position during the mid-systolic phase, often in direct apposition with the left ventricular septal surface. It returns to its usual posterior position only at the end of systole (Figure 59.18) (Williams and Tucker, 1977; Feigenbaum 1981a). Although considered an indication of a dynamic outflow obstruction, the abnormality in itself is not pathognomonic for hypertrophic cardiomyopathy. Other echographic signs suggesting the presence of a dynamic outflow obstruction are partial mid-systolic closure of the aortic leaflets (Figure 59.18b), often with a coarse flutter, and close apposition during diastole of the aortic leaflet of the mitral valve and the left ventricular septal surface.

Cross-sectional echocardiography is the non-invasive investigation that allows more cases to be diagnosed, and it complements measurements that can be made with standard and digitized M-mode echocardiography. The site and extent of hypertrophy is better assessed than with M-mode echocardiography, thus avoiding false-negative diagnosis. The thickening of the ventricular septum is often extensive and usually involves also the anterior wall of the left ventricle. The abnormality, however, can be discrete (Figure 59.19). Hence, echographic examination should include imaging of the entire length of both right and left septal surfaces (Williams and Tucker, 1977). In patients with hypertrophic cardiomyopathy of a more concentric nature, the posterior wall of the left ventricle may also be thick (Figure 59.20). The ratio of the septal thickness to the posterior wall may then no longer be abnormal. This may occur in patients with both the obstructive and non-obstructive varieties of the disease.

The myocardial echo intensity has been shown to be higher in those with hypertrophic cardiomyopathy than in normals. This is presumably caused by the fibrosis, a finding also seen in other forms of secondary left ventricular hypertrophy (Gibson, 1985). More recently, Vitale and colleagues (1996) studied ultrasonic reflectivity of the

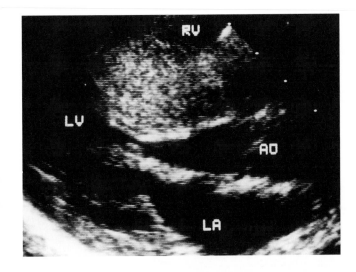

Figure 59.19. Parasternal left ventricular long-axis echocardiographic section obtained from an asymptomatic 3-year-old child with marked asymmetric septal hypertrophy. AO, aorta; LA, left atrium; LV, left ventricle; RV, right ventricle.

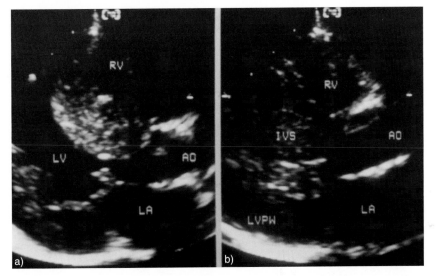

Figure 59.20. Parasternal left ventricular echocardiographic section obtained from a patient in diastole (a) and systole (b) with hypertrophic cardiomyopathy. Note thickening of both the ventricular septum and left ventricular posterior wall (a) and cavity obliteration during systole (b). IVS, muscular ventricular septum; other abbreviations as in Figure 59.19.

myocardium, showing it to be significantly increased in adults with hypertrophic cardiomyopathy compared with normals, but not in children with the disease who were less than 10 years of age, perhaps in agreement with different clinical manifestations in the two age groups.

Doppler interrogation of the atrioventricular and arterial valves is useful in the assessment of gradients across both ventricular outflow tracts (Figures 59.21 and 59.22) as well as for valvar regurgitation. Doppler investigations in hypertrophic cardiomyopathy, however, have concentrated more on the assessment of diastolic function (see Chapter 13).

CARDIAC CATHETERIZATION AND ANGIOGRAPHY

Cardiac catheterization and angiography have been used less often over recent years because of the availability of non-invasive techniques able to demarcate ventricular hypertrophy and estimate intraventricular pressure gradients. If needed, left-sided studies are mainly performed in retrograde fashion. The decrease in diastolic compliance of the left ventricle leads to a rise in left ventricular end-diastolic pressures and left atrial pressures. The elevated end-diastolic pressure is mainly caused by the 'atrial kick' (Figure 59.23). Obstruction across the left ventricular outflow tract can be demonstrated by withdrawing from the left ventricle to the aorta. The experienced investigator may notice that the level of obstruction is located at a greater distance from the aortic valve than usually seen in discrete subvalvar aortic stenosis. Considerable variations in the pressure gradient may be recorded during the same investigation. The pressure tracing in the subvalvar low-pressure chamber often has a typical rectangular configuration, with coarse vibrations on the horizontal plateau. The pressure tracing

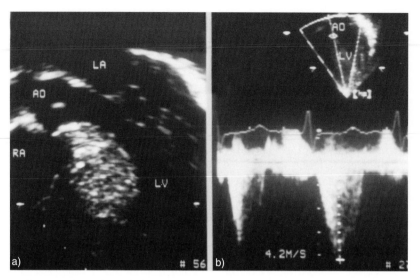

Figure 59.21. Hypertrophic cardiomyopathy with marked septal hypertrophy. (a) Apical four chamber view incorporating the aortic root. (b) The pulsed wave Doppler signal shows a maximal instantaneous peak systolic velocity of 4.2 m/s, corresponding to an instantaneous systolic gradient of 70 mmHg across the left ventricular outflow tract. Abbreviations as in Figure 59.19.

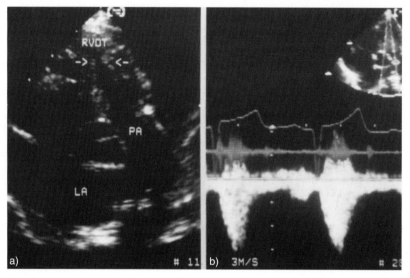

Figure 59.22. Echocardiography in a patient with hypertrophic cardiomyopathy. (a) Parasternal short-axis view at the level of the aortic root shows marked narrowing in the subpulmonary area (arrows). (b) The corresponding pulsed wave Doppler signal shows a maximal instantaneous velocity of 3 m/s across the right ventricular outflow tract. LA, left atrium; PA, pulmonary artery; RVOT, right ventricular outflow tract.

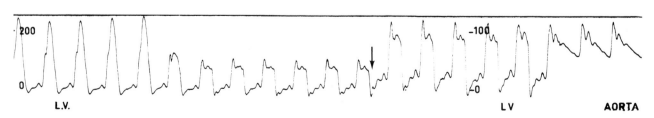

Figure 59.23. A withdrawal tracing from the left ventricle (LV) to the aorta in a 10-year-old boy with hypertrophic cardiomyopathy and severe left ventricular outflow obstruction. The tracing from the apical to the subvalvar region demonstrates a gradient of about 100 mmHg. The tracing from the subvalvar region to the aorta does not show any gradient (note the change in calibration: arrow). The ventricular pressure curves show a high end-diastolic pressure resulting from the 'atrial kick'. The pressure tracing from the cavity of the left ventricle shows a notch approximately at the height of the peak pressure of the subvalver region of the left ventricle. The pressure curve of this subvalvar region has a rectangular configuration with some coarse vibrations on the horizontal plateau. The tracings from the aorta demonstrate a tidal wave. (See also Figure 59.13b.)

of the cavity of the left ventricle sometimes shows a notch in the upstroke approximately at the height of the peak pressure in the subvalvar chamber (Soulie et al, 1962; Braunwald et al, 1964). The aortic pressure tracing shows a characteristic 'spike-and-dome' appearance. A rapid rise is followed by a dip in pressure, and a second dome-shaped wave. No increase in pulse pressure is noted with a postextrasystolic beat. It is argued by some that the pressure differences recorded between the aorta and the inflow portion of the left ventricle may not always reflect a true obstruction; they could rather be caused by 'trapping' of the catheter tip or could reflect the virtual elimination of the left ventricular cavity during systole (Criley et al, 1965, 1976; Goodwin, 1980, 1982; Murgo et al, 1980, 1983). The pressure gradient may vary spontaneously. It is affected by many circumstances, such as the position of the body, respiration, exercise, Valsalva manoeuvres, extrasystoles, circulating blood volume and various drugs. Should signs of obstruction be absent during the invasive study, inotropic drugs such as isoprenaline (isoproterenol) may be used to provoke a gradient over the outflow tract of the left ventricle (Braunwald et al, 1964). Right-sided studies may demonstrate the same haemodynamic features as described for the left side of the heart. More accurate assessment of diastolic function is possible if measurements of pressure and volume are made simultaneously.

Angiocardiography shows a distorted and irregular contour of the ventricles due to massive hypertrophy of the septum, the papillary muscles and the apical muscular trabeculations. When seen in the frontal projection, the left ventricular cavity exhibits an inward concavity during diastole at the mid-portion of its superior margin, caused by the hypertrophic ventricular septum. A similar indentation can be seen in the posteroinferior margin, caused by hypertrophy of the posteromedial papillary muscle. This biconcave configuration produces an hourglass appearance (Figures 59.24 and 59.25). An elongated and narrowed left ventricular outflow tract may be seen during systole, either in the subvalvar region or in the mid-portion of the ventricle (Figure 59.24b). If apical hypertrophy is the predominant feature, a spade-shaped appearance can be seen at end-diastole (Yamaguchi et al, 1979).

Another important feature of hypertrophic cardiomyopathy is the virtual elimination of the left ventricular cavity during systole. Contrast material is frequently pressed into the apical trabecular part of the ventricle, which, therefore, appears isolated from the body of the main cavity (Figure 59.25b) (Goodwin, 1982). Mitral insufficiency is easily demonstrated by angiocardiography. Left ventricular dilation is rare. When present, it is almost always associated with severe and widespread disease, mitral regurgitation or massive myocardial

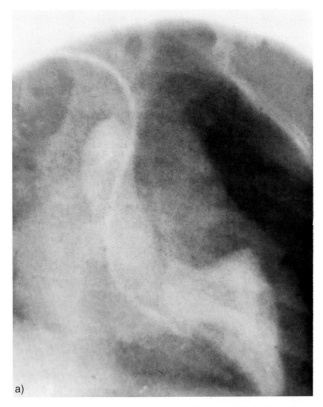 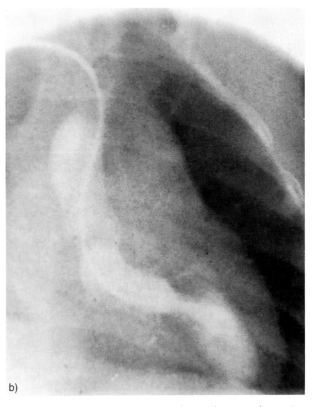

a) b)

Figure 59.24. Cineangiocardiogram of the left ventricle in frontal projection in an 8-year-old child with hypertrophic cardiomyopathy. (a) In diastole, the left ventricular cavity is distorted, with impressions on the superior and inferior border. (b) In systole, the cavity is divided into two compartments.

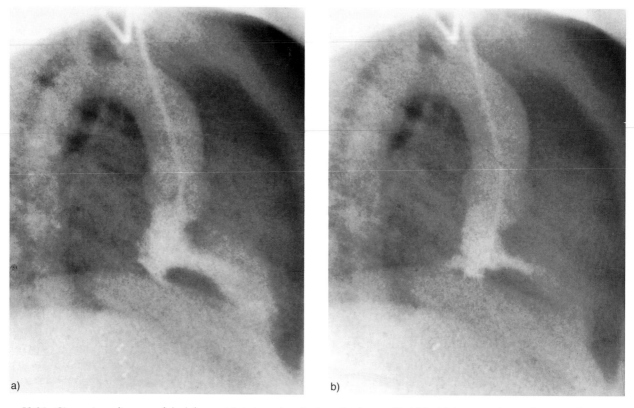

Figure 59.25. Cineangiocardiogram of the left ventricle in lateral projection of a 6-year-old child with hypertrophic cardiomyopathy. (a) In diastole, indentations in the superior and inferior margins give the left ventricular cavity an hour-glass appearance. (b) During systole, the left ventricular cavity is nearly eliminated.

infarction. Right ventricular angiocardiograms can demonstrate bulging of the hypertrophied septum into the right ventricular outflow tract (Figure 59.26). The coronary arteries are often dilated. The angiographic appearance of the ascending aorta and the sinuses of Valsalva is almost always within the normal range. There is no direct correlation between the angiocardiographic features and the haemodynamic findings.

OTHER IMAGING MODALITIES

Magnetic resonance imaging is an alternative non-invasive imaging modality that allows good demarcation of the myocardial wall (Higgins et al, 1985), and hence measurements of wall thickness. It is considered by some a better method in the assessment of degree and extension of hypertrophy (Pons-Llado et al, 1997; Posma et al, 1996), partly because of the poor ultrasonic window found in some patients. It is particularly useful for measurements of the right ventricular free wall (Suzuki et al,

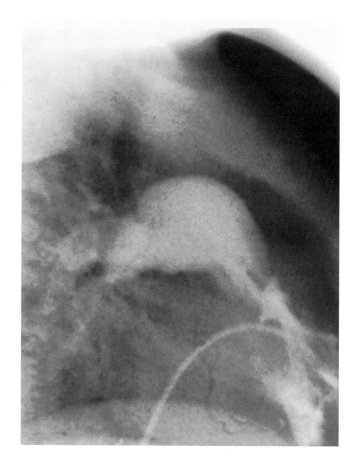

Figure 59.26. Cineangiocardiogram of the right ventricle in lateral projection of a 14-year-old child with hypertrophic cardiomyopathy and right ventricular outflow obstruction. The outflow tract is significantly narrowed by bulging of the hypertrophied ventricular septum.

1988), left ventricular mass (Allison et al, 1993), and in the evaluation of apical hypertrophic cardiomyopathy (Casolo et al, 1989; Soler et al, 1997). More recently, sophisticated techniques such as three-dimensional studies (Dong et al, 1994), cine resonance imaging (Schwammenthal et al, 1994; Nakatani et al, 1996; Sato et al, 1996; Yamanari et al, 1996; Ishino and Nakata, 1997) and gadolinium-enhanced resonance imaging (Koito et al, 1995) have concentrated mainly on the assessment of regional ventricular function. Their place in the clinical assessment of children with hypertrophic cardiomyopathy, however, is limited. Echocardiography is a routine investigation in most institutions worldwide, thus negating the need for further, more expensive, investigations to be carried out.

Myocardial imaging with thallium-201 at rest and during exercise also enables the demonstration of an increased thickness of the ventricular septum and posterior wall, as well as the contour and size of the ventricular chambers. Because the technique also enables demonstration of areas of myocardial ischaemia, it has been used to study pathophysiological implications of ischaemia in patients with hypertrophic cardiomyopathy. Dilsizan and colleagues (1993) showed that exercise-induced ischaemia was a frequent finding in children who had previously suffered cardiac arrest or syncope, whereas Elliot et al (1996) found no association between reversible thallium-201 perfusion defects and exertional chest pain or electrocardiographic changes.

MANAGEMENT

The therapeutic measures in patients with hypertrophic cardiomyopathy are mainly symptomatic. Both medical and surgical treatment appear effective in relieving symptoms in at least a number of patients. In those who are symptomatic, treatment may improve quality of life by relieving symptoms, providing the treatment itself does not have important side effects. In symptom-free patients, however, 'to treat or not to treat' can be a clinical dilemma. It is necessary to balance risks and benefits of introducing therapy. In general, medical therapy is aimed at improving diastolic filling and reducing myocardial contractility. These manoeuvres, therefore, not only reduce the degree of outflow tract obstruction but also reduce myocardial ischaemia by decreasing consumption of oxygen. Consequently, in the presence of strikingly severe ventricular hypertrophy, or outflow tract obstruction, the physician might feel it appropriate to treat even those patients who are asymptomatic. It is important to look for evidence to support the use of drugs based on their haemodynamic effects. It is also important to consider if any of these effects, the control or prevention of arrhythmias or possible effects of the drugs on the extent of hypertrophy might possibly decrease the occurrence of sudden death, stop progression of the disease, or improve

long-term survival. All these issues become even more relevant since a larger number of asymptomatic patients are now frequently recognized, either through screening programmes or from studies of unselected populations. The latter show many patients to be completely asymptomatic or else to have only minor symptoms (Shapiro and Zezulka, 1983; Kofflard et al, 1993; Spirito et al, 1994; Cannan et al, 1995; Cecchi et al, 1995).

MEDICAL TREATMENT

Beta blockade

The use of β-blockers may improve symptoms from one third (Maron et al, 1987a,b) to half (Bonow et al, 1988) of patients. Exercise endurance has also been shown to improve when compared with those using a placebo (Rosing et al, 1985). The presumed mechanism for these effects appears to be related both to the negative inotropic and chronotropic effects on the heart and to vasoconstriction from peripheral β-blockade when noncardioselective blocking agents are used (Webb-Peploe, 1985). Propranolol, by decreasing contractility, increasing afterload and prolonging diastole, decreases gradients across the left ventricular outflow tract and hence reduces myocardial demand for oxygen and, the level of ischaemia (Bonow et al, 1988; Webb-Peploe, 1985). It has no direct effect on myocardial metabolism (Thompson et al, 1980).

Earlier studies suggested that propranolol improved left ventricular filling and relaxation, as evidenced by an increase in left ventricular dimensions, faster diastolic rate of closure of the mitral valve and reduction of isovolumic relaxation time (Saenz de la Calzada et al, 1976). It also ameliorated diastolic distensibility, shown by a decrease in the ratio of diastolic change in pressure to diastolic change in volume (Swanton et al, 1977; Webb-Peploe, 1985). The latter change, however, was not a consistent finding (Speiser and Krayenbuehl, 1981). Although propranolol increases passive ventricular filling by prolongation of the diastolic phase (Harrison et al, 1964; Cohen and Braunwald, 1967; Thompson et al, 1980), it has been shown not to have a direct effect on the active process of relaxation. During isovolumic relaxation, decay of left ventricular pressure resembles an exponential and can be expressed by a time constant of relaxation ('tau'). This time constant has been shown to be prolonged in patients with hypertrophic cardiomyopathy (Thompson et al, 1983) and is not improved by acute use of propranolol (Hess et al, 1983; Thompson et al, 1983). In individual patients, however, by decreasing myocardial ischaemia or heart rate, diastolic function may improve (Bonow et al, 1988).

In standard doses, propranolol has not been shown to decrease the incidence of arrhythmia (Ingham et al, 1978; McKenna et al, 1980), to prevent sudden death (Maron et al, 1982a; Pelliccia et al, 1990) or to affect the magnitude or progression of hypertrophy (Domenicucci et al,

1985). Initial observations on its use in very high doses in children suggested that it might favourably affect progression of hypertrophy (Ostman-Smith, 1991). More recently, Ostman-Smith and Wetrell (1997) presented their retrospective review of young patients with hypertrophic cardiomyopathy, comparing those receiving no treatment, β-blockade or verapamil. They showed better survival, and less morbidity, in the group receiving propranolol in doses varying between 5 and 18 mg/kg. Further prospective studies are needed to confirm these observations.

Calcium antagonists: verapamil

Symptomatic improvement that is superior to that obtained with the use of propranolol (Maron et al, 1985; Rosing et al, 1985), and increased exercise endurance, have been reported with the use of verapamil (Rosing et al, 1979, 1981; Hanrath et al, 1983; Bonow et al, 1985). In adults who were only mild to moderately symptomatic, a recent randomized, double-blind cross-over trial of nadolol, verapamil and placebo has shown neither drug to improve exercise capacity, although symptomatic benefit was reported (Gilligan et al, 1993). Children treated with oral verapamil for a period of up to 20 months have shown similar response to that with propranolol; they also showed less exercise-induced depression of the ST segment (Spicer et al, 1984).

Similarly to β-blockade, verapamil may well exert its beneficial effects by having negative inotropic and chronotropic effects. Decreased contractility, and reduced gradients across the left ventricular outflow tract, therefore, may be responsible for symptomatic improvement (Anderson et al, 1984). Myocardial consumption of oxygen is reduced by lowered blood pressure, either by its negative inotropic effect or because of peripheral vasodilatation (Wilmshurst et al, 1986).

Verapamil seems to enhance left ventricular relaxation and filling when used intravenously or orally (Hanrath et al, 1980a; Bonow et al, 1981, 1983; Hess et al, 1986). Exercise-induced changes in left ventricular peak rate of filling were associated with increased exercise capacity; in patients without improvement in diastolic parameters, no substantial change was noted in the exercise parameters (Bonow et al, 1985). Improvement of left ventricular filling, and better exercise tests, have also been demonstrated in children receiving oral verapamil (Shaffer et al, 1988). Reduction of regional asynchrony after its use may also account for some of its beneficial effects (Bonow et al, 1987). It is not clear if these measured changes in ventricular diastolic function are the result of a direct effect on transarcolemmal influx of calcium or are caused by an indirect action on loading conditions, sympathetic reflexes or myocardial consumption and supply of oxygen (Lorell and Barry, 1984; Walsh, 1989). Fan and colleagues (1995) showed that verapamil, when used acutely in adult patients with diastolic dysfunction,

appeared to improve left ventricular filling by reducing left ventricular afterload.

Despite reports claiming that verapamil might have reduced septal hypertrophy (Troesch et al, 1979) and left ventricular muscle mass (Kaltenbach et al, 1979), differences in measurements were not clinically or statistically significant. Spicer et al (1984) showed significant change in septal thickness in young patients treated with verapamil, but posterior left ventricular wall measurements, although also significantly reduced, varied by only 1 mm. Others have shown no difference in measurements of septal or posterior wall thickness following its use for at least 1 year (Rosing et al, 1981).

In one study, verapamil appeared more effective than propranolol in preventing sudden death, although it was associated with a greater incidence of side effects and the occurrence of non-sudden cardiac deaths caused by progressive myocardial deterioration despite withdrawal of medication (Pelliccia et al, 1990). Death from pulmonary oedema has also been reported (Rosing et al, 1981), based on which its use was contraindicated in patients with a history suggestive of an elevated pulmonary venous pressure. Ostman-Smith and Wetrell (1997) have also shown a higher mortality associated with verapamil compared with propranolol or no treatment.

Further to its haemodynamic effects, the electrophysiological action of verapamil in prolonging conduction in the atrioventricular node must also be considered. In children under the age of 1 year, there are additional medicolegal implications (Garson, 1987). Metabolic clearance increases with age, and metabolism of the drug seems to improve during the first year of life (Piovan et al, 1995). Marked variations in clearance and bioavailability are observed (Echizen and Eichelbaum, 1986), and levels of verapamil in the plasma in children show wide intersubject variability at any given daily dose (Piovan et al, 1995). In a study of nine selected children with hypertrophic cardiomyopathy who were given intravenous verapamil, one went into a junctional escape rhythm and eight had prolongation of the PR interval. Despite these findings, it was suggested that verapamil might be an effective choice for children with this condition, providing there is careful monitoring of levels in the plasma (Spicer et al, 1983). In a subsequent study using oral verapamil, the same group reported no need to discontinue the drug because of side effects (Spicer et al, 1984). Death associated with complete heart block, however, has been reported in children receiving verapamil chronically (Moran and Colan, 1998).

Other calcium antagonists: nifedipine and diltiazem

Results on the use of nifedipine in adults with hypertrophic cardiomyopathy are conflicting and probably reflect the heterogeneity of the populations studied and the status of ventricular function (Ludbrook et al, 1982). Improvement in left ventricular relaxation, diastolic filling and distensibility have been shown by some (Lorell et al, 1982; Paulus et al, 1983), while others have shown no change in diastolic parameters but rather significant reduction of afterload in some. This has potential deleterious effects, with an increase in gradients across the outflow tracts (Betocchi et al, 1985). Yamakado and colleagues (1990) studied symptom-free or minimally symptomatic patients and also showed no advantage from the use of nifedipine.

Diltiazem appears to have beneficial effects on left ventricular relaxation and filling, when used either intravenously or orally (Nagao et al, 1983; Suwa et al, 1984; Betocchi et al, 1996b). Toshima et al (1986) showed similar symptomatic relief with the use of diltiazem. They also showed similar changes on echocardiographic and exercise test variables to those seen with verapamil, but a tendency to have less serious side effects. Its potential use in hypertrophic cardiomyopathy has not been extensively studied, and its systematic use in childhood is not yet reported.

Disopyramide

Disopiramide is a class Ia antiarrhythmic drug, but it also has antagonistic effects against calcium. It has been suggested as an optional drug in the treatment of patients with outflow tract obstruction, since it appears to reduce the gradient significantly (Pollick et al, 1988; Pollick, 1988; Sherrid et al, 1988; Duncan et al, 1991), probably through a negative inotropic effect. It also appears to affect diastolic properties of the myocardium. Echocardiographic indexes of assessing diastolic filling have been shown to improve after intravenous infusion of the drug (Nagashima, 1991; Sumimoto et al, 1992). Matsubara and colleagues (1995), nonetheless, showed that disopyramide only shortened the time constant of left ventricular pressure fall (tau) measured at cardiac catheterization in patients with outflow tract obstruction, and this correlated with a fall in the gradient, suggesting that improved diastolic function is secondary to a reduction in ventricular afterload. Its use in children with hypertrophic cardiomyopathy has not been assessed systematically.

Amiodarone

Amiodarone, a class III antiarrhythmic drug, is effective in treating arrhythmias frequently seen in adults with hypertrophic cardiomyopathy (McKenna et al, 1981b, 1984). It appears to improve survival of those patients manifesting episodes of ventricular tachycardia (McKenna et al, 1985). Amiodarone is used essentially as an antiarrhythmic drug (Delahaye and Azzano, 1994) but is not without adverse effects (Fananapazir and Epstein, 1991; Fananapazir et al, 1991). In patients with hypertrophic cardiomyopathy, QT dispersion on the standard electrocardiogram has been shown to be associated with sudden death (Buja et al, 1993). Dritsas and colleagues (1992) have shown that amiodarone reduced QTc dispersion despite increasing maximum QTc (Fei et al, 1994). As far as ventricular function

is concerned, some studies have suggested that it does not impair systolic function significantly if its use is relatively short term (Sugrue et al, 1984). Others have shown an increase in mean pulmonary capillary wedge pressure and mean pulmonary arterial pressure, both at rest and during exercise (Paulus et al, 1986). It also seems to have a better therapeutic profile than other antiarrhythmic drugs in adults with complex arrhythmias (Antiarrhythmic Drug Evaluation Group, 1992), but side effects are clearly described (Harris et al, 1983). In childhood, despite a higher risk of sudden death, arrhythmias are less common. Its empirical use, therefore, does not appear justified. Its use should be restricted to the patients considered to be at 'very high risk'.

NON-SURGICAL INTERVENTION

The use of dual-chamber pacing has gained favour over recent years as an alternative to surgery for symptomatic adults who are resistant to drug therapy (McDonald et al, 1988; Fananapazir et al, 1992, 1994; Jeanrenaud et al, 1992). The gradient across the outflow tract is probably decreased by altering the sequence of ventricular contraction, but this can also affect ventricular filling and cardiac output (Betocchi et al, 1996a; Nishimura et al, 1996). Furthermore, in a recent randomized, double-blind, crossover study, subjective and objective assessment of exercise endurance were shown to be similar in both treated and untreated groups (Nishimura et al, 1997). Sigwart (1995) recently described an interventional catheter technique by which alcohol injected through the first major septal artery produced a localized area of myocardial infarct, reduced the thickness of the ventricular septum and decreased the gradient across the outflow tract. Further studies are needed to assess long-term results.

SURGICAL TREATMENT

Surgery is contemplated in patients who, despite medical therapy, remain symptomatic. Some asymptomatic patients have also had operations. Reported operative mortality is relatively low (Williams et al, 1987; Mohr et al, 1989; Cohn et al, 1992; Heric et al, 1995), and there is a suggestion that survival is improved (Mohr et al, 1989; Seiler et al, 1991). Most series consist of adults. Symptoms improve, and approximately two thirds are symptom free after the procedure (Mohr et al, 1989). The occurrence of arrhythmias remains a frequent persistent cause of problems in about a quarter of patients (Williams et al, 1987).

CURRENT DILEMMAS ─────────

TO TREAT OR NOT TO TREAT AND HOW?

The need still exists for large longitudinal, population-based studies in asymptomatic and symptomatic children with hypertrophic cardiomyopathy to assess the effects of medical therapy and surgery on symptoms and outcome. The feasibility of such trials, however, is questionable. Symptomatic patients are treated to relieve symptoms. At the Royal Brompton Hospital, medical therapy, mainly propranolol, has been used in a number of children with some improvement of symptoms. Surgery has been carried out in only a small number. For those who remain asymptomatic, there is no standard management. It may seem reasonable to introduce treatment if there is a strong family history of sudden death, or a severe gradient across the outflow tract, in the hope that treatment will change survival. It is also prudent to limit intense or competitive physical activities (Maron et al, 1985), although sudden death may still occur even if physical exercise is minimal (Romeo et al, 1990). As arrhythmias appear to be infrequent in children, and in the lack of evidence that sudden death will be prevented, it seems unreasonable to give drugs to an asymptomatic infant.

TO SCREEN OR NOT TO SCREEN AND HOW?

During family screening for hypertrophic cardiomyopathy, clinical assessment and counselling is difficult, as a normal echocardiogram does not exclude an abnormal genotype. Furthermore, although the electrocardiogram appears to be a more sensitive test, both examinations can be normal in patients who carry the mutation (al-Mahdawi et al, 1994; Ryan et al, 1995). Those with the mutation, however, amounted to only 3% of adults known to have hypertrophic cardiomyopathy, or identified as having a mutation of β-myosin (Ryan et al, 1995). The clinical significance for an individual who is normal clinically yet carries the mutation is unknown. This emphasizes the dilemmas surrounding genetic screening, particularly when considering for the possibility of prenatal or preclinical diagnosis of carrier status (Rosenzweig et al, 1991).

Dilemmas also occur if a positive clinical diagnosis is made during screening programmes of patients who are completely asymptomatic, particularly when such diagnosis is made at a very young age. Parents, in particular, must consider the implications for themselves and their offspring should the diagnosis be made. Although many patients might want to know their own status, it is arguable when that decision is made for their children. Other aspects than medical ones of making a positive diagnosis in an asymptomatic child need to be discussed prior to generalized screening. Screening for hypertrophic cardiomyopathy has, and will, generate much more discussion (Clark and Coats, 1993; Harper and Clarke, 1993; McLatchie et al, 1993; Marteau and Michie, 1995).

——RESTRICTIVE CARDIOMYOPATHY——

Of all types of cardiomyopathy, the restrictive one is the least common. It is defined by the presence of an abnor-

mal diastolic function, with restriction to ventricular filling and consequent reduction of diastolic volume of the right, the left or both ventricles. Typically, systolic function and ventricular wall thickness are normal, or nearly so (WHO/ISFC, 1996). By definition, therefore, the main characteristic of a restrictive cardiomyopathy is a haemodynamic change. Although it can be an idiopathic condition, a variety of pathological processes may generate similar abnormal haemodynamic status. Restriction may be related to an abnormal endocardium, the myocardium or both. It may also be associated with cardiac infiltration and obliteration. Specific disease processes include amyloidosis, a condition that is the most common cause of restrictive cardiomyopathy in adults but is not seen in childhood. Historically, however, two main pathological conditions have been associated with the clinical and haemodynamic features of restrictive cardiomyopathy. These are endomyocardial fibrosis and Loffler's endocarditis (Loffler, 1936).

In 1948, Davies described the presence of extensive fibrosis of the endocardium and myocardium in a population of Africans. The condition, named endomyocardial fibrosis, was initially thought to be confined to Africa. Since then, it has been reported in other tropical countries in different continents, but also in the United States of America and the United Kingdom (Clark et al, 1956; Dissanayake, 1959; Nakajima et al, 1961; Faruque, 1963; Andrade and Guimaraes, 1964; Contreras et al, 1971; Puigbo et al, 1983). In 1936, Loffler described a condition named parietal fibroplastic endocarditis, thought to occur in temperate zones and to be associated with eosinophilia. It is also referred to as Loffler's eosinophilic endocarditis. These two entities were believed initially to be different diseases. Decades have now passed since their initial description and, although far from understanding the whole pathological process, evidence seems to show that there is a connection between hypereosinophilia and endomyocardial disease (Gerbaux et al, 1956; Ive et al, 1967; Roberts et al, 1969). Following Loffler's description, others have reported patients with similar clinical and pathological features who were considered to have 'eosinophilic leukaemia' (Evans and Nesbit, 1949; Fadell et al, 1957; Bentley et al, 1961). Subsequently, further patients have been identified with associated eosinophilia with endomyocardial fibrosis (Roberts et al, 1969; Brockington et al, 1970). It is now considered that Loffler's endocarditis and Davies' endomyocardial fibrosis are simply the same disease process seen at different stages (Roberts et al, 1970). The various causes of high numbers of eosinophils in the blood, including the idiopathic form, are encompassed under the name 'hypereosinophilic syndrome' (Hardy and Anderson, 1968). In the presence of cardiac involvement, the term 'endomyocardial disease with or without eosinophilia' is used (Paquet and Hanna, 1990). A comprehensive review of the association between eosinophilia and endomyocardial disease was provided by Olsen and Spry (1985).

Apart from these associations, restrictive cardiomyopathy can also be an idiopathic condition. Clinically and haemodynamically, it may simulate constrictive pericarditis, and differentiation of the two can be difficult. Its rarity, not only in adults but also in children, accounts for the paucity of data on the subject. Histology may show interstitial myocardial fibrosis. Recent descriptions of electron microscopical findings in patients with the haemodynamics of restrictive cardiomyopathy also suggest that restrictive and hypertrophic cardiomyopathies may share some of the morphological changes of myocardial disarray (Angelini et al, 1997).

PREVALENCE AND EPIDEMIOLOGY

Idiopathic restrictive cardiomyopathy is rare in adults. It accounted for less than 0.5% of all patients undergoing diagnostic cardiac catheterization in Boston between 1975 and 1978, this corresponding to about 11% of all patients diagnosed as having cardiomyopathy (Benotti et al, 1980). As with all other types of cardiomyopathy, it is difficult to ascertain prevalence in the general population. It appears to be even rarer in childhood. In hospital environments, an average of about one patient with the condition was seen every 2 years (Lewis, 1992; Cetta et al, 1995). Denfield et al (1997) recently reported 12 patients seen over nearly 30 years, but only a proportion of these seemed to be truly 'idiopathic'. It is uncommon for the idiopathic variant to present in the first year of life. Age at presentation in different reported series ranges from 0.9 to 15 years (Mehta et al, 1984; Gewillig et al, 1992; Lewis, 1992; Cetta et al, 1995; Denfield et al, 1997). Median age at diagnosis is reported by some to be about 3 years (Lewis, 1992; Denfield et al, 1997), and by others to be around 11 years (Mehta et al, 1984; Cetta et al, 1995). This difference probably reflects the heterogeneity of the hospital-based populations studied. The disease appears to affect both sexes in a similar way (Mehta et al, 1984; Lewis, 1992; Cetta et al, 1995). Most cases seem to be sporadic, but familial cases are reported (Aroney et al, 1988; Fitzpatrick et al, 1990; Lewis, 1992; Angelini et al, 1997), including one family with Noonan syndrome (Cooke et al, 1994). Katritsis and colleagues (1991) suggest that restrictive cardiomyopathy may have dominant inheritance with incomplete penetrance.

NATURAL HISTORY

Benotti and colleagues (1980) suggested that the prognosis is poor in adults if there is a specific infiltrative or fibrotic process leading to restrictive cardiomyopathy. In nine patients with the idiopathic form, they observed symptomatic improvement and no deaths during a mean follow-up period of 22 months. Similarly, Siegel et al (1984) also encountered adults with a restrictive haemodynamic profile without any associated infiltrative process who exhibited stable and prolonged clinical course extending up to 14 years.

A worse prognosis, however, with poor response to medical therapy and progressive deterioration, is reported in children (Gewillig et al, 1992; Lewis, 1992; Cetta et al, 1995; Denfield et al, 1997). All presented series are small. Clinical presentation is usually with heart failure, but absence of pulmonary venous congestion predicts a longer survival (Cetta et al, 1995). Embolic episodes are relatively common and occurred in one third of patients in one series (Denfield et al, 1997). Marked elevation of pulmonary vascular resistance may also develop relatively early in the course of the disease (Denfield et al, 1997), with further clinical deterioration and worsening outcome. Lewis (1992) found actuarial survival at 1.5 years to be 44%, falling to 29% at 4 years. Cetta and colleagues (1995) followed eight children with idiopathic restrictive cardiomyopathy. Of these, over half died during the median follow-up time of 11.5 years, with half of these dying in the first year after presentation. Denfield et al (1997) also observed a high mortality, with three quarters of the children dying within 6 years of presentation.

AETIOLOGY AND PATHOGENESIS

The intrinsic mechanisms that ultimately lead to abnormal relaxation and impaired filling in idiopathic restrictive cardiomyopathy are unknown. In some patients, there are morphological changes of interstitial fibrosis, but normal myocardial appearances have also been documented in patients with the diagnostic haemodynamic profile (Benotti et al, 1980).

As discussed previously, there are a number of diseases, especially infiltrative processes, that are known to affect the myocardium and lead to altered ventricular compliance (see above).

The exact role of eosinophils in pathogenesis is uncertain. The eosinophil itself appears to have a direct causal effect in the pathological process, ultimately leading to endomyocardial fibrosis, possibly related to an immunological reaction (Libanoff and McMahon, 1976) or a direct toxic effect on the endocardium (Spry and Tai, 1976).

PATHOLOGY

The heart is usually of normal size, but with ventricular cavities that are markedly obliterated by extensive endocardial thickening. The tension apparatus of the atrioventricular valves is usually incorporated within the obliterative process. Histology reveals endomyocardial fibrosis. In early stages of the disease, it may be possible to find an eosinophilic cellular infiltration, often accompanied by an early proliferative endocardial reaction. These changes may be seen in biopsy samples.

PATHOPHYSIOLOGY

The various pathological processes that involve the myocardium and endocardium lead to a restrictive physiology owing to decreased ventricular diastolic compliance. Compliance relates changes in pressure that occur in response to a certain change in volume. If it is reduced, a small increase in volume results in a much higher than expected increase in pressure. With this disturbance in the pressure–volume characteristics, there is a sudden elevation in pressure as the ventricular cavity fills. This starts in early diastole and is maintained throughout this phase of the cardiac cycle. Elevated left and right ventricular end-diastolic pressures lead to an increase in left and right atrial pressures, with consequent pulmonary venous congestion, pulmonary hypertension, and systemic venous hypertension, respectively.

CLINICAL FEATURES

Symptoms are the rule in patients with restrictive cardiomyopathy. Clinical manifestation may vary depending on whether the left, right, or both ventricles are involved in the process. In the series of Lewis and colleagues (Lewis, 1992), comprising eight children with idiopathic restrictive cardiomyopathy, all had marked systemic venous congestion and hepatomegaly. In nine adults (Benotti et al, 1980), dyspnoea on exertion and fatigue were the most common complaints, followed by peripheral oedema and atypical chest pain. Murmurs are common (Benotti et al, 1980; Lewis, 1992). They were observed in the majority of children and found to be caused by atrioventricular valvar regurgitation. A gallop rhythm may also be present (Lewis, 1992). In some patients, an associated skeletal myopathy has been reported (Fitzpatrick et al, 1990; Katritsis et al, 1991).

INVESTIGATIONS

ELECTROCARDIOGRAPHY

The electrocardiogram shows marked atrial enlargement in virtually all patients. ST segment and T wave changes are also a common finding, although left ventricular hypertrophy is seen in less than half (Lewis, 1992). Impaired atrioventricular conduction is frequently reported (Mehta et al, 1984; Lewis, 1992). and may vary from first-degree block to complete heart block requiring pacemaker implantation. Although children are usually in sinus rhythm, it is of interest that, in the series of Siegel

and colleagues (1984), all adults were in atrial fibrillation. All required insertion of pacemakers during follow-up, either because of atrioventricular block or sick sinus syndrome. Heart block has also been documented in a family with restrictive cardiomyopathy (Fitzpatrick et al, 1990).

CHEST RADIOGRAPHY

A cardiothoracic ratio greater than 0.5 on the chest radiograph is frequently seen both in children (Lewis, 1992) and adults (Benotti et al, 1980; Siegel et al, 1984). Pulmonary venous congestion is a common finding (Siegel et al, 1984; Lewis, 1992; Cetta et al, 1995).

ECHOCARDIOGRAPHY

The most striking reported finding on the echocardiogram of a child with restrictive cardiomyopathy is atrial dilation associated with normal or near normal ventricular dimensions and systolic function (Figure 59.27). M-mode measurements of wall thickness shows normal or mildly increased values (Mehta et al, 1984). Both the left and right atriums were affected in all children studied by Lewis and colleagues (Lewis, 1992), and also in those reported by Cetta and colleagues (1995). Left atrial enlargement was also a constant feature in those reviewed by Mehta et al (1984). Conversely, in a series of adults in which patients were selected subsequent to catheterization and fulfilled the haemodynamic criteria for restrictive physiology, there was great variability on the echocardiographic findings, including two patients reported to be normal. Only one out of nine adults in this series showed an enlarged left atrium (Benotti et al, 1980). Although this discrepancy might result, in some part, from different criteria for inclusion, the lack of

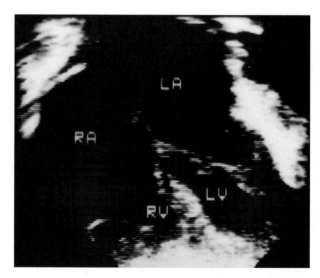

Figure 59.27. Apical four chamber view obtained from a child with restrictive cardiomyopathy. Note the gross dilation of both atriums. Abbreviations as in Figure 59.19.

reported similar series in children possibly reflects the fact that atrial dilatation occurs much earlier in the course of the disease in children compared with adults, leading to a worse outlook for children with restrictive cardiomyopathy.

The echocardiographic findings encountered in patients with endomyocardial disease with or without eosinophilia have certain diagnostic characteristics. Abnormal high-intensity echoes were observed in some patients and seemed to correspond to known areas of fibrosis, namely the apical ventricular portions, the inflow tract of the right ventricle and the posterior wall and papillary muscles of the mitral valve (Davies et al, 1982). Apical obliteration with hyperechoic endocardial surface and involvement of the papillary muscles and leaflets of the atrioventricular valves was also observed by others (Acquatella et al, 1983). The echocardiographic findings also seem to correlate well with clinical presentation. Gottdiener et al (1983) found that, in those patients who have mitral regurgitation clinically, there was an abnormal thickening of the posterior wall of the left ventricle behind the mural leaflet of the mitral valve, as well as impaired excursion of this leaflet. Similarly, echodense structures suggestive of thrombus were identified in the apical region and inflow tract of the left ventricle, or in both in those patients who had clinical manifestations of systemic embolism.

Doppler assessment is consistent with a restrictive filling pattern and elevated end-diastolic pressures, showing short atrioventricular deceleration time and increased E/A ratio (Figure 59.28) (Appleton et al, 1988; Cetta et al, 1995; Cohen et al, 1996). Atrioventricular valvar regurgitation can be documented in a significant number (Figure 59.29) (Lewis, 1992).

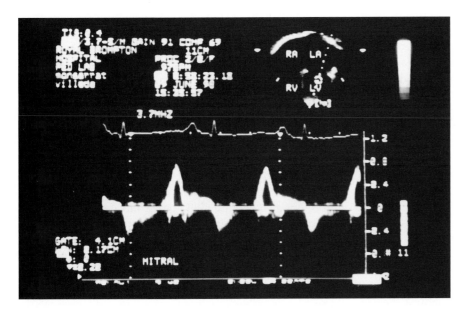

Figure 59.28. Pulsed wave Doppler signal across the mitral valve obtained from a child with restrictive cardiomyopathy. There is a rapid deceleration slope during early ventricular filling (E wave) but no demonstrable flow in late diastole.

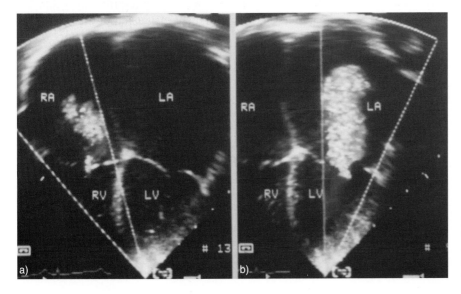

Figure 59.29. Apical four chamber view (a) with additional colour flow mapping (b) obtained from a child with restrictive cardiomyopathy. Note obvious regurgitation of both atrioventricular valves.

CARDIAC CATHETERIZATION

The haemodynamic profile of restriction owing to abnormal ventricular compliances is well demonstrated by cardiac catheterization. There is a significant fall in ventricular pressure at the onset of diastole with a rapid and abrupt rise in the early phase of diastole. This is known as a 'dip-and-plateau' pattern, corresponding to a prominent descent and rapid rise and plateau in the atrial pressure recording. The sharp rise in ventricular pressure and abrupt plateau in early diastole gives rise to the so-called 'square root sign' (Benotti et al, 1980). This pattern is characteristic of either restrictive cardiomyopathy or constrictive pericarditis. Right and left ventricular end-diastolic pressures may be very close to each other, differing by only 3–4 mmHg, or may be almost superimposable, again simulating constrictive pericarditis. Benotti and colleagues (1980) found that left ventricular end-diastolic pressure exceeded the corresponding right ventricular pressure by at lest 5 mmHg in nearly four fifths of their patients. In some patients, based on haemodynamic criterions, differential diagnosis between the two conditions was difficult. In the children studied by Lewis and colleagues (Lewis, 1992), mean left ventricular end-diastolic pressure was significantly higher than the right-sided pressure. In two patients, however, they differed by only 4–5 mmHg.

Various invasive and non-invasive methods have been used to differentiate between restriction and constriction (Aroney et al, 1989; Gerson et al, 1989; Hatle et al, 1989; Morgan et al, 1989; Klein et al, 1993; Garcia et al, 1996; Akasaka et al, 1997). As pointed out by Vaitkus and Kussmaul (1991), many of the proposed indexes are complex, limiting their clinical use. Although distinction between the two groups might be possible, only endomyocardial biopsy (Schoenfeld et al, 1987) or exploratory thoracotomy is likely to give the answer in many cases. Endomyocardial biopsy may show a specific infiltrative process (Schoenfeld et al, 1987), but a normal result does not entirely rule out an idiopathic restrictive cardiomyopathy (Benotti et al, 1980).

MANAGEMENT

Management of restrictive cardiomyopathy in childhood is difficult, as there is poor response to medical therapy in all reported series. Cardiac transplantation should be considered early in the course of the disease (Lewis, 1992). Conventional treatment of heart failure with diuretics may produce hypotension owing to a decrease in preload (Paquet and Hanna, 1990). Haemodynamic measurements at cardiac catheterization after oral captopril showed no increase in cardiac output but revealed systemic hypotension. This drug, therefore, should not be used in children with restrictive cardiomyopathy (Bengur et al, 1991). Because of the similarity in the haemodynamics to hypertrophic cardiomyopathy, the use of calcium-blocking agents such as verapamil has been suggested because of its effects on diastolic function (Benotti et al, 1980). This, however, has still to be fully evaluated.

Resection of subendocardial fibrosis with or without valvar replacement can lead to symptomatic improvement in some patients (Moraes et al, 1983; da Costa et al, 1989). Replacement of the mitral valve has also been reported in idiopathic hypereosinophilic syndrome (Blake et al, 1985; Hendren et al, 1988; Boustany et al, 1991).

DIFFERENTIAL DIAGNOSIS OF CARDIOMYOPATHY

In childhood, one usually faces a long list of systemic disorders that might affect the myocardium and simulate the clinical and echocardiographic picture of cardiomyopathy. These are, in general, uncommon or rare disorders. In many instances, there will be involvement of other organs that will give a clue to any possible association with other disease processes. When facing a new patient whose echocardiogram resembles cardiomyopathy, and particularly in the child in the first year of life, it may be appropriate to perform basic investigations for certain known conditions. If present, they might give further insight into prognosis for the particular child and help in counselling the families.

We have tried over the years to develop a protocol of investigations for such cases. This has proven difficult, in part because of the numerous rarities reported in the literature but also because many of the metabolic tests can be difficult to interpret. Interpretation of the profile of organic acids, for example, often depends on the clinical condition of the child. Because of the complexity of metabolic pathways, advice from an expert in metabolic disorders is desirable. Many of the tests require a large amount of blood. This is often difficult to obtain in a small child, particularly for what usually turns out to be a negative investigation. Nevertheless, we have tried to simplify this approach. We acknowledge that the guidelines which follow are far from complete but may be more practical. Others (Lombes et al, 1987) who routinely perform complex investigations have found a high prevalence of mitochondrial and respiratory chain defects associated with cardiomyopathies in childhood. These investigations are not, however, without a risk to the patient (Matthys et al, 1991).

The protocol that appears in Table 59.2 and 59.3 is a guideline to provide minimal investigations for a child with cardiomyopathy, yet it aims at excluding conditions such as aortic coarctation or anomalous left coronary artery from the pulmonary trunk before submitting the child to a long list of investigations for a possible cardiomyopathy. It should be tailored to the individual child and particular hospital where investigations are carried out.

Some of the suggested investigations are common routine tests such as full blood count, electrolytes and

Table 59.2. Protocol for investigating a child with suspected cardiomyopathy.

ECHOCARDIOGRAPHIC APPEARANCES

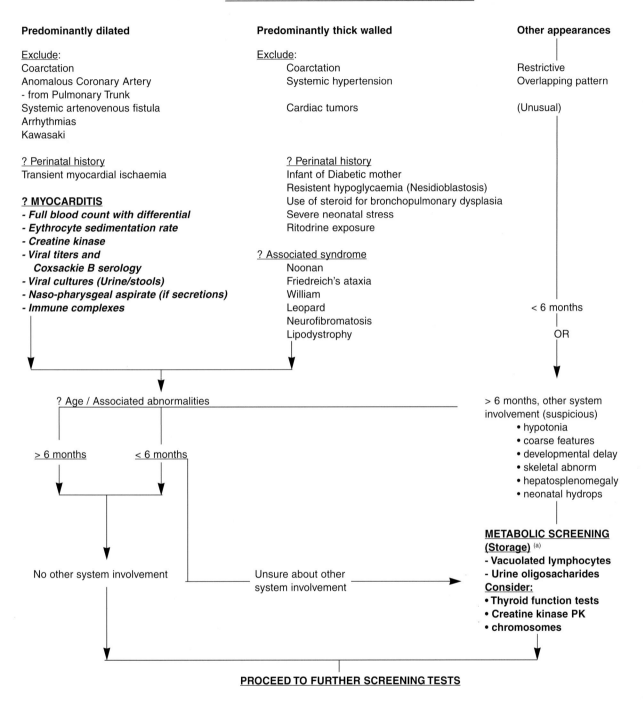

Predominantly dilated

Exclude:
Coarctation
Anomalous Coronary Artery
- from Pulmonary Trunk
Systemic artenovenous fistula
Arrhythmias
Kawasaki

? Perinatal history
Transient myocardial ischaemia

? MYOCARDITIS
- Full blood count with differential
- Eythrocyte sedimentation rate
- Creatine kinase
- Viral titers and
 Coxsackie B serology
- Viral cultures (Urine/stools)
- Naso-pharysgeal aspirate (if secretions)
- Immune complexes

? Age / Associated abnormalities

> 6 months   < 6 months

No other system involvement

Predominantly thick walled

Exclude:
Coarctation
Systemic hypertension

Cardiac tumors

? Perinatal history
Infant of Diabetic mother
Resistent hypoglycaemia (Nesidioblastosis)
Use of steroid for bronchopulmonary dysplasia
Severe neonatal stress
Ritodrine exposure

? Associated syndrome
Noonan
Friedreich's ataxia
William
Leopard
Neurofibromatosis
Lipodystrophy

Unsure about other
system involvement

Other appearances

Restrictive
Overlapping pattern

(Unusual)

< 6 months

OR

> 6 months, other system
involvement (suspicious)
• hypotonia
• coarse features
• developmental delay
• skeletal abnorm
• hepatosplenomegaly
• neonatal hydrops

**METABOLIC SCREENING
(Storage)** [a]
- Vacuolated lymphocytes
- Urine oligosacharides
Consider:
• Thyroid function tests
• Creatine kinase PK
• chromosomes

PROCEED TO FURTHER SCREENING TESTS

[a]Storage diseases:

• Glycogen storage: Pompe's disease (dilated ventricle with thick wall and poor function)
• mucopolysaccharidoses: Hurler, Marateaux–Lamy (similar to hypertrophic cardiomyopathy or dilated, endocardial fibroelastosis)
• gangliosidosis: GM1 generalized gangliosidosis (dilated)
• sialic acid storage (dilated, poor function, thickened ventricular wall).

liver function tests. Other tests, such as chromosomal as analysis and assessment of thyroid function, may be indicated based on individual findings. Analysis of the blood film for the presence of vacuolated lymphocytes constitutes a useful screening test in the young infant. The main diagnosis of concern Pompe's disease, but other storage diseases may also present white cells with abnormal vacuoles. Although these metabolic conditions are rare, it is important to exclude them, not only for the child's prognosis but also for family counselling. The blood film must,

Table 59.3. Further screening tests after preliminary assessment of a child with suspected cardiomyopathy.

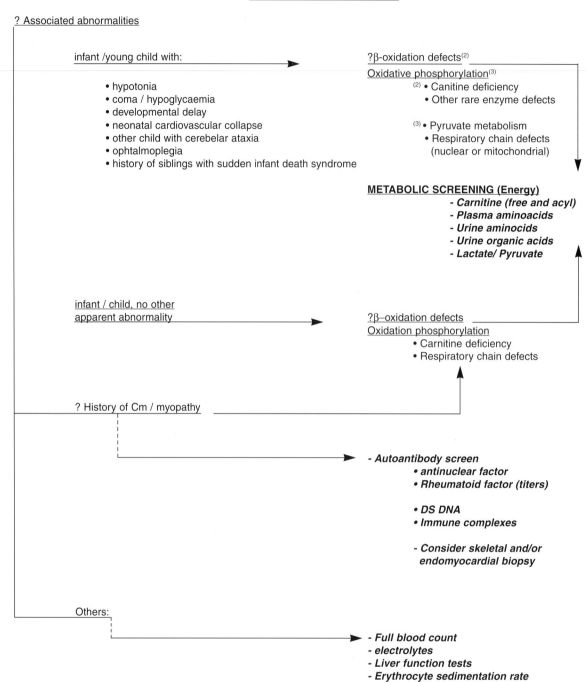

FURTHER SCREENING TESTS

? Associated abnormalities

infant /young child with:

?β-oxidation defects[2]

Oxidative phosphorylation[3]

- • hypotonia
- • coma / hypoglycaemia
- • developmental delay
- • neonatal cardiovascular collapse
- • other child with cerebelar ataxia
- • ophtalmoplegia
- • history of siblings with sudden infant death syndrome

[2] • Canitine deficiency
 • Other rare enzyme defects

[3] • Pyruvate metabolism
 • Respiratory chain defects
  (nuclear or mitochondrial)

METABOLIC SCREENING (Energy)
 - *Carnitine (free and acyl)*
 - *Plasma aminoacids*
 - *Urine aminocids*
 - *Urine organic acids*
 - *Lactate/ Pyruvate*

infant / child, no other
apparent abnormality

?β–oxidation defects
Oxidation phosphorylation
 • Carnitine deficiency
 • Respiratory chain defects

? History of Cm / myopathy

- *Autoantibody screen*
  • *antinuclear factor*
  • *Rheumatoid factor (titers)*

  • *DS DNA*
  • *Immune complexes*

 - *Consider skeletal and/or
  endomyocardial biopsy*

Others:

 - *Full blood count*
 - *electrolytes*
 - *Liver function tests*
 - *Erythrocyte sedimentation rate*

however, be interpreted by an experienced investigator. The investigation for urinary glycosaminoglycans used to be part of our routine screening tests for metabolic disorders, aimed mainly at excluding one of the mucopolysaccharidoses. These conditions should always be considered, particularly in the young infant with a predominantly dilated ventricle and poor ventricular function. Disorders of mucopolysaccharides should be picked up when check-ing vacuolated lymphocytes, but if the search for vacuolated lymphocytes is negative, and/or there is strong suspicion of a storage disorder, other investigations are indicated, including, for example, analysis of specific white cell enzymes. Such analysis is more than just a screening test. If there is strong suspicion of a metabolic abnormality, such as mucopolysacharidoses, this might be a more appropriate and straightforward test. It should not be a routine test for all children with cardiomyopathy, as it is not cost effective.

Certain investigations, such as taking samples for measurements of pyruvate, may require special arrangements with local laboratories in order for these to be processed adequately. Testing for creatine kinase is usually a routine test in the laboratory. Analysis of the myocardial fraction, however, is usually requested separately. It is, therefore, appropriate to discuss the protocol with the different laboratories involved. In small children, one should try to use the minimal feasible amount of blood for carrying out the investigations. This should be discussed and organized well in advance to avoid taking repeated blood samples in small children.

Several investigations are considered under special circumstances only, either on the basis of results of previous investigations and/or based on family history. Skeletal/endomyocardial biopsies, and screening for autoantibodies, could be done as part of the routine tests but may require another 3 ml of blood. Measurement of iron requires an extra 2 ml of blood and it might not be justified to use this as a routine test. If there is a history of multiple blood transfusions, then secondary haemochromatosis is a diagnostic possibility and should, therefore, be investigated. Primary haemochromatosis is rare. If it is thought necessary to assay white cell enzymes or take a liver or skin biopsy, then it is appropriate to refer the child to a specialized metabolic unit.

REFERENCES

Acquatella H, Schiller N B, Puigbo J J et al 1983 Value of two-dimensional echocardiography in endomyocardial disease with and without eosinophilia. A clinical and pathologic study. Circulation 67: 1219–1226

Ades L C, Gedeon A K, Wilson M J et al 1993 Barth syndrome: clinical features and confirmation of gene localisation to distal Xq28. American Journal of Medical Genetics 45: 327–334

Agaki T, Benson L N, Lightfoot N E et al 1991 Natural history of dilated cardiomyopathy in children. American Heart Journal 121: 1502–1503

Agnoletti G, Donzelli C, Benetti A et al 1995 The finding of endocardial fibroelastosis in a 20-week-old fetus. Cardiologia 40: 515–517

Agostini P G, de Cesare N, Doria E et al 1986 Afterload reduction: A comparison of captopril and nifedipine in dilated cardiomyopathy. British Heart Journal 55: 391–399

Akasaka T, Yoshida K, Yamamuro A et al 1997 Phasic coronary flow characteristics in patients with constrictive pericarditis: comparison with restrictive cardiomyopathy. Circulation 96: 1874–1881

al-Mahdawi S, Chamberlain S, Chojnowska L et al 1994 The electrocardiogram is a more sensitive indicator than echocardiography of hypertrophic cardiomyopathy in families with a mutation in the MYH7 gene. British Heart Journal 72: 105–111

Alboliras E T, Shub C, Gomez M R et al 1986 Spectrum of cardiac involvement in Friedreich's ataxia: clinical, electrocardiographic and echocardiographic observations. American Journal of Cardiology 58: 518–524

Allison J D, Flickinger F W, Wright J C et al 1993 Measurement of left ventricular mass in hypertrophic cardiomyopathy using MRI: comparison with echocardiography. Magnetic Resonance Imaging 11: 329–334

Anderson D M, Raff G L, Ports T A et al 1984 Hypertrophic obstructive cardiomyopathy. Effects of acute and chronic verapamil treatment on left ventricular systolic and diastolic function. British Heart Journal 51: 523–529

Anderson J L, Carlquist J F, Hammond E H 1982 Deficient natural killer cell activity in patients with idiopathic dilated cardiomyopathy. Lancet ii: 1124–1127

Anderson J L, Carlquist J F, Lutz J R et al 1984 HLA A, B and DR typing in idiopathic dilated cardiomyopathy: A search for immune response factors. American Journal of Cardiology 53: 1326–1330

Andrade Z A, Guimaraes A C 1964 Endomyocardial fibrosis in Bahia, Brazil. British Heart Journal 26: 813–820

Angelini A, Calzolari V, Thiene G et al 1997 Morphologic spectrum of primary restrictive cardiomyopathy. American Journal of Cardiology 80: 1046–1050

Antiarrhythmic Drug Evaluation Group 1992 A multicentre, randomized trial on the benefit/risk profile of amiodarone, flecainide and propafenone in patients with cardiac disease and complex ventricular arrhythmias. European Heart Journal 13: 1251–1258

Appleton C P, Hatle L K, Popp R L 1988 Demonstration of restrictive ventricular physiology by Doppler echocardiography. Journal of American College of Cardiology 11: 757–768

Aretz H T 1987 Myocarditis: the Dallas criteria. Human Pathology 18: 619–624

Aroney C, Bett N, Radford D 1988 Familial restrictive cardiomyopathy. Australian and New Zealand Journal of Medicine 18: 877–878

Aroney C N, Ruddy T D, Dighero H et al 1989 Differentiation of restrictive cardiomyopathy from pericardial constriction: assessment of diastolic function by radionuclide angiography. Journal of American College of Cardiology 13: 1007–1014

Artman M, Parrish M D, Appleton S et al 1987 Hemodynamic effects of hydralazine in infants with idiopathic dilated cardiomyopathy and congestive heart failure. American Heart Journal 113: 144–150

Bahl O P, Massie F 1972 Electrocardiographic and vectorcardiographic patterns in cardiomyopathy. Davis, Philadelphia, PA 95–112

Barr P A, Celermajer J M, Bowdler J D et al 1973 Idiopathic hypertrophic obstructive cardiomyopathy causing severe right ventricular outflow tract obstruction in infancy. British Heart Journal 35: 1109–1115

Barth P G, Scholte H R, Berden J A et al 1983 An X-linked mitochondrial disease affecting cardiac muscle, skeletal muscle and neutrophil leucocytes. Journal of the Neurological Sciences 62: 327–355

Barth P G, van den Bogert C, Bolhuis P A et al 1996 X-linked cardioskeletal myopathy and neutropenia (Barth syndrome): respiratory-chain abnormalities in cultured fibroblasts. Journal of Inherited Metabolic Disease 19: 157–160

Becker A E, Caruso G 1982 Myocardial disarray. A critical review. British Heart Journal 47: 527–538

Beekman R H, Rocchini A P, Dick M II et al 1984 Vasodilator therapy in children: acute and chronic effects in children with left ventricular dysfunction or mitral regurgitation. Pediatrics 73: 43–51

Benchimol A, Legler J F, Dimond E J 1963 The carotid tracing and apex cardiogram in subaortic stenosis and idiopathic myocardial hypertrophy. American Journal of Cardiology 11: 427–435

Bender J R 1991 Idiopathic dilated cardiomyopathy. An immunologic, genetic, or infectious disease, or all of the above? Circulation 83: 704–706

Bengur A R, Beekman R H, Rocchini A P et al 1991 Acute hemodynamic effects of captopril in children with a congestive or restrictive cardiomyopathy. Circulation 83: 523–527

Bennett M J, Hale D E, Pollitt R J et al 1996 Endocardial fibroelastosis and primary carnitine deficiency due to a defect in the plasma membrane carnitine transporter (clinical conference). Clinical Cardiology 19: 243–246

Benotti JR, Grossman W, Cohn PF 1980 Clinical profile of restrictive cardiomyopathy. Circulation 61: 1206–1212

Benson L N 1992 Dilated cardiomyopathies of childhood. Progress in Pediatric Cardiology 1: 13–36

Bentley H P, Jr, Reardon A E, Knoedler J P et al 1961 Eosinophilic leukemia. Report of a case with review and classification. American Journal of Medicine 30: 310–312

Bercu B A, Diettert G A, Danforth W H et al 1958 Pseudoaortic stenosis produced by ventricular hypertrophy. American Journal of Medicine 25: 814–825

Berheim P I 1910 De l'asystolie veneiuse dans l'hypertrophie du coeur gauche, par stinose concomitant du ventricule droit revue. Medicine (Paris) 30: 785

Berko B A, Swift M 1987 X-linked dilated cardiomyopathy. New England Journal of Medicine 316: 1186–1191

Betocchi S, Cannon R O, Watson R M et al 1985 Effects of sublingual nifedipine on hemodynamics and systolic and diastolic function in patients with hypertrophic cardiomyopathy. Circulation 72: 1001–1007

Betocchi S, Losi M A, Piscione F et al 1996a Effects of dual-chamber pacing in hypertrophic cardiomyopathy on left ventricular outflow tract obstruction and on diastolic function. American Journal of Cardiology 77: 498–502

Betocchi S, Piscione F, Losi M et al 1996b Effects of diltiazem on left ventricular systolic and diastolic function in hypertrophic cardiomyopathy. American Journal of Cardiology 78: 451–457

Bhargava H, Donner R M, Sanchez G et al 1987 Endomyocardial biopsy after heart transplantation in children. Journal of Heart Transplantation 6: 298–302

Bjorkhem G, Lundstrom N R, Wallentin I et al 1981 Endocardial fibroelastosis with predominant involvement of left atrium. Possibility of diagnosis by non-invasive methods. British Heart Journal 46: 331–337

Blake D P, Palmer T E, Olinger G N 1985 Mitral valve replacement in idiopathic hypereosinophilic syndrome. Journal of Thoracic and Cardiovascular Surgery 89: 630–632

Bleyl S B, Mumford B R, Brown-Harrison M C et al 1997 Xq28-linked noncompaction of the left ventricular myocardium: prenatal diagnosis and pathologic analysis of affected individuals. American Journal of Medical Genetics 72: 257–265

Bloom K R 1978 Muscular subaortic stenosis, Vol. 3. McMillan, New York, 710–719

Bonow R O, Rosing D R, Bacharach S L et al 1981 Effects of verapamil on left ventricular systolic function and diastolic filling in patients with hypertrophic cardiomyopathy. Circulation 64: 787–796

Bonow R O, Ostrow H G, Rosing D R et al 1983 Effects of verapamil on left ventricular systolic and diastolic function in patients with hypertrophic cardiomyopathy: pressure–volume analysis with a nonimaging scintillation probe. Circulation 68: 1062–1073

Bonow R O, Dilsizian V, Rosing D R et al 1985 Verapamil-induced improvement in left ventricular diastolic filling and increased exercise tolerance in patients with hypertrophic cardiomyopathy: short-and long-term effects. Circulation 72: 853–864

Bonow R O, Vitale D F, Maron B J et al 1987 Regional left ventricular asynchrony and impaired global left ventricular filling in hypertrophic cardiomyopathy: effect of verapamil. Journal of the American College of Cardiology 9: 1108–1116

Bonow R O, Maron B J, Leon M B et al 1988 Medical and surgical therapy of hypertrophic cardiomyopathy. Cardiovascular Clinics 19: 221–239

Boustany C W, Jr., Murphy G W, Hicks G L, Jr. 1991 Mitral valve replacement in idiopathic hypereosinophilic syndrome. Annals of Thoracic Surgery 51: 1007–1009

Bowles N E, Richardson P J, Olsen E G et al 1986 Detection of Coxsackie-B-virus-specific RNA sequences in myocardial biopsy samples from patients with myocarditis and dilated cardiomyopathy. Lancet i: 1120–1123

Bowles N E, Rose M L, Taylor P et al 1989 End-stage dilated cardiomyopathy. Persistence of enterovirus RNA in myocardium at cardiac transplantation and lack of immune response. Circulation 80: 1128–1136

Brachfeld N, Gorlin R 1961 Functional subaortic stenosis. Annals of Internal Medicine 54: 1–11

Braudo M, Wigle E D, Keith J D 1964 A distinctive electrocardiogram in muscular subaortic stenosis due to ventricular septal hypertrophy. American Journal of Cardiology 14: 599–607

Braunwald E, Morrow A G, Cornell W P et al 1960 Idiopathic hypertrophic subaortic stenosis. Clinical, hemodynamic, and angiographic manifestations. American Journal of Medicine 29: 924–945

Braunwald E, Lambrew C T, Rockoff S D et al 1964 Idiopathic hypertrophic subaortic stenosis. I. A description of the disease based upon analysis of 64 patients. Circulation 30 (suppl IV): 3–119

Brock R C 1957 Functional obstruction of the left ventricle (acquired aortic subvalvar stenosis). Guy's Hospital Report 106: 221–238

Brock R C 1959 Functional obstruction of the left ventricle (acquired subaortic stenosis). Guy's Hospital Report 108: 126–143

Brockenbrough E C, Braunwald E, Morrow A G 1961 A hemodynamic technique for the detection of hypertrophic subaortic stenosis. Circulation 23: 189–194

Brockington I F, Luzzatto L, Osunkoya B O 1970 The heart in eosinophilic leukaemia. African Journal of Medical Sciences 1: 343–352

Buja G, Miorelli M, Turrini P et al 1993 Comparison of QT dispersion in hypertrophic cardiomyopathy between patients with and without ventricular arrhythmias and sudden death. American Journal of Cardiology 72: 973–976

Bulkley B H, D'Amico B, Taylor A L 1983 Extensive myocardial fiber disarray in aortic and pulmonary atresia. Relevance to hypertrophic cardiomyopathy. Circulation 67: 191–198

Burch M, Mann J M, Sharland M et al 1992 Myocardial disarray in Noonan syndrome. British Heart Journal 68: 586–588

Burch M, Siddiqi S A, Celermajer D S et al 1994 Dilated cardiomyopathy in children: determinants of outcome. British Heart Journal 72: 246–250

Burn J, Camm J, Davies M J et al 1997 The phenotype/genotype relation and the current status of genetic screening in hypertrophic cardiomyopathy, Marfan syndrome, and the long QT syndrome. Heart 78: 110–116

Caforio A L, Bonifacio E, Stewart J T et al 1990 Novel organ-specific circulating cardiac autoantibodies in dilated cardiomyopathy. Journal of American College of Cardiology 15: 1527–1534

Cannan C R, Reeder G S, Bailey K R et al 1995 Natural history of hypertrophic cardiomyopathy. A population-based study, 1976 through 1990. Circulation 92: 2488–2495

Carceller A M, Maroto E, Fouron J et al 1990 Dilated and contracted forms of primary endocardial fibroelastosis: a single fetal disease with two stages of development. British Heart Journal 63: 311–313

Carlquist J F, Menlove R L, Murray M B et al 1991 HLA class II (DR and DQ) antigen associations in idiopathic dilated cardiomyopathy: Validation study and meta-analysis of published HLA association studies. Circulation 83: 515–522

Carrier L, Hengstenberg C, Beckmann J S et al 1993 Mapping of a novel gene for familial hypertrophic cardiomyopathy to chromosome 11. Nature Genetics 4: 311–313

Carvalho J S, Markiewicz M 1997 Dilated endocardial fibroelastosis: unusual late finding with congenital hydrops. Pediatric Cardiology 18: 389–391

Carvalho J S, Silva C M C, Shinebourne E A et al 1996 Prognostic value of posterior wall thickness in childhood dilated cardiomyopathy and myocarditis. European Heart Journal 17: 1233–1238

Casolo G C, Trotta F, Rostagno C et al 1989 Detection of apical hypertrophic cardiomyopathy by magnetic resonance imaging. American Heart Journal 117: 468–472

Cecchi F, Olivotto I, Montereggi A et al 1995 Hypertrophic cardiomyopathy in Tuscany: clinical course and outcome in an unselected regional population. Journal of the American College of Cardiology 26: 1529–1536

Cetta F, O'Leary P W, Seward J B et al 1995 Idiopathic restrictive cardiomyopathy in childhood: diagnostic features and clinical course. Mayo Clinic Proceedings 70(7): 634–640

Chan K Y, Iwahara M, Benson L N et al 1991 Immunosuppressive therapy in the management of acute myocarditis in children: a clinical trial. Journal of American College of Cardiology 17: 458–460

Chandar J S, Wolff G S, Garson A, Jr et al 1990 Ventricular arrhythmias in postoperative tetralogy of Fallot. American Journal of Cardiology 65: 655–661

Chen S, Nouri S, Balfour I et al 1990 Clinical profile of congestive cardiomyopathy in children. Journal of American College of Cardiology 15: 189–193

Chen S, Thompson M W, Rose V 1971 Endocardial fibroelastosis: family studies with special reference to counseling. Journal of Pediatrics 79(3): 385–392

Chow L H, Gauntt C J, McManus B M 1991 Differential effects of myocarditic variants of coxsackievirus B3 in inbred mice: a pathologic characterisation of heart tissue damage. Laboratory Investigation 64: 55–64

Ciro E, Nichols P F, Maron B J 1983 Heterogeneous morphologic expression of genetically transmitted hypertrophic cardiomyopathy. Two-dimensional echocardiographic analysis. Circulation 67(6): 1227–1233

Clark A L, Coats A J 1993 Screening for hypertrophic cardiomyopathy. British Medical Journal 306: 409–410

Clark G M, Valentine E, Blount S G 1956 Endocardial fibrosis simulating constrictive pericarditis. New England Journal of Medicine 254: 349–355

Cochrane H R, May F E B, Ashcroft T et al 1991 Enterovirus and idiopathic dilated cardiomyopathy. Journal of Pathology 163: 129–131

Codd M B, Sugrve D D, Gersch B J et al 1989 Epidemiology of idiopathic dilated and hypertrophic cardiomyopathy: a population based study in Olmsted County, Minesota, 1975–1984. Circulation 80(3): 564–572

Cohen G I, Pietrolungo J F, Thomas J D et al 1996 A practical guide to assessment of ventricular diastolic function using Doppler echocardiography. Journal of the American College of Cardiology 27(7): 1753–1760

Cohen J, Effat H, Goodwin J F et al 1964 Hypertrophic obstructive cardiomyopathy. British Heart Journal 26: 16–32

Cohen L S, Braunwald E 1967 Amelioration of angina pectoris in idiopathic hypertrophic subaortic stenosis with beta-adrenergic blockade. Circulation 35(5): 847–851

Cohn L H, Trehan H, Collins J J, Jr. 1992 Long-term follow-up of patients undergoing myotomy/myectomy for obstructive hypertrophic cardiomyopathy. American Journal of Cardiology 70(6): 657–660

Colan S D, Spevak P J, Parness I A et al 1992 Cardiomyopathies. Mosby-Year Book, St. Louis, MO, p 329–361

CONSENSUS Trial Study Group 1987 Effect of enalapril on mortality in severe congestive heart failure: results of the Cooperative North Scandinavian Enalapril Survival Study (Consensus). New England Journal of Medicine 316: 1429–1435

Contreras R, Bialostozky D, Medrano G et al 1971 African or tropical endomyocardial fibrosis. Report of the 1st case seen in Mexico. Archivos del Instituto de Cardiologia de Mexico 41(4): 476–489

Cooke R A, Chambers J B, Curry P V 1994 Noonan's cardiomyopathy: a non-hypertrophic variant. British Heart Journal 71(6): 561–565

Criley J M, Lewis K B, White R I, Jr et al 1965 Pressure gradients without obstruction. A new concept of 'hypertrophic subaortic stenosis'. Circulation 32(6): 881–887

Criley J M, Lennon P A, Abbasi A et al 1976 Hypertrophic cardiomyopathy. Grune & Stratton, NY, p 771–826

Cripps T R, Counihan P J, Frenneaux M P et al 1990 Signal-averaged electrocardiography in hypertrophic cardiomyopathy. Journal of the American College of Cardiology 15(5): 956–961

D'Adamo P, Fassone L, Gedeon A et al 1997 The X-linked gene G4.5 is responsible for different infantile dilated cardiomyopathies. American Journal of Human Genetics 61(4): 862–867

da Costa F D, Moraes C R, Rodriques J V et al 1989 Early surgical results in the treatment of endomyocardial fibrosis. A Brazilian cooperative study. European Journal of Cardiothoracic Surgery 3(5): 408–413

Davies J N P 1948 Endomyocardial necrosis. A heart disease of obscure aetiology in Africans. MD Thesis, University of Bristol

Davies J, Gibson D G, Foale R et al 1982 Echocardiographic features of eosinophilic endomyocardial disease. British Heart Journal 48(5): 434–440

Davies M J, McKenna W J 1994 Dilated cardiomyopathy: an introduction to pathology and pathogenesis. British Heart Journal 72(suppl): 24

Davies M J, Ward D E 1992 How can myocarditis be diagnosed and should it be treated? British Heart Journal 68: 346–347

Dec G W, Palacios I, Yasuda T et al 1990 Antimyosin antibody cardiac imaging: its role in the diagnosis of myocarditis. Journal of the American College of Cardiology 16: 97–104

Delahaye J P, Azzano O 1994 Hypertrophic obstructive cardiomyopathy: current treatment, indications and results. Presse Medicale 23(20): 925–927

Denfield S W, Rosenthal G, Gajarski R J et al 1997 Restrictive cardiomyopathies in childhood. Etiologies and natural history. Texas Heart Institute Journal 24(1): 38–44

Devi A S, Eisenfeld L, Uphoff D et al 1995 New syndrome of hydrocephalus, endocardial fibroelastosis, and cataracts (HEC syndrome). American Journal of Medical Genetics 56: 62–66

Di Lenarda A, Secoli G, Perkan A et al 1995 Changing mortality in dilated cardiomyopathy. The Heart Muscle Disease Study Group. British Heart Journal 72: S46–S51

Dilsizian V, Bonow R O, Epstein S E et al 1993 Myocardial ischemia detected by thallium scintigraphy is frequently related to cardiac arrest and syncope in young patients with hypertrophic cardiomyopathy. Journal of the American College of Cardiology 22(3): 796–804

Dincsoy M Y, Dincsoy H P, Kessler A D et al 1965 Generalised glycogenosis and associated fibroelastosis; report of three cases with biochemical studies. Journal of Pediatrics 67: 728–740

Doi Y L, McKenna W J, Gehrke J et al 1980 M mode echocardiography in hypertrophic cardiomyopathy: diagnostic criteria and prediction of obstruction. American Journal of Cardiology 45(1): 6–14

Domenicucci S, Lazzeroni E, Roelandt J et al 1985 Progression of hypertrophic cardiomyopathy. A cross sectional echocardiographic study. British Heart Journal 53(4): 405–411

Dong S J, MacGregor J H, Crawley A P et al 1994 Left ventricular wall thickness and regional systolic function in patients with hypertrophic cardiomyopathy. A three-dimensional tagged magnetic resonance imaging study. Circulation 90(3): 1200–1209

Dritsas A, Gilligan D, Nihoyannopoulos P et al 1992 Amiodarone reduces QT dispersion in patients with hypertrophic cardiomyopathy. International Journal of Cardiology 36(3): 345–349

Drucker N A, Colan S D, Lewis A B et al 1994 Gamma-globulin treatment of acute myocarditis in the pediatric population. Circulation 89: 252–257

Duncan W J, Tyrrell M J, Bharadwaj B B 1991 Disopyramide as a negative inotrope in obstructive cardiomyopathy in children. Canadian Journal of Cardiology 7(2): 81–86

Durand J B, Bachinski L L, Bieling L C et al 1995 Localization of a gene responsible for familial dilated cardiomyopathy to chromosome 1q32. Circulation 92: 3387–3389

Echizen H, Eichelbaum M 1986 Clinical pharmacokinetics of verapamil, nifedipine and diltiazem. Clinical Pharmacokinetics 11(6): 425–449

Edwards J E 1954 Functional pathology of congenital heart disease. Pediatric Clinics of North America 2: 13–50

Ehlers K H, Engle M A, Levin A R et al 1972 Eccentric ventricular hypertrophy in familial and sporadic instances of 46 XX, XY Turner phenotype. Circulation 45(3): 639–652

Elliott P M, Kaski J C, Prasad K et al 1996 Chest pain during daily life in patients with hypertrophic cardiomyopathy: an ambulatory electrocardiographic study. European Heart Journal 17(7): 1056–1064

Epstein S E, Maron B J 1982 Hypertrophic cardiomyopathy. An overview. Springer-Verlag, Berlin, p 5–18

Evans T S, Nesbit R 1949 Eosinophilic leukemia. Report of a case with autopsy confirmation: review of the literature. Blood 4: 603

Factor S M 1978 Endocardial fibroelastosis: myocardial and vascular alterations associated with viral-like nuclear particles. American Heart Journal 96(6): 791–801

Fadell E J, Crone R I, Leonard M et al 1957 Eosinophilic leukemia. Archives of Internal Medicine 99: 819–823

Fan J, Zhang Y, Zhang M 1995 Effects of verapamil on left ventricular diastolic dysfunction. Chinese Journal of Internal Medicine 34(6): 378–380

Fananapazir L, Epstein S E 1991 Value of electrophysiologic studies in hypertrophic cardiomyopathy treated with amiodarone. American Journal of Cardiology 67(2): 175–182

Fananapazir L, Leon M B, Bonow R O et al 1991 Sudden death during empiric amiodarone therapy in symptomatic hypertrophic cardiomyopathy. American Journal of Cardiology 67(2): 169–174

Fananapazir L, Cannon R O, Tripodi D et al 1992 Impact of dual-chamber permanent pacing in patients with obstructive hypertrophic cardiomyopathy with symptoms refractory to verapamil and beta-adrenergic blocker therapy. Circulation 85: 2149–2161

Fananapazir L, Epstein N D, Curiel R V et al 1994 Long-term results of dual-chamber (DDD) pacing in obstructive hypertrophic cardiomyopathy. Evidence for progressive symptomatic and hemodynamic improvement and reduction of left ventricular hypertrophy. Circulation 90: 2731–2742

Farrell D J, Skinner J R 1992 Restrictive endocardial fibroelastosis in a neonate without other cardiac pathology. Journal of Clinical Pathology 45(11): 1042–1043

Faruque A A 1963 Adult endomyocardial fibrosis in Britain. Lancet ii: 331–333

Fei L, Slade A K, Grace A A et al 1994 Ambulatory assessment of the QT interval in patients with hypertrophic cardiomyopathy: risk stratification and effect of low dose amiodarone. Pacing & Clinical Electrophysiology 17: 2222–2227

Feigenbaum H 1981a Echocardiography, 3rd edn. Lea & Febiger, Philadelphia, p 452–465

Feigenbaum H 1981b Endomyocardial fibrosis. In: Echocardiography, 3rd edn. Lea & Febiger, Philadelphia, p 472–471

Ferencz C, Neill C A 1992 Cardiomyopathy in infancy: observations in an epidemiologic study. Pediatric Cardiology 13(2): 65–71

Fiddler G I, Tajik A J, Weidman W et al 1978 Idiopathic hypertrophic subaortic stenosis in the young. American Journal of Cardiology 42(5): 793–799

Fischer J H 1962 Primary endocardial fibroelastosis: a review of 15 cases. Canadian Medical Association Journal 87: 105–109

Fitchett D H, Sugrue D D, MacArthur C G et al 1984 Right ventricular dilated cardiomyopathy. British Heart Journal 51: 25–29

Fitzpatrick A P, Shapiro L M, Rickards A F et al 1990 Familial restrictive cardiomyopathy with atrioventricular block and skeletal myopathy. British Heart Journal 63(2): 114–118

Fontana R S, Edwards J E 1962 Congenital cardiac disease: a review of 357 cases studied pathologically. Saunders, Philadelphia, PA, p 141–146

Forfar J O, Miller R A, Bain A D et al 1964 Endocardial fibroelastosis. British Medical Journal 2: 7–12

Fowles R E, Bieber C P, Stinson E B 1979 Defective in vitro suppressor cell function in idiopathic congestive cardiomyopathy. Circulation 59: 483–491

Frank S, Braunwald E 1968 Idiopathic hypertrophic subaortic stenosis. Clinical analysis of 126 patients with emphasis on the natural history. Circulation 37(5): 759–788

Friedman R A, Moak J P, Garson A, Jr. 1991 Clinical course of idiopathic dilated cardiomyopathy in children. Journal of the American College of Cardiology 18: 152–156

Friedman R A 1995 Myocarditis. In: Garson Jr, A, Bricker J T, McNamara D G (eds) The science and practice of pediatric cardiology. Lea & Fabiger, Philadelphia, PA, p 1577–1589

Fuster V, Gersh B J, Giuliani E R et al 1981 The natural history of idiopathic dilated cardiomyopathy. American Journal of Cardiology 47: 525–531

Garcia M J, Rodriguez L, Ares M et al 1996 Differentiation of constrictive pericarditis from restrictive cardiomyopathy: assessment of left ventricular diastolic velocities in longitudinal axis by Doppler tissue imaging. Journal of the American College of Cardiology 27(1): 108–114

Garson A, Jr. 1987 Medicolegal problems in the management of cardiac arrhythmias in children. Pediatrics 79(1): 84–88

Geisterfer-Lowrance A A, Kass S, Tanigawa G et al 1990 A molecular basis for familial hypertrophic cardiomyopathy: a beta cardiac myosin heavy chain gene missense mutation. Cell 62(5): 999–1006

Gerbaux A, DeBrux J, Bennaceur M et al 1956 L'endocardite parietale fibroplastique avec esinophilie sanguine (endocardite de Loffler). Bulletins et Memories de la Societe Medicale des Hopitaux de Paris 72: 456–466

Gerli R, Rambotti P, Spinozzi F et al 1986 Immunologic studies of peripheral blood from patients with idiopathic dilated cardiomyopathy. American Heart Journal 112: 350–355

Gerson M C, Colthar M S, Fowler N O 1989 Differentiation of constrictive pericarditis and restrictive cardiomyopathy by radionuclide ventriculography. American Heart Journal 118(1): 114–120

Gersony W M, Katz S L, Nadas A S 1966 Endocardial fibroelastosis and mumps virus. Endocardial fibroelastosis and the mumps virus. Pediatrics 37(3): 430–434

Gewillig M C, Moerman P, Dumoulin M et al 1992 Restrictive cardiomyopathy in childhood. Pediatric Cardiology 13: 258

Gibson D G, Traill T A, Hall R J et al 1979 Echocardiographic features of secondary left ventricular hypertrophy. British Heart Journal 41(1): 54–59

Gibson D G 1985 Clinical significance of myocardial intensity in hypertrophic cardiomyopathy and other forms of left ventricular hypertrophy. (In: Cardiomyopathies – the message for the 1980s.) Postgraduate Medical Journal 61: 1105–1135

Gilligan D M, Chan W L, Joshi J et al 1993 A double-blind, placebo-controlled crossover trial of nadolol and verapamil in mild and moderately symptomatic hypertrophic cardiomyopathy. Journal of the American College of Cardiology 21: 1672–1679

Glancy D L, O'Brien K P, Gold H K et al 1970 Atrial fibrillation in patients with idiopathic hypertrophic subaortic stenosis. British Heart Journal 32(5): 652–659

Glasgow G A, Gardin J M, Burn C S et al 1980 Echocardiographic and Doppler flow observations in hypertrophic subaortic stenosis. Circulation 62(Suppl III): 99

Goldblatt J, Melmed J, Rose G 1987 Autosomal recessive inheritance of idiopathic dilated cardiomyopathy in a Madeira portuguese kindred. Clinical Genetics 31: 249–254

Goodwin J F 1980 Hypertrophic cardiomyopathy: a disease in search of its own identity. American Journal of Cardiology 45(1): 177–180

Goodwin J F 1982 The frontiers of cardiomyopathy. British Heart Journal 48(1): 1–18

Gottdiener J S, Maron B J, Schooley R T et al 1983 Two-dimensional echocardiographic assessment of the idiopathic hypereosinophilic syndrome. Anatomic basis of mitral regurgitation and peripheral embolization. Circulation 67(3): 572–578

Graham T P, Jr, Jarmakani M M, Canent R V, Jr. et al 1968 Characterization of left heart volumes and mass in normal children and in infants with intrinsic myocardial disease. Circulation 38(5): 826–837

Grasso M, Arbustini E, Silini E et al 1992 Search for coxsackie B3 RNA in idiopathic dilated cardiomyopathy using gene amplification by polymerase chain reaction. American Journal of Cardiology 69: 658–664

Greaves S C, Roche A H, Neutze J M et al 1987 Inheritance of hypertrophic cardiomyopathy: a cross sectional and M mode echocardiographic study of 50 families. British Heart Journal 58(3): 259–266

Greenwood R D, Nadas A S, Fyler D C 1976 The clinical course of primary myocardial disease in infants and children. American Heart Journal 92: 549–560

Griffin M L, Hernandez A, Martin T C et al 1988 Dilated cardiomyopathy in infants and children. Journal of the American College of Cardiology 11(1): 139–144

Grossman W 1986 Profiles in dilated (congestive) and hypertrophic cardiomyopathies In: Cardiac catheterisation and angiography, 3rd edn. Lea & Fabiger, Philadelphia, PA, p 412–426

Gutgesell H P, Speer M E, Rosenberg H S 1980 Characterization of the cardiomyopathy in infants of diabetic mothers. Circulation 61(2): 441–450

Hada Y, Sakamoto T, Amano K et al 1987 Prevalence of hypertrophic cardiomyopathy in a population of adult Japanese workers as detected by echocardiographic screening. American Journal of Cardiology 59(1): 183–184

Hanrath P, Mathey D G, Kremer P et al 1980a Effect of verapamil on left ventricular isovolumic relaxation time and regional left ventricular filling in hypertrophic cardiomyopathy. American Journal of Cardiology 45(6): 1258–1264

Hanrath P, Mathey D G, Siegert R et al 1980b Left ventricular relaxation and filling pattern in different forms of left ventricular hypertrophy: an echocardiographic study. American Journal of Cardiology 45(1): 15–23

Hanrath P, Schluter M, Sonntag F et al 1983 Influence of verapamil therapy on left ventricular performance at rest and during exercise in hypertrophic cardiomyopathy. American Journal of Cardiology 52(5): 544–548

Hardarson T, De la Calzada C S, Curiel R et al 1973 Prognosis and mortality of hypertrophic obstructive cardiomyopathy. Lancet ii (7844): 1462–1467

Hardy W R, Anderson R E 1968 The hypereosinophilic syndromes. Annals of Internal Medicine 68(6): 1220–1229

Harper P S, Clarke A J 1993 Screening for hypertrophic cardiomyopathy. British Medical Journal 306(6881): 859–860

Harris L, McKenna W J, Rowland E et al 1983 Side effects of long-term amiodarone therapy. Circulation 67(1): 45–51

Harrison D C, Braunwald E, Glick P L et al 1964 Effects of beta adrenergic blockade on the circulation, with particular reference to observations in patients with hypertrophic subaortic stenosis. Circulation 29: 84–98

Hashimoto T, Yano K, Matsumoto Y et al 1988 Contracted form of primary endocardial fibroelastosis in a young adult without congestive heart failure. Japanese Heart Journal 29(1): 121–126

Hastreiter A R, Fisher E A 1977 Endocardial fibroelastosis. In: Moss A J, Adams F H and Emmanouillides G C (eds) Heart disease in infants, children and adolescents. Williams & Wilkins, Baltimore, p 496–505

Hatle L K, Appleton C P, Popp R L 1989 Differentiation of constrictive pericarditis and restrictive cardiomyopathy by Doppler echocardiography. Circulation 79(2): 357–370

Hendren W G, Jones E L, Smith M D 1988 Aortic and mitral valve replacement in idiopathic hypereosinophilic syndrome. Annals of Thoracic Surgery 46(5): 570–571

Henry W L, Clark C E, Epstein S E 1973a Asymmetric septal hypertrophy (ASH): the unifying link in the IHSS disease spectrum. Observations regarding its pathogenesis, pathophysiology, and course. Circulation 47(4): 827–832

Henry W L, Clark C E, Epstein S E 1973b Asymmetric septal hypertrophy. Echocardiographic identification of the pathognomonic anatomic abnormality of IHSS. Circulation 47(2): 225–233

Heric B, Lytle B W, Miller D P et al 1995 Surgical management of hypertrophic obstructive cardiomyopathy. Early and late results. Journal of Thoracic and Cardiovascular Surgery 110(1): 195–206

Hernandez R R, Greenfield J C, Jr, McCall B W 1964 Pressure-flow studies in hypertrophic subaortic stenosis. Journal of Clinical Investigation 34: 401

Hess O M, Grimm J, Krayenbuehl H P 1983 Diastolic function in hypertrophic cardiomyopathy: effects of propranolol and verapamil on diastolic stiffness. European Heart Journal 4(Suppl F): 47–56

Hess O M, Murakami T, Krayenbuehl H P 1986 Does verapamil improve left ventricular relaxation in patients with myocardial hypertrophy? Circulation 74(3): 530–543

Higgins C B, Byrd B F, Stark D et al 1985 Magnetic resonance imaging in hypertrophic cardiomyopathy. American Journal of Cardiology 55(9): 1121–1126

Hollman A, Goodwin J F, Teare R D et al 1960 A family with obstructive cardiomyopathy (asymmetrical hypertrophy). British Heart Journal 22(449): 456

Hsu D T, Addonizio L J, Hordof A J et al 1991 Acute pulmonary embolism in pediatric patients awaiting heart transplantation. Journal of the American College of Cardiology 17: 1621–1625

Huber S A, Lodge P A 1986 Coxsackievirus B3 myocarditis: identification of different pathogenic mechanisms in DBA/2 and Balb/c mice. American Journal of Pathology 122: 284–291

Hutchins G M, Moore G W, Jones J F et al 1981 Postnatal endocardial fibroelastosis of the valve of the foramen ovale. American Journal of Cardiology 47(1): 90–94

Hutchins G M, Vie S A 1972 The progression of interstitial myocarditis to idiopathic endocardial fibroelastosis. American Journal of Pathology 66(3): 483–496

Ingham R E, Mason J W, Rossen R M et al 1978 Electrophysiologic findings in patients with idiopathic hypertrophic subaortic stenosis. American Journal of Cardiology 41(5): 811–816

Ino T, Benson L N, Freedom R M et al 1988 Natural history and prognostic risk factors in endocardial fibroelastosis. American Journal of Cardiology 62(7): 431–434

Ishino Y, Nakata H 1997 Evaluation of left ventricular systolic function using cine MRI – application to hypertrophic cardiomyopathy. Japanese Journal of Clinical Medicine 55(7): 1805–1810

Ive F A, Willis A J, Ikeme A C et al 1967 Endomyocardial fibrosis and filariasis. Quarterly Journal of Medicine 36(144): 495–516

Jarcho J A, McKenna W, Pare J A et al 1989 Mapping a gene for familial hypertrophic cardiomyopathy to chromosome 14q1. New England Journal of Medicine 321(20): 1372–1378

Jarrar M, Vaksmann G, Godart F et al 1994 Natural history and prognostic factors in primary endocardial fibroelastosis in infants. Archives des Maladies du Coeur et des Vaisseaux 86(5): 653–656

Jeanrenaud X, Goy J J, Kappenberger L 1992 Effects of dual-chamber pacing in hypertrophic obstructive cardiomyopathy. Lancet 339(8805): 1318–1323

Jin O, Sole M J, Butany J W et al 1990 Detection of enterovirus RNA in myocardial biopsies from patients with myocarditis and cardiomyopathy using gene amplification by polymerase chain reaction. Circulation 82: 8–16

Johnson F R 1952 Anoxia as cause of endocardial fibroelastosis in infancy. American Medical Association Archives of Pathology 54: 237–247

Kaltenbach M, Hopf R, Kober G et al 1979 Treatment of hypertrophic obstructive cardiomyopathy with verapamil. British Heart Journal 42(1): 35–42

Kandolf R, Hofschneider P H 1989 Enterovirus-induced cardiomyopathy. In: Notkins AL, Oldstone MBA (eds) Concepts in viral pathogenesis III. Springer-Verlag, New York, p 282–290

Katritsis D, Wilmshurst P T, Wendon J A et al 1991 Primary restrictive cardiomyopathy: clinical and pathologic characteristics. Journal of the American College of Cardiology 18(5): 1230–1235

Keeling P J, Jeffery S, Caforio A L et al 1992 Similar prevalence of enteroviral genome within the myocardium from patients with idiopathic dilated cardiomyopathy and controls by the polymerase chain reaction. British Heart Journal 68: 554–559

Keith J D, Rose V, Manning J A 1978 Endocardial fibroelastosis. In: Keith J D, Rowe R D, Vlad P (eds) Heart disease in infancy and childhood, 3rd edn. McMillan, New York, p 941–957

Kishimoto C, Abelman W H 1989 Monoclonal antibody therapy for prevention of acute coxsackievirus B3 myocarditis in mice. Circulation 79: 1300–1308

Klein A L, Cohen G I, Pietrolungo J F et al 1993 Differentiation of constrictive pericarditis from restrictive cardiomyopathy by Doppler transesophageal echocardiographic measurements of respiratory variations in pulmonary venous flow. Journal of the American College of Cardiology 22(7): 1935–1943

Kline I K, Miller A J, Pick R et al 1964 The relationship between human endocardial fibroelastosis and obstruction of cardiac lymphatics. Circulation 30: 728–735

Klues H G, Schiffers A, Maron B J 1995 Phenotypic spectrum and patterns of left ventricular hypertrophy in hypertrophic cardiomyopathy: morphologic observations and significance as assessed by two-dimensional echocardiography in 600 patients. Journal of the American College of Cardiology 26: 1699–1708

Kofflard M J, Waldstein D J, Vos J et al 1993 Prognosis in hypertrophic cardiomyopathy observed in a large clinic population. American Journal of Cardiology 72(12): 939–943

Koito H, Suzuki J, Nakamori H et al 1995 Clinical significance of abnormal high signal intensity of left ventricular myocardium by gadolinium-diethylenetriaminepenta-acetic acid enhanced magnetic resonance imaging in hypertrophic cardiomyopathy. Journal of Cardiology 25(4): 163–170

Lambert E C, Vlad P 1958 Primary endocardial disease. Pediatric Clinics of North America 5: 1057–1085

Latif N, Baker C S, Dunn M J et al 1993 Frequency and specificity of antiheart antibodies in patients with dilated cardiomyopathy detected using SDS-PAGE and western blotting. Journal of the American College of Cardiology 22: 1378–1384

Leatherbury L, Chandra R S, Shapiro S R et al 1988 Value of endomyocardial biopsy in infants, children and adolescents with dilated or hypertrophic cardiomyopathy and myocarditis. Journal of the American College of Cardiology 12: 1547–1554

Levin S 1980 Parvovirus: a possible etiologic agent in cardiomyopathy and endocardial fibroelastosis. Human Pathology 11(5): 404–405

Lewis A B, Neustein H B, Takahashi M et al 1985 Findings on endomyocardial biopsy in infants and children with dilated cardiomyopathy. American Journal of Cardiology 55: 143–145

Lewis A B 1992 Clinical profile and outcome of restrictive cardiomyopathy in children. American Heart Journal 123(6): 1589–1593

Lewis A B, Chabot M 1991 Outcome of infants and children with dilated cardiomyopathy. American Journal of Cardiology 68: 365–369

Lewis A B, Chabot M 1993 The effect of treatment with angiotensin-converting enzyme inhibitors on survival of pediatric patients with dilated cardiomyopathy. Pediatric Cardiology 14: 9–12

Libanoff A J, McMahon N J 1976 Eosinophilia and endomyocardial fibrosis. American Journal of Cardiology 37(3): 438–441

Liljeqvist J A, Bergstrom T, Holmstrom S et al 1993 Failure to demonstrate enterovirus aetiology in Swedish patients with dilated cardiomyopathy. Journal of Genetics and Virology 39: 6–10

Liu P, McLaughlin P R, Sole M J 1992 Treatment of myocarditis: current recommendations and future frontiers. Heart Failure 8: 33–40

Liu P P 1992 New concepts in myocarditis. Crossroads in the 1990s. Progress in Pediatric Cardiology 1: 37–47

Loffler W 1936 Endocarditis parietalis fibroplastic mit Bluteosinophilie Schweizer. Medizine Wochenschrift 66: 817–820

Lombes A, Herve F, Ogier H et al 1987 Apparently idiopathic primary myocardiopathies in children. The role of metabolic etiology. Archives Francaises de Pediatrie 44(8): 569–578

Lorell B H, Paulus W J, Grossman W et al 1982 Modification of abnormal left ventricular diastolic properties by nifedipine in patients with hypertrophic cardiomyopathy. Circulation 65(3): 499–507

Lorell B H, Barry W H 1984 Effects of verapamil on contraction and relaxation of cultured chick embryo ventricular cells during calcium overload. Journal of the American College of Cardiology 3(2: Pt 1): 341–348

Ludbrook P A, Tiefenbrunn A J, Reed F R et al 1982 Acute hemodynamic responses to sublingual nifedipine:

dependence on left ventricular function. Circulation 65(3): 489–498

Lurie P R, Fujita M, Neustein H B 1978 Transvascular endomyocardial biopsy in infants and small children: description of a new technique. American Journal of Cardiology 42: 453–457

Lurie P R 1988 Endocardial fibroelastosis is not a disease. American Journal of Cardiology 62(7): 468–470

MacRae C A, Ghaisas N, Kass S et al 1995 Familial hypertrophic cardiomyopathy with Wolff-Parkinson-White syndrome maps to a locus on chromosome 7q3. Journal of Clinical Investigation 96: 1216–1220

Mandel R I, Bruner J P 1995 Endocardial fibroelastosis: an unusual cause of pulmonary hypertension in pregnancy. American Journal of Perinatology 12(5): 319–321

Marles S L, Chudley A E 1990 Ulnar agenesis and endocardial fibroelastosis. American Journal of Medical Genetics 37(2): 258–260

Maron B 1983 Cardiomyopathies. In: Adams F, Emmanouilides G C (eds) Moss' Heart disease in infants, children and adolescents, 3rd edn. Williams & Wilkins, Baltimore, MD, p 757–780

Maron B J, Lipson L C, Roberts W C et al 1978 'Malignant' hypertrophic cardiomyopathy: identification of a subgroup of families with unusually frequent premature death. American Journal of Cardiology 41(7): 1133–1140

Maron B J, Sato N, Roberts W C et al 1979 Quantitative analysis of cardiac muscle cell disorganization in the ventricular septum. Comparison of fetuses and infants with and without congenital heart disease and patients with hypertrophic cardiomyopathy. Circulation 60(3): 685–696

Maron B J, Roberts W C, Epstein S E 1982a Sudden death in hypertrophic cardiomyopathy: a profile of 78 patients. Circulation 65(7): 1388–1394

Maron B J, Tajik A J, Ruttenberg H D et al 1982b Hypertrophic cardiomyopathy in infants: clinical features and natural history. Circulation 65(1): 7–17

Maron B J, Nichols P F, Pickle L W et al 1984 Patterns of inheritance in hypertrophic cardiomyopathy: assessment by M-mode and two-dimensional echocardiography. American Journal of Cardiology 53(8): 1087–1094

Maron B J, Gaffney F A, Jeresaty R M et al 1985 Cardiovascular abnormalities in the athlete: recommendations regarding eligibility for competition. Task force III: hypertrophic cardiomyopathy, other myopericardial diseases and mitral valve prolapse. Journal of the American College of Cardiology 6(6): 1215–1217

Maron B J, Bonow R O, Cannon R O et al 1987a Hypertrophic cardiomyopathy. Interrelations of clinical manifestations, pathophysiology, and therapy (1). New England Journal of Medicine 316(13): 780–789

Maron B J, Bonow R O, Cannon R O et al 1987b Hypertrophic cardiomyopathy. Interrelations of clinical manifestations, pathophysiology, and therapy (2). New England Journal of Medicine 316(14): 844–852

Maron B J, Gardin J M, Flack J M et al 1995 Prevalence of hypertrophic cardiomyopathy in a general population of young adults. Echocardiographic analysis of 4111 subjects in the CARDIA Study. Coronary Artery Risk Development in (Young) Adults. Circulation 92: 785–789

Maron B J, Roberts W C 1979 Quantitative analysis of cardiac muscle cell disorganization in the ventricular septum of patients with hypertrophic cardiomyopathy. Circulation 59(4): 689–706

Maron B J, Roberts W C 1981a Cardiomyopathies in the first two decades of life. Davis, Philadelphia, p 35–78

Maron B J, Roberts W C 1981b Cardiomyopathies in the first two decades of life. Cardiovascular Clinics 11(2): 35–78

Marteau T, Michie S 1995 Genetic testing for familial hypertrophic cardiomyopathy in newborn infants. A positive screening test for an untreatable condition provides psychological relief from uncertainty. British Medical Journal 311: 58–59

Mason J W, Billingham M E, Ricci D R 1980 Treatment of acute inflammatory myocarditis assisted by endomyocardial biopsy. American Journal of Cardiology 45: 1037–1044

Matitiau A, Perez-Atayde A, Sanders S P et al 1994 Infantile dilated cardiomyopathy. Relation of outcome to left ventricular mechanics, hemodynamics, and histology at the time of presentation. Circulation 90: 1310–1318

Matsubara H, Nakatani S, Nagata S et al 1995 Salutary effect of disopyramide on left ventricular diastolic function in hypertrophic obstructive cardiomyopathy. Journal of the American College of Cardiology 26: 768–775

Matthys D, Van Coster R, Verhaaren H 1991 Fatal outcome of pyruvate loading test in child with restrictive cardiomyopathy. Lancet 338(8773): 1020–1021

McDonald K, McWilliams E, O'Keeffe B et al 1988 Functional assessment of patients treated with permanent dual chamber pacing as a primary treatment for hypertrophic cardiomyopathy. European Heart Journal 9(8): 893–898

McKenna W, Deanfield J, Faruqui A et al 1981 Prognosis in hypertrophic cardiomyopathy: role of age and clinical, electrocardiographic and hemodynamic features. American Journal of Cardiology 47(3): 532–538

McKenna W J, Chetty S, Oakley C M et al 1980 Arrhythmia in hypertrophic cardiomyopathy: exercise and 48 hour ambulatory electrocardiographic assessment with and without beta adrenergic blocking therapy. American Journal of Cardiology 45(1): 1–5

McKenna W J, England D, Doi Y L et al 1981a Arrhythmia in hypertrophic cardiomyopathy. I: Influence on prognosis. British Heart Journal 46(2): 168–172

McKenna W J, Harris L, Perez G et al 1981b Arrhythmia in hypertrophic cardiomyopathy. II: Comparison of amiodarone and verapamil in treatment. British Heart Journal 46(2): 173–178

McKenna W J, Harris L, Rowland E et al 1984 Amiodarone for long-term management of patients with hypertrophic cardiomyopathy. American Journal of Cardiology 54(7): 802–810

McKenna W J, Oakley C M, Krikler D M et al 1985 Improved survival with amiodarone in patients with hypertrophic cardiomyopathy and ventricular tachycardia. British Heart Journal 53(4): 412–416

McKenna W J, Franklin R C, Nihoyannopoulos P et al 1988a Arrhythmia and prognosis in infants, children and adolescents with hypertrophic cardiomyopathy. Journal of the American College of Cardiology 11(1): 147–153

McKenna W J, Kleinebenne A, Nihoyannopoulos P et al 1988b Echocardiographic measurement of right ventricular wall thickness in hypertrophic cardiomyopathy: relation to clinical and prognostic features. Journal of the American College of Cardiology 11(2): 351–358

McKenna W J, Spirito P, Desnos M et al 1997 Experience from clinical genetics in hypertrophic cardiomyopathy: proposal for new diagnostic criteria in adult members of affected families. Heart 77: 130–132

McKenna W J, Camm A J 1989 Sudden death in hypertrophic cardiomyopathy. Assessment of patients at high risk. Circulation 80(5): 1489–1492

McKenna W J, Deanfield J E 1984 Hypertrophic cardiomyopathy: an important cause of sudden death. Archives of Disease in Childhood 59(10): 971–975

McLatchie G R, Pedoe D S, McKenna W J et al 1993 Screening for hypertrophic cardiomyopathy. British Medical Journal 306(6881): 860

McLoughlin T G, Schiebler G L, Krovetz L J 1968 Hemodynamic findings in children with endocardial fibroelastosis. Analysis of 22 cases. American Heart Journal 75(2): 162–172

Meerschwam I S 1968 Hypertrophic obstructive cardiomyopathy Excerpta Medica, Amsterdam

Mehta A V, Ferrer P L, Pickoff A S et al 1984 M-mode echocardiographic findings in children with idiopathic restrictive cardiomyopathy. Pediatric Cardiology 5(4): 273–279

Menapace F J, Hammer W J, Kessler K K et al 1977 Echocardiographic measurements of left ventricular free wall thickness in weight lifters: a problem with the definition of ASH American. Journal of Cardiology 39: 276

Mestroni L, Krajinovic M, Severini G M et al 1995 Familial dilated cardiomyopathy. British Heart Journal 72: S35–S41

Michels V V 1993 Genetics of idiopathic dilated cardiomyopathy. Heart Failure 10: 87–94

Michels V V, Driscoll D J, Miller F A, Jr. 1985 Familial aggregation of idiopathic dilated cardiomyopathy. American Journal of Cardiology 55: 1232–1233

Michels V V, Moll P P, Miller F A et al 1992 The frequency of familial dilated cardiomyopathy in a series of patients with dilated cardiomyopathy. New England Journal of Medicine 326: 77–82

Michels V V, Moll P P, Rodeheffer R J et al 1994 Circulating heart autoantibodies in familial as compared with nonfamilial idiopathic dilated cardiomyopathy. Mayo Clinic Proceedings 69: 24–27

Milasin J, Muntoni F, Severini G M et al 1996 A point mutation in the 5′ splice site of the dystrophin gene first intron responsible for X-linked dilated cardiomyopathy. Human Molecular Genetics 5(1): 73–79

Miller G, Partridge A 1983 Mucopolysaccharidosis type VI presenting in infancy with endocardial fibroelastosis and heart failure. Pediatric Cardiology 4: 61–62

Mitchell S C, Froehlich L A, Banas J S, Jr. et al 1966 An epidemiologic assessment of primary endocardial fibroelastosis. American Journal of Cardiology 18(6): 859–866

Mohr R, Schaff H V, Danielson G K et al 1989 The outcome of surgical treatment of hypertrophic obstructive cardiomyopathy. Exprience over 15 years. Journal of Thoracic and Cardiovascular Surgery 97(5): 666–674

Moller J H, Lucas R V, Jr., Adams P, Jr. et al 1964 Endocardial fibroelastosis. A clinical and anatomical study of 47 patients with emphasis on its relationship to mitral insufficiency. Circulation 30: 759–782

Moller P, Lunde P, Hovig T et al 1979 Familial cardiomyopathy. Autosomally, dominantly inherited congestive cardiomyopathy with two cases of septal hypertrophy in one family. Clinical Genetics 16: 233–243

Moraes C R, Buffolo E, Lima R et al 1983 Surgical treatment of endomyocardial fibrosis. Journal of Thoracic & Cardiovascular Surgery 85(5): 738–745

Morgan J M, Raposo L, Clague J C et al 1989 Restrictive cardiomyopathy and constrictive pericarditis: non-invasive distinction by digitised M mode echocardiography. British Heart Journal 61(1): 29–37

Muir P, Nicholson F, Jhetam M et al 1993 Rapid diagnosis of enterovirus infection by magnetic bead extraction and polymerase chain reaction detection of enterovirus RNA in clinical specimens. Journal of Clinical Microbiology 31: 31–38

Muntoni F, Cau M, Ganau A et al 1993 Brief report: deletion of the dystrophin muscle-promoter region associated with X-linked dilated cardiomyopathy. New England Journal of Medicine 329(13): 921–925

Muntoni F, Di Lenarda A, Porcu M et al 1997 Dystrophin gene abnormalities in two patients with dilated cardiomyopathy. Heart 78(6): 608–612

Murgo J P, Alter B R, Dorethy J F et al 1980 Dynamics of left ventricular ejection in obstructive and nonobstructive hypertrophic cardiomyopathy. Journal of Clinical Investigation 66(6): 1369–1382

Murgo J P, Alter B R, Dorethy J F et al 1983 The effects of intraventricular gradients on left ventricular ejection dynamics. European Heart Journal 4(Suppl F): 23–38

Nagao M, Omote S, Takizawa A et al 1983 Effect of diltiazem on left ventricular isovolumic relaxation time in patients with hypertrophic cardiomyopathy. Japanese Circulation Journal 47(1): 54–58

Nagaratnam N, Dissanayake R V P 1959 Endomyocardial fibrosis in the Ceylonese. British Heart Journal 21: 167–173

Nagashima J 1991 Doppler and echocardiographic assessments of effects of diisopyramide on non-obstructive hypertrophic cardiomyopathy. Journal of Cardiology 21(1): 75–86

Nakajima K, Okada R, Ueda H 1961 A case report of endomyocardial fibrosis. Japanese Heart Journal 2: 265–275

Nakatani S, White R D, Powell K A et al 1996 Dynamic magnetic resonance imaging assessment of the effect of ventricular wall curvature on regional function in hypertrophic cardiomyopathy. American Journal of Cardiology 77(8): 618–622

Nellen M, Beck W, Vogelpoel L et al 1971 Auscultatory phenomena in hypertrophic obstructive cardiomyopathy In: Wolstenholme G E W, O'Connor M (eds) Ciba Foundation study group 37. Churchill, London, p 77–103

Newbould M J, Armstrong G R, Barson A J 1991 Endocardial fibroelastosis in infants with hydrops fetalis. Journal of Clinical Pathology 44(7): 576–579

Ni J, Bowles N E, Kim Y H et al 1997 Viral infection of the myocardium in endocardial fibroelastosis. Molecular evidence for the role of mumps virus as an etiologic agent. Circulation 95(1): 133–139

Nishimura R A, Hayes D L, Ilstrup D M et al 1996 Effect of dual-chamber pacing on systolic and diastolic function in patients with hypertrophic cardiomyopathy. Acute Doppler echocardiographic and catheterization hemodynamic study. Journal of the American College of Cardiology 27: 421–430

Nishimura R A, Trusty J M, Hayes D L et al 1997 Dual-chamber pacing for hypertrophic cardiomyopathy: a randomized, double-blind, crossover trial. Journal of the American College of Cardiology 29(2): 435–441

Noren G R, Adams P, Anderson R C 1963 Positive skin reactivity to mump virus antigen in endocardial fibroelastosis. Journal of Pediatrics 62: 604–609

Nydegger U E 1984 Selected pathophysiological aspects of autoimmune diseases as the basis for transfusion therapy with polyclonal antibody mixtures. Triangle 23: 133–140

O'Connell J B, Robinson J A, Henkin R E et al 1981 Immunosuppressive therapy in patients with congestive cardiomyopathy and myocardial uptake of gallium-67. Circulation 64: 780–786

O'Connell J B, Henkin R E, Robinson J A et al 1984 Gallium-67 imaging in patients with dilated cardiomyopathy and biopsy-proven myocarditis. Circulation 70: 58–62

Oldfors A, Eriksson B O, Kyllerman M et al 1994 Dilated cardiomyopathy and the dystrophin gene: an illustrated review. British Heart Journal 72(4): 344–348

Olsen E G, Spry C J 1985 Relation between eosinophilia and endomyocardial disease. Progress in Cardiovascular Disease 27(4): 241–254

Orstavik K H, Skjorten F, Hellebostad M et al 1993 Possible X linked congenital mitochondrial cardiomyopathy in three families. Journal of Medical Genetics 30(4): 269–272

Ostman-Smith I 1991 Regression of cardiac hypertrophy achieved by high dose propranolol treatment in children and adults with hypertrophic cardiomyopathy. British Heart Journal 66: 76

Ostman-Smith I, Wetrell G 1997 Benefit from high-dose beta-adrenoceptor antagonist therapy on both survival and morbidity in childhood hypertrophic cardiomyopathy. In: Imai Y, Momma K (eds) Proceedings of the Second World Congress of Pediatric Cardiology and Cardiac Surgery, Futura Publishing Company, Inc. Armonk, New York, p 241–245

Paasch L H, Zook B C 1980 The pathogenesis of endocardial fibroelastosis in Burmese cats. Laboratory Investigation 42(2): 197–204

Paquet M, Hanna B D 1990 Myocardial disease. In: Garson Jr, A, Bricker J T, McNamara D G (eds) The science and practice of pediatric cardiology. Lea & Fabiger, Philadelphia, PA, p 1634–1646

Parrilo J E, Cunnion R E, Epstein S E et al 1989 A prospective randomised trial of prednisone for dilated cardiomyopathy. New England Journal of Medicine 321: 1061–1068

Paulus W J, Lorell B H, Craig W E et al 1983 Comparison of the effects of nitroprusside and nifedipine on diastolic properties in patients with hypertrophic cardiomyopathy: altered left ventricular loading or improved muscle

inactivation? Journal of the American College of Cardiology 2(5): 879–886

Paulus W J, Nellens P, Heyndrickx G R et al 1986 Effects of long-term treatment with amiodarone on exercise hemodynamics and left ventricular relaxation in patients with hypertrophic cardiomyopathy. Circulation 74(3): 544–554

Pelliccia F, Cianfrocca C, Romeo F et al 1990 Hypertrophic cardiomyopathy: long-term effects of propranolol versus verapamil in preventing sudden death in 'low-risk' patients. Cardiovascular Drugs & Therapy 4(6): 1515–1518

Perloff J K 1980 Neurological disorders and heart disease. In: Braunwald E (Ed.) Heart disease. Saunders, Philadelphia, PA, p 180

Pierce G E, Morrow A G, Braunwald E 1964 Idiopathic hypertrophic subaortic stenosis; intraoperative studies of the mechanism of obstruction and its hemodynamic consequence. Circulation 40(Suppl IV): 152–206

Piovan D, Padrini R, Svalato Moreolo G et al 1995 Verapamil and norverapamil plasma levels in infants and children during chronic oral treatment. Therapeutic Drug Monitoring 17(1): 60–67

Pollick C, Morgan C D, Gilbert B W et al 1982 Muscular subaortic stenosis: the temporal relationship between systolic anterior motion of the anterior mitral leaflet and the pressure gradient. Circulation 66(5): 1087–1094

Pollick C 1988 Disopyramide in hypertrophic cardiomyopathy. II. Noninvasive assessment after oral administration. American Journal of Cardiology 62(17): 1252–1255

Pollick C, Kimball B, Henderson M et al 1988 Disopyramide in hypertrophic cardiomyopathy. I. Hemodynamic assessment after intravenous administration. American Journal of Cardiology 62(17): 1248–1251

Pongpanigh B, Iasraprasart S 1985 Congestive cardiomyopathy in infants and children. Clinical features and natural history. Japanese Heart Journal 27: 11–15

Pons-Llado G, Carreras F, Borras X et al 1997 Comparison of morphologic assessment of hypertrophic cardiomyopathy by magnetic resonance versus echocardiographic imaging. American Journal of Cardiology 79(12): 1651–1656

Posma J L, Blanksma P K, van der Wall E E et al 1996 Assessment of quantitative hypertrophy scores in hypertrophic cardiomyopathy: magnetic resonance imaging versus echocardiography. American Heart Journal 132: 1020–1027

Puigbo J J, Combellas I, Acquatella H et al 1983 Endomyocardial disease in South America – report on 23 cases in Venezuela. Postgraduate Medical Journal 59(689): 162–169

Rao P S 1995 Afterload reduction for dilated cardiomyopathy. Pediatric Cardiology 16: 51

Revel A, Ariel I, Rein A J J T et al 1994 Fetal endocardial fibroelastosis. Journal of Clinical Ultrasound 22: 355–356

Rios B, Nihill M R, Mullins C E 1984 Left ventricular endomyocardial biopsy in children with the transseptal long sheath technique. Catheterization and Cardiovascular Diagnosis 10: 417–423

Roberts W C, Liegler D G, Carbone P P 1969 Endomyocardial disease and eosinophilia. A clinical and pathologic spectrum. American Journal of Medicine 46(1): 28–42

Roberts W C, Buja L M, Ferrans V J 1970 Loffler's fibroplastic parietal endocarditis, eosinophilic leukemia, and Davies' endomyocardial fibrosis: the same disease at different stages? Pathologia et Microbiologia 35(1): 90–95

Robinson K, Frenneaux M P, Stockins B et al 1990 Atrial fibrillation in hypertrophic cardiomyopathy: a longitudinal study. Journal of the American College of Cardiology 15(6): 1279–1285

Romeo F, Pellicia F, Cianfrocca C et al 1989 Determinants of end-stage idiopathic dilated cardiomyopathy: a multivariate analysis of 104 patients. Clinical Cardiology 12: 387–392

Romeo F, Cianfrocca C, Pelliccia F et al 1990 Long-term prognosis in children with hypertrophic cardiomyopathy: an analysis of 37 patients aged less than or equal to 14 years at diagnosis. Clinical Cardiology 13(2): 101–107

Roper N 1987 Pocket medical dictionary, 14th edn. Churchill Livingstone, Edinburgh, p 180

Rosenzweig A, Watkins H, Hwang D S et al 1991 Preclinical diagnosis of familial hypertrophic cardiomyopathy by genetic analysis of blood lymphocytes. New England Journal of Medicine 325(25): 1753–1760

Rosing D R, Kent K M, Maron B J et al 1979 Verapamil therapy: a new approach to the pharmacologic treatment of hypertrophic cardiomyopathy. II. Effects on exercise capacity and symptomatic status. Circulation 60(6): 1208–1213

Rosing D R, Condit J R, Maron B J et al 1981 Verapamil therapy: a new approach to the pharmacologic treatment of hypertrophic cardiomyopathy: III. Effects of long-term administration. American Journal of Cardiology 48(3): 545–553

Rosing D R, Idanpaan-Heikkila U, Maron B J et al 1985 Use of calcium-channel blocking drugs in hypertrophic cardiomyopathy. American Journal of Cardiology 55(3): 185B–195B

Ross J, Jr, Braunwald E, Gault J H et al 1966 The mechanism of the intraventricular pressure gradient in idiopathic hypertrophic subaortic stenosis. Circulation 34(4): 558–578

Rowe R D, Freedom R M, Mehrizi A et al 1981a Cardiomyopathies. In: The neonate with congenital heart disease. WB Saunders, Philadelphia, PA, 397–442

Rowe R D, Freedom R M, Mehrizi A et al 1981b Endocardial fibroelastosi. In: The neonate with congenital heart disease. Saunders, Philadelphia, PA, p 422–428

Rowe R D, Benson L N, Wilson G et al 1987 Clinical diagnosis of left ventricular endocardial fibroelastosis (EFE) of the dilated type: the Keith criteria and tissue confirmation. Paper presented at the 23rd Annual General Meeting, Association of European Paediatric Cardiologists, Hamburg

Ruesch S, Krahenbuhl S, Kleinle S et al 1996 Combined 3-methylglutaconic and 3-hydroxy-3-methylglutaric aciduria with endocardial fibroelastosis and dilatative cardiomyopathy in male and female siblings with partial deficiency of complex II/III in fibroblasts. Enzyme and Protein 49(5–6): 321–329

Ryan M P, Cleland J G, French J A et al 1995 The standard electrocardiogram as a screening test for hypertrophic cardiomyopathy. American Journal of Cardiology 76: 689–694

Saenz de la Calzada C, Ziady G M, Hardarson T et al 1976 Effect of acute administration of propranolol on ventricular function in hypertrophic obstructive cardiomyopathy measured by non-invasive techniques. British Heart Journal 38(8): 798–803

Sakakibara S, Konno S 1962 Endomyocardial biopsy. Japanese Heart Journal 3: 537–542

Sato T, Yamanari H, Ohe T et al 1996 Regional left ventricular contractile dynamics in hypertrophic cardiomyopathy evaluated by magnetic resonance imaging. Heart and Vessels 11(5): 248–254

Savage D D, Castelli W P, Abott R D et al 1983 Hypertrophic cardiomyopathy and its markers in the general population: the great masquerader revisited: the Framingham study. Journal of Cardiovascular Ultrasonography 2: 41–47

Schaffer M S, Freedom R M, Rowe R D 1983 Hypertrophic cardiomyopathy presenting before 2 years of age in 13 patients. Pediatric Cardiology 4(2): 113–119

Schmaltz A A, Apitz J, Hort W 1982 Endomyocardial biopsy in infants and children: technique, indications and results. European Heart Journal 138: 211–215

Schmaltz A A, Apitz J, Hort W 1987 Dilated cardiomyopathy in childhood: problems of diagnosis and long-term follow-up. Dilated cardiomyopathy in childhood: problems of diagnosis and long-term follow-up. European Heart Journal 8(2): 100–105

Schoenfeld M H, Supple E W, Dec G W, Jr. et al 1987 Restrictive cardiomyopathy versus constrictive pericarditis: role of endomyocardial biopsy in avoiding unnecessary thoracotomy. Circulation 75(5): 1012–1017

Schulz R, Vogt J, Voss W et al 1987 Mucolipidosis type II (I-cell disease) with unusually severe heart involvement. Monatsschrift Kinderheikunde 135(10): 708–711

Schwammenthal E, Wichter T, Joachimsen K et al 1994 Detection of regional left ventricular asynchrony in obstructive hypertrophic cardiomyopathy by magnetic resonance imaging. American Heart Journal 127(3): 600–606

Seiler C, Hess O M, Schoenbeck M et al 1991 Long-term follow-up of medical versus surgical therapy for hypertrophic cardiomyopathy: a retrospective study. Journal of the American College of Cardiology 17(3): 634–642

Sellers F J, Keith J D, Manning J A 1964 The diagnosis of primary endocardial fibroelastosis. Circulation 29: 49–59

Shaddy R E, Bullock E A 1993 Efficacy of 100 consecutive right ventricular endomyocardial biopsies in pediatric patients using the right internal jugular venous approach. Pediatric Cardiology 14: 5–8

Shaffer E M, Rocchini A P, Spicer R L et al 1988 Effects of verapamil on left ventricular diastolic filling in children with hypertrophic cardiomyopathy. American Journal of Cardiology 61(6): 413–417

Shapiro L M, Zezulka A 1983 Hypertrophic cardiomyopathy a common disease with a good prognosis. Five year experience of a district general hospital. British Heart Journal 50(6): 530–533

Sherrid M, Delia E, Dwyer E 1988 Oral disopyramide therapy for obstructive hypertrophic cardiomyopathy. American Journal of Cardiology 62(16): 1085–1088

Siegel R J, Shah P K, Fishbein M C 1984 Idiopathic restrictive cardiomyopathy. Circulation 70(2): 165–169

Sigwart U 1995 Non-surgical myocardial reduction for hypertrophic obstructive cardiomyopathy. Lancet 346(8969): 211–214

Skinner J R, Manzoor A, Hayes A M et al 1997 A regional study of presentation and outcome of hypertrophic cardiomyopathy in infants. Heart 77: 229–233

Sobaniec-Zotowska M, Sulkowski S, Sobaniec W et al 1991 Endocardial fibroelastosis in children to one year of age. Polski Tygodnik Lekarski 46(6–7): 118–120

Soler R, Rodriguez E, Rodriguez J A et al 1997 Magnetic resonance imaging of apical hypertrophic cardiomyopathy. Journal of Thoracic Imaging 12(3): 221–225

Solomon S D, Geisterfer-Lowrance A A, Vosberg H P et al 1990 A locus for familial hypertrophic cardiomyopathy is closely linked to the cardiac myosin heavy chain genes, CRI-L436, and CRI-L329 on chromosome 14 at q11-q12. American Journal of Human Genetics 47(3): 389–394

Soulie P, Joly F, Carlotti J 1962 Les stenoses idiopathique de la chambre de chase du ventricule gauche (A propos de 10 observations). Acta Cardiologica (Bruxelles) 17: 335–378

Speiser K W, Krayenbuehl H P 1981 Reappraisal of the effect of acute betablockade on left ventricular filling dynamics in hypertrophic obstructive cardiomyopathy. European Heart Journal 2(1): 21–29

Spicer R L, Rocchini A P, Crowley D C et al 1983 Hemodynamic effects of verapamil in children and adolescents with hypertrophic cardiomyopathy. Circulation 67(2): 413–420

Spicer R L, Rocchini A P, Crowley D C et al 1984 Chronic verapamil therapy in pediatric and young adult patients with hypertrophic cardiomyopathy. American Journal of Cardiology 53(11): 1614–1619

Spirito P, Rapezzi C, Autore C et al 1994 Prognosis of asymptomatic patients with hypertrophic cardiomyopathy and nonsustained ventricular tachycardia. Circulation 90(6): 2743–2747

Spirito P, Maron B J 1990 Relation between extent of left ventricular hypertrophy and occurrence of sudden cardiac death in hypertrophic cardiomyopathy. Journal of the American College of Cardiology 15(7): 1521–1526

Spry C J, Tai P C 1976 Studies on blood eosinophils. II. Patients with Loffler's cardiomyopathy. Clinical & Experimental Immunology 24(3): 423–434

St John Sutton M G, Lie J T, Anderson K R et al 1980 Histopathological specificity of hypertrophic obstructive cardiomyopathy. Myocardial fibre disarray and myocardial fibrosis. British Heart Journal 44(4): 433–443

Stafford W J, Trohman R G, Bilsker M et al 1986 Cardiac arrest in an adolescent with atrial fibrillation and hypertrophic cardiomyopathy. Journal of the American College of Cardiology 7(3): 701–704

Stein H, Shnier M H, Wayburne S et al 1964 Cardiomyopathy in African children. Archives of Diseases in Childhood 39: 610–617

Stephan M J, Stevens E L, Jr, Wenstrup R J et al 1989 Mucopolysaccharidosis I presenting with endocardial fibroelastosis of infancy. American Journal of Diseases of Children 143(7): 782–784

Sugrue D D, Dickie S, Myers M J et al 1984 Effect of amiodarone on left ventricular ejection and filling in hypertrophic cardiomyopathy as assessed by radionuclide angiography. American Journal of Cardiology 54(8): 1054–1058

Sumimoto T, Hamada M, Ohtani T et al 1992 Effect of disopyramide on left ventricular diastolic function in patients with hypertrophic cardiomyopathy: comparison with diltiazem. Cardiovascular Drugs & Therapy 6(4): 425–428

Suomalainen A, Paetau A, Leinonen H et al 1992 Inherited idiopathic dilated cardiomyopathy with multiple deletions of mitochondrial DNA. Lancet 340: 1319–1320

Sutton M G, Tajik A J, Gibson D G et al 1978 Echocardiographic assessment of left ventricular filling and septal and posterior wall dynamics in idiopathic hypertrophic subaortic stenosis. Circulation 57(3): 512–520

Suwa M, Hirota Y, Kawamura K 1984 Improvement in left ventricular diastolic function during intravenous and oral diltiazem therapy in patients with hypertrophic cardiomyopathy: an echocardiographic study. American Journal of Cardiology 54(8): 1047–1053

Suzuki J, Sakamoto T, Takenaka K et al 1988 Assessment of the thickness of the right ventricular free wall by magnetic resonance imaging in patients with hypertrophic cardiomyopathy. British Heart Journal 60(5): 440–445

Swanton R H, Brooksby I A, Jenkins B S et al 1977 Hemodynamic studies of beta blockade in hypertrophic obstructive cardiomyopathy. European Journal of Cardiology 5(4): 327–341

Taliercio C P, Seward J B, Driscoll D J et al 1985 Idiopathic dilated cardiomyopathy in the young: clinical profile and natural history. Journal of American College of Cardiology 6: 1126–1131.

Taliercio C P 1988 Dilated cardiomyopathy in children. Journal of American College of Cardiology 11: 145–146

Teare R D 1958 Asymmetrical hypertrophy of the heart in young adults. British Heart Journal 20: 1–8

Ten Cate F J 1978 Asymmetric septal hypertrophy (ASH): echocardiographic manifestations. Theses, Brander-Offset, Rotterdam

Thierfelder L, Watkins H, MacRae C et al 1994 Alpha-tropomyosin and cardiac troponin T mutations cause familial hypertrophic cardiomyopathy: a disease of the sarcomere. Cell 77(5): 701–712

Thompson D S, Naqvi N, Juul S M et al 1980 Effects of propranolol on myocardial oxygen consumption, substrate extraction, and haemodynamics in hypertrophic obstructive cardiomyopathy. British Heart Journal 44(5): 488–498

Thompson D S, Wilmshurst P, Juul S M et al 1983 Pressure-derived indices of left ventricular isovolumic relaxation in patients with hypertrophic cardiomyopathy. British Heart Journal 49(3): 259–267

Toshima H, Koga Y, Nagata H et al 1986 Comparable effects of oral diltiazem and verapamil in the treatment of hypertrophic cardiomyopathy. Double-blind crossover study. Japanese Heart Journal 27(5): 701–715

Towbin J A, Heijtmancik J F, Brink P et al 1993 X-linked dilated cardiomyopathy: molecular genetic evidence of linkage to the Duchenne muscular dystrophy (dystrophin) gene at Xp21 locus. Circulation 87: 1854–1865

Tripp M E, Katcher M L, Peters H E et al 1981 Systemic carnitine deficiency presenting as familial endocardial fibroelastosis. A treatable cardiomyopathy. New England Journal of Medicine 305: 385–390

Troesch M, Hirzel H O, Jeni R et al 1979 Reduction of septal thickness in patients with asymmetric septal hypertrophy (ASH). Circulation 60(suppl II): 155

Vaitkus P T, Kussmaul W G 1991 Constrictive pericarditis versus restrictive cardiomyopathy: a reappraisal and update of diagnostic criteria. American Heart Journal 122(5): 1431–1441

Vitale D F, Bonow R O, Calabro R et al 1996 Myocardial ultrasonic tissue characterization in pediatric and adult patients with hypertrophic cardiomyopathy. Circulation 94: 2826–2830

Walsh R A 1989 The effects of calcium entry blockade on normal and ischemic ventricular diastolic function. Circulation 80 (suppl IV): 52–58

Watkins H, Seidman C E, MacRae C et al 1992a Progress in familial hypertrophic cardiomyopathy: molecular genetic analyses in the original family studied by Teare. British Heart Journal 67(1): 34–38

Watkins H, Thierfelder L, Hwang D S et al 1992b Sporadic hypertrophic cardiomyopathy due to de novo myosin mutations. Journal of Clinical Investigation 90(5): 1666–1671

Watkins H, Conner D, Thierfelder L et al 1995 Mutations in the cardiac myosin binding protein-C gene on chromosome 11 cause familial hypertrophic cardiomyopathy. Nature Genetics 11(4): 434–437

Webb-Peploe M M 1985 Beta-blockade in the treatment of hypertrophic cardiomyopathy. (In: Cardiomyopathies – the message for the 1980s) Postgraduate Medical Journal 61: 1105–1135

Webber S A, Sandor G G S, Farquharson D et al 1993 Diagnosis and outcome of dilated cardiomyopathy in the fetus. Cardiology in the Young 3: 27–33

Webber S A, Boyle G J, Jaffe R et al 1994 Role of right ventricular endomyocardial biopsy in infants and children with suspected or possible myocarditis. British Heart Journal 72: 360–363

Wellens H J J, Cubbers W J, Losekoot T G 1977 Preexcitation. In: Robert N K, Gelband H (eds) Cardiac arrhythmias in the neonate, infant and child. Appleton-Century Crofts, NY, p. 231–263

Weller A H, Hall M, Huber S A 1992 Polyclonal immunoglobulin therapy protects against cardiac damage in experimental coxsackievirus-induced myocarditis. European Heart Journal 13: 115–119

Westwood M, Harris R, Burn J L et al 1975 Heredity in primary endocardial fibroelastosis. British Heart Journal 37(10): 1077–1084

Westwood M 1977 Endocardial fibroelastosis and Niemann-Pick disease. British Heart Journal 39(12): 1394–1396

WHO/ISFC (World Health Organization/International Society and Federation of Cardiology) Task Force 1980 Report on the definition and classification of cardiomyopathies. British Heart Journal 44: 672–673

WHO/ISFC (World Health Organization/International Society and Federation of Cardiology) Task Force 1996 Report on the definition and classification of cardiomyopathies 1995. Circulation 93: 841–842

Wigle E D 1962 Idiopathic ventricular septal hypertrophy causing muscular subaortic stenosis. Circulation 26: 325–340

Wigle E D 1964 Muscular subaortic stenosis. The clinical syndrome, with additional evidence of ventricular septal hypertrophy. In: Wolstenholme G E W, O'Connor M (eds) Cardiomyopathies. Ciba Foundation Symposium 49. Churchill, London

Wilensky R L, Yudelman P, Cohen A I et al 1988 Serial electrocardiographic changes in idiopathic dilated cardiomyopathy confirmed at necropsy. American Journal of Cardiology 62: 276–283

Wiles H B, McArthur P D, Taylor A B et al 1991 Prognostic features of children with idiopathic dilated cardiomyopathy. American Journal of Cardiology 68: 1372–1376

Williams R G, Tucker C R 1977 Echocardiographic diagnosis of congenital heart disease. Little Brown, Boston, MA, 201–211

Williams W G, Wigle E D, Rakowski H et al 1987 Results of surgery for hypertrophic obstructive cardiomyopathy. Circulation 76 (Suppl V): 104–108

Wilmshurst P T, Thompson D S, Juul S M et al 1986 Effects of verapamil on haemodynamic function and myocardial metabolism in patients with hypertrophic cardiomyopathy. British Heart Journal 56(6): 544–553

Wong C Y, Woodruff J J, Woodruff J F R 1977 Generation of cytotoxic T lymphocytes during coxsackievirus B-3 infection: II. Characterisation of effector cells and demonstration of cytotoxicity against viral-infected myofibers. Journal of Immunology 118: 1165–1169

Wong P, Cotter L, Gibson D G 1980 Early systolic closure of the aortic valve. British Heart Journal 44(4): 386–389

Yamaguchi H, Ishimura T, Nishiyama S et al 1979 Hypertrophic nonobstructive cardiomyopathy with giant negative T waves (apical hypertrophy): ventriculographic and echocardiographic features in 30 patients. American Journal of Cardiology 44(3): 401–412

Yamakado T, Okano H, Higashiyama S et al 1990 Effects of nifedipine on left ventricular diastolic function in patients with asymptomatic or minimally symptomatic hypertrophic cardiomyopathy. Circulation 81(2): 593–601

Yamanari H, Morita H, Nakamura K et al 1996 Assessment of regional early diastolic function using cine magnetic resonance imaging in patients with hypertrophic cardiomyopathy. Japanese Circulation Journal 60(12): 917–924

Yoshizato T, Edwards W D, Alboliras E T et al 1990 Safety and utility of endomyocardial biopsy in infants, children and adolescents: a review of 66 procedures in 53 patients. Journal of American College of Cardiology 15: 436–442

Yukihito S, Maruyama S, Kawai C et al 1992 Effect of immunostimulant therapy on acute viral myocarditis in an animal model. American Heart Journal 124: 428–434

Zosmer N, Bajoria R, Weiner E et al 1994 Clinical and echographic features of in utero cardiac dysfunction in the recipient twin in twin–twin transfusion syndrome. British Heart Journal 72(1): 74–79

60

Arterio-venous fistulas and related conditions

S. A. Qureshi and J. F. Reidy

INTRODUCTION

An arterio-venous fistula is an abnormal connection between an artery and a vein without an intervening capillary bed. As a result of the low resistance in the veins, a large shunt can occur through the fistula. There is shunting throughout the cardiac cycle and conse- quently, a continuous murmur is produced. Arterio- venous fistulas can involve either the pulmonary or sys- temic circulations. These are separate entities. They will, therefore, be considered separately.

EXTRACARDIAC SYSTEMIC ARTERIO-VENOUS MALFORMATIONS

Arterio-venous malformations and fistulas can affect any part of the body. They have a wide range of pathologies, ranging from malformations consisting of abnormal capillaries and dilated venous spaces to direct fistulous communications between a major artery and vein.

Such systemic arterio-venous malformations and fistulas can be subdivided into those within and those outside the heart. Extracardiac systemic arterio-venous malformations are only of importance to the paediatric cardiologist when they are haemodynamically significant and are associated with a large left-to-right shunt. This is a rare situation. Such abnormalities are usually congenital in origin. Any large systemic malformation may present with high-output cardiac failure in later life but rarely in childhood. When a neonate or infant presents with high-output cardiac failure, the most likely extracardiac cause is an aneurysm of the vein of Galen.

ANEURYSM OF THE VEIN OF GALEN

Aneurysm of the vein of Galen is an intracerebral arterio- venous malformation. It is the most frequent haemo- dynamically significant extracardiac arterio-venous malformation. It is an uncommon cause of severe cardiac failure in infancy. Affected neonates and infants present with congestive cardiac failure that suggests a cardiac cause and can, therefore, give rise to diagnostic problems. One or multiple feeding arteries directly communicate with the vein. The massive dilation of the vein is then the result of large volume of flow through the fistula, as it is the preferred site of venous drainage.

CLINICAL PRESENTATION

Aneurysm of the vein of Galen is an uncommon mal- formation. Between 1964 and 1982, at Great Ormond Street Hospital in London, 16 patients were encountered (Stanbridge et al, 1983), while only 29 patients were seen with such aneurysms at the Hospital for Sick Children in Toronto between 1950 and 1980 (Hoffman et al, 1982). Review of the English literature from 1937 to 1981 showed 128 cases.

Clinical presentation was characteristic for neonates, infants and older children and adults. Of the 128 patients, 45 presented in the neonatal period, 36 were seen between 3 weeks and 11 months, and 47 were older children and adults. Of the 45 neonates, all but two presented with heart failure; these two presented with subarachnoid haemor- rhage and hydrocephalus respectively. In addition to heart failure, which is often refractory to treatment, these neonates showed features of pulmonary hypertension and myocardial ischaemia, as well as cerebral ischaemia resulting from the cerebral 'steal' effect. Compared with the neonates, only 2 of the 36 patients presenting as infants had heart failure. The majority had hydrocephalus, although one patient presented with a subarachnoid haemorrhage. In the 47 older children and adults, only one had heart failure, with the most common presentation being subarachnoid haemorrhage (in 18). Hydrocephalus developed in 14; venous hypertension resulting in epistaxis and distended veins occurred in seven, while, in a further seven, there was generalized neurological deterioration thought to be caused by the steal effect of the fistula. In the neonate, if the pul- monary vascular resistance remains high, right-to-left shunting and cyanosis can occur as a result of the grossly increased systemic return. As the run-off from the arterial to venous circulations is of low resistance, there may be bounding pulses, particularly in the carotid arteries, as well as tachycardia. The neck veins may be engorged, and a continuous murmur is typically heard over the skull vault.

DIAGNOSIS

When the fistula is large, the chest radiograph usually shows cardiac enlargement with marked pulmonary plethora (Figure 60.1). If there is significant right-to-left shunting as a result of an elevated pulmonary vascular resistance, then pulmonary oligaemia may also be present. The electrocardiogram usually shows biventricular hypertrophy. Echocardiography demonstrates enlargement of all four chambers and excludes a cardiac cause for heart failure. Prior to the availability of ultrasound, the diagnosis was often made with difficulty, and angiography was usually necessary. Ultrasonic scanning of the head via the anterior fontanelle now demonstrates the centrally situated aneurysmal vein of Galen; it also often shows the presence of the feeding arteries (Figure 60.2). Doppler ultrasound, and in particular colour Doppler, more readily demonstrates the direction of blood flow.

Angiography

Although no longer necessary to make the diagnosis, detailed angiography is needed to plan the management of these patients. Right-sided intracardiac pressures are often elevated, especially when there is cardiac failure or when the pulmonary vascular resistance is elevated. The presence of a raised superior caval venous oxygen

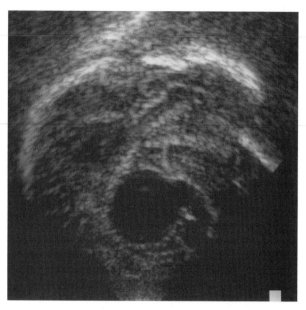

Figure 60.2. A transfontanelle ultrasound shows a large central circular echo-free abnormality (black circle) typical of a vein of Galen aneurysm. A large vein is seen draining from the right side. Colour Doppler should demonstrate arterial flow.

saturation reflects the degree of left-to-right shunting. Four-vessel cerebral angiography is necessary to give a detailed assessment of the arterial supply prior to any subsequent intervention. Digital angiography reduces the amount of contrast medium needed. Non-ionic contrast media should always be used. Detailed selective angiography is necessary to plan treatment by surgery or transcatheter embolization (Figure 60.3).

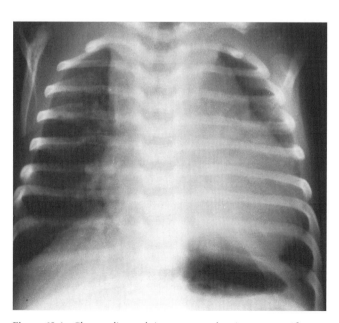

Figure 60.1. Chest radiograph in a neonate showing non-specific features of marked cardiac enlargement and pulmonary plethora. The absence of any intracardiac abnormality on echocardiography should suggest the diagnosis of a vein of Galen aneurysm.

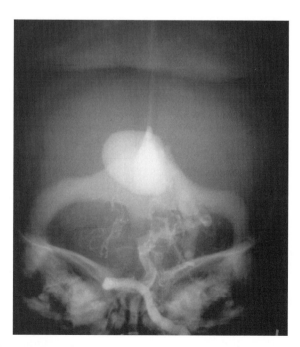

Figure 60.3. A selective carotid arteriogram (anteroposterior view) shows the vein of Galen aneurysm rapidly filling via multiple small arterial branches. It gained a further supply from the contralateral carotid artery.

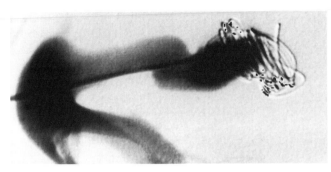

Figure 60.4. Percutaneous catheterization of a vein of Galen aneurysm via the transtorcular approach (lateral view). The catheter tip is in the vein of Galen aneurysm and multiple large 0.038 inch (0.95 mm) steel coils have been positioned within it. Injection of contrast demonstrates the large straight sinus draining to the lateral sinuses.

Four patterns of angiographic findings have been described. In neonates, multiple arteries arise from the internal carotid arterial branches and feed the aneurysm at its anterosuperior border. The aneurysm then drains by very large straight and lateral sinuses (Figure 60.4). Most commonly in infants, the feeding artery is situated inferiorly and laterally and consists of a single posterior choroidal artery. In infants and older children, the feeding arteries are usually located anteriorly and superiorly and consist of one or two posterior choroidal arteries, as well as anterior cerebral arteries. In older children, most commonly the feeding vessels consist of a network of branches arising from the posterior choroidal and thalamic perforating arteries.

MANAGEMENT

Interest in these aneurysms has increased in recent years because of their earlier detection with ultrasound and the availability of new methods of treatment, such as transcatheter embolization. In neonates, the two major problems are the cerebral damage caused by the steal effect, and the marked degree of shunting that may result in myocardial ischaemia and infarction. If the flow on the arterial side can be reduced, these effects may diminish. Both the aneurysm and the vein of Galen may then become smaller, or even return to normal. It is then not necessary to resect the aneurysm, unlike other arteriovenous malformations in which there is a tendency for recurrence. The outlook in the neonates treated medically is grim. In the Toronto series, seven out of eight children treated medically died (Hoffman et al, 1982). Only one of seven surgically treated neonates survived, but this child had a residual hemiparesis.

Embolization

Transcatheter embolization has been employed since the late 1980s, during which time digital angiography, and increasingly sophisticated techniques, have enabled it to

be developed into an effective alternative to surgery (Ciricillo et al, 1990; Friedman et al, 1991; Lasjaunias et al, 1991). There are three main approaches. Using a transfemoral arterial approach, the feeding arteries to the aneurysm can be selectively catheterized and embolized with liquid agents such as bucrilate. This poses technical problems in neonates in catheterizing the small intracerebral branches. An alternative, and more direct, route is a torcular approach. A small craniectomy is made over the region of the torcular, and the straight sinus is directly entered percutaneously (Figure 60.4) (Mickle and Quisling, 1986; Hanner et al, 1988; Nelson et al, 1988). The third approach is to employ retrograde venous access (Dowd et al, 1990). Great care must be taken not to create too dramatic a disturbance in the intracerebral haemodynamics, and risks of intracerebral bleeding should be avoided during manipulation of the catheter. One centre has evaluated its experience with 43 patients, with transarterial embolization with bucrilate used in 34 patients (Lasjaunias et al, 1991). Occlusion of the lesion was confirmed by follow-up angiography in 47% when the child was 6 months of age or older. The overall mortality in the neonates was 28%, with a total of 18.6% for all ages. Of all the referred cases, three quarters were considered clinically normal or showed only moderate mental retardation, which was diminishing. These results represent a significant advance in management.

Infants have a much better outlook than neonates. Of eight infants in the Toronto series, six were treated surgically, and five of these were reported to be normal after the procedure (Hoffman et al, 1982). Transcatheter embolization is an attractive alternative therapy in these older children, as there is usually a single feeding artery. The progress that has been made in treatment is well summarized in the experience from two centres (Edwards et al, 1988; Friedman et al, 1991). In a review of 12 years' experience at one of these centres, only five of the first eleven patients survived, four having seizures, and three with marked mental retardation (Friedman et al, 1991). In contrast, six of the last eleven patients survived, five still with seizures, but only one with mental retardation.

CORONARY ARTERIO-VENOUS FISTULAS

Coronary arterio-venous malformations, or fistulas, are direct connections between one or more of the coronary arteries and a cardiac chamber or great vessel. They are rare, especially in the absence of other additional intracardiac defects such as pulmonary atresia with intact ventricular septum (Levin et al, 1978). They are, however, the most common coronary arterial anomaly that is haemodynamically significant (Effler et al, 1967; Baltaxe and Wilson 1977; Wilde and Watt, 1980). Although usually congenital, they have been noted after cardiac surgery, such as valvar replacement, coronary artery

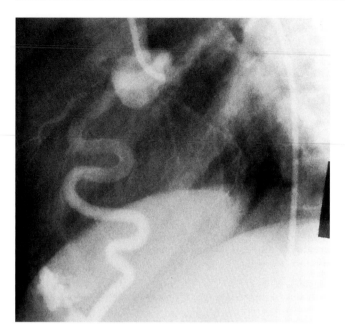

Figure 60.5. A non-selective left coronary angiogram in the left anterior oblique projection showing a coronary arterio-venous fistula originating from a dilated diagonal branch of the left anterior descending coronary artery; the fistula has a long and tortuous course and terminates in the right ventricle.

bypass grafting or after repeated myocardial biopsies in cardiac transplantation (Jebara et al, 1991; Marin-Neto et al, 1991; Reidy et al, 1991; Somers and Varney, 1991).

Typically, the fistula consists of a dilated artery that has a long and tortuous course around the heart before terminating in a chamber or a vessel (Figure 60.5). The fistula may drain a major coronary artery, or one or several branches of a coronary artery, to either a cardiac chamber or a nearby vessel. Multiple feeding arteries to a single coronary arterio-venous fistula may also occur (Podolsky et al, 1991; Reidy et al, 1991). More than half of the fistulas originate from the right coronary artery, the left anterior descending coronary artery being next most frequently involved (McNamara and Gross, 1969). Origin from both the right and left coronary arteries is rare, with an incidence of about 5% (Babb and Field, 1977; Baim et al, 1982). Nine tenths of the fistulas from either coronary artery drain to the right side of the heart. The remainder drain to either the left atrium or the left ventricle (Levin et al, 1978). The sites of drainage in the right heart include right atrium or its tributaries, the right ventricle or the pulmonary trunk. Multiple fistulas between the three major coronary arteries and the left ventricle have also been reported (Black et al, 1991).

PATHOPHYSIOLOGY

When coronary arteriovenous fistulas drain to the right side of the heart, or its venous tributaries, the volume load is increased to the right heart, as well as to the pulmonary vascular bed, the left atrium and the left ventricle. When the fistulas connect with the left atrium or the left ventricle, there is volume overloading of these chambers but no increase in the flow to the lungs.

CLINICAL FEATURES

Although the fistulas are congential, they do not usually cause symptoms or complications in the first two decades of life. After this age, the frequency of both symptoms and complications increases (Liberthson et al, 1979). The aneurysmal section of the fistula may slowly and progressively dilate, and the feeding artery may become more tortuous with time (Takahashi et al, 1994). The important complications include 'steal' from the adjacent myocardium, resulting in ischaemia and angina, atherosclerotic changes at points of stress, thrombosis and embolism, cardiac failure, atrial fibrillation, rupture, endocarditis, endarteritis and arrhythmias (Haberman et al, 1963; McNamara and Gross, 1969; St John Sutton et al, 1980; Wilde and Watt 1980; Moro-Serrano et al, 1992; Skimming and Walls, 1993; Alkhulaifi et al 1995). Recently, recurrent septic pulmonary embolism has been reported as a complication of endocarditis of the tricuspid valve in association with a coronary arterial fistula (Ong, 1993). Jet lesions may be found on the wall of the coronary sinus opposite the site of entry of the fistula, on the tricuspid valve or at the orifice of the coronary artery (Tsagaris and Hecht 1962; Symbas et al, 1967; Ong, 1993). Thrombosis within the fistula may, on occasions, result in acute myocardial infarction, paroxysmal atrial fibrillation and ventricular arrhythmias (Ramo et al, 1994; Roughneen et al, 1994; Shirai et al, 1994). Spontaneous rupture of the aneurysmal fistula, resulting in haemopericardium, has also been reported (Bauer et al, 1996).

Some fistulas may be large in the newborn period, but others may increase in size over time. They vary from simple short and direct connections between a coronary artery and a chamber or a large vessel (such as fistula from a coronary artery to the pulmonary trunk) to complex aneurysmal cavities in which blood may stagnate, clot and calcify. The largest shunts tend to occur in those fistulas in which the coronary artery connects to the right side of the heart rather than to the left. Even with these, the left-to-right shunt is rarely more than 3:1; usually it is less than 2:1.

In many of the early reported cases, the fistula was discovered incidentally at postmortem. Now presentation is usually with an asymptomatic continuous murmur, or occasionally with various symptoms related to the cardiovascular system (Vavuranakis et al, 1995). Coronary arterio-venous fistulas have been discovered in 0.1% of over 33 000 patients who had coronary angiography (Vavuranakis et al, 1995). The majority of the patients are asymptomatic, with normal exercise tolerance.

Symptoms, when present, include exercise intolerance because of dyspnoea, angina and arrhythmias. Patients with large left-to-right shunts may have symptoms of congestive cardiac failure, especially in infancy, and occasionally in the neonatal period (Bosi et al, 1992). Presentation with congestive cardiac failure has also been reported in the elderly (Kugelmass et al, 1992). Some may have angina and electrocardiographic evidence of myocardial ischaemia (Reidy et al, 1991). The mechanism of angina produced by congenital coronary arterial fistulas has been discussed by several authors (Swank and Koepke, 1972; Rittenhouse et al, 1975; Liberthson et al, 1979; Ahmed et al, 1982; Urrutia et al, 1983). It may occur because of a 'steal phenomenon', similar to that which is thought to occur when the coronary arteries arise anomalously from the pulmonary arteries. The fact that exercise-stress thallium scintigraphy has shown the presence of reversible ischaemia supports the phenomenon of 'coronary steal' (Oshiro et al, 1990). In an isolated case report of a patient with atypical chest pain, however, stress scintigraphy and multigated ventriculography failed to reveal any direct evidence of 'coronary steal' (Said et al, 1992).

The single most important physical sign that results in referral to paediatric cardiologists is the detection of an asymptomatic continuous murmur over the precordium. The murmur, while sounding similar to that of a patent arterial duct, has to be differentiated from it. The murmur is heard over the mid-chest rather than below the left clavicle, even to the right of the sternal border, and typically peaks in mid-diastole rather than systole, as occurs when the murmur originates from the arterial duct. Such findings should alert the physician to the possibility of a coronary arterio-venous fistula. The patient is then referred for echocardiographic assessment.

DIFFERENTIAL DIAGNOSIS

The differential diagnoses include patency of the arterial duct, ruptured aneurysm of a sinus of Valsalva, ventricular septal defect with aortic regurgitation, venous hums and other systemic and pulmonary arterio-venous fistulas. Indeed, when it became possible to operate upon patent arterial ducts, similarities in physical findings led to unintentional surgical exploration of a few patients with coronary arterial fistulas.

INVESTIGATIONS

The electrocardiogram and chest radiograph are unlikely to help in the diagnosis and assessment. The electrocardiogram may show the effects of left ventricular volume overload and ischaemic changes. If the electrocardiogram is normal, and the patient is old enough to exercise either on the treadmill or a bicycle with electrocardiographic

monitoring, ST segment changes indicative of ischaemia may become apparent. Generally a chest radiograph is normal, but occasionally moderate cardiomegaly may be present.

Coronary arterio-venous fistulas can usually be demonstrated by cross-sectional echocardiography (Reeder et al, 1980; Agatston et al, 1984; Satomi et al, 1984; Cooper et al, 1985). When the proximal coronary artery that feeds the fistula is dilated and tortuous in the presence of a large shunt, cross-sectional echocardiography is helpful in making an accurate diagnosis. When the fistula and the resulting shunt are small, colour Doppler echocardiography may be diagnostic. This may clearly show the chamber or the vessel into which the fistula drains. Conventional pulsed and continuous wave Doppler can then confirm the high-velocity flow through the fistula. If a dilated coronary artery can be traced from its origin from the aorta into the fistula, the diagnosis can be confirmed with certainty by conventional Doppler, and in particular by colour flow mapping (Reeder et al, 1980). In some studies, single or biplane transoesophageal echocardiography has been employed for better definition of the fistulas (Rubin et al, 1992; Sunaga et al, 1992; Prewitt et al, 1994).

Assessment by nuclear cardiological techniques is not necessary for the diagnosis but may provide additional information that may aid subsequent management. A first-pass radionuclide scan, which has been shown to be superior to cardiac catheterization in quantifying the shunt (Baker et al, 1985), will estimate the size of the left-to-right shunt. In patients who are able to exercise, and especially those who complain of angina or dyspnoea, stress thallium scanning may demonstrate reversible ischaemia; it may also determine the size of the territory under threat of ischaemia (Oshiro et al, 1990). In older patients, other areas of acquired coronary arterial disease may be discovered that influence the subsequent management. In these older patients, if a coronary arterial fistula is discovered, even if the coronary arteries are free of atheromatous disease, closure of such a fistula may relieve the symptoms (Prakash et al, 1993).

Selective coronary angiography is essential to confirm the diagnosis, and to demonstrate the detailed anatomy of the fistula (Figure 60.6). This should only be performed when definitive treatment is planned and now should rarely be required to make the diagnosis. Cardiac catheterization also determines the size of the shunt. While clues will be available from the cross-sectional and colour Doppler echocardiograms, a preliminary root aortogram helps to determine which coronary artery to catheterize selectively. Visualization of the fistula may be improved by using the 'laid-back' aortogram (Hofbeck et al, 1993). This is obtained by adding a 45 degrees caudal angulation to the frontal view with slight left or right anterior oblique orientation. A more important reason for detailed selective coronary angiographic assessment is to investigate the possibility of multiple

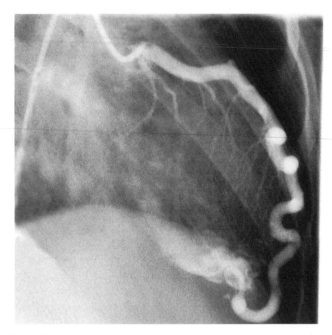

Figure 60.6. A selective left coronary arteriogram (same patient as in Figure 60.5) in the right anterior oblique projection showing the anatomy of the fistula more clearly. The normal coronary arterial branches are less well filled. There appears to be a single feeding artery draining to the right ventricle.

feeding vessels to the fistula (Figure 60.7). Coronary angiography in several planes then assumes great importance; it should be performed as in adults. These views include right anterior oblique, straight anteroposterior, left anterior oblique, left anterior oblique with caudocranial angulation, and left lateral projections.

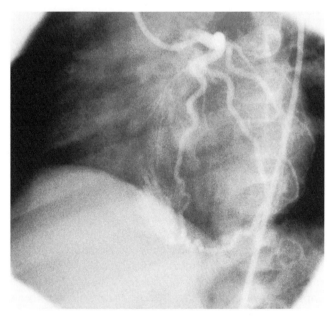

Figure 60.7. A selective left coronary arteriogram in the left anterior oblique projection showing two feeding arteries (left anterior descending and its diagonal branch) draining into the right ventricle. Often the second feeding artery only becomes obvious when the first one has been occluded.

MANAGEMENT

SURGERY

As techniques for accurately diagnosing coronary arteriovenous fistulas have improved, open heart surgery has become safer, making it even more unlikely that the natural history will ever be clearly defined. Most authors have advocated surgery in view of the low operative mortality (Blanche and Chaux, 1990; Davis et al, 1994; Carrel et al, 1996; Mavroudis et al, 1997). Liberthson et al (1979) showed that symptomatic patients over 20 years of age had considerably more problems, as well as more postoperative complications. They concluded that all significant coronary arterial fistulas should be closed, even in the absence of symptoms, to prevent potential complications such as bacterial endarteritis, progressive enlargement, secondary atherosclerotic involvement with rupture, and thromboembolism. Early surgery also avoids postoperative problems that can complicate later operations. This policy has to be balanced against the well-documented reports of spontaneous regression, or closure, in some younger children with relatively small fistulas draining into the right ventricle (Jaffe et al, 1973; Liberthson et al, 1979; Griffiths et al, 1983; Hackett and Hallidie-Smith, 1984; Muthusamy et al, 1990; Nakatani et al, 1991).

The aim of surgery is to close the fistula while preserving the flow of blood through normal coronary branches. Different surgical techniques have been used, and all of them appear to be adequate. The fistula is closed at the point of entry into the heart, without interrupting the continuity of the more proximal coronary artery. Closure can be achieved, without extracorporeal circulation, by clamping and suturing the fistulous channels on the outside of the heart. This approach does not require opening the fistula, the cardiac chambers or the great vessels, and the technique may be performed with the heart beating. More frequently, however, cardiopulmonary bypass is needed. This may be essential if it becomes necessary to enter a chamber to close the fistula from within, or if insertion of a bypass graft is necessary to maintain viability of the myocardium distal to the ligated artery. A small proportion of patients may develop complications postoperatively. These include ischaemia or infarction downstream from the point of ligation. This may be especially significant when a fistula from the right coronary artery drains to the right atrium or superior caval vein. Ligation of such a vessel may interrupt the artery of the sinus node.

Surgical treatment is associated with some morbidity but a low mortality rate, ranging from 0 to 6% (Abott et al, 1961; Hallman et al, 1966; Meyer et al, 1975; Rittenhouse et al, 1975; Wilde and Watt 1980; Macri et al, 1982; Kirklin and Barrat-Boyes, 1987; Muthusamy et al, 1990; Carrel et al, 1996; Mavroudis et al, 1997). Myocardial infarction has been reported in less than 5%

of patients (Rittenhouse et al, 1975), and there is a low but significant risk of persistence or recurrence of the fistula (Abott et al, 1961; Hallman et al, 1966; Meyer et al, 1975; Rittenhouse et al, 1975; Urrutia et al, 1983). The true incidence of recurrence, however, is unknown. Median sternotomy and cardiopulmonary bypass also have their own associated morbidity (Kirklin and Barrat-Boyes, 1987). Little has been said about the possibility of developing arteriosclerosis in the region of the fistula either subsequent to or prior to surgical treatment.

TRANSCATHETER EMBOLIZATION

Until recently, surgery was the only definitive treatment available for coronary arterio-venous fistulas. Recently, percutaneous transcatheter embolization has emerged as an effective and safe alternative. When available, it should be considered the treatment of choice (Reidy et al, 1983, 1985, 1990, 1991; Bennett and Maree 1989; Hartnell and Jordan, 1990; Issenberg, 1990; Perry et al, 1992; van den Brand, 1992).

The aim of embolization is to occlude the fistulous artery as distally as possible, or as close to its termination as possible. This should preclude any possibility of occluding branches to normal myocardium. If, however, embolization is effected too distally, the device employed could pass beyond the fistula into the draining vessel or chamber, and thence into the pulmonary circulation. Consequently, it is important that, whatever technique is used, the occlusion is effected at a very precise point. In practice, this means using different types of material for embolization, such as detachable balloons, stainless steel coils or platinum microcoils (Hartnell and Jordan, 1990; Issenberg, 1990; Reidy et al, 1991; Perry et al, 1992; van den Brand, 1992; de Wolf et al, 1994; Skimming et al, 1995).

The particular technique employed will depend on the age of the patient and the arrangement of the feeding arteries, their size, degree of tortuosity and the location of the fistulous connection. The arteries to these fistulas, even in small children, may be both large and tortuous. Detachable balloons have been effectively deployed as they can be floated out with arterial flow. They effect immediate occlusion that is reversible until the balloon is detached. They are, however, complex to use and require large non-tapered catheters for their introduction, which presents a limitation to their use in infants and young children (Reidy et al, 1983, 1985, 1991; Skimming et al, 1995). Early deflation and premature detachment of these balloons are further problems. Generally they are little used.

Steel coils (0.038 inch (0.95 mm)) have been widely used for embolization elsewhere in the vascular system. Standard non-tapered catheters of 5 or 6 French size are required for delivery. Positioning such catheters satisfactorily in a distal location in the fistula may be both difficult and hazardous. In such circumstances, platinum

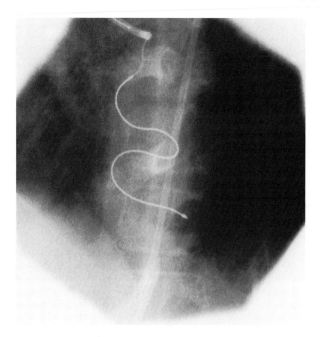

Figure 60.8. A cine frame in the left anterior oblique projection showing a guiding catheter at the origin of the main stem of the left coronary artery. Through this, a 3 Fr Tracker catheter has been passed along the tortuous coronary arterio-venous fistula and placed in a distal location (same patient as in Figures 60.5 and 60.6). A controlled release coil is just protruding through the tip of the Tracker catheter.

microcoils (0.018 inch (0.45 mm)) are safer, particularly when a coaxial 3 French catheter is used. Such catheters, used with steerable guidewires, can be manipulated safely through tortuous arteries into very distal locations (Figure 60.8). Moreover, the high flow that is usually encountered in coronary arterial fistulas can be difficult to occlude. Using a mass of platinum coils is frequently necessary. Recently, new coils that can be delivered with control have become available. They are now being evaluated clinically (de Wolf et al, 1994; Qureshi et al, 1996). The procedure has become safer with their use, and coils as long as 30 cm can now be positioned, with the added advantage of being withdrawable back into the catheter if the final position is not satisfactory. These coils are not fibred, and this results in very little resistance to their passage through the microcatheters. Even if these coils embolize inadvertently, they are easy to retrieve. Fistulous arteries permitting very high flow present a particular problem, but temporary occlusion of the proximal artery with a balloon occlusion catheter has allowed an occluding mass of these coils (Figure 60.9) to be safely and satisfactorily positioned (Quek et al, 1996; Qureshi et al, 1996). This technique should now be regarded as optimal.

Arteriography will usually have demonstrated the fistula prior to embolization. Further detailed and more selective coronary angiography may be necessary to obtain more details of the normal coronary arterial branches, which may be small but are at risk during occlusion. The 'steal' effect from a fistula permitting high

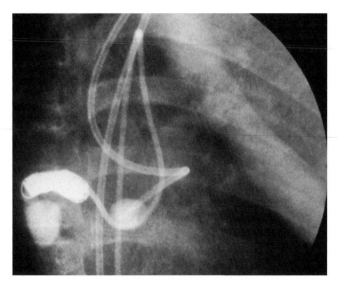

Figure 60.9. In a patient with a large fistula from the right coronary artery to the right atrium, a 5 Fr Berman balloon has been inflated in the proximal dilated feeding artery in order to stop the flow in the fistula. This has allowed multiple coils to be placed distally and packed to produce occlusion of the fistula. Once the balloon is deflated, the nest of coils should stay in place.

flow usually results in poor opacification of the normal branches. Their presence and size may consequently be underestimated.

Whatever method is used, occlusion or near occlusion should have been effected soon after the embolization. Sometimes, a small second branch feeding the fistula may only become opacified when the main feeding vessel has been occluded (Figure 60.10). It is vital to select a technique of embolization that is suitable for the size and the location of the fistula. A wide range of equipment should

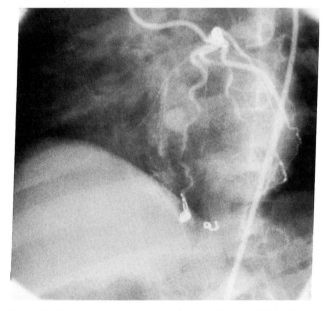

Figure 60.10. In the same patient as shown in Figure 60.7, both the feeding arteries were occluded by selective catheterization of each vessel by a Tracker catheter and placement of controlled release coils.

be available to cope with the great variety of fistulas, as well as possible complications of the techniques.

In our early experience, reported in 1991, correct positioning and occlusion was achieved in six out of seven patients (Reidy et al, 1991). Since then we have occluded successfully an additional 16 fistulas. In 13 of the patients, a combination of conventional and controlled delivery coils was used (Qureshi et al, 1996). Complete occlusion was achieved in nine tenths of the patients. Coils embolized in nearly one quarter of patients but were retrieved in all cases. Some of the inadvertent embolizations occurred as a result of high flow in the large fistulas. We attempted to avoid or reduce the possibility of these complications occurring by using the technique of temporary balloon occlusion to arrest the flow in the fistula. No other major complications were encountered, but minor complications included transient T wave inversion in one patient, and transient right bundle branch block in one further patient. No patient had myocardial infarction. Therefore, excellent results are achieved by embolization. Furthermore, the techniques of catheter closure allow a further arterial feeding vessel to be discovered by selective coronary angiography at the end of the procedure. If such a dual supply is noted, this vessel can also be occluded. Nowadays, no patient should be referred for surgical ligation before transcatheter closure has been considered.

AORTO–LEFT VENTRICULAR TUNNEL

Aorto–left ventricular tunnel is an extremely rare defect. It consists of an endothelialized communication between the aorta and the left ventricle. The abnormal channel, described usually as a tunnel, but better considered as a defect (Serino et al, 1983), originates in the ascending aorta, bypasses the aortic valve and terminates in the left ventricle (Figure 60.11). The incidence is higher in males than females, with a ratio of 2–3:1 (Levy et al, 1982; Hucin et al, 1989).

Although Edwards (1961) originally believed that the lesion was acquired, Levy et al (1963) subsequently described the tunnel as a congenital entity. The tunnel is usually present at birth and has been detected prenatally by fetal echocardiography (Sharland 1992; Sousa-Uva et al, 1996). The earliest prenatal detection was at 19 weeks of gestation, when a dilated aortic root and left ventricle were noted (Sharland, 1992). The most important clue for the diagnosis was provided by the presence, on colour Doppler echocardiography, of marked aortic regurgitation. It has been suggested that aorto–left ventricular tunnel results from the rupture of an aneurysm of a sinus of Valsalva into the left ventricle during fetal life.

The origin of the tunnel is usually above the right sinus of Valsalva and the orifice of the right coronary artery.

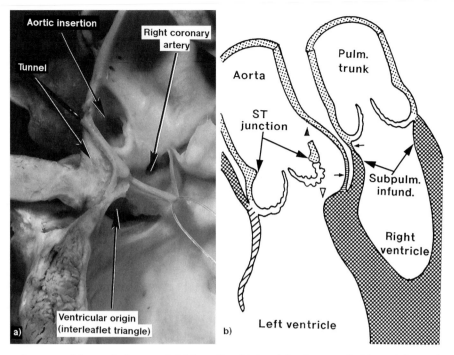

Figure 60.11. The structure of an aorto–left ventricular tunnel. (a) In reality, this is a defect between the hinge of the aortic valve and the valvar sinus, with the tunnel running through the tissue plane between the aortic sinus and the free-standing muscular subpulmonary infundibulum (subpulm, infund). (b) The diagram shows the arrangement as it would be seen in section viewed from the right side. Pulm, pulmonary; ST, sinotubular junction.

Both of these structures can remain normal, although the artery can originate from the tunnel. There is usually a sharp ridge separating the sinus below and the orifice of the tunnel above (Figure 60.11). The tunnel courses in the tissue plane between the free-standing muscular right ventricular infundibulum and the aortic sinus; it then usually enters the left ventricle through the fibrous triangle between the right and left coronary leaflets of the aortic valve (Ho et al, 1998). Occasionally, a tunnel may originate above the origin of the left coronary artery (Figure 60.12) (Grant et al, 1985). The tunnel itself may be dilated aneurysmally through part or the whole of its course. Associated cardiac defects include aortic valves with two leaflets, with aortic stenosis or regurgitation seen in the majority of patients. Other defects include patency of the arterial duct, ventricular septal defect, pulmonary stenosis, infundibular right ventricular obstruction, aneurysm of the membranous septum and critical aortic stenosis (Webber et al, 1991; Knott-Craig et al, 1992). Distortion of the aortic valve occurs because of the lack of support of its right coronary leaflet. The haemodynamic effect is that of severe regurgitation.

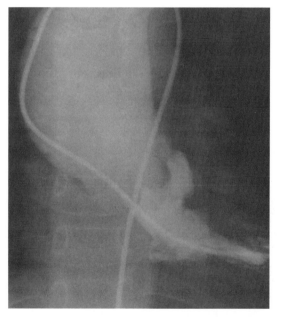

Figure 60.12. This left ventricular angiogram profiled in anteroposterior projection shows an aorto–left ventricular tunnel originating above the left coronary artery. The ascending aorta and the aortic root are very dilated. (Reproduced by kind permission of Dr Wolfgang Kohler, Erfurt, Germany.)

CLINICAL FEATURES

The symptoms and signs depend on the size of the tunnel and the severity of aortic regurgitation. Patients with severe aortic regurgitation usually present with symptoms of congestive cardiac failure. The presentation can occur at any point from birth to adult life (Akalin et al, 1989; Hucin et al, 1989). Afflicted patients frequently have a wide pulse pressure, and loud systolic and diastolic to-and-fro murmurs are heard at the base of the heart, usually with a short interval separating them. It is essential to consider the possibility of aorto–left ventricular tunnel in any neonate or infant who has systolic and diastolic murmurs along with the signs of aortic regurgitation. It may produce congestive cardiac failure in the neonate or infant. There may be associated left ventricular enlargement and overactivity, and a dilated ascending aorta may be obvious on a chest radiograph. In the fetus, the presence of aortic regurgitation may provide a clue to the presence of a tunnel. Left ventricular dysfunction may be present; it may be associated with hydrops (Sharland, 1992; Sousa-Uva, 1996).

INVESTIGATIONS

The electrocardiogram shows left ventricular hypertrophy in the majority of patients. Cross-sectional echocardiography and colour Doppler usually confirms the diagnosis. In the occasional patient in whom the diagnosis is difficult, magnetic resonance imaging or cardiac catheterization may be helpful (Humes et al, 1986). Angiography in the aortic root usually confirms the diagnosis. There may be gross dilation and distortion of the right aortic sinus, ascending aorta and the left ventricle. Angiography may also show normal origin of the coronary arteries, thus differentiating an aorto–left ventricular tunnel from a fistula from the coronary artery to the left ventricle. The anterior location of the abnormal tunnel, and the demonstration of a normal aortic sinus of Valsalva, distinguishes the tunnel from ruptured aneurysm of a sinus of Valsalva into the left ventricle.

MANAGEMENT

Levy et al (1963) first reported aorto–left ventricular tunnel presenting at birth and requiring surgery in early life. Usually the clinical presentation is with severe regurgitation at or soon after birth with early congestive cardiac failure (Perez-Martinez et al, 1973; Hucin et al, 1989). Symptoms of congestive cardiac failure may appear later in the second or third decade of life (Levy et al, 1982; Akalin et al, 1989). Some patients may die despite medical treatment (Levy et al, 1982). Others may survive to undergo successful surgical repair. The presence of congestive cardiac failure is a clear indication for surgery. In asymptomatic neonates, or in those patients in whom cardiac failure is well controlled, surgery can be delayed for a few weeks or months. Early surgical intervention may be needed in order to prevent progressive damage to the aortic valvar leaflets or deformity of the aortic root (Tuna and Edwards, 1988; Sreeram et al, 1991). When the presentation is with severe aortic stenosis rather than regurgitation, early surgery may be required (Weldner et al, 1996).

SURGERY

The technique of surgical repair depends on the type of tunnel. For those with a small aortic opening, closure of the orifice in two layers was advocated by Levy et al (1963). With larger openings, the aortic end is closed with a patch (Horvath et al, 1991). Other approaches include closure of both the aortic and left ventricular ends of the tunnel. In all the techniques, it is imperative to avoid distortion of the aortic valve and damage to the right coronary artery or the conduction system. In a recent series covering a period of 20 years and including 13 children who had surgical repair, the tunnel originated from the right coronary aortic sinus in 12 of the patients, and from the left coronary sinus in one (Horvath et al, 1991). Both ends of the tunnel were closed in the majority, while only one end was closed in the remainder. One child died after surgery. In a smaller series of four children undergoing surgery in the first 2 years of life, there were no deaths and, at late assessment, only trivial aortic regurgitation was present (Sreeram et al, 1991). Consequently, the reported operative mortality ranges between 0 and 20% (Hovaguimian et al, 1988; Horvath et al, 1991; Sreeram et al, 1991; Sousa-Uva et al, 1996). Late complications include aortic regurgitation in up to three quarters of patients after repair of the tunnel (Hovaguimian et al, 1988; Sreeram et al, 1991). This may necessitate reoperation on the aortic valve. Occasionally, it may not be possible to preserve the native aortic valve. This may occur when the aortic valve is severely stenotic. Replacement of the aortic root with an aortic homograft may then be required to repair both the tunnel and the stenotic aortic valve (Weldner et al, 1996).

It is important to suspect this rare anomaly in the differential diagnosis of any neonate, infant or a child with signs of severe aortic regurgitation. Early diagnosis, and subsequently early surgery, is important to prevent dilation of the aortic root and distortion of the aortic valvar leaflets.

ANEURYSMS OF THE SINUSES OF VALSALVA

Aneurysm of one of the aortic sinuses of Valsalva is a rare defect that may be congenital or acquired. Congenital aneurysms result from a weakness in the sinus, which produces a downward prolapse. The dilated sinus may bulge into an atrium or ventricle and may rupture. It is rare in infancy and childhood, being more commonly seen in adults. Aneurysms may be acquired through bacterial endocarditis, but in this setting, it is also possible that endocarditis may have occurred on a congenital aneurysm. It can be difficult, therefore, to distinguish between congenital and acquired aneurysms, although frequently the congenital ones are associated with a ventricular septal defect and aortic coarctation. Most aneurysms are single, and most commonly affect the right coronary aortic sinus. Less commonly, the non-coronary aortic sinus is involved. The left coronary aortic sinus is rarely involved. Aneurysms of the right coronary aortic sinus usually prolapse into the right ventricle or right atrium, and those from the non-coronary sinus into the right atrium. Aneurysms of the left coronary aortic sinus prolapse into the left ventricle. The most common aneurysm, from the right coronary aortic sinus prolapsing into the right ventricle, may be associated with a ventricular septal defect. Rupture frequently occurs into the right heart chambers rather than the left. The right sinus of Valsalva may rupture into the right ventricle or the right atrium (Figure 60.13). Aneurysms of the non-coronary aortic sinus tend to rupture into the right or left atrium, whilst aneurysms of the left coronary aortic sinus may rupture into the left ventricle or the left atrium (Glock et al, 1990; Rothbart and Chahine, 1990; Cabanes et al, 1992). Rupture can also occur through the septal leaflet of the tricuspid valve (Kallis et al, 1993). There is an increased incidence of rupture when an aneurysm occurs in the presence of a doubly committed subarterial ventricular septal defect (Momma et al, 1984). Those aneurysms of the sinus of Valsalva that occur with Marfan's syndrome are considered as a separate entity. Other associated lesions include an aortic valve with two leaflets, and aortic coarctation. Rupture of a sinus has been reported in a patient with Behçet's disease (Koh et al, 1994), and as a late complication after repair of dissection of the ascending aorta in one series of 33 patients, in whom aneurysm of a sinus of Valsalva was present in one third (Simon et al, 1994).

CLINICAL FEATURES

When the aneurysm has not ruptured, it usually produces no symptoms. It may only be discovered as a chance finding on echocardiography or angiography performed for another lesion, such as ventricular septal defect. The natural history of an unruptured aneurysm is not known, and although rupture has been reported in the neonatal period (Perry et al, 1991), it occurs more frequently in the third or fourth decade of life. Rupture may produce central precordial chest pain and sudden dyspnoea because of a large left-to-right shunt combined with aortic regurgitation. Very occasionally, rupture may not produce any symptoms. Even rarer still is rupture into the pericardial cavity (Brabham and Roberts, 1990). Unruptured aneurysms may cause angina, which may be intractable, especially when the aneurysm causes distortion of the coronary arterial origins (Tami et al, 1993). Myocardial infarction may occur by compression of the coronary arteries, and this may occasionally be fatal (Bashour et al, 1996; Ferreira et al, 1996). Other possible complications include transient ischaemic attacks and cerebral embolism (Wortham et al, 1993; Steinberg et al, 1996; Stollberger et al, 1996). Physical examination may reveal a wide pulse pressure and left or right ventricular overactivity. The murmurs vary from ejection systolic combined with early but long diastolic murmurs to continuous murmurs heard at the right or left lower sternal borders. Obstruction of the right ventricular outflow tract has occasionally been reported, with or without the presence of a ventricular septal defect (D'Silva et al, 1992; Liang et al, 1996).

INVESTIGATIONS

The electrocardiogram usually shows left ventricular hypertrophy and occasionally biventricular hypertrophy. Cross-sectional combined with colour Doppler echocardiography is helpful in the diagnosis (Missault et al, 1995). It frequently shows dilation of the aortic root and left ventricular volume overload. A ruptured right sinus may protrude anteriorly, caudally and leftwards. Severe aortic regurgitation may be present, with turbulent flow into the right ventricle or right atrium seen on colour Doppler (Rothbart and Chahine, 1990). Echocardiography will also show the presence or absence of a ventricular septal defect. Transoesophageal echocardiography shows the anatomy in more detail and is perhaps superior to the transthoracic approach (McKenney et al, 1992). Frequently, surgery can be performed without cardiac catheterization (Sahasakul et al, 1990; Steinberg et al, 1996). Cardiac catheterization and angiography merely confirm these findings but may show the deformed sinus more convincingly. Although filling of the right heart chambers, into which the aneurysm may have ruptured, is frequently seen, occasionally the rapid

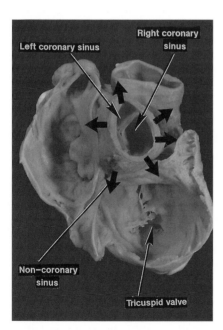

Figure 60.13. The sites of potential rupture of aneurysms of the aortic sinuses of Valsalva, indicated by arrows, have been superimposed on this picture of the short axis of the normal heart viewed from the atrial aspect.

heart rate and the high cardiac output prevent their opacification. Apart from conventional echocardiography, magnetic resonance imaging in isolation and combined with cine phase contrast imaging have been used for non-invasive diagnosis (Ho et al, 1995; Kulan et al, 1996).

MANAGEMENT

Corrective surgery is performed on cardiopulmonary bypass. Direct closure can be carried out through an aortotomy, through the right ventricle or via the right atrium. Sometimes both the aorta and the chamber of entry need to be explored for effective repair (Gupta et al, 1994). Closure of a ventricular septal defect, if present, is required. The aortic valvar leaflets may need resuspension in order to reduce the severity of aortic regurgitation, which may determine the outcome. Even after successful surgical repair, the prognosis is guarded. Recurrence, or an increase, of aortic regurgitation is frequently seen and may require further surgery. It is debatable whether an aneurysm discovered incidentally in an asymptomatic child should be surgically repaired.

Lukacs and colleagues (1992) have described their experience with 15 patients, ranging in age between 15 and 54 years, who underwent surgery between 1969 and 1989. The most frequent site of rupture was from the right coronary aortic sinus to the right ventricle, while in some it was into the right atrium. The aortic valve needed to be replaced at operation, and the aneurysms were repaired via an aortotomy, through the right ventricle or the right atrium. There were no early or late deaths. In a larger series of 31 patients reported from the Mayo Clinic (van Son et al, 1994), the majority of the aneurysms originated in the right coronary aortic sinus and entered the right ventricle or the right atrium. Almost half the patients had an associated ventricular septal defect, most commonly doubly committed and subarterial. Aortic regurgitation was present in about two fifths. The overall survival was 95% at 20 years. Reoperation was needed in one sixth of the patients for replacement of the aortic valve, recurrence of the fistula or recurrence of a ventricular septal defect.

AORTOPULMONARY WINDOW

This is a rare defect found between the ascending components of the aorta and the pulmonary trunk. It results from incomplete separation of the arterial segment of the heart tube by the aortopulmonary septum. It can be differentiated from common arterial trunk, where there is a common truncal valve, by the presence of two separate arterial valves arising from separate subarterial ventricular outflow tracts (Figure 60.14). The window usually occurs between the left lateral wall of the aorta and the

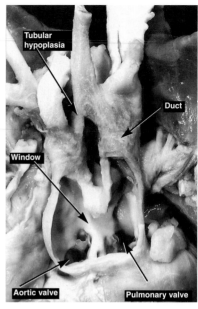

Figure 60.14. This dissection shows a circular aortopulmonary window between the ascending portions of the aorta and the pulmonary trunk. Note the separate arterial valves, each supported by its own ventricular outflow tract. Note also the association of tubular hypoplasia of the aortic arch, with the descending aorta fed through an arterial duct.

right wall of the pulmonary trunk. The size varies from small to large, and this determines the magnitude of the shunt through it, the pulmonary arterial pressures and the clinical features.

Kutsche and Van Mierop (1987) reported on the pathological features and associated cardiac defects. Three variants were described: a circular-shaped defect midway between the arterial valves and the bifurcation of the pulmonary trunk, a helical-shaped defect in a similar position, and a large defect without posterior or distal borders. Since then, a tunnel-like window (Figure 60.15) has been described by Ho and her associates (1994). In about half the patients, the aortopulmonary window is an isolated finding; in the others associated defects are found, such as ventricular septal defect, anomalous origin of the right or left coronary arteries from the pulmonary trunk, aortic coarctation, interruption of the aortic arch, tricuspid atresia, aortic origin of one pulmonary artery and tetralogy of Fallot (Brouwer et al, 1990; Carminati et al, 1990; Ding et al, 1990; Qureshi et al, 1990; Redington et al, 1991; Sreeram and Walsh, 1991; Backer et al, 1992; Boonstra et al, 1992; Geva et al, 1992; Horimi et al, 1992; Ingram and Ott, 1992; van Son et al, 1993; Chopra et al, 1994; Donofrio et al, 1995; Kim et al, 1995; Tkebuchava et al, 1997). Di George syndrome is not usually present in these patients. A traumatic aortopulmonary window has been reported after balloon dilation of branch pulmonary arterial stenosis (Preminger et al, 1994).

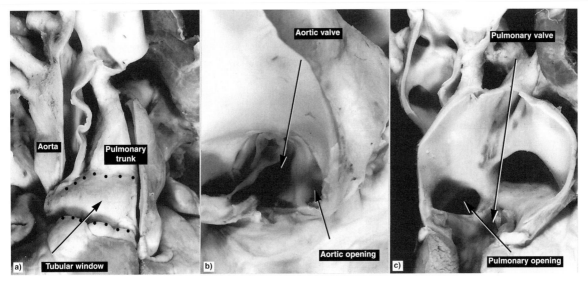

Figure 60.15. This aortopulmonary window was in the form of a tubular tunnel across the anterior parts of the arterial trunks (a). The ends of the tunnel are shown from the aortic (b) and the pulmonary (c) aspects.

CLINICAL FEATURES

The haemodynamic findings are similar to those found with common arterial trunk. The neonates or infants may have congestive cardiac failure in the presence of signs suggestive of a patent arterial duct, but with a clinical suspicion of common arterial trunk. As the pulmonary vascular resistance falls during the first few weeks of life, the left-to-right shunt through the window increases. Pulmonary hypertension is a frequent complication, depending on the size of the window. The peripheral pulses are bounding, and there may be a systolic murmur at the base, rather than a continuous murmur, because of the high pulmonary arterial pressures. When the shunt is large, there is often a mid-diastolic murmur owing to increased flow across the mitral valve. The pulmonary component of the second sound is frequently accentuated. If the window is small, there may be a continuous murmur similar to that generated by an arterial duct. If the window is left uncorrected, pulmonary vascular disease may develop within the first few years. Concomitant reversal of the shunt through the window may then cause cyanosis.

INVESTIGATIONS

The electrocardiogram may show left atrial hypertrophy resulting from increased flow. Frequently there is biventricular hypertrophy. The chest radiograph may show generalized cardiomegaly with plethoric lung fields in those with large windows, but may be normal in those with small windows. The diagnosis is usually easily made with cross-sectional echocardiography (Balaji et al, 1991; Horimi et al, 1992). Parasternal long- and short-axis views are needed to identify two arterial valves, thus excluding a common arterial trunk. A high left parasternal long-axis view will demonstrate the presence of an arterial duct. In between these views, a high parasternal short-axis view of aorta and the pulmonary trunk will show the window when the transducer is tilted superiorly (Figure 60.16). Although it is often possible to see the sharp margins of the window on echocardiography, colour Doppler is an essential complementary technique that confirms flow of blood through the window.

Cardiac catheterization is not usually needed unless there is some doubt about the presence of pulmonary vascular disease, or it is performed to delineate other additional defects. If the window is small, the right heart

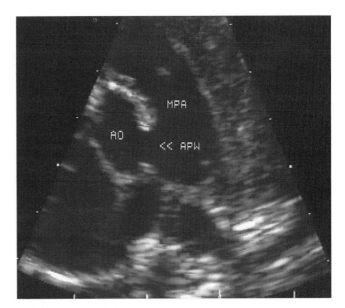

Figure 60.16. A high parasternal short-axis cross-sectional echocardiogram showing an aortopulmonary window (APW). AO, aorta; MPA pulmonary trunk.

pressures may be normal. They may be equal to systemic pressures if the window is large. Operability may need to be determined by calculation of the pulmonary vascular resistance in air and 100% oxygen. Aortography in the anteroposterior and lateral projections usually demonstrates the window. The main differential diagnoses include common arterial trunk and a large patent arterial duct. Other angiograms may be needed to confirm other additional defects, such as anomalous origin of one of the coronary arteries. Magnetic resonance imaging seems a better alternative method for diagnosing aortopulmonary window and other additional defects (Kim et al, 1995).

MANAGEMENT

Because of the rarity of aortopulmonary windows, no large series of patients are available to determine the natural history. In the recent experience reported by Tkebuchava and colleagues (1997), 13 patients underwent surgical repair over the period from 1971 to 1993. One patient died early after surgery, and there were no late deaths. In the series of 19 patients reported by van Son et al (1993), the operative mortality was 21%, but all the deaths occurred in patients undergoing surgery in the 1960s. The risk factors identified for death, in addition to those of surgery, included high pulmonary vascular resistance. Some patients may survive to early adult life without surgery but will have established pulmonary vascular disease. Once a patient presents with suspected aortopulmonary window, medical treatment is initially needed to control congestive cardiac failure. If cardiac failure cannot be controlled, there is no need to delay surgery. When the window is large, surgery should be carried out at presentation in the first few months, and preferably before 6 months of age.

Repair can usually be performed with cardiopulmonary bypass via a thoracotomy or a sternotomy (Deverall et al, 1969; van Son et al, 1993; Kawata et al, 1996; Tkebuchava et al, 1997). Technically, the windows are easy to repair by direct suture when small, or with a patch if large. Direct suture is usually achieved using a transpulmonary approach, while a patch is inserted via either the transpulmonary or a transaortic approach (van Son et al, 1993; Tkebuchava et al, 1997). An inverted flap of pulmonary trunk has been used to repair the window (Messmer et al, 1994). The risks of surgery should be low and the long-term outlook excellent. Repair of a window has been performed without cardiopulmonary bypass in a baby weighing 758 g, the window being ligated with a clip (Kawata et al, 1996). When a window is associated with other complex defects, then primary repair of all the additional defects is usually undertaken in the neonatal period or in early infancy (Ding et al, 1990; Qureshi et al, 1990; Sreeram and Walsh, 1991; Boonstra et al, 1992; Geva et al, 1992;

Ingram and Ott, 1992; van Son et al, 1993; Donofrio et al, 1995; Tkebuchava et al, 1997; Di Bella and Gladstone, 1998). It is essential to evaluate the coronary arterial anatomy preoperatively in order to avoid missing anomalous origin of either coronary artery from the pulmonary trunk. If present, this association may have an important influence on the outcome (Kutsche and Van Mierop, 1987). A patient has been found, nonetheless, to have anomalous origin of the circumflex coronary artery from the pulmonary trunk 14 years after repair of the window (Chopra et al, 1994).

Non-surgical closure has been performed using a double umbrella occluding device, but this method is likely to be suitable only for small windows (Stamato et al, 1995; Tulloh and Rigby, 1997).

PULMONARY ARTERIO-VENOUS MALFORMATIONS

Pulmonary arterio-venous malformations are congenital malformations providing an abnormal communication between a pulmonary artery and vein that bypasses the normal pulmonary capillary bed. They may occur as an isolated anomaly or as multiple lesions. Rarely, such an abnormality is acquired, but it is then described not as a pulmonary arterio-venous malformation but as an arterio-venous fistula. Interest in pulmonary arterio-venous malformations has increased since the mid-1980s with the realisation that they cause more clinical problems and a greater morbidity than had been previously recognized, together with the emergence of transcatheter embolization as an effective and safe alternative therapy to surgery (Pennington et al, 1992; Puskas et al, 1993; Pollak et al, 1994; Dutton et al, 1995).

INCIDENCE

Pulmonary arterio-venous malformations are rare. Only 60 cases were found in a 20-year survey of the experience at the Mayo Clinic, four of them in children (Dines et al, 1974). At the Johns Hopkins Hospital, three pulmonary arterio-venous malformations were found in 15 000 consecutive postmortems (Sloan and Cooley, 1953). In a survey at the Hospital for Sick Children in Toronto, only six cases were found in 15 104 cases of congenital heart disease (Keith, 1978). These figures probably represent an underestimate, as small lesions may easily be missed at postmortem, as well as on routine investigations. It is now also realised that relatives of patients known to have pulmonary arterio-venous malformations, even in the absence of hereditary haemorrhagic telangiectasia, can have incidental and asymptomatic pulmonary arterio-venous malformations.

Pulmonary arterio-venous malformations may occur as an isolated vascular anomaly or in association with hereditary haemorrhagic telangiectasia. In some reported series, pulmonary arterio-venous malformations are more commonly associated with hereditary haemorrhagic telangiectasia (White et al, 1988; Dutton et al, 1995), but in others the majority are sporadic cases (Dines et al, 1983). Now that the relatives of patients with pulmonary arterio-venous malformations are being actively screened, it appears that they too are more commonly afflicted with hereditary haemorrhagic telangiectasia (White, 1992; Dutton et al, 1995). When pulmonary arterio-venous malformations are multiple, there is a more common association with hereditary haemorrhagic telangiectasia (Dines et al, 1983; McCue et al, 1984). An incidence of up to one third has been described in those with hereditary haemorrhagic telangiectasia, and there is also an increased incidence in the apparently unaffected relatives of these patients.

The malformations can be solitary, multiple of varying size, multiple of uniform size and diffuse (Higgins and Wexler, 1976). The lesions can also be classified according to their structure (White et al, 1983). This is simpler, and more appropriate for assessment and evaluation prior to embolization. Based on angioarchitectural criteria, four fifths consist of a single pulmonary artery communicating directly with the vein via the malformation, which is usually aneurysmal and non-septated (Figure 60.17a). This so-called simple type (Figures 60.18 and 60.19) can usually be cured by appropriate embolization of the feeding artery. The remaining one fifth of the lesions are complex (Figures 60.17b, 60.20 and 60.21), consisting of two or more connecting pulmonary arterial branches feeding aneurysmal and septated malformations, often cirsoid, with two or more

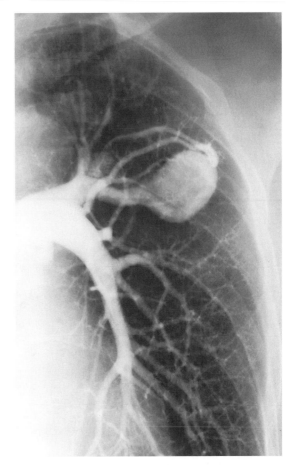

Figure 60.18. A selective injection into the left pulmonary artery shows a pulmonary arterio-venous malformation supplied by a single large feeding artery. The draining vein has not yet opacified (the same patient is shown in Figures 60.19 and 60.25).

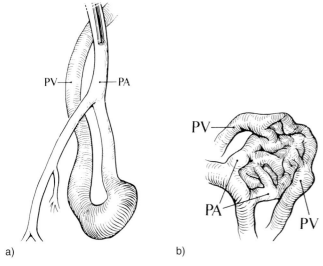

Figure 60.17. Pulmonary arterio-venous malformations can be considered simple (a) or complex (b). In the most common form (a), a large single feeding artery (PA) is seen with a single pulmonary vein (PV) draining the non-septated malformation. In the less common complex type (b), multiple arteries and veins supply and drain from the septated malformation.

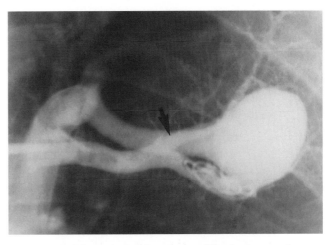

Figure 60.19. The angiographic anatomy of the simple type of pulmonary arterio-venous malformation is best shown on this film with the injection directly into the feeding artery. Despite a collection of coils immediately proximal to the malformation, and further coils within it, the malformation has not been occluded. Note the artery (black arrow) supplying normal lung immediately proximal to the coils and the single large vein draining to the left atrium (same patient as Figures 60.18 and 60.25).

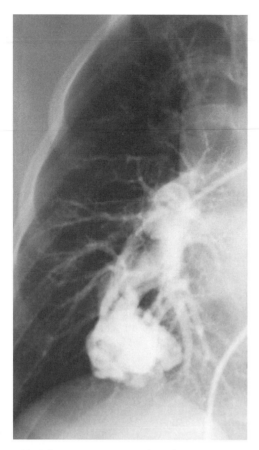

Figure 60.20. Selective injection into the right pulmonary artery shows a complex type of pulmonary arterio-venous malformation with multiple feeding arteries.

draining veins. Rarely, pulmonary arterio-venous malformations can be diffuse; in this case, most of the lungs contain multiple small arterio-venous communications (Figures 60.22 and 60.23). In diffuse liver disease such as cirrhosis, right-to-left shunting has sometimes been associated with multiple very small arterio-venous fistulas (Hansoti and Sharma, 1989). Similar multiple fistulas can develop after construction of cavopulmonary

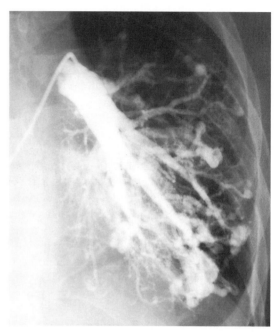

Figure 60.22. A 35-year-old patient with hereditary telangiectasia also had very extensive pulmonary arterio-venous malformations, revealed by an injection into the left descending pulmonary artery.

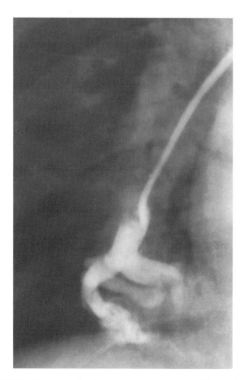

Figure 60.21. A more selective injection into the malformation shown in Figure 60.19 reveals the presence of several feeding arteries.

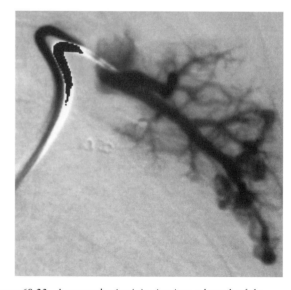

Figure 60.23. A superselective injection into a branch of the pulmonary artery shows that there are relatively normal appearing arteries arising side by side with abnormal arteries to small pulmonary arterio-venous malformations. This would make selective embolization very difficult, as normal branches would also be occluded.

connections that exclude hepatic flow from the lungs (Amodeo and Marino, 1998).

Most commonly, pulmonary arterio-venous malformations are found in the lower lobes or the right middle lobe. Overall, they are described more commonly in the right lung (Moyer et al, 1962; Gomes et al, 1969). They do not generally show much of a tendency to increase in size, but long-term follow-up studies with measurements are not available. Studies using computed tomography, however, together with serial measurements of arterial blood gases, have shown that there is little change in the degree of right-to-left shunting or in the size of the malformations over a period of 3 to 4 years (Remy et al, 1992; White, 1992). In one patient followed for 24 years, serial chest radiographs showed that the fistulas in both lungs had been increasing gradually in size but at different rates (Teragaki et al, 1988). Several reports have described increase in size of the malformation during pregnancy, or the occurrence of significant complications (Swinburne et al, 1986; Gammon et al, 1990; Laroche et al, 1992). It has been suggested that it is particularly important to screen young female relatives of affected patients or members of families with hereditary haemorrhagic telangiectasia for the presence of asymptomatic pulmonary arterio-venous malformations (Laroche et al, 1992), and that this should be carried out before puberty.

CLINICAL PRESENTATION

Pulmonary arterio-venous malformations present very rarely in neonates and infants (Hall et al, 1965; Clarke et al, 1976), when cyanosis, respiratory distress and severe heart failure result. Echocardiography is needed to rule out congenital heart disease. More commonly, they present in older children, although it is quite common for the malformations to go undetected until mid-adult life. Sometimes the diagnosis is made as an incidental finding on a routine chest radiograph (Figure 60.24). Patients may present with symptoms of dyspnoea and fatigue, which may have been present for some years, even from childhood. Often there is a history of cyanosis on exercise, sometimes with surprisingly good exercise tolerance. A quite common presentation is for the patient to develop neurological problems (Desai et al, 1992; Dutton et al, 1995). This is now recognized to be a major cause of morbidity. It is the single most important reason why such malformations should be actively looked for and treated in patients with hereditary haemorrhagic telangiectasia (White, 1992). Some form of cerebrovascular accident, such as a stroke or transient ischaemic attack, may be the initial presenting feature. White (1991, 1992) has suggested that up to half of patients are at risk either from some form of paradoxical embolism leading to transient ischaemic attacks or strokes, or from an intra-cerebral abscess. Such an ischaemic episode may be

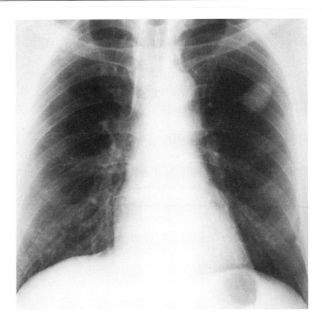

Figure 60.24. Chest radiograph of a 45-year-old man shows a smooth oval density on the left upper zone. It was just possible to see a tubular structure connecting this with the hilum, suggesting the diagnosis of a pulmonary arterio-venous malformation.

caused by thrombosis associated with polycythaemia or may be caused by a paradoxical embolism related to venous thrombosis and right-to-left shunting. There was an 18% incidence of strokes and a 37% incidence of transient ischaemic attacks in his 78 patients. White also drew attention to the presence on tomographic scans of evidence of strokes not necessarily associated with any symptoms. Haemoptysis rarely occurs from rupture of a pulmonary arterio-venous malformation, or alternatively may be caused by bleeding from telangiectasia involving the airways (Prager et al, 1983). Haemothorax is another rare form of presentation. Bleeding from hereditary haemorrhagic telangiectasia involving the nose and lips may result in an iron deficiency anaemia, and such lesions can affect other parts of the body, including the gut and abdominal organs.

The clinical examination may reveal central cyanosis and clubbing. In the presence of anaemia, the cyanosis may not be obvious. Evidence of hereditary haemorrhagic telangiectasia may be seen involving the nails, skin and mucous membranes of the mouth, but such changes are rare in children. Examination of the heart and chest will be normal, except that a murmur may be heard associated with a large superficially placed pulmonary arterio-venous malformation. The murmur is usually systolic or continuous.

INVESTIGATIONS

The electrocardiogram is usually normal except in infancy. The echocardiogram, which may also be normal, is important to exclude any intracardiac disease. In many instances, a chest radiograph will either diagnose or strongly suggest a pulmonary arterio-venous malformation. The heart is usually of normal size and the malformations may be seen in the lungs. Typically they are round, well-defined homogeneous opacities, often peripherally situated (Figure 60.24). Though not always obvious, especially when at the lung bases and behind the heart, abnormal vessels connecting the malformation to the hilum can usually be discerned. Sometimes the chest radiograph will be normal (Love et al, 1992), when small pulmonary arterio-venous malformations are not visible or, rarely, in the presence of diffuse and very small lesions (MacNee et al, 1985). Computed tomography is currently the best modality for demonstrating pulmonary arterio-venous malformations (Remy et al, 1992). If the diagnosis is in doubt, then computed tomography, with intravenous contrast, will confirm the diagnosis. High-resolution scans through the lungs, and the availability of fast spiral scanners, will now mean that more, and even very small, lesions will be demonstrated. In a recent study, nearly half the small lesions were missed on routine angiography, whereas only two were missed by tomographic scanning (Remy et al, 1992). If obvious lesions are seen on the chest radiograph, and the clinical diagnosis is not in doubt, there would seem little point in doing any further tomography, as detailed angiography is necessary to plan for any embolization of the larger lesions. When a pulmonary arterio-venous malformation is diagnosed or strongly suspected, the measurement of arterial blood gases is useful to confirm the presence of hypoxaemia and to quantify any right-to-left shunting (Pennington et al, 1992; White, 1992; Dutton et al, 1995). The arterial oxygen saturation should be measured breathing room air in the erect or sitting position and, after 20 minutes, while breathing 100% oxygen (Terry et al, 1983). Orthodeoxia is a term used when arterial oxygen saturations significantly drop in the standing or sitting positions. This is related to the predominantly basal location of pulmonary arterio-venous malformations and the gravitational shifts of flow that result, as well as the increase in lung volume. Quantitative assessment of the degree of right-to-left shunting can be made from nuclear medicine studies (Seto et al, 1985; Chilvers et al, 1988). Following an injection of technetium-labelled microspheres, counts may be made over part of the systemic circulation such as the kidney. This technique can be used to assess the effectiveness of embolization, particularly when there are multiple malformations. A further technique to detect right-to-left shunting is to use echocardiography to look for evidence of microcavitation in the left atrium after a peripheral injection of saline (Barzilai et al, 1991).

PULMONARY ANGIOGRAPHY

It makes sense to perform angiography and embolization on the same occasion especially if there are multiple lesions that may need several attempts at embolization. Detailed pulmonary angiography is necessary to demonstrate clearly the angioarchitecture of the malformations. Initially, selective right or left pulmonary angiograms are performed with either film or digital angiography (Figures 60.18 and 60.20). With the availability of large-field image intensifiers, and with the quality of digital angiography that can now be obtained, conventional film techniques are no longer needed. Selective catheterization is then needed to demonstrate the feeding artery and its relationship to the adjacent normal lung branches (Figures 60.19 and 60.23). Locating the feeding artery may be difficult, especially in the lower zones where many vessels are closely related. Specialized catheter techniques, together with digital angiography, are essential requirements. Injections in varying degrees of obliquity may be needed to show the arterial anatomy.

TREATMENT

SURGERY

Until 1978, the only treatment available was surgery. The various operations performed included pneumonectomy (Charbon et al, 1952), transection of the pulmonary trunk (Toombes et al, 1984), lobectomy, segmentectomy, ligation of feeding vessels, intra-aneurysmal obliteration of the malformation (Shumacker and Waldhausen, 1963) and wedge resection (Bosher et al, 1959; Prager et al, 1983). The aim was to be as conservative as possible, for at least two reasons. First, any lung tissue removed is likely to have normal function. Second, the greater the amount of the normal pulmonary circulation that is obliterated, the greater the flow to the rest of the lungs. It may be that such high flows then cause enlargement of other malformations (Hodgson and Kaye, 1963). Complications of surgery were unusual even in children (Bosher et al, 1959; Shumaker and Waldhausen, 1963; Puskas et al, 1993).

EMBOLIZATION

Transcatheter occlusion of a pulmonary arterio-venous malformation was first described by Porstmann in 1977. Many series have now confirmed the initial encouraging response (White et al, 1988; Puskas et al, 1993; Pollak et al, 1994; Dutton et al, 1995). Whenever embolization is planned, it is essential to obtain informed consent. The aim is to occlude either the feeding artery or the malformation itself (Figures 60.25 and 60.26). It is vital that techniques are used that prevent any possibility of the material used for embolization passing through the malformation and ending up in the systemic circulation. Embolization of pulmonary arterio-venous malformations should not be attempted unless the operator is experienced with embolization elsewhere in the body.

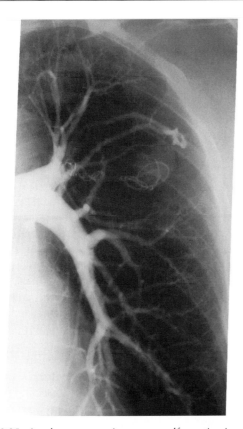

Figure 60.25. A pulmonary arterio-venous malformation is supplied by a single large feeding artery (see earlier catheterization in the same patient shown in Figure 60.18). At this second embolization procedure, further coils have been positioned more proximally in the feeding artery. This has occluded the pulmonary arterio-venous malformation, but at the cost of occluding also a small branch supplying normal lung.

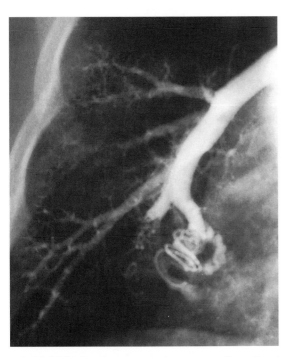

Figure 60.26. Multiple pulmonary arterio-venous malformations in the right lower lobe. These were separately embolized with coils. The film taken after the procedure confirms occlusion of the malformations.

Embolization of the pulmonary arteries is unique in that, unlike systemic arterial embolization where the lungs act as very effective filters for any material that crosses to the venous circulation, the consequences can be catastrophic with a pulmonary arterio-venous malformation. Even with all the necessary precautions, there has to be a very small risk of some systemic embolism, and the patient should be warned of this. If polycythaemia of significant degree is present, then venesection should be performed prior to embolization. It is also advisable to give a bolus of heparin, approximately 5000 units, at the start of the procedure.

Techniques for embolization

All symptomatic pulmonary arterio-venous malformations, and those associated with hypoxia in the sitting or standing position, should be treated. The risk of paradoxical embolism in small pulmonary arterio-venous malformations in the absence of these problems is very difficult to predict. It has been suggested that, when the feeding artery is greater than 3 mm in diameter, embolotherapy should be advocated, but this will be influenced by the age of the patient. Embolization was first described by Porstmann in 1977, who used steel coils. In practice, only two techniques are now available for the occlusion of pulmonary arterio-venous malformations. These are the use of either detachable balloons or metallic coils (Pollak et al, 1994). Both methods have advantages and disadvantages.

In the simple malformation with a single feeding artery, the aim should be to occlude the artery just before it enters the aneurysmal part of the malformation (Figure 60.19). More proximal occlusion will occlude some branches supplying normal parenchyma and result in pulmonary infarction (Remy et al, 1992). It is important to assess the diameter of the artery, as this must not be bigger than the diameter of the coil or balloon intended to be used to occlude it. A small coil or balloon could pass through the malformation and into the single draining vein, which is usually larger than the artery. Whichever technique is used, it is important that the tip of the catheter is precisely placed and that, prior to detaching a balloon or pushing out a coil, this position and its relationship to the feeding artery is confirmed. Though detachable balloons have been advocated (White et al, 1988), it is now coils that are most commonly used for occlusion. Until recently, the range of coils was limited, but now platinum microcoils with complex helical shapes and of large diameter are available. Unlike balloons, conventional coils have a major disadvantage in that, once the coil protrudes from the tip of the catheter, there is no control in its positioning. The embolization is then irreversible.

Recent developments with electrolytic coils, and coils inserted with the facility for controlled release, allow for complete control and reversibility should the position of the extruded coil be unsatisfactory (Dutton et al, 1995).

Large arteries may need multiple coils to effect occlusion. If occlusion is going to occur, it will have happened within 15 to 20 minutes of insertion. A large vessel may need several coils of larger diameter to form an anchor point on which several smaller coils can then be trapped to form a 'nest' of coils (Figure 60.25). Very large coils, up to 20 mm in diameter, are now available. These can be placed directly into the aneurysmal part of the malformation (Figure 60.25) rather than in the feeding artery (Coley and Jackson 1996). If the malformation itself is occluded, there is then no risk of revascularization from opening of unseen small collaterals. Moreover, no branches to normal lung parenchyma would then be occluded. A theoretical disadvantage in the use of coils, not shared by detachable balloons, is that, when the coil is partially occluding the feeding artery, a thrombus may form that could embolize into the systemic circulation. There is no evidence to suggest that this occurs.

Balloon embolization is a specialized technique that has its advocates (Barth et al, 1982; Pollak et al, 1994). Detachable balloons produce precise and immediate occlusion. An advantage is that, until the balloon is detached, the technique is reversible and its position can be readily adjusted. Balloons, however, are more complex to use and require large and non-tapered catheters. This is a particular problem for use in infants and young children. Other problems are early detachment and premature deflation, as the balloons are usually filled with contrast medium.

The feeding artery to a pulmonary arterio-venous malformation will also supply some normal lung parenchyma. Even with very careful and precise embolization, there is the likelihood of a small amount of normal lung being infarcted (see Figures 60.23 and 60.25) (Remy et al, 1992). The more proximal the occlusion, the greater the amount of infarction that will occur. In the experience of White and his colleagues (1988), who embolized a total of 276 pulmonary arterio-venous malformations in 78 patients, six patients had pleurisy, which lasted up to 5 days. One of these patients had a significant effusion that required thoracocentesis.

Pulmonary arterio-venous malformations are not common, and there are few detailed results. In the series reported by White and his colleagues (1988), all malformations fed by arteries exceeding 3 mm were occluded, though multiple catheterizations were necessary in some. Failure to restore the arterial oxygen saturations to normal values resulted from persistence of residual malformations too small to be considered for occlusion. Patients with multiple malformations will sometimes have one small lesion that is jointly supplied with a segment of normal lung parenchyma. Occluding the malformation would mean losing that segment of normal lung. In the simple type of malformation, be they single or multiple, embolization is an effective technique that is safe and usually curative. Embolization is now the treatment of choice, and surgery should be reserved for those occasions when embolization is felt to be not technically possible, or when embolization has failed. Unlike arterio-venous malformations elsewhere in the body, these lesions do not recanalize. In the more complex and diffuse pulmonary arterio-venous malformations, it is much more difficult to eradicate completely all the lesions. However, by embolizing the larger ones, significant clinical improvement can be achieved (Figure 60.22). It is always possible to repeat embolizations with no increased risk. Careful monitoring of the effects of embolization by measuring blood gases and, possibly, by nuclear medicine studies is essential.

REFERENCES

Abott O A, Rivarola C H, Logne R B 1961 Surgical correction of coronary arteriovenous fistula. Journal of Thoracic and Cardiovascular Surgery 42: 660–671

Agatston A S, Chapman E, Hildner F J, Samet P 1984 Diagnosis of a right coronary artery–right atrial fistula using two-dimensional and Doppler echocardiography. American Journal of Cardiology 54: 238–239

Ahmed S S, Harder B, Regan T J 1982 Silent left coronary artery–cameral fistula: probable cause of myocardial ischemia. American Heart Journal 104: 869–870

Akalin H, Erd C, Oral D et al 1989 Aortic left ventricular tunnel: successful diagnostic and surgical approach to the oldest patient in the literature. Journal of Thoracic & Cardiovascular Surgery 97: 804–805

Alkhulaifi A M, Horner S M, Pugsley W B, Swanton R H 1995 Coronary artery fistulas presenting with bacterial endocarditis. Annals of Thoracic Surgery 60: 202–204

Amodeo A, Marino B 1998 Pulmonary arteriovenous fistulas in patients with left isomerism and cardiac malformations. Cardiology in the Young 8: 283–284

Babb J D, Field J M 1977 Double coronary arteriovenous fistula. Chest 72: 656–658

Backer C L, Stout M J, Zales V R et al 1992 Anomalous origin of the left coronary artery. A twenty-year review of surgical management. Journal of Thoracic & Cardiovascular Surgery 103: 1049–1057

Baim D S, Kline H, Silberman J F 1982 Bilateral coronary arteriopulmonary artery fistulas. Circulation 65: 810–815

Baker E J, Ellam S V, Lorber A, Jones O D H, Tynan M J, Maisey M N 1985 Superiority of radionuclide over oximetry measurement of left to right shunts. British Heart Journal 53: 535–540

Balaji S, Burch M, Sullivan I D 1991 Accuracy of cross-sectional echocardiography in diagnosis of aortopulmonary window. American Journal of Cardiology 67: 650–653

Baltaxe A H, Wixson D 1977 The incidence of congenital anomalies of the coronary arteries in the adult population. Radiology 122: 47–52

Barth K H, White R I, Kaufman S L, Terry P B, Roland J M 1982 Embolotherapy of pulmonary arteriovenous malformations with detachable balloons. Radiology 142: 599–606

Barzilai B, Waggoner A D, Spessert C, Picus D, Goodenberger D 1991 Two-dimensional echocardiography in the detection and follow up of congenital pulmonary arteriovenous malformations. American Journal of Cardiology 68: 1507–1510

Bashour T T, Chen F, Yap A, Mason D T, Baladi N 1996 Fatal myocardial ischemia caused by compression of the left coronary system by a large left sinus of Valsalva aneurysm. American Heart Journal 132: 1050–1052

Bauer H H, Allmendinger P D, Flaherty J, Owlia D, Rossi M A, Chen C 1996 Congenital coronary arteriovenous fistula: spontaneous rupture and cardiac tamponade. Annals of Thoracic Surgery 62: 1521–1523

Bennett J M, Maree E 1989 Successful embolization of a coronary artery fistula. International Journal of Cardiology 23: 405–406

Black I W, Loo C K, Allan R M 1991 Multiple coronary artery–left ventricular fistulae: clinical, angiographic, and pathologic findings. European Journal of Cardiothoracic Surgery 23: 133–135

Blanche C, Chaux A 1990 Long-term results of surgery for coronary fistulas. International Surgery 75: 238–239

Boonstra P W, Talsma M, Ebels T 1992 Interruption of the aortic arch, distal aortopulmonary window, arterial duct and aortic origin of the right pulmonary artery in a neonate: report of a case successfully repaired in a one-stage operation. International Journal of Cardiology 34: 108–110

Bosher L H Jr, Blake A, Byrd B R 1959 An analysis of the pathologic anatomy of pulmonary arteriovenous aneurysms with particular reference to the applicability of local excision. Surgery 45: 91–104

Bosi G, Milanesi O, Scorrano M, Pellegrino P A, Lintermans J P 1992 Doppler and 2D echocardiographic diagnosis of congenital coronary artery fistulae to the right cardiac chambers: report of 3 cases. European Journal of Pediatrics 151: 555–557

Brabham K R, Roberts W C 1990 Fatal intrapericardial rupture of sinus of Valsalva aneurysm. American Heart Journal 120: 1455–1456

Brouwer M H, Beaufort-Krol G C, Talsma M D 1990 Aortopulmonary window associated with an anomalous origin of the right coronary artery. International Journal of Cardiology 28: 384–386

Cabanes L, Garcia E, van Damme C et al 1992 Aneurysm of the non-coronary sinus of Valsalva ruptured into the left atrium. American Heart Journal 124: 1659–1661

Carminati M, Borghi A, Valsecchi O et al 1990 Aortopulmonary window coexisting with tetralogy of Fallot: echocardiographic diagnosis. Pediatric Cardiology 11: 41–43

Carrel T, Tkebuchava T, Jenni R, Arbenz U, Turina M 1996 Congenital coronary fistulas in children and adults: diagnosis, surgical technique and results. Cardiology 87: 325–330

Charbon B C, Adams W E, Carlson R F 1952 Surgical treatment of multiple arteriovenous fistulas in the right lung in a patient having undergone a left pneumonectomy seven years earlier for the same disease. Journal of Thoracic and Cardiovascular Surgery 23: 188–196

Chilvers E R, Peters A M, George P, Hughes J M, Allison D J 1988 Quantification of right to left shunt through pulmonary arteriovenous malformation using ^{99}Tc albumin microspheres. Clinical Radiology 39: 611–614

Chopra P S, Reed W H, Wilson A D, Rao P S 1994 Delayed presentation of anomalous circumflex coronary artery arising from pulmonary artery following repair of aortopulmonary window in infancy. Chest 106: 1920–1922

Ciricillo S F, Edwards M S, Schmidt K G et al 1990 Interventional neuroradiological management of vein of Galen malformations in the neonate. Neurosurgery 27: 22–28

Clarke C P, Goh T H, Blackwood A, Venables A W 1976 Massive pulmonary arteriovenous fistula in the newborn. British Heart Journal 38: 1092–1095

Coley S C, Jackson J E 1996 Venous sac embolisation of pulmonary arteriovenous malformations in two patients. American Journal of Roentgenology 167: 452–454

Cooper M J, Bernstein D, Silverman N H 1985 Recognition of left coronary artery fistula to the left and right ventricles by contrast echocardiography. Journal of American College of Cardiology 6: 923–926

Davis J T, Allen H D, Wheller J J et al 1994 Coronary artery fistula in the pediatric age group: a 19-year institutional experience. Annals of Thoracic Surgery 58: 760–763

Desai S P, Rees C, Jinkins J R 1991 Paradoxical cerebral emboli associated with pulmonary arteriovenous shunts: report of three cases. American Journal of Neuroradiology 12: 355–359

Deverall P B, Aberdeen E, Bonham-Carter R E, Waterston D J 1969 Aorticopulmonary window. Journal of Thoracic and Cardiovascular Surgery 57: 479–486

de Wolf D, Terriere M, de Wilde P, Reidy J F 1994 Embolization of a coronary fistula with a controlled delivery platinum coil in a 2-year old. Pediatric Cardiology 15: 308–310

Di Bella I, Gladstone D J 1998 Surgical management of aortopulmonary window. Annals of Thoracic Surgery 65: 768–770

Dines D E, Arms R A, Bernatz P E, Gomes M R 1974 Pulmonary arteriovenous fistulas. Mayo Clinic Proceedings 49: 460–465

Dines D E, Seward J B, Bernatz P E 1983 Pulmonary arteriovenous fistulas. Mayo Clinic Proceedings 58: 176–181

Ding W X, Su Z K, Cao D F, Jonas R A 1990 One-stage repair of absence of the aortopulmonary septum and interrupted aortic arch. Annals of Thoracic Surgery 49: 664–666

Donofrio M T, Ramaciotti C, Weinberg P M, Murphy J D 1995 Aortic atresia with interruption of the aortic arch and an aortopulmonary fistulous tract: case report. Pediatric Cardiology 16: 147–149

Dowd C F, Halbach V V, Barnwell S L, Higashida R T, Edwards M S, Hieshima G B 1990 Transfemoral venous embolization of vein of Galen malformations. American Journal of Neuroradiology 11: 643–648

D'Silva S A, Dalvi B V, Lokhandwala Y Y, Kale P A, Tendolkar A G 1992 Unruptured congenital aneurysm of the left sinus of Valsalva presenting as acute right ventricular failure. Chest 101: 578–579

Dutton J A, Jackson J E, Hughes J M et al 1995 Pulmonary arteriovenous malformations: results of treatment with coil embolisation in 53 patients. American Journal of Roentgenology 165: 1119–1125

Edwards J E 1961 Atlas of acquired disease of the heart and great vessels, Vol. III. Saunders, Philadelphia, PA, p 1142

Edwards M S B, Heishima G, Higashida R, Halbach V 1988 Management of vein of Galen malformations in the neonate. International Paediatrics 3: 184–188

Effler D B, Sheldon W C, Turner J J, Groves L K 1967 Coronary arteriovenous fistulas: diagnosis and surgical management: report of fifteen cases. Surgery 61: 41–50

Ferreira A C, de Marchena E, Mayor M, Bolooki H 1996 Sinus of Valsalva aneurysm presenting as myocardial infarction during dobutamine stress test. Catheterization and Cardiovascular Diagnosis 39: 400–402

Friedman D M, Madrid M, Berenstein A, Choi I S, Wisoff J H 1991 Neonatal vein of Galen malformations: experience in developing a multidisciplinary approach using an embolisation treatment protocol. Clinical Paediatrics 30: 621–629

Gammon R B, Miksa A K, Keller F S 1990 Osler–Weber–Rendu disease and pulmonary arteriovenous fistulas. Deterioration and embolotherapy during pregnancy. Chest 98: 1522–1524

Geva T, Ott D A, Ludomirsky A, Argyle S J, O'Laughlin M P 1992 Tricuspid atresia associated with aortopulmonary window: controlling pulmonary blood flow with a fenestrated patch. American Heart Journal 123: 260–262

Glock Y, Ferrarini J M, Puel J, Fauvel J M, Bounhourne J P, Puel P 1990 Isolated aneurysm of the left sinus of Valsalva. Rupture into the left atrium, left ventricle, and dynamic coronary constriction. Journal of Cardiovascular Surgery 31: 35–38

Gomes M R, Bernatz P E, Dines D E 1969 Pulmonary arteriovenous fistulas. Annals of Thoracic Surgery 7: 582–593

Grant P, Abrams L D, de Giovanni J V, Shah K J, Silove E D 1985 Aortic left ventricular tunnel arises from the left aortic sinus. American Journal of Cardiology 55: 1657–1658

Griffiths S P, Ellis K, Hordof A J, Martin E, Levine O R, Gersony W N 1983 Spontaneous complete closure of a congenital coronary fistula. Journal of American College of Cardiology 2: 1169–1171

Gupta R, Khanna S K, Akhtar M et al 1994 Dual exposure and repair technique for ruptured aneurysms of aortic sinus of Valsalva. Indian Heart Journal 46: 31–36

Haberman J H, Howard J L, Johnson E S 1963 Rupture of the coronary sinus with hemopericardium. Circulation 28: 1143–1144

Hackett D, Hallidie-Smith K A 1984 Spontaneous closure of coronary artery–cardiac chamber fistula. British Heart Journal 54: 477–479

Hall R J, Nelson W P, Blake H A, Geiger J P 1965 Massive pulmonary arteriovenous fistula in the newborn: a correctable form of 'cynanotic heart disease', an additional cause of cyanosis with left axis deviation. Circulation 31: 762–767

Hallman G L, Cooley D E, Singer D B 1966 Congenital anomalies of the coronary arteries: anatomy, pathology and surgical treatment. Surgery 59: 133–144

Hanner J S, Quisling R G, Mickle J P, Hawkins J S 1988 Gianturco coil embolisation of vein of Galen aneurysms: Technical aspects. Radiographics 8: 935–946

Hansoti R C, Sharma S 1989 Cirrhosis of the liver simulating congenital cyanotic heart disease. Chest 96: 843–848

Hartnell G G, Jordan S C 1990 Balloon embolisation of a coronary arterial fistula. International Journal of Cardiology 29: 381–383

Higgins C B, Wexler L 1976 Clinical and angiographic features of pulmonary arteriovenous fistulas in children. Radiology 119: 171–175

Ho S Y, Gerlis L M, Anderson C, Devine W A, Smith A 1994 The morphology of aortopulmonary windows with regard to their classification and morphogenesis. Cardiology in the Young 4: 146–155

Ho S Y, Muriago M, Cook A C, Thiene G, Anderson R H 1998 Surgical anatomy of aorto-left ventricular tunnel. Annals of Thoracic Surgery 65: 509–514

Ho V B, Kinney J B, Sahn D J 1995 Ruptured sinus of Valsalva aneurysm: cine phase-contrast MR characterization. Journal of Computer-assisted Tomography 19: 652–656

Hodgson C H, Kaye R L 1963 Pulmonary arteriovenous fistulas: physiologic and clinical considerations. Disease of the Chest 43: 449–455

Hofbeck M, Wild F, Singer H 1993 Improved visualisation of a coronary artery fistula by the 'laid-back' aortogram. British Heart Journal 70: 272–273

Hoffman C H, Kaye R L 1963 Pulmonary arteriovenous fistulas: physiologic and clinical considerations. Disease of the Chest 43: 449–455

Hoffman H J, Chuang S, Hendrick B, Humphreys R P 1982 Aneurysms of the vein of Galen. Journal of Neurosurgery 57: 316–322

Horimi H, Hasegawa T, Shiraishi H, Endo H, Yanagisawa M 1992 Detection of aortopulmonary window with ventricular septal defect by Doppler color flow imaging. Chest 101: 280–281

Horvath P, Balaji S, Skovranek S, Hucin B, de Leval M R, Stark J 1991 Surgical treatment of aortico–left ventricular tunnel. European Journal of Cardiothoracic Surgery 5: 113–116

Hovaguimian H, Cobanoglu A, Starr A 1988 Aortic left ventricular tunnel; a clinical review and new surgical classification. Annals of Thoracic Surgery 45: 106–112

Hucin B, Morvath P, Skovranek J, Reich O, Samanek M 1989 Correction of aortic left ventricular tunnel during the first day of life. Annals of Thoracic Surgery 47: 254–256

Humes R A, Hagler D G, Julsrud P R, Levy S M, Feldt R M, Schaff H V 1986 Aortic left ventricular tunnel: diagnosis based on two-dimensional echocardiography, color flow Doppler imaging and magnetic resonance imaging. Mayo Clinic Proceedings 61: 401/417

Ingram M T, Ott D A 1992 Concomitant repair of aortopulmonary window and interrupted aortic arch. Annals of Thoracic Surgery 53: 909–911

Issenberg H J 1990 Transcatheter coil closure of a congenital coronary arterial fistula. American Heart Journal 120: 1441–1443

Jaffe R B, Glancy D L, Epstein S E, Brown B G, Morrow A G 1973 Coronary arterial–right heart fistulae: long-term observations in seven patients. Circulation 47: 133–143

Jebara V A, Sarkis A, Acar C et al 1991 Coronary artery–left ventricle fistulas after cardiac surgery. American Heart Journal 122: 1759–1762

Kallis P, de Belder M, Smith E E 1993 Rupture of a sinus of Valsalva aneurysm through the tricuspid septal leaflet. Annals of Thoracic Surgery 55: 1247–1248

Kawata H, Kishimoto H, Ueno T, Nakajima T, Inamura N, Nakada T 1996 Repair of aortopulmonary window in an infant with extremely low birth weight. Annals of Thoracic Surgery 62: 1843–1845

Keith J D 1978 Pulmonary arteriovenous aneurysms. In: Keith J D, Rowe R D, Vlad P (eds) Heart disease in infancy and childhood. Macmillan, New York, p 887–889

Kim T K, Choe Y H, Kim H S et al 1995 Anomalous origin of the right pulmonary artery from the ascending aorta: diagnosis by magnetic resonance imaging. Cardiovascular Interventional Radiology 18: 118–121

Kirklin J W, Barrat-Boyes B G 1987 Cardiac surgery. John Wiley, New York, p 945–955

Knott-Craig C J, van der Merwe P L, Kalis N N, Hunter J 1992 Repair of aortico–left ventricular tunnel associated with subpulmonary obstruction. Annals of Thoracic Surgery 54: 557–559

Koh K K, Lee K H, Kim S S, Lee S C, Jin S H, Cho S W 1994 Ruptured aneurysm of the sinus of Valsalva in a patient with Behcet's disease. International Journal of Cardiology 47: 177–179

Kugelmass A D, Manning W J, Piana R N, Weintraub R M, Baim D S, Grossman W 1992 Coronary arteriovenous fistula presenting as congestive heart failure. European Journal of Cardiothoracic Surgery 26: 19–25

Kulan K, Kulan C, Tuncer C, Komsuoglu B, Zengin M 1996 Echocardiography and magnetic resonance imaging of sinus of Valsalva aneurysm with rupture into the ventricle. Journal of Cardiovascular Surgery 37: 639–641

Kutsche L M, Van Mierop L H S 1987 Anatomy and pathogenesis of aorticopulmonary septal defect. American Journal of Cardiology 59: 443–447

Laroche C M, Wells F, Shneerson J 1992 Massive hemothorax due to enlarging arteriovenous fistula in pregnancy. Chest 101: 1452–1454

Lasjaunias P, Garcia-Monaco R, Rodesch G et al 1991 Vein of Galen malformation. Endovascular management of 43 cases. Childs Nervous System (Germany) 7: 360–367

Levin D C, Fellows K E, Abrams H L 1978 Hemodynamically significant primary anomalies of the coronary arteries. Circulation 58: 25–34

Levy M J, Lillehei C W, Anderson R C, Amplatz K, Edwards J E 1963 Aortico–left ventricular tunnel. Circulation 27: 841–853

Levy M J, Schachner A, Blieden L C 1982 Aortic left ventricular tunnel–collective review. Journal of Thoracic and Cardiovascular Surgery 84: 102–109

Liang C D, Chang J P, Kao C L 1996 Unruptured sinus of Valsalva aneurysm with right ventricular outflow tract obstruction associated with ventricular septal defect. Catheterization and Cardiovascular Diagnosis 37: 158–161

Liberthson R R, Sagar K, Berkoben J P, Weintraub R M, Levine F H 1979 Congenital coronary arteriovenous fistula: report of 13 patients, review of the literature and delineation of management. Circulation 59: 849–854

Love B B, Biller J, Landas S K, Hoover W W 1992 Diagnosis of pulmonary arteriovenous malformations by ultrafast chest computed tomography in Rendu–Osler–Weber syndrome with cerebral ischaemia – a case report. Angiology 43: 522–528

Lukacs L, Bartek I, Haan A, Hankoczy J, Arvay A 1992 Ruptured aneurysms of the sinus of Valsalva. European Journal of Cardiothoracic Surgery 6: 15–17

MacNee W, Buist T A S, Finlayson N D C et al 1985 Multiple microscopic pulmonary arteriovenous connections in the lungs presenting as cynanosis. Thorax 40: 316–318

Macri R, Capulzini A, Fazzini L, Cornali M, Verunelli F, Reginato E 1982 Congenital coronary artery fistula. Thoracic and Cardiovascular Surgeon 30: 167–171

Marin-Neto J A, Simoes M V, Vicente W V 1991 Acquired aorto–coronary vein fistula after bypass graft surgery: report of two cases with long-term follow-up. International Journal of Cardiology 30: 121–124

Mavroudis C, Backer C L, Rocchini A P, Muster A J, Gevitz M 1997 Coronary artery fistulas in infants and children: a surgical review and discussion of coil embolization. Annals of Thoracic Surgery 63: 1235–1242

McCue C M, Hartenberg M, Nance W E 1984 Pulmonary arteriovenous malformations related to Rendu–Osler–Weber syndrome. American Journal of Medical Genetics 19: 19–27

McKenney P A, Shemin R J, Wiegers S E 1992 Role of transesophageal echocardiography in sinus of Valsalva aneurysm. American Heart Journal 123: 228–229

McNamara J J, Gross R E 1969 Congenital coronary artery fistula. Surgery 65: 59–69

Messmer B J 1994 Pulmonary artery flap for closure of aortopulmonary window. Annals of Thoracic Surgery 57: 498–501

Meyer J, Reul G J, Mullins C E, McCoy J, Hallman G L, Cooley D E 1975 Congenital fistulae of the coronary arteries. Journal of Cardiovascular Surgery 16: 506–511

Mickle J P, Quisling R G 1986 The transtorcular coil embolisation of vein of Galen aneurysms. Journal of Neurosurgery 64: 731–735

Missault L, Callens B, Taeymans Y 1995 Echocardiography of sinus of Valsalva aneurysm with rupture into the right atrium. International Journal of Cardiology 47: 269–272

Momma K, Toyama K, Takao A et al 1984 Natural history of subarterial infundibular ventricular septal defect. American Heart Journal 108: 1312–1317

Moro-Serrano C, Martinez J, Madrid A H et al 1992 Ventricular tachycardia in a patient with congenital coronary arteriovenous fistula. American Heart Journal 124: 503–505

Moyer J H, Glantz G, Brest A N 1962 Pulmonary arteriovenous fistulas: physiologic and clinical considerations. American Journal of Medicine 32: 417–435

Muthusamy R, Gupta G, Ahmed R A, de Giovanni J, Singh S P 1990 Fistula between a branch of left anterior descending coronary artery and pulmonary artery with spontaneous closure. European Heart Journal 11: 954–956

Nakatani S, Nanto S, Masuyama T, Tamai J, Kodama K 1991 Spontaneous near disappearance of bilateral coronary artery–pulmonary artery fistulas. Chest 99: 1288–1289

Nelson M, Dickinson D F, Wilson N 1988 Transtorcular coil embolisation of malformation of the vein of Galen – rapid resolution of heart failure in neonates. International Journal of Cardiology 18: 437–441

Ong M L 1993 Endocarditis of the tricuspid valve associated with congenital coronary arteriovenous fistula. British Heart Journal 70: 276–278

Oshiro K, Shimabukuro M, Nakada Y et al 1990 Multiple coronary LV fistulas: demonstration of coronary steal phenomenon by stress thallium scintigraphy and exercise haemodynamics. American Heart Journal 120: 217–219

Pennington D W, Gold W M, Gordon R L, Steiger D, Ring E J, Golden J A 1992 Treatment of pulmonary arteriovenous malformations by therapeutic embolisation. Rest and exercise physiology in 8 patients. American Review of Respiratory Disease 145: 1047–1051

Perez-Martinez V, Quero M, Castro C, Moreno F, Brito J M, Merino G 1973 Aortico–left ventricular tunnel. A clinical and pathologic review of this uncommon entity. American Heart Journal 85: 237–245

Perry L W, Martin G R, Galioto F M Jr, Midgley F M 1991 Rupture of congenital sinus of Valsalva aneurysm in a newborn. American Journal of Cardiology 68: 1255–1256

Perry S B, Rome J, Keane J F, Baim D S, Lock J E 1992 Transcatheter closure of coronary artery fistulas. Journal of American College of Cardiology 20: 205–209

Podolsky L, Ledley G S, Goldstein J, Kotler M N, Yazdanfar S 1991 Bilateral coronary artery to left ventricular fistulas. Catheterization and Cardiovascular Diagnosis 24: 271–273

Pollak J S, Egglin T K, Rosenblatt M M, Dickey K W, White R I 1994 Clinical results of transvenous systemic embotherapy with a neuroradiologic detachable balloon. Radiology 191: 477–482

Portsmann W 1977 Therapeutic embolisation of arteriovenous pulmonary fistula by catheter technique. In: Kelopo (ed.) Current concepts in paediatric radiology. Springer, Berlin, p 23–31

Prager R L, Laws K H, Bender H W 1983 Arteriovenous fistula of the lung. Annals of Thoracic Surgery 36: 231–239

Prakash A, Reidy J F, Holt P M 1993 Correction of myocardial ischaemia after transcatheter embolisation of a small left coronary artery venous fistula. British Heart Journal 69: 270–271

Preminger T J, Lock J E, Perry S B 1994 Traumatic aortopulmonary window as a copmplication of pulmonary artery balloon angioplasty: transcatheter occlusion with a covered stent. A case report. Catheterization and Cardiovascular Diagnosis 31: 286–289

Prewitt K C, Smolin M R, Coster T S, Vernalis M N, Bunda M, Wortham D C 1994 Coronary artery fistula diagnosed by transesophageal echocardiography. Chest 105: 959–961

Puskas J D, Allen M S, Moncure A C et al 1993 Pulmonary arteriovenous malformation: therapeutic options. Annals of Thoracic Surgery 56: 253–257

Quek S C, Wong J, Tay J S, Reidy J, Qureshi S A 1996 Transcatheter embolization of coronary artery fistula with controlled release coils. Journal of Paediatrics and Child Health 32: 542–544

Qureshi S A, Maruszewski B, McKay R, Arnold R, West C A, Hamilton D I 1990 Determinants of survival following repair of interrupted aortic arch in infancy. International Journal of Cardiology 26: 303–312

Qureshi S A, Reidy J F, Alwi M B et al 1996 Use of interlocking detachable coils in embolization of coronary arteriovenous fistulas. American Journal of Cardiology 78: 110–113

Ramo O J, Totterman K J, Harjula A L 1994 Thrombosed coronary artery fistula as a cause of paroxysmal atrial fibrillation and ventricular arrhythmia. Cardiovascular Surgery 2: 720–722

Redington A N, Rigby M L, Ho S Y, Gunthard J, Anderson R H 1991 Aortic atresia with aortopulmonary window and interruption of the aortic arch. Pediatric Cardiology 12: 49–51

Reeder G S, Tajik A J, Smith H C 1980 Visualization of coronary artery fistula by two-dimensional echocardiography. Mayo Clinic Proceedings 55: 185–189

Reidy J F, Sowton E, Ross D N 1983 Transcatheter occlusion of coronary to bronchial anastomosis by detachable balloon combined with coronary angioplasty at the same procedure. British Heart Journal 49: 284–287

Reidy J F, Jones O D H, Tynan M J, Baker E J, Joseph M C 1985 Embolization procedures in congenital heart disease. British Heart Journal 54: 184–192

Reidy J F, Tynan M J, Qureshi S A 1990 Embolisation of a complex coronary arterio-venous fistula in a 6 year old child: the need for specialised embolisation techniques. British Heart Journal 63: 246–248

Reidy J F, Anjos R T, Qureshi S A, Baker E J, Tynan M J 1991 Transcatheter embolization in the treatment of coronary artery fistulas. Journal of American College of Cardiology 18: 187–192

Remy J, Remy-Jardin M, Wattinne L, Deffonthines C 1992 Pulmonary arteriovenous malformations: evaluation with CT of the chest before and after treatment. Radiology 182: 809–816

Rittenhouse E A, Doty D B, Ehrenhaft J L 1975 Congenital coronary artery–cardiac chamber fistula. Annals of Thoracic Surgery 20: 468–485

Rothbart R M, Chahine R A 1990 Left sinus of Valsalva aneurysm with rupture into the left ventricular outflow tract: diagnosis by color-encoded Doppler imaging. American Heart Journal 120: 224–227

Roughneen P T, Bhattacharjee M, Morris P T, Nasser M, Reul G J 1994 Spontaneous thrombosis in a coronary artery fistula with aneurysmal dilatation of the sinus of Valsalva. Annals of Thoracic Surgery 57: 232–234

Rubin D A, Zaki A M, Zaghlol S, Abdala S, Fahmy A R, Ziady G 1992 Visualization of coronary artery fistula with transesophageal echocardiography. Journal of the American Society of Echocardiography 5: 173–175

Sahasakul Y, Panchavinnin P, Chaithiraphan S, Sakiyalak P 1990 Echocardiographic diagnosis of a ruptured aneurysm of the sinus of Valsalva: operation without catheterisation in seven patients. British Heart Journal 64: 195–198

Said S A, Bucx J J, van de Weel F A 1992 Stress MIBI scintigraphy in multiple coronary-pulmonary fistula: failure to demonstrate 'steal' phenomenon. International Journal of Cardiology 35: 270–272

Satomi G, Nakamura K, Narai S, Takao A 1984 Systematic visualization of coronary arteries by two-dimensional echocardiography in children and infants: evaluation in

Kawasaki's disease and coronary arteriovenous fistulas. American Heart Journal 107: 497–505

Serino W, Andrade J, Ross D, de Leval M, Somerville J 1983 Aorto–left ventricular communication after closure. Late post-operative problems. British Heart Journal 49: 501–506

Seto H, Futatsuya R, Kamei T et al 1985 Pulmonary arteriovenous malformation: radionucleide detection and quantification of right to left shunting. Radiation Medicine 3: 33–37

Sharland G K 1992 Left heart disease in the fetus. MD thesis, University of London, p 190

Shirai K, Ogawa M, Kawaguchi H, Kawano T, Nakashima Y, Arakawa K 1994 Acute myocardial infarction due to thrombus formation in congenital coronary artery fistula. European Heart Journal 15: 577–579

Shumacker H B, Waldhausen J A 1963 Pulmonary arteriovenous fistulas in children. Annals of Surgery 158: 713–720

Simon P, Owen A N, Moidl R et al 1994 Sinus of Valsalva aneurysm: a late complication after repair of ascending aortic dissection. Thoracic and Cardiovascular Surgeon 42: 29–31

Skimming J W, Walls J T 1993 Congenital coronary artery fistula suggesting a 'steal phenomenon' in a neonate. Pediatric Cardiology 14: 174–175

Skimming J W, Gessner I H, Victorica B E, Mickle J P 1995 Percutaneous transcatheter occlusion of coronary artery fistulas using detachable balloons. Pediatric Cardiology 16: 38–41

Sloan R D, Cooley R N 1953 Congenital pulmonary arteriovenous aneurysm. American Journal of Roentgenology 70: 183–210

Somers J M, Verney G I 1991 Coronary cameral fistulae following heart transplantation. Clinical Radiology 44: 419–421

Sousa-Uva M, Touchot A, Fermont L et al 1996 Aortico–left ventricular tunnel in fetuses and infants. Annals of Thoracic Surgery 61: 1805–1810

Sreeram N, Walsh K 1991 Aortopulmonary window with aortic origin of the right pulmonary artery. International Journal of Cardiology 31: 249–251

Sreeram N, Franks R, Arnold R, Walsh K 1991 Aortico–left ventricular tunnel: long-term outcome after surgical repair. Journal of American College of Cardiology 17: 950–955

St John Sutton M G, Miller G A, Kerr I H, Traill T A 1980 Coronary steal via large coronary artery to bronchial artery anastomosis successfully treated by operation. British Heart Journal 44: 460–463

Stamato T, Benson L N, Smallhorn J F, Freedom R M 1995 Transcatheter closure of an aortopulmonary window with a modified double umbrella occluder system. Catherization and Cardiovascular Diagnosis 35: 165–167

Stanbridge R D, Westaby S, Smallhorn J, Taylor J F N 1983 Intracranial arteriovenous malformation with aneurysm of the vein of Galen as a cause of heart failure in infancy. Echocardiographic diagnosis and results of treatment. British Heart Journal 49: 157–162

Steinberg E, Wun H, Bosco J, Kronzon I 1996 Spontaneous echocardiographic contrast within an unruptured sinus of Valsalva aneurysm: a potential embolic source diagnosed by transesophageal echocardiography. Journal of the American Society of Echocardiography 9: 880–881

Stollberger C, Seitelberger R, Fenninger C, Prainer C, Slany J 1996 Aneurysm of the left sinus of Valsalva. An unusual source of cerebral embolism. Stroke 27: 1424–1426

Sunaga Y, Taniichi Y, Okubo N et al 1992 Biplane transesophageal echocardiographic study of left coronary artery to right atrium fistula. American Heart Journal 123: 1058–1060

Swank M, Koepke D E 1972 Coronary artery to left atrium fistula requiring revascularisation: case report and literature review. Thorax 37: 376–380

Swinburne A J, Fedullo A J, Gangemi R, Mijangos J A 1986 Hereditary telangiectasia and multiple pulmonary arteriovenous fistulas. Clinical deterioration during pregnancy. Chest 89: 459–460

Symbas P N, Schlant R C, Hatcher C R et al 1967 Congenital fistula of the right coronary artery to right ventricle complicated by *Actinobacillus actinomycetemcomitans* endarteritis. Journal of Thoracic and Cardiovascular Surgery 53: 379–384

Takahashi M, Sekiguchi H, Fujikawa H et al 1994 Multicystic aneurysmal dilatation of bilateral coronary artery fistula. Catheterization and Cardiovascular Diagnosis 31: 290–292

Tami L F, Turi Z G, Arbulu A 1993 Sinus of Valsalva aneurysms involving both coronary ostia. Catheterization and Cardiovascular Diagnosis 29: 304–308

Teragaki M, Akioka K, Yasuda M et al 1988 Hereditary haemorrhagic telangiectasia with growing pulmonary arteriovenous fistulas followed for 24 years. American Journal of Medical Science 295: 545–547

Terry P B, White R I, Barth K H, Kaufman S L, Mitchell S E 1983 Pulmonary arteriovenous malformations. New England Journal of Medicine 308: 1197–1200

Tkebuchava T, von Segesser L K, Vogt P R et al 1997 Congenital aortopulmonary window: diagnosis, surgical technique and long-term results. European Journal of Cardiothoracic Surgery 11: 293–297

Toombes H, Paul K, Vogt-Moykopf I 1984 Treatment of multiple unilateral arteriovenous fistulae by transection of the pulmonary artery. Thoracic and Cardiovascular Surgeon 32: 60–63

Tsagaris T J, Hecht H H 1962 Coronary artery aneurysm and subacute bacterial endocarditis. Annals of Internal Medicine 57: 116–121

Tulloh R M, Rigby M L 1997 Transcatheter umbrella closure of aortopulmonary window. Heart 77: 479–480

Tuna I C, Edwards J E 1988 Aortic left ventricular tunnel and aortic insufficiency. Annals of Thoracic Surgery 45: 5–6

Urrutia S C O, Falaschi G, Ott D A 1983 Surgical management of 56 patients with congenital coronary artery fistulas. Annals of Thoracic Surgery 35: 300–307

Van den Brand M, Pieterman H, Suryapranata H, Bogers A J 1992 Closure of a coronary fistula with a transcatheter implantable coil. Catheterization and Cardiovascular Diagnosis 25: 223–226

van Son J A, Puga F J, Danielson G K et al 1993 Aortopulmonary window: factors associated with early and late success after surgical treatment. Mayo Clinic Proceedings 68: 128–133 van Son J A, Danielson G K, Schaff H V, Orszulak T A, Edwards W D, Seward J B 1994 Long-term outcome of surgical repair of ruptured sinus of Valsalva aneurysm. Circulation 90 (suppl II): 20–29

Vavuranakis M, Bush C A, Boudouloas H 1995 Coronary artery fistulas in adults: incidence, angiographic characteristics, natural history. Catheterization and Cardiovascular Diagnosis 35: 116–120

Webber S, Johnston B, LeBlanc J, Patterson M 1991 Aortico–left ventricular tunnel associated with critical aortic stenosis in the newborn. Pediatric Cardiology 12: 237–240

Weldner P, Dhillon R, Taylor J F, de Leval M R 1996 An alternative method for repair of aortico–left ventricular tunnel associated with severe aortic stenosis presenting in a newborn. European Journal of Cardiothoracic Surgery 10: 380–382

White R I 1991 Case 16-1990: brain abscess and pulmonary arteriovenous malformation. New England Journal of Medicine 324: 1439–1440

White R I 1992 Pulmonary arteriovenous malformations: how do we diagnose them and why is it important to do so? Radiology 182: 633–635

White R I, Mitchell S E, Barth K H et al 1983 Angio-architecture of pulmonary arteriovenous malformations: an important consideration before embolotherapy. American Journal of Roentgenology 140: 681–686

White R I, Lynch-Nyhan A, Terry P et al 1988 Long term outlook of embolotherapy. Radiology 169: 663–669

Wilde P, Watt I 1980 Congenital coronary artery fistulae: six new cases with a collective review. Clinical Radiology 31: 301–311

Wortham D C, Gorman P D, Hull R W, Vernalis M N, Gaither N S 1993 Unruptured sinus of Valsalva aneurysm presenting with embolization. American Heart Journal 125: 896–898

61

══ Cardiac tumours ══

M. A. Gatzoulis and A. E. Becker

─────────────── INTRODUCTION ───────────────

Cardiac tumours in infants and children are rare. Their atypical clinical presentation prevented timely diagnosis in the past, when cardiac tumours were often a post-mortem finding. The widespread use of echocardiography and other non-invasive diagnostic methods in recent years, however, has resulted in a marked increase in the detection of children, and indeed fetuses, with cardiac tumours, many of whom may be asymptomatic. In turn, early recognition of cardiac tumours has resulted in better understanding of their natural history and, combined with advances in surgical techniques, an improved overall outcome (Hwa et al, 1994; Marx, 1995).

It is difficult to ascertain the true incidence of cardiac tumours because of the tendency so far to base estimates on postmortem studies, case reports and single institutional experiences. The lack of non-invasive diagnostic imaging in earlier reports was another limiting factor. Reported incidence varied from 0.027% amongst 11 000 paediatric postmortem specimens (Nadas and Ellison, 1968) to 0.49% amongst 2251 infants surveyed with congenital heart disease (New England Regional Infant Cardiac Program – Fyler, 1980). A large published series of primary tumours and cysts of the heart and pericardium, from the files of the Armed Forces Institute of Pathology, showed that among a total number of 533 tumours and cysts, 48 occurred in infants and 89 in children (15 years of age or younger) (McAllister and

Fenoglio, 1978). Of these, only 10 (7.5%) tumours were considered malignant. The relative incidence of cardiac tumours in these 137 children is shown in Table 61.1.

Table 61.1. Relative incidence of cardiac tumours in infants and children in a postmortem series of 444 primary tumours of the heart and pericardium

	Infants (47)	Children (86)
Benign tumours		
Rhabdomyoma	28	35
Teratoma	9	11
Fibroma	6	12
Haemangioma	1	4
Mesothelioma (of the atrioventricular node)	1	3
Myxoma	0	12
Neurofibroma	0	1
Total	45	78
Malignant tumours		
Fibrosarcoma	1	1
Rhabdomyosarcoma	1	2
Malignant teratoma	0	4
Neurogenic sarcoma	0	1
Total	2	8

Source: McAllister and Fenoglio (1978).

─────────────── GENERAL ASPECTS ───────────────

CLINICAL SIGNS AND SYMPTOMS ─────────

Although cardiac tumours are usually benign in children, they may induce even life-threatening symptoms. Their clinical manifestations are often non-specific. They may mimic many other diseases of the heart and lungs. Classically, the clinical presentation is divided into three major groups: systemic, embolic and cardiac effects.

SYSTEMIC MANIFESTATIONS

The systemic manifestations of tumours of the heart are manifold and include findings such as fever and general malaise. Digital clubbing, Raynaud's phenomenon, myalgia and arthralgia are usually associated with myxomas. Abnormal laboratory findings include an elevated erythrocyte sedimentation rate, hypergamma-globulinaemia, thrombocytosis or thrombocytopenia, polycythaemia, leucocytosis and anaemia. These features are reversible when the tumour is removed (Willman et al, 1965). The mechanisms underlying these systemic manifestations are, as yet, not fully understood. There is some evidence that secretory products of the tumour, necrosis of the tumour and immune reactivity may all play a role (MacGregor and Cullen, 1959; Curry et al, 1967; Steinke et al, 1972; Burnes et al, 1982).

EMBOLIC MANIFESTATIONS

These events can all be caused by embolization of either fragments of the tumour itself or thrombuses aggregated at the surface of the tumour. The distribution of such emboluses depends largely on the localization of the primary tumour itself and the presence or absence of additional cardiac malformations (such as additional shunts or abnormal patterns of flow). Embolization of tumour fragments can occur only when the tumour itself has an intracavitary extension (Burton and Johnson, 1970). Thromboembolic formation, however, can occur also with primary intramural tumours that compromise the endocardium of the cardiac chamber, either by mechanical compression or by inducing a functional disturbance.

Generally speaking, left-sided tumours embolize to the systemic circulation. Hence, they may affect almost any organ. Sudden occlusion of a peripheral artery should always alert to the possibility of embolization from a primary intracardiac tumour. Moreover, multiple systemic emboluses may mimic systemic vasculitis or infective endocarditis, particularly when they produce systemic manifestations.

Primary tumours in the right-sided heart chambers may cause pulmonary emboluses. These may be indistinguishable from those occurring secondary to venous thromboembolism. It is significant in this respect that the perfusion defect in the lung when caused by an embolus from a tumour does not usually resolve within a few weeks. Tumour embolization is also suggested by complete absence of flow to one lung in the presence of a normal perfusion scan of the opposite lung. This is most unusual in patients with recurrent pulmonary venous thromboembolism.

CARDIAC MANIFESTATIONS

The cardiac events are largely dependent on the location and the extent of the tumour within the heart. Tumours that are localized within the myocardium may occasionally pass unnoticed clinically. They may then be discovered as incidental findings at echocardiography or postmortem. When located in the region of the atrioventricular node and conduction tissues, however, even small tumours may produce disturbance of atrioventricular conduction. Complete atrioventricular block and sudden death are seen as the extreme. Moreover, the intramural location of primary tumours of the heart may underlie a

wide variety of disturbances of rhythm, including atrial fibrillation or flutter, paroxysmal atrial tachycardia, atrioventricular junctional rhythm, atrial and ventricular premature beats, ventricular tachycardia and ventricular fibrillation (Harvey, 1968; van der Hauwaert, 1971; Engle et al, 1974; Filiatrault et al, 1991; Mulher et al, 1994). Infiltrative tumours of the myocardium can cause haemodynamic compromise. This tends to occur late in the clinical course when there is substantial involvement of the myocardium or of the pericardium, producing symptoms of cardiac failure consequent to systolic and or diastolic dysfunction. In some instances, the clinical presentation may mimic that of dilated, restrictive or hypertrophic obstructive cardiomyopathy (Chapter 59). Pericardial exudate, eventually with cardiac tamponade, may be the first symptom of the epicardial location of the tumour. This is mainly seen in malignant and in secondary lesions.

Primary cardiac tumours with an intracavitary extension may cause obstruction or may interfere with valvar closure. The signs and symptoms are then highly dependent upon the chamber involved and the size of the tumour. The embolic effects, which are a frequent complication of such tumours, similarly relate directly to the site of the tumour. Left atrial tumours may produce mitral stenosis or insufficiency and, hence, may mimic valvar disease. The symptoms and signs may have a sudden onset, particularly in the case of a pedunculated highly mobile left atrial tumour.

Such findings are often intermittent and related to the patient's position. They are of paramount significance and should always alert to the possibility of a tumour.

Intracavitary tumours within the right atrium frequently produce symptoms of right heart failure. The manifestations may result from either obstruction of the tricuspid orifice or tricuspid valvar insufficiency, the latter secondary to interference from the tumour with valvar closure. The localization of the tumour may produce caval venous obstruction as the leading feature.

Right ventricular intracavitary tumours may produce signs and symptoms of inflow or outflow obstructions and of atrioventricular valvar insufficiency. Right heart failure is often the leading manifestation. As with all heart tumours, the physical signs may vary considerably depending upon its site and size. The picture may be further complicated by pulmonary embolization and secondary pulmonary hypertension. Tumours in the right ventricle, therefore, may mimic congenital pulmonary stenosis, restrictive cardiomyopathy or even cyanotic heart disease (Marin-Garcia et al, 1984).

Intracavitary left ventricular tumours may also cause inflow or outflow obstruction or atrioventricular valvar insufficiency, with all their accompanying signs and symptoms. Syncope and sudden unexpected death may be the first manifestations. Atypical chest pain may occur. This is caused by coronary arterial obstruction, either from compression by the tumour itself or because of coronary arterial embolism. Hence, intracavitary left ventricular tumours may mimic other conditions such as aortic and subaortic stenosis, asymmetric septal hypertrophy and endocardial fibroelastosis (Selzer et al, 1972).

INVESTIGATIONS

Physical examination and the usual laboratory studies are non-conclusive. Murmurs, when present, are in themselves non-specific, but certain atypical findings may suggest a cardiac tumour rather than primary valvar or myocardial disease. Such findings include postural variation in the intensity of the murmur and the presence of a so-called tumour 'plop'. The plop has been described particularly in patients with left atrial myxoma, being characteristic of a pedunculated and highly sessile tumour. It most likely results from sudden tension on the stalk of the tumour as it prolapses during diastole into the left ventricular cavity. The auscultatory findings are otherwise highly variable. Differentiation from organic valvar disease is often impossible.

ELECTROCARDIOGRAPHY

The electrocardiogram is non-specific. All kinds of rhythm and conduction disturbances, or voltage and ST–T wave segmental abnormalities may be seen (Cola et al, 1992; Muhler et al, 1994). The electrocardiogram may also display the typical pattern of atrial dilation or ventricular hypertrophy. Incidental low-voltage complexes may be registered, indicating possible pericardial involvement. Occasionally a pre-excitation pattern is present (Milner et al, 1980; Biancaniello et al, 1982).

CHEST RADIOGRAPHY

Cardiac tumours may alter the contour of the heart, but the changes in themselves are non-specific. The cardiac contour may be normal or may display enlargement of either the entire heart size or any particular chamber. Gross and bizarre distortions of the cardiac contour occasionally occur that are then suggestive of a tumour. The overall picture may be further complicated by the presence of pericardial fluid. Radiographic signs of pulmonary venous obstruction may be observed in patients with obstructive left-sided heart tumours (Steiner, 1968). Calcification of a primary heart tumour may occasionally be so intense that it can be noted on the chest radiograph (Waaler et al, 1972; Williams et al, 1982).

ECHOCARDIOGRAPHY

Echocardiographic examination of cardiac tumours is universally established as the main, and usually the only, diagnostic modality required for children. It allows accurate determination of the extent and location of the lesion, its haemodynamic consequences and for most patients obviates the need for cardiac catheterization and angiography (Arciniegas et al, 1980; Come et al, 1981; de Pace et al, 1981; Riggs et al, 1981; Bini et al, 1983; Marx et al, 1984; Hwa et al, 1994) (Figure 61.1a, b). Fyke et al (1985) reported not only a dramatic increase in the annual incidence of cardiac neoplasms over a 5-year period since the advent of cross-sectional echocardiography, but also an equally dramatic reduction in unexpected intraoperative findings.

The sensitivity of echocardiography is greatest for endocardial lesions, where the contrast between tumour and an echolucent cavity is most apparent and permits characterization of the size and mobility of these masses. In contrast, echocardiographic assessment of the pericardium for tumours may be quite limited because of its echo density or farfield position. While involvement of the pericardium and extracardiac mediastinum by the tumour may be examined by scanning from multiple transducer positions (and, incidentally, is a mandatory examination in any pericardial effusion of unknown aetiology), magnetic resonance imaging is a more capable and reliable technique for this task. Texture may be inferred by the gray scale appearance, although interpretation remains subjective (Green et al, 1983). Colour processing of the cross-sectional gray scale image has also been applied to distinguish tumour mass from endocardium (Allan et al, 1983). B-colour has been reported to assist in definition of the edge of tumours and in recognizing small masses, particularly when intramural (Hwa et al, 1994).

Echocardiography also gives information as to whether the tumour is encapsulated or not, and whether the tumour is solid or cystic (Farooki et al, 1977; Biancaniello et al, 1982). Cardiac tumours have the tendency to occur at multiple sites. Hence, echocardiographic evaluation should be thorough, encompassing the whole heart. Pericardial fluid may be present, especially in malignant and metastatic lesions.

Transoesophageal echocardiography can be used as a useful adjunct to transthoracic imaging, notably in patients with suboptimal transthoracic windows, and is ideally suited for the examination of suspected tumours involving the atriums, interatrial septum, caval veins, atrioventricular valves and, to a lesser extent, the great arteries (Cohen et al, 1990; Mugge et al, 1991). Another important application is the differentiation of true pathology from normal, or variants of normal, anatomy. For example, a prominent terminal crest may simulate a mass during transthoracic imaging of the morphologically right atrium; transoesophageal echocardiography can demonstrate this to be a normal structure. In addition, transoesophageal imaging can be used intraoperatively to assist with surgical excision of cardiac tumours.

Dynamic three-dimensional echocardiography has been recently employed in the preoperative assessment of cardiac tumours as it may yield important additional

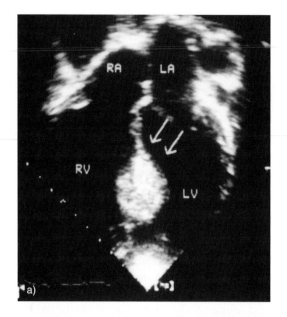

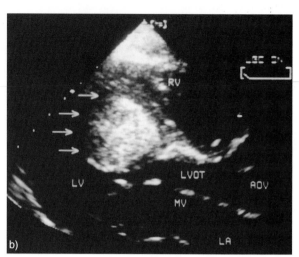

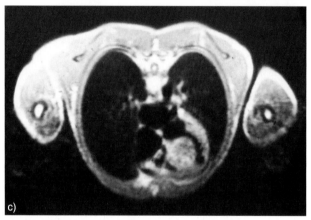

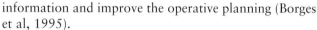

Figure 61.1. Imaging of a patient with a fibroma. (a) Apical four chamber cross-sectional echocardiogram showing a solitary, whitish tumour in the ventricular septum (arrows), typical of fibroma. (b) Parasternal long-axis echocardiographic view (diastolic frame). Note the circumscript appearance of the fibroma, suggesting an encapsulated nature. However, microscopic studies often reveal intermingling of the tumour with the adjacent myocardium. Pulsed and continuous Doppler interrogation with colour Doppler mapping were employed to exclude significant left ventricular inflow and outflow abnormalities in this case. (c) The magnetic resonance image has a wider field of view encompassing the pericardium, mediastinum and the lungs. The absence of additional intracardiac tumours or of any extracardiac extension, strongly supports the initial diagnosis of fibroma. AoV, aortic valve; LA, left atrium; LV, left ventricle; LVOT, left ventricular outflow tract; MV, mitral valve; RA, right atrium; RV, right ventricle.

information and improve the operative planning (Borges et al, 1995).

Prenatal echocardiographic screening, performed usually for the assessment of intrauterine growth or occasionally as part of investigations for fetal arrhythmias or nonimmune hydrops and high risk pregnancies, has led to fetal tumours being diagnosed as early as 20 weeks of gestation (de Vore et al, 1982; Birnbaum et al, 1985; Cyr et al, 1988; Rheuban et al, 1991; Holley et al, 1995). These tumours are usually rhabdomyomas. Although most of these patients are, and remain, asymptomatic (Wallace et al, 1990; Holley et al, 1995), prior knowledge of the tumour/s in the few patients who may be critically ill at birth can optimize their postnatal care (de Geeter et al, 1983). Spontaneous regression of even symptomatic fetal cardiac tumours has also been described (Brand and Friedberg, 1992).

MAGNETIC RESONANCE IMAGING

Magnetic resonance imaging, when gated using the electrocardiogram, can identify a variety of tumours primar-

ily involving the cardiac chambers and, therefore, may complement echocardiography (Brown et al, 1989; Rienmuller et al, 1989). The wide field of view achieved with magnetic resonance imaging, which encompasses the lungs, mediastinum, pericardium, great vessels and of course the heart itself, is a great advantage over that in echocardiography (White and Zisch, 1991) (Figure 61.1c). The inherent natural contrast between the intracardiac and vascular spaces and the surrounding walls of cardiovascular structures enables sharp delineation of the myocardium with negligible interference by bony or lung tissue (Boxer et al, 1985).

Resonance imaging is unquestionably the superior investigative approach in pericardial lesions, with or without extension into contiguous structures, areas often poorly visualized by echocardiography. In addition, a limited degree of tissue characterization is possible with the latter technology. Contrast-enhanced imaging with paramagnetic agents and radiofrequency labelling have been employed in that respect for further differentiation of tumour from viable myocardium (Niwa et al, 1989; Bouton et al, 1991). Spin echo and cine gradient echo techniques may provide additional valuable information concerning the mobility of cardiac tumours, a better appreciation of the site of attachment and their effects on myocardial and valvar function (Sechtem et al, 1987).

The use of resonance imaging in children, nonetheless, is not free of limitations. Heavy sedation is often required to suppress deep respiration and other movements, and in those with arrhythmias, interference can still cause significant motion artifact despite electrocardiographic gating; this compromises the quality of imaging. In addition, and in contrast to echocardiography, the machine is not portable and, therefore, is not suitable for patients requiring intensive care.

CATHETERIZATION AND ANGIOCARDIOGRAPHY

Once accepted as the gold standard for diagnosis, angiocardiography has waned in importance as the result of the availability and reliability of the non-invasive methods of imaging discussed above. Angiocardiography does not demonstrate extension of tumour into the ventricular walls but only the presence of the tumour within the cavities, as demonstrated by filling defects. The possibility of diagnosis by endomyocardial biopsy has been suggested (Bini et al, 1983). This is hardly ever necessary today, as a firm diagnosis can be established using non-invasive imaging alone; diagnosis is confirmed by perioperative biopsy when surgical excision of the tumour is justified. Pressure measurements can be obtained with catheterization, although this has the inherent risk of placing a catheter near or across a friable tumour, a process that may lead to embolization (Ludomirski et al, 1985).

SUMMARY

Transthoracic echocardiography remains the procedure of choice in screening for cardiac tumours. Magnetic resonance and transoesophageal echocardiographic imaging clearly complement one another, and the choice between these techniques depends upon various factors including the transthoracic echogenicity of the patient, the site of the possible tumour, the availability of these methods, cost, and the physical status and age of the patient.

TUMOUR TYPES

RHABDOMYOMA

Rhabdomyomas may present as circumscribed non-encapsulated lesions. Their size may vary from a few millimetres to several centimetres. Occasionally, the lesion may outgrow the size of the heart. Rhabdomyomas are usually multiple and have a distinct preference for the

ventricular septum and the adjacent ventricular walls (Arciniegas et al, 1980). The lesions may be limited to the myocardium, often leading to compression and deformity of the cardiac chambers. Alternatively, they may extend from their intramural location into an intracavitary position. Such lesions are characterized histologically by grotesquely swollen myocytes, which present an almost 'empty' cytoplasm traversed by tiny strands of cross-striated sarcoplasm. The nucleus may thus appear suspended within the cell, giving rise to the so-called 'spider cell'. Spontaneous regression is possible, as was demonstrated by Marx et al (1984) by echocardiographic follow-up, and can occur within a period as short as 6 weeks (Webb et al, 1993). Tuberous sclerosis is present in over one half of the patients found to have rhabdomyomas (Webb et al, 1993; Nir et al, 1995). Rhabdomyomas are by far the most frequent tumours found in fetuses, infants and children. They occur almost exclusively in patients under the age of 15 years. The lesions most likely represent hamartomas rather than true neoplasms (Fenoglio et al, 1977; Bruni et al, 1980).

Two main clinical categories can be distinguished. In some patients, the rhabdomyoma is found as an incidental postmortem finding. Among these patients, the clinical profile has often been dominated by signs and symptoms of tuberous sclerosis. In other patients, however, rhabdomyoma is the immediate cause of morbidity and/or mortality. In some, the cardiac tumour may have led to stillbirth, or death within a few days of birth. In others, the rhabdomyoma may become clinically manifest (usually because of cardiomegaly, congestive heart failure, cyanosis and cardiac arrhythmias) and death may occur suddenly and unexpectedly (Nadas and Ellison, 1968; Engle et al, 1974; Arciniegas, 1980; Milner et al, 1980). In general, the prognosis of children with a symptomatic rhabdomyoma is bad. In the series of McAllister and Fenoglio (1978), over three quarters of the children died before the age of 1 year. A literature review in 1982 indicated that, of all patients with a rhabdomyoma, two fifths died before the age of 6 months, three fifths before 1 year of age and four fifths before the age of 5 years (Spooner et al, 1982). These results have to be interpreted with caution in the current era of improved diagnostic ability, followed by an increasing prevalence of cardiac tumours reported in paediatric patients. Of symptomatic patients, nearly three quarters have an intracavitary rhabdomyoma, with marked obstruction to blood flow in at least one cardiac chamber (Shaher et al, 1972; Harinck et al, 1974; McAllister and Fenoglio, 1978; Spooner et al, 1982). It has been suggested, with good reason, that the demonstration of an intracardiac mass in a symptomatic child under 5 years of age strongly suggests the diagnosis of rhabdomyoma. This is important, particularly in view of the concept that the rhabdomyoma represents a hamartoma rather than a true neoplasm, and since it has been shown that intracavitary rhabdomyomas are only rarely associated with tuberous sclerosis. This group of patients, therefore, may be amenable to surgical treatment. Complete removal, however, is not always possible (Arciniegas et al, 1980; Bini et al, 1983).

FIBROMA

Cardiac fibromas, found in one sixth of cases, ranked second in frequency amongst tumours identified at postmortem in hearts of children between 1 and 15 years of age (McAllister and Fenoglio, 1978); the reported prevalence in clinical series has been higher, at one quarter (Marx, 1995). Fibromas are seen throughout childhood, although they are less common in fetuses and newborns (Freedom and Benson, 1992; Holley et al, 1995).

The gross appearance of cardiac fibromas is relatively uniform (Figure 61.1a, b). They present as solid, firm, whitish lesions with a distinct fibromatous architecture on cut sections. They may vary in size, but when they have led to functional impairment they are usually several centimetres in size. Their circumscript appearance suggests an encapsulated nature, but microscopic studies reveal intermingling of the tumour with the adjacent myocardium. Moreover, satellite nodules may be present. Calcification within the lesions is not at all uncommon (Waaler et al, 1972; Williams et al, 1982).

Cardiac fibromas, in practical terms, are slow-growing but potentially aggressive lesions. Spontaneous regression has not been observed, and surgical excision is often required. Signs and symptoms are largely dependent on the location of the tumour (Burke et al, 1994). There is a distinct predilection for the ventricular septum and left ventricular wall. This preference may underlie the presentation of cardiac fibromas with sudden and unexpected death. Cardiac arrhythmias and atrioventricular conduction disturbances can occur. The position within the ventricular septum may also lead to compression of the cardiac chambers and, hence, may cause obstruction. Cardiomegaly is often the leading sign when the lesion is localized in the ventricular or atrial free wall. As fibromas and rhabdomyomas may have similar appearances on imaging, complete evaluation for tuberous sclerosis is warranted. Successful surgical excision of large tumours has been reported in children of all ages (Williams et al, 1972; 1982; Parmley et al, 1988), with no recurrence of disease over follow-up of several years (Yamaguchi et al, 1990; Brown et al, 1990).

MYXOMA

Myxomas are the most common type of cardiac tumours in the overall population. They make up approximately one quarter of all primary tumours of the heart, but their incidence is much lower in infants and children. Myxomas may have a familial trait (Siltanen et al, 1976).

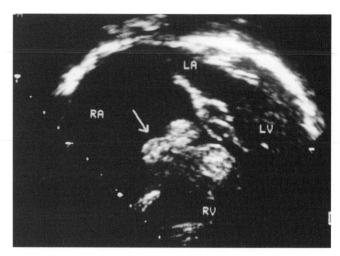

Figure 61.2. Subcostal four chamber echocardiographic view from a patient presenting with syncope. Note the pedunculated mass (arrow) with a smooth, lobulated surface, attached to the right atrial aspect of the atrial septum, protruding into the tricuspid valve during diastole, causing almost complete right ventricular inflow obstruction. Although these features were suggestive of an atrial myxoma, histology revealed the diagnosis of synovial sarcoma. Abbreviations as in Figure 61.1.

Cardiac myxomas are usually attached to the atrial septum in the region of the oval fossa. Their gross appearance is that of a pedunculated mass, either with a villous surface (often harbouring adherent thrombus) or with a smooth and lobulated surface. Highly sessile atrial tumours may protrude into the atrioventricular orifice during ventricular diastole (Figure 61.2). The surface of the myxoma may serve as a source of thromboembolus. The friable appearance of the villous surface may easily cause detachment and embolization of myxomatous fragments. The stalk usually contains vessels of large calibre, which can occasionally be seen on coronary angiograms.

The tumours are composed of polygonal 'myxoma' cells, embedded with a mucoid ground substance rich in glycosaminoglycans. The cellular make-up within the tumour is quite variable. Although the pathogenesis has been controversial, presently there is convincing evidence that the lesions cannot be considered an organized thrombus but represent a true neoplasm originating from multipotential subendocardial mesenchymal cells (Ferrans and Roberts, 1973). Most myxomas are pedunculated and extend into a cardiac chamber. Approximately 95% arise from the endocardial surface of one of the atriums, with the left atrium being involved in three quarters of patients. The remaining myxomas arise from the right or left ventricular endocardium with almost equal incidence. Multiple myxomas occur in approximately 5% of patients. In such instances, the left atrial myxoma usually dominates the clinical picture. Hence, the possibility of additional right atrial myxomas should always be carefully evaluated.

The systemic, embolic and cardiac manifestations, as previously described, may dominate the clinical profile, although most experience in this respect is based on adults rather than children (Steinke et al, 1972). In general terms, the signs and symptoms relate directly to the site and size of the tumour. In overall series, signs and symptoms of mitral valvar disease dominate the clinical presentation. Other features (such as embolic phenomena, signs and symptoms of tricuspid valvar disease, sudden and unexpected death, pericarditis, myocardial infarction, signs and symptoms of pulmonary valvar disease and fever of undetermined origin) may also be the leading manifestation (Steinke et al, 1972; Chandraratna et al, 1977). In a proportion of patients there are no cardiac symptoms. The tumour may then be detected as an incidental finding. Removal of an intracardiac myxoma is a standard procedure with good results. The stalk should be removed completely or else there may be recurrence. Follow-up evaluation for recurrence of disease is warranted.

TERATOMA

Teratomas, by definition, contain elements derived from all three germ layers of the body. In the collection of the Armed Forces Institute of Pathology, teratomas were the second most frequent lesions found in infancy (McAllister and Fenoglio, 1978). Most are extracardiac, albeit intrapericardial. They are located at the base of the heart, usually being attached to the root of the arterial pedicle. Intracardiac teratomas do occur but are exceptionally rare. The intrapericardial teratomas may grow to bizarre dimensions. They may then impair cardiac function or lead to compression of airways. Sudden death, severe encroachment by the tumour on the heart and great vessels, tamponade and infectious pericarditis have all been reported (Marsten et al, 1966; White et al, 1968; Lintermans et al, 1973).

Infants with intrapericardial teratoma frequently present with tamponade and cardiovascular collapse. Early and accurate diagnosis is of paramount importance in such critically ill patients, as surgical excision and decompression of the pericardial effusion can be achieved successfully. Furthermore, diagnosis during fetal life allows prompt postnatal surgical intervention before cardiopulmonary distress develops (de Geeter et al, 1983). In older, asymptomatic children surgical removal of the tumour is recommended because of the risk of sudden death and its potential for malignant transformation (Agozzino et al, 1984).

HAEMANGIOMA

Haemangiomas arising from the heart are extremely rare but are otherwise identical to those occurring elsewhere in the body (McAllister and Fenoglio, 1978). They have a slight tendency to occur in the atrial walls and epicardium and may cause haemopericardium and tamponade. Intracardiac haemangiomas may also occur. The clinical presentation may be diverse, ranging from no manifestations whatsoever to cardiomegaly with pericardial effusion and congestive heart failure.

Gross inspection will usually readily identify the true nature of the lesion. They usually intermingle extensively with adjacent cardiac structures, thus hampering surgical excision. Nevertheless, when the tumour produces symptoms, the treatment of choice is surgical excision (Ilbawi et al, 1982).

MESOTHELIOMA OF THE ATRIOVENTRICULAR NODE

Mesothelioma of the atrioventricular node is an exceedingly rare condition. The lesion consists of slit-like spaces covered by a uniform layer of polygonal cells embedded in a fibrous stroma, which usually replace part of the atrioventricular node. The majority of patients have partial or complete atrioventricular block, and often die either of complete heart block or ventricular fibrillation (McAllister and Fenoglio, 1978). It seems impossible to make this diagnosis on purely clinical grounds. Mesothelioma of the atrioventricular node has been described as occurring at almost any age, occurring from 11 months to 71 years in the series from the Armed Forces Institute of Pathology (McAllister and Fenoglio, 1978). In symptomatic patients, a pacemaker is usually implanted to maintain normal ventricular function. In some patients, however, pacing is not well tolerated and ventricular fibrillation may ensue.

PURKINJE CELL TUMOURS

Tumours of the Purkinje cells are known under a variety of terms, including oncocytic cardiomyopathy, histiocytoid cardiomyopathy and foamy myocardial transfusion (Becker, 1995). These are rare lesions, the nature of which remains uncertain, but they are associated with tachyarrhythmias and, so far, have been reported only in young infants. They may give rise to incessant ventricular tachycardia and may occur as discrete subendocardial nodules, or they may present diffusely throughout the ventricles (Garson et al, 1987).

The overall worldwide experience with this peculiar abnormality is limited and usually based on single case reports; the largest series that we are aware of is the series of 14 'Purkinje cell tumours' reported by Garson et al (1987). Our own experience is limited to four infants, each of whom died suddenly and unexpectedly (see also Becker, 1995). The histopathology of the lesion is characterized by clusters or sheaths of myocardial cells transformed into swollen rounded or polyhydral shapes, with a slightly granular eosinophilic and often vacuolated cytoplasm; this provides the foamy appearance of the lesions. Ultrastructurally the cells contain an increased number of mitochondria. The findings of our fourth case, however, were particularly interesting. Referred by Dr Joe de Giovanni, from Birmingham, UK, the heart came from an infant who died suddenly. Sectioning of the atrioventricular junction revealed multiple accessory atrioventricular connections (Figure 61.3a), all composed of typically oncocytic myocardial cells (Figure 61.3b). Similar hearts with virtually identical accessory atrioventricular connections have previously been described by Keller et al (1987). The fascinating arrangement of the conduction system in these cases adds to the mystery surrounding this entity.

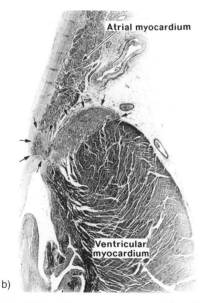

a)

☆ = nodule of foamy cells

b)

Figure 61.3. A Purkinje cell tumour presenting with sudden death. (a) Diagram of the atrioventricular (AV) junction demonstrating the presence of multiple accessory atrioventricular connections. (Courtesy of Dr S. Y. Ho.) (b) Histologic section from the patient shows clusters of oncocytic myocardial cells transformed into cells with swollen rounded or polyhydral cytoplasm, providing the foamy appearance accessory pathway (arrows) connecting atrial to ventricular myocardium. (Courtesy of Drs J. de Giovanni and S. Y. Ho.)

PRIMARY MALIGNANT TUMOURS

Primary malignant tumours of the heart are extremely rare in infancy and childhood (see Table 61.1). They are characterized clinically by a rapidly downhill course, with death occurring shortly following the onset of symptoms. This is caused by the rapid growth of the tumour, systemic dissemination and unfavourable response to medical therapy (Mahar et al, 1979; Schmaltz and Apitz, 1982). These malignant tumours have a tendency to invade the myocardium and to extend within the cardiac chambers (Figure 61.2). The signs and symptoms relate to their precise position and extent.

SECONDARY MALIGNANT TUMOURS

These are also very rare in children but are more frequent than the primary type. The clinical picture is nearly always dominated by the underlying disease, but occasionally the cardiac symptoms constitute the basis for the presenting complaints. Lymphosarcoma is the most common underlying disease, but solid tumours may also metastasize or grow into the heart (Farooki et al, 1975; Riggs et al, 1981). The symptoms produced by the metastatic lesions depend on the site and extent of the tumours. Pericardial involvement may give rise to pericardial effusion, which is often blood stained. Cardiac compression may be caused by either an effusion or a solid tumour encasing the heart.

SURGICAL THERAPY

The planning of surgical treatment must be based on the accurate assessment of the number, location, size and extent of the tumour or tumours, on the haemodynamic status of the patient and on the histological nature of the lesions. The advances in cross-sectional echocardiography provide most of this information. Although endomyocardial biopsy has been promoted as a means of histological diagnosis (Bini et al, 1983), in many cases the histological nature of the tumour may be predicted accurately from the clinical investigations. In infants, multiple nodules nearly always point to a rhabdomyoma (by far the most common tumour of the heart in children) (Figure 61.4). The presence of tuberous sclerosis in the infant, or in the family, confirms the diagnosis. A large and well-circumscribed tumour in the septum or ventricular wall is likely to be a fibroma or an intracardiac teratoma (Figure 61.5). Primary malignant tumours are extremely uncommon and early death is the rule.

Surgical resection is indicated in all symptomatic patients, in those with significant obstruction of either the ventricular inlet or outlet (Arciniegas et al, 1980) or in the setting of life-threatening arrhythmias (Engle et al, 1974). Single lesions amenable to surgical resection should always

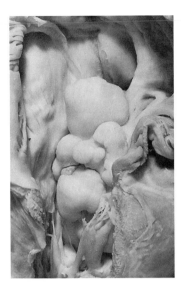

Figure 61.4. A nodular rhabdomyoma originating from the ventricular septum. It extends through the tricuspid orifice into the right atrium.

be removed because of the possibility of arrhythmias and even sudden death. In the presence of multiple lesions, and in the absence of symptoms, surgery is better postponed. The aim must be complete resection. Incomplete removal may result later in arrhythmias, and the potential for sudden death will remain. Even large solitary intramural and extramural lesions may be resected successfully if they are well circumscribed and benign (Bini et al, 1983). Following successful and complete resection of cardiac fibromas, patients have an excellent probability of remaining free of disease (Williams et al, 1982). Partial resection for relief of obstruction and amelioration of an increase in chamber size may be indicated when there are significant haemodynamic alterations. This may be compatible with long-lasting relief of symptoms (Arciniegas et al, 1980). Extensive myocardial involvement may militate against complete removal of the tumour or may make it unre-

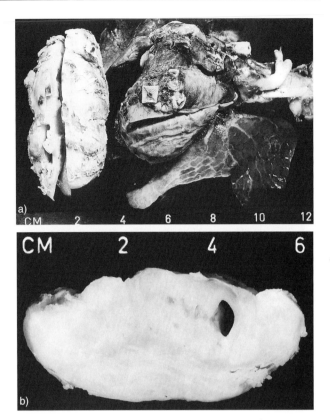

Figure 61.5. Cardiac fibroma. (a) The heart lung specimen is shown following surgical removal of cardiac fibroma, which is shown separately. (b) a cross-section through the fibroma reveals its fibrous architecture.

sectable. In this case, transplantation may be an alternative (Jamieson et al, 1981).

After resection of an extensive septal cardiac tumour, repair of the septum can usually be accomplished by apposition of the myocardial layers. In the setting of myxomas, careful examination of the entire heart is necessary to remove concurrent sites of myxomatous tissue (Figure 61.6). Small residual septal defects may

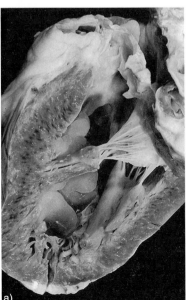
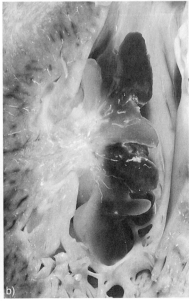

Figure 61.6. Cardiac myxoma. (a) The left ventricular septal origin of the myxoma obliterates the left ventricular cavity. (b) A detail of the tumour can be seen.

close spontaneously, whereas larger defects require reconstruction with a prosthetic patch (Williams et al, 1982; Mustafa et al, 1978). Defects of the atrial and ventricular free wall can usually be closed directly.

Occasionally, however, reconstruction with prosthetic material or autogenous pericardium may be necessary (Culliford et al, 1978; Ilbawi et al, 1982; Williams et al, 1982).

REFERENCES

Agozzino L, Vosa C, Arciprete P, de Leva F, Cotrufo M 1984 Intrapericardial teratoma in the newborn: review of literature and report of successful surgery in infant with intrapericardial teratoma. International Journal of Cardiology 5: 21–28

Allan L D, Joseph M C, Tynan M 1983 Clinical value of echocardiographic colour image processing in two cases of primary cardiac tumour. British Heart Journal 49: 154–156

Arciniegas E, Hakim M, Farooki Z Q, Truccone J M, Green E W 1980 Primary cardiac tumours in children. Journal of Thoracic and Cardiovascular Surgery 79: 782–591

Becker A E 1995 Tumours of the heart and pericardium. In: Fletcher C D M (ed.) Diagnostic histopathology of tumours. Edinburgh, Churchill Livingstone, p 7–41

Biancaniello T M, Meyer R A, Gaum W E, Kaplan S 1982 Primary benign intramural ventricular tumours in children. Pre- and postoperative electrocardiographic, echocardiographic and angiocardiographic evaluation. American Heart Journal 103: 852–857

Bini R M, Westaby S, Bargeron L M Jr, Pacifico A D, Kirklin J W 1983 Investigation and management of primary cardiac tumours in infants and children. Journal of the American College of Cardiology 2: 351–357

Birnbaum S E, McGahan J P, Janos G G, Meyers M 1985 Fetal tachycardia and intramyocardial tumors. Journal of American College of Cardiology 6: 1358–1361

Borges A C, Witt C, Bartel T, Muller S, Konertz W, Baumann G 1995 Preoperative two- and three-dimensional transeosophageal echocardiographic assessment of heart tumours. Annals of Thoracic Surgery 61: 1163–1167

Bouton S, Yang A, McCrindle B W, Kidd L, McVeigh E R, Zerhouni E A 1991 Differentiation of tumour from viable myocardium using cardiac tagging with MRI imaging. Journal of Computer Assisted Tomography 15: 676–678

Boxer R A, LaCorte M A, Singh S et al 1985 Diagnosis of cardiac tumors in infants by magnetic resonance imaging. American Journal of Cardiology 56: 831–832

Brown J J, Barakos J A, Higgins C B 1989 Magnetic resonance imaging of cardiac and pericardial masses. Journal of Thoracic Imaging 4: 58–64

Brown I W, McGoldrick J P, Robles A, Curella G W, Gula G, Ross D N 1990 Left ventricular fibroma: echocardiographic diagnosis and surgical excision in three cases. Journal of Cardiovascular Surgery 31: 536–540

Brand J M, Friedberg D Z 1992 Spontaneous regression of a primary cardiac tumor presenting as fetal tachyarrhythmias. Journal of Perinatology 12: 48–50

Bruni C, Prioleau P G, Ivey H H, Nolan S P 1980 New fine structural features of cardiac rhabdomyoma. Report of a case. Cancer 46: 2068–2073

Burke A P, Rosado-de-Cristenson R, Templeton P A, Virmani R 1994 Cardiac fibroma: clinicopathological correlates and surgical treatment. Journal of Thoracic and Cardiovascular Surgery 108: 862–870

Burnes E R, Schulman I C, Murphy M J 1982 Hematologic manifestations and etiology of atrial myxoma. American Journal of Medical Science 284: 17–21

Burton C, Johnson J 1970 Multiple cerebral aneurysms and cardiac myxoma. New England Journal of Medicine 282: 35–36

Chandraratna P A N, San Pedro S, Elkins R C, Grantham N 1977 Echocardiographic, angiocardiographic and surgical correlations in right ventricular myoxma simulating valvar pulmonic stenosis. Circulation 55: 619–622

Cohen G I, Klein A L, Chan K-L, Schiavone W A 1990 Transesophageal echocardiographic imaging of right heart masses in patients with venous lines. Circulation 82(suppl III): 32

Cola H, Hoffman R, Borrega N G, Lazzari J O 1992 Left posterior hemiblock related to an interventricular septum tumour. European Heart Journal 13: 574–575

Come P C, Riley M F, Markis J E, Malagold M 1981 Limitations of echocardiographic techniques in evaluation of left atrial masses. American Journal of Cardiology 48: 947–953

Culliford A T, Isom O W, Trehan N K, Doyle E, Gorstein F, Spencer F C 1978 Benign tumours of right atrium necessitating extensive resection and reconstruction. Journal of Thoracic and Cardiovascular Surgery 76: 178–182

Curry H F L, Mathews J A, Robinson J 1967 Right atrial myxoma mimicking a rheumatic disorder. British Medical Journal i: 547–548

Cyr D R, Guntheroth W G, Nyberg D A, Smith J R, Mudelman S R, Ek M 1988 Prenatal diagnosis of an intrapericardial teratoma. Journal of Ultrasound Medicine 7: 87–90

De Geeter B, Kretz J G, Nisand I, Eisenmann B, Kieny M T, Kieny R 1983 Intrapericardial teratoma in a newborn infant: use of fetal echocardiography. Annals of Thoracic Surgery 35: 664–666

De Pace N L, Soulen R L, Kotler M N, Mintz G S 1981 Two dimensional echocardiographic detection of intraatrial masses. American Journal of Cardiology 48: 954–960

De Vore G R, Hakim S, Kleinman C S, Hobbins J C 1982 The in utero diagnosis of an interventricular septal cardiac rhabdomyoma by means of real-time-directed, M-mode echocardiography. American Journal of Obstetrics and Gynecology 143: 967–969

Engle M A, Ebert P A, Pedo S G 1974 Recurrent ventricular tachycardia due to resectable cardiac tumour. Circulation 50: 1050–1057

Farooki Z Q, Henry J G, Green E W 1975 Echocardiographic diagnosis of right atrial extension of Wilm's tumour. American Journal of Cardiology 36: 363–365

Farooki Z Q, Adelman S, Green E W 1977 Echocardiographic differentiation of a cystic and a solid tumor of the heart. American Journal of Cardiology 39: 107

Fenoglio J Jr, Diana D J, Bower T E, McAllister H A Jr, Ferrans V J 1977 Ultrastructure of cardiac rhabdomyoma. Human Pathology 8: 700–706

Ferrans V J, Roberts W C 1973 Structural features of cardiac myxomas. Histology, histochemistry and electromicroscopy. Human Pathology 4: 111–146

Filiatrault M, Beland M J, Neilson K A, Paquet M 1991 Cardiac fibroma presenting with clinically significant arrhythmias in infancy. Pediatric Cardiology 12: 118–120

Freedom R M, Benson L N 1992 Cardiac neoplasms. In: Freedom R M, Benson L N, Smalhorn J F (eds) Neonatal heart disease. Springer-Verlag, London, p 723–730

Fyke F E, Seward J B, Edwards W D 1985 Primary cardiac tumors: experience with 30 consecutive patients since the introduction of two-dimensional echocardiography. Journal of American College of Cardiology 5: 1465–1473

Fyler D C 1980 Report of the New England Regional Infant Cardiac Program. Paediatrics 65(suppl): 376–461

Garson A, Smith R T, Moak J P et al 1987 Incessant ventricular tachycardia in infants: myocardial hamartomas and surgical cure. Journal of American College of Cardiology 10: 619–626

Green S E, Joynt L F, Fitzerald P J, Rubenson D S, Popp R L 1983 In vivo ultrasonic characterization of human intracardiac masses. American Journal of Cardiology 51: 231–236

Harinck E, Moulaert A J, Rohmer J, Brom A G 1974 Cardiac rhabdomyoma in infancy. Acta Pediatrica Scandinavica 63: 283–286

Harvey W P 1968 Clinical aspects of cardiac tumours. American Journal of Cardiology 21: 328–343

Holley D G, Martin G R, Brenner J I 1995 Diagnosis and management of fetal cardiac tumors: a multicenter experience and review of published reports. Journal of American College of Cardiology 26: 516–520

Hwa J, Ward C, Nunn G, Cooper S, Lau K C, Sholler G 1994 Primary intraventricular cardiac tumors in children: contemporary diagnostic and management options. Pediatric Cardiology 15: 233–237

Ilbawi M, Deleon S, Riggs T, Hemandez R 1982 Primary vascular tumour of the heart in infancy. Chest 81: 511–512

Jamieson S W, Gaudiani V A, Reitz B A, Oyer P E, Stinson E B, Shumway N E 1981 Operative treatment of an unresectable tumor of the left ventricle. Journal of Thoracic and Cardiovascular Surgery 81: 797–799

Keller B B, Mehta A V, Shamszadeh M et al 1987 Oncocytic cardiomyopathy of infancy with Wolff–Parkinson–White syndrome and ectopic foci causing tachydysrhythmias in children. American Heart Journal 114: 782–792

Lintermans J P, Schoevaertds J C, Fiasse L, Renoirte-Monjoie A M 1973 Intrapericardial teratoma: a curable cause of cardiac tamponade in infancy. Clinical Pediatrics 12: 316–318

Ludomirski A, Vargo T A, Murphy D J, Gresik M V, Ott D A, Mullins C E 1985 Intracardiac undifferentiated sarcoma in infancy. Journal of American College of Cardiology 6: 1362–1364

McAllister H A, Fenoglio J J Jr 1978 Atlas of tumor pathology, second series: Tumors of the cardiovascular system. Armed Forces Institute of Pathology, Washington DC

MacGregor G A, Cullen R A 1959 The syndrome of fever, anaemia, and high sedimentation rate with an atrial myxoma. British Medical Journal 2: 991–993

Mahar L J, Lie J T, Groover R V, Sewer J B, Puga F J, Feldt R H 1979 Primary cardiac myxosarcoma in a child. Mayo Clinic Proceedings 54: 261–266

Marin-Garcia J, Fitch C W, Shenefelt R E 1984 Primary right ventricular tumor (fibroma) simulating cyanotic heart disease in a newborn. Journal of the American College of Cardiology 3: 868–871

Marsten J L, Cooper A G, Ankeney J L 1966 Acute cardiac temponade due to perforation of a benign mediastinal teratoma into the pericardial sac. Review of cardiovascular manifestations of mediastinal teratomas. Journal of Thoracic and Cardiovascular Surgery 51: 700–707

Marx G R 1995 Cardiac tumors. In: Emmanouilides G C, Riemenschneider T A, Allen H D, Gutgesell H P (eds) Moss and Adams heart disease in infants, children and adolescents including the fetus and young adult. Williams & Wilkins, Baltimore, MD, p 1773–1786

Marx G R, Bierman F Z, Matthews E, Williams R 1984 Two dimensional echocardiographic diagnosis of intracardiac masses in infancy. Journal of the American College of Cardiology 3: 827–832

Milner S, Abramowitz J A, Levin S E 1980 Rhabdomyoma of the heart in a newborn infant. Diagnosis by echocardiography. British Heart Journal 44: 224–227

Mugge A, Daniel W G, Haverich A et al 1991 Diagnosis of noninfective cardiac mass lesions by two-dimensional echocardiography: comparison of the transthoracic and transesophageal approaches. Circulation 83: 70–78

Mulher E G, Kienast W, Turniski-Harder V, von Bernuth G 1994 Arrhythmias in infants and children with primary cardiac tumours. European Heart Journal 15: 915–921

Mustafa I, Shinebourne E A, Lincoln C 1978 Successful replacement of the interventricular septum following excision of a large intramural fibroma. Journal of Cardiovascular Surgery 19: 411–416

Nadas A S, Ellison R C 1968 Cardiac tumors in infancy. American Journal of Cardiology 21: 363–366

Nir A, Tajik A J, Freeman W K et al 1995 Tuberous sclerosis and cardiac rhabdomyoma. American Journal of Cardiology 76: 419–421

Niwa K, Tashima K, Terai M, Okajima U, Makajima H 1989 Contrast-enhanced magnetic resonance imaging of cardiac tumors in children. American Heart Journal 118: 424–425

Parmley L F, Salley R K, Williams J P, Head G B 1988 The clinical spectrum of cardiac fibroma with diagnostic and surgical considerations: noninvasive imaging enhances management. Annals of Thoracic Surgery 45: 455–465

Rheuban K S, McDaniel N L, Feldman P S, Mayes D C, Rodgers B M 1991 Intrapericardial teratoma causing non-immune hydrops fetalis and pericardial tamponade: a case report. Pediatric Cardiology 12: 54–56

Rienmullar R, Lloret J L, Tiling R et al 1989 MR imaging of pediatric cardiac tumors previously diagnosed by echocardiography. Journal of Computer Assisted Tomography 13: 621–626

Riggs T, Paul M H, de Leon S, Ilbawi M 1981 Two dimensional echocardiography in the evaluation of right atrial masses; five cases in pediatric patients. American Journal of Cardiology 48: 961–966

Schmaltz A A, Apitz J 1982 Primary rhabdomyosarcoma of the heart. Pediatric Cardiology 2: 73–75

Sechtem U, Pflugfelder P W, White R D et al 1987 Cine MR imaging: Potential for the evaluation of cardiovascular function. American Journal of Roentgenology 148: 239–246

Selzer A, Sakai E J, Popper R W 1972 Protean clinical manifestation of primary tumours of the heart. American Journal of Medicine 52: 9–18

Shaher R M, Minizer J, Farina M, Alley R, Bishop M 1972 Clinical presentation of rhabdomyoma of the heart in infancy and childhood. American Journal of Cardiology 30: 95–103

Siltanen P, Tuuteri L, Norio R, Tala P, Ahrenberg P, Halonen P I 1976 Atrial myxoma in a family. American Journal of Cardiology 38: 252–256

Spooner E W, Farina M A, Shaher R M, Foster E D 1982 Left ventricular rhabdomyoma causing subaortic stenosis – two dimensional echocardiographic appearance. Pediatric Cardiology 2: 67–71

Steiner R E 1968 Radiological aspects of cardiac tumours. American Journal of Cardiology 21: 344–356

Steinke W E, Perry L W, Gold H R, McClenathan J E, Scott L P 1972 Left atrial myxoma in a child. Pediatrics 49: 580–589

van der Hauwaert L G 1971 Cardiac tumors in infancy and childhood. British Heart Journal 33: 125–132

Waaler P E, Svendson S, Halvorsen J F 1972 Intramural calcified fibroma of the heart. Acta Pediatrica Scandinavica 61: 217–222

Wallace G, Smith H C, Rimmer S, D'Souza S W 1990 Tuberous sclerosis presenting with fetal and neonatal cardiac tumors. Archives of Disease of Childhood 65: 367–370

Webb D W, Thomas R D, Osborne J P 1993 Cardiac rhabdomyomas and their association with tuberous sclerosis. Archives of Disease of Childhood 68: 367–370

White J J, Kaback M M, Haller J A Jr 1968 Diagnosis and excision of an intrapericardial teratoma in an infant. Journal of Thoracic and Cardiovascular Surgery 55: 153–156

White R D, Zisch R J 1991 Magnetic resonance imaging of pericardial disease and paracardiac and intracardiac masses. In Elliot L P (ed) The fundamentals of cardiac imaging in infants, children, and adults. Lippincott, Philadelphia, PA, p 420–433

Willman V L, Symbas P N, Mamiya R T, Cooper T, Hanlon C R 1965 Unusual aspects of intracavity tumors of the heart. Diseases of the Chest 47: 669–671

Williams D B, Danielson G K, McGoon D C, Feldt R H, Edwards W D 1982 Cardiac fibroma: long-term survival after excision. Journal of Thoracic and Cardiovascular Surgery 84: 230–236

Williams W G, Trusler G A, Fowler R S, Scott M E, Mustard W T 1972 Left ventricular myocardial fibroma. A case report and review of cardiac tumors in children. Journal of Pediatric Surgery 7: 324–328

Yamaguchi M, Hosokawa Y, Ohashi H, Imai M, Oshima Y, Minamiji K 1990 Cardiac fibroma: long-term fate after excision. Journal of Thoracic and Cardiovascular Surgery 103: 140–145

62

Kawasaki disease

W. H. Neches

INTRODUCTION

In 1967, Tomisaku Kawasaki described 50 infants and children with an unusual illness that was characterized by prolonged fever, skin rash and lymphadenopathy. He termed this illness mucocutaneous lymph node syndrome (Kawasaki, 1967). In 1974, reports of mucocutaneous lymph node syndrome, which has subsequently become known as Kawasaki disease, appeared in the English language literature (Kawasaki et al, 1974; Yanagisawa et al, 1974). Although patients with this disease have been described subsequently in most other parts of the world, the greatest prevalence is still in Japan, where about 2000 new patients are seen annually and almost 100 000 cases have been described since it was initially reported.

In the first 25 years after the description of Kawasaki disease, over 500 reports have described the epidemiology, pathology and clinical features of the disease. The aetiology and pathogenesis remain unknown. A specific diagnostic test to confirm the clinical diagnosis is unavailable; consequently, the diagnosis, as well as the management, remains controversial. Although this chapter describes the features of Kawasaki disease that are currently known, a great deal more remains to be discovered about this puzzling disease.

AETIOLOGY AND EPIDEMIOLOGY

The incidence of Kawasaki disease in Japan greatly exceeds that in the rest of the world. In the USA, cases were first recognized during the 1970s in California and Hawaii, states with a large Oriental population, particularly of Japanese ancestry. This would suggest that particular genetic factors may increase susceptibility to this disease. The disease has been reported, however, throughout the world in individuals of various races and socioeconomic backgrounds. Among Caucasians, the incidence of Kawasaki disease appears higher in the USA than in Europe and this probably represents the true occurrence of the disease rather than merely reflecting the number of reports appearing in English. A 7-year survey of the incidence of Kawasaki disease in the USA, from 1984–1990 (Taubert et al 1991), suggested an attack rate of 9/100 000 in children less than 5 years of age. In contrast, during a 5-year period from 1981–1985 in Japan, the attack rate varied from 77 to 195/100 000 in children less than 5 years of age (Fukushige et al, 1991).

Kawasaki disease is an illness that is found essentially in infants and young children. As the disease has become more widely recognized, there have been some reports of adult cases. There is a well-documented acute case in a 33-year-old Japanese woman physician who was visiting our insti-tution. Cases in older children, adolescents and adults, however, represent only a small proportion of the total. Over 80% of patients with Kawasaki disease are 4 years or less; about 60% of patients are less than 2 years of age, and 20–25% of patients are less than 1 year of age at the time of their acute illness. More males than females are found to have the disease, with a ratio of 1.4:1 to 1.7:1.

Kawasaki disease is seen throughout the year, although some seasonal increments have occurred occasionally in Japan during the spring months (Yanagawa et al, 1987). At our institution, Kawasaki disease has a greater prevalence during the winter and spring months. Most cases occur sporadically, but occasional clusters of cases have been reported in a number of communities. In our institution, two major clusters occurred, one in 1978 and the other in 1983. In Japan, three major outbreaks of Kawasaki disease have occurred in 1979, 1982 and 1986 (Naoe et al, 1991).

Despite extensive epidemiological investigations in Japan and in clustered cases in the USA, no specific pattern has been found. Even during these periods of increased occurrence, the cases usually appear randomly with no consistent geographic or socioeconomic predilection. The disorder is not familial, and no relationship has been found with other illnesses or factors in the patient's history. Person-to-person or secondary transmission are not found and children with Kawasaki disease generally do not live in the same neighbourhood. It is extremely uncommon to find Kawasaki disease in siblings; in the 1–2% when this does occur, siblings usually have the illness within a few weeks of each other. Although the occurrence of mini-epidemics or clusters of Kawasaki disease suggests an infectious cause, on the one hand, the lack of familial or community clustering does not support this hypothesis. On the other hand, the outbreaks could be traced retrospectively, in the three epidemics that occurred in Japan, to certain geographic areas, with the incidence increasing progressively in areas distant from the initial outbreak. Poisoning with heavy metals or other environmental toxins has also been suggested as a cause but is also unlikely in the absence of close grouping of cases. This disease could represent a form of collagen vascular disease; however, its sudden emergence in almost epidemic proportions in Japan suggests some external influencing factor. A possible relationship to household mites was suggested in Japan (Hamashima et al, 1983), while in the USA, an association with recent shampooing of carpets in the home was also reported (Patriarca et al, 1982; Rauch et al, 1991). These could explain sporadic cases but not those cases occurring in clusters. Many other viral, bacterial and immunological theories have been presented; however to date, the cause of this disease remains illusive. Currently, the belief is that this syndrome represents an immunological response of an individual to an external agent: infectious, antigenic or toxic.

PATHOLOGY

When death occurs during the acute or subacute phase of Kawasaki disease, the major pathological changes are found in the coronary arteries. There is necrotizing coronary arteritis, formation of aneurysms and thrombosis of a major branch of a coronary artery (Figure 62.1). Acute myocardial infarction is usually the immediate cause of death, while, rarely, death is from rupture of a coronary arterial aneurysm (Naoe et al, 1991). There is often mild and variable involvement of other medium-sized muscular arteries; occasionally, aneurysms are found in brachiocephalic, renal, mesenteric or iliac arteries. Surprisingly, aneurysms are almost never found in the cerebrovascular system.

The pathological stages of Kawasaki disease (Table 62.1) closely follow the clinical stages (Fujiwara and Hamashima 1978; Hamashima et al, 1983). In the first stage, pancarditis and extensive involvement of small vessels is found. During the second stage, which corresponds to the early subacute clinical phase, vasculitis progressively involves medium-sized vessels and coronary arterial aneurysms develop. The third stage represents the early convalescent phase, and the acute inflammatory process begins to disappear. The fourth stage is the one of convalescence and later. Inflammation is absent and coronary arterial and myocardial lesions are present.

Coronary arterial lesions appear to resolve in many patients (Kato et al, 1996). It is presumed, therefore, that Kawasaki disease may not be a serious problem for most patients once recovery has occurred. In fact, abnormalities of vascular endothelial function persist many years after resolution of Kawasaki disease, even in patients with no detectable coronary involvement (Dhillon et al, 1996). In addition, myocardial involvement was found in each of 201 patients who underwent endomyocardial biopsy during cardiac catheterization, although coronary arterial aneurysms were present in only 12.9% (Yutani et al, 1981). The period after the onset of the disease for which patients were studied varied; about 10% of the group were studied for 2 to 5 years and another 10% for more than 5 years. Yonesaka et al (1991) found myocardial changes of interstitial fibrosis, degeneration and inflammatory cell infiltrates in about half of a small group of patients who underwent serial endomyocardial biopsy 2.5 to 10 years

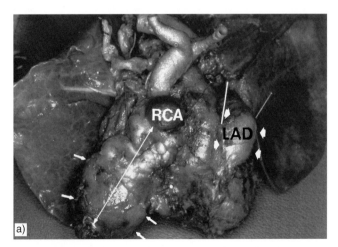
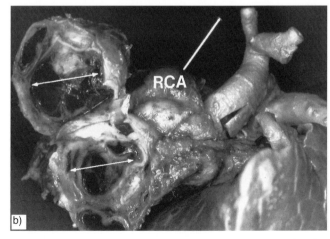

Figure 62.1. Kawasaki disease. (a) Aneurysms of major coronary arteries. The left anterior descending (LAD) coronary artery is indicated with thick arrows. The right coronary artery (RCA) is shown with thin arrows. (b) Cross-section through massive right coronary arterial aneurysm (arrows) showing intraluminal thrombosis.

Table 62.1 Classification of states of angiitis in Kawasaki disease

Stage	Time scale (days)	Characteristics
I	0–9	Perivasculitis and vasculitis of arterioles, venules, capillaries and small arteries Perivasculitis and endarteritis of large arteries without inflammation of media Pericarditis, interstital myocarditis Endocarditis with valvitis
II	12–25	Panvasculitis and perivasculitis of large arteries Appearance of aneurysms in stems of main coronary arteries Severe stenosis or obstruction of large arteries owing to thrombus or proliferative changes of intima Pericarditis, myocarditis with valvitis, coagulation necrosis
III	28–31	Granulation of larger arteries with slight cell infiltration of perivascular area Disappearance of vasculitis of small arteries and arterioles Myocarditis and coagulation necrosis
IV	Over 40	Scars of large arteries with calcification and recanalization Severe stenosis or obstruction of larger arteries owing to thickening of intima Coagulation necrosis, fibrosis of the heart muscle, endocardial fibroelastosis

Source: Hamashima et al (1983).

following Kawasaki disease. Naoe et al (1987) described a group of five patients who had recovered from Kawasaki disease, were felt to have normal coronary arteries and who died of unrelated causes such as leukaemia, meningitis or accident. Examination of the coronary arteries revealed scarring, intimal thickening and disruption of the internal elastic lamina in each patient. No inflammation, thrombosis or recanalization was present. Therefore, children who have had Kawasaki disease may be at greater risk of future problems with myocardial and/or coronary arterial disease than had previously been thought.

Since its first description, there has been a question as to whether Kawasaki disease is a new disease or merely a new expression of an old disease. Congenital coronary arterial aneurysms, usually discovered at postmortem, have been reported for many years (Mattern et al, 1972; Wilson et al, 1975). In most of these cases, no preceding illness suggested Kawasaki disease. About 25 cases of periarteritis nodosa occurring in infancy were described prior to 1972 (Ahlstrom et al, 1977; Landing and Larson, 1977). This disease, primarily affecting infants, had a fulminant course and usually was not diagnosed before death. Periarteritis nodosa as seen in infancy shares many clinical features with Kawasaki disease except desquamation of the fingertips and toes. Both the gross and the microscopic pathological features of Kawasaki disease and infantile periarteritis nodosa are virtually identical. These are probably not separate entities but merely different patterns of clinical expression of the same pathological disorder.

CLINICAL FEATURES

Kawasaki disease is primarily a disease of young children, with more than half of the cases occurring before 2 years of age and over 80% of cases in children less than 4 years of age. There are six major clinical features that characterize Kawasaki disease including: fever of over 5 days' duration, conjunctival congestion, changes in the oral mucosa, changes in the extremities, a polymorphous rash to the trunk and swelling of the cervical lymph nodes. The diagnostic guidelines for Kawasaki disease have been described by the Japan Kawasaki Disease Research Committee and the fourth revision, from 1984, is shown in Table 62.2 (Yanagawa et al, 1987). In this fourth revision, it was indicated that Kawasaki disease could be diagnosed only if four of the principal symptoms occurred, providing the patient subsequently was found to have coronary arterial aneurysms. In our experience, at least 75% of patients manifest all of the principal symptoms. An increasing number of patients, however, have been found to have coronary arterial aneurysms some time after an acute febrile illness that, in retrospect, may have been Kawasaki disease. Some adolescents and young adults have been seen with coronary arterial aneurysms whose family had no recall of an illness resembling Kawasaki disease. The use of intravenous gammaglobulin has further clouded the clinical diagnosis of Kawasaki disease. Increasingly, patients in the USA receive a course of intravenous gammaglobulin after only 3 or 4 days of fever and clinical findings that suggest, but do not meet, the criterions for the diagnosis of Kawasaki disease. In many of these patients, the illness subsides within 24 to 48 hours after the administration of gammaglobulin; consequently, the patients never meet the criterions required for the diagnosis of Kawasaki disease. Each of these principal symptoms, as well as the other significant symptoms or findings, may occur independently in many other disorders. It is the specific and characteristic sequence of events and a combination of these features that characterizes Kawasaki disease (Figure 62.2).

Table 62.2 Diagnostic guidelines for Kawasaki disease: fourth revised edition

A Principal symptoms

1. Fever persisting 5 days or more
2. Changes of peripheral extremities:
   a. initial stage: reddening of palms and soles, indurative oedema
   b. convalescent stage: membranous desquamation from fingertips
3. Polymorphous exanthema
4. Bilateral conjunctival congestion
5. Changes of lips and oral cavity: reddening of lips, strawberry tongue, diffuse injection of oral and pharyngeal mucosa
6. Acute non-purulent cervical lymphadenopathy

At least five items should be satisfied for diagnosis of Kawasaki disease. However, if four items of the principal symptoms are present, Kawasaki disease can be diagnosed when coronary aneurysm is recognized by cross-sectional echocardiography or coronary angiography.

B. Other significant symtoms or findings for clinical consideration

1. Cardiovascular: auscultation (heart murmur, gallop rhythm, distant heart sounds), electrocardiographic changes (prolonged PR–QT intervals, abnormal Q wave, low voltage ST–T changes, arrhythmias), chest radiograph findings (cardiomegaly), cross-sectional echocardiographic findings (pericardial effusion, coronary aneurysms) aneurysm of peripheral arteries other than coronary (axillary etc.), angina pectoris or myocardial infarction
2. Gastrointestinal tract: diarrhoea, vomiting, abdominal pain, hydrops of gallbladder, paralytic ileus, mild jaundice, slight increase of serum transaminase
3. Blood: leucocytosis with shift to the left, thrombocytosis, increased erythrocyte sedimentation rate, positive C-reactive protein, hypoalbuminaemia, increased α_2-globulin, slight decrease in erythrocyte and haemoglobin levels
4. Urine: proteinuria, increase of leucocytes in urine sediment
5. Skin: redness and crust at the site of BCG inoculation, small pustules, transverse furrows of the finger nails
6. Respiratory: cough, rhinorrhoea, abnormal shadow on chest radiograph
7. Joints: pain, swelling
8. Neurological: pleocytosis of mononuclear cells in cerebrospinal fluid, convulsions, unconsciousness, facial palsy, paralysis of the extremities

Remarks

1. For item (2) under principal symptoms, convalescent stage is considered important
2. Male to female ratio 1.3–1.5:1; 80–85% patients less than 5 years of age; fatality rate 0.3–0.5%
3. Recurrence rate 2–3%; proportion of sibling cases: 1–2%

Source: Japan Kawasaki Disease Research Committee (1984).

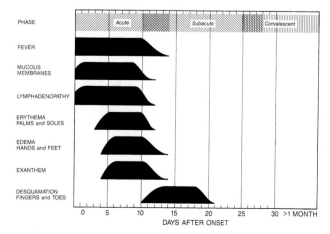

Figure 62.2. The time sequence of the major clinical features of Kawasaki disease.

FEVER

Fever is one of the major clinical features of the illness and has an abrupt onset. Characteristically, temperature spikes in excess of 104°F (40°C) occur several times each day. Prior to the use of gammaglobulin, and even with salicylate therapy, the high fever generally lasted about 10 days and often persisted for about 2 weeks. Occasionally, the febrile course lasted 3 weeks or longer, although the temperature in such patients was generally much lower than during the early acute phase. In a few patients, the acute febrile phase lasted less than 10 days; as discussed above, at least 5 days of fever are required to fulfil the criterion on which diagnosis of Kawasaki disease is based.

CONJUNCTIVAL CONGESTION

Bilateral congestion (injection) of the ocular conjunctivas occurs during the acute phase, usually within 24 to 48 hours after the onset of fever. This extensive hyperaemia is not associated with the discharge or other findings associated with conjunctivitis from other causes.

ORAL MUCOSA

The changes in the mouth are also apparent within 24 to 48 hours of the onset of fever. There is considerable erythema of the entire oral mucosa, redness of the lips and tongue and enlargement of the papillas of the tongue (resulting in a 'strawberry tongue'). The lips become dry and fissured, often interfering with the intake of food and fluid. The changes in the mucous membranes of the eye and mouth generally persist until the ninth day of illness and usually subside by the twelfth day in those patients who have not received gammaglobulin therapy.

CHANGES IN THE EXTREMITIES

Erythema of the palms and soles generally appears on the third to fifth day of illness and is accompanied by indurative oedema of the hands and feet. These findings begin to disappear around the tenth day. The characteristic clinical feature that distinguishes Kawasaki disease from other similar disorders is the desquamation of the fingertips and toes (Figure 62.3). Desquamation generally occurs towards the second week of illness in the period of transition from the febrile, acute phase to the subacute phase. During the subacute phase, which occurs during the third and fourth weeks after the onset of illness, the periungual desquamation progresses to involve the remainder of the finger tips and toes and usually the palms and soles. In some cases, transverse furrows (Bow's lines) appear across the middle of the nails during the convalescent phase, approximately 2 months after the onset of the illness.

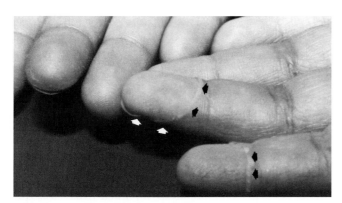

Figure 62.3. Desquamation of the fingertips (arrows).

SKIN

A polymorphous exanthematous rash begins within a few days of the onset of the fever, about the same time as changes in the extremities appear. The rash may be generalized but usually has a truncal distribution. It is usually non-pruritic and shows large irregular erythematous areas or is a fine maculopapular morbilliform rash similar to rubeola. The rash usually lasts for about 5 to 7 days.

LYMPHADENOPATHY

Cervical lymphadenopathy with lymph nodes greater than 1.5 cm in diameter is present in over 75% of patients. The lymphadenopathy is not suppurative or tender and rarely shows redness. It generally begins within a day or two of the onset of the illness and persists until about the tenth day (the end of the acute phase).

OTHER MANIFESTATIONS

A number of other symptoms or clinical features can be present in patients with Kawasaki disease. Cardiovascular involvement will be discussed separately. Although other organs may be involved, the combination varies among patients. The presence of many other signs and symptoms suggests that widespread involvement of multiple systems occurs in patients with Kawasaki disease.

GASTROINTESTINAL SYSTEM

Gastrointestinal involvement occurs in one quarter to one third of the patients and presents as abdominal pain or diarrhoea. Vomiting is an occasional but unusual feature. Hepatocellular involvement is found in 10 to 20% of patients and is evident as a mild or moderate elevation of bilirubin and serum transaminase during the acute phase. Right upper quadrant abdominal pain and a mass caused by gallbladder hydrops has occurred in about 5% of our patients. These findings usually disappear with the end of the acute phase.

GENITOURINARY SYSTEM

Urinary abnormalities occur in about one third of patients. Proteinuria is commonly present, with a non-specific urethritis and a sterile pyuria.

MUSCULOSKELETAL SYSTEM

Arthralgia or arthritis is present in about one third of patients, occurring toward the end of the acute phase and during the early subacute phase. The large joints of the extremities are more commonly involved. Findings subside toward the end of the subacute phase.

CENTRAL NERVOUS SYSTEM

Central nervous system involvement with aseptic meningitis was found in about 15% of patients early in our experience. Since the cerebrospinal fluid has not been examined routinely in patients with this disease since the 1980s, the true prevalence at the end of the 1990s of involvement of the central nervous system is unknown. Almost all patients are strikingly irritable, often lethargic and generally appear moderately to severely ill even without evidence of aseptic meningitis.

LABORATORY DATA

The laboratory findings in patients with Kawasaki disease are non-specific and consistent with an acute inflammatory process. Leucocytosis, frequently in excess of 20×10^9 cells/l and with a shift to the left, is present. The test for C-reactive protein is positive in over three quarters of patients and the erythrocyte sedimentation rate is often significantly elevated, in some in excess of 100 mm/hour. Immunoglobulin E and α_2-globulin levels may be increased.

Striking thrombocytosis is a characteristic, but not diagnostic feature of Kawasaki disease. The platelet count usually begins to rise toward the end of the acute phase, reaching levels between 600×10^9 and 1000×10^9 cells/l. This peak usually occurs toward the end of the third week of illness and is followed by a fall to normal during convalesence.

CARDIAC INVOLVEMENT

Kawasaki disease was first considered a severe but self-limiting disorder since all patients were thought to recover. During the 1980s and 1990s, 10 national surveys on Kawasaki disease have been conducted by Yanagawa, Shigematsu and the Japan Kawasaki Disease Research-Committee (Naoe et al, 1991). A fatality rate of 0.4% was reported (363 of 94 330). This death rate is lower than the 1–2% reported in the 1970s (Kawasaki et al, 1974). Since most of these data represent patients seen prior to the era of the use of gammaglobulin, it is likely that this represents increased recognition of milder disease rather than the result of specific therapy. Of deaths, 70% are in infants less than 1 year of age, with 90% occurring suddenly, usually during the convalescent phase, 3 to 7 weeks after the onset of illness (Fujiwara and Hamashima, 1978). Fatalities have increasingly been reported many years after the onset of Kawasaki disease, occasionally in patients not considered to have cardiac involvement (Kato et al, 1986; Suzuki et al, 1988; Naoe et al, 1991; Buns et al, 1996).

Whether early or late, death is of cardiovascular origin. Most fatalities occur suddenly, usually from thrombosis of coronary arterial aneurysms. Consequently, involvement of the cardiovascular system in Kawasaki disease is important, since the deaths in this disease result from cardiovascular complications.

In most current reports of Kawasaki disease in Japan, cardiac involvement with the development of coronary arterial aneurysms occurs in 15–25% of patients (Yanagawa et al, 1987; Nakamura et al, 1991; Kato et al, 1996). All patients have tachycardia during the acute phase of the illness, although the presence of a gallop rhythm is unusual in our series. A soft, non-specific systolic ejection murmur at the upper left sternal border is common and is considered to be functional. Although a significant percentage of electrocardiographic abnormalities have been reported, our experience has been that the chest radiograph and electrocardiogram usually are normal even in patients who subsequently are documented to have coronary arterial involvement. When the electrocardiogram is abnormal, the changes are usually non-specific, occurring during the first 2 weeks of illness and then regressing. A decrease in the R wave amplitude, prolonged PR and/or QT interval, and minor ST segment changes have been found (Hiraishi et al, 1981).

In patients with Kawasaki disease, several clinical features correlate with the presence of cardiac involvement: a prolonged febrile course greater than 14 days in duration or a recurrence of fever, rash, or desquamation after these findings have disappeared; persistent elevation of acute phase reactants for more than 1 month (white blood cell count, erythrocyte sedimentation rate and C-reactive protein level); or elevation of cardiac specific enzymes (Asai, 1983). In our experience, the presence of marked thrombocytosis, (platelet counts greater than 1000×10^9 cells/l) is also associated with coronary arterial aneurysms.

Cardiac abnormalities may appear at any time during the course of the illness, especially towards the end of the acute febrile phase. Cardiac findings include the presence of an apical systolic murmur of mitral regurgitation, cardiomegaly, congestive heart failure, pericarditis or pericardial effusion. Major electrocardiographic abnormalities (including first-, second- or third-degree atrioventricular block; premature ventricular contractions; or atrial or ventricular tachyarrhythmias) appearing after the end of the second week of illness strongly suggest cardiac involvement. Electrocardiographic signs of myocardial ischaemia or infarction, or the presence of cardiogenic shock, have ominous implications.

A clinical scoring system (Asai, 1983) was developed to identify patients with coronary arterial aneurysms (Table 62.3). The maximum number of points that a patient can have with this modified Asai scoring system is 23. A score greater than 9 strongly indicates the presence of coronary arterial involvement. Although most patients subsequently found to have coronary aneurysms would be considered to be at high risk based on the modified Asai scoring system, false positives (patients

Table 62.3 Clinical scoring system for Kawasaki disease

Clinical features	Score[a]		
	0	1	2
Sex	Female	Male	
Age (years)	<1	>1	
Duration of fever (days)	<14	14–15	16
Recurrent fever	No		Yes
Recurrent rash	No		Yes
Recurrent desquamation	No		Yes
Anaemia (haemoglobulin, <10 g/dl)	No	Yes	
Maximum white blood cell count (× 10⁹ cells/l)	<26	26–30	>30
Maximum sedimentation rate (mm/h)	<60	60–100	>100
Prolonged acute reactants[b] (months)	<1		>1
Cardiomegaly	No	Yes	
Arrhythmia	No	Yes	
Ischaemic signs and symptoms	No		Yes
Pericarditis	No	Yes	Yes (with effusion)

[a] Modified from the scoring system developed by Asai (1983).
[b] Acute reactants are erythrocyte sedimentation rate and C-reactive protein.

who have a high clinical score but who do not have coronary arterial aneurysms) occur. False negatives can also occur.

INVESTIGATION

ECHOCARDIOGRAPHIC FEATURES

Cross-sectional echocardiography has become an essential tool for the diagnosis and management of children with Kawasaki disease. It is important to remember that the irritability of infants and small children with this disease often interferes with an adequate echocardiographic examination, since a considerable amount of cooperation from the patient is necessary to visualize the coronary arterial anatomy adequately. It is usually worthwhile to sedate irritable patients prior to echocardiographic evaluation. In our experience, chloral hydrate (50 to 75 mg/kg) is safe and effective.

Cross-sectional echocardiography has been used for the detection of coronary arterial aneurysms since 1979 (Hiraishi et al, 1979; Yoshikawa et al, 1979). Arjunan et al (1986) described the calibre of coronary arteries in normal children and in children with Kawasaki disease without coronary aneurysms. In both groups, the size of the proximal coronary arteries showed little variability in the first centimetre from the ostium. The diameters varied from 2 mm in infants up to 5 mm in teenagers, with a progressive increase in size with increasing age. Aneurysms are seen as saccular or fusiform dilations in a coronary artery (Figure 62.4).

The main coronary arteries are usually visualized adequately from the parasternal short-axis view. Specific techniques were developed for imaging the peripheral

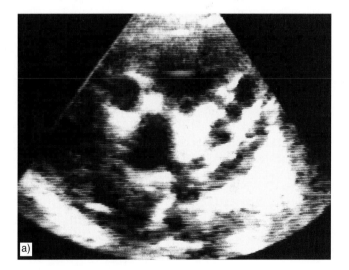
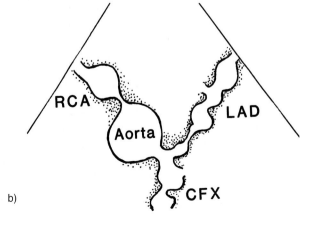

Figure 62.4. Cross-sectional echocardiography can show coronary arterial aneurysms. (a) An echocardiogram showing extensive aneurysms. (b) Diagram of echocardiogram. CFX, circumflex coronary artery; LAD, left anterior descending coronary artery; RCA, right coronary artery.

segments of the right and left coronary arteries from the subcostal position in order to add to the information obtained from the parasternal approach (Yoshida et al, 1982; Maeda et al, 1983). Adoption of a systematic approach towards imaging of the coronary arteries from multiple projections, together with technological improvement in the resolution of images, has led to consistent and accurate imaging of the majority of the coronary arterial tree (Satomi et al, 1984).

With increasing experience, the sensitivity of cross-sectional echocardiography in detecting aneurysms in the proximal portion of the coronary arteries is nearly 100%, with a specificity of 97% (Capanari et al, 1986). The sensitivity for detection of aneurysms located distally, however, may be as low as 50% (Figure 62.5) (Capanari et al, 1986). Serial echocardiographic evaluation throughout the different stages of Kawasaki disease has demonstrated that the aneurysms usually appear during the second week after the onset of the illness (Hiraishi et al, 1981; Yanagisawa et al, 1985). True aneurysmal formation can be saccular or fusiform. Abnormalities such as perivascular brightness, which is an increased echogenicity of the walls of the coronary artery; and transient dilation of the coronary artery, can also be noted.

Aneurysms have a tendency to regress spontaneously in as many as 50% of patients. Large aneurysms are more likely to persist, or even develop stenosis (Figure 62.6) (Pahl et al, 1989). Although coronary arterial aneurysms are readily seen with cross-sectional echocardiography, especially in the proximal coronary arteries, it is not possible to detect the presence of obstructive lesions echocardiographically (Ettedgui et al, 1991). Consequently,

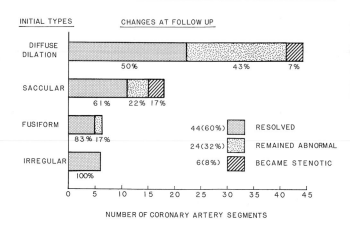

Figure 62.6. Fate of 75 coronary lesions classified by type of abnormality found at initial catheterization in 15 patients with Kawasaki disease who underwent follow-up study.

to rely exclusively on echocardiography for long-term follow-up of coronary aneurysms, as suggested by some authors (Chung et al, 1988), might lead to missing patients with coronary arterial stenoses. It is these patients who have the highest risk of myocardial infarction or sudden death. Echocardiography, therefore, should be used in conjunction with coronary angiography to provide optimal long-term care of the child with Kawasaki disease and coronary arterial involvement. Echocardiography should be used as a screening tool for detection of aneurysms in the acute stages of the disease and to monitor resolution or reduction in their size. The presence of coronary stenoses and distal lesions of the coronary arteries, can be established with cineangiography (Figure 62.7) (Pahl et al, 1989; Pahl-Schuette et al, 1991; Takahashi and Mason, 1991).

Our current recommendation is to perform an echocardiogram within 2 weeks of the acute illness, to repeat the study at 4 to 6 weeks from acute onset and to repeat it again in 1 year. If no abnormality of the coronary arteries is detected, then echocardiography during follow-up is oriented toward assessing valvar insufficiency and ventricular function and should be used as best suited to each individual patient. If a coronary arterial abnormality is discovered, such as coronary arterial aneurysms, or whenever there is concern about coronary arterial stenosis, coronary angiography is warranted (Ettedgui et al, 1991).

ANGIOCARDIOGRAPHY

Routine cardiac catheterization and angiocardiography are not recommended for evaluation of every patient with Kawasaki disease. When coronary arterial aneurysms are present, they are usually found in the proximal portion of one of the major coronary arteries. Cross-sectional echocardiography is an extremely valuable screening tool for coronary arterial involvement, since the proximal portions of the coronary arteries are the

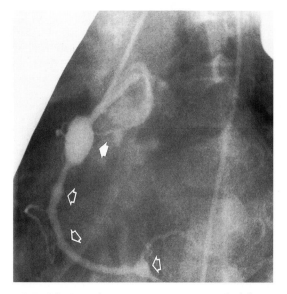

Figure 62.5. Selective right coronary arteriogram in the left anterior oblique view demonstrating a large saccular aneurysm (solid arrow) in the proximal segment. Diffuse irregularity and an additional aneurysm (open arrows) seen distally were not apparent echocardiographically.

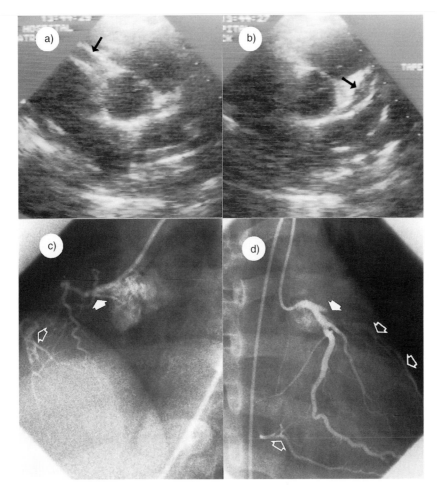

Figure 62.7. Echocardiograms in a short-axis view demonstrating an aneurysm (arrows) in both the right (a) and left (b) coronary arteries. However, coronary arterial stenosis or obliteration was not apparent and was only visualized by selective coronary angiography in the left anterior oblique view of the right coronary arteriogram (c) and right anterior oblique view of the left coronary arteriogram (d). These showed complete obliteration (solid arrows) of the coronary arteries with retrograde filling (open arrows). Both echocardiographic and angiographic studies were done on the same day.

areas most readily visualized with this technique. Angiocardiography is indicated for patients who have coronary arterial aneurysms demonstrated by cross-sectional echocardiography (Nakano et al, 1985; Pahl et al, 1989; Suzuki and Kamiya, 1991). We also recommend angiography for any patient who has signs of cardiac involvement during the acute or subacute phase of the illness, and in those at high risk for cardiac involvement even when cross-sectional echocardiography is negative.

Cross-sectional echocardiography and coronary angiography are complementary in the evaluation of coronary arterial abnormalities. Angiocardiography is important for demonstration of the extent and severity of coronary arterial lesions since quantification of the size, number and location of coronary arterial aneurysms is not possible with echocardiography (Pahl et al, 1989). Angiography performed within a few months of the acute disease provides a valuable baseline, which is important in the ongoing management of patients with cardiac involvement. Aneurysms demonstrated angiographically may be either fusiform or saccular and may either be soli-

tary or occur as multiple lesions with extensive involvement of both coronary arteries (Figure 62.8). A system for quantification of the severity of coronary arterial lesions based upon the findings of coronary angiography has been described that can be used to indicate the nature and extent of coronary arterial lesions and to evaluate factors that affect the eventual outcome (Table 62.4) (Nakano et al, 1985).

Table 62.4 Quantitative grading for coronary aneurysm

Grade[a]	Size (maximal diameter, mm)	Description
0 (normal)	–	No aneurysms
1 (mild)	>4	Localized, proximal lesions
2 (moderate)	4–8	Solitary, multiple or extensive
3 (severe)	>8	Extensive, diffuse, multiple vessels

[a] Modified from Nakano et al (1985).

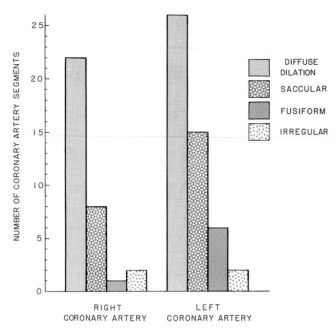

Figure 62.8. Incidence and types of coronary arterial abnormalities in 82 segments in patients with Kawasaki disease who had cardiac catheterization after their acute illness.

The presence of extremely sluggish coronary blood flow has been demonstrated in patients undergoing angiography within a few months following their episode of Kawasaki disease (Pahl et al, 1989). When an aortogram is performed, the coronary arteries normally fill during the first diastolic cycle. As soon as the injection ceases, the contrast material is rapidly cleared from the ascending aorta and the coronary arteries remain visualized for only three or four additional cardiac cycles. In contrast, when the coronary arteries are involved in Kawasaki disease, even when there is only mild dilation, clearing is markedly delayed. Contrast material commonly remains in the coronary arteries for as many as 12 to 15 cardiac cycles thereafter. Although the clinical significance of this finding is unclear, the presence of dilation and aneurysms of the coronary arteries, extremely sluggish blood flow and marked thrombocytosis would seem to combine to make those patients with all three features at considerable risk for the development of thrombosis.

MANAGEMENT

Since the aetiology of Kawasaki disease is unknown, no preventative measures or specific treatments are available. Current therapy has two major goals: treatment of the acute phase and prevention of coronary arterial thrombosis. During the acute inflammatory stage, agents with anti-inflammatory properties are used. At the end of the acute phase and during the subacute phase of the illness, significant thrombocytosis is present. Since this may enhance the potential for thrombosis of a coronary arterial aneurysms with subsequent myocardial infarc-

tion or death, the second therapeutic goal is the prevention of thrombosis.

ASPIRIN

Acetylsalicylic acid (aspirin) is the most widely used drug in the management of Kawasaki disease (Koren et al, 1985). The dose recommended in the literature has varied widely, making it difficult to compare the outcome of various series. The daily dose of aspirin (80 to 100 mg/kg) used in the management of patients with rheumatic fever or rheumatoid arthritis often has been used as the standard for anti-inflammatory therapy. This dose generally achieves a blood salicylate level of 20–30 mg/dl, which is considered to be in the therapeutic range. In patients with Kawasaki disease, absorption of salicylate is impaired and, as a result, administration of salicylate in this dosage during the acute phase often achieves a level well below 20 mg/dl, which may be subtherapeutic (Koren et al, 1985). The daily dose of aspirin recommended during the acute phase has ranged from 30 to 200 mg/kg (the level achieved with these doses generally has not been reported). It is impossible, therefore, to assess the effectiveness of different forms of therapy, especially when the therapeutic range for salicylate is unknown in patients with Kawasaki disease. Previously, we recommended a daily dose of 100 to 150 mg/kg during the acute phase, with monitoring of the serum salicylate level and adjustment of the dosage to achieve a peak serum concentration of 20 mg/dl. Since the advent of the use of intravenous gammaglobulin therapy, the associated use of salicylate therapy has become even more confusing. In most institutions, 50 or 100 mg/kg of aspirin is used daily during the acute phase of the disease. This arbitrary dosage is used without monitoring blood levels and without any attempt to achieve a specific concentration in the serum. After the acute stage, low-dose salicylates are used to prevent thrombosis, as will be described below.

CORTICOSTEROIDS

Corticosteroids are among the most potent anti-inflammatory agents, and yet their use is generally considered to be contraindicated in patients with Kawasaki disease. In fact, only one study (Kato et al, 1979) has evaluated the use of corticosteroid therapy in Kawasaki disease. This study has been quoted widely and used as a rationale for the contraindication to the use of steroids. In the report, 92 patients were evaluated and were treated by five different protocols at five different hospitals. The study was poorly controlled and the series relatively small. Considerable bias may have been introduced in assignment of patients to the different protocols, since three of the five hospitals used only three of the protocols. About 65% of the patients receiving only prednisolone (11 of 17), 11% of the patients receiving aspirin alone (4 of 36), and 20% of the patients receiving antibiotics alone (5 of 25) were found to have coronary arterial aneurysms. The conclusion that has been perpetuated in the literature is that the use of steroids in this group of patients was associated with an extremely high incidence of aneurysms. Of the remaining patients, one small group received prednisolone and warfarin; in this group two of seven (29%) developing a coronary arterial aneurysm. The other group of seven patients' was treated with prednisolone plus aspirin, and these patients did not develop coronary arterial aneurysms. Although this last group was small, it is a striking comparison with the 17 patients in the group receiving prednisolone of which 11 developed coronary arterial aneurysms. The authors of the article disregarded the small group of patients who were treated with prednisolone and aspirin and in whom coronary arterial aneurysms were not demonstrated. They concluded that steroids act adversely to cause a progression of the coronary arterial lesions in Kawasaki disease. Although this conclusion may be correct, it is not justified by their data. Cremer, in Germany (1989), has been using steroids and aspirin given in low doses in the treatment of patients with Kawasaki disease with results comparable to those for patients treated with intravenous gammaglobulin. The results of this small series should provide a strong stimulus for future investigation to re-evaluate the use of this potent anti-inflammatory agent in the treatment of Kawasaki disease.

GAMMAGLOBULIN

Landmark studies in Japan and the USA in the mid 1980s (Furusho et al, 1984; Iwasa et al, 1985; Newburger et al, 1986) demonstrated that the administration of high-dose intravenous gammaglobulin reduces the incidence of coronary arterial aneurysms in patients with Kawasaki disease. High-dose intravenous gammaglobulin (400 mg/kg daily for 4 consecutive days) and 50 or 100 mg/kg aspirin daily have been used in most studies. In the early 1990s many centres began using a single high dose of intravenous gammaglobulin of 2000 mg/kg administered over 10 to 12 hours rather than the 4-day course (Rowley and Shulman, 1991). A small percentage of patients with Kawasaki disease who received intravenous gammaglobulin have persistent or recurrent fever; in these patients the treatment may not have had the anti-inflammatory effect generally seen in other patients. When this occurs, it has been recommended that these patients should be retreated with intravenous gammaglobulin, although no data exist on which to make recommendations (Rowley and Shulman 1991; Sundel et al, 1991).

There are a number of concerns about treatment with gammaglobulin as used in the USA and Japan. Aside from the high cost of thousands of dollars and a few days of hospitalization for each patient, over 80% of patients who are treated probably would not have developed coronary arterial aneurysms. In addition, over 50% of coronary arterial abnormalities (dilation, small aneurysms) that do occur resolve spontaneously within 1 year following the acute illness. Furthermore, there are those patients who do not have Kawasaki disease but who receive intravenous gammaglobulin on the third or fourth day of a febrile illness before all clinical criterions have developed. On the basis of this, Kawasaki and others have stated that in the United States and now in Japan, 150% of patients with Kawasaki disease will receive intravenous gamma globulin therapy. Other concerns regarding the use of gammaglobulin include the risk of acquiring hepatitis, AIDS or potentially altering the immune system in a negative manner such that routine childhood immunizations are ineffective. Anaphylaxis and serum sickness may also occur, as well as hypotension if given to a child with myocardial dysfunction. It is also not known whether the various types of intravenous gammaglobulin have the same effect in the treatment of Kawasaki disease. The various commercial forms of gammaglobulin are prepared in different manners and, therefore, may have varying degrees of effectiveness and different rates of adverse reactions (Silverman et al, 1991). No data are available in a substantial series comparing the effectiveness and safety of these different preparations.

PLATELET-INHIBITING DRUGS

Since coronary thrombosis is the usual cause of death from Kawasaki disease, long-term therapy is directed towards the prevention of this serious complication. Once the acute phase has passed, and the fever has subsided, the dose of aspirin is reduced to a level that will inhibit aggregation of platelets. Aspirin is used in a daily dose of 5 mg/kg for a period of 1 month after signs of the acute illness have subsided, or until the platelet count and erythrocyte sedimentation rate have returned to normal. In a patient with coronary arterial lesions, daily dipyridamole 5 mg/kg is added to the regimen. This combination of aspirin and dipyridamole is continued until it has been demonstrated by angiography that coronary arterial, abnormalities have resolved.

LONG-TERM FOLLOW-UP

At the Children's Hospital of Pittsburgh, all patients with Kawasaki disease undergo clinical examination and non-invasive studies, including cross-sectional echocardiography, during the acute, subacute and convalescence phases of their illness (Figure 62.9). Patients at the lowest risk for cardiac involvement (a short-term illness with no signs of cardiac involvement) undergo cross-sectional echocardiography 1 month after the acute illness has subsided and again 1 year later. If the echocardiographic studies are normal, these patients are not seen again routinely. We plan to evaluate these patients again in late childhood with clinical examination, echocardiography and stress exercise testing.

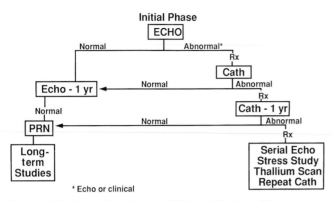

Figure 62.9. Protocol used at the Children's Hospital of Pittsburgh for the management of patients following the acute phase of Kawasaki disease. Cath, catheterization; ECHO, echocardiography; PRN, as required; Rx, treatment with aspirin and dipyridamole.

Patients at high risk because of a prolonged or recurrent illness, or with evidence of cardiac involvement, undergo catheterization and angiocardiography during the convalescent phase. If the coronary arteries are normal, and the acute illness has subsided, aspirin is discontinued and periodic cross-sectional echocardiography is performed yearly for a few years. When coronary arterial aneurysms have been documented by angiography, antiplatelet therapy (aspirin and dipyridamole) is continued until the coronary arterial abnormalities have resolved. Angiocardiography is performed 1 year later regardless of the echocardiographic findings. If the echocardiogram is normal, resolution of the coronary arterial lesions is best documented angiographically. If resolution has occurred, medications are discontinued and the patient subsequently is followed clinically and noninvasively. If the lesions persist as shown by echocardio-

graphy, angiography will show the extent and status of coronary arterial aneurysms and provide quantitative evaluation of changes that have occurred, in particular the presence or absence of stenosis (Figure 62.10). Decisions about follow-up angiocardiography are made on an individual basis. Thallium radionuclide studies are generally normal at rest even in patients who have significant coronary arterial stenosis. Exercise stress testing, with or without thallium, can be performed when the patient reaches an appropriate age. Perfusion abnormalities are better demonstrated by single photon emission tomography. Positron emission tomography has shown that patients in whom the coronary arteries appear normal angiographically may still have a diminished flow reserve (Muzik et al, 1996). Stress echocardiography may be useful to identify patients with decreased myocardial perfusion who may appear normal at rest (Pahl et al, 1995). This technique can also be utilized successfully in small children with the use of intravenous dobutamine, eliminating the necessity for treadmill exercise.

Sudden death has been increasingly reported to occur some years following the acute episode of Kawasaki disease (Kato et al, 1986). Signs and symptoms of coronary arterial insufficiency, or the finding of substantial coronary arterial stenosis with abnormal myocardial blood flow even in an asymptomatic patient, are indications for the use of coronary arterial bypass surgery (Kitamura, 1991).

SUMMARY

Kawasaki disease is now recognized throughout the world. Its aetiology, natural history, and relationship to

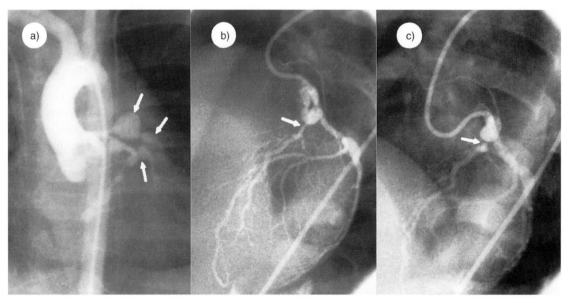

Figure 62.10. Serial angiograms showing progression of stenosis in the left anterior descending coronary artery. (a) Initial aortogram in anteroposterior view showing multiple large aneurysms (arrows). (b,c) Selective left coronary angiograms 15 months (b) and 26 months (c) after initial study in the left anterior view demonstrating progressive stenosis (arrows) in the left anterior descending branch.

other previously described entities are unknown. In most patients, the disease is self-limited and resolves spontaneously. Cardiac involvement may be more widespread than previously suspected and, eventually, may result in significant long-term cardiovascular abnormalities. The overall mortality is 0.4% in Kawasaki disease, and death is always a result of cardiac complications. Death usually occurs in the first month or so following the illness, although death has been reported many years later. Coronary arterial abnormalities occur in 15 to 20% of patients. Their significance is unknown, since these lesions resolve in many and the reported mortality is far lower than the reported incidence of the compli-

cation. Since the aetiology is unknown, specific treatment is unavailable. Most centres currently use intravenous gammaglobulin therapy along with salicylates, but the most effective regimen remains to be established. The use of corticosteroids needs to be re-evaluated in light of concerns about the validity of the study that suggested their contraindication. In the absence of any specific treatment of the cardiac complications, long-term treatment with medication to suppress aggregation of platelets is indicated for patients with coronary arterial abnormalities. The long-term outlook, even for those without apparent cardiac involvement, is currently unknown.

REFERENCES

Ahlstrom H, Lundstrom N R, Mortensson W, Ostberg G, Lantorp K 1977 Infantile periarteritis nodosa or mucocutaneous lymph node syndrome. Acta Paediatrica Scandanavica 66: 193–198

Arjunan K, Daniels S, Meyer R, Schwartz D, Barron H, Kaplan S 1986 Coronary artery caliber in normal children and patients with Kawasaki disease but without aneurysms: an echocardiographic and angiographic study. Journal of the American College of Cardiology 8: 1119–1124

Asai T 1983 Evaluation method for the degree of seriousness in Kawasaki disease. Acta Paediatrica Japonica 25: 170–175

Burns J C, Shike H, Gordon J B, Malhotra A, Schoenwetter M, Kawasaki T 1996 Sequelae of Kawasaki disease in adolescents and young adults. Journal of the American College of Cardiology 28: 253–257

Capanari T, Daniels S, Meyer R, Schwartz D, Kaplan S 1986 Sensitivity, specificity and predictive value of two-dimensional echocardiography in detecting coronary artery aneurysms in patients with Kawasaki disease. Journal of the American College of Cardiology 7: 355–360

Chung K, Fulton D, Lapp R, Spector S, Sahn D 1988 One-year follow-up of cardiac and coronary artery disease in infants and children with Kawasaki disease. American Heart Journal 115: 1263–1267

Cremer H 1989 Considerations on treatment of Kawasaki disease. Presented at the third international Kawasaki disease symposium, Tokyo, Japan

Dhillon R, Clarkson P, Donald A E et al 1996 Endothelial dysfunction late after Kawasaki disease. Circulation 94: 2103–2106

Ettedgui J A Neches W H, Pahl E 1991 The role of cross-sectional echocardiography in Kawasaki disease. Cardiology in the Young 1: 221–224

Fujiwara H and Hamashima Y 1978 Pathology of the heart in Kawasaki disease. Pediatrics 61: 100–107

Fukushige J, Takahashi N, Ueda K 1991 Presented at the Fourth international Kawasaki disease symposium, Wailea, Hawaii

Furusho K, Kamiya T, Nakano H et al 1984 High-dose intravenous gammaglobulin for Kawasaki disease. Lancet ii: 1055–1058

Hamashima Y, Tasaka K, Fujiwara H, Hoshino T, Matsuda S, Kao T 1983 Kawasaki's disease – its pathological features and possible pathogenesis. Acta Paediatrica Japonica 25: 108–117

Hiraishi S, Yashiro K, Kusano S 1979 Noninvasive visualization of coronary arterial aneurysm in infants and young children with mucocutaneous lymph node syndrome with two dimensional echocardiography. American Journal of Cardiology 43: 1225–1233

Hiraishi S, Yashiro K, Oguchi K, Kusano S, Ishii K, Nakazawa K 1981 Clinical course of cardiovascular involvement in the mucocutaneous lymph node syndrome. Relation between clinical signs of carditis and development of coronary arterial aneurysms. American Journal of Cardiology 47: 323–330

Iwasa M, Sugiyama K, Kawase A et al 1985 Prevention of coronary artery involvement in Kawasaki disease by early intravenous high dose gammaglobulin. In: Proceedings of the second world congress of pediatric cardiology. Springer-Verlag, New York, p 26

Kato H, Koike S, Yokoyama T 1979 Kawasaki disease: effect of treatment on coronary artery involvement. Pediatrics 63: 175–179

Kato H, Ichinose E, Kawasaki T 1986 Myocardial infarction in Kawasaki disease: Clinical analyses of 195 cases. Journal of Pediatrics 108: 923–927

Kato H, Sugimura T, Akagi T et al 1996 Long-term consequences of Kawasaki disease. A 10–21 year follow-up study of 594 patients. Circulation 94: 1379–1385

Kawasaki T 1967 Febrile oculo-oro-cutaneo-acrodesquamatous syndrome with or without acute non-suppurative cervical lymphadenitis in infancy and childhood. Clinical observation of 50 cases. Japanese Journal of Allergy 16: 178–222 (In Japanese)

Kawasaki T, Kosaki F, Okawa S, Shigematsu I, Yanagawa H 1974 A new infantile acute febrile mucocutaneous lymph node syndrome (MLNS) prevailing in Japan. Pediatrics 54: 271–276

Kitamura S 1991 Surgical management for cardiovascular lesions in Kawasaki disease. Cardiology in the Young 1: 240–253

Koren G, Rose V, Lavi S, Rowe R 1985 Probable efficacy of high-dose salicylates in reducing coronary involvement in Kawasaki disease. Journal of the American Medical Association 254: 767–769

Landing B H, Larson E J 1977 Are infantile periarteritis nodosa with coronary artery involvement and fatal mucocutaneous lymph node syndrome the same? Comparison of 20 patients from North American with patients from Hawaii and Japan. Pediatrics 59: 651–662

Maeda T, Yoshida H, Funabashi T et al 1983 Subcostal 2-dimensional echocardiographic imaging of peripheral left coronary artery aneurysms in Kawasaki disease. American Journal of Cardiology 52: 48–52

Mattern A L, Baker W P, McHale J J, Lee D E 1972 Congenital coronary aneurysms with angina pectoris and myocardial infarction treated with saphenous vein bypass graft. American Journal of Cardiology 30: 906–909

Muzik O, Paridon S M, Singh T P, Morrow W R, Dayanikli F, Di Carli M F 1996 Quantification of myocardial blood flow and flow reserve in children with a history of Kawasaki disease and normal coronary arteries using positron emission tomography. Journal of the American College of Cardiology 28: 757–762

Nakamura Y, Fujita Y, Nagai M et al 1991 Cardiac sequelae of Kawasaki disease in Japan: statistical analysis. Pediatrics 88: 1144–1147

Nakano H, Ueda K, Saito A, Nojima K 1985 Repeated quantitative angiograms in coronary arterial aneurysm in Kawasaki disease. American Journal of Cardiology 56: 846–851

Naoe S, Takahaski K, Masuda H, Tanaka N 1987 Coronary findings post Kawasaki disease in children who died of other causes. In: Shulman S T (ed.) Kawasaki disease. Alan R. Liss, New York, 341–346

Naoe S, Takahaski K, Masuda H, Tanaka N 1991 Kawasaki disease with particular emphasis on arterial lesions. Acta Pathologica Japonica 41: 785–797

Newburger J W, Takahashi M, Burns J C et al 1986 The treatment of Kawasaki syndrome with intravenous gamma globulin. New England Journal of Medicine 315: 341–347

Pahl E, Ettedgui J A, Neches W H, Park S C 1989 The value of angiography in the follow-up of coronary involvement in mucocutaneous lymph node syndrome (Kawasaki disease). Journal of the American College of Cardiology 14: 1318–1325

Pahl E, Sehgal R, Chrystof D et al 1995 Feasibility of exercise stress echocardiography for the follow-up of children with coronary involvement secondary to Kawasaki disease. Circulation 91: 122–128

Pahl-Schuette E, Neches W H, Beerman L B, Ettedgui J A, Park S C 1991 Coronary angiography to assess progression of coronary stenosis after Kawasaki disease. Presented at the fourth international Kawasaki disease symposium, Wailea, Hawaii

Patriarca P A, Rogers M F, Morens D M et al 1982 Kawasaki syndrome: association with the application of rug shampoo. Lancet ii: 578–580

Rauch A M, Glode M P, Wiggins J W et al 1991 Outbreak of Kawasaki syndrome in Denver, Colorado: association with rug and carpet cleaning. Pediatrics 87: 663–669

Rowley A H, Shulman S T 1991 Current therapy for acute Kawasaki syndrome. Journal of Pediatrics 118: 987–991

Satomi G, Nakamura K, Narai S, Takao A 1984 Systematic visualization of coronary arteries by two-dimensional echocardiography in children and infants: evaluation in Kawasaki's disease and coronary arteriovenous fistulas. American Heart Journal 107: 497–505

Silverman E D, Rose V, Dyck J, Smallhorn J, Laxer R M 1991 Comparison of different intravenous gammaglobumin preparations in the treatment of Kawasaki disease. Presented at the fourth international Kawasaki disease symposium, Wailea, Hawaii

Sundel R P, Belser A S, Baker A, Burns J C, Newburger J W 1991 Gamma Globumin retreatment in Kawasaki disease. Presented at the fourth international Kawasaki disease symposium, Wailea, Hawaii

Suzuki A, Kamiya T 1991 Visualization of the coronary arterial lesions in Kawasaki disease by coronary angiography. Cardiology in the Young 1: 225–233

Suzuki A, Kamiya T, Kuwahara N, Ono Y, Takamiya M 1988 Myocardial ischemia in Kawasaki disease: follow-up study by cardiac catheterization and coronary angiography. Pediatric Cardiology 9: 1–5

Takahaski M, Mason W 1991 Can echocardiogram predict coronary angiographic findings: aneurysm size, thrombisis and stenosis? Presented at the fourth international Kawasaki disease symposium, Wailea, Hawaii

Taubert K A, Rowley A H, Shulman S T 1991 A seven year (1984–1990) US Nationwide hospital survey of Kawasaki disease (KD). Presented at the fourth international Kawasaki disease symposium, Wailea, Hawaii

Wilson C S, Weaver W F, Zeman E D, Forker A D 1975 Bilateral nonfistulous congenital coronary arterial aneurysms. American Journal of Cardiology 35: 319–323

Yanagawa H, Kawasaki T, Shiegematsu I 1987 Nationwide survey on Kawasaki disease in Japan. Pediatrics 80: 58–62

Yanagisawa M, Kobayaski N, Matsuya S 1974 Myocardial infarction due to coronary thromboarteritis following acute febrile mocucutaneous lymph node syndrome (MLNS) in an infant. Pediatrics 54: 277–280

Yanagisawa M, Yano S, Shiraishi H, Nakajima Y, Fujimoto T, Itoh K 1985 Coronary aneurysms in Kawasaki disease: follow-up observation by two dimensional echocardiography. Pediatric Cardiology 6: 11–16

Yonesaka S, Tomimoto K, Takahashi T, Furukawa H, Oura H 1991 Clinical studies on long-standing Kawasaki disease with special reference to myocardial changes using endomyocardial biopsy. Presented at the fourth international Kawasaki disease symposium, Wailea, Hawaii

Yoshida H, Maeda T, Funabashi T, Nakaya S, Takabatake S, Taniguchi N 1982 Subcostal two-dimensional imaging of peripheral right coronary artery in Kawasaki disease. Circulation 65: 956–961

Yoshikawa J, Yanagihara K, Owaki T et al 1979 Cross sectional echocardiographic diagnosis of coronary artery aneurysms in patients with the mucocutaneous lymph node syndrome. Circulation 59: 133–139

Yutani C, Go S, Kamiya K et al 1981 Cardiac biopsy of Kawasaki disease. Archives of Pathology and Laboratory Medicine 105: 470–473

PART VI

GENERAL PAEDIATRIC CARDIOLOGICAL DISEASE

63
—— Non-rheumatic inflammatory —— heart disease

E. Baker

—— INTRODUCTION ——

In this chapter we will discuss inflammatory diseases of the heart excluding rheumatic fever (Chapters 64 and 65), Kawasaki disease (Chapter 62) and infectious endocarditis (Chapter 66). Although the heart may be the primary target organ, inflammatory heart disease of non-rheumatic origin is often more generalized in nature. Usually such diseases affect various structures of the heart in combination. Only rarely will they be limited to the endocardium, the myocardium or the pericardium. To clarify our discussion, however, we will distinguish between myocarditis and pericarditis.

——MYOCARDITIS——

Myocarditis is defined as an inflammatory response within the myocardium. The aetiology and pathogenesis of the disease are most variable. In many patients, the precise mechanisms involved still remain unclear. The clinical consequences of myocarditis are largely determined by the degree and extent of myocardial injury. The disease may first present with pump failure or with abnormalities of rhythm and conduction. In the acute stage, sudden death may occur, often before the diagnosis is made.

The heart is often dilated, and histological studies will reveal myocardial necrosis with accompanying inflammatory reactions (Figure 63.1). The degree and extent of myocardial necrosis may vary considerably, as may the type of inflammation. Usually, neither one of these histological findings is diagnostic as far as aetiology and pathogenesis are concerned. In more advanced stages of the disease, part of the damaged myocardium may be replaced by scar tissue. Eventually, the histology of the affected heart may be dominated by interstitial fibrosis. In such instances, the term 'chronic myocarditis' is often used. Histological grading of myocarditis has been described by several authors (Fenoglio et al, 1983; Daly et al, 1984). The most recent consensus is the Dallas criterions (Aretz et al, 1987). In children, two main classes of non-

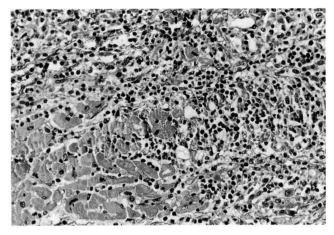

Figure 63.1. Micrograph of myocarditis. There is massive leucocytic infiltration with myocardial cell necrosis. (Haematoxylin–eosin stain, × 230.)

rheumatic myocarditis can be recognized: infectious myocarditis and generalized autoimmune myocarditis.

INFECTIOUS MYOCARDITIS ——

EPIDEMIOLOGY AND PREVALENCE

Infectious myocarditis can occur as a complication of almost any infectious disease. Viral infections are by far the most important in the industrialized Western World, but in other parts of the world, protozoal infections may rank highest (see Chapter 69). Many acute bacterial infections can result in myocarditis, and it can occur as a complication of tuberculosis, Lyme disease and haemolytic uraemic syndrome (Abu-Arafeh et al, 1995; Horowitz and Belkin, 1995; Nagi et al, 1996; Baysal et al, 1998). Infectious myocarditis is a frequent complication of opportunistic infections in patients with immune deficiencies, either primary or secondary, such as those that occur in patients treated with cytostatic or immunosuppressive drugs. Obviously, therefore, the type and incidence of infectious myocarditis will vary considerably from one part of the world to the other. Moreover, the 'true' prevalence of infectious myocarditis in any given population is, as yet, unknown. This is because the disease may take a subclinical course in many patients, and, hence, will go undetected. In others, the presence of an infectious myocarditis may be completely masked by the more overt signs and symptoms of other affected organs. Depending on the histological criterions used, evidence of myocarditis has been found in up to one twentieth of postmortems (Passarino et al, 1997).

VIRAL MYOCARDITIS

The majority of the cases of myocarditis seen in the Western World are of viral origin. Almost any viral disease can be complicated by myocarditis. Hence, the clinician should always be alert to this possibility. The most important viruses are coxsackie virus BI-5, A4 and 16, echovirus and those producing influenza, mumps and rubella (Shimizu et al, 1995; Baboonian et al, 1997). Human immunodeficiency virus also commonly infects the heart (Barbaro et al, 1998). In children, it can cause myocarditis and pericarditis, often presenting with the picture of a dilated cardiomyopathy (Lipschultz et al, 1990; Luginbuhl et al, 1993; Lipshultz et al, 1998).

The viral infection may be acquired transplacentally or by contacts in the nursery. Infection with coxsackievirus B may present in neonates and infants with myocarditis as the leading abnormality. Such infections in older children often cause pericarditis as the dominant feature. The mechanisms involved in producing the myocardial injury are still obscure. Invasion of the myocardial cells by viruses, or elaboration of toxins, may play an important role. Alternatively, cellular immune mechanisms may be of great importance. Immune reactions may continue after the viral infection of the heart has run its course and produce chronic myocardial damage.

CLINICAL FEATURES

The clinical onset of myocarditis usually occurs after a latent period following the onset of a systemic viral infection. The signs and symptoms of myocarditis are highly variable but are principally the result of heart failure or disturbances of rhythm. It is understandable, therefore, that there is no single characteristic clinical profile for myocarditis. Indeed, a whole spectrum of abnormalities may exist. At the one end, a child may develop an infectious myocarditis that remains completely unnoticed. At the other end, a child may become acutely ill with signs of both left- and right-sided heart failure and low cardiac output, often further complicated by disturbances of rhythm and sudden death.

All signs and symptoms, even the most subtle ones, that indicate failing pump function or abnormalities in rhythm and conduction should alert the physician to a cardiac complication. This is particularly so when noticed in the setting of a viral disease. In this respect, the important features that may give a clue to the diagnosis are cardiac enlargement, heart failure, tachycardia, gallop rhythm, tachypnoea, dyspnoea, fatigue and the appearance of an apical murmur indicating mitral insufficiency. There may be chest pain from the accompanying pericarditis. Non-specific symptoms, such as fever, diarrhoea, problems with feeding, pallor, mild jaundice and lethargy, often mark the clinical onset of the principal disease. Occasionally, the clinical picture may be dominated by severe respiratory distress secondary to left ventricular failure (Figure 63.2), so much so that initially a respiratory infection is mistakenly diagnosed. The clinical picture of heart failure in a previously well child with, often a minor, preceding viral infection is typical.

LABORATORY FINDINGS

The sedimentation rate is usually elevated but may be normal. The white cell count is variable, as are the levels of the cardiac enzymes, all depending on the severity of the disease and the nature of the infection.

All available diagnostic procedures should be used, including close collaboration with the bacteriological laboratory, in an attempt to identify the microorganism. Blood cultures, as well as swabs from nose, throat and rectum, should be taken in an attempt to isolate the infectious agent. Cultures from stool, urine and, eventually, from cerebrospinal fluid are essential. Acute and convalescent serum, with an interval of 2 to 4 weeks, should be drawn for assessment of antibodies. Specific IgM antibodies may indicate a recent viral infection. Despite all studies, however, the diagnosis of 'viral' myocarditis is often based on circumstantial evidence along with the exclusion of other possible aetiologies, rather than positive identification of an aetiological agent.

INVESTIGATIONS

Radiology

The size of the heart may be normal, particularly in the early period of the disease. More frequently, the heart will be enlarged with normal lung fields. Occasionally, pulmonary venous congestion will be evident (Figure 63.2).

Electrocardiography

Electrocardiographic abnormalities are common in myocarditis but are non-specific. There is often a sinus tachycardia, with lowering of the QRS complexes in the standard leads and/or precordial leads, flattening or inversion of the T waves and changes in the ST segment. Arrhythmias are often present and may lead to unexpected death. Occasionally, conduction disturbances are seen, with varying degrees of heart block. Complete

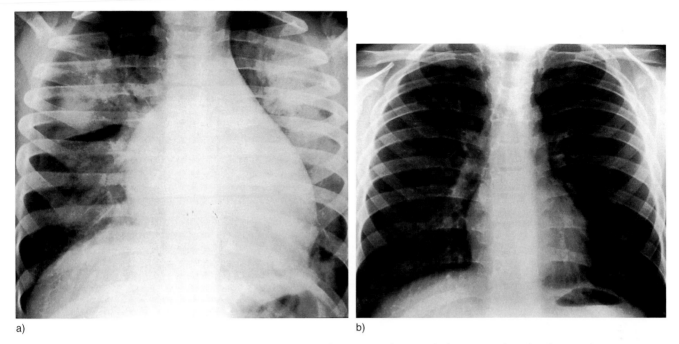

Figure 63.2. Chest radiograph of a 9-year-old boy with viral myocarditis. (a) At admission the heart was enlarged with signs of severe venous congestion of the lungs; clinically he was in respiratory distress. (b) After 30 days the heart was of normal size and configuration and the lung fields were clear.

atrioventricular block is rare. The QRS complexes may be broadened with left or right bundle branch block configuration (Figure 63.3) (Sevy et al, 1968; Scott et al, 1970; Morales et al, 1971; Forfang and Lippested, 1974; van Kirk et al, 1974). The electrocardiographic changes may disappear during the course of the disease or they may show a progressive evolution to overt abnormalities. The abnormalities may persist after the patient has

recovered clinically, most likely because of myocardial fibrosis.

Echocardiography

Echocardiography may demonstrate important, albeit non-specific, features. There is nearly always dilation of the heart chambers, usually the left ventricle. The left

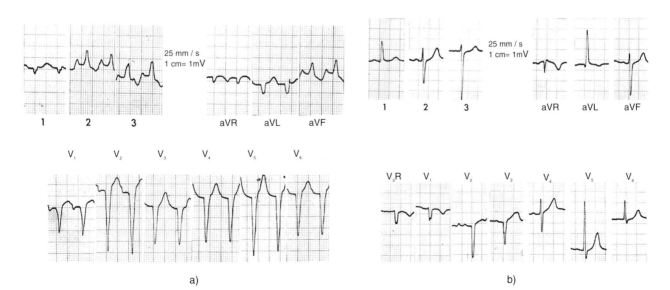

Figure 63.3. Electrocardiogram of a 9-year-old boy with viral myocarditis. (a) The electrocardiogram on admission showed first-degree atrioventricular block with broad QRS complexes. There is an infarction pattern with QS complexes in all precordial leads. (b) After 30 days the electrocardiogram had normalized, but there was left-axis deviation with slightly broadened QRS complexes (incomplete left bundle branch block). After 4 years the electrocardiogram had not changed in any important way.

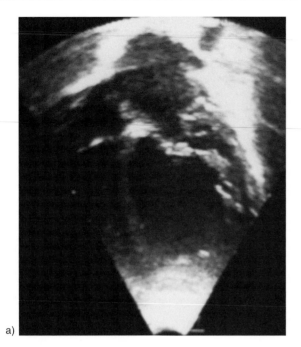

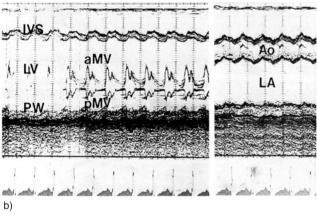

Figure 63.4. Echocardiograms of a child with acute myocarditis. (a) This cross-sectional echocardiogram is an apical four chamber view. The left ventricle (LV) and left atrium (LA) are markedly dilated. (b) In an M-mode echocardiogram, the severely dilated left ventricle can be seen, with reduced motion of both the interventricular septum (IVS) and the posterior wall (PW). The left ventricular shortening fraction is low, 16%. aMV, anterior leaflet of mitral valve; Ao, aorta; pMV, posterior leaflet of mitral valve.

atrium may also be enlarged, especially in the presence of mitral insufficiency (Figure 63.4). The motion of the ventricular septum and of the ventricular walls may be reduced and abnormal, and the ejection fraction may be decreased. The echocardiogram is of great importance in demonstrating or excluding a pericardial effusion. Identical echocardiographic findings are found in chronic myocarditis and dilated cardiomyopathy.

Radionuclide angiography

Radionuclide scans have been used for the detection of myocarditis either using gallium-67 scans or indium-111-labelled monoclonal antimyosin antibody (O'Connell

et al, 1984; Rezkalla et al, 1989). In practice, the most valuable role of radionuclide imaging is the serial measurement of left ventricular function, where it provides a more reproducible measurement of function than echocardiography (Chapter 15).

Endomyocardial biopsy

The place of routine endomyocardial biopsy in suspected myocarditis is still controversial. The histological changes of myocarditis are patchy, and so there can never be total confidence that a negative biopsy excludes myocarditis. There is no evidence that biopsy is of value in determining prognosis or in helping further management (Grogan et al, 1995). After many years of pursuing a policy of routine biopsy in suspected cases, we have been unable to demonstrate any benefit and have abandoned the practice.

TREATMENT

If an infectious agent has been identified as the cause of the myocarditis, and a specific treatment is available, then that should be started. In most cases, the causative agent is not identified. Treatment will then be non-specific, aiming at lowering the cardiac pre- and after-load, and at preventing and controlling complications such as heart failure and disturbances of rhythm.

Bedrest is considered mandatory for at least 14 days in the acute stage in order to reduce the workload of the heart. Prolonged bedrest is necessary in patients with longstanding heart failure, or a recurrence following an initial favourable response. A good response is characterized by a sleeping pulse rate of less than 100 beats per minute in children, and of less than 12 beats per minute in infants (Rowe et al, 1981). Restlessness and hypoxic stress should be avoided; oxygen is administered if necessary.

Cardiac failure should be treated with diuretics and inhibitors of angiotensin-converting enzyme, such as captopril (Rezkalla et al, 1996). Digoxin is still sometimes used but may induce ventricular arrhythmias. Other orally active inotropic agents, such as enoximone, are preferred in patients with very poor left ventricular function. Diuretics and inotropic agents may well need to be given intravenously in the initial stages of treatment.

Patients should be closely monitored for the occurrence of arrhythmias. When present, these disturbances should be treated if they have a deleterious haemodynamic effect. Many antiarrhythmic drugs will further depress myocardial contractility and should be used with care. Drugs that spare ventricular function, such as amiodarone, are preferred.

Thrombosis can occur in those with a very dilated left atrium and ventricles. In such patients, transoesophageal echocardiography is needed to exclude intracardiac thrombosis with confidence. Anticoagulation should always be considered in these circumstances. If evidence of intracardiac thrombosis is seen echocardiographically, anticoagulation should be continued until the left ventricular function has improved.

The value of prescribing drugs that suppress the inflammatory reaction is unclear. This approach was advocated in the expectation that immunosuppressive therapy would resolve the cellular infiltrate in the myocardium and, hence, reduce mortality and morbidity. The use of steroids is contraindicated in the acute phase (Maisch et al, 1996). They have long been used in the extremely ill and rapidly deteriorating child (Lambert et al, 1968; Rowe et al, 1981). They are still advocated for patients with biopsy-proven disease who fail to respond to conventional therapy (Brown and O'Connell, 1995). Steroids have been reported to help in the treatment of heart block or ventricular tachycardia brought on by myocarditis (Lambert et al, 1968; Ino et al, 1995). Despite this anecdotal evidence, a recent trial has shown no benefit from the routine use of prednisolone combined with either cyclosporin A (cyclosporine) or azothioprine (Mason et al, 1995). Recently, it has been suggested that immunoglobulin given intravenously in high doses may be beneficial in improving the recovery of ventricular function (McNamara et al, 1997). This is, as yet, unproven.

Children may die during the acute phase of the illness. In those whose left ventricular function is very poor, who fail to improve (remaining dependent on diuretics or inotropic agents given in high doses intravenously to control heart failure) or who develop intractable life-threatening arrhythmias, the option of cardiac transplantation should be considered. Transplantation may also be necessary for those who recover from the acute phase of myocarditis but continue to have poor left ventricular function over the longer term.

PROGNOSIS

Many children make a full recovery from myocarditis. In sporadic cases observed in childhood, death has been recorded in half the patients (Lerner et al, 1975; Rowe et al, 1981). Much myocarditis is, however, subclinical; consequently, such accounts tell little about the overall prognosis for the disease. The clinical signs and symptoms usually subside within a few weeks or months. It may take a little longer for the size of the heart and the electrocardiogram parameters to normalize. In some patients, this may take a year or more. Occasionally, the heart may remain enlarged, or episodes of cardiac failure may recur after an initial favourable response. The prognosis in these patients is usually poor.

DIFFERENTIAL DIAGNOSIS

Myocarditis needs to be distinguished from other anomalies that present with signs and symptoms of acute heart failure early in life. In glycogen storage disease, the clinical features and the electrocardiogram are typical. Enzymic studies will lead to the correct diagnosis. Anomalous origin of the left coronary artery from the pulmonary trunk is characterized by electrocardiographic signs of an anterolateral myocardial infarction. The diagnosis can be confirmed echocardiographically, or by angiocardiography (see Chapter 17). Enlargement of the heart and heart failure may also be caused by longstanding and severe anaemia of various causes. Dilation of the heart may occur also as a secondary phenomenon in patients with systemic arterio-venous fistulas. Occasionally, a child may present with all the signs and symptoms of dilated cardiomyopathy without a history of an infectious disease. Acute heart failure accompanied by mitral insufficiency is often the leading symptom. From a clinical viewpoint, there is no difference from 'chronic' myocarditis. Indeed, a direct correlation between the two conditions has been suggested (Mason et al, 1980; Goodwin, 1982; Shapiro et al, 1983).

GENERALIZED AUTOIMMUNE MYOCARDITIS—

Generalized autoimmune myocarditis encompasses a heterogeneous group of diseases. Some cause myocarditis as the dominant feature, while others have an arteritis as the leading pathology. These diseases are also known as 'collagen diseases' or 'connective tissue diseases'. Only the cardiac aspects of the most important diseases relevant to children will be discussed.

SYSTEMIC LUPUS ERYTHEMATOSUS

In systemic, or disseminated, lupus erythematosus, the myocardial lesions consist mainly of fibrinoid changes in the connective tissue with a cellular reaction. Similar changes may affect the valves, notably the mitral and aortic valves. The lesions may heal leaving fibrous scars. Libman and Sacks (1924) described a distinctive type of valvar and mural endocarditis that occurs in this condition. It is characterized by verrucous lesions along the line of closure of the valves, as well as along the under surface of the leaflets extending onto the mural endocardium. The disease usually has a systematized character and involves many systems, including the heart. Cardiovascular manifestations are infrequent in children.

Cardiac manifestations

The dominating cardiac feature is pericarditis. A pericardial friction rub is often present, and the chest radiograph will show an enlarged heart. Myocardial involvement may underscore heart failure. The latter feature may be complicated further by valvar dysfunction, either as part of the disease or secondary to the ventricular volume overload and accompanying dilation of the chambers. Mitral insufficiency is the most frequent valvar abnormality, although significant aortic insufficiency has been described (Oh et al, 1974). The electrocardiogram will usually show non-specific changes of the ST segment. Disturbances of rhythm and conduction are frequent.

Treatment

The treatment of choice is corticosteroids, which also have a favourable effect on the management of cardiac dysfunction. Deleterious effects on the heart have been described, nonetheless, from chronic administration of suppressive doses of prednisone (Bulkley and Roberts, 1975).

DERMATOMYOSITIS

Pathology

Dermatomyositis is a multisystemic disease of uncertain aetiology that is characterized by diffuse non-suppurative inflammation of striated muscle and skin (Sullivan, 1982). It is initially characterized by oedema of the subendothelial connective tissue, with collection of inflammatory changes round cells in both skin and muscle. Hyalinized material is found in the media of the arterioles, with inflammatory reaction in and around the vessels. In the phase of healing, there may be deposition of calcium salts in skin, subcutaneous tissue and interfascial planes of muscle. The myocardium may show loss of striations, fragmentation and vascularization of muscle fibres. The interstitial tissues of the heart may show swelling and oedema.

Cardiac involvement

Tachycardia is the most common finding. The electrocardiogram may be normal, although occasionally abnormal T waves may be encountered. Complete heart block and arrhythmias have been reported. Murmurs are heard in about one tenth of cases. Cardiac enlargement and heart failure are uncommon. Acute myocarditis, and pericarditis with a pericardial friction rub, have been described.

Treatment and prognosis

Long-term treatment with prednisone is beneficial in the majority. Other immunosuppressive agents are rarely required (Dubowitz, 1978; Sullivan, 1982). Most children will recover, and medication can be discontinued over 1 or 2 years. Functional ability is good in most patients.

——— PERICARDITIS ———

Pericarditis is defined as an inflammatory reaction of the pericardium in response to injury, whether infectious or non-infectious in nature. Its precise incidence is unknown, but there is evidence that, clinically, pericarditis may often pass unnoticed. Indeed, clinical recognition will depend heavily upon the type and severity of the pericardial reaction. When limited, it may easily resolve without attracting notice. It often coexists with myocarditis. As with myocarditis, the aetiology of pericarditis differs considerably from one part of the world to the other. Infectious causes, such as tuberculosis, and pericarditis caused by a generalized autoimmune disease, such as rheumatic fever, are rare in the Western World. They still form a major threat in other parts of the world.

PATHOPHYSIOLOGY ——————

The pericardium is a double layered sack lined by mesothelial cells and lubricated by a thin film of fluid. This construction enables the heart to move freely without friction. An accumulation of fluid within the sack, however, may cause cardiac dysfunction, particularly when it occurs over a short period of time. Likewise, a fibrous change within the pericardial layers may have an effect upon cardiac function.

An inflammatory response of pericardium may cause exudation as part of the reaction. This may lead, in turn, to an excessive accumulation of fluid within the pericardial sack. This can cause a rise in intrapericardial pressure. Compression of the heart by the pericardial fluid can cause a decrease of cardiac output, stroke volume and systolic arterial pressure, resulting in cardiac tamponade. The pericardium is relatively inelastic and, as a result, the pressure–volume relationship of the heart has a progressively rising slope. An initial increase in intrapericardial fluid does not result in a substantial rise in pressure, whereas additional accumulation of fluid will very soon result in a significant elevation of pressure (Holt, 1970; Shabetai, 1976). Likewise, in patients with signs and symptoms of cardiac tamponade owing to excessive intrapericardial fluid, evacuation of a small amount may cause a marked decrease in pressure.

The time during which the fluid accumulates plays a major role. Slow accumulation of fluid will stretch the pericardium gradually. This is much better tolerated than conditions that lead to a rapid increase, and hence equally rapid build-up of pressure. In more severe forms of pericarditis, the increased pressures will lead to impaired venous return during ventricular diastole. This results in a decline in cardiac output (Shabetai et al, 1970; Shabetai, 1976). During inspiration, the blood pressure may fall abnormally over more than 10 mmHg, leading to a paradoxical pulse. In its most severe form, no further filling of the cardiac chambers is possible, and the patient will die with signs of electromechanic dissociation. Acute cardiac tamponade is rare in infants and children.

In patients with a haemodynamically significant build-up of pressure within the pericardial sack, several compensatory mechanisms develop in an attempt to maintain an adequate cardiac output. An increase in heart rate, together with peripheral vasoconstriction, increases the afterload of the heart. This results in a higher mean pressure at the expense of a narrow pulse pressure. These compensatory mechanisms are vital. They should not be corrected, as cardiac output may then drop even further (Nadas and Fyler, 1972). Injudicious use of diuretics in such circumstances can make matters worse rather than better.

Constrictive pericarditis was once most commonly seen as a complication of tuberculous pericarditis. Acute viral or idiopathic pericarditis is now a more common antecedent (Cameron et al, 1987). It is uncommon in childhood.

CLINICAL FEATURES

In adults with acute fibrinous pericarditis, precordial pain is often the dominant symptom. In childhood, this symptom is less important. When it does occur, the site, radiation, severity and character of the pain are highly variable. The discomfort may be diminished by sitting up and leaning forward. Other manoeuvres, such as inspiration, deep breathing and coughing, may increase the sensation of discomfort. At this stage, the pericarditis does not necessarily interfere with the circulation.

At physical examination, the friction rub is the most typical and diagnostic finding, although its absence does not exclude the presence of pericarditis. The rub is maximal along the left sternal border but is often audible over the entire precordium. It is best heard with the patient sitting up or leaning forward. When the pericardial effusion increases, the friction rub may be heard intermittently, or it may disappear totally. The presence of a pericardial rub, however, does not exclude the presence of a large effusion. With marked effusions, the heart sounds are often muffled, and they may become extremely faint. It should be noted that the development of a pericardial effusion does not always produce symptoms and, hence, may escape clinical notice.

With an increase of fluid, cardiac tamponade will develop. This is characterized by a rise in venous pressure, an enlargement of the liver and the presence of peripheral oedema. The systolic blood pressure is low, and the pulse pressure is narrow. A paradoxical pulse is often present. The patient usually appears sick, anxious and distressed and is cyanosed and dyspnoeic. Moreover, fever, tachycardia and tachypnoea are commonly present. Signs and symptoms of toxicity are often present when the pericarditis is caused by bacterial infection. This condition should be considered an emergency, requiring prompt medical or surgical treatment.

In the presence of a large pericardial effusion the lower part of the lung may be compressed. This can result in dullness on percussion and bronchial breathing laterally and at the back, a combination known as Ewart's sign.

INVESTIGATIONS

ECHOCARDIOGRAPHY

Cross-sectional echocardiography is the most important diagnostic technique. If a pericardial effusion is suspected as a cause of haemodynamic compromise, the examination should be undertaken urgently. In the normal heart, the pericardial sack is hardly identified. The anterior right ventricular wall of the heart is in direct contact with the anterior chest wall, and the inferior and posterior left ventricular walls are in direct contact with the diaphragm, posterior mediastinal structures and the pleura.

A pericardial effusion will widen the space because of the accumulation of fluid, which does not reflect ultrasound (Figure 63.5). Echocardiography will show this echo-free space around the heart. Thickening of the pericardium is an uncommon finding. A combination of M-mode and cross-sectional echocardiography permits a rough estimation of the quantity of the collected fluid.

The majority of patients with small-to-moderate effusions demonstrate essentially normal cardiac motion. Patients with an acute small-volume tamponade produced by a small volume of fluid may demonstrate a limited motion of the cardiac walls. In the presence of large effusions, excessive cardiac displacement may occur. This is observed mainly in benign viral pericarditis and malignancies, but it is rare in children. Cardiac tamponade is primarily a clinical and not an echocardiographic diagnosis (Spodick, 1996). The echocardiographic differentiation of a haemodynamically insignificant effusion from one with tamponade is not easy, but the findings indicating tamponade are diastolic collapse of the right atrial, right ventricular and left atrial walls (Shiina et al, 1979; Armstrong et al, 1982; Reddy et al, 1990). In addition, when there is tamponade, Doppler interrogation of the superior caval vein will show an absence of diastolic flow (Byrd and Linden, 1990).

RADIOLOGY

The cardiac silhouette may be normal as long as a sizeable effusion is absent. Fluid in the pericardial sack manifests itself radiologically as an enlarged silhouette. In borderline cases, comparison with a previous radiography can be most helpful. As fluid accumulates, the cardiac silhouette increases. This manifests as blunting of the cardiophrenic angles, and disappearance of the sharp angulations between contiguous structures of the heart and great vessels. The cardiac silhouette assumes the overall shape of a water bottle (Figure 63.6a). In infants, nonetheless, the configuration of the heart may be atypical (Figure 63.6b).

Changes in the configuration of the cardiac silhouette are occasionally observed when the patient is changed from a recumbent to an upright position. In children, this is not a very reliable finding.

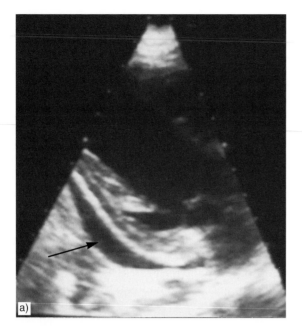

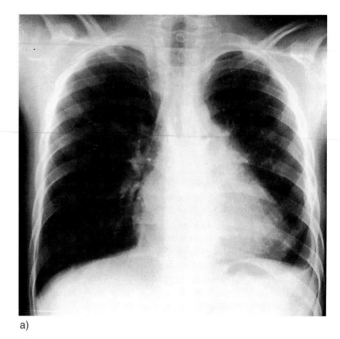

a)

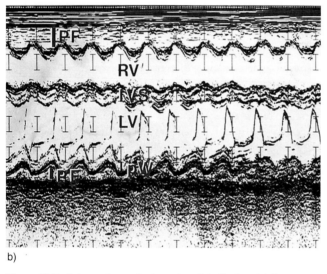

b)

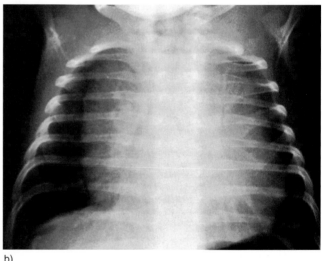

b)

Figure 63.5. Echocardiography in pericardial effusion. (a) A parasternal long-axis view shows an echo-free space posterior to the left ventricular posterior wall (arrow). (b) M-mode echocardiogram shows a pericardial effusion (PF). It is seen anterior to the right ventricle (RV) and posterior to the posterior wall of the left ventricle (pW). LV, cavity of left ventricle.

Figure 63.6. (a) Chest radiograph in a boy with viral pericarditis. The heart is slightly enlarged; the sharp angulations between contiguous structures of the heart have disappeared. (b) Chest radiograph of a 3-month-old infant with a large pericardial effusion. The heart shadow is greatly enlarged and the vascular pedicle is broadened by the accumulation of mediastinal fluid.

ELECTROCARDIOGRAPHY

Sequential electrocardiographic changes are observed in most patients with pericarditis (Figure 63.7) (Spodick, 1974; Liebman, 1982; Baljepally and Spodick, 1998). They are the result of subepicardial myocardial damage. In the initial stage of the disease, the ST segment is elevated in almost all leads except for leads V_I and aVR, which often remain unaltered. After a few hours to days, the ST segments may return to the baseline, and the T waves may become flat (Figure 63.8). In a later stage, the T waves may become inverted. The electrocardiogram

may return to normal during convalescence, although the T waves may remain inverted for several months; occasionally they may remain in this form as a permanent change.

In patients with pericardial effusion, the electrocardiogram may have a generalized low voltage. A shift of the PQ segment has also been described as an important feature (Spodick, 1973). Sinus tachycardia unrelated to fever or other cardiac problems may be present in the initial phase. Supraventricular tachycardias, and ventricular ectopic beats, are a regular phenomenon (Dunn and Rinkenberger, 1976). None of these changes, however,

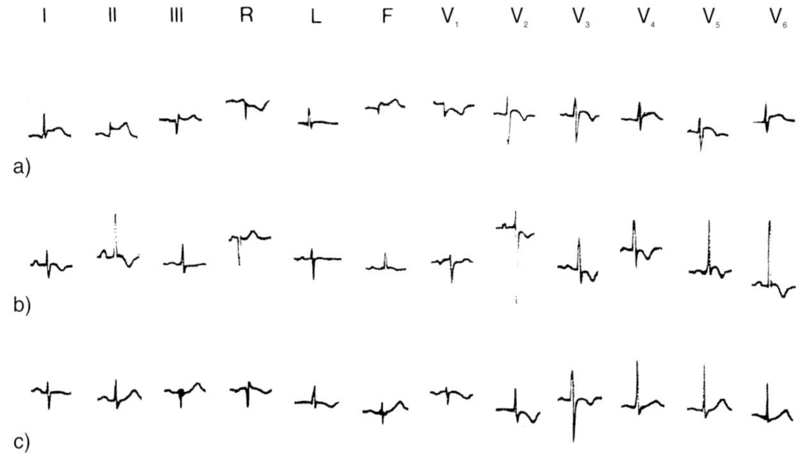

I   II   III   R   L   F   V₁   V₂   V₃   V₄   V₅   V₆

a)

b)

c)

Figure 63.7. Electrocardiograms of a 7-year-old boy with pericarditis. (a) On the first day of fever and precordial pain there is ST elevation in nearly all leads. (b) After 4 weeks, there are negative T waves, especially in the leads I, II, V₄–V₆. (c) After 1 year, the electrocardiogram is nearly normal but there is still a flat T wave in lead I.

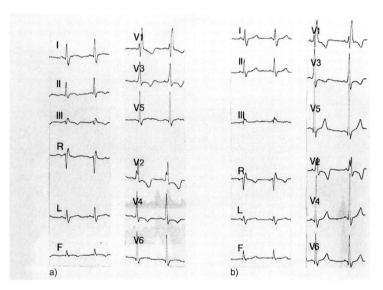

Figure 63.8. Electrocardiogram of a 14-year-old girl with pericarditis. (a) On admission, 1 week after onset of the disease, the T waves are flat in the leads I, II, V₅ and V₆ and negative in II, III, ACF and V₄. (b) After 4 weeks, the electrocardiogram is normal again.

can be considered specific for pericarditis. Indeed, the electrocardiogram may occasionally remain completely normal.

PERICARDIOCENTESIS

Where there is tamponade, or where the pericardial fluid needs to be drained for diagnostic reasons, the choice is between percutaneous aspiration and surgical evacuation. The echocardiographic appearances are of critical importance in determining the correct approach.

Where there is tamponade, with a large, tense collection of non-loculated fluid, aspiration is usually the quickest and safest approach. This should always be done with echocardiographic guidance. Screening with

X-ray and electrocardiographic guidance are also of value. The safest approach is sub-xiphoid. Ideally, the patient should be tilted head up, thus encouraging the pericardial fluid to collect anteriorly and inferiorly. Under local anaesthesia, a needle is inserted at about 45 degrees to the abdominal wall. It should be angled cranially and slightly toward the left. The needle is aspirated as it is advanced. As the pericardium is entered, it is felt to give and the pericardial fluid will fill the syringe. If the needle is connected to the V lead of an electrocardiogram, the signal will indicate if it has been advanced too far and touched the heart. Radiography can be used, or echocardiographic contrast can be injected, if there is doubt about the position of the tip of the needle.

Once the pericardium is entered, it is best to exchange the needle for a soft pigtail catheter over a wire, using the

Seldinger technique. The pericardial fluid can then be aspirated. If the accumulation is recurrent, the pigtail catheter can be left in place as a pericardial drain. The fluid should be sent for bacteriology and cytology.

Percutaneous aspiration is a straightforward and safe procedure where there is a large anterior collection of fluid. Where the collection is small, or predominantly posterior, aspiration is more difficult and more dangerous. Under these circumstances, or when the fluid is loculated or the accumulation is recurrent, surgical evacuation with the creation of a pericardial window should be considered.

SPECIFIC SYNDROMES

ACUTE BACTERIAL PERICARDITIS

Since the introduction of antibiotics, the incidence of acute bacterial pericarditis has declined drastically. In the Western World, it has become a rare condition. Nevertheless, it remains an important disease from the point of view of therapy and prognosis.

In most instances, bacterial pericarditis is caused by septicaemia or direct spread from another site of infection, although such a primary site may pass unnoticed. Well-known sources for bacterial pericarditis are pyelonephritis, osteomyelitis, tonsillitis, bacterial pneumonia and left-sided empyema. Pericarditis may complicate a bacterial endocarditis; it is then usually caused by direct spread from the valvar lesions into the epicardium (see Chapter 66).

The microorganisms most commonly involved are *Haemophilus influenzae*, *Staphylococcus*, *Pneumococcus*, *Meningococcus*, and *Streptococcus* spp. Almost any microorganism, however, may cause pericarditis (Brook and Frazier, 1996). In children in particular, involvement of the pericardium used to be a most hazardous complication of the tuberculous infection.

Usually the disease has an acute onset with pain, high fever, tachycardia and tachypnoea. The children often present with signs and symptoms of toxicity. Indeed, the clinical findings of pericardial tamponade and sepsis are highly suggestive of bacterial pericarditis (Nadas and Fyler, 1972). A friction rub may be present but, on other occasions, the heart may be enlarged with a rapid rate without a friction rub. These findings in the presence of high fever are, nevertheless, most suggestive for the presence of bacterial pericarditis. The patient may rapidly deteriorate, and prompt and adequate therapy is required.

Since bacterial pericarditis is often secondary to another infection elsewhere, an intensive search is always necessary for such a primary source. Whenever possible, the medical treatment of bacterial pericarditis should be based on the identification of the primary organism, so that the most effective treatment can be selected. Any previous antibacterial treatment may interfere with this

goal. Microbiological and chemical investigations of the pericardial fluid are essential. Cytological studies should be performed to exclude a malignancy.

Blood cultures are important, and from three to five sets should be taken in the first 1 or 2 days after admission. In two fifths to four fifths of patients, these cultures will be positive, depending on the organism involved. Specific stains for acid-fast bacteria in the sputum, gastric contents or urine may disclose tuberculosis as the primary disease. Lumbar puncture may be necessary to prove or eliminate concomitant meningitis.

Treatment

Appropriate treatment consists of prompt and adequate antibiotic therapy, together with evacuation of the pericardial fluid (Feldman, 1979; Morgan et al, 1983).

The antibiotic therapy should be guided by the sensitivity of the causative organism. Broad-spectrum antibiotics should be avoided if possible. The duration of the therapy depends upon the clinical response, but a total antibiotic therapy of at least 4 to 6 weeks is necessary. The fever curve, sedimentation rate and white blood count may be helpful in evaluating the effectiveness of the treatment. A pericardial tap may be sufficient for diagnostic purposes, but a needle or a small-bore pericardiocentesis tube is inadequate for the evacuation of the pericardial fluid. This is because the pus is often loculated or thick. Subxiphoid surgical drainage with a large-bore pericardiostomy tube or a pericardiectomy should be performed to obtain the optimal results (Driscoll and Rhodes, 1983; Morgan et al, 1983).

ACUTE VIRAL PERICARDITIS

Viral pericarditis is almost always accompanied by a myocarditis, and it is the latter that usually dominates the clinical manifestations. The precise incidence of viral myopericarditis is unknown, but it is probably much higher than can be distilled from the reports in the literature. This is because it is likely that many cases of viral myopericarditis will pass unnoticed. In approximately four fifths of patients with the typical signs and symptoms of acute pericarditis, the aetiology cannot be established, even after extensive laboratory studies. In many instances, therefore, the viral origin of an acute pericarditis will never be proven. Such cases are better termed 'acute benign' or 'idiopathic' pericarditis. Isolated instances of acute pericarditis have been documented with almost all known viruses. The most frequently encountered cardiotrophic viruses are coxsackievirus (group B), echovirus, adenovirus and those producing influenza (van Reken et al, 1974).

The typical signs and symptoms of acute viral pericarditis are a low-grade temperature, chest pain and a friction rub. They often develop after an infection of the upper respiratory tract. The children appear less toxic than those seen with bacterial pericarditis. The white cell count is usually not elevated, and a relative lymphocytosis may be present. Malaise, feeding problems, tachycardia and tachypnoea are often the presenting symptoms in infants.

Pericardial effusion may develop rapidly, but tamponade is rare with a viral pericarditis in the acute stage. Every attempt should be made to unravel the aetiology of the pericarditis. A definite diagnosis of viral pericarditis requires the isolation of the virus. For this, cultures of throat washings, blood, urine and stools should be obtained. A two- to fourfold rise of neutralizing antibodies is a relatively easy screening method to find out whether or not the patient has had a viral infection. Direct proof, however, that the virus is the immediate cause of the pericarditis can only be obtained when the virus is isolated from the pericardium itself. Hence, a diagnostic pericardiocentesis must be considered. Pericardial fluid should be cultured for all types of organism, and extensive biochemical and cytological investigations should be performed.

The therapy of acute pericarditis is symptomatic. It includes bedrest, particularly in those who have myocardial involvement, until the evidence of the infection has disappeared. Precordial pain may be relieved by salicylates, codeine and other drugs. When there are arrhythmias, antiarrhythmic drugs may be used with care. The use of steroids is best avoided, as it is thought to increase the risk of the development of chronic relapsing pericarditis. Pericardiocentesis is indicated in patients showing signs and symptoms of tamponade.

The prognosis is usually favourable. The disease is often self-limiting, with complete recovery in 3 to 4 weeks. In infants and children with diffuse myocardial involvement, nonetheless, the disease may lead to death. In the fullness of time, a recurrent chronic pericarditis, probably related to a cellular immune mechanism, or a constrictive pericarditis may develop and require surgical intervention.

POSTPERICARDECTOMY SYNDROME

Any episode of acute pericarditis may be followed by recurrent pericarditis. This includes the acute pericarditis that accompanies myocardial infarction, when the recurrence is called Dressler's syndrome. Of more relevance in children is the sequence following cardiac surgery with opening of the pericardium, when it is called the postpericardiotomy syndrome. Cardiac surgery is followed by an acute illness, with fever and pericardial and pleural inflammatory reactions. The symptoms develop mostly in the first week after operation, but a febrile period of 2 to 3 weeks is not uncommon. Further relapses are also uncommon but can appear as long as months or years after the initial event.

The pathogenesis of the disease is unclear. Development of anti-heart antibodies in a high percentage of the patients suggests a secondary autoimmune response, possibly in association with a viral infection. There is often an eosinophilia (Engle et al, 1980; Prince and Cunha, 1997).

The earliest clinical manifestation is a sustained or spiked fever, usually between 38 and 39°C. Sometimes the children feel ill, with symptoms of general malaise. All the features of pericarditis may be present, including the typical precordial pain. A friction rub is often present. Cardiac tamponade may require pericardiocentesis. Initially, the fluid withdrawn is serosanguineous, but at a later stage only serous fluid is obtained. The fluid is sterile. The chest radiograph and the electrocardiogram show the features of pericarditis. The echocardiogram is indispensable in demonstrating the pericardial fluid, and in differentiating the syndrome from cardiac failure of other causes. Signs and symptoms of pleural involvement are common, especially on the left.

The disease is self-limiting in 2 to 3 weeks. The most important therapeutic measure is bedrest until the fever has disappeared. Salicylates or indomethacin (indometacin) are useful in lowering the temperature and diminishing the precordial pain. In the severely ill child, a course of prednisolone, starting at 2 mg/kg per day and reducing over 2 weeks, is very effective in normalizing body temperature and reducing the pain. Colchicine has been used in adults with this condition and has been found to be effective in the treatment of flare-ups and in the prevention of recurrences (Alder et al, 1998). There have been reports of its use in children (Yazigi and Abou-Charaf, 1998). Diuretics may be useful in reducing the effusion, but should be used with caution. Prompt pericardiocentesis is indicated in patients who develop cardiac tamponade.

REFERENCES

Abu-Arafeh I, Gray E, Youngson G, Auchterlonie I, Russell G 1995 Myocarditis and haemolytic uraemic syndrome. Archives of Disease in Childhood 72: 46–47

Alder Y, Guindo J, Finkelstein Y et al 1998 Colchicine for large pericardial effusion. Clinical Cardiology 21: 143–144

Aretz H T, Billingham M E, Edwards W D 1987 Myocarditis, a histological definition and classification. American Journal of Cardiovascular Pathology 1: 3–13

Armstrong W F, Schilt B P, Helper D J, Dillon J C, Feigenbaum H 1982 Diastolic collapse of the right ventricle with cardiac tamponade: an echocardiographic study. Circulation 65: 1491–1497

Baboonian C, Davies M J, Booth J C, McKenna W J 1997 Coxsackie B viruses and human heart disease. Current Topics in Microbiology and Immunology 223: 31–52

Baljepally R, Spodick D H 1998 PR-segment deviation as the initial electrocardiographic response in acute pericarditis. American Journal of Cardiology 81: 1505–1506

Barbaro G, Di Lorenzo G, Grisorio B, Barbarini G 1998 Incidence of dilated cardiomyopathy and detection of HIV in myocardial cells of HIV-positive patients. New England Journal of Medicine 339: 1093–1099

Baysal K, Sancak R, Ozturk F, Uysal S, Gurses N 1998 Cardiac involvement due to *Salmonella typhi* infections in children. Annals of Tropical Paediatrics 18: 23–25

Brook I, Frazier E H 1996 Microbiology of acute purulent pericarditis. A 12-year experience in a military hospital. Archives of Internal Medicine 156: 1857–1860

Brown C A, O'Connell J B 1995 Myocarditis and idiopathic dilated cardiomyopathy. American Journal of Medicine 99: 309–314

Bulkley B H, Roberts W C 1975 The heart in systemic lupus erythematosus and the changes induced by corticosteroid therapy. A study of 36 necropsy patients. American Journal of Medicine 58: 243–264

Byrd B F III, Linden R W 1990 Superior vena cava Doppler flow velocity patterns in pericardial disease. American Journal of Cardiology 65: 1464

Cameron J, Oesterle S N, Baldwin J C, Hancock E W 1987 The aetiology spectrum of constrictive pericarditis. American Heart Journal 113: 354–360

Daly K, Richardson P J, Olsen E G J et al 1984 Acute myocarditis – role of histological and virological examination in the diagnosis and assessment of immunosuppressive treatment. British Heart Journal 51: 30–35

Driscoll D J, Rhodes K H 1983 Treatment of purulent carditis – a comment. Journal of Thoracic and Cardiovascular Surgery 85: 531

Dubowitz V 1978 Muscle disorders in childhood. Saunders, Philadelphia, PA

Dunn M, Rinkenberger R L 1976 Clinical aspects of acute pericarditis. In: Spodick D H (ed.) Pericardial diseases. Cardiovascular clinics 7, 3rd edn. Davis, Philadephia, PA, p 131–147

Engle M A, Zabriskie J B, Senterfit L B, Gay W A Jr, O'Loughlin J E, Ehlers K A 1980 Viral illness and the post pericardiotomy syndrome. A prospective study in children. Circulation 62: 1151–1158

Feldman W 1979 Bacterial etiology and mortality of purulent pericarditis in paediatric patients. American Journal of Diseases of Children 133: 641–644

Fenoglio J J Jr, Ursell P C, Kellogg C F, Drusin R E, Wiss M B 1983 Diagnosis and classification of myocarditis by endomyocardial biopsy. New England Journal of Medicine 308: 12–18

Forfang K, Lippest C T 1974 Transient left posterior hemiblock in acute myocarditis. Journal of Electrocardiography 7: 83–85

Goodwin J F 1982 The frontiers of cardiomyopathy. British Heart Journal 48: 1–18

Grogan M, Redfield M M, Bailey K R et al 1995 Long-term outcome of patients with biopsy-proved myocarditis: comparison with idiopathic dilated cardiomyopathy. Journal of the American College of Cardiology 26: 80–84

Holt J P 1970 The normal pericardium. American Journal of Cardiology 26: 455–465

Horowitz H W, Belkin R N 1995 Acute myopericarditis resulting from Lyme disease. American Heart Journal 130: 176–178

Ino T, Okubo M, Akimoto K, Nishimoto K, Yabuta K, Kawai S 1995 Corticosteroid therapy for ventricular tachycardia in children with silent lymphocytis myocarditis. Journal of Pediatrics 126: 304–308

Lambert E C, Moore A A D, Hohn A R 1968 Myocarditis. In: Watson H (ed.) Pediatric cardiology. Lloyd-Luke, London, p 741–749

Lerner A M, Wilson F M, Reyes P 1975 Enteroviruses and the heart (with special emphasis on the probable role of coxsackieviruses, group B, types 1–5). Epidemiological and experimental studies. Modern Concepts in Cardiovascular Diseases 44: 7–11

Libman E, Sacks B 1924 A hitherto undescribed form of valvular and mural endocarditis. Archives of Internal Medicine 33: 701–737

Liebman I 1982 S T and T abnormalities due to various 'primary' causes. In: Liebman J, Plonsey R, Gillette P C (eds) Pediatric electrocardiography. Williams & Wilkins, Baltimore, MD, p 192–201

Lipshultz S E, Fox C H, Perez-Atayde A R 1990 Identification of human immunodeficiency virus-1 RNA and DNA in the heart of a child with cardiovascular abnormalities and congenital acquired immune deficiency syndrome. American Journal of Cardiology 66: 246–250

Lipschultz S E, Easley K A, Orav E J et al 1998 Left ventricular structure and function in children infected with human immunodeficiency virus: the prospective P2C2 HIV Multicenter Study. Pediatric Pulmonary and Cardiac Complications of Vertically Transmitted HIV Infection (P2C2 HIV) Study Group. Circulation 97: 1246–1256

Luginbuhl L M, Orav E J, McIntosh K, Lipschultz S E 1993 Cardiac morbidity and related mortality in children with HIV infection. Journal of the American Medical Association 269: 2869–2875

Maisch B, Herzum M, Hufnagel G, Schonian U 1996 Immunosuppressive and immunomodulatory treatment for myocarditis. Current Opinion in Cardiology 11: 310–324

Mason J W, Billingham M E, Ricci D R 1980 Treatment of acute inflammatory myocarditis assisted by endomyocardial biopsy. American Journal of Cardiology 45: 1037–1044

Mason J W, O'Connell J B, Herskowitz A et al 1995 A clinical trial of immunosuppresive therapy for myocarditis. The Myocarditis Treatment Trial Investigators. New England Journal of Medicine 333: 269–275

McNamara D M, Rosenblum W D, Janosko K M et al 1997 Intravenous immune globulin in the therapy of myocarditis and acute cardiomyopathy. Circulation 95: 2476–2478

Morales A R, Adelman S, Fine G 1971 Varicella myocarditis: a case of sudden death. Archives of Pathology 91: 29–31

Morgan R J, Stephenson L W, Woolf P K, Eda R N, Edmunds L H 1983 Surgical treatment of purulent pericarditis in children. Journal of Thoracic and Cardiovascular Surgery 85: 527–531

Nadas A S, Fyler D C 1972 Pediatric cardiology: diseases of the pericardium. Saunders, Philadelphia, PA, p 249–261

Nagi K S, Joshi R, Thakur R K 1996 Cardiac manifestations of Lyme disease. Canadian Journal of Cardiology 12: 503–506

O'Connell J B, Henlan R E, Robinson J A et al 1984 Gallium-67 imaging in patients with dilated cardiomyopathy and biopsy proven myocarditis. Circulation 70: 58–62

Oh W M C, Taylor R T, Olsen E G J 1974 Aortic regurgitation in systemic lupus erythematosus requiring aortic valve replacement. British Heart Journal 36: 413–416

Passarino G, Burlo P, Ciccone G et al 1997 Prevalence of myocarditis at autopsy in Turin, Italy. Archives of Pathology and Laboratory Medicine 121: 619–622

Prince S E, Cunha B A 1997 Postpericardectomy syndrome. Heart and Lung 26: 165–168

Reddy P S, Curtiss E I, Uretsky B F 1990 Spectrum of haemodynamic changes in cardiac tamponade. American Journal of Cardiology 66: 1487–1491

Rezkalla S, Kloner R A, Khaw B A et al 1989 Detection of experimental myocarditis by monoclonal antimyosin antibody FAB fragments. American Heart Journal 117: 391–395

Rezkalla S H, Raikar S, Kloner R A 1996 Treatment of viral myocarditis with focus on captopril. American Journal of Cardiology 77: 634–637

Rowe R D, Freedom R M, Mehrizi A, Bloom K R 1981 The neonate with congenital heart disease: myocarditis. Saunders, Philadelphia, PA, p 409–412

Scott L P, Gutelius M F, Parrott R H 1970 Children with acute respiratory tract infections: an electrocardiographic survey. American Journal Diseases of Children 119: 111–113

Sevy S, Kelly J, Ernst H 1968 Fatal paroxysmal tachycardia associated with focal myocarditis of the Purkinjie system in a fourteen month old girl. Journal of Pediatrics 72: 796–800

Shabetai R 1976 Pericardial diseases. In: Spodick D H (ed.) Cardiovascular clinic 7, 3rd edn. Davis, Philadelphia, PA, p 67–89

Shabetai R, Fowler N O, Guntheroth W G 1970 The hemodynamics of cardiac tamponade and constrictive pericarditis. American Journal of Cardiology 26: 480

Shapiro L M, Rozkovec A, Cambridge G, Hallidie-Smith K A, Goodwin J F 1983 myocarditis in siblings leading to chronic heart failure. European Heart Journal 4: 742–746

Shiina S, Yaginuma T, Kondok K, Kawai N, Hosoda S 1979 Echocardiographic evaluation of impending cardiac tamponade. Journal of Cardiography 9: 555–557

Shimizu C, Rambaud C, Cheron G et al 1995 Molecular identification of viruses in sudden death associated with myocarditis and pericarditis. Pediatric Infectious Disease Journal 14: 584–588

Spodick D H 1973 Diagnostic electrocardiographic sequences in acute pericarditis: significance of PR segment and PR vector changes. Circulation 48: 575–581

Spodick D H 1974 Electrocardiogram in acute pericarditis: distributions of morphologic and axial changes by stages. American Journal of Cardiology 33: 470–474

Spodick D H 1996 Bedside diagnosis of cardiac tamponade. Texas Heart Institute Journal 23: 239

Sullivan D B 1982 Dermatomyositis. In: Cassidy J T (ed.) Textbook of pediatric rheumatology. Wiley, New York, p 407–432

van Kirk J E, Simons A B, Armstrong W R 1974 Candida myocarditis causing complete atrioventricular block. Journal of the American Medical Association 227: 931–933

van Reken D, Strauss A, Hernandez A, Feigin R D 1974 Infectious pericarditis in children. Journal of Pediatrics 85: 165–169

Yazigi A, Abou-Charaf L C 1998 Colchicine for recurrent pericarditis in children. Acta Paediatrica 87: 603–604

64

Acute rheumatic fever

E. E. Ortiz[1]

INTRODUCTION

Rheumatic fever is an acute, non-suppurative inflammatory disease that follows group A streptococcal infection of the throat. At the beginning of the 21st century, and 400 years after the first report, it has remained the most common cause of acquired heart disease in children and young adults. It has continued to be a major public health problem worldwide, but particularly in developing countries. The World Health Organization, in 1990, estimated that 12 million people are affected, with more than 400 000 deaths occurring annually and with hundreds of thousands more, mainly children, left disabled. Although the incidence has declined significantly in developed countries, the emergence of significant outbreaks of rheumatic fever in the USA and Europe suggests that all factors involved in the disease process have not yet been fully elucidated.

HISTORICAL BACKGROUND

Although the manifestations of rheumatic fever were described separately in the latter half of the 17th century, the full clinical syndrome was appreciated only near the end of the 19th century.

Acute migratory polyarthritis, then known as 'acute articular rheumatism' was the first major manifestation described by Guilleaume de Baillou in France. Almost simultaneously, Thomas Syndenham of England in 1605 distinguished this form of arthritis from gout. The following year, he also described 'St Vitus dance', the disorder of movement that is now called Syndenham's chorea.

In 1761, Morgagni of Italy first described abnormalities in the valves of hearts at postmortem from patients with acute articular rheumatism. The subcutaneous nodules were first described in 1813 by William C. Wells of London, when he published 16 cases of 'rheumatism of the heart' (Benedek, 1984).

Five years later (1818), the first clinical description of rheumatic heart disease was reported by Rene T. Laennec when he introduced the stethoscope. Numerous reports on the association of rheumatic arthritis with involvement of the heart followed, but the unification of carditis, polyarthritis, chorea, subcutaneous nodules and erythema marginatum as the full syndrome of rheumatic fever was made only in 1886 by Cheadle. The 'Aschoff nodule', the pathognomonic microscopic lesion of rheumatic carditis, was described by Ludwig Aschoff in 1904 (Benedek, 1984).

The correlation between the history of streptococcal sore throat and rheumatic fever was strongly suspected in the early 1900s. It was not until 1931, however, that the connection was firmly established by means of convincing bacteriological and epidemiological studies done by Coburn in the United States of America (Coburn, 1931) and Collis in England (Collis, 1938). This was further confirmed by studies that showed that recurrence of rheumatic fever could be prevented by continuous use of antibiotics against streptococcus (Coburn and Moore, 1939). In 1951, Wannamaker went one step further and showed that the first attack could be prevented by adequate treatment of the streptococcal pharyngitis with penicillin.

EPIDEMIOLOGY

In general, the epidemiology of acute rheumatic fever seems to follow that of streptococcal pharyngitis. It occurs with equal frequency in males and females, with the peak age of onset occurring from 5 to 15 years of age. Although very uncommon before the age of 4 years, we have seen 12 children younger than this age during the

---

[1] Adapted from the chapter prepared for the 1st edition by the late I. P. Sukumar.

last 5 years with acute rheumatic fever complicated by carditis. The syndrome is usually associated with poverty, malnutrition and overcrowding, although its occurrence among the middle class communities in the United States did not follow this historical association. It is also more common in urban centres than rural communities.

It occurs in all races, and in all parts of the world, although the higher prevalence in certain groups are well documented, such as the Maoris of New Zealand (Caughey et al, 1975). Although it is traditionally considered to be a disease of the temperate climate, it is now more commonly reported in tropical climates, particularly in developing countries.

The general decline in the incidence of rheumatic fever in many areas of the world has been attributed to improved economic standards, decreased crowding at home, wider provision of health care and antibiotic therapy, and change in the virulence of the causative organisms (Stollerman, 1975). This decline is best exemplified in the United States of America where the annual incidence per 100 000 population, decreased from 100–200 in the early 1900s, to 12.3 in the 1930s, 2.9 in the late 1960s and 0.5 in the mid-1980s (Gordis, 1985; Markowitz, 1985; WHO, 1988; Ferguson et al, 1991). In most developing countries, however, it has remained a major problem of public health. The most recent compilation of epidemiological data shows that the incidence of acute attacks ranges from less than 5 to more than 100 per 100 000 population. Among school children, the incidence ranged from 0.1 to 22 per 1000, with prevalence generally higher in countries with large proportions of the population having low incomes (Achutti and Achutti, 1992). It must be stated, however, that the reported decline in incidence and prevalence may be underesti-

mated because of inherent difficulties in obtaining epidemiological data, particularly in developing countries where social and health care services are less than adequate.

The prevalence of the group A streptococcus in the upper respiratory tract of healthy school children ranges from 10 to 50%. This may reflect either an acute infection or a carrier state. In acute infections, the patient harbours the organism and develops antibodies as a response, whereas, in the carrier state, the involved person does not develop antibodies. The incidence of rheumatic fever following documented streptococcal pharyngitis varies, ranging from 0.3 to 3.0%. The rate of 'attack' has been shown to be considerably higher in individuals who have had a previous rheumatic episode than in the normal population (Taranta, 1967).

PATHOGENESIS

Whereas the relationship between group A streptococcal pharyngitis and the development of acute rheumatic fever had been established firmly as early as the 1930s, the exact mechanism of pathogenesis remains elusive. Recent epidemiological data and research seem to show that the disease is found only in humans, and that the acute episode only occurs in genetically susceptible patients after infection by certain rheumatogenic strains of group A streptococcus. Hypersensitivity appears to be the common ground. Currently accepted evidences regarding this relationship can be considered in terms of the genetic susceptibility of the host, the nature of the streptococcal structure, the influence of copathogens, and the immunological reactions initiated (Figure 64.1).

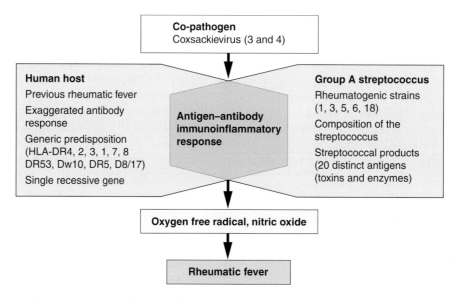

Figure 64.1 The interactions between the susceptible human host and rheumatogenic group A streptococcus to produce the clinical syndrome of rheumatic fever.

THE GENETIC SUSCEPTIBILITY OF THE HUMAN HOST

Relatively few individuals (2–3%) will develop rheumatic fever after acute streptococcal pharyngitis (Siegel et al, 1961). However, in those who have had previous episodes of rheumatic fewer, recurrence will occur in approximately half (Rammelkamp, 1957).

Children who develop rheumatic fever demonstrate an exaggerated antibody response to toxins produced by the streptococcus (such as antistreptodysin O) compared with other patients who recovered from streptococcus pharyngitis and did not develop rheumatic fever (Taranta et al, 1964; Schulman et al, 1974; Morell et al, 1990).

Genetic predisposition is evidenced by high concordance (20%) among monozygotic twins, and by high incidence among the Maoris of New Zealand compared with their Caucasian neighbours irrespective of their economic and social status (Caughey et al, 1975). Further evidence is provided by the association of the disease with inheritance of HLA antigen markers (HLA-DR4,2,3,1,78-DR-53, Dw10) among different populations and ethnic groups (Anastasiou-Nana et al, 1986; Ayoub et al, 1986; Jhinghan et al, 1986; Maharaj et al, 1987; Rajapakse et al, 1987; Guilherme, 1991), by the protective effect of HLA-DR5 (Carlquist et al, 1995) and by the association with high level of expression of a B cell alloantigen D8/17 (Taneja et al, 1989). The genetic susceptibility to rheumatic fever is mediated by a single recessive gene (Read et al, 1938; Wilson and Schweitzer, 1954).

THE RHEUMATOGENIC GROUP A STREPTOCOCCUS

Among the group A β-haemolytic streptococcuses, there are nephritogenic strains (49, 58, 57, 60 and 63) causing pyodermas and impetigo and rheumatogenic strains (1, 3, 5, 6 and 18) causing rheumatic fever (Wannamaker, 1970).

The group A streptococcus is a Gram-positive chain-forming coccus which may have an outer hyaluronic acid capsule when freshly isolated from clinical material (Figure 64.2). The mucoid appearance on culture is probably a result of hydrolysis of the capsule hyaluronidase that is produced during the growth of the organism.

Past and recent outbreaks of both infection by the group A streptococcus and rheumatic fever showed highly mucoid colonies in samples grown in blood agar (Kaplan et al, 1989a; Johnson et al, 1992). Below the outer capsule is the protein layer, which consists of two major protein antigens, the M and T proteins. An R protein may be seen in some strains. The M proteins are type specific and are thought to be important in virulence (Lancefield, 1962). They also provide protection against subsequent streptococcal infection. Nearly 70 distinct antigenic types of this protein exist. Most M types of group A streptococcus are 'rheumatogenic' (Stollerman, 1969; Wannamaker, 1970). T proteins constitute the other major antigenic system of the group A streptococcus and serve as an extremely useful epidemiological marker (Dillon, 1967; Parker, 1969). Another protein associated with the cell wall is the M-associated protein, which is antigenic but not type specific (Widdowson et al, 1971). Inner to the protein layer is a layer of carbohydrates that is specific to the streptococcal group. These carry specific immunological groups designated A to U, with a further provisional group V to Z (excluding I and J). Purified group A carbohydrate has been shown to be non-toxic to animals when given intravenously (Schmidt, 1952; Ginsburg, 1972). The carbohydrate has also been shown to cross-react with the structural glycoproteins of cardiac valves (Goldstein et al, 1968) and epithelial cells of the thymus (Lyampert et al, 1976). The peptidoglycan (mucopeptide) is the basal layer of the cell wall and has been shown to have many properties in common with the endotoxins of Gram-negative bacteria (Krause, 1972). When given intravenously, it causes extensive granulomatous lesions in the heart. In combination with carbohydrate, it seems to have arthropathic properties (Rotta and Bednar, 1969; Cromartie et al, 1977). Another cell-associated component (lipoteichoic

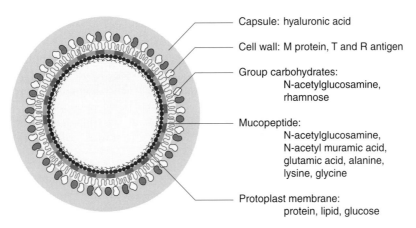

Capsule: hyaluronic acid

Cell wall: M protein, T and R antigen

Group carbohydrates:
N-acetylglucosamine,
rhamnose

Mucopeptide:
N-acetylglucosamine,
N-acetyl muramic acid,
glutamic acid, alanine,
lysine, glycine

Protoplast membrane:
protein, lipid, glucose

Figure 64.2 The components of streptococcus that can cross-react with the human host.

Table 64.1 Immunological cross-reactions between streptococcal components and mammalian constituents

Streptococcal component	Mammalian tissue constituent
Steptococcal hyaluronic acid	Mammalian hyaluronic acid and protein polysaccharide
Group A carbohydrate	Glycoproteins of heart valves
Protein cell wall	Sarcolemma of cardiac and skeletal muscle
Protein of cell membrane	Sarcolemma of cardiac and skeletal muscle
Glycoprotein of cell membrane	Glycoprotein of glomerular basement membrane
Antigen of cell membrane	Histocompatibility antigen

Adapted from McCarty, 1972.

acid) is located on the fimbrias of the organism and seems to be important in the colonization of the human oropharyngeal mucosa (Beachey and Ofek, 1976). The protoplast membrane of the group A streptococcus has been shown to cross-react with the sarcolemma of the myocardial muscle fibre (Zabriskie and Freimer, 1966). Various streptococcal components overall, however, are known to cross-react with the tissue components of the host (Table 64.1) (McCarty, 1972).

The group A streptococcus produces a large number of extracellular products that include at least 20 distinct antigens including toxins and enzymes (Halbert and Keatinge, 1961). The organism also produces two distinct haemolysins. One is an oxygen-labile, heat-labile, sulphydryl-dependent and highly antigenic component: so-called streptolysin O (Bernheimer, 1972). This is toxic to a whole range of mammalian cells, and in particular to the myocardial cells (Ginsburg, 1972). The other haemolysin (streptolysin S) is an oxygen-stable, non-antigenic component that is highly toxic to a wide variety of mammalian cells. This substance is strongly inhibited by certain non-immunoglobulin serum components (Cuppari et al, 1972; Ginsburg, 1972). Most of the members of group A elaborate fibrinolytic substances that are antigenic. There are two recognized antigenic types of streptokinase. The role for these substances in virulence is minimal. Four immunologically distinct types of deoxyribonucleases (A, B, C and D) are also produced. These substances are non-toxic to mammalian cells because they do not penetrate living cells. Deoxyribonuclease B is highly immunogenic and is the most important product in terms of measurement of serological response. Another extracellular substance is the 'spreading factor', or hyaluronidase, which is highly antigenic (Ginsburg, 1972). In addition to these substances, the group A streptococcus produces nicotinamide adenine dinucleotide glycohydrolase, opacity factor and pyrogenic exotoxins. It is the last that are also thought to be responsible for the skin rash of scarlet fever. These toxins have also been shown to induce production of lymphokines (tumour necrosis factor 2 and interleukins 3 and 6) and are thought to be superantigens (Stevens, 1992).

COPATHOGENS

Burch et al (1970) postulated the possible aetiological role of coxsackieviruses in a proportion of cases of valvar heart disease otherwise grouped as 'rheumatic' heart disease. This is especially so in those in whom an antecedent history of rheumatic fever or serological evidence of streptococcal infection is lacking. Pongpanich (1976) found serological evidence of coxsackie virus B infections in a significant number of patients with acute rheumatic fever and rheumatic heart disease. Recently, the demonstration of antibodies against coxsackie virus B3 and 4 in chronic valvar disease has raised the possibility of a role for these viruses in the pathogenesis. Such findings, however, have not been corroborated in acute rheumatic fever, or in patients with rheumatic heart disease and a definite history of antecedent streptococcal infection. Whether such viral infection acts as a copathogen in rheumatic fever will need further elucidation.

THE IMMUNOLOGICAL REACTION

The various streptococcal components and the formed antibodies have been found to cross-react with antigens found not only in the cardiac muscles and valves but also in the joints, skin and brain (Baird et al, 1991; Todome et al, 1992).

These antiheart antibodies have been demonstrated in atrial tissues removed at the time of mitral valvar surgery (Goldstein et al, 1968). The toxins produced by the organism may also cause damage to the tissues; this, in turn, may lead to formation of antibodies to altered host antigens (Gray et al, 1981; Hafez et al, 1990; Kotb et al, 1990). Such interactions may precipitate, or activate, an antigen–antibody immunoinflammatory response (humoral or cell mediated). Recent studies have shown that the damage seen in heart valves can be linked to activated helper T cells, production of cytokines, damage to tissues from cytotoxic T cells, subsequent activation of macrophages and neutrophils and generation of oxygen free radicals and nitric oxide.

The roles of viral copathogens, the M protein and various pyogenic and pyrogenic exotoxins, acting as superantigens, are being investigated. Such reactions may explain the period of latency of 1 to 5 weeks (on average, 3 weeks) from the time of streptococcal pharyngitis to the clinical manifestations of the disease.

PATHOLOGY

During the acute rheumatic process, pathological inflammatory changes commonly occur in the heart, blood vessels, joints and subcutaneous tissues. The inflammatory reaction of the acute rheumatic process seems to be mediated by an unusual type of immune reaction against both the components of the streptococcus, and against cardiac components (Kaplan and Suchy, 1964; Kaplan and Svec, 1964). It is possible that regional variations in the distribution of these components of cardiac tissue may be at least partly responsible for the preferential distribution of the inflammatory process in certain sites of the heart. Ferrans and Roberts (1980) have emphasized that endocarditis is the most important component of the acute pancarditis. Severe involvement of the mitral annulus is an important factor in the pathogenesis of mitral regurgitation, which results from a combination of valvitis, annular dilation and dysfunction of the papillary muscles. The early exudative changes involve oedema, haemorrhage, tissue necrosis and infiltration by round cells. The myocardium is particularly affected, and damage to the cardiac muscle is often accompanied by interstitial oedema. The proliferative reaction occurs later, and consists essentially of scar formation, production of specific granulomas and thrombosis. The proliferative reaction is found most frequently in the heart, blood vessels, lungs, periarticular spaces, tendons and the central nervous system. Inflammation of the valvar endocardium is manifested by oedema and cellular infiltration. Verrucose lesions composed of fibrinoid and thrombotic material are found predominantly at the line of closure of the valves and on the tendinous cords. The valves are swollen, oedematous and distorted. The parietal endocardium, however, is not usually involved. Involvement of the pericardium may vary from serofibrinous pericarditis to a predominantly exudative form. It seldom leads to chronic pericardial disease. The evolution of these lesions produces the anatomical basis of rheumatic valvar disease. The verrucose lesions become more adherent and the valves develop fibrotic thickening of the leaflets, which tend to adhere to each other. The papillary muscles and tendinous cords, initially thick and oedematous, become scarred and shortened. When recurrences of the rheumatic process occur, fresh vegetations and exudates are deposited on the already affected surfaces.

The Aschoff body, or nodule (Figure 64.3), is the specific principal feature of myocardial involvement in the acute rheumatic process that helps to differentiate this process from a number of similar disorders of collagen (von Glahn, 1947). This lesion, generally considered to be a form of granuloma, occurs mainly in the mural endocardium but may also occur in the interstitium of the myocardium and the epicardium. The Aschoff bodies follow a cycle of development. This starts with an exudative degenerative phase, followed by a granulomatous phase characterized by the presence of typical Aschoff cells. They ultimately heal by fibrosis (Saphir, 1959). Mature Aschoff bodies consist of Aschoff cells, Antischkow cells, plasma cells, lymphocytes, fibrinoid material and hypereosinophilic and fragmented bundles

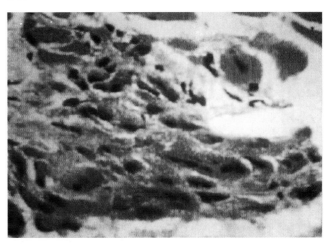

Figure 64.3 The Aschoff nodule in a right ventricular endomyocardial biopsy specimen from a 17-year-old girl with congestive heart failure caused by recurrence of rheumatic fever. This fully developed Aschoff nodule (haematoxylin–eosin, × 330) has a central ill-defined area of oedematous interstitial connective tissue with fraying, fragmentation and disintegration of collagen fibres that stain deeply eosinophilic (fibrinoid necrosis). (From Massell and Narula (1995) with permission.)

of collagen. In the early stages, they contain neutrophilic and eosinophilic leucocytes. The classical concept that Aschoff bodies represent a response of the connective tissue was challenged by Murphy (1959), who postulated that the bodies may develop as a consequence of injury to cardiac muscle or to endocardial smooth muscle. The classical concept, nonetheless, is well supported by most ultrastructural studies and has found wide acceptance among pathologists (Lannigan and Zaki, 1963, 1968). Recent works have demonstrated that components of Aschoff lesions are monocytic and macrophagic in nature, they probably function as antigen-presenting cells, with important pathogenetic roles in the development of carditis (Ros Reis et al, 1982).

The earlier concept that Aschoff bodies are shortlived is contradicted by the finding of Aschoff bodies in left atrial appendages excised in patients undergoing mitral valvotomy who did not have any other evidence of the active rheumatic process (Pai and Kinare, 1969). It is now evident that Aschoff bodies can persist in some patients for a long period following the earlier acute rheumatic process. The presence of Aschoff bodies in atrial biopsies suggests that these bodies may be indicative of either a continuing subclinical rheumatic activity or that they represent a slowly healing residue of the earlier activity, with no relationship to continuing activity. Virmani and Roberts (1977) found that Aschoff bodies occurred more frequently in younger than older patients, were more common in mitral stenosis than in mitral regurgitation in adults and were not necessarily indicative of a recent rheumatic carditis.

Histopathological examinations done on surgical and necropsy specimens from patients with rheumatic fever/rheumatic heart disease in Sao Paulo, Brazil showed mild inflammatory infiltrations in the myocardium or in the valves, but granulation tissue was always present. In contrast, specimens from India showed very prominent inflammatory infiltrations and calcifications (Assis and Higuchi, 1992). These histopathological variations may again be an indication of genetic differences among hosts or, possibly, may depend upon virulence of the infecting streptococcus.

Synovial membranes of joints affected by the acute rheumatic process show oedema, fibrinoid necrosis and granulomatous infiltration with large mononuclear cells. Aschoff bodies may be found in the periarticular tissue and the synovium. These lesions usually heal without any scarring or residual deformity of the joints. Rheumatic subcutaneous nodules show granulation tissue with a central area of fibrinoid necrosis and a surrounding zone with cellular infiltration and proliferative endarteritis in the blood vessels. These nodules also heal without any residual scarring.

Erythema marginatum is caused by vasculitis. This may also be the pathological process responsible for Syndenham's chorea. The lesions, which consist of cellular changes with lymphocytic perivascular infiltrates, are usually located in the basal ganglia and the cerebellum.

DIAGNOSIS

The diagnosis of the acute rheumatic process can be difficult because of the wide variations in the symptomatology and presentation of the disease, the varying severity of the manifestations and its resemblance to other disease processes, especially in the initial stages. The presenting features may be general or specific. The general manifestations are mostly an expression of an underlying active inflammatory process and are considered as minor criterions. The specific manifestations, considered as major criterions, are based on objective clinical findings by a careful and critical physical examination.

THE CLINICAL MANIFESTATIONS

The onset of symptoms usually occurs 2 to 3 weeks after the streptococcal pharyngitis. It involves multiple systems of organs, and the symptomatology varies greatly not only in its presentation but also in severity. The clinical manifestations may vary from apparently symptomless activity to a fulminant illness with severe cardiac involvement resulting in acute heart failure and death in days or weeks.

Thomas Duckett Jones, in 1944, proposed a set of guidelines for the diagnosis of rheumatic fever, now known as the Jones' criterions (Jones, 1944). His objective was to provide a uniform diagnostic reference for research programmes and to avoid overdiagnosis and treatment. He organized the important features into

major and minor categories. The clinical findings that were most useful diagnostically were designated major manifestations, while other less characteristic findings were listed as minor manifestations. The presence of two major, or one major and two minor manifestations, indicated a high probability of rheumatic involvement. Since there was no specific diagnostic test, the criterions became accepted worldwide. Although the initial proposals have been altered several times (Rutstein et al, 1955; Stollerman et al, 1965; Jones, 1984; Dajani et al, 1992), the basic concepts have remained intact.

Other than the major and minor criterions, there are other clinical features that may suggest the possibility of an acute rheumatic process but are not common or specific enough to justify inclusion as specific findings. Tachycardia, which occurs in any febrile illness, is common, and may be disproportionate to the degree of fever. Anaemia may be present but is not specific to the disease. Usually it does not become evident until other manifestations of the rheumatic process are well established. Feinstein and Spagnuolo (1962) reported the occurrence of epistaxis in up to one-tenth of patients. Nosebleeds, however, are common in children, with many other causes. A detailed workup in every case of nosebleed is not, therefore, justified unless there are other specific features to suggest acute rheumatism. Acute abdominal pain severe enough to mimic acute appendicitis may be one of the early manifestations of acute rheumatic fever. This has been attributed to mesenteric adenitis.

The latest version of the guidelines was drafted to emphasize the diagnosis of the initial attack (Table 64.2) (Dajani et al, 1992). It was not meant to diagnose recurrences and rheumatic activity, nor to predict the course or severity of the disease.

It is to be emphasized that these criterions are not meant as substitutes for the judgement of the clinician; they are intended only as guidelines to help to restrict the diagnosis to an acceptable clinical group. They are

Table 64.2 Jones' criteria 1992 update: guidelines for the diagnosis of initial attack of rheumatic fever

Major manifestations	Minor manifestations
Carditis	Clinical findings
Polyarthritis	Fever
Chorea	Arthralgia
Erythema marginatum	Laboratory findings
Subcutaneous nodules	Elevated erythrocytic sodimentation rate
	C-Reactive protein
	Prolonged PR interval on electrocardiogram

Supporting evidence for an antecedent group A streptococcal infection: positive throat culture or rapid streptococcal antigen test; elevated or rising streptococcal antibody titre

Adapted from Dajani et al (1992) with permission.

divided into major and minor features and, by themselves, carry no prognostic significance.

MAJOR MANIFESTATIONS

MIGRATORY POLYARTHRITIS

Polyarthritis is the most common major manifestation. It occurs in about three quarters of all initial episodes, and in more than one half of recurrences. It is encountered more frequently in older children, adolescents and adults. It is uncommon under the age of 3 years, and is fairly rare below the age of 5. Polyarthritis is classically migratory and non-suppurative, involving usually two or more joints, although occasionally it may be limited to one joint. The larger joints, such as knees, wrist, ankles and elbows, are more frequently involved but occasionally the small joints, including the temperomandibular joint and those of the vertebras, may be affected. Joints, particularly the large ones in the lower limbs, are affected in quick succession, each one usually for only a few days or a week at the most, so that there is an overlapping in time of the involvement of several joints. In the absence of anti-inflammatory treatment, the arthritis may last for up to 4 weeks, usually leaving no residual deformity. The arthritis is of shorter duration and less severe in children than in adults. The affected joints while the disease is active are red, swollen, tender to touch and very painful on movement (McDonald and Weisman, 1978). In rheumatic, as opposed to rheumatoid, arthritis, larger joints are affected for a shorter time, and in more migratory fashion, It has been suggested that, in general, the more severe the polyarthritis the less likely may be the involvement of the heart. Feinstein and Spagnuolo (1962) found that there was evidence of carditis in only one-quarter of patients when the joints were red and swollen, while this proportion increased to two-fifths when the joints were only tender, and to over nine-tenths when only polyarthralgia was present with no objective evidence of involvement of the joints. Conversely, classical rheumatic polyarthritis may occur and recur in the same individual without any evidence of cardiac involvement. It is important to emphasize the need to withhold anti-inflammatory drugs until the signs and symptoms have been fully observed and found compatible with rheumatic migratory polyarthritis.

Although it is the most common manifestation, it is also the least specific, as it is a feature of many other disease conditions.

CARDITIS

Carditis is seen in up to half of patients with rheumatic fever and is the usual cause of admission to hospital, although incidence could be higher in developing countries, as demonstrated by the recent outbreaks in the United States of America. Carditis is the most serious manifestation of the acute rheumatic process, since it is the only one that can cause death during the acute attack or produce residual disability and late mortality. Rheumatic carditis is a pancarditis. The involvement of the endocardium, and the resulting valvar malfunction, accounts for the clinical signs. Cardiac failure is usually the result of the associated myocarditis. Pericarditis may also occur either in its fibrinoid form or as a pericardial effusion of varying severity. It does not occur as an isolated finding, and cardiac tamponade is uncommon. Cardiac involvement tends to appear early in the acute process and is rarely delayed by as long as 3 weeks after the onset. At times, the carditis may initially be subclinical even if the acute rheumatic process is recognized, and it may become overt only during a recurrent episode. A history of rheumatic fever without overt carditis does not confer immunity from future rheumatic heart disease (Kuttner and Mayer, 1963).

The important murmurs in patients with acute rheumatic carditis are the apical holosystolic murmur of mitral incompetence, the early diastolic decrescendo murmur of aortic incompetence and the mid-diastolic murmur at the apex, the Carey–Coombs murmur. In patients who have had earlier rheumatic heart disease, or are known to have had past rheumatic fever, documentation of a change in the established murmurs or the appearance of a new murmur is of considerable value. Murmurs resulting from valvar stenosis are seldom seen in an initial attack of active carditis. Considerable care is needed in assessing apical systolic murmurs. The soft mitral regurgitant murmur is the most frequent. This may be pansystolic, or it may peak during late systole. The intensity and the duration of this murmur can wane towards recovery. These murmurs fill most of systole and are often transmitted to the axilla. The patient who has borderline murmurs needs to be watched and assessed at subsequent examinations. The early diastolic murmur of aortic incompetence may occasionally be heard only intermittently. The development of a low-pitched apical mid-diastolic murmur, the Carey–Coombs murmur, attributed to mitral valvitis, helps to confirm the organic significance of an apical systolic murmur. The diastolic murmur does not usually persist and tends to disappear during recovery from the acute episode. Unlike the mitral murmurs that may disappear on recovery, the murmur of aortic regurgitation tends to be more persistent and indicates permanent valvar injury, although the development of severe aortic incompetence during a single episode of rheumatic carditis is unusual. The murmurs in acute rheumatic carditis typically change from day to day, depending on the alteration in the myocardial and valvar function with or without treatment. Considerable care and critical clinical evaluation is necessary, nonetheless, before changing murmurs alone are accepted as a sign of carditis. The importance of this sign in those known to have rheumatic heart disease should be evaluated in conjunction with their earlier documentation. The first heart sound may be diminished in about half the children with mitral insufficiency in the presence of carditis. It is attributed to a lengthened conduction time, which permits early closure of the mitral valve and thus diminishes the valvar component of the first heart sound (Dock, 1933; Keith, 1937).

Congestive heart failure occurs with varying frequency, presenting with cardiomegaly, persistent evaluation of the sleeping pulse rate and gallop rhythm. The sudden onset of congestive heart failure, with cardiomegaly on a chest radiograph, may occasionally be the first sign of active carditis in a person known to have rheumatic valvar disease. Other causes, such as arryhthmias, respiratory infections, lack of adherence to a given medical regimen, and bouts of increased physical activity, can equally precipitate cardiac failure.

Pericarditis as part of active carditis is always associated with evidence of valvar involvement. It commonly manifests as a friction rub heard over the precordium, especially near the sternum, with a to-and-fro character in systole and diastole. In rheumatic carditis, the pericardial rub lasts from a few days to a week, unlike in pyogenic infection where it is more transient. Pericardial effusion is not uncommon, but the size of the effusion is variable. In the presence of congestive heart failure with underlying myocarditis, this effusion may go unrecognized. Echocardiography has become an invaluable tool in assessing the presence and magnitude of the pericardial effusion. Cardiac tamponade is uncommon, and pericardial aspiration is rarely required. Abnormalities in the electrocardigram, such as abnormal ST segments and T wave changes in the left pericardium, may occur (Keith et al, 1967). Cherian (1979) reported that typical electrocardiographic evidence of pericarditis is infrequent in rheumatic compared with viral pericarditis, probably because of the concomitant involvement of the myocardium and the changes resulting from valvar involvement.

During the active phase of carditis, the chest radiograph may show rapid changes in the heart size, significant pulmonary congestion or even frank pulmonary oedema. The pulmonary congestion is usually the result of left ventricular failure caused by myocarditis. It does not always carry a grave prognosis, either for the immediate future or for later valvar dysfunction. The fluctuations in heart size may be caused by the myocarditis alone with development of heart failure or by the accumulation of pericardial fluid (Oakley, 1980). The electrocardiogram may show disproportionate sinus tachycardia, a prolonged PR interval or a prolonged QT interval. Conduction defects with atrioventricular block or fascicular blocks may develop transiently but are rarely permanent.

At present, the medical literature is replete with articles describing findings of cardiac involvement on echocardiography in patients with rheumatic fever with no heart murmurs (see discussion on echocardiography, below).

SUBCUTANEOUS NODULES

Subcutaneous nodules are seen in less than one-twentieth of patients. They are hard and shot-like nodules found particularly over the occipital region, the vertebral spines and over the external surfaces of the elbows, knees and wrists. They are smaller and shorter lived than those of rheumatoid arthritis. They are particularly uncommon below the age of 3 years and in adults. Interestingly, they occur more frequently in the presence of active carditis than as an isolated manifestation, Oakley (1980) reported that carditis is usually present when nodules occur, and that nodules may coexist with chorea in patients with subacute or chronic rheumatic activity, who may have shown no clinical evidence of carditis.

SYDENHAM'S CHOREA

Chorea, also known as Sydenham's chorea or St Vitus' dance, is a neurological disorder characterized by abnormal involuntary and purposeless movements, grimacing, muscular weakness and emotional instability. The last may be an initial presenting sign. Chorea must be differentiated from fits, athetosis and fidgeting caused by behavioural problems. It occurs mostly in children, particularly in females, and is unusual in adults except during pregnancy (chorea gravidarum). Chorea occurs in one sixth of patients with the acute rheumatic process and it can occur unaccompanied by other major manifestations of rheumatic fever. The latency period is long, varying from 1–6 months with an average of 3 months. Spasticity is a feature but tendon jerks remain normal. Incoordination is shown when the patient is asked to perform specific actions. The involuntary movements disappear during sleep. Patients who develop chorea as an isolated rheumatic manifestation have a relatively higher incidence of cardiac involvement in later years this being found in up to one-quarter after 20 years (Bland, 1961). These patients may have had a mild transient carditis before the onset of chorea but soon after the streptococcal infection that caused it. This may have been asymptomatic but sufficient to establish chronic valvar disease. Because of the prolonged period of latency, the erythrocytic sedimentation rate, C-reactive protein, and even the antistreptolysin O titre, may all be normal.

ERYTHEMA MARGINATUM

Erythema marginatum is a non-pruritic, painless, pink evanescent skin rash that occurs mainly on the trunk, the buttocks or the proximal part of the limbs, but not the face. The individual lesions expand centrifugally while the skin in the centre returns to normal. It occurs mainly in patients in the early phase of active carditis, but it may reappear later, even during convalescence. It is seen in less than 3% of patients. Although it is uncommon now in the acute phase, it is seen so infrequently in other diseases that it has been granted major status in the modified Jones' criterions.

The lack of itching and induration helps to distinguish this condition from drug reactions and serum sickness.

MINOR MANIFESTATIONS

The so-called minor manifestations, both clinical and laboratory in origin, are so characterized because they are relatively non-specific. Although common in the acute rheumatic process, they may be found in other diseases. Fever, which is present in more than half the patients at some time or other except in those with chorea, is of low grade and tends to subside even without treatment within 1 to 2 weeks. It is associated with anorexia, listlessness and, when prolonged, with weight loss. The temperature ranges between 100 and 103°F (37.8–39.5°C) and is rarely accompanied by chills or seizures. The presence of fever in untreated patients with either polyarthritis or active carditis is so common that its absence demands careful reconsideration of the diagnosis. Laboratory indexes of persistence of rheumatic activity do continue after the fever has completely subsided; consequently, the absence of fever does not exclude rheumatic activity.

Prolongation of the PR interval has been reported to occur in two-fifths of patients (Di Sciascio and Taranta, 1980). It is useful in the diagnosis of the acute rheumatic process, but not in that of clinically significant carditis, since it does not correlate with organic murmurs, the prognosis or with residual heart disease. Cherian (1979) reported that a prolonged PR interval was less frequent than a prolonged QT interval. A prolonged PR interval is rather non-specific, however, and may occur in many infectious diseases besides rheumatic fever. It is now generally agreed that the diagnosis of carditis cannot be made on this finding alone. Arthralgia, without objective joint findings, although common in the acute rheumatic process, may be found in many other diseases. Even with a careful history and physical examination, it may be difficult to differentiate from non-specific growing pains. It has been reported (Roy, 1960; Cherian, 1979) that polyarthralgia may be as common as polyarthritis in patients with a definite acute rheumatic process. It has also been claimed that, at least in the regions where rheumatic fever is endemic, polyarthralgia supported by evidence of a preceding β-haemolytic streptococcal infection can be considered a major criterion without causing overdiagnosis. Apart from the first attacks, this practice will be particularly useful in deciding on the presence of rheumatic activity, both in patients with a past history of rheumatic fever and in those with established rheumatic heart disease.

INVESTIGATIONS

LABORATORY EXAMINATIONS

There is no laboratory test specific for rheumatic fever. Two groups of tests are commonly used. Identification of the acute phase reactants provides evidence of a recent inflammatory process. The most commonly used acute phase reactants are the erythrocytic sedimentation rate and the test for C-reactive protein. The leucocytosis may occur but is not sufficiently constant to be of diagnostic value. Both the erythrocytic sedimentation rate and the level of C-reactive protein may be normal in patients with isolated chorea or erythema marginatum, but they are usually elevated in presence of the other clinical manifestations of rheumatic fever and are modified by anti-inflammatory therapy. The sedimentation rate can be elevated merely as a result of any infection or associated anaemia. It can be low in the presence of congestive heart failure in carditis. In general, it remains high far longer than the other signs and is useful in deciding how long the patient should be kept in bed or how to modify suppressive therapy. The C-reactive protein can be an oversensitive indication of the acute inflammatory process, this being a drawback to its usefulness, but it is not influenced by anaemia or by heart failure. A positive C-reactive protein test has been shown to be less useful or reliable than an elevated sedimentation rate (Cherian, 1979). Both these tests are non-specific, and abnormal findings may occur in many other conditions.

THROAT CULTURES

Throat cultures have traditionally been the gold standard with which to determine the presence of streptococcal infection. A positive culture, however, may not distinguish between acute streptococcal infection and streptococcal carriers having a concomitant viral infection. A negative result after 24 hours may allow the physician to withhold antibiotic therapy in the majority of patients with sore throats. Incubatation for another 24 hours may be needed to maximize sensitivity for detection of the group A streptococcus.

In the absence of a positive culture, antigen detection tests or streptococcal antibody tests are requested. More than nine-tenths of patients with rheumatic fever when first seen show an elevation of antibodies to one or more of the streptococcal antigens (Wannamaker and Ayoub, 1960). At present, many of the tests for these antigens are available commercially. Most are very specific, but their sensitivity in clinical pratice is quite low. Newer tests are currently being developed that will increase their sensitivity (optical immunoassay, gene probe test). Be that as it may, positive rapid response to a streptococcal antigen test indicates that a patient with acute pharyngitis must be treated.

Of the streptococcal antibody titre determinations, antistreptolysin O is the most commonly requested. It provides reliable confirmation of recent streptococcal infection involving group A. Only three to four-fifths of patients, however, give positive reactions. When judging the results, a value of 330 todd units or greater in children, or 250 todd unit for adults, is considered significant. A fourfold rise in titre in two samples taken 10 days apart is preferred. A high titre is not diagnostic by itself in the absence of other manifestations.

Timing of the determination is also necessary when interpretating the result. The titre usually becomes elevated 2 weeks after the streptococcal infection, peaks at 4–6 weeks and decreases after another 2 weeks.

If the titre is not elevated, an anti-DNAase B test may be requested. This stays elevated for a longer period of time than does antistreptolysin O titre. Streptozyme test (Wampole Laboratories, Stamford, CT, USA), a rapid commercially available slide agglutination test to detect antibodies to several streptococcal antigens, has been developed to increase the rate of detection. It is, however, less well standardized. It is also important to remember that these tests should not be used to differentiate an infection from a carrier state.

The titres are likely to be normal in patients with chorea, in those in the early phase of the disease or in those with chronic carditis, since in the last the titres may have returned to normal. The antibody response can be suppressed by antibiotic or steroid therapy. While normal titres do not exclude the diagnosis of rheumatic activity, absence of elevated titres calls for very careful reconsideration of the diagnosis. This sign is useful in eliminating disease states that simulate rheumatic fever. This is especially true in differentiating between other forms of myocarditis and arthropathies that clinically resemble the acute rheumatic process. When the manifestations of the acute process are typical, the diagnosis is often made with confidence. In a number of instances, it is made with difficulty because of the wide variation in the clinical manifestations. Such patients may need to be observed for weeks before a final diagnosis can be established. The careful use of the updated Jones' criteria, along with streptococcal antibody tests, does help to minimize incorrect diagnosis.

Subclinical or smoldering carditis may exist in the absence of other major manifestations. Neither over- nor underdiagnosis of carditis are uncommon. Considering the number of adults who still present with established rheumatic valvar disease without any preceding history of rheumatic fever, underdiagnosis is particularly common. Overdiagnosis can be equally detrimental when children with innocent murmurs or murmurs caused by congenital heart defects associated with sore throats or arthralgia are wrongly labelled as having rheumatic heart disease. There are many other disease processes that may currently fulfil the Jones' criteria in their early stage or mimic the acute rheumatic process very closely. The differential diagnosis includes rheumatoid arthritis, serum sickness, other arthropathies, infective endocarditis, Henoch–Schönlein purpura, acute leukaemia, viral myocarditis, viral pericarditis, systemic lupus erythematosus and other collagen disorders that may affect both joints and the heart, poliomyelitis and acute appendicitis.

ECHOCARDIOGRAPHY

The advent of echocardiography has paved the way for a clearer understanding of the pathophysiological findings observed in the hearts of patients with rheumatic fever with or without carditis. Results of this diagnostic modality have shown that as many as three-fifths of patients without clinical evidence of carditis had significant findings of mitral valvar prolapse, annular dilation, chamber enlargement and multiple valvar regurgitation (Ty and Ortiz, 1992).

These studies have also documented that the presence of congestive heart failure in patients with carditis was related more to the severity of valvar regurgitation and the number of valves involved than to myocardial dysfunction. Although mitral valvar regurgitation is the most common abnormal feature, aortic and tricuspid valvar regurgitation are more commonly seen than previously thought. Other studies have advocated that Doppler evidence of valvar regurgitation be accepted as carditis even in the absence of a murmur (Dajani et al, 1993; Wilson and Neutze, 1995).

Veasy, in 1995, proposed that Doppler evidences for mitral and aortic regurgitations be included as one of the minor manifestations in the revised Jones' criteria provided that rigid echocardiographic rules are employed. For mitral regurgitation, these are that the regurgitant jet should be holosystolic, followed back to the left atrial wall, accompanied by a mosaic pattern and seen in two planes. For aortic regurgitation the regurgitant jet should be holodiastolic and extend into the left ventricle to the tip of the aortic leaflet of the mitral valve.

Analysis of current data on the use of echocardiography has made Narula and colleagues move one step further (Narula et al, 1999) and conclude that echocardiography and Doppler may have a place as a major criterion in the Jones' criteria in the United States of America and possibly in other developed countries provided strict criterions are established. Implementation of this modification to the Jones' criteria may not be practicable at this point in developing countries unless prospective well-controlled studies are done that will demonstrate distinctly superior treatment and prognostic value of detecting carditis in this manner.

MANAGEMENT

Treatment of rheumatic fever depends on the major manifestation(s) present. Apart from a therapeutic course of penicillin to eradicate the causative streptococcal infection, there is no universally approved or accepted treatment that has been shown by careful scientific trial to be definitely superior to any other. The choice of suppressive medication, duration of bedrest, and subsequent restriction of physical activity, is best decided on an individual basis. Medical treatment is still based on salicylates, steroids and bedrest. It is very important to defer the starting of anti-inflammatory or suppressive drug treatment until a definitive diagnosis has been established. It is unwise to start a therapeutic trial of either salicylates or steroids prematurely, since this may suppress the disease process sufficiently to make a firm diagnosis almost impossible. All patients should be evaluated carefully for the first 2 to 3 weeks, basically to detect whether carditis develops. Treatment to prevent congestive heart failure, however, must be started at once if heart failure becomes manifest. A careful record of the sleeping pulse rate is important. An unexplained tachycardia during sleep in a patient who is afebrile may be an indication of the onset of carditis. Laboratory evaluation should include tests for haemoglobin, haematocrit, acute phase reactants, streptococcal antibody titres and preferably more than one or two throat cultures taken before penicillin therapy is started. A chest radiograph is indicated to determine the heart size, and an electrocardiogram and echocardiogram are justified.

It is generally accepted that, within a week or 10 days after the onset of streptococcal pharyngitis, an attack of rheumatic fever can be avoided This is of value not only for the individual patient, but for preventing the chance of infection spreading to others. In this light, a case can be made for giving penicillin to every child who is suspected of having a haemolytic streptococcal infection. Theoretically, this approach would help to eliminate rheumatic fever and overcome the practical logistic difficulties of obtaining throat cultures from all patients in order to select those who specifically require penicillin treatment. After all, in the dosage recommended for treating acute pharyngitis, serious side reactions and major sensitive reactions to penicillin are unusual. In endemic areas with a high incidence of rheumatic fever and poor bacteriological support, it is quite acceptable to recommend such treatment of all sore throats of unknown or uncertain aetiology. As far as is possible, however, throat cultures should be obtained. Patients with any manifestation of the acute rheumatic process,

including chorea, should be given a therapeutic course of antimicrobial agents for 10 days to eradicate residual streptococcal infection that may be difficult to isolate. Eradication is dependent on the choice of the drug and length of time for which effective blood levels of drug are maintained. The recommendation of the American Heart Association Rheumatic Fever Committee (Dajani et al, 1995) is widely accepted (Table 64.3). Intramuscular benzathine penicillin (benzathine penicillin G) is the drug of choice, especially for those patients who are unlikely to complete an adequate course of oral therapy. For patients weighing less than 60 lbs (27 kg), one intramuscular injection of 600 000 units is recommended. For patients weighing more than 60 lbs (27 kg), the dosage should be increased to 1 200 000 units (1200 ku). The oral antibiotic of choice is phenoxy methylpenicillin (penicillin V). Oral penicillin has the reported advantage of a lower incidence of allergic reactions; however, the disadvantage is that the tablets may be taken irregularly, leading to an inadequate blood level. The dosage for both children and adults is 250 mg three or four times daily for a full 10 days. It is important to emphasize to patients that they must continue to take the penicillin regularly for the entire period, even though they will probably be completely asymptomatic after the first few days. Drugs other than penicillin offer no advantage for treatment of streptococcal infection. Their use should be limited to patients who are allergic to penicillin. Erythromycin is the drug of choice for such patients. It should also be given in divided doses for 10 days at a dose of 40 mg/kg body weight per day (not to exceed 1 g daily). Although very rare strains of group A β-haemolytic streptococcus have been reported to be resistant to erythromycin, this seems to be of little general clinical significance at the present time. The new macrolide azithromycin has a similar antibacterial spectrum to that of erythromycin against the group A streptococcus, but has less gastrointestinal side effects. It can be given once a day for 5 days. The recommended dosage is 500 mg as a single dose on the first day, followed by 250 mg once daily for

Table 64.3 Primary prevention of rheumatic fever (treatment of streptococcal tonsillopharyngitis)[a]

Agent	Dose	Mode	Duration
Benzathine penicillin	600 000 units for patients <27 kg (60 lb)	Intramuscular	Once
or	1200 000 units for patients >27 kg (60 lb)		
Phenoxymethylpenicillin (penicillin V)	Children: 250 mg 2–3 times daily Adolescents and adults: 500 mg 2–3 times daily	Oral	10 days
For individuals allergic to penicillin			
Erythromycin			
Estolate	20–40 mg/kg per day in 2–4 doses (maximum 1 g/day)	Oral	10 days
or			
Ethylsuccinate	40 mg/kg per day in 2–4 doses (maximum 1 g/day)	Oral	10 days

[a]For other acceptable alternatives, see text. The following are not acceptable: sulphonamides, trimethoprim, tetracyclines and chloramphenicol. From Dajani et al (1995) with permission.

4 days for those 16 years of age or older. It has been shown to produce high tonsillar tissue concentration. Another acceptable alternative for patients allergic to penicillin is an oral cephalosporin, like cephalexin (cefalexin) or cefadroxil, which has a narrower spectrum of activity. Care must be observed, as some who are allergic to penicillin may also be allergic to cephalosporins. The drawback of these alternatives is their cost.

Certain antimicrobials are not recommended for treatment of streptococcal infection. Tetracycline should not be used because of the very high prevalence of strains that are resistant to this antibiotic. The sulphonamide drugs, although effective as continuous prophylaxis for the prevention of recurrent attacks of rheumatic fever, should not be used for the treatment of streptococcal infection because they will not eradicate the streptococcus. For patients who have already had rheumatic fever, there can be little argument against prescription of penicillin for atypical or undiagnosed sore throats. Secondary prophylaxis should be started as soon as the diagnosis is established, the appropriate cultures have been taken and soon after a therapeutic eradication course of penicillin has been given. The risk of acquiring a new streptococcal infection may be especially high in the hospital environment. As such, initiation of prophylaxis should not be delayed until the patient is discharged.

BEDREST

The recommended duration and strictness of bedrest is variable depending on the manifestations. The general trend is towards a shorter hospital stay, as the value of prolonged bedrest has not been scientifically established. Patients without overt carditis may be allowed up as soon as the fever and local symptoms have subsided and laboratory evidence of inflammation has begun to regress. In those with carditis, the duration of bedrest depends on the severity of the carditis and the speed of regression of the acute episode. The recommendation of prolonged bedrest is based primarily on reducing cardiac work in those with carditis, and avoiding as much as possible the use of involved joints in those with arthritis. Massell et al (1958) recommend that patients should be in bed for the first 2 to 3 weeks of the illness, since carditis, if it is not already evident, may appear during this period. Strict bedrest should be limited to patients with arthritis of the lower limbs, and to those with carditis and a large heart. Those with polyarthritis or polyarthralgia are usually asymptomatic by the second or third week, and may then be gradually allowed to start moving around while they continue on antisuppressive drugs. Patients with cardiac murmurs, but no definite cardiomegaly or congestive heart failure with or without polyarthritis, should be kept in bed for about a month, but the bedrest need not be strict. In the third or fourth week, they may have supervised ambulation for a few hours daily. Patients with carditis and cardiomegaly but without definite congestive failure should be kept in bed for at least 6 weeks, rest being strictly enforced over the first 4 weeks. Patients with carditis and congestive heart failure should be kept on absolute rest until the failure is completely controlled, and they should maintain modified bedrest for about 4 weeks after the anti-inflammatory treatment has been stopped, provided there is no rebound. If there is a rebound, they need to return to bedrest until 2 weeks after this has subsided (Di Sciascio and Taranta, 1980).

ANTI-INFLAMMATORY DRUGS

Anti-inflammatory drugs, such as salicylates and steroids, are now widely used during the acute rheumatic process and are dramatically effective in suppressing the acute signs of inflammation. Arthritis and fever subside quickly, usually within a few days. The acute phase reactants may remain abnormal for weeks after the disappearance of fever and joint manifestations. These drugs have very little or a doubtful effect on erythema marginatum, chorea or subcutaneous nodules, or in preventing the development of valvar heart disease. Steroids have been shown to suppress acute manifestations more rapidly than salicylates, but there is a greater tendency for the manifestations to reappear after discontinuation of treatment (United Kingdom and United States Joint Report, 1955, 1965). The as yet unsettled controversy in the choice between salicylate or steroids in the treatment of the acute rheumatic process is based primarily on their possible effect on the cardiovascular manifestations, especially in relation to prevention or modification or residual rheumatic heart disease. There are several studies that have been designed to compare salicylates with steroids (Illingworth et al, 1957; Cooperative Rheumatic Fever Study Group, 1960, 1965; United Kingdom and United States Joint Report, 1965). Salicylate therapy does not alter the incidence of residual heart disease (Alexander and Smith, 1962). The increased consumption of oxygen with high doses of salicylates may have a possible deleterious effect by increasing the workload of the heart and may promote the development of congestive heart failure. It is now agreed that salicylates exert no specific effect on the lesions of the acute rheumatic process at any site, but they do produce excellent symptomatic relief of arthritis and fever. There is, as yet, no clear evidence that steroids reduce the incidence and severity of residual rheumatic heart disease. Yet steroids are used in patients with carditis, especially those with severe carditis and congestive heart failure, since there is a definite impression that death during the acute attack may be prevented and the overall morbidity appears to be reduced.

In the most recent review of the literature, a meta-analysis on the advantage of corticosteroid treatment over salicylates in treating rheumatic carditis showed no statistically significant difference in preventing development of pathological murmur at 1 year after treatment (Albert et al, 1995).

Patients who present only with arthralgia, or with mild arthritis and no carditis, require only analgesics for symptomatic relief and a full course of aspirin is not required. Patients with established arthritis but without carditis respond well to treatment with salicylates. An effective, safer but non-toxic dose of aspirin for children is 75–100 mg/kg body weight per day in four divided doses. This produces a blood salicylate level of not more than 20 mg, which is well below the toxic range. The full dose is given for the first 2 weeks and subsequently gradually reduced over the next 4 to 6 weeks. A larger or a smaller dose can be used depending on the response to treatment. If more massive doses of salicylates are given, salicylate toxicity is common. Hyperpnoea is one of the early signs of salicylate toxicity. Nausea, vomiting, tinnitus, lassitude and occasionally delirium, convulsion and coma can occur.

Carditis in most instances is treated with steroids. Those with carditis but without overt cardiac failure may be started on aspirin. In patients with cardiomegaly, aspirin alone is often insufficient to control the symptoms or does so only at toxic or near toxic levels. This situation may require a change to steroids. Patients with carditis and congestive heart failure should be given steroids. Prednisone is usually preferred as it produces less retention of sodium and loss of potassium. Adrenocorticotrophic hormone and hydrocortisone are rarely used now. The initial dose of prednisone is 2 mg/kg per day in three divided doses, which may be increased if heart failure is not controlled quickly. Those with severe heart failure presenting acutely may be given intravenous methyl prednisolone followed by oral prednisone. After 2 or 3 weeks, prednisone should be gradually withdrawn, decreasing the daily dose once in 3 or 4 days and adding aspirin at standard doses. Aspirin should be continued for 3 to 4 weeks after the prednisone is stopped. This overlap therapy reduces the incidence of post-therapeutic clinical rebounds (Di Sciascio and Taranta, 1980). Steroids are usually used in the amount just sufficient to suppress the acute inflammatory manifestations. Occasionally, high doses of steroids need to be given on a prolonged basis, although usually a low suppressive dose can be achieved. Prednisone can be tapered off and stopped as soon as the fever has subsided, the acute phase reactants are normal and cardiac signs have become stable. In some patients with severe carditis, it may become necessary to continue steroids for months, since a reduction of the dose may be followed by reappearance of signs of activity. Under these circumstances, it is acceptable to continue maintenance therapy at a lower dose until all signs of activity have fully regressed.

Congestive heart failure in rheumatic carditis is often controlled with bedrest and steroids alone. Digitalis was previously considered to be contraindicated in the presence of carditis, since some patients may be unusually sensitive to the glycoside. It is now generally agreed that digitalis can be used in patients with rheumatic heart disease and heart failure regardless of the presence or absence of active carditis, but caution is required in monitoring the dosage. The sleeping pulse rate is a more useful index to assess digitalis dosage than is tachycardia present during waking hours. Diuretics are used as and when indicated. Patients with moderate to severe mitral regurgitation or aortic incompetence may be given drugs to reduce afterload.

TREATMENT OF CHOREA

Isolated chorea is treated symptomatically, since neither salicylates nor steroids have any effect on the course. Chorea when associated with other rheumatic manifestations should be treated with salicylates. These patients should be kept on bedrest in a quiet area to protect them from external stimulation, and given appropriate sedation. Besides barbiturates and chlorpromazine, diazepam has been shown to be of value in the management of chorea (Lockman, 1975). Haloperidol and, more recently, sodium valproate (valproic acid) have been shown to be effective in controlling chorea (Daoud et al, 1990). The need for a course of penicillin to eradicate the streptococcus, and subsequent regular chemoprophylaxis, is as important in chorea as in any other rheumatic manifestation.

REBOUNDS

Rebounds are not uncommon after cessation of anti-inflammatory treatment and usually occur within 2 to 3 weeks. They vary in intensity. Some patients show only laboratory abnormalities. Those with clinical rebounds usually show arthralgia, fever and occasionally arthritis, but severe cardiac manifestations may also occur. Rebounds occur more often after steroid therapy than with salicylates. Laboratory rebounds, and most of the clinical rebounds, do not require any treatment except for analgesics or small doses of aspirin, and they usually subside spontaneously within a few days. It is preferable to use salicylates rather than steroids for more severe rebounds since a second rebound is less likely with salicylates. Only the very severe clinical rebounds need a full reinstitution of the earlier treatment (Feinstein and Spagnuolo, 1962).

PREVENTION

The single most important achievement in rheumatic fever has been the success of chemoprophylaxis in preventing recurrences and, to some extent, the initial attacks. Two types of prevention are advocated for rheumatic fever: primary and secondary.

PRIMARY PREVENTION ————————————

The effective treatment of streptococcal throat infections to prevent the occurrence of rheumatic fever is termed primary prevention. A clinical diagnosis of streptococcal sore throat often poses a problem because of the difficulty in ruling out other bacterial and viral causes. Table 64.4 summarizes the clinical characteristics that may be helpful in identifying a streptococcal tonsillopharyngitis. Patients with fever (usually of 101–104°F, 38.3–40.0°C), red throat with exudate and tender anterior cervical lymph nodes are more likely to have streptococcal pharyngitis (Kaplan et al, 1971). The same clinical picture may also be associated, nonetheless, with viral infections (Kaplan, 1972). Hoarseness, conjunctivitis, cough and coryza are usually not associated with streptococcal infections (Di Sciascio and Taranta, 1980). Streptococcal infections may not always manifest as a severe pharyngitis. A clinically mild sore throat is not uncommon with streptococcal infections and may still lead to rheumatic fever. In order to avoid the risk of underdiagnosis, it is safer to perform throat cultures on all patients with pharyngitis and treat those with a positive culture (Wannamaker, 1976) Penicillin is the antimicrobial agent of choice for the treatment of group A streptococcal pharyngitis. The details of drug regimens used in primary prevention (initial therapeutic streptococcal eradicating dose or courses of antibiotics) have been given above. Caution should be exercised in continuing erythromycin without checking on the drug sensitivity of the group A streptococcus, since a small proportion of strains are resistant (Stollerman, 1982). Early studies by Morris et al (1956) have shown the inadequacy of sulphadiazine (sulfadiazine) in primary prevention. This is because only bactericidal drugs can eliminate the streptococcus from the throat, a primary requisite in the prevention of rheumatic fever. Tetracyclines are not recommended for the same reason (Brink et al, 1951). Large-scale mass prophylaxis has been shown to be effective in populations with epidemics of streptococcal pharyngitis (Chancey et al, 1955).

Table 64.4 Clinical characteristics of acute pharyngitis caused by group A β-haemolytic streptococcal infection ('strep throat')

Most common in 5–15 year group
Sudden onset of acute pharyngeal pain and malaise
Headache
Fever of 102–104°F (39–40°C)
Pharyngeal erythema and exudate, soft palatal petechias
Enlarged tender cervical lymph nodes
    Scabby erosions on the edges of nostrils
    Presence of constitutional signs and symptoms
Acute otitis media
Vomiting
Suppurative sinusitis

Treatment failures recognized by bacteriological examination may occur in about one tenth of patients. Such 'bacteriologic relapse' occurs more often in patients treated with oral penicillin. This could possibly result from the presence of penicillinase-producing staphylococcuses in the oropharynx (Bernstein et al, 1964). The relapses may also be caused by infection by a new type or the same type of staphylococcus as a result of suppression of type-specific antibodies by penicillin.

Individuals with streptococcal pharyngitis, or those who have recently acquired group A streptococcal infection, are the ones more likely to spread the infection to contacts. Young children appear to spread the infection more often than adults (Wannamaker et al, 1954; Breese and Disney, 1956). Nasal carriers usually become negative for group A streptococcus in the nose within a week, in contrast to asymptomatic throat carriers in whom the organisms persist for weeks or months in the absence of treatment (Rammelkamp, 1957). Throat carriers can be transient, convalescent or chronic. Chronic carriers may not show any clinical or serological evidence of infection and, with progression of time, may reveal the organisms in the throat only intermittently ('spotty' carriers). The nasal carriers usually are refractory to treatment and harbour less virulent strains of streptococcus; which show a difference in type from the strains from those with acute infections (Krause et al, 1962). The treatment of carriers has questionable value, especially in the absence of clinical or epidemiological evidence of active streptococcal infection in them or their contracts (Krause et al, 1962; American Heart Association, 1977). In contrast, family contacts, especially siblings of patients with acute pharyngitis, are at high risk and should have cultures of throat swabs made and receive treatment if these are positive (Di Sciascio and Taranta, 1980).

SECONDARY PREVENTION ————————————

The institution of continuous chemoprophylactic regimens to prevent recurrences in patients who have already had an attack of rheumatic fever is referred to as secondary prevention. Secondary prophylaxis is an absolute must to reduce the morbidity and mortality in rheumatic individuals. It is markedly effective in reducing, and practically eliminating recurrences when benzathine penicillin is used. Moreover, the success of secondary prophylaxis is beyond a purely numerical reduction of attacks of rheumatic fever because a disproportionate number of deaths and disabilities are caused by recurrences rather than first attacks.

In 1995, an update of the 1988 statement on the treatment of streptococcal pharyngitis and rheumatic fever was made. The current recommendations are shown in Table 64.5. As early as 1964, intramuscular benzathine penicillin, once every 4 weeks at a dose of 1 200 000 units, has been shown to be the most effective form of

Table 64.5 Secondary prevention of rheumatic fever (prevention of recurrent attacks)[a]

Agent	Dose	Mode
Benzathine penicillin (benzathine penicillin G) or	1 200 000 U every 4 weeks[a]	Intramuscular
Phenoxymethyl penicillin (penicillin V) or	250 mg twice daily	Oral
Sulphadiazine (sulfadiazine)	0.5 g once daily for patients less than 60 lb (27 kg) 1.0 g once daily for patients over 60 lb (27 kg)	Oral
For individuals allergic to penicillin and sulphadiazine Erythromycin	250 mg twice daily	Oral

[a] In high-risk situations, administration every 3 weeks is justified and recommended.
From Dajani et al (1995) with permission.

prophylaxis (Alban et al, 1964) and is still currently advocated (Dajani et al, 1995). This long-acting penicillin is more effective than oral prophylaxis because lack of compliance with continuous oral medication is not uncommon. In countries where the incidence of rheumatic fever is particularly high, in special circumstances or in certain high-risk individuals, such as patients with residual rheumatic carditis, the administration of benzathine penicillin every 3 weeks is justified and recommended (Lue et al 1986; Kaplan et al, 1989b). The recommended dosage for oral sulphadiazine as prophylaxis is 0.5 g once daily for patients weighing less than 60 lb (27 kg) and 1 g once daily for patients weighing more than this. For prophylaxis using oral penicillin, the recommended dose is 250 mg twice daily for phenoxymethylpenicillin. Patients sensitive to both penicillin and sulphonamides may be given erythromycin 250 mg twice daily.

DURATION OF PROPHYLAXIS

The most effective protection from rheumatic recurrences is provided by long-term continuous prophylaxis maintained for the lifetime of the patient. Lifetime prophylaxis is particularly important in those with established rheumatic heart disease (Di Sciascio and Taranta, 1980; Stollerman, 1982). It is known, however, that the risk of

recurrences declines with the age of the patient and with the interval since the most recent attack. Patients without heart disease are at less risk of recurrences than those with cardiac lesions. Considering the difficulties of maintaining lifetime prophylaxis, exceptions may be made for maintaining prophylaxis, especially in older patients. These exceptions are determined on an individual basis. In coming to a decision, the physician should carefully take into account a number of factors, such as the patient's risk of acquiring a streptococcal infection, the anticipated recurrence rate per infection and the consequences of recurrence. Current recommendations by the American Heart Association are given in Table 64.6. Adults at an increased risk, such as parents of young children, school teachers, medical and paramedical personnel and military cadets and servicemen, necessarily need prophylaxis over a longer period of time. The greatest risk of rheumatic recurrences is in the disadvantaged, which includes those with established rheumatic heart disease, those who have had a recent attack of rheumatic fever (within the last 3 years), those who have had multiple attacks in the past, children and adolescents and those suffering crowding at home. Prophylaxis should be continued for a long time in individuals who have had valvar surgery for rheumatic heart disease, even after valvar replacement with prosthetic valves, since they continue to be at risk. In countries with poor socioeconomic development, the cost factor and poor compliance of

Table 64.6 Duration of secondary rheumatic fever prophylaxis

Category	Duration
Rheumatic fever with carditis and residual heart disease (persistent valvar disease[a])	At least 10 years since last episode and at least until age 40 years; sometimes lifelong prophylaxis
Rheumatic fever with carditis but no residual heart disease (no valvar disease[a])	10 years or well into adulthood, whichever is longer
Rheumatic fever without carditis	5 years or until age 21 years whichever is longer

[a]Clinical or echocardiographic evidence.
From Dajani et al (1995) with permission.

patients weighs heavily against effective programmes for secondary prophylaxis.

STREPTOCOCCAL VACCINE

Immunoprophylaxis is still in the exploratory stage. The need for a streptococcal vaccine may not be so acute in the developed countries where there is a low incidence of the rheumatic sequels. The quest for a safe and effective vaccine is much needed for populations of the under-developed countries where rheumatic fever is endemic, and the chance of an improvement in living standards and chemoprophylaxis is small (Stollerman, 1980). With the increase of resistance to drugs other than penicillin, the danger of resistance also emerging to this drug adds further impetus to the search for a safe immunization. The 'pep M-type' vaccines initially have been shown to be useful in eliciting protective immunity both in animals and humans by producing antibodies against the amino-terminal end of the M protein; these vaccines enable specific opsonization of the streptococcus (Beachey et al, 1979, 1984; Dale et al, 1983, 1986; Beachey and Seyer, 1986; Dale and Beachey, 1986). At least three such vaccines (pep M5, M6 and M24) have proven successful (Beachy et al, 1979, 1981). A restricted polyvalent vaccine incorporating the limited number of rheumatogenic types may prove even more successful. These vaccines have been observed to be safe without the danger of inducing a cross-reactive autoimmune response (Stollerman, 1982). It was initially thought that immunity was related to the accommodation of antibodies to the many different M serotypes. Current observations, however, have shown that the M protein is constantly changing and peptides representing serotype M5, M6, M24 with variable amino-terminal sequences were poorly recognized in samples from adults living in an endemic area (Pruhsakorn et al, 1994). These same authors were able to develop human antibodies to peptide 145 (within the conserved region of the carboxy-terminal of the protein) that were able to opsonize isolates of streptococcus from Thai and Australian aborigines. They hope soon to develop a vaccine derived from this highly conserved part of the M protein that will facilitate rapid development of protective antibodies and prevent streptococcal infections and their consequences, including rheumatic fever. With this, and other advances in immunogenetics (Patarryo et al, 1979), we look forward to greater progress in eradicating the disease in the 21st century.

REFERENCES

Achutti A, Achutti V R 1992 Epidemiology of rheumatic fever in the developing world. Cardiology in the Young 2: 206–215

Albani B, Epstein J A, Feinstein A R et al 1964 Rheumatic fever in children and adolescents: a long term epidemiologic study of subsequent prophylaxis, streptococcal infections and clinical sequence. Annals of Internal Medicine 60(suppl 5)

Albert D A, Harel L, Karrison T 1995 The treatment of rheumatic carditis: a review and meta-analysis. Medicine 74: 1–12

Alexander W D, Smith G 1962 Disadvantageous circulatory effects of salicylate in rheumatic fever. Lancet i: 768–771

American Heart Association 1955 Report of Rheumatic Fever Committee. Jones criteria (modified) for guidance in diagnosis of rheumatic fever. Modern Concepts of Cardiovascular Diseases 24: 291–293

American Heart Association 1977 Committee on rheumatic fever and bacterial endocarditis. Prevention of rheumatic fever. Circulation 55: 1

Anastasiou-Nana M I, Anderson J L, Carlquist J F, Nanas J N 1986 HLA-DR typing and lymphocyte subset evaluation in rheumatic heart disease: a search for immune response factors. American Heart Journal 112: 992–997

Assis R V C, Higuchi M L 1992 New pathological aspects of rheumatic heart disease. Cardiology in the Young 2: 216–221

Ayoub E M, Barret D J, Maclaren N K, Krischer J P 1986 Association of class II human histocompatibility leukocyte antigens with rheumatic fever. Journal of Clinical Investigation 77: 2019–2025

Baird R W, Bronze M S, Kraus W et al 1991 Epitopes of group A streptococcal M protein shared with antigens of articular cartilage and synovium. Journal of Immunology 146: 3132–3137

Beachey E H, Ofek I 1976 Epithelial cell binding of group A streptococci by lipoteichoic acid on fimbriae denuded of M protein. Journal of Experimental Medicine 143: 759–771

Beachey E H, Seyer J M 1986 Protective and nonprotective epitopes of chemically synthesized peptides of the NH$_2$-terminal region of type 6 streptococcal M protein. Journal of Immunology 136: 2287–2292

Beachey E H, Stollerman G H, Johnson R H, Ofek I, Bisno A L 1979 Human immune response to immunization with a structurally defined polypeptide fragment of streptococcal M protein. Journal of Experimental Medicine 150: 862–877

Beachey E H, Seyer J M, Dale J B, Simpson W A, Kang A H 1981 Type-specific protective immunity evoked by synthetic peptide of streptococcus pyogenes M protein. Nature 292: 457–459

Beachey E H, Tartar A, Seyer J M, Chedid L 1984 Epitope-specific protective immunogenicity of chemically synthesized 13-18-, and 23-residue peptide fragments of streptococcal M protein. Proceeding of the National Academy of Sciences of the USA State of America 81: 2203–2207

Beachey E H, Seyer J M, Dale J B 1987 Protective immunogenicity and T lymphocyte specificity of a trivalent hybrid peptide containing NH$_2$-terminal sequence of types 5, 6, and 24 M protein synthesized in tandem. Journal of Experimental Medicine 166: 647–656

Benedek T G 1984 Subcutaneous nodules and the differentiation of rheumatoid arthritis from rheumatic fever. Seminar in Arthritis and Rheumatism 13: 306–321

Bernheimer A W 1972 Hemolysins of streptococci: characterization and effects on biological membranes In: Wannamaker L W, Matsen J M (eds) Streptococci and streptococcal diseases. Academic Press, New York, p 19–31

Bernstein S H, Stollerman M, Allerhand J 1964 Demonstration of penicillin inhibition by pharyngitis. Journal of Laboratory and Clinical Medicine 63: 14–22

Bland E F 1961 Chorea as a manifestation of rheumatic fever: a long-term perspective. Transactions of American Clinical Climatology Association 73: 209–313

Breese B B, Disney F A 1956 Factors influencing spread of beta-hemolytic streptococcal infections within family group. Pediatrics 17: 834–838

Brink W R, Rammelkamp C H Jr, Denny F W, Wannamaker L W 1951 Effect of penicillin and aureomycin on the natural course of streptococcal tonsillitis and pharyngitis. American Journal of Medicine 10: 300–308

Burch G E, Giles T D, Colcolough H L 1970 Pathogenesis of 'rheuamtic' heart disease: critique and theory. American Heart Journal 80: 556–561

Carlquist J F, Ward R H, Meyer K J, Husebye D, Feolo M, Anderson J L 1995 Immune response factors in rheumatic heart disease: meta-analysis of HLA-DR associations and evaluation of additional class II alleles. American College of Cardiology 26: 452–457

Caughey D E, Douglas R, Wilson W, Hassal I B 1975. HLA antigens in Europeans and Maoris with rheumatic fever and rheumatic heart disease. Journal of Rheumatology 2: 319–322

Chancey R L, Morris A J, Conner R H, Cantanzaro F J, Chamovitz R, Rammelkamp C H Jr 1955 Studies of streptococcal prophylaxis; comparison of oral penicillin and benzathine penicillin. American Journal of Medical Sciences 229: 165–171

Cherian G 1979 Acute rheumatic fever–the Jones' criteria–a review and a case for polyarthralgia. Journal of Association of Physicians of India 27: 453–457

Coburn A F 1931 The factor of infections in the rheumatic state. Williams & Wilkins, Baltimore, MD

Coburn A F, Moore L V 1939 The prophylactic use of sulfanilamide in streptococcal respiratory infections with especial reference to rheumatic fever. Journal of Clinical Investigation 18: 147

Collis W R F 1938 Bacteriology of rheumatic fever. Lancet ii: 817

Cooperative Rheumatic Fever Study Group 1960 A comparison of the effect of prednisone and acetyl salicylic acid on the incidence of residual rheumatic heart disease. New England Journal of Medicine 262: 895–902

Cooperative Rheumatic Fever Study Group (eds) 1965 A comparison of short-term intensive prednisone and acetyl salicylic acid therapy in the treatment of acute rheumatic fever. New England Journal of Medicine 272: 63–70

Cromartie W J, Craddock J G, Schwab J H, Anderle S K, Yang C H 1977 Arthritis in rats after systemic injection of streptococcal cells or cell walls. Journal of Experimental Medicine 146: 1585–1602

Cuppari G, Quagliata F, Ieri A, Taranta A 1972 Lymphocyte transformation with streptolysin S preparations and inhibition of streptolysin S by serum in rheumatic fever and other rheumatic diseases. Journal of Laboratory and Clinical Medicine 80: 165–178

Dajani A S, Ayoub E, Bierman F Z et al 1992 Special writing group of the Committee on Rheumatic Fever, Endocarditis and Kawasaki disease of the Council of Cardiovascular Disease in the Young of the American Heart Association. Guidelines for the diagnosis of rheumatic fever: Jones, criteria: 1992 update. Journal of the American Medical Association 268: 2069–2073

Dajani A, Allen A D, Taubert K A 1993 Echocardiography for the diagnosis and management of rheumatic fever. Journal of the American Medical Association 269: 2084–2093

Dajani A, Taubert K, Ferrieri P, Peter G, Shulman S 1995 Treatment ofacute streptococcal pharyngitis and prevention of rheumatic fever: a statement for health professionals health professionals. Pediatrics 96: 758–764

Dale J B, Beachey E H 1986 Localization of protective epitomes of the amino terminus of type 5. Streptococcal M protein. Journal of Experimental Medicine 163: 1191–1202

Dale J B, Seyer J M, Beachey E H 1983 Type-specific immunogenicity of a chemically synthesized peptides fragment of type 5 streptococcal M protein. Journal of Experimental Medicine 158: 1727–1732

Dale J B, Seyer J M, Beachey E H 1986 Protective and nonprotective epitomes of chemically synthesized peptides of the NH2-terminal region of type streptococcal M protein. Journal of Immunology 136: 2287–2292

Daoud A S, Zalci M, Shaki R, Al-Salch Q 1990 Effectiveness of sodium valproate in the treatment of Syndenham's chorea. Neurology 40: 1140–1141

Denny F W Jr, Wannamaker L W, Brink W R, Rammerlkamp C H Jr, Cruster E A 1950 Prevention of rheumatic fever. Treatment of the preceding streptococcal infection. Journal of American Medical Association 143: 151–153

Dillon H C Jr 1967 Pyoderma and nephritis. Annual Review of Medicine 18: 207–218

Di Sciascio G, Taranta A 1980 Rheumatic fever in children. American Heart Journal 99: 635–658

Dock W 1933 Mode of production of first heart sound. Archives of Internal Medicine 51: 737–746

Dos Reis G A, Gaspar M I, Barcinski M A 1982 Immune recognition in the streptococcal carditis of mice: the role of macrophages in the generation of heart-reactive lymphocytes. Journal of Immunology 128: 1514–1521

Feinstein A R, Spagnuolo M 1962 The clinical pattern of acute rheumatic fever: a reappraisal. Medicine 41: 279–305

Ferguson G W, Shultz J M, Bisno A L 1991 Epidemiology of acute rheumatic fever in a multiethnic, multirural urban community. The Miami–Dale Country experience. Journal of Infectious Diseases 164: 720–725

Ferrans V J, Roberts W C 1980 Pathology of rheumatic heart disease. In: Borman J B, Gotsman M S (eds) Rheumatic valvular disease in children. Springer-Verlag, Berlin, p 28–58

Ginsburg I 1972 Mechanisms of cell and tissue injury induced by group A streptococci: relation to post-streptococcal sequelae. Journal of Infectious Diseases 126: 294–340, 419–456

Goldstein I, Rebeyrotte P, Parlebos T, Halpen B 1968 Isolation from heart valve of glycopeptides which share immunological properties with streptococcus hemolyticus group A polysaccharides. Nature 219: 866–869

Gordis L 1985 The virtual disappearance of rheumatic fever in the United States: lessons in the rise and fall of the disease. Circulation 72: 1155–1162

Gray E D, Wannamaker L W, Ayoub E M, el Kholy A, Abdin Z H 1981 Cellular immune responses to extracellular streptococcal products in rheumatic heart disease. Journal of Clinical Investigations 68: 665–671

Guilherme L, Weidebach W, Kiss M H, Snitcowsky R, Kalil J 1991 Association of human leukocyte class II antigens with rheumatic fever or rheumatic heart disease in a Brazilian population. Circulation 83: 1995–1998

Hafez M, Abdalla A, el-Shennawy F et al 1990 Immunogenetic study of the response to streptococcal carbohydrate antigen of the cell wall in rheumatic fever. Annals of Rheumatic Disease 9: 708–714

Halbert S P, Keatinge S L 1961 The analysis of streptococcal infections. Journal of Experimental Medicine 113: 1013–1028

Illingworth R S, Lorber J, Holt K S, Rendle-Short J, Jowett G H, Gibson W M 1957 Acute rheumatic fever in children. A comparison of six forms of treatment in 200 cases. Lancet ii: 653–659

Jhinghan B, Mehra N K, Reddy K S, Taneja V, Vaidya M C, Bhatia M L 1986 HLA, blood groups and secretor status in patients with established rheumatic fever and rheumatic heart disease. Tissue Antigens 27: 172–178

Johnson D R, Stevens D L, Kaplan E L 1992 Epidemiologic analysis of group A streptococcal serotypes associated with severe systemic infections, rheumatic fever or uncomplicated pharyngitis. Journal of Infections Diseases 166: 374–382

Jones T D 1944 Diagnosis of rheumatic fever. Journal of the American Medical Association 126: 481–484

Jones Criteria (Revised) 1984 for guidance in the diagnosis of rheumatic fever. Circulation 69: 203A–208A

Kaplan E L 1972 Unresolved problems in diagnosis and epidemiology of streptococcal infection In: Wannamaker L W, Matsen J M (eds) Streptococci and streptococcal diseases. Academic Press, New York, 557–570

Kaplan M H Suchy M L 1964 Immunologic relation of streptococcal and tissue antigens II. Cross reactions of antisera to mammalian heart tissue with a cell wall constituent of certain strains of group A streptococci. Journal of Experimental Medicine 119: 643–649

Kaplan M H, Svec K H 1964 Immunologic relation of streptococcal and tissue antigens III. Presence in human sera of streptococcal antigen cross-reactive with human heart tissue. Association with streptococcal infection, rheumatic fever and glomerulonephritis. Journal of Experimental Medicine 119: 651–666

Kaplan E L, Top F H Jr, Dudding B A, Wannamaker L W 1971 Diagnosis of streptococcal pharyngitis: The problem of differentiating active infection from the carrier state in the symptomatic child. Journal of Infectious Diseases 123: 490–501

Kaplan E L, Johnson D R, Cleary P P 1989a Group A streptococcal serotypes isolated from patient and sibling contacts during the resurgence of rheumatic fever in the United States in the mid-1980s Journal of Infectious Diseases 159: 101–103

Kaplan E L, Berrios X, Speth J, Siefferman T, Guzman B, Quesny F 1989b Pharmacokinetics of benzathine penicillin G: serum levels during the 28 days after intramuscular injection of 1 200 000 units. Pediatrics 115: 146–150

Keith J D 1937 Variations in the first heart sound and the auriculoventricular conduction time in children with rheumatic fever. Archives of Diseases in Childhood 12: 217–224

Keith J D, Rowe R D, Vlad P (eds) 1967 Rheumatic fever and rheumatic heart disease. In: Heart disease in infancy and childhood, 2nd edn. McMillan, New York, p 893–931

Kobt M, Majumdar G, Tomai M, Beachey E H 1990 Accessory cell-independant stimulation of human T cells by streptococcal M protein superantigen. Journal of Immunology 145: 1332–1336

Krause R M 1972 The streptococcal cell: relationship of structure, function and pathogenesis. In: Wannamaker L W, Matsen J M (eds) Streptococci and streptococcal diseases. Academic Press, New York, p 3–18

Krause R M, Rammelkamp C H Jr, Deny F W Jr, Wannamaker L W 1962 Studies of the carrier state following infection with group A streptococci In Effect of climate. Journal of Clinical Investigation 41: 568–574

Kuttner A G, Mayer E F 1963 Carditis during second attack of rheumatic fever. Its incidence in patients without clinical evidence of cardiac involvement in their initial rheumatic episode. New England Journal of Medicine 268: 1259–1261

Lancefield R G 1962 Current knowledge of type-specific M antigens of group A streptococci. Journal of Immunology 89: 307–313

Lannigan R, Zaki S 1963 Electron microscopic appearances of rheumatic lesions in the left auricular appendage in mitral stenosis. Nature 198: 898–899

Lannigan R, Zaki S 1968 An electron-microscope study of acid mucopolysaccharide in rheumatic heart lesions. Journal of Pathology and Bacteriology 96: 305–309

Lockman L A 1975 Movement disorders. In: Swainman K, Wright F (eds) Practice of pediatric neurology. Mosby, St Louis, MO

Lue H C, Wu M H, Hsieh K H et al 1986 Rheumatic fever recurrences: controlled study or 3-week versus 4-week benzathine penicillin prevention program. Journal of Pediatrics 108: 299–304

Lyampert I M, Belatskaya L V, Borodiyuk N A, Gnezditskaya E V, Rossokhina I I, Danilova T A 1976 A cross-reactive antigen of thymus and skin epithelial cells common with the polysaccharide of group A streptococci. Immunology 31: 47–55

Maharaj B, Hammond M G, Appadoo B et al 1987 HLA-A, B, DR, and DQ antigens in black patients with severe chronic rheumatic heart disease. Circulation 76: 259–261

Markowitz M 1985 The decline of rheumatic fever: role of medical intervention. Journal of Pediatrics 106: 545–550

McCarty M 1972 Theories of pathogenesis of streptococcal complications. In: Wannamaker L W, Matsen J M (eds) Streptococci and streptococcal disease. Academic Press, New York, p 517–526

McDonald E C, Weisman M H 1978 Articular manifestation of rheumatic fever in adults. Annals of Internal Medicine 89: 917–920

Massell B F, Flyer D C, Roy S B 1958 The clinical picture of rheumatic fever–diagnosis, immediate prognosis, course and therapeutic implications. American Journal of Cardiology 1: 436–449

Morell A, Doran J E, Skvaril F 1990 Outgoing of the humoral response to group A streptococcal carbohydrate: class and IgG subclass composition of antibodies in children. European Journal of Immunology 20: 1513

Morris A J, Chamovitz R, Catanzaro F J, Rammelkamp C H Jr 1956 Prevention of rheumatic fever by treatment of previous streptococci infections. Effect of sulphadiazine. Journal of American Medical Association 160: 114–166

Murphy G E 1959 On muscle cells, Aschoff bodies and cardiac Failure in rheumatic heart disease. Bulletin of the New York Academy of Medicine 35: 619–651

Narula J, Chandrasekhar Y, Rahimtoola S 1999 Diagnosis of active rheumatic carditis the echoes of change. Circulation 100: 1576–1581

Oakley C M 1980 Acute rheumatic carditis. In: Borman J B, Gotsman M S (eds) Rheumatic valvular disease in children. Springer-Verlag, Berlin, p 15

Pai A M, Kinare S G 1969 Auricular biopsies in rheumatic mitral stenosis. A histopathologic study of 264 cases. Journal of Postgraduate Medicine 14: 176–186

Parker M T 1969 streptococcal skin infection and acute glomeralonephritis. British Journal of Dermatology 81(suppl 1): 37–46

Patarryo M E, Winchester R J, Vejerano A et al 1979 Association of a B-cell alloantigen with susceptibility to rheumatic fever. Nature 278: 173–174

Pongpanich B 1976 The possible role of coxsackie group B virus in the pathogenesis of rheumatic fever and rheumatic heart disease in Thailand. (Abstract) 2nd southeast Asian conference on rheumatic fever and rheumatic heart disease, Philippines, p 21

Pruksakorn S, Curric B, Brandt E et al 1994 Towards a vaccine for rheumatic fever: identification of a conserved target epitome on M protein of group A streptococci. Lancet 344: 639–642

Rajapakse C N A, Halim K, Al-Orainey I, AI-Nozha M, AI-Aska A K 1987 A genetic marker for rheumatic heart disease. British Health Journal 58: 659–662

Rammelkamp C H Jr 1957 Epidemiology of streptococcal infections. Harvey Lectures 51: 113–142

Rammelkamp C H Jr, Denny F W, Wannamaker L W 1952 Studies on the epidemiology of rheumatic fever in the Armed Services. In: Thomas L (ed.) Rheumatic Fever. University of Minnesota Press, Minnesota, p 72–89

Read F E M, Ciocco A, Taussig H B 1938 Frequency of rheumatic manifestations among siblings, parents, uncles, aunts and grandparents of rheumatic and congenital patients. American Journal of Hygiene. 27: 719–737

Rotta J, Bednar B 1969 Biological properties of cell wall mucopeptide of hemolytic streptococci. Journal of Experimental Medicine 130: 31–47

Roy S B 1960 The diagnosis of rheumatic fever. Journal of Indian Medical Association 35: 344–351

Rutstein D D, Baver W, Dorfman A et al 1955 Jones, criteria (modified) for guidance in the diagnosis of rheumatic fever. Modern Concepts in Cardiovascular Disease 24: 291–293

Saphir O 1959 The Aschoff nodule. American Journal of Clinical Pathology 31: 534–539

Schmidt W C 1952 Group A streptococcus polysaccharide: Studies on its preparation, chemical composition and cellular localization after intravenous injection into mice. Journal of Experimental Medicine 95: 105–118

Schulman S T, Ayoub E M, Victoria B E et al 1974 Difference in antibody response to streptococcal antigens in children with rheumatic and non-rheumatic mitral valve disease. Circulation 50: 1244–1251

Siegel A C, Johnson E E, Stollerman G H 1961 Controlled studies of streptococcal pharyngitis in a pediatric population. I. Factors related to the attack rate of rheumatic fever. New England Journal of Medicine 265: 559–564

Stevens D L 1992 Invasive group A streptococcus infections. Clinical Infections Diseases 14: 2–13

Stollerman G H 1969 Nephritogenic and rheumatogenic group A streptococci. Journal of Infectious Diseases 120: 258–263

Stollerman G 1975 Epidemiology of rheumatic fever. In: Rheumatic fever and streptococcal infections. Grune and Stratton, New York, p 66

Stollerman G H 1980 Streptococcal vaccines and global strategies for prevention of rheumatic fever. American Journal of Medicine 68: 636–638

Stollerman G H 1982 Global changes in group A streptococcal diseases and strategics for their prevention. Advances in Internal Medicine 27: 373–406

Stollerman G H, Markowitz M, Taranta A, Wannamaker L W, Whitemore R 1965 A Jones, criteria (revised) for guidance in the diagnosis of rheumatic fever. Circulation 32: 664–668

Taneja V, Mehra N K, Reddy K S et al 1989 HLA-DR/DQ and reactivity to B cell alloantigen D8/17 in Indian patients with rheumatic heart disease. Circulation 80: 335–340

Taranta A 1967 Factors influencing recurrent rheumatic fever. Annual Review Medicine 18: 159–172

Taranta A, Wood H F, Feinstein A R et al 1964 Rheumatic fever in children and adolescents. IV. Relation of the rheumatic fever recurrence rate per streptococcal infection to the titers of streptococcal antibodies. American Internal Medicine 60: 47–57

Todome Y, Ohkuni H, Mizuse M et al 1992 Detection of antibodies against streptococcal peptidoglycan and the peptide subunit (synthetic tetra-D-alanyl-bovine serum albumin complex) in rheumatic diseases. International Archives of Allergy and Immunology 97:301–307

Ty E T, Ortiz E E 1992 M-mode, cross-sectional and color flow doppler echocardiographic findings in acute rheumatic fever. Cardiology in the Young 2: 229–235

United Kingdom and United States Joint Report 1955 The treatment of acute rheumatic fever in children. A cooperative clinical trial of ACTH, cortisone and aspirin. Circulation 11: 343–377

United Kingdom and United States Joint Report 1965 The natural history of rheumatic fever and rheumatic heart disease: Ten year report of a cooperative clinical trial of ACTH, cortisone and aspirin. Circulation 32: 445–456

Veasy L G 1995 Rheumatic fever–T. Duchett Jones and the rest of the story. Cardiology of the Young 5: 293–301

Virmani R, Roberts W C 1977 Aschoff bodies in operatively excised atrial appendages and in papillary muscles. Frequency and clinical significance. Circulation 55: 559–563 von Glahn W C 1947 The pathology of rheumatism. American Journal of Medicine 2: 76–85

Wannamaker L W 1951 Prophylaxis of acute rheumatic fever by treatment of the preceding streptococcal infection with various amounts of depot penicillin. American Journal of Medicine 10: 673–685

Wannamaker L W 1970 Medical progress: Differences between streptococcal infections of the throat and the skin. New England Journal of Medicine 282: 23–31, 78–85

Wannamaker L W 1976 A penicillin shot without culturing the child's throat. Journal of the American Medical Association 235: 913–914

Wannamaker L W, Ayoub E M 1960 Antibody in acute rheumatic fever. Circulation 21: 598–614

Wannamaker L W, Wyo C, Denny W, Perry W D, Siegal A C, Rammelkamp C H Jr 1954 Studies on immunity to streptococcal infections in man. American Journal of Diseases in Children 86: 347–348

Widdowson J P, Maxted W R, Pinney A M 1971 An M-associated protein antigen (MAP) of group A streptococci. Journal of Hygiene 69: 533–564

Wilson M G, Schweitzer M 1954 Pattern of hereditary susceptibility in rheumatic fever. Circulation 10: 699–704

Wilson N J, Neutze J M 1995 Echocardiographic diagnosis of subclinical carditis in acute rheumatic fever. International Journal of Cardiology 50: 1–6

WHO Study Group 1988 Rheumatic fever and rheumatic heart disease. World Health Organization Technical Report Series 764: 21–25

Zabriskie J B, Freimer E H 1966 An immunological relationship between the group A streptococcus and mammalian muscle. Journal of Experimental Medicine 124: 661–678

65

Chronic rheumatic valvar disease

E. E. Ortiz and R. H. Anderson*

INTRODUCTION

Permanent damage to the valves of the heart is the most important sequel of the acute rheumatic process. It is the major cause of morbidity and mortality and requires medical or surgical treatment. The clinical presentation, the mortality, as well as the frequency and speed of development of established valvar disease after the acute rheumatic process, vary considerably geographically, influenced primarily by the socioeconomic and medical backgrounds of the populations involved. In North America and Western Europe, the incidence and virulence of the acute process, and the residual development of chronic valvar disease, was declining by the end of the 1970s (Markowitz, 1977). In most developed countries, therefore, severe rheumatic valvar disease is now uncommon in children, and treatment for the advanced form of the disease is usually limited to adults. In contrast, in most developing countries in Asia, Africa, Central and South America, the rheumatic process frequently has a much more malignant effect on the heart than in adults, resulting in severe pathological changes that lead to well-established and severe valvar disease. The accelerated time course, and the high incidence of severe disease seen in the developing countries, has been attributed to more frequent recurrent streptococcal infections, and to recurrences of the acute rheumatic process, as well as a generalized decrease in the resistance of the host. Chronic disease, involving the mitral valve in particular, occurs frequently in children. Many of these children die in consequence of the valvar disease before the age of 20 years (Borman et al, 1961; Gotsman and van der Horst, 1975). Mitral stenosis is a common lesion, and percutaneous balloon valvoplasty, or closed mitral commissurotomy, are frequent procedures carried out in children in these regions. Mitral incompetence, aortic incompetence and tricuspid valvar disease may also be sufficiently severe to cause life-threatening haemodynamic effects. These complications may require major cardiac surgery, either electively or even occasionally as an emergency. The progress in diagnostic methods, catheter interventions, surgical expertise and techniques, and the development of improved valvar prostheses, has encouraged the increased use of non-surgical and surgical techniques for the treatment of rheumatic valvar disease in these areas in children and young adults, with encouraging long-term results.

The healing process of rheumatic carditis results in varying degrees of fibrosis and valvar damage. Besides this, subacute, subclinical or chronic carditis may, and does, modify the course of the disease by aggravating the myocardial damage. This adds to the haemodynamic effects of the valvar lesions themselves. Acute rheumatic pericarditis usually heals to give a normal pericardium. Though, in some instances, fusion and thickening of the pericardium may occur with adhesions, this rarely affects the ultimate cardiac performance. Rheumatic carditis may heal with minimal residue, involving minor degrees of thickening of the valves and tendinous cords, and some fibrosis of the valvar endocardium. It is generally felt that these minor lesions are usually non-progressive and are unlikely to produce subsequent abnormal haemodynamic effects. These valves are, however, susceptible to infective endocarditis, which, should it occur, will significantly alter the cardiac status. In endemic areas, particularly in developing countries, progression does occur over a fairly short period of time from mild lesions to significant ones. It is likely that episodes of subclinical carditis result in more significant chronic rheumatic valvar disease. The fact that many adults present with rheumatic heart disease without an earlier history of an acute episode supports this view, although the exact incidence, diagnosis and recognition of subclinical attacks is difficult to evaluate. More recent studies, using echocardiography, have consistently documented that subclinical carditis does occur, and that the true incidence of carditis is probably much higher than previously thought.

---

*Adapted from a chapter prepared for the First Edition by the late I. P. Sukumar.

The incidence of chronic rheumatic valvar disease is higher in those who have had severe cardiac involvement during the initial episode or, more importantly, in those who develop recurrences of acute rheumatic process over a short period of time. There is a characteristic distribution of pathological lesions. The relative frequency with which each individual valve is affected may be related to the pressure load against which it normally operates. Multiple involvement is common (Wood, 1968). The mitral valve is most commonly affected, followed by a combination of mitral and aortic valves, isolated aortic valvar disease, usually incompetence, and combined mitral, aortic and tricuspid disease (Figure 65.1). Chronic rheumatic involvement of the pulmonary valve is rare. For example, in all patients seen with chronic rheumatic valvar disease in childhood and adolescence, Kaplan (1977) reported an overall involvement of the mitral valve in 85%, the aortic valve in 54% and the tricuspid and pulmonary valves in less than 5%. The most common rheumatic lesion in developing countries is pure mitral incompetence, which occurs as an isolated lesion in about two fifths of children. Mixed mitral valvar disease is common, while pure mitral stenosis is present in one tenth. This is in contrast to the distribution of mitral valvar lesions in the United State of America and the United Kingdom, where pure mitral stenosis is more common. The aortic valvar is involved in between one tenth and half the patients, but this is seen more often in the older subjects in Western populations. Most of those with aortic valvar disease have associated mitral valve disease. Isolated rheumatic aortic valvar disease is uncommon, and when encountered it usually produces valvar incompetence. Tricuspid valvar disease occurs in about one eighth of patients, invariably accompanying mitral and or aortic valvar lesions. The pulmonary valve is involved in only 1% (Wood, 1968; Spencer and Makene, 1972; McLaren et al, 1975). A higher incidence of mitral stenosis in the young has been reported from many tropical countries (Cherian et al, 1964; Paul, 1967; Gotsman & van der Horst, 1975).

PATHOLOGY OF CHRONIC VALVAR DISEASE

CHANGES WITHIN THE HEART

There is no single pathological change that is responsible for the development of chronic valvar disease following the acute rheumatic process. The mechanisms by which acute valvitis results in chronic deformity include continuing endocardial inflammation, neovascularization of the valvar leaflets, scarring by deposition of new fibrous connective tissue and degeneration of pre-existing fibrous connective tissue that has been involved in the earlier inflammatory process. Little is known of the factors that influence the progression of these pathological changes. A strong correlation exists, nonetheless, between the severity and the number of episodes of carditis, the number of valves damaged and the extent of this damage. As the valves become deformed, there is considerable remodelling of the entire valvar and subvalvar apparatus, which involves synthesis of large amounts of new collagen. Additionally, there is replacement of normally arranged collagen that has been broken down as a result of inflammation. The new collagen is then arranged in a different pattern. Several distinct types of collagen are known to exist, but the relative extent of involvement of each type in the fibrotic process is not fully determined. Fibrils of mature collagen, as well as finer fibrils and fragmentation and degeneration of collagen, have been demonstrated in leaflets from rheumatic valves (Fenoglio and Wagner, 1973).

Rheumatic heart disease may well be viewed as a disease of the mitral valve (Ferrans and Roberts, 1980). The other valves are involved anatomically and functionally, but anatomically the mitral valve is always involved. Aschoff bodies have never been found in hearts without anatomical disease of the mitral valve. In isolated mitral stenosis, the leaflets are diffusely thickened by fibrous tissue, the commissures are fused and the tendinous chords are shortened and fused. The entire valvar mechanism becomes funnel-shaped, with its apex in the left ventricular cavity, where the greatest obstruction occurs. The entrance to the valvar funnel at the level of the atrioventricular junction is usually less narrowed. Fusion of the leaflets invariably takes place at both ends of their zone of apposition. Occasionally, one end may be more fused than the other, the anterolateral end more often than the posteroinferior. Should fusion involve only

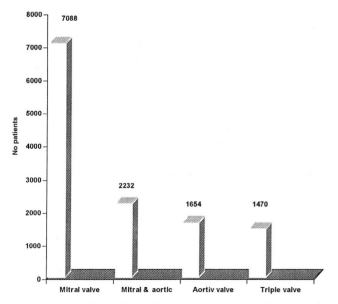

Figure 65.1. Analysis of the valves involved in the overall experience of the Christian Medical College, Vellore, India, with patients having chronic rheumatic heart disease. Only a minority of these patients were children or young adults (see Figure 65.2).

one end, the stenotic orifice is eccentric. With symmetrical fusion, the narrowed distal orifice is more centrally located. The so-called 'fish-mouth' appearance of the valvar orifice occurs in lesions that produce both stenosis and incompetence. The tendinous cords can be retracted; as a result, the leaflets appear to insert almost directly into the papillary muscles. This aggravates the degree of obstruction through obliteration of the intercordal spaces. The extent and progression of calcification is largely time dependent, and hence it is less frequent in children and adolescents. An earlier commissurotomy does not necessarily predispose the valvar leaflets to deposition of calcium. In terms of the haemodynamic effects, subvalvar fusion and cordal shortening are as important as commissural fusion. The pathological anatomy of mitral incompetence involves the valvar leaflets, particularly their attachments at the atrioventricular junction, and the tendinous cords. The leaflets are scarred and contracted. The mural leaflet is more frequently involved than the aortic leaflet. Valvar shortening means that the leaflets are not able to coapt. With left atrial enlargement, further separation of the leaflets occurs, widening the atrioventricular junction and thus increasing the degree of mitral incompetence. The tendinous cords then restrain the mural leaflet, which is displaced posteriorly over the base of the left ventricular wall. Since the left atrium is also displaced downwards and posteriorly, the mural leaflet is pulled across as the left atrium enlarges. Rupture of cords is usually caused by infective endocarditis but can also occur in acute rheumatic valvitis. Shortening of the papillary muscles, and dilation of the atrioventricular junction, aggravates the degree of mitral incompetence. Structural alterations in the purely incompetent mitral valve are markedly different from those in the stenotic valve. Deposition of calcium, commissural fusion, thickening of the cords and cordal fusion are far less frequent in mitral incompetence. The left atrial dilation is a result of the earlier rheumatic inflammation. The cause of the so-called 'giant left atrium' in some patients with mitral incompetence is uncertain. It is possible that these patients have had more frequent or more severe attacks of rheumatic carditis, with severe destruction of atrial myocardial fibres.

Chronic rheumatic aortic stenosis occurs through fusion of the commissures, and thickening and fibrosis of the leaflets, and, as a result the valve becomes transformed into a rigid structure with a central triangular orifice. As anticipated, typically the valve retains its trifoliate template, but the rheumatic process can also involve aortic valves with only two leaflets. It is unusual, however, for the valve to be purely stenotic. More frequently it is incompetent, or incompetent and stenotic. When incompetent, the valvar leaflets are thickened, fibrosed and contracted and are unable to coapt centrally during diastole. Alternatively, one or more of the leaflets may be severely retracted. Sometimes, only a small remnant of the original leaflet is identifiable. In a purely regurgitant rheumatic aortic valve, calcification is uncommon. The aorta may dilate but is of normal thickness and the intima is not affected. Associated fibrous thickening of the mitral valve is invariably found (Roberts, 1970a).

Rheumatic tricuspid stenosis is the result of diffuse thickening of the valvar leaflets. This is usually because of proliferation of fibrous tissue and commissural fusion, but cordal shortening and fibrosis may also occur. Calcification is uncommon. Tricuspid regurgitation is most commonly functional, as a consequence of severe right ventricular dilation, rather than organic. Sclerosis of the valvar leaflets, fibrosis with cordal thickening and some commissural fusion and increased vascularity with perivascular fibrosis have all been described in addition to the dilated atrioventricular junction (Banerjee et al, 1982). Organic disease of the pulmonary valve is an extreme rarity.

CHANGES IN THE LUNGS

With chronic rheumatic valvar disease, especially mitral stenosis and incompetence, secondary changes occur in the lungs. The changes in the pulmonary veins may include intimal, medial and adventitial fibrous proliferation. The lymphatics may show marked dilation, and the interlobular septums may show considerable thickening, through oedema, dilated lymphatic channels or formation of fibrous tissue. The alveolar septums may have thickened initially by dilation of alveolar capillaries, and later by fibrous tissue. The alveolar sacks accumulate serum and erythrocytes, the latter resulting in the deposition of haemosiderin-laden macrophages. The pulmonary changes are far more obvious and common in mitral stenosis than in any other valvar lesion, although many of them do occur with mitral regurgitation and severe aortic regurgitation. With the typical involvement of the mitral valve occurring precociously in children in the tropics, severe pulmonary hypertension with pulmonary arterial and arteriolar changes are common.

CLINICAL MANIFESTATIONS

Chronic rheumatic valvar disease, when encountered at any age, usually exists in the combinations discussed above. Valvar lesions that are purely stenotic or incompetent certainly do occur, but combinations are more common. For the sake of simplicity, subsequent description of the clinical findings, and the treatment, will be made as though the individual lesion existed as an isolated entity. As also emphasized, although significant rheumatic valvar disease of sufficient severity to present as a therapeutic or surgical problem is now uncommon in children and adolescents in developed countries, this is not the case in those countries that are less developed.

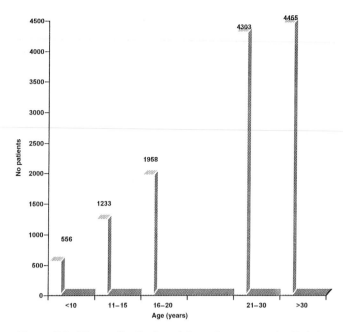

Figure 65.2. The age distribution of the patients seen at the Christian Medical College, Vellore, India, with chronic rheumatic heart disease. Only three tenths were less than 20 years of age.

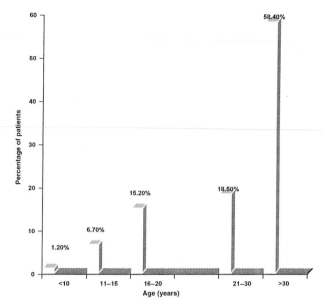

Figure 65.3. The age distribution of the patients seen at Christian Medical College, Vellore, India, in whom a closed mitral valvotomy was carried out. Just under one quarter were young adults or children.

When the first edition of this book appeared, of the patients admitted with established chronic severe rheumatic valvar disease at Vellore, in India, one third were below the age of 20 yearss (Figure 65.2). Since clinically important chronic rheumatic heart disease continues to occur in children in the developing countries, descriptions of the disease entity will be given as seen in those areas. The diagnosis of established rheumatic valvar disease in childhood and adolescents is not particularly difficult. The management of the individual patient, however, is determined not only by the severity of the valvar lesions, but also by the association of intercurrent arrhythmias, other disease processes and the presence of additional myocardial dysfunction. Myocardial dysfunction definitely influences the severity, the clinical progress and the prognosis of rheumatic valvar disease.

—————— MITRAL STENOSIS ——————

Mitral stenosis is a common chronic rheumatic valvar lesion. In developed countries, however, this finding is rare in children and adolescents, probably involving less than one twentieth of those with rheumatic heart disease. If the mitral valve is involved, a number of years usually elapse before the narrowing of the valvar orifice reaches a level sufficient to produce symptoms. In the United States of America, 5 to 10 years were said to be required for this progression (Nadas and Fyler, 1972). Wood (1954), from an even earlier era, described a latent period of 19 years for the development of significant mitral stenosis. In contrast, in most developing countries, mitral stenosis requiring surgical treatment can still occur from

6 months to 3 years after the initial rheumatic episode. Out of a consecutive series of 579 closed mitral valvotomies performed in young patients in India (Sukumar, 1982), one third had symptoms lasting for less than 12 months, and in another third the symptoms lasted less than 3 years, with a mean duration of 2 years. Similar data have been reported from other neighbouring countries. Paul (1967) found that in one quarter of patients the interval between the initial rheumatic episode and surgery was less than 1 year, and in almost another half it was less than 2 years. Analysis of the surgical experience with closed mitral valvotomy in Vellore, involving almost 4000 procedures (Sukumar, 1982), shows that almost one quarter were undertaken in patients aged less than 20 years (Figure 65.3). Although females are said to be more frequently involved when adult (Wood, 1954), the incidence is nearly equal between the genders in children seen in India (Cherian et al, 1964) and Sri Lanka (Paul, 1967). The major difference between mitral stenosis as seen in adults and that in children, at least as seen in the developing countries, is the accelerated rapid progression of the rheumatic process in the latter. This produces sufficient valvar disorganization to require early surgical treatment. Critical or significant mitral stenosis is present when the area of the valvar orifice is reduced to about one quarter of the expected normal for the age.

PHYSIOLOGY ——————

The obstruction of the valvar orifice produces a barrier in diastolic left ventricular filling from the left atrium. Gorlin et al (1951a,b, 1955) showed that the pressure in the left atrium has to be elevated to overcome the obstruction at the site of the mitral valve. Thus, a gradient is established between the left atrial and left ventricular end-diastolic pressures. The elevated left atrial pressure is reflected in the elevated pulmonary capillary or pulmonary wedge pressure. The severity of mitral stenosis determines both the gradient and the left atrial and pulmonary venous pressures. With critical mitral stenosis, that is with valvar areas less than one quarter of the expected normal, there is severe left atrial and pulmonary venous hypertension. The pulmonary arterial pressure rises correspondingly to maintain an adequate pulmonary flow. Pulmonary arteriolar constriction, a result of a combination of vasospasm and pulmonary arteriolar disease, results in an elevated pulmonary vascular resistance. With persistent significant pulmonary hypertension, right ventricular failure occurs. With mild-to-moderate elevation of left atrial pressure, exercise or sudden tachyarrhythmias may diminish the diastolic filling period, resulting in an abrupt elevation of the left atrial pressure. Pulmonary oedema may then occur. Pulmonary hypertension in the beginning is passive. With alteration of pulmonary exchange of gases, and associated hypoxia and arteriolar vasoconstriction, obliterative pulmonary hypertension develops. Since the pulmonary venous pressure in critical mitral stenosis may exceed the oncotic plasma pressure of 30 mmHg, the increased pulmonary vascular resistance is to a large extent a protective mechanism. Thickening of the capillary walls, interstitial tissue and alveolar membranes produces a barrier at the interface between the capillaries and the alveolar sacks. In isolated mitral stenosis, the relationships of pulmonary pressure and flow are not constant. In some patients, the pulmonary circulation is maintained with only modest elevation of pulmonary arterial pressure, while in others established pulmonary vascular disease occurs with severe pulmonary hypertension and pressures above systemic level. Most patients with mild-to-moderate mitral stenosis are able to maintain an adequate cardiac output with moderate exercise. In the presence of critical mitral stenosis, the cardiac output is low at rest. Exercise does not increase the cardiac output, which may even fall in the presence of significant pulmonary hypertension. The latter also causes tricuspid incompetence. In patients who have had repeated episodes of rheumatic carditis, the severity and frequency of congestive heart failure is out of proportion to the severity of the valvar disease alone.

CLINICAL FEATURES

The symptoms, physical signs and the amount of clinical disability parallel the severity of mitral stenosis. Those with minimal stenosis may be completely asymptomatic. The common symptoms in critical stenosis are effort dyspnoea, orthopnoea, paroxysmal nocturnal dyspnoea and episodes of pulmonary oedema. These symptoms may be aggravated by recurrence of carditis, intercurrent infections, uncontrolled tachycardia or atrial fibrillation on undue exertion. Congestive heart failure usually occurs with severe stenosis and more than moderate pulmonary hypertension. This may also be aggravated or precipitated by the above-mentioned conditions. Haemoptysis can occur, either during bouts of paroxysmal dyspnoea or as a result of rupture of bronchial or pleurohilar veins. Occasionally, it happens because of peripheral pulmonary infarction. Atrial fibrillation and systemic embolization are uncommon in children. In the presence of a low cardiac output and a high pulmonary vascular resistance, peripheral cyanosis and a malar flush have been described. The volume of the pulses is small or normal. The systemic venous pressure is elevated in the presence of heart failure and pulmonary hypertension. This elevation is proportional to the severity of stenosis, and it becomes marked with the onset of cardiac failure or atrial fibrillation. The cardiac impulse is usually right ventricular, characteristically described as 'tapping' in nature. When pulmonary hypertension is present, a parasternal lift is found, and pulmonary arterial pulsations, as well as closure of the pulmonary valve, are palpable. There are classic auscultatory findings in mitral stenosis. The first heart sound is accentuated because of an abrupt closure of the leaflets, which are held open until the beginning of ventricular systole. There is a loud, sharp and high-pitched opening snap caused by a sudden tensing of the leaflets at the limit of their excursion of opening in diastole. A long, rumbling, low-pitched mid-diastolic murmur is heard at the apex, often with presystolic accentuation. The interval between closure of the aortic valve and the onset of the opening snap correlates with the severity of stenosis (Wells, 1954). In the absence of associated mitral incompetence, the duration of the diastolic murmur is directly proportional to the severity of the stenosis. The duration of the murmur, however, may be altered by a fast ventricular rate or by the presence of congestive heart failure. The murmur is best appreciated in the lateral position, listening with the bell of the stethoscope. It is augmented by inhalation of amyl nitrite, and by exercise. The onset of the atrial fibrillation tends to abolish the presystolic accentuation. The presence of a pulmonary ejection click and an accentuated pulmonary component of the second sound, along with murmurs of pulmonary and tricuspid incompetence, indicate severe pulmonary hypertension. So-called 'silent' mitral stenosis occurs in severe disease with a low cardiac output, or with severe calcification.

The electrocardiogram shows evidence of left atrial enlargement. Broad notched P waves are seen in the limb leads, or a biphasic P wave in V_1 and V_2, with a marked negative component. Right atrial enlargement, right-axis deviation, and right ventricular hypertrophy of varying degrees reflect the severity of the pulmonary hypertension (Figure 65.4). Atrial fibrillation is uncommon in children and adolescents. In mild stenosis, the tracing may be

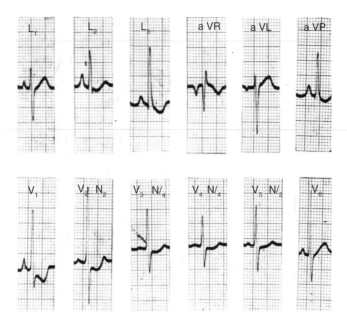

Figure 65.4. The electrocardiogram of an 11-year-old child with tight mitral stenosis and severe pulmonary hypertension. There is evidence of right-axis deviation, right ventricular hypertrophy and enlargement of both atrial chambers.

completely normal. The chest radiograph shows varying degrees of left atrial enlargement which displaces the oesophagus backwards, with elevation of the left main bronchus and widening of the carina. The enlarged left atrial appendage may be visible on the left cardiac border (Figure 65.5). In the presence of pulmonary hypertension, the pulmonary trunk and the chambers of the right heart are enlarged. The aorta is usually normal or small. Valvar calcification is best seen by cine-fluoroscopy. The degree

of left atrial enlargement is usually less in isolated mitral stenosis than in mitral incompetence. With mild pulmonary venous hypertension, there is initially distension only of the pulmonary veins from the lower lobes, which may be difficult to identify clearly. Once there is significant pulmonary venous hypertension, usually with a pressure of more than 15 mmHg, there is interstitial oedema in the lower zone and vasoconstriction in the veins supplying them. The flow of pulmonary blood is then increased in the veins to the upper lobes, which are dilated, producing differential pulmonary venous circulation. Kerley's A and B lines are seen because of interstitial oedema and small interlobar effusions. Acute pulmonary oedema is recognized by a typical perihilar opacity with radiations to the periphery.

The echocardiogram has, over the last few years, become the most useful diagnostic tool in the assessment of mitral stenosis in the preoperative phase, and even more so during postoperative follow-up. M-mode interrogation still provides considerable information. The valvar leaflets move anteriorly during diastole rather than posteriorly as in the normal situation. The EF slope is decreased, as is the rate of diastolic closure of the aortic mitral leaflet, generally in relation to the severity of the mitral stenosis. Exact correlations between the EF slope and the calculated area of the mitral valvar orifice are lacking. The slope ranges from 10 to 25 mm/s in mild-to-moderate stenosis, and is less than 10 mm/s in severe stenosis. The mural leaflet is frequently tethered to the aortic leaflet, and both can move in parallel fashion during diastole. The amplitude of opening of the aortic leaflet is decreased. Echoes may occur as a result of heavy fibrosis or calcification. The left atrial dimension is

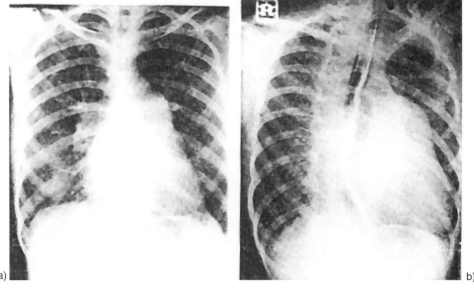

Figure 65.5. The chest radiograph, shown in posteroanterior and right anterior oblique views, the latter with a barium swallow, from a 12-year-old child with severe mitral stenosis and pulmonary hypertension. (a) The frontal view shows cardiomegaly, with an enlarged left atrium, seen as a double density, a dilated pulmonary trunk and venous congestion in the upper lobes of the lungs. (b) The oblique view demonstrates the backward displacement of the barium-filled oesophagus caused by left atrial enlargement.

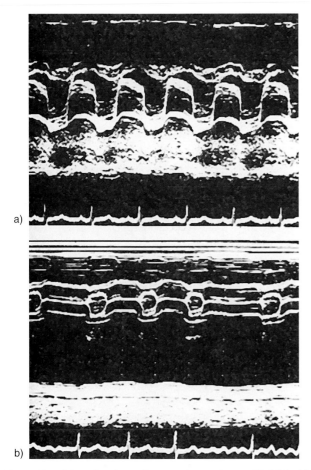

a)

b)

Figure 65.6. M-mode echocardiograms from a 9-year-old child with severe mitral stenosis. The upper trace shows a decreased EF slope of the aortic leaflet of the mitral valve, and abnormal movement of the mural leaflet. Both leaflets are thickened and move forward parallel to each other during diastole. The lower trace shows that the aortic valve and aortic root are normal, but the left atrial diameter is increased.

increased. Left ventricular and aortic dimensions are usually normal (Figure 65.6). As expected, cross-sectional echocardiograms provide considerably more information. The parasternal long-axis view demonstrates the mitral valve, the subvalvar apparatus, the left atrium, the aortic valve and the aortic root. Thickening and tethering of the stenotic leaflets can be seen. Severe fibrosis or calcification, which may also involve the subvalvar apparatus, reduces the mobility of the leaflets. Left ventricular contraction is usually normal, but there may be a reduced rate of filling. The short-axis view provides a more accurate assessment of the anatomy of the valvar orifice and the thickness of the leaflets. Areas measured using this view show good correlation with measurements made using Gorlin's formula (Henry et al, 1975). The relative size and relations of the ventricles and atriums are better seen in the apical four-chamber view. Besides left atrial enlargement, there may be evidence of right ventricular dilatation, paradoxical septal motion and deviation of the septum into the left ventricle seen with the onset of pulmonary hypertension, especially in the presence of tricuspid incompetence.

In the majority of patients with isolated mitral stenosis, where the clinical, electrocardiographic, radiological and echocardiographic appearances are characteristic, cardiac catheterization and angiography are not required. These techniques are needed in the presence of associated valvar lesions, or when the clinical features are atypical. They make it possible to exclude associated mitral incompetence, which may preclude a closed mitral valvotomy, to assess the degree and severity of associated aortic and tricuspid valvar lesions, and to assess left ventricular dysfunction in a patient with congestive heart failure. Associated incompetence can occasionally be excluded in patients with severe pulmonary hypertension and tricuspid regurgitation, in whom the signs of mitral stenosis may be atypical. The cardinal abnormality at catheterization is the diastolic gradient across the mitral valve, measured by simultaneous recording of pressures in the left ventricle and either in the pulmonary capillary wedge or directly in the left atrium. Simultaneous measurements are more useful than measuring pulmonary capillary wedge pressures alone (Figure 65.7). The severity of obstruction shown by the degree of the diastolic gradient correlates well with calculated areas of the mitral valve. In sinus rhythm, the late diastolic 'post-A' gradient is the most important measurement. In the presence of atrial fibrillation, however, the A wave disappears. The C-wave then becomes prominent and an X descent is not usually clearly seen. It is useful to calculate

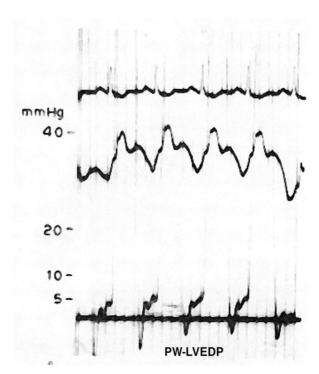

Figure 65.7. Simultaneously recorded pulmonary capillary wedge and left ventricular pressures reveal a gradient across the mitral valve in a 10-year-old child with severe mitral stenosis. The wedge pressure is markedly elevated, with a high end-diastolic gradient between the pulmonary wedge (PW) and left ventricular end-diastolic pressure (LVedp).

the gradient in six or seven consecutive cycles and take an average. The level of pulmonary hypertension can be measured from the peak and the mean pulmonary arterial pressure and the calculated index of pulmonary vascular resistance. In those who have apparently mild mitral stenosis, as shown by a small gradient, but with significant symptoms, measurement of the gradient is useful subsequent to exercise. If performing angiography, the mitral valve is best profiled by selective left ventricular angiography in the 30 degree right anterior oblique position. In mitral stenosis with a mobile valve, a clear non-opacified crescent is clearly visualized (Figure 65.8). This view is also the best for assessing the degree of mitral incompetence and the function of the left ventricle. Aortic root angiography in the left anterior oblique view is usually performed to exclude or assess the degree of associated aortic incompetence. In most cases, nonetheless, these measurements and other necessary data can now be obtained with a high degree of accuracy by echocardiography.

The profile of mitral stenosis in younger patients as seen in the developing countries, as mentioned earlier, appears to be different from that seen in the developed countries. In developing countries, it is characterized by a short duration and rapid progression of symptoms, with significant pulmonary hypertension and congestive

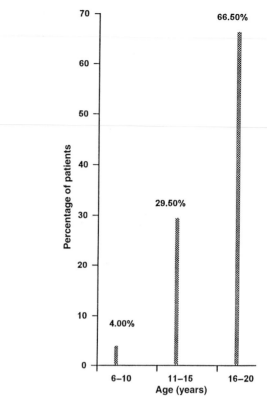

Figure 65.9. The age distribution of almost 600 children and young adults with mitral stenosis who underwent closed mitral valvotomy at the Christian Medical College, Vellore, India. Mean age 16.4 years; youngest (5 patients) 8 years of age. See text for further discussion.

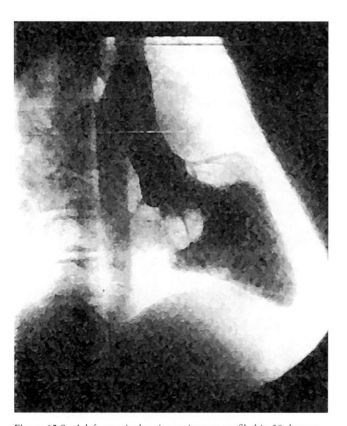

Figure 65.8. A left ventricular cineangiogram profiled in 30 degrees right anterior oblique projection in a patient with tight mitral stenosis. The left ventricular function is normal. A clear crescent is produced by the non-opacified blood from the left atrium crossing a mobile but stenotic valve.

heart failure, requiring surgery at an earlier age. In the patients with mitral stenosis undergoing surgery at Vellore, and reported by Sukumar in 1982 (Figure 65.9), one third were below the age of 15 years, one fifth were between 16 and 17, and almost half were between 18 and 20 years. Of these patients, one quarter came from a low socioeconomic group and over a fifth had clinical evidence of malnutrition. A past rheumatic history was available in only half. Assessment of the preoperative functional status, using the criterions of the New York Heart Association, showed that only one sixth were in grade 1, with one third in grade 2, and half in grades 3 or 4. Clinical evidence of an enlarged heart was found in two thirds, and one third had paroxysmal nocturnal dyspnoea or congestive cardiac failure. Haemoptysis was noticed in one fifth, but embolic manifestations were uncommon. Clinical signs of pulmonary hypertension were present in almost all. Nearly one third had murmurs of tricuspid regurgitation, and one tenth had pulmonary incompetence. Increased heart size was noted on the chest radiography in three quarters, with evidence of left atrial enlargement in virtually all. A prominent pulmonary trunk, and differential flow through the pulmonary veins to the upper lobes, were virtually ubiquitous. Atrial fibrillation, however, was very rare. Of the patients, 90 had undergone haemodynamic investigations. The right atrial A wave was more than 8 mmHg in one third, and right ventricular end-diastolic pressure was more than 8 mmHg in two fifths. The peak systolic pulmonary arterial pressure was normal in only one twentieth, ranging from 25 to 150 mmHg, with a mean of 72.6 mmHg. The pulmonary arterial peak pressure was suprasystemic in one tenth. Pulmonary vascular resistance index was more than 6 units in two thirds. The pulmonary capillary wedge pressure ranged from 14 to 43 mmHg, with a mean of 26.8 mmHg. In two thirds, the wedge pressure was more than 21 mmHg.

The gradient across the mitral valve ranged from 10 to 35 mmHg, with a mean of 19.2 mmHg. In one third, it was above 21 mmHg. The systemic index was less than 1.6 l/min m^{-2} in two thirds. At surgery, the mitral valvar diameter was found to be less than 5 mm in almost four fifths, and between 6 and 10 mm in another fifth. Both ends of the zone of apposition between the valvar leaflets were fused in over nine tenths. Shrinkage of the valvar leaflets, and subvalvar fusion, was noted in almost half. Calcification, however, was uncommon. Aschoff bodies were found in the left atrial appendage of almost three fifths, but organized thrombus in the left atrium or its appendage was discovered in only one tenth.

MANAGEMENT

The management of isolated mitral stenosis has traditionally been surgical. Since the 1980s, advances in interventional cardiology have dramatically changed the options for management. The potential surgical strategies include open and closed mitral commissurotomy or replacement of the valve, while intervention involves use of special catheters with balloons and other devices. But whether the options are interventional or surgical, the timing and indications have remained the same.

The timing is determined by the effects of obstruction, and by symptoms, rather than by age. Clinical indications include effort intolerance of grade 2 or more, haemoptysis, pulmonary oedema, signs of significant pulmonary hypertension, systemic embolization, atrial fibrillation and the presence of functional tricuspid incompetence with or without congestive heart failure.

Laboratory indications include an electrocardiogram showing right-axis deviation with right ventricular hypertrophy, radiological evidence of significant pulmonary venous or arterial hypertension or cardiomegaly, an echocardiographic mitral EF slope of less than 15 mm/s or a valvar diameter of less than 1 cm^2 on cross-sectional echocardiography. With increased experience in the use of catheters, and improved techniques in surgery and anaesthesia, at least in areas where the disease process is endemic and rapidly progressive, and mortality and morbidity both at and after surgery are related to the preoperative status, a case can be made for advocating closed mitral valvotomy, either by surgery or catheter, in patients with mild symptoms who have clinical signs of critical mitral stenosis.

The advent of percutaneous valvotomy has revolutionized the management of rheumatic mitral valvar stenosis. Balloon valvoplasty is now an acceptable alternative to surgery in the treatment of selected patients. Since its introduction by Inoue et al (1984), it has gained wide acceptance in both developed and developing countries. Several studies that followed showed that the mitral valvar area could be safely and effectively increased, with significant short (Lock et al, 1985; Nobuyoshi, 1989; NHLBIBVR, 1992) and mid-term (Block et al, 1992; Desideri et al, 1992; Essop et al, 1995) clinical improvement. The results obtained are comparable with those from open and closed surgical mitral commisurotomy (Turi et al, 1991; Reyes et al, 1994).

The balloon is introduced through the right femoral vein and advanced to the left atrium using an anterograde transeptal approach. Although Inoue and his colleagues (1984) used only a single balloon, subsequent investigators suggested the use of a double balloon catheter (Palacios et al, 1989; Vahanian et al, 1989). The size of the balloon is calculated by assuming the circumference surrounding the balloon, or the continuity of the circumference of separate balloons, and is normalized for body surface area and mitral valvar diameter at the atrioventricular junction as measured on the echocardiogram. Left ventriculography in the 45 degree right anterior oblique projection is performed in patients before and after the valvotomy. It is important to check for mitral regurgitation subsequent to the procedure. Severe postprocedural regurgitation is defined as an increase of two or more grades in regurgitation as seen on the angiogram obtained immediately after the procedure, with a final degree of mitral regurgitation equal to 3+ or 4+ as judged in the system for grading proposed by Sellers et al (1964).

So as better to select patients for balloon dilation, Wilkins et al (1988) proposed an echocardiographic scoring index based on the mobility and thickness of the leaflets, coupled with subvalvar thickening and the presence of calcification. The index has now been widely accepted. For mobility gradation, leaflets that are highly mobile, with restricted motion only at the tips, make up the first grade. In the second grade, the mid and basal portions have normal mobility. In the third grade, the leaflets continue to move forward in diastole, mainly from the base, while in the fourth, and most severe, grade there is no or only minimal forward movement of the leaflets in diastole. Gradation of thickening groups leaflets of near normal thickness (4 to 5 mm) as first grade. In the second grade, the middle of the leaflet is normal, but there is marked thickening of the margins, up to 8 mm. In the third grade, this degree of thickening extends through the entire leaflet, while marked thickening of the entirety of both leaflets gives the most severe fourth grade. Gradation of the tension apparatus has the first grade with minimal thickening just below the leaflets. Thickening of cordal structures along one third of their length makes up the second grade, with extensive thickening up to the distal third representing the third grade. The most severe fourth grade involves thickening and shortening of all cordal structures extending to the papillary muscles. For calcification, the first grade is a single area of increased echocardiographic brightness. In the second grade, there are scattered areas of brightness confined to the leaflet margins, while brightness extending into the mid-portion of the leaflets makes up the third grade. In the fourth, and most severe, grade, there is extensive brightness throughout most of the tissue of the leaflets.

By adding the score for all four components, giving a range from 0 to 16 points, a normal value would be scored as 0, and a mitral valve with severe subvalvar thickening extending into the papillary muscles, severe calcification of both ends of the zone of apposition between the leaflets, and heterogenous thickening of both leaflets, would be scored at 16. A score of greater than 8 is considered to represent severe morphological abnormality and to make the patient less suitable for balloon intervention. A successful outcome has been defined as a gain in the mitral valvar area of a least 1.5 cm², or an increase by more than half from the baseline area. In the study reported by Wilkins et al (1988), and in subsequent reports (Come et al, 1988; Vahanian et al, 1989), dilation at least doubled the valvar area from an initial mean of about 1 cm². Although mild regurgitation is reported in about two fifths of those undergoing balloon dilation, development of severe regurgitation remains one of the most important complications. This has been encountered in between one hundredth and one fifth of patients (McKay et al, 1987; Abascal et al, 1988). Observations at surgery and postmortem have shown that the mechanism underscoring severe incompetence is, in most cases, tearing of either the aortic or mural leaflet, with less frequent causes being excessive separation of the ends of the zone of apposition or rupture of the papillary muscles or tendinous cords with and without prolapse of the leaflets (Essop et al, 1991).

The results of these studies prompted Padial and colleagues (1996), and Mueller (1998), to develop another diagnostic scoring index to predict the development of severe mitral regurgitation. These scoring indexes are currently being validated. Suffice it to say that, as more evidence accrues, eccentricity of the distal valvar orifice, fusion of the ends of the zone of apposition of the leaflets and calcifications that were not included in the original index developed by Wilkins et al (1988), but which have significant bearing in the development of postprocedural regurgitation, are all coming under increased scrutiny.

At present, percutaneous balloon valvoplasty can be advocated as the procedure of choice for isolated rheumatic mitral stenosis, especially in developing countries where economic considerations play a major role in deciding the options for management.

SURGERY

The techniques for surgical relief of mitral stenosis are a closed commissurotomy through the left atrium, which is the oldest method, transventricular closed valvotomy, valvotomy under direct vision using cardiopulmonary bypass, or replacement of the mitral valve. Closed valvotomy in young patients through the left ventricle is well documented (Paul, 1967; John et al, 1975). With this technique, John et al (1975) reported an overall mortality of 5.8%, which had fallen to 2% in the last 150 patients, with an excellent functional improvement achieved in almost nine tenths. Restenosis occurred in less than one twentieth in the initial 5 years, and in no more than one tenth in the subsequent 5 years. An adequate valvotomy was achieved in 96.5% of patients. Mortality was shown to be directly related to preoperative functional status. Those who had severe pulmonary hypertension, and significant congestive heart failure, had a higher mortality rate than the others. Improvement of three or more grades in the classification of the New York Heart Association was achieved in almost all of those in functional classes III and IV prior to the operation. Associated mild aortic incompetence was not considered a contraindication to a closed valvotomy. Open valvotomy under direct vision using cardiopulmonary bypass has also been advocated (Iraj Aryanpur et al, 1977) as the only effective way of relieving the obstruction. The excellence of the results reported by John et al (1975) and Paul (1967) over the long term, nonetheless, have demonstrated the efficacy of the simple transventricular closed valvotomy. Extreme valvar distortion, and calcification, is uncommon in children and adolescents. Therefore, it is not surprising that a closed valvotomy yields excellent immediate and late results. By the same token, equally good results in such patients might now be anticipated from balloon valvoplasty (Essop et al, 1995; Frater, 1995). Contraindications to closed mitral valvotomy are the presence of calcification, associated mitral incompetence and more than moderately severe aortic incompetence. These findings, of course, also contraindicate catheter intervention.

Even in the presence of mitral restenosis, good functional results have been reported following a closed transventricular revalvotomy (John et al, 1975; Suri et al, 1996), but there is an increasing tendency to opt for an open procedure in the presence of restenosis. Replacement of the mitral valve, regardless of the type of the valve used, is a much more serious undertaking. Besides the higher operative and late mortality, there is the problem of long-term or lifetime anticoagulation, the question of how long the prosthetic valve will last and the incidence of embolic as well as late prosthetic complications. Replacement of the valve, therefore, should be performed only as a life-saving measure in children with intractable heart failure with associated mitral incompetence. The results of mitral valvotomy, regardless of the technique used, have been gratifying in children with mitral stenosis. There is usually marked symptomatic relief, and significant regression of pulmonary hypertension. The earlier fear of a higher frequency of mitral restenosis has not been confirmed on long-term follow-up. In fact, there is a lower incidence of restenosis than in adults, probably because of the pliable nature of the valves, which are less frequently calcified. Indeed, it has been suggested that, in young patients, restenosis is not the result of the relentless progression of the disease (John et al, 1975).

———— MITRAL INCOMPETENCE ————

Mitral incompetence is probably, at all ages, the most common valvar defect resulting from the acute rheumatic process. It occurs either as an isolated lesion or in combination with other valvar defects. Unlike mitral stenosis, where there is a variable latent period between the acute rheumatic process and the establishment of the valvar defect, mitral incompetence is frequently present from the onset of the active process itself. Mitral incompetence may either progress or decrease depending on recurrences and the initial severity of the lesion. Tomkins et al (1972) found that only one quarter of their patients who initially had mitral incompetence still had regurgitation 9 years later. Of patients who have been on chemoprophylaxis, between one and three quarters with mitral regurgitation may lose the systolic murmur within the first decade following the acute episode (Massell et al, 1961; Wilson, 1962). In contrast, in developing countries, mitral incompetence can be a rapidly progressive process, and it frequently requires early surgery. The severity of the initial incompetence, and the number of subsequent episodes, determine the course of the disease. A systolic murmur of mild mitral incompetence may well persist throughout the lifetime of the patient without any symptoms or further complications. In contrast, significant mechanical mitral insufficiency may progress, rapidly leading on to congestive heart failure. In general, mild-to-moderate mitral incompetence is better tolerated than similar degrees of mitral stenosis. Isolated mitral incompetence affects men more often than women, although John et al (1983) reported a higher incidence among female patients undergoing valvar replacement.

PHYSIOLOGY ————————————

There is an increased volume overload of the left ventricle and left atrium as a result of the regurgitation occurring during systole. Left ventricular end-diastolic volume is increased so that, despite the regurgitation into the left atrium, an adequate forward flow is maintained into the aorta during left ventricular systole. The important haemodynamic consequences are dilatation and hypertrophy of both the left ventricle and the left atrium. There is a rise in the left atrial pressure, mainly owing to a prominent V wave, which ultimately causes pulmonary venous and pulmonary arterial hypertension. With increasing regurgitation, there is decreased forward stroke volume, and lowering of the cardiac output. In young children, and in older patients, the ventricular function may be impaired, partly as a result of active inflammation because of ventricular fibrosis (Eckberg et al, 1973). Mild mitral incompetence does not significantly alter the haemodynamics for a considerable length of time. With moderate-to-severe mitral incompetence, though pulmonary arterial hypertension does occur, it does not reach the levels found in tight mitral stenosis. It has been shown that severe mitral regurgitation is tolerated very much better than an equal degree of aortic regurgitation.

The size of the left atrium is an important determinant of the rise in pressure in the left atrium and the pulmonary veins. In chronic rheumatic heart disease, since the left atrium has time to dilate, the rise in pressure is relatively low. In contrast, in acute mitral regurgitation with a normally sized left atrium, the left atrial pressure rises suddenly to a marked degree. With aneurysmal dilation of the left atrium and florid mitral incompetence, the left atrial pressure may be near normal (Braunwald and Awe, 1963). This factor, coupled with the earlier-mentioned lower energy cost of ventricular work, probably explain why moderate-to-severe mitral regurgitation is tolerated for a number of years in many patients. In diastole, the left ventricle has a rapid high filling pressure. It dilates to accommodate the blood that has regurgitated during the previous systole, in addition to the normal pulmonary venous return. In chronic mitral incompetence, as the left ventricle enlarges, there is an apparent increase in left ventricular diastolic compliance. The increased end-diastolic volume brings in the Frank–Starling mechanism, allowing a larger stroke output and increased left ventricular compliance. The increase in end-diastolic fibre length, without a corresponding increase in end-diastolic pressure, prevents a marked increase in pulmonary venous pressure (Rappaport, 1975). In moderate mitral incompetence, regurgitant flow from the left ventricle to atrium during systole is approximately half of the total ventricular stroke output. In chronic mitral incompetence, with progressive dilatation of the left ventricle, which tends to normalize the ejection fraction, the ventricle can dilate to an end-diastolic volume of 140 ml/m^2. It can then eject a total stroke volume of 90 ml/m^2, with an end-systolic volume of 50 ml/m^2. Left ventricular dilation is proportional to the severity of mitral incompetence, and the compliance of the ventricle increases. Hypertrophy of the muscle normalizes left ventricular wall stress and is appropriate for both the degree of volume load and the degree of dilatation (Lewis and Gotsman, 1975). Elevation of the left atrial pressure is caused by the prominent V wave resulting from the systolic jet of mitral incompetence. The relation of the height of the V wave to the rate of the descent of the Y descent is a relatively crude index of the degree of mitral regurgitation. The height of the V wave is related to the regurgitant volume as well as to the compliance and volume of the left atrium. Despite the large left atrium, giant V waves of 50–80 mmHg have been reported in children as a result of the severity of the mechanical lesion (Lewis and Gotsman, 1974). The mean left atrial and pulmonary venous pressures rise, leading to a decreased pulmonary compliance and subsequently pulmonary vasoconstriction. The mean pulmonary venous pressure is the major determinant of the resulting pulmonary arterial hypertension. As discussed, this is less marked than in corresponding mitral stenosis, but severe pulmonary venous and arterial hypertension do occur in severe mitral incompetence. Ventricular function is usually normal in children with mitral incompetence. The ejection fractions are maintained, left ventricular end-diastolic pressure increases relatively slightly because of the compensatory change in left ventricular compliance, and left ventricular pressure–time relations remain normal. The forward stroke volume is maintained until late in the disease, when the regurgitant volume becomes so large that most of the stroke output empties into the left atrium. The forward stroke volume and cardiac output then decrease. A direct relationship exists between the regurgitant volume, the reduction in the forward stroke output, the elevation of the left atrial pressure and the degree of clinical disability (Lewis and Gotsman, 1974).

CLINICAL FEATURES

The severity, and to a lesser extent the chronicity, of the mitral incompetence mainly determine the symptoms. Those with mild lesions are completely asymptomatic. In adults and adolescents with even moderate mitral incompetence, symptoms may be relatively unimpressive. In those with severe incompetence, in contrast, there is effort dyspnoea, easy fatiguability, poor weight gain, palpitations on effort, paroxysmal nocturnal dyspnoea and, finally, congestive heart failure. A dilated left atrium can press on the recurrent laryngeal nerve and produce hoarseness of the voice. Paroxysmal or chronic atrial fibrillation and infective endocarditis are more common than in mitral stenosis. The jugular venous pressure is normal when there is no congestive heart failure, while normal blood pressure is associated with a slightly widened pulse pressure, giving a brisk pulse. The apical impulse is usually normal in mild lesions with no major precordial pulsations. In significant mitral incompetence, a hyperdynamic forcible left ventricular heaving apex is palpable, being displaced downwards and laterally. Systolic expansion of the large left atrium may be palpable along the left sternal edge. The first heart sound is usually normal in intensity or somewhat soft. The second heart sound is markedly split because of the shortening of left ventricular systole. The most important clinical feature is the characteristic apical systolic murmur. The murmur is pan- or holosystolic. Starting with the first

sound, which is often muffled, the murmur occupies all of systole. Indeed, it may well extend to the sound of closure of the aortic valve. It is heard best at the apex, radiates to the left axilla and left sternal edge, is unaffected by respiration and has a blowing quality with no accentuation in mid- or late-systole. In mild mitral incompetence, there may be a localized murmur maximally audible at the apex and conducted to the axilla. This 'classical' murmur is not always present. Some patients with significant mitral incompetence have a musical seagull murmur. The late systolic murmur of mild mitral incompetence is often indistinguishable from that of late systolic murmur found with the prolapsing mitral valve (Barlow and Pocock, 1975). Occasionally, especially in the presence of acute valvitis, the murmur may be short, occurring in early' mid- or late-systole. Rarely, despite florid mitral incompetence, there may be absence of the characteristic murmur (Schrire et al, 1961). There is no definite correlation between the severity of the lesion and the length or the intensity of the apical systolic murmur. With severe mitral incompetence, a mid-diastolic blowing murmur is audible at the apex caused by increased diastolic flow through the mitral valve and the turbulence created at the end of the rapid ventricular phase. This murmur, while it may be rumbling, does not extend to late diastole and is usually shorter than the murmur heard in mitral stenosis. A low-pitched third heart sound, which is often palpable and is caused by the considerable early diastolic filling of the ventricle, is heard in those with significant mitral incompetence. The presence of a loud third heart sound excludes the coexistence of significant mitral stenosis. When there is associated pulmonary hypertension, its signs are present. These include a right ventricular parasternal lift, a loud palpable pulmonary competent and murmurs of pulmonary and or tricuspid incompetence. It needs to be emphasized that the clinical signs of mitral incompetence are much less clear-cut than those of mitral stenosis.

The electrocardiogram may be normal when the incompetence is mild. Even with moderate incompetence, the features may be inconclusive. The P wave is broad, bifid or notched, usually best seen in II or VI. A more reliable sign of left atrial enlargement is a terminal negative deflection of the P wave in lead V_1, of more than 4 ms in width and 1 mm in depth. Left ventricular hypertrophy occurs when mitral incompetence is more than moderate. There may be changes in the ST and T waves over the lateral chest leads when the incompetence is severe. In the presence of associated pulmonary hypertension, right ventricular hypertrophy and right atrial enlargement are not uncommon (Figure 65.10). Atrial fibrillation occurs in severe disease, and in those with long-standing chronic mitral incompetence. While it is uncommon in children and adolescents, atrial fibrillation is more common in the younger age group of those with mitral incompetence than in those with mitral stenosis. Nearly half of younger patients undergoing replacement of the mitral valve had

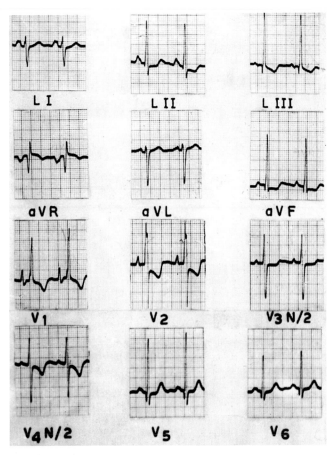

Figure 65.10. The electrocardiogram from an 8-year-old child with isolated and severe mitral incompetence complicated by pulmonary hypertension. There is evidence of biventricular hypertrophy and enlargement of both atriums.

atrial fibrillation, compared with only 2% of those undergoing closed mitral valvotomy for mitral stenosis (John et al, 1975, 1983).

The chest radiograph may be normal in patients with mild lesions. With well-established mitral incompetence, the left atrium is enlarged. Giant and aneurysmally dilated left atriums are seen in those with isolated and severe incompetence. The size of the left atrium reflects to a certain extent the severity of the incompetence. There is left ventricular enlargement from dilation, and the size of the left ventricle is proportional to the degree of mitral regurgitation. There is pulmonary venous engorgement, especially in the upper lobes (Figure 65.11). With the onset of pulmonary hypertension and right ventricular failure, the pulmonary trunk becomes prominent, and there is dilation of the right ventricle and right atrium. Septal lines appear with the onset of cardiac failure. The M-mode echocardiogram is not diagnostic, as opposed to that in mitral stenosis, but does reflect the consequences of the disease (Feigenbaum, 1972). The left ventricle and atrium are dilated. The EF slope of diastolic closure is not specific nor does it indicate the severity of incompetence. It probably reflects the compliance of the left ventricle. There is increase in the left ventricular septal and posterior wall

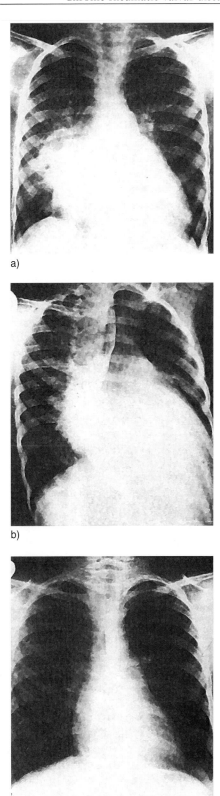

a)

b)

c)

Figure 65.11. Pre- and post-operative radiographs from an 11-year-old child with severe isolated mitral incompetence. (a) The frontal view shows cardiomegaly, marked enlargement of the left atrium with a prominent appendage, and venous congestion of the upper lobes of the lungs. (b) The barium swallow profiled in right oblique projection confirms the dilatation of the left atrium, with posterior displacement of the oesophagus. (c) After replacement of the mitral valve, there is regression of all the abnormal features.

movement because of the large stroke volume. Thickening of the mitral valve, shown by multiple echoes on the mitral leaflets, may be seen. Although the rheumatic leaflets may prolapse, the echocardiogram is useful in differentiating rheumatic disease from other causes of valvar prolapse, such as papillary muscle dysfunction, functional mitral incompetence caused by severe cardiac dilatation in primary cardiac muscle disease, and ruptured tendinous cords. The cross-sectional echocardiogram in the long-axis view reveals a large dilated well-contracting left ventricle and a dilated pulsatile left atrium. It also provides important information about the pathology of the mitral valve. The leaflets of the rheumatic valve are thickened and rigid. Cordal rupture, vegetations of infective endocarditis or the presence or absence of left atrial thrombuses can all be recognized. The precise diagnosis of valvar incompetence has been facilitated by the availability of Doppler and colour-flow mapping. The valvar orifice is interrogated for signals indicating a jet with high velocity occurring during systole. Colour imaging visualizes the severity, direction and velocity of the abnormal pattern of flow into the left atrium. These features permit highly sensitive and specific diagnosis of the degree of incompetence. The increased sophistication of modern machines, however, means that mild or trivial incompetence can be seen in up to two fifths of normal subjects. It is wise, therefore, to take note of the criterions suggested by Minich et al (1997) to avoid overdiagnosis.

Cardiac catheterization and angiography are not indicated in children and adolescents unless they are symptomatic enough to be seriously considered for valvar surgery. They are useful in the presence of multiple valvar lesions, in patients who may not be that symptomatic but where the diagnosis is in doubt, and to exclude congenital heart disease with associated intracardiac shunts and valvar incompetence. The techniques are also of value in severely symptomatic patients to document the presence and severity of myocardiac dysfunction. The mean left atrial or pulmonary capillary pressure is usually elevated, but in a small number an aneurysmally dilated left atrium can produce a normal left atrial pressure despite significant regurgitation (Braunwald and Awe, 1963). With significant mitral incompetence, the left atrial pressure is elevated, with a large V wave and a sharp Y descent. Giant V waves, with left atrial pressures more typical of ventricular levels, have been described (Werko, 1962). A diastolic pressure gradient across the mitral valve can be found even in the absence of significant mitral stenosis. It results from the large diastolic flow across the mitral valve (Neustadt and Shaffer, 1959). The left ventricular systolic pressures are usually normal, and end-diastolic pressure is normal unless there is left ventricular failure. The cardiac index is reduced when there is significant disease. Calculation of the valvar area by Gorlin's formula is less reliable in the setting of valvar incompetence. Regurgitant volume is measured as the difference between angiographically determined total left ventricular volume and

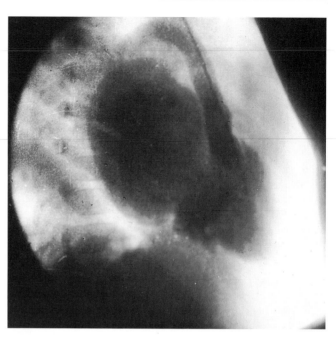

Figure 65.12. A left ventricular angiogram is profiled in 30 degrees right anterior oblique orientation, from the same patient as shown in Figure 65.11. There is severe regurgitation with a wide jet across the mitral valve, producing dense opacification of the entire left atrium. The aorta appears relatively hypoplastic as a result of the low cardiac output.

the forward stroke volume measured by the Fick method, fibreoptic technique, or indicator dilution technique (Sandler et al, 1963; Sauter et al, 1964; Tyrrell et al, 1970). It can also be achieved by calculating the angiographically measured difference between the right and the left ventricular stroke volumes (Sulayman et al, 1975). Selective left ventricular angiography in the 30 degree right anterior oblique projection profiles the left ventricle, left atrium and the mitral valve (Figure 65.12). From the practical point of view, a qualitative estimation of the severity of incompetence from the amount of regurgitation into the left atrium of material injected into the left ventricle has been found useful. The degree of opacification of the left atrium does depend on the quantity of blood in the left atrium and the rate of left atrial emptying, as well as on the severity of regurgitation. The width of the jet of mitral incompetence is a good guide to the size of the regurgitant orifice. The left ventricular size, wall thickness and function, and the degree of movements of the leaflets, can also be assessed. In most children, the ventricular function is usually normal. A decreased left ventricular ejection fraction indicates poor myocardial function. Most patients with this finding have an increased end-diastolic volume.

MANAGEMENT

Medical treatment essentially consists of frequent follow-up with adequate chemoprophylaxis for a long enough period, treatment of congestive heart failure when it occurs, and management of arrhythmias, infections and recurrences of the acute rheumatic process. Antibiotic prophylaxis against infective endocarditis is also necessary.

Curative treatment for mitral incompetence is surgical, either by replacement of the valve or repair. This is seldom necessary in children or adolescents in the developed countries where the disease process remains relatively stable. In the developing countries, children and young adolescents with mitral incompetence present frequently with a severe progressive downhill course, marked disability and congestive heart failure. Surgery is then required as a life-saving measure. Despite the advances in the surgical techniques, and improved early and later mortality, the indications for surgery in children with mitral incompetence need to be more strict than for closed mitral valvotomy. The accepted indications for surgery in mitral incompetence are the presence of severe regurgitation with significant disability and symptoms, presence of recurrent or persistent congestive heart failure, progressive or severe pulmonary hypertension, increasing cardiomegaly on the chest radiograph, progressive left ventricular hypertrophy on the electrocardiogram and the presence of atrial fibrillation. The last feature is usually indicative of severe disease. Some children have clinical features of severe mitral incompetence, with marked cardiomegaly on the electrocardiogram and echocardiogram, but may be apparently not that symptomatic. Surgery has to be considered in these patients. Children who deteriorate during the acute phase of rheumatic activity may require surgery as an emergency procedure.

While the indications for surgery are now generally accepted, the controversy regarding the specific surgical technique still remains unsettled. The currently available procedures are valvar replacement using prosthetic valves, tissue valves, which can be heterografts or homografts, and repair using various techniques of annuloplasty or valvoplasty with or without specially designed prosthetic frames. Reconstructive annuloplasty is attractive in children since it avoids the need for anticoagulation, along with long-term complications from prosthetic valves, such as thromboembolism, infection and haemolysis. This technique is still not so popular, probably since the operation is more complex. Carpentier (1980) reported good results with reconstructive valvar surgery with a low mortality and good functional improvement, including some who underwent surgery during an episode of acute theumatic fever. Chauvaud and colleagues (1986), however, in the follow-up of these patients, found that one fifth required reoperation within 10 years. Despite this, others have reported encouraging results for valvar reconstruction. Al Jubair and his colleagues (1988), working in Saudi Arabia, repaired incompetent valves in 42 children, with no hospital mortality. Over the period of follow-up, albeit relatively short, the valve needed replacement in seven children, while another three had severe regurgit-

ation controlled by medical therapy. Their conclusion was that, while repair was not as durable as for the congenitally malformed valve, the effort of preserving the native valve was well worthwhile, delaying vlavar replacement by at least 5 years.

If the valve is to be replaced, then heterograft tissue valves are attractive in children and adolescents. They do not require anticoagulants yet have a low rate of thromboembolization, along with haemodynamically good characteristics of flow because of their relatively low profile. In adults, substantial durability and low mortality rates were reported for such valves (Davila and Magilligan, 1977; Ionescu et al, 1977; Stinson et al, 1977), but there were disquietingly worrying sequels, such as fibrocalcific obstructions and early degeneration (Kutsche et al, 1978; Geha et al, 1979). All prosthetic valves have their advantages and disadvantages, and the ideal prosthesis is not currently available. The Starr–Edwards ball valve prosthesis has been most extensively used for a long period (Barnhorst, 1975; John et al, 1983, 1990). Low profile disc valves, such as the Bjork–Shiley, have the advantage of being insertable in children with a small left ventricular cavity but have a high propensity for thromboembolism and show a tendency to clot (Ben-Zvi et al, 1974; Roberts and Hammer, 1976). John and his colleagues (1990) have now reported experience with almost 200 patients undergoing surgery below the age of 20 years. Overall mortality was 9.6%, and actuarial survival at 20 years was 59.3%. In the last 5 years of the analysis, operative mortality was less than 3%. The survivors showed excellent improvement. The incidence of thromboembolism was only 0.41 per 100 patient-years. Young women who subsequently married were not disadvantaged in terms of child-bearing. Therefore, regardless of the technique used, results of surgery are now generally excellent, with good clinical improvement, regression of symptoms, signs and cardiomegaly (Figure 65.11c), acceptable hospital mortality and relatively favourable long-term results. Considering the rapid deterioration and high mortality associated with severe mitral incompetence in children (Harris et al, 1966), a more aggressive approach to surgery is now tenable. Surgery should not be recommended automatically, but the hazards of undue delay should be recognized and kept in mind. While the controversy between the various types of valve is unsettled, and there appears to be a continuing enthusiasm for valvar repair and for the use of tissue valves, the excellence of the results reported by John and colleagues (1990) bear testament to the durability of the Starr–Edwards prosthesis. Frequent follow-up and medical management is necessary after any type of valvar surgery, since later morbidity and mortality do occur. If a prosthetic valve is used, long-term anticoagulation is required. The later complications are thromboembolism, haemorrhage from over-anticoagulation, valvar failure or dysfunction, and infective endocarditis.

AORTIC STENOSIS

Isolated rheumatic aortic stenosis is rare in childhood. Since rheumatic aortic stenosis develops slowly and insiduously, it usually presents at a much later age. Consequently, aortic stenosis occurring as an isolated lesion in children is usually considered to be congenital in origin (Roberts, 1970b). In a study of 111 hearts from patients with aortic stenosis, Pomerance (1972) did not find a single case of congenital aortic stenosis in the setting of a trifoliate valve. Roberts (1970a), however, reported that it was reasonable to conclude that the aetiology was rheumatic when aortic stenosis with a trifoliate valve was associated with anatomical disease of the mitral valve. These discussions, of course, reflect disease as encountered in developed countries. In the developing countries, rheumatic aortic stenosis, like rheumatic mitral stenosis, can occur at a much earlier age. Vijayaraghavan et al (1977) reported 30 patients under the age of 30 years with rheumatic aortic stenosis combined with mitral stenosis, of whom 12 were below the age of 20. In the experience of the Institute of Cardiology in São Paulo, Brazil, nonetheless, isolated aortic stenosis made up less than one-twentieth of the valvar disease seen as a consequence of the chronic rheumatic process (Aiello, Tanaka, and Pomerantzeff, personal communication, 1999). Similarly, in the experience reported by John and colleagues (1990), only 6 of 57 aortic valves were replaced because of pure stenosis.

CLINICAL FEATURES

The mild lesions usually cause no symptoms. In moderate aortic stenosis, there may be effort intolerance of some degree, along with palpitations and angina on extreme effort. With severe stenosis, dyspnoea is always present. Palpitations and angina on effort or at rest, and syncope, are common. Since rheumatic aortic stenosis is most usually seen in association with other lesions, it tends to be the clinical findings of those lesions that dominate the clinical picture. The peripheral pulse volume is low, with an anacrotic slow rising pulse. The apical impulse is left ventricular in type with a sustained thrust with little cardiomegaly. Presystolic pulsation from left atrial contraction may be palpable. A systolic thrill of varying intensity and duration is felt in the aortic area, often radiating to the suprasternal notch and into both carotid arteries. The characteristic murmur is rough, coarse and long, being ejection and systolic in type, and it is best heard in the aortic area or in the third left intercostal space. It radiates to the neck. An ejection click may be audible. In severe aortic stenosis, the ejection click may be inaudible, the long ejection systolic murmur may have a late systolic accentuation and a loud fourth heart sound may be audible.

The electrocardiogram shows left ventricular hypertrophy of varying degree. With severe disease, there are changes in the ST–T waves. The chest radiography may appear normal in the early stage of the disease. Left ventricular enlargement is apparent with severe disease, and poststenotic dilatation of the aorta can be seen. Pulmonary venous congestion indicates the presence of ventricular failure. The echocardiogram shows hypertrophy of the left ventricle, with increased thickness of the free wall and septum with good contraction. The ratio of the left ventricular cavity to the ventricular wall thickness can be related to the severity of the aortic stenosis and the transventricular gradient (Aziz et al, 1977). Movements of the leaflets are limited, and multiple echoes may be obtained from the thickened leaflets. Unlike congenital aortic stenosis, it is unusual to find an eccentric position of the leaflets.

Cardiac catheterization and angiography are required to measure the gradient across the valve (Figure 65.13), to calculate the valvar area, assess left ventricular function and exclude other lesions. The left ventricular pressure, besides being elevated, may show an a-wave impression on the upstroke. In severe disease, the left ventricular end-diastolic pressures are elevated. Pulmonary hypertension is uncommon, and pulmonary capillary pressures are usually normal or only minimally elevated. Left ventricular angiography shows a relatively normal or small cavity with vigorous contraction. Selective aortic root angiography can demonstrate the presence of three valvar leaflets and document presence or absence of associated aortic incompetence. A gradient across the aortic valve of more than 50 mm, in the absence of other lesions, indicates significant stenosis.

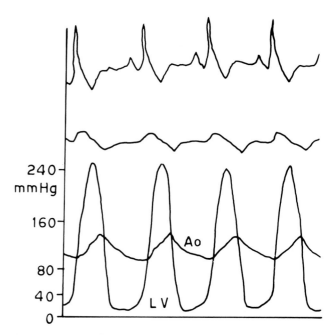

Figure 65.13. Simultaneously recorded left ventricular and aortic pressures in a 15-year-old child with aortic stenosis. There is a peak-to-peak systolic gradient across the aortic valve of nearly 100 mmHg. This patient had associated severe mitral stenosis (Ao, aorta; LV, left ventricle).

The calculated valvar area is usually less than 0.7 cm/m² in these cases.

MANAGEMENT

Those with mild-to-moderate aortic stenosis should be treated conservatively, with chemoprophylaxis against further rheumatic disease and infective endocarditis. They should be advised to avoid vigorous exercise or active sports. Surgical treatment is indicated in children with severe disease who have definite severe symptoms, although occasionally patients with a significant gradient across the aortic valve may be apparently symptom free. The electrocardiogram provides a good guide to the severity. Severe left ventricular hypertrophy with changes in the ST–T segments, reflects severe disease, as does an increasing cardiothoracic ratio on the chest radiograph. Haemodynamically, a peak-to-peak systolic gradient across the aortic valve of 50 mm or more at rest, and/or a valvar area of less than 0.7 cm/m², are indications for surgery.

Commissurotomy of the aortic valve under direct vision using cardiopulmonary bypass is the treatment of choice (Paul et al, 1998). The pathology of the valve in some patients may necessitate valvar replacement. Besides the problems discussed above regarding the various types of valve, aortic stenosis has an additional important technical disadvantage in that the aortic root is often small; consequently only prostheses of smaller size can be used. This results in residual gradients and a higher frequency of reoperations. One important advance in the surgical treatment of aortic stenosis has been the technique described by Konno et al (1975) for enlarging the aortic root. Despite the recent advances, there are still considerable limitations in the prostheses available. The prosthetic mechanical valves, which have the advantage of durability, have the disadvantage of being thrombogenic despite the use of anticoagulant therapy (Perez-Alvarez et al, 1968). Tissue valves, which are relatively free of the problems of thromboembolism, have a limited durability (Hirshfeld et al, 1974). An important factor in the timing of the operation is the ability of the myocardium to cope with the haemodynamic load. There are no absolute methods for assessing left ventricular function. There is rough correlation between the end-diastolic pressure and the preoperative heart size with late results of aortic valve replacement. Significant worsening of the late results has been shown when these measurements are increasingly abnormal (McGoon, 1976). The timing of valvar replacement in a child, therefore, has to be based not only on the severity but on other factors as well. The early results following aortic valvar replacement have been good (Bloodwell et al, 1968; Vidne and Levy, 1970; Berry et al, 1974). The preoperative mortality and morbidity are relatively low, and periprosthetic leaks and heart blocks are uncommon (John et al, 1990). Late complications are infective endocarditis and the possibility of

another operation being required owing to valvar failure or an increasing gradient caused by the relatively small size of the valve. Although thromboembolism is a concern, John and colleagues (1990) encountered only 0.56 episodes per 100 patient-years. In view of the problems with replacing the aortic valve, it is not surprising that surgeons have attempted to use the Ross procedure for patients with rheumatic disease, albeit more frequently for those with aortic incompetence (see below). The results are conflicting. Kumar and colleagues (1993) reported the procedure as a 'near perfect' solution. Choudhary and associates (1999), in contrast, struck a much more cautious note, finding that the autograft was itself susceptible to rheumatic disease. This will be discussed further in relation to aortic valvar incompetence.

AORTIC REGURGITATION

Aortic regurgitation is the most common consequence of rheumatic aortic valvitis. It frequently occurs in combination with mitral valvar disease. Bland and Jones (1951) reported that over half of patients who developed rheumatic heart disease had evidence of aortic valvar involvement. Isolated aortic involvement, which was almost exclusively incompetence, was found in less than one tenth. Arora et al (1981) found isolated aortic regurgitation in only one twentieth of a large series of patients, with regurgitation combined with aortic stenosis in another one twentieth. Isolated aortic regurgitation accounted for about one eighth of the patients with rheumatic heart disease seen at Vellore (Sukumar, 1982).

Unlike mitral disease, the disappearance of the aortic murmur is relatively uncommon, although Massell et al (1961) have quoted the disappearance of aortic murmurs with time. Aortic regurgitation may range in severity from minimal regurgitation with only a faint murmur to severe free aortic regurgitation. It is more common in men. The usual natural history is a long asymptomatic period in which mild-to-moderate incompetence is well tolerated and produces no symptoms (Goldschlager, 1973; Smith et al, 1976). Patients who have recurrent rheumatic episodes may have a more rapid progress, and severe incompetence may become established over a period of 10 years. In developing countries, however, as with juvenile mitral valvar disease, severe aortic incompetence may become established within 1 or 2 years of the initial infective episode. Infective endocarditis can also produce acute incompetence, which may rapidly be fatal unless treated. Those with associated mitral valvar disease, especially mitral incompetence, have a more progressively rapid downhill course.

PHYSIOLOGY

Aortic regurgitation results in a volume overload on the left ventricle, which leads to dilation and hypertrophy of the ventricle. The degree of left ventricular dilation is proportional to the severity of the regurgitant volume. There are additional factors such as the size of the regurgitant opening, the phasic nature of the regurgitation, the duration of diastole, the peripheral resistance, the reaction of the left ventricle in diastole, and myocardial perfusion (Reichek et al, 1974). To maintain an adequate forward stroke output in the presence of a normal ejection fraction, the left ventricle has to have a large end-diastolic volume, which accommodates the regurgitant flow. In chronic aortic incompetence, since the left ventricle is able to dilate over a period of time, the increase in diastolic compliance permits the left ventricle to accommodate a large regurgitant fraction without a corresponding increase in end-diastolic pressure. The ventricular stress is kept within the normal range through associated ventricular hypertrophy and reduced aortic impedance (Rappaport, 1975). Peripheral vasodilation is almost invariably present with significant aortic incompetence. The rapid dissipation of blood into the dilated peripheral vascular bed augments the central aortic regurgitation, resulting in a low diastolic pressure. The lowering of the diastolic pressure has two ill-effects. These are reduction of coronary arterial flow and inadequate nutrition of the peripheral tissues. The peak systolic pressure rises as a compensatory mechanism, resulting in a higher mean arterial pressure. The elevated systolic pressure adds a pressure overload to the already existing volume overload of the left ventricle. Both the preload and the afterload are altered, with a significant increase in the total work of, and consumption of oxygen by, the left ventricle (Braunwald, 1969). The wide peripheral arterial pulse pressure in severe incompetence is the result of a combination of the peripheral vasodilatation and central aortic regurgitation. The peripheral pulse curve shows a rapid rise to a high peak, with a sharp descending limb and a relatively unimportant dicrotic notch, with a low diastolic pressure and a high systolic peak pressure. The central aortic pressure, however, differs from the peripheral arterial pulse in that there is a sharp early peak followed by a second peak of varying amplitude. Left ventricular coronary arterial perfusion is dependent both on the duration of diastole and on the gradient between the left ventricular end-diastolic pressure and aortic diastolic pressure. In severe aortic incompetence, there is a low aortic diastolic pressure and increasing left ventricular end-diastolic pressures. The diastolic filling period may be altered by tachycardia. This, added to the progressive left ventricular hypertrophy, produces an inadequate coronary arterial flow. Compensatory hypertrophy may be limited because of ischaemia, which leads to ventricular fibrosis and failure. With the onset of left ventricular failure, the end-diastolic pressure rises, with an appropriate rise in the left atrial and pulmonary venous pressures, and subsequently of the pulmonary arterial pressures. Severe pulmonary hypertension is not common in chronic aortic incompetence. In contrast, when the aortic regurgitation occurs acutely, there is a sudden rise in the ventricular diastolic pressure and a sharp rise in pulmonary venous pressure because the left ventricle is relatively unprepared. A sharp and high rise of the end-diastolic pressure may further markedly decrease the flow of blood in the coronary arteries. All these factors add to the systolic dysfunction of the left ventricle and result in a low cardiac output with pulmonary oedema and severe congestive heart failure.

CLINICAL FEATURES

Patients with mild aortic incompetence are asymptomatic. In some, apart from the murmur, even the peripheral signs may be lacking. Those with moderate incompetence may remain relatively asymptomatic despite cardiac dilatation, as the ventricle is able to increase the cardiac output appropriately on exercise (Goldschlager et al, 1973). In severe aortic incompetence, there may be palpitations on rest or on effort. Effort dyspnoea occurs early and progresses. With the onset of left ventricular failure, orthopnoea and pulmonary oedema occur. Angina is found in those with more severe disease. The presence of nocturnal angina indicates a poor prognosis. Children and adolescents with severe disease may have nocturnal sweating, tachycardia and nightmares. Sudden death may occur in the late stage of the disease. The blood pressure shows elevated systolic and low diastolic pressures, with a wide pulse pressure. The width of the pulse pressure, and the low diastolic pressure, are roughly proportional to the severity of the lesion. In those with moderate incompetence, however, the width of the pulse pressure does not always correlate with the severity. With severe incompetence, a collapsing water-hammer pulse is present. Other peripheral signs of a wide pulse pressure are increased and marked carotid pulsations (Corrigan's sign), 'pistol shot' sounds over the femoral pulses, Duroziez's sign of a systolic and diastolic murmur becoming audible when critical pressure is applied to a large artery, visible capillary pulsations in the nail beds (Quincke's sign) and the sign of the nodding head (named for de Musset, one of the few signs named in honour of the patient!). Cardiac enlargement is related to the severity of regurgitation. The apex beat is hyperdynamic and forcible, and there may be expandable pulsations over the entire precordium, with prominence of the left chest. The diagnostic sign of aortic incompetence is an early diastolic high-pitched blowing decrescendo murmur heard best at the mid left sternal border or the right sternal border. It is best heard with the diaphragm of the stethoscope, with the patient leaning forwards in full expiration. The length and loudness of the murmur are poorly correlated with the severity of the incompetence. An aortic systolic ejection flow murmur radiating to the neck, occasionally preceded by an ejection click, is present with severe incompetence, and the apical mid- and late-diastolic murmur named for Austin Flint often occurs. This is indistinguishable from that of mitral stenosis, but it is usually not accompanied by a thrill. This murmur results from fluttering of the aortic leaflet of the mitral valve and antegrade flow of blood through a closing mitral orifice. Amyl nitrite decreases the intensity of the early diastolic as well as the Austin Flint murmur, but it increases the loudness of the murmur of organic mitral stenosis. Premature closure of the mitral valve may occur in severe regurgitation, producing a decreased intensity of the first heart sound. Fourth heart sounds are uncommon, and a third sound indicates ventricular failure. In the presence of severe congestive failure, particularly in acute aortic regurgitation, the peripheral signs are diminished, and murmurs may not be easily audible. Acute aortic incompetence presents with acute pulmonary oedema and gross congestive heart failure. The electrocardiogram may be normal with a mild lesion. Left ventricular hypertrophy is present, with deep Q waves over the left chest leads with severe regurgitation. In advanced disease, left atrial P waves and changes in the ST–T segments are present. The chest radiograph shows considerable enlargement of the left ventricle with moderate or severe incompetence. The ascending aorta and arch are prominent. With advanced disease, enlargement of the left atrium and pulmonary venous congestion are found. The echocardiogram shows a dilated left ventricular cavity, usually with a normal left atrium and increased movements of the ventricular septum and the left ventricular posterior wall. Wide fluttering of the aortic leaflet of the mitral valve usually occurs in patients who have an Austin Flint murmur. Absence of mitral flutter does not exclude aortic incompetence. The echocardiogram easily resolves the issue of presence or absence of organic mitral stenosis. In severe aortic regurgitation, premature closure and delayed opening of the mitral valve are seen. Cross-sectional echocardiography provides a more dynamic view of the size of the ventricle, the degree of ventricular hypertrophy and abnormal movement of the mitral valve. The echocardiogram is also useful in assessing left ventricular function. Doppler interrogation is similarly helpful. Spatial mapping of the regurgitant jet permits estimation of the degree of severity of regurgitation. If signals are recorded only within a localized region of the outflow tract just beneath the aortic valvar leaflets, the regurgitation is considered mild. When the signal extends to the tip of the aortic leaflet of the mitral valve, then regurgitation is held to be moderate, whereas severe regurgitation is accompanied by signals extending towards the apex (Zhang et al, 1986).

Cardiac catheterization and angiography are indicated only in patients with severe or progressive lesions, and when surgical treatment is contemplated. Details of abnormal pressures and flows have been discussed above. In severe aortic incompetence, the aortic tracings reveal a wide pulse pressure and a low diastolic pressure. The left ventricular end-diastolic pressure may be slightly elevated or high, and the pulmonary capillary wedge pressure usually reflects the left ventricular end-diastolic pressure unless there is associated mitral valvar disease. Pulmonary arterial hypertension is uncommon, unless there is chronic long-standing disease, additional mitral valvar disease or acute aortic incompetence. The cardiac output is relatively normal or slightly decreased. Left ventriculography is useful in assessing the size and the function of the left ventricle, and the presence or absence of additional mitral incompetence. Quantification of the regurgitant fraction and volume can be made with the combination of the dye dilution technique with angiography (Strober et al 1968; Tyrell et al, 1970). The left ventricular end-diastolic volume has a close correlation with the regurgitant volume. In the absence of myocardial failure, it is a good index of the severity of the regurgitation (Reichek et al, 1974). Regurgitation fractions of more than 50%, and an ejection fraction of less than 40%, indicate severe left ventricular dysfunction. Selective aortography in the right and the left anterior oblique projections provides details of the size of the aortic root and the aortic valve, and the degree of regurgitation. In moderate aortic incompetence, the entire left ventricle is opacified for several beats; in severe regurgitation, the ventricle is opacified for more than 10 beats.

MANAGEMENT

Medical treatment consists of continuing prophylaxis against rheumatic disease and infective endocarditis, and management of congestive heart failure when present. In patients who have more than moderate aortic incompetence despite their apparent lack of symptoms, competitive games and sports are to be restricted. Since the underlying problem is mechanical, medical therapy is of limited value once congestive failure develops. When myocardial function is impaired, any delay in performing surgery courts the risk of poorer subsequent surgical results. Those with acute aortic incompetence require urgent valvar replacement, since few of these patients survive medical therapy alone. The indications for replacement of the valve in a child with chronic aortic regurgitation need to be stringent. Those who are significantly symptomatic are candidates for surgery, especially children who have angina either on effort or at rest, nocturnal dyspnoea, chronic or recurrent congestive heart failure or evidence of severe aortic regurgitation with regurgitation fractions of more than 50%, an ejection fraction of less than 40% and more than moderately severe aortic regurgitation on angiography. Occasionally, there are children who apparently have mild symptoms but with signs of severe aortic regurgitation. The timing of surgery in these children is more difficult. It should be based on the severity of incompetence, judged not only by the clinical, radiographic, echocardiographic and electrocardiographic signs but also by the haemodynamic criterions mentioned above.

Surgical treatment in aortic regurgitation consists primarily of replacement by a prosthetic, tissue or homograft valve. The evidence is still conflicting concerning the role of autograft replacement using the patient's own pulmonary valve. Unlike the situation with the incompetent mitral valve, reconstructive surgery is not feasible. The problems, advantages and disadvantages of the prosthetic versus the tissue valves have already been mentioned. Because of the problems with the valves currently available, the Ross procedure would seem to offer many advantages. Indeed, as already mentioned, Kumar and his colleagues (1993) used the Ross procedure in 38 patients with incompetent rheumatic aortic valves. There were no early or late deaths. Only one patient required reoperation because of valvar regurgitation over their short follow-up. Choudhary and colleagues (1999), in contrast, despite low surgical mortality in a series of 75 patients with rheumatic incompetence, found severe regurgitation of the pulmonary valve in its neoaortic position in 13 of their patients. All these patients were children or young adults. Morphological assessment of the explanted autograft showed features compatible with rheumatic valvitis. Despite the attraction of the Ross procedure, therefore, they recommended a cautious approach. Fortunately, unlike the situation in aortic stenosis, the aortic root in aortic regurgitation is usually dilated. This permits insertion of a relatively large prosthetic valve. The largest and longest experience has been with the caged-ball valve. Use of this prosthesis continues to provide excellent results (John et al, 1990). It has long been suggested that, in isolated aortic valvar disease, unmounted aortic homografts are superior to mechanical prostheses, since these are both non-thrombogenic and haemodynamically superior (Barratt-Boyes and Roche, 1969). Sudden death from failure of the leaflets is uncommon. Early and late mortality compare well with the other types of valve (Weir et al, 1978). At present, therefore, the best type of valve for replacement has still to be determined. Irrespective of the valve used, subsequent to valvar replacement there is usually dramatic improvement in the clinical status, and most patients improve with corresponding reduction in their heart size. The late complications mentioned above, such as thromboembolism, infective endocarditis and the need for reoperation, still exist. Since there is no consensus yet as to the type of valve to be used, it is appropriate that a conservative approach is continued to be used for aortic valvar replacement in children.

TRICUSPID INCOMPETENCE

In rheumatic heart disease, tricuspid incompetence practically never occurs as an isolated lesion. It is frequently functional, with right ventricular dilation occurring as a result of severe pulmonary hypertension, though occasionally it can be organic. Banerjee et al (1982), in a post-mortem study, found evidence of organic valvitis in one third of patients who had clinical tricuspid regurgitation. Tricuspid regurgitation is most commonly associated with severe mitral valvar disease, most frequently mitral stenosis followed by mitral stenosis and incompetence, although it does also occur in combination with mitral and aortic valvar disease. Just over one tenth of the patients at Vellore (see Figure 65.1) had tricuspid incompetence as part of triple valvar disease. In the surgical experience of the King Faisal Hospital in Riyadh, Saudi Arabia, however, one quarter of all patients required operations on the tricuspid valve, with half of these valves showing evidence of organic disease, albeit with very few presenting in childhood (Prabhakar et al, 1993). When the tricuspid valve is incompetent, there is right atrial volume load, and the increase in the mean right atrial pressure is transmitted to both superior and inferior caval veins.

The symptoms in these patients, nonetheless, are dominated by the associated mitral and/or aortic disease. Occasionally, in some patients, the onset of tricuspid regurgitation tends to decrease the degree of dyspnoea and orthopnoea. Hepatic enlargement, which is usually present, can produce discomfort or pain in the right upper quadrant of the abdomen. The jugular venous pressure is always elevated, sometimes markedly so, with a dominant V wave and a rapid Y descent. A large C wave may also be seen in the absence of atrial fibrillation. Since the jugular venous pressure represents right atrial pressure, the height of the V wave and the Y descent are good indicators of the severity of tricuspid regurgitation. The liver is enlarged, tender and pulsatile in systole. The murmur of tricuspid incompetence is pan-systolic, blowing in nature, best audible in the fourth left intercostal space, and characteristically increases on inspiration. With mild incompetence, the murmur may be audible only during inspiration. In moderately severe incompetence, it is present throughout the respiratory cycle yet shows the increase with inspiration. With severe incompetence, the right ventricle is already maximally overloaded. Inspiration cannot then alter the flow of blood across the tricuspid valve. Respiratory variation may not be present. The murmur may then be loud and audible over a large area of the pericardium, including the axilla, and may produce diagnostic difficulties in excluding associated mitral incompetence. A right ventricular third heart sound may be audible. Mid-diastolic flow murmurs in the tricuspid area are less frequent than in the setting of mitral incompetence, since the cardiac output is usually low. With severe tricuspid incompetence, ascites, oedema and emaciation may be present, as well as hepatomegaly. With chronic gross hepatomegaly, clinical and laboratory signs of hepatic dysfunction can occur. A protein-losing enteropathy, resulting from the elevated splanchnic venous pressure, has been described (Strober et al, 1968). The combination of a low cardiac output and renal congestion can result in a decreased glomerular filtration rate, marked retention of fluid and elevated blood urea. With severe incompetence, a hypodynamic high-amplitude right ventricular parasternal lift, with retraction along the right sternal border, produces a seesaw rocking motion of the entire precordium (Armstrong and Gotsman, 1974).

The electrocardiogram usually shows right ventricular hypertrophy, right atrial enlargement and the effects of the left-sided lesions. Atrial fibrillation is common. The chest radiograph usually shows considerable generalized cardiomegaly, with right atrial and caval venous engorgement in addition to the signs of underlying mitral and/or aortic valvar disease. The echocardiogram shows a dilated right ventricular cavity, with paradoxical motion of the ventricular septum and exaggerated movement of the tricuspid valve. While the echocardiogram is fairly typical, it is not diagnostic, since a similar appearance may be seen in right ventricular volume overload from other conditions, such as atrial septal defects (Diamond et al, 1971). Cardiac catheterization shows an elevated right atrial mean pressure, with a dominant V wave and sharp rapid Y descent. The right ventricular end-diastolic pressure is usually elevated. Right ventricular angiography in the 30 degree right anterior oblique projection profiles the tricuspid valve. It shows a dilated right ventricle, with regurgitation of contrast medium into the right atrium, but the valvar leaflets are not usually easy to visualize.

MANAGEMENT

Intensive medical therapy using anticongestive measures produces regression of the functional tricuspid incompetence, and occasionally even disappearance of the physical signs. In tight mitral stenosis, the tricuspid incompetence is mostly functional. Mitral valvar surgery alone is sufficient to produce the required fall in the pulmonary arterial and right ventricular pressure and regression of tricuspid incompetence. These patients may require continued maintenance therapy with digitalis and diuretics for some time. Annuloplasty is rarely required. In patients with severe mitral incompetence and mild-to-moderate tricuspid regurgitation, replacement of the mitral valve alone is again usually sufficient. Those with severe tricuspid incompetence may occasionally require annuloplasty or other reparative procedures. Patients who have severe tricuspid regurgitation together with mitral and aortic valve disease more often require surgical intervention (Prabhakar et al, 1993).

TRICUSPID STENOSIS

Tricuspid stenosis is the least common lesion in rheumatic heart disease. It is even less common in children, being extremely rare as an isolated lesion (Morgan et al, 1971).

Even when seen in combination with disease of the mitral and aortic valves, tricuspid stenosis in association with incompetence is more common than pure stenosis alone. The presence of tricuspid stenosis adds an additional increment to the right atrial and systemic venous pressure.

The symptoms are commonly related to those of the associated lesions. With tricuspid obstruction, a sudden increase in pulmonary flow is less likely, and dyspnoea or orthopnoea may be less prominent. In the presence of severe mitral stenosis and low cardiac output, especially in those with atrial fibrillation, the signs of tricuspid stenosis may be masked unless they are looked for carefully. A high sharp A wave indicates increased atrial contraction, and the slow Y descent results from impairment of the right ventricular filling (Gibson and Wood, 1955). With significant tricuspid stenosis, there is a sharp A wave in the jugular venous pressure, and a slow Y descent is found in those patients in sinus rhythm. The large A wave is caused by increased atrial contraction, and the slow Y descent reflects impairment of the right ventricular filling with inspiration. The murmur of tricuspid stenosis usually has a higher pitch than that of mitral stenosis, which it closely resembles. When there is atrial fibrillation, the murmur occurs earlier in diastole. A tricuspid opening snap is often present, but it may be difficult to differentiate it from that of the associated mitral stenosis. When atrial fibrillation is present, atrial contraction is obliterated. The prominent A wave, as well as the presystolic murmur, will then disappear. Clinical diagnosis becomes difficult.

The electrocardiogram in patients with sinus rhythm shows severe right atrial enlargement with tall peaked P waves, in addition to the changes produced by the associated lesions. Similarly, the radiological abnormalities are basically those of the associated lesions but, in addition, show an enlarged right atrium and a distended superior caval vein. The echocardiogram shows a thickened tricuspid valve, with a marked decrease in its rate of diastolic closure. More importantly, it documents the presence or absence of associated mitral stenosis.

At cardiac catheterization, a diastolic gradient can be demonstrated across the tricuspid valve. The right atrial pressure is increased. Those with sinus rhythm show a giant A wave and a slow Y descent. It is preferable to record simultaneous right atrial and right ventricular pressures using a double lumen catheter rather than make a withdrawal from right ventricle to right atrium (Figure 65.14). A selective right atrial angiogram in the 30 degrees right anterior oblique projection demonstrates the doming effect of the tricuspid valve into the right ventricle, with the narrow jet of dye passing through the stenosed orifice.

MANAGEMENT

Since most patients with tricuspid stenosis require surgery for the associated lesions, the valve can be surgically corrected at the same time. Commissurotomy under direct vision usually yields good results. Occasionally, with very deformed valves, and in those with mixed disease, replacement of the valve becomes necessary, although primary repair was feasible in the greater number of patients undergoing surgery in Riyadh (Prabhakar et al, 1993). If replacement is essential, a low-profile prosthesis or tissue valve should be used.

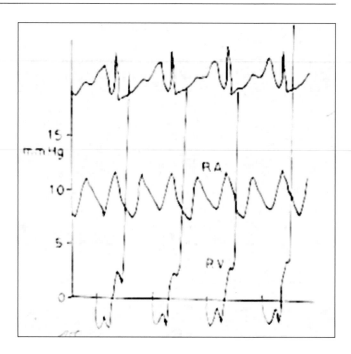

Figure 65.14. Simultaneously recorded right atrial (RA) and ventricular (RV) pressures in a 16-year-old patient with severe tricuspid stenosis showing the gradient across the valve. There is a prominent A wave with a sharp Y descent in the right atrial tracing, and the gradient is seen at end-diastole. The patient had, in addition, significant mitral and aortic stenosis.

REFERENCES

Abascal V M, Wilkins G T, Choong C Y, Block P C, Palacios I, Weyman A E 1988 Mitral regurgitation after percutaneous balloon mitral valvuloplasty in adults: evaluation by pulsed Doppler echocardiography. Journal of the American College of Cardiology 11: 257–263

Al Jubair K A, Javalla A, Fadala M et al 1998 Repair of the mitral valve because of pure rheumatic mitral valvar incompetence in the young. Cardiology in the Young 8: 90–93

Armstrong T G, Gotsman M S 1974 The left parasternal lift in tricuspid incompetence. American Heart Journal 88: 183–190

Arora A, Subramanyam G, Khalilullah M, Gupta M P 1981 Clinical profile of rheumatic fever and rheumatic heart disease: A study of 2500 cases. Indian Heart Journal 33: 264–273

Aziz KU, van Grondelle A, Paul M H, Muster A J 1977 Echocardiographic assessment of the relation between left ventricular wall and cavity dimensions and peak systolic pressure in children with aortic stenosis. American Journal of Cardiology 40: 775–780

Banerjee A, Khanna S K, Beohar P C, Narayanan P S, Malhotra V, Mehta V K et al 1982 Tricuspid regurgitation associated with mitral stenosis: a clinicopathological study. Indian Heart Journal 34: 8–12

Barlow J B, Pocock W A 1975 The problems of non-ejection systolic clicks and associated mitral systolic murmurs: emphasis on the billowing mitral leaflet syndrome. American Heart Journal 90: 636–655

Barnhorst D A, Oxman H A, Connolly D C, Pluth J R, Danielson G K, Wallace R B, McGoon DC 1975 Longterm followup of isolated replacement of the aortic or mitral valve with the Starr–Edwards prosthesis. American Journal of Cardiology 35: 228–233

Barratt-Boyes B G, Roche A H C 1969 A review of aortic valve homografts over a six and one half year period. Annals of Surgery 170: 483–490

Ben-Zvi J, Hildner FJ, Chandraratna P A, Samet P 1974 Thrombosis on Bjork–Shiley aortic valve prosthesis. Clinical arteriographic, echocardiographic and therapeutic observations in seven cases. American Journal of Cardiology 34: 538–544

Berry B E, Ritter D G, Wallace R B, McGoon D C, Danielson G K 1974 Cardiac valve replacement in children. Journal of Thoracic and Cardiovascular Surgery 68: 705–710

Bland E F, Jones T D 1951 Rheumatic fever and rheumatic heart disease. A twenty year report on 1000 patients followed since childhood. Circulation 4: 836–843

Block P C, Palacios I F, Block E H, Tuzcu E M, Griffin B 1992 Late (two year) follow-up after percutaneous balloon mitral valvotomy. American Journal of Cardiology 69: 537–541

Bloodwell R D, Hallman G L, Cooley D A 1968 Cardiac valve replacement in children. Surgery 63: 77–89

Borman JB, Stern S, Shapira T, Milwidsky H, Braun K 1961 Mitral valvotomy in children. American Heart Journal 61: 763–769

Braunwald E 1969 Mitral regurgitation, physiologic, clinical and surgical considerations. New England Journal of Medicine 281: 425–433

Braunwald E, Awe W C 1963 The syndrome of severe mitral regurgitation with normal left atrial pressure. Circulation 27: 29–35

Carpentier A 1980 Reconstructive surgery of rheumatic valvular disease in children under 12 years of age. In: Borman J B, Gotsman M S (eds) Rheumatic valvular disease in children. Springer-Verlag, Berlin, p 149–159

Chauvaud S, Perier P, Toutati G et al 1986 Long-term results of valve repair in children with acquired mitral valve incompetence. Circulation 74 (suppl 1): 104–109

Cherian G, Vytilingam K I, Sukumar I P, Gopinath N 1964 Mitral valvotomy in young patients. British Heart Journal 26: 157–166

Choudhary S K, Mathur A, Sharma R et al 1999 Pulmonary autograft: should it be used in young patients with rheumatic disease? Journal of Thoracic and Cardiovascular Surgery 118: 483–490

Come P C, Riley M F, Diver D J, Morgan J P, Safian R D, McKay R G 1988 Non invasive assessment of mitral stenosis before and after percutaneous balloon mitral valvuloplasty. American Journal of Cardiology 61: 817–825

Davila J C, Magilligan 1977 Experience with the Hancock porcine xenograft for mitral replacement. In: Davila J C (ed) 2nd Henry Ford symposium on cardiac surgery. Appleton Century Crofts, New York, p 485

Desideri S, Vanderperren O, Serra A et al 1992 Long term (9 to 33 months) echocardiographic follow-up after successful percutaneous mitral valvotomy. American Journal of Cardiology 69: 1602–1606

Diamond M A, Dillon J C, Haine C L, Chang S C, Feigenbaum H 1971 Echocardiographic features of atrial septal defect. Circulation 43: 129–135

Eckberg D L, Gault J H, Bouchard R L, Karliner J S, Ross J Jr 1973 Mechanics of left ventricular contraction in chronic severe mitral regurgitation. Circulation 47: 1252–1259

Essop M R, Rothlisberger C, Dullabh A, Sareli P 1995 Can the long term outcomes of percutaneous balloon mitral valvotomy and surgical commissurotomy be expected to be similar? Journal of Heart Valve Disease 4: 446–452

Essop M R, Wisenbaugh T, Skoularigis J, Middlemost S, Sareli P 1991 Mitral regurgitation following mitral balloon valvotomy. Differing mechanisms for severe versus mild-to-moderate lesions. Circulation 84: 1669–1679

Feigenbaum H 1972 Echocardiography. Lea & Febiger, Philadelphia, P A

Fenoglio J J Jr, Wagner B M 1973 Studies in rheumatic fever VI. Ultrastructure of chronic rheumatic heart disease. American Journal of Pathology 73: 623–640

Ferrans V J, Roberts W C 1980 Pathology of rheumatic heart disease. In: Borman J B, Gotsman MS (eds) Rheumatic valvular disease in children. Springer-Verlag, Berlin, p 28–58

Frater R W 1995 Balloon versus surgical commissurotomy. Journal of Heart Valve Disease 4: 444–445

Geha A S, Laks H, Stansel H C et al 1979 Late failure of porcine valve heterografts in children. Journal of Thoracic and Cardiovascular Surgery 78: 351–364

Gibson R V, Wood P 1955 The diagnosis of tricuspid stenosis. British Heart Journal 17: 552–562

Goldberg S J, Allen H D, Marx G R, Connersten R L 1988 Doppler echocardiography. Lea & Febiger, Philadelphia, p. 293–301

Goldschlager N, Pfeifer J, Cohn K, Popper R, Selzer A 1973 The natural history of aortic regurgitation. A clinical and hemodynamic study. American Journal of Medicine 54: 577–588

Gorlin R, Lewis B M, Haynes F W, Spiegl R J, Dexter L 1951a Factors regulating pulmonary 'capillary' pressure in mitral stenosis IV. American Heart Journal 41: 834–854

Gorlin R, Sawyer C G, Haynes F W, Goodale W T, Dexter L 1951b Effects of exercise on circulatory dynamics in mitral stenosis III. American Heart Journal 41: 192–203

Gorlin R, McMillan I K, Meed W E, Mathews M B, Dalby R 1955 Dynamics of the circulation in aortic valvular disease. American Journal of Medicine 18: 855–870

Gotsman M S, van der Horst R L 1975 Surgical management of severe mitral valve disease in childhood. American Heart Journal 90: 685–687

Harris L C, Nghiem O X, Schreiber M H 1966 Rheumatic mitral insufficiency in children: Course, prognosis and effect of valve replacement. American Journal of Cardiology 17: 194–202

Henry W L, Griffith J M, Michaelis L L, McIntosh C L, Morrow A G, Epstein SE 1975 Measurement of mitral orifice area in patients with mitral valve disease by real-time, two dimensional echocardiography. Circulation 51: 827–831

Hirshfeld J W Jr, Epstein S E, Roberts A J, Glancy D L, Morrow AG 1974 Indices predicting long-term survival after valve replacement in patients with aortic stenosis. Circulation 50: 1190–1191

Inoue K, Owaki T, Makamura T, Kitamura F, Miyamoto N 1984 Clinical application of transvenous mitral commissurotomy by a new balloon catheter. Journal of Thoracic and Cardiovascular Surgery 87: 394–402

Ionescu M I, Tandon A P, Mary D A S, Abid A 1977 Heart valve replacement with the Ionescu Shiley pericardial xenograft. Journal of Thoracic and Cardiovascular Surgery 73: 31–42

Iraj Aryanpur, Iraj Nazarian, Bijan Siassi 1977 Rheumatic heart disease in developing countries. In: Moss A J, Adams F H, Emmanouilides G C (eds) Heart disease in infants, children and adolescents. Williams & Wilkins, Baltimore, M D, ch 34, p 547–557

John S, Krishnaswami S, Jairaj P S, Cherian G, Muralidharan S, Sukumar I P, Cherian G 1975 The profile and surgical management of mitral stenosis in young patients. Journal of Thoracic and Cardiovascular Surgery 69: 631–638

John S, Bashi V V, Jairaj P S et al 1983 Mitral valve replacement in the young patient with rheumatic heart disease: Early and late results in 118 subjects. Journal of Thoracic and Cardiovascular Surgery 86: 209–216

John S, Ravikumar E, Jairaj P S, Chowdhury V, Krishnaswami S 1990 Valve replacement in the young patient with rheumatic heart disease. Preview of a twenty-year experience. Journal of Thoracic and Cardiovascular Surgery 99: 631–638

Kaplan S 1977 Chronic rheumatic heart disease. In: Moss A J, Adams F H, Emmanouilides G C (eds) Heart disease in infants, children and adolescents. Williams & Wilkins, Baltimore, M D, Ch 33, p 533–547

Konno S, Imai Y, Iida Y, Nakajima M, Tatsuno K 1975 A new method for prosthetic valve replacement in congenital aortic stenosis associated with hypoplasia of the aortic valve ring. Journal of Thoracic and Cardiovascular Surgery 70: 909–917

Kumar N, Prabhakar G, Gometza B, at Halees Z, Duran C M 1993 The Ross procedure in a young rheumatic population: early clinical and echocardiographic profile. Journal of Heart Valve Disease 2: 376–379

Kutsche L M, Oyer P, Shumway N, Baum D 1979 An important complication of Hancock mitral valve replacement in children. Circulation 60(suppl I): 98–103

Lewis B S, Gotsman M S 1974 Left ventricular function during systole and diastole, in mitral incompetence. American Journal of Cardiology 34: 635–643

Lewis B S, Gotsman M S 1975 Cardiac hypertrophy and left ventricular end-diastolic stress. Israel Journal of Medical Sciences 11: 299–303

Lock J E, Khalilullah M, Shrivasta S, Bahl V, Keane J F 1985 Percutaneous catheter commissurotomy in rheumatic mitral stenosis. New England Journal of Medicine 313: 1515–1518

McGoon D C 1976 Valvular replacement and ventricular function. Journal of Thoracic and Cardiovascular Surgery 72: 326–327

McKay R, Lock J E, Safian R D et al 1987 Balloon dilation of mitral stenosis in adult patients: postmortem and percutaneous mitral valvuloplasty studies. Journal of the American College of Cardiology 9: 723–731

McLaren M J, Hawkins D , Koornhof H J 1975 Epidemiology of rheumatic heart disease in black school children of Soweto, Johannesburg. British Medical Journal 3: 474–478

Markowitz M 1977 The changing picture of rheumatic fever. Arthritis and Rheumatism 20: 369–374

Massell B F, Jhaveri S, Czoniczer G, Barnet R 1961 Treatment of rheumatic fever and rheumatic carditis: observations providing a basis for the selection of aspirin or adrenocortical steroids. Medical Clinics of North America 45: 1349–1368

Minich LL, Tani L Y, Pagotto L T, Shaddy R E, Veasy L G 1997 Doppler echocardiography distinguishes between physiologic and pathologic 'silent' mitral regurgitation in patients which rheumatic fever. Clinical Cardiology 20: 924–926

Morgan J R, Forker A D, Coates J R, Myers W S 1971 Isolated tricuspid stenosis. Circulation 44: 729–732

Mueller U K, Sareli P, Essop M R 1998 Anterior mitral leaflet retraction – a new echocardiographic predictor of severe mitral regurgitation following balloon valvuloplasty by the Inoue technique. American Journal of Cardiology 81: 656–659

Nadas A S, Fyler D C (eds) 1972 Acute rheumatic fever and rheumatic heart disease. In: Paediatric cardiology. Saunders, Philadelphia, P A, Ch 7, p 141–181

Neustadt J E, Shaffer A B 1959 Diagnostic value of the left atrial pressure pulse in mitral valvular disease. American Heart Journal 58: 675–688

NHLBIBVR (The National Heart, Lung and Blood Institute Balloon Valvuloplasty Registry) 1992 Multicenter experience with balloon mitral commissurotomy: NHLBI Balloon Valvuloplasty Registry report on immediate and 30-day follow-up results. Circulation 85: 448–461

Nobuyoshi M, Hamasaki N, Kimura T et al 1989 Indications, complications, a short-term clinical outcome of percutaneous transvenous mitral commissurotomy. Circulation 80: 782–792

Padial L R, Freitas N, Sagie A et al 1996 Echocardiography can predict which patients will develop severe mitral regurgitation after percutaneous mitral valvulotomy. Journal of the American College of Cardiology 27: 1225–1231

Palacios I F, Block P C, Brandi S et al 1989 Percutaneous balloon valvotomy for patients with severe mitral stenosis. Circulation 75: 778–784

Paul A T S 1967 The problem of mitral stenosis in childhood. Annals of Royal College of Surgeons of England 41: 387–402

Paul P, Mokracek A, Cerny S, Musilova B 1998 Reconstructive surgery of the aortic valve in rheumatic stenosis. Rozhledy V Chirugii 77: 150–153

Perez-Alvarez J J, Perez-Trevino C, Reta-Villalobos A, Jiminez-Martinez M, Arguero-Sanchez R, Lopez-Cellular M 1968 Valvular prosthesis in children. Surgery 65: 668–675

Pomerance 1972 Pathogenesis of aortic stenosis and its relation to age. British Heart Journal 34: 569–574

Prabhakar G, Kumar N, Gometza B, at Halees Z, Duran C M 1993 Surgery for organic rheumatic disease of the tricuspid valve. Journal of heart valve Disease 2: 561–566

Rappaport E 1975 Natural history of aortic and mitral valve disease. American Journal of Cardiology 35: 221–227

Reichek N, Shelburne J C, Perloff J K 1974 Clinical aspects of rheumatic valvular disease. In: Sonnenblick E H, Lesch M (eds) Valvular heart disease. Grune & Stratton, New York, p 131

Reyes V P et al 1994 Percutaneous balloon valvuloplasty compared with open surgical commissurotomy for mitral stenosis. New England Journal of Medicine 331: 961–967

Roberts W C 1970a Anatomically isolated aortic valvular disease. The case against its being of rheumatic etiology. American Journal of Medicine 49: 151–159

Roberts W C 1970b The structure of the aortic valve in clinically isolated aortic stenosis. An autopsy study of 162 patients over 15 years of age. Circulation 42: 91–97

Roberts W C, Hammer W J 1976 Cardiac pathology after valve replacement with a tilting disc prosthesis (Bjork–Shiley type): a study of 46 necropsy patients and 49 Bjork–Shiley prostheses. American Journal of Cardiology 37: 1024–1033

Sandler H, Dodge H T, Hay R E, Rackley C E 1963 Quantitation of valvular insufficiency in men by angiocardiography. American Heart Journal 65: 501–507

Sauter HJ, Dodge H T, Johnston R R, Graham T P 1964 The relationship of left atrial pressure and volume in patients with heart disease. American Heart Journal 67: 635–641

Schrire V, Vogelpoel L, Nellen M, Swanepoel A, Beck W 1961 Silent mitral incompetence. American Heart Journal 61: 723–729

Sellers R D, Levy M J, Amplatz K, Zellehe C W 1964 Left retrograde cardioangiography in acquired cardiac disease: technique, indications and interpretation of 700 cases. American Journal of Cardiology 14: 437–447

Smith H J, Neutze J M, Roche A H G, Agnew T M, Baratt-Boyes BG 1976 The natural history of rheumatic aortic regurgitation and the indications for surgery. British Heart Journal 38: 147–154

Spencer S S, Makene W J 1972 Rheumatic heart disease in Tanzanie. East African Medical Journal 49: 909–920

Stinson E B, Griepp R B, Oyer P E, Shumway N E 1977 Longterm experience with porcine aortic valve xenografts. Journal of Thoracic and Cardiovascular Surgery 73: 54–63

Strober W, Cohen L S, Waldman T A, Braunwald E 1968 Tricuspid regurgitation: a newly recognized cause of protein-losing enteropathy, lymphcytopenia and immunologic deficiency. American Journal of Medicine 44: 842–850

Sukumar IP 1982 Rheumatic heart disease in the young with special reference to juvenile mitral stenosis. Presidential address of the Cardiological Society of India. Proceedings of the International Congress on Tropical Cardiology, Bombay (India), October 1982

Sulayman R, Mathew R, Thilenius O G, Replogle R, Arcilla R A 1975 Hemodynamics and annuloplasty in isolated mitral regurgitation in children. Circulation 52: 1144–1151

Suri R K, Pathania R, Jha N K et al 1996. Closed mitral valvotomy for mitral restenosis: experience in 113 consecutive cases. Journal of Thoracic and Cardiovascular Surgery 112: 727–730

Tomkins D G, Boxerbaum B, Lichman J 1972 Longterm prognosis of rheumatic fever patients receiving regular intramuscular benzathine penicillin. Circulation 45: 543–551

Turi Z G et al 1991 Percutaneous balloon versus surgical closed commissurotomy for mitral stenosis: a prospective randomized trial. Circulation 83: 1179–1185

Tyrrell M J, Ellison R C, Hugenholtz P G, Nadas A S 1970 Correlation of degree of the left ventricular volume overload with clinical course in aortic and mitral regurgitation. British Heart Journal 32: 683–690

Vahanian A, Michel P L, Cormier B et al 1989 Results of percutaneous mitral commissurotomy in 200 patients. American Journal of Cardiology 63: 847–852

Vidne B, Levy M J 1970 Heart valve replacement in children. Journal of Thoracic and Cardiovascular Surgery 78: 123–127

Vijayaraghavan G, Cherian G, Krishnaswami S, Sukumar I P, John S 1977 Rheumatic aortic stenosis in young patients presenting with combined aortic and mitral stenosis. British Heart Journal 39: 294–298

Weir N M, Matisonn R E, Mitha A S, Le Roux B T, Rogers N M, Chesler E 1978 Valve replacement for rheumatic aortic incompetence in adolescents. Thorax 33: 608–615

Wells B 1954 The assessment of mitral stenosis by phonocardiography. British Heart Journal 16: 261–266

Werko L 1962 The dynamics and consequence of stenosis or insufficiency of the cardiac valves. In: Handbook of physiology, Section 2, Vol 1. American Physiological Society, Washington, D C

Wilkins G T, Weyman A E, Abascal V M, Block P C, Palacios IF 1988 Percutaneous balloon dilatation of mitral valve: an analysis of echocardiographic variables related to outcome and the mechanism of dilatation. British Heart Journal 60: 299–308

Wilson M G 1962 The life history of systolic murmurs in rheumatic heart disease. Progress in Cardiovascular Diseases 5: 145–151

Wood P 1954 An appreciation of mitral stenosis. British Medical Journal i: 1051, 1113

Wood P 1968 Diseases of the heart and circulation, 3rd edn. Eyre & Spottiswoode, London, p 600

Zhang Y, Nitter-Hauge S, Ihlen H et al 1986 Measurement of aortic regurgitation by Doppler echocardiography. British Heart Journal 55: 32–38

66

Infective endocarditis

E. A. Shinebourne

INTRODUCTION

The term 'infective' is preferable to 'bacterial' endocarditis, since fungal, rickettsial and probably viral agents can also initiate endocarditis. As reported by Major (1945), the first description of endocarditis was by Lazare Riviere in 1646. The patient developed heart failure with pulmonary oedema and died. Large vegetations occluding the aortic valve were found at postmortem. In 1883, Eischorst (cited by Major, 1945) made the distinction between acute and subacute endocarditis, and in 1885 Osler noted the association between prior damage to cardiac valves and endocarditis. In his Goulstonian lecturers, Osler described the clinical and pathological features of the disease and noted that micrococci were frequently found in the vegetations.

The distinction between acute and subacute endocarditis is less useful than describing the disease according to the infecting organism. While organisms with low virulences, such as the viridans group of streptococci, usually give rise to a subacute form of the illness, and pyogenic bacteriums such as *Staphylococcus aureus* cause a more virulent illness, this is not invariable. Host defence factors, a history of recent cardiac surgery or interventional cardiac catheterization, and prolonged intensive care can all modify the clinical picture. By definition, infective endocarditis is a microbial infection of the endocardium, but this term may be used loosely to describe infections of the arterial duct, surgically created shunts such as a classical or modified Blalock–Taussig anastomosis, or infection at the site of aortic coarctation. An infective endarteritis would be a more accurate term for this latter group. As will be discussed later, underlying structural heart disease is usual. In developed countries, the anomalies are principally congenital, while rheumatic heart disease still forms the substrate in many poorer countries. Infective endocarditis can develop in the setting of a normal heart, with drug addicts being at particular risk (Dressler and Roberts, 1989). Infective endocarditis may uncommonly affect infants and neonates, especially those undergoing intensive care with long-term indwelling venous catheters (Blieden et al, 1972; Saiman et al, 1993).

The disease was exclusively fatal prior to introduction of sulphonamides, when a small proportion of patients were successfully treated. It was not until the introduction of penicillin (Florey and Florey, 1943) that a large proportion was cured, and the mortality rapidly fell to about 30% (Vogler et al, 1962). The overall mortality, however, remained much the same in the next decade (Shinebourne et al, 1969; Hayward, 1973), perhaps with a further fall in the more recent decades. In adults, this relates in part to early replacement of damaged valves (Lowes et al, 1980), although those who advocate early surgical intervention in children, for instance to remove vegetations (Citak et al, 1992; Nomura et al, 1995), do not provide convincing evidence of a lower mortality than those using a more conservative approach. There is evidence, nonetheless, of a declining mortality in some recently reported series (Awadallah et al, 1991). In our own institution, amongst 21 children treated for infective endocarditis since January 1990, only two have died. One of these had a normal heart but was severely immune deficient, while the other had undergone surgery to replace an infected conduit containing a pulmonary homograft. In general, not only has the mortality remained high, but, despite greater knowledge of aetiology and pathogenesis, the overall incidence has also remained constant (Weinstein, 1972). Older patients, however, are now the most frequently affected. In the 1930s, the peak age affected was 32 years (Hamburger, 1963). In the 1940s, this had risen to 40–42 years (Wedgwood, 1955) and to 50–54 years by the 1960s (Kerr, 1964). Bacterial endocarditis is currently extremely uncommon in children, being more a disease of those aged 50 to 80 years. Analysis of prevalence at our own institution since 1990 shows a similar distribution, with 21 cases occurring under 15 years, 40 between 16 and 40 years, and 82 cases occurring in those over 40 years. When children are affected, it is again the older children, and in particular adolescents, who predominate. The disease is more common in males than in females.

One might now expect that infective endocarditis would carry a low risk. It is well recognized and should always be suspected in patients with known cardiac lesions who develop a persistent febrile illness. Techniques for culturing organisms have also much improved, and there is now a wide variety of antimicrobial agents available for therapeutic use. The disease should be recognized earlier and treated earlier and more effectively than ever before (Zuberbuhler, 1997). But for all that, mortality remains unacceptably high.

MICROBIOLOGY

Infective or, more specifically, bacterial endocarditis has traditionally been described as acute or subacute, the inference being that the virulence of the infecting organism determines both the severity and course of the disease. Acute bacterial endocarditis was thought to be caused by *Staphylococcus aureus*, *Streptococcus pyogenes* (β-haemolytic streptococci) or *Neisseria gonorrhoeae*. All of these agents cause an acute, severe illness with rapid destruction of valvar tissue and production of septic embolus and pyaemic abscesses. In contrast, subacute bacterial endocarditis was thought to be caused by less virulent organisms, such as *Streptococcus viridans* or *Streptococcus faecalis*. These distinctions, though useful clinically, do not always hold. Therefore, the clinical features of subacute bacterial endocarditis may be caused by *Staphylococcus aureus*, while *Streptococcus viridans* can, under some circumstances, cause a fulminating disease (Uwaydah and Weinberg, 1965). For these reasons, Lerner and Weinstein (1966) suggested that the terms 'acute' and 'subacute' be abolished. In paediatric practice, however, the clinical distinctions are still useful, perhaps more so in this age range than in the elderly. Nonetheless, as Cole (1975) has pointed out, modern concepts of any disease with an infective basis demand consideration of the system available for host defence, as well as of the virulence of the infecting organism. The defences of the host profoundly affect the clinical manifestations of infection with a particular organism. For example, in subacute bacterial endocarditis, it is the immune response of the subject to the infection that dominates the clinical picture. Lack of adequate resistance to infection accounts for the prevalence of acute bacterial endocarditis in debilitated patients, or in those with leukaemia or other malignant disease, in whom the heart may well be normal. In older patients, the types of infecting organism may have changed over the years. This is not so in children. Similar organisms have predominated since the 1970s (Johnson et al, 1975; Zuberbuhler et al, 1994).

The clinical presentation of infective endocarditis, therefore, depends not only on the causative organism but also on other factors. These include the valve infected, whether it is native or prosthetic, whether the infection was acquired in the community or in hospital and whether previous antimicrobial therapy may have modified the disease.

GRAM-POSITIVE ORGANISMS

GRAM-POSITIVE COCCI

The Gram-positive cocci include *Staphylococcus*, *Streptococcus* and *Pneumococcus* species.

Alpha-haemolytic streptococci

The α-haemolytic organisms exhibit α-haemolysis on blood agar plates and include the viridans group of streptococci. They caused more than nine tenths of infective endocarditis in the pre-antibiotic era (Tompsett, 1964). This proportion has fallen to about half of all cases of infective endocarditis with positive blood cultures (Moulsdale et al, 1980), which accounts for almost three quarters of subacute infections. The viridans group, however, remains the most common infecting organism (Lowes et al, 1980). Their names are confusing and not helpful from the clinical point of view. They include the *mitis*, *salivarius*, *sanguis*, *mitior*, *mutans* and *bovis* species, and some group D enterococci, or faecal streptococci, including *Streptococcus faecalis*. Microbiologically, they are a complicated group, but this should not affect therapy. Even when there are mixed organisms, one of the *Streptococcus* species is nearly always one of those involved (Pankey, 1961). Streptococci form part of the normal flora of the mouth, as well as the upper respiratory tract. They cause most, but not all, attacks of bacterial endocarditis following dental treatment. It is of note that these streptococci rarely cause other forms of infection in humans. Why they should be the most common cause of bacterial endocarditis remains incompletely explained.

Bacterial studies during dental extractions show a bacteraemia that lasts usually for 15–20 minutes. It consists principally of *Streptococcus mutans*, which is the dominant organism in the mouth. *Streptococcus sanguis*, however, is the commonest cause of subacute bacterial endocarditis (Elliot, 1973). Probably the crucial factor is the ability of *Streptococcus sanguis* to synthesize a sticky surface that gives the organism particular adhesive properties (Gibbons, 1972). Bacterial adhesiveness may result from sticky polysaccharides, but some bacterial wall membranes are inherently stickier than others. Other bacteriums have hair-like structures that enhance adhesiveness (Swanson et al, 1971). Further consideration of the relationship of dental treatment to infective endocarditis, and its prevention, will be dealt with later.

Enterococci

Faecal streptococci, which cause up to one-fifth of cases of infective endocarditis, are normal commensals in the gut, genitourinary tract and, sometimes, the mouth.

Endocarditis may follow manoeuvres in the genito-urinary tract such as urethral catheterization, abortion, normal delivery (Mandell et al, 1970) or even insertion of an intrauterine contraceptive device (de Swiet et al, 1975). All these precipitating factors tend to be more important in older patients. As more patients with complex cyanotic heart disease reach adult life, more cases of endocarditis will be expected following insertion of intrauterine contraceptive devices or following delivery. This is especially so since, in the polycythaemic patient with cyanotic congenital heart disease, most oral contraceptives are contraindicated because of the risks of thrombosis. Enterococci also include organisms such as *Streptococcus zymogenes* and *Streptococcus liquefaciens*. These organisms may produce α- or β-haemolysis or no haemolysis on blood agar plates. Particular care, therefore, is necessary in their precise identification.

Other streptococci

Streptococcus bovis, like *Streptococcus faecalis*, is a member of Lancefield group D. It is not an enterococcus but tends to produce a typical subacute course of disease, albeit with a more favourable prognosis (Moellering et al, 1974).

Streptococcus pyogenes is a group A haemolytic bacterium. It is used to cause an acute fulminating infection, often following erysipelas. Infection from this organism is now fortunately uncommon, probably because of the early use of antibiotics for acute cellulitis.

Streptococcus pneumoniae, the pneumococcus, was also commoner until the introduction of antibiotics. Pneumococcal endocarditis previously tended to develop as a complication of pneumococcal meningitis or lobar pneumonia. The group of patients with congenital heart disease most at risk nowadays from infection with this organism are probably those with right isomerism and asplenia (Chapter 31).

Anaerobic and microaerophilic streptococci cause approximately 5% of cases of infective endocarditis (Wedgwood, 1955), the disease being either acute or subacute. Special techniques of culture are required for their identification (Lerner and Weinstein, 1966). As culture of these organisms can be difficult, aerobic and anaerobic cultures should be made in all suspected cases of endocarditis.

Staphylococci

Staphylococcus aureus is coagulase-positive and often resistant to penicillin; it is the most common cause of acute endocarditis. The organism may affect normal valves, especially in immunologically depressed individuals. It is frequently found as the cause of right-sided endocarditis affecting the tricuspid valve in abusers of intravenous drugs. In children, it is more likely to complicate cardiac catheterization, cardiac surgery or, at least, insertion of a venous cannula.

GRAM-POSITIVE BACILLI

Gram-positive bacilli are uncommon causes of bacterial endocarditis. They affect immune depressed or debilitated patients. Many such organisms have been documented as causing infective endocarditis, including *Listeria monocytogenes* (Elston et al, 1969; Bayer et al, 1977), lactobacilli, which are normal commensals in the mouth, colon and vagina (Axelrod et al, 1973), diphtheroids (van Scoy et al, 1977), *Bacillus subtilis* and *Nocardia israelii*.

GRAM-NEGATIVE ORGANISMS

Neisseria gonorrhoeae can cause a fulminating endocarditis, but, even in the current era, it is not a major problem in children. Gram-negative bacilli are seldom the cause of endocarditis in children or, for that matter, in older people despite the high frequency of bacteraemia they produce (Uwaydah and Weinberg, 1965). This is probably because these organisms are not particularly sticky and do not adhere easily to abnormal endocardium or damaged valves (Holmes and Ramirez-Ronda, 1977). *Escherichia coli* and *Enterobacter* and *Klebsiella* species are again very rare causes of bacterial endocarditis in children. They are more common in older patients, intravenous drug addicts or patients with prosthetic valves.

Pseudomonas aeroginosa is a particular problem in patients requiring long-term intensive care and needing indwelling cannulas. In particular, the combination of indwelling cannulas and the use of multiple antibiotics during inpatient hospital stay sets the scene for infection with *Pseudomonas* species. *Haemophilus influenzae* or *Haemophilus parainfluenzae* rarely cause endocarditis in children. Virtually all of these organisms are far more likely to affect prosthetic valves.

YEASTS AND FUNGI

Endocarditis caused by candidal infection usually develops after previous antimicrobial therapy. It is rare as a spontaneous infection. As with most of the less virulent organisms, infection is particularly a problem after insertion of artificial materials, such as a valve or conduit. It is probable that access to the circulation is gained from infected sites of intravenous access rather than from spores in imperfectly sterilized valves (Darell, 1975). Candidal infection may also complicate adequately treated bacterial infection as a superinfection (Seelig et al, 1974). *Histoplasma coccidioides* and *Aspergillus* species are other rare non-bacterial causes of endocarditis.

VIRUSES

Evidence for a viral aetiology for infective endocarditis in humans, though persuasive, is circumstantial. Endocarditis has been produced in mice (Burch et al, 1966) and in monkeys (de Pasquale et al, 1966) by infection with coxsackievirus B4. These workers have also demonstrated coxsackieviral antigens within the valves and myocardium in humans (Burch et al, 1967). Viral infections in humans, nonetheless, are common. It is possible that virally induced endocardial change may occur that could act as a focus for subsequent bacterial infection (Cole, 1975).

RICKETTSIA AND CHLAMYDIA SPECIES

Q fever endocarditis caused by *Coxiella burnetii* is uncommon in children. It has been described affecting the aortic or mitral valve in teenagers (Kristinsson and Bentall, 1967). Infective endocarditis may also occur during an episode of psittacosis caused by *Chlamydia psittaci* or by *Chlamydia trachomatis* (van der Bel-Kahn et al, 1978).

UNDERLYING CARDIAC DISEASE AND SITE OF INFECTION

Half the cases of infective endocarditis in adults is still superimposed on chronic rheumatic heart disease. It is the mitral or aortic valves that are most usually affected (Lerner and Weinstein, 1966). Congenital heart disease is the usual underlying cause in children, the commonest lesions (Johnson et al, 1975) being a small ventricular septal defect, aortic stenosis or incompetence, tetralogy of Fallot (especially when palliated by construction of a shunt (Blumenthal et al, 1960)) or persistent patency of the arterial duct. No case of bacterial endocarditis has been described in patients with an isolated atrial septal defect, although patients with an atrioventricular septal defect and separate valvar orifices (primum defect) may be affected. Review of the more recent literature gives slightly conflicting information as to whether there is or is not a 'changing pattern' of endocarditis. In some centres, up to one fifth of cases occurred within a few days or weeks of cardiac surgery (Sholler et al, 1986; Karl et al, 1987), but not in our own or the Pittsburgh series (Zuberbuhler et al, 1994). Probably the most comprehensive population-based data are those of van der Meer et al (1992). They reported an incidence in the Netherlands of 19 cases per million per year, of which 7% occurred within 30 days of a procedure in a patient with known heart disease. Inevitably, however, as more children with congenital heart disease survive surgical interventions, the proportion at risk of developing endocarditis increases (Awadallah et al, 1991; Nomura et al, 1995). In the series reported by Zuberbuhler and his colleagues (1994), in our own series and in many others, ventricular or atrioventricular septal defects, aortic valvar disease and tetralogy of Fallot, especially when palliated with a modified Blalock–Taussig shunt, remain

the commonest underlying conditions. Mitral valvar prolapse (Lachman et al, 1975; Awadallah et al, 1991) also remains important as an underlying cause in children in whom no cardiac anomaly had been suspected prior to development of endocarditis, as does a bicuspid aortic valve in older subjects. As more children with complete transposition survive either the arterial switch or construction of a shunt when a ventricular septal defect is associated with obstruction of the left ventricular outflow tract, so this group provides the substrate for endocarditis, as do patients with common arterial trunk before and after corrective surgery (Nomura et al, 1995).

Other groups particularly at risk are those with prosthetic valves or a conduit from the ventricle to the pulmonary arteries (Awardallah et al, 1991). Infective endocarditis has been reported in patients with hypertrophic cardiomyopathy, but not during childhood (Alessandri et al, 1990). It remains extremely rare in isolated pulmonary valvar stenosis, with only 1 of 28 patients having the congenital abnormality as the sole risk factor in the series reported by Cassling et al (1985).

The risk of bacterial endocarditis in children aged between 5 and 14 years with a ventricular septal defect has been estimated as 1 in 500 patient-years, or 2 infections per 100 over a period of 10 years (Shah et al, 1966). The incidence is considerably higher when aortic incompetence complicates the picuture (Hallidie-Smith et al, 1969), or in those defects producing a shunt from left ventricle to right atrium (Mellins et al, 1964). Data from the North American multicentred long-term follow-up study of congenital heart disease known as NHS-2 has further refined the risk of infective endocarditis for aortic stenosis, pulmonary stenosis and ventricular septal defects (Gersony et al, 1993). The risk for aortic stenosis was 27.1 per 10 000 person-years, being 15.7 per 10 000 person-years for those treated medically and 40.9 per 10 000 person-years for those managed surgically. The increased risk for those managed surgically was thought to be a function of severity rather than of postoperative aortic incompetence, although the data are not totally convincing on this matter. For ventricular septal defect, the risk was 14.5 per 10 000 person-years, approximately half that for aortic stenosis. The risk of endocarditis in the patients with a ventricular septal defect was not related to the size of the defect but was halved after surgical closure. The risk of infective endocarditis was very low in patients with pulmonary stenosis, at 0.9 per 10 000 person-years, representing only one patient amongst the 592 followed. For subjects under 18 years of age with ventricular septal defect, the risk per year was 0.1%, but this almost doubled in those over 18 years (to 0.18%). The risks for those with aortic stenosis are 0.02% following cardiac catheterization, 1.8% if untreated and 3.8% following surgery. When bacterial endocarditis complicates tetralogy of Fallot with pulmonary atresia, it is usually the aortic valve that is affected (Figure 66.1) (Blumenthal et al, 1960). This is

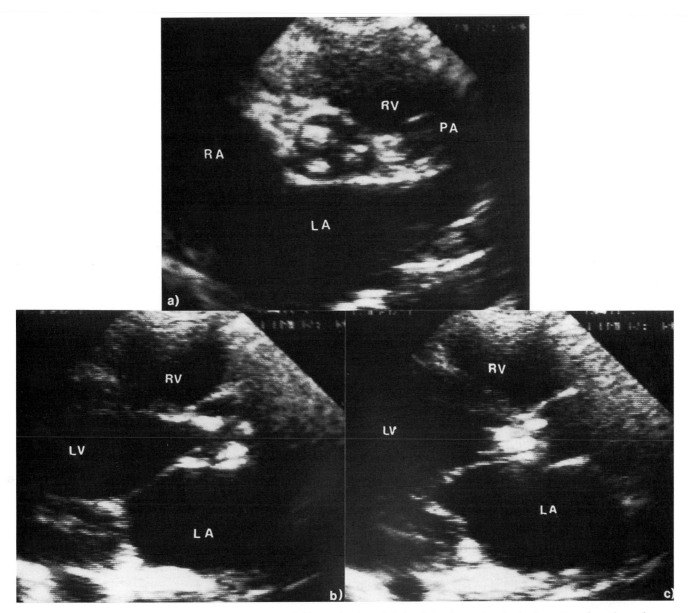

Figure 66.1. Cross-sectional echocardiogram in a patient with bacterial endocarditis involving the aortic valve in the setting of tetralogy of Fallot. (a) Parasternal short-axis view showing the three normally thin aortic valvar leaflets replaced by echodense masses consisting of vegetations and thrombus. Compare with the anatomical specimen shown in Figure 66.2 from the same patient. The patient died from acute obstruction of the orifice of the left coronary artery by vegetations attached to the left coronary aortic valvar leaflet. The parasternal long-axis views from the same patient show the thickened valvar leaflets in systole (b) and diastole (c).

usually also the case in tetralogy with pulmonary stenosis, although then the pulmonary valve itself may be affected.

What factors determine the higher prevalence of infective endocarditis in certain anomalies, and what is the site in the heart at which infective endocarditis commences? Lepeschkin (1952) first stressed the importance of hydrodynamic factors in the site of endocarditis when he noted that infection was most common on the mitral valve. The next commonest site was the aortic valve, followed some way behind by the tricuspid and, very rarely, the pulmonary valve. It is the elegant work of Rodbard (1963) that still best answers these questions. He assembled the

data to show that endocarditis occurs when a high-pressure source, such as the left ventricle or aorta, drives blood at high velocities through a narrow orifice, such as an aortic coarctation, a small ventricular septal defect or arterial duct or a regurgitant aortic or mitral valve, into a low-pressure sink, such as the atrium, pulmonary trunk or right ventricle. The high velocity of the stream of blood immediately beyond the orifice leads to a marked drop in lateral hydrostatic pressure; consequently, perfusion of the intima at this site in the vessel or cardiac chamber is reduced. This is then the characteristic site of the infective process. This Venturi effect accounts for the finding that it is the left atrial side of the mitral valve that is affected in mitral incompetence, while, in a ventricular septal defect, infection is centred on the right ventricular surface of the septum. Small defects are nearly always involved, as large defects rapidly dissipate any differences in pressure. Similarly, in an arterial duct, it is the pulmonary arterial end that is infected, while in aortic incompetence it is the ventricular surface of the leaflets that is involved. In experiments using bacterial aerosols in a Venturi tube, Rodbard also showed that organisms were deposited downstream in an analogous fashion to that postulated for endocarditis.

In addition to a Venturi effect accounting for the siting of primary infective lesions, secondary, or even primary, jet lesions may be the focus for infection. The presumed mechanism is that jets of blood at high pressure impinge on the endocardium. This causes damage or provokes endocardial thickening, with subsequent deposition of fibrin and the production of thrombotic vegetations. This accounts for McCallum's patch as a secondary site of endocarditis in the left atrial wall in mitral incompetence. It similarly explains the involvement of the free wall of the right ventricle with an infection involving a ventricular septal defect, and the involvement of the tendinous cords or the aortic leaflet of the mitral valve when endocarditis affects an incompetent aortic valve.

PATHOLOGY

Vegetations consisting of craggy friable masses of thrombus measuring up to 1 or 2 cm in diameter (Figure 66.2)

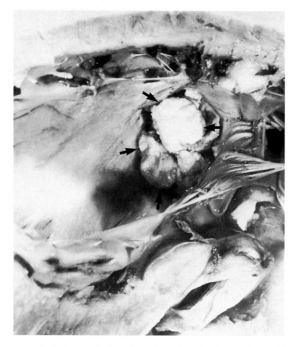

Figure 66.2. Left ventricular view of aortic valve in a patient with bacterial endocarditis. The valve is trileaflet and friable vegetations are seen (arrowed) on all three leaflets. The cross-sectional echocardiogram from this patient is shown in Figure 66.1.

are the characteristic pathological feature of infective endocarditis (Osler, 1885). They are typically attached to valvar leaflets, often at their lines of closure, to the endocardium of the ventricles or to the left atrium.

When rheumatic heart disease is present, the aortic and mitral valves are commonly involved. The vegetations may spread from the leaflets of the aortic valve to the aortic leaflet of the mitral valve, or to the aortic root with occlusion of a coronary artery. The vegetations may be sufficiently large to occlude either the aortic or mitral valve (Roberts et al, 1967). This complication is most common with fungal infections. Other complications include ruptured papillary muscles, perforation of valvar leaflets, aneurysms of the sinus of Valsalva and formation of mycotic aneurysms in the aortic root. Ulceration of valvar leaflets, in addition to perforations, are more typical of acute than subacute endocarditis. Abscesses of the valvar rings may be found. These may predispose to haemorrhagic pericarditis and tamponade (Arnett and Roberts, 1976). They also increase the likelihood of paravalvar leaks following insertion of a valvar prosthesis. Myocardial abscesses can also be produced. These may account for minor disturbances in conduction, while pathological Q waves probably indicate coronary embolization (Shinebourne et al, 1969).

Histological examination of vegetations reveals platelet and fibrin thrombuses with varying numbers of infectious organisms. Masses of polymorphonucleocytes are seen in acute endocarditis, and the valvar endothelium is ulcerated. Fewer organisms are seen following a more subacute course. Mononuclear cells and lymphocytes predominate with few polymorphs. Giant cells are occasionally seen containing phagocytosed organisms. The underlying valve becomes vascularized and invaded by capillaries and fibroplasts, which grow into and organize the thrombus. Widespread changes may also be seen in the myocardium, consisting of diffuse or localized collections of lymphocytes and mononuclear cells with degeneration of muscle fibres. While large coronary arteries may show discrete embolization, the smaller vessels exhibit endothelial swelling and proliferation, with perivascular cellular infiltrates. This is all strongly suggestive of an immune process.

CLINICAL FEATURES

HISTORY

In past decades, a history of rheumatic fever has been found in a high proportion of patients with infective endocarditis. In Europe and America, however, rheumatic fever has become uncommon. Chronic rheumatic heart disease is now rare in these countries as the substrate for infective endocarditis in children. This is not the case in many poor or underdeveloped parts of the world, where rheumatic fever is rife. In Africa, the Indian subcontinent, Central and South America and parts of the Middle and Far East, rheumatic mitral or aortic valvar disease still remains the most common basis for infective endocarditis.

Congenital heart disease forms the anatomical substrate for most cases of infective endocarditis in our own practice. Included within this group should be patients with a possibly previously unsuspected bicuspid aortic valve.

A subacute course of infection is unusual under the age of 2 years, and most patients with endocarditis below this age will have an acute fulminating disease. In infants in particular, endocarditis may be found in the setting of an otherwise normal heart, where the disease may be part of an overwhelming septicaemia (Zakrzewski and Keith, 1965). In many children with infective endocarditis, no precipitating event or focus of infection will be found. Where one is found, dental extractions, orthodontic procedures or other dental manipulations are the most common. Bacteraemia is found in between a quarter and three quarters of cases following extraction of an infected tooth (Everett and Hirschman, 1977). Extractions of non-diseased primary teeth and healthy secondary teeth, as well as scaling or vigorous brushing, also give rise to significant bacteraemia (Peterson and Peacock, 1976). Common surgical procedures such as tonsillectomy and adenoidectomy may also cause bacteraemia, while even non-surgical manipulations of the upper respiratory tract, such as endotracheal intubation, nasotracheal suction or bronchoscopy, are hazardous (Le Frock et al, 1976). Abdominal surgery, such as an appendicectomy, also gives rise to bacteraemia, although bacterial endocarditis does not so commonly follow such procedures. This is probably because the organisms liberated into the circulation are less likely to adhere to damaged or abnormal endocardium.

Cardiac catheterization rarely causes endocarditis, although staphylococcal infection may occur, especially at the site of entry of the catheter. Pacing wires are also associated with this problem. Endocarditis may follow cardiac surgery. The patient is at particular risk when artificial material, such as an external conduit or prosthetic valve, is inserted, or, for that matter, if a permanent pacemaker is needed. Childbirth is another occasion when bacteraemia may occur. Those addicted to heroin are always at particular risk, as virtually any organism may be inadvertently injected. The only other special groups of children at risk are those with a ventriculo-atrial shunt constructed to treat hydrocephalus, and possibly children with artificial vascular shunts inserted to facilitate renal haemodialysis.

It is helpful to think of the clinical manifestations of infective endocarditis as having three phases, each varying in time depending on the virulence of the organism and the immunological response of the patient (Cole, 1975). There is first an acute infective phase. A relatively latent phase ensues with little to find clinically or, for that matter, bacteriologically (Libman, 1913). There is then a chronic immunological phase, where many of the classical signs of subacute bacterial endocarditis become apparent.

SYMPTOMS

Fever, manifest as sweating, chills, shivering or rigors, is the commonest presenting feature. While initially continuous, the fever may become recurrent with relatively symptomless intervals. This is particularly so when short non-bactericidal courses of antibiotics have been given, often for short non-specific pyrexial illnesses. The indiscriminate proferring of antibiotics to children with congenital heart disease is ill-advised unless a genuine cause of illness or pyrexia is found.

Toxaemia, manifest as malaise, tiredness, weakness, anorexia, generalized lethargy, aches and pains, usually accompanies fever. Weight loss completes the picture of a severely unwell patient with varied and non-specific symptoms. As the diagnosis may not be made for some weeks, abnormal behavioural causes may sometimes be sought for a child's apathy. Atypical presentation of infective endocarditis should, therefore, be considered in any lethargic child with a known cardiac abnormality.

An embolic episode may be a further mode of presentation. This is perhaps more common in adults than in children. Any organ of the body may be affected. Renal infarcts caused by embolization of relatively large renal arteries may cause frank haematuria. Splenic infarcts may give pain in the left loin. Occlusion of limb vessels may cause localized symptoms. Right heart endocarditis, though uncommon in children, may present with haemoptysis or even as recurrent 'chest infections' owing to pulmonary embolization. Cerebral infarcts may present as a stroke, while blindness in one eye may be caused by embolic retinal arterial occlusion. Although gross embolization may occur, it is now realised that many of the features previously attributed to microembolization are caused by immunological phenomenons (Bacon et al, 1974) (see below).

Increasing breathlessness and tachycardia may reflect heart failure and/or anaemia. The latter may present as pallor and contributes to the general feeling of malaise. Heart failure may be caused by both mechanical and myocardial factors. Destruction of valves can give rise to severe aortic or mitral incompetence, while coronary embolization may produce myocardial infarction. A diffuse myocarditis may also contribute to heart failure.

Neurological manifestations or complications of infective endocarditis are extremely common, being found in over one third of patients (Jones et al, 1969). A diffuse cerebral vasculitis is found that can result in confusional states, headaches, psychiatric disturbances and any of the features of meningoencephalitis. Subarachnoid haemorrhage from rupture of a mycotic aneurysm may occur but is uncommon in children. A stroke or acute hemiparesis from a major embolus or ruptured aneurysm, convulsions or features of peripheral neuropathy may be present. The prognosis is worse in those with neurological symptoms, the mortality being two (Jones et al, 1969) or three times (Pruitt et al, 1978) greater than in other patients with endocarditis.

Arthralgia may be a presenting symptom. Sometimes there is arthritis of a single joint, but more commonly there is a generalized arthralgia (Doyle et al, 1962). Rheumatoid arthritis may be simulated since, owing to high levels of gammaglobulin in the plasma, latex fixation tests may also be positive (Bacon et al, 1974). Abdominal pain, nausea and diarrhoea are other nonspecific manifestations of infective endocarditis.

PHYSICAL FINDINGS

The child usually appears ill, pyrexial and anaemic. Splenomegaly will be present in at least two thirds. It is often painless, but the spleen may be tender when it is greatly enlarged. Hepatomegaly and other signs of heart failure may be evident. Auscultation of the heart should reveal signs of the underlying cardiac anomaly. The early diastolic murmur of aortic incompetence should be carefully sought, as the aortic valve is so commonly affected. Likewise, the recent development of mitral or tricuspid regurgitation may arouse suspicion. Indeed, when any of the auscultatory findings have changed since a previous examination, infective endocarditis should be suspected. Such a change is one of the classical features of the disease. Finger clubbing may develop or be present when there is a subacute course to the disease. In some patients it will simply reflect cyanotic heart disease.

In underdeveloped or poor countries, anaemia and fever are extremely common in the general population of children and may have many causes apart from infective endocarditis, including malaria or other parasitic infestations. In these circumstances, differential diagnosis of the ill, pale, pyrexial, clubbed child with a heart murmur is difficult. It may be impossible to determine the true cause without laboratory aids, which, under just these circumstances, may simply not be available.

Other classical features of 'subacute' bacterial endocarditis are splinter haemorrhages, petechial lesions, Osler's nodes, Janeway lesions and Roth's spots. Splinter haemorrhages are linear haemorrhages present or beneath the fingernails and, occasionally, the toenails. They are variable in number and can be distinguished from traumatic lesions or real splinters by the fact that their distal end does not reach the distal edge of the nail bed. The petechial lesions found in infective endocarditis characteristically have a pale centre. They are seen in the conjunctivas, the backs of the hands, in the oral mucous membranes and, occasionally, on the anterior aspect of the chest or abdomen. Osler's nodes, which are uncommon in

children (Zahrzewski and Keith, 1965), are small raised red or purple nodules. They are tender or painful, being found in the pulp of the terminal phalanx of the fingers. Rarely, they exist on the backs of the toes, the soles of the feet or the thenar or hypothenar eminences. Janeway lesions are small, irregular, flat, macular non-tender lesions that blanch with pressure. They are typically also found on the thenar or hypothenar eminence but may coalesce to form a diffuse macular erythematous rash. Roth's spots are cotton wool-like exudates in the retina. They are not specific for infective endocarditis. They consist of aggregations of cytoid bodies made up of perivascular collections of lymphocytes in the nerve layer of the retina, with oedema and sometimes haemorrhage.

IMMUNE COMPLEX PHENOMENONS

Cordeiro et al (1965) assembled evidence to suggest that many of the symptoms and signs of infective endocarditis formerly attributed to microembolization were caused by deposition of complexes of antibody, antigen and complement. Cole (1975) listed multiple lesions as examples of immune complex phenomenons (Table 66.1). Similarly, the diffuse myocarditis often found could be caused by an immunological disturbance.

The evidence of widespread vascular fragility, anaemia, changes in circulating gammaglobulins and diffuse glomerulonephritis support this concept. Furthermore, as Hamer and O'Grady (1977) point out, the presence of splinter haemorrhages and diffuse renal disease in patients with right-sided cardiac lesions (in which embolization is confined to the pulmonary vascular bed) makes unlikely an embolic explanation for these phenomenons.

The best supporting evidence for the concept that immune complex phenomenons play a major role in endocarditis is that the pathological changes in the kidneys, both in acute and subacute bacterial endocarditis, may be identical to the changes found in acute or chronic proliferative glomerulonephritis (Tu et al, 1969; Gutman et al, 1972).

The subacute phase of infective endocarditis has many clinical and pathological features similar to those of so-called autoimmune diseases such as systemic lupus

Table 66.1. Immune complex phenomenons

Petechial rash
Roth's spots
Osler's nodes
Janeway lesions
Haematuria (microscopic)
Retinal haemorrhage
Cerebral vasculitis
Arthralgia
Splinter haemorrhages (possible)
Mycotic aneurysms (possible)

erythematosus or polyarteritis nodosa. Latex fixation tests are positive in half of the patients with infective endocarditis (Williams and Kunkel, 1962). Antiglobulins such as rheumatoid factor are also commonly found.

Circulating immune complexes can be demonstrated in the serum of patients with endocarditis. The levels have been positively correlated with longer duration of illness, extracardiac features of the illness and a low level of complement in the serum. Bayer et al (1976) also showed that the levels of circulating immune complexes fell to zero when therapy was successful, as evidenced by negative blood cultures, regression of peripheral non-cardiac signs and a rise in complement in the serum. In the group of patients studied by these workers, some patients remained unwell despite negative blood cultures. Surgical removal of the infected valve was then thought necessary. Only after removal of the valve did the levels of immune complex fall and the complement rise in the serum. This suggests that monitoring these entities may indicate efficacy of treatment. As a further development, this group later suggested that the presence of circulating immune complexes would be a useful way of deciding if a patient with septicaemia and positive blood cultures did indeed have active endocarditis (Bayer et al, 1979).

Other evidence for immune mechanisms in endocarditis is found in studies demonstrating cross-reactivity between heart cells and serums obtained from subjects immunized with constituents of streptococcal cell wall (Kaplan, 1963a,b) or between streptococci and glomerular basement membrane (Markowitz and Lange, 1964).

Autoimmune mechanisms may also play a part in pathogenesis. Cole (1975) postulated that persistence of antigenic material from the infecting agent may produce a delayed hypersensitivity response. This then causes further damage, possibly with alteration in host tissue antigens. Immune responses are further activated if the defences of the host no longer recognize its own tissues as self. This phase is characterized by high levels of immunoglobulin G, and of antibody against the bacterium (Phair et al, 1972).

The pathological lesions produced by immune complexes are determined by the ratio of antigen to antibody. Those formed when antigen is in excess cause increased capillary permeability, possibly by immune complexes acting on platelets and causing them to release vasoactive amines (Kniker and Cochrane, 1968). These allow plasma to filter through the vessel wall with deposition of complexes. When antigen and antibody are present in equivalence, granulomas are formed (Spector and Heeson, 1969). The principal antibodies involved in the phagocytosis and killing of organisms in infective endocarditis are immunoglobulin G-opsonins (Laxdal et al, 1968). There is evidence that some of the other antibodies detected during the immunological phase of bacterial endocarditis, such as antiglobulins, are antiopsonic and may reduce phagocytosis (Meissner et al, 1968). Cole (1975) suggested that, in addition to antibiotics, or

surgery, there may be a place for suppression of immunity in the therapy of infective endocarditis. This intriguing suggestion remains to be tested.

ECHOCARDIOGRAPHY

Cross-sectional echocardiography (Gilbert et al, 1977) demonstrates well vegetations attached to valvar structures in patients with infective endocarditis (Figure 66.1). Studies show that four fifths of patients or more will have vegetations that are demonstrated by cross-sectional echocardiography (Martin et al, 1980; Stewart et al, 1980). Those with positive echocardiographic features are more likely to have complications such as major embolization, congestive heart failure and the need for emergency valvar replacement, which may be performed on the basis of the echocardiographic features alone (Davis et al, 1980). However, while the echocardiographic demonstration of vegetations confirms the diagnosis of endocarditis, lack of demonstration does not rule out the diagnosis. Ongoing management should not in any way be based solely on echocardiographic features (Stewart et al, 1980).

LABORATORY DIAGNOSIS

BLOOD CULTURES

Isolation of the infecting organism by culturing blood is of paramount importance, both in making the diagnosis and in planning treatment. The technique used to obtain blood cultures should be designed to avoid contamination with skin commensals. The skin should be cleaned with an alcoholic solution, and the vein entered directly. Optimal sterile techniques should be used, and preferably disposable sterile gloves. Depending on size of the patient, 5–10 ml of blood should be withdrawn, and half injected into each of two containers through the rubber seals.

Three samples of blood for culture are probably adequate in order to isolate the organism in the majority of patients and to clarify whether or not an organism grown is a contaminant (Hamer and O'Grady, 1977). The time at which blood is taken for culture is not critical. Although 'showers' of organisms may precede an acute rise in temperature (Weiss and Ottenberg, 1932), bacteraemia is constant (Bennett and Beeson, 1954). There is no advantage of arterial over venous sampling to obtain the blood used for culture (Bennet and Beeson, 1954), although culturing bone marrow may be useful for some resistant or unusual organisms (Finland, 1954). Once in the laboratory, the bottles are incubated, inspected and subcultured after 24 and 48 hours, and weekly thereafter. Aerobic and anaerobic cultures are made.

ERYTHROCYTIC SEDIMENTATION RATE

Another useful, if non-specific, laboratory finding is a raised erythrocytic sedimentation rate. This may also be elevated during active rheumatic fever, but a normal value makes diagnosis of either condition extremely unlikely. During antibiotic therapy, reversion of a raised sedimentation rate to normal makes it probable that therapy is effective.

HAEMATOLOGICAL FINDINGS

Anaemia is the rule. It is usually normocytic but may be microcytic, especially if infection has been long-standing. Nucleated red cells may be seen in the peripheral film. The total white cell count is typically elevated with a preponderance of polymorphonucleocytes, although the white cell count may be normal or low, especially in the setting of staphylococcal infections (Fisher et al, 1955).

HAEMATURIA

More than nine tenths of patients will have at least microscopic haematuria. Its absence makes diagnosis unlikely (Shinebourne et al, 1969).

NEGATIVE BLOOD CULTURES

The problem of negative blood cultures remains important, as not only is mortality higher in this group (Cates and Christie, 1951), but rational and controlled therapy is impossible to achieve. Contrary to many of the earlier views on this topic, infective endocarditis with negative blood cultures is usually caused by infection with the common or usual organisms such as the viridans group of streptococcus (Pesanti and Smith, 1979). The problem is that the organisms contained within the vegetations are unexposed, being encased by depositions of fibrin and thrombus. This is particularly the case in patients with clinical features of immune complex phenomenons. It is more often a problem in adults with endocarditis than in children. Previous, often cavalier, treatment with antibiotics is another cause for negative cultures. We cannot stress strongly enough the need for taking blood samples for culture prior to commencement of antibiotics.

Rickettsial infections, such as Q fever, can be diagnosed by serological studies, as can chlamydial infections such as psittacosis.

In practice, Candida species are the one common group for which standard techniques for culturing blood are negative. This diagnosis, therefore, should be considered in any patient with persistent infection who has had prolonged periods of intravenous cannulation, or else who has had artificial material inserted at surgery.

Modern technological methods of culturing blood, such as Bactec or Organon–Technika, are more efficient than previous techniques. Culturing blood on Sabourand's medium may be successful after 10 days to 3 weeks but may take longer. While serological tests are specific for *Candida* (Remington et al, 1972), care must be taken in interpreting results, as positive results may be obtained in patients with bacterial endocarditis and no other evidence of candidal infection (Bacon et al, 1974).

THE RELATIONSHIP OF DENTAL PROCEDURES TO INFECTIVE ENDOCARDITIS

Various species of α-haemolytic streptococci, particularly *S. sanguis*, *S. minor*, and *S. mutans*, constitute the most common cause of infective endocarditis. These organisms are found principally in the mouth. Much evidence exists to indicate that dental procedures are an important precipitating factor in the disease. McGowan (1978) found that dental procedures were implicated in one eighth of nearly 5000 cases of endocarditis published between 1909 and 1975. The risk of developing endocarditis, nonetheless, even in patients with a known cardiac anomaly, is low. It has been being estimated at 1 in 5000 dental procedures (Hilson, 1970). In practice, infective endocarditis is the only direct complication of dental surgery that may prove fatal. Few would argue about the need for antibiotic prophylaxis, at least in susceptible individuals. More extreme views are that, whether or not they have cardiac disease, everyone should have antibiotic prophylaxis for dental extractions (Oakley, 1979), or that susceptible patients should be rendered edentulous (Beeley, 1969). It seems to us more sensible to identify the patients at excess risk carefully as discussed above, along with the particular dental procedures producing bacteraemia. These include extractions (Baumgartner et al, 1977), scaling (Lineberger and de Marco, 1973), major root fillings (Baumgartner et al, 1976) and any surgical procedure in which a mucoperiosteal flap is raised (Baumgartner et al, 1977). All these interventions warrant prophylaxis (McGowan, 1982).

Streptococcal bacteraemia, however, may also occur in patients with poor oral hygiene in the absence of dental procedures simply through chewing (Okell and Elliot, 1935), brushing the teeth (Cobe, 1954) or using dental floss (Carroll and Seybor, 1980). Guntheroth (1984) reviewed in detail the relationship of previous dental extractions to development of infective endocarditis. From the literature, he estimated that, of 1322 patients with the disease, only 47 (3.6%) had undergone a prior extraction. While two fifths of patients have a positive blood culture after an extraction, this only lasts for up to 30 minutes. Bacteraemia was found in 38% of patients as a result of chewing, and in 11% with poor oral hygiene and no intervention. Consequently, in a hypothetical situation ending with a dental extraction, bacteraemia will be present 1000 times more frequently owing to activities other than the extraction itself. The principal conclusion to be drawn from this study is that the importance of good oral hygiene should be stressed, as well as the additional need for prophylaxis following dental extractions. During extractions, it is possible that the number of organisms entering the circulation in a short space of time will be greater. If antibiotic cover is to be given, it is necessary to weigh up the risks of complications of the antibiotic against the risks of infection. Our own preference is to err on the side of giving prophylactic antibiotics. This is indicated by our clinical experience that it is rare to find a child who has not, on some previous occasion, already safely received antibiotics for a trivial or even speculative bacterial infection! There is no evidence of which we are aware to indicate that the spontaneous shedding of deciduous teeth in children is accompanied either by significant bacteraemia or risk of endocarditis. Antibiotic prophylaxis is not, therefore, indicated in this situation.

A prophylactic measure that should, perhaps, be used in all cases is the use of local antiseptic applications (Jones et al, 1970). This presumably works by killing organisms in the mouth prior to their possible liberation into the circulation. Jones and colleagues (1970) showed that prior rinsing of the mouth with a phenolated mouthwash significantly reduced subsequent bacteraemia. Reports have now emerged of infective endocarditis developing even when appropriate antibiotic prophylaxis has been given against infection with a resistant organism (Thekekera et al, 1994; O'Sullivan et al, 1996), thus reinforcing still further the need for good dental care.

PROPHYLAXIS

EXPERIMENTAL MODELS

The efficacy of prophylactic antibiotic regimens has been tested using an experimental model for infective endocarditis developed by Garrison and Freedman (1970). They placed plastic catheters in the right atrium or left ventricle of rabbits via the jugular vein or carotid artery. Where the catheters impinged on and damaged the endocardium, this then acted as the site for formation of sterile thrombotic vegetations, previously suggested by Angrist and Oka (1963) as the site of adherence and trapping of organisms in the bloodstream of humans. These non-infective thrombotic vegetations were then shown to have an extremely high affinity for certain members of the viridans group, in particular for *Streptococcus sanguis*, the commonest cause of infective endocarditis in humans (Durack and Beeson, 1972). Using this model, a single high dose of benzylpenicillin (penicillin G) was shown to produce high peak bactericidal levels of antibiotic but

failed to prevent endocarditis (Durack and Petersdorf, 1973). Later work comparing regimens using single and multiple doses of different antibiotics against different innoculations of streptococci indicated that high levels were necessary in the plasma for a long period to provide adequate protection (Pelletier et al, 1975).

Antibiotic prophylaxis for infective endocarditis has become complicated and varied between different countries. Many of the suggested regimens are either painful or toxic. Leport and colleagues (1988) have, however, produced a consensus in an excellent review of the national recommendations, those cardiac conditions requiring antibiotic prophylaxis, the risk factors involved and the agents that should be used. In short, where the risk is low, one dose of amoxycillin (amoxicillin) (or clindamycin if the patient is allergic to penicillin) is sufficient. This should be given 1 hour before the procedure. In patients at higher risk, amoxycillin, or vancomycin with gentamicin given intravenously, should be employed.

PRINCIPLES AND SPECIFIC RECOMMENDATIONS

Good dental hygiene must be encouraged, with regular visits to the dentist to detect and treat caries. When antibiotic prophylaxis is required, bactericidal rather than bacteriostatic drugs should be used. Otherwise organisms may survive and become adherent to damaged or abnormal endothelium (Pelletier et al, 1975). Antibiotic prophylaxis should be given within 1 hour of the dental procedure. If therapy is started even 12 hours earlier, resistant organisms in the flora of the mouth will multiply and constitute a high proportion of any subsequent bacteraemia (Garrod and Waterworth, 1962). Bactericidal levels of antibiotic should be present in the serum for at least 9 or 10 hours if organisms that may have become adherent to cardiac lesions are to be eradicated.

The regimen used must be acceptable to patients, therefore preferably given by mouth, and its application simple. Amoxycillin is preferable to penicillin (Shanson et al, 1978). The drug is more completely absorbed, higher peak levels are reached for equivalent dosages and the levels in the serum are sustained for longer. Although, in adults, a single dose of 3 g amoxycillin given orally does produce levels in the serum that are bactericidal to *Streptococcus viridans* for at least 10 hours (Shanson et al, 1980), it is still probably safer to give a second oral dose 6 to 8 hours after the procedure.

Patients at special risk are those with artificial valves or those who have external valved conduits. This group should have parenteral therapy prior to dental treatment, they are best dealt with in hospital. The regimen that we recommend is that published in the British National Formulary, 1998, based on the recommendations of a Working Party of the British Society for Antimicrobial Chemotherapy (1990, 1992, 1997).

ROUTINE ORAL PROPHYLAXIS OUTSIDE HOSPITAL

For those above the age of 10 years who have not received more than a single dose of penicillin in the previous month, 3 g amoxycillin (the adult dose) should be given 1 hour before the procedure as routine oral prophylaxis. This should be given under supervision in the dental surgery, so that the dental practitioner is certain the child has received prophylaxis. Children aged from 5 to 10 years should receive half the adult dose, and those under 5 years one quarter the adult dose, namely 750 mg.

Patients allergic to penicillin, or who have received more than a single dose of penicillin in the previous month, should be given clindamycin. For those aged over 10 years, 600 mg clindamycin is given orally 1 hour before the procedure. This must be taken under supervision. Those aged from 5 to 10 years should receive 300 mg, and those aged under 5 years one quarter the adult dose, namely 150 mg.

PARENTERAL PROPHYLAXIS FOR PATIENTS RECEIVING GENERAL ANAESTHESIA BUT AT NO OTHER SPECIAL RISK

At induction, the patient is given 1 g amoxycillin intravenously, then another 500 mg amoxycillin orally 6 hours later (adult dosage). Children aged from 5 to 10 years receive half the adult dose, and those under 5 years one quarter the adult dose.

For patients who are allergic to penicillin, or who have received more than a single dose of penicillin in the previous month, 1 g vancomycin is given by slow intravenous injection over at least 100 minutes, followed by 120 mg gentamycin at induction, with children under 10 years receiving vancomycin 20 mg/kg and gentamicin 2 mg/kg body weight.

Alternative recommended regimens for this group are 400 mg teicoplanin given intravenously, together with 120 mg gentamicin at induction. Children under 14 years receive teicoplanin 6 mg/kg and gentamicin 2 mg/kg, or 300 mg clindamycin given intravenously over 10 minutes at induction with 150 mg clindamycin given orally or intravenously 6 hours later. Children aged from 5 to 10 years receive half this adult dose, and those under 5 years one quarter the adult dose. For patients at special risk, such as those with a prosthetic valve or previous history of endocarditis, 1 g amoxycillin and 120 mg gentamicin are given intravenously at induction, then 500 mg amoxycillin is given orally 6 hours later. Again, children aged from 5 to 10 years receive half this dosage, and those under 5 years one quarter the adult dose of amoxycillin, with gentamicin given at 2 mg/kg body weight.

Vancomycin is particularly effective, probably because, in addition to its bactericidal effect, it also has a rapid effect on the stickiness of the streptococcal cell wall resulting in a reduced tendency for adhesion of organisms to damaged endothelium (Bernard et al, 1981).

Unfortunately, it is also extremely irritant and rather toxic.

Other circumstances should be mentioned. For children undergoing orthodontic procedures, many visits are frequently necessary before a suitable result has been achieved. In those undergoing such treatment, it is sensible to give single doses of 3 g amoxycillin (or 1.5 g if under 12 years of age) on each occasion. In the penicillin-sensitive person, clindamycin should be used. When glandular fever is present or suspected, clindamycin or erythromycin is preferable to amoxycillin in view of the risk of allergic responses.

AWARENESS OF THE NEED FOR PROPHYLAXIS AND COMPLIANCE OF THE PATIENT

Infective endocarditis is more common in adolescents and young adults than in young children. The reason for this remains speculative. Poor dental hygiene, especially as teenagers reject the need for, or outgrow, parental guidance, may be a factor. It could also be that paediatric cardiologists are more likely to remind parents of the need for good dental care than are adult cardiologists, who spend most of their time looking after patients with ischaemic or hypertensive heart disease. Be that as it may, an important study by van der Meer et al (1992) showed poor adherence to guidelines. Of 455 families surveyed on their awareness of need for and use of prophylaxis, 82% responded. Of these, 70% remembered receiving some form of advice, but only 22% received antibiotic prophylaxis for a dental procedure.

——— TREATMENT ———

CHOICE, ADMINISTRATION AND MONITORING OF ANTIMICROBIAL THERAPY

Isolation of the infecting organism is of such paramount importance that blood for cultures must always be taken before commencing therapy. Unless the condition of the patient is deteriorating, initiation of therapy can usually be delayed until the organism has been identified, or more importantly, its antibiotic sensitivities determined.

If 'blind' therapy is required, we would usually start in children with a combination of drugs suitable for culture-negative endocarditis. This combination should be adequate for both streptococci and staphylococci. The combination we usually choose is teicoplanin given intravenously with rifampicin (rifampin) given orally or intravenously.

Once an organism has been isolated, antibiotic therapy is commenced using bactericidal agents, such as one of the penicillins, an aminoglycoside, sodium fucidate, clindamycin, lincomycin, vancomycin, teicoplanin or one of the cephalosporins. Bacteriostatic agents, such as the sulphonamides, tetracyclines or chloramphenicol, should be avoided. Although they may suppress fever, the infection is not eradicated and progressive damage to valves may occur (Cates and Christie, 1951). It is our practice to use at least two, preferably synergistic, agents to which the organism is sensitive. This is because of the risks of development of bacterial resistance, and to ensure that persistent or persisting organisms are eradicated. Because of uncertainties in oral absorption of antibiotics, and because of the possibility of non-compliance by children or their families, therapy is always carried out in hospital, and drugs are administered parenterally. As multiple intramuscular injections are painful and distressing to the child, antibiotics are given intravenously through indwelling venous cannulas that have been carefully inserted percutaneously using full sterile precautions. The cannulas, and their site of insertion, are changed if possible every 5 days. They are never left more than 7 days. The risk of superinfection with candida through the sites of cannulation can best be avoided by twice weekly flushing of the drips with a fungostatic agent such as amphotericin (amphotericin B) (Brennan et al, 1972). In general, antibiotics are given by intermittent 4-, 6- or 8-hourly injections into the cannula rather than by continuous infusion. This is because many antibiotics such as penicillin lose some of their efficacy when dissolved in dextrose (Simberkoff et al, 1970). This technique has the additional advantage of producing higher peak levels, although renal excretion may be accelerated and more frequent administration of antibiotics may be required. Therapy is continued for a minimum of 4 weeks, but usually for 6 weeks. We prefer to discontinue therapy while the child is still in hospital to see if there is any recurrence of fever or other evidence of infection. We accept there are advocates of shorter periods of therapy, particularly for penicillin-sensitive streptococcal endocarditis (Tan et al, 1971; Wilson et al, 1982). Economic factors can also be a major consideration. But our preference remains for longer courses of therapy (Cates and Christie, 1951). There are also strong advocates of oral rather than parenteral therapy (Gray et al, 1964; Gray, 1975) for 'very' penicillin-sensitive organisms. Even in these cases, one cannot always be certain in the individual child that some of the organisms are not more resistant.

It is also essential to confirm that the organism originally isolated from the patient is killed by the patient's serum while treatment is in progress. Blood is taken from the patient when levels of the antibiotic will be lowest in the plasma. This is just before the next dose of antibiotic. Tube dilutions of serum are then 'put up' against the originally isolated organism. After overnight incubation, the tubes that show no growth are subcultured to see whether the serum is bactericidal or merely bacteriostatic. If the serum is bactericidal at a dilution of 1 in 4, it is considered that adequate antibiotic therapy is being achieved (Schlichter and MacLean, 1947; Jawetz, 1962).

As discussed, the choice of antibiotic depends essentially on the sensitivities of the organisms isolated. For viridans streptococci, the synergistic combination of penicillin and gentamicin is generally used. For *Streptococcus faecalis* and other enterococcal infections, a combination of ampicillin, or amoxycillin, and gentamicin is usually, but not always, effective. Endocarditis caused by staphylococci is frequently penicillin resistant. Flucloxacillin (floxacillin) with gentamicin, and/or fucidate, is a useful combination under these circumstances. Sodium fucidate is one of the few agents we may give orally rather than intravenously, as it is so well absorbed. We would reiterate, however, that constant back titration of the patient's serum against the originally isolated organisms is of paramount importance in monitoring the efficacy of antimicrobial therapy. Further discussion of the various antibiotic combinations that may be used is beyond the scope of this chapter. We should perhaps add that, when penicillin-sensitive organisms are involved, probenecid may be used to retard excretion of penicillin and to elevate levels in the blood.

Candidal endocarditis is difficult to treat. A combination of amphotericin with flucytosine should be effective (Darell, 1975). Q fever endocarditis, not that it is common in children, should probably be treated with co-trimoxazole (Freeman and Hodson, 1972).

Effective treatment of endocarditis should result in abolition of fever, along with return to normal of the sedimentation rate and the white blood cell count, although the latter may not always be elevated prior to treatment (Fisher et al, 1955).

INDICATIONS FOR SURGERY

In 1939, Tubbs successfully closed a persistent arterial duct that remained infected despite use of sulphonamides (Bourne et al, 1941). Touroff and Vessell (1940) had reported similar success in a patient who had not received antibiotics. Subsequent experience indicated that mortality, previously total, could be more than halved in this way (Tubbs, 1944). Of interest in this context is the documentation by Morhous (1958) of spontaneous cure in a patient with infective endocarditis on a persistent arterial duct. The murmur disappeared, presumably because of ductal occlusion by the inflammatory process or vegetations. With it, the haemodynamic basis for endocarditis and endarteritis was removed. Nowadays, surgical closure of an arterial duct is standard practice, but it was the results of this early experience that influenced current thinking, as the risk of endocarditis was thereby avoided. In similar fashion, a cure was reported of endocarditis caused by *Candida albicans*, at a time when antifungal agents were not well developed, by surgical closure of the underlying ventricular septal defect.

Acute aortic incompetence owing to perforation or rupture of a leaflet, or acute mitral incompetence caused by ruptured tendinous cords, produces rapid and severe heart failure with pulmonary oedema as the left ventricle is unprepared for the sudden volume overload. The aortic valve is affected more commonly than the mitral valve (Stason et al, 1968; Wise et al, 1971). Emergency valvar replacement may be necessary. This tends, however, to be a problem more in adults than in children. Excellent results are now achieved with early valvar replacement in patients with deteriorating haemodynamic function (Stason et al, 1968; Wise et al, 1971), although 'cutting out' of sutures attaching a valvar prosthesis to friable tissue may lead to paravalvar leaks (Manhas et al, 1970). Not only may acute valvar incompetence occur, but surgery may be required to remove a mass of vegetations, which can cause valvar obstruction, particularly of the aortic valve (Figure 66.2).

Surgical removal of infected left-sided vegetations is advocated when there are embolic phenomenons and large vegetations remain (Yokochi et al, 1986; Nomura et al, 1995). Some would intervene aggressively in the absence of embolic phenomenons or serious haemody-namic deterioration (Citak et al, 1992). At this stage, the role for surgical intervention whenever sizeable vegetations are seen is not clear, but published surgical results do not show a significant advantage over more conservative management in patients without evidence of haemodynamic decompensation. When required, nonetheless, surgical intervention is now yielding gratifying results, even in the developing world (Sharma et al, 1997).

Perhaps the major indication for surgical intervention in children with infective endocarditis is when foreign material has been previously inserted. Infection around the patch inserted for closure of a ventricular septal defect may cause it to become detached, with subsequent progressive heart failure. This may be a particular problem in patients with tetralogy of Fallot who have had relief of right ventricular outflow tract obstruction, since the pulmonary vascular bed is unprotected and acute pulmonary oedema may ensue. As in adults, endocarditis occurring after insertion of a valvar prosthesis, or conduit, may require removal of the foreign material before treatment becomes successful.

REFERENCES

Alessandri N, Pannarale G, del Monte F, Moretti F, Marino B, Reale A 1990 Hypertrophic obstructive cardiomyopathy and infective endocarditis: a report of seven cases and a review of the literature. European Heart Journal 11: 1041–1048

Angrist A A, Oka M 1963 Pathogenesis of bacterial endocarditis. Journal of the American Medical Association 183: 249–252

Arnett E N, Roberts W C 1976 Valve ring abscess in active infective endocarditis. Frequency, location and clues to clinical diagnosis from the study of 95 necropsy patients. Circulation 54: 140–145

Awadallah S M, Kavey R E, Byrum C J, Smith F C, Kveselis D A, Blackman M S 1991 The changing pattern of infective endocarditis in childhood. American Journal of Cardiology 68: 90–94

Axelrod J, Keusch G T, Bottone E S M, Hirschman S Z 1973 Endocarditis caused by Lactobacillus plantarum. Annals of Internal Medicine 78: 33–37

Bacon P A, Davidson C, Smith B 1974 Antibodies to candida and autoantibodies in subacute bacterial endocarditis. Quarterly Journal of Medicine 43: 537–550

Baumgartner J C, Heggers J P, Harrison J W 1976 The incidence of bacteremias related to endodontic procedures. I. Non-surgical endodontics. Journal of Endodontics 2: 135–140

Baumgartner J C, Heggers J P, Harrison J W 1977 Incidence of bacteremias related to endodontic procedures. II. Surgical endodontics. Journal of Endodontics 3: 399–402

Bayer A S, Theofilopoulos A N, Eisenberg R, Dixon F J, Guze L B 1976 Circulating immune complexes in infective endocarditis. New England Journal of Medicine 295: 1500–1505

Bayer A S, Chow A N, Guze L B 1977 Listeria monocytogenes endocarditis: report of a case and review of the literature. American Journal of Medical Science 273: 319–323

Bayer A S, Theofilopoulos A N, Tillman D B, Dixon F J, Guze L B 1979 Use of circulating immune complex levels in the serodifferentiation of endocarditic and non endocarditic septicaemias. American Journal of Medicine 66: 58–62

Beeley L 1969 Teeth, Streptococcus viridans and subacute bacterial endocarditis. British Dental Journal 127: 424

Bennett I L Jr, Beeson P B 1954 Bacteremia: consideration of some experimental and clinical aspects. Yale Journal of Biology and Medicine 26: 241–262

Bernard J P, Francioli I, Glauser M P 1981 Prophylaxis of endocarditis due to vancomycin tolerant Strep. sanguis: study on the mechanism of protection by vancomycin. Paper read at the 12th International Congress of Chemotherapy, Florence, Italy, 24 July

Blieden L C, Morehead R R, Burke B, Kaplan E L 1972 Bacterial endocarditis in the neonate. American Journal of Diseases of Children 124: 747–749

Blumenthal S, Griffiths S P, Morgan B C 1960 Bacterial endocarditis in children with heart disease. Pediatrics 26: 933–1017

Bourne G, Keele K D, Tubbs O S 1941 Ligation and chemotherapy for infection of patient ductus arteriosus. Lancet ii: 444–446

Brennan M F, Goldman M H, O'Connell R C, Kundsin R B 1972 Prolonged parenteral alimentation: candida growth and prevention of candidaemia by amphotericin installation. Annals of Surgery 176: 265–272

Burch G E, de Pasquale N P, Sun S C, Hale A R, Mogabgab W J 1966 Experimental coxsackie virus endocarditis. Journal of the American Medical Association 196: 349–352

Burch G E, Sun S C, Colcolough H L, Sohal R S, de Pasquale N P 1967 Coxsackie B viral myocarditis and valvulitis identified in routine autopsy specimens by immunofluorescent techniques. American Heart Journal 74: 13–23

Carroll G C, Seybor R I 1980 Dental tossing and its relationship to transient bacteremia. Journal of Periodontology 51: 691–692

Cassling R S, Rogler W C, McMann B M 1985 Isolated pulmonic valve in infective endocarditis: A diagnostically elusive entity. American Heart Journal 109: 558–567

Cates J E, Christie R V 1951 Subacute bacterial endocarditis. Quarterly Journal of Medicine 20: 93–130

Citak M, Rees A, Mavroudis C 1992 Surgical management of infective endocarditis in children. Annals of Thoracic Surgery 54: 755–760

Cobe H M 1954 Transitory bacteraemia. Oral Surgery 7: 609–615

Cole P 1975 The enigma of infective endocarditis. Hospital Update 128–138, 152–159

Cordeiro A, Costa H, Lagenha F 1965 Immunologic phase of subacute bacterial endocarditis. A new concept and general considerations. [Editorial] American Journal of Cardiology 16: 477–481

Darell J H 1975 Candida endocarditis. British Medical Journal 3: 632–633

Davis R S, Strom J A, Frishman W et al 1980 The demonstration of vegetations by echocardiography in bacterial endocarditis. An indication for early surgical intervention. American Journal of Medicine 69: 57–63

de Pasquale N P, Burch G E, Sun S C, Hale A R, Mogabgab W J 1966 Experimental coxsackie virus B4 valvulitis in cynomolgus monkeys. American Heart Journal 71: 678–683

de Swiet M T, Ramsay I, Rees G M 1975 Bacterial endocarditis after insertion of an intrauterine contraceptive device. British Medical Journal 3: 76–77

Doyle E F, Spagnuolo M, Taranta A, Kuttner A G, Markowitz M 1962 The risk of bacterial endocarditis during antirheumatic prophylaxis. Journal of the American Medical Association 201: 807–812

Dressler F A, Roberts W C 1989 Infective endocarditis in opiate addicts: analysis of 80 cases studied at necropsy. American Journal of Cardiology 63: 1240–1257

Durack D T, Beeson P B 1972 Experimental bacterial endocarditis. I. Colonisation of a sterile vegetation. II. Survival of bacteria in endocardial vegetations. British Journal of Experimental Pathology 53: 44–49

Durack D T, Petersdorf R F 1973 Chemotherapy of experimental streptococcal endocarditis. I. Comparison of commonly recommended prophylactic regimes. Journal of Clinical Investigation 52: 592–598

Elliott S D 1973 The incidence of group H-streptococci in blood cultures from patients with subacute bacterial endocarditis (SBE). Journal of Medical Microbiology 6: 14

Elston H R, Zencka A E, Sketch M H 1969 Listeria monocytogenes endocarditis: a clinical and bacteriological report. Archives of Internal Medicine (Chicago) 124: 488–491

Everett E D, Hirschman J V 1977 Transient bacteremia and endocarditis: A review. Medicine 56: 61–77

Finland M 1954 Treatment of bacterial endocarditis. New England Journal of Medicine 250: 419–428

Fisher A M, Wagner H N, Ross R S 1955 Staphylococcal endocarditis: some clinical and therapeutic observations on thirty-eight cases. Archives of Internal Medicine 95: 427–437

Florey M E, Florey H W 1943 General and local administration of penicillin. Lancet i: 387–397

Freeman R, Hodson M E 1972 Q fever endocarditis treated with trimethoprim and sulphamethoxazole. British Medical Journal 1: 419–420

Garrison P K, Freedman L R 1970 Experimental endocarditis. I. Staphylococcal endocarditis in rabbits resulting from placement of a polythene catheter in the right side of the heart. Yale Journal of Biology and Medicine 42: 394–410

Garrod L P, Waterworth M M 1962 The risks of dental extraction during penicillin treatment. British Heart Journal 24: 39–46

Gersony W M, Hayes C J, Driscoll D J et al 1993 Second natural history study of congenital heart defects. Quality of life of patients with aortic stenosis, pulmonary stenosis, or ventricular septal defect. Circulation 87: 152–165

Gibbons R J 1972 In: Wannamaker L W (ed.) Streptococci and streptococcal diseases. Edward Arnold, London, p 371

Gilbert B W, Haney R S, Crawford F et al 1977 Two-dimensional echocardiographic assessment of vegetative endocarditis. Circulation 55: 346–353

Gray I R 1975 The choice of antibiotic for treating infective endocarditis. Quarterly Journal of Medicine 44: 449–458

Gray I R, Tai A R, Wallace J G, Calder J H 1964 Oral treatment of bacterial endocarditis with penicillins. Lancet ii: 110–114

Guntheroth W G 1984 How important are dental procedures as a cause of infective endocarditis? American Journal of Cardiology 54: 797–801

Gutman R A, Striker G E, Gilliland B C, Cutler R E 1972 The immune complex glomerulonephritis of bacterial endocarditis. Medicine (Baltimore) 51: 1–25

Hallidie-Smith K A, Olsen E G, Oakley C M, Goodwin J F, Bentall H B, Cleland W P 1969 Ventricular septal defect and aortic regurgitation. Thorax 24: 257–275

Hamburger M 1963 Acute and subacute bacterial endocarditis. Archives of Internal Medicine (Chicago) 112: 1–2

Hamer J, O'Grady F W 1977 Infective endocarditis. In: Hamer J (ed.) Recent advances in cardiology. Churchill Livingstone, Edinburgh, p 447–471

Hayward G W 1973 Infective endocarditis: a changing disease. British Medical Journal ii: 706–709

Hilson G R F 1970 Is chemoprophylaxis necessary? Proceedings of the Royal Society of Medicine 63: 267–271

Holmes R K, Ramirez-Ronda C H 1977 Adherence of bacteria to the endothelium of heart valves. Infective endocarditis, an American Heart Association Symposium. American Heart Association Monograph 52: 12–13

Jawetz E 1962 Assay of antibacterial activity in serum: useful guide for antimicrobial therapy. American Journal of Diseases of Childhood 103: 81–84

Johnson D H, Rosenthal A, Nadas A S 1975 A forty-year review of bacterial endocarditis in infancy and childhood. Circulation 51: 581–588

Jones H R, Siekert R G, Geraci J E 1969 Neurologic manifestations of bacterial endocarditis. Annals of Internal Medicine 71: 21–28

Jones J C, Cutcher J L, Goldberg J R, Lilly G E 1970 Control of bacteremia associated with extraction of teeth. 1. Oral Surgery, Oral Medicine and Oral Pathology 30: 454–459

Kaplan M H 1963a Immunologic relationship of group A streptococcal strains and human heart tissue. Possible significance for the pathogenesis of rheumatic fever. American Heart Journal 65: 426–427

Kaplan M H 1963b Immunologic relation of streptococcal and tissue antigens. I. Properties of an antigen in certain strains of group A streptococci exhibiting an immunologic cross-reaction with human heart tissue. Journal of Immunology 90: 595–606

Karl T, Wensley D, Stark J, de Leval M, Rees P, Taylor J F 1987 Infective endocarditis in children with congenital heart disease: comparison of selected features in patients with surgical correction or palliation and those without. British Heart Journal 58: 57–65

Kerr A Jr 1964 Bacterial endocarditis – revisited. Modern Concepts of Cardiovascular Disease 33: 831–836

Kniker W T, Cochrane C G 1968 The localisation of circulating immune complexes in experimental serum sickness. The role of vasoactive amines and hydrodynamic forces. Journal of Experimental Medicine 127: 119–136

Kristinsson A, Bentall H H 1967 Medical and surgical treatment of Q-fever endocarditis. Lancet ii: 693–697

Lachman A S, Branwell-Jones D M, Lakier J B, Pocock W A, Barlow J B 1975 Infective endocarditis in the billowing mitral leaflet syndrome. British Heart Journal 37: 326–330

Laxdal T, Messner R P, Williams R C Jr, Quie P G 1968 Opsonic, agglutinating, and complement fixing antibodies in patients with subacute bacterial endocarditis. Journal of Laboratory Clinical Medicine 71: 638–653

Le Frock J L, Klainer A S, Wu W-H, Turndorf H 1976 Transient bacteremia associated with nasotracheal suctioning. Journal of the American Medical Association 236: 1610–1611

Lepeschkin E 1952 On the relation between the site of valvular involvement in endocarditis and blood pressure resting on the valve. American Journal of the Medical Sciences 224: 318–319

Leport C and the Endocarditis Working Group of the International Society of Chemotherapy 1998 Microbiology and Infection 4: 3556–3561

Lerner P I, Weinstein L 1966 Infective endocarditis in the antibiotic era. New England Journal of Medicine 274: 199–206, 259–266, 323–331, 388–393

Libman E 1913 The clinical features of cases of subacute bacterial endocarditis that have spontaneously become bacteria-free. American Journal of Medicine Science 146: 625–630

Lineberger L T, De Marco T J 1973 Evaluation of transient bacteremia following routine periodontal procedures. Journal of Periodontology 44: 757–762

Lowes J A, Hamer J, Williams G et al 1980 10 years of infective endocarditis at St Bartholomew's Hospital: analysis of clinical features and treatment in relation to prognosis and mortality. Lancet i: 133–136

Major R H 1945 Notes on the history of endocarditis. Bulletin of the History of Medicine 17: 351–359

Mandell G L, Kaye D, Levison M E, Hook E W 1970 Enterococcal endocarditis: an analysis of 38 patients observed at the New York Hospital–Cornell Medical Center. Archives of Internal Medicine 125: 258–264

Manhas D R, Hessel E A, Winterscheid L C, Dillard D H, Merendino K A 1970 Open heart surgery in infective endocarditis. Circulation 41: 841–848

Markowitz A S, Lange C F Jr 1964 Streptococcal related glomerulonephritis I. Isolation, immunochemistry and comparative chemistry of soluble fractions from type 12 nephritogenic streptococci and human glomeruli. Journal of Immunology 92: 565–575

Martin R P, Meltzer R S, Chia B L, Stinson E G, Rakowski H, Popp R L 1980 Clinical utility of two dimensional echocardiography in infective endocarditis. American Journal of Cardiology 46: 379–385

McGowan D A 1978 Failure of prophylaxis of infective endocarditis following dental treatment. Journal of Antimicrobial Chemotherapy 4: 486–488

McGowan D A 1982 Experimental evidence on the prevention of infective endocarditis in dentistry. In: The nature and prevention of bacterial endocarditis. Medicine Publishing Foundation, London, p 15–21

Meissner R P, Laxdal T, Quie P G, Williams R C 1968 Rheumatoid factor in subacute bacterial endocarditis – bacterium, duration of disease or genetic predisposition. Annals of Internal Medicine 68: 746–749

Mellins R B, Cheng G, Ellis K, Jameson A G, Maim J R, Blumenthal S 1964 Ventricular septal defect with shunt from left ventricle to right atrium: bacterial endocarditis as a complication. British Heart Journal 26: 584–591

Moellering R C Jr, Watson B K, Kunz L J 1974 Endocarditis due to group D streptococci. Comparison of disease by Streptococcus bovis with that produced by enterococci. American Journal of Medicine 57: 239–250

Moulsdale M T, Eykyri S J, Phillips I 1980 Infective endocarditis 1970–1979. A study of culture-positive cases in St Thomas's Hospital. Quarterly Journal of Medicine 49: 315–328

Mourhous E J 1958 Subacute bacterial endocarditis of a patent ductus arteriosus. Virginia Medical Monthly 85: 565–567

Nomura F, Penny D J, Menahem S, Pawade A, Karl T R 1995 Surgical intervention for infective endocarditis in infancy and childhood. Annals of Thoracic Surgery 60: 90–95

Oakley C M 1979 Prevention of infective endocarditis. Thorax 34: 711–712

Okell C C, Elliott S D 1935 Bacteraemia and oral sepsis with special reference to the aetiology of subacute endocarditis. Lancet ii: 869–872

Osler W 1885 Malignant endocarditis. Goulstonian lecturers. Lancet i: 459–464

O'Sullivan J, Anderson J, Bain H 1996 Infective endocarditis in children following dental extraction and appropriate antibiotic prophylaxis. British Dental Journal 181: 64–65

Pankey G A 1961 Subacute bacterial endocarditis at University of Minnesota Hospitals (1939–1959). Annals of Internal Medicine 55: 550–561

Pelletier L L Jr, Rack D T, Petersdorf R G 1975 Chemotherapy of experimental streptococcal endocarditis. IV. Further observations on prophylaxis. Journal of Clinical Investigation 56: 319–330

Pesanti E L, Smith I M 1979 Infective endocarditis with negative blood cultures. American Journal of Medicine 66: 43–50

Peterson L J, Peacock R 1976 The incidence of bacteremia in pediatric patients following tooth extraction. Circulation 53: 676–679

Phair J P, Kippel T, MacKenzie M R 1972 Antiglobulins in endocarditis. Infection and Immunity 5: 24–26

Pruitt A A, Rubin R H, Karchmer A W, Duncan G W 1978 Neurologic complications of bacterial endocarditis. Medicine 57: 329–343

Remington J S, Gaines J P, Gilmer M A 1972 Demonstration of Candida precipitations in human sera by immunoelectrophoresis. Lancet i: 413–418

Roberts W C, Ewy G A, Glancy D L, Marchus F I 1967 Valvular stenosis produced by active infective endocarditis. Circulation 36: 449–451

Rodbard S 1963 Blood velocity and endocarditis. Circulation 27: 18–28

Saiman L, Prince A, Gersony W M 1993 Pediatric infective endocarditis in the modern era. Journal of Pediatrics 122: 847–853

Schlichter J G, MacLean H 1947 A method of determining the effective therapeutic level in the treatment of subacute bacterial endocarditis with penicillin: a preliminary report. American Heart Journal 34: 209–211

Seelig M S, Speth C P, Kozinn P J, Taschdjian C L, Toni E F, Goldberg P 1974 Patterns of candida endocarditis following cardiac surgery: importance of early diagnosis and therapy (an analysis of 91 cases). Progress in Cardiovascular Diseases 17: 125–160

Shah P, Singh W S A, Rose V, Keith J D 1966 Incidence of bacterial endocarditis in ventricular septal defects. Circulation 34: 127–131

Shanson D C, Cannon P, Wilks M 1978 Amoxycillin compared with penicillin V for the prophylaxis of dental bacteremia. Journal of Antimicrobial Chemotherapy 4: 431–436

Shanson D C, Ashford R F U, Singh J 1980 High dose oral amoxycillin for preventing endocarditis. British Medical Journal 280: 446–448

Sharma M, Saxena A, Kothari S S et al 1997 Infectious endocarditis in children: changing patterns in a developing country. Cardiology in the Young 7: 201–206

Shinebourne E A, Cripps C M, Hayward G W, Shooter R A 1969 Bacterial endocarditis 1956–1965: analysis of clinical features and treatment in relation to prognosis and mortality. British Heart Journal 5: 536–542

Sholler G F, Hawker R E, Celermajer J M 1986 Infective endocarditis in childhood. Pediatric Cardiology 6: 183–186

Simberkoff M S, Thomas L, McGregor D, Shenkein I, Levine B 1970 Inactivation of penicillins by carbohydrate solutions at alkaline pH. New England Journal of Medicine 283: 116–119

Spector W G, Heesom N 1969 The production of granulomata by antigen–antibody complexes. Journal of Pathology 98: 31–39

Stason W B, De Sanctis R W, Weinberg A N, Austen W G 1968 Cardiac surgery in bacterial endocarditis. Circulation 38: 514–523

Stewart J A, Silimperi D, Harris P, Kentwise N, Fraker T D, Kisslo J A 1980 Echocardiographic documentation of vegetative lesions in infective endocarditis: clinical implications. Circulation 61: 374–380

Swanson J, Kraus S J, Gotschlich E C 1971 Studies on gonococcus infection. I. Pili and zones of adhesion: their relation to gonococcal growth patterns. Journal of Experimental Medicine 134: 886–906

Tan J S, Terhune C A Jr, Kaplan S, Hamburger M 1971 Successful two-week treatment schedule for penicillin-

susceptible Streptococcus viridans endocarditis. Lancet ii: 1340–1343

Thekekara A G, Denham B, Duff D F 1994 Eleven year review of infective endocarditis. Irish Medical Journal 87: 80–82

Tompsett R 1964 Diagnosis and treatment of bacterial endocarditis. Disease-A-Month, vol. 1. PH Kay, Chicago, 1–32

Touroff A S W, Vessell H 1940 Subacute Streptococcus viridans endarteritis complicating patent ductus arteriosus. Journal of the American Heart Association 115: 1270–1272

Tu W-H, Shearn M A, Lee J C 1969 Acute diffuse glomerulonephritis in acute staphylococcal endocarditis. Annals of Internal Medicine 71: 335–341

Tubbs O S 1944 Effect of ligation on infection of the patent ductus arteriosus. British Journal of Surgery 32: 1–12

Uwaydah M M, Weinberg A N 1965 Bacterial endocarditis – a changing pattern. New England Journal of Medicine 273: 1231–1235

van der Bel-Kahn J M, Watanakunakorn C, Menefee M G, Long H D, Dicter R 1978 Chlamydia trachomatis endocarditis. American Heart Journal 95: 627–636

van der Meer J T M, van Wijk W, Thompson J, Valkenburg H A, Michel M F 1992 Awareness of need and actual use of prophylaxis: lack of patient compliance in the prevention of bacterial endocarditis. Journal of Antimicrobial Chemotherapy 29: 187–194

van Scoy R E, Cohen S N, Geraci J E, Washington J A 1977 Coryneform bacterial endocarditis. Mayo Clinic Proceedings 52: 216–219

Vogler W R, Dorney E R, Bridges H A 1962 Bacterial endocarditis: a review of 148 cases. American Journal of Medicine 32: 910–921

Wedgwood J 1955 Early diagnosis of subacute bacterial endocarditis. Lancet ii: 1058–1063

Weinstein L 1972 Infective endocarditis: past, present and future. Journal of Royal College of Physicians, London 6: 161–174

Weiss H, Ottenberg R 1932 Relation between bacteria and temperature in subacute bacterial endocarditis. Journal of Infectious Diseases 50: 61–68

Williams R C, Kunkel H G 1962 Rheumatoid factor, complement and conglutinin aberrations in patients with subacute bacterial endocarditis. Journal of Clinical Investigation 41: 666–675

Wilson W R, Giuliani E R, Geraci J C 1982 Treatment of penicillin-sensitive streptococcal infective endocarditis. Mayo Clinic Proceedings 57: 95–100

Wise J R, Bentall H H, Cleland W P, Goodwin J F, Hallidie-Smith K A, Oakley C M 1971 Urgent aortic valve replacement for acute aortic regurgitation due to infective endocarditis. Lancet ii: 115–121

Working Party of the British Society for Antimicrobial Chemotherapy 1990 Antibiotic prophylaxis of infective endocarditis. Lancet 335: 88–89

Working Party of the British Society for Antimicrobial Chemotherapy 1992 Antibiotic prophylaxis of infective endocarditis. Lancet 339: 1292–1293

Working Party of the British Society for Antimicrobial Chemotherapy 1997 Changes in recommendations about amoxycillin prophylaxis for prevention of endocarditis. Lancet 350: 1100

Yokochi K, Sakamoto H, Mikajima T, Ichinose E, Kato H, Eto Y 1986 Infective endocarditis in children: a current diagnostic trend and the embolic complications. Japanese Circulation Journal 50: 1294–1297

Zakrzewski T, Keith J D 1965 Bacterial endocarditis in infants and children. Journal of Pediatrics 67: 1179–1193

Zuberbuhler J R 1997 The changing face of bacterial endocarditis. Cardiology in the Young 7: 129–130

Zuberbuhler J R, Neches W H, Park S C 1994 Infective endocarditis – an experience spanning three decades. Cardiology in the Young 4: 244–251

67

Cardiological aspects of systemic disease

J. A. Ettedgui and J. M. Tersak

INTRODUCTION

Cardiac involvement in systemic disease can be broadly divided into those conditions in which the heart is involved in the disease process itself and those in which a structural or functional cardiac abnormality is associated with other anomalies, usually in a recognizable syndrome. Many of the conditions in this latter group have been dealt with in sections on aetiology and genetics. These will not be dealt with again, although they may be mentioned (or the discussion amplified) as seems necessary. For vignettes of syndromes with cardiac involvement, the reader is referred to the Appendix to Chapter 7. This Appendix is as comprehensive as possible but still leaves a vast number of systemic diseases that may involve the heart during childhood. It is these latter diseases that will be summarized in this chapter (Table 67.1).

Table 67.1. Systemic diseases with cardiac involvement

Metabolic diseases
Storage diseases
Glycogen storage disease
    Type I: von Gierhe's disease
    Type II: Pompe's disease
    Type III: Cori's disease,
    Type IV: Andersen's disease
    Type V: McArdle's disease
    Type VI: liver phosphorylase deficiency
    Type VII: Tarui's disease
Ethanolominosis
Mucopolysaccharidoses
    Type I: Hurler's syndrome, Sheie syndrome, intermediate (Hurler–Scheie) syndrome
    Type II: Hunter syndrome
    Type III: Sanfilippo syndrome
    Type IV: Morquio's syndrome
    Type VI: Maroteaux–Lamy syndrome
    Type VII: Sly syndrome
Mucolipidoses
    Type II: inclusion cell disease
    Type III: pseudo-Hurler polydystrophy
Disorders of glycoprotein degradation
    Mannosidosis
    Fucosidosis
    Sialidosis
    Aspartoglycosaminuria
Acid lipase deficiency: Wolman's disease, cholesterol ester storage disease
Sphingolipidoses
    Sphingomyelin lipidosis: Niemann–Pick disease
    Glucosylceramidosis: Gaucher's disease

    α-Galactosidase A deficiency: Fabry's disease
Gangliosidoses
    GM_1 gangliosidosis
    GM_2 gangliosidosis: Tay–Sachs disease, Sandhoff disease

Inherited disorders of endocrine function
Diabetes mellitus
Pituitary gigantism and acromegaly
Disorders of thyroid function
    Hypothyroidism
    Hyperthyroidism

Disorders of collagen synthesis
Ehlers–Danlos syndrome
Cutis laxa
Osteogenesis imperfecta
Marfan's syndrome

Neuromuscular diseases
Muscular dystrophies
    Duchenne's muscular dystrophy
    Childhood muscular dystrophy
    Myotonic muscular dystrophy: Steinert's disease
    Autosomal dominant scapuloperoneal myopathy
    Becker's muscular dystrophy
    Facioscapulohumeral muscular dystrophy;
        Landouzy–Déjérine syndrome
    X-linked humeroperoneal myopathy: Emery–Dreifuss disease
Centronuclear myopathy
Friedreich's ataxia
Arthrogryopsis multiplex congenita

Continued on next page

1777

Table 67.1. Systemic diseases with cardiac involvement (*contd*)

Peroneal muscular atrophy: Charcot–Marie–Tooth disease
Juvenile spinal muscular atrophy: Kugelberg–Welander syndrome
Heredopathia atactica polyneuritiformis (diseases): Refsum's disease
Mitochondrial myopathies

Deficiencies
Selenium: Keshan disease
Carnitine
Thiamine: beri-beri

Depositions
Haemochromatosis

Connective tissue diseases
Juvenile rheumatoid arthritis: Still's disease
Systemic lupus erythematosus

Disease induced by toxic mechanisms
Adverse reactions to drugs
Toxic substances
Radiation

Miscellaneous systemic disorders
Progeria
Arteriohepatic dysplasia: Alagille syndrome
Sickle cell haemoglobinopathy

METABOLIC DISORDERS: STORAGE DISEASES

We have chosen to group together here the glycogen storage diseases, ethanolaminosis, the mucopolysaccharidoses, the mucolipidoses, disorders of glycoprotein degradation, acid lipase deficiency, the sphingolipidoses and the gangliosidoses.

GLYCOGEN STORAGE DISEASES

Glycogen storage diseases can be due to various disorders. There may be an inability to synthesize normal glycogen. Alternatively, there may be an inability to break down glycogen. In the extreme form, abnormal glycogen is synthesized but cannot be broken down. There are twelve described types within this range of disease. Cardiac involvement has been documented in types I to VIII.

GLYCOGEN STORAGE DISEASE TYPE I (VON GIERHE'S DISEASE, GLUCOSE 6-PHOSPHATASE DEFICIENCY)

Clinical manifestations of type I glucogen storage disease are profound hypoglycaemia, associated with hyperlipidaemia, hyperuricaemia and lactic acidosis. It presents in childhood and primarily involves liver, kidneys and small intestinal mucosa. Pulmonary hypertension in association with type I glycogen storage disease has been described recently. Postulated mechanisms include chronic stimulation of the smooth muscle of the pulmonary arterioles by the persistent hepatic metabolism of circulating catecholamines (Furukawa et al, 1990; Hamaoka et al, 1990).

GLYCOGEN STORAGE DISEASE TYPE II (POMPE'S DISEASE)

Pompe's disease is a generalized glycogen storage disease in which glycogen of normal structure is accumulated in the myocardium, skeletal muscle and the liver. The disease is progressive and is associated with deficiency of lysosomal maltase (α-1,4-glucosidase). The connection between the accumulation of glycogen in the lysosome and the cytoplasmic accumulation that characterizes the disease is not clear. There is, however, generalized accumulation of glycogen in the heart (including in the conduction tissues), in skeletal muscle (notably the tongue and diaphragm) and in the liver. Central and peripheral neurones and smooth muscle are also affected. Appropriate staining methods demonstrate the excessive glycogen. Estimates of glycogen content of between 5 and 10% of the wet weight of affected tissues represent an increase of two- to sixfold over normal levels. The results are cardiomegaly, hepatomegaly, a thick diaphragm and a large thick tongue. In the heart, the glycogen is deposited mainly in ventricular muscle. There is gross thickening of the ventricular walls, with impairment of both diastolic and systolic performance. The babies appear normal at birth. Muscle weakness and hypotonia are noted during the first 6 months of life, together with signs of congestive cardiac failure. Additional presenting features are aspiration pneumonia and respiratory failure. Although there is excess glycogen in the liver, hepatomegaly is not a feature until heart failure sets in. The disease is progressive, and most affected babies die before the age of 1 year. The clinical course may be complicated by arrhythmias. Since patients with Pompe's disease appear very sensitive to digoxin, this drug must be used with extreme caution. Irritability and poor feeding often draw attention to the disease, and some abnormality is usually noted by the age of 1 month. The cardiac physical signs are not characteristic, variable murmurs being heard. Unexplained cardiomegaly and congestive cardiac failure in a generally 'floppy' baby should suggest the diagnosis.

The chest radiograph may be normal at birth, but in all affected infants the heart becomes enlarged within a few weeks. There is no specific cardiac silhouette, but rather a generalized smooth enlargement of the contour. The characteristic electrocardiographic features are a short PR interval, wider than normal QRS complexes and voltage evidence of left or biventricular hypertrophy. In addition, in the majority there are Q waves and inverted T waves in leads I, II and the left chest leads (Ehlers et al, 1962). Electrophysiological studies have shown a short AH interval (Gillette et al, 1974). Both M-mode and cross-sectional echocardiograms demonstrate gross increase in the thickness of the ventricular free walls and the ventricular septum (Figure 67.1). An impairment of ventricular filling in diastole has been noted (Buckley and Hutchins, 1978), together with reduction of the rate and extent of systolic shortening. Angiocardiography is rarely performed nowadays, since it adds nothing to the diagnosis.

When the complete clinical picture is present, this (together with the characteristic electrocardiogram) will lead immediately to the definitive diagnostic investigation. This is the demonstration of deficiency of lysosomal α-1,4-glucosidase in fibroblasts grown from a skin biopsy. Sometimes the skeletal muscle abnormalities are less evident. The presentation is then as a cardiomyopathy alone. Pompe's disease should be considered in any such case and skin biopsy performed. The disease is progressive and the majority die before reaching their first birthday. No specific treatment is available, but supportive and decongestive measures are indicated. Since the disease appears to be inherited in an autosomal recessive fashion, parents should be advised of the availability of prenatal diagnosis via culture of amniocytes obtained by amniocentesis. An 'adult' form of α-1,4-glucosidase deficiency also exists (sometimes called type IIb). In these patients, the heart is spared. In only one reported family have both types been found in different individuals (Busch et al, 1979). The relationship between the two forms is unclear.

GLYCOGEN STORAGE DISEASE TYPE III (CORI'S DISEASE, AMYLO-1,6-GLUCOSIDASE (DEBRANCHER) DEFICIENCY)

In Cori's disease, an autosomal recessive condition, glycogen accumulates in skeletal muscle, the liver and in cardiac muscle (Miller et al, 1972; Labrune et al, 1991). Although the electrocardiogram may show biventricular hypertrophy, there is usually no obvious cardiac decompensation. Sudden death has been reported.

GLYCOGEN STORAGE DISEASE TYPE IV (ANDERSEN'S DISEASE, α-1,4-GLUCAN-6-GLUCOSYLTRANSFERASE (BRANCHER) DEFICIENCY)

Andersen's disease is a rare glycogen storage disease characterized by deposition of glycogen of abnormal structure in the liver, leading to cirrhosis. There is also deposition of polysaccharide in the heart. Non-specific electrocardiographic changes and death in heart failure have been reported.

GLYCOGEN STORAGE DISEASE TYPE V (MCARDLE'S DISEASE, MUSCLE PHOSPHORYLASE DEFICIENCY)

McArdle's disease is usually recognized in adolescence or adult life. Its main clinical features are muscle fatiguability, muscle cramps and myoglobinuria. Rare variants have been reported causing death in infancy from respiratory failure. No clinical cardiac manifestations have been reported, but on occasion the electrocardiogram has features similar to those seen in Pompe's disease (Salter, 1968).

GLYCOGEN STORAGE DISEASE TYPE VI (PHOSPHORYLASE b KINASE DEFICIENCY OR LIVER PHOSPHORYLASE DEFICIENCY)

Type VI glycogen storage disease involves both X-linked and autosomal recessive modes of inheritance. Both have

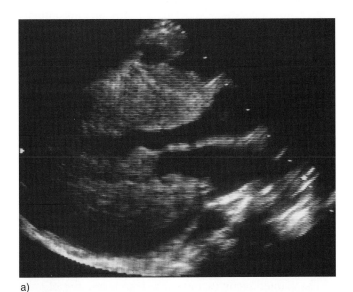

a)

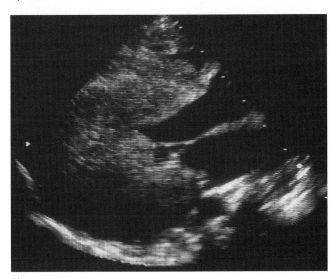

b)

Figure 67.1 Typical echocardiographic findings in glycogen storage disease type II. (a) Diastolic frame in long axis shows severe concentric left ventricular hypertrophy. (b) The systolic frame from the same child shows the absence of subaortic obstruction.

involvement of the liver in childhood, whereas involvement of muscles occurs in young adults with the autosomal recessive form of the disease. Rare forms of phosphorylase b kinase deficiency have been described in which deposition of glycogen is limited to the heart. Echocardiography demonstrates a hypertrophic cardiomyopathy (Eishi et al, 1985; Servidie et al, 1988).

GLYCOGEN STORAGE DISEASE TYPE VII (TARUI'S DISEASE, MUSCLE PHOSPHOFRUCTOKINASE I DEFICIENCY)

Type VII is a rare form of glycogen storage disease that presents in early childhood or adult life with fatiguability, muscular weakness that can be progressive, muscle cramps and myoglobinuria. An infantile form of the disease has also been described in the members of one family. Cardiomyopathy occurred in addition to the progressive muscular weakness, and abnormal deposition of glycogen has been noted in the cardiac muscle at autopsy (Amit et al, 1992).

ETHANOLAMINOSIS

Ethanolaminosis is a generalized storage disease involving accumulation of ethanolamine. It leads to early death with muscular hypotonia, cerebral dysfunction and failure to thrive. Affected infants also have cardiac enlargement (Vietor et al, 1977).

MUCOPOLYSACCHARIDOSES

The mucopolysaccharidoses result from deficiency of lysosomal enzymes involved in the degradation of mucopolysaccharides. The incompletely degraded mucopolysaccharides then accumulate in the tissues. The substances accumulated are dermatan sulphate, heparan sulphate or keratan sulphate. They can accumulate alone or in combinations. In all forms, there is skeletal involvement. In most there is clouding of the cornea and glaucoma. Retinal pigmentation frequently occurs. Deafness is a feature of all types. In most, there is hepatosplenomegaly. Involvement of the central nervous system is common, usually with cervical myelopathy as a consequence of pachymeningitis or atlanto-occipital subluxation.

Cardiovascular involvement is a feature of all types. The mucopolysaccharides are deposited in arterial walls, producing lesions similar to atherosclerosis (Taylor et al, 1991). Deposition in cardiac valves leads to valvar stenosis or regurgitation. The various forms of these diseases are brought about by deficiencies of ten identifiable lysosomal enzymes. Specific deficiency can be demonstrated in cultured fibroblasts, and prenatal diagnosis from culture of amniocytes is possible. The availability of such diagnosis is important, since there is great genetic variability within different forms of mucopolysaccharidosis.

MUCOPOLYSACCHARIDOSIS TYPE I (DEFICIENCY OF α-L-IDURONIDASE)

The three major clinical forms of α-L-iduronidase deficiency are Hurler's syndrome, the Scheie's syndrome, and a syndrome intermediate between the two, the Hurler–Scheie's syndrome.

Hurler's syndrome

The defect in Hurler's syndrome is virtual absence of lysosomal α-L-iduronidase. This enzyme is responsible for breakdown of heparan sulphate and dermatan sulphate to heparan and hyaluronic acid, respectively. The enzyme is completely absent in fibroblasts, but some activity is present in the liver. Consequently, traces of the breakdown products of heparan and dermatan may be found in the urine. As a consequence of this enzymic deficiency, both heparan and dermatan sulphates accumulate in the lysosomes of many tissues. When seen in neurones, the lesions bear some resemblance to those found in Tay–Sachs disease. Deposition in the arterial walls is associated with proliferation of smooth muscle cells, and the lesions are described as 'pseudo-atheromatosis'. There is proliferation of both elastic fibres and collagen accompanying the lysosomal accumulation of mucopolysaccharides. This results in meningeal thickening (pachymeningitis). The thickening of collagen leads in turn to carpal tunnel syndrome and stiff joints, which may result in claw hand if the fingers are involved.

Pathological findings in the heart include deposition of muocopolysaccharide in structures such as the sinus and atrioventricular nodes as well as in the myocardium and endocardium. The last can lead to endocardial fibroelastosis (Stephan et al, 1989; Chow and Chow, 1992).

The babies seem to be normal at birth, the clinical features appearing after the age of 1 year when the facial features become coarse. Premature closure of the skull sutures, and hydrocephalus as a consequence of pachymeningitis lead to cranial deformities. The characteristic lumbar lordosis develops because of stiff joints. Growth retardation then becomes evident after the age of 2 or 3 years; deafness, corneal clouding and (sometimes) glaucoma subsequently develop. The liver and spleen are always enlarged; although the heart is rarely spared, clinical evidence of cardiac involvement is seen only in half the patients. Angina pectoris is an occasional symptom, but more frequently attention is drawn by the finding of a cardiac murmur or systemic hypertension. The murmurs are variable and usually not loud. Rarely the murmur of aortic or mitral insufficiency may be heard. Cardiac failure as the presenting feature associated with endocardial fibroelastosis has been reported (Donaldson et al, 1989; Stephan et al, 1989).

There are typical skeletal radiological features. The clavicles have wide medial ends. The lower thoracic and upper lumbar vertebras have a flared and hook-shaped appearance. There are also changes in the skull and long bones, the latter being more severely affected in the upper limbs. The heart is usually enlarged but with no specific silhouette, although left atrial enlargement will occur with severe mitral regurgitation. Similarly, there are no specific electrocardiographic features, although combined ventricular hypertrophy is frequent. A long QT interval has been reported in most patients (Krovetz et al, 1965).

Thickening of the leaflets of the mitral valve and its annulus is seen echocardiographically. Left ventricular volume load and diastolic flutter of the mitral valve are seen when aortic regurgitation is present. Cardiac catheterization and angiocardiography add little to the diagnostic findings, which include systemic and mild pulmonary hypertension. When present, the haemodynamics and angiography will reflect the severity of valvar insufficiency. The disease progresses inexorably, death occurring by the age of 10 years from heart failure, sudden death or from chest infection. No treatment has yet proved satisfactory in rectifying the enzymic deficiency.

Scheie's syndrome

Patients with Scheie's syndrome are less severely affected and have normal stature and intellect. They also have a near normal lifespan. The most striking features are corneal clouding and stiff joints. Typical cardiac manifestations are aortic stenosis and regurgitation or mitral regurgitation. These should be managed in a similar fashion to that employed in otherwise normal subjects. Scheie's syndrome is inherited in autosomal fashion.

Hurler–Scheie's syndrome

Hurler–Scheie's syndrome (or the intermediate syndrome) falls in severity between the two extremes of α-L-iduronidase deficiency. The patients are of short stature with mental retardation and multiple bony defects. There is clouding of the cornea and stiff joints, claw-hand being particularly common. Aortic and mitral valvar involvement are responsible for the cardiac problems. Asymmetric septal hypertrophy has also been reported (Gross et al, 1988). The clinical course is intermediate between Hurler's and Scheie's syndromes, patients living into adolescence or even to the third decade. The genetics were thought to be a compound of the two extreme syndromes, comparable to that seen in the three forms of sickle cell disease (SS, CC and SC, the last being the compound form). Reports of Hurler–Scheie's syndrome in consanguinous families, however, suggest that a third allele is responsible. The basic differences between the three forms of mucopolysaccharidosis type I are unclear at present.

MUCOPOLYSACCHARIDOSIS TYPE II (HUNTER'S SYNDROME, IDURONATE SULPHATE DEFICIENCY)

Deficiency of iduronate sulphate results in block of degradation of dermatan sulphate. The difference in clinical profile between this and Hurler's and Sheie's syndromes (for example, the absence of corneal clouding in Hunter's syndrome) may result from specific variability in the degree of blockage of degradation of the mucopolysaccharide. This could be caused by tissue accumulation of a single sulphated iduronic acid. Furthermore, it may be that the block to degradation caused by the accumulation of idurone sulphate may be bypassed by hyaluronidase. The severe and mild forms of Hunter's syndrome both have total (or near total) deficiency of iduronate sulphate.

The condition can occur with a wide variety in severity, which tends to breed true in any given family. Apart from the extreme rarity of corneal clouding in Hunter's syndrome, the clinical features are those of Hurler's syndrome, although usually less severe. A positive distinguishing physical sign pointed out by Hunter himself (1916) is the occurrence of pebble-like ivory-coloured skin lesions. These are seen over the scapulas, and occasionally on the pectoral regions.

Cardiac involvement produces all the manifestations so far mentioned, namely aortic and mitral regurgitation or stenosis, ischaemic changes and evidence of myocardial dysfunction. Echocardiography is a useful method for evaluating cardiac involvement in Hunter's syndrome. The clinical course is extremely varied. Severely affected individuals die before the age of 15 years. At the opposite end of the spectrum, however, survival beyond the sixth decade has been reported. Death in younger patients is usually associated with progressive neurological deterioration. The disease is inherited as an X-linked recessive trait. Since the reproductive fitness of the Hunter gene is low, a large minority of cases must result from new mutations.

MUCOPOLYSACCHARIDOSIS TYPE III (SANFILIPPO SYNDROME)

Residues have to be removed during the degradation of heparan sulphate and N-sulphated or N-acetylated α-linked glucosamine. Deficiency of one of four enzymes required for this degradation results in the Sanfilippo syndrome. Consequently, there are four biochemically distinct types of the disease (designated A to D) although they all present the same clinical features.

The onset is usually evident in the first few years of life with 'behavioural' problems. Mental and neurological deterioration are severe and lead to death in the first two decades. Bone, joint and cardiac involvement are generally less severe than in Hurler's syndrome. Corneal clouding is never seen.

There is wide variation in the severity and age at death in all four forms, but type A (heparan N-sulphatase deficiency) is likely to be the most severe (van de Kamp, 1979; Matalon et al, 1980). Inheritance is in autosomal recessive fashion. Because of the minor musculoskeletal involvement, the Sanfilippo syndrome is probably the most underdiagnosed of the mucopolysaccharidoses.

MUCOPOLYSACCHARIDOSIS TYPE IV (MORQUIO'S SYNDROME)

Morquio's syndrome results from defective degradation of keratan sulphate. It occurs in two biochemically distinct forms. So-called type A is presumed to be a deficiency of N-acetylgalactosamine-6-sulphatase while type B results from deficiency of β-galactosidase. The two types have similar clinical features, but type B is less severe, sometimes called the 'long-legged' variant. Keratan sulphate is excreted in the urine in type A but is less evident in type B.

Keratan sulphate is found in cartilage, intervertebral discs and the cornea. Thus, skeletal involvement with dwarfism, pectus and bow-legs are the most obvious manifestations. Corneal clouding is the rule. In contrast to the monopolysaccharidoses described above, the joints in Morquio's syndrome are hyperextensible. Absence or severe hypoplasia of the odontoid process, together with laxity of its associated ligaments, leads to atlanto-occipital subluxation and consequent cervical myelopathy. The heart is clinically involved only in the severe type. Valves of the heart are primarily involved, with thickening of mitral and aortic leaflets. Concentric left ventricular hypertrophy and, rarely, asymmetric septal hypertrophy have been described (Gross, 1988; John, 1990). Survival beyond the third or fourth decade is usual. The effects of the cervical myelopathy and respiratory problems are the usual cause of death.

MUCOPOLYSACCHARIDOSIS TYPE VI (MAROTEAUX–LAMY SYNDROME)

Deficiency of N-acetylgalactosamine-4-sulphatase results in an inability to hydrolyse the sulphate groups in dermatan sulphate. The clinical picture is similar to that of Hurler's syndrome, but normal intelligence is maintained. Although severe in its classical form, milder variations exist. Affected infants can present with an acute cardiopathy (Hayflick, 1992). Thickened mitral and aortic leaflets necessitating valvar replacement has been noted in young adults (Marwick et al, 1992). Death usually occurs in the third decade. The condition is inherited in an autosomal recessive fashion.

MUCOPOLYSACCHARIDOSIS TYPE VII (SLY SYNDROME)

Deficiency of β-glucuronidase results in a clinical syndrome of extremely variable severity. Included in the features are coarse facies, corneal clouding, abdominal and inguinal hernias, puffy hands and feet, hepatosplenomegaly and a small thoracolumbar hump. The cardiovascular manifestations are hypertension, aortic aneurysm, aortic regurgitation and obstructive arterial disease. This extremely rare condition is inherited in autosomal recessive fashion. Duration of survival varies widely and depends on the severity of the disease. Death

as early as 30 months has occurred in one child with severe disease.

MUCOLIPIDOSES

The mucolipidoses present with clinical features similar to the mucopolysaccharidoses but are biochemically distinct. Leroy and Demars (1967) observed inclusions in cultured fibroblasts that occupied the whole cytoplasmic space apart from the Golgi apparatus. It was because of this that the name inclusion cell or I-cell disease was coined. The cause of the lysosomal storage defect is deficiency of several acid hydrolases in the lysosome. But this is not the primary problem, since the plasma abounds in these acid hydrolases (albeit in unstable forms). The problem is failure to locate the hydrolases within the lysosome. It is suggested that failure of phosphorylation of mannose residues of the hydrolases is the primary defect. Hydrolases without mannose 6-phosphate components are then not recognized by the lysosome and are not transported across the lysosomal membrane, particularly of connective tissue. In this way, inclusion cell disease and pseudo-Hurler polydystrophy differ from sialidosis (previously called mucolipidosis type I) where there is a single lysosomal enzyme defect. We, therefore, follow Neufeld and McKusick (1983) in limiting the designation of inclusion cell disease to the two conditions with absence of lysosomal hydrolase.

MUCOLIPIDOSIS TYPE II (INCLUSION CELL DISEASE)

The patients with inclusion cell disease present clinical features very similar to those with Hurler's syndrome. Hepatosplenomegaly is not so obvious, however, while striking gingival hypertrophy is a feature not encountered in Hurler's syndrome. Furthermore, the disease becomes evident earlier than does Hurler's syndrome. Corneal clouding is the rule. The skeletal and joint abnormalities, together with myocardial infiltration, usually lead to death by the age of 5 years either from respiratory causes or cardiac failure.

MUCOLIPIDOSIS TYPE III (PSEUDO-HURLER POLYDYSTROPHY)

Mucolipidosis type III is less severe than type II. Patients usually present with joint stiffness at the age of 4 or 5 years. Growth is moderately retarded and corneal clouding is present by the age of 7 or 8 years. The patients are disabled by carpal tunnel syndrome and destruction of the hip joints. Cardiac involvement (particularly aortic regurgitation) does occur but is usually not sufficiently severe to give clinical problems. Patients with pseudo-Hurler polydystrophy survive into the fourth decade. The mucolipidoses are inherited in autosomal recessive fashion. Diagnosis is suggested by clinical features resembling mucopolysaccharidoses but without their biochemical abnormalities. Findings of high serum levels of β-hexosaminidases, iduronate sulphatase and arylsulphatase A are diagnostic. The characteristic enzymic deficiencies in fibroblasts can be identified in cultured cells.

DISORDERS OF GLYCOPROTEIN DEGRADATION

Specific lysosomal enzymic deficiencies result in failure of degradation of glycoproteins, with consequent accumulation of glycoproteins in many tissues, especially the nervous system. They became recognized when patients with appearances similar to the mucopolysaccharidoses were found to have biochemically distinct diseases.

The four known disorders of glycoprotein degradation, mannosidosis, fucosidosis, sialidosis and aspartoglycosaminuria, can all be diagnosed by demonstration of the enzyme defect in cultured fibroblasts. Prenatal diagnosis has been accomplished in the first three and should be possible in aspartoglycosaminuria.

MANNOSIDOSIS

Deficiency of α-mannosidase results in the accumulation of mannose-containing substances, predominantly in liver cells and neurones. Oligosaccharides are excreted in the urine. The patients present with features suggestive of mucopolysaccharidosis but have an increased susceptibility to infections. Early onset of the disease shown as type I is associated with increased severity. Death occurs between 3 and 10 years of age. Late-onset disease (type II) runs a more benign course. The cardiac manifestation is a short PR interval, with the Wolff–Parkinson–White syndrome being seen on one occasion (Mehta and Desnick, 1978).

FUCOSIDOSIS

Deficiency of fucosidase results in the accumulation of oligosaccharides and some lipid material. Two clinical types are recognized. The first type presents in infancy with coarse facies, growth retardation, mental retardation and neurological deterioration. Hepatosplenomegaly and cardiomegaly are usually present. Convulsions and respiratory infections often occur. The second type has a more benign course and a later onset. Apart from cardiomegaly, arrhythmias have been reported.

SIALIDOSIS

The basic defect in sialidosis is deficiency of α-neuraminidase, with accumulation of presumed sialopolysaccharides. Two forms exist. The first is of late onset and patients are of normal appearance but develop the 'cherry red spot myoclonus syndrome'. Decreased visual accuity is associated with a cherry red spot in the macular region. Neurological (and occasional renal) manifestations dominate the clinical picture. The second type has an early onset, even on occasion being obvious at birth. This is seen in subjects of Japanese origin. The patients have coarse features and enlargement of various organs including the heart. Echocardiography has shown a thickened left ventricular wall along with thickening of the mitral valve (Kelley et al, 1981). There is great variability in the spectrum of severity even in the group with early onset. Survival beyond 20 years is rare, while, occasionally, affected subjects are still-born. Sialidosis is inherited in autosomal recessive fashion.

ASPARTOGLYCOSAMINURIA

Aspartoglycosaminuria is a rare disease characterized by excretion of aspartoglycosamine in the urine. It is associated with coarse features, joint laxity, short stature and mental retardation. It has on one occasion been shown to have cardiac involvement evidenced by mitral regurgitation.

ACID LIPASE DEFICIENCY (WOLMAN'S DISEASE AND CHOLESTEROL ESTER STORAGE DISEASE)

Deficiency of lysosomal acid lipase results in accumulation of cholesterol in most tissues of the body. The disease occurs in two forms. Wolman's disease is a disease of infancy presenting with vomiting, diarrhoea, hepatosplenomegaly, anaemia and calcification of the adrenal glands. Cardiac manifestations are not usually evident but microscopic examination of the arteries shows excess fatty deposits. Hepatomegaly is frequently the only sign in the milder form of the disease – cholesterol ester storage disease. Early atherosclerosis, aortic stenosis and pulmonary vascular obstructive disease have all been reported. The diagnosis of Wolman's disease is suggested by the association of hepatosplenomegaly with adrenal calcification. Definitive diagnosis of either disease can be made by assessing acid lipase activity in cultured skin fibroblasts. The disease is inherited in autosomal recessive fashion.

SPHINGOLIPIDOSES

SPHINGOMYELIN LIPIDOSIS (NIEMANN–PICK DISEASE)

In Niemann–Pick disease, there is accumulation of sphingomyelin in the cells as a result of deficiency of sphingomyelinase. At least four variants exist, but the most frequently encountered is the infantile acute neuronopathic form. The majority of such patients are of

Askenazy Jewish heritage. The disease is characterized by hepatosplenomegaly and the occurrence of 'foam' storage cells in many tissues. The heart is not usually affected, but one infant with acute neuronopathic disease had endocardial fibroelastosis (Westwood, 1977). Since there were no storage cells in the heart, however, this may have been a chance association. Niemann–Pick disease in most of its forms is inherited as an autosomal recessive trait.

GLUCOSYLCERAMIDOSIS (GAUCHER'S DISEASE)

Gaucher's disease is the most common inherited disorder of glycolipid metabolism. In his original description, Phillippe Gaucher (1882) ascribed the changes to a primary epithelioma of the spleen. There is excessive accumulation of glucosylceramide in cells of the reticulo-endothelial system in organs throughout the body resulting from deficiency of the enzyme glucocerebrosidase, which cleaves glucose from glucocerebroside. The disease occurs in three varieties. The first (the chronic non-neuronopathic form) can occur at any age. It is characterized by enlargement of the spleen with hypersplenism, hepatomegaly (with evidence of abnormal liver function) and skeletal lesions (including aseptic necrosis of the head of the femur). Other long bones and vertebras may also be eroded. In patients with this type of disease, cardiac involvement may be seen with myocardial infiltration or restrictive pericardial disease. The most frequently encountered cardiac problem, however, is cor pulmonale secondary to pulmonary involvement. Mitral and aortic stenosis and insufficiency can also be seen (Saraçlar et al, 1991). The course is variable. Death may occur in early childhood or, particularly when onset is late, there may be a normal life expectancy. Further variability is apparently the consequence of the non-neuronopathic form at onset changing to one of the other forms with poorer prognosis.

The acute neuronopathic form (the second type) is usually recognized within the second half of the first year of life. Neurological involvement is evident early, afflicting particularly the cranial nerves and extrapyramidal tracts. The mechanism of death is usually a respiratory infection, since aspiration is common owing to incoordination of the nasopharynx.

The subacute neuronopathic form (the final variant) falls between the acute and chronic forms. The neurological involvement renders it less benign than the chronic variant, but its course usually stretches over many years.

The diagnosis of Gaucher's disease is confirmed by the finding of typical storage cells in the bone marrow or by liver biopsy. The Gaucher cell is large and lipid laden. The cytoplasm is described as having a 'wrinkled tissue paper' or 'crumpled silk' appearance. The nucleus is eccentric. These cells have to be differentiated from cells found in multiple myeloma, leukaemia, thalassaemia and congenital dyserythropoietic anaemia. Demonstration of the enzymic deficiency in cultured skin fibroblasts or in leucocytes confirms the diagnosis. Approaches to treatment have included organ transplantation and administration of the purified enzyme. The results are as yet unpredictable. All three variants are inherited as autosomal recessive traits. Intrauterine diagnosis is available and heterozygotes can be identified at least for the acute and chronic types.

ALPHA-GALACTOSIDASE A DEFICIENCY (FABRY'S DISEASE)

Deficiency of α-galactosidase, a lysosomal enzyme, results in accumulation of phosphosphingolipids in the lysosomes of many tissues and also in the body fluids. The most frequently affected tissue is the vascular endothelium. The disease is of X-linked inheritance, but heterozygous women do show some manifestations of the disease. The gene locus for the enzyme is on the long arm of the X chromosome.

The disease usually presents in childhood in the male homozygote, often with periodic crises of severe pain of burning character, which usually start in the hands and feet. Crises occur most usually in the afternoon. Development of crises, which become less frequent and severe with time, may, however, be followed by eruption of skin lesions, by angiokeratomas and by typical opacities of the cornea and the lens. The angiokeratomas are clusters of dark red to purple punctate lesions, which are usually flat or slightly raised. They occur most frequently between the umbilicus and the knees. They do not blanch on pressure. Hyperkeratosis and hypohydrosis usually accompany the angiokeratomas. Occular lesions include typical creamy whorl-like opacities in the cornea. They are frequently found in the female heterozygote as well as the male homozygote. Cardiac disease is manifest with increasing age. Myocardial ischaemia and infarction are common and are secondary to the vascular lesions. Mitral regurgitation and aortic stenosis are the most frequently encountered valvar lesions (Desnick et al, 1976). Infiltration of the conduction tissues occurs. This results in progressive shortening of the PR interval, as in other storage diseases that affect the specialized atrioventricular conduction axis (Mehta et al, 1977). Myocardial deposition can be detected echocardiographically by demonstration of septal and left ventricular wall thickening (Bass et al, 1980). Progressive deposition of glycosphingolipid means that the cardiac problems themselves are also progressive. Since concomitant renal involvement occurs, the cardiac effects are exacerbated by, for example, renal hypertension. The clinical course in the male homozygote is one of steady deterioration during early adult life, death being from cardiac or renal disease. The heterozygote female experiences little limitation of style and length of life. The diagnosis can be confirmed (and heterozygotes identified) by demonstrating the enzymic deficiency in leucocytes and by an abnormally high content of accumulated substrates in tears or urinary sediment. Prenatal diagnosis is available. Treatment at present is only supportive. Enzyme replacement therapy, although at an early stage of development, appears promising.

THE GANGLIOSIDOSES

The gangliosidoses are lysosomal storage diseases characterized by accumulation of gangliosides GM_1 or GM_2 (or related conjugates) owing to deficiency of specific lysosomal hydrolases. The enzyme deficient in GM_1 gangliosidoses is acid β-galactosidase. Deficiency of hexosaminidase A or B (or both) or a deficiency of an enzyme activator results in GM_2 gangliosidoses.

GM₁ GANGLIOSIDOSES

There are many enzymatic and clinical subdivisions of GM_1 gangliosidosis. The gene locus is on the short arm of chromosome 3. Mutation at this locus results in absence of enzyme activity for acid β-galactosidase. The wide variation in clinical picture has resulted in a broad classification of infant, juvenile and adult forms. All forms of GM_1 gangliosidosis are inherited as autosomal recessive traits.

The infant form is a rapidly progressive disease characterized by hypotonia, poor feeding and failure to make motor or intellectual progress. Progressive neurological deterioration results in spastic quadriplegia or decerebrate rigidity. Rarified bones and beaked vertebras are some of the skeletal lesions encountered. As in Tay–Sachs disease (see below), a cherry red spot is seen in the macular region of the retina. Death usually occurs by the age of 2 years, frequently from bronchopneumonia. The heart is typically involved in the infant but not the juvenile or adult forms. Cardiac involvement usually includes cardiomegaly on chest radiography, left ventricular hypertrophy on the echocardiogram and congestive cardiac failure (Rosenberg et al, 1985).

GM₂ GANGLIOSIDOSES

The GM_2 gangliosidoses include Tay–Sachs disease (severe deficiency of hexosaminidase A) and Sandhoff disease (severe deficiency of both types A and B of the enzyme). The juvenile and adult (chronic) GM_2 gangliosidoses result from less-severe deficiencies of hexosaminidase type A.

Tay–Sachs disease

Tay–Sachs disease is the most common of the gangliosidoses; it presents with motor weakness in the first 6 months of life. There is progressive motor and mental deterioration, with convulsions, spasticity and decerebrate rigidity. Death usually occurs by the age of 3 years, the most frequent cause being bronchopneumonia. The children have doll-like facies. Examination of the retina shows the typical cherry red macula, which later becomes brown. Cardiac accumulation of substrate is usual; however, save for a prolonged QT interval and nonspecific T wave changes, cardiac manifestations are rare.

Sandhoff disease

Sandhoff disease is similar to Tay–Sachs disease in its presentation and course but is biochemically distinct. A cardiomyopathy (Blieden et al, 1974) has been described along with thickening of the mitral valve and its tension apparatus. The coronary arteries may also be narrowed (Blieden and Moller, 1974). As with GM_1 gangliosidoses, the inheritance is autosomal recessive. Prenatal diagnosis is available for the gangliosidoses but is not absolutely reliable.

METABOLIC DISORDERS: INHERITED ENDOCRINE DYSFUNCTION

DIABETES MELLITUS

The annual incidence of juvenile diabetes is between 8 and 10 per 100 000 of the population at risk (Bloom et al, 1975; Crossley and Upsdell, 1980). New cases are half as frequent under the age of 10 years as they are between 10 and 20 years of age. Since cardiovascular complications are manifested later in the disease, they are exceedingly rare in childhood (Fisher et al, 1989). Nonetheless, there will be problems presented to the paediatric cardiologist by diabetes because fetal mortality is high in pregnant diabetics. Furthermore, there is an increased risk of congenital cardiac anomalies in the offspring of diabetic women. Isolated ventricular septal defects and complete transposition are particularly frequent. The most obvious complication, however, is macrosomia. Even in the absence of congenital heart disease, babies of diabetic mothers have a host of problems. The syndrome is seen both in mothers with established diabetes and in those who develop the disease later. The babies have a characteristic appearance, with high birthweight, plumpness and puffy plethoric facies. They are 'jittery' owing to hypoglycaemia secondary to hyperinsulinism. The organs, including the heart, are enlarged. The babies are frequently tachypnoeic, but this may not be of cardiac aetiology. Respiratory distress syndrome is quite common. Cardiac murmurs are frequent and approximately 1 in 10–20 exhibit signs of congestive cardiac failure. Approximately one third have radiological cardiomegaly. The electrocardiogram is rarely diagnostic.

Echocardiography shows thickening of the right and left ventricular walls together with the septum. Indeed, the ventricular septum is usually thicker than the free walls. Septal thickness, is, in general, most pronounced in those infants in congestive cardiac failure (Mace et al, 1979). A spectrum of abnormality exists from that of hypertrophy to hypertrophic obstructive cardiomyopathy. Left ventricular outflow tract obstruction can occur, as demonstrated by cardiac catheterization. The subvalvar pressure gradient in one patient diminished on administration of propanolol (Way et al, 1979). Treatment of congestive cardiac failure should be by the use of diuretics. Digitalis is contraindicated since enhancement of contractile performance may cause worsening of the condition. The clinical and echocardiographic signs of hypertrophic cardiomyopathy resolve over the early weeks of life and patients appear to be left with no permanent cardiac disorder.

More important than diagnosis and treatment is prevention. It is suggested that the most severely affected newborns are those in whom maternal control of diabetes has been poor. This certainly conforms to our experience of a well-controlled diabetic population, in which, although the echocardiographic stigmas are present, no case of severe cardiac disease has been encountered. Therefore, good control of maternal diabetes is essential.

PITUITARY GIGANTISM AND ACROMEGALY

Adenomas of the pituitary that secrete growth hormones cause gigantism in growing children and acromegaly in adults. A cardiomyopathy owing to myocardial hypertrophy and interstitial fibrosis is known to occur in the late stages of the adult illness but is very rare in the juvenile forms.

DISORDERS OF THYROID FUNCTION

HYPOTHYROIDISM

Congenital hypothyroidism

Congenital hypothyroidism has many aetiologies. The most common cause is congenital thyroid dysplasia, present in approximately 1 in 6000 livebirths. There are rarer causes, including endemic iodine deficiency, diminished responsiveness to thyrotrophin in familial goitre and administration of antithyroid drugs to pregnant mothers. The cardiac features of cretinism are not dramatic. Normal or slow heart rates and radiological cardiomegaly are usually the only ones. The latter is usually caused by pericardial effusion, which is an extremely common feature. Cardiac performance is usually well preserved. Heart rate abnormalities and pericardial effusions resolve when substitution treatment of the hypothyroidism is successful. A pericardial effusion can be detected by echocardiography in approximately one half of these patients (Rondanini et al, 1991).

Juvenile hypothyroidism

As with congenital forms, juvenile hypothyroidism has multiple aetiologies. It is generally the result of autoimmune thyroiditis (Hashimoto's disease). Growth retardation is the most common form of presentation. It can lead to delayed sexual maturation. Cardiac signs and symptoms are few and heart failure is very rare. Bradycardia, low pulse pressure, poor peripheral circulation and non-specific heart murmurs may be present. Pericardial effusions (with no evidence of pericarditis) occur in some patients. Tamponade is rarely seen because of the slow rate of fluid accumulation. About one half of the patients with pericardial effusions have associated pleural effusions. Establishment of an euthyroid state reverses the cardiac manifestations.

HYPERTHYROIDISM

Juvenile hyperthyroidism

The most common cause of juvenile hyperthyroidism is diffuse toxic goitre (Grave's disease). This is an autoimmune disease in which IgG immunoglobulins, which stimulate excessive production of thyroid hormones, can be demonstrated. It is more common in girls, with a female to male ratio of approximately 5:1. Its greatest incidence is between the ages of 11 and 19 years, and it is rarely seen in children under the age of 3 years. Presenting symptoms include restlessness, poor performance at school, irritability, weight loss and occasionally diarrhoea. On examination, patients have warm skin, and a fine tremor is visible in outstretched hands. Thyroid enlargement is always present, and bruits are audible over the enlarged gland because of its increased vascularity. Exophthalmos is common but is not marked. Cardiovascular involvement is secondary to an increased adrenergic drive and to direct myocardial stimulation by thyroid hormones. The pulse is fast with a wide pulse pressure. The systolic blood pressure is increased and the apical impulse is hyperdynamic. On auscultation, the first heart sound is accentuated and non-specific systolic murmurs may be present. A high incidence of mitral valvar prolapse has been reported in adults with Grave's disease (Channick et al, 1981; Brauman et al, 1985) but has not been demonstrated in children (Carceller et al, 1984). This suggests that the appearance of the prolapse is related to the duration of the disease.

The electrocardiogram is atypical. Sinus tachycardia, first-degree atrioventricular block and non-specific ST segment and T wave changes may be present. Signs of atrial and left ventricular enlargement are more common in children than in adults (Pilapil and Watson, 1970). Although atrial fibrillation is quite common in adults, it is extremely rare in children. Radiographic cardiomegaly, and a slight increase in pulmonary vascular markings, may be seen, especially in the setting of cardiac failure. The echocardiogram reveals hyperdynamic contractions of the ventricular septum and the left ventricular posterior wall.

Evaluation of cardiac function by radionuclide angiography in the presence of hyperthyroidism has shown a fall in left ventricular ejection fraction with exercise. Upon restoration of a normal thyroid state, the ejection fraction shows its normal exercise-induced increase (Forfar et al, 1982). In general, the cardiovascular system in childhood tolerates well the effects of hyperthyroidism. In the presence of heart failure, however, concomitant cardiovascular lesions must be excluded. Cardiovascular manifestations of hyperthyroidism are reversible with treatment but, if long-standing or poorly treated, the disease may predispose to irreversible cardiac dysfunction (Cavallo et al, 1984).

The clinical diagnosis is confirmed by demonstrating increased levels of triiodothyronine (T_3) and thyroxine (T_4). The initial therapeutic approach is generally medical treatment. The most commonly used drugs, carbimazole and propylthiouracil, inhibit thyroxine synthesis. Potassium perchlorate blocks iodine uptake by the thyroid and a normal thyroid state is obtained. Treatment is maintained for 2 years before attempting discontinuation. Surgery is indicated only in the presence of poor medical control or relapse when medical treatment is stopped. The procedure performed is subtotal thyroidectomy. The risk of malignancies after the use of radioactive iodine in children has yet to be clarified. For this reason, its routine use in childhood is not currently advocated.

DISORDERS OF COLLAGEN SYNTHESIS

The group of disorders of collagen synthesis includes several diseases with cardiac involvement. Included in this discussion are Ehlers–Danlos syndrome, cutis laxa, osteogenesis imperfecta and Marfan's syndrome. Alcaptonuria also comes into this general group but, as yet, cardiac disease has not become manifest in childhood. Direct cardiac involvement does not occur in epidermolysis bullosa, but the heart may be affected when the condition is complicated by amyloidosis.

EHLERS–DANLOS SYNDROME

Phenotypical features unite the biochemically and genetically heterogeneous group of disorders included in Ehlers–Danlos syndrome. The stigmas are hyperextensible skin and joints, easy bruising and poor healing of wounds. A distinctive facial appearance includes epicanthic folds, a flat bridge of the nose and prominent downward pointing ears. The skin, apart from the palms and soles, is smooth and rubbery. In later life it may hang in folds from the elbows. Premature death is common in the most severe form and the babies have poor muscular

tone. In addition to the epicanthic folds, ocular signs include easy eversion of the upper eyelid (Meterier's sign), blue scleras and a dislocated lens. A variety of congenital heart defects have been reported (Beighton, 1969; Antani and Srinivas, 1973; Leier et al, 1980). Prolapse of the mitral or tricuspid valves is more characteristic. Life-threatening haemorrhage from arterial or aortic rupture in response to relatively minor trauma is rarer.

CUTIS LAXA

Cutis laxa is, again, a genetically heterogeneous group of conditions characterized in the phenotype by the skin being so loose that it appears too large for the body. Unlike the Ehlers–Danlos syndrome, the lax skin is slow to recoil after being stretched. Cutis laxa has some features in common with the Ehlers–Danlos syndrome, such as fragility of the skin, hypermobile joints and easy bruising. There are characteristic facies, including a long upper lip, a hooked nose and a short columella. The defect of connective tissue also results in a deep voice owing to lax vocal cords. Hernias and rectal or vaginal prolapse are all common. From the cardiac standpoint, peripheral pulmonary stenosis and aortic dilation have been reported. The major problem, however, is cor pulmonale, since emphysema is frequently progressive and severe. Patients with the neonatal variant of cutis laxa can have severe mitral regurgitation with dysplastic valvar leaflets (Bonneau et al, 1991).

OSTEOGENESIS IMPERFECTA

Bone fragility is the main clinical feature of this condition. Although the fractures are subperiostial with little displacement, the multiplicity of fractures leads to bowing of the long bones. Additionally, the vertebras are biconcave, with the disc sometimes perforating the vertebral body to give the appearance known as Schmorl's nodes. The skull is frequently made up largely of Wormian bones and shows frontal and parietal bossing. The skeletal deformities lead to short stature. The skin is thin but not lax. The scleras are blue in most types; however, in the so-called type III variant of the disease, they become less blue with age, while in type IV they are never blue. The cardiovascular manifestations include aortic and mitral regurgitation owing to dilation of the valvar rings or, in the latter, to prolapse from ruptured cords. Medial necrosis of the aorta also occurs (White et al, 1983). Congenital cardiac abnormalities such as atrial septal defects and tetralogy of Fallot have been seen (Vetter et al, 1989).

MARFAN'S SYNDROME

Marfan's syndrome is transmitted as an autosomal dominant disease with variable clinical expression.

Immunohistologic studies suggest that a defect in the microfibrillar fibre system accounts for the pathological changes in these patients (Boucek et al, 1981; Hollister et al, 1990). The prevalence is estimated at 4–6 per 100 000 (Pyeritz and McKusick, 1979). Over 70% of those affected are diagnosed before the age of 10 years. Physical features of the syndrome are present at birth (Phornphutkul et al, 1973). Affected persons are usually very tall, with an increase in the length of the limbs compared with the trunk. Their arm span exceeds their height. They have long, thin fingers, hypermobile joints, kyphoscoliosis and chest deformities. Inguinal hernias are very common. Ocular abnormalities occur in about three quarters of patients. The most frequent are subluxation of the lenses and myopia.

Cardiac manifestations in childhood are less severe than in adults. Mitral valvar disease in the form of valve prolapse and incompetence are the most frequent abnormalities. They are present in approximately three quarters of the patients (Bruno et al, 1984; Chen et al, 1985). Dilation of the aortic root and fusiform aneurysms of the ascending aorta are also common and are prevalent in males (Phornphutkul et al, 1973; Roberts and Honig, 1982). The major consequences of these aortic lesions are valvar regurgitation, aortic rupture and dissection. Aortic involvement is progressive with age and is probably a result of the effects of pressure on a predisposed wall (Roberts and Honig, 1982). Histopathological examination of the ascending aorta reveals degeneration of the elastic fibres (cystic medial necrosis), which is most severe in patients with aneurysms. The leaflets of the aortic valves have increased amounts of acid mucopolysaccharide material. The mitral valvar annulus is dilated and may become calcified (Roberts and Honig, 1982). Nonetheless, diagnosis is basically clinical. It is centred around four major criterions: family history, ocular, skeletal and cardiovascular manifestations. The presence of any two of these criterions makes the diagnosis (Pyeritz and McKusick, 1979).

The electrocardiogram will show signs of left ventricular and left atrial enlargement when there is significant valvar insufficiency. Rhythm disturbances such as first-degree atrioventricular block, atrial ectopic beats, atrial flutter, fibrillation and tachycardia are common. Ventricular arrhythmias are present in about one third of the patients during childhood. Progressing with age, they appear to be closely related to mitral valvar prolapse and prolonged ventricular repolarization (Chen et al, 1985). Radiographic examination of the cardiac shadow is difficult in the presence of thoracic skeletal deformities. Cardiac enlargement may be seen in the presence of valvar insufficiency and dilation of the ascending aorta. Echocardiographic evaluation is essential. Mitral valvar prolapse is a very frequent finding. Dilation of the aortic root, sometimes with paradoxical motion of the posterior aortic wall, is common. Mitral and aortic incompetence will lead to left atrial and left ventricular volume overload. Doppler echocardiography should increase the early diagnosis of the valvar abnormalities. Cardiac catheterization is useful for further assessment of these lesions. Aortic angiography will reveal the dilation of the aortic root. Evaluation with magnetic resonance imaging has demonstrated decreased aortic distensibility and increased stiffness in children with Marfan's syndrome (Savolainen et al, 1992).

Life expectancy is very variable. Death usually occurs in the fourth decade, mainly from cardiovascular causes (Roberts and Honig, 1982). Heart failure, dissection or aneurysms of the aorta, and sudden death are the most frequent causes. Incompetence of both mitral and aortic valves carries a poor prognosis. There is no specific treatment for this condition. Valvar abnormalities require antibiotic prophylaxis for bacterial endocarditis. The benefits in children of prophylactic propranolol to delay the dilation of the aorta through its negative inotropic effects have not been proven (Ose and McKucick, 1977; Pyeritz and McKusick, 1979). Heart failure is best treated with diuretics and vasodilators, since the positive inotropic effects of digitalis may further damage the aortic root. Surgical replacement of the mitral and/or aortic valves, and of the ascending aorta, may be necessary.

The timing of such surgery must be decided in the light of the risks of surgery and the known life expectancy (Table 67.2). It must then be remembered that the data shown in the table are from all the patients referred to a particular centre specializing in this syndrome. This is unlikely to correspond to similar data for patients referred to a cardiologist or cardiac surgeon. Roberts and Honig (1982) have suggested (on rather slender evidence) that treatment of patients with fusiform ascending aortic aneurysms should be directed at elimination or prevention of aortic regurgitation and in preventing aneurysmal rupture, rather than at preventing dissection, because the last is an infrequent complication in such patients. Unfortunately, dissection is not all that uncommon (Pyeritz et al, 1982; Crawford, 1983). Certainly, the original operative technique of replacement of the ascending aorta above the sinuses is inadequate. This is because further dilation of the sinuses themselves may occur, with dissection, rupture, obstruction to coronary flow or dehiscence of the prosthesis used to replace the aortic valve (Pyeritz et al, 1982). Consequently, the first line of treatment should be replacement of the entire aortic root with a composite graft consisting of the aortic valve and the ascending aorta. The native coronary arteries are then implanted into this graft (Bentall and DeBono, 1968). The distal end of the graft is sutured just short of the brachiocephalic artery. Mitral valvar replacement may be needed at the same time, and repair of more distal aneurysms may become necessary at a later date (Crawford, 1983). Hospital mortality has been variously reported as between 0 and 12% (Donaldson et al, 1980; McDonald et al, 1981; Crawford, 1983). Overall survival was reported as 61% at 3 years (McDonald et al, 1981),

Table 67.2. Probability of surviving additional years at a given age for patients with Marfan's syndrome

Attained age (years)	Probability of survival of males for further years					Probability of survival of females for further years				
	6	10	16	20	26	6	10	16	20	26
10	0.97	0.93	0.84	0.78	0.56	0.95	0.95	0.87	0.85	0.80
20	0.90	0.84	0.60	0.55	0.47	0.92	0.90	0.84	0.81	0.67
30	0.72	0.66	0.57	0.38	0.33	0.94	0.90	0.74	0.61	0.31
40	0.86	0.58	0.50	0.32	–	0.82	0.67	0.34	–	–

From Murdoch et al (1972).

77% at 6 years (Donaldson et al, 1980) and 62% at 15 years (Crawford, 1983). Given that many of these operations were carried out on acutely ill patients with, for example, aortic dissection, this must represent a considerable improvement on the natural history of the condition. In 1983, Crawford pointed out that two thirds of the late deaths in his series were from lesions that could successfully have been avoided by presently available methods of treatment. Since late deaths are rather uncommon following replacement of the aortic root, it does seem that an aggressive surgical approach is justified. Therefore, we recommend replacement for all symptomatic patients with aortic regurgitation and for all patients, even without symptoms, who exhibit aortic regurgitation that is more than moderate or that is associated with T wave abnormalities on the electrocardiogram. We advise replacement of the mitral valve for more-or-less isolated mitral regurgitation where symptoms persist despite medical treatment. Aortic dissection or rupture requires urgent operation, and we would recommend careful follow-up of the size of the aortic root by echocardiography in asymptomatic patients. It is rare, though possible (Roberts and Honig, 1982), for dissection to occur in an aorta of normal size. Among 13 patients who experienced aortic rupture or dissection, the aorta was 5.5 cm or more in diameter in all but two, and in these no echocardiogram had been obtained in the previous 6 months (McDonald et al, 1981). Consequently, it seems reasonable to advocate elective replacement of the aortic root in patients whose aortic diameter is 5.5 cm or greater.

INFANTILE MARFAN'S SYNDROME

Vary rarely, an infantile variant of Marfan's syndrome is seen. The skeletal and ocular manifestations are similar to the adult forms but the cardiovascular features are distinct (Geva et al, 1990). There is marked myxomatous thickening and redundancy of the leaflets of the mitral and tricuspid valves, with elongation of the tendinous cords leading to severe valvar insufficiency. Morbidity and mortality are primarily related to mitral and tricuspid valvar disease, as opposed to aortic dissection and rupture in the adult form. Affected infants present in congestive heart failure that responds poorly to con-

ventional therapy. Death often occurs within the first 2 years of life. A family history of Marfan's syndrome is much less common in infants who present with severe cardiovascular symptoms early in life (El Habbal et al, 1992).

—— NEUROMUSCULAR DISEASES ——

MUSCULAR DYSTROPHIES ——

DUCHENNE'S MUSCULAR DYSTROPHY

Duchenne's muscular dystrophy is an X-linked recessive disease. Because of this, it almost always afflicts males. Its incidence in male children is calculated at 13–33 per 100 000 livebirths. Since females with Turner syndrome have only one X chromosome, they too can inherit the disease, and it is seen rarely in this setting. The disease is believed to be caused by a defect in the sarcolemmal membrane of muscular cells. This permits an unknown substance (possibly calcium) to enter the cell and activate catabolic processes leading to necrosis (Walton and Gardner-Medwin, 1981).

The earliest symptoms are clumsiness in walking, a tendency to fall and an inability to run. Those with the disease also have difficulty in climbing stairs and getting up from the floor. Clinical onset is usually manifest before 4 years of age. Deterioration is continuous. Most are unable to walk by the age of 10 years and few survive beyond 25 years. Intellectual retardation is common, verbal ability being most severely affected (Walton and Gardner-Medwin, 1981). Muscular weakness and atrophy initially affect the proximal muscle groups of the upper limbs. Leg involvement extends from the quadriceps and gluteal muscles to the anterior tibial muscles. Weakness later affects other muscle groups. More power is generally retained in the distal muscles. Slight facial weakness occurs in the late stages. Scapular 'winging' is also a later phenomenon. Muscular hypertrophy of calves, masticatory muscles and deltoids is followed by a pseudohypertrophic phase of fatty replacement. Tendon reflexes are lost in the weak muscles. Contractures of the calves and hip flexor muscles develop around the age of 8 years. Contractures appear in the hips, knees, elbows and wrist when the patients are confined to wheelchairs. Severe spinal and thoracic deformities are seen late in the disease. Kyphoscoliosis is common. These result from disuse and abnormal posture. Generalized decalcification of the bones leads to frequent pathological fractures.

Myocardial involvement is very common. It is uncertain at what stage it begins, since the physical incapacity limits its expression (Evans, 1983). Latent failure may be precipitated by exercise. The cardiac dysfunction is progressive (Goldberg et al, 1983) and has been shown to parallel the skeletal muscle dysfunction (Hunsaker et al, 1982). Chest radiography reveals spinal and thoracic deformities, but there is no specific abnormality of the cardiac shadow. In contrast, there is a distinct and almost diagnostic electrocardiographic trace in 50–90% of patients. This includes tall R waves over the right precordial leads with increased R:S amplitude ratios, together with narrow and deep Q waves in the limb and left precordial leads. Female carriers may also have the abnormal electrocardiogram (Evans, 1983). These findings correspond to pathological observations. There is fatty and fibrous tissue replacement of the myocardium with selective scarring of the posterolateral wall of the left ventricle and, sometimes, involvement of the posterolateral papillary muscle (Evans, 1983). Conduction abnormalities are also frequently seen. Among these are prolonged intra-atrial conduction, right bundle branch block, a superior QRS axis and a short PR interval. Histological studies of the conduction system show multifocal areas of fibrosis, vacuolization and fatty infiltration (Sanyal and Johnson, 1982). The echocardiogram reveals impairment of both systolic (Hunsaker et al, 1982) and diastolic function. Thickness of the left ventricular wall is decreased, and this is not related to physical inactivity (Goldberg et al, 1983). The end-diastolic and end-systolic dimensions of the left ventricle increase as systolic function deteriorates. There is a strong correlation between left ventricular and premature ventricular contractions (Mori et al, 1990).

The diagnosis is made from the clinical characteristics, the high levels of creatine kinase activity and biopsy of the skeletal muscles. Creatine kinase activity is 100–300 times the normal at 1–5 years of age. Other muscle enzymes like aldolase, glutamic oxalic transaminase, lactic dehydrogenase and pyruvate kinase are also grossly elevated. Creatine kinase levels diminish later in the disease but still remain well above normal limits (Walton and Gardner-Medwin, 1981). Muscle biopsy shows scattered hyaline fibres with active muscle necrosis and regeneration. There is splitting of the muscle fibres, with fatty replacement. The nucleases are of varied size. The muscle fascicles also become surrounded by perimysial and endomysial connective tissue (Walton and Gardner-Medwin, 1981). Electromyography reveals a decrease in the mean action potential voltage and its duration. An increase in the number of polyphasic potentials is also seen.

There is no specific treatment. Since bedrest is harmful, regular physical activity and exercise are to be encouraged. Avoidance of obesity is an important general measure, along with prevention of muscle contractures by passive stretching. Because of the risks of anaesthesia and immobilization, the benefit from major orthopaedic procedures must be carefully considered. Prevention of scoliosis and thoracic deformities in the wheelchair phase help to avoid respiratory impairment and slow the deterioration of respiratory function. Death is usually from respiratory infections and insufficiency, heart failure or cardiac arrhythmias. Detection of carriers is important for appropriate genetic counselling. Over half the carriers can be identified by their elevated creative kinase levels, electromyography and muscle biopsy. The analysis of the pedigree is particularly useful.

CHILDHOOD MUSCULAR DYSTROPHY

Childhood muscular dystrophy is a very rare disorder resembling Duchenne's muscular dystrophy. It is inherited in autosomal recessive fashion and the general prognosis is better than in Duchenne's disease. Symptoms generally appear between 5 and 10 years of age. The disease is slowly progressive, the patients becoming unable to walk by their twenties. Death occurs in the fifth decade. The proximal muscles of upper and lower limbs are affected. Facial involvement and muscular hypertrophy are present in some patients. The heart is rarely affected and the electrocardiogram is usually normal. QRS changes identical to those seen in Duchenne's muscular dystrophy have occasionally been described (Jackson and Carey, 1961). The creatine kinase levels are mildly elevated and the histological appearance of the muscle biopsy cannot be distinguished from the other muscular dystrophies (Walton and Gardner-Medwin, 1981).

MYOTONIC MUSCULAR DYSTROPHY (STEINERT'S DISEASE)

The involvement of systemic tissues together with the presence of myotonia and muscular atrophy separate myotonic muscular dystrophy from the other muscular dystrophies. It has a high incidence, calculated at 13.5 per 100 000 livebirths. Onset is usually between 20 and 50 years of age, but many cases are clinically apparent during childhood. It is probably caused by widespread dysfunction of cell membranes related to decreased permeability to chloride ions. It is transmitted in an autosomal dominant fashion (Walton and Gardner-Medwin, 1981).

Myotonia is the presenting clinical feature in one third of cases. Others present with weakness of the hands, foot drop or a tendency to fall. The heart may occasionally become involved prior to diagnosis of the neuromuscular disorder. The facial, masticatory, sternomastoid, forearm, anterior tibial and peroneal muscles are those first affected by weakness. Later it extends to neighbouring muscle groups. The typical facies are characterized by lack of facial expression and difficulty in closing the eyes and moving the mouth. Ptosis and dysarthria are frequent. Myotonia is often limited to the tongue, forearms and hands, but it may be generalized. The tendon reflexes in the affected muscle groups are reduced.

Cataracts are present in almost all those affected. All have impaired pulmonary vital capacity and maximum breathing capacity. Abnormal contractions of the oesophagus are thought to be the cause of dysphagia and pulmonary aspiration. Testicular atrophy, diabetes mellitus, increased metabolism of immunoglobin G with low serum levels, progressive dementia and subnormal intelligence are frequent associations (Walton and Gardner-Medwin, 1981). The heart is involved in two thirds, mainly with conduction defects and arrhythmias. No relationship exists between the degree of involvement of the cardiac and the skeletal muscle. Chest radiography will show the associated deformities of the bony thorax together with elevated hemidiaphragms. The cardiac silhouette is normal. Death from cardiac involvement is almost always caused by complete atrioventricular block or ventricular tachycardia. It is very rarely caused by myocardial failure (Evans, 1983; Perloff et al, 1984).

The most common abnormalities in the electrocardiogram are low amplitudes of the P wave, atrioventricular block of any degree, right and left bundle branch block, abnormal Q waves and changes in the ST segment and T wave. It is believed that regional myocardial dystrophy is responsible for the abnormal Q waves (Bharati et al, 1984; Perloff et al, 1984). Rhythm disturbances include sinus brachycardia, premature atrial beats, atrial fibrillation, atrial flutter, ventricular premature beats and ventricular tachycardia (Evans, 1983; Bharati et al, 1984; Perloff et al, 1984). Four fifths of the patients have electrophysiological evidence of disease of the atrioventricular conduction axis. A further one fifth have evidence of intra-atrial conduction disturbances (Prystowsky et al, 1979; Gottdiener et al, 1982a; Bharati et al, 1984; Perloff et al, 1984). Disease of the atrioventricular conduction axis progresses with time (Prystowsky et al, 1979). A correlative study revealed fibrosis of the right and left bundle branches and fatty infiltration and degeneration around the atrioventricular node, which corresponded accurately with the electrocardiographic and electrophysiological evaluation performed during life (Bharati et al, 1984).

Mitral valvar prolapse is frequently associated with myotonic muscular dystrophy and is diagnosed echocardiographically. It is present in approximately one third of patients. There is no relationship, however, between mitral valvar prolapse and the arrhythmias. Systolic and diastolic function are normal (Gottdiener et al, 1982a; Perloff et al, 1984). Normal ejection fractions at rest are recorded with radionuclide angiography. Some patients fail to show an increase with exercise. Apical hypokinesia

may be present but is of doubtful significance (Perloff et al, 1984).

Careful clinical examination and a high degree of suspicion are required for an early diagnosis. Electromyography and muscle biopsy are useful techniques, as is slit lamp examination for cataracts. Cardiological evaluation is required in all patients because of the frequent association of heart disease. The diseases shows progressive deterioration, with physical incapacity 15–20 years after the onset of muscular symptoms. Death is usually from respiratory infections, aspiration, cardiac arrhythmias or anaesthetic complications (Walton and Gardner-Medwin, 1981).

There is no specific treatment for the condition. Active exercise and weight control are important general therapeutic measures. Systemic complications are treated as they arise. Myotonia is relieved by the use of procainamide or phenytoin (diphenylhydantoin). Caution must be exerted, however, since procainamide exacerbates pre-existing conduction disturbances (Walton and Gardner-Medwin, 1981). Electrophysiological studies are warranted in symptomatic patients presenting with syncope or presyncope. A ventricular pacemaker is needed when there are significant abnormalities in the formation or conduction of the cardiac impulse (Prystowsky et al, 1979).

Myotonic muscular dystrophy appears and progresses during early adult life in the majority of those affected. In a proportion, however, the disease is present at birth. Such congenital cases are often treated as a separate entity. Indeed, as will be seen, they have a totally different presentation and clinical picture. Nonetheless, in the fullness of time they come to resemble the adult form. The congenital form is characterized by bilateral facial weakness, hypotonia and mental retardation with delayed motor and speech development. Neonatal respiratory distress is very frequent. Such infants have a high incidence of feeding difficulties owing to muscle weakness. Talipes are a common association. Clinical myotonia is absent but can be demonstrated electromyographically. The adult features of the disease appear during late childhood and adolescence. Cardiac involvement takes the form of a dilated cardiomyopathy. Non-specific electrocardiographic abnormalities appear with progression of the disease (Harper, 1979). Mortality is high in the neonatal period as a result of respiratory distress. Beyond this time, there is a tendency to improve, only for the patients to deteriorate as the adult characteristics of the disease appear (Walton and Gardner-Medwin, 1981). The condition is transmitted by the mother. Her clinical involvement has often failed previously to be noted (Harper, 1979; Walton and Gardner-Medwin, 1981).

AUTOSOMAL DOMINANT SCAPULOPERONEAL MYOPATHY

Scapuloperoneal myopathy is a very rare form of muscular dystrophy. Two distinct groups are recognized according to the age of onset. They share an autosomal dominant form of inheritance and involve the same muscle groups. Weakness and atrophy affects the neck, shoulder girdle and upper arm muscles, together with the tibial and peroneal muscles in the legs. Foot drop and an awkward gait are frequent early symptoms. Deep tendon reflexes are commonly absent. Serum levels of creatine kinase are slightly elevated. Electromyography and muscle biopsy show the changes common to muscular dystrophies.

The group of patients with early onset generally present under the age of 10 years, and in these the disease takes a rapid course. Patients develop early contractures and are severely incapacitated by their late teens. They frequently have clinical and electrocardiographic signs of a dilated cardiomyopathy with congestive cardiac failure (Chakrabarti and Pearce, 1981). Those patients having a late onset present over the age of 40 years and the clinical course is slow. They seldom develop contractures. Cardiac involvement, usually late, could well be a result of ischaemic heart disease (Thomas et al, 1975; Chakrabarti and Pearce, 1981).

BECKER'S MUSCULAR DYSTROPHY

Becker's muscular dystrophy is one of the most frequent types of muscular dystrophy and is inherited in X-linked recessive fashion. The incidence is of the order of 3–6 per 100 000 male births. The muscular groups involved are very similar to those in Duchenne's muscular dystrophy. The peroneal and anterior tibial muscles are also affected in the Becker form of dystrophy. The facial muscles are not involved. Calf hypertrophy and muscle cramps are frequent early symptoms. Club feet are often seen. Contractures appear in the final stages and scoliosis is rare. Developmental delay is uncommon. The onset of the symptoms is between 5 and 15 years of age, with inability to walk being present by the third decade and death occurring in the fifth. The individual range, however, is very wide (Gardner-Medwin, 1980). The diagnosis is basically clinical. Serum creatine kinase activity is 25–200 times the normal. The electromyogram and the muscle biopsy are unspecific but help to rule out other conditions.

Cardiac abnormalities are infrequent in childhood and consist of atrial arrhythmias and conduction system abnormalities (Evans, 1983). Q waves, increased R:S ratios and T wave changes are seen on the electrocardiogram (Walton and Gardner-Medwin, 1981). A dilated cardiomyopathy associated with Becker's muscular dystrophy has also been described (Katiyar et al, 1977). Most patients are asymptomatic from a cardiac standpoint (Steare et al, 1992), with abnormalities noted on the electrocardiogram and/or echocardiogram. Severe left ventricular dysfunction, leading to orthotopic heart transplantation, has been reported (Donofrio et al, 1989).

FASCIOSCAPULOHUMERAL MUSCULAR DYSTROPHY (LANDOUZY–DÉJÉRINE SYNDROME)

Fascioscapulohumeral muscular dystrophy is inherited in an autosomal dominant fashion. It is uncommon, with an incidence of 0.4–0.5 per 100 000 live births. Facial and shoulder weakness generally develop in the second or third decade and progress very slowly. Patients with severe forms of this disease will occasionally present early in life, and progression is then rapid. Characteristically, there are no facial lines and the eyelids are very weak. Winging of the scapulas is seen when the arms are abducted and there is a marked thoracolumbar lordosis. Affected muscles include the neck flexors, the serrate and pectoral muscles, biceps and triceps in the upper limbs, the hip flexors and the anterior tibial muscles; in the late stages, the quadriceps and sartorius in the lower limbs are also affected. The intellect is normal (Gardner-Medwin, 1980). The serum levels of creatine kinase are normal or else only mildly elevated.

Ventricular function is rarely affected. Electromechanical atrial paralysis has been described (Baldwin et al, 1973). It has been postulated more recently that the electromechanical atrial paralysis occurs in patients with Emery–Dreifuss disease, which is phenotypically similar to fascioscapulohumeral muscular dystrophy. These latter patients have more benign cardiac involvement, consisting of abnormalities in function of the sinus and atrioventricular nodes in approximately one third of patients (Stevenson et al, 1990).

X-LINKED HUMEROPERONEAL MYOPATHY (EMERY–DREIFUSS DISEASE)

Emery–Dreifuss disease is a very rare condition that presents around 5 to 15 years of age. It is inherited in an X-linked recessive fashion. The biceps and triceps are more severely affected than the deltoid muscle. The peroneals are more involved than the proximal musculature of the legs. Contractures generally develop at the elbows, posterior cervical muscles and the Achilles' tendon. Pseudohypertrophy is absent. Creatine kinase levels are 3–10 times above normal. Progression is very slow, and the physical limitations are minimal. There is normal intellectual function (Hopkins et al, 1981).

Cardiac involvement is manifest by atrial arrhythmias and atrioventricular block. Any degree of atrioventricular block can be present, slow junctional escape rhythms being associated with complete block. Severe bradycardia is seen in patients with permanent atrial paralysis or complete atrioventricular block. This group is at high risk of syncopal episodes and sudden death. When occurring, these are the main causes of mortality (Waters et al, 1975; Hassan et al, 1979; Dickey et al, 1984). Ventricular function is usually normal, but progressive left ventricular dysfunction can occur in young adults

(Yoshioka et al, 1989). Those with bradycardia may have hypertrophied and dilated left ventricles, probably as a compensatory physiological response. Electrophysiological studies show prolonged HV intervals and, on some occasions, a complete absence of the His potential. This finding, together with the very slow junctional escape rhythms, suggests that the myopathic process extends into the atrioventricular conduction axis (Waters et al, 1975). The high risk of sudden death in this variety of muscular dystrophy makes early recognition important, since insertion of a ventricular pacemaker in patients with bradycardia will improve survival (Waters et al, 1975; Hassan et al, 1979). Genetic variants of this disease have been described with similar cardiac and muscular involvement but with autosomal dominant and recessive inheritance (Fenichel et al, 1982; Takamoto et al, 1984).

CENTRONUCLEAR MYOPATHY

This uncommon muscular disorder is characterized by ptosis, strabismus, generalized muscle wasting and weakness, together with absent or reduced deep tendon reflexes. Developmental delay and dysarthria are common (Gardner-Medwin & Tizard, 1981). The association of a dilated cardiomyopathy is well recognized. Patients have a prolonged PR interval and a superior axis on the electrocardiogram. Heart failure improves with diuretics and digitalis (Verheist et al, 1976). The diagnosis is based on clinical findings, raised levels of creatine-kinase in blood, evidence of a myopathy on electromyography, and a typical histological picture. This consists of central location of the nucleus, with variation of muscle fibre diameter and a tendency for predominance of type 1 fibres. Inheritance is autosomal recessive, but families with autosomal dominant and X-linked transmission have been described (Gardner-Medwin & Tizard, 1981).

FRIEDREICH'S ATAXIA

Friedreich's ataxia is a rare spinocerebellar neuromyelopathy. Children present around the age of 6 years. The most frequent early symptom is an abnormal gait. Neurological signs include the ataxic gait, absent tendon reflexes, incoordination and a positive Romberg test (Ackroyd et al, 1984). Lower limb weakness and muscular atrophy are common, as are dysarthria and loss of vibration and positional sense and extensor plantar responses. Some patients have nystagmus. The presence of brisk tendon reflexes makes the diagnosis of Friedreich's ataxia very unlikely (Ackroyd et al, 1984). Skeletal involvement is common, with club feet and scoliosis among the most frequent manifestations. Apart from the clinical aspects of the disease, nerve conduction studies are essential to support the diagnosis. Motor con-

duction velocity is normal and sensory conduction is absent or markedly reduced (Ackroyd et al, 1984). Since clinical, electrocardiographic and radiographic examination of the heart are non-specific for the evaluation of cardiac involvement in Friedreich's ataxia, an echocardiogram is necessary in every patient.

The heart is involved in a very high percentage, and cardiac symptoms are an integral part of the clinical spectrum of the disease. Most usually, the heart exhibits a symmetrical, concentric and slowly progressive hypertrophic cardiomyopathy (St John Sutton et al, 1980; Gottdiener et al, 1982b; Evans, 1983; Harding and Hewler, 1983; Ackroyd et al, 1984). Obstructive forms have been described frequently (Evans, 1983; Pentland and Fox, 1983). Very rarely acute dilated cardiomyopathies are seen (Berg et al, 1980). Cardiac involvement may occasionally precede the onset of neurological manifestations (Harding and Hewler, 1983). Cardiac symptoms are present in approximately one third of the patients and consist mainly of exertional dyspnoea, palpitations and angina. Clinical findings of cardiac disease are not present in every case patient. When they are, they include systolic murmurs at the left sternal border and apex, together with third and fourth heart sounds. The pulse may have a rapid upstroke. Evaluation of the severity of heart disease by physical examination is often difficult because of the presence of scoliosis and the lack of consistent cardiovascular signs.

Pathological studies reveal cardiac dilation with ventricular hypertrophy. Histologically, there is a degeneration of myocardial cells with myocardial fibrosis. Intracellular granular deposits of calcium and iron are seen. Surprisingly, the anticipated myofibrillar disarray of hypertrophic obstructive cardiomyopathy has not been reported (St John Sutton et al, 1980; Evans, 1983). Electrocardiographic changes are present in over two thirds of patients and they progress in relation to the duration of the disease (Harding and Hewler, 1983). The most frequent changes involve the ST segments and T waves. These are non-specific and are presumably caused by repolarization disturbances from the underlying myocardial fibrosis. Signs of ventricular hypertrophy are also frequent, and right- or left-axis deviation is common. Arrhythmias are not frequent. When present they include supraventricular and ventricular premature beats, supraventricular tachycardia, atrial flutter and atrial fibrillation (Harding and Hewler, 1983; Pentland and Fox, 1983). The onset of fibrillation presages a very poor prognosis (Harding and Hewler, 1983).

The presence of scoliosis makes radiographic evaluation of the heart difficult. Heart size is usually normal. Practically every patient has an abnormal echocardiogram. The most common anomalies reflect the presence of symmetrical concentric hypertrophic cardiomyopathy. There is an increase in left ventricular wall and septal thickness. Asymmetrical septal hypertrophy with systolic anterior motion of the mitral valve has been reported

(Evans, 1983; Pentland and Fox, 1983). Features of a dilated cardiomyopathy are occasionally seen (Berg et al, 1980; Gottdiener et al, 1982b). Impaired left ventricular function has also been shown echocardiographically. Reduced fractional shortening of the left ventricle is common (St John Sutton et al, 1980; Pentland and Fox, 1983). The systolic function of the posterior wall is more severely affected than that of the septum. Abnormal diastolic function may antedate systolic abnormalities. A constant feature is the delay in mitral valvar opening. The late appearance of systolic dysfunction may explain the delay in finding cardiac signs and symptoms (St John Sutton et al, 1980).

Haemodynamic and angiographic studies confirm the presence of concentric left ventricular hypertrophy and also demonstrate the presence of asymmetrical obstructive hypertrophic cardiomyopathy (Evans, 1983).

The clinical course is marked by steadily progressive deterioration. Cardiac failure, which appears late in the course of the disease, has a poor prognosis and is often a preterminal event (Harding and Hewler, 1983). It is thought that heart failure represents the end stage of progression of the concentric hypertrophic form of cardiomyopathy to a dilated one (Gottdiener et al, 1982b). Most patients with Friedreich's ataxia die from cardiac causes. Heart failure accounts for half of the deaths. Cardiac arrhythmias and respiratory complications are the other major causes of death.

There is no specific treatment. Congestive cardiac failure is generally treated with diuretics and digitalis. The latter drug must be administered with extreme care in those patients with obstructive hypertrophic cardiomyopathy. Calcium antagonists may be useful in modifying the progression of the cardiomyopathy (Berg et al, 1980). Friedreich's ataxia is transmitted as an autosomal recessive condition, the cardiac and neurological abnormalities being the expression of a single gene (Pentland and Fox, 1983).

ARTHROGRYPOSIS MULTIPLEX CONGENITA

Arthrogryposis multiplex congenita presents with joint contractures at birth in at least two different areas of the body. A typical presentation includes equinovarus deformities of the feet, abducted hips, incompletely extended knees and elbows, pronated forearms and claw hands. The majority of those affected have a neurogenic cause with patchy loss of anterior horn cells. They seem to result from environmental factors occurring in utero rather than from a familial condition. A myopathic form also exists with autosomal recessive inheritance (Walton and Gardner-Medwin, 1981).

The heart is rarely involved. A report of the myopathic form of arthrogryposis multiplex congenita revealed congenital heart disease in one quarter (Lebenthal et al, 1970). Patency of the arterial duct and congenital aortic

stenosis are the most frequently reported associations (Friedman et al, 1965; Lebenthal et al, 1970).

PERONEAL MUSCULAR ATROPHY (CHARCOT–MARIE–TOOTH DISEASE)

Peroneal muscular atrophy is a rare neuromuscular disorder inherited in an autosomal dominant fashion. It is predominantly a motor neuropathy that produces atrophy and weakness of the feet and peroneal muscles. This determines the typical 'inverted bottle' appearance of the legs. Bilateral club foot is a frequent association. The hand and forearm muscles may also be involved. There is a decrease or loss of the deep tendon reflexes. Electromyographic studies show slowing of nerve conduction velocity or signs of denervation. It has minimal effect on longevity.

The cardiac involvement has classically been related to supraventricular arrhythmias and conduction system abnormalities. Sick sinus syndrome, right bundle branch block, complete heart block, Wolff–Parkinson–White syndrome, atrial fibrillation and atrial flutter have been described (Littler, 1970; Bowers, 1973; Evans, 1983; Lowry and Littler, 1983). It has been postulated that there is a primary degeneration of the conduction system rather than changes secondary to a cardiomyopathy (Littler, 1970). A large prospective study (Isner et al, 1979) failed to show any difference between the incidence of these abnormalities among patients with peroneal muscular atrophy and the general population. Nearly a third of their patients, however, had clinical or echocardiographic evidence of mitral valvar prolapse. The echocardiographic studies failed to show dilation of the chambers of the heart or myocardial dysfunction.

The Roussy–Lévy syndrome shares many features with peroneal muscular atrophy. Heart disease in this condition consists of a dilated cardiomyopathy (Lascelles et al, 1970).

JUVENILE SPINAL MUSCULAR ATROPHY (KUGELBERG–WELANDER SYNDROME)

Juvenile spinal muscular atrophy appears in childhood or adolescence. Initially it is manifest by weakness and atrophy of the proximal limb muscles, which is later followed by distal disease. The usual presentation is with difficulty in walking, climbing stairs and lifting the arms. Fasciculation is seen in half those affected. The clinical course is slowly progressive. There is evidence from electromyography and muscle biopsy to indicate lower motor neurone disease (Campbell and Liversedge, 1981). Some patients have an associated dilated cardiomyopathy. Rhythm disturbances are very frequent and include atrial premature beats, atrial fibrillation, atrial flutter and advanced degrees of atrioventricular block. Some patients require the implantation of a pacemaker (Tanaka et al, 1976). The syndrome is transmitted in autosomal recessive fashion.

HEREDOPATHIA ATACTICA POLINEURITIFORMIS (REFSUM'S DISEASE)

Refsum's disease is a rare neurological disorder produced by a primary deficiency of phytanic acid oxidase. This leads to accumulation of phytanic acid (3-7-11-15-hexadecanoic acid) in blood and tissues. Symptoms appear in the first and second decade of life and initial presentation is with weakness, unsteady gait and night blindness. These patients have a diagnostic tetrad: retinitis pigmentosa, peripheral polyneuropathy with diminished or absent deep tendon reflexes, cerebellar ataxia, and high protein levels in cerebrospinal fluid without pleocytosis. Other frequent signs are nerve deafness, an inability to smell, nystagmus and abnormalities of the pupils (Walton and Gardner-Medwin, 1981; Steinberg, 1983). The heart is rarely affected. Conduction abnormalities, especially advanced degrees of atrioventricular block requiring pacemaker therapy, have been described (Lewis et al, 1966). Cardiomyopathy is a rare association (Poulos et al, 1984).

Diets low in phytanic acid produce clinical improvement. Complete recovery is rarely obtained, but treatment will slow the progression of the disease. The association of plasmapheresis to the diet reduces the levels of phytanic acid more rapidly (Steinberg, 1983). This disorder is inherited in an autosomal recessive fashion.

MITOCHONDRIAL MYOPATHIES

The mitochondrial myopathies are muscle and systemic disorders characterized by the presence of mitochondria with abnormal structure, number and/or function (Sengers et al, 1984). Chronic progressive ophthalmoplegia (Kearns–Sayre syndome, ophthalmoplegia plus syndrome) is frequently encountered among these diseases. It is associated with pigmentary degeneration of the retina, lack of coordination, facial and limb weakness, short stature and endocrine anomalies. The disease appears in childhood and has a progressive course.

The most frequently reported cardiac anomaly is progressive heart block. Electrocardiograms should be performed frequently for early recognition and appropriate pacemaker insertion (McComish et al, 1976; Darsee et al, 1980; Egger et al, 1981). Cardiomyopathy and mitral valvar prolapse have also been described (Neustein et al, 1979; Bogousslavsky et al, 1982).

The presence of ragged red fibres on muscle biopsy is a constant finding. These result from peripheral aggregates of abnormal mitochondrions. These patients also have high blood levels of lactate and pyruvate. They usually have enzymatic defects in the pyruvate dehydrogenase complex or in the respiratory chain (Sengers et al, 1984). Apart from their abnormal size, number and distribution, the mitochondrions show abnormal cristas and paracrystalline inclusions (Egger et al, 1981; Sengers et al, 1984). A recent report suggests that Kearns–Sayre syndrome results from a disorder in folate and carnitine metabolism (DiMauro and Coulter, 1983).

Nearly all mitochondrial DNA is maternally transmitted. Inheritance, therefore, follows non-Mendelian patterns (Egger and Wilson, 1983). Families with mitochondrial myopathies showing autosomal dominant, recessive and X-linked transmission have also been described (Neustein et al, 1979; Sengers et al, 1984).

DEFICIENCIES

SELENIUM

Selenium is a trace element that is an essential component of glutathione peroxidase. The enzyme removes organic hydroperoxides from the cell. Absence of selenium, possibly associated with absence of vitamin E, would permit damage to the cell membrane by lipid peroxides. Deficiency of selenium, also known as 'Keshan disease', affects children living in areas with a poor content of selenium in the soil (or with a poor diet) (Collip and Chen 1981). It gives rise to an endemic cardiomyopathy that affects children between 1 and 9 years of age, living in an area extending from the northeast to the southwest of China, where the content of selenium in the soil and food is very low. The incidence has been significantly reduced by supplementing oral sodium selenite in the diet (1–5 years with 0.5 mg daily and 6–9 years with 1 mg/daily) with no adverse side effects (Editorial, 1979). Once fully developed, the cardiomyopathy is irreversible (Johnson et al, 1981). Histopathological features of the heart are areas of myocytic loss with replacement fibrosis in the subepicardial surface of the ventricles (Johnson et al, 1981; Fleming et al, 1982). Two cases of cardiomyopathy very similar to this deficiency have been described in association with prolonged parenteral nutrition and low levels of selenium in the heart and the erythrocytes (Johnson et al, 1981; Fleming et al, 1982). Selenium deficiency can occur in children with phenylketonuria, who then present with ventricular tachycardia (Greeves et al, 1990).

CARNITINE

L-Carnitine (hydroxytrimethylammonium butyrate) is an essential cofactor in the transfer of long-chain fatty acids across the inner mitochondrial membrane. Depletion of carnitine blocks the mitochondrial oxidation of fatty acids and leads to cytoplasmic accumulation of lipids. Cardiac and skeletal muscles use fatty acids as their main substrate and, therefore, are very sensitive to carnitine deficiency (Tripp et al, 1981; Waber et al, 1982; Rebouche and Engel, 1983). Primary carnitine deficiency syndromes are divided into myopathic and systemic forms. Patients with muscular deficiency present with progressive weakness and are thought to have abnormal transport of carnitine into skeletal muscle. They have normal plasma levels but low muscle concentrations of carnitine. Systemic deficiency presents early in life, with encephalopathy, hypoglycaemia, liver failure and cardiomyopathy (Chapoy et al, 1980). Muscle weakness and developmental delay are common. Hypotheses for the cause of systemic deficiency include defects in synthesis, renal handling, gastrointestinal absorption and cellular transport or excessive degradation (Waber et al, 1982; Rebouche and Engel, 1983). Accumulation of triglycerides in muscle often occurs since fatty acids are not transported effectively into the mitochondrions for oxidation. Patients have low plasma and tissue concentrations of carnitine.

Cardiomyopathy has frequently been reported in association with either systemic or myopathic deficiency (Hart et al, 1978). Many patients are in heart failure when they come to medical attention (Stanley et al, 1991). The electrocardiogram is non-specific, with signs of left ventricular hypertrophy. Very tall and peaked T waves, like those seen in hyperkalaemia, have been described (Tripp et al, 1981; Waber et al, 1982). The echocardiogram reveals left ventricular and left atrial dilation with signs of poor left ventricular function. The last can also be demonstrated by nuclear angiography. Heart failure responds poorly to conventional therapy. Endocardial fibroelastosis as a result of systemic carnitine deficiency has been described (Tripp et al, 1981). The diagnosis is dependent on the demonstration of low levels of carnitine in the tissues or blood. Muscle biopsy shows large amounts of lipids in type I muscle fibres and abnormal mitochondrions. The disease is usually fatal without treatment. Oral L-carnitine at a daily dose of 0.1–0.2 mg/kg in divided doses has produced clinical improvement in some patients (Chapoy et al, 1980; Tripp et al, 1981; Waber et al, 1982). Others fail to respond to therapy (Hart et al, 1978). Diarrhoea is the main side effect. Diets with only 20% of calories from fat are also useful in long-term treatment. Carnitine deficiency is inherited in autosomal recessive fashion.

Sudden death in the neonatal period has been described in other disorders of fatty acid metabolism (Honat et al, 1985; Harpey et al, 1987, 1990). Pathological examination has revealed vacuolation of the myocytes consistent with high lipid content (Tonsgard et al, 1991). The clinical manifestations may resemble Reye's syndrome and may be precipitated by a viral illness or stress.

THIAMINE DEFICIENCY (BERI-BERI)

Thiamine (vitamin B_1) is a water-soluble vitamin that is absorbed from the small intestine. In its active form of thiamine pyrophosphate, it is an essential coenzyme in the metabolism of pyruvate and in the transketolase reaction (Neal and Sauberlich, 1980). Thiamine deficiency produces a disease known as beri-beri, which has been related to diets consisting of polished rice in oriental societies and to alcoholism in occidental ones (Sandstead, 1980). Classically, the disease has been divided into two major types. In dry beri-beri, the patients have peripheral neuropathy with varied disorders of sensation sometimes amounting to anaesthesia, muscle weakness and atrophy; reduced deep tendon reflexes; fatigue; and difficulty in concentrating. In contrast, in wet beri-beri, where the presenting features are a high output cardiac failure with peripheral oedema, the patients have diminished peripheral vascular resistance as a result of muscular arteriolar vasodilatation, a wide pulse pressure and a warm skin (McIntyre and Stanley, 1971). The mechanism leading to a reduction of peripheral vascular resistance is believed to be directly related to the lack of thiamine, since after treatment this parameter returns rapidly to normal (Attas et al, 1978). Despite high cardiac output, oliguria is present owing to reduction of renal blood flow and glomerular filtration rate. Increased jugular venous pressure results from peripheral venoconstriction and from an increase in the circulating blood volume (Kawai et al, 1980). Cutaneous vasoconstriction becomes evident with progression of heart failure, and this results in cold hands and peripheral cyanosis. It is not clear whether heart failure results from primary myocardial involvement or whether it is secondary to the vascular changes. In some patients, the additional toxic effects of alcohol make this differentiation very difficult (Editorial, 1982). Current evidence suggests that it results from a combination of both mechanisms (Attas et al, 1978). Histological studies of the heart have shown hydropic degeneration, interstitial and perivascular oedema, fibrosis and necrosis of myocardial tissue.

An acute variant of the disease with vascular collapse, metabolic acidosis and variable cardiac output is known as Shoshin beri-beri. Patients present in severe biventricular failure. They have renal dysfunction leading to metabolic acidosis. There is a high arterial oxygen saturation secondary to tachypnoea, which contrasts with peripheral cyanosis caused by cutaneous vasoconstriction (Engbers et al, 1984). Cardiac catheterization reveals increased right and left atrial pressures and a low peripheral vascular resistance (Pereira et al, 1984). Early diagnosis is necessary because patients die rapidly if left untreated. The presentation varies with age. Affected infants are very rarely seen in Western countries. It appears in nursing babies of thiamine-deficient mothers around 1–4 months of age. Sometimes the clinical onset is sudden. Acute congestive cardiac failure may then appear in apparently healthy babies following a minor illness. In others, signs and symptoms mimicking meningitis are seen. Administration of thiamine produces a rapid recovery. If not, death occurs (Sandstead, 1980).

Beyond infancy, the dry form is seen in children fed polished rice. Signs and symptoms are of peripheral neuropathy. Cardiovascular involvement and oedema are rare. When presenting in adolescence, alcohol consumption must be considered in addition to poor dietary intake. Patients present with malaise, fatigue, palpitations, dyspnoea and peripheral oedema. They have an increased jugular venous pressure, a high pulse pressure, a gallop rhythm with non-specific apical systolic murmurs and a loud pulmonary component to the second sound. There is cardiomegaly on the chest radiograph in half and the electrocardiogram shows non-specific T wave changes. Haemodynamic studies reveal high cardiac index, stroke index, circulating blood volume and low peripheral vascular resistance (Kawai et al, 1980).

Clinical suspicion and a dietary history of poor thiamine intake and/or excessive alcohol consumption are necessary for diagnosis. Patients with beri-beri exhibit low transketolase activity in erythrocytes, which increases after the administration of thiamine pyrophosphate. Patients have low thiamine levels in blood and urine (Sandstead, 1980). An acute response to intravenous thiamine during cardiac catheterization, with an increase in peripheral vascular resistance and a reduction in cardiac output, has also been used as a diagnostic test (Ikram et al, 1981).

Beri-beri is a treatable cause of heart failure. There is a rapid response to administration of thiamine. Parenteral therapy (50 mg intravenously) is necessary in extreme cases. Administration can later be continued orally. Bedrest, oxygen, diuretics and digitalis are useful therapeutic adjuncts. Shoshin beri-beri is a medical emergency that is fatal without aggressive medical management. Correction of the acidosis with sodium bicarbonate is essential, together with the measures already described.

A balanced diet, with an adequate intake of meat, fresh vegetables and whole grains will supply the daily requirements of thiamine and prevent beri-beri. The recommended daily intakes are 0.3 mg in infants under 6 months and 0.5 mg in those 6–12 months of age. Older children will require between 0.7 and 1.4 mg depending on age. Adult males need 1.4 mg and females 1.1 mg, which should increase by 0.3 mg during pregnancy and lactation (Neal and Sauberlich, 1980). Thiamine toxicity has not been reported.

DEPOSITIONS

The major disease caused by deposition that gives problems in childhood is haemochromatosis. The other depositions, such as amyloidosis, do not usually produce difficulties prior to adulthood.

HAEMOCHROMATOSIS

Haemochromatosis results from deposition of iron; it may be primary or secondary. Idiopathic (or primary) haemochromatosis is a rare disease resulting from excessive iron absorption from the diet for unknown causes. It is inherited in autosomal recessive fashion. There is an association with HLA groups A3 and B14 (Bothwell et al, 1983). Secondary haemochromatosis is generally the result of excessive administration of iron through multiple blood transfusions in chronic transfusion-dependent non-haemorrhagic anaemias. The most frequent of these is β-thalassaemia. Each 250 ml of blood delivers approximately 200 mg of iron (Buja and Roberts, 1971; Mitchell, 1983). Cardiac dysfunction generally occurs after 100 units of blood have been transfused (Leon et al, 1979). Though the primary and secondary diseases are quite different, the damaging effects of iron are similar (Mitchell, 1983). The excess iron in the tissues weakens the lysosomal membranes and produces damage to the cells (Bothwell et al, 1983).

Idiopathic haemochromatosis appears between 40 and 60 years of age and is extremely rare in childhood (Perkins et al, 1965). The secondary form may be clinically apparent in the second decade or earlier, depending on the frequency of transfusions. There is widespread deposition of iron in the liver, spleen, pancreas, gonads, skin and heart, which leads to the clinical manifestations. The classic triad consists of hepatic cirrhosis, bronze pigmentation of the skin and diabetes mellitus. Splenomegaly is present in approximately half the patients with idiopathic haemochromatosis and in virtually every patient with β-thalassaemia. Cardiac involvement results from excessive deposits of haemosiderin in the heart. This produces a dilated cardiomyopathy with heart failure. A restrictive cardiomyopathy has also been described (Cutler et al, 1980).

The heart is rusty-brown at postmortem with dilation of all cardiac chambers. Concentration of iron is greater in the subepicardial part of the heart; therefore, limiting the use of endomyocardial biopsies (Fitchett et al, 1980). Iron in the form of haemosiderin initially adopts a perinuclear distribution and then extends peripherally as the amount of deposits increase (Buja and Roberts, 1971; Fitchett et al, 1980). These are greater in the ventricles than in the atriums and the conduction tissues (Vigorita and Hutchins, 1979).

Low-voltage QRS complexes are seen electrocardiographically with non-specific ST segments and T wave changes. A prolonged QT interval may be present. There may be evidence of right or left ventricular hypertrophy. Rhythm disturbances are common; these include atrial and ventricular premature contractions, supraventricular and ventricular tachycardias and varying degrees of atrioventricular block. There is a correlation between deposits of iron in the conduction tissue and rhythm disturbances (Vigorita and Hutchins, 1979).

Cardiac enlargement and signs of heart failure (when present) are seen in the chest radiograph. Echocardiography shows increased left ventricular wall thickness, signs of increased left ventricular and left atrial dimensions, and a reduction in fractional shortening and ejection fraction (Borow et al, 1982; Dabestani et al, 1984).

Equilibrium-gated blood pool studies reveal poor left ventricular performance with a low ejection fraction, which is present before clinical evidence of heart failure appears (Dabestani et al, 1984). Laboratory studies should include measurements of plasma iron, ferritin and saturation of transferrin. These are always elevated. Measurement of iron content of samples obtained by needle biopsy of the liver allow accurate estimations of total body iron (Bothwell et al, 1983; Mitchell, 1983).

Cardiac failure is the cause of death in about one third of the patients. Early onset of heart failure and ventricular arrhythmias have a poor prognosis. Malignant hepatoma is an important late complication in the older patients. Removal of iron by repeated venesection, or by chelation with desferrioxamine reverses all the cardiac manifestations except the conduction disturbances (Short et al, 1981; Candell-Riera et al, 1982). Symptomatic heart block requires insertion of a pacemaker (Mitchell, 1983). Conventional treatment with diuretics, digitalis and antiarrhythmic drugs are valuable therapeutic adjuncts when required.

———CONNECTIVE TISSUE DISEASES———

JUVENILE RHEUMATOID ARTHRITIS (STILL'S DISEASE)———————————————

Still's disease is the most common form of chronic juvenile arthritis. It is characterized by the absence of positive serological tests. The aetiology is unknown, but HLA-B27 histocompatibility antigen is found in approximately a quarter of patients (Resnick and Niwayama, 1981). According to its form of presentation, it is classified as the systemic, polyarticular or pauci-articular type of disease.

Patients with the systemic disease have a febrile illness accompanied by an evanescent rash, hepatosplenomegaly and generalized lymphadenopathy. Arthritis may or may not be present. Pleuritis with interstitial pulmonary disease, pericarditis and myocarditis are frequently seen.

The polyarticular disease is characterized by symmetrical involvement of the wrist, knee, and ankle joints. The cervical spine is frequently affected. Systemic manifestations are of a milder nature. Rash, splenomegaly, and lymphadenopathy may be present.

The pauci-articular variety affects small children. The joints involved are the knees, ankles, elbows or wrists. Systemic manifestations are infrequent. Such patients are at risk of blindness from iridocyclitis. This form has the best prognosis. Pericarditis is the most common form of cardiac involvement, being seen in approximately one third of patients (Bernstein et al, 1974; Svantesson et al, 1983). The group with systemic onset is most commonly affected. Many patients may be asymptomatic from the cardiovascular point of view. Others may have signs and symptoms of acute pericarditis with chest pain, friction rub, fever, tachycardia and dyspnoea (Bernstein et al, 1974; Svantesson et al, 1983; Marin-Garcia et al, 1984). A small group may exhibit pericardial tamponade (Scharf et al, 1976; Majeed and Kvasnicka, 1978; Allukal et al, 1984). Some patients with systemic disease may develop myocarditis during the acute phase of the illness (Miller and French, 1977; Svantesson et al, 1983). Valvitis is very rarely seen. Myocarditis may be the cause of death. Both pericarditis and myocarditis may be of recurrent nature and reappear with flare-ups of the disease. The risk of recurrence is highest in the first 5 years of the disease (Svantesson et al, 1983). Chronic constrictive pericarditis has not been described. Non-specific ST segment and T wave changes are the most frequent electrocardiographic signs. Cardiomegaly with a globular-shaped heart may be seen on the chest radiograph. The echocardiogram has greatly increased the diagnosis of pericardial disease since small pericardial effusions can now be detected. Ventricular dilation is seen when myocarditis is present. Laboratory studies reveal anaemia, leucocytosis and an elevated erythrocytic sedimentation rate. Rheumatoid factor and antinuclear antibodies are very rarely seen. Analysis of the pericardial fluid shows a characteristically low level of glucose and elevation of gammaglobulins, acid phosphatase and lactic dehydrogenase (Scharf et al, 1976; Majeed and Kvasnicka, 1978).

Treatment of pericarditis is with high-dose salicyclates or indomethacin (indometacin) and steroids. The last seem to reduce the risk of tamponade (Svantesson et al, 1983; Marin-Garcia et al, 1984). Patients with myocarditis benefit from high doses of steroids and from diuretics. Digoxin must be used with extreme care because of the high risk of toxic effects (Miller and French, 1977). In the presence of tamponade, pericardial fluid must be drained urgently, either by pericardiocentesis (Scharf et al, 1976; Majeed and Kvasnicka, 1978) or pericardiectomy (Allukal et al, 1984).

SYSTEMIC LUPUS ERYTHEMATOSUS———————

Systemic lupus erythematosus is a generalized, progressive, multisystem connective tissue disease of unknown aetiology. During childhood, the mean age of onset is 12 years. Very rarely is it present before the age of 5 years (Fish et al, 1977; King et al, 1977). The cutaneous, osteoarticular, renal, haematopoietic, central nervous, pulmonary and gastrointestinal systems are commonly affected. Cardiac involvement is also very frequent and can be present at any time during the course of the disease. The most common manifestations are pericarditis, myocarditis, Libman–Sacks endocarditis leading to valvar stenosis and/or incompetence, rhythm disturbances, coronary arterial disease, and systemic and pulmonary hypertension. Any of these can lead to congestive cardiac failure, which carries a poor prognosis (Fish et al, 1977; King et al, 1977; Englund and Lucas, 1983; Ansari et al, 1985). Deposition of immune complexes and complement activation have a major pathogenetic role in these lesions.

Pericarditis is the most common cardiac manifestation. Up to three quarters of patients have echocardiographic evidence of pericardial disease. Clinical involvement is seen in one third, generally as acute pericarditis, which may have a recurrent nature. Serous effusions are common, and complement levels in the fluid are very low. Cases of chronic constrictive pericarditis and tamponade are rare.

Evidence of myocarditis can be seen in about half the patients at postmortem, but clinical involvement is generally silent. Dyspnoea is the most common symptom. The presence of a gallop rhythm, cardiomegaly on the chest radiograph and ventricular dilation on the echocardiogram complete the clinical picture. The electrocardiogram is non-specific. T wave inversion, ventricular premature beats and first-degree atrioventricular block may all be present. In approximately half the patients, the presence of non-bacterial verrucous vegetations (known as Libman–Sacks endocarditis) is noted. These are clumps of fibrin with lymphocytes and plasma cell infiltrates, which are most frequently seen on the mitral and/or aortic valves. They measure 0.1–4 mm in diameter. Fibrous tissue (which may later become calcified) appears during the healing process. This whole process leads to valvar dysfunction. Mitral and aortic incompetence (and, less frequently, stenosis) are the most common lesions. Echocardiographic evaluation is a useful non-invasive method for assessment of valvar dysfunction. Doppler examination should increase the sensitivity of early detection of valve disease. The presence of Libman–Sacks vegetations predisposes to bacterial endocarditis. Peripheral embolism is rare.

The coronary arteries can be affected by an acute inflammatory arteritic process or, less frequently in childhood, by atherosclerosis. Coronary arteritis can lead to aneurysmal dilation of the arteries, thrombosis and myocardial infarction. This is an uncommon cause of death.

Rhythm and conduction disturbances are common. Atrial fibrillation or flutter may be seen during acute pericarditis, whereas ventricular ectopic beats and first-degree atrioventricular block are seen in the course of active myocarditis. Complete heart block may result from vasculitis of small vessels, and fibrosis of the conduction system has been described in adults. Systemic hypertension is very frequent. It is generally caused by lupic nephritis or by prolonged steroid therapy.

The revised criteria for the diagnosis of systemic lupus erythematosus require the presence of at least four of the following manifestations: malar rash, discoid rash, photosensitivity, oral ulcers, arthritis, serositis (pleuritis or pericarditis), renal disorders (proteinuria, cellular casts), neurological disorders (seizures, psychosis), haematological disorders (haemolytic anaemia, leucopenia, lymphopenia, thrombocytopenia), immunological disorders (positive lupus erythematosus cell preparations, antibodies against double-stranded DNA (anti-dsDNA) or Smith protein (anti-Sm)) or antinuclear antibodies (Tan et al, 1982).

Long-term prognosis is variable. Boys seem to have a more severe form of the disease than girls. Ten-year survival rates of 86% have been reported (Fish et al, 1977). The most common causes of death are renal involvement and sepsis. Death from cardiac lesions is not frequent. Steroid therapy is the basis of treatment. Prednisolone (or an equivalent) is started at 50–75 mg/m^2 daily for 3–6 weeks and then tapered to a dose sufficient to suppress activity of the disease. Immunosuppressive therapy with azathioprine or cyclophosphamide can be used as a supplement where there is no response to high doses of steroids, or when there is severe renal or central nervous system involvement.

Apart from this systemic form of therapy, the management of specific lesions does not differ from the patient without lupus erythematosus. The presence of Libman–Sacks endocarditis requires antibiotic prophylaxis for bacterial endocarditis (Englund and Lucas, 1983).

Neonatal lupus erythematosus is a rare variety of the systemic disease. It is frequently associated with maternal lupus. It is characterized by cutaneous lesions with or without congenitally complete heart block and systemic manifestations (Reed et al, 1983; Korkij and Soltani, 1984; Lane and Watson, 1984). Skin lesions develop within the first 3 months of life and occur mainly in areas exposed to light, thus suggesting photosensitivity. They consist of erythematous macules, papules or plaques that may exhibit the characteristics of discoid lupus (scaling, atrophy, follicular plugging or telangiectasia). Later, they have residual hyper- or hypopigmentation and completely resolve within 12 months with minimal atrophy or scarring.

Systemic manifestations include hepatosplenomegaly, anaemia, leucopenia and thrombocytopenia. They occur within the first weeks of life and tend to be self-limiting. Specific treatment is rarely necessary. Congenitally complete heart block, unlike the cutaneous and systemic manifestations, is irreversible. There is a high correlation with the presence of anti-SS-A/Ro antibodies in maternal serum, these having been demonstrated in over three quarters of patients (Scott et al, 1983). The autoantibodies are frequently found in patients with systemic lupus erythematosus and Sjögren's syndrome, but they are rarely encountered in the general population. Anti-SS-A/Ro antibodies are immunoglobulin G forms that reach the fetus by transplacental transfer (Reed et al, 1983; Scott et al, 1983). They can be detected in babies with congenitally complete heart block before 3 months of age, but not after they are 6 months old. The underlying mechanism producing heart block is not clear, but it produces fibrosis of the atrial component of the atrioventricular conduction axis. Pacing may be required. In some infants, the antibodies may also affect the muscle and result in a dilated cardiomyopathy.

HEART DISEASE INDUCED BY TOXIC MECHANISMS

Adverse reactions to drugs and other substances can affect the heart in different ways. These can be classified as hypersensitivity myocarditis, toxic myocarditis, cardiomyopathy or endocardial fibrosis (Tables 67.3–67.5) (Billingham, 1980).

The list of drugs in which hypersensitivity myocarditis has been described is very long (Table 67.3). The true incidence is unknown, since it is rarely recognized clinically and, therefore, tends to be a postmortem finding. Inappropriate sinus tachycardia, mild radiographic cardiomegaly and ST segment and T wave changes on the electrocardiogram in the presence of other allergic reactions and hypereosinophilia should raise suspicion for clinical diagnosis. Diagnosis is important since sudden death from heart block or ventricular tachycardia can occur (Taliercio et al, 1985). Hypersensitivity myocarditis is not dose dependent and can occur at any time during administration of drugs. A delayed hypersensitivity reaction is the accepted mechanism. Histopathological examination reveals an interstitial inflammatory infiltrate with eosinophils, atypical lymphocytes and plasma cells, which mainly affects the ventricles. Myocytic damage is seen, but necrosis is uncommon. Severe cases may exhibit a non-necrotizing vasculitis (Billingham, 1980). These

Table 67.3. Drugs producing hypersensitivity myocarditis

Acetazolamide
Amitryptiline
Amphotericin (amphotericin B)
Carbamazepine
Chloramphenicol
Indomethacin (indometacin)
Isoniazid
Methyldopa
Para-aminosalycilic acid
Penicillin
Phenindione
Phenylbutazone
Phenytoin (diphenylhydantoin)
Smallpox vaccine
Spironolactone
Streptomycin
Sulphonamides
Sulphonylureas
Tetracyclines
Thiazide diuretics
Tetanus toxoid

Adapted from Billingham (1980) and Taliercio et al (1985).

Table 67.4. Drugs and agents producing toxic myocarditis

Antimony
Anthracycline antibiotics
Arsenicals
Barbiturates
Caffeine
Catecholamines
Cyclophosphamide
Emetine
5-Fluoruracil
Lithium carbonate
Hydralazine
Paraquat
Phenothiazines
Plasmocid
Quinidine
Rapeseed oil

Adapted from Billingham (1980).

Table 67.5. Drugs and agents producing endocardial fibrosis

Serotonin
Methysergide
Mercury
Busulfan
Radiation

Adapted from Billingham (1980).

lesions are reversible upon stopping the drug; therefore, fibrosis is not seen. Treatment is centred around discontinuing the offending drug and use of corticosteroids or immunosuppressive therapy (Taliercio et al, 1985).

Many substances have been implicated in the production of toxic myocarditis (Table 67.4). This is a dose-related condition in which the effects are cumulative. Clinical presentation is that of acute myocarditis. Extensive cellular necrosis occurs over a short period. Histopathological signs include myocardial damage, inflammatory infiltrate and acute necrotizing vasculitis (Billingham, 1980). Upon recovery, there can be multiple focal scars with residual myocardial dysfunction.

Drug-induced cardiomyopathies are most commonly attributed to alcohol, cobalt and the anthracycline antibiotics (Billingham, 1980). They produce a dilated cardiomyopathy with poor contractility, leading to congestive cardiac failure. Of these drugs, the anthracycline antibiotics, especially adriamycin, are important in childhood. Chronic cardiotoxic effects of adriamycin result in a dose-related cardiomyopathy, which generally appears at a cumulative dose exceeding 450–550 mg/m^2. There is great individual variation (Kantrowitz and Bristow, 1984). Cardiac function should be continually monitored by echocardiography and/or radionuclide angiography. Echocardiography and systolic time intervals have also been used (Brockmeier et al, 1984). If these tests are abnormal, cardiac catheterization and biopsy are warranted before discontinuing the drug (Kantrowitz and Bristow, 1984). Pathological lesions are focal and disseminated throughout the left ventricular wall and ventricular septum. Myocytes exhibit vacuolar degeneration and/or myofibrillar loss, which may progress to necrosis and interstitial fibrosis. Inflammatory infiltrates are not present (Billingham, 1980; Kantrowitz and Bristow, 1984). The formation of free radicals and the release of cardio- and vasoactive substances are the most accepted pathogenetic hypotheses. It has been postulated that the use of anthracycline antibiotics in children impairs myocardial growth, this leading to a progressive increase in afterload that may be accompanied by decreased systolic function (Lipshultz et al, 1991).

Cardiac irradiation during radiotherapy can produce a dose-related heart disease. This appears with doses greater than 4000–6000 rad, depending on the amount of cardiac surface exposed. The most common lesion is a delayed pericarditis, which generally appears within the first year of radiation. It adopts the form of an acute pericarditis with fever, pleuritic chest pain and a pericardial friction rub. Alternatively, it may produce a chronic, generally asymptomatic, pericardial effusion. Treatment is supportive and the disease tends to resolve spontaneously. Some patients develop tamponade requiring pericardiocentesis, and some progress to a chronic constrictive pericarditis that needs pericardiectomy (Stewart and Fajardo, 1984). Pancarditis is the most severe form of radiation-induced heart disease. There is pericardial and myocardial fibrosis with or without endocardial fibrosis. Patients present in intractable heart failure with the clinical and haemodynamic features of a restrictive cardiomyopathy. Irradiation and adriamycin have additive cardiotoxic effects that appear at much lower doses of each agent when both forms of therapy are used simultaneously or sequentially (Kantrowitz and Bristow, 1984; Stewart and Fajardo, 1984).

MISCELLANEOUS SYSTEMIC DISORDERS

PROGERIA

Progeria is a disease of unknown cause in which there is premature ageing. Survival beyond the second decade is rare. Affected children are normal during the first months of life, exhibiting evidence of the disease in the second year with failure to thrive, loss of subcutaneous fat, scleroderma, alopecia and development of a typical facies. This consists of a disproportionately large head for the face, 'beaked' nose, micrognathia, thin lips and prominent eyes. Skeletal abnormalities include dystrophic clavicles, thoracic deformities, knock-knees, persistent patency of the fontanelle and osteoarthritis.

Intellectual development is normal (DeBusk, 1983). The cardiovascular system is affected by premature atherosclerosis of the coronary arteries and the aorta. Most patients have ischaemic heart disease and die from myocardial infarctions. Some present with a dilated cardiomyopathy and heart failure with normal coronary arteries. Calcification of the mitral and aortic valves is common (Baker et al, 1981). Endocrine function of adrenal, thyroid, parathyroid and pituitary glands is normal. There is, however, resistance to insulin and abnormal serum lipids, with an increase in total lipids, pre-beta and beta lipoproteins. Dietary treatment with reduction of the serum lipids to within normal range does not seem to alter the course of the disease (MacNamara et al, 1970).

ARTERIOHEPATIC DYSPLASIA (ALAGILLE SYNDROME)

Arteriohepatic dysplasia is characterized by chronic cholestasis. It usually becomes apparent within the first 3 months of life with prolonged jaundice. Involved infants may present later with a heart murmur (Alagille et al, 1975; Levin et al, 1980). The other features making up this syndrome are a typical facies, vertebral malformations, peripheral pulmonary stenosis and ocular involvement. Delayed physical, mental and sexual development have not been consistently reported (Watson and Miller, 1973; Alagille et al, 1975; Greenwood et al, 1976; Levin et al, 1980; Mueller et al, 1984).

The characteristic facial appearance consists of a prominent forehead, deep-set eyes with mild hypertelorism and a small pointed chin (Watson and Miller, 1973; Alagille et al, 1975; Levin et al, 1980; Mueller et al, 1984). Ophthalmological examination reveals chorioretinal atrophy and pigment clumping, which may be pathognomonic (Mueller et al, 1984). Peripheral pulmonary stenosis is the typical cardiovascular anomaly (Watson and Miller, 1973; Alagille et al, 1975; Greenwood et al, 1976; Levin et al, 1980; Mueller et al, 1984). On physical examination, there is a prominent left parasternal impulse and an ejection systolic murmur at the upper left sternal border radiating to the back, where it may be heard extending into diastole. The electrocardiogram shows right ventricular hypertrophy. Heart size may be normal or increased on the chest radiograph and the lung fields may appear normal or oligaemic. Cardiac catheterization and angiography confirm the peripheral pulmonary stenosis, which may be single or multiple. The most frequent accompanying cardiovascular lesions are patency of the arterial duct, valvar pulmonary stenosis, and atrial and ventricular septal defects (Watson and Miller, 1973; Alagille et al, 1975; Greenwood et al, 1976; Levin et al, 1980).

Many patients have vertebral arch anomalies, usually with a butterfly appearance of the dorsal vertebras

(Alagille et al, 1975; Levin et al, 1980; Mueller et al, 1984). Xanthomas of the palms, extensor surfaces and skin creases of the hands are seen when hyperlipidaemia is present. Elevated serum lipids and cholesterol are controlled by the use of cholestyramine (colestyramine) and by the addition of corn oil to the diet (Alagille et al, 1975; Greenwood et al, 1976). Arteriohepatic dysplasia is confirmed by liver biopsy, which shows the bile ducts to be absent from most portal areas. Periportal fibrosis is absent or mild, and the extrahepatic system is patent (Alagille et al, 1975; Levin et al, 1980; Mueller et al, 1984). Additional laboratory findings include elevated 5'-nucleotidase, alkaline phosphatase, transaminases and bilirubin. Serum lipids and cholesterol are also frequently elevated (Alagille et al, 1975; Greenwood et al, 1976).

The peripheral pulmonary stenosis is not progressive, and it does not influence the long-term prognosis of the disease. Half the deaths are from hepatic or cardiac causes (Alagille et al, 1975; Greenwood et al, 1976; Mueller et al, 1984). The aetiology of the syndrome remains unknown. Intrauterine viral infections have been postulated but not proven. The tendency to appear in families suggests autosomal transmission with variable expression and reduced penetrance (Watson and Miller, 1973; Alagille et al, 1975; Greenwood et al, 1976; Levin et al, 1980; Mueller et al, 1984).

SICKLE CELL HAEMOGLOBINOPATHY

Sickle cell haemoglobulinopathy is a chronic haemolytic anaemia that predominantly affects the Black population. The underlying abnormality is the substitution of glutamic acid by valine in the sixth position of the β-chain of haemoglobin. This results in the formation of haemoglobin S. When oxygen tension is reduced, the haemoglobin S molecules polymerize and produce a crescent, sickle-shape deformity in the red cells. The pathophysiological consequences of this are vaso-occlusive phenomenons and chronic haemolysis. Organs affected by this process are the kidneys, lungs, liver, spleen, central nervous system and bones. There are a host of cardiovascular signs and symptoms in patients with sickle cell anaemia, but there is no histopathological evidence of a specific sickle cell cardiomyopathy (Gerry et al, 1978). Cardiac output is increased, with an increase in stroke volume and afterload reduction. The most common symptoms are exertional dyspnoea and palpitations. Physical examination reveals signs of a hyperdynamic circulation.

Peripheral pulses are full and the apex beat is prominent and displaced laterally. Heart sounds are loud. The second heart sound is widely split and the pulmonary component is often increased. Ejection systolic murmurs are usually present. A third heart sound may be heard, but its presence does not imply cardiac failure. Signs of congestive heart failure are rare. Peripheral oedema,

pulmonary rales and hepatomegaly may be secondary to venous stasis, pulmonary disease and cholestasis, respectively, and this can confuse the issue (Falk and Hood, 1982).

The electrocardiogram is non-specific. Signs of left ventricular hypertrophy are usually present. First-degree atrioventricular block and ST segment and T wave changes are common. Right ventricular hypertrophy is usually secondary to pulmonary vaso-occlusive disease and is more frequent in older patients. Cardiac enlargement and increased pulmonary vascular markings resembling those seen with a left-to-right shunt are the most frequent radiographic signs. Pulmonary infiltrates produced by infarction and infection may also be present. Echocardiographic examination reveals left atrial and ventricular dilation as a result of the volume overload of chronic anaemia. Left ventricular contraction is very dynamic (Falk and Hood, 1982; Balfour et al, 1984). Mitral valvar prolapse has been found in one quarter of patients with sickle cell anaemia (Lippmann et al, 1985).

Congestive cardiac failure is more common in adults than children. It appears to be secondary to coexisting renal or cardiovascular disease (Gerry et al, 1978). Myocardial dysfunction with, and abnormal response to, exercise has been demonstrated in children (Covitz et al, 1983; Deneberg et al, 1983; Balfour et al, 1984; Alpert et al, 1984). There is no clear explanation for this. Correlation analysis has shown that the most important determinants of exercise performance are haemogloblin and the haematocrit (Covitz et al, 1983; Alpert et al, 1984). Cardiac function has been shown to normalize following transfusion of packed red cells, further supporting the notion that cardiac abnormalities are related to chronic anaemia and not specific to sickle cell anaemia (Lester et al, 1990). There is no specific treatment. Transfusion of packed cells and exchange transfusions have been used. Diuretics and digitalis are rarely required. Infections are the most common cause of death in childhood (Gerry et al, 1978).

REFERENCES

Ackroyd R S, Finnegan J A, Green S H 1984 Friedreich's ataxia. A clinical review with neurophysiological and echocardiographic findings. Archives of Disease in Childhood 59: 217–221

Alagille D, Odievre M, Gautier M, Dommergues J P 1975 Hepatic ductular hypoplasia associated with characteristic facies, vertebral malformations, retarded physical, mental and sexual development and a cardiac murmur. Journal of Pediatrics 86: 63–71

Allukal M K, Costello P B, Green F A 1984 Cardiac tamponade in systemic juvenile rheumatoid arthritis requiring emergency pericardiectomy. Journal of Rheumatology 11: 222–225

Alpert B S, Dover V, Strong W B, Covitz W 1984 Longitudinal exercise hemodynamics in children with sickle cell anemia. American Journal of Diseases of Childhood 138: 1021–1024

Amit R, Bashan N, Abarbanel J M, Shapira Y, Sofer S, Moses S 1992 Fatal familial infantile glycogen storage disease: multisystem phosphofructokinase deficiency. Muscle and Nerve 15: 455–458

Ansari A, Larson P H, Bates H D 1985 Cardiovascular manifestations of systemic lupus erythematosus: current perspective. Progress in Cardiovascular Diseases 27: 421–434

Antani J, Srinivas H V 1973 Ehlers–Danlos syndrome and cardiovascular abnormalities. Chest 63: 214–217

Attas M, Hanley H G, Stultz D, Jones M R, McAllister R G 1978 Fulminant beriberi heart disease with tactic acidosis: presentation of a case with evaluation of left ventricular function and review of pathophysiologic mechanisms. Circulation 58: 566–572

Baker P B, Baba N, Boesel C P 1981 Cardiovascular abnormalities in progeria. Case report and review of the literature. Archives of Pathology and Laboratory Medicine 105: 384–386

Baldwin B J, Talley R C, Johnson C, Nutter D O 1973 Permanent paralysis of the atrium in a patient with facioscapulohumeral muscular dystrophy. American Journal of Cardiology 31: 649–653

Balfour I C, Covitz W, Davis H, Rao P S, Strong W B, Alpert B S 1984 Cardiac size and function in children with sickle cell anemia. American Heart Journal 108: 345–350

Bass J L, Shrivastava S, Grabowski G A, Desnick R J, Moller J H 1980 The M-mode echocardiogram in Fabry's disease. American Heart Journal 100: 807–812

Beighton P 1969 Cardiac abnormalities in Ehlers–Danlos syndrome. British Heart Journal 31: 227–232

Bentall H, DeBono A 1968 A technique for complete replacement of the ascending aorta. Thorax 23: 338–339

Berg R A, Kaplan A M, Jarret P B, Moltham M E 1980 Friedreich's ataxia with acute cardiomyopathy. American Journal of Diseases of Childhood 134: 390–393

Bernstein B, Takahashi M, Hanson V 1974 Cardiac involvement in juvenile rheumatoid arthritis. Journal of Pediatrics 85: 313–317

Bharati S, Bump F T, Bauernfiend R, Lev M 1984 Dystrophica myotonia. Correlative electrocardiographic, electrophysiologic and conduction system study. Chest 86: 444–450

Billingham M E 1980 Morphologic changes in drug induced heart disease. In: Bristow M R (ed.) Drug induced heart disease. Elsevier, Amsterdam, p 127–149

Blieden L B, Moller J H 1974 Cardiac involvement in inherited disorders of metabolism. Progress in Cardiovascular Diseases 16: 615–631

Blieden L C, Desnick R J, Carter J B, Krivit W, Moller J H, Sharp H L 1974 Cardiac malformations in Sandhoff's disease. Inborn error of glycosphyngolipid metabolism. American Journal of Cardiology 34: 83–88

Bloom A, Hayes T M, Gamble D R 1975 Registry of newly diagnosed diabetic children. British Medical Journal 3: 580–583

Bogousslavsky J, Perentes E, Deruaz J P, Regli F 1982 Mitochondrial myopathy and cardiomyopathy with neurodegenerative features and multiple brain infarcts. Journal of Neurological Sciences 55: 351–357

Bonneau D, Huret J L, Godeau G et al 1991 Recurrent Ctb(7)(q31.3) and possible laminin involvement in a neonatal cutis laxa with a marfan phenotype. Human Genetics 87: 317–319

Borow K M, Propper R, Bierman F Z, Grady S, Inati A 1982 The left ventricular end-systolic pressure-dimension relation in patients with thalassemia major. A new noninvasive method for assessing contractile state. Circulation 66: 980–985

Bothwell T H, Charlton R W, Motulsky A G 1983 Idiopathic hematochromatosis. In Stanbury J B Wyngarden J, Frederickson D, Golstein J, Brown M (eds) The metabolic basis of inherited disease, 5th edn. McGraw Hill, New York p 1269–1298

Boucek R J, Noble N L, Gunja-Smith Z, Butler W T 1981 The Marfan syndrome: a deficiency in chemically stable collagen cross-links. New England Journal of Medicine 305: 988–991

Bowers D 1973 Charcot–Marie–Tooth disease. Wolff–Parkinson–White syndrome and abnormal intracardiac conduction. American Heart Journal 86: 535–538

Brauman A, Algom M, Gilboa Y, Ramot Y, Golik A, Stryjer D 1985 Mitral valve prolapse in hyperthyroidism of two different origins. British Heart Journal 53: 374–377

Braunlin E A, Hunter D W, Kriuit W et al 1992 Evaluation of coronary artery disease in the Hurler syndrome by angiography. American Journal of Cardiology 69: 1487–1489

Brockmeier F K, Rosland G A, Finne P H 1984 Cardiomyopathy induced by anthracycline derivatives. Acta Paediatrica Scandinavica 73: 387–391

Bruno L, Tredici S, Mangiavacchi M, Colombo V, Mazzota G F, Sirtori C R 1984 Cardiac, skeletal and ocular abnormalities in patients with Marfan's syndrome and in their relatives. Comparison with the cardiac abnormalities in patients with kyphoscoliosis. British Heart Journal 51: 220–230

Bulkley B H, Hutchins G M 1978 Pompe's disease presenting as hypertrophic cardiomyopathy with Wolff–Parkinson–White syndrome. American Heart Journal 96: 246–252

Buja L M, Roberts W C 1971 Iron in the heart. Etiology and clinical significance. American Journal of Medicine 51: 209–221

Busch H F M, Koster J F, van Weerden T W 1979 Infantile and adult onset acid maltase deficiency occurring in the same family. Neurology 29: 415–416

Campbell M J, Liversedge L A 1981 The motor neuron diseases (including the spinal muscular atrophies). In: Walton J (ed.) Disorders of the voluntary muscle. Churchill Livingstone, Edinburgh, p 725–752

Candell-Riera J, Lu L, Seres L et al 1982 Cardiac hematochromatosis: beneficial effects of iron removal therapy: an echocardiographic study. American Journal of Cardiology 52: 824–829

Carceller A M, Fouron J C, Letarte J et al 1984 Absence of mitral valve prolapse in juvenile hyperthyroidism. American Journal of Cardiology 54: 455–456

Cavallo A, Joseph C J, Casta A 1984 Cardiac complications in juvenile hyperthyroidism. American Journal of Diseases of Childhood 138: 479–482

Chakrabarti A, Pearce J M S 1981 Scapuloperoneal syndrome with cardiomyopathy: report of a family with autosomal dominant inheritance and unusual features. Journal of Neurology, Neurosurgery and Psychiatry (London) 44: 1146–1152

Channick R J, Adlin E V, Marks A D et al 1981 Hyperthyroidism with mitral valve prolapse. New England Journal of Medicine 305: 497–500

Chapoy P, Angelini C, Brown W J, Stiff J, Shug A, Cederbaum S D 1980 Systemic carnitine deficiency – a treatable inherited lipid storage disease presenting as Reye's syndrome. New England Journal of Medicine 303: 1389–1394

Chen S, Fagan L F, Nouri S, Donahoe J L 1985 Ventricular dysrhythmias in children with Marfan's syndrome. American Journal of Diseases of Childhood 139: 273–276

Chow L T, Chow W 1992 The cardiac conduction system in Hurler syndrome: pathological features and clinical implications. Cardiology of the Young 2: 196–199

Collip P S, Chen S Y 1981 Cardiomyopathy and selenium deficiency in a two year old girl. New England Journal of Medicine 304: 1305–1306

Covitz W, Eubig C, Balfour I C, Alpert B S, Strong W B, Durant R H 1983 Exercise induced cardiac dysfunction in sickle cell anemia. A radionuclide study. American Journal of Cardiology 51: 571–575

Crawford E S 1983 Marfan's syndrome. Broad spectral surgical treatment of cardiovascular manifestations. Annals of Surgery 198: 487–505

Crossley J R, Upsdell M 1980 The incidence of juvenile diabetes mellitus in New Zealand–34. Diabetologia 18: 29

Cutler D J, Isner J M, Bracey A W et al 1980 Hemochromatosis heart disease: an unemphasized cause of potentially reversible restrictive cardiomyopathy. American Journal of Medicine 69: 923–928

Dabestani A, Child J S, Henze E et al 1984 Primary hemochromatosis: anatomic and physiologic characteristics of the cardiac ventricles and their response to phlebotomy. American Journal of Cardiology 54: 153–159

Darsee J R, Miklozek C L, Heymsfield S B, Hopkins L C, Wenger N K 1980 Mitral valve prolapse and ophthalmoplegia: a progressive cardioneurologic syndrome. Annals of Internal Medicine 92: 735–741

DeBusk F 1983 Progeria. In Behrman R E, Vaughan V C (eds) Nelson's textbook of pediatrics. Saunders, Philadelphia, PA, p 1776–1777

Deneberg B S, Criner G, Jones R, Spann J F 1983 Cardiac function in sickle cell anemia. American Journal of Cardiology 51: 1674–1678

Desnick R J, Blieden L D, Sharp H L, Moller J H 1976 Cardiac valvular anomalies in Fabry's disease: clinical, morphologic and biochemical studies. Circulation 54: 818–825

Dickey R P, Ziter F A, Smith R A 1984 Emery–Dreifuss muscular dystrophy. Journal of Pediatrics 104: 555–559

DiMauro S, Coulter D 1983 Kearn–Sayre syndrome. A possible disorder of folate and carnitine metabolism. Pediatric Research 17: 268–271

Donaldson M D C, Pennock C A, Berry P J, Duncan A W, Cawdery J E, Leonard J V 1989 Hurler syndrome with cardiomyopathy in infancy. Journal of Pediatrics 114: 429–430

Donaldson R M, Emanuel R W, Olsen E G J, Ross D N 1980 Management of cardiovascular complications in Marfan syndrome. Lancet i: 1178–1179

Donofrio P D, Challa V R, Hackshaw B T, Mills S A, Cordell R 1989 Cardiac transplantation in a patient with muscular dystrophy and cardiomyopathy. Archives of Neurology 46: 705–707

Editorial 1979 Selenium in the heart of China. Lancet ii: 889–890

Editorial 1982 Cardiovascular beriberi. Lancet i: 1287

Egger J, Wilson J 1983 Mitochondrial inheritance in a mitochondrially mediated disease. New England Journal of Medicine 309: 142–146

Egger J, Lake B D, Wilson J 1981 Mitochondrial cytopathy. A multisystem disorder with ragged red fibres on muscle biopsy. Archives of Disease in Childhood 56: 741–752

Ehlers K H, Hagstrom J W C, Lukas D S, Redo S F, Engle M A 1962 Glycogen storage disease of the myocardium with obstruction of the left ventricular outflow. Circulation 25: 96–109

Eishi Y, Takemura T, Sone R et al 1985 Glycogen storage disease confined to the heart with deficient activity of cardiac phosphorylase kinase: a new type of glycogen storage disease. Human Pathology 16: 193–197

El-Habbal M H 1992 Cardiovascular manifestations of Marfan's syndrome in the young. American Heart Journal 123: 752–757

Engbers J G, Molhoek G P, Carntzenius A C 1984 Shoshin beriberi: a rare diagnostic problem. British Heart Journal 51: 581–582

Englund J A, Lucas R V 1983 Cardiac complications in children with systemic lupus erythematosus. Pediatrics 72: 724–730

Evans T 1983 Cardiac abnormalities associated with hereditary neuromuscular diseases: In: Symons C, Evans T (eds) Specific heart muscle disease. P S G Wright, Boston p 46–61

Falk R H, Hood W B 1982 The heart in sickle cell anemia. Archives of Internal Medicine 142: 1680–1684

Fenichel G M, Sul Y C, Kilroy A W, Blouin R 1982 An autosomal dominant dystrophy with humeropelvic distribution and cardiomyopathy. Neurology 32: 1399–1401

Fish A J, Blau E B, Westberg N G, Burke B A, Vernier R L, Michael A F 1977 Systemic lupus erythematosus within the first two decades of life. American Journal of Medicine 62: 99–117

Fisher B M, Cleland J G F, Dargie H J, Frier B M 1989 Non-invasive evaluation of cardiac function in young patients with type 1 diabetes. Diabetic Medicine 6: 677–681

Fitchett D H, Coltart D J, Littler W A et al 1980 Cardiac involvement in secondary haemochromatosis: a catheter biopsy study and analysis of myocardium. Cardiovascular Research 14: 719–724

Fleming C R, Lie T J, McCall J T, O'Brien J F, Baillie E E, Thistle J L 1982 Selenium deficiency and fatal cardiomyopathy in a patient on home parenteral nutrition. Gastroenterology 83: 689–693

Forfar J C, Muir A L, Sawers S A, Toft A D 1982 Abnormal left ventricular function in hyperthyroidism. Evidence for a possible reversible cardiomyopathy. New England Journal of Medicine 307: 1165–1170

Friedman W, Mason D, Braunwald E 1965 Arthrogyropsis multiplex congenita associated with congenital aortic stenosis. Journal of Pediatrics 67: 682–685

Furukawa N, Kinugasa A, Inoue S, Imashuku, Takamatsu T, Sawada T 1990 Type 1 glycogen storage disease with vasoconstrictive pulmonary hypertension. Journal of Inherited Metabolic Disease. 13: 102–107

Gardner-Medwin D 1980 Clinical features and classification of the muscular dystrophies. British Medical Bulletin 36: 109–115

Gardner-Medwin D, Tizard J P M 1981 Neuromuscular disorders in infancy and early childhood. In: Walton J (ed.) Disorders of voluntary muscle. Churchill Livingstone, Edinburgh, p 625–663

Gaucher P C E 1882 De l'epitheliome primitif de la rate. These de Paris

Gerry J L, Bulkley B H, Hutchins G M 1978 Clinicopathologic analysis of cardiac dysfunction in 52 patients with sickle cell anemia. American Journal of Cardiology 42: 211–216

Geva T, Sanders S P, Diogenes M S, Rockenmacher S, Van Praagh R 1990 Two-dimensional and Doppler echocardiographic and pathologic characteristics of the infantile Marfan syndrome. American Journal of Cardiology 65: 1230–1237

Gillette P C, Nihill M R, Singer D B 1974 Electrophysiological mechanism for the short PR interval in Pompe's disease. American Journal of Diseases of Childhood 128: 622–626

Goldberg S J, Stern L Z, Feldman L, Sahn D J, Allen H D, Valdes-Cruz L M 1983 Serial left ventricular wall measurements in Duchenne's muscular dystrophy. Journal of the American College of Cardiology 2: 136–142

Gottdiener J S, Hawley R J, Gay J A, DiBanco R, Fletcher R D, Engel W K 1982a Left ventricular relaxation, mitral valve prolapse and intracardiac conduction in myotonia atrophica: assessment by digitized echocardiography and non-invasive His bundle recording. American Heart Journal 104: 77–85

Gottdiener J S, Hawley R J, Maron B J, Bertorini T F, Engle W K 1982b Characteristics of the cardiac hypertrophy in Friedreich's ataxia. American Heart Journal 103: 525–531

Greenwood R D, Rosenthal A, Crocker A C, Nadas A S 1976 Syndrome of intrahepatic binary dysgenesis and cardiovascular malformations. Pediatrics 58: 243–247

Greeves L G, Carson D J, Craig B G, McMaster D 1990 Potentially life-threatening cardiac dysrhythmia in a child with selenium deficiency and phenylketonuria. Acta Paediatrica Scandinavica 79: 1259–1263

Gross D M, Williams J C, Caprioli C, Domingues B, Howell R R 1988 Echocardiographic abnormalities in the mucopoly sacchande storage diseases. American Journal of Cardiology 61: 170–176

Hamaoka K, Nakagawa M, Furukawa N, Sawada T 1990 Pulmonary hypertension in type 1 glycogen storage disease. Pediatric Cardiology 11: 54–56

Harding A E, Hewler R L 1983 The heart disease of Friedreich's ataxia: a clinical and electrocardiographic study of 115 patients, with an analysis of serial electrocardiographic changes in 30 cases. Quarterly Journal of Medicine 208: 489–502

Harper P 1979 Myotonic dystrophy. Saunders, Philadelphia

Harpey J, Charpentier C, Coudé M, Diury P, Paturneau-Jouas M 1987 Sudden infant death syndrome and multiple acyl-coenzyme A dehydrogenase deficiency, ethylmalonic–adipic aciduria, or systemic carnitine deficiency. Journal of Pediatrics 110: 881–883

Harpey J, Charpentier C, Peturneau-Jouas M 1990 Sudden infant death syndrome and inherited disorders of fatty acid β-oxidation. Biology of Neonates 58: 70–80

Hart Z H, Chang C, DiMauro S, Farooki Q, Ayyar R 1978 Muscle carnitine deficiency and fatal cardiomyopathy. Neurology 28: 147–151

Hassan Z U, Fastabend C P, Mohanty P K, Isaacs E R 1979 Atrioventricular block and supraventricular arrhythmias with X-linked muscular dystrophy. Circulation 60: 1365–1369

Hayflick S, Rowe S, Kavanaugh-McHugh A, Olson J L, Valle D 1992 Acute infantile cardiomyopathy as a presenting feature of mucopolysaccharidosis VI. Journal of Pediatrics 120: 269–272

Hollister D W, Godfrey M, Sakai L Y, Pyeritz R E 1990 Immunohistologic abnormalities of the microfibrillar-fiber system in the Marfan syndrome. New England Journal of Medicine 323: 152–159

Hopkins L C, Jackson J A, Elsas L J 1981 Emery–Dreifuss humeroperoneal muscular dystrophy and X-linked myopathy with unusual contractures and brachycardia. Annals of Neurology 10: 230–237

Howat A J, Bennett M J, Variend S, Shaw L, Engel P C 1985 Defects of metabolism of fatty acids in the sudden infant death syndrome. British Medical Journal 290: 1771–1773

Hunsaker R H, Fulkerson P K, Barry F J, Lewis R P, Leier C V, Unverferth D V 1982 Cardiac function in Duchenne's muscular dystrophy. Results of a 10 year follow-up study and non-invasive tests. American Journal of Medicine 73: 235–238

Hunter C 1916 A rare disease in two brothers. (Elevation of scapula, limitation of movement of joints and other skeletal abnormalities.) Proceedings of the Royal Society of London 104–116

Ikram H, Maslowski A H, Smith B L, Nicholls M G 1981 The haemodynamic, histopathological and hormonal features of alcoholic cardiac beriberi. Quarterly Journal of Medicine 200: 359–375

Isner J M, Hawley R J, Weintraub A M, Engel W K 1979 Cardiac findings in Charcot–Marie–Tooth disease: a prospective study for 68 patients. Archives of Internal Medicine 139: 1161–1165

Jackson C, Carey J 1961 Progressive muscular dystrophy: autosomal recessive type. Pediatrics 28: 77–84

John R M, Hunter D, Swantan R H 1990 Echocardiographic abnormalities in type IV mucopolysaccharidosis. Archives of Disease in Childhood 65: 746–749

Johnson R A, Baker S S, Fallon J T et al 1981 An occidental case of cardiomyopathy and selenium deficiency. New England Journal of Medicine 304: 1210–1212

Kantrowitz N E, Bristow M R 1984 Cardiotoxicity of antitumor agents. Progress in Cardiovascular Diseases 27: 195–200

Katiyar B C, Misra S, Somani P N, Chaterji A M 1977 Congestive cardiomyopathy in a family of Becker's X-linked muscular dystrophy. Postgraduate Medical Journal 53: 12–15

Kawai C, Wakagayashi A, Matsumura T, Yui Y 1980 Reappearance of beriberi heart disease in Japan. A study of 23 cases. American Journal of Medicine 69: 383–386

Kelley T E, Bartoshesky L, Harris D J, McCauley R G K, Feingold M, Schott G 1981 Mucolipidosis I (acid neuraminidase deficiency). Three cases and delineation of the variability of phenotype. American Journal of Diseases of Childhood 135: 703–708

King K K, Kornreich H K, Bernstein B H, Singsen B H, Hanson V 1977 The clinical spectrum of systemic lupus erythematosus in childhood. Arthritis and Rheumatism 20: 2:287–294

Korkij W, Soltani K 1984 Neonatal lupus erythematosus: a review. Pediatric Dermatology 1: 189–195

Krovetz L J, Lorincz A E, Schiebler G I 1965 Cardiovascular manifestations of the Hurler syndrome: hemodynamic and angiocardiographic observations in 15 patients. Circulation 31: 132–141

Labrune P, Huguet P, Odieure M 1991 Cardiomyopathy in glycogen storage disease type III: clinical and echographic study of 18 patients. Pediatric Cardiology 12: 161–163

Lane A T, Watson R M 1984 Neonatal lupus erythematosus. American Journal of Diseases of Childhood 138: 663–666

Lascelles R G, Baker I A, Thomas P K 1970 Hereditary polyneuropathy of Roussy–Lévy type with associated cardiomyopathy. Guys Hospital Reports 119: 253–262

Lebenthal E, Shochet S B, Adam A et al 1970 Arthrogryopsis multiplex congenita: twenty three cases in an Arab kindred. Pediatrics 46: 891–899

Leier C V, Call T D, Fulkerson P K, Wooley C F 1980 The spectrum of cardiac defects in Ehler–Danlos syndrome types I and III. Annals of Internal Medicine 92: 171–178

Leon M B, Borer J S, Bacharach S L et al 1979 Detection of early cardiac dysfunction in patients with severe beta-thalassemia and chronic iron overload. New England Journal of Medicine 301: 1143–1148

Leroy J G, Demars R I 1967 Mutant enzymatic and cytological phenotypes in cultured human fibroblasts. Science 157: 804–806

Lester L A, Sodt P C, Hutcheon N, Arcilla R A 1990 Cardiovascular effects of hypertransfusion therapy in children with sickle cell anemia. Pediatric Cardiology 11: 131–137

Levin S E, Zarvos P, Milner S, Schmaman A 1980 Arteriohepatic dysplasia: association of liver disease with pulmonary arterial stenosis as well as facial and skeletal abnormalities. Pediatrics 66: 876–883

Lewis D, White H, Dunn M 1966 Refsum's syndrome. A neurological disease with interesting cardiovascular manifestations. American Journal of Cardiology 17: 128–129

Lippman S M, Ginzton L E, Thigpen T, Tanaka K R, Laks M M 1985 Mitral valve prolapse in sickle cell disease. Presumptive evidence for a linked connective tissue disorder. Archives of Internal Medicine 145: 435–438

Lipshulttz S E, Colan S D, Gelber R D, Perez-Atayae A R, Sallen S E, Sanders S P 1991 Late cardiac effects of doxorubicin therapy for acute lymphoblastic leukemia in childhood. New England Journal of Medicine 324: 808–815

Littler W A 1970 Heart block and peroneal muscular atrophy. Quarterly Journal of Medicine 155: 431–439

Lowry P J, Littler W A 1983 Peroneal muscular atrophy associated with cardiac conducting tissue disease: further observations. Postgraduate Medical Journal 59: 530–532

Mace S, Hirschfield S, Riggs T, Fanaroff A, Merkatz J R 1979 Echocardiographic abnormalities in infants of diabetic mothers. Journal of Pediatrics 95: 1013–1019

MacNamara B G P, Farn K T, Mitra A K, Lloyd J F, Fosbrooke A S 1970 Progeria. Case report with long term studies of serum lipids. Archives of Diseases in Childhood 45: 553–560

McComish M, Compston A, Jewitt D 1976 Cardiac abnormalities in chronic progressive external ophthalmoplegia. British Heart Journal 38: 526–529

McDonald G R, Schaff H V, Pyeritz R E, McKusick V A, Gott V L 1981 Surgical management of patients with the Marfan syndrome and dilatation of the ascending aorta. Journal of Thoracic and Cardiovascular Surgery 81: 180–186

McIntyre N, Stanley N N 1971 Cardiac beriberi: two modes of presentation. British Medical Journal 3: 567–569

Majeed H A, Kvasnicka J 1978 Juvenile rheumatoid arthritis with cardiac tamponade. Annals of the Rheumatic Diseases 37: 273–276

Marin-Garcia J, Sheridan R, Hanissian A S 1984 Echocardiographic detection of early cardiac involvement in juvenile rheumatoid arthritis. Pediatrics 73: 394–397

Marwick T H, Bastian B, Hughes C F, Bailey B P 1992 Mitral stenosis in the Maroteaux–Lamy syndrome: a treatable cause of dyspnoea. Fellowship of Postgraduate Medicine 68: 287–288

Matalon R, Deanching M, Nakamura F, Bloom A 1980 A recessively inherited lethal disease in a caribbean isolate. A sulfamidase deficiency. Pediatric Research 14: 542–545

Mehta J, Desnick R J 1978 Abbreviated PR interval in mannosidosis. Journal of Pediatrics 92: 599–601

Mehta J, Tuna N, Moller J H, Desnick R J 1977 Electrocardiographic and vectorcardiographic abnormalities in Fabry's disease. American Heart Journal 93: 699–705

Miller C G, Alleyne G A, Broons S E H 1972 Gross cardiac involvement in glycogen storage disease type III. British Heart Journal 34: 862–864

Miller J J, French J W 1977 Myocarditis in juvenile rheumatosis arthritis. American Journal of Diseases of Childhood 131: 205–209

Mitchell A G 1983 Cardiac disease associated with iron overload. In: Symons C, Evans T (eds) Specific heart muscle disease. P S G Wright, Boston p 33–45

Mori H, Utsunomiya T, Ishiyima M, Shibuya N, Oku Y, Hashiba K 1990 The relationship between 24 hour total heart beats or ventricular arrhythmias and cardiopulmonary function in patients with Duchenne's muscular dystrophy. Japanese Heart Journal 5: 599–608

Moses S W, Wanderman K L, Myroz A, Frydman M 1989 Cardiac involvement in glycogen storage disease type III. European Journal of Pediatrics 148: 764–766.

Mueller R F, Pagon R A, Pepin M G et al 1984 Arteriohepatic dysplasia: phenotypic features and family studies. Clinical Genetics 25: 323–331

Murdoch J L, Walker B A, Halpern B L, Kuzma J W, McKusick V A 1972 Life expectancy and causes of death in the Marfon syndrome. New England Journal of Medicine 13: 804–808

Neal R A, Sauberlich H E 1980 Thiamine. In: Goodhart R S, Shils M E (eds) Modern nutrition in health and disease. Lea & Febiger, Philadelphia, PA, p 191–197

Neufeld E F, McKusick V A 1983 Disorders of lysosomal enzyme synthesis and location: 1-cell disease and pseudo-Hurler polydystrophy. In: Stanbury J B, Wyngaarden J B, Fredrickson D S, Goldstein J L, Brown M S (eds) The metabolic basis of inherited disease, 5th edn. McGraw-Hill, New York, p 778–787

Neustein H B, Lurie P R, Dahms B, Takahashi M 1979 An X-linked recessive cardiomyopathy with abnormal mitochondria. Pediatrics 64: 24–29

Ose L, McKusick V A 1977 Prophylactic use of propranolol in the Marfan syndrome to prevent aortic dissection. Birth Defects: Original Article Series 13: 163–169

Pentland B, Fox K A A 1983 The heart in Friedreich's ataxia. Journal of Neurology, Neurosurgery and Psychiatry (London) 46: 1138–1142

Pereira V G, Masuda Z, Katz A, Tronchini V 1984 Shoshin beriberi: report of two successfully treated patients with hemodynamic documentation. American Journal of Cardiology 53: 1467–1471

Perkins K W, McInnes I W S, Blackburn C R B, Beal R W 1965 Idiopathic haemochromatosis in children. Report of a family. American Journal of Medicine 39: 118–126

Perloff J K, Stevenson W G, Roberts N K, Cabeen W, Weiss J 1984 Cardiac involvement in myotonic muscular dystrophy (Steinert's disease): a prospective study of 25 patients. American Journal of Cardiology 54: 1074–1081

Phornphutkul C, Rosenthal A, Nadas A S 1973 Cardiac manifestations of Marfan syndrome in infancy and childhood. Circulation 47: 587–596

Pilapil V R, Watson D G 1979 Electrocardiogram in hyperthyroid children. American Journal of Diseases of Childhood 119: 245–248

Poulos A, Pollard A C, Mitchell J D, Wise G, Mortimer G 1984 Patterns of Refsum's disease. Archives of Disease in Childhood 59: 222–229

Prystowsky E N, Pritchett E L, Roses A D, Gallagher J 1979 The natural history of conduction system disease in myotonic muscular dystrophy as determined by serial electrophysiologic studies. Circulation 60: 1360–1364

Pyeritz R E, McKusick V A 1979 The Marfan syndrome: diagnosis and management. New England Journal of Medicine 300: 772–777

Pyeritz R E, Gott V L, McDonald G R et al 1982 Surgical repair of the Marfan aorta: technique, indications and complications. Johns Hopkins Medical Journal 151: 71–82

Rebouche C J, Engel A G 1983 Carnitine metabolism and deficiency syndromes. Mayo Clinic Proceedings 58: 533–540

Reed B R, Lee L A, Harmon C et al 1983 Autoantibodies to SS-A/RO in infants with congenital heart block. Journal of Pediatrics 103: 889–891

Resnick D, Niwayama G 1981 Juvenile chronic arthritis. In: Resnick D, Niwayama G (eds) Diagnosis of bone and joint disorders. Saunders, Philadelphia, PA, p 1008–1039

Roberts W C, Honig H S 1982 The spectrum of cardiovascular disease in the Marfan syndrome: a clinics–morphologic study of 18 necropsy patients and comparison to 151 previously reported necropsy patients. American Heart Journal 104: 115–135

Rondanini G F, de Danizza G, Bollati et al 1991 Congenital hypothyroidism and pericardial effusion. Hormone Research 35: 41–44

Rosenburg H, Frewen T C, Li M D et al 1985 Cardiac involvement in diseases characterized by β-galactosidase deficiency. Journal of Pediatrics 106: 78–80

Salter R H 1968 The muscle glycogenoses. Lancet i: 1301–1304

Sandstead H H 1980 Clinical manifestations of certain classical deficiency diseases. In Goodhart R S, Shils M E (eds) Modern nutrition in health and disease. Lea & Febiger, Philadelphia, PA, p 685–696

Sanyal S K, Johnson W W 1982 Cardiac conduction abnormalities in children with Duchenne's progressive muscular dystrophy: electrocardiographic features and morphologic correlates. Circulation 66: 853–863

Saradar M, Atalay S, Koçak N, Özkutlu S 1991 Gaucher's disease with mitral and aortic involvement: echocardiographic findings. Pediatric Cardiology 13: 56–58

Savolainen A, Keto P, Hakal P et al 1992 Aortic distensibility in children with Marfan syndrome. American Journal of Cardiology 70: 691–692

Scharf J, Levy J, Benderly A, Nahir M 1976 Pericardial tamponade in juvenile rheumatoid arthritis. Arthritis and Rheumatism 19: 760–762

Scott J S, Maddison P J, Taylor P V, Esscher E, Scott O, Skinner R P 1983 Connective tissue disease, antibodies to ribonucleoprotein and congenital heart block. New England Journal of Medicine 309: 209–212

Sengers R C, Stadhouders A M, Trijbels J M 1984 Mitochondrial myopathies. Clinical, morphological and biochemical aspects. European Journal of Pediatrics 141: 192–207

Servidei S, Metlay L A, Chodosh J, Di Mavro S 1988 Fatal infantile cardiopathy caused by phosphorylase β-kinase deficiency. Journal of Pediatrics 113: 82–85

Short E M, Winkle R A, Billingham M E 1981 Myocardial involvement in idiopathic hemochromatosis. Morphologic and clinical improvement following venesection. American Journal of Medicine 70: 1275–1279

St John Sutton M G, Olukotun A Y, Tajik A J, Lovett J L, Giuliani E R 1980 Left ventricular function in Friedreich's ataxia. An echocardiographic study. British Heart Journal 44: 309–316

Stanley C A, DeLeeuw S, Coates P M et al 1991 Chronic cardiomyopathy and weakness or acute coma in children with a defect in carnitine uptake. Annals of Neurology 30: 709–716

Steare S E, Dubowitz V, Benatar A 1992 Subclinical cardiomyopathy in Becker muscular dystrophy. British Heart Journal 68: 304–308

Steinberg D 1983 Phytanic acid storage disease (Refsum's disease). In Stanbury J B, Wyngarden J, Frederickson D, Golstein J, Brown M (eds) The metabolic basis of inherited disease, 5th edn. McGraw-Hill, New York, p 731–747

Stephan M J, Stevens E L, Wenstrup R J et al 1989 Mucopolysaccharidosis I presenting with endocardial fibroelastosis of infancy. American Journal of Diseases of Childhood 143: 782–784

Stevenson W G, Perloff J K, Weiss J N, Anderson T L 1990 Facioscapulohumeral muscular dystrophy: evidence for selective genetic electrophysiologic cardiac involvement. Journal of the American College of Cardiology 15: 292–299

Stewart J R, Fajardo L F 1984 Radiation induced heart disease: an update. Progress in Cardiovascular Diseases 27: 173–194

Svantesson H, Bjorkhem G, Elborgh R 1983 Cardiac involvement in juvenile rheumatoid arthritis. A follow-up study. Acta Paediatrica Scandinavica 72: 345–350

Takamoto K, Hirose K, Uono M, Nonaka I 1984 A genetic variant of Emery–Dreifuss disease. Muscular dystrophy with humeropelvic distribution, early joint contracture and permanent atrial paralysis. Archives of Neurology 41: 1293–1294

Taliercio C P, Olney B A, Lie J T 1985 Myocarditis related to drug hypersensitivity. Mayo Clinic Proceedings 60: 463–468

Tan C T T, Schaff H V, Miller F A, Edwards W D, Karnes P S 1992 Valvular heart disease in four patients' with Maroteaux–Lamy Syndrome. Circulation 85: 188–195

Tan E M, Cohen A S, Fries J F et al 1982 The 1982 revised criteria for the classification of systemic lupus erythematosus. Arthritis and Rheumatism 25: 1217–1277

Tanaka H, Uemeura N, Toyama Y, Kudo A, Ohkatsu Y, Kanehisa T 1976 Cardiac involvement in the Kugel–Welander syndrome. American Journal of Cardiology 38: 528–532

Taylor D, Blaser S I, Burrows P E, Stringer D A, Clarke J T R, Thorner P 1991 Arteriopathy and coarctation of the abdominal aorta in children with mucopolysaccharidosis: imaging findings. American Journal of Roentgenology 157: 819–823

Thomas P K, Schott G D, Morgan-Hughes J A 1975 Adult onset of scapuloperoneal myopathy. Journal of Neurology, Neurosurgery and Psychiatry, London 38: 1008–1015

Tonsgard J H, Stephens J K, Rhead W J et al 1991 Defect in fatty acid oxidation: laboratory and pathologic findings in a patient. Pediatric Neurology 7: 125–130

Tripp M E, Ketcher M L, Peters H A, et al 1981 Systemic carnitine deficiency presenting as familial endocardial fibroelastosis. New England Journal of Medicine 305: 385–390

van de Kamp J J P 1979 The Sanfillipo syndrome: a clinical genetical study of 75 patients in the Netherlands. Doctoral Thesis. S-Gravenhage J H Pasmans

Verheist W, Brucher J M, Goddeeris P, Lauweryns J, de Geest H 1976 Familial centronuclear myopathy associated with cardiomyopathy. British Heart Journal 38: 504–509

Vetter U, Maierhoter B, Müller M et al 1989 Ostenogensis imperfecta in childhood: cardiac and renal manifestations. European Journal of Pediatrics 149: 184–187

Vietor K W, Haysteen B, Harms D, Busse H, Heyne K 1977 Ethanolaminosis: a newly recognized generalized storage disease with cardiomegaly, cerebral dysfunction and early death. European Journal of Pediatrics 126: 61–75

Vigorita V J, Hutchins G M 1979 Cardiac conduction system in hemochromatosis: clinical pathologic features of six patients. American Journal of Cardiology 44: 418–423

Waber L J, Valle D, Neill C, DiMauro S, Shug A 1982 Carnitinas familial cardiomyopathy: a treatable defect in carnitine transport. Journal of Pediatrics 101: 700–705

Walton J N, Gardner-Medwin D 1981 Progressive muscular dystrophy and the myotonic disorders. In: Walton J (ed.) The disorders of voluntary muscle. Churchill Livingstone, Edinburgh, p 481–524

Waters D D, Nutter D O, Hopkins L C, Dorney E R 1975 Cardiac features of an unusual X-linked humeroperoneal neuromuscular disease. New England Journal of Medicine 293: 1017–1022

Watson G H, Miller V 1973 Arteriohepatic dysplasia. Familial pulmonary stenosis with neonatal liver disease. Archives of Disease in Childhood 48: 459–466

Way G L, Wolfe R R, Eshaghpour E, Bender R L, Jaffe R B, Ruttenberg H D 1979 The natural history of hypertrophic cardiomyopathy in infants of diabetic mothers. Journal of Pediatrics 95: 1020–1025

Westwood M 1977 Endocardial fibroelastosis and Niemann–Pick disease. British Heart Journal 39: 1394–1396

White N J, Winearls C G, Smith R 1983 Cardiovascular abnormalities in osteogenesis imperfects. American Heart Journal 106: 1416–1420

Yoshioka M, Saida K, Itagaki Y, Kamiya T 1989 Follow up study of cardiac involvement in Emery–Dreifuss muscular dystrophy. Archives of Disease in Childhood 64: 713–715

68
Systemic hypertension

C. Reid and C. Chantler

INTRODUCTION

Persistent systemic hypertension is a major cause of morbidity and mortality in adults. Early recognition and appropriate treatment are associated with a considerably improved prognosis. Essential hypertension is the most common form of hypertension in adults, but it is becoming increasingly clear that the origin of this condition is in childhood. Secondary hypertension is clinically much more important in children and is commonly caused by renal disease. Detection and control not only reduce the general morbidity of hypertension but also protect the function of the already damaged kidney. Recent pharmacological advances fortunately enable the blood pressure to be controlled in all patients with a minimum of undesirable side effects. Consequently, the management of hypertension is particularly rewarding for the practising paediatrician.

THE MEASUREMENT OF SYSTEMIC BLOOD PRESSURE

Probably the most common cause of apparent hypertension is inadequate measurement of blood pressure.

CUFF SIZE

The most common error in measurement of blood pressure is the selection of the wrong size of cuff. The inflatable bladder, rather than the cloth envelope which surrounds it, should be the correct width and length. In this respect, a plastic non-distensible cuff or bladder is probably more reliable than the usual cloth cuff with a separate rubber bladder (Steinfeld et al, 1978). The bladder should be centred over the brachial artery and should encircle most (at least three quarters) of the upper arm. The width should be two thirds of the length of the upper arm. In practice, the widest cuff that will still enable auscultation of the antecubital fossa is used. Appropriate sizes are shown in Table 68.1. The most common error

Table 68.1. Sizes of sphygmomanometer cuffs

	Width of bladder (cm)	Length of bladder (cm)
Newborns	4	5–10
Infants	6	12
1–5 years	8	15
6–9 years	10	20
10 years and over	13	23
Obese adults	15	30
Adult thigh	18	36

Adapted from Leuman (1979).

with babies is to choose a cuff that is too short to encircle the arm. It is important when comparing pressures in the arms and legs of a child with suspected aortic coarctation to use a large leg cuff applied to the thigh or above the ankle (Elseed et al, 1973). The size of the cuff used should be recorded so that sequential pressures can be compared.

TECHNIQUE OF MEASUREMENT

Mercury sphygmomanometers are preferred to aneroid manometers, which, while less bulky, require regular calibration. Random zero sphygmomanometers, which eliminate digit preference bias by the observer, are preferred in epidemiological studies in children (Nuutinen et al, 1992), though their use has been questioned recently in adults (Conroy et al, 1993). The child should be relaxed and quiet when the recording is made. It is useless to measure the blood pressure in a crying infant. The infant of 6 weeks, when awake, has a systolic pressure, on average, 7 mmHg higher than when asleep (de Swiet et al, 1980). The child should sit comfortably, with the right arm fully exposed resting on a table at the level of the heart. Rolling up the sleeve of shirts or pullovers in order to fit the cuff is not satisfactory. The sphygmomanometer should be placed at the level of the observer's eye to eliminate error from parallax. It is important to inflate the cuff about 20 mmHg above the point at which the radial pulse disappears. In some patients with hypertension, a 'silent gap' exists between the systolic and diastolic pressures. Simply inflating the cuff until the sounds disappear in such individuals will produce a sometimes serious underestimation of systolic blood pressure. After inflation, the cuff is deflated at a rate of 2–3 mmHg/s while auscultating over the brachial artery. The sudden distension of the collapsed artery at the systolic pressure is associated with a clear tapping sound, defined as phase 1 of the Korotkoff sounds. The murmur of turbulent blood flowing through the partially occluded artery is phase 2. Phase 3 is a high-pitched sound produced when the artery, closed during diastole, opens in systole. When the artery no longer closes during diastole, the tapping sounds are low pitched and muffled and quieter. This is phase 4. Phase 5, when the sounds disappear, is variable and may not occur in some children. Phase 4 tends to overestimate the diastolic pressure while phase 5 underestimates it. Phase 4 has generally been preferred in the United Kingdom (Short, 1976) and was recommended by the Task Force Reports on Blood Pressure Control in Children (NHLBI, 1977, 1987). Phase 5, nonetheless, was recommended by an international committee in 1987 (Scharer, 1987), and the 1996 update on the Task Force Recommendations also advocates using phase 5 (NHBPEP, 1996). Recording the systolic pressure by palpation of the radial artery underestimates the pressure by 11 ± 8 mmHg (Elseed et al, 1973).

The measurement of blood pressure in infants, and in some older children, is sometimes difficult because the sounds are inaudible. The old flush technique is unreliable. It has now been superseded by the use of Doppler ultrasound, using an ultrasonic beam to detect motion of the arterial wall when the cuff is deflated. This technique is remarkably reliable for measurement of the systolic pressure and corresponds to the intra-arterial pressure better than any other method, including auscultation (Elseed et al, 1973). It is less reliable in the measurement of diastolic pressure, even when machines specifically designed for diastolic pressure are used (Whyte et al, 1975). All hospital paediatric departments, especially those specializing in paediatric cardiology, should have an ultrasound machine for measurement of blood pressure. It is particularly useful in determining pressure in the legs in children with suspected aortic coarctation (Elseed et al, 1973). Automatically inflated cuffs have recently been introduced; these measure both systolic and diastolic blood pressure and record the results at preset time intervals by detecting oscillations in the pressure from the cuff. They are especially useful in the care of the critically ill child because they save nursing time and reduce disturbance of the patient. The calibration needs to be checked frequently if the result is to be regarded as accurate, but they are useful in detecting changes. Indeed, they will alarm automatically if preset parameters are exceeded.

AMBULATORY MEASUREMENT OF BLOOD PRESSURE

Recently, ambulatory monitoring of blood pressure using a small, portable, programmable monitor has become a well-accepted method for the diagnosis of hypertension and assessment of treatment in adults. There is now an expanding literature derived from children, providing normal values based on sex and age (Krull et al, 1993; Harshfield et al, 1994; Reusz et al, 1994; Reichert et al, 1995; Soergel et al, 1997) and using measurements in different disease states (Lingens et al, 1995, 1997). The monitors typically use an oscillometric technique. They can be programmed to record the blood pressure frequently, for example every 30 minutes during the day and hourly at night. The readings are stored for later downloading, display and analysis by personal computer. The monitor can be worn on the belt or in the pocket, and the recording is made as the children carry on their normal daytime and night-time activities. This method avoids observer error and bias and is more reproducible than readings of blood pressure made in the clinic. It identifies those patients who have high blood pressure readings when seen in clinic but whose blood pressure is normal in their everyday environment (so-called 'white coat hypertension', discussed below). Ambulatory monitoring provides a better measure of total blood pressure load than does casual blood pressure readings (Zachariah et al, 1988). The result correlates more closely with measures of damage to the heart (Devereux et al, 1983; White et al, 1989) and kidneys (Giaconi et al, 1989) induced by blood pressure. Perhaps the main reservation about the method is that none of the major trials of intervention and drug treatment in hypertension have been based on ambulatory readings, and there is still relatively little information on the long-term prognostic value of these readings.

NORMAL BLOOD PRESSURE IN CHILDHOOD

A large number of studies have been undertaken to establish the range of blood pressure found in normal children (Leuman, 1979). The results for boys are summarized in Figure 68.1. As a general rule, a steady increase in blood pressure with age has been observed, with no significant difference between the sexes during childhood. Most studies, unfortunately, differ in some respect: in the sizes of cuff used, whether measurements are taken with the patient sitting or supine, different end-points used for diastolic pressure and so on. These differences in technique make apparent differences between ethnic groups difficult to interpret. Nigerian children were found to have higher pressures than Black-American children (Aderele and Seriki, 1974). Higher values for Black than White children might be expected in view of the higher

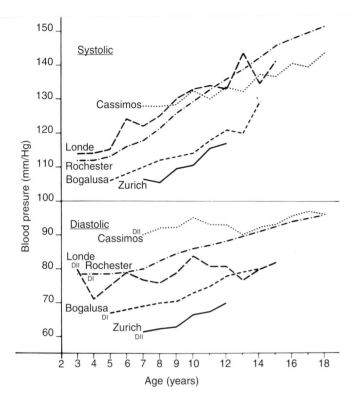

Figure 68.1. The 95th percentile for systolic and diastolic blood pressure in boys taken from various sources. Data were from the Rochester (Minnesota) study (NHLBI, 1977), including data from the Muscatine (Iowa) study (Clark et al, 1978); a Scandinavian study (Cassimos et al, 1977); the Bogalusa study (Voors et al, 1976); the Zurich study (Leuman et al, 1979); and the Londe study (Londe, 1968). The conditions and measurement parameters varied. Children were seated, except in the study of Londe, where they were supine. The cuff widths used were 9 and 13 cm (Scandinavian study), two thirds of the upper arm (Londe study), at least two thirds of upper arm (Rochester), mostly 10 and 12.5 cm (Bogalusa) and the largest possible (Zurich). Standard mercury sphygmomanometers were used except in the Zurich study, where random zero manometers were used. There is an overlap between diastolic I (DI, muffling, phase 4) and diastolic II (DII, cessation of sounds, phase 5). (Reprinted with permission of the author and publisher from Leuman, 1979.)

prevalence of hypertension in Black adults. These were reported by the Bogalusa study (Voors et al, 1976), but similar (NHLBI, 1987; Harshfield et al, 1993) or lower (Londe et al, 1977) values have also been found. A significant increase in the proportion of hypertensive 18-year-old Black adolescents has been reported (Kilcoyne et al, 1974a; Roberts and Maurer, 1977). Harshfield et al (1993) found no difference in the renin–angiotensin–aldosterone system when comparing black and white children and adolescents.

Burlage (1923), in an early study, suggested that height rather than age was the appropriate standard to which blood pressure should be related. After controlling for height, the effect of age on blood pressure disappears. Voors et al (1977) suggested that evaluation of blood pressure in an individual should be based on both height and weight rather than age. It is not clear whether sexual maturation has an effect, independent of body mass, on blood pressure (Leuman, 1979). Obesity poses special problems because of the essential requirement for an adequate cuff in making measurements. Where adequate sizes have been used, obese adolescents have been found to have a higher incidence of hypertension (Levine et al, 1976; Londe et al, 1977a,b). Maxwell et al (1982) have derived corrections according to the circumference of the arm and the size of the cuff used in the measurement. These are shown in Table 68.2. Values of serum cholesterol and triglyceride do not show much relation to blood pressure (Voors et al, 1976), but levels of glucose in the plasma 1 hour after a glucose load were found to correlate with blood pressure independently of weight (Florey et al, 1976). Reliable data concerning salt intake and

blood pressure in children are not yet available. Children in an area with drinking water that contained a large amount of salt, however, had higher blood pressures (Calabrese and Tuthill, 1977). No relation between blood pressure and preference for salt was noted in the Muscatine study (Lauer et al, 1976). No difference was apparent in blood pressure between bottle- and breast-fed infants (de Swiet et al, 1980).

The practising clinician requires standards with which to compare the blood pressure of individual patients. These are provided by Figures 68.2–68.4, which show centile charts developed by the Second Task Force on Blood Pressure Control in Children (NHLBI, 1987). An update on this 1987 Task Force Report has been published, giving very comprehensive charts of 90th and 95th percentile blood pressure values for seven different height centiles at each age from 1 to 17 years (NHBPEP, 1996).

NORMAL VALUES FOR AMBULATORY MONITORING OF BLOOD PRESSURE

Data on 24-hour ambulatory monitoring in normal children and adolescents have now been published by several authors (Krull et al, 1993; Harshfield et al, 1994; Reusz et al, 1994; Reichert et al, 1995; Soergel et al, 1997). These publications contain detailed tables and graphs of mean and standard deviation for systolic and diastolic blood pressure, for day and night, and by sex, height and age. There are some common findings in all the series. An important pattern in normal children and adolescents is

Table 68.2. Correction of systolic and diastolic readings of blood pressure, obtained with cuffs of different sizes according to arm circumference

Arm circumference (cm)	Correction (mmHg) for varying cuff size					
	12 cm × 23 cm		15 cm × 30 cm		18 cm × 36 cm	
	S	D	S	D	S	D
20	+11	+7	+11	+7	+11	+7
22	+9	+6	+9	+6	+11	+6
24	+7	+9	+8	+5	+10	+6
26	+5	+3	+7	+5	+9	+5
28	+3	+2	+5	+4	+8	+5
30	0	0	+4	+3	+7	+4
32	−2	−1	+3	+2	+6	+4
34	−4	−3	+2	+1	+5	+3
36	−6	−4	0	+1	+5	+3
38	−8	−6	−1	0	+4	+2
40	−10	−7	−2	−1	+3	+1
42	−12	−9	−4	−2	+2	+1
44	−14	−10	−5	−3	+1	0
46	−16	−11	−6	−3	0	0
48	−18	−13	−7	−4	−1	−1
50	−21	−14	−9	−5	−1	−1
52	−23	−16	−10	−6	−2	−2
54	−25	−17	−11	−7	−3	−2

Adapted from Maxwell et al (1982).
D, diastolic; S, systolic.

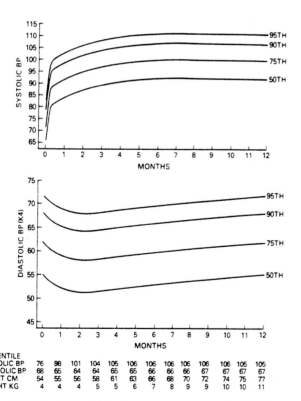

90TH PERCENTILE												
SYSTOLIC BP	76	98	101	104	105	106	106	106	106	106	106	105	105
DIASTOLIC BP	68	65	64	64	65	65	66	66	66	67	67	67	67
HEIGHT CM	54	55	56	58	61	63	66	68	70	72	74	75	77
WEIGHT KG	4	4	4	5	5	6	7	8	9	9	10	10	11

Figure 68.2. Percentiles of blood pressure measurement in girls from birth to 12 months of age. (Reprinted from the second report of the Task Force on Blood Pressure Control in Children (1987), with permission. Copyright American Academy of Pediatrics.)

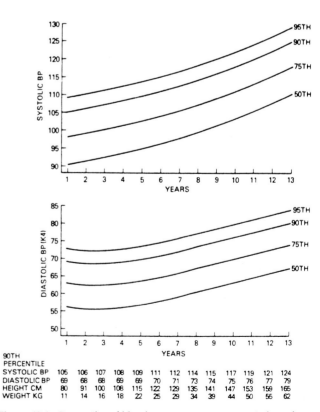

90TH PERCENTILE												
SYSTOLIC BP	105	106	107	108	109	111	112	114	115	117	119	121	124
DIASTOLIC BP	69	68	68	69	69	70	71	73	74	75	76	77	79
HEIGHT CM	80	91	100	108	115	122	129	135	141	147	153	159	165
WEIGHT KG	11	14	16	18	22	25	29	34	39	44	50	55	62

Figure 68.3. Percentiles of blood pressure measurement in boys from 1 to 13 years of age. (Reprinted from the second report of the Task Force on Blood Pressure Control in Children (1987), with permission. Copyright American Academy of Pediatrics.)

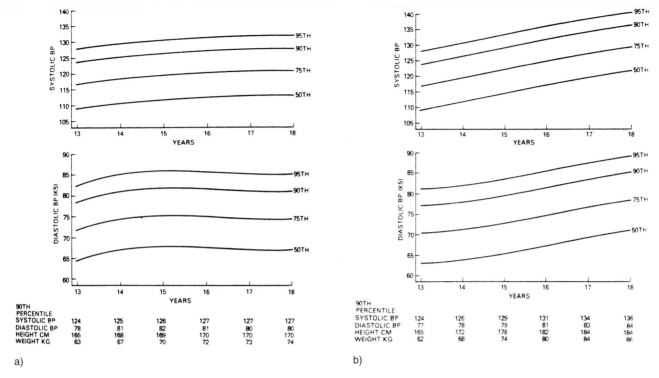

Figure 68.4. Percentiles of blood pressure measurement in girls (a) and boys (b) aged 13 to 18 years. (Reprinted from the second report of the Task Force on Blood Pressure Control in Children (1987) with permission. Copyright American Academy of Pediatrics.)

the nocturnal fall in blood pressure relative to daytime values. The average fall is 12–13% for systolic blood pressure and 21–23% for diastolic blood pressure (Krull et al, 1993; Reusz et al, 1994; Soergel et al, 1997). Mean ambulatory systolic and diastolic blood pressures are higher during the daytime than casual readings for the same age and height. Consequently, normal values based on casual measurements, such as the Task Force data described above, should not be used for assessment of readings obtained by ambulatory monitoring. While Krull et al (1993) and Reusz et al (1994) found no differences in blood pressure between the sexes for the age range 6 to 14 years, Harshfield et al (1994) found higher values for boys at all ages from 10 to 18 years, and Soergel et al (1997) found higher values for boys at all heights. Harshfield et al (1994) found higher values for Black teenagers when sleeping compared with White teenagers, though there was no daytime difference. Alpert and Daniels (1997) speculate that this reduced nocturnal fall in blood pressure in Black children may represent an increased blood pressure load, which might contribute to the excess morbidity and mortality from essential hypertension seen in Black-Americans.

VARIABILITY OF BLOOD PRESSURE

Serial determinations of blood pressure are necessary before concluding that a child is hypertensive. Kilcoyne

(1974a) found that the proportion of children with a systolic blood pressure greater than 140 mmHg fell from 5.4 to 1.2% on repeat determination. In the Muscatine study (Rames et al, 1978), the proportion of 6600 children with a blood pressure higher than the 95th percentile fell from 13% to less than 1% when restudied. Similarly, Falkner et al (1981) found 11.2% of boys of high school age had blood pressures above the 90th percentile on first measurement. Hypertension defined as a blood pressure higher than the 95th percentile was found in only 1.8% of 13–14 year olds, 4.2% of 14–15 year olds and 7.9% of 15–16 year olds when measured 12 months later. A higher proportion, therefore, of older boys had persistent hypertension. Many who were originally on the 90th per centile remained at that level. There is a general tendency for initially high blood pressures to regress towards the mean. This tendency is greatest in those with the highest pressures. It is not clear whether the initial recording or the later basal record is the better predictor of hypertensive disease (Beevers, 1982). It is important to recognize that most people have a highly labile blood pressure (Pickering, 1968). Only one fifth of those identified as having a labile blood pressure when young will have definite hypertension in later life (Julius, 1977). It seems reasonable, at least in children, only to follow up those whose blood pressure is persistently raised. General advice in relation to weight, smoking and other risk factors (see below) should be given to those adolescents who are persistently borderline.

TRACKING

The tendency of the blood pressure of an individual to rise with time along the percentile of the initial determination has been called 'tracking'. Miall and Lovell (1967) followed the blood pressure of two cohorts from South Wales over a period of 8 to 10 years. They showed that the rise noted was significantly related to mean pressure at first determination but only indirectly related to age. This conclusion was confirmed in a larger study extending over 30 years (Harlan et al, 1973). Tracking indicates that the blood pressure of an individual is determined from an early age. Any rise that occurs becomes steeper with time and is related to the initial starting pressure. Blood pressure does not rise with age in everyone. Indeed, in some populations it does not rise at all (Peart, 1980). This emphasizes the pathological nature of a raised blood pressure, and of tracking. The importance of tracking in children is, first, whether it occurs and, if it does so, at what age. Second, whether tracking would enable individuals at risk of development of hypertensive disease to be identified with reasonable reliability early in life. A number of studies have demonstrated tracking in childhood (Clarke et al, 1978; Zinner et al, 1978; Leuman, 1979). The phenomenon is not so marked as in adults, but the relation between initial and later pressures increases significantly as the population passes through adolescence. In the study of Zinner et al (1978), two thirds of 88 children with systolic blood pressures more than one standard deviation above the mean at the initial evaluation were above the mean at follow-up. In the Muscatine study (Clarke et al, 1978), the correlation coefficient for systolic pressures measured 6 years apart was 0.30. The correlation in adults is about 0.7, and this is achieved by about 18 years of age (Zinner et al, 1978). Rosner et al (1977) demonstrated tracking from 5 years of age. De Swiet et al (1980a,b) have shown, in a careful study following babies from birth, that it starts between 1 and 5 years of age. By 4 years, the correlation in repeated measurements was 0.47. It is not yet clear, however, with what confidence it will be possible to predict those individuals who will be at risk from hypertension when they become adults. The realization that the rise in blood pressure with age is not inevitable, and that individuals at risk might be identified early so that appropriate avoidance of risk factors might ameliorate their future morbidity, is of considerable potential importance. Further research is required to identify those risk factors (see below) to show that their avoidance alters prognosis and to demonstrate the reliability of early identification of a raised blood pressure in predicting future disease.

FAMILIAL CLUSTERING

The tendency for parents and children and siblings to have similar blood pressures is well recognized amongst adults. This clustering is apparent in children, with a correlation between siblings of 0.33 at the age of 2–14 years (Zinner et al, 1971). Significant, though less strong, correlations have been found between mothers and infants as young as 1 week (Biron and Mongeau, 1978). Studies on adopted children, compared with other members of the family, including non-adopted siblings, have shown no correlation between the blood pressure of adopted children and other members of the family. The blood pressure of the parents and the non-adopted children, in contrast, correlated significantly (Biron and Mongeau, 1978). This implies that, at least in children, inheritance is more important than environment in determining blood pressure. Environment is not without influence, however, and the duration of adoption rather than age at adoption, as well as resemblance in body weight, was linked to the small positive aggregation of blood pressure observed in adoptees living in the same home (Biron et al, 1977; Biron and Mongeau, 1978).

EXERCISE, TRACTION AND HYPERTENSION

Isometric rather than dynamic exercise is associated with a greater rise in diastolic pressure (Strong et al, 1978). The Task Force Group (NHLBI, 1977) expressed doubt concerning the advisability of isometric exercise, such as weight lifting, body building and so on, in hypertensive children. Fixler et al (1979), however, demonstrated no dangerous rise in either diastolic or systolic pressure during either dynamic or isometric exercise in hypertensive adolescents. Nudel (1980) concluded that maximal exercise testing was safe in hypertensive adolescents. Their exercise performance was normal, though systolic and diastolic pressures were higher than in children with labile hypertension. They suggested that exercise testing should be recommended to identify those with an excessive response (blood pressure greater than 230/120 mmHg). This finding might indicate caution in allowing full participation in physical activity such as competitive sports. With this caveat, exercise is recommended for hypertension because it is associated with a useful reduction in peripheral vascular resistance and blood pressure (McEnery and Davis, 1978). Children undergoing orthopaedic immobilization with plaster casts, or those in traction, have a fourfold greater incidence of hypertension (Turner et al, 1979). The rise in blood pressure averaged 33 mmHg in one study, being maximal on the fourth day of treatment. It resolved when the treatment was stopped (Linshaw et al, 1979). The cause is not known, but it has been related to increased sympathetic activity from stretching of the sciatic nerve, to retention of salt and water from immobilization, and to increased production of catecholamines causing increased output of renin from the kidney (Linshaw et al, 1979).

HYPERTENSION

'When I use a word,' Humpty Dumpty said in a rather scornful tone, 'it means just what I choose it to mean, neither more nor less.' 'The question is,' said Alice, 'whether you can make words mean different things.' 'The question is,' said Humpty Dumpty, 'which is to be master, that's all.'
(*Alice Through The Looking Glass*, Lewis Carroll).

DEFINITION

There is no agreed definition of what constitutes hypertension (Peart, 1980). Blood pressure is a continuous variable within a population. Any decision to regard a certain level as pathological must, therefore, be arbitrary (Pickering, 1968). It is possible, nonetheless, to define the statistical likelihood of a pathological event occurring at a given level of blood pressure. If the generally observed rise in blood pressure with advancing age in adult life is itself pathological, then the appropriate cut-off point might be the mean +2 standard deviations for a young adult (140/90 mmHg). Alternatively, an even lower value of 125/75 mmHg might be taken, since this represents the mean. The rise with age in childhood discussed previously is probably related to body size. It is, therefore, to be regarded as physiological. In children, the normal can be defined in relation to the population. Values above the 95th percentile are then regarded as being more likely to represent abnormality. This approach necessarily defines 5% of the population as being hypertensive. Such an approach is probably not relevant in adult life, because the population used to establish normality is not itself normal, at least in Western societies. The most appropriate definition, therefore, is the level above which there is an associated significant risk of developing an increased morbidity and mortality in the future (Peart, 1980). For example, men aged from 40 to 69 years with a blood pressure of 160/100 mmHg are four times more likely to die than those with a blood pressure of 120/80 mmHg (Office of Health Economics, 1980). A man with a blood pressure of 150/100 mmHg at the age of 45 years can expect to live 11 years less than a man with a blood pressure of 120/80 mmHg (Metropolitan Life Insurance Company, 1961).

The next question to be asked is whether treatment to lower blood pressure will be associated with a reduction in the excess morbidity and mortality. It is now generally accepted that treatment should be given to an adult with a diastolic blood pressure persistently above 110 mmHg. Trials have been conducted (Management Committee 1980, 1982; Hypertension Detection and Follow-Up Programme Cooperative Group, 1982; Medical Research Council, 1985) to evaluate the effect of lowering blood pressure in adults with diastolic pressures between 90 and 109 mmHg, and to judge the associated costs and benefits (Office of Health Economics, 1980). There was a significant decrease in the incidence in stroke, though not all studies found a decrease in mortality from all causes. Current recommendations for patients with mild hypertension include starting non-pharmacological treatment, such as exercise and modification of diet, in all and targeting groups at high risk, such as those with diabetes or pre-existing cardiovascular disease, and patients over 60 years of age for pharmacological treatment (Black, 1993; Langer, 1995; Swales, 1995; Ramsay et al, 1996). It is still too early, nonetheless, to determine general policy or, indeed, to recommend mass screening.

It will be apparent, therefore, that any definition of hypertension is to some extent arbitrary and no universally acceptable definitions are available. For children, we offer the following suggestions. A child up to adolescence with either systolic and/or diastolic pressures persistently at or above the 95th percentile for height and age can be said to have mild hypertension. After adolescence, the value exceeding the 95th percentile for an adolescent may be regarded as abnormal. This may be taken as a blood pressure greater than 140/90 mmHg. In contrast, a child whose blood pressure, either systolic and/or diastolic, persistently exceeds the 95th percentile by at least 15 mmHg can be said to have severe hypertension (Leuman, 1979). Malignant hypertension can then be defined as the presence of hypertensive retinopathy, this reflecting severe vascular damage secondary to hypertension.

CLASSIFICATION

Primary, or essential, hypertension is a term used to describe hypertension for which no obvious cause is apparent. This is the most common type of mild hypertension found in children. Secondary hypertension, where the raised blood pressure is caused by primary disease or abnormality in other organs, usually the kidneys, is the most common cause of severe hypertension in children. Increasing knowledge has enabled some children with severe hypertension previously regarded as primary now to be classified as secondary.

Systolic and diastolic hypertension may be present simultaneously. Isolated systolic hypertension, with a wide pulse pressure, may be a feature of hyperthyroidism, aortic valvar incompetence, patency of the arterial duct or an arterio-venous shunt. Stress may cause a rise in both systolic and diastolic pressure, or in systolic pressure alone.

White-coat hypertension is the term coined for measurements that are higher when taken in the clinic than in self-measurement at home or in ambulatory monitoring. It is well known that the presence of medical personnel influences blood pressure (Mancia et al, 1983). From one fifth to two fifths of individuals with borderline hypertension measured in the clinic can be reclassified as normotensive during daytime ambulatory monitoring (Pickering et al, 1988). There is debate over the risk of cardiovascular morbidity for this group of patients. Glen et al (1996) found abnormalities of arterial elasticity and diastolic ventricular function similar to those found in persistently hypertensive patients. Furthermore, white-coat hypertension may evolve to sustained hypertension (Bidlingmeyer et al, 1996). McGrath (1996) maintains that white-coat hypertension probably carries a cardiovascular risk somewhere between that of sustained hypertension and normotension. The natural history of this group of patients, and the effect of treating them, will require very long-term large clinical studies.

The severity of the vascular changes observed on retinal examination permits grading of hypertension. Grade I changes occur with mild venous narrowing at the site of arterial crossing, with slight thickening of the arterial wall. In grade II, there is obvious arteriolar thickening – the so-called 'copper wire' appearance. Grade III changes exist when the arteriolar wall is so thick that no column of blood is visible – the 'silver wire' appearance with marked venous compression. Grade IV changes are described when the arterioles are thin fibrous cords with no distal flow. Retinal haemorrhages and exudates are additionally present in grade III, while papilloedema is a feature of grade IV retinopathy. Malignant hypertension is associated with grade IV retinopathy. Severe retinal changes are less common in children, though papilloedema is observed in hypertensive encephalopathy with headache, drowsiness and convulsions (Balfe and Rance, 1978).

PREVALENCE

The overall prevalence of mild hypertension must be about 5%, because this is determined by the definition. The definition, however, requires that the raised blood pressure be persistent. This will tend to lower the prevalence, while the inclusion of systolic or diastolic pressure within the definition will tend to raise it. Kilcoyne et al (1974a), after repeated screening of adolescents, identified 1.2% (for systolic) and 2.4% (for diastolic) as having mild hypertension. Results from various surveys (Leuman, 1979) range from 13 and 2% at initial screening to about 1% with persistent mild hypertension.

The prevalence rate for severe hypertension is difficult to ascertain. It can only be determined from surveys of populations. Detailed diagnoses are not always provided in such studies. Prevalence rates for secondary hypertension vary between zero and 0.2% in various surveys (Leuman, 1979). They vary according to the type of survey, and the selection and referral to hospital for investigations. Some studies of normal populations covering thousands of children have revealed no cases of severe secondary hypertension (Dube et al, 1975; Leuman, 1979). In the Muscatine study (Rames et al, 1978), 0.1% had secondary hypertension. Results

obtained from other surveys were Pistulkova et al (1976) 0.07%, Gill (1977) 0.11%, Strunge and Trostmann (1978) 0.17% and Bridigkeit (1978, quoted by Leuman, 1979) 0.2%.

CAUSES OF HYPERTENSION

Table 68.3 lists some of the conditions that may be associated with hypertension. The list is not exhaustive, and the selection and classifications somewhat arbitrary. In contrast, Table 68.4 shows the final diagnosis of 100 children referred with severe hypertension to a specialized

Table 68.3. Causes of hypertension in children

System	Condition
Renovascular	Renal artery stenosis, neurofibromatosis, thrombosis, trauma, fistula, external compression, haemolytic uraemic syndrome
Parenchymal renal disease	Nephritis, nephrosis, pyelonephritis (reflux nephropathy), trauma, Wilms' tumour, haemangiopericytoma, cystic disease, obstructive uropathy, dysplasia, hypoplasia, radiation nephritis, cortical necrosis, Henoch–Schönlein disease, post-transplantation, collagen disease, heavy metal poisoning, amyloidosis, Fabry's disease, nephrocalcinosis, uric acid nephropathy
Cardiovascular	Aortic coarctation, polycythaemia, anaemia, pseudoxanthoma elasticum, Takayasu's arteritis, patent arterial duct, arterio-venous fistula, leukaemia, subacute bacterial endocarditis, aortic incompetence, salt and water overload
Endocrine	Phaeochromocytoma, neuroblastoma, hyperthyroidism, congenital adrenal hyperplasia, Conn's syndrome, Cushing's syndrome, Liddle's syndrome, hyperparathyroidism, ovarian tumours, dexamethasone-suppressive hyperaldosteronism, 17-hydroxylase deficiency, 11-hydroxylase deficiency, idiopathic mineralocorticoid excess
Metabolic and drugs	Porphyria, hypercalcaemia, vitamin D intoxication, liquorice ingestion, diabetes mellitus, hypernatraemia, steroid administration, amphetamine or sympathomimetic overdosage (including nose-drops), contraceptive pills
Central nervous system	Raised intracranial pressure, dysautonomia, Guillain–Barré syndrome, poliomyelitis, convulsions, anxiety
Miscellaneous	Essential, burns, traction, dehydration, Stevens–Johnson syndrome

Table 68.4. Final diagnosis in 100 children referred consecutively over a 5-year period, according to age

	Age (years)			
	0–1	1–5	6–15	All
Chronic glomerulonephritis		2	33	35
Reflux nephropathy			14	14
Obstructive uropathy	1	1	4	6
Haemolytic uraemic syndrome	1	2	3	6
Renovascular	1	3	2	6
Polycystic (infantile and adult)		1	3	4
Dysplastic kidneys			3	3
Cystinosis			3	3
Hypoplastic kidneys		1	1	2
Juvenile nephronophthisis			2	2
Wilms' tumour				2
Papillary necrosis		1		1
Essential hypertension			1	1
Obesity			1	1
Aortic coarctation	8	5	2	15
Total	12	16	72	100

From Gill et al (1976).

centre. Results from other surveys of secondary hypertension are similar (Still and Cotton, 1967; Buehlmeyer, 1974; Uhari and Koskimies, 1979). On average in these four series, 67% of the children had renal disease, 7% had renal vascular hypertension, 22% had aortic coarctation, 1.5% had an endocrine cause and 2.5% had some other disorder. In practice, the daunting list of conditions in Table 68.3 is hardly relevant. If the primary condition is not obvious, and coarctation is excluded, renal disease accounts for the vast majority of cases.

Table 68.4 also shows the age distribution of the different causes identified. Aortic coarctation, renovascular hypertension (mainly from thrombosis of the renal artery following umbilical arterial catheterization) and intracranial haemorrhage are common causes in neonates and infants. In the pre-school child, aortic coarctation, renovascular causes, congenital renal abnormalities, tumours and haemolytic uraemic syndrome predominate. In the older child, chronic nephritis, reflux nephropathy and end-stage renal disease are more common.

CLINICAL FEATURES AND COMPLICATIONS

The presenting symptom of hypertension varies according to the severity of the causative disease, the severity of the hypertension and the age of the child. The raised blood pressure may be an unexpected cause of a common childhood symptom, such as recurrent abdominal pain or headache. Alternatively, it may be an incidental and apparently unconnected finding on physical examination in a child with another complaint. In our series of 100

consecutive cases, 16% were being examined for a cardiac murmur. In a further 17%, the hypertension was an incidental finding (Gill et al, 1976). One child with a blood pressure of 240/130 mmHg at the age of 5 years presented with recurrent abdominal pain and had severe bilateral renal arterial stenosis. The renal function was normal, however, largely because of an extensive anastomotic blood supply to the kidneys (Figure 68.5). Table 68.5 shows the major clinical symptoms of 45 infants and 600 children with hypertension reported in the literature and analysed by Leuman (1979). Anorexia and haematuria, respectively, were the presenting features in another two of our children. Inspection of this list emphasizes the need to exclude hypertension in any sick child. It is tragic, therefore, to note that the measurement of blood pressure is often not included in the physical examination. Our experience includes the development of hypertensive encephalopathy, convulsions, residual permanent neurological disability, blindness, end-stage renal failure and other complications in children previously treated at home or in hospital for headaches, facial palsy, poor growth, abdominal pain and so on, but all without their blood pressures being determined.

Congestive cardiac failure with fluid overload is a common feature in severe hypertension caused by renal disease. Cardiac dilation with mitral incompetence may be present and this will disappear after control of the hypertension. Pulmonary oedema may be life threatening and require immediate positive pressure ventilation. The fluid overload is treated with intravenous frusemide (furosemide; 5 mg/kg body weight) to induce diuresis, or

Table 68.5. Clinical syndromes of hypertension

Syndromes	Percentage
Infants	
Congestive cardiac failure	56
Respiratory distress	36
Failure to thrive, vomiting	29
Irritability	20
Convulsions	11
Children	
Headache	30
Nausea, vomiting	13
Hypertensive encephalopathy	10.6
Polydipsia, polyuria	7.4
Visual problems	5.2
Tiredness, irritability	4.5
Cardiac failure	4.5
Facial palsy	3.4
Epistaxis	3.0
Growth retardation, weight loss	2.7
Cardiac murmur	2.7
Abdominal pain	1.8
Enuresis	1.2

Data from 645 infants and children.
From Leuman (1979).

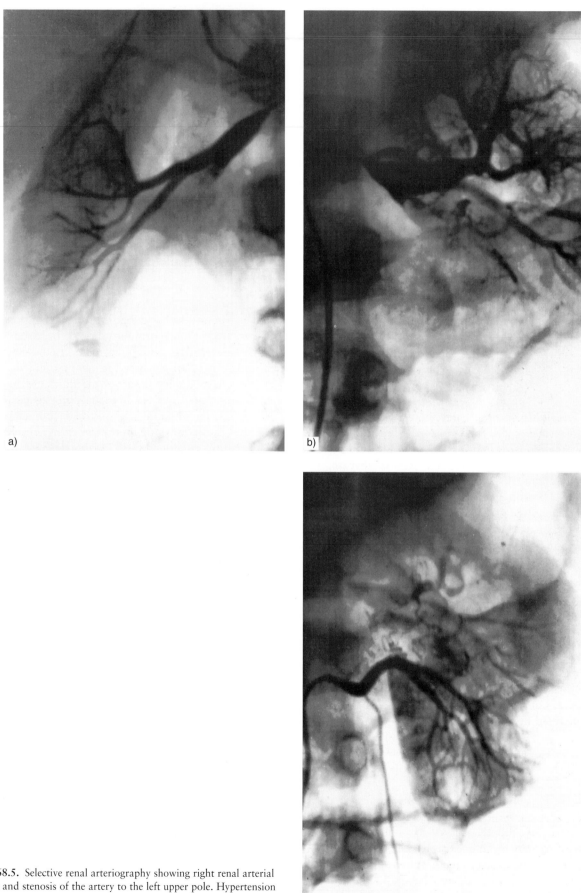

Figure 68.5. Selective renal arteriography showing right renal arterial stenosis and stenosis of the artery to the left upper pole. Hypertension was cured by placing a saphenous vein graft from the aorta to beyond the stenosis on the left, and by autotransplantation of the right kidney.

with dialysis if renal failure is present. Malignant hypertension may be associated with a cardiac myopathy (see Chapter 59), with improvement in ventricular function as the vasculitis subsides following hypotensive therapy. Obstructive cardiomyopathy with septal hypertrophy has been described in children on chronic dialysis (Drukker, 1981). It is probably related, at least in part, to chronic hypertension. The decision whether to treat borderline hypertension is often difficult. Evidence of associated disease should be sought. The features that may be present include minor retinal changes; cardiac enlargement; altered ventricular function (such as increased left ventricular stroke work) associated with a raised afterload, which leads to concentric ventricular hypertrophy and can be detected by echocardiography (Savage et al, 1979; Messerli, 1982), and left ventricular hypertrophy, which is detected by electrocardiography.

About one tenth of children with hypertension have neurological symptoms and complications (Gill et al, 1976; Uhari et al, 1979). In such children, the neurological problem is frequently the presenting feature. A review of 45 children with neurological features associated with hypertension showed that convulsions were the most frequently encountered complication, occurring in 92% of the children (Trompeter et al, 1982). Facial palsy and an altered level of consciousness were each encountered in 4%. Cuneo and Caronna (1977) proposed that the neurological complications could be classified into three syndromes: hypertensive encephalopathy, lacunar infarction and cerebral haemorrhage. In hypertensive encephalopathy, there is focal damage to cerebral arterioles. This increases capillary permeability and results in cerebral oedema. Headache is a common feature. Visual complaints range from blurring of vision to transient blindness. Nausea and vomiting are often present; convulsions, both focal and general, occur more frequently in children. Papilloedema alone or with retinal haemorrhages is often present. Long-term follow-up suggests that the prognosis is good with no permanent neurological deficit. No focal abnormality is found on computed tomography of the brain following a single episode of hypertensive encephalopathy (Trompeter et al, 1982). Magnetic resonance imaging of the brain, nonetheless, may reveal characteristic changes (Hinchey et al, 1996). A tendency to convulsions may continue, however, and infarction or cerebral haemorrhage may lead to permanent disability. One of the patients described by Uhari and co-workers (1979) had impaired vision and apraxia following infarction. Two more with cerebral haemorrhage were left with a hemiplegia, while one child died from cerebral haemorrhage. In spite of the relatively good prognosis in survivors, hypertensive encephalopathy is potentially fatal and requires urgent treatment.

Visual disturbances may be caused by retinal involvement; cortical blindness associated with cerebral oedema, which usually resolves leaving no residual impairment; vitreous haemorrhage; and infarction of the anterior visual pathways (Hulse et al, 1979). The last leads to permanent disability with absent pupillary responses to light, defects in the visual field and optic atrophy. It probably results from vasculitis of the small vessels. One of the patients described by Hulse et al (1979) also had a transverse myelopathy, probably related to hypotension following treatment. The prevention of cerebral haemorrhage in patients with malignant hypertension requires a rapid reduction in blood pressure. Hypotension must not occur if cerebral, spinal or optic nerve infarction is to be avoided (see Treatment, below). The blood pressure that should be considered as hypotensive is a relative figure because a higher level of pressure may be required to maintain adequate cerebral perfusion in the chronically hypertensive.

DIAGNOSIS

At diagnosis, it is necessary to establish the severity of the effects of the hypertension and the cause. A complete family history is important. Essential hypertension is often familial. Some types of renal disease are inherited (Chantler, 1983). Diabetes mellitus has a familial predisposition, congenital adrenal hyperplasia is an autosomal recessive disorder and neurofibromatosis has a dominant inheritance. Renal disease is a common cause of death in sickle cell disease, and so on. The blood pressure of the parents and siblings should be measured. The past history must include conditions or events that could have been related to renal disease. In this list, events may be included such as trauma to the kidneys; urinary tract infection; polyuria or polydipsia; perinatal asphyxia, which may have caused renal infarction or renal venous thrombosis; congenital rubella; abdominal radiation; proteinuria; haematuria; and so on. The present history will include drug ingestion and symptoms associated with hypertension, such as headaches, epistaxis or blurred vision. The periodicity of the symptoms should be elicited. Intermittent episodes of headache, flushing, sweating and palpitations may suggest a phaeochromocytoma. The physical examination should include measurement of blood pressure both standing and lying, the determination of blood pressure in the legs, a record of height and weight, palpation of all peripheral pulses, examination for bruits particularly over the carotid arteries and renal areas, a full cardiac and neurological examination, and palpation for abdominal masses or enlargement of the bladder. Evidence for neurofibromatosis, such as café-au-lait patches, Cushing's disease, the depigmented areas of tuberous sclerosis, systemic lupus erythematosus and so on should be sought. Longstanding renal insufficiency is often associated with poor growth, delayed skeletal and sexual maturation, anaemia and renal osteodystrophy.

A strong indication of the cause of the hypertension is often present from the history and examination. The

15–30% of children with secondary hypertension caused by aortic coarctation should certainly be identified. As a general rule, essential hypertension is usually mild while secondary hypertension is severe. Routine investigations, and those designed to establish the severity of the hypertension, will include a full blood count, measurement of the blood electrolytes, chest radiograph, electrocardiogram and an echocardiogram (Laird and Fixler, 1981; Berenson et al, 1989). The urine should be examined for blood, protein, cells, and casts, and it should be cultured. Unless the cause is obvious, urinary vanillylmandelic acid (see below) is usually determined to exclude either a phaeochromocytoma or hypertension caused by neuroblastoma. An intravenous urogram or an alternative (see below) investigation is usually performed.

Renal disease, or renal arterial stenosis, is by far the commonest cause of secondary hypertension in childhood. This will usually be apparent as the cause after these routine investigations. Specific investigations required for the exact renal diagnosis are discussed below under the relevant section. A raised level of plasma renin taken while supine is a useful indicator of renal disease. It may also be raised, however, when renal damage is sustained from hypertension from a non-renal cause. The necessary control of the hypertension with drugs prior to investigation frequently invalidates the determination of plasma renin. A hypokalaemic alkalosis suggests a mineralocorticoid syndrome, but secondary hyperaldosteronism from hyper-reninism will produce similar electrolytic disturbances. Unless the hypertension is mild, the initial control and diagnosis requires admission to hospital.

PROGNOSIS

The prognosis for hypertension in children depends on many factors, but particularly on the nature of the underlying disease. The prognosis for severe hypertension that is untreated or inadequately controlled is extremely poor. Of 55 children seen between 1954 and 1964, one third were dead within 14 months, and uraemia was responsible for 18 of the fatalities (Still and Cotton, 1967). The advent of effective hypotensive agents has improved the outcome. Only 17 of 100 children seen between 1970 and 1975 died, though an additional 34 children were alive on dialysis or following renal transplantation (Gill et al, 1976). Only 11 of 164 children reviewed by Uhari and Koskimies (1979) died over a period of follow-up of 1 to 17 years (mean 4 years).

SCREENING

Controversy exists as to whether normal children should be screened for hypertension. The Task Force examining blood pressure in children in the United States of America (NHLBI, 1977) concluded that children aged 3 years and older should have their blood pressure measured annually as part of their continuing health care. More recent reports from the United States have questioned the usefulness of routine blood pressure measurement (Gillman et al, 1993). British editorial opinion has been that screening of blood pressure in children is unjustified because the technique is laborious and the results difficult to interpret. Blood pressure in children is very variable, and the correlation between initial and follow-up measurements is not sufficiently strong to allow predictions of future blood pressure levels to be made from initial recordings (Houtman and Dillon, 1991; de Swiet, 1992). One could add that the rate of identification of severe hypertension is too low to justify the expense (Editorial, 1973, 1977). For mild hypertension, the dilemma is considerable, because a predictably large number of such children would necessarily be identified by a screening programme. To label an apparently well child as hypertensive could, and probably would, cause great harm. To treat mild hypertension is expensive and may be dangerous. But to leave hypertensive children undiagnosed, who may become hypertensive adults, may also be undesirable (Editorial, 1979).

The issues with severe hypertension are more clear cut. Early diagnosis allows effective treatment, prevents complications and improves life expectancy. While screening of a normal population of children for hypertension is not cost-effective (NHLBI, 1987), the measurement of blood pressure should be part of the normal physical examination of a child. Children with a blood pressure higher than the 95th percentile for age or height should be recalled for further measurement. If found to be normal, no further follow-up is required, though general advice concerning weight reduction, diet and so on should be given. The child with severe hypertension is investigated immediately. The infrequent child with mild hypertension should be followed (see below). Ambulatory monitoring may help to establish whether the child with mild hypertension found in the clinic also has mild but sustained hypertension at home or at school, or whether they have white-coat hypertension (see above).

HYPERTENSION IN INFANTS

The diagnosis of hypertension in infancy requires knowledge of the normal limits for blood pressure. Data in premature and term neonates, and in infants in the first year of life, are limited (de Swiet et al, 1980; Hegyi et al, 1996). A particular obstacle to establishing normal ranges in premature neonates has been obtaining a sufficient number who could be considered normal and healthy. A simple guide is that repeated systolic pressure above 90 mmHg in neonates at term and above 80 mmHg in preterm neonates defines hypertension (Adelman, 1988). Systemic hypertension in the newborn that is not related to aortic coarctation appears to be increasing. This may partly be because of improved detection using Doppler ultrasound to measure blood pressure in the infant; however, an increase in thromboembolic occlusions of the renal vasculature has been recorded. Adelman (1978) reported an incidence of 2.5% in an intensive care nursery over a period of 3 years. Embolic occlusion of the renal artery, with the thrombus originating in the arterial duct, is well recognized (Dimmick et al, 1979). A more common source for an embolus is an umbilical arterial catheter: 80% of reported cases of renal arterial thrombosis were associated with indwelling umbilical arterial catheters (Adelman, 1978). Aortic thrombosis has been demonstrated in up to 30% of neonates with long-dwelling catheters (Jackson et al, 1987). It is important to check that the tip of the catheter is left below the level of the renal artery (T_9 to L_1) and immediately to withdraw it below this level if it is found to be incorrectly positioned. A relatively common cause of neonatal hypertension is bronchopulmonary dysplasia (Abman et al, 1984). Other rarer causes of neonatal hypertension include congenital renal arterial stenosis (Rahill et al, 1974), renal venous thrombosis, structural renal disorders, raised intracranial pressure from space-occupying lesions, phaeochromocytoma, congenital adrenal hyperplasia and autosomal recessive polycystic kidney disease. Cole et al (1987) found that all nine infants they reviewed with this last diagnosis had established hypertension by 3 months of age. Infants requiring extracorporeal membrane oxygenation are also at risk of hypertension (Boedy et al, 1990).

Neonates with hypertension are often severely ill, with tachypnoea, cyanosis and congestive cardiac failure. Neurological symptoms are common, with lethargy, fits, coma, apnoea and hemiparesis. These symptoms may be related to intracranial bleeding or to hypertensive encephalopathy. One quarter of affected infants, however, may be asymptomatic (Adelman, 1978). Renal enlargement is uncommon except with renal venous thrombosis. Haematuria and proteinuria occur in about half the children, but can be present without hypertension. Raised blood urea or plasma creatinine is common. A consumptive coagulopathy with a microangiopathic haemolytic anaemia may be present, with thrombocytopenia, fragmented red cells and prolonged prothrombin and partial thromboplastin times. Plasma renin activity is usually raised. The most useful investigation is dynamic renal scintigraphy with technetium-99m mercaptoacetyltriglycine or dimercaptosuccinic acid, which will show a non-functioning or poorly functioning kidney with diminished blood flow. The diagnosis can be confirmed with an aortogram and selective renal arteriogram.

Control of the hypertension is vital. It can usually be achieved with medications, though nephrectomy has been recommended (Plumer et al, 1976). Hydralazine (up to 10 mg/kg per day) and propranolol (up to 2 mg/kg per day) are usually successful, though a diuretic may also be required. More potent vasodilator agents, such as minoxidil or the angiotensin-converting enzyme inhibitor cap-

topril, may be required. Acute control of severe hypertension can usually be obtained with an intravenous infusion of labetalol (1–3 mg/kg per hour) or nitroprusside (2.5–5 µg/kg per minute).

Neonatal hypertension is a serious condition. One third of all infants reported before 1977 died (Adelman, 1978). Pharmacological control of the raised blood pressure is now possible, however, and all 17 neonates observed by Adelman (1978) responded, with medication eventually being discontinued in 13. At follow-up of 12 of these infants to a mean duration of 5.8 years, blood pressure had normalized in all and had remained normal off medication. Of these 12, 10 had normal creatinine clearance, though five had unilateral renal atrophy (Adelman, 1987). Friedman and Hustead (1987) followed up 17 babies found to be hypertensive after discharge from a neonatal intensive care unit. Of the 12 requiring drug treatment, all were able to discontinue medication by 24 months of age. Improvement in function of the embolized kidney can occur. Removal of a non-functioning kidney is, therefore, best delayed.

ESSENTIAL (PRIMARY) HYPERTENSION

Cardiovascular disease accounts for the majority of deaths between the ages of 30 and 69 years (Hypertension Detection and Follow Up Programme Cooperative Group, 1979). Hypertension is a contributing factor in many. About 90% of adults with raised blood pressures have essential or primary hypertension (Brest and Bower, 1966). Estimates of the prevalence of hypertension in adults, defined as a blood pressure greater than 140/90 mmHg (range 15–20%), though in some populations, for example, Black-Americans, the prevalence is higher (Hypertension Study Group, 1971). Previous trials (Office of Health Economics, 1980) suggest that identification and treatment of hypertensive males over the age of 50 years could prevent between 12 000 and 40 000 early deaths over a 5-year period, mainly from reduction in cerebrovascular disease and myocardial infarction. The importance of essential hypertension, and its related morbidity and mortality, in adults has led to increasing interest in the early characteristics seen during childhood that are associated with the development of hypertension in adult life. The prevalence of essential hypertension in children is probably similar to that of mild hypertension. It affects about 1% of school children (Leuman, 1979) and has a slightly higher prevalence in adolescents, especially Black males. Unfortunately, few epidemiological studies have involved rigorous exclusion of secondary hypertension as a cause of the persistently raised blood pressure before concluding that essential hypertension was present. Therefore, estimates for the frequency of essential hypertension as the cause of raised blood pressure in children range from 50 to 90% (Loggie, 1971; Londe et al, 1971;

Kilcoyne et al, 1974b; Silverberg et al, 1975; Levine et al, 1976; Rames et al, 1978) Conversely, most severe hypertension in children is secondary.

PATHOGENESIS

The cause of essential hypertension is not known (Peart, 1980). Certain features are thought to be related, though their relative importance is controversial. The rise in blood pressure with age is well documented and is probably pathological (see above), at least after childhood. Familial clustering of hypertension is also well known (see above) and is related more to inheritance than to environment. Parental hypertension is present in 30–80% of hypertensive children (Aschinberg et al, 1977; Londe et al, 1977a,b). The prevalence of hypertension in the offspring of hypertensive adults, however, is not known. It is probably low (Kaplan et al, 1978).

The prevalence of hypertension varies amongst populations. It is almost zero in Eskimos but affects over a third of Northern Japanese, this fact correlating with intake of salt (Knudsen and Dahl, 1966). About a third of Black-Americans are hypertensive (Wilber, 1972). Black workers with similar social and dietary backgrounds to white workers in London have higher blood pressures (Sever et al, 1979). This suggests that, while environment is a major factor determining the susceptibility to hypertension, the racial inheritance is also important. There is evidence that the same abnormality of production of growth factor and responsiveness in skin fibroblasts that leads to formation of keloid in black people may also be manifest as an abnormal response of nephron vascular smooth muscle cells, leading to excessive formation of fibrous tissue and nephrosclerosis (Dustan, 1995).

There is good evidence that essential hypertension may have its origins in fetal and infant life. Recent studies have shown a strong link between fetal growth and birthweight, and later risk of coronary arterial disease, stroke and hypertension (Barker et al, 1989, 1990, 1993; Law et al, 1993). Death rates from coronary arterial disease and stroke, and systolic and diastolic blood pressure levels, fell progressively between those with the lowest and those with the highest birthweights. This inverse relationship between systolic blood pressure and birthweight is apparent in the early months of life. It grows progressively stronger with age, implying that the association is initiated in fetal life and amplified throughout life (Law et al, 1993). The underlying explanation for this clear association is still debated. Mackenzie and Brenner (1995) suggest that the link is a deficiency of nephrons at birth in babies with low birthweight. A deficiency of nephrons may then progress, through hyperfiltration injury in the remaining nephrons, to further glomerulosclerosis and hypertension (Hostetter et al, 1981). Mackenzie and Brenner (1995) point out that demographic groups with a high prevalence of hypertension, such as Black-Americans and Japanese, have a smaller ratio of kidney to body size. Low birthweight resulting from intrauterine growth retardation in humans is also associated with a reduction in the number of nephrons in the baby (Hinchcliffe et al, 1992). Some strains of inbred spontaneously hypertensive rats have reduced nephron counts (Brenner et al, 1988) and restriction of dietary protein in pregnant rats led to offspring with fewer nephrons and hypertension in maturity (Langley and Jackson, 1994).

Even allowing for the overestimate of blood pressure that is common in obese patients (see above), hypertension is common in obesity. Between 20 and 86% of hypertensive children are overweight (Leuman, 1979). An excess of adipose tissue augments cardiac output, stroke volume and intravascular volume but lowers peripheral vascular resistance. In contrast, essential hypertension is associated with a normal cardiac output, a contracted intravascular volume and a raised peripheral vascular resistance (Messerli, 1982). The combination of obesity and essential hypertension, therefore, increases both preload and afterload, thus increasing the risk of congestive cardiac failure. The fall in blood pressure with loss of weight is associated with a decrease in cardiac output without any change in vascular resistance.

Stress, however defined, has been thought to contribute to the development of hypertension (Harris and Forsyth, 1973). Social cultural analyses have studied a number of factors such as the effect of urban as opposed to rural life, employment creating nervous tension and the effect of lack of sleep (Lieberman, 1974). Although individuals exposed to external pressure may be more susceptible, there is no consistent evidence that such stress causes hypertension.

Systemic arterial hypertension may result from an increase in cardiac output or peripheral vascular resistance, or both (Guyton, 1976). Increased peripheral vascular resistance is present in most patients with hypertension, but cardiac output may be normal even with volume loading hypertension in end-stage renal failure, Cushing's syndrome, or aldosteronism. Tachycardia is common in all forms of hypertension, which suggests that arterial and cardiac baroreceptors are disturbed, probably by being 'reset' to function at a higher basal level of pressure. In volume-loading hypertension, there is a direct correlation between plasma volume and mean arterial pressure. In essential hypertension, renin-dependent hypertension and with phaeochromocytoma, in contrast, there is an inverse relationship between diastolic pressure and plasma volume. In essential hypertension, cardiac output is often increased early in the disease but later falls to normal.

The strong genetic component in essential hypertension has been discussed. Dahl and Schakow (1964) developed two strains of rats, one of which became hypertensive when fed excessive salt, whereas the other remained normotensive. Once established, the hypertension in the strain fed with salt was self-perpetuating. The genetic nature of essential hypertension, and its self-perpetuation, are perhaps the two most recognized characteristics of the condition. Thus, the rise in peripheral vascular resistance leads to hypertension, which causes arteriosclerosis, further hypertension and, finally, culminates in cerebrovascular disease and myocardial infarction. Many explanations have been proposed for the initiation of the process. These include the neurogenic theory of Folkow (1978), who showed that a thickened arteriolar wall with a constricted lumen is a universal feature of hypertension. These changes occur rapidly and are self-maintaining, such that a variety of stimuluses will then produce an increased vasoconstrictor response.

Borst (1963) demonstrated that loading with salt raised blood pressure, venous pressure, extracellular fluid volume and body weight. The rise in blood pressure was maintained after the salt retention ceased. He proposed that the kidney in essential hypertension required a higher blood pressure and that, initially, salt and water were retained by the kidney, thus causing a rise in cardiac output and blood pressure. The rise in blood pressure under these circumstances is dependent on either an increase or a steady maintenance of peripheral vascular resistance. If the compliance of the arteriolar bed increased with the salt and water overload, pressure would remain steady. Guyton (1976) has developed the theory of long-term control of blood pressure that relates blood volume, cardiac output and renal function so that a rise in blood volume will produce a corresponding increase in urinary output, thus returning both cardiac output and blood pressure to normal. He has emphasized two important features of this theoretical model. First, only small changes in the volume of fluid in the body will produce substantial variation in arterial pressure. Second, the system controlling renal function relative to body fluid shows infinite gain. If peripheral vascular resistance rises, the arterial pressure will rise to whatever degree is required to generate the necessary urinary output. This theory suggests, therefore, that essential hypertension begins as a deficiency in excretion of sodium by the kidneys and continues because of the obligatory relation between arterial pressure, peripheral vascular resistance and urinary output.

People with essential hypertension excrete a salt load more rapidly than do normal subjects, and this abnormality is present in normotensive young relatives (Wiggins et al, 1978). These observations suggest that a renal abnormality may precede the development of essential hypertension in susceptible people. The relation between the prevalence of hypertension in a population and the cultural preference for salt in the diet is well established (Elliott et al, 1996), though correlations between intake of salt and blood pressure within communities are less obvious (Editorial 1981). It had been demonstrated that strains of rats that develop hypertension when fed a diet high in salt have kidneys that are less able to excrete sodium, and that the hypertension is mediated by a humoral factor (Dahl et al, 1967). Bianchi et al (1975) have suggested that the hypertensive rats retain sodium with an increase in blood volume but then overproduce a substance that promotes excretion by the kidney and also causes hypertension. Natriuretic hormone has been extracted from normal urine (Clarkson et al, 1979), and de Wardener and MacGregor (1980) have suggested that it is responsible for the rise in peripheral vascular resistance in essential hypertension by its effects not just in promoting excretion of sodium in the proximal tubule but also by affecting transport of sodium into the arteriolar cell. There is evidence for decreased flux of sodium, and an increased potassium flux, in erythrocytes from patients with essential hypertension (Garay and Meyer, 1979). This abnormality is familial (Woods et al, 1981). The content of sodium in arteries is increased in essential hypertension. Moreover, serum from patients with essential hypertension diminished sodium transport in normal white blood cells (Poston et al, 1981).

In summary, therefore, essential hypertension has a strong genetic component, and abnormalities of excretion of sodium by the kidney (and diminished cellular sodium flux) are apparent in people with essential hypertension and in their young relatives without hypertension. These changes could account, first, for the susceptibility of certain individuals to diets high in salt, second, for the circulatory changes recognized in early and established essential hypertension and, finally, for the raised peripheral vascular resistance, which is then perpetuated and becomes permanent according to the theories advanced by Folkow (1978) and Guyton (1976).

These ideas have important implications for children. If they are confirmed, then the genesis of eventual hypertensive disease is in childhood (de Swiet, 1982). It seems reasonable to advise families with a history of hypertension to restrict intake of sodium by avoiding foods high in salt, reducing salt in cooking and banning extra salt from the table. Salt is, to some extent, an acquired taste. Children of parents with hypertension would be less likely to acquire the taste if they consumed the parents' restricted sodium diet. Even for those children who do not have a family history of hypertension, the persistent consumption of a diet high in salt is best avoided. Take-away and 'fast' foods are a particular problem. The average Chinese take-away meal contains 225 mmol sodium, while a hamburger and chips has 95 mmol (de Swiet et al 1982). Processed food accounts for 80% of the salt intake in the average Western diet, and it is argued that the manufacturers of this processed food should reduce its content of salt (Antonios and MacGregor, 1996).

The association of hypercholesterolaemia and hypertension with coronary arterial disease is well recognized (Kannel and Dawber, 1973). Lowering serum cholesterol by avoidance of animal fat and the substitution of polyunsaturated for saturated fatty acids would seem to be indicated for those with raised levels, especially if they are hypertensive or have a family history of hypertension. Obesity should likewise be treated by exercise and reduction in caloric intake, particularly carbohydrate, which is related to hypertriglyceridaemia. Whether the type of carbohydrate ingested is related to atherosclerosis and hypertension is not clear. The avoidance of refined sugar with the substitution of starch and the consumption of a diet high in fibre, nonetheless, is recommended for those with hypertension. Again, the alteration of the diet of susceptible families may provide advantages for the children in later life.

The relation between smoking and cardiovascular disease is well known. Heavy, as opposed to moderate, drinkers also have higher blood pressure, though it is sometimes difficult to separate the effects of smoking and drinking, which are frequently associated (Peart, 1980).

MALIGNANT HYPERTENSION

Malignant hypertension implies a condition which, if untreated, will lead to death within a few weeks (Kincaid Smith, 1981). The appearance of haemorrhages, exudates and papilloedema on retinal examination in someone with previously uncomplicated severe hypertension denotes the onset of vasculitis. It is accompanied by weakness, wasting and debilitation, usually leading to death from progressive uraemia with the vasculitis involving the renal vessels. It has been proposed that the high systemic blood pressure associated with critical circulating levels of vasoactive hormones, such as angiotensin II, vasopressin and noradrenaline, leads to the onset of a pressure natriuresis, in other words massive loss of salt and water leading to hypovolaemia. The hypovolaemia causes a further rise in production of vasoactive hormone, intense vasoconstriction and damage to the arteriolar endothelium, causing activation of platelets and release of thromboxane. This, in turn, leads to further vasoconstriction and is associated with marked intimal hyperplasia, deposition of fibrin and formation of thrombus. All this contributes to the established vicious circle (Kincaid Smith, 1981).

It is clear from this analysis that depletion of salt and vasoconstriction are key features in the progression of malignant hypertension. Treatment with peripheral vasodilator agents to lower blood pressure should, therefore, be accompanied by judicious replacement of salt and not by further sodium restriction unless there is clear evidence of salt and water overload.

INVESTIGATION AND DIAGNOSIS

The majority of children with essential hypertension have only mild elevations of blood pressure with no clinical signs of hypertension. Only 2 of 74 children reported by Londe et al (1971) had left ventricular hypertrophy. Severe hypertension can result from essential hypertension, with 3 of 41 patients reported by New et al (1976) having diastolic blood pressures greater than 122 mmHg.

Adults with essential hypertension have been classified according to their plasma renin activity (Brunner et al, 1972) though the significance of this is not established (Dunn and Tanner, 1974). Low levels of renin are common in Blacks with hypertension, and there is some evidence that cardiovascular complications, such as cerebrovascular accidents or myocardial infarcts, are rarer if the plasma renin activity is low. Plasma renin activity, however, is usually normal in children with essential hypertension (Londe et al, 1971; Levine et al, 1976; Leuman, 1979). Occasional instances of low renin and essential hypertension in children have been reported (Leuman et al, 1975).

The diagnosis of essential hypertension depends on the exclusion of all known causes of secondary hypertension (see Table 68.3). Cardiovascular causes are usually excluded during the clinical history and examination. Similarly, the problems produced by the central nervous system, or hypertension related to drugs or metabolic causes, do not pose diagnostic difficulties. Renal disease may be apparent from the clinical evaluation, from the examination of urine or from the measurement of plasma electrolytes. A hypokalaemic alkalosis, which suggests either primary or secondary excess of mineralocorticoids, should be excluded in all cases. Plasma renin activity should be carefully determined (see below) and would be expected to be normal in essential hypertension. An intravenous urogram, with the early films taken in rapid sequence from 1 minute after injection of the contrast medium, is usually appropriate to exclude major structural abnormalities of the kidneys and to identify some cases of renal vascular hypertension. If the clinical history and examination, full blood count, plasma electrolytes, examination of urine, urinary excretion of catecholamine metabolites, thyroid function, intravenous urogram, renal scintigraphy scans to detect hypoperfusion and renal scarring, plasma renin activity and urine steroid excretion are all normal, and the hypertension is not severe, then a diagnosis of essential hypertension is usually appropriate. Severe hypertension, particularly with a raised plasma renin activity, will necessitate a careful search for a renal or renovascular cause. This will involve a renal arteriogram, usually with selective sampling from the renal vein to measure levels of renin in the plasma (see below).

MANAGEMENT

There is no question about the desirability of treating children with severe hypertension. Appropriate treatment is discussed under Medical therapy. About 1% of children will have mild hypertension, defined as a blood pressure persistently more than 2 standard deviations (95th percentile) above the mean for children of the same age and sex (see Figures 68.2–68.4). The upper values for normal are, therefore, 110/65 mmHg from 0 to 3 years of age, 120/70 mmHg from 4 to 7 years of age, 130/75 mmHg from 8 to 10 years of age, 140/80 mmHg from 11 to 15 years of age and 140/90 mmHg thereafter. The decision to attempt to lower the blood pressure in such children is controversial (see above). It must depend, to some extent, on the assessment by the physician of the circumstances of each child. The psychosocial effects on an adolescent of forcing a confrontation with the implications of long-term management for hypertension may exacerbate the problem, as well as causing undesirable alterations in behavioural growth. Compliance, particularly with medication, may be unsatisfactory. Indeed, the benefits of early treatment may be outweighed by the possibility of chronic damage from the side effects of the drugs (Londe and Goldring, 1972).

General dietary and health advice should initially be given. The avoidance of risk factors such as smoking should be encouraged. Obesity should be treated with caloric reduction, and regular exercise encouraged. A reduced intake of salt (50 mmol/day; no added salt to cooking or at table) and a diet high in potassium (Skrabal et al, 1981) can be instituted. A high ratio of polyunsaturated to saturated fats should be encouraged, while foods rich in cholesterol should be avoided, refined carbohydrate reduced and dietary fibre content increased. Such advice may seem a counsel of perfection, but much can usually be achieved by a minimum of intervention and without generating excessive anxiety or food fads. Compounds known to exacerbate hypertension, such as liquorice, sympathomimetics, corticosteroids and oral contraceptives, should be avoided.

Such measures are probably all that is required initially, together with a relaxed but reliable follow-up to check the blood pressure. If the blood pressure remains obviously unacceptably raised (more than 3 standard deviations above the mean), or continues to be mildly raised over a period of 1 to 2 years, then a decision may be required to institute drug therapy. A thiazide such as bendrofluazide (bendroflumethiazide) (see below) is a reasonable first choice. In this case, the plasma electrolytes, uric acid and blood glucose should be checked at intervals. If this is insufficient, then a β-blocker such as atenolol can be added. Further drugs are rarely required. The decision to start therapy is a serious one. Treatment must be long term and careful supervision, including a regular check for side effects, is imperative. Attempts should be made at regular intervals to reduce, and even to discontinue, the medication. Information currently available suggests that while many hypertensive children will continue to have elevated blood pressures (Kilcoyne, 1978) some will become normotensive.

Caution regarding treatment of mild hypertension is advisable, not withstanding the reports of successful intervention. (Hypertension Detection and Follow Up Programme Cooperative Group, 1979; Management Committee, 1980). This is because some studies have failed to demonstrate a significant difference in morbidity from coronary arterial disease between a control group and a group undergoing treatment that involved the reduction in known risk factors and the treatment of hypertension (Editorial, 1982). A reasonable interpretation of available evidence would allow advice concerning smoking, hypercholesterolaemia, obesity and exercise (Choquette and Ferguson, 1973). The creation of undue anxiety should always be avoided. Treatment with drugs to reduce blood pressure is more controversial but seems reasonable, as indicated above, as long as careful follow-up is guaranteed. Hypertension induced by oral contraceptives is common, with an incidence of 7.5%. Furthermore, oral contraceptives will exacerbate hypertension in a similar proportion of individuals (Finerty, 1978). The mechanism is thought to involve stimulation of the renin–aldosterone release, a direct effect of oestrogen on retention of salt and water and sensitization of smooth muscle to vasoconstriction produced by angiotensin II. Cardiac output may also increase. Decisions regarding individual patients will need to take account of individual factors, not least the assessment of the risk of pregnancy. It would seem advisable, however, to discontinue oral contraception if hypertension occurs but not to preclude its use in the presence of pre-existing mild hypertension. A low-oestrogen pill should be used. A further rise in blood pressure would then be an indication for stopping treatment.

Up to half of the adults receiving antihypertensive therapy become non-compliant. This is probably equally common in children, especially adolescents (Ruley, 1978). The quality of the relationship between doctor and patient, the degree of knowledge of the patient and participation and the ease of consultation are important factors. The ease of drug administration, including a reduction in the number of drugs and frequency of ingestion, is important. Long-acting formulations requiring once daily dosage are preferred. Alterations in life style, including diet, must be introduced slowly. Changing habits is often resisted and may also lead to non-compliance in other areas.

RENAL HYPERTENSION

PATHOPHYSIOLOGY

Renin is a proteolytic enzyme that is produced by the juxtaglomerular cells and stored in the afferent arteriole. After release into the blood, it reacts with a plasma substrate produced by the liver, angiotensinogen, to form the decapeptide angiotensin I. Angiotensin I is further acted upon by converting enzyme in the lung to produce the octapeptide angiotensin II, which raises blood pressure by direct vasoconstriction and by its indirect effects on the nervous system. It stimulates secretion of aldosterone, promotes retention of sodium by the kidney and stimulates thirst and the release of catecholamines and vasopressin (Brown et al, 1979). Baroreceptors located in the afferent arteriole control the release of renin. This is also affected by other factors, including delivery of sodium in the distal tubule to the macula densa, sympathetic activity, catecholamines and hypokalaemia. Activity of the renin–angiotensin system is intrinsically related to sodium balance and the volume of extracellular fluid. Specimens for determination of plasma renin activity need to be obtained under controlled circumstances, with the patient supine and relaxed, and interpreted in relation to sodium balance. A highly significant inverse correlation exists between plasma renin activity and total exchangeable sodium (Davies et al, 1973). In children, studies of the relationship between plasma renin activity and both age and sodium excretion have given conflicting results. Dillon and Ryness (1975) demonstrated an inverse correlation between plasma renin activity and age, but no clear relationship with urinary excretion of sodium (Table 68.6). Harshfield et al (1993), in contrast, found no correlation with age, but a highly significant inverse relationship with urinary excretion of sodium.

The importance of renal ischaemia in the generation of hypertension has been appreciated since the classic experiments of Goldblatt using dogs (1934). The detailed mechanisms remain controversial (Brown et al, 1979). Unilateral renal arterial constriction in the rat will produce hypertension. If the constriction is removed within a few weeks, the hypertension subsides. If the clip is left for longer and then removed, the hypertension often persists. Removal of the non-clipped kidney, but not the previously clipped kidney, will often result in a fall in blood pressure. Concentrations of angiotension II rise in the plasma with the initial unilateral renal arterial constriction, and this is probably responsible for the initial rise in blood pressure. Thereafter, the concentration slowly decreases even though the hypertension persists. It is likely that the renin–angiotensin system is still responsible for the hypertension at this stage. This is partly through its vasoconstrictive action, and partly because of retention of salt (Brown et al, 1979). Later, after months or years, removal of the abnormal kidney in humans fails to reduce blood pressure. It is likely that renin is not involved in the maintenance of the hypertension. The mechanism by which retention of salt causes hypertension is not certain. It would be expected that a rise in arterial pressure would lead to a pressure natriuresis. If hypertension is maintained without depletion of sodium, therefore, the relation between blood pressure and renal excretion of salt must be reset at a higher level (Guyton et al, 1973). This is perhaps a result of the effect of angiotensin II in reducing renal perfusion and increasing retention of sodium by the kidney, both directly and by release of aldosterone (Brown et al, 1979). The persistence of hypertension after the removal of the initial cause in experimental animals has its clinical counterpart in phaeochromocytoma, Cushing's syndrome, Conn's syndrome and aortic coarctation. In these instances, the blood pressure does not always return to normal after removal of the cause.

The persistent hypertension may be related to damage to the renal vasculature of the non-experimental kidney. This can, in some way which is not yet clear, cause retention of sodium. The mechanism may be similar to that involved in the later stages of essential hypertension (see above) and to the increased peripheral vascular resistance caused by medial and intimal hypertrophy of peripheral arterioles (Folkow, 1978). The complexities of experimental renal hypertension are such that it can cause no surprise that the amelioration of renal ischaemia in the human does not always lead to a reduction in hypertension (Ingelfinger, 1993). Fortunately, in children, perhaps because the period of hypertension is shorter, the results of surgery for renovascular hypertension are more predictable.

RENOVASCULAR HYPERTENSION

Renovascular hypertension can be defined as hypertension resulting from obstruction to flow of blood in the

Table 68.6. Plasma renin activity and plasma aldosterone concentration in normal children

Age (years)	Mean daily sodium excretion (mmol/kg)	Supine plasma renin activity (ngAI/l per hour)		Supine plasma aldosterone concentrations (pmol/l)	
		Mean	Range	Mean	Range
<1	1.2	1459	472–3130	788	164–2929
1–4	3.8	757	110–2610	294	69–946
5–9	2.5	417	131–834	147	28–616
10–15	2.5	321	55–899	211	72–577
Adult	2.1	85	22–311	230	39–422

After Dillon and Ryness (1975).

renal artery or its branches. The obstruction may be caused by intrinsic disease of the artery or by compression on the artery from outside. Overall, fibromuscular dysplasia (fibromuscular non-atherosclerotic stenosis of the renal vessels) is classified according to the arterial layer in which the lesions predominate (Youngberg et al, 1977). Intimal fibroplasia is a rare cause in adults but occurs primarily in children, whereas fibromuscular dysplasia, or hyperplasia of the media, is more common and predominates in adolescents and adults. Overall, the condition is most common in middle-aged females (sex ratio 1.3:1; average age 38 years) (Leuman 1979). The lesion in adults is commonly situated in the middle or distal part of the renal artery; whereas stenosis occurs more frequently at the origin of the vessel in children. The aetiology of the condition is unknown, but a cellular reaction to altered dynamics of pressure and flow in the artery has been proposed (Youngberg et al, 1977; Twigg and Palmisano, 1965). The prevalence of the condition is unknown, but large series have been reported (Stanley and Fry, 1981). It is important to recognize that the condition may be progressive (Aurell, 1979) and may also involve arteries other than the renal vessels (Pesonen et al, 1980). A careful search for the involvement of other arteries is mandatory, with particular note taken of absent peripheral pulses or the presence of bruits, especially over the carotids.

A number of cases are associated with neurofibromatosis (Muller-Wiefel, 1978). A careful family history, and clinical examination for other features of the condition, are, therefore, important. The renal arterial stenosis in neurofibromatosis is usually caused by intimal proliferation or neurofibromatotic proliferation in the arterial wall (Leuman, 1979). Associated coarctation of the abdominal aorta is common. Occasionally, compression on the artery from outside by a neurofibroma or ganglion neuroma is responsible for hypertension. Other space-occupying lesions that may involve compression of the renal artery include tumours, fibrous bands, haematomas and phaeochromocytomas. Coarctation of the abdominal aorta without neurofibromatosis is often accompanied by renal arterial stenosis (Juncos et al, 1976). Other vessels originating from the abdominal aorta are usually involved. Decisions regarding treatment are extremely difficult, because surgical correction of the renal arterial stenosis by vascular shunts from above the coarctation may compromise flow to other organs, including the spinal arteries. Correction of the coarctation by refashioning of the abdominal aorta with a vascular prosthesis is a massive procedure that probably will require reimplantation of all major vessels that are stenosed. Autotransplantation of the kidney below the coarctation may not improve renal blood flow. Acquired narrowing of the abdominal aorta has been observed following radiotherapy for intra-abdominal malignant disease (Da Hae Lee et al, 1976).

Takayasu's arteritis is an important cause of renovascular hypertension in non-white children (Wiggelinkhuizen and Cremin, 1978). The arteritis affects the aorta, the proximal portions of its major branches and the pulmonary arteries. The onset of the vasculitis is associated with an acute systemic illness, which usually subsides after a few weeks but may recur. The aetiology is unknown, though a link with tuberculosis has been suggested (Morrison et al, 1989; Milner et al, 1991). A raised sedimentation rate and elevated levels of immunoglobulin indicate active disease. The prognosis is, to some extent, dependent on the severity of the vasculitis and the resultant damage. Following this, management is mainly concerned with the control of the hypertension. Other miscellaneous causes may be found. Renal arterial stenosis can be present in some cases of infantile hypercalcaemia syndrome (Chantler et al, 1966). Thrombosis or embolism of the renal artery is an important cause of hypertension in infants (see above). Stenosis of arterial branches within the kidney may lead to severe hypertension and is difficult to diagnose (Bennett et al, 1974). Diffuse renal arteriolar stenotic lesions can occur in polyarteritis nodosa, haemolytic uraemic syndrome, and following renal radiation (Vidt, 1977). Renal venous thrombosis in infancy can lead to the development of hypertension (Arneil et al, 1973). Hypertension is common after renal transplantation but only rarely is caused by renal arterial stenosis. Renal hypertension can occur after traumatic injury to the kidney, causing renal arterial thrombosis or intrarenal vascular damage, or from perinephric inflammation causing constriction on the kidney (Leuman, 1979). Arterio-venous fistulas, either congenital or acquired, following trauma, surgery, or renal biopsy, can all cause hypertension.

A bruit over the renal artery is a useful diagnostic sign; this is often absent in children with renovascular hypertension. A hypokalaemic alkalosis resulting from secondary hyperaldosteronism is common with severe hypertension, and the concentration of renin in plasma from fasting patients obtained while supine is raised in 80% (Robson, 1978). This measurement is often invalidated by the existing treatment for the hypertension. A carefully performed intravenous urogram with early films taken in rapid sequence is always required, if only to exclude parenchymal renal damage. In renal arterial stenosis, the urogram should demonstrate a small kidney with late but dense opacification of the nephrogram. This is caused by increased fractional tubular reabsorption of sodium and water in the affected kidney. Unfortunately, these signs are often absent. Doppler ultrasound is not a sensitive technique for detecting renal arterial stenosis (Kliewer et al, 1993; Postma et al, 1996). Dynamic renal scintigraphy using diethylenetriaminepentaacetic acid labelled with technetium-99m (Tc-DTPA) may show reduced renal blood flow to the affected kidney, but again this scan is often normal. Performing the scan before and then after a dose of an inhibitor of angiotensin-converting enzyme, such as captopril, may reveal a significant reduction in function of the affected kidney on the second scan. This technique has been found to have sensitivity and specificity of around 90% in adult patients (Jonker et al, 1993). A study in children of captopril-primed scans with dimercaptosuccinic acid labelled with technetium-99m (^{99m}Tc-DMSA) gave a sensitivity and specificity of 80% and 89% respectively, when compared with renal arteriography (Minty et al, 1993).

Direct evidence of renal ischaemia with stimulation of the renin–angiotensin system is derived from the differential determination of renal venous renin. A ratio of 1.5 or more between the affected and the non-affected kidney may predict unilateral renal ischaemia, and an anticipated positive response to surgery (Dillon et al, 1978; Dillon, 1980). Using this ratio to predict unilateral disease, however, does not always correlate with the arteriographic findings (Deal et al, 1992) and in no way removes the need for arteriography. The level of renin in the renal vein of the non-affected kidney is usually suppressed to the level of the systemic plasma renin concentration. A ratio of less than 1.5 suggests either bilateral disease or non-renovascular hypertension, though renovascular hypertension and successful surgery has been reported in some patients (Godard, 1977). A normal renal arteriogram, with similar activities of renin in both renal veins, will certainly exclude a renal cause for hypertension in most, if not all, cases.

The main investigation for renal arterial stenosis is selective renal arteriography (Figure 68.5) and estimation of renal venous renin. The investigation carries a morbidity and mortality, though the incidence of severe complications should be less than 1% in experienced units (Robson, 1978). If the hypertension is mild and easily controlled, and if the other investigations do not suggest renovascular hypertension, it is reasonable not to recommend arteriography, though careful follow-up is essential. The blood pressure should be carefully controlled before attempting arteriography. The procedure is usually performed under sedation or general anaesthesia, with access to the renal artery and vein from puncture of the femoral vessels. The amount of contrast injected should be the minimum required, because acute renal failure complicating the procedure is well recognized. Adequate hydration should be maintained and the blood pressure monitored throughout the procedure.

Newer less invasive techniques that await full evaluation include magnetic resonance angiography (Debatin et al, 1991) and computed tomographic and spiral angiography (Rubin et al, 1994).

The rate of cure for surgery in renovascular hypertension in children is high (Dillon et al, 1978; Leuman, 1979; Stanley and Fry, 1981; Stanley et al, 1982). It varied between 85 and 100% in various series of properly selected patients, with no operative deaths in many series (Stanley et al, 1982). Surgery is usually preferable to medical treatment for children with severe renovascular hypertension. The operative techniques vary according to the nature of the disease. They include renal arterial reconstruction, autotransplantation and pros-

thetic bypass of the stenosis (Orcutt et al, 1974; Stanley et al, 1982). The role of percutaneous angiographic balloon dilation of the renal arterial stenosis is not fully defined in children, but the technique is less successful with ostial stenosis or the long segment renal arterial stenosis seen in neurofibromatosis (Ingelfinger 1993). Good results have been obtained in other cases, though restenosis is common (Robinson et al 1991) and stenosis may develop in the contralateral previously normal renal artery (Kurien et al, 1997). The progressive nature of fibromuscular dysplasia in children suggests that every attempt should be made to preserve renal function. Nephrectomy should be performed only if the kidney is small or scarred and has very poor function (less than 10–20% of total function).

RENAL PARENCHYMAL DISEASE

The renal disease causing hypertension is usually evident from the initial clinical and laboratory evaluation (Table 68.4). Reflux nephropathy is the predominant cause of chronic pyelonephritis. Perhaps 10–20% of such children will develop hypertension (Savage et al, 1978; Goonasekera et al, 1996). Chronic pyelonephritis accounts for over half the children with severe hypertension in some series (Still and Cotton, 1967). A careful search for renal scarring is, therefore, mandatory in any child with severe hypertension. There is debate over whether intravenous urography or ^{99m}-technetium DMSA scan is the better investigation for the demonstration of renal scars (Goldraich et al, 1989; Smellie, 1989). If scarring is demonstrated, a micturating cystourethrogram should be performed. Dynamic or static renal scintigraphy using ^{99m}Tc-DMSA is often helpful in showing small scars. It is likely that most cases of segmental renal hypoplasia, or the Ask–Upmark kidney (Rosenfell et al, 1973), are secondary to vesicoureteric reflux. In some cases, the segmental hypoplasia may be the consequence of dysplasia, with disordered renal development during fetal life, again usually associated with reflux. Alternatively, it may be acquired after birth from damage caused by reflux and infection. Treatment of hypertension is medical, as the damage is often bilateral and affects more than one segment of the kidney. Removal of the affected area, therefore, is not possible. Sometimes, especially with apparently unilateral disease, estimations of renal venous renin will demonstrate that the cause of hypertension is a small, scarred and poorly functioning kidney. This can then be removed with resolution of the hypertension. Alternatively, hyper-reninaemia may only be present in a branch of the renal vein draining a small scarred segment. This again can be removed by partial nephrectomy. Obstruction at the pelviureteric junction is occasionally associated with hypertension, which can be cured in some instances by a pyeloplasty (Chapman and Douglas, 1975; Carella and Silber, 1976).

Hypertension is common in acute nephritic syndrome. Indeed, this diagnosis has to be considered in any child with unexplained acute hypertension. Plasma renin is low because of the retention of sodium (Powell et al, 1974). Hypertension is also common in chronic glomerulonephritis (Table 68.5) and is almost invariable when renal function declines.

Diseases associated with widespread arteriolar damage, such as haemolytic uraemic syndrome, systemic lupus erythematosus and polyarteritis nodosa, are often accompanied by hypertension. Careful control of the raised blood pressure is associated with a better prognosis.

Polycystic kidneys are an important cause of hypertension. This occurs early in the autosomal recessive form of the condition seen in childhood (Rahill and Rubin, 1972). Hypertension may also develop in childhood in the more common autosomal dominant polycystic kidney disease. Multicystic dysplastic kidneys can cause hypertension in later life and are, therefore, usually removed in infancy (Webb et al, 1997). Hypertension has also been described in a child with medullary sponge kidneys associated with the Beckwith–Wiedemann syndrome (Virdis et al, 1979).

It is the case that hypertension can occur with all forms of renal disease. It is less common with primary interstitial tubular diseases, such as the Fanconi syndrome or juvenile nephronophthisis, and with the diseases associated with salt wasting, such as renal dysplasia or obstructive uropathy in infancy. When renal insufficiency supervenes, however, even children with these conditions may develop hypertension. In the majority of patients with end-stage renal failure, the hypertension responds to removal of salt and water by dialysis. However, even intensive ultrafiltration occasionally fails to ameliorate the hypertension. Indeed, it can make it worse, with high concentrations of plasma renin–angiotensin causing intense vasoconstriction. Such patients are often thirsty and have large weight gains between dialyses. Until recently, nephrectomy was required to cure the hypertension. The introduction of captopril, a blocker of angiotensin-converting enzyme, now enables many cases to be managed medically.

PRIMARY HYPER-RENINISM

Severe hypertension is uncommon in children with nephroblastoma (Wilms' tumour). It can occur when renal ischaemia is present or after haemorrhage into the tumour. Occasionally, production of renin by the tumour has been described (Sheth et al, 1978). Tumours of the juxtaglomerular cells (haemangiopericytomas) are extremely rare. With these tumours, the plasma renin activity is elevated, and there is often evidence of secondary hyperaldosteronism. The tumours are single, benign and small, measuring 0.8–4.0 cm (Leuman, 1979). They are suspected when a raised level of renin is found in the

renal vein in association with a normal intravenous urogram. They may be apparent as a translucent area seen during the nephrographic phase of a selective renal arteriogram (Brown et al, 1973). Computed tomography may assist in the diagnosis of these lesions (McVicar et al, 1993). Surgical removal of the tumour is indicated.

AORTIC COARCTATION

PATHOPHYSIOLOGY

Aortic coarctation is found in over 20% of those suffering from secondary hypertension in childhood (Leuman, 1979). It is, therefore, the second most important cause, after renal disease, of severe hypertension in children. Cardiovascular causes, such as cerebral haemorrhage, dissection or rupture of the ascending aorta or congestive heart failure, are responsible for the majority of deaths in untreated patients (Goldring, 1978). The cause of the hypertension in patients with coarctation is complex and not fully explained (Gruskin, 1977). The majority of experimental models simulating coarctation have required the constriction to be placed above the origin of the renal arteries. Even when hypertension has occurred with a constriction below the renal arteries, an alteration in renal function has been observed. It seems reasonable, therefore, to implicate the kidney in the genesis or maintenance of the hypertension, although the important role of the mechanical obstruction cannot be disregarded (Gupta and Wiggers, 1951). Glomerular filtration rate is often normal in children with coarctation. Renal plasma flow may be reduced, however, causing an increase in filtration fraction. Measurements of the distribution of blood flow between the renal cortex and medulla have shown a reduction in blood flow in the outer cortex (Gruskin, 1977). These changes suggest an increase in renal vascular resistance. These alterations in renal haemodynamics usually return to normal after surgery. Aperia et al (1973) found that the rate of excretion of an oral sodium load was reduced in children with coarctation and improved after surgery. The rate of excretion correlated with the changes in renal haemodynamics.

The involvement of the renin–angiotensin system in the hypertension of aortic coarctation is also controversial. Concentrations of renin are usually normal in the plasma of children with established coarctation (Strong et al, 1970) but rise abnormally with restriction of sodium. Plasma renin activity increases after experimental production of coarctation but then returns to normal (van Way et al, 1976). Saralasin, an agent which blocks angiotensin, caused a significant fall in blood pressure in patients with coarctation (Ribeiro and Krakoff, 1976). Alpert et al (1979) have suggested that the hypertension in coarctation resembles the hypertension produced in the 'one kidney, one clip' model of Goldblatt (Brown et al, 1979; see also above). In this form of experimental hypertension, the initial rise in blood pressure is associated with a rise in renin–angiotensin, which later falls to normal. The maintenance of hypertension at this stage is associated with an increase in peripheral vascular resistance. This may be related to an alteration in distribution of sodium and water unrelated to the kidneys, but it is accompanied by a change in handling of sodium and water by the kidneys, perhaps associated with a change in renal haemodynamics. Removal of the renal arterial constriction, or the aortic coarctation, usually leads to a reversal of the hypertension. In long-standing cases, however, the blood pressure fails to fall because of a fixed raised peripheral vascular resistance. In this respect, it is of interest that only 6% of patients with coarctation aged between 1 and 5 years had residual hypertension, whereas 30% of those undergoing surgery between 6 and 18 years, and 47% of those aged from 19 to 40 years, had hypertension following surgery (Goldring, 1978). The incidence of residual hypertension was high in infants, but it was then related to persistence or recurrence of the coarctation.

MANAGEMENT

The diagnosis and treatment of the hypertension associated with coarctation is discussed in detail in Chapter 56. The treatment of the hypertension is surgical removal of the coarcted segment. If the hypertension persists, then reinvestigation is required to ensure that an adequate aortic lumen has been created (Goldring, 1978). If the lumen is satisfactory, then medical management is indicated (see below).

Preoperative congestive cardiac failure is present in over two thirds of infants. Neonates may present severely ill with renal insufficiency, pulmonary oedema and hyperkalaemia. Careful assessment, with collaboration between different specialists, is required in the management of such children. Peritoneal dialysis, with correction of the metabolic acidosis and hyperkalaemia and removal of fluid, is frequently required prior to cardiac catheterization and surgery.

ENDOCRINE DISORDERS

ADRENOCORTICAL HYPERTENSION

The adrenal gland synthesizes mineralocorticoids, glucocorticoids and sex hormones from cholesterol. Plasma cortisol feeds back to the pituitary to control the output of adrenocorticotrophic hormone, which stimulates the rate of conversion of cholesterol to pregnenalone. This is an intermediate in the production of all three classes of adrenocortical hormone. Any failure of the normal feedback control by cortisol will produce an increase in adrenocorticotrophic hormone, giving rise to congenital adrenal hyperplasia. The most useful investigations in the diagnosis of adrenocortical hypertension are a determination of plasma renin activity (which is usually suppressed) and plasma aldosterone, the exclusion of a hypokalaemic alkalosis and a careful analysis of the urinary excretion of steroids.

11β-HYDROXYLASE DEFICIENCY

11-Hydroxylation is the final step in the production of cortisol (compound F) from its immediate precursor corticosterone (compound S). It is also an essential step in the production of aldosterone from desoxycorticosteroid. Adrenal hyperplasia results from the decreased production of cortisol with an increase in plasma levels of compound S and its urinary metabolites (tetrahydro-S, desoxycorticosteroid and tetrahydrodesoxycorticosteroid, adrenal androgens and urinary 17-ketosteroids). Virilization is a prominent clinical feature and hypertension is present in many patients. This is in contrast to the more common variety of congenital adrenal hyperplasia associated with a deficiency in 21-hydroxylase. Hypertension is thought to be caused by an excess of desoxycorticosteroid, which has mineralocorticoid effects. There is evidence of hyperaldosteronism with a hypokalaemic alkalosis and a low concentration of renin in the plasma.

17α-HYDROXYLASE DEFICIENCY

17-Hydroxylation is required for the conversion of pregnenalone to 17-hydroxypregnenalone in the production of cortisol and sex hormones. A defect in this process, therefore, results in the diminished secretion of all glucocorticoids and sex hormones, with an increased secretion of mineralocorticoids, leading to hypertension and hypokalaemia. Clinical features include hypogonadism, ammenorrhoea and male pseudohermaphroditism. The production of 17-desoxysteroids, including desoxycorticosteroid and compound B, is increased but secretion of aldosterone is low, perhaps because of the low plasma levels of renin, which is required for the synthesis of aldosterone. It is suppressed by the high plasma concentration of desoxycorticosteroid (New and Levine, 1978). The hypertension in both varieties of congenital adrenal hyperplasia resolves with treatment with a glucocorticoid.

CUSHING'S SYNDROME

Cushing's syndrome is caused either by excessive production of adrenocorticotrophic hormone, leading to adrenal hyperplasia, or by an adrenal tumour. Hypertension occurs in 80% of patients (Loridan and Senior, 1969). Clinical features include obesity, short stature, hirsutism and acne. The cause of the hypertension is not clear. Levels of aldosterone in the plasma are not elevated. Two mechanisms have been considered, either retention of sodium with extracellular fluid expansion or peripheral vasoconstriction, the latter resulting from increased activity of the renin–angiotensin system caused by increased hepatic production of renin substrate (Krakhoff et al, 1975). Hypertension may persist after surgery. This has been attributed to chronic renal damage from long-standing hypertension. Cushing's syndrome in children is more commonly related to an adrenal carcinoma and is accompanied by virilization more frequently than by adrenal hyperplasia.

HYPERALDOSTERONISM AND LOW-RENIN HYPERTENSION

Concentration of aldosterone in the plasma is high in infancy and decreases to adult values by 5 years of age (Table 68.6) (Dillon and Ryness, 1975; Kowarski and Migeon, 1977). Urinary aldosterone excretion is related to excretion of sodium (New et al, 1976). The cardinal features of hyperaldosteronism are retention of sodium, hypokalaemia, hypertension and suppressed plasma renin activity. These changes are seen in a variety of hypertensive syndromes; these share the common feature of low plasma renin activity, but some conditions have high levels of aldosterone and others have low (Table 68.7). Several of these syndromes are inherited as single Mendelian traits, including dexamethasone-suppressible hypertension and Liddle's syndrome, which are autosomal dominant, and apparent mineralocorticoid excess, which is autosomal recessive. The molecular defect has been established for each of these conditions, enabling genetic diagnosis. In addition, the urinary steroid profiles of these conditions are characteristic and can aid in diagnosis (Shackleton, 1993).

PRIMARY HYPERALDOSTERONISM

Primary hyperaldosteronism is extremely rare in children and is usually related to nodular hyperplasia rather than to Conn's syndrome, where there is an aldosterone-producing tumour. Hypertension may be severe and is associated with a low plasma concentration of renin and hypokalaemia. Oedema is either absent or minimal. Surgery is recommended for adrenal adenomas. Hypertension frequently recurs after operative treatment for nodular hyperplasia, which may, therefore, respond more satisfactorily to long-term treatment with the aldosterone antagonist spironolactone.

DEXAMETHASONE-SUPPRESSIBLE HYPERALDOSTERONISM

The hypertension in dexamethasone-suppressible hyperaldosteronism, a dominantly inherited condition that is also known as glucocorticoid-remediable aldosteronism or familial hyperaldosteronism type I, is variable and resistant to normal drug treatment; however, it responds to treatment with dexamethasone. Plasma renin activity is profoundly low, and serum aldosterone levels are usually, but not always, raised. The genetic defect is an unequal cross-over event between genes encoding 11β-hydroxylase and aldosterone synthase. This results in a chimeric gene duplication containing the regulatory elements of 11β-hydroxylase and the coding sequence of aldosterone synthase (Lifton et al, 1992). Consequently, aldosterone is ectopically synthesized in the adrenal zona fasciculata under the regulation of adrenocorticotrophin hormone, rather than its usual secretagogue, angiotensin II. This chimeric gene product converts cortisol to its 18-oxo and 18-hydroxy metabolites, leading to a pathognomonic profile of urinary steroids, with a raised ratio of 18-oxotetrahydrocortisol to tetrahydroaldosterone (Rich et al, 1992). Treatment with dexamethasone leads to

Table 68.7. Syndromes of low-renin hypertension

Condition	Inheritance	Aldosterone	Potassium	Mechanism
11β-Hydroxylase deficiency	Autosomal recessive	Decreased	Low	11β-Hydroxylase deficiency
17α-Hydroxylase deficiency	Autosomal recessive	Decreased	Low	17α-Hydroxylase deficiency
Primary hyperaldosteronism	Sporadic	Increased	Low	Adrenocortical hyper or tumour
Dexamethasone-suppressible gene hyperaldosteronism	Autosomal dominant	Increased	Low	11β-Hydroxlyase/aldosterone synthase chimeric gene duplication
Liddle's syndrome	Autosomal dominant	Decreased	Low	Mutations in β/γ-subunits of epithelial sodium channel conferring increased activity
Apparent mineralocorticoid excess	Autosomal recessive	Decreased	Low	11β-hydroxysteroid dehydrogenase deficiency with impaired conversion of cortisol to cortisone
Gordon's syndrome	Autosomal dominant	Decreased	High	Increased proximal tubular NaCl reabsorption; genetic defect unknown

suppression of adrenocorticotrophic hormone, and hence suppression of the ectopically produced aldosterone. Direct aldosterone antagonists, such as spironolactone, have also been successful and may avoid the side effects of dexamethasone (Yiu et al, 1997).

LIDDLE'S SYNDROME

Liddle's syndrome is an autosomal dominant condition with a clinical presentation typical of primary hyper-aldosteronism, and yet levels of aldosterone in the serum and urine, as well as plasma renin activity, are suppressed (Liddle et al, 1963; Aarskog et al, 1967). Patients have constitutive activation of the amiloride-sensitive distal renal epithelial sodium channel as a result of mutations in the β- or γ-subunit of the epithelial sodium channel (Shimkets et al, 1994; Hansson et al, 1995; Schild et al, 1995). Analysis of urinary steroids reveals negligible aldosterone. Treatment with triamterine or amiloride is successful.

APPARENT MINERALOCORTICOID EXCESS

A number of children have been observed with hypertension associated with suppressed plasma renin activity, subnormal levels of aldosterone, hypokalaemia with alkalosis, and a reduced excretion of all known steroids (New and Levine, 1978; Shackleton et al, 1980). Deficiency of 11β-hydroxysteroid dehydrogenase appears to be the primary defect, though the cause of the hypertension remains obscure (Edwards et al, 1988). DiMartino-Nardi and New (1987) postulate that the enzymic defect results in impaired peripheral conversion of cortisol to cortisone. Analysis of urinary steroids by mass spectrometry gas chromatography shows a ratio of cortisone to cortisol of less than 1, the normal ratio being greater than 1. The cortisol leads to suppression of adrenocorticotrophic hormone, and hence reduced excretion of other corticosteroids. In addition, reduced conversion of cortisol to cortisone in the mineralocorticoid receptor leads to accumulated cortisol, having an unusually active mineralocorticoid effect. The condition responds to treatment with spironolactone, an antagonist of the mineralocorticoid receptor.

GORDON'S SYNDROME

Gordon's syndrome is an autosomal dominant condition that is also known as pseudohypoaldosteronism type II. It is characterized by hypertension with low plasma renin activity, hyperkalaemia, metabolic acidosis and normal glomerular filtration rates (Gordon et al, 1970). The underlying mechanism is probably increased proximal tubular reabsorption of sodium and chloride, although the genetic defect has not yet been established. The condition responds to restriction of sodium and therapy with thiazide diuretics.

LOW-RENIN ESSENTIAL HYPERTENSION

Essential hypertension with low renin is rare in children (Leuman et al, 1975) though more common in adults. While no defect of mineralocorticoid metabolism has been detected, the suggestion has been made that such a defect exists (Hollifield et al, 1977).

PHAEOCHROMOCYTOMA

Benign phaeochromocytomas, and the malignant phaeochromoblastomas, develop from chromaffin tissue in the adrenal gland or sympathetic ganglions. These tumours produce excessive amounts of catecholamines and lead to an increase in the excretion of their metabolites in the urine. Abnormal production of catecholamines is also observed with neuroblastomas, and occasionally with ganglion neuromas. Adrenaline and noradrenaline are the principle biologically active catecholamines. Noradrenaline is synthesized from tyrosine via dihydroxyphenylalanine and dopamine. It is then methylated to produce adrenaline, this being the main hormone of the adrenal medulla. Noradrenaline is principally produced by postganglionic sympathetic nerves. Noradrenaline acts mainly on sympathetic α-adrenoceptors, while adrenaline stimulates both α- and β-adrenoceptors. The catecholamines are metabolized to metadrenaline and normetadrenaline and then oxidized to the principle urinary metabolite 3-methoxy-4-hydroxymandelic acid, also called vanillylmandelic acid. The urine also contains homovanillic acid, produced from dopamine, as well as adrenaline and noradrenaline. Malignant tumours excrete dopamine and homovanillic acid. Normal values for urinary catecholamine excretion are shown in Table 68.8. Bananas, and drugs and foods containing vanilla, should be eliminated from the diet before collecting the urine. Methyldopa, clofibrate and inhibitors of monoamine oxidase will reduce excretion of catecholamines. Excretion is usually raised in children with phaeochromocytomas, especially if the urine is collected when the patient is hypertensive. Because of the practical difficulties in obtaining accurately timed 24-hour urine collections in small children, spot urine samples may be used, expressing the excretion of vanillylmandelic acid relative to urinary creatinine (Niehaus et al, 1979). Nonetheless, 24-hour collections may be necessary if the hypertension is episodic. Occasionally, in the small number of cases in which the tumours are small, the excretion of vanillylmandelic acid may be low. Plasma adrenaline and noradrenaline should also be measured. Typically, adrenal tumours produce a rise predominantly in adrenaline, while extra-adrenal tumours lead to raised noradrenaline levels. Consequently, in suspicious cases, the test should be repeated when the child is hypertensive and the noradrenaline and adrenaline determined in addition to the levels of vanillylmandelic acid.

Table 68.8. Urinary catecholamine excretion

Age (years)	Excretion in 24 hour (mean ± SD; µg/m²)			
	Dopamine	Noradrenaline	Adrenaline	VMA (HMMA)
0–1	221 ± 93	41 ± 15	4.7 ± 3.3	2021 ± 1121
1–5	187 ± 53	28 ± 9	4.9 ± 4.4	2001 ± 571
6–15	145 ± 55	31 ± 16	4.3 ± 1.9	2133 ± 378
>15	151 ± 44	30 ± 8	4.3 ± 1.9	1931 ± 389

From Voorhess (1967).
SD, standard deviation; VMA, vanillylmandelic acid; HMMA, 3-methoxy-4-hydroxymandelic acid.

The hypertension is usually ascribed to the increased secretion of noradrenaline. Thus, administration of phentolamine, which blocks α-adrenoceptors, will lower the blood pressure by more than 20 mmHg. A starting dose of 0.01 mg/kg body weight is increased to 0.1 mg/kg if no effect is observed. False positive results are common. The majority of children also have high plasma renin concentrations with secondary aldosteronism. This has been ascribed to depletion of fluid volume, direct stimulation of renin secretion by adrenaline, compression on the renal artery by the tumour, or associated renal arterial disease in those with neurofibromatosis (Leuman, 1979).

The adrenal medulla is the common site for the tumours, which vary in size from 1 to 10 cm. They are more common on the right and are bilateral in one fifth. In one third, tumours are situated in both the adrenal and extra-adrenal areas or only in an extra-adrenal site. Boys are affected twice as often as girls, and the incidence is highest between the ages of 11 and 15 years. The most common extra-adrenal site is the aortic bifurcation or the vicinity of the renal hilus. Bladder tumours are described, which cause paroxysmal hypertension during micturition and, sometimes, haematuria (Das et al, 1983). A dominant mode of inheritance is apparent in some families, and more than half of the patients have multiple tumours. Phaeochromocytoma is frequently associated with other conditions, such as neurofibromatosis, or von Hippel–Lindau disease, and with the autosomally dominant multiple endocrine neoplasia syndrome, which includes medullary thyroid carcinoma, islet cell adenoma and hyperparathyroidism (Stackpole et al, 1963). Hypertension is less common with other neurogenic tumours and only affects about one tenth of children with neuroblastomas. An increase in urinary dopamine and its metabolite homovanillic acid is a characteristic of neuroblastomas.

Clinical features relate to the hypertension, which is sustained in 88% of cases. Headaches, sweating, nausea and vomiting, visual disturbances, abdominal pain, polyuria and polydipsia, convulsions and acrocyanosis occur with diminishing frequency (Stackpole et al, 1963).

The location of the tumour(s) can be established with a variety of imaging techniques including ultrasound, [131I]-metaiodobenzylguanidine, computed tomography and magnetic resonance imaging (Boland and Lee, 1995). More invasive techniques involve sampling of blood at different levels from the inferior caval vein for determination of plasma catecholamines and arteriography (Lewis et al, 1987). Invasive investigations should only be performed after full α- and β-adrenoceptor blockade to control the hypertension and after correction of hypovolaemia. This latter is essential in any case before surgery. Safe anaesthesia and surgery require careful preoperative preparation. Phenoxybenzamine (1 mg/kg per day) is used to block α-adrenoceptors, and propranolol (1 mg/kg per day) is used for blockade of β-adrenoceptors. Monitoring of arterial and central venous pressures is required during surgery. Intravenous adrenergic blocking agents should be readily available. Occasionally blockade of α-adrenceptors is unsuccessful. In such cases, α-methyltyrosine, an inhibitor of tyrosine hydroxylase, has proved useful in reducing secretion of catecholamines (Robinson et al, 1977).

Surgical removal of the tumours(s) results in cure, but the frequency of multiple tumours suggests that long-term follow-up is indicated.

MISCELLANEOUS ENDOCRINE CAUSES

Primary hyperthyroidism is a rare cause of hypertension in children (Mosier, 1975). Hypertension is also rare in children with primary hyperparathyroidism and is probably related to nephrocalcinosis (Vasquez, 1973) and to hypercalcaemia, which raises peripheral vascular resistance (see below).

NEUROLOGICAL DISORDERS

Severe hypertension can occur in a variety of acute neurological disorders, for example Guillain Barré syndrome (Stapleton et al, 1978), poliomyelitis, intracranial lesions such as tumours, trauma, asphyxia and encephalitis (Eden et al, 1977). Autonomic dysfunction with overactivity of the sympathetic system is thought to be involved in the pathogenesis in these disorders and in the Riley–Day syndrome of familial dysautonomia (Ziegler et al, 1976), though raised intracranial pressure may be a particular precipitating factor.

MISCELLANEOUS CAUSES OF HYPERTENSION

DRUGS

Oral contraceptives have been discussed above. Glucocorticoids and mineralocorticoids are potent causes of hypertension, particularly in children with pre-existing renal disease. Sympathomimetic agents can raise the blood pressure even when used as topical preparations (Borromeo McGrail et al, 1973) or in nose drops. Mercury poisoning causing acrodynia (pink disease) is associated with hypertension. Poisoning with heavy metals, such as cadmium and lead; overdosage of reserpine, methyldopa and phenylcyclidine; and cough syrup containing ephredine have all caused hypertension (Leuman, 1979).

BURNS

Systemic hypertension occurs in one third of children with severe burns (Douglas and Broadfoot, 1972). Excessive production of catecholamine, increased renin–angiotensin stimulation, volume expansion and hypercalcaemia have been considered in the pathogenesis (Leuman, 1979).

HYPERCALCAEMIA

Hypercalcaemia is associated with hypertension, probably because of a rise in peripheral vascular resistance (Scholz, 1977). The syndrome of infantile hypercalcaemia (Chantler et al, 1966) may be associated with renal arterial stenosis and hypertension.

OTHER CAUSES

Hypertension occurs in acute intermittent porphyria (Stein and Tschudy, 1970). It can be associated with Turner syndrome, even in the absence of aortic coarctation (Engel and Forbes, 1965), and with Marfan's syndrome (Kuehl and Fricke, 1973). It has been described in pseudoxanthoma elasticum (Parker et al, 1964), Stevens–Johnson syndrome (Loggie, 1969) and with acrodermatitis enteropathica (Aberg et al, 1976). It also occurs during sickle cell crisis (Sellers, 1978; see Chapter 67). Ingestion of liquorice, which contains a substance with a mineralocorticoid effect, may cause hypertension that is similar to the hypertension induced by desoxycorticosteroid (Epstein et al, 1977).

MEDICAL THERAPY

The importance of non-pharmacological interventions (Kaplan, 1981) in the management of hypertension has been discussed above, as have the indications for treatment and for surgery. Pharmacological treatment is considered here. Maintenance treatment of chronic hypertension and emergency management of severe hypertension will be discussed separately.

MAINTENANCE THERAPY OF CHRONIC HYPERTENSION

Maintenance therapy for chronic hypertension is intended to control the blood pressure at the 90th percentile or less for height, age and sex (Table 68.9). Reference should, therefore, be made to the available percentile tables of blood pressure during childhood so that a clear target range for treatment is identified. Compliance is promoted by using the fewest drugs in the lowest dosage frequency. Long-acting formulations requiring once or twice daily dosage are increasingly available for a range of drugs. If more than one drug is required, the additional drug(s) should act through a different, and hence complimentary, mechanism.

The availability of inhibitors of angiotensin-converting enzyme and blockers of the calcium channel provides the majority of hypertensive children with effective and simple treatment that is relatively free of serious side effects. These drugs increasingly are becoming first choice of therapy and have largely displaced the 'stepped-care' approach (Chalmers, 1981), which involved the gradual introduction of diuretics, β-blockers, and vasodilators. It should be noted that information on the use of some of the available antihypertensive drugs is limited.

INHIBITORS OF ANGIOTENSIN-CONVERTING ENZYME

The angiotensin-converting enzyme inhibitors are effective antihypertensive agents (Friedman et al, 1981), particularly in renin-mediated hypertension. They also have other benefits in specific situations, such as proteinuric renal impairment and diabetes mellitus (Kamper et al, 1992; Louis et al, 1993). The hypotensive effect is not usually seen until some 90% of the enzymic activity has been inhibited; consequently, there may not be a graded dose–response effect. Captopril is useful initial treatment as the half-life is short (2 hours), allowing fairly rapid modification of dose until control is achieved. The recommended dose by body weight for neonates and infants is smaller, as the potency is greater in this group. It is recommended that a small initial test dose be given while the patient is closely observed, as some people show a profound fall in blood pressure; with postural hypotension, after a single dose. Enalapril has a long

Table 68.9 **Antihypertensive drugs for oral use**

Drug	Major side effects	Precautions	Dose
Angiotensin-2 converting enzyme inhibitors			
Captopril	Hypotension, rash, cough, agranulocytosis	Avoid in renal artery stenosis	Children: 0.1–0.5 mg/kg (maximum 2 mg/kg) three times a day Neonates: 0.01–0.05 mg/kg three times a day
Enalapril	Hypotension, cough	Avoid in renal artery stenosis	0.1 mg/kg (maximum 1.0 mg/kg) once daily (enalapril has been substituted for captopril as 1 mg enalapril per 7.5 mg captopril)
Calcium channel blocker			
Nifedipine	Flushing, tachycardia, headache	–	Capsule: 5–10 mg three times a day Modified release tablets: 10–20 mg twice a day Slow release tablets: 30–60 mg once a day
Diuretics			
Chlorothiazide	Hypokalaemia, hyperuricaemia	Renal insufficiency	10 mg/kg (maximum 40 mg/kg) per day
Frusemide	Hypokalaemia		1–4 mg/kg once or twice a day
Spironolactone	Hyperkalaemia, gynaecomastia	Renal insufficiency	1 mg/kg twice or three times a day
β-Adrenoceptor blockers			
Propranolol	Reduced cardiac output, bradycardia	Cardiac failure, asthma	0.2–2.0 mg/kg three times a day
Atenolol	As propranolol	As propranolol	1–2 mg/kg (maximum 8 mg/kg) once a day
α-Adrenoceptor blocker			
Prazosin	Hypotension after first dose, dizziness	First dose reaction	0.01 mg/kg three times a day; increase to a maximum of 0.5 mg/kg three times a day
Mixed α- and β-adrenoceptor blocker			
Labetolol	Rash, dry eyes, dizziness	Cardiac failure, asthma	1–2 mg/kg three or four times a day
Vasodilators			
Minoxidil	Fluid retention, tachycardia, hirsutism	–	0.1 mg/kg bd twice daily; increase by 0.1 mg/kg per dose every 3 days to a maximum of 0.5 mg/kg twice a day
Hydralazine	Flushing, tachycardia, lupus syndrome	–	0.2–1.0 mg/kg

half-life of 12 hours, enabling once daily dosage, which helps compliance in long-term therapy. The reduction in production of aldosterone associated with these drugs may lead to an increase in serum potassium, especially with pre-existing renal impairment. Rash, neutropenia, loss of taste, and cough are rare side effects. This class of drugs is relatively contraindicated in renal arterial stenosis, as they inhibit the angiotensin II-mediated compensatory efferent arteriolar vasoconstriction, with the risk of a precipitous fall in glomerular filtration rate (Hricick and Dunn, 1990).

CALCIUM CHANNEL BLOCKERS

The calcium channel blockers are most effective in low-renin, volume-dependent hypertension. They interfere with the inward displacement of calcium ions through voltage-dependent slow channels in the cell membrane, and reduce blood pressure by causing vasodilatation. Nifedipine has been widely used, both in its short-acting form for the rapid lowering of blood pressure in urgent situations, and in its slow-release forms for maintenance treatment of chronic hypertension. Side effects are related to vasodilatation and include tachycardia and flushing. Amlodipine is a newer agent that requires only single daily dosage. It is not officially licensed for use in children but has been used successfully in this age group.

DIURETICS

The diuretics are particularly useful in patients with renal disease. They are often required as a second agent to control the fluid retention associated with long-term use of vasodilators. Thiazide diuretics are effective if the glomerular filtration rate is over 50% of normal, but a loop diuretic such as frusemide will be needed for more severe degrees of renal impairment. Side effects include hypokalaemia with both groups of diuretic, and ototoxicity with loop diuretics. The mineralocorticoid antagonist spironolactone is useful in conditions of mineralocorticoid excess. It may also be used in addition to a loop or thiazide diuretic for its potassium-sparing effect. Triamterene and amiloride are used specifically for Liddle's syndrome.

BLOCKERS OF β-ADRENOCEPTORS

The β-blockers have been used as first-line therapy for a long time and are effective in many patients. Cardiac output is reduced, peripheral release of noradrenaline is impaired, release of renin is inhibited and there is centrally mediated reduction in peripheral sympathetic activity. There is a relatively poor correlation between the antihypertensive effect of the drug and the level of drug in the plasma. Side effects are numerous and include exacerbation of asthma and cardiac failure, depressed mood, nightmares and disturbed lipid and glucose metabolism. Propranolol is the best known agent, while atenolol has a long half-life and need only be given once daily.

BLOCKERS OF α-ADRENOCEPTORS

Prazosin is an α_1-adrenoceptor blocker and has few serious side effects in children. The antihypertensive effect is through vasodilation. Caution should be observed with the first dose, as this may cause marked postural hypotension. This class of drug is useful in treating catecholamine-induced hypertension. Recently, a long-acting α-adrenoceptor blocker, doxazosin, has been available for once daily dosage. It is not officially licensed for use in children.

BLOCKERS OF BOTH α- AND β-ADRENOCEPTORS

Labetolol (Frick and Porste, 1976) is a non-selective β-blocker, with less potent α-adrenoceptor blocking properties. Its main use is as an intravenous infusion in the treatment of hypertensive emergencies.

VASODILATING AGENTS

The vasodilators are a group of pharmacologically diverse drugs that have vasodilation as their common effect. Some drugs with this effect have already been described above. Hydralazine and minoxidil act directly on the vascular smooth muscle to reduce peripheral vas-cular resistance. Hydralazine is most often used as an intravenous bolus for rapid control of severe hypertension. Minoxidil is a powerful vasodilator and is usually used as an added agent in resistant hypertension. It causes marked hirsutism. As mentioned above, long-term use of vasodilating drugs is often associated with retention of salt and water, and a diuretic may, therefore, need to be used in addition.

HYPERTENSIVE CRISIS

The rapid but controlled lowering of blood pressure is essential in children who present with hypertensive encephalopathy. Similarly, severely elevated blood pressure that has not yet led to symptomatic damage to target organs should be urgently controlled before an adverse event occurs. Clinical improvement is often seen with a relatively small reduction of blood pressure, and the initial aim should not be rapid reduction of blood pressure to normal levels. Sudden massive falls in blood pressure have to be avoided if neurological complications are to be prevented (Deal et al, 1992). These complications are more likely if the hypertension has been long standing, though the chronicity of hypertension may not be apparent at initial clinical assessment of a child presenting with hypertensive crisis. A selection of drugs for use in hypertensive emergencies is shown in Table 68.10. An intravenous line should always be established. Some children with malignant hypertension are depleted for salt and fluid and have intense vasoconstriction. They may be especially sensitive to vasodilation and require considerable quantities of saline to maintain and control the blood pressure. The controlled reduction in blood pressure over 96 hours is important, and intravenous infusion of labetalol is now our first choice. If it proves insufficient, then sodium nitroprusside is added. The latter is especially useful because of its short duration of action. Constant monitoring of the rate of infusion and blood pressure is required during its use. Thiocyanate toxicity can occur with long-term therapy or with renal insufficiency. Although nitroprusside has been used without ill effects for up to 10 days (Luderer et al, 1977), plasma thiocyanate should be monitored after 24 hours and treatment discontinued if the concentration exceeds 12 mg/dl (Gordillo Paniagtia et al, 1975). Less severe hypertensive crisis is often managed very successfully with oral nifedipine in rapid-acting capsule form. Children should be instructed to bite the capsule, as most absorption occurs after swallowing the contained liquid. In small children, the liquid may be aspirated from the capsule by syringe and fine needle and then administered orally. Intravenous hydralazine may also be used as a rapid acting vasodilator. These agents, however, give less precise control over the rate of fall of blood pressure, and intravenous infusion treatment is preferred where there is symptomatic severe hypertension.

Table 68.10. Drugs for treatment of hypertensive emergencies

Drug	Onset of action	Dose and route	Mode of action	Comments
Labetolol	Minutes	1–3 mg/kg per h as i.v. infusion	Vasodilator	Titrate rate of constant infusion against change in blood pressure
Sodium nitroprusside	Seconds	0.5 µg/kg per min i.v.; increase by 0.2 µg/kg per min to a maximum of 8 µg/kg per min	Vasodilator	1. Titrate rate of constant infusion against change in blood pressure 2. Stop treatment if plasma thiocyanate exceeds 12 mg/dl
Hydralazine	Minutes	1. 0.3–0.5 mg/kg as i.v. slow bolus dose; maximum 4-hourly 2. 0.025–0.05 mg/kg per h i.v. to maximum of 3 mg/kg in 24 h	Vasodilator	Titrate rate of constant infusion against change in blood pressure
Nifedipine (capsules)	Minutes	0.25–0.5 mg/kg orally	Vasodilator	1. Effect is less controllable than with i.v. infusion 2. Child must bite and swallow capsule, or liquid contents should be removed via a needle and syringe and then swallowed
Minoxidil	Minutes	0.1–0.2 mg/kg orally	Vasodilator	See (1) for nifedipine
Frusemide	Minutes	2–5 mg/kg i.v. over 20 min	Loop diuretic	For severe intravascular volume expansion states Rapid administration of large doses may be ototoxic

i.v., intravenous.

It is important initially to assess clinically the adequacy of the extracellular fluid volume. If there is evidence of overload with increased venous pressure or pulmonary oedema, then removal of fluid by a frusemide-induced diuresis or by dialysis is required. The hypertension of acute nephritic syndrome often settles rapidly if an adequate diuresis can be obtained. A child with severe hypertension requires constant supervision over the first 96 hours of treatment by both medical and nursing staff if the steady reduction in blood pressure is to be achieved without cardiovascular or neurological catastrophes.

REFERENCES

Aarskog D, Sta K F, Thorsen T, Wefring K W 1967 Hypertension and hypokalaemic alkalosis associated with underproduction of aldosterone. Pediatrics 39: 884–890

Aberg H, Michaelsson G, Walldius G 1976 Hypertension in a patient with acrodermatitis enteropathica. Acta Paediatrica Scandinavica 65: 757–759

Abman S H, Warady B A, Lum G M, Koops B L 1984 Systemic hypertension in infants with bronchopulmonary dysplasia. Journal of Pediatrics 104: 928–931

Adelman R D 1978 Neonatal hypertension. Pediatric Clinics of North America 25: 99–110

Adelman R D 1987 Long-term follow-up of neonatal renovascular hypertension. Pediatric Nephrology 1: 35–41

Adelman R D 1988 The hypertensive neonate. Clinics in Perinatology 15: 567–585

Aderele W I, Seriki O 1974 Hypertension in Nigerian children. Archives of Disease in Childhood 49: 413–417

Alpert B S, Daniels S R 1997 Twenty-four-hour ambulatory blood pressure monitoring: now that technology has come of age – we need to catch up. Journal of Pediatrics 130: 167–169

Alpert B S, Bain H H, Balfe J W, Kidd B S L, Olley P M 1979 Role of the renin–angiotensin–aldosterone system in hypertensive children with coarctation of the aorta. American Journal of Cardiology 43: 828–834

Antonios T F T, MacGregor G A 1996 Salt–more adverse effects. Lancet 348: 250–251

Aperia A, Berg U, Broberger O, Soderlund S, Thoren C 1973 The renal response to an oral salt and fluid load in children with coarctation of the aorta. Acta Paediatrica Scandinavica 62: 241–247

Arneill G G, MacDonald A M, Murphy A V, Sweet E M 1973 Renal venous thrombosis. Clinical Nephrology 1: 119–131

Aschinberg L S, Zeis P M, Miller R A, John E G, Chan L L 1977 Essential hypertension in childhood. Journal of American Medical Association 238: 322–324

Aurell M 1979 Fibromuscular dysplasia of the renal arteries. British Medical Journal i: 1180–1181

Balfe J W, Rance C P 1978 Recognition and management of hypertensive crises in childhood. Pediatric Clinics of North America 25: 159–174

Barker D J P, Winter P D, Osmond C, Margetts B, Simmonds S J 1989 Weight in infancy and death from ischaemic heart disease. Lancet 334: 577–580

Barker D J P, Bull A R, Osmond C, Simmonds S J 1990 Fetal and placental size and risk of hypertension in adult life. British Medical Journal 301: 259–262

Barker D J P, Osmond C, Simmonds S J, Wield G A 1993 The relation of small head circumference and thinness at birth to death from cardiovascular disease in adult life. British Medical Journal 306: 422–426

Beevers D G 1982 Blood pressures that fall on rechecking. British Medical Journal 284: 71

Bennett S P, Levine L S, Siegal E J et al 1974 Juvenile hypertension caused by overproduction of renin within a renal segment. Journal of Pediatrics 84: 689–695

Berenson G S, Lawrence M, Soto L 1989 The heart and hypertension in childhood. Seminars in Nephrology 9: 236–246

Bianchi G, Baer P G, Fox U et al 1975 Changes in renin, water balance and sodium balance during development of high blood pressure in genetically hypertensive rats. Circulation Research 36/37(suppl 11): 153–161

Bidlingmeyer I, Burnier M, Bidlingmeyer M, Waeber B, Brunner H R 1996 Isolated office hypertension: a prehypertensive state? Journal of Hypertension 14: 327–332

Biron P, Mongeau J G 1978 Familial aggregation of blood pressure and its components. Pediatric Clinics of North America 25: 29–33

Biron P, Mongeau J G, Bertrand D 1977 Familial resemblance of body weight and weight/height in 374 homes with adopted children. Journal of Pediatrics 91: 555–558

Black H R 1993 Treatment of mild hypertension: the more things change. Journal of the American Medical Association 270: 757–759

Boedy R F, Goldberg A K, Howell C G, Hulse E, Edwards E G, Kanto W P Jr 1990 Incidence of hypertension in infants on extracorporeal membrane oxygenation. Journal of Pediatric Surgery 25: 258–261

Boland G W, Lee M J 1995 Magnetic resonance imaging of the adrenal gland. Critical Reviews in Diagnostic Imaging 36: 115–174

Borromeo McGrail V, Bordiuk J M, Keitel H 1973 Systemic hypertension following ocular administration of 10% phenylalamine in the neonate. Pediatrics 51: 1032–1036

Borst J G G, Borst de Geus A 1963 Hypertension explained by Starling's theory of circulatory homeostasis. Lancet i: 677–682

Brenner B M, Garcia D L, Anderson S 1988 Glomeruli and blood pressure. Less of one, more of the other? American Journal of Hypertension 1: 335–347

Brest A N, Bower R 1966 Renal arterial hypertension incidence, diagnosis and treatment. American Journal of Cardiology 17: 612–616

Brown J J, Fraser R, Lever A F et al 1973 Hypertension and secondary hyperaldosteronism associated with a renin secreting renal juxtaglomerular cell tumour. Lancet ii: 1228–1232

Brown J J, Lever A F, Robertson J I S 1979 Renal hypertension: aetiology, diagnosis and treatment. In: Black D, Jones N F (eds) Renal disease, 4th edn. Blackwell, London, p 731–765

Brunner H R, Laragh J H, Baer L et al 1972 Essential hypertension: renin aldosterone, heart attack and stroke. New England Journal of Medicine 286: 441–449

Buehlmeyer K 1974 Differential diagnose des hypertoniebe fundes im kindesalter. Munchen Medische Wochenschrift 116: 711–716

Burlage S R 1923 The blood pressure and heart rate in girls during adolescence. American Journal of Physiology 64: 252–284

Calabrese E J, Tuthill R W 1977 Elevated blood pressure and high sodium levels in the public drinking water. Archives of Environmental Health 32: 200–202

Carella J A, Silbeir I 1976 Hyperreninaemic hypertension in an infant secondary to pelviureteric junction obstruction treated successfully by surgery. Journal of Pediatrics 88: 987–989

Cassimos C, Varlgmis G, Karamperis S, Katsouyannopoulos V 1977 Blood pressure in children and adolescents. Acta Paediatrica Scandinavica 66: 439–443

Chalmers J P 1981 Rational basis for drug treatment of hypertension. Australian and New Zealand Journal of Medicine 2(suppl 1): 69–72

Chantler C 1983 Familial renal disease. In: Weatherall D J, Ledingham J G G, Warrell D A, (eds) Oxford textbook of medicine. Oxford University Press, Oxford p 18.75–18.81

Chantler C, Joseph M C, Davies H 1966 Cardiovascular and other associations of infantile hypercalcaemia. Guy's Hospital Reports 115: 221–241

Chapman W S, Douglas A S 1975 Hypertension and unilateral hydronephrosis in children successfully treated by pyeloplasty, report of two cases. Journal of Paediatric Surgery 10: 281–282

Choquette G, Ferguson R J 1973 Blood pressure reduction in borderline hypertensives following physical training. Canadian Medical Association Journal 108: 699–703

Clarke W R, Schrott H G, Leaverton P E, Connor W E, Lauer R M 1978 Tracking of blood lipids and blood pressures in school age children: the Muscatine study. Circulation 58: 626–634

Clarkson E M, Raw S M, de Wardener H E 1979 Further observations on a low molecular weight natriuretic substance in the urine of normal man. Kidney International 16: 710–721

Cole B R, Conley S B, Stapleton F B 1987 Polycystic kidney disease in the first year of life. Journal of Pediatrics 111: 693–699

Conroy R M, O'Brien E, O'Malley K, Atkins N 1993 Measurement error in the Hawksley random zero sphygimomanometer; what damage has been done and what can we learn? British Medical Journal 306: 1319–1322

Cuneo R A, Caronna J J 1977 Neurological complications of hypertension. Medical Clinics of North America 61: 565–580

Da Hae Lee, Sapire D, Markowitz R, Gruskin A 1976 Radiation injury to abdominal aorta and iliac artery sustained in infancy. South African Medical Journal 50: 658–660

Dahl L K, Schakow E 1964 Effects of chronic excess salt ingestion: experimental hypertension in the rat. Canadian Medical Association Journal 90: 155–160

Dahl L K, Knudsen K D, Heine M, Leitl G 1967 Effects of chronic excess salt ingestion: genetic influences on the development of salt hypertension in parabiotic rats, evidence for a humoral factor. Journal of Experimental Medicine 126: 687–699

Das S, Bulusu N V, Lowe P 1983 Primary vesical phaeochromocytoma. Urology 21: 20–25

Davies D L, Beevers D G, Briggs J D et al 1973 Abnormal relation between exchangeable sodium and the renin angiotensin system in malignant hypertension and in hypertension in chronic renal failure. Lancet i: 683–687

Deal J E, Barratt T M, Dillon M J 1992 Management of hypertensive emergencies. Archives of Disease in Childhood 67: 1089–1092

Deal J E, Snell M F, Barratt T M, Dillon M J 1992. Renovascular disease in childhood. Journal of Pediatrics 121: 378–384

Debatin S F, Spritzer C E, Crist T M et al 1991 Imaging of renal arteries: value of MR angiography. American Journal of Roentgenology 157: 981–990

de Swiet M 1982 Blood pressure, sodium and take away food. Archives of Disease in Childhood 57: 645–646

de Swiet M, Fayers P, Shinebourne E A 1980a Value of repeated blood pressure measurements in children – the Brompton study. British Medical Journal i: 1567–1568

de Swiet M, Fayers P, Shinebourne E A 1980b Systolic blood pressure in a population of infants in the first year of life: the Brompton study. Paediatrics 65: 1028–1035

de Swiet M, Fayers P, Shinebourne E A 1982 Blood pressure in the first 10 years of life: the Brompton study. British Medical Journal 304: 23–26

de Wardener H E, MacGregor G A 1980 Dahl's hypothesis that a saliuretic substance may be responsible for a sustained rise in arterial pressure: its possible role in essential hypertension. Kidney International 18: 1–9

Devereux R B, Pickering T G, Harshfield G A et al 1983 Left ventricular hypertrophy in patients with hypertension: importance of blood pressure response to regularly recurring stress. Circulation 68: 470–476

Dillon M J 1980 Renin angiotensin aldosterone system. European Journal of Clinical Pharmacology 18: 105–108

Dillon M J, Ryness J M 1975 Plasma renin activity and aldosterone concentration in children. British Medical Journal 4: 316–319

Dillon M J, Shah V, Barratt T M 1978 Renal vein renin measurements in children with hypertension. British Medical Journal 2: 168–170

DiMartino-Nardi J, New M I 1987 Low-renin hypertension of childhood. Pediatric Nephrology 1: 99–108

Dimmick J E, Patterson M W H, Wu H W A 1979 Systemic hypertension in a newborn infant. Journal of Pediatrics 95: 321–324

Douglas B S, Broadfoot M J 1972 Hypertension in burnt children. Australia and New Zealand Journal of Surgery 42: 194–196

Drukker A 1981 Hypertrophic cardiomyopathy in children with end stage renal disease and hypertension. Proceedings EDTA 18: 542–555

Dube S K, Kapoor S, Ratner H, Tunick F L 1975 Blood pressure studies in black children. American Journal of Diseases in Childhood 129: 1177–1180

Dunn M J, Tanner R L 1974 Low renin hypertension. Kidney International 5: 317–325

Dustan H P 1995 Does keloid pathogenesis hold the key to understanding black/white differences in hypertension severity? Hypertension 26: 858–862

Eden O B, Sills J A, Brown J K 1977 Hypertension in acute neurological diseases of childhood. Developmental Medicine and Child Neurology 19: 437–445

Editorial 1973 Detection of hypertension in children. British Medical Journal 3: 356

Editorial 1977 Childhood hypertension. British Medical Journal 2: 76–77

Editorial 1979 Hypertension in childhood. Lancet ii: 833–834

Editorial 1981 New evidence linking salt and hypertension. British Medical Journal 282: 1993–1994

Editorial 1982 Does control of risk factors prevent coronary artery disease? British Medical Journal 285: 1065–1066

Edwards C R, Stewart P M, Burt D et al 1988 Localisation of 11β-hydroxysteroid dehydrogenase – tissue specific protector of the mineralocorticoid receptor. Lancet 332: 986–989

Elliott P, Stamler J, Nichols R et al for the Intersalt Cooperative Research Group 1996 Intersalt revisited: further analysis of 24 hour sodium excretion and blood pressure within and across populations. British Medical Journal 312: 1249–1253

Elseed A M, Shinebourne E A, Joseph M C 1973 Assessment of techniques for measurement of blood pressure in infants and children. Archives of Disease in Childhood 48: 932–936

Engel E, Forbes A P 1965 Cytogenetic and clinical findings in 48 patients with congenitally defective or absent ovaries. Medicine (Baltimore) 44: 135–164

Epstein M T, Espiner E A, Donald R A, Hughes H 1977 Liquorice toxicity and the renin angiotensin aldosterone axis in man. British Medical Journal i: 209–210

Falkner B, Hamstra B, Lombardo R, Shirk J 1981 Blood pressure variability in adolescent males. International Journal of Paediatric Nephrology 2: 177–180

Finerty F A 1978 Contraception and pregnancy in the young female hypertensive patient. Pediatric Clinics of North America 25: 119–126

Fixler D E, Laird P E, Browne R 1979 Response of hypertensive adolescents to dynamic and isometric exercise stress. Paediatrics 64: 579–583

Florey C, Du V, Uppal S, Lowy C 1976 Relation between blood pressure weight and plasma sugar and serum insulin levels in school children aged 9–12 years in Westland, Holland. British Medical Journal i: 1368–1371

Folkow B 1978 The fourth Volhard lecture: cardiovascular structural adaptation: its role in the initiation and maintenance of primary hypertension. Clinical Science and Molecular Medicine 55(suppl 4): 3S–22S

Frick M H, Porste P 1976 Combined alpha and beta adrenoceptor blockade with labetalol in hypertension. British Medical Journal i: 1046–1048

Friedman A L, Hustead V A 1987 Hypertension in babies following discharge from a neonatal intensive care unit: A 3-year follow-up. Pediatric Nephrology 1: 30–34

Friedman A, Chesney R W, Ball D, Goodfriend T 1981 Effective use of captopril (angiotensin I converting enzyme inhibitor) in severe childhood hypertension. Journal of Pediatrics 97: 664–667

Garay R P, Meyer P 1979 A new test showing abnormal net Na⁺ and K⁺ fluxes in erythrocytes of essential hypertensive patients. Lancet i: 349–352

Giaconi S, Levanti C, Fommei E et al 1989 Microalbuminuria and casual and ambulatory blood pressure monitoring in normotensives and in patients with borderline and mild essential hypertension. American Journal of Hypertension 2: 259–261

Gill D G 1977 Blood pressure in Dublin school children. Irish Medical Journal 146: 255–259

Gill D G, Mendes de Costa B, Cameron J S et al 1976 Analysis of 100 children with severe and persistent hypertension. Archives of Disease in Childhood 51: 951–956

Gillman M W, Cook N R, Rosner B et al 1993 Identifying children at high risk for the development of essential hypertension. Journal of Pediatrics 122: 837–846

Glen S K, Elliott H L, Curzio J L, Lees K R, Reid J L 1996 White-coat hypertension as a cause of cardiovascular dysfunction. Lancet 348: 654–657

Godard C 1977 Predictive value of renal vein renin measurements in children with various forms of renal hypertension. Helvetica Paediatrica Acta 32: 49–57

Goldblatt H, Lynch J, Hanzal R H, Summerville W W 1934 Studies on experimental hypertension 1. The production of persistent elevation of systolic blood pressure by means of renal ischaemia. Journal of Experimental Medicine 59: 347–379

Goldraich N P, Ramos O L, Goldraich I H 1989 Urography versus DMSA scan in children with vesicoureteric reflux. Pediatric Nephrology 3: 1–5

Goldring D 1978 Treatment of the infant and child with coarctation of the aorta. Pediatric Clinics of North America 25: 111–119

Goonasekera C D A, Shah V, Wade A M, Barratt T M, Dillon M J 1996 15-year follow-up of renin and blood pressure in reflux nephropathy. Lancet 347: 640–643

Gordillo Paniagua G, Velasquez Jones L, Martini R, Vaidez Bolanos E 1975 Sodium nitroprusside treatment of severe arterial hypertension in children. Journal of Pediatrics 87: 799–802

Gordon R D, Geddes R A, Pawsey C J K et al 1970 Hypertension and severe hyperkalaemia associated with suppression of renin and aldosterone and completely reversed by dietary sodium restriction. Australian Annals of Medicine 19: 287–294

Gruskin A B 1977 The kidney in congenital heart disease: an overview. In: Barness L A (ed.) Advances in pediatrics, vol 24. Year Book Medical, Chicago, IL, p 133–189

Gupta T C, Wiggers C J 1951 Basic haemodynamic changes produced by aortic coarctation of different degrees. Circulation 3: 17–31

Guyton A C 1976 Textbook of medical physiology, 5th edn. Saunders, Philadelphia, PA

Guyton A C, Cowley A W, Coleman T G et al 1973 Post tubular versus tubular mechanisms of renal hypertension. In: Mechanisms of hypertension. Excepta Medica, Amsterdam, p 16

Guyton A C, Cowley A W, Young D B et al 1976 Integration and control of circulatory function. In: Guyton A C, Cowley A W (eds) Cardiovascular physiology 11, vol 9. International Review of Physiology. Baltimore University Park Press, Baltimore, MD

Hansson J H, Nelson-Williams C, Suzuki H et al 1995 Hypertension caused by a truncated epithelial sodium channel γ subunit: genetic heterogeneity of Liddle syndrome. Nature Genetics 11: 76–82

Harlan W R, Obermon A, Mitchell R E, Graybiel A 1973 In: Onesti G, Kim K E, Moyer J H (eds) Hypertension: mechanisms and management. Grutie & Stratton, New York, p 85

Harris R E, Forsyth R P 1973 Personality and emotional stress in essential hypertension in man. In: Onesti G, Kim K E, Moyer J H (eds) Hypertension: mechanisms and management. Grune & Stratton, New York, p 902

Harshfield G A, Alpert B S, Pulliam D A 1993 Renin–angiotensin–aldosterone system in healthy subjects aged ten to eighteen years. Journal of Pediatrics 122: 563–567

Harshfield G A, Alpert B S, Pulliam D A, Somes G W, Wilson D K 1994 Ambulatory blood pressure recordings in children and adolescents. Pediatrics 94: 180–184

Hegyi T, Anwar M, Carbone M T et al 1996 Blood pressure ranges in premature infants: II the first week of life. Pediatrics 97: 336–342

Hinchcliffe S A, Lynch M R, Sargent P H, Howard C V, Van V D 1992 The effect of intrauterine growth retardation on the development of renal nephrons. British Journal of Obstetrics and Gynaecology 99: 296–301

Hinchey J, Chaves C, Appignani B 1996 A reversible posterior leukoencephalopathy syndrome. New England Journal of Medicine 334: 494–500

Hollifield J W, Slaton P E, Wilson H et al 1977 Are there unknown mineralocorticoids in low renin essential hypertension? Mayo Clinic Proceedings 52: 329–333

Hostetter T H, Olson J L, Rennke H G, Venkatachalam M A, Brenner B M 1981 Hyperfiltration in remnant nephrons: a potentially adverse response to renal ablation. American Journal of Physiology 241: F85–F93

Houtman P N, Dillon M J 1991 Routine measurement of blood pressure in schoolchildren. Archives of Disease in Childhood 66: 567–568

Hricik D E, Dunn M J 1990 Angiotensin-converting enzyme inhibitor-induced renal failure: causes, consequences, and diagnostic uses. Journal of the American Society of Nephrology 1: 845–858

Hulse J A, Taylor D S I, Dillon M J 1979 Blindness and paraplegia in severe childhood hypertension. Lancet ii: 553–556

Hypertension Detection and Follow Up Programme Cooperative Group 1979 Five year findings of the hypertensive detection and follow up program. Journal of the American Medical Association 242: 2562–2571

Hypertension Detection and Follow Up Programme Cooperative Group 1982 The effect of treatment on mortality in 'mild' hypertension. New England Journal of Medicine 307: 976–980

Hypertension Study Group 1971 Intersociety commission for heart disease resources. Guidelines for the detection, diagnosis and management of hypertensive populations. Circulation 263(suppl A): 44

Ingelfinger J R 1993 Renovascular disease in children. Kidney International 43: 453–505

Jackson J C, Truog W E, Watchko J F, Mack L A, Cyr D R, van Belle G 1987 Efficacy of thromboresistant umbilical artery catheters in reducing thrombosis and related complications. Journal of Pediatrics 110: 102–105

Jonker G J, Huisman R M, de Zeeuw D 1993 Enhancement of screening tests for renovascular hypertension by angiotensin converting enzyme inhibitors. Nephrology, Dialysis and Transplantation 8: 798–807

Julius S 1977 In: Garest J, Kouiw E, Kuchel O (eds) Hypertension. McGraw Hill, New York, p 630

Juncos L I, Deture F A, Walker R D, Maclovsky M L 1976 Renin dependent renovascular hypertension in an infant with abdominal aortic atresia. Urology 7: 628–631

Kamper A L, Strandgaard S, Leyssac P P 1992 Effect of enalapril on the progression of chronic renal failure: a randomized control trial. American Journal of Hypertension 5: 423–430

Kannel W B, Dawber T R 1973 Hypertensive cardiovascular disease in Framingham Study. In: Onesti G, Kim K E, Moyer J H (eds) Hypertension: mechanisms and management. Grune & Stratton, New York, p 902

Kaplan B S, Fox H, Seidman E, Drummond K N 1978 Normal blood pressure in offspring of persons with essential hypertension. Canadian Medical Association Journal 118: 1415–1417

Kaplan N M 1981 Non drug treatment of hypertension. Australian New Zealand Journal of Medicine 11(suppl 1): 73–75

Kilcoyne M M 1978 Natural history of hypertension in adolescents. Pediatric Clinics of North America 25: 47–53

Kilcoyne M M, Richter R W, Alsop P A 1974a Adolescent hypertension I. Detection and prevalence. Circulation 50: 758–764

Kilcoyne M M, Richter R W, Alsop P A 1974b Adolescent hypertension II. Characteristics and response to treatment. Circulation 50: 1014–1019

Kincaid Smith P 1981 Understanding malignant hypertension. Australia and New Zealand Journal of Medicine 11(suppl 1): 64–68

Kliewer M A, Tupler R H, Carroll B A et al 1993 Renal artery stenosis: analysis of Doppler waveform parameters and tardus–parvus pattern. Radiology 189: 779–787

Knudsen K D, Dabl L K 1966 Essential hypertension: inborn error of sodium metabolism? Postgraduate Medical Journal 42: 148–152

Kowarski A A, Migeon C J 1977 Aldosterone in childhood. In: New M I, Levine L S (eds) Juvenile hypertension. Kroc Foundation Series 8. Raven, New York, p 97

Krakhoff L, Nicolis F, Amsel B 1975 Pathogenesis of hypertension in Cushings syndrome. American Journal of Medicine 58: 216–220

Krull F, Buck T, Offner G, Brodehl J 1993 Twenty-four hour blood pressure monitoring in healthy children. European Journal of Pediatrics 152: 555–558

Kuehl I, Fricke G 1973 Kardiovaskulare manifestationen forem des Marfan Syndroms. Klinische Wochenschrift 51: 1129–1142

Kurien A, John P R, Milford D V 1997 Hypertension secondary to progressive vascular neurofibromatosis. Archives of Disease in Childhood 76: 454–455

Laird W P, Fixler D E 1981 Left ventricular hypertrophy in adolescents with elevated blood pressure: assessment by chest roentgenography, electrocardiography, and echocardiography. Pediatrics 69: 255–259

Langer R D 1995 The epidemiology of hypertension control in populations. Clinical and Experimental Hypertension 17: 1127–1144

Langley S C, Jackson A A 1994 Increased systolic blood pressure in adult rats induced by fetal exposure to maternal low protein diets. Clinical Science 86: 217–222

Lauer R M, Filer L J Jr, Reiter M A, Clarke W R 1976 Blood pressure, salt preference, salt threshold and relative weight. American Journal of Disease in Childhood 130: 493–497

Law C M, de Swiet M, Osmond C et al 1993 Initiation of hypertension in utero and its amplification throughout life. British Medical Journal 306: 24–27

Leuman E P 1979 Blood pressure and hypertension in childhood and adolescence. In: Frick P, von Harneck G A, Martini G A, Prader A, Schoen P, Wolff H P (eds) Advances in internal medicine and pediatrics. Springer, Berlin, p 109–183

Leuman E P, Nussberger J, Vetter W 1975 Low renin essential hypertension in a child. Helvetia Paediatrica Acta 30: 357–363

Leuman E P, Bodmer H G, Vetter W, Epstein F H 1979 Studies of blood pressure in school children of Zurich, Switzerland. International Symposium on Juvenile Hypertension, Parma, June

Levine L S, Lewy J E, New M I 1976 Hypertension in high school students, evaluation in New York City. New York State Journal of Medicine 76: 40–44

Lewis D, Dalton N, Rigdon S P A 1987 Phaeochromocytoma: report of three cases. Pediatric Nephrology 1: 46–49

Liddle G W, Bledsoe T, Coppage W S 1963 A familial renal disorder simulating primary aldosteronism but with negligible aldosterone secretion. Transactions of the Association of American Physicians 76: 199–213

Lieberman E 1974 Essential hypertension in children and youth. A pediatric perspective. Journal of Pediatrics 85: 1–11

Lifton R P, Dluhy R G, Powers M et al 1992 Chimeric 11β-hydroxylase/aldosterone synthase gene causes GRA and human hypertension. Nature 355: 262–265

Lingens S, Soergel M, Loirat C, Busch C, Lemmer B, Scharer K 1995 Ambulatory blood pressure monitoring in pediatric patients treated by regular haemodialysis and peritoneal dialysis. Pediatric Nephrology 9: 167–172

Lingens S, Freund M, Seeman T, Witte K, Lemmer B, Scharer K 1997 Circadian blood pressure changes in untreated children with kidney disease and conserved renal function. Acta Paediatrica 86: 719–723

Linshaw M A, Stapleton F B, Gruskin A B, Baluarte J, Harbin G L 1979 Traction related hypertension in children. Journal of Pediatrics 95: 994–996

Loggie J M H 1969 Hypertension in children and adolescents 1. Causes and diagnostic studies. Journal of Pediatrics 74: 331–355

Loggie J M H 1971 Systemic hypertension in children and adolescents. Causes and treatment. Pediatric Clinics of North America 18: 1273–1310

Londe S 1968 Blood pressure standards for normal children as determined under office conditions. Clinical Pediatrics (Philadelphia) 7: 400–403

Londe S, Goldring D 1972 Hypertension in children. American Heart Journal 84: 1–4

Londe S, Bourgoignie J J, Robson A M, Goldring D 1971 Hypertension in apparently normal children. Journal of Pediatrics 78: 569–577

Londe S, Gollub S W, Goldring D 1977a Blood pressure in black and white children. Journal of Pediatrics 90: 93–95

Londe S, Goldring D, Gollub S W, Hernandez A 1977b Blood pressure and hypertension in children: studies, problems and perceptives. In: New M I, Levine L S (eds) Juvenile hypertension. Raven, New York, p 13–23

Loridan L, Senior B 1969 Cushings syndrome in infancy. Journal of Pediatrics 75: 349–359

Louis E J, Hunsicker L G, Bain R P, Rohde R D 1993 The effect of angiotensin-converting-enzyme inhibition on diabetic nephropathy. New England Journal of Medicine 329: 1456–1462

Luderer J R, Hayes A H, Dubysisky O, Berlin C M 1977 Longterm administration of sodium nitroprusside in childhood. Journal of Pediatrics 91: 490–491

Mackenzie H S, Brenner B M 1995 Fewer nephrons at birth: a missing link in the etiology of essential hypertension? American Journal of Kidney Diseases 26: 91–98

McEnery P T, Davis C A 1978 Non pharmacologic interventions in hypertension. Pediatric Clinics of North America 1978: 127–136

McGrath B 1996 Is white coat hypertension innocent? Lancet 348: 630

McVicar M, Carman C, Chandra M, Abbi R J, Teichberg S, Kahn E 1993 Hypertension secondary to renin-secreting juxtaglomerular cell tumor: case report and review of 38 cases. Pediatric Nephrology 7: 404–412

Management Committee 1980 Australian Therapeutic Trial in mild hypertension. Lancet i: 1261–1267

Management Committee 1982 Australian Therapeutic Trial in mild hypertension. Lancet i: 185–191

Mancia G, Bertineri G, Grassi G et al 1983 Effects of blood pressure measurement by the doctor on patient's blood pressure and heart rate. Lancet ii: 695–697

Maxwell M H, Waks A U, Schroth P C, Karam M, Dornfield L P 1982 Error in blood pressure measurement due to incorrect cuff size in obese patients. Lancet ii: 33–35

Medical Research Council Working Party on Mild to Moderate Hypertension 1985 MRC trial of treatment of mild hypertension: principal results. British Medical Journal 291: 97–104

Messerli F H 1982 Cardiovascular effects of obesity and hypertension. Lancet i: 1166–1168

Metropolitan Life Insurance Company 1961 Blood pressure: insurance experience and its implications. Metropolitan Life, New York

Miall W E, Lovell H G 1967 Relation between change of blood pressure and age. British Medical Journal ii: 660–664

Milner L S, Jacobs D W, Thomson P D et al 1991 Management of severe hypertension in childhood Takayasu's arteritis. Pediatric Nephrology 5: 38–41

Minty I, Lythgoe M F, Gordon I 1993 Hypertension in paediatrics: can pre and post captopril technetium-99 m dimercaptosuccinic acid scans exclude renovascular disease? European Journal of Nuclear Medicine 20: 699–702

Morrison R, Milner L S, Jacobs D et al 1989 The role of mycobacteria in Takayasu's arteritis (TA). Kidney International 35: 913

Mosier H D 1975 Hyperthyroidism. In: Gardner L I (ed.) Endocrine and genetic aspects of childhood and adolescence, 2nd edn. Saunders, Philadelphia, PA, p 285–317

Mueller Wiefel D E 1978 Renovasculare Hypertension bei Neurofibromitose von Recklinghausen. Monatsschrift Kinderheilkubde 126: 113–118

National High Blood Pressure Education Program (NHBPEP) Working Group on Hypertension Control in Children and Adolescents 1996 Update on the 1987 task force report on high blood pressure in children and adolescents: a working group report from the National High Blood Pressure Education Program. Pediatrics 98: 649–658

New M I, Levine L S 1978 Adrenocortical hypertension. Pediatric Clinics of North America 25: 67–81

New M I, Baum C J, Levine L S 1976 Nomograms relating aldosterone excretion to urinary sodium and potassium in the pediatric population: their application to the study of childhood hypertension. American Journal of Cardiology 37: 658–666

NHLBI (National Heart, Lung and Blood Institute of the USA) 1977 Task force on blood pressure control in children. Pediatrics 59(suppl): 797–820

NHLBI (National Heart, Lung and Blood Institute of the USA) 1987 Task force on blood pressure control in children (second report). Pediatrics 79: 1–25

Niehaus C E, Ersser R S, Atherden S M 1979 Routine laboratory investigation of urinary catecholamine metabolites in sick children. Annals of Clinical Biochemistry 16: 38–43

Nudel D B, Goutman N, Brunson S C et al 1980 Exercise performance of hypertensive adolescents. Paediatrics 65: 1073–1078

Nuutinen M, Turtinen J, Uharim 1992 Randon Zcro Sphygomanometer, Rose's tape, and the accuracy of the blood pressure measurements in children. Pediatric Research 32: 243–247

Office of Health Economics 1980 Briefing No. 12: hypertension. Office of Health Economics, London

Orcutt T W, Foster J H, Richie R E, Wilson J P, Warner H E 1974 Bilateral ex vivo renal artery reconstruction with autotransplantation. Journal of the American Medical Association 228: 493–495

Parker J C, Friedmann Kien A E, Levin S, Bartter F C 1964 Pseudoxanthema elasticum and hypertension. New England Journal of Medicine 271: 1204–1206

Peart W S 1980 Concepts in hypertension. The Croonian Lecture, 1979 Journal of the Royal College of Physicians of London 14: 141–152

Pesonen E, Koskimies O, Rapola J, Jaaskelainen J 1980 Fibromuscular disease in a child with generalised arterial disease. Acta Paediatrica Scandinavica 69: 563–566

Pickering G W 1968 High blood pressure, 2nd edn. Churchill, London, p 35

Pickering T G, James G D, Boddie C, Harshfield G A, Blank S, Laragh J H 1988 How common is white coat hypertension? Journal of the American Medical Society 259: 225–228

Pistulkova H, Blaha J, Skodova I 1976 Prevalence of hypertension in children and adolescents. Cor Vasa 18: 237–240

Plumer L B, Koplan G W, Mendoza S A 1976 Hypertension in infants – a complication of umbilical arterial catheterisation. Journal of Pediatrics 89: 802–805

Postma C T, Bijlstra P J, Rosenbusch G, Thien T 1996 Pattern recognition of loss of early systolic peak by Doppler ultrasound has a low sensitivity for the detection of renal artery stenosis. Journal of Human Hypertension 10: 81–184

Poston L, Sewell R B, Wilkinson S P et al 1981 Evidence for a circulating sodium transport inhibitor in essential hypertension. British Medical Journal 282: 874–849

Powell H R, Rotenberg E, Williams A L, McCredie D A 1974 Plasma renin activity in acute post streptococcal glomerulonephritis and the haemolytic uraemic syndrome. Archives of Disease in Childhood 49: 802–807

Rahill W J, Rubin M I 1972 Hypertension in infantile polycystic renal disease. The importance of early recognition and treatment of severe hypertension in polycystic renal disease. Clinical Pediatrics (Philadelphia) 11: 232–235

Rahill W J, Molteni A, Hawkin K M, Koo J H, Menon V A 1974 Hypertension and narrowing of the renal arteries in infancy. Journal of Pediatrics 84: 39–44

Rames L K, Clarke W R, Connor W E, Reiter M A, Lauer R M 1978 Normal blood pressures and the evaluation of sustained blood pressure elevation in childhood: the Muscatine Study. Pediatrics 61: 245–251

Ramsay L E, ul Haq I, Yeo W W, Jackson P R 1996 Interpretation of prospective trials in hypertension: do treatment guidelines accurately reflect current evidence? Journal of Hypertension Suppl 14: S187–S194

Reichert H, Lindinger A, Frey O et al 1995 Ambulatory blood pressure monitoring in healthy schoolchildren. Pediatric Nephrology 9: 282–286

Reusz G S, Hobor M, Tulassay T, Sallay P, Miltenyi M 1994 24 hour blood pressure monitoring in healthy and hypertensive children. Archives of Disease in Childhood 70: 90–94

Ribeiro A V, Krakoff L R 1976 Angiotensin blockade in coarctation of the aorta. New England Journal of Medicine 295: 148–150

Rich G, Ulick S, Cook S, Wang J, Lifton R P, Dluhy R G 1992 GRA in a large kindred: clinical spectrum and diagnosis using a characteristic biochemical phenotype. Annals of Internal Medicine 116: 813–820

Roberts J, Maurer K 1977 Blood pressure levels of persons 6–74 years, United States, 1971–74. Vital and Health Statistics series 11, no 203. DHEW Publ No (HRA) 78–1648. US Government Printing Office, Washington, DC

Robinson N, Gedroye W, Reidy J, Saxton H M 1991 Renal artery stenosis in children. Clinical Radiology 376–382

Robinson R G, de Quattro V, Grushkin C, Kieberman E 1977 Childhood phaeochromocytoma: treatment with alpha methyl tyrosine for resistant hypertension. Journal of Pediatrics 91: 143–147

Robson A M 1978 Special diagnostic studies for the detection of renal and renovascular forms of hypertension. Pediatric Clinics of North America 25: 83–98

Rosenfell J B, Cohen L, Garty I, Ben Bassat M 1973 Unilateral renal hypoplasia with hypertension (Ask Upmark Kidney). British Medical Journal ii: 217–218

Rosner B, Hennekens C H, Kass E H, Miall W E 1977 Age specific correlation analysis of longitudinal blood pressure data. American Journal of Epidemiology 106: 306–313

Rubin G D, Dake M F, Napel S et al 1994 Spiral CT of renal artery stenosis: comparison of three-dimensional rendering techniques. Radiology 190: 181–189

Ruley E J 1978 Compliance in young hypertensive patients. Pediatric Clinics of North America 25: 175–182

Savage D D, Drages J I, Henry W L et al 1979 Echocardiographic assessment of cardiac anatomy and function in hypertensive subjects. Circulation 623–628

Savage J M, Dillon M J, Shah V, Barratt T M, Williams D I 1978 Renin and blood pressure in children with renal scarring and vesicoureteric reflux. Lancet ii: 441–444

Scharer K 1987 Hypertension in children and adolescents – 1986. Pediatric Nephrology 1: 50–58

Schild L, Canessa C M, Shimkets R A, Gautschi I, Lifton R P, Rossier B C 1995 A mutation in the epithelial sodium channel causing Liddle disease increases channel activity in the *Xenopus laevis* oocyte expression system. Proceedings of the National Academy of Sciences USA 92: 5699–5703

Scholz D A 1977 Hypertension and hyperparathyroidism. [Editorial] Archives of Internal Medicine 137: 1123–1124

Sellers B B 1978 Intermittent hypertension during sickle cell crisis. Journal of Pediatrics 92: 941–943

Sever P S, Peart W S, Meade T W, Davies I B, Gordon D 1979 Ethnic differences in blood pressure with observations on noradrenaline and renin, part I and II. Working population and hospital hypertensive population. Clinical and Experimental Hypertension 1: 733–761

Shackleton C H 1993 Mass spectrometry in the diagnosis of steroid-related disorders and in hypertension research. Journal of Steroid Biochemistry and Molecular Biology 45: 127–140

Shackleton C H L, Honour J W, Dillon M J, Chantler C, Jones R W A 1980 Hypertension in a 4 year old child; gas chromatographic and mass spectrometric evidence for deficient hepatic metabolism of steroids. Journal of Clinical Endocrinology and Metabolism 50: 786–792

Sheth K H, Tang T T, Blaedel M E, Good T A 1978 Polydipsia, polyuria and hypertension associated with renin secreting Wilm's Tumour. Journal of Paediatrics 92: 921–924

Shimkets R A, Warnock D G, Bositis C M et al 1994 Liddle's syndrome: heritable human hypertension caused by mutations in the beta subunit of the epithelial sodium channel. Cell 79: 407–414

Short D 1976 The diastolic dilemma. British Medical Journal ii: 685–686

Silverberg D S, van Nostrand C, Juckli B, Smith E S O, van Dorsser E 1975 Screening for hypertension in a high school population. Canadian Medical Association Journal 113: 103–108

Skrabal F, Aubock J, Hortnagel H 1981 Low sodium/high potassium diet for prevention of hypertension: probable mechanism of action. Lancet ii: 895–900

Smellie J M 1989 The DMSA scan and intravenous urography in the detection of renal scarring. Pediatric Nephrology 3: 6–8

Soergel M, Kirschstein M, Busch C et al 1997 Oscillometric twenty-four-hour ambulatory blood pressure values in healthy children and adolescents: a multicentre trial including 1141 subjects. Journal of Pediatrics 130: 178–184

Stackpole R H, Melicow M M, Uson A C 1963 Phaeochromocytoma in children. Report of 9 cases and review of the first 100 published cases with follow up studies. Journal of Pediatrics 63: 315–330

Stanley J C, Fry W J 1981 Pediatric renal artery occlusive disease and renovascular hypertension. Archives of Surgery 116: 669–676

Stanley J C, Whitehouse W M, Graham L M et al 1982 Operative therapy of renovascular hypertension. British Journal of Surgery 69(suppl): S63–S66

Stapleton F B, Skoglund R R, Daggett R B 1978 Hypertension associated with Guillain-Barré syndrome. Pediatrics 62: 588–590

Stein J A, Tschudy D P 1970 Acute intermittent porphyria. A clinical and biochemical study of 46 patients. Medicine (Baltimore) 49: 1–16

Steinfeld L, Dimich I, Reder R, Cohen M, Alexander H 1978 Sphygmomanometry in the pediatric patient. Journal of Pediatrics 92: 934–938

Still J L, Cotton D C 1967 Severe hypertension in childhood. Archives of Disease in Childhood 42: 34–39

Strong W B, Botti R E, Silbert D R, Liebman J 1970 Peripheral and renal vein plasma renin activity and coarctation of the aorta. Pediatrics 45: 254–259

Strong W B, Miller M D, Striplin M et al 1978 Blood pressure response to isometric and dynamic exercise in healthy black children. American Journal of Diseases in Childhood 132: 587–591

Strunge P, Trostmann A F 1978 Serum lipids blood pressure, skin folds, height and weight in 580 Danish school children aged 8–17 years. Danish Medical Bulletin 25: 166–171

Swales J D 1995 Management guidelines for hypertension: is anyone taking notice? Journal of Human Hypertension 9(Suppl 2): S9–S13

Trompeter R S, Smith R L, Neville B C R, Chantler C 1982 Neurological complications of arterial hypertension in children. Archives of Disease in Childhood 57: 913–917

Turner M C, Ruley E J, Buckley K M, Strife C F 1979 Blood pressure elevation in children with orthopedic immobilisation. Journal of Pediatrics 95: 988–992

Twigg H L, Palmisano P J 1965 Fibromuscular hyperplasia of the iliac artery. American Journal of Roentgenology 95: 418–423

Uhari M, Koskimies O 1979 A survey of 164 Finnish children and adolescents with hypertension. Acta paediatrica Scandinavica 68: 193–198

Uhari M, Saukkonen A L, Koskimies O 1979 Central nervous system involvement in severe arterial hypertension of childhood. European Journal of Paediatrics 132: 141–146

Van Way C W, Michelakis A M, Anderson W J, Manlove A, Oates J A 1976 Studies of plasma renin activity in coarctation of the aorta. Annals of Surgery 183: 229–238

Vasquez A M 1973 Nephrocalcinosis and hypertension in juvenile primary hyperparthyroidism. American Journal of Disease in Childhood 125: 104–106

Vidt D G 1977 Hypertension induced by irradiation to the kidney. Archives of Internal Medicine 137: 840–841

Virdis R, Drayer J I M, Montolia J, Levine L S, Laragh J H 1979 Hypertension and medullary sponge kidneys in an adolescent with Beckwith–Wiedemann syndrome. Journal of Paediatrics 91: 761–763

Voorhess M L 1967 Urinary catecholamine excretion by healthy children. Pediatrics 39: 252–257

Voors A W, Foster T A, Frerichs R R, Webber L S, Berenson G S 1976 Studies of blood pressure in children aged 5–14 years in a total biracial community. The Bogalusa Heart Study. Circulation 54: 319–327

Voors A W, Webber L S, Frerichs R R, Berenson G S 1977 Body height and body mass as determinants of basal blood pressure in children – the Bogalusa Heart Study. American Journal of Epidemiology 106: 101–108

Webb N J A, Lewis M A, Bruce J et al 1997 Unilateral multicystic dysplastic kidney: the case for nephrectomy. Archives of Disease in Childhood 76: 31–34

White W B, Schulman P, McCabe E J, Dey H M 1989 Average daily blood pressure, not office blood pressure, determines cardiac function in patients with hypertension. Journal of the American Medical Association 261: 873–877

Whyte R K, Elseed A M, Fraser C B, Shinebourne E A, de Swiet M 1975 Assessment of Doppler ultrasound to measure systolic and diastolic blood pressures in infants and young children. Archives of Disease in Childhood 50: 542–544

Wiggelinkhuizen J, Cremin B J 1978 Takayusu arteritis and renovascular hypertension in children. Pediatrics 62: 209–217

Wiggins R C, Basar I, Slater J D H 1978 Effect of arterial pressure and inheritance on the normal sodium excretory capacity in normal young men. Clinical Science and Molecular Medicine 54: 639–647

Wilber J A 1972 Atlanta community high blood pressure programme methods of community hypertension screening. Circulation Research 31(suppl 2): 101–109

Woods K L, Beavers D G, West M 1981 Familial abnormality of erythrocyte cation transport in essential hypertension. Lancet 282: 1186–1188

Yiu V W Y, Dluhy R P, Lifton R P, Guay-Woodford L M 1997 Low peripheral plasma renin activity as a critical marker in pediatric hypertension. Pediatric Nephrology 11: 343–346

Youngberg S P, Sheps S G, Strong C G 1977 Fibromuscular disease of the renal arteries. Medical Clinics of North America 61: 623–641

Zachariah P K, Sheps S G, Ilstrup D M et al 1988 Blood pressure load – a better determinant of hypertension. Mayo Clinic Proceedings 63: 94–98

Ziegler M G, Lake C R, Kopin I J 1976 Deficient sympathetic nervous responses in familial dysautonomia. New England Journal of Medicine 294: 630–633

Zinner S H, Levy P S, Kass E H 1971 Familial aggregation of blood pressure in childhood. New England Journal of Medicine 284: 401–404

Zinner S H, Margolitis H S, Rosner B, Kass E J 1978 Stability of blood pressure rank and urinary kallikrein concentration in childhood: an eight year follow up. Circulation 58: 908–915

69

Paediatric cardiology in the tropics

M. Bertrand and D. Metras

INTRODUCTION

Paediatric cardiology in the tropics has, for long, received little attention, notably in the tropics themselves. Because of this, a chapter such as this must address many unanswered questions. The contributions of South African cardiologists, and happenings such as the opening of the Institute of Cardiology in Abidjan, and the advent in Abidjan of cardiac surgery, offered definite steps forward. More attention in these countries and in others, has now been paid to congenital heart diseases. Indeed, in Abidjan the majority of the cardiac surgical cases in one unit has involved patients under 15 years of age, including surgery for rheumatic heart disease and also for endomyocardial fibrosis (Metras et al, 1982a). Antia (1976) had considered that the main cardiac disorders as reported from many parts of the African continent were congenital heart disease, rheumatic heart disease, idiopathic cardiomegaly, endomyocardial fibrosis and a miscellaneous group made up of viral, tuberculous, pyogenic myocarditis, anaemic, renal disease and so on. This opinion was endorsed by our experience in Abidjan (Bertrand, 1979; Multiple African Collaborative Study, 1982).

This chapter will not deal with rheumatic heart disease. Although very common in tropical countries, and particularly in Africa (Caddell et al, 1966), this topic is dealt with in chapters 64–65. We will deal with the cardiac manifestations of the other important conditions or diseases encountered with frequency in children in the tropics, notably parasitic diseases, such as schistosomiasis, malaria and trypanosomiasis, and the sickle cell haemoglobinopathies. We will also consider several cardiac diseases confined more specifically to childhood, such as cardiomyopathies, endomyocardial fibrosis and congenital heart diseases. Finally, we will deal with the special problems produced by hypertension in children in tropical areas.

CARDIAC SIGNS IN SCHISTOSOMIASIS

Schistosomiasis, or bilharziasis is a parasitic disease produced by trematode worms. The adult worms, or schistosomes, live in the blood vessels, particularly in the vascular plexuses of the bladder and rectum. The pathogenic action of the schistosomes is produced by their eggs, which are eliminated through the walls of the bladder, the sigmoid colon or the rectum. This results in lesions of the urinary or digestive systems. The eggs stimulate inflammation, which becomes fibrous and, in time, induces formation of a calcified lesion in the walls of the urinary or digestive tracts. These result in deformations and stenoses. The eggs also migrate into the systemic system to create lesions within the liver (giving portal hypertension), the lung and probably the myocardium. Direct involvement of the heart, however, is rare (Gelfand et al, 1959). Nonetheless, in the evolution of the disease, cardiac signs may result from pulmonary arterial hypertension or from indirect causes such as anaemia, systemic hypertension or iatrogenic complications.

PULMONARY ARTERIAL HYPERTENSION

Pulmonary arterial hypertension results from the migration of eggs to the lung. Inflammatory or fibrous lesions can be produced either in the arterial walls or in the lung parenchyma (Figures 69.1 and 69.2). The pulmonary arteritis thus produced causes precapillary hypertension and sometimes produces shunts with hypoxaemia. In our experience (Bertrand et al, 1978a), we found pulmonary hypertension in up to one-fifth of patients undergoing catheterization, but only a small proportion of these had clinical signs related with the hypertension. In Brasil (Guimaraes 1982), pulmonary hypertension was found in one-eight. Chest radiography may reveal dilatation of the pulmonary trunk and its branches, with sometimes an increase in size of the right heart (Figure 69.3). The peripheral lung fields can be normal, or can present a pseudomiliary or micronodular appearance. We have observed the 'dead-tree' appearance of the pulmonary

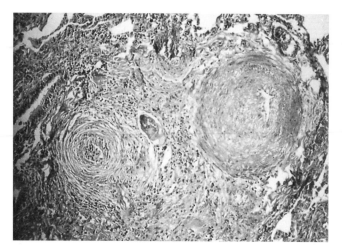

Figure 69.1. Pulmonary schistosomiasis, lesions of obliterative arteritis (right) and an inflammatory granuloma (left) can be seen.

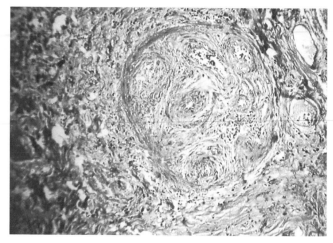

Figure 69.2. Pulmonary schistosomiasis. Lesion of pulmonary arteries with recanalization.

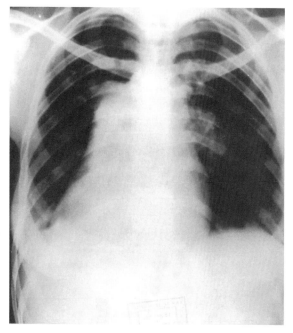

Figure 69.3. Pulmonary schistosomiasis. The frontal chest radiograph of a patient with pulmonary hypertension. Note the prominent pulmonary trunk and its main branches.

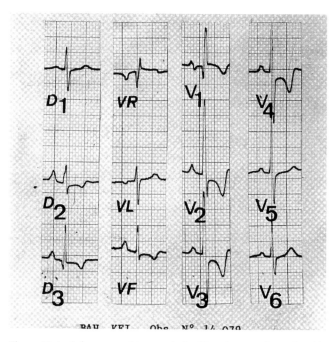

Figure 69.4. Pulmonary schistosomiasis. Chronic cor pulmonale with electrocardiographic signs of right atrial and right ventricular hypertrophy.

arterial branches in pulmonary angiograms. The electrocardiogram reveals signs of right atrial and ventricular enlargement (Figure 69.4) and of chronic cor pulmonale. Badawi (1961) observed features of right ventricular hypertrophy. In our experience (Bertrand et al, 1978a), these signs were observed when the systolic pulmonary arterial pressures were elevated but the capillary wedge pressures were normal. For treatment, it is necessary to destroy the parasites. This must be undertaken with caution if there are signs of right ventricular involvement. Some medications may be toxic for the myocardium, such as nitrothiazol or dehydroemetine. Others may lead to destruction of the parasites, with liberation of antigens and immunological risk.

BILHARZIAL MYOCARDITIS

The myocarditis that may accompany schistosomiasis is less well documented than the pulmonary arteritis. Evidence in experimental animals is equivocal (Pifano and Marcuzzi, 1950; Lobo et al, 1952; Menezes, 1954; Sadeler, 1973). Pathological observations are rare (Clark and de Graeffe, 1935; Jaffe, 1937; Africa and Sta-Cruz, 1948, Zahawi and Shukri, 1956; Williams, 1958; Stransky and Quiant, 1959). These various workers have described finding isolated eggs in the myocardium, inflammatory granulomas, congestion and interstitial oedema, and myofibrillary alterations. As a whole, these lesions are not well understood. One cannot question their existence, but their parasitic or immunological origin remains uncertain.

Signs of congestive heart failure may be observed among young patients with severe infection. In the absence of clinical signs, we have observed electrocardiographic anomalies such as flat or negative T waves or atrioventricular dissociation (Bertrand et al, 1971). The diagnosis of bilharzial myocarditis is a diagnosis of probability if there are clinical, echographic or electrocardiographic signs without pulmonary arterial hypertension, an active schistosmiasis and in the absence of all other aetiologies. We have made a positive diagnosis in only one tenth of potential cases. Nitrothiazol or dehydroemetine must be used with caution, since the toxic effects of these drugs can exacerbate the cardiac failure, although newer antischistosomic drugs do not have this effect.

OTHER CARDIAC SIGNS IN SCHISTOSOMIASIS

Other cardiac manifestations are relatively frequent and were seen in two fifths of 37 patients in one series (Bertrand et al, 1978b). Myocarditis can be observed, secondary to anaemia, the anaemia itself being caused by digestive or urinary haemorrhage, haemolysis or malnutrition. Hypertensive myocardiopathy was observed only once in these 37 patients and occurred secondary to chronic bilharzial nephropathy. Renal involvement can be interstitial, when produced by *Schistosoma haematobium*, or glomerular as seen with *Schistosoma mansonii*. The studies of Pobbee (1968) and Le Bras (1974) have shown that hypertension is no more frequent in those with renal involvement than in the overall group with schistosomiasis. Acute cor pulmonale, or coronary obstruction produced by the adult worm, are exceedingly rare. Iatrogenic myocarditis was induced in less than one-third of the 37 patients (Bertrand et al 1978b). In these however, abnormalities were observed on the electrocardiogram during treatment with nitrothiazol or dihydroemetine. It is our opinion that schistosomiasis could also be one of the causes of endomyocardial fibrosis. Most of the patients with this disease in the Ivory Coast come from a geographic area where schistosomiasis is endemic.

CARDIAC SIGNS DURING ATTACKS OF MALARIA

Cardiac involvement in malaria is rare, but a few cases have been reported (Rey et al, 1992). In a series of 50 patients with observed attacks of malaria, functional symptoms were seen in seven; these were not significant, usually being atypical chest pains and palpitations (Bertrand et al, 1975a). Chest pain with feelings of tightness has also been described. Among the most interesting clinical signs is the dissociation of heart rate and fever, with a relative bradycardia in up to one half of the

patients. A cardiac systolic murmur has been noted in a few patients, probably related to anaemia. The electrocardiogram shows non-specific changes. Usually, there are flat or negative T waves. In two patients having co-existing cardiac disease, namely cardiomyopathy and valvar disease, atrial fibrillation and transient second-degree atrioventricular block was observed. The cardiothoracic ratio was increased on the radiograph in one third of patients (Bertrand et al, 1975a) but without signs of cardiac failure, which was observed in Dakar, (Sankalé et al, 1969). The pulmonary symptoms and signs present in some patients, such as congestion, asthmatic crises, pleural effusion and acute pulmonary oedema, must be distinguished from congestive heart failure. Usually benign, these manifestations have led to death in a few cases.

The cause of the cardiovascular signs in malaria is not well known. Myocardial lesions (Sankalé et al, 1969) and capillary obstructions (Herrera, 1960) have been described. The roles of anaemia, anoxia, electrolytic imbalance, modifications of capillary permeability, microthrombosis and competition between host and parasite for glucose have all been implicated. The prognosis of cardiovascular anomalies is good. Herrera (1960), however, reported the death of an 8-year-old child in cardiac failure. At necropsy, coronary occlusion was found along with micro-infarctions. The treatment is as for malaria in general. We must emphasize the efficacy and the good tolerance of intravenous quinine at right dosage (although it is now largely superseded by infusion because of the hazard attached to intravenous injection). Halofautrine can be associated with lengthening of the QTc interval and observation of late potentials (Guidicelli, 1996).

Cardiovascular signs should always be sought, and even anticipated, during a malarial attack, particularly the relative bradycardia and electrocardiographic abnormalities. A malarial attack occurring in a patient with heart disease can lead to, or reveal, arrhythmias and disturbances of conduction. The prognosis is good. Treatment must be started rapidly and watched carefully, particularly in patients with abnormal hearts. Good antimalarial prophylaxis is optimal.

CARDIAC SIGNS IN TRYPANOSOMIASIS

Cardiac lesions are well recognized in American trypanosomiasis better known as Chagas' disease. Although they have been less well studied, they are also present in African trypanosomiasis.

ACUTE MYOCARDITIS

This phase is often overlooked among individuals having a chronic myocardiopathy. In other patients, the myocarditis is severe, most commonly in young children. There is congestive heart failure with hepatic enlargement and oedema of the legs. Sometimes, there is cardiovascular collapse. Auscultation reveals tachycardia with faint heart sounds, and sometimes a functional systolic murmur. The chest radiograph demonstrates a grossly enlarged heart. The electrocardiogram shows non-specific ST–T abnormalities (de Souza Amorium 1979). Arrhythmias, and disturbance of conduction, can occur during this acute phase. The appearance of intraventricular block is considered a poor prognostic sign. Echocardiograms show dilatation of the cardiac chambers with diffuse hypocontractility (Rocha et al, 1993). An acute pericardial effusion was found in the majority of patients seen by Chapuis (1976). Death occurs in one tenth. The diagnosis is made by the discovery of the parasite in the peripheral blood or fluids. The treatment includes the use of nifurtimox (Lampit). At pathology, the myocardial cells contain great numbers of the parasite. There is also fragmentation and degeneration of the myocardial fibres, with interstitial inflammatory infiltrates.

CHRONIC MYOCARDIOPATHY

The pathogenesis of chronic chagasic myocarditis remains incompletely understood. Several hypotheses have been proposed. These include direct destruction of tissues, a neurogenic theory, immune reactions, and microvascular disease.

This disease predominates in members of rural populations during their third or fourth decade. It is, therefore, a disease of adulthood. Half of all infected patients are said to suffer cardiac involvement, even if they had no history of acute myocarditis during childhood. There are symptoms and signs of cardiac failure, along with chest pain and palpitations. Auscultation reveals decreased intensity of the heart sounds, sometimes with a gallop rhythm and a systolic murmur resulting from mitral or tricuspid insufficiency. The chest radiograph reveals cardiomegaly. Arrhythmias and conduction disturbances are common (Rosenbaum, 1964) and make the outcome worse (Guerrero et al, 1991). There is a great danger of syncope and sudden death. The electrocardiogram shows abnormalities of the T and P wave, and sometimes signs of left ventricular hypertrophy. Echocardiography shows dilated and diffusely hypokinetic ventricles. Thallium-201 scintigraphy shows abnormalities of myocardial perfusion (Marin-Neto et al, 1992). The disease is progressive, and the reported survival after the occurrence of congestive heart failure is less than 2 years (Prata et al, 1974). The treatment is only symptomatic, since the parasites are beyond eradication at this stage. At pathology, there is an interstitial fibrosis with infiltrates of monocytes, lymphocytes and plasmocytes. There is often a microaneurysm at the cardiac apex. Parasites are rarely present in the myocardium.

AMERICAN TRYPANOSOMIASIS

Chagas' disease, produced by *Trypanosoma cruzi*, is transmitted by insects that live in thatched roofs. They drop during the night onto the sleeping victims, biting them on uncovered areas. The bite produces the so-called chagoma at the site of inoculation, followed by the Romana sign of conjunctivitis and enlargement of lymph nodes. Early signs are not specific. Thus fever, dyspnoea, cough, cyanosis and/or pallor, irritability, restlessness and anorexia can all occur. There is often a fever during the period of acute dissemination. Cardiac, meningitis, encephalitic and respiratory problems can all ensue. Mortality is high in children. A latent phase follows the acute attack. Its duration is variable, often lasting for several years. A minority of the patients exhibit lesions during the chronic phase. These may be chronic cardiomyopathy, or lesions in the digestive tract. Exceptionally, encephalopathy can occur. It is suggested that these changes result from the effect of either toxins or immunoglobins on the parasympathetic neurones (Koberle, 1968).

AFRICAN TRYPANOSOMIASIS

African trypanosomiasis, produced by *Trypanosoma rhodesiense* or *T. gambiense*, is transmitted to humans by various species of the tsetse fly, which live in the forest galleries and the savanna areas. The natural history may be divided into three periods. The period of incubation usually has no clinical manifestations. The bite of the fly is often overlooked, although sometimes there is a local inflammatory reaction. During the period of invasion, the trypanosomes can be isolated in the peripheral blood and in the lymph nodes. The invasive period is characterized by an infectious syndrome with fever, lymphadenopathy, hepatosplenomegaly, and cutaneous signs. The third, neurological, period involves a parasitic meningoencephalitis. This causes difficulty in sleeping, along with sensory, motor, psychic and neuroendocrinological problems. It leads to a state of marasmus with encephalitis. Cardiovascular manifestations have been described during the two last stages. The evolutionary history of the various periods is either progressive over several years with periods of stabilization or short, with a duration of some months. It is a continuous evolution with subacute periods, rather than a chronic one. Infection with *Trypanosoma gambiense* gives a longer evolution than does *Trypanosoma rhodesiense*. The diagnosis is usually made by the discovery of the parasite in the blood, the lymph nodes or the spinal fluid. Indirect evidence is obtained from serological reactions, particularly immunofluorescence. The drug usually employed for treatment is suramine (Moranyl), pentamidine or melarsoprol (Arsobal). These drugs may themselves produce cardiovascular signs. Melarsoprol can be followed by a lethal arsenical encephalopathy. Administration of steroids is useful. Difluoromethylornithine (eflornithine) can be used in the presence of cardiac signs (Bertrand et al, 1995). Whether it is indicated in the absence of cardiac signs has yet to be studied.

RHODESIAN SLEEPING SICKNESS

Cardiac signs occur during the stage of invasion in Rhodesian sleeping sickness and are sometimes responsible for death even before the neurological stage is reached. Tachycardia, decreased heart sounds, gallop rhythm and often a low blood pressure are observed. Cardiomegaly is sometimes seen. Acute pericarditis has been described by Hawking and Greenfield (1941). Electrocardiographic studies (Schylns and Jansen 1955; Jones et al, 1975) showed changes in one half of the patients examined before, during, or after treatment. They were mostly anomalies of repolarization, or else first-degree atrioventricular block. Left ventricular hypertrophy, intraventricular block, Q waves, U waves, and anomalies of the QT segment were more rarely observed. Evolution towards congestive heart failure has been observed and can lead to death (de Raadt and Koten, 1968), although there is the possibility of cure after specific treatment. Inflammatory infiltrates (Hawking and Greenfield, 1941) or interstitial haemorrhages with cellular infiltration (de Raadt and Koten, 1968) have been seen in the myocardium and pericardium.

GAMBIAN SLEEPING SICKNESS

The cardiac signs of Gambian sleeping sickness include palpitations or atypical precordial pain. There are some-times signs of cardiac failure (Bertrand et al, 1974). At auscultation, the heart sounds are decreased, and there is sometimes a systolic murmur. Rarely, a gallop sound is heard. The pulse pressure is decreased, especially in the upright position. A pericardial effusion may be present (Figure 69.5). The heart size, as seen on the chest radiograph, can be normal, increased or decreased. Small hearts can have concentric muscular hypertrophy, observable at angiocardiography (Figure 69.6), echocardiography or postmortem. The electrocardiogram shows changes in up to one half of patients. The voltages are decreased, and there are diffusely flat or negative T waves, with modifications of the ST-T segment, signs of ischaemia and signs of right or left ventricular hypertrophy (Bertrand et al, 1969; Poltera et al, 1976). Disturbances of conduction have been observed (Figure 69.7), with a small incidence of complete heart block (Bertrand et al, 1969). Heart block is much less frequent than in American trypanosomiasis. When found, it probably a consequence of an inflammatory process, since it is spontaneously variable and sensitive to treatment with steroids. Specific treatment directed against the parasite, and occasional treatment with steroids, produce favourable results based on cardiac signs (Bertrand et al, 1995). The treatment of the trypanosomiasis itself may lead to a lethal encephalopathy that is unrelated to the occasional cardiac involvement. At pathology, thickening of the myocardium has been found, with infiltrations of plasma cells, histiocytes, and lymphocytes (Figure 69.8) throughout the heart wall. There were also areas of fibrosis (Figure 69.9). The conduction tissues can be involved (Bertrand et al, 1969; Poltera et al, 1976). In the pathological study of Adams et al, (1986), all three children examined had myocarditis.

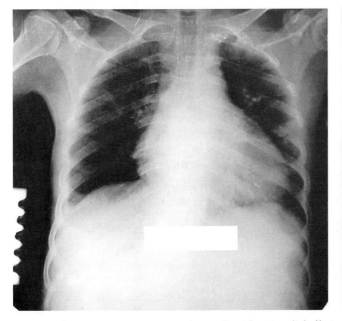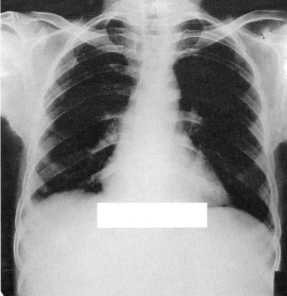

Figure 69.5. African trypanosomiasis. Cardiomegaly with pericardial effusion (left) which regressed after treatment of the trypanosomiasis (right).

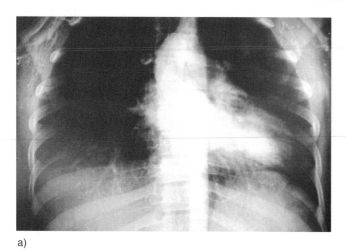

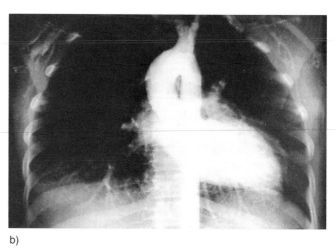

a)   b)

Figure 69.6. African trypanosomiasis. Cineangiogram has been taken in (a) systole and (b) diastole. There is a muscular concentric hypertrophy of the left ventricle.

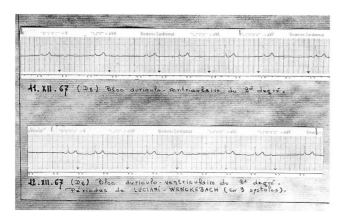

Figure 69.7. African trypanosomiasis. There is variable atrioventricular block. The electrocardiogram returned to normal after specific treatment of the trypanosomiasis together with steroid treatment.

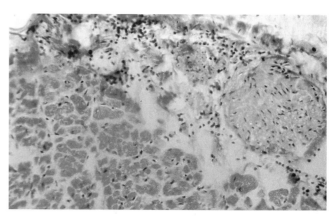

Figure 69.8. African trypanosomiasis. This section of the myocardium shows an inflammatory infiltrate around a small nerve.

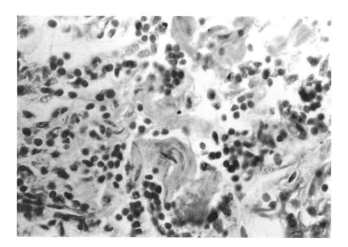

Figure 69.9. African trypanosomiasis. There is a myocardial inflammatory infiltrate with beginnings of fibrosis.

CARDIAC PROBLEMS WITH SICKLE-CELL HAEMOGLOBINOPATHIES

The cardiac signs are well documented in homozygous (SS) or double heterozygous (SC) patients with sickle cell disease. They are less well documented in heterozygous patients with only the sickle cell trait (AS). The great number of individuals with the heterozygous state, however, means that this remains a real problem, particularly when open heart surgery is performed in such patients.

PATHOPHYSIOLOGY

There is a decrease in the affinity of the red cells for oxygen, and it is this change that results in sickling. This phenomenon increases the viscosity of the blood, with resulting capillary obstruction and haemolysis. The tissue hypoxia and acidosis that ensue further enhance the phenomenon. Exceptionally, obstruction can occur in the coronary or pulmonary capillaries. Hypoxia can also be responsible for myocardial dysfunction.

CARDIAC MANIFESTATIONS

FREQUENCY

In tropical Africa, between one-fifth and one-third of the population are compromised by sickle cell haemoglobinopathy. The homozygous, and doubly heterozygous patients have frequent cardiac manifestations, occuring in up to four-fifths of cases (Bertrand et al, 1975b). However, because only a small number of such patients are admitted to hospital, they make up a very small group of patients. The patients with the sickle cell trait have fewer cardiac manifestations but they make up a much larger number of hospitalized patients.

CLINICAL CARDIAC MANIFESTATIONS

Anaemia occurs when the haemoglobin is below 7 g/dl but this is rare in heterozygotes. This signs are fatigue, dyspnoea on exertion, palpitations, and atypical chest pain. The physical findings may sometimes include cardiac failure, but more commonly they are the signs of increased output (Brinsfield et al, 1963; Lindsay et al, 1974; Bertrand et al, 1975b). The electrocardiogram reveals abnormalities of the ST–T segment, sometimes with signs of ventricular hypertrophy and a prolonged QT interval. Diagnosis of ischaemic manifestations is valid only in the absence of anaemia (Botreau Roussel et al, 1977). Chest pains can occur, which may have the character of angina pectoris. The electrocardiogram then shows signs of localized ischaemia, although the possibility of myocardial infarction with normal coronary arteries has been reported (three times, but not in children). A myocardiopathic presentation is more frequent in heterozygous individuals. There is a cardiomegaly with non-specific repolarization changes in the electrocardiogram. Sometimes, there are only electrocardiographic abnormalities. Pulmonary arterial hypertension, and cor pulmonale (Bertrand et al, 1975b), is seen more frequently in the adult, but we have seen this once in an 11-year-old girl. Capillary pulmonary thrombosis is held to be responsible. There are the usual signs of pulmonary hypertension. Children usually die before puberty because of pulmonary problems, measles, or malaria. The main problem in diagnosis is to relate the cardiac signs, usually obvious, to the sickle disorder and to rule out any other cause. Prevention is the best treatment. For symptomatic relief, oxygen and alkalinization are often necessary. Vasodilators are useful, but some medications that act on the red cell are efficient. An example

is oxpentifylline (pentoxifylline) given intravenously during the acute manifestations, and orally for prophylaxis. Platelet antiaggregants are increasingly used.

SICKLE CELL HAEMOGLOBINOPATHY AND OPEN HEART SURGERY

Sickle cell haemoglobinopathies, with an incidence of 11% in Ivory Coast, present particular problems while performing open heart surgery. De Leval et al (1974) and Leachman et al (1976) have outlined the potential dangers in the use of cardiopulmonary bypass in sickle cell trait, disease and syndrome. A significant decrease in the saturation of oxygen, and the development of acidosis, can initiate the sickling phenomenon. This is initially reversible but then becomes irreversible. As already stated, the viscosity of the blood increases under these conditions, and capillary stasis occurs. Consequent capillary thrombosis, with tissue ischaemia and hypoxaemia, initiates a vicious circle. Sickle cells mechanically are more fragile; consequently haemolysis can occur during bypass. Any decrease in body temperature increases blood viscosity and further augments sickling. During surgery, therefore, it is essential to achieve optimal oxygenation, to avoid acidosis, to reduce the percentage of S-haemoglobin S by pre- or intraoperative exchange transfusions and priming the pump with blood, to avoid systemic or local hypothermia and to avoid aortic cross-clamping. All these techniques are the opposite of modern techniques for bypass and myocardial protection and are contrary to the usual routine employed in our institution. We undertook a study of bypass in 20 patients, including nine children with various cardiac anomalies, who exhibited either the sickle cell trait or sickle cell syndromes (SC, S-Thal). There were two postoperative deaths in the group, which were unrelated to the sickle cell disorder. Open heart surgery could be achieved safely in these patients using haemodilution (Metras et al, 1982b). The use of blood was limited to anaemic patients and 6 of the 20 patients underwent surgery without the use of blood throughout their entire hospital stay. We further used moderate systemic hypothermia at 28°C, and topical hypothermia, together with aortic cross-clamping and cold cardioplegia. In none of the patients did these techniques give problems. In particular, there was no significant haemolysis or sickling of the red cells. A similar observation concerning hypothermia and cardioplegia has been reported in one patient by Hudson et al (1981). Haemodilution, according to some authors, improves capillary perfusion. Hypothermia should decrease the risks of sickling, since the dissociation curve of haemoglobin is directly influenced by the temperature (Lonsdorfer et al, 1979). A decrease in the temperature increases the oxygen saturation at an equivalent partial pressure, thus influencing the polymerization of haemoglobin S. Cardiopulmonary bypass, therefore, can safely be achieved in all patients with the sickle cell trait or syndrome when using modern techniques of myocardial preservation.

PRIMARY CARDIOMYOPATHY IN CHILDREN

Primary cardiomyopathy is considered here to cover primary involvement of the myocardium, as opposed to those cardiomyopathies that are secondary to congenital or acquired lesions or that are infectious, parasitic, toxic, inflammatory and metabolic forms of myocarditis. In Africa, however, investigations concerning aetiology are usually poor. Some of the patients thought to have primary cardiomyopathy probably have parasitic or infectious myocardiopathies. With these caveats in mind, cardiomyopathies as here defined represent up to one-tenth of all cardiac diseases seen in children. In Africa, they are in fourth position after congenital heart disease, valvar diseases and endomyocardial fibrosis (Antia et al, 1968; Antia, 1976, 1978). Cardiomyopathies without hypertrophy are more numerous in Africa than in Europe. The heart is dilated, but the walls are not hypertrophic.

Clinically, acute or subacute types are seen more often in children less than 5 years of age. The chronic types are more frequent in children over the age of 5 years. It is the chronic forms seen in older children that are more likely to be hypertrophic. The clinical pattern of obstructive cardiomyopathy is rare. In the history, premonitory infectious symptoms, or digestive or pulmonary symptoms, are found at or shortly before the onset of the disease (Antia, 1976). Various initial features are signs of cardiac failure, arrhythmias, cardiomegaly, systolic murmur, or even acute symptoms of arterial embolism. The blood pressure is normal or low. The chest radiography reveals cardiomegaly with pulmonary vascular engorgement. Electrocardiography usually demonstrates signs of left ventricular hypertrophy or diffuse changes in the ST–T segment. The condition must be distinguished from ventricular hypertrophy secondary to arterial hypertension or aortic coarctation, and from the non-hypertrophic forms of myocardial disease occurring secondary to abnormal origin of the left coronary artery from the pulmonary trunk, or to an infectious process. Some cardiomyopathies identified at postmortem are found to be associated with fibroelastosis (Casasoprano, 1973; Ribierre et al, 1982). Ribierre and colleagues (1982) have argued that fibroelastosis is a non-specific reaction of the endocardium, and is probably genetically determined. They argue it can be secondary to congenital heart disease or can occur in a primary cardiomyopathic form in infancy. It is difficult to evaluate the evolution of these cardiomyopathies. In Ivory Coast, the mortality is high, occurring in up to half the young children seen with acute disease. In the chronic types, seen in older children, the risk is of arrhythmias and sudden death rather than

cardiac insufficiency. It is difficult to establish a long-term prognosis, since most of the patients are lost to follow-up. The treatment is purely symptomatic. Antiarrhythmic (anticoagulant in the embolic type), diuretic and vasoactive medications are used, along with digitalis. Beta-blockers are used in the setting of obstructive hypertrophy. The use of steroids is controversial for acute disease. Their general usefulness had not been demonstrated, although some have recommended use for a period of 2 months (Ribierre et al, 1982).

ENDOMYOCARDIAL FIBROSIS

The constrictive or restrictive forms of endomyocardial fibrosis can be distinguished from the chronic cardiomyopathies by several features. First, the anatomical lesion predominates on the endocardium, and has a restrictive effect. Second, the pathophysiology and symptomatology are those of restrictive cardiac failure. Third, the treatment nowadays is essentially surgical. It is probably that endomyocardial fibrosis can be also distinguished from chronic cardiomyopathies by its aetiology. This is essentially unknown, although immunological and/or eosinophilic factors seem likely to be involved.

WORLDWIDE OCCURRENCE

Endocardial fibrosis was first described in Europe, where Loeffler (1936) recognized the eosinophilic form, calling it parietal fibroplastic endocarditis. Later, the restrictive variant was described by Davies in Africa (1948). The subsequent descriptions of the disease came essentially from tropical Africa, where it was studied in Uganda, Nigeria and Ivory Coast. Some cases have also been observed in Benin, Central Africa, Gabon, Zaire, Mozambique and Senegal. Since 1950, endomyocardial fibrosis has been observed in the Americas, notably Brasil, Venezuela, Colombia, Mexico and Cuba, and in tropical Asian areas such as Sri-Lanka, Vietnam and India. It has also been seen in temperate areas like the United States of America, the United Kingdom, Japan, Denmark, Switzerland and France. It has now become accepted that the endomyocardial and parietal fibroplastic forms are two different stages of the same disease (Bertrand, 1979; Olsen and Spry, 1979; Goodwin, 1982). The parietal fibroplastic type is mostly seen in older individuals living in temperate areas. Its features are hypereosinophilia, inflammatory signs and development of visceral lesions. By comparison, endomyocardial fibrosis is seen mostly in tropical areas and affects children and adolescents rather than adults. Hypereosinophilia, inflammatory signs and visceral lesions are less common.

Epidemiological studies have shown the disease to be more prevalent in tropical than in temperate areas. It is responsible for one sixth of cardiac failure in Uganda,

Table 69.1 Prevalence of rheumatic heart disease and cardiomyopathy in the Ivory Coast

	Rheumatic heart disease (%)	Cardiomyopathy (including endomyocardial fibro elastosis) (%)
Forest	10.2–16.4	12.9–30.5
Savannah	12.9–20.5	7.6–9.0

and one tenth in Nigeria. In Ivory Coast, it produces one fifth of all instances of primary cardiac failure in patients under 40 years, and half in children under 16 years. In tropical regions, the prevalence is greater in forest areas. In these areas, some groups of population are more commonly affected, such as the Akan groups in Ivory Coast. This is probably a result of ecological rather than genetic factors. It seems that there is a balance between the prevalence of rheumatic heart disease, which predominate in certain populations, and endomyocardial fibrosis, which predominates in other populations. This has been seen in Uganda, and is similar in Ivory Coast (Table 69.1).

In the multiple African Collaborative Study (1982), there was a decreasing prevalence of rheumatic heart disease from Maghreb to the intertropical forest area, falling from just under half of cardiovascular consultations and admissions in Maghreb, to one-fifth in Sahel and one-sixth in the areas of tropical forest. In contrast, cardiomyopathies are found essentially in the forested areas, accounting for one-sixth of cardiovascular morbidity, whereas they represent less than one-tenth in Sahel and only one-hundreth in Maghreb. The patients with cardiomyopathy are mostly children, adolescents or young adults. Their age is lower in tropical than in temperate areas. In patients undergoing surgery, ages are lower in Africa than in India or Brasil. In the Ivory Coast, the mean age is 15.5 years (with a range from 2 to 54 years). Endomyocardial fibrosis is seen mostly in men, who made up seven-tenths of the series of Brockington and Olsen (1978). Similarly, more than two-thirds of those seen in the Ivory Coast are male.

PATHOLOGY

The heart in endomyocardial fibrosis shows a moderate increase in volume and weight. When the right ventricle is severely diseased, there is a retraction with a notch at the apex, the infundibulum being enlarged. The right atrium is enlarged, sometimes being aneurysmal. When the left ventricle is affected, the external appearance is unremarkable, although the left atrium is sometimes dilated. It is the appearance of the endocardium that permits an easy diagnosis. Macroscopically, the fibrosis is white, like mother-of-pearl, with a variable thickness. It is retractile and sometimes calcified. The fibrosis can be confined to either the right or left ventricles, but most often it affects both. It can occur mostly at the apex

(Figure 69.10), or in the ventricular inlet and the area of the papillary muscles. When the fibrosis affects the papillary muscles and tendinous cords, it can retract the leaflets of the atrioventricular valves. The atrial endocardium is usually unaffected. Organized thrombuses can be found in the ventricles or the atriums. Two layers are seen with the microscope, the myocardium making a third layer (Figure 69.11). The superficial layer is formed of connective tissue, with collagen fibres, a few cells and vessels but no elastic fibres. Calcification is seen in one third of hearts, sometimes with ossification. The deep layer is formed of younger connective tissue with numerous fibroblasts, few collagen fibres and no elastic fibres.

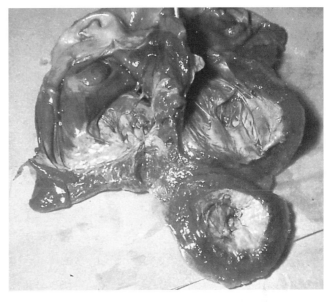

Figure 69.10. Endomyocardial fibrosis. Specimen of bilateral fibrosis. The right ventricular apex is retracted (left) with extensive fibrosis. The left ventricular apex is also retracted (right) with extensive fibrosis reaching the mitral papillary muscles. The tricuspid and mitral valvar leaflets are normal.

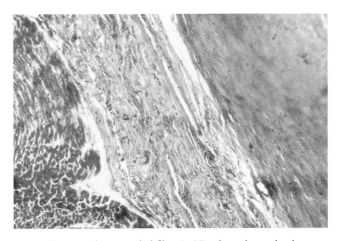

Figure 69.11. Endomyocardial fibrosis. Histology shows the three typical layers. From left to right are the normal myocardium, the deep layer with 'young' conjunctive tissue (fibroblasts, collagen fibres, capillaries) and the superficial layer (collagen fibres, few cells).

The capillary vessels in this layer are dilated and numerous. Eosinophilic infiltrates are sometimes found, but rarely in Africa according to Olsen and Spry (1979), the evolution involves an acute necrotic stage, then a thrombotic stage and finally a fibrotic stage. The myocardium itself is relatively untouched. About one third of the patients observed in Abidjan presented with fibrous bands localized to the subendocardial area of the ventricular wall. This fibrosis may sometimes affect a greater part of the mural thickness. In Europe, myocardial involvement is more frequent. A pericardial effusion is seen in seven-tenths of patients, being of a serous or serohaemorrhagic nature. Moderate inflammatory signs are present on the epicardium in one fifth. The peripheral, systemic and coronary arteries may present signs of inflammatory arteritis, especially in the parietal variant. In Africa, this finding is exceptional. With this in mind, it must be emphasized that the lesions start (Figure 69.12) and predominate on the endocardium. They often affect the pericardium. In our experience, they tend to spare the myocardium. This anatomical finding is one of the arguments in favour of surgical treatment.

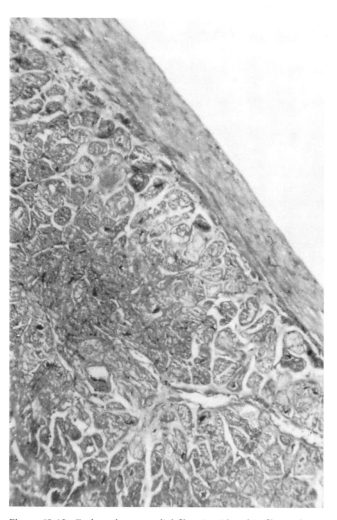

Figure 69.12. Early endomyocardial fibrosis with a thin fibrotic layer covering the myocardium.

PATHOPHYSIOLOGY

The presence of a diffuse endocardial fibrosis reduces the ventricular compliance and leads to a restrictive syndrome. Where there is localized ventricular fibrosis, the global compliance can be conserved. If fibrosis is localized to a papillary muscle, atrioventricular valvar incompetence may ensue, particularly when the mitral valve is involved. When the right ventricle is involved, the dilated ventricle and atrium are often transformed into a widely communicating cavity through a dilated tricuspid orifice. This explains the similar pressures found in the right-sided chambers and the caval veins. The reduction of the velocity, and the stagnation of the blood in the right heart cavities, leads to the reduction in the intensity of murmurs.

SYMPTOMS AND SIGNS

GENERAL SYMPTOMATOLOGY

Patients with endomyocardial fibrosis are more often male. In tropical Africa, they are usually children, adolescents or young adults, with the mean age being 15.5 years in Abidjan. In India and Brazil, in contrast, the mean age is 25–30 years. In Europe, patients tend to be still older. The period between onset of symptoms and diagnosis in patients in Abidjan was of the order of 4 and 5 years. The general condition of most patients is poor. There is reduction in weight and size coupted with retardation of puberty, pointing to long-standing disease. Recurrent ascites, or subclinical jaundice or cyanosis, is sometimes present. Usually there is no fever apart from that resulting from coincidental causes. A febrile, pseudoinfectious onset of the disease has been described in Nigeria.

RIGHT VENTRICULAR ENDOMYOCARDIAL FIBROSIS

Clinical examination reveals important venous stasis. There is hepatomegaly, often with systolic pulsation of the liver. The jugular veins are prominent, and sometimes recurrent ascitis and lower limb oedema are observed. At auscultation, a protodiastolic sound described as an 'endocardial snap' is heard, sometimes with a murmur of tricuspid, or more rarely pulmonary, insufficiency. There is sometimes a palpable beating of the subpulmonary infundibulum. There is no pulmonary stasis in the isolated right ventricular type. Atrial arrhythmias are present in three quarters of patients and may vary spontaneously in the same patient. Conduction disturbances of varying degree can be present. Of great diagnostic interest is the presence of Q waves in leads V_1 and V_2 (Ikeme and Uzodike, 1971; Bertrand et al, 1978a). Along with Sodi-Pallares (1951), we think these are a manifestation of right atrial dilatation. The presence of right atrial hypertrophy without signs of ventricular hypertrophy is a good sign, but right ventricular hypertrophy can also be observed. The pattern of the protodiastolic endocardial snap can readily be shown with phonocardiography. The sound is of low frequency and occurs contemporaneously with the dip and ascension seen in the mechanogram (Bertrand and Renambot, 1975). The sound seems to be related to the transmission of the atrial wave to the right ventricle. Using M-mode echocardiography, it is possible to see endocardial thickening and paradoxal septal motion (Dienot, 1981). With cross-sectional studies (Touza, 1985, Okereke et al, 1991), the characteristic pattern is apical obliteration, dilation of the right ventricular outflow and the tricuspid valvar annulus and poor coaption of tricuspid valvar leaflets with regurgitation. The right atrium is very large, but rarely contains thrombus. The chest radiograph shows a large right atrium. Sometimes the dilated subpulmonary infundibulum may be seen forming the left heart border. Linear or curved calcifications may be seen near the apex in a minority of patients. The angiocardiogram (Figure 69.13) shows a dilated, and often huge, right atrium, with a long period of emptying. There is amputation of the right ventricular apex (Cockshott, 1965), often with a dilated infundibulum. In one third of patients, there are filling defects or irregularities of the ventricular border (Bertrand, 1979). The pulmonary trunk can be normal, or large and pulsatile. The haemodynamic signs (Figure 69.14) include dip plateau pressure curves. Guimaraes et al (1974) have observed early pulmonary valvar closure before the Q wave of the electrocardiogram, as if the atrium propelled the blood towards the pulmonary trunk to compensate for the lack of ventricular propulsion. We have also seen this feature.

LEFT VENTRICULAR ENDOMYOCARDIAL FIBROSIS

The clinical signs of endomyocardial fibrosis affecting the left ventricle are more variable than when the right ventricle is affected. They may mimic isolated mitral insufficiency in a young subject, exceptionally showing signs of mitral stenosis (Nagagaratnam and Dissannayake, 1959). Left ventricular failure sometimes occurs, with a subsequent rapid downhill course. In all patients, there is

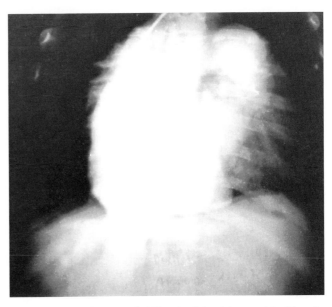

Figure 69.13. Endomyocardial fibrosis of the right ventricle. There is an amputation of the apex, with a somewhat dilated infundibulum and irregularities of the ventricular border. The right atrium is grossly dilated with reflux in the inferior caval vein.

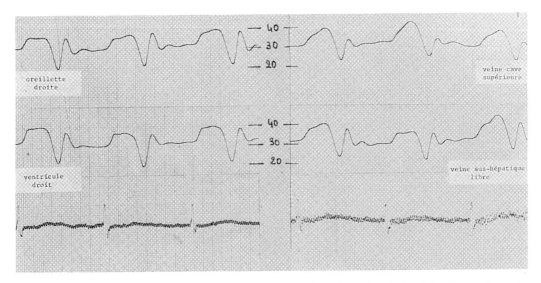

Figure 69.14. Endomyocardial fibrosis of the right ventricle. Pressure recordings have been taken in the right atrium and superior caval vein (top), and the right ventricle and hepatic veins (bottom). The aspect is similar in all the cavities, with elevated pressure (mean 30 mmHg) and a diastolic dip-plateau.

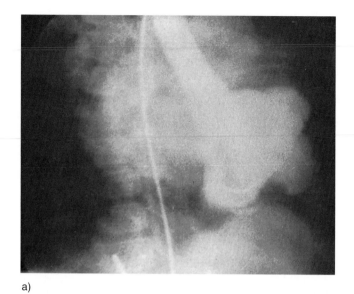

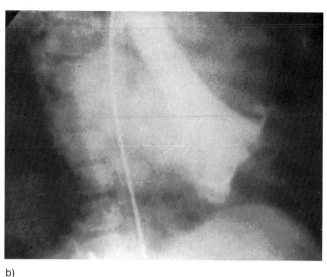

a)   b)

Figure 69.15. Endomyocardial fibrosis of the left ventricle, as illustrated by cineangiography in the right anterior oblique projection for (a) systolic and (b) diastolic frames. There is a severe amputation of the cavity in systole. In diastole, the outflow tract is dilated. There is also marked mitral insufficiency. (Courtesy of Metras et al 1982 Journal of Thoracic and Cardiovascular Surgery 83: 52.)

important pulmonary stasis, with the tendency towards right ventricular failure. Arrhythmias are frequent, but disturbances of conduction are less well documented. Signs of left atrial and ventricular hypertrophy, or left anterior hemiblock, can be observed. There may be reduction in the duration of the R wave in leads V_5 and V_6. The phonomechanogram shows a murmur of mitral insufficiency. Exceptionally, there is a diastolic murmur. The endocardial snap is observed in many patients. Endocardial thickening and a rigid square septal motion is seen on M-mode examination (Dienot et al 1981). Apical obliteration is seen on cross-sectional examination (Touza et al, 1985). The mitral valvar leaflets can be normal, but their motion is very often impeded by thickening and distortion of the subvalvar apparatus. The chest radiograph is not diagnostic. The left ventricle is enlarged, and there are signs of pleural and pulmonary stasis. The pulmonary arteries are dilated. Sometimes the features are suggestive of mitral stenosis. Calcifications can be observed near the apex in up to one tenth of patients. Angiocardiography shows retraction of the apex of the left ventricle, the feature of the playing card 'heart' or an 'apple stalk' (Cockshott, 1965; Bertrand et al, 1980). Often there is dilatation of the outflow portion, giving a 'mushroom' (Figure 69.15) or 'boxing glove' formation. Mitral insufficiency is seen in two thirds of patients. There are filling defects or diverticulums of the ventricular contour in half and hypertrophy of the papillary muscles in one third of patients. The ascending aorta is superimposed on the descending aorta in one third. A pericardial effusion is present in half. The haemodynamic signs include dip-plateau pressure curves in the left ventricle (Figure 69.16), with elevated pulmonary capillary and arterial pressures.

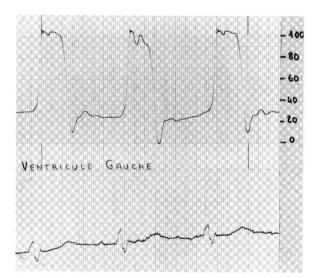

Figure 69.16. Endomyocardial fibrosis of the left ventricle: pressure recording in the left ventricle. There is a dip-plateau aspect in diastole, with an elevated end-diastolic pressure.

BIVENTRICULAR ENDOMYOCARDIAL FIBROSIS

Endomyocardial fibrosis most frequently affects both ventricles and this form occurs in from half to three quarters of patients. It associates the signs of right and left ventricular disease. Most of the time, one ventricle is predominantly involved, usually the right.

VARIATIONS IN SYMPTOMS

An atrial variant can occur in which a succession of atrial arrhythmias leads to cardiovascular collapse. In this pattern, the right atrium is often very large. Death by arrhythmia is possible. The pericardial type presents with an effusion, rarely accompanied by a friction rub, which is serohaemorrhagic or inflammatory. The exudale is rich in cells and poor in albumin. This pericardial effusion can complicate the postoperative period. A variant pseudo-cirrhotic is often seen in young people. Ascites is very abundant and recurrent, but is not inflammatory. The liver is hard, with a sharp edge, and exhibits systolic pulsations. Some of our patients with this variant have shown neither true cirrhosis nor signs of portal hypertension. A febrile type is sometimes observed. In Nigeria and Brazil, a febrile onset of the disease has been described with an infectious aspect. Calcifications are observed in one tenth of patients, with endocardial calcifications along the pulmonary infundibulum or at the apex of the left ventricle.

LABORATORY DATA

In some series, especially from Europe, hypereosinophilia is reported in up to one-third of patients. In our experience, there is marked variability in the eosinophil count. We will discuss this fact below in the section devoted to aetiology. A systematic search for parasites has incriminated filariasis in Gabon and Nigeria; schistosomiasis in Ivory Coast, Brasil; and distomatosis in Europe. In Uganda, elevated titres of antistreptolysin were reported, but in our series they were normal. The rate of crythrocylic sedimentation is usually accelerated. The serum protein is elevated (Carlisle et al, 1972), with the globulins, mostly gamma and beta, being increased. Rarely a decrease in albumin is observed. Anti-cardiac antibodies were found in just over half by van der Geld et al (1966). Shaper et al (1967) have shown that patients often have other antibodies, particularly antimalarial, and suggested a tendency to autoimmunity. The data concerning coagulation cannot properly be interpreted because they are ill-assorted. In some cases of long-standing hepatic stasis, a decreased prothrombin time is observed, together with other signs of hepatic cellular insufficiency. An elevation of serum creatinine can be observed in those with advanced cardiorenal insufficiency.

COURSE OF THE DISEASE

Generally signs are progressively more severe and the patients die in months or years, but the disease seems to run with pauses, some patients experiencing periods without aggravation, and others even improving on treatment. These pauses can last several years. Ventricular fibrosis, in contrast, seems to be a non-changing process that is a consequence of previous disease. In Brazil (Mady et al, 1991), no progression was

seen in patients who had undergone two or more ventriculographies at intervals varying from 5 to 122 months, with a mean of 47.5 months .

DIAGNOSIS

The diagnosis is suggested by the clinical and non-invasive data, mainly echocardiography. It is confirmed by catheterization and angiography. Alternate diagnoses which can be considered for right ventricular or biventricular disease are chronic constrictive pericarditis restrictive fibrous cardiomyopathies, Ebstein's malformation, and right ventricular dysplasia. The possible alternatives to left ventricular disease are primary cardiomyopathies, valvar mitral insufficiency, and mitral stenosis. Diagnosis may be very difficult if the fibrosis is limited to the base of a papillary muscle, thus producing severe mitral insufficiency but without accompanying restrictive pressure recordings, and without obvious angiographic signs. In such cases, the diagnosis is made only at surgery. Endomyocardial biopsy can be positive, but owing to the localized nature of the disease, its benefits are debatable. The endocavitary electrocardiogram is a means of diagnosis, since the large monophasic wave seen in normal people, and in those with pericarditis or cardiomyopathy, is absent in those with endomyocardial fibrosis.

TREATMENT AND PROGRESS

Our experience is based on the 65 patients undergoing surgery in Abidjan and Marseilles, the recent experience at the Abidjan Institute of Cardiology (Kacou-Guikahue, 1991) and on our earlier study of 31 patients who underwent surgery compared with 30 patients who did not (Bertrand et al 1982b; Bertrand, 1985). Of those undergoing surgery, three quarters were children under 15 years of age. The patients not undergoing surgery received digitalis and diuretics. The medical treatment had a favourable effect but a limited action. Treatment of arrhythmias was useful, in particular the conversion of an atrial fibrillation. Atrial contraction, when present, palliates the deficient ventricular contraction. The fibrotic layer, however may, render endocavitary stimulation difficult. The role of anticoagulants, antiaggregants, steroids and immunosuppressants have not been evaluated at the stage of fibrosis. In patients submitted to medical therapy, there are improvements combined with periods of stabilization. These periods may last months or years. The patients die in months or years as a result of irreducible cardiac failure, arrhythmias, or thrombosis. Acute pulmonary oedema is rare in left ventricular disease. Surgical treatment was introduced by Dubost and Deloche in 1971. The principle of treatment is based upon creating a plane of cleavage between the fibrotic layer and the normal myocardium. Thus, an endocardiectomy can be performed. For several years, it was our belief that the subvalvar apparatus had to be resected together with the fibrotic layer, and the procedure was, therefore, completed by valvar replacement. In more recent years, we have achieved limited endocardiectomies combined with conservative valvar procedures (Metras et al, 1983). More recently, systematic salvage of the valvar apparatus has been advocated by a group from Brasil (de Oliveria et al, 1990). In patients with extensive fibrosis, this has been achieved not only in the right, but also in the left ventricle. Although technically demanding, this approach is an important advance, since valvar replace-

ment produces major problems in the tropics. The postoperative course is usually difficult, being complicated by low cardiac output, and the mortality is high. In our experience, mortality occurred mainly with left ventricular and biventricular disease. In spite of a complicated postoperative period, the late results are favourable. In terms of objective improvement such as size of the heart, intracardiac pressures, cineangiograms, and so on, we have achieved better results with left ventricular (Figure 69.17) than with right ventricular disease. In those with right ventricular involvements, the heart remains large, with persistent atrial arrhythmias and persistent hepatic enlargement.

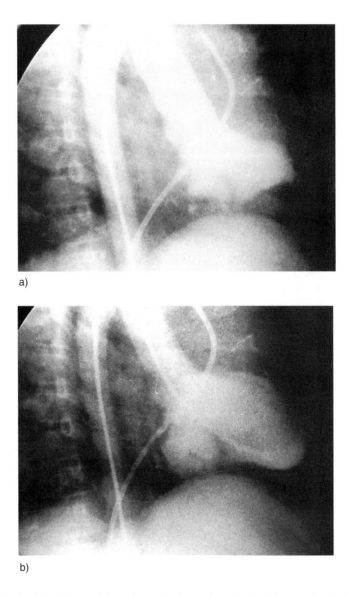

a)

b)

Figure 69.17. Endomyocardial fibrosis of the left ventricle as shown by cineangiography in right anterior oblique b view. (a) Systolic and (b) Diastolic frames. Postoperative results 1 year after endocardiectomy and mitral valve replacement (same patient as Fig. 56.15). There is an almost normal ventricular cavity and contraction. There is no mitral insufficiency. (Courtesy of Metras et al 1982 Journal of Thoracic and Cardiovascular Surgery 83: 52.)

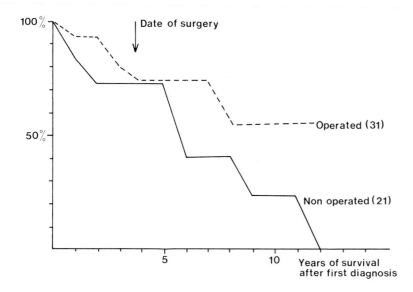

Figure 69.18. Endomyocardial fibrosis. Actuarial survival curves after first diagnosis in 31 patients undergoing surgery compared with 30 who did not have surgery.

Study of those with and without surgical treatment (Bertrand et al, 1985) has confirmed that overall survival is better after surgery (Figure 69.18). Our experience suggests that left ventricular lesions must be resected when there is evidence of restriction and/or a severe mitral insufficiency. Right ventricular disease requires surgery when there are signs of restriction, which is usually associated with a tricuspid insufficiency. Surgery is favourable in the biventricular form, but the prognosis is poorer than in the unilateral types. No factor has thus far been identified as being of prognostic value. In all types, there are some general contraindications that must be respected. Surgery must be postponed when there are signs of abundant pericardial effusion, evidence of evolution of the disease such as fever, laboratory tests of inflammation, or hypereosinophilia or association with another disease. Surgery must be rejected when there is abundant ascites with hepatic fibrosis.

Because of the marked postoperative mortality, it seems prudent to verify whether or not the patient is in a stable stage, adopting a conservative approach in patients with minimal symptoms who have a good prognosis (Mady et al, 1990). For patients with more severe problems, and for most children, surgical treatment remains the best approach.

The good long-term results of endocardiectomies with valvar replacement confirm the notion that the disease is essentially endocardial, since such positive responses would be unexpected had the myocardium been involved. These long-term results have been confirmed by other studies that showed that endomyocardial fibrosis did not progress (Mady et al, 1991).

AETIOLOGY

Several theories have been proposed to account for development of endomyocardial fibrosis. A genetic factor specific to tropical populations can be ruled out, since the disease is seen in other populations. No systematic study has been done of genetic status. Infections have been incriminated. Regardless of the type–cutaneous, pulmonary, urinary, bacterial or viral – they are all frequent in Africa. No precise correlation has been demonstrated. Shaper et al (1974) argued that streptococcal rheumatic disease could affect the valvar endocardium in some populations and the parietal endocardium in others. It was mentioned above that an inverse relation exists in Africa between rheumatic heart disease and endomyocardial fibrosis. It is noteworthy that both diseases affect children and adolescents. Parasitosis has been thought to be a possible cause by several authors. *Loa loa* filariasis was suggested by Gerbaux (1962) and by Ive et al (1967). In Uganda, Connor et al (1967, 1968) observed microfilaria in one myocardial specimen and serologic tests for filaria were proved positive in nearly one half of the patients seen in Abidjan. Schistosomiasis has been implicated as a possible cause in the Ivory Coast, Brazil and in Egypt (Rashwan et al, 1995). Most of the patients come from an endemic area. In these, the serology is positive in over one half, and the rectal mucosal biopsy is positive in almost two thirds. Guimaraes et al (1971) also noted this coexistence. Distomatosis was identified in the patients of Dallochio et al (1975) and Potier et al (1978). African trypanosomiasis has been incriminated by Poltera et al (1976). We think that this last disease is more likely to give a myocardial involvement, although we have once noted a lymphocytic infiltration confined to the endocardium. Bowel parasitosis has been observed in two thirds of the patients, with one quarter having polyparasitosis. No difference has been noted, however, compared with the general population. No direct role can be attributed to malaria, a disease common to most patients.

Metabolic causes have also been incriminated. Thus, elevated total levels of protien have been found in the blood, notably hyperglobulinaemia (Carlisle et al, 1972).

These changes, however, are again often found in the general African population, and are by no means specific. In protein deficiency, or kwashiorkor, seen in children, Thomas et al (1971) noted that endocardial fibrosis was observed only once in 103 postmortems. There were also four cases of fibroelastosis. Arnott (1959) has suggested that a diet rich in plantains seems to lead to a hyperserotonic serum. Experimentally, these diets do not lead to endocardial lesions, except in some exceptional conditions of deficiency and hepatic insufficiency.

The immunological hypothesis is based upon the fact that anticardiac antibodies had been found in over one half of the patients (Van der Geld et al, 1966; Shaper et al 1967). Their presence was more frequent when antimalarial antibodies were also elevated. Deposits of fibrin and immunoglobin were found on the surface of the heart, or at the level of the endocardium and the myocardium. The antibodies could result either from the liberation of endocardial antigens following a lesion of the endocardium or from the production of anti-cardiac antibodies in the presence of various antigens, for example parasitic, viral or bacterial antigens. In both cases, the circulating immune complexes could deposit on the endocardium and the vascular endothelium. Fibrous proliferation of the endocardium would result. The genetic or acquired characteristics are still to be determined. The tendency of Africans to develop cheloid scars should also be remembered.

The possibility of an hypereosinophilic syndrome has been raised by several groups (Roberts et al, 1969; Chusid et al, 1975; Olsen and Spry, 1979; Parrillo et al, 1979). Cardiac failure is one of the causes of death in various hypereosinophilic syndromes, such as leukaemia, Hodgkin's disease and cancer. In these, the most characteristic lesion is endomyocardial fibrosis. Eosinophilia may well be a factor of irritation for the endocardium. Some anomalies of eosinophils favour this hypothesis, notably the increased fixation of Fc fragments of immunoglobulin G, the degranulated and vacuolized cells and their prolonged half-life. Olsen and Spry (1979) have suggested that these 'activated' eosinophils could secrete cytotoxic components and produce inflammation of the endothelium and endocardium. This hypothesis can certainly explain the hypereosinophilic forms. But many variants of the disease do not exhibit hypereosinophilia. If these variants are to be explained on the same basis, it becomes necessary to postulate a stage of hypereosinophilia existing at the initial stage of the disease, with subsequent endocardial inflammation. Certainly in the patient seen late, which is frequent in Africa, the hypereosinophilia could have disappeared with the endocardial lesion then transformed to an advanced stage of fibrosis.

In India (Valiathan and Kartha, 1990), a geochemical hypothesis has been advanced, since patients have been noted with nutritional deficits, notably with lack of magnesium. A deficiency of magnesium with high concentrations of cerium and thorium (both abundant in the soil) have been found in affected hearts. Such a conjunction could trigger cellular dysfunction, but could it explain endomyocardial fibrosis?

PROPOSED PREVENTIVE MEANS

Preventive means are possible only in those areas where the disease is important in terms of morbidity or mortality. The first step is to determine the exposed areas, especially in the tropical forest. The necessary epidemiologic research has been done in Ivory Coast. The most threatened group is the Akan group, four fifths of the patients coming from these areas. In these threatened areas, general measures can be taken against parasitosis. Another feasible preventive method could be based on the hypothesis of hypereosinophilia. Because the patients are young, prophylaxis could be offered to children less than 15 years of age. A yearly school consultation could be done, and the discovery of hypereosinophilia would result in commencement of antiparasitic treatment. The indications for steroid therapy or hydroxyurea remain debateable. Nonetheless, using corticosteroids or hydroxyurea, Parrillo et al (1979) were able to demonstrate regression of cardiac signs in hypereosinophilic patients. The discovery of established cardiac diseases should then be the trigger for rapid medical or surgical treatment. Should the hypothesis of lack of magnesium be confirmed, prevention could also be achieved by supplementation of the deficient element.

CONGENITAL HEART DISEASES IN THE TROPICS

Congenital heart diseases in tropical areas have been studied in various parts of the world, notably Central America (Espino-Vela, 1974), Southeast Asia (Walooppillai and Jayasinghe, 1970) and Africa (Gupta and Antia, 1967; Wood et al, 1969; Adetuyibi et al, 1976; van der horst, 1985; Chauvet et al, 1986).

GENERAL FREQUENCY

It is difficult to be precise concerning the frequency of congenital heart diseases in tropical countries. In the study by Espino-Vela (1974) for Central America congenital cardiac malformations were found in 2.2% of 1 000 000 unselected patients. In Asia, a necropsy study of 19 415 cases showed a 2.1% incidence of congenital heart disease. In Nigeria (Gupta and Antia, 1967), the incidence of congenital heart disease was 0.35 per 100 births, and 0.2% among 4568 necropsies (Adetuyibi et al, 1976). It was 0.64% among 9432 necropsies in Uganda (Wood et al, 1969). The true incidence of congenital cardiac disease cannot be decided from these studies since many were conducted in selected hospital patients. As pointed out by Espino-Vela (1974), the overall frequency in tropical countries is almost certainly similar to the 0.3–0.6% quoted for occidental countries (Nadas and Fyler 1972). In Abidjan, congenital cardiac malformations make up 1.55% of all cardiac diseases seen in patients admitted to hospital.

AETIOLOGICAL FACTORS

The climate and the geographical situation are not considered to have an influence on the incidence of congenital cardiac malformations and certainly no particular condition found in tropical areas has been shown to cause such diseases. Furthermore, no differences have been shown between the different ethnic groups. High altitude, however, has been shown to be an aetiological factor in the incidence of persistent patency of the arterial duct and pulmonary hypertension, particularly in Mexico and some parts of Peru (Espino-Vela, 1974).

FREQUENCY OF THE MOST COMMON CONGENITAL MALFORMATIONS

Whwn we compare the order and frequency of congenital cardiac malfomations in three main occidental series and two tropical series. The five major diseases prove to be the same, albeit that the order varies (Table 69.2). One main difference is the relative rarity of aortic coarctation in tropical countries. In the series of Nadas and Fyler (1972) in the USA it was third at 8.1%, and in Wood's series (1968) it was fourth with 10%. In several

tropical series it has been rare, seen in only about 2%. In a series of 555 cases confirmed by catheterization (Walooppillai and Jayasinghe, 1970), it was even lower, being found in less than 1%. This malformation is generally rare in Black people, whether in tropical areas or not. Indeed, it is rare in all races other than Caucasians (Hernandez et al, 1969; Maron et al, 1973). Another difference is the rarity of subvalvar aortic stenosis in tropical countries. In the occidental series, the incidence is around 6%. It was not encountered, however, among the 555 patients seen in Sri-Lanka (Walooppillai and Jayasinghe, 1970). Amongst our 612 patients undergoing catheterization at the Abidjan Institute of Cardiology (Chauvet et al 1986), the distribution of the different diseases is very close to that observed in Europe, apart from the absence of severe congenital malformations such as complete transposition, aortic coarctation or aortic stenosis, which are probably lethal prior to their discovery (Table 69.3).

PROBLEMS OF DIAGNOSIS

There were no unusual findings in the clinical signs. The only diagnostic problem is the difficulty in recognizing cyanosis in Black people. The gums and the nails are frequently pigmented, and the cyanotic colour is easily overlooked. Anaemia is a common finding in tropical Africa, thus decreasing still further the amount of reduced haemoglobin and rendering the cyanosis even less obvious. Because of late consultation and late diagnosis, the general cardiac status of patients is usually severe, both in Africa and in tropical countries in general.

Table 69.2 Frequency of the main congenital heart diseases in tropical and temperate

	Tropical areas (%)			Temperate areas (%)		
	Africa[1]	South Africa[2]	Singapore[3]	UK[4]	USA[5]	France[6]
Ventricular septal defect	25.8	18.8	23.1	12	19.4	20
Atrial septal defect	15	5.9	11.9	23.5	4.5	7
Tetralogy of Fallot	14.9	16.1	8	9.5	6	10
Valvar pulmonary stenosis	5.2	4.7	8	11	7.5	10
Patent arterial duct	17.8	16.1	11.4	9	15.5	15
Atrioventricular septal defect	3.5	2.6				
Complete transposition	1.6	3.3	5		4.7	9
Aortic coarctation	1.6	4.9	4.6	10	8.1	9
Aortic stenosis	1.5	2.4		6	5.5	6
Eisenmenger's syndrome			3.9	7		
Others	13.1	25.2				

From [1] Chauvet et al (1986); [2] van der Horst (1985); [3] Muir (1960); [4] Wood et al (1968); [5] Nadas and Fyler (1972); [6] Dupois (1981).

Table 69.3 The results of catheterization in 612 patients with congenital cardiac disease in Abidjan

Cardiac disease	Number
Left to right shunt	
Ventricular septal defect	158 (25.8%)
Persistent arterial duct	109 (17.8%)
Atrial septal defect	92 (15.0%)
Atrioventricular septal defect	22 (3.5%)
Cyanotic lesions	
Tetralogy of Fallot	91 (14.9%)
Double outlet ventricle	15 (2.5%)
Pulmonary atresia with intact ventricular septum	12 (2%)
Double inlet ventricle	11 (1.8%)
Tricuspid atresia	10 (1.6%)
Complete transposition	10 (1.6%)
Common arterial trunk	8 (1.3%)
Anomalous pulmonary venous connection	3 (0.5%)
Obstructive lesions	
Pulmonary stenosis or atresia with intact ventricular septum	32 (5.2%)
Aortic stenosis	9 (1.5%)
Aortic Coarctation	10 (1.6%)
Ebstein's malformation	1 (0.1%)
Obstructive cardiomyopathies	1 (0.1%)
Others	18 (2.9%)
Total	612 (100%)

HYPERTENSION IN CHILDREN

Arterial hypertension is a problem of public health in Africa. The prevalence in the general population varies from 4.96 to 15.34% (Bertrand, 1979). In the Ivory Coast, the prevalence is 13.9% (Bertrand et al, 1976). The deleterious effect of the raised blood pressure on society (Bertrand et al, 1981a) cannot be evaluated precisely, but it is probably considerable, since hypertension is responsible for 9.5% of the deaths, and 7.8% of hospital admissions. Cerebral complications, left ventricular insufficiency and renal insufficiency are frequent. Sick-leave as a consequence of hypertension is considerable. Treatment and follow-up of patients is essential. But the cost is also considerable. In tropical areas, this often cannot be achieved within the existing system of social service. The discovery and the follow-up of children at risk, therefore, must be seen as the major means of combating hypertension (Bertrand, 1995). Such a system requires establishment of normal pressures, identification of children to be followed, and elucidation of the required prophylactic or therapeutic measures.

DETERMINATION OF THE NORM

In view of the variation in environmental factors and genetic factors, these norms must, if possible, be determined for every area (see also Chapter 68). In the Ivory Coast, two types of study have been made. One was concerned with the relation of sex and age. The other combined these features with size and weight. The first study involved over 15 000 pupils from 11 to 18 years old (Bertrand et al, 1981b). The measurements were done in the sitting position after several minutes of rest (Table 69.4). The diastolic pressure used was that measured at phase V of Korotkof. (In the UK, it is more usual to take phase IV as the value for diastolic pressure.) To establish norms that are of value in regular medical practice, the numbers obtained were approximated to the nearest 5 mmHg and took account of weight or excess weight and size. A statistical study allowed the best correlated parameter to be identified. The second study concerned 1803 individuals aged from 10 to 25 years (Bertrand et al, 1982a). The method of measurement was the same

Table 69.4 Norms for blood pressure[a] related to age in the Ivory Coast

Age (years)	Average BP (mmHg)		Average BP + 1SD (mmHg)		Average BP + 2SD (mmHg)	
	S	D	S	D	S	D
Boys						
11–12						
13–14	120	70	130	80	150	90
15–16						
17–18	125	70	140	85	155	95
Girls						
11–12						
13–14	120	70	130	80	150	90
15–16						
17–18						

BP, blood pressure; S, systolic; D, diastolic; SD, standard deviation.
[a] Values approximated to nearest 5 mmHg.

Table 69.5 Norms for blood pressure[a] related to weight for children in the Ivory Coast

Weight (kg)	Average BP (mmHg)		Average BP + 1SD (mmHg)		Average BP + 2SD (mmHg)	
	S	D	S	D	S	D
Males						
30–34	110	65	120	75	135	85
35–39	110	70	125	75	140	85
40–44	115	70	130	80	140	90
45–49	120	70	130	80	145	90
50–54	120	75	135	80	145	90
55–59	125	75	135	85	150	90
60–64	125	75	140	85	155	95
65–69	130	75	145	85	155	95
70–74	135	75	145	90	160	95
75 or greater	135	75	150	90	160	100
Females						
30–34	110	65	125	75	135	80
35–39	115	65	125	75	135	85
40–44	115	70	125	75	135	85
45–49	115	70	130	75	140	85
50–54	120	70	130	80	140	85
55–59	120	70	130	80	140	85
60–64	120	70	130	80	145	90
65–69	125	75	135	80	145	90
70–74	125	75	135	80	145	90
75 or greater	125	75	135	85	150	90

From Bertrand et al (1982a).
BP, blood pressure; S, systolic; D, diastolic; SD, standard deviation.
[a] Values approximated to nearest 5 mmHg.

as in the previous study, but with the aim also of correlating blood pressure with weight and size. As had been shown by the previous studies of Heyden et al (1969), Froment (1970), Dube et al (1975), Voors et al (1976) and Aullen (1980), the best correlation was with weight (Table 69.5). The relation with excess weight appeared to be less close, a link appearing only for a weight index greater than 100% in both sexes. We also observed the correlation between blood pressure and age found previously by most authors. We obtained this correlation in both sexes, but it disappeared when age and size were suppressed, except in boys for the diastolic pressure. Size does not appear to be a determinant parameter in Ivory Coast. This is in contradiction to the observations of Andre et al (1980). In our study, girls have a less elevated blood pressure, but the link with weight is still present. These facts persuaded us to propose norms in relation with weight. They seem better adjusted than age-related norms. These are the norms given in Table 69.5. We have indicated the average pressures and the numbers corresponding to average norms plus one or two standard deviations having approximated the numbers to the nearest 5 mmHg). Norms have now also been determined in Nigeria (Akinkugbe, 1990) with regard to sex and age (Table 69.6) and in Benin (Frances, 1995).

Table 69.6 Mean blood pressure in Nigerian children

	Systolic BP (mmHg) at age		Diastolic BP (mmHg) at age	
	2–5 years	6–12 years	2–5 years	6–12 years
Males	96.3	102.2	60.6	67.4
Females	98.5	105.3	62.3	68.5
ALL	97.4	103.7	61.5	67.9

BP, blood pressure.
From Akinkugbe et al (1990).

WHICH CHILDREN SHOULD BE FOLLOWED?

Whatever the chosen norm, it seems useful to establish the groups to follow, taking account of the epidemiological partitioning of blood pressure. 'Normal' individuals are those in whom the pressure is inferior or equal to one standard deviation of the mean blood pressure. 'Limit' individuals are those in whom the pressure is between one or two standard deviations of the mean. Those 'at risk for hypertension' have a blood pressure superior or equal to two standard deviations from this mean pressure. In our study involving 1155 individuals (Bertrand et al, 1981), just over four-fifth of the children were 'normal', one-seventh were 'limit' and just under one-twentieth were at risk for hypertension. If we accept the hypothesis of tracking, the follow-up of the children in the two last groups should lead to avoidance of hypertension in the adult. Those children to be followed can also be identified by an investigation for family history of hypertension. The study of other risk factors can also lead to a better selection of those children to be followed.

HOW SHOULD THE PATIENTS BE TREATED? ──

The measures for prophylaxis are the same in tropical areas as in other parts of the world. We have tried to adapt them to the observations made in sub-Saharan Africa. 'Normal' individuals are examined every 3 years, and they are not submitted to any prophylaxis. 'Limit' individuals must be examined every 2 years. They are advised to reduce intake of salt to a minimum, to avoid excessive gain in weight, not to smoke, to practise a sport and not to use oral contraceptives. Those individuals considered at risk of hypertension must be examined every year. The same advice is given. It is also necessary to record their blood pressure repeatedly. If these repeated measurements show a pressure greater than two standard deviations above the mean plus 2 standard deviations, then appropriate investigations must be done to search for the cause. Treatment must be discussed.

REFERENCES

Adams J H, Haller L, Boa F Y et al 1986 Human African trypanosomiasis (*T. B. Gambiense*): a study of 16 fatal cases of sleeping sickness with some observations on acute active arsenical encephalopathy. Neuropathology and Applied Neurobiology 12: 81–94

Adetuyibi A, Akisanya J B, Onadeko 1976 Analysis of the causes of death on the medical wards of the University college hospital, Ibadan over a 14 year period (1960–1973). Transactions of the Royal Society of Tropical Medicine and Hygiene 70: 466–473

Africa A, Sta-Cruz J Z 1948 Eggs of *Schistosoma japonicum* in the human heart. [Quoted by Faust E C: An inquiry into the ectopic lesions in schistosomiasis.] American Journal of Tropical Medicine 28: 165–199

Akinkugbe F M, Akinwolere O A O, Oyewole A I M 1990 Blood pressure in 3 socio-economic groups of Black children. Tropical Cardiology 16: 7–16

André J L, Deschamp J P, Gueguen R 1980 Tension artérielle chez l'enfant et chez l'adolescent. Valeurs rapporochées à l'âge et al taille chez 17067 sujets. Archives Françaises de Pédiatrie 37: 477–482

Antia A U 1976 Paediatric cardiology in Africa. In: Akinkugbe O O (ed.) Cardiovascular disease in Africa. Ciba Geigy, p 308–312

Antia A U, Talbert J L, Paplanus S H 1968 Etiology of endomyocardial fibrosis: an experimental evaluation of plantain ingestion and chronic lymphatic obstruction. Johns Hopkins Medical Journal 122: 87–93

Antia A U, Effiong C E, Dawadu A H 1978 The pattern of acquired heart disease in Nigerian children. African Journal of Medical Science 3: 1–6

Arnott W N 1959 A problem of tropical cardiology. British Medical Journal 2: 1273–1275

Aullen J P 1980 Hypertension artérielle. Obésité. Une étude étude épidémiologique sur 7002 sujets dans un département français. Annales de Cardiologie et d'Angdéologie 29: 463–470

Badawi 1961 Mechanism of pulmonary in bilharzial cor pulmonale. Alexandria Medical Journal 7: 523–535

Bertrand E 1979 Fibrose endomyocardique constrictive. In: Précis de pathologie cardiovasculaire tropicale. Sandoz Rueil Malmaison, France, p 46–70

Bertrand E 1995 Hypertension arterielle des populations originaires d'Afrique Noire. P Pradel, Paris

Bertrand E, Renambot J 1975 Intérât diagnostique des signes phonomécanographiques de la fibrose endomyocardique constrictive. Acta Cardiologica 30: 405–418

Bertrand E, Sentilhes L, Baudin L, Barabé P, Aye H 1969 Troubles de conduction cardiaque dans la trypanosomiase humaine Africaine. Archives des Maladies du Coeur 62: 247–253

Bertrand E, Barabé P, Carrie J, Rive J 1971 Le coeur bilharzien à Abidjan. Archives des Maladies du Coeur 64: 727–741

Bertrand E, Serie F, Rive J et al 1974 Aspects actuels des signes cardiaques de la trypanosomiase humaine à *Tr. gambiense* (à propos de 194 malades). Acta Cardiologica 29: 363–381

Bertrand E, Clerc M, Renambot J, Odi Assamoi M, Chauvet J 1975a 50 cas de paludisme aigu: étude symptomatologique et notamment cardiaque. Bulletin de la Société de Pathologie Exotique 68: 456–466

Bertrand E, Chauvet J, Le Bras M, Renambot J 1975b Les signes cardiaques chez les sujets porteurs du trait drépanocytaire. Bulletin de l'Institut National des Statistiques et de la Recherche Medicale (Paris) 44: 99–104

Bertrand E, Serie F, Kong I et al 1976 Etude de la prevalence et de certains aspects épidémiologiques de l'hypertension artérielle en Côte d'Ivoire. Bulletin de l'Organisation Mondiale de la Santé 54: 449–454

Bertrand E, Dalger J P, Ramiara J P, Renambot J, Attia Y 1978a L'hypertension artérielle pulmonaire bilharzienne. Etude clinique et hémodynamique chez 37 malades. Archives des Maladies du Coeur 71: 216–221

Bertrand E, Dalger J P, Ramiara J P, Renambot J, Attai Y 1978b Les signes cardiaques dans la bilharziose en dehors de toute hypertension artérielle pulmonaire. Archives des Maladies du Coeur 71: 676–680

Bertrand E, Cailleau G, Ekra A, Calvy H, Chauvet J, Metras D 1980 Diagnostic angiocardiographique de la fibrose endomyocardique constrictive A propos de 47 cas observés à Abidjan. Coeur 11: 15–25

Bertrand E, Ravinet L, Odi Assamoi M 1981a L'hypertension artérielle envisagée comme un problème de santé publique en Côte d'Ivoire. Cardiologie Tropicale 7: 155–160

Bertrand E, Ravinet L, Coly M 1981b Determination des normes tensionnelles chez 15756 écoliers africains de 11 à 18 ans en Côte d'Ivoire. Archives des Maladies du Coeur 74(no. spédial): 15–25

Bertrand E, Bertrand C, Ravinet L et al 1982a Etude des normes tensionnnelles chez 1803 jeunes ivoiriens de 10 à 25 ans: détermination des normes par rapport au poids. Cardiologie Tropicale 8: 93–102

Bertrand E, Chauvet J, Odi Assamoi M et al 1982b Evaluation des résultats du traitement chirurgical de la fibrose endomyocardique. Etude de 31 malades opérés et 30 malades non opérés. Bulletin de l'Académie de Médecine (Paris) 166: 1179–1186

Bertrand E, Chauvet J, Ekra A, Apea G J 1985 Etude hémodynamique de 74 cas de fibrose endomyocardique. Seminars de Hopiteaux de Paris 61: 1073–1076

Bertrand E, Levy S, Frances Y, LaFay V, Dreuilhe J L 1995 Trypanosomiase humaine africaine et myocardite. Traitement par difluoromethylornithine. Medecine Malades Infection 25: 1–3

Botreau Roussel P, Drobinski G, Levy R, Vachon J M, Niver M, Grosgogeat Y 1977 Infarctus du myocarde et drépanocytose hétédrozygote. A propos de 2 cas. Archives des Maladies du Coeur 70: 141–147

Brinsfield D F, Edwards K, Watkins L W 1963 Sickle cell trait and abnormal cardiovascular findings. South African Medical Journal 56: 1443–1453

Brokington I F, Olsen E G 1978 Loeffler's endocarditis and Davies' endomyocardial fibrosis. American Heart Journal 85: 308–322

Caddell J L, Workley A, Connor D H, D'Arbela P G, Billinghurst J R 1966 Acquired heart disease in Ugandan children. British Heart Journal 28: 759–764

Carlisle R, Ogunba E O, Farlane, H, Onayemi O A, Oyeleye U O 1972 Immunoglobins and antibody to loa-loa in Nigerians with endomyocardial fibrosis and heart diseases. British Heart Journal 34: 678–680

Casasoprano A 1973 Myocardites, fibroelastose de l'endocarde, maladies de surcharge. In: Gerard C, Louchet E (eds) Precis de cardiologie de l'enfant. Masson, Paris, p 540–554

Chapuis Y 1976 La myocardite aiguë de la maladie de Chagas chez l'enfant. Cardiologie Tropicale 2: 179–183

Chauvet J, Kacou-Guikahue' M, Séka R et al 1986 – Etude de 612 cardiopaties congenitales cathéterizées à Abidjan. Les Conditions du dépistage. Cardiologe Tropicale 12: 119–124

Chusid M, Dales D C, West B C et al 1975 The hypereosinophilic syndrome: analysis of 14 cases with review of the literature. Medicine (Baltimore) 54: 1–27

Clark, de Graeffe 1935 Chronic pulmonary arteries in schistosomiasis mansoni with right ventricular hypertrophy. American Journal of Pathology 11: 693–705

Cockshott W P 1965 Angiocardiography of endomyocardial fibrosis. British Journal of Radiology 38: 192–200

Connor D H, Somers K, Hutt M S R, Mannion W C, Darbela P G 1967 Endomyocardial fibrosis in Uganda. American Heart Journal 74: 687–709

Connor D H, Somers K, Hutt M S R, Mannion W C, Darbela P G 1968 Endocardial fibrosis in Uganda. American Heart Journal 75: 107–124

Dallochio M, Clementy J, Mullon P, Bricaud H, Brousset P 1975 Fibrose endomyocardique et distomatose. Archives des Maladies du Coeur 68: 329–332

Davies J N P 1948 Endocardial fibrosis in East African. East African Medical Journal 25: 10–14

de Leval M, Taswell H F, Bowie E J W, Danielson G K 1974 Open-heart surgery in patients with inherited haemoglobinopathies red-cell dyscrasias and coagulopathies. Archives of Surgery 109: 618–622

de Oliveira S A, Barreto A C P, Mady C et al 1990 Surgical treatment of endomyocardial fibrosis: a new approach. Journal of the American College of Cardiology 16: 1246–1251

de Raadt P, Koten J W 1968 Myocarditis in I. *rhodesiene* trypanosomiasis. East African Medical Journal 45: 128–132

de Souza Amorium D 1979 Chagas disease. In: Yu P N, Goodwin J F (eds) Progress in Cardiology. Lea & Febiger PA, Philadelphia 235–279

Dienot B, Ekra A, Bertrand E 1981 Diagnostic échocardiographique de la fibrose endomyocardique constrictive (à propos de 45 cans). Cardiologie Tropicale 9: 107–114

Dubé S K, Dapoo'c R, Ratner H 1975 Blood pressure studies in black children. American Journal of Diseases of Children 129: 1177–1180

Dubost C H, Deloche A 1971 Fibrose endomyocardiques. In: Actualités de chirurgie cardio-vasculaire de l'Hôpital Broussais. Masson, Paris, p 149–158

Espino-Vela J 1974 Congenital heart disease. In: Shaper A G, Hutt M S R, Fejfar Z (eds) Cardiovascular diseases in the tropics. p 324–329

Frances Y 1995 Methodes de mesure de la pression arterielle. In: Bertrand E (ed.) Hypertension arterielle des populations originaires d'Afrique Noire. Pradel, Paris

Froment A 1970 La pression artérielle chez l'enfant d'âge scolaire: relations avec quelques variables. Bulletin de l'Institut National des statistiques et de la Recherche Médicale 25: 1227–1236

Gelfand M, Alves W, Woods R W 1959 The frequency of schistosomal ovi deposition in the heart. Transactions of the Royal Society of Tropical Medicine and Hygiene 53: 282–284

Gerbaux A 1962 L'endocardite pariétale fibroplastique. Coeur et et Médecine Interne 2: 139–149

Goodwin S F 1982 The frontiers of cardiomyopathy. British Heart Journal 48: 1–18

Guerrero L, Carracso H, Parada H, Molina C, Chuecos R 1991 Mecanica ventricular y arritmias cardiacas in patientes chagasicos y con miocardiopatias dilatadas primarias. Seqimiento eco-electrocardiographico. Arquivos Brasileiros Cardiologia 56: 465–469

Guidicelli C P, Touze J E, Bernard J 1996 Modifications electrocardiographiques dues a l'halofantizne dans le traitement du paludisine: implications thérapeutiques. Bulletin de l'Académie Nationale de Médecine 180: 71–82

Guimaraes A C 1982 Situagao actual dos conhecimentos sobre O envolvimento cardiopulmonar na esquistossomose mansonica. Arquivos Brasilieros Cardiologia 38: 301–309

Guimaraes A C, Esteves F P, Filho A S, Macedo V 1971 Clinical aspects of endomyocardial fibrosis in Bahia (Brazil). American Heart Journal 81: 7–19

Guimaraes A C, Filho A S, Esteves J P, Vinhaes L S, Abreu W N 1974 Hemodynamics in endomyocardial fibrosis. American Heart Journal 88: 294–303

Gupta B, Antia A U 1967 Incidence of congenital heart disease in Nigerian children. British Heart Journal 29: 906–909

Hawking F, Greenfield 1941 Two autopsies on rhodesiene sleeping sickness: visceral lesions and significance of changes in cerebrospinal fluid. Transactions of the Royal Society of Tropical Medicine and Hygiene 35: 155–161

Hernandez F A, Miller R H, Schiebler G L 1969 Rarity of coarctation of the aorta in the American negro. Journal of Paediatrics 74: 623–626

Herrera J M 1960 Cardiac lesions in vivax malaria: study of a case with coronary and myocardial damage. Archives of the Institute of Cardiology, Mexico 30: 26–36

Heyden S, Bartel A G, Hames C G 1969 Elevated blood pressure levels in adolescents, Evans Country, Georgia. Seven years of follow-up of 30 patients and 30 controls. Journal of the American Medical Association 209: 1683–1689

Hudson I, Davidson I A, McGregor C G A 1981 Mitral valve replacement using cold cardioplegia in a patient with sickle cell trait. Thorax 36: 151–152

Ikeme A C, Uzodike V O 1971 The electrocardiogram in endomyocardial fibrosis. West African Medical Journal 20: 345–351

Ive F A, Willis A S P, Ikeme Ac, Brockington I F 1967 Endomyocardial fibrosis and filariasis. Quarterly Journal of Medicine 36: 495–516

Jaffe R 1937 Sobre la miocarditis cronica, como causa de la muerte en Venezuela. Bulletao de las Hospitales 3: 112–115

Jones I G, Lowenthal M N, Buyst H 1975 Electrocardiographic changes in African trypanosomiasis caused by *Trypanosomia bruce rhodesiense*. Transactions of the Royal Society of Tropical Medicine and Hygiene 69: 388–395

Kacou G M, Chauvet J, Zabsonre P et al 1991 Endocarditis parietale chronique chez l'enfant: indications chirurgicales, résultats et évolution post-opératoire chez 98 énfants (dont 55 opérés) Cardiologie Tropicale 17(no. special): 71–79

Koberle F 1968 Chagas disease. In: Dawes B (ed.) Advances in parasitology, vol 6. Academic Press, London, p 63

Leachman R D, Millet W T, Atios I M 1976 Sickle cell trait complicated by sickle cell thrombi after open heart surgery. American Heart Journal 74: 268–270

Le Bras 1974 Incidence de la bilharziose dans l'hypertension d'origine rénale. Afrique Médicale 13: 1021–1025

Lindsay J, Meshel J C, Patterson R H 1974 The cardiovascular manifestations of sickle cell disease. Archives of Internal Medicine 133: 643–653

Lobo J, Coutinho, Filho J 1952 Ovo de Schistosoma mansoni no miocardio de Camundonga albino. Publicacoes Medicas Sao Paulo 22: 9–12

Loeffler W 1936 Endocarditis parietalis fibroplastica mit bluteosinophile. Schweizerische Medizinische Wochenschrift 36: 817

Lonsdorfer J, Boutros-Toni F, Clermont L, Cabannes R 1979 Etude in vitro de l'influence des gaz du sang sur la falciformation. Société Biologique Clinique de Côte d'Ivoire: March 8th

Mady C, Bardetto A C P, de Oliveira S A et al 1990 Endomyocardiol fibrosis: follow-up of clinically and surgically treated patients Arquivos Brasilieros Cardiologia 55: 241–244

Mady C, Barretto A C P, de Oliveira S A et al 1991 Evolution of the endocardial fibrotic process in endomyocardial fibrosis American Journal of Cardiology 68: 402–403

Marin-Neto J A, Marzullo P, Marcassa C et al 1992 Myocardial perfusion abnormalities in chronic Chagas' disease as detected by thallium-201 scintigraphy. American Journal of Cardiology 69: 780–784

Maron B J, Applefeld J M, Krovetz L J 1973 Racial frequencies in congenital heart disease. Circulation 47: 359–363

Menezes H 1954 Estudo histologico das les oes cardiacas con cobaios infestados experimentalmente pelo Schistosoma mansoni. Anais de Faculdade de Medicina da Universidade do Recife 14: 171–187

Metras D, Ouattara K, Ekra A, Bertrand E 1982a Endomyocardial fibrosis: early and late results of surgery in 20 patients. Journal of Thoracic and Cardiovascular Surgery 83: 52–64

Metras D, Ouezzin Coulibaly A, Ouattara K, Longechaud A, Millet P, Chauvet J 1982b Open-heart surgery in sickle-cell haemoglobinopathies: A report of 15 cases. Thorax 37: 486–491

Metras D, Ouattara K, Coulibaly A O, Touze S E 1983 Left endomyocardial fibrosis with severe mitral insufficiency. The case for mitral valve repair. Report of 4 cases. Thoracic and Cardiovascular Surgeon 3: 297

Muir C S 1960 Incidence of congenital heart disease in Singapore. British Heart Journal 22: 243–254

Multiple Africa Collaborative Study 1982 African multicentric research on cardiovascular diseases. Tropical Cardiology 8: 87–90 145–146

Nadas A S, Fyler D C 1972 In: Paediatric cardiology, 3rd edn. Saunders, Philadelphia, PA, p 683

Nagaratnam N, Dissanayake R V P 1959 Endomyocardial fibrosis in Ceylonese. British Heart Journal 21: 167–173

Okereke O U J, Chickwendu V C, Henacho H N C, Ikeh V O 1991 Non-invasive diagnosis of endomyocardial fibrosis in Nigeria using 2D echocardiography. Tropicale Cardiologie 17: 97–110

Olsen E S G, Spry C S F 1979 The pathogenesis of Loeffler's endomyocardial disease and its relationship with endomyocardial fibrosis. In: Yu P N, Goodwin S F (eds) Progress in cardiology, vol 8. Lea & Febiger, Philadelphia, PA, p 281–303

Parrillo J E, Borer J S, Henry W L, Wolff S W, Fancy A S 1979 The cardiovascular manifestations of the hypereosinophilic syndrome. American Journal of Medicine 67: 572

Pifano F, Marcuzzi G 1950 Contribution al estudio experimental de las miocardiopathias parasitarias de la region neo-tropica. Rachivos Venezuela Patologia Tropicale Parasitologica Medicina 2: 175–182

Pobbee J O M 1968 The aetiology of hypertension with special reference to renal disease and schistosomiasis. In: Hypertension in Africa. Literam, Ireja, Lagos, p 15–31

Poltera A A, Cox J N, Owor R 1976 Pancarditis affecting the conduction system and all valves in human African trypanosomiasis. British Heart Journal 38: 927–837

Potier S C, Khayat A, Foucault S P 1978 Distomatose et cardiopathie (à propos de 2 nouvelles observations). Archives des Maladies du Coeur 71: 1299–1306

Prata A, Andrade Z, Guimaraes A 1974 Chagas' heart disease in cardiovascular diseases in the tropics. In: Shaper A G (ed.) Cardiovascular disease in the tropics. British Medical Association, London, p 264–282

Ribierre M, Landau J F, Fermont L, Batisse A, Kachaner J 1982 Myocardites aiguës infectieuses. Semaine des Hôpitaux de Paris 58: 485–492

Rashwan M A, Ayman M, Ashour S, Hassanin M H, Abouzeina A 1995 Endomyocardial fibrosis in Egypt: an illustrated review. British Heart Journal 73: 284–289

Rey D, Monlun E, Christman D, Kremer M, Storck D 1992 L'aitente myocardique au cours du paludisme. Revue Medecine Interne Suppl 13: 265–268

Roberts W C, Leigler D G, Carbone P P 1969 Endomyocardial disease and eosinophilia. A clinical and pathological spectrum. American Journal of Medicine 46: 28–42

Rocha A, Da Cunha J A, David W et al 1993 Cardiopathia chagasica cronica causando insufficiencia cardiaca congestiva na infancia. Revista Sociedad Brasilieros Medicina Tropicao 26: 243–249

Rosenbaum M D 1964 Chagasic myocardiopathy. Progress in Cardiovascular Diseases 7: 199–205

Sadeler B C 1973 Electrocardiogramme et fréquence cardiaque de mesocricetus auratus aux différentes phases de l'infestation bilharzienne à Schistosoma mansoni. Médecine Tropicale 33: 579–594

Sankalé M, Quenum C, Koaté P 1969 L'atteinte myocardique au cours du paludisme. Vie Médicale 50: 2729–2734

Schylns C, Jansen P 1955 Recherches électrocardiographiques dans la maladie du sommeil. Acta Cardiologica 10: 26–32

Shaper A G, Kaplan M H, Foster W D, MacIntosh D M, Wilks N E 1967 Immunological studies in endomyocardial fibrosis and other forms of heart disease in the tropics. Lancet i: 598–600

Shaper A G, Hutt M S R, Fesfar Z 1974 Endomyocardial fibrosis. In: Shaper A G (ed.) Cardiovascular disease in the tropics. British Medical Association, London, p 22

Sodi-Pallares D 1951 Nuevas bases de la electrocardiographia. Prensa Medica Mexicans, Mexico City

Stransky E, Quiant N L 1959 On generalized schistosomiasis with special consideration to changes in the lungs and the heart in childhood. Pediatria Internazionale 9: 715–730

Thomas J, Sagnet H, Chastel C, Le Vourgh C 1971 Le kwashiorkor de famine (ou de guerre). Reflexions à propos de 1900 observations. Presse Médicale 79: 1681–1684

Touza J E, Ekra A, Mardelle T et al 1985 L'echocardiograhie dans 17 cas de fibrose andomyocardique–confrontation angiocardiographique et chirurgicale. Coeur 15: 161–168

Valiathan S M, Kartha C C 1990 Endomyocardial fibrosis, the possible connection with myocardial levels of magnesium and cerium. International Journal of Cardiology 28: 1–5

Van Der Geld H, Peetoom F, Somers K, Kanyerezi B R 1966 Immuno-histological and serological studies in endomyocardial fibrosis. Lancet ii: 1210–1214

Van der Horst R L 1985 The pattern and frequency of congenital heart diseases among Blacks. South African Medical Journal 68: 375–378

Voors A W, Foster T A, Frerichs R R, Webber L S, Berenson G S 1976 Studies of blood pressures in children, age 5–14 years, in a total biracial community. The Bogolusa Heart Study. Circulation 54: 319–327

Wallooppilai N J, Jayasinghe M de S 1970 Congenital heart disease in Ceylon. British Heart Journal 32: 304–306

Williams A W 1958 Cor pulmonale in schistosomiasis. East African Medical Journal 35: 1–6

Wood P 1968 In: Diseases of the heart and circulation, 3rd edn. Eyre & Spottiswoode, London

Wood J B, Serumager J, Lewis M G 1969 Congenital heart disease at necropsy in Uganda. A 16-year survey at Mulago Hospital, Kampala. British Heart Journal 31: 76–79

Zahawi S, Shukri N 1956 Ectopic schistosomiasis and bilharzial myocarditis. Transactions of the Royal Society of Tropical Medicine and Hygiene 50: 166–168

PART VII

RISK FACTORS
AND FOLLOW-UP

70

Cardiovascular risk factors in infancy and childhood

M. de Swiet

INTRODUCTION

Epidemiological studies performed in adults allow precise quantification of the risks of vascular disease. The Framingham Study has shown that 'An efficient practical set of variables for this purpose is a casual blood test for cholesterol and sugar, a blood pressure determination, an electrocardiogram and a cigarette smoking history. With this set of variables, the risk of coronary heart disease can be estimated over a 30-fold range and 10% of the asymptomatic population identified, in whom 25% of the coronary heart disease, 40% of the occlusive peripheral arterial disease and 50% of the strokes and congestive heart failure will evolve.' (Kannel, 1976). This is of particular importance because treatment of some risk factors, particularly hypertension in asymptomatic individuals, has been shown to decrease the subsequent incidence of vascular disease (Veterans Administration Co-operative Study, 1967, 1970; Hypertension, Detection and Follow-up Co-operative Program Group, 1979; Management Committee, 1980).

A further incentive to the identification of risk factors in children is that intervention might be more successful at this age than in adults. For example, it is possible that a short period of treatment of hypertension in infancy might prevent the patient developing hypertension in later life and might obviate the necessity for lifelong antihypertensive therapy starting in middle age. There is evidence that intimal thickening of coronary arteries starts in the first month of life (Neufeld et al, 1962; Jaffe et al, 1971), and fatty streaks can be demonstrated in childhood. If there is a group of children particularly at risk from vascular disease and/or abnormalities of lipid metabolism, perhaps treatment by dietary manipulation should be started in childhood rather than in later life, where the results have either been ineffective or only effective under strict control (Dayton et al, 1969). More recently, Barker and his colleagues in Southampton have presented data that suggest that the intrauterine environment has a profound influence on long-term development. Specifically, those individuals who had a low birthweight are more likely to have hypertension in later

life (Barker et al, 1989, 1990; Law et al, 1993). A low ratio between birthweight and placental weight is also a predictor of hypertension in later life (Barker et al, 1990), suggesting that intrauterine malnutrition is an important factor. Consequently, intervention could start in fetal life rather than after birth.

Unfortunately, measurement of risk factors in infancy does not approach the precision achieved in adults for three reasons. First, measurement of risk factors in adults can be initiated in a retrospective manner and then subsequently confirmed in prospective studies. For example, in a retrospective study, the significance of a risk factor such as hypertension is assessed by comparing its incidence in a representative group suffering from myocardial infarction with its incidence in the general population. If the incidence of hypertension is higher in the former group, hypertension is thought to be a risk factor for myocardial infarction. This approach to identifying potential risk factors cannot be employed in infancy, since the vascular diseases concerned, such as myocardial infarction and cerebrovascular accidents, are virtually unknown in infancy. Although the risk factors usually studied in infancy are those that are known to be risk factors in adults, prospective studies are essential.

The second difficulty is that such prospective studies must be very long. The longer the study, the more difficult it is to perform, since the subjects become dispersed and are difficult to trace and observe. In the United States of America, the annual incidence of coronary arterial disease is still small in the age group from 35 to 44 years (40/10 000 population), although it approximately doubles with each 10-year increase in age, until it reaches 209/1000 in the age group 55 to 64 years (Margolis et al, 1976). The ideal prospective study of risk factors in infancy, therefore, should last at least 50 years, which is a formidable undertaking. An alternative approach is to examine the persistence of known risk factors from one age group to the next. This approach has been best documented in the study of blood pressure in childhood and is further discussed below. For example, the 'Thousand

Aviator Study' (Oberman et al, 1967) showed that those airforce pilots who had hypertension at the age of 20 years were likely to have hypertension when their blood pressures were measured 10 and 20 years later, at the ages of 30 and 40 years. The group of investigators led by Kass has shown that blood pressure at 2–14 years of age is related to blood pressure measured 4 years later in the same population (then aged 8–16 years; Zinner et al, 1974) and 8 years later (when aged 10–22 years; Zinner et al, 1978). If these observations are taken together, it may be assumed that the hypertensive children, in whom Kass and his colleagues measured the blood pressure (Zinner et al, 1974, 1978), would have become the hypertensive young adults of the Thousand Aviator Study. These would be the individuals at risk from cardiovascular disease in later life, but this is only an assumption. The ideal study would examine the evidence of vascular disease and risk factors in the same individuals both as children and adults.

The third problem affecting the precision of measurement of risk factors in children is the variability of the risk factors themselves, in particular the measurement of blood lipids and blood pressure. It is well known that blood pressure varies throughout the day in adults. It is not so well known that blood pressure also varies in children (de Swiet et al, 1975). Both true variability and measurement artefact move casual measurements of blood pressure away from those that are representative of the subject's true status.

BLOOD PRESSURE

Numerous prospective surveys have demonstrated the potency of hypertension in adults as a risk factor for cardiovascular disease. Only within the 1990s, however, has it been possible to measure blood pressure accurately and non-invasively in infants. For example, it has been shown that the Doppler technique can be used by either doctors or nurses with considerable accuracy, in contrast with previous methods such as flush, auscultation or palpation, which underestimate systolic blood pressure by as much as 45 mmHg (Elseed et al, 1973). It is not yet possible to measure diastolic blood pressure with accuracy in infancy using the Doppler technique (Whyte et al, 1975). Although measurement of diastolic blood pressure may be of clinical value, it gives no additional information as a risk factor, since cardiovascular morbidity is more closely related to systolic than to diastolic blood pressure (Kannel and Dawber, 1974).

NORMAL VALUES

The most extensive study of blood pressure starting from birth is the Brompton Study (de Swiet et al, 1976, 1980a,b 1981, 1992; Earley et al, 1980). This is a population study of blood pressure that was started in the neonatal period;

previous studies were either based on small selected groups of neonates (Hennekens et al, 1976; Lee et al, 1976) or on larger populations of older children (Johnson et al, 1965; Uppal, 1974; Zinner et al, 1974; Lauer et al, 1975; Voors et al, 1976; Beaglehole et al, 1977). The purpose of the study is to establish the normal range of blood pressure in infants and young children in order to be able to categorize infants as normotensive or hypertensive.

There is considerable variability in blood pressure in children, not only within a 24-hour period (de Swiet et al, 1975) but also when blood pressure is measured over a longer interval. Kilcoyne et al (1974) showed that the prevalence of systemic hypertension (blood pressure greater than 140 mmHg) fell from 5.4 to 1.2% after repeat screening. In the Muscatine Study (Rames et al, 1978), the incidence of a similar elevation in blood pressure fell from 13 to 1% on rescreening. The existence of this degree of variability has emphasized the necessity for longitudinal studies to define precisely how closely measurements of blood pressure made at one age are related to those made as children grow older (see below).

Figure 70.1 gives the data of the Brompton Study and shows that the 50th percentile for systolic blood pressure rises rapidly from 75 mmHg at age 4 days to 95 mmHg at age 6 weeks. It then remains stable until at least age 5 years. It also shows the pooled data derived from the Miami, Muscatine and Rochester Studies of the American Task Force for Blood Pressure Control (1977). Blood pressure appears to rise after 5 years according to the data of the Task Force. These Task Force data need checking, however, since they are based on two different populations: infants of the Miami Study aged 1–5 years and of the Iowa Study using children aged 5–18 years. The apparent rise in blood pressure after age 5 years may, therefore, be caused by methodological differences. The normal range for systolic blood pressure varying by age (from 4 days to 10 years) and cuff size is shown in Table 70.1 (de Swiet et al 1992).

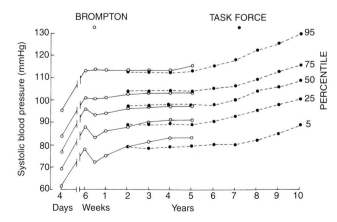

Figure 70.1 Blood pressure in children aged 4 days to 5 years (Brompton study) compared with the data of the Task Force for Blood Pressure Control in Infancy (aged 2–10 years). (From Blumenthal et al, 1977).

Table 70.1.   Systolic blood pressures in children awake by age and cuff size.

Infant age	Systolic blood pressure (mmHg)					
	Cuff 4 cm		Cuff 8 cm		Cuff 12 cm	
	Mean ± SD (No. observations)	95%[a]	Mean ± SD (No. observations)	95%[a]	Mean ± SD (No. observations)	95%[a]
4 days[b]	76.2 ± 9.9 (171)	95				
6 weeks	95.7 ± 10.7 (1129)	113				
6 months	104.8 ± 10.7 (129)	124	88.5 ± 12.3 (738)	109		
1 year			93.4 ± 11.1 (1323)	112		
2 year			95.5 ± 10.6 (1322)	115		
3 year			96.8 ± 9.7 (1218)	115		
4 year			97.4 ± 9.3 (1149)	113		
5 year			96.2 ± 9.4 (777)	114	89.1 ± 9.3 (218)	107
6 year			95.8 ± 9.1 (449)	112	90.0 ± 8.2 (626)	104
7 year			97.3 ± 9.2 (187)	114	90.0 ± 8.6 (881)	104
8 year			96.2 ± 8.6 (55)	110	91.9 ± 8.4 (1042)	105
9 year					92.3 ± 8.7 (963)	106
10 year					94.3 ± 8.8 (449)	111

[a] 95th percentile.
[b] Most of the neonates were asleep at the time of blood pressure measurement at this age.

BLOOD PRESSURE TRACKING

In adults, the correlation coefficient of an individual's blood pressure measured on one occassion and 1 year later is about 0.7 (Rosner et al, 1977). This correlation coefficient (tracking coefficient) is reached by the age of 18 years. What evidence is there that significant tracking occurs before the age of 18? The Brompton Study has demonstrated significant tracking from age of 1 year, when the correlation coefficient with blood pressure at the age of 2 years is 0.24 (de Swiet et al, 1980a). The 1- and 2-year tracking correlations increase with age (Figure 70.2). By the age of 10 years, the 1-year tracking coefficient has increased to 0.59 (de Swiet et al, 1992).

These data would suggest that the presence of relative hypertension with a systolic blood pressure in excess of the 95th percentile (113 mmHg) in the first years of life is a risk factor for hypertension in later life and, therefore, for cardiovascular disease in general.

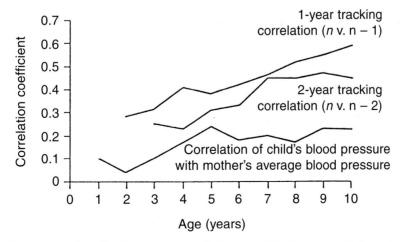

Figure 70.2 Correlation coefficients for tracking blood pressure and mother's average blood pressure with increasing age. (De Swiet et al 1992. With permission.)

In an older age-group, Zinner et al (1974) showed that there was a significant positive correlation between initial measurements and follow-up, the measurements separated by 4 years in a group of American children aged 2–14 years at first investigation. Beaglehole et al (1977) have confirmed this observation for systolic but not diastolic blood pressure in 332 Polynesian children aged initially 5–14 years, follow-up for 1.5–3.7 years. It is important to note that these, and the Brompton studies, showed that the follow-up blood pressure was still correlated after correction for weight, which they also found was related to blood pressure. Beaglehole et al (1977) also corrected for length of follow-up and found that the relationship was still significant. Buck (1973) re-examined 28 children whose blood pressures had been found to be beyond 1 standard deviation above the mean when they were first studied at the age of 5 years. She found that, at age 12 years, their blood pressures were still significantly elevated when compared with age-matched controls.

Heyden et al (1969), in the Evans County Georgia Study, reinvestigated 30 individuals who had been found to have hypertension (blood pressure greater than 140 mmHg systolic, 90 mmHg diastolic) between the ages of 15 and 25 years. At repeat examination 7 years later, five had persistent hypertension (each of three readings greater than 160 mmHg systolic or 93 mmHg diastolic) and seven more had borderline hypertension (mean of these three readings greater than 140 mmHg systolic or 90 mmHg diastolic). In addition, there were two deaths from cerebral haemorrhage, and four patients had developed symptomatic hypertension. This study is one of the earliest to demonstrate that hypertension between the ages of 15 and 25 years is a risk factor for symptomatic hypertension later in life.

In the Muscatine Study (Lauer et al, 1975), schoolchildren in Iowa aged 6–18 years had their blood pressure measured three times in 5 years (Clarke et al, 1976). The correlation coefficients between the individual pairs from three readings varied between 0.17 and 0.36, confirming other studies of the power of the tracking coefficient.

In summary, there are several studies in which the tracking of blood pressure has been investigated, measurements starting as early as 4 days after birth in one study. It would appear that tracking starts to be demonstrable in the first year of life, but that the correlation in serial measurements made at this age is weak. If it is assumed that high blood pressure in childhood is a risk factor for subsequent adult cardiovascular disease, the relationship is likely to be weaker than that between blood pressure measured in adult life and the development of cardiovascular disease. The correlation coefficient between successive measurements increases with age until, at 20 years, it has reached its adult level. At present, only in the Evans County Georgia Study (Heyden et al, 1969) has high blood pressure existing before the age of 25 years been shown to be associated with subsequent cardiovascular morbidity and mortality.

It is probable that other studies will show a similar association if the period of follow-up is sufficiently long.

FAMILIAL AGGREGATION OF BLOOD PRESSURE

The familial aggregation of blood pressure has been well documented in adults (Miall and Oldham, 1955; Platt, 1963; Miall et al, 1967). This is thought to be a consequence of a combination of genetic and environmental factors (Feinlieb et al, 1977). Because of the difficulty in performing longitudinal studies of blood pressure from infancy to adult life, it has been inferred that the age at which familial aggregation can first be demonstrated is the age at which children first have blood pressures representative of those that they will have in adult life. Stated another way, this is the age at which tracking begins. To demonstrate familial aggregation, it is only necessary to make measurements of more than one member of the family at one single time. Follow-up measurements, which have inherent practical difficulties, are, therefore, not necessary.

Lee et al (1976) demonstrated a weak correlation between the diastolic blood pressure of neonates and their mothers. Hennekens et al (1976), in the Miami Study, demonstrated familial aggregation of systolic and diastolic blood pressure at the age of 1 month, but not in newborns. Neither of these studies have shown very strong familial correlations. This probably accounts for the discrepancies regarding the age at which correlations can first be demonstrated – or whether systolic or diastolic blood pressure is the more important determinant. In the Brompton Study (de Swiet et al, 1992), correlation of the child's systolic blood pressure with the mother's average blood pressure was first shown between the ages of 2 and 3 years and increased in strength until the age of 5 years (Figure 70.2). Addition of the father's blood pressure did not increase the strength of the correlation.

BLOOD LIPIDS

Since the levels of various lipids in the blood have been shown to be related to cardiovascular morbidity and mortality, similar epidemiological studies to those already quoted for hypertension have been performed in the lipid field. Although there are several cross-sectional studies available, there are fewer data on longitudinal correlations of blood lipid content. Yet, if elevated blood lipid levels in childhood are to be considered risk factors, their consistency must be demonstrated. For example, in the excellently documented Muscatine Study, Lauer et al (1975) extrapolate from adult data to define cardiovascular risk factors as levels greater than, or equal to, 5.69 mmol/l for cholesterol, 140 mmHg systolic or 90 mmHg diastolic for blood pressure, and relative weight greater than 130%

mean. They then state that, using these criterions, 1% of children aged 14–18 years have three risk factors positive, 4.6% two risk factors and 22.7% one risk factor. But this approach is not appropriate for two related reasons. First, as with blood pressure, the relationship between elevated levels of blood lipid in infancy and the subsequent development of adult cardiovascular disease is not known. Second, there is little evidence concerning the 'tracking' of blood lipids. Do those children with elevated blood lipids become adults with elevated blood lipids? Lloyd (1976) believes that it is not clear if levels of lipid in the serum in adult life can be predicted from estimations made during infancy and childhood. She has shown a weak correlation ($r = 0.4$) between lipid levels measured at birth and those measured 1 year later (Darmady et al, 1972). Cholesterol levels also show considerable variability. For example, Uppal, in the Westland Study of 2388 schoolchildren in Holland (Uppal, 1974; Uppal et al, 1974), found a mean blood cholesterol of 4.66 mmol/l. Although 5% of the children had a blood cholesterol in excess of 6.21 mmol/l, only 40% of these children still had a blood cholesterol in excess of 6.21 mmol/l when re-examined 6 months later.

NORMAL VALUES FOR BLOOD LIPIDS

In order to discuss the possible implications of abnormal lipid levels, it is essential to define normality. This is not easy because there are relatively few population studies of blood lipids. Furthermore, in the affluent populations with a high dietary intake of fat, where studies are usually made, the normal range of blood lipids may not be what is desirable. Even the normal range of blood lipids may be too high to minimize the risk of ischaemic heart disease. At birth, levels of cholesterol are low (about 1.94 mmol/l) and independent of variables such as maternal hyperlipidaemia, gestation or ethnic origin (Drash, 1972). The level then rises within the first year of life to become the value for the rest of childhood (Lloyd, 1976).

It has been suggested on the basis of epidemiological studies by Drash (1972) and Godfrey et al (1972) that 5.17 mmol/l should be the upper limit of normal for cholesterol. Yet Uppal et al (1974), reviewing studies of levels of blood lipids in children throughout the world, show that up to 30% of the Westland population may have a serum cholesterol level greater than 5.17 mmol/l.

The data for serum tryglyceride are even more difficult to obtain, for there are wide fluctuations related to the time of feeding. A fast of between 8 and 12 hours is necessary to obtain repeatable and constant values. Using these criterions, the suggested upper limit for children is 140 mg/dl (1.4 g/l) (Godfrey et al, 1972; Lloyd, 1976).

PRIMARY HYPERLIPOPROTEINAEMIA

The relatively modest increases in blood lipids discussed so far are probably associated with diet or other secondary conditions, such as diabetes mellitus. Much greater increases in blood lipids occur in the primary hyperlipoproteinaemias, particularly in the homozygous forms. For example, in homozygous familial hypercholesterolaemia, the serum cholesterol may be as great at 26 mmol/l, and the affected children rarely live beyond adolescence (Fredrickson and Levy, 1972). Even heterozygotes have an increased risk of ischaemic heart disease compared with unaffected relatives (Stone et al, 1974). The subject has been well reviewed by Lloyd (1976).

It can be concluded that levels of cholesterol persistently exceeding 6.47 mmol/l (1 mmol/l = 38.7 mg/dl or 387 mg/l) or of tryglyceride exceeding 140 mg/dl are likely to be abnormal in children, and probably indicate primary hyperlipoproteinaemia. Both hetero- and homozygotes have an unequivocal increased risk of vascular disease. More modest increases in the concentrations of blood lipids are much more common. Their potencies as cardiovascular risk factors still remain unknown.

OBESITY

Evidence from the Framingham Study (Kannel and Dawber, 1974) suggests that much of the risk of obesity comes from its association with other risk factors. Obesity is correlated with raised levels of blood pressure and cholesterol, and with glucose intolerance. When allowance has been made for these risks, obesity has little additional contribution to make to the cardiovascular risk profile.

It is likely that there is a similar relationship between obesity in childhood and cardiovascular risk in adult life. We have found in the Brompton Study that blood pressure is related to weight at all ages studied. Voors et al (1977), in the Bogalusa Study, have found that the index of weight to height accounts for about 40% of the variability in blood pressure between the ages of 5 and 15 years. These authors believe that the increase in body mass is the major determinant of the increase in blood pressure associated with age in this age group.

Only long-term studies will show whether obesity in childhood makes any further contribution to cardiovascular risk apart from its relationship with blood pressure. It is unlikely that neonatal obesity will be a very strong risk factor, since approximately 70% of babies overweight in the first year of life are of normal weight by the age of 4 to 7 years (Lloyd, 1976). Older children track rather better for weight (13% of overweight women aged 26 years had been overweight at the age of 7 years: Stark et al, 1981).

SALT

Is high salt intake related to the development of hypertension and, therefore, a risk factor for coronary arterial disease? Two possible ways in which sodium might be involved in the initiation of hypertension are by primary increase in blood volume, and hence cardiac output (Guyton, 1980), or by an increase in the peripheral resistance associated with increased stiffness of blood vessels related to their intracellular content of sodium (Blaustein, 1977; Tobian, 1981).

Studies of the relationship between hypertension and sodium flux across red cell membranes in hypertensives and their first-degree relatives implicates sodium in the pathogenesis of hypertension (Garay and Meyer, 1979; Garay et al, 1980; Woods et al, 1981). This relationship between dietary sodium and hypertension is seen in populations, as well as in individuals. There are several epidemiological studies in South Africa (Trusell et al, 1972), Polynesia (Prior et al, 1968), the West Indies (Kohlstaedt et al, 1958) and South America (Oliver et al, 1975) that link a low-salt diet with the absence of hypertension. Dahl et al (1962) have shown, in spontaneously hypertensive rats, that intake of salt interacts with genetic factors to cause hypertension. Miall (1959), in contrast, found no relationship between blood pressure and sodium excretion in the population he studied in the Rhondda Valley. The relationship between sodium intake and blood pressure could similarly not be demonstrated in individuals in a community (Hollander et al, 1961). But there is evidence that a modest reduction of sodium intake, from a mean of 162 mmol/h to a mean of 90 mmol in 24 hours, will reduce blood pressure in mildly hypertensive subjects (MacGregor et al, 1982). The reduction of 7 mmHg is comparable to that seen with treatment with β-adrenergic blocking agents (MacGregor et al, 1982).

It is likely, therefore, that sodium intake is related to blood pressure in individuals who are susceptible for other (unknown) reasons. It is important to be aware that the sodium content of processed food can vary considerably, and be markedly in excess of a similar diet cooked at home from raw ingredients. The consumer may not necessarily be aware of this, because the sodium is present as sodium glutamate added to improve flavour or as sodium nitrite as a preservative, rather than as sodium chloride. For example, a well-known brand of hamburger and chips contains 97 mmol sodium per portion, and one of fried chicken contains 75 mmol per portion (MacGregor et al, 1982). One small Chinese takeaway meal can contain 225 mmol sodium, or nearly twice the average adult intake (MacGregor et al, 1982).

Paediatricians have long been aware of the risks of excessive content of sodium in infant feeds. They should now realise that the content in the diets of older children is also important, particularly if they have other risk factors, such as hypertension or obesity.

BIRTHWEIGHT AND ITS RELATION TO PLACENTAL WEIGHT

Barker and colleagues measured the blood pressures of 459 men and women in Preston, United Kingdom

(Barker et al, 1990) at a mean age of 50 years and 1231 men and women in Hertfordshire, United Kingdom between the ages of 59 and 71 years (Hales et al, 1991). Detailed records had been kept of their birthweights and their mother's pregnancies. Surprisingly, blood pressure in the later half of life was found to be related inversely to birthweight: small babies grew up to be hypertensive adults. Since hypertension is a risk factor for cardiovascular disease, it must also be inferred that low birthweight is a risk factor for cardiovascular disease. The direct association between low birthweight and cardiovascular disease, however, has yet to be shown. The data of the Brompton Study have been used to examine the development of this effect (Law et al, 1993). Figure 70.3 shows that, in the first 10 years of life, a 1 kg decrease in birthweight from the mean is associated with a 2 mmHg increase in blood pressure from the mean. By the age of 67, this same change in birthweight increases blood pressure by 6 mmHg. It is not clear how this amplification of effect occurs with increasing age.

The ratio of birthweight to placental weight could be considered a measure of the intrauterine environment, since the uterus grew a relatively large fetus with only a small placenta. This ratio is inversely related to blood pressure in adult life (Barker et al, 1990). In other words, a 'bad' intrauterine environment is associated with the subsequent development of hypertension. These associations will have to be considered by obstetricians when they contemplate interventions that influence fetal growth, such as aggressive lowering of blood glucose to produce smaller babies in mothers with diabetes.

SMOKING

There is clear evidence that smoking is a cardiovascular risk factor in adults (Kannel, 1976). Smoking habits tend to be acquired early in life and are often familial (Bewley, 1978). It would, therefore, seem desirable to dissuade 'at risk' families from smoking for the sake of their children's health. It remains to be seen whether this will be a significant additional reason for giving up the habit.

THE CONTRACEPTIVE PILL

When women under the age of 45 years take the contraceptive pill, it has been shown that the pill interacts significantly with smoking, hypertension, diabetes and type II hyperlipoproteinaemia as risk factors for myocardial infarction (Mann and Inman, 1975; Mann et al, 1975). It is unlikely that taking the pill would add any risk in the absence of the above risk factors. But, on the above evidence, adolescents who are obese and who have elevated blood pressures should be counselled against using the contraceptive pill.

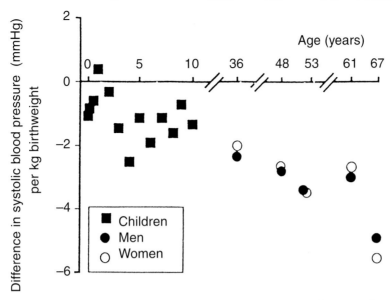

Figure 70.3 Relation between systolic blood pressure and birthweight at different ages. (Low et al 1993. With permission.)

CONCLUSIONS AND RECOMMENDATIONS

As yet, there are no hard data linking cardiovascular risk with risk factors present in infancy. Some potential risk factors, such as smoking or taking the contraceptive pill, are voluntarily accepted. Susceptible children and adolescents should be actively discouraged from accepting them. Other possible risk factors, such as hypertension and raised levels of lipid in the blood, are more related to the genetic make-up and environment of the child. More drastic steps are necessary, therefore, to alter them. In these circumstances, it would seem prudent to manipulate only the extreme examples until further evidence is forthcoming concerning the power of each individual risk factor. In the future, we will also have to consider the relation of the intrauterine environment to the subsequent development of cardiovascular disease, as well as to the development of other conditions such as diabetes.

REFERENCES

Barker D, Osmond C, Golding J, Kuh D, Wadsworth M 1989 Growth in utero, blood pressure in childhood and adult life, and mortality from cardiovascular disease. British Medical Journal 298: 564–567

Barker D, Bull A, Osmond C, Simmonds S 1990 Fetal and placental size and risk of hypertension in adult life. British Medical Journal 301: 259–262

Beaglehole R, Salmond C E, Eyles E F 1977 A longitudinal study of blood pressure in Polynesian children. American Journal of Epidemiology 105: 87–89

Bewley B R 1978 Smoking in Childhood. Postgraduate Medical Journal 54: 197–198

Blaustein M P 1977 Sodium ions, cation ions, blood pressure regulation and hypertension: a reassessment and a hypothesis. American Journal of Physiology 232: C165–C173

Blumethal S, Epps R P, Heavenrich R et al 1977 Report of the task force on blood pressure control in children. Pediatrics 59(Suppl): 797–820

Buck, C W 1973 The persistence of elevated blood pressure first observed age five. Journal of Chronic Diseases 26: 101–104

Clarke W, Woolson R, Schrott H, Wiebe D, Lauer R 1976 Tracking of blood pressure, serum lipids and obesity in children: The Muscatine Study. Circulation, 53/54 (Suppl II): 23

Dahl L K, Heine M, Tassinari L 1962 Role of genetic factors in susceptibility to experimental hypertension due to chronic excess salt ingestion. Nature 194: 480–482

Darmady J M, Fosbrooke A S, Lloyd J K 1972 Prospective study of serum cholesterol levels during the first year of life. British Medical Journal 2: 585–688

Dayton S, Pearce M L, Hashimoto S, Dixon W J, Tomiyasu V 1969 A controlled clinical trial of a diet high in unsaturated fat in preventing complications of atherosclerosis. Circulation 40 (Suppl II): 163

de Swiet M, Fancourt R, Pete J 1975 Systolic blood pressure variation during the first 6 days of life. Clinical Science and Molecular Medicine 49: 557–561

de Swiet M, Fayers P, Shinebourne E A 1976 Blood pressure survey in a population of newborn infants. British Medical Journal 2: 911

de Swiet M, Fayers P, Shinebourne E A 1980a The value of repeated blood pressure measurements in children: the Brompton Study. British Medical Journal 280: 1567–1569

de Swiet M, Fayers P, Shinebourne E A 1980b Systolic blood pressure in a population of infants in the first year of life: the Brompton Study. Pediatrics 65: 1028–1035 de Swiet M, Earley A, Fayers P, Shinebourne E A 1981 Epidemiological study of blood pressure in infancy. In: Giovannelli G, New M J, Gorini S (eds) Hypertension in children and adolescents. Raven Press, NY, p 283–286

de Swiet M, Fayers P, Shinebourne E A 1992 Blood pressure in first 10 years of life: The Brompton Study. British Medical Journal 304: 23–26

Drash A 1972 Atherosclerosis, cholesterol and the paediatrician. Journal of Pediatrics 80: 693–696

Earley A, Fayers P, Ng S, Shinebourne E A, de Swiet M 1980 Blood pressure in the first six weeks of life. Archives of Diseases in Childhood 55: 755–757

Elseed A M, Shinebourne E A, Joseph M C 1973 Assessment of techniques for measurement of blood pressure in infants and children. Archives of Diseases in Childhood 48: 932–936

Feinlieb M, Garrison R J, Fabsitz R et al 1977 The NHLBI twin study of cardiovascular disease risk factors: methodology and summary of results. American Journal of Epidemiology 106: 284–295

Fredrickson D S, Levy R I 1972 Familial hyperlipoproteinaemia. In: Stanbury J B, Wyngarden J B, Fredrickson D S (eds) Metabolic basis of inherited disease, 3rd edn. McGrawHill, NY p 545–614

Garay R P, Meyer P 1979 A new test showing abnormal net Na$^+$ and K$^+$, fluxes in erythrocytes of essential hypertensive patients. Lancet i: 349–353

Garay R P, Elghozi J L, Dagher G, Meyer P 1980 Laboratory distinction between essential and secondary hypertension by measurement of erythrocyte cation fluxes. New England Journal of Medicine 302: 769–771

Godfrey R C, Stenhouse N S, Cullen K J, Blackman V 1972 Cholesterol and the child: studies of the cholesterol levels of Busselton schoolchildren and their parents. Australian Pediatric Journal 8: 72–78

Guyton A C 1980 Arterial pressure and hypertension. Saunders, Philadelphia

Hales C, Barker D, Clarke P et al 1991 Fetal and infant growth and impaired glucose tolerance at the age 64. British Medical Journal 303: 1019–1022

Hennekens C H, Jesse M J, Klein B E, Gourley J E, Blumenthal S 1976 Aggregation of blood pressure in infants and their siblings. American Journal of Epidemiology 103: 457–463

Heyden S, Bartel A G, Hames C G, McDonough J R 1969 Elevated blood pressure levels in adolescents, Evans County, Georgia. Seven year follow up of 30 patients and 30 controls. Journal of American Medical Association 209: 1683–1689

Hollander W, Chobanian A V, Burrows B A 1961 Body fluid and electrolyte composition in arterial hypertension. 1. Studies in essential, renal and malignant hypertension. Journal of Clinical Investigation 40: 408–422

Hypertension, Detection and Follow-up Cooperative Program Group 1979 Five-year findings of the hypertension detection and follow-up program. 1. Reduction in mortality of persons with high blood pressure, including mild hypertension. Journal of American Medical Association 242: 2562–2571

Jaffe D, Hartcroft W S, Manning M, Eleta G 1971 Coronary arteries in newborn children Acta Paediatrica Scandinavica (Suppl) 219: 328

Johnson B C, Epstein F H, Kjelsberg M O 1965 Distributions and familial studies of blood pressure and serum cholesterol levels in a total community Tecumseh, Michigan. Journal of Chronic Diseases 18: 147–160

Kannel W B 1976 Some lessons in cardiovascular epidemiology from Framingham. American Journal of Cardiology 37: 269–282

Kannel W B, Dawber T R 1974 Hypertension as an ingredient of a cardiovascular risk profile. British Journal of Hospital Medicine 11: 508

Kilcoyne M M, Richter R W, Alsup P A 1974 Adolescent hypertension. 1 Detection and prevalence. Circulation 50: 758–764

Kohlstaedt K C, Moser M, Francis T, Neel J, Moore F 1958 Panel discussion on genetic and environmental factors in human hypertension. Circulation 17: 728–742

Lauer R M, Connor W E, Leaverton P E, Reiter M A, Clarke W R 1975 Coronary heart disease risk factors in schoolchildren: the Muscatine Study. Journal of Pediatrics 86: 697–706

Law C M, de Swiet M, Osmond C et al 1993 Initiation of hypertension in utero and its amplification throughout life. British Medical Journal 306: 24–27

Lee Y, Rosner B, Gould J B, Kass E H 1976 Familial aggregation of blood pressures of newborn infants and their mothers. Pediatrics 58: 722–729

Lloyd J K 1976 Hyperlipoproteinaemia and atherosclerosis. In: Hull D (ed.) Recent advances in paediatrics. Churchill Livingstone, Edinburgh

MacGregor G A, Markandu N D, Best F E et al 1982 Double blind randomised crossover trial of moderate sodium restriction in essential hypertension. Lancet i: 351–355

Management Committee 1980 The Australian therapeutic trial in mild hypertension Lancet i: 1261–1267

Mann J I, Inman W H W 1975 Oral contraceptives and death from myocardial infarction. British Medical Journal 2: 245–248

Mann J I, Vessey M P, Thorogood M, Doll R 1975 Myocardial infarction in young women with special reference to oral contraceptive practice. British Medical Journal 2: 241–245

Margolis J R, Gillum R F, Feinleib M, Brasch R, Fabbitz R 1976 Community surveillance for coronary heart disease: the Framingham cardiovascular disease study. American Journal of Cardiology 37: 61–67

Miall W E 1959 Follow-up study of arterial pressure in the population of a Welsh mining valley. British Medical Journal 161: 1204–1210

Miall W E, Oldham P O 1955 A study of arterial blood pressure and its inheritance in a sample of the general population. Clinical Science 14: 459–488

Miall W E, Hencage P, Knosia T, Lovell H G, Moore F 1967 Factors influencing the degree of resemblance in arterial pressure of close relations. Clinical Science 33: 271–283

Neufeld H N, Wagenvoort C H, Edwards J E 1962 Coronary arteries in fetuses, infants, juveniles and young adults. Laboratory Investigation 11: 837–844

Oberman A, Lane N E, Harlan W, Graybiel A, Mitchell R E 1967 Trends in systolic blood pressure in the thousand aviator cohort over a twenty-four year period. Circulation 36: 812–822

Oliver W J, Cohen E L, Neel J V 1975 Blood pressure, sodium intake and sodium related hormones in the

Yanomano Indian, a 'no salt' culture. Circulation, 52: 146–151

Platt R 1963 Heredity in hypertension. Lancet i: 899–904

Prior I A M, Grimley Evans J, Harvey H P B, Davidson F, Lindsey M 1968 Sodium intake and blood pressure in two Polynesian populations. New England Journal of Medicine 279: 515–520

Rames L K, Clarke W R, Connor W E, Reiter M A, Lauer R M 1978 Normal blood pressures and the evaluation of sustained blood pressure elevation in childhood: the Muscatine Study. Pediatrics 61: 245–251

Rosner B, Hennekens C H, Kass E H, Miall W E 1977 Age-specific correlation analysis of longitudinal blood pressure data. American Journal of Epidemiology 106: 306–313

Stark O, Atkins E, Wolff O H, Douglas J W B 1981 Longitudinal study of obesity in the National Survey of Health and Development. British Medical Journal 283: 13–17

Stone N J, Levy R I, Fredrickson D S, Verter J 1974 Coronary artery disease in kindred with familial type II hyperlipoproteinaemia. Circulation 49: 476–488

Tobian L 1981 Salt and hypertension. Annals of New York Academy of Science 304: 178–202

Trusell A S, Kennelly B M, Hansen J D L, Lee R B 1972 Blood pressure of the Kung Bushmen in Northern Botswana. American Heart Journal 84: 512

Uppal S C 1974 Coronary heart disease, risk patterns in Dutch youth. New Rhine, Leiden

Uppal S C, De Haas J H, Arntzenius A C 1974 Westland Schoolchildren, Surrey. A preliminary report on risk factors for CHD. Heart Bulletin Aug: 95–98

Veterans Administration Cooperative Study Group on Antihypertensive Agents 1967 Effects of treatment on morbidity in hypertension: results in patients with diastolic blood pressures averaging 115 through 129 mmHg. Journal of American Medical Association 202: 1028–1034

Veterans Administration Cooperative Study Group on Antihypertensive Agents 1970 Effects of treatment on morbidity in hypertension. II. Results in patients with diastolic blood pressure averaging 90 through 114 mmHg. Journal of American Medical Association 213: 1143–1152

Voors W A, Foster T A, Frerichs R R, Webber L S, Berenson G S 1976 Studies of blood pressure in children, ages 5–14 years in a total biracial community: the Bogalusa Heart Study. Circulation 54: 319–327

Voors A W, Webber L S, Frerichs R R, Berenson G S 1977 Body height and body mass as determinants of basal blood pressure in children: the Bogalusa Heart Study. American Journal of Epidemiology 106: 101–108

Whyte R K, Elseed A M, Fraser C B, Shinebourne E A, de Swiet M 1975 Assessment of Doppler ultrasound to measure systolic blood pressures in infants and young children. Archives of Diseases in Childhood 50: 542–544

Woods K L, Beavers D G, West M 1981 Familial abnormality of erythrocyte cation transport in essential hypertension. British Medical Journal 282: 1186–1188

Zinner S H, Martin L F, Sacks F, Rosner B, Kass E H 1974 A longitudinal study of blood pressure in childhood. American Journal of Epidemiology 100: 437–442

Zinner S M, Margolius H S, Rosner B, Kass E H 1978 Stability of blood pressure rank and urinary kallikrein concentration in childhood: and eight-year follow-up. Circulation 58: 908–915

71

Management of congenital heart disease in pregnancy

M. de Swiet

INTRODUCTION

Most patients and their families know that pregnancy can be dangerous for those who have heart disease. The paediatric cardiologist will, therefore, be asked questions about the possible effects of pregnancy by the parents of his female patients. No doubt the children will ask these questions too as they grow older. In the absence of specialized centres for the 'grown-up' survivors of congenital heart disease (Somerville, 1990; Celermajer and Deanfield, 1991), obstetric, adult cardiological and general medical colleagues will turn to the paediatric cardiologist for advice about the management of pregnancy in patients with congenital heart disease. It is for these reasons that this section

on the management of pregnancy has been included in this text relating to paediatric cardiology.

The natural history of congenital heart disease in pregnancy is considered initially, then general measures applicable to all patients with heart disease in pregnancy, and finally some specific conditions where there is information and usually concern about the outcome in pregnancy. Counselling of the mother with congenital heart disease concerning the risks of congenital heart disease in her infant is considered in Chapter 73. For general reviews see Elkayam and Gleicher (1982) and de Swiet (1995).

NATURAL HISTORY

INCIDENCE

The stated incidence of congenital heart disease in pregnancy varies between 0.1% or less (Mendelson, 1960; Sugrue et al, 1981) and 0.5% (de Swiet and Fidler, 1981). It may be misleading to quote such data, since they would depend on diagnostic criterions that change with time (such as the change in diagnosis of mitral regurgitation from rheumatic to congenital owing to mitral valvar prolapse) and according to the different referral populations of different hospitals. In general, the overall prevalence of acquired (largely rheumatic) heart disease in pregnancy is declining, and that of congenital heart disease is increasing. This occurs both relatively and also absolutely as survivors of congenital heart disease in childhood become pregnant.

At present, the most experience of congenital heart disease in pregnancy is limited to relatively simple defects, which usually have not been corrected. Five representative series are shown in Table 71.1. Although the numbers involved in each series are very different, the overall pattern is similar. The most common lesions are atrial and ventricular septal defects and patency of the arterial duct, together accounting for about 60%

of cases. These are followed by pulmonary stenosis, Fallot's tetralogy, and aortic coarctation, which, together, contribute another 24%. Isolated lesions, such as aortic stenosis and Ebstein's malformation, account for the remainder (Copeland et al, 1963; Neilson et al, 1970; Ong and Puraviappan, 1975; Sugrue et al, 1981). It is likely that these data reflect no more than the incidence of congenital heart disease in the general female population. Three of the series are quite old and date from 1963–1975. In the series from Dublin (1969–1978), and Leicester (1985), we see the effect of surgery. More cases of patent arterial duct and atrial septal defect have been corrected.

MATERNAL MORTALITY

The one physiological condition with an undoubtedly high maternal mortality is an elevation in pulmonary vascular resistance (Jewett, 1979). This occurs most frequently in Eisenmenger's syndrome, where the maternal mortality is between 26 and 50% (Morgan Jones and Howitt 1965; Neilson et al, 1970; Pitts et al, 1977; Gleicher et al, 1979; Stoddart and O'Sullivan 1993). The

Table 71.1.   The prevalence of various forms of congenital heart disease in pregnancy

	Prevalence (%)					
	Ohio	Queensland	Dublin	Connecticut[a]	Leicester	Total
Total number	125	93	74	482	73	847
Patent arterial duct	24	27	9	22	11	21
Atrial septal defect	29	26	38	14	22	20
Pulmonary stenosis	4	12	6	10[b]	11	9
Ventricular septal defect	22	14	13	20	16	19
Tetralogy of Fallot	4	4	13	8	8	8
Aortic coarctation	10	6	6		7	7
Aortic valve disease	3	4	6	12	7	5
Mitral valve disease				7	14	5
Other	2	2		7	4	5
Unclassified	5	5				4
						1

[a] Expressed as percentage of all 233 mothers who became pregnant (some had more than one pregnancy).
[b] Includes all pregnancies where mother had obstruction to right ventricular outflow.
Source: Ohio, Copeland et al (1963); Queensland, Neilson et al (1970); Dublin, Sugrue et al (1981); Connecticut, Ohio, Whittemore et al (1982); Leicester MacNab and MacAfee (1985).

Confidential Enquiries into Maternal Mortality in England and Wales indicate that Eisenmenger's syndrome was the most frequent form of congenital heart disease to be associated with maternal mortality and was responsible for 17 of the 47 deaths from congenital heart disease between 1961 and 1975 (Department of Health and Social Security, 1979). Between 1985 and 1990, there were four maternal deaths in the United Kingdom from Eisenmenger's syndrome and six from other causes of pulmonary hypertension out of a total of 19 deaths from congenital heart disease (Department of Health and Social Security, 1991, 1994). Only Batson (1974) has reported a series of 23 pregnancies with no maternal deaths. The reason for this unusual success is not clear. An elevation in pulmonary vascular resistance is also seen, though less frequently, in primary pulmonary hypertension, when the reported maternal mortality is 40–50% (Morgan Jones and Howitt, 1965; Sinnenberg, 1980; Nelson et al, 1983).

In contrast, in Fallot's tetralogy, where the pulmonary vascular resistance is normal, the reported maternal mortality varies between 4 and 20% (Mendelson, 1960; Jacoby, 1964; Morgan Jones and Howitt, 1965). Furthermore, the figure of 20% is based on one maternal death in five pregnancies reported in the study of Jacoby (1964).

The maternal mortality is said to be high in Marfan's syndrome (Pyeritz and McKuisick, 1979; Hall, 1981), and in the arterial and classic forms of Ehlers–Danlos syndrome (Rudd et al, 1983). Ehler–Danlos syndrome is now classified in up to ten subtypes depending on the nature of the biochemical abnormality of the connective tissue. It is type IV disease that has a particularly high maternal mortality (Peaceman and Cruikshank, 1987).

Apart from the risk of aortic dissection, Ehlers–Danlos syndrome and Marfan's syndrome (Irons and Pollard, 1993), like pseudoxanthoma elasticum (Berde et al, 1983), predispose to the additional risk of bleeding from poor healing of obstetric lacerations and operative wound scars. The exact risk has not been stated. The incidence of these conditions in the general obstetric population is unknown. In contrast, Espino Vela and Alvarado-Toro (1971) have reported a series of 105 patients with atrial septal defect (confirmed by catheter in 41 patients) who had up to 10 or more pregnancies with no maternal mortality.

FETAL OUTCOME

In the five series of patients with congenital heart disease in pregnancy cited in Table 71.1, there was no excess fetal mortality except in the group with cyanotic congenital heart disease, whether associated with pulmonary hypertension or not. Here the babies are generally growth retarded (Schaefer et al, 1968; Batson, 1974), and the fetal loss, including abortion, may be as high as 40% (Copeland et al, 1963; Batson, 1974; Gleicher et al, 1979). Even in tetralogy of Fallot, which does not have a particularly high maternal mortality, the fetal loss rate may be as high as 57%, and most of the babies are growth retarded (Jacoby, 1964). This is hardly surprising in view of the inefficient mechanisms of placental exchange, which cannot compensate for the maternal systemic hypoxaemia. It is likely that the fetus dies because of inadequate supply of oxygen or because of prematurity (Gleicher et al, 1979), which may be iatrogenic.

Uncorrected aortic coarctation has also been associated with a 13% fetal loss rate (Burwell and Metcalfe, 1958) and intrauterine growth retardation (Benny et al, 1980), presumably because of inadequate placental perfusion. Severe aortic occlusion requiring axillary femoral grafting, in contrast, may be compatible with a normally grown fetus (Socol et al, 1981).

GENERAL PRINCIPLES OF MANAGEMENT

The general principles concerning the management of heart disease in pregnancy are well known (de Swiet, 1995). Diagnosis and assessment of severity of the condition are described elsewhere in this book. Nonetheless, certain aspects of the problem should be emphasized.

All patients with heart disease who are pregnant should be managed in a combined obstetric/cardiac clinic by one obstetrician and one cardiologist who are both interested in the other's problems. In this way, the number of hospital visits by the patient is kept to a minimum, and the obstetrician and cardiologist obtain the maximum expertise in the management of relatively rare conditions. With regard to the management of congenital heart disease in pregnancy, the cardiologist should ideally be one who is specialized in the care of 'grown-up' survivors of congenital heart disease (Somerville, 1990; Celermajer and Deanfield, 1991). There are profound changes in the normal maternal cardiovascular system in pregnancy, the most important being a 40% increase in the cardiac output with a corresponding fall in peripheral vascular resistance (de Swiet, 1991). It has not been established to what extent these changes occur in patients with abnormal or damaged hearts, but it is clear that pregnancy may distort many of the physical signs of heart disease. At the initial visit of the patient, the severity of the cardiac condition should be assessed or reassessed, and decisions made about the necessity for termination of pregnancy or cardiac surgery. In patients with well-managed congenital heart disease, these decisions should have been made before the patient became pregnant. Inevitably, some patients present for the first time in pregnancy, or have been lost to follow-up before pregnancy.

Only Eisenmenger's syndrome and primary pulmonary hypertension are absolute indications for termination of pregnancy. In all other cases, the decision as to whether the pregnancy should continue depends on an individual assessment of the risk of pregnancy compared with the patient's desire to have children.

Cardiac surgery in pregnancy is more often considered in acquired (particularly rheumatic heart disease) than in congenital heart disease. In aortic coarctation, the risk of dissection in pregnancy has probably been exaggerated (see below). Repair would, therefore, not be advised unless hypertension could not be controlled medically. Valvar replacement, which might be considered in some cases of Marfan's syndrome, has a similar good maternal result in pregnancy compared with the non-pregnant state, but the fetal loss is high, almost certainly related to inadequate perfusion of the uterus during cardiopulmonary bypass (Lamb et al, 1981). Valvoplasty, often as a palliative procedure, may well become the preferred intervention for stenotic lesions in pregnancy (Lao et al, 1993).

After the initial assessment of the patient, the remainder of medical management during pregnancy is associated with avoiding, if possible, those factors which increase the risk of heart failure, and with treating heart failure vigorously if it occurs. Risk factors for heart failure include infections (particularly urinary tract infection in pregnancy), hypertension (both pregnancy-associated and pregnancy-induced), obesity, multiple pregnancy, anaemia, the development of arrhythmias and, very rarely, the development of hyperthyroidism.

Labour should not be induced because of heart disease. Indeed, the risk of failed induction and of possible sepsis are contraindications. Nevertheless, these risks are slight, and induction should not be withheld if it is necessary for obstetric reasons. Furthermore, induction near term may be justified to plan delivery in daylight hours in complicated cases requiring optimal medical support.

Most patients with heart disease do have relatively rapid and uncomplicated labours. In the majority, analgesia is best given by epidural anaesthesia, which decreases cardiac output and heart rate, since it is an effective analgesic, and also decreases cardiac output by causing peripheral vasodilation and decreasing venous return. The use of epidural anaesthesia is questioned in Eisenmenger's syndrome and contraindicated in hypertrophic cardiomyopathy. Most obstetric emergencies arising in labour, including the need for Caesarean section, can be managed using epidural anaesthesia. If this is not available, or if elective Caesarean section is advised, general anaesthesia probably causes less haemodynamic derangement than does epidural anaesthesia. But there are few adequate comparisons of these forms of anaesthesia in comparable patients, and more depends on the skill and preference of the anaesthetist.

The use of oxytocic drugs in the third stage of labour is much debated. The theoretical disadvantage is that ergometrine (ergonovine) and oxytocin will cause a tonic contraction of the uterus, expressing about 500 ml of blood into the circulation. However, the management of postpartum haemorrhage in a patient with heart disease is not easy. Our practice is to give oxytocin in the third-stage by infusion in all patients unless they are in heart failure. The oxytocin can be accompanied by intravenous frusemide (furosemide).

ENDOCARDITIS AND ITS PREVENTION IN PREGNANCY

The Confidential Enquiries into Maternal Death in England and Wales show that there have been 10 maternal deaths from endocarditis in England and Wales between 1970 and 1975 (Department of Health and Social Security, 1979), and a further four deaths between 1985 and 1990 (Department of Health and Social Security, 1991). The case for antibiotic prophylaxis in labour, however, has not been proved. There are several large series of patients with heart disease in pregnancy where no antibiotics have been given, and where no endocarditis has been observed (Smith et al, 1976; Fleming, 1977; Sugrue et al, 1981). It is difficult (Burwell and Metcalfe, 1958), though not impossible (Redleaf and Farell 1954; McCormack et al, 1975), to document bacteraemia in labour. Several authors have argued persuasively against antibiotic prophylaxis (Fleming, 1977). The British Society for Antimicrobial Chemotherapy (Endocarditis Working Party, 1990) only recommends antibiotic prophylaxis in childbirth for those with prosthetic heart valves. Yet, from the data of the Confidential Maternal Mortality series, it would seem that women are at increased risk from endocarditis in pregnancy. What is not clear from the data of these reports is whether the endocarditis was contracted during labour and was potentially preventable by antibiotics, or whether endocarditis arose at some other time. The one patient who is described in detail in the 1973–1975 report did appear to develop endocarditis during a normal delivery, and other non-fatal cases have been reported (de Swiet et al, 1975). Until more details are available, we will continue to use antibiotic prophylaxis (ampicillin 500 mg intramuscular and gentamicin 80 mg intramuscular) in the form of three injections given 8 hourly at the onset or induction of labour (Durack, 1975). The patient who is penicillin sensitive receives one intravenous injection of teicoplanin 6 mg/kg plus gentamicin 2 mg/kg (Simmons et al, 1992).

TREATMENT OF HEART FAILURE AND ARRHYTHMIAS DURING PREGNANCY

The principles of treatment of heart failure in pregnancy are the same as in the non-pregnant state. Because of concern about maternal and fetal wellbeing, such patients should be treated in hospital.

DIGOXIN

The indications for the use of digoxin are the need to control the heart rate in atrial fibrillation and some other supraventricular tachycardias, and to increase the force of contraction (when given acutely in heart failure). If patients do develop atrial fibrillation in pregnancy, consideration should be given to anticoagulation with warfarin (see below) because of the risk of systemic embolism (Szekely and Snaith, 1953).

Requirements for digoxin are believed to be the same in pregnancy as in the non-pregnant state (Conradsson and Werkö, 1974). Both digoxin (Rogers et al, 1972) and digitoxin (Okita et al, 1956) cross the placenta and produce similar drug levels in the fetus to those seen in the mother (Rogers et al, 1972; Saarikoski, 1976). Digoxin enters the umbilical circulation within 5 minutes of intravenous administration to the mother (Saarikoski, 1976). In general, there is no evidence that therapeutic maternal drug levels of digoxin affect the neonatal electrocardiograph parameters (Mendelson, 1960; Rogers et al, 1972) or cause any harm to the fetus.

Digoxin is also secreted in breast milk, but since the total daily excretion in a mother with therapeutic blood levels would not exceed 2 mg (Levy et al, 1977), this too is unlikely to cause any harm to the neonate unless it has any other predisposing causes of digitalis toxicity, such as hypokalaemia.

DIURETIC THERAPY

Frusemide is the most commonly used, rapidly acting, loop diuretic for the treatment of pulmonary oedema. Ethacrynic acid (etacrynic acid) has also been used successfully in the management of pulmonary oedema associated with mitral stenosis in labour (Young and Heft, 1970). In congestive cardiac failure, where speed of action is not so important, oral thiazides are usually used in the first instance, although the extra potency of the loop diuretics may be necessary in a few patients. Andersen (1970) showed that the use of thiazide in late pregnancy was not associated with any significant depletion of salt or water in the neonate.

There are no risks in the use of diuretics in the treatment of heart failure that are specific to pregnancy; however, as in the non-pregnant state, hypokalaemia is an important complication in a patient who may also be taking digoxin. Treatment of pulmonary oedema should also include opiates, such as morphine, which reduce anxiety and decrease venous return by causing venodilation.

VASODILATORS

Vasodilating drugs should be withheld unless absolutely necessary. Nitrates are preferable to inhibitors of angiotension-converting enzyme, even though they cause reduced variability of fetal heart rate (Cotton et al, 1986). The enzyme inhibitors cause renal failure in newborn infants, which has been fatal (Hanssens et al, 1991).

TREATMENT OF ARRHYTHMIAS

Most 'malignant' arrhythmias result from ischaemic heart disease, which usually presents in women after their childbearing years and is rare in pregnancy (Ginz, 1970; Husaini, 1971). There is limited experience, therefore, in the treatment of arrhythmias during pregnancy.

Nevertheless, the problem does exist, particularly in patients who have non-ischaemic abnormalities of the cardiac conduction tissues, such as are believed to occur in the Wolff–Parkinson–White, Lown–Ganong–Levine and long QT syndromes (Wilkinson et al, 1991). Arrhythmias are also frequently late complications following surgical construction of shunts for complete transposition, the Fontan procedure and correction of Fallot's tetralogy. Paroxysmal and persistent atrial tachycardias are said to occur more frequently in pregnancy than in the non-pregnant state (Szekely and Snaith, 1953; Hubbard et al, 1983). The antiarrhythmic drugs that have been used most frequently in pregnancy are digoxin (discussed above), quinidine, and β-adrenergic blocking agents, in particular propranolol and oxprenolol. The indications for the use of these drugs are unaltered by pregnancy. Isolated case reports of intrauterine growth retardation, acute fetal distress in labour and hypoglycaemia in the neonate in patients taking propranolol were followed by reports of a significant further retardation of growth in the fetuses of women taking atenolol (Butters et al, 1990) in early pregnancy. Atenolol should, therefore, be avoided at this time. It is not clear whether this risk is specific to atenolol, or whether it applies to all β-blocking drugs (Gladstone et al, 1975; Cotrill et al, 1977; Habib and McArthy, 1977).

Quinidine is used to maintain or induce sinus rhythm in patients after conversion using direct current, or digoxin therapy, respectively. It is well tolerated in pregnancy (Ueland et al, 1981), and has only minimal oxytocic effect (Mendelson, 1956).

Procainamide has been electively given to one patient in order to treat supraventricular tachycardia in the fetus. The outcome was successful, even though it was suggested that relatively little procainamide had crossed the placenta (Dumesic et al, 1982).

There is much less experience of other antiarrhythmic drugs, such as verapamil, bretylium tosylate (bretylium tosilate), amiodarone or disopyramide. One case report has documented the safety of mexiletine in pregnancy for the treatment of ventricular arrhythmia (Timmis et al, 1980). The use of disopyramide has been associated with hypertonic uterine activity on one occasion (Leonard et al, 1978). It should, therefore, only be used with extreme caution. Verapamil is excreted in breast milk, although it is controversial whether the amounts involved are significant (Inoue and Unno, 1983; de Swiet, 1984). The use of amiodarone has been reviewed in at least 30 pregnancies (Barrett and Penn, 1986; Foster and Love, 1988). There is no evidence of teratogenicity in the relatively few pregnancies reported (Pitcher et al, 1983). Amiodarone contains large quantities of iodine, is known to affect the maternal thyroid and might affect also the fetal thyroid, producing hypo- or hyperthyroidism. Although neonatal hypothyroidism has been noted in one poorly documented case (Haffeje, 1983), other abnormalities have been mild and transient (Penn et al, 1985; Robson et al,

1985). In addition, neonatal bradycardia, and prolongation of the QT intervals in infants, have also been found (McKenna et al, 1983; Penn et al, 1985). These abnormalities have been transient and do not seem to have caused any harm. Amiodarone, nonetheless, is a potentially dangerous drug. On the basis of these reports, it would seem reasonable to recommend its use in arrhythmias seen in late pregnancy that are resistant to all other therapies. Patients should not breast feed when they are taking amiodarone.

Adenosine is rapidly becoming the agent of choice for the acute management of tachyarrhythmias, in preference to verapamil (Camm and Garratt, 1991). There is very little published experience with this drug in pregnancy but it is most unlikely to affect the fetus adversely, since it has a short plasma half-life of less than 2 seconds (Camm and Garratt, 1991). Conversion of tachyarrhythmias using direct current is safe in pregnancy and does not harm the fetus (Finlay and Edmonds, 1979).

The difficulty arises in considering long-term prophylactic treatment with antiarrhythmic drugs that have not been extensively used in pregnancy. Here, each case must be considered on its own merits, paying particular attention to the frequency and severity of the attacks of arrhythmia. A single short episode of supraventricular tachycardia associated with no other symptoms does not require prophylactic treatment. Frequent attacks of ventricular tachycardia associated with syncope would require prophylaxis, whatever the outcome in the fetus.

ANTICOAGULANT TREATMENT

Anticoagulation is a major problem in the management of patients with heart disease in pregnancy. Anticoagulation may be necessary in patients with congenital heart disease who have pulmonary hypertension owing to pulmonary vascular disease, in those who have artificial valves and in those with atrial fibrillation. For conditions such as pulmonary embolus, we believe that subcutaneous heparin is safer than warfarin (Howell et al, 1983). There appears to be less maternal bleeding and less fetal risk of abortion and congenital abnormalities such as chondrodysplasia punctata or optic atrophy. Where there is a risk of systemic thromboembolism, subcutaneous treatment does not seem to be adequate (Sbarouni and Oakley, 1994), as is the case in most cases of heart disease. Indeed, there are reports of artificial valves that have thrombosed during pregnancy when the mother has been managed with subcutaneous heparin (Bennett and Oakley, 1968; Antunes et al, 1984). There is no ideal solution to this problem. Even though the risk of fetal malformations, such as optic atrophy, persists after 16 weeks of gestation (Shaul and Hall, 1977), we believe that the fetal risks are relatively small (Chong et al, 1984; Sbarouni and Oakley, 1994) and that warfarin should be used until about 37 weeks of gestation. At this time, when the risk of fetal bleeding associated with labour seems to be too great, the patient should be admitted to hospital and given continuous intravenous heparin to produce a level of heparin as assayed by neutralization of protamine sulphate of 0.4–0.6 units/ml (Dacie, 1975). Heparin does not cross the placenta and will not, therefore, cause bleeding in the fetus. It is believed that the clotting system of the fetus will return to normal after warfarin has been withheld for 1 week. At that time, maternal dosage of heparin should be reduced to give a heparin level of 0.4 units/ml, and labour should be induced.

If the patient inadvertently goes into labour taking warfarin, she should be given vitamin K to reverse the action of warfarin in the fetus and started on subcutaneous treatment with heparin. In extreme cases, vitamin K has been given intramuscularly to the fetus by transamniotic injection (Larsen et al, 1978).

After delivery, because of the risk of maternal postpartum haemorrhage, the patient should continue to receive heparin for 7 days. Warfarin may then be recommenced. This is not a contraindication to breast feeding (Orme et al, 1977), although dindevan is excreted in breast milk (Eckstein and Jack, 1970), and patients taking dindevan should not breast feed. In the future, use of high-dose subcutaneous low-molecular-weight heparins may obviate the need for warfarin therapy.

SPECIFIC CONDITIONS OF CONCERN

EISENMENGER'S SYNDROME

As we have seen, Eisenmenger's syndrome has a high maternal mortality. Most patients die with Eisenmenger's syndrome in the puerperium. Although deaths are occasionally sudden owing to thromboembolism, this is not usually so. More frequently, these patients die through a slowly falling level of systemic oxygenation, with associated decrease in the cardiac output. A consideration of the haemodynamics involved (Figure 71.1) suggests how this might occur, and how it could be managed. In a large defect such as ventricular septal defect, the blood is freely mixed in the right and left ventricles, and the ratio of flow of blood in the pulmonary circuit (Q_p) to that in the systemic circuit (Q_s) is inversely proportional to the ratio of the pulmonary resistance (R_p) to the systemic resistance (R_s). This can be expressed as

$$Q_p/Q_s \propto R_s/R_p$$

Pulmonary blood flow is also proportional to cardiac output (CO) so

$$Q_p \propto Q_s \times CO \times R_s/R_p$$

Consequently, any fall in the ratio R_s/R_p will cause a fall in pulmonary blood flow. For example, in pre-eclamptic toxaemia, the resistance to flow of pulmonary blood

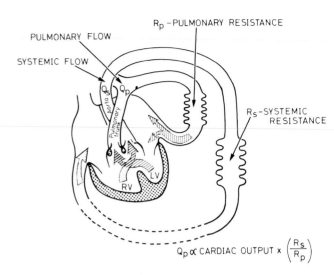

Figure 71.1. Pulmonary and systemic blood flows and resistances in Eisenmenger's syndrome associated with ventricular septal defect. RV, right ventricle; LV, left ventricle. (Reproduced with permission from de Swiet and Fidler, 1981.)

increases, and the cardiac output falls (Littler et al, 1973). These factors would, therefore, decrease pulmonary blood flow. This could account for the observed deterioration in Eisenmenger's syndrome associated with hypertensive pregnancy (Morgan Jones and Howitt, 1965).

What can be offered to the pregnant patient with Eisenmenger's syndrome? Unfortunately, abortion would appear to be the answer. The maternal mortality associated with abortion is only 7% compared with 30% for continuing the pregnancy (Gleicher et al, 1979). The place of anticoagulation is not clear. Although these women are at risk of pulmonary and systemic embolism, they have also died from bleeding subsequent to prophylactic anticoagulation (Kahn, 1993). Labour should not be induced unless there are good obstetric reasons. Induced labour carries a higher risk of Caesarean section, which is associated with a particularly high maternal mortality in Eisenmenger's syndrome (Gleicher et al, 1979). There is controversy concerning the place of epidural anaesthesia for the management of labour. Although epidural anaesthesia could decrease the Q_p/Q_s ratio by decreasing the systemic vascular resistance, this does not appear to occur, at least in the one patient studied by Midwall et al (1978). On balance, a carefully administered elective epidural anaesthetic at the beginning of labour is probably preferable to emergency epidural or general anaesthesia should it suddenly be decided that instrumental delivery is necessary (Crawford et al, 1971; Gleicher et al, 1979; McMurray and Kenny, 1982).

If the patient does become hypotensive, with increasing cyanosis and decreasing cardiac output, it has recently been shown that delivery of high inspired concentrations of oxygen will decrease pulmonary vascular resistance, increase the Q_p/Q_s ratio, and increase peripheral oxygen saturation (Midwall et al, 1978). In addition, α-sympathomimetic agents such as phenylephrine, methoxamine and noradrenaline (norepinephrine) will increase R_s and, thus, increase pulmonary blood flow (Devitt and Noble, 1980). Drugs such as tolazoline, phentolamine, nitroprusside and isoprenaline (isoproterenol), which have been used to decrease pulmonary vascular resistance in other clinical situations, probably should not be given, since they will also decrease the systemic vascular resistance (Devitt and Noble, 1980). If systemic resistance decreases more than pulmonary resistance, pulmonary blood flow will decrease rather than increase. The same problem occurs with dopamine and β-sympathomimetic drugs, which have been given to increase cardiac output. They, too, will decrease systemic resistance. If this decreases more than the cardiac output increases, pulmonary blood flow will fall. As a result, the management of the deteriorating patient with Eisenmenger's syndrome depends on giving oxygen and α-sympathomimeticamines.

More recently, inhaled nitric oxide has been shown to act selectively as a pulmonary vasodilator (Pepke-Zaba et al, 1991) in some cases of pulmonary hypertension. Delivery and monitoring of the gas is a problem, but it has also been used in neonates (Roberts et al, 1992). Expertise in treatment using nitric oxide, therefore, may be available near to some obstetric services.

AORTIC COARCTATION AND MARFAN'S SYNDROME

In both aortic coarctation and Marfan's syndrome, the maternal risk is of dissection of the aorta associated with the hyperdynamic circulation of pregnancy, and possibly an increased risk of medial degeneration owing to the hormonal environment of pregnancy (Konishi et al, 1980). The maternal mortality in coarctation has been stated to be as high as 17% (Mendelson, 1940). It has, therefore, been suggested that all patients with coarctation presenting in pregnancy should either have an abortion or have the defect repaired before delivery. Mendelson's series, however, dates from 1858–1939, and there have only been 14 maternal deaths reported in the whole literature, none of which occurred in the 83 patients studied since 1960 (Deal and Wooley, 1973). The risk of dissection has probably been exaggerated, and good obstetric care and effective antihypertensive therapy will decrease the risk still further. It is probable that we no longer see patients similar to those of Mendelson's series, since most patients with severe coarctation undergo surgery in infancy.

It is suggested that only those patients who already have evidence of dissection should have the coarctation repaired in pregnancy. Any hypertension as detected in the arms should be treated aggressively with antihypertensive drugs (Benny et al, 1980). If there is gross widening of the ascending aorta, suggesting intrinsic disease of the aorta, the patient should be delivered by elective Caesarean section to reduce the risk of dissection associated with labour.

Some authors also consider the risk of dissection to be so high in Marfan's syndrome that they advise avoidance of pregnancy, or termination if there is any degree of aortic dilation (Pyeritz and McKusick, 1979). Again, this seems an extreme attitude. The gene responsible for abnormal fibrillin synthesis on chromosome 15 has now been discovered (Tsipouras et al, 1992). Some patients and families with Marfan's syndrome have formes frustes of the condition (atypical mild form), where there may be arachnodactyly, a high arched palate, abnormalities of lens and long patella tendons, with no evidence of disease of the aorta or aortic valves. There may only be minor abnormalities of the mitral valve if there is any cardiac disease at all. These families tend to 'breed true', and pregnancy would confer no extra risk. There cannot, therefore, be an overall condemnation of pregnancy in all cases of Marfan's syndrome. Even if the patient does have involvement of the aorta, the number of cases of dissection reported in pregnancy is extremely small. It is unlikely that the risk is very high, and I believe that pregnancy should be allowed to continue in all but those with the most severe disease. As in aortic coarctation any associated hypertension should be treated aggressively, and delivery should be by Caesarean section if there is evidence of aortic disease.

HYPERTROPHIC OBSTRUCTIVE CARDIOMYOPATHY

Extensive experience of the management of hypertrophic obstructive cardiomyopathy in pregnancy has been reported by Oakley and colleagues (1979) from the Hammersmith Hospital. These authors originally advocated β-adrenergic blockade in all patients to reduce the risk of syncope, resulting from obstruction of the left ventricular outflow tract (Turner et al, 1968). This treatment is now reserved for symptomatic patients only. These patients should not be allowed to become hypovolaemic, since this too increases the risk of obstruction of the left ventricular outflow tract. Particular care should be taken in fluid replacement if these patients have an antepartum haemorrhage, and care should be taken to avoid postpartum haemorrhage. During labour, patients with hypertrophic obstructive cardiomyopathy should not have epidural anaesthesia, since this causes relative hypovolaemia by increasing venous capacitance in the legs.

CONGENITAL HEART BLOCK

Maternal congenital heart block is usually no problem in pregnancy. Although part of the normal response to pregnancy includes an increase in heart rate to increase the cardiac output, this is not obligatory. There are many records of successful pregnancy in patients with heart block, both paced (Ginns and Holinrake, 1970) and not paced (Szekely and Snaith, 1974). Presumably, patients are able to increase stroke volume sufficiently at the end of pregnancy or during labour (Bowman and Millar-Craig, 1980). They may require temporary pacing at this time.

TRICUSPID ATRESIA AND THE FONTAN PROCEDURE

In tricuspid atresia, there is no communication between the right atrium and the right ventricle. If the child or fetus survives, blood exits the right atrium via an atrial septal defect and perfuses the lungs via a ventricular septal defect. In the Fontan procedure, the right atrium is connected directly to the pulmonary arteries to improve pulmonary blood flow, and the atrial and ventricular septal defects are closed. There have been a number of reports of pregnancies in patients with tricuspid atresia, both corrected and uncorrected (Novy et al, 1968; Collins et al, 1977; Hatjis et al, 1983). In general, the maternal outcome depends on her state of health at the beginning of the pregnancy, and the fetal outcome on the degree of maternal cyanosis. In addition, these patients have a high thromboembolic risk. In part, this results from the polycythaemia of cyanosis. In addition, the Fontan procedure is associated with an acquired thrombotic state caused partly by deficiencies in the production of protein C, antithrombin III and protein S (Cromme-Dijkhuis et al, 1990). It is likely that these deficiencies result from impaired hepatic function, possibly owing to the high venous pressure resulting from the Fontan procedure. Protein C, antithrombin III, and protein S should be estimated in all patients following the Fontan operation, particularly if they are contemplating pregnancy. Suitable thromboprophylaxis should be used if there are significant abnormalities. Subcutaneous heparin would be the obvious choice if treatment is required in pregnancy.

MISCELLANEOUS CONDITIONS

Pregnancy has been described in a number of patients with so-called univentricular hearts (univentricular) atrioventricular connection with concordant or discordant ventriculo-arterial connections); usually these patients have already undergone a surgical procedure for the heart

condition (Yuzpe et al, 1970; Levy et al, 1977; Leibbrand et al, 1982; Baumann and Huch, 1986; Johnston and de Bono, 1989; Walsh et al, 1990). The maternal outcome depends on the degree of pulmonary vascular disease, her symptoms, whether she has been in congestive heart failure and the nature of other abnormalities. The fetal outcome depends on the degree of maternal cyanosis.

There is a single report of pregnancy following the Mustard operation for complete transposition. The patient was delivered at 37 weeks of gestation when she developed pulmonary oedema owing to atrial flutter, but the pregnancy was otherwise uneventful (Neukermanns et al, 1988). In Ebstein's malformation, the tricuspid valve is displaced into the right ventricle. The malformation, which can be diagnosed by echocardiography, is often treated with lithium. The major risks are right-sided heart failure and arrhythmias, but successful pregnancies have been reported (Littler et al, 1973; Kahler, 1975).

HEART TRANSPLANTS

Heart or heart–lung transplants are increasingly being used for the treatment of congenital heart disease, either as the first procedure in patients with pulmonary vascular disease or, occasionally, as an elective primary procedure in the knowledge that previous cardiothoracic surgery prejudices the outcome of subsequent transplantation (Somerville, 1990; Celermajer and Deanfield, 1991).

A series of 30 pregnancies in recipients of heart transplants has been described (Scott et al, 1993). The problems of immunosuppression are no different than those in other organ transplants, particularly renal transplants, for which there is extensive experience in pregnancy. In general, these patients have good haemodynamic function and the transplanted heart copes well with the extra work of pregnancy (Kossoy et al, 1988). Nevertheless, the pregnancies are frequently complicated by pre-existing hypertension, pre-eclampsia and preterm labour (Scott et al, 1993).

CONCLUSION

The outlook for most patients with simple congenital heart disease in pregnancy is generally good. Eisenmenger's syndrome is the one condition that has a particularly high maternal mortality. Patients who have more complex heart disease and have undergone surgery should also do well, providing they are not in heart failure before pregnancy and they do not have pulmonary vascular disease. Anticoagulant therapy is an additional hazard that requires very careful management.

REFERENCES

Andersen J B 1970 The effect of diuretics in late pregnancy on the new born infant. Acta Paediatrica Scandinavica 59: 659–663

Antunes M J, Myer I G, Santos L P 1984 Thrombosis of mitral valve replacement: management by simultaneous Caesarean section and mitral valve replacement. British Journal of Obstetrics and Gynaecology 91: 716–718

Barrett P A, Penn I M 1986 Amiodarone in pregnancy. Clinical Progress in Electrophysiology 4: 158–159

Batson G A 1974 Cyanotic congenital heart disease and pregnancy. British Journal of Obstetrics and Gynaecology 81: 549–553

Baumann H, Huch R 1986 Altitude exposure and staying at high altitude in pregnancy: effects on the mother and fetus. Zentralblatt Für Gynakologie 108: 889–899

Bennett G G, Oakley C M 1968 Pregnancy in a patient with a mitral valve prosthesis. Lancet i: 616–619

Benny P S, Prasao J, MacVicar J 1980 Pregnancy and coarctation of the aorta. Case Report. British Journal of Obstetrics and Gynaecology 87: 1159–1161

Berde C, Willis D C, Sandberg E C 1983 Pregnancy in women with pseudoxanthoma elasticum. Obstetrical and Gynaecological Survey 38: 339–344

Bowman P R, Millar-Craig H W 1980 Congenital heart block and pregnancy: a further case report. Journal of Obstetrics and Gynaecology 1: 98–99

Burwell C S, Metcalfe J 1958 Heart disease and pregnancy; physiology and management. Churchill, London

Butters L, Kennedy S, Rubin P C 1990 Atenolol in essential hypertension during pregnancy. British Medical Journal 301: 587–589

Camm A J, Garratt C J 1991 Adenosine and supraventricular tachycardia. New England Journal of Medicine 325: 1621–1629

Celermajer D S, Deanfield J E 1991 Adults with congenital heart disease. British Medical Journal 303: 1413–1414

Chong M K B, Harvey D, de Swiet M 1984 Follow-up study of children whose mothers were treated with warfarin during pregnancy. British Journal of Obstetrics and Gynaecology 91: 1070–1073

Collins M L, Leal J, Thompson N J 1977 Tricuspid atresia and pregnancy. Obstetrics and Gynaecology 50: 72–73

Conradsson T B, Werkö L 1974 Management of heart disease in pregnancy. Progress in Cardiovascular Disease 16: 407–419

Copeland W E, Wooley C F, Ryan J M, Runco V, Levin H S 1963 Pregnancy and congenital heart disease. American Journal of Obstetrics and Gynecology 86: 107–110

Cotrill C M, McAllister R G Jr, Gettes L, Noonan J A 1977 Propranolol therapy during pregnancy, labour and delivery: evidence for transplancental drug transfer and impaired neonatal drug disposition. Journal of Pediatrics 91: 812–814

Cotton D B, Longmire S, Jones M M et al 1986 Cardiovascular alterations in severe pregnancy-induced hypertension: effects of intravenous nitroglycerin coupled with blood volume expansion. American Journal of Obstetrics and Gynecology 145: 1053–1059

Crawford J S, Mills W G, Pentecost B L 1971 A pregnant patient with Eisenmenger's syndrome. British Journal of Anaesthesia 43: 1091–1094

Cromme-Dijkhuis A H, Henkens C M A, Bijleveld C M A et al 1990 Coagulation factor abnormalities as possible thrombotic risk factors after Fontan operations. Lancet 336: 1087–1090

Dacie J 1975 Practical haematology. Churchill Livingstone, Edinburgh, p 413–414

Deal K, Wooley C F 1973 Coarctation of the aorta and pregnancy. Annals of Internal Medicine 78: 706–710

Department of Health and Social Security 1979 Report on confidential enquiries into maternal deaths in England and Wales 1973–1975. HMSO, London

Department of Health 1991 Report on confidential enquiries into maternal deaths in the United Kingdom 1985–1987. HMSO, London

Department of Health 1994 Report on confidential enquiries into maternal deaths in the United Kingdom 1988–1990. HMSO, London

de Swiet M 1984 Excretion of verapamil in human milk. British Medical Journal 288: 644–645

de Swiet M 1991 The cardiovascular system. In: Hytten F, Chamberlain G (eds) Clinical physiology in obstetrics 2nd edn. Blackwell, Oxford, p 3–38

de Swiet M 1995 Heart disease in pregnancy. In: de Swiet M (ed.) Medical disorders in obstetric practice 3rd edn Blackwell, Oxford, p 116–148

de Swiet M, Fidler J 1981 Heart disease in pregnancy. Some controversies. Journal of the Royal College of Physicians 15: 183–186

de Swiet M, de Louvois J, Hurley R 1975 Failure of cephalosporins to prevent bacterial endocarditis during labour. [Letter] Lancet ii: 186

Devitt J H, Noble W H 1980 Eisenmenger's syndrome and pregnancy. New England Journal of Medicine 302: 751

Dumesic D A, Silverman N H, Tobias S, Golbus M S 1982 Transplacental cardioversion of fetal supraventricular tachycardia with procainamide. New England Journal of Medicine 307: 1128–1131

Durack D T 1975 Current practice in prevention of bacterial endocarditis. British Heart Journal 37: 478–481

Eckstein H, Jack B 1970 Breast feeding and anticoagulant therapy. Lancet i: 672–673

Elkayam V, Gleicher N 1982 Cardiac problems in pregnancy. Diagnosis and management of maternal and fetal disorders. Alan R Liss, New York, p 5–27

Endocarditis Working Party 1990 Antibiotic prophylaxis of infective endocarditis. Recommendations for the Endocarditis Working Party of the British Society for Antimicrobial Chemotherapy. Lancet 355: 88–89

Espino Vela J, Alvarado-Toro A 1971 Natural history of atrial septal defect. Cardiovascular Clinics 2: 104–125

Finlay A Y, Edmunds V 1979 D C cardioversion in pregnancy. British Journal of Clinical Practice 33: 88–94

Fleming H A 1977 Antibiotic prophylaxis against infective endocarditis after delivery. Lancet i: 144–145

Foster C J, Love H G 1988 Amiodarone in pregnancy. Case report and review of literature. International Journal of Cardiology 20: 307–316

Ginns H M, Holinrake K 1970 Complete heart block in pregnancy treated with an internal cardiac pacemaker.

Journal of Obstetrics and Gynaecology of the British Commonwealth 77: 710–719

Ginz B 1970 Myocardial infarction in pregnancy. Journal of Obstetrics and Gynaecology of the British Commonwealth 77: 610

Gladstone G R, Hordof A, Gersony W M 1975 Propranolol administration during pregnancy: effects on the fetus. Journal of Pediatrics 86: 962–964

Gleicher N, Midwall J, Hochberger D, Jaffin H 1979 Eisenmenger's syndrome and pregnancy. Obstetrical and Gynaecological Survey 34: 721–741

Habib A, McArthy J S 1977 Effects on the neonate of propranolol administered during pregnancy. Journal of Pediatrics 91: 808–811

Haffeje E 1983 In discussion–amiodarone pharmacokinetics. American Heart Journal 106: 847

Hall J G 1981 Disorders of connective tissue and skeletal dysplasia. In: Simpson J L, Shulman J D (eds) Genetic disorders in pregnancy. Academic Press, New York, p 57–87

Hanssens M, Keirse M J, Vankelecom F, van Assche F A 1991 Fetal and neonatal effects of treatment with angiotensin-converting enzyme inhibitors in pregnancy. Obstetrics and Gynaecology 78: 128–135

Hatjis C G, Gibson M, Capeless E L et al 1983 Pregnancy in a patient with tricuspid atresia. American Journal of Obstetrics and Gynecology 145: 114–115

Howell R, Fidler J, Letsky E, de Swiet M 1983 The risks of antenatal subcutaneous heparin prophylaxis: a controlled trial. British Journal of Obstetrics and Gynaecology 90: 1124–1128

Hubbard W N, Jenkins B A G, Ward D E 1983 Persistent atrial tachycardia in pregnancy. British Medical Journal 287: 327

Husaini M H 1971 Myocardial infarction during pregnancy: report of two cases and review of the literature. Postgraduate Medical Journal 47: 660–665

Inoue H, Unno N 1983 Excretion of verapamil in human milk. [Unreviewed report] British Medical Journal 287: 1596

Irons D W, Pollard K P 1993 Postpartum haemorrhage secondary to Marfan's disease of the uterine vasculature. British Journal of Obstetrics and Gynaecology 100: 279–281

Jacoby W J 1964 Pregnancy with tetralogy and pentalogy of Fallot. American Journal of Cardiology 14: 866–873

Jewett J F 1979 Pulmonary hypertension and pre-eclampsia. New England Journal of Medicine 301: 1063–1064

Johnston T A, de Bono D 1989 Single ventricle and pulmonary hypertension. A successful pregnancy. Case report. British Journal of Obstetrics and Gynaecology 96: 731–734

Kahler R L 1975 Cardiac disease In: Burrow G N, Ferris (eds) Medical compications during pregnancy. Saunders, Philadelphia, PA, p 105–145

Khan M L 1993 Eisenmenger's syndrome in pregnancy New England Journal of Medicine 329: 887

Konishi Y, Tatsuta N, Kumada K et al 1980 Dissecting aneurysm during pregnancy and the puerperium. Japanese Circulation Journal 44: 726–732

Kossoy L R, Herbert C M, Wentz A C 1988 Management of heart transplant recipients: guidelines for the obstetrician–gynecologist. American Journal of Obstetrics and Gynecology 159: 490–499

Lamb M P, Ross K, Johnstone A M, Manners J M 1981 Fetal heart monitoring during open heart surgery. British Journal of Obstetrics and Gynaecology 88: 669–674

Lao T T, Adelman A G, Sermer M, Colman J M 1993 Balloon valvoplasty for congenital aortic stenosis in pregnancy. British Journal of Obstetrics and Gynaecology 100: 1141–1142

Larsen J F, Jacobsen B, Holm H H, Pedersen J F, Mantoni M 1978 Intrauterine injection of vitamin K before the delivery during anticoagulant treatment of the mother. Acta Obstetrica Gynecologica Scandinavica 57: 227–230

Leibbrand G, Muench U, Gander M 1982 Two successful pregnancies in a patient with single ventricle and transposition of the great arteries. International Journal of Cardiology 1: 257–262

Leonard R F, Braun T E, Levy A M 1978 Initiation of uterine contractions by disopyramide during pregnancy. New England Journal of Medicine 299: 84–85

Levy M, Grait L, Laufer N 1977 Excretion of drugs in human milk. [Letter] New England Journal of Medicine 297: 789

Littler W A, Redman C W G, Bonnar J, Berkin L S, Lee G de J 1973 Reduced pulmonary arterial compliance in hypertensive pregnancy. Lancet i: 1274–1278

MacNab G, MacAfee C A J 1985 A changing pattern of heart disease associated with pregnancy. Journal of Obstetrics of Gynaecology 5: 139–142

McCormack W M, Rosner B, Lee Y H, Rankin J S, Lin J S 1975 Isolation of mycoplasma from blood obtained shortly after vaginal delivery. Lancet i: 596–599

McKenna W J, Harris L, Rowland E, Whitelaw A, Storey G C A, Holt D W 1983 Amiodarone therapy during pregnancy. American Journal of Cardiology 51: 1231–1233

McMurray T J, Kenny N T 1982 Extradural anaesthesia in parturients with severe cardiovascular disease. Anaesthesia 37: 442–445

Mendelson C L 1940 Pregnancy and coarctation of the aorta. American Journal of Obstetrics and Gynecology 39: 1014–1021

Mendelson C L 1956 Disorders of the heart beat during pregnancy. American Journal of Obstetrics and Gynecology 72: 1268–1301

Mendelson C L 1960 Cardiac disease in pregnancy. Davis, Philadelphia, PA

Midwall J, Jaffin H, Herman M V, Kuper Smith J 1978 Shunt flow and pulmona haemodynamics during labour and delivery in the Eisenmenger syndrome. American Journal of Cardiology 42: 299–303

Morgan Jones A, Howitt G 1965 Eisenmenger syndrome in pregnancy. British Medical Journal 1: 1627–1631

Neilson G, Gale E G, Blunt A 1970 Congenital heart disease and pregnancy. Medical Journal of Australia 1: 1086–1088

Nelson D M, Main E, Crafford W, Ahumada G G 1983 Peripartum heart failure due to primary pulmonary hypertension. Obstetrics and Gynaecology 62: 58S–63S

Neukermans K, Sullivan T J, Pitlick P T 1988 Successful pregnancy after the mustard operation for transposition of the great arteries. American Journal of Cardiology 62: 838–839

Novy M J Peterson E N, Metcalfe J 1968 Respiratory characteristics of maternal and fetal blood in cyanotic congenital heart disease. American Journal of Obstetrics and Gynecology 100: 821

Oakley G D G, McGarry K, Limb D G, Oakley C M 1979 Management of pregnancy in patients with hypertrophic cardiomyopathy. British Medical Journal 1: 1749–1750

Okita G T, Plotz E J, Davis M E 1956 Placental transfer of radioactive digitoxin in pregnant woman and its fetal distribution. Circulation Research 4: 376–380

Ong H C, Puraviappan A P 1975 Congenital heart disease and pregnancy in the tropics. Australia and New Zealand Journal of Obstetrics and Gynaecology 15: 99–103

Orme M L'E, Lewis P J, de Swiet M et al 1977 May mothers given warfarin breast-feed their infants? British Medical Journal 1: 1564–1565

Peaceman A M, Cruikshank D P 1987 Ehler–Danlos syndrome and pregnancy: association of type IV disease with maternal death. Obstetrics and Gynaecology 69: 428–431

Penn I M, Barrett P A, Pannikote V, Barnaby P F, Campbell J B, Lyons N R 1985 Amiodarone in pregnancy. American Journal of Cardiology 56: 196–197

Pepke-Zara J, Higenbottam T W, Diha-Xuan A T et al 1991 Inhaled nitric oxide as a cause of selective pulmonary vasodilatation in pulmonary hypertension. Lancet 338: 1173–1174

Pitcher D, Leather H M, Storey G C A, Holt D W 1983 Amiodarone in pregnancy, Lancet i: 597–598

Pitts J A, Crosby W M, Basta L C 1977 Eisenmenger's syndrome in pregnancy. American Heart Journal 93: 321–326

Pyeritz R E, McKuisick V A 1979 The Marfan syndrome: diagnosis and management. New England Journal of Medicine 300: 772–777

Redleaf P D, Farrell E J 1954 Bacteremia during parturition–prevention of subacute bacterial endocarditis. Journal of the American Medical Association 169: 1284–1285

Roberts J D, Polander D M, Lang P, Zapol W M 1992 Inhaled nitric oxide in persistent pulmonary hypertension of the newborn. Lancet 340: 818–819

Robson D J, Raj M V, Storey G C A, Holt D W 1985 Use of amiodarone during pregnancy. Postgraduate Medical Journal 61: 75–77

Rogers M E, Willerson J T, Goldblatt A, Smith T W 1972 Serum digoxin concentrations in the human fetus, neonate and infant. New England Journal of Medicine 287: 1010–1013

Rudd N L, Nimrod C, Holbrook K A, Byers P H 1983 Pregnancy complications in type IV Ehlers–Danlos syndrome. Lancet i: 50–53

Saarikoski S 1976 Placental transfer and fetal uptake of ^{3}H-digoxin in humans. British Journal of Obstetrics and Gynaecology 83: 879–884

Sbarouni E, Oakley C M 1994 Outcome of pregnancy in women with valve prostheses. British Heart Journal 71: 196–201

Schaefer G, Arditi L I, Solomon H A, Ringland J E 1968 Congenital heart disease and pregnancy. Clinical Obstetrics and Gynaecology 11: 1048–1063

Scott J R, Wagoner L E, Olsen S L et al 1993 Pregnancy in heart transplant recipients: management and outcome. Obstetrics and Gynaecology 82: 324–327

Shaul W L, Hall J G 1977 Multiple congenital anomalies associated with anticoagulants. American Journal of Obstetrics and Gynecology 127: 191–198

Simmons N A, Ball A P, Cawson R A et al 1992 Antibiotic prophylaxis and infective endocarditis. Lancet 339: 1292–1293

Sinnenberg R J 1980 Pulmonary hypertension in pregnancy. Southern Medical Journal 73: 1529–1531

Smith R H, Radford D J, Clark R A, Julian D G 1976 Infective endocarditis: a summary of cases in the South-East Region of Scotland 1969–1972. Thorax 31: 373–379

Socol M L, Conn J, Frederiksen M C 1981 Pregnancy associated with partial aortic occlusion. American Journal of Obstetrics and Gynecology 139: 965–967

Somerville J 1990 'Grown-up' survivors of congenital heart disease: who knows? who cares? British Journal of Hospital Medicine 43: 132–136

Stoddart P, O'Sullivan G 1993 Eisenmenger's syndrome in pregnancy: a case report and review. International Journal of Obstetric Anesthesia 2: 159–168

Sugrue D, Blake S, MacDonald D 1981 Pregnancy complicated by maternal heart disease at the National Maternity Hospital, Dublin, Ireland, 1969 to 1978. American Journal of Obstetrics and Gynecology 139: 1–6

Szekely P, Snaith L 1953 Paroxysmal tachycardia in pregnancy. British Heart Journal 15: 195–198

Szekely P, Snaith L 1974 Heart disease and pregnancy. Churchill Livingstone, Edinburgh

Timmis A D, Jackson G, Holt O W 1980 Mexiletine for control of ventricular dysrhythmias in pregnancy. Lancet ii: 647–648

Tsipouras P, Del Mastro R, Sarfarazi M et al 1992 Genetic linkage of the Marfan syndrome, ectopia lentis and congenital contractural arachnodactyly to the fibrillin genes on chromosones 15 and 5. New England Journal of Medicine 326: 905–909

Turner G M, Oakley C M, Dixon H G 1968 Management of pregnancy complicated by hypertrophic obstructive cardiomyopathy. British Medical Journal 4: 281–284

Ueland K, McAnulty J H, Ueland F R, Metcalfe J 1981 Special considerations in the use of cardiovascular drugs. Clinical Obstetrics and Gynaecology 24: 809–823

Walsh T, Savage R, Bakersmith Hess D 1990 Successful pregnancy in a patient with a double inlet left ventricle treated with a septation procedure. Southern Medical Journal 83: 358–359

Whittmore R, Hobbins J C, Engle M A 1982 Pregnancy and its outcome, in women with and without surgical treatment of congenital heart disease. American Journal of Cardiology. 50: 641–651

Wilkinson C, Gyaneshwar R, McCusker C 1991 Twin pregnancy in a patient with idiopathic long QT syndrome. Case report. British Journal of Obstetrics and Gynaecology 98: 1300–1302

Young B K, Heft J I 1970 Treatment of pulmonary oedema with ethacrynic acid during labour. American Journal of Obstetrics and Gynecology 107: 330–331

Yuzpe A A, Sanghvi V R, Johnson F L, Robinson J G 1970 Successful pregnancy in a patient with single ventricle and other congenital cardiac anomalies. Canadian Medical Association Journal 108: 1073–1075

72

Congenital heart disease in adolescents and adults

J. E. Deanfield, S. Cullen and D. S. Celermajer

INTRODUCTION

Without early treatment, the majority of patients with congenital heart disease would die in infancy or childhood, with only less than one-sixth surviving until puberty (MacMahon et al, 1953). Advances in surgical treatment, however, from ligation of a persistent arterial duct (Gross and Hubbard, 1939) to the innovations of the 1990s, as well as advances in medical treatment, have transformed the outlook for children, even with complex defects; consequently, the majority now survive into adolescence and adult life. This story of success has radically altered both the size of the population of young adults with congenital heart disease and the complexity of the disease. In the United States of America, it has been estimated that well over 500 000 patients with functionally important congenital cardiac malformations have reached adulthood since the 1960s (Perloff, 1989). This population will inevitably continue to grow with ongoing improvements in medical and surgical management. Specialized long-term care is now required to match the standards of excellence set in childhood. Currently, this is not widely available; as a result, patients who outgrow the paediatric clinic are often lost to follow-up, or managed as 'one-off' cases by adult physicians who are more experienced in dealing with acquired heart disease.

Despite the fact that most patients now surviving to adult life will have undergone surgery during childhood, 'total correction' is not the rule (Stark 1989a). The majority, if not all, require long-term surveillance, and many need reoperations. This is demanding, and carries a high risk, particularly when undertaken by surgeons who do not have specific training or experience. Other adults may require their first operation for congenital lesions in the heart that were well tolerated during childhood. Arrhythmia is common, as are residual lesions, haemodynamic problems and endocarditis. Although adult cardiologists may be expert in one or more of these areas, the critical relationship between rhythm and haemodynamic status in hearts with complex circulations may result in catastrophic errors of treatment being made by those who lack experience with congenital malformations.

Newer non-invasive diagnostic techniques, such as transoesophageal imaging and magnetic resonance imaging, are often required for the serial evaluation of complex lesions. Interventional procedures have proved an important modality of treatment, either instead of or as an adjunct to surgery. As well as medical problems, psychosocial issues, such as the search for employment, life and health insurance, participation in sports and socialization are of great importance to adolescents and young adults with congenital heart disease. Many of the 'normal' ordeals of growing up are more difficult for this group, for whom chronic illness, embarrassing scars and/or exercise limitation may inhibit normal social intercourse and maturation.

In addition to provision of care, long-term follow-up data is crucial as a 'feedback' to improve strategies for initial management in childhood. Such data have already changed the surgical approach to common defects such as complete transposition (see Chapter 48). The ratio of risk to benefit for currently favoured surgical procedures, such as the Ross procedure for aortic valvar disease, will be judged by their long-term results in comparison with other surgical approaches. Late complications encountered in older patients, such as the disappointing survival of replaced homograft conduits, will also be the stimulus for new research. One of the major roles of any centralized service provided for young adults with heart disease should be to collect data on the functional capability and long-term outcomes of those whose disease is congenital, both for the medical speciality and for use by governments.

Over the last few years, appreciation of the importance of this group of complex patients has led to international efforts to improve organization of care. Specific working groups have been established within countries and major cardiac societies, such as the European Society of Cardiology and the American College of Cardiology, to coordinate care and to facilitate collaboration and research. In this respect, the Canadian Cardiovascular Society has also been a pioneer. In 1996, it sponsored a consensus conference on adult congenital heart disease, the recommendations of which have been published (Canadian Cardiovascular Society, 1996). This first attempt at evidence-based medicine will be followed by further international updates, including one from a Task Force of the European Society of Cardiology.

Clearly, optimal organization of care for patients who have grown up with congenital heart disease will depend on national systems for health care. Regional referral centres are required to consolidate clinical research, to enable training of personnel and to ensure maintenance of special skills. These should be staffed by adult cardiologists with specific expertise in interventional catheterization, imaging, electrophysiology and pacing, by paediatric cardiologists and, ideally, by newly trained staff with experience both in congenital and acquired heart disease. Surgeons and cardiac anaesthetists trained in congenital heart disease and transplantation are also essential, as is a pathologist with special knowledge of congenital cardiac malformations. Ideally, this team should work within a multidisciplinary institute and have access at least to specialists in obstetrics and gynaecology, genetics, nephrology, respiratory medicine, infectious disease, neurology and psychiatry.

MEDICAL ASPECTS

Many young adults with congenital cardiac disease have mild lesions that have not, and may not ever, require surgery. The most common defects in this category are small ventricular septal defects, mild pulmonary or aortic valvar stenosis and prolapse of the mitral valve (Table 72.1). Such patients need infrequent follow-up, being seen about every second year, to assess any progression in severity of the lesion, to reinforce the need for antibiotic prophylaxis against infective endocarditis, and to discuss psychosocial issues. Other patients reach adult life with more complex defects which are still 'uncorrected'. Some may still be candidates for palliative or definitive surgery. In others, surgery may no longer be possible, often because of irreversible pulmonary vascular disease. The survivors of surgery in childhood, however, now form the largest group of patients reaching adult life (Table 72.2). Like the patient who has not undergone surgery, the majority need continuing medical surveillance. This is because late cardiovascular problems may result from haemodynamic deterioration, from onset of arrhythmia or from endocarditis. Some survivors to adulthood may have important associated syndromes, such as Down's syndrome, 22q11 deletion or the CHARGE (coloboma, heart disease, atresia, choanas, retarded growth and/or central nervous system anomalies, genital hypoplasia and ear anomalies) association. They may also have significant extracardiac disabilities and may need special care by allied health professionals and other physicians. In addition, all adults with congenital cardiac malformations are susceptible to the

Table 72.1. Common congenital cardiac defects compatible with survival to adult life without surgery or intervention catheterization

Mild pulmonary valvar stenosis
Peripheral pulmonary stenosis
Bicuspid aortic valve
Mild subaortic stenosis
Mild supravalvar aortic stenosis
Small atrial septal defect
Small ventricular septal defect
Small persistent arterial duct
Mitral valvar prolapse
Ebsteins's malformation
Congenitally corrected transposition
Balanced complex lesions (such as double inlet ventricle with pulmonary stenosis)
Defects with pulmonary vascular obstructive disease (Eisenmenger's syndrome)

Table 72.2. Common congenital cardiac diseases compatible with survival to adult life after surgery or interventional catheterization

Atrial septal defect
Ventricular septal defect
Atrioventricular septal defect
Pulmonary stenosis
Aortic valvar disease
Aortic coarctation
Tetralogy of Fallot with pulmonary stenosis or atresia
Complete transposition
Totally anomalous pulmonary venous connection
Mitral valvar disease
Ebstein's malformation
Fontan procedure for complex congenital heart disease
Congenitally corrected transposition

potential acquired cardiac and non-cardiac 'medical problems' of adulthood.

HAEMODYNAMICS

Late haemodynamic deterioration may occur in the setting of operated or unoperated disease. Progressive congestive cardiac failure secondary to myocardial deterioration is the most common cause of disability and death in young adults with congenital heart disease, in whom the ventricles may have been subjected to many years of volume and pressure loading, often in the presence of chronic hypoxaemia. Furthermore, in the early era of paediatric cardiac surgery, many children were repaired at an older age than is the current surgical practice, with greater consequent preoperative damage. Myocardial protection may have been less than optimal, especially for lengthy procedures, resulting in further myocardial damage.

Residual haemodynamic defects are often present in patients who have undergone repair, and these may cause problems even many years after surgery. These may be amenable to further surgery or may require long-term medical treatment. Standard medical therapy for the failing ventricle includes digitalis, diuretics and, increasingly, agents that reduce the afterload. In addition, post-operative circulations created by the definitive repair of many congenital defects often result in an adequate physiological repair, with oxygenated blood going to the body and deoxygenated blood to lungs, but still fail to reproduce normal anatomy. For example, after intra-atrial repair for complete transposition, the morphologically right ventricle remains on the systemic side of the circulation (Graham et al, 1975). There are concerns about long-term function in such patients when the right ventricle supports the systemic circulation (Gelatt et al, 1997; Deanfield, 1999). Similarly, after the Fontan operation and its many modifications, systemic ventricular performance may be a determinant of late morbidity and mortality. The different morphology and loading conditions for these ventricles means that standard tests of ventricular function, derived from studies of structurally normal hearts, may be inappropriate for evaluation of these patients (Redington et al, 1989). The development of load-independent indexes of cardiac performance is improving understanding of atrioventricular and ventriculo-arterial coupling, as well as of intrinsic myocardial properties (Brookes et al, 1998; White et al, 1998). This should enable examination of changes in cardiovascular function during long-term follow-up and serve as a guide to therapy.

Many important questions remain about dynamic changes in the circulation of adults with congenital heart disease. For example, what is the likely long-term effect of non-pulsatile flow on the pulmonary vasculature after certain modified Fontan operations (Mathur and Glenn, 1973; de Leval et al, 1988)? What is the effect of a relatively low volume non-compliant atrium on ventricular filling, as after a Mustard operation? How will the coronary circulation develop after an arterial switch operation? Suitable follow-up should provide the answers to these questions.

ARRHYTHMIAS

Arrhythmias, and conduction defects, have a major impact on the prognosis and management of both un-operated and operated patients. They are the major cause of morbidity and the need for hospitalization in grown-up patients with congenital cardiac disease. They have been linked to sudden death in a number of conditions (Godman et al, 1974; Stevenson et al, 1991; Saul and Alexander, 1999). In patients who have not undergone surgery, chamber dilation, myocardial hypertrophy and fibrosis may all contribute to the genesis of arrhythmia

(Sullivan et al, 1987). In patients who have undergone surgery, additional damage to the sinus or atrioventricular nodes and conduction tissues, together with myocardial scarring, may cause electrophysiological problems. Not only is the aetiology multifactorial, but the clinical significance of the arrhythmia depends very much on the haemodynamic context in which it occurs. Disturbances of rhythm that might be benign in a structurally normal heart may be life threatening in one that is congenitally malformed.

BRADYARRHYTHMIA

Injury to the sinus node occurs most frequently in patients who have had atrial surgery (Garson, 1990). Abnormalities of sinus nodal function are common in patients after the Mustard or Senning operations (Deanfield et al, 1988). Sinus nodal dysfunction has also been reported after surgery for tetralogy of Fallot, and after the Fontan procedure (Weber et al, 1989; Gewillig et al, 1992). Clinical manifestations include sinus bradycardia, sinuatrial block, sinus arrest and occasionally the tachy–bradycardia syndrome with paroxysmal atrial flutter and fibrillation. Although bradycardia has been postulated as the cause of sudden death in some conditions, current evidence indicates that tachyarrhythmia is usually a more likely explanation in the majority of patients (Balaji et al, 1991).

In patients with sinus nodal disease, insertion of a pacemaker is indicated for patients with bradycardia-related symptoms such as tiredness, dizziness or syncope. It is also indicated when the heart rate is extremely low, for example less than 30 beats per minute. The indications for insertion in asymptomatic individuals, however, are still controversial. In many cases, the arrhythmia is benign but may have detrimental effects on long-term cardiac performance. Pacing may prove difficult because of complex underlying anatomy, and consequent lack of a suitable site for fixation of an endocardial lead. The choice of pacemaker will depend on the precise indication. The simplest VVI pacemaker may be adequate to prevent bradycardia-related sudden death. Rate-responsive pacemakers, nonetheless, are preferable. The increasingly sophisticated dual chamber systems for pacing may be indicated in most patients if the best haemodynamic results are to be obtained (Ward et al, 1983; Kratz et al, 1992; Nathan and Davies, 1992).

Injury to the atrioventricular node, and to the proximal ventricular conduction tissues, may result from any operation in the region of the atrioventricular junction. Even temporary postoperative complete atrioventricular block has been shown to have an adverse prognostic significance, particularly if the site of damage is below the bundle of His. In a 30-year follow-up of surgical repair of ventricular septal defect, the development of transient complete heart block for longer than 72 hours, followed by resumption of sinus rhythm, was a strong independent predictor of late mortality (Murphy et al, 1989). Postoperative right bundle block is extremely common after ventriculotomy. It may be related to closure of the ventricular septal defect or to interruption of the distal conduction pathways by ventriculotomy or resection of muscle (Vetter and Horowitz, 1982). Occasionally, the electrocardiographic pattern of right bundle branch block with left-axis deviation occurs, giving so-called bifascicular block. There may also be prolongation of the PR interval, or trifascicular block (Kulbertus et al, 1969; Deanfield et al 1980). While early reports suggested that these lesions may predispose to late sudden cardiac death (Wolff et al, 1972), numerous more recent studies have failed to substantiate this adverse prognosis (Cullen et al, 1994). Fortunately, permanent high-grade atrioventricular block is much less common than in the early surgical era (Fryda et al, 1971). It does still occasionally, nonetheless, complicate some repairs, such as closure of ventricular septal defect in the setting of congenitally corrected transposition (Lundstrom et al, 1990).

TACHYARRHYTHMIA

Evidence is accumulating that tachyarrhythmias, particularly in the context of abnormal underlying haemodynamics, are potentially life threatening. Late sudden death has been reported in several lesions, both before and after repair. In general, the worse the disease (in other words with the most complex anatomy and/or the most extensive surgery) the greater is the incidence of sudden death (Garson, 1990). The identification of patients at risk and their management are important and controversial issues. After the Mustard and Senning procedures, atrial flutter, often with rapid ventricular response, is dangerous, especially when it occurs in association with right ventricular dysfunction or obstruction of the venous pathways (Gewillig et al, 1991). Medical or electrical cardioversion should be attempted to restore sinus rhythm. Drug therapy may need to be accompanied by insertion of a pacemaker, and/or by anticoagulation, if there is recurrent arrhythmia.

Surgical treatment, or radiofrequency ablation, has been advocated for certain cases of atrial flutter (Dorostkar et al, 1998). Atrial tachyarrhythmias are also common after the Fontan operation, probably related to injury to the sinus node, atrial suturing and/or presence of a dilated hypertensive right atrium (Gewillig et al, 1992). Modification of the operation to exclude the right atrium from the Fontan circuit, the so-called 'total cavopulmonary connection', may reduce the incidence of potentially serious early and late disturbances of rhythm (Balaji et al, 1991; Gardiner et al, 1996). Superiority over the atriopulmonary connection, however, has yet to be clearly demonstrated.

Ventricular arrhythmia is known to occur after open-heart surgery, particularly repair of tetralogy of Fallot (Quattlebaum et al, 1976; Garson et al, 1979; Kavey et al, 1982; Gatzoulis et al, 1997). Studies using ambulatory electrocardiographic monitoring in postoperative patients have documented asymptomatic complex ectopy, and non-sustained ventricular tachycardia, in up to half of patients (Vaksmann et al, 1990; Cullen et al, 1994). Up to one third have inducible ventricular tachycardia when studied electrophysiologically (Garson et al, 1985). Experimental and clinical studies have shown that the electrical substrate for re-entry is in the right ventricle (Deanfield et al, 1985). In several analyses, older age at surgery emerged as a predisposing factor (Deanfield et al, 1984; Vaksmann et al, 1990). This suggests that preoperative factors, present at the time of repair, may be involved in the genesis of postoperative arrhythmia, in addition to the myocardial damage occurring at the time of surgery or during postoperative follow-up (Sullivan et al, 1987). This is consistent with morphological studies that documented increasing fibrosis of the right ventricle as part of the natural history of defects such as tetralogy of Fallot (Hegerty et al, 1988; Jones and Ferrans, 1989). The current approach of early surgical repair for tetralogy of Fallot may reduce the incidence of postoperative ventricular arrhythmia (Walsh et al, 1988). Other risk factors include elevated right ventricular systolic pressure, reduced right ventricular ejection fraction, pulmonary regurgitation and a ventriculotomy scar (Horowitz et al, 1980; Koboyashi et al, 1984).

The interaction between vulnerability to serious ventricular arrhythmia and the mechanical properties of the circulation has long been known. This has received considerable recent attention after repair of tetralogy of Fallot. The duration of the QRS complex has been related to right ventricular size. Prolongation beyond 180 ms has been proposed as a marker of risk of sudden death (Gatzoulis et al, 1995a). Risk stratification may be further refined by evaluation of the temporal pattern of the prolongation during follow-up, and by more detailed analysis of abnormalities of repolarization. Identification of cohorts of patients at high-risk for major arrhythmias or sudden death, and indications for treatment, remain a problem. Ambulatory monitoring has proved of limited value because, in some conditions, particularly tetralogy of Fallot, there is a disparity between the high frequency of arrhythmia and the much lower incidence of sudden death. No association between non-sustained ventricular arrhythmia on ambulatory electrocardiography monitoring and late sudden death has been found on prospective evaluation (Cullen et al, 1994). Furthermore, prophylactic antiarrhythmic therapy has not been shown to be of value in asymptomatic patients with congenital heart defects. Indeed, such treatment may have pro-arrhythmic potential (Greene et al, 1992), be negatively inotropic or have serious extracardiac side effects (Thorne et al, 1999). Any patient with symptoms, prolongation of the QRS complex and who demonstrates sustained ventricular tachycardia should be evaluated and treated actively. This should include detailed haemodynamic study, as treatment of residual cardiac abnormalities such as pulmonary regurgitation may be the best way of improving morbidity and mortality (d'Udekem et al, 1998; Oechslin et al, 1999). Undoubtedly, in the next few years, stratification for risk of sudden death in patients with congenital cardiac lesions will be refined. It will involve a combination of haemodynamic and electrophysiological testing, both at rest and after exercise, as well as newer measurements such as heart rate variability derived from measures used in acquired heart disease.

CYANOSIS

Adults with congenital heart disease may have central cyanosis from right-to-left shunting secondary to their uncorrected cardiac defect (such as those with tetralogy of Fallot with pulmonary atresia) or from pulmonary vascular disease (as in Eisenmenger's syndrome). The last complication should be seen less frequently in the years ahead because of its early recognition coupled with more frequent repair of congenital heart disease in infancy. A significant number of patients, nonetheless, currently reach adult life with pulmonary vascular disease as a result of lesions such as large ventricular septal defect, atrioventricular septal defects and common arterial trunk. In some, the pulmonary vascular resistance may already have been too high at the time of diagnosis, while in others pulmonary vascular disease may have progressed despite complete repair of the underlying defect.

Although 'incurable', the prognosis for the patient with the Eisenmenger's syndrome depends to a great extent on non-pharmacological management, such as judicious venesection and avoidance of potentially dangerous medications or anaesthetics (Jones and Patel, 1996; Daliento et al, 1998; Ammesh et al, 1999). Although a number of drugs have been tried, including calcium channel blockers, inhibitors of angiotensin-converting enzyme, and nitrates, no treatment has been shown to alter the progression of the disease (Packer, 1985a,b; Rich et al, 1992). Death may result from right heart failure, pulmonary haemorrhage or arrhythmia (Morrison et al, 1983; Rounds and Hill, 1984).

Cyanotic patients are prone to specific extracardiac medical problems. Haematological adaptations to maintain transport of oxygen to metabolizing tissues include excessive erythropoiesis, which may lead to polycythaemia and hyperviscosity (Rudolph et al, 1953). Many patients with cyanotic disease establish a stable high haematocrit and exhibit few symptoms of hyperviscosity. These patients have a low risk of stroke and do not require venesection (Perloff et al, 1988; Territo et al, 1991). In others, the haematocrit may rise progressively. Once it exceeds 65%, they may suffer from symptoms of hyperviscosity, such as headache, dizziness and fatigue. They are then at risk from cerebrovascular thrombosis (Thorne, 1998). Symptoms may be improved by judicious venesection (Oldershaw and St John Sutton, 1980). At phlebotomy, no more than 500 ml should be removed. This should be combined with volume replacement, especially in the patient with pulmonary hypertension. Overzealous venesection may result in iron deficiency. This is highly undesirable because of the consequent decrease in the capacity to carry oxygen, the hyperviscosity in its own right and the increased high risk of stroke. The paradoxical iron deficiency of polycythaemic patients is often overlooked. It can be diagnosed by examination of the peripheral blood film, or by measurement of the levels of ferratin in the serum. Iron supplements may be required, especially when iron deficiency is anticipated, such as in phlebotomy or menorrhagia. The results should be carefully monitored by frequent measurement of haemoglobin, the haematocrit and reticulocyte counts.

Patients with chronic cyanosis also develop defective haemostasis from abnormalities in the number and function of the platelets, and in the coagulative and fibrinolytic systems (Lusher, 1987). This is particularly marked in those who are polycythaemic and may cause bruising or epistaxis. The risk of haemorrhage, especially at surgery, is well recognized and may be fatal.

Progressive kyphoscoliosis may complicate the course for both cyanotic and acyanotic adolescents with congenital heart disease (Jordan et al, 1972). It is more common in those who received a previous thoracotomy. The degree of deformity, if left untreated, may become profound, and it can then compromise cardiopulmonary function. Treatment with bracing, or by insertion of Harrington rods, may be indicated even if the patient has an uncorrectable cardiac lesion, since the kyphoscoliosis may significantly reduce both the quality and duration of life.

Hyperuricaemia is common because of the increased turnover of erythrocytes and renal dysfunction (Young, 1980). Arthralgia is well recognized, but gouty arthritis is rare and often misdiagnosed. Other important problems include acne, particularly in adolescents, and renal impairment, which may deteriorate to renal failure as a result of relatively minor interventions such as injection of contrast medium at angiography (Ross et al, 1966). Gallstones and cholecystitis are more common in polycythaemic patients because of production of calcium bilirubinate. Patients with right-to-left shunts are also at risk of paradoxical embolus, which may cause a cerebral or renal infarction. A cerebral abscess is a well-known complication of a septic embolus. This must always be considered in the cyanotic patient who develops headaches of sudden onset, somnolence, other neurological symptoms or a low-grade fever.

ENDOCARDITIS

Patients with both unoperated and operated disease are at risk from infective endocarditis, particularly those with prosthetic valves and systemic-to-pulmonary arterial shunts (Kaplan et al, 1979). The wide variety of potential portals of entry may not be appreciated by the patient or the physician. In addition to dental work, they include skin sepsis, obstetric and gynaecological procedures, genitourinary and gastrointestinal interventions and all forms of surgery (Sande et al, 1969; Sullivan et al, 1973; de Swiet et al, 1975; Shull et al, 1975; Gorge et al, 1990). Fibreoptic or flexible endoscopy and cardiac catheterization do not, in normal circumstances, result in bacteraemia. Endocarditis prophylaxis is not recommended for these procedures. There is, however, a risk of bacteraemia, and therefore infective endocarditis, in young adults who elect to have body piercing, including the ears, or have a tattoo.

Patients at risk must be educated. They need to be aware of the importance of good oral, skin and nail hygiene, as well as the circumstances of risk. Preferably they should carry an information card with them. The symptoms of endocarditis may be subtle; consequently, the diagnosis must be considered in any patient who experiences unexplained malaise or fever. Unfortunately, injudicious prescription of antibiotics without previous blood culture may mask the problem, thus making difficult bacteriological diagnosis and subsequent appropriate treatment.

Lifelong antibiotic prophylaxis is recommended for susceptible patients, whether or not they have undergone cardiac surgery, but the specific indications and optimal regimens are still debated. The special report from the American Heart Association on Prevention of Infective Endocarditis has stratified groups at risk for the various lesions (Shulman et al, 1984; Ad-hoc Working Party, 1998). In the United States, prophylaxis is advocated for all lesions except atrial septal defects within the oval fossa closed by direct suture or a divided persistent arterial duct. Infective endocarditis, however, is extremely rare in lesions such as uncorrected atrial septal defect within the oval fossa, pulmonary valvar stenosis or spontaneously closed ventricular septal defect. In order to ensure compliance, the chosen antibiotic regimen should be simple. The recommendation in the United Kingdom of a single large oral dose of amoxycillin (amoxicillin) has proved very effective for dental prophylaxis (Oakley and Somerville, 1981).

PREGNANCY

With the decreasing prevalence of rheumatic heart disease, congenital lesions currently account for an important proportion of the cases of maternal heart disease in pregnancy (de Swiet, 1987; McFaul et al, 1988). Advice is sought on both maternal and fetal risk, as well as on the incidence of congenital cardiac malformations anticipated in the offspring. Firm recommendations for many conditions are difficult, as most experience has been gathered for patients with relatively simple defects such as atrial septal defect and persistent

arterial duct (Copeland et al, 1963; Neilson et al, 1970). In patients undergoing continuing care for congenital heart disease, discussions about contraception, pregnancy, and the risk of recurrence should start at an early age, preferably before conception.

In general, mothers with congenital cardiac disease should be managed jointly throughout pregnancy by a cardiologist and an obstetrician, both experienced in this area. Before prescribing any cardiovascular drug during pregnancy, the effects on both mother and fetus must be considered. Management of labour should be specifically directed for avoidance of rapid changes in circulatory volume, blood pressure or cardiac output. The American Heart Association no longer recommends prophylaxis against endocarditis for vaginal delivery (Shulman et al, 1984; Dajani et al, 1997). This, however, is not based on controlled data, and most cardiologists recommend antibiotics during delivery for almost all patients with congenital cardiac defects. Labour should be conducted in the left lateral position, thus avoiding haemodynamic fluctuations caused by compression of the great vessels in the abdomen by the contracting uterus. Careful epidural anaesthesia usually allows good relief of pain with reasonable haemodynamic control. Spontaneous vaginal delivery is favoured, with caesarean section reserved for obstetric indications.

MATERNAL RISK

There are profound changes in the maternal cardiovascular system during pregnancy, including an increase in blood volume of up to two-fifths, a fall in peripheral vascular resistance and an increase in cardiac output, also of about two-fifths (Perloff, 1991). In general, women with left-to-right shunts, or those with valvar regurgitation, tolerate pregnancy well. Those with right-to-left shunts, or valvar stenosis, do less well. Asymptomatic young women with small-to-moderate left-to-right shunts, and normal pulmonary arterial pressures, can expect an uncomplicated pregnancy and labour. In the presence of a large left-to-right shunt, however, heart failure may be provoked or aggravated by pregnancy.

An elevated pulmonary vascular resistance is the only clear contraindication to pregnancy. In this setting, maternal mortality is high, up to half of those with Eisenmenger's syndrome even with meticulous management in the best centres (Daliento et al, 1998). Although successful outcome is possible, the latest advice is to avoid pregnancy. If such patients are seen late in pregnancy, and termination is not feasible, management should concentrate on maintenance of adequate preload and avoidance of vasodilation.

Patients with Marfan's syndrome and dilated aortic roots (Hall, 1981), and those with severe aortic stenosis, are also at increased risk. They should be counselled to consider elective surgical intervention prior to conception (Elkayam et al, 1995). While very early reports suggested a high risk for aortic coarctation (Mendelson, 1940), with complications of aortic rupture and cerebral haemorrhage, subsequent data have been more encouraging (Deal and Colley, 1973).

FETAL RISK

Placental insufficiency may result from maternal cyanosis, or from poor perfusion in those with obstructive lesions in the left heart. Patients with cyanosis have the most problems in carrying a fetus to term and have a high incidence of early spontaneous abortion. A clear relationship has now been demonstrated between the degree of hypoxaemia, rather than hyperviscosity, and fetal loss (Presbitero et al, 1992). Meticulous care during pregnancy and delivery minimized the rate of maternal complications, but complications still occurred in nearly one quarter of pregnancies. Such patients require rest, a short labour and should avoid vasodilators, dehydration and sepsis. Fetal risk is also increased if the mother has aortic coarctation (Benny et al, 1980). This results from compromised placental blood supply. In these patients, the decision as to whether to attempt to continue with pregnancy depends on an assessment of the risk to the mother and fetus compared with the desire of the patients to have children.

ANTICOAGULANTS

Special problems exist in the management of pregnant women with atrial arrhythmias or prosthetic cardiac valves and conduits. This is because of the risk to the mother of thromboembolism, and the risk to the fetus of potentially teratogenic oral anticoagulants, such as warfarin, which cross the placenta (Limet and Grondin, 1977; Lutz et al, 1978; Hall et al, 1980; Hurbe-Alessio et al, 1986; Oakley, 1995). There is no ideal solution. Even subcutaneous administration of heparin does not completely protect the mother from thromboembolic complications (Antunes et al, 1984). Some difficulties may be prevented by the elective use of bioprosthetic valves, rather than mechanical prostheses, for teenaged girls needing surgery.

Depending on the condition involved, and the maternal motivation and compliance, the use, if possible, of subcutaneous heparin at the time of conception and in the first trimester, followed by warfarin in mid-trimester and heparin in late pregnancy and throughout delivery is one option for treatment. Warfarin may be recommenced one week after delivery. It is not a contraindication to breast-feeding (Canadian Cardiovascular Society, 1996)

——————SURGICAL ASPECTS——————

INITIAL OPERATIONS FOR CONGENITAL CARDIAC DISEASE IN ADULTS

The first surgical repair for a congenital cardiac lesion may be required in the teenager or adult. This may be

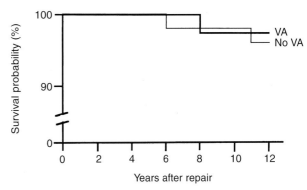

Figure 72.1. Actuarial survival curves plotting the survival probability against years followed up for two similar groups of patients who had been followed for 12 years after successful repair of tetralogy of Fallot: 47 patients who had no significant ventricular arrhythmia (VA) at baseline Holter monitor and 39 patients who had significant ventricular arrhythmia (< Lown grade 2). These two survival curves are not significantly different.

because the lesion has been mild and of little haemodynamic significance in childhood but has progressed in severity with time. Examples include a bicuspid aortic valve, which becomes progressively stenotic, Marfan's syndrome with dilation of the aortic root and Ebstein's malformation with worsening symptoms. Alternatively, lesions such as small-to-moderate atrial septal defect, or aortic coarctation, may have been missed or misdiagnosed until adult life. In certain complex congenital cardiac malformations, the combination of lesions produces a balanced haemodynamic state compatible with prolonged survival without intervention. Patients with double inlet ventricle and pulmonary stenosis, or tetralogy of Fallot with pulmonary atresia and systemic-to-pulmonary collateral arteries, may remain well until the second and even third decades of life before deteriorating (Figure 72.1) (Franklin et al, 1991). The contemplation of cardiac surgery in an adolescent or young adult is often terrifying, implying the acceptance of the presence of a serious problem by the patient and the immediate friends and family. The scar on the chest may cause embarrassment, and the patient may suffer discrimination both socially and at work. All these issues must be dealt with sympathetically by the physician.

REOPERATION ——————————

Reoperations in adults with congenital cardiac malformations provide a particular challenge to surgeon, anaesthetist and physician (Table 72.3) (Stark and Pacifico, 1989). The need for reoperation often comes as a shock to patients and relatives, who may have believed that the surgery undertaken in childhood was curative. As a result, resentment is frequent and tact is needed when handling such patients.

The risks are almost always higher than for primary procedures, for reasons that are both avoidable and

Table 72.3. Indications for reoperation in adults with congenital cardiac disease

---

Staged repair of complex defects, such as tetralogy of Fallot with pulmonary atresia

Residual defects after definitive repair such as ventricular septal defect after tetralogy of Fallot or left atrioventricular valvar regurgitation after atrioventricular septal defect

New or recurrent defects after definitive repair such as: subaortic stenosis, restenosis of aortic valve, pulmonary regurgitation in tetralogy of Fallot

Inevitable reoperation after definitive repair in childhood such as: prosthetic valves, extracardiac conduits

Unexpected complications such as: infective endocarditis

Transplantation for uncorrectable congenital cardiac disease

---

unavoidable. Careful preoperative planning should include complete understanding of the anatomy of the heart and its relations, particularly to the chest wall and sternum, as well as a study of previous operative reports, which may have been performed at another institution by another surgeon. Re-entry to the chest should not be left to junior members of the team, as this part of the operation often carries considerable risk. Major haemorrhage has been reported as a complication of a repeated sternotomy, with a high mortality (Dobell and Jain, 1984). The risk is particularly high when the ventricle immediately posterior to the sternum is at high pressure, or when an extracardiac conduit lies in this position. Re-entry via a different approach will avoid adhesions and, thus, minimize bleeding. On occasion, it may be necessary to establish femoro–femoral bypass with cooling before the chest is opened. The current use of Goretex membranes under the sternum may reduce the difficulties of future repeat procedures (Iyer et al, 1993). Postoperative haemodynamic and respiratory problems are particularly common after reoperation because of the prolonged duration of previous surgery, previous damage to the myocardium and greater use of blood products.

STAGED REPAIR

For complex congenital cardiac disease, several palliations may be required into adolescence or adulthood. This course may be necessary for patients with tetralogy of Fallot with pulmonary atresia, hypoplastic pulmonary arteries and with multifocal pulmonary blood supply (Puga et al, 1989). Palliative procedures to increase flow to the central pulmonary arteries, and to unifocalize the sources of pulmonary flow by direct or indirect anastomosis of collateral vessels to the pulmonary arteries, may eventually result in the ability to perform a repair. This is usually achieved by insertion of a conduit between the right ventricle and the pulmonary arteries and closure of the ventricular septal defect. If properly performed, it results in an acceptable postoperative ratio

of the right and left ventricular pressures (Sullivan et al, 1988; Puga et al, 1989; Reddy et al, 1995). Excellent surgical results have been reported for staged repair starting with central shunting and followed by unifocalization (Watterson et al, 1991), but the long-term outcome is not yet available, particularly with regard to late right ventricular haemodynamics.

Other situations in which definitive repair may be indicated in the young adult are complex defects with one functioning ventricle, such patients having been palliated by construction of a systemic-to-pulmonary arterial shunt or banding of the pulmonary trunk in childhood. In those patients who fulfil the anatomical and physiological criterions for a Fontan operation, it is likely that long-term results will be better after this type of operation than after construction of a systemic-to-pulmonary arterial shunt, the latter resulting in a chronically increased load to the ventricle (Gewillig et al, 1990b). Disconcerting late problems, however, have begun to become apparent after the Fontan operation. Indeed, some centres have moved away from the Fontan procedures, regarding construction of a bidirectional cavopulmonary anastomosis combined with a systemic-to-pulmonary shunt as the best definitive palliation (Bonnet et al, 1998). No long-term results are yet available for this approach, which is likely to give a long-term outcome similar to that found in patients with only a systemic-to-pulmonary arterial shunt. More long-term data are needed for the type of Fontan operation currently being performed (Fontan et al, 1990; Driscoll et al, 1992; Gentles et al, 1997). The Fontan procedure, nonetheless, should always be presented to families as a definitive palliative operation for a complex cardiac deficit, rather than as a complete repair.

RESIDUAL OR RECURRENT DEFECTS

Residual or recurrent defects may be difficult to distinguish unless careful assessment has been performed after the original repair. They may have a major impact on morbidity and mortality, such as when major regurgitation across the left atrioventricular valve persists after repair of an atrioventricular septal defect (Studer et al, 1982). Much more long-term follow-up data are needed before guidelines for reoperation for relatively minor residual abnormalities, such as mild left atrioventricular valvar regurgitation in this situation, can be established.

The reported need for reoperation after 'corrective' surgery for tetralogy of Fallot varies between 1.8 and 13% over a follow-up of up to 31 years (Poirier et al, 1977; Zhao et al, 1985; Murphy et al, 1993). Residual interventricular communications, obstruction in the right ventricular outflow tract and pulmonary regurgitation are the most common residual abnormalities. Indeed, pulmonary regurgitation is particularly frequent, especially after the use of a transjunctional patch at the repair. The determinants include not only the procedure on the right ventricular outflow tract but also the presence of restrictive physiology of the right ventricle. The latter complication may provide 'paradoxical' benefit in the long-term by limiting pulmonary regurgitation (Gatzoulis et al, 1995b). The haemodynamic consequences on right ventricular function are greater in the presence of residual obstruction and residual interventricular communications (Chaturvedi et al, 1997). Replacement of the pulmonary valve has not often been required in the first two decades after repair but may become increasingly necessary because of late right ventricular dysfunction (d'Udekem et al, 1998). Current indications include progressive right ventricular dilation and a decrease in exercise tolerance (Wessel et al, 1980). This may also become part of the management of patients who present with clinically manifested arrhythmia (Oechslin et al, 1999). When performed prior to the supervention of right ventricular failure, often with tricuspid regurgitation and atrial flutter or fibrillation, both clinical status and right ventricular function have been shown to improve (Ilbawi et al, 1981; Oechslin et al, 1999). It is likely that, in future, indications for reoperation will become more liberal. The optimal method for assessing the severity of pulmonary regurgitation, however, is still not well established. Insertion of conductance catheters is invasive. Echo Doppler interrogation provides information on ventriculo–arterial coupling. Mapping of its velocity using cinemagnetic imaging is an excellent technique for volumetric quantitation (Rebergen et al, 1992).

INEVITABLE REOPERATIONS

Repair of malformations that have involved insertion of a prosthetic valve, or an extracardiac conduit, results in an inevitable need for reoperation, because the prostheses have either become too small or have undergone degeneration. Extracardiac conduits are commonly used for repair of tetralogy of Fallot with pulmonary atresia, common arterial trunk and complete or corrected transposition with obstruction of the left ventricular outflow tract. Development of obstruction is influenced by the type of conduit used, the technique of its insertion and the timing of the original operation. Heterografts have shown a high incidence of early obstruction. In an early study, replacement of two-thirds of heterograft conduits was required following repair of common arterial trunk in infancy. The mean interval between original operation and replacement was 4 years (Ebert et al, 1984). Jonas and colleagues (1985) found that all their survivors required replacement of the conduit with 10 years. Ross and Somerville (1966) described the first use of a homograft aortic valve for the repair of tetralogy of Fallot with pulmonary atresia, but these also inevitably require replacement. Irradiated and frozen homografts have performed poorly, with early calcification and obstruction (Merin and McGoon, 1973; Park et al, 1973). Fresh homografts or homografts preserved in antibiotic nutrients have fared much better. They are the current con-

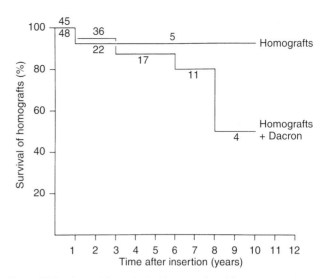

Figure 72.2. Actuarial survival of homografts without reoperation, showing that 93% of homografts used alone remain free of obstruction 2–10 years after insertion, whereas only 52% of those extended with woven Dacron were free of obstruction at 10 years.

duits of choice (Shabbo et al, 1980; de Carlo et al, 1984). Besides the conduit itself, operative technique and the use of a large conduit have clear beneficial influence on the need for early replacement.

Patients with right-sided conduits need careful follow-up, particularly towards the end of the anticipated period of acceptable performance (Figure 72.2). The clinical signs of severe obstruction may be subtle and are often underestimated. As a result, replacement may be performed too late. The consequent major deleterious effects on right ventricular function increase the risk of surgery. They may not be fully reversible. Regular non-invasive evaluation using cross-sectional echocardiography, transoesophageal echocardiography and magnetic resonance imaging is indicated. This now provides the information previously obtained by cardiac catheterization with angiography. Reoperation is mandated if the right ventricular pressure is near systemic, or if there is evidence of deteriorating ventricular function (Stark, 1989b). The life expectancy of the replaced homograft conduit is of major concern. It had been hoped that insertion of an 'adult' size conduit in teenagers would provide excellent survival for decades, and that further replacement would not be required. Data from a large study at Great Ormond Street, however, has shown that, in some groups at least, survival of the second conduit may even be shorter than that used at the first operation (Stark, 1998). The prospect is worrying for patients returning for multiple replacements for conduits at shorter intervals, with associated higher surgical morbidity and mortality. The development of medical and surgical strategies to preserve conduits is a high priority.

Several studies have emphasized the palliative nature of aortic valvotomy in childhood (Presbitero et al, 1982; Stewart et al, 1978; Heish et al, 1986). Isolated stenosis occurs most frequently in the bicuspid valve, although in symptomatic neonates and infants the structural abnormality of the valve may be more severe, and the results of surgery even worse. In a series of infants undergoing open aortic valvotomy, actuarial survival was 94% at 5 years, but only 77% at 22 years. Reoperation was carried out in one third, and the actuarial probability of reoperation was 44% at 22 years (Rao et al, 1989; Mullins et al, 1990). When serious events such as death, reoperation and endocarditis were grouped together, 92% were free of events at 5 years, but only 39% at 22 years. Balloon aortic valvotomy as the initial procedure for aortic stenosis has produced results equivalent to those of surgery, although rigorous trials to compare the approaches have not, and likely will not, be performed. Balloon valvotomy has a high chance of successful relief of stenosis in young patients with bicuspid valves (Sholler et al, 1988; Rao et al, 1989; Borghi et al, 1999). It is the treatment of choice in most, in contrast to the disappointing impact of this technique in elderly patients (Safian et al, 1988).

UNEXPECTED REOPERATIONS

Unexpected reoperation may be required for sudden failure or thrombosis of a prosthetic valve, for infective endocarditis and for thrombosis in circulations with low flow, such as after construction of an atriopulmonary connection. Endocarditis is particularly difficult to diagnose in those with complex malformations, where the site of vegetations may not be easy to image, for example in a Blalock–Taussig shunt. Reoperation in the patient with uncontrolled endocarditis or endarteritis carries a high risk.

TRANSPLANTATION OF THE HEART OR HEART AND LUNGS

A significant number of adolescents and young adults with congenital cardiac disease develop late cardiorespiratory problems that are unresponsive to medical therapy and not amenable to further palliation or repair. These patients often have severe myocardial dysfunction, pulmonary vascular disease or multiple previous chest incisions and complex anatomy. In these patients, the only remaining prospect may be transplantation of the heart in isolation, the heart together with the lungs, or transplantation of the lungs with cardiac repair.

Cardiac transplantation has become an accepted therapy for selected patients with refractory cardiac failure, with current actuarial survival rates of greater than 80% and 5-year survival close to 70% (Hosenpud et al, 1999). Long-term hazards include late occlusive graft coronary arterial disease (Sharples et al, 1991), systemic hypertension, diabetes, renal dysfunction, hyperlipidaemia and susceptibility to infection and malignancy (Hosenpud et al, 1999). The operation itself may be more complicated in adults with congenital cardiac disease because of adhesions from previous procedures and unusual anatomy.

Transplantation of the heart and lungs is an option for those with cardiac disease and high pulmonary vascular resistance, or very abnormal pulmonary arterial blood supply. Patients with congenital cardiac disease make up about one quarter of the transplant recipients (Hosenpud et al, 1999). Outcome is worse than for transplantation of the heart alone. One year survival is from 60 to 70% with 5-year survival of only 40% (Hosenpud et al, 1999). Recent data from a single institution, nonetheless, showed 1- and 5-year survival rates for Eisenmenger's syndrome of 83% and 74%, respectively (Harringer et al, 1999). Bleeding in surgery is a major problem in patients with complex congenital cardiac disease and chronic cyanosis, who often have acquired collateral vasculature in the chest wall either as a result of palliation with one or more thoracotomies or from the disease process itself. As with cardiac transplantation, shortage of donors is an important factor. This has stimulated interest in double lung transplantation for patients with primary pulmonary hypertension or Eisenmenger's syndrome, in conjunction with surgical correction of the cardiac defect.

NON-CARDIAC SURGERY

Non-cardiac surgery in adults with congenital heart disease, when performed without adequate preparation, is a major cause of avoidable morbidity and mortality. All the risks of anaesthesia encountered for cardiac reoperation apply equally to non-cardiac surgery, but in the latter instance the patient is often managed by medical and anaesthetic staff who may be unfamiliar with the significance of the congenital heart disease or may even be unaware of it. For example, in patients with pulmonary vascular disease, a sudden fall in systemic vascular resistance related to general anaesthesia may have disastrous consequences (Jones and Patel, 1996; Ammesh et al, 1999). Similar haemodynamic changes may induce a severe hypercyanotic spell in a patient with uncorrected tetralogy of Fallot. Meticulous pre-, intra- and postoperative haemodynamic monitoring is mandatory, with avoidance of vasodilating anaesthetic agents, hypoxia, hypoventilation and important loss of blood or volume.

Many patients with congenital cardiac malformations may be at increased risk from arrhythmia, and from agents that even temporarily depress ventricular function. The surgeon must be aware of the presence of a pacemaker or pacing leads, which may affect the safe use of diathermy. Cyanotic patients also have impaired haemostasis, as will any patient receiving anticoagulants. Intravenous lines, drugs and infusions must be managed carefully in patients with intracardiac shunts, as air or other embolic agents may reach the systemic circulation. Prophylaxis against infective endocarditis is usually indicated. The choice of the antibiotic regimen is dictated by the surgical procedure or intervention being undertaken. The safety of non-cardiac surgery in adults with congenital cardiac disease could be greatly increased if physicians, anaesthetists and surgeons were familiar with these issues, sought specialized advice and, if necessary, referred the patient to a team with more experience.

PSYCHOSOCIAL ASPECTS

A crucial transition occurs for the patient with congenital cardiac disease during adolescence. Previously, the child is legally dependent on his or her parents and is cared for in the compassionate environment of a children's hospital. By the end of the teenage years, the search for social and financial independence has begun, and the young adult needs to understand the nature and implications of his or her cardiac problems.

Many adolescents resent the idea that they need ongoing care after childhood. They may then deny the presence or relevance of their malformation, fail to comply with treatment or fail to attend for follow-up. Others remain dependent on their parents and physicians and are overly anxious about relatively trivial residual problems. Even a 'small hole in the heart' may seem ominous. Sympathetic and sensible advice and guidance must be available, especially regarding exercise and sport, employment, insurance, socialization, contraception and genetic counselling. Optimal management of care during this difficult adolescent phase is often best achieved by a clinic that is managed jointly by the team of paediatric cardiologists familiar to the patient and family and the team that will take responsibility for long-term care.

EXERCISE AND SPORTS

Exercise is of both physical and psychosocial benefit. It leads to improved cardiovascular fitness, and to decreased likelihood of obesity, hypertension and ischaemic heart disease (Mayer and Bullen, 1974; Rocchini et al, 1988; Must et al, 1992). Participation in exercise and sport is also part of normal socialization.

Exercise capacity is diminished in many adults with congenital cardiac disease, even after surgery. This may result from a number of factors, such as an inability to increase the heart rate appropriately, for example after atrial surgery with damage to the sinus node. Alternatively, there may be an inability to increase myocardial contractility, as may occur with chronic volume or pressure overload on the heart, chronic hypoxaemia or damage from suboptimal myocardial protection at surgery. A third possibility is an inability to maintain appropriate cardiac filling, as after the Fontan procedure or after intra-atrial repair of complete transposition. An inability to increase delivery of oxygen to exercising muscles, for example to the legs in aortic coarctation or in patients with cyanosis

and/or hyperviscosity, may also limit exercise performance. In any event, reduced performance may also reflect lack of regular exercise in overprotected individuals with congenital cardiac defects. This is often reinforced by doctors, who, if in doubt, tend to proscribe exercise.

It remains difficult to make dogmatic recommendations (Maron et al, 1985; Cullen et al, 1991; Soni and Deanfield, 1997). In some cases, exercise capacity is clearly normal and the risk is minimal, such as after closure of a small arterial duct. In others, exercise capacity is limited or the risk is high, as in aortic stenosis with severe left ventricular hypertrophy. Between these extremes is a grey area in which recommendations must take into account the individual, the underlying cardiac defect, the haemodynamic status and the type of sport or exercise contemplated. This may be isotonic or isometric, social or competitive, contact or non-contact. Formal testing should be performed, preferably with measurement of uptake of oxygen, both as a measure of the effects of submaximal and maximal exercise and as a reassurance to the patient. A walking test over 12 minutes gives a good guide to functional capacity, whereas a treadmill protocol with more strenuous effort is employed to assess risk by revealing occult arrhythmia, ischaemia or fall in blood pressure. Subjective estimates of exercise capacity are almost always inaccurate (Cullen et al, 1991).

In general, subjects with volume overload, valvar regurgitation and left-to-right shunts have good tolerance to exercise. Those with pressure overload, valvar stenosis, and right-to-left shunts do not. Recommendations for individual lesions are given in Table 72.4. Patients with fixed and elevated pulmonary vascular resistance have limited exercise capacity. In these, exercise carries considerable risk. As a result, most forms of active exercise should be avoided. Otherwise, these recommendations should be considered only as guidelines, as adequate information with which to assess both capacity and the associated risk is not yet available for many conditions. In patients with aortic stenosis, isometric exercise, such as rowing or weightlifting, should certainly be avoided. We currently recommend unrestricted regular exercise for those with mild disease, and formal exercise testing for those with moderate disease, with particular attention to changes in blood pressure and the ST segments.

Supervised programmes of training for adults with congenital cardiac disease can improve aerobic fitness and increase the safe and appropriate level at which such individuals can participate in sport. By providing support and encouragement, such programmes also improve psychological adjustment and self-esteem.

EMPLOYMENT

Most patients can work. They should have access to employment appropriate to their physical and intellectual capabilities. In the United States of America, patients

Table 72.4. Recommendations concerning exercise for those with residual heart lesions

Exercise	Residual lesion
Not limited	Left-to-right shunts without ventricular dysfunction or pulmonary vascular disease Mild-to-moderate valvar regurgitation Mild valvar stenosis Most arrhythmias in the structurally normal heart, including Wolff–Parkinson–White syndrome Postoperative patients with excellent haemodynamic repairs, such as closure of atrial septal defect or some cases of tetralogy of Fallot
Strenuous sport should be restricted (but lesser levels of exercise should be permitted)	Mild left ventricular outflow tract obstruction Ventricular dysfunction with ejection fraction <40% Postoperative atrial redirection for complete transposition Hearts with univentricular atrioventricular connection (preoperative and postoperative) Some arrhythmias Some treated hypertensive patients after coarctation repair
All moderate and strenous exercise should be restricted	Moderate and severe pulmonary vascular disease Severe valvar stenosis Long QT syndrome with exercise-induced ventricular tachycardia Postoperative patients with exercise-induced ventricular tachycardia

with ventricular septal defect and pulmonary or aortic stenosis have been shown to achieve levels of education comparable with the normal population (Weidman et al, 1988). No similar data are yet available for large groups of patients with more complex defects, although their situation will undoubtedly prove worse. Despite the excellent potential of many adults with congenital cardiac disease, job discrimination is frequently encountered, even when a patient has been cleared by a cardiologist. In the United States, legislation has been passed that seeks to prevent discrimination. Employers are obliged to consider only the capacity to perform the given job and not to anticipate future deterioration. In other countries, including the United Kingdom, some employers take into account not only the present ability but also future prospects for absenteesim or premature curtailment of the career (Celermajer and Deanfield, 1993). In such circumstances, young adults with congenital cardiac disease are at a disadvantage, particularly if they apply for jobs with a long apprenticeship or period of training.

Restrictions for employment exist when the safety of others is the direct responsibility of the individual with congenital cardiac disease. This includes possession of a licence to drive a heavy goods or public service vehicle. In the United Kingdom, drivers in these categories are required to hold vocational, in addition to their ordinary, driving licences. Although the only legal bar is epilepsy, individuals with congenital cardiac disease are not considered if they have a history of paroxysmal arrhythmia, a pacemaker, a prosthetic heart valve or conduit, a markedly abnormal electrocardiogram, hypertension or abnormal haemodynamics with the need for chronic medications. The armed services exclude most applicants with a previous history of cardiac disease. The regulations for commercial airline

pilots are also clear and state that a risk of sudden cardiac death or acute disability of 1% per annum is the maximum considered acceptable for multicrew flights and 0.1% for solo flights (Tunstall-Pedoe, 1988). The number of congenital cardiac malformations in which such rates of low risk are clearly defined remains small (Deanfield, 1992).

LIFE AND HEALTH INSURANCE

Insurance companies are, of necessity, fiscally conservative. In the absence of adequate long-term data of survival for many operated and unoperated congenital lesions, life insurance may be difficult to obtain. A survey in the United States of America revealed that only patients with very simple lesions were insured at regular rates (Truesdell, 1986). These included mild pulmonary valvar stenosis, surgically corrected defects within the oval fossa, ventricular septal defect and persistent arterial duct. The results of a similar survey of British life insurance companies (Celermajer and Deanfield, 1993) revealed an even more restrictive policy (Table 72.5). There were significant inconsistencies in ratings between companies. Young adults declined by one company, therefore, should be advised to 'shop around'. Inability to gain affordable life insurance can make it difficult for many young adults with congenital cardiac disease to buy their own home, as mortgage companies often require applicants to hold life insurance as collateral.

Availability of health insurance varies greatly between countries, and practice is likely to change considerably in the next few years. In general, health insurance may be obtained by most young adults with congenital cardiac disease, but the policy often excludes benefits for medical

Table 72.5. Life insurability of those with congenital cardiac defects

Defect	Normal	High rates	Not offered
Aortic regurgitation			
Mild		*	
Moderate		*	
Severe			*
Aortic stenosis			
Mild		*	
Moderate		*	
Severe			*
Mitral regurgitation			
Mild		*	
Moderate		*	
Severe			*
Mitral stenosis			
Mild		*	
Moderate		*	
Severe			*
Prolapsed mitral valve (no regurgitation)	*		
Mitral valvar replacement		*a	
Aortic valvar replacement		*a	
Double valvar replacement			*
Pulmonary stenosis			
Mild		*	
Moderate		*	
Severe			*
Ebstein's malformation			
Mild			*
Moderate			*
Severe			*
Postoperative			*
Atrial septal defect			
QP/QS <2		*	
QP/QS >2		*	
Postoperative		*b	
Ventricular septal defect			
QP/QS <2		*	
QP/QS >2		*	
Postoperative normal		*b	
Postoperative with raised PVR			*
Patent arterial duct			*
Preoperative			*
Postoperative	*		
Aortic coarctation			
Mild			*
Moderate			*
Severe			*
Postoperative normal	*		
Postoperative with raised BP		*	
Tetralogy of Fallot			
Preoperative		*	
Postoperative		*c	
Complete transposition			
Post-Mustard/Senning			*
Post-arterial switch			*d
Totally anomalous pulmonary venous connection: postoperative		*	

Table 72.5. Life insurability of those with congenital cardiac defects (*contd*)

Defect	Normal	High rates	Not offered
Common arterial trunk:			
Postoperative			*
Fontan procedure			*
Complete heart block		*	

BP, blood pressure; PVR, pulmonary vascular resistance; QP/QS, pulmonary to systemic shunt.
aPolicy limited to 25 years postoperative by one company.
bReducing to normal rates after 4 years by two companies.
cHigh-rate policy for short duration only by two companies.
dHigh-rate policy for limited duration by one company.

or surgical treatment of the cardiac condition itself (Allen et al, 1992; Celermajer and Deanfield, 1993). Patients are at particular disadvantage with systems of health care based on insurance, as they may have formidable obstacles when they outgrow the insurance policy that covered their medical care in childhood.

SOCIAL AND INTELLECTUAL DEVELOPMENT —

Large controlled longitudinal studies of the psychosocial consequences of congenital heart disease are rare. Those which exist are difficult to interpret (Mahoney et al, 1991). Most patients with congenital cardiac disease appear well adjusted but have subtle feelings of 'difference' from their peers. Lack of self-esteem and fear of isolation are common (Kellerman et al, 1980). These feelings are often compounded by limitation of activities compared with others by the presence of scars, cardiac symptoms, hospital visits and family anxiety. As a result, adolescents and adults with congenital cardiac disease should be encouraged to lead as normal a life as possible and openly to discuss their fears and anxieties. Anxiety about sexual activity, including fear of death during intercourse, marriage and childbirth are common. Patients often find these aspects difficult to discuss, particularly with the doctor in a regular clinic (Zelter et al, 1980). These issues must be handled with sensitivity by the team caring for the patient, which may include a nurse, social worker and psychologist.

Assessment of the impact of congenital cardiac disease on intellectual development remains controversial. Interpretation of testing must take into account the very abnormal childhood experienced by many patients, with absence from schooling for medical reasons as well as decreased social interaction. In addition, patients have often had an overprotected childhood, and their attitude to testing may be different. All studies of intellect exclude patients with genetic syndromes, and other dysmorphic, somatic or neurological defects, but subtle abnormalities are easily missed (Myers-Vando et al, 1979). In the Second

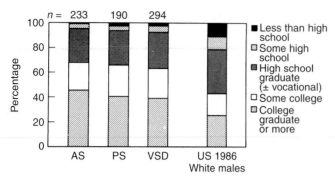

Figure 72.3. Bar graph of the educational achievement in male patients at least 25 years of age, grouped by underlying congenital heart lesion. Age- and sex-adjusted rates from the general population are also presented. AS, aortic stenosis; PS, pulmonary stenosis; VSD, ventricular septal defect.

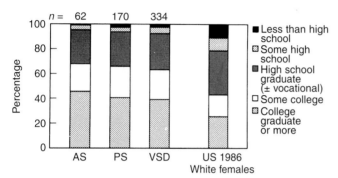

Figure 72.4. Bar graph of the educational achievement in female patients at least 25 years of age at study contact, grouped by underlying congenital heart lesion. Age- and sex-adjusted rates from the general population are also presented. AS, aortic stenosis; PS, pulmonary stenosis; VSD, ventricular septal defect.

Joint Study on the Natural History of Congenital Heart Defects (1993), investigators from North America reported similar educational achievements in young adults surviving with aortic stenosis, pulmonary stenosis and ventricular septal defect, including patients who had required surgery (Figures 72.3 and 72.4) (Keane et al, 1996). As access to health care in the study centres may not have been universal throughout the period of study, these data may not be truly representative for all patients.

Certain aspects of development may be more specifically affected by congenital cardiac disease. For example, walking is delayed in cyanotic children, but speech is not (Silbert et al, 1969). This will affect the relevance of early testing on later performance. Currently, data suggest that cyanosis is associated with mild intellectual impairment (Newberger et al, 1984; Aram et al, 1985). This may be reduced by early corrective surgery, even involving cardiopulmonary bypass.

CONTRACEPTION

Most young people in Europe and North America become sexually active during their teenage years. Adolescents and young adults, therefore, should be given appropriate advice about contraception from an early age (Huffman, 1981). In general, the low-dose oestrogen oral contraceptive pill is safe for young women with congenital cardiac disease (Rabajoli et al, 1992). Exceptions include those with hypertension (for example when associated with aortic coarctation), those with pulmonary vascular disease and those with cyanosis with associated polycythaemia. In such cases, a preparation using progesterone only is an alternative, albeit with a lower contraceptive efficacy and more side effects (Fraser, 1988). Intrauterine devices should not be used because of the risk of endocarditis (Whittemore, 1989). Barrier methods, either using condoms or diaphragms, are safe and effective. Laparoscopic sterilization should be considered in women with severe pulmonary vascular disease or lesions in which pregnancy would result in high maternal risk (Snabes et al, 1991).

GENETIC COUNSELLING

Genetic counselling should be provided for all potential parents with congenital heart disease. Risks of recurrence in siblings of patients with congenital heart disease are well documented, and range between 1 and 8% (Allan et al, 1986). For affected potential parents, however, the recurrence risk in offspring is the key information, and fewer data currently exist. Early reports showed very high apparent recurrent risks compared with studies involving siblings, with figures up to 16%. These studies are difficult to interpret. Criterions for inclusion varied, and most had significant potential ascertainment bias. In general, risks of recurrence are considerably higher than those for siblings (Burn, 1987). In a recent large study carried out in the United Kingdom, the risk of recurrence was determined as 4.1% in 727 individuals with 393 live offspring. Interestingly, the risk was significantly higher in offspring whose mother, rather than father, had congenital cardiac disease. Certain forms of disease clearly recur more frequently than others, particularly obstructive lesions of the left heart, such as subaortic stenosis, and atrioventricular septal defects. The genetic basis for these lesions is likely to become clearer over the next few years. Fetal echocardiography should be offered to all affected couples in the early stages of pregnancy. This can provide great reassurance for the majority. Accurate detection of most important congenital cardiac anomalies (Allan et al, 1997) enables appropriate counselling of those with abnormal babies.

SPECIFIC LESIONS

GENERAL ASPECTS

The spectrum of congenital abnormalities seen in adults is determined by the incidence of the abnormalities at birth, their natural history in childhood and the impact of medical and surgical intervention on outcome (Tables 72.1 and 72.2).

Interpretation of the limited literature on long-term outcome of congenital heart defects is often difficult, especially as many groups report the outcome of highly selected patients seen only at tertiary referral centres. In many series, follow-up is still short and numbers of survivors are small. The era of open heart surgery for congenital defects began only in the 1950s, and definitive repair has only been attempted much more recently for many types of lesion, as in the Fontan operation (Fontan and Baudet, 1971). In addition, surgical practice has undergone a process of evolution during this time, with new operations for some lesions (as with complete transposition) or major change in operative technique for others (such as atriopulmonary and cavopulmonary connections). Advances in cardiopulmonary bypass, and myocardial protection, have accompanied improved preoperative diagnosis and recognition of intracardiac anatomy, particularly with regard to the disposition of the conduction tissues. For almost all lesions, the philosophy of management has changed, with a trend to early primary correction where possible as opposed to initial palliation. Consequently, for many defects, the important long-term outcome relevant to current practice is not yet known.

INVESTIGATIONS

Although transthoracic echocardiography and cardiac catheterization are the major diagnostic investigations in paediatric cardiology, these may be more difficult to perform and less informative in adolescents and young adults with congenital cardiac disease. Transthoracic ultrasound is more difficult in adults because of increasing chest size, and thus reduction in the ultrasound window, and the need for lower-frequency, lower-resolution transducers. Furthermore, deformities of the chest wall, scoliosis, cardiac malposition and dense adhesions following previous surgery (some or all of which are often found in this group of patients) may impair the quality of the images obtained. Diagnostic catherization may be difficult to perform because of problems in vascular access. Angiographic images may be poor in overweight adults, or in subjects with abnormal chest wall geometry. Difficulties in vascular access have been reported in one-third of subjects previously catheterized, especially those who had undergone cut-down procedures or multiple previous studies (Celermajer et al, 1993).

Transoesophageal echocardiography, and magnetic resonance imaging, can provide excellent pictures in adults with repaired or unrepaired congenital cardiac malformations (Figures 72.5 and 72.6; Plate 72.1). Both techniques appear to be sensitive and specific and may be repeated serially. They have gained acceptance as important tests in cases where transthoracic echocardio-

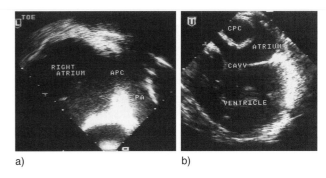

a)   b)

Figure 72.5. Transoesophageal echocardiographic pictures taken from patients who have had modified Fontan procedures for complex congenital cardiac disease. In both cases, the pictures obtained by transthoracic echocardiography were of suboptimal quality. (a) A longitudinal view of an unobstructed atriopulmonary connection (APC). (b) A transverse view of a cavopulmonary connection. CPC indicates the pathway from the inferior caval vein to the pulmonary arteries. CAVV, common atrioventricular valve; PA, pulmonary artery.

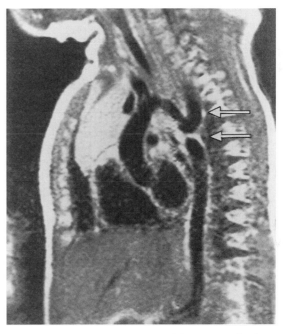

Figure 72.6. Magnetic resonance image of the aortic arch, showing aortic coarctation (lower arrow) just distal to the origin of the left subclavian artery (top arrow).

graphy provides inadequate information (Hirsch et al, 1994). Clinics dealing with adults with congenital cardiac disease must have access to both techniques.

Transoesophageal echocardiography, together with colour Doppler, allows optimal visualization of the morphology of the atrial appendages, atrial pathways, the Fontan circulation, the atrioventricular junctions and valves, the subaortic region and the ascending and descending aorta. It is also useful for study of prosthetic mitral valvar function and the assessment of endocarditis and its complications.

Magnetic resonance imaging can provide high-quality pictures of the heart and great vessels (Didier et al, 1999; Roest et al, 1999). Function, and patterns of flow, can also be studied, with potential for quantification of regurgitant volumes and shunting. Acquisition and resolution of the images have advanced rapidly, and realtime imaging is now feasible. Three-dimensional reconstruction, with peripheral venous injection of gadolinium contrast, is now routine. This is particularly useful for visualization of the complex anatomy of the great vessels and their spacial relationships within the chest. Postacquisition processing of scans of the heart can provide detailed three-dimensional information to supplement that obtained by ultrasound. Despite early concerns about scanning patients with pacemakers, prosthetic valves or prosthetic clips, useful information can be obtained safely, including prosthetic valvar function. Magnetic resonance imaging is likely to prove indispensable for non-invasive study of the great vessels, including coarctation, conduits, pulmonary veins and arteries, and to reduce the need for invasive evaluation still further.

Other imaging modalities, such as ultrafast computed tomography and radionuclide scanning, may also provide useful additional information, but their role in clinical practice is less well established.

INTERVENTIONAL CATHETERIZATION

Interventional catheterization has had an enormous impact on the management of congenital cardiac disease in the 1990s. The range of procedures of value in adults has expanded with developments in the design of catheters and the introduction of new devices (Redington et al, 1994; Gibbs, 2000).

Balloon dilation has become the treatment of choice for many patients with aortic stenosis, pulmonary arterial stenosis, aortic recoarctation and narrowed venous pathways after intratrial repair of complete transposition. Such techniques can obviate the need for cardiac surgery. The introduction of vascular stents has further expanded the indications for interventional treatment, with greatly improved long-term results in many situations. Closure of a patent arterial duct is occasionally indicated in adults, and a range of devices permit non-surgical closure of patent oval foramens and defects within the oval fossa. Other valuable indications, which may provide definitive treatment or simplify surgical treatment, include closure of residual ventricular septal defects and embolization of aortopulmonary collateral arteries or systemic-to-pulmonary arterial shunts.

ATRIAL SEPTAL DEFECT ———————

Atrial septal defect is among the most common congenital anomalies encountered in adolescents and adults, accounting for up to one third of lesions in this population (Borow and Braunwald, 1988; Child and Perloff, 1991). Approximately three quarters are within the oval fossa, one fifth are atrioventricular septal defects with only atrial shunting, one twentieth are sinus venosus defects, and defects at other sites are rare (Kirklin and Barratt-Boyes, 1986; Warnes et al, 1991a). Associated lesions include pulmonary stenosis, mitral valvar prolapse and mitral regurgitation. Atrial septal defects may be associated with other syndromes, including the Holt–Oram syndrome (Massumi et al, 1966), and may be familial (Nora et al, 1967). In the latter situation, conduction disease manifesting as prolongation of the PR interval and, rarely, heart block have been described.

NATURAL HISTORY

Survival into adulthood is the rule, and patients living into their ninth and tenth decade have been reported (St John Sutton et al, 1981; Perloff, 1984). Life expectancy, however, is not normal. Death during the first 20 years of life is infrequent, but after the age of 40 years, the mortality increases to about 6% per year (Craig and Selzer, 1968; Campbell, 1970a). Defects may go unrecognized for many years because symptoms are rare until later life, and physical signs may be subtle. Later, the natural history is characterized by progressive symptoms and cardiomegaly, the development of atrial arrhythmias, right ventricular hypertrophy and pulmonary hypertension.

The mechanisms for the development of symptoms are multifactorial. They include the change in left ventricular compliance from superimposed hypertension or coronary arterial disease and long-standing right ventricular volume overload. Supraventricular arrhythmias, particularly atrial fibrillation and flutter, may precipitate cardiac failure. Progressive pulmonary vascular disease may develop after the third decade of life. Rarer complications include systemic and pulmonary embolization, recurrent chest infections and infective endocarditis.

MANAGEMENT

Surgical closure, either by direct suture or use of a patch, has been performed since the 1960s. Surgery may be performed by a median sternotomy or, alternatively, via a right thoracotomy or submammary incision. The last may be more cosmetically acceptable in young females. Although there has been some controversy about the indications for closure in asymptomatic subjects, most agree that all haemodynamically significant defects (in other words those with ratios of pulmonary-to-systemic flow greater than 2:1) should be repaired, even in the absence of symptoms. Surgery carries a low risk, with less than 1% operative mortality, provided the pulmonary vascular resistance is not significantly elevated (Kirklin and Barratt-Boyes, 1986). Closure may also be carried out by use of a variety of devices inserted at cardiac catheterization (Hellenbrand et al, 1990). These have now gone through an evolution in design from the early devices, which had problems such as strut fracture and embolization. New devices, such as the Amplatzer device, are relatively simple to insert. The attraction of closing such defects without open heart surgery is obvious (Chan et al, 1999; Dhillon et al, 1999).

LATE RESULTS

In a large study from the Mayo Clinic of patients undergoing surgical repair of an atrial septal defect between 1956 and 1960, late survival of patients undergoing operation before 24 years of age was not significantly different from that of an age- and sex-matched control population. Late survival in patients aged from 25 to 41 years was still good, but less than that of the control population, whereas repair after the age of 41 years was associated with significantly poorer late survival (Figure 72.7). The combination of older age at operation, and pulmonary hypertension, had an additive effect on late mortality (Murphy et al, 1990). In this, and other series, the propensity for atrial fibrillation and flutter increased as a function of age, both before and after operation (Brandenburg et al, 1983; Murphy et al, 1990). One fifth of late deaths were from stroke, and all occurred in patients with postoperative atrial fibrillation or flutter. These data support the current policy of repair at a preschool age, or as early as the diagnosis is made in those presenting as young adults. A separate study of patients who underwent closure of atrial septal defect between 60 and 78 years of age revealed a benefit in survival in patients discharged from hospital compared with historical controls without surgery matched for age and sex (St John Sutton et al, 1981). In very old patients, the indication for closure may be less clear, as additional cardiovascular disease increases the early morbidity and mortality of surgery. Long-term benefit is less easy to demonstrate. Pulmonary vascular disease may preclude surgery, but this is rare. Supraventricular arrhythmia is the main cause of late morbidity in patients who undergo closure as adults. As a result, more aggressive treatment has been recommended, including a modified Maze operation (Gatzoulis et al, 1999).

The near normal survival, and low morbidity, in patients undergoing repair within the first two decades of life have important implications for employment and insurance. Such patients should be encouraged to lead a normal life. Competitive sports should not be restricted in the absence of haemodynamic or electrophysiological sequals. Patients who have undergone repair in the third decade of life, or later, require regular surveillance. Although late survival is good, the development of supraventricular arrhythmia, and the risk of cerebrovascular accident, are of concern. Anticoagulation is indicated in patients with atrial fibrillation.

VENTRICULAR SEPTAL DEFECT ————————

Isolated ventricular septal defect, although one of the commonest congenital abnormalities in infants and children, is less frequent in adolescents and adults. Most patients with a haemodynamically significant defect will have undergone repair in childhood, and spontaneous

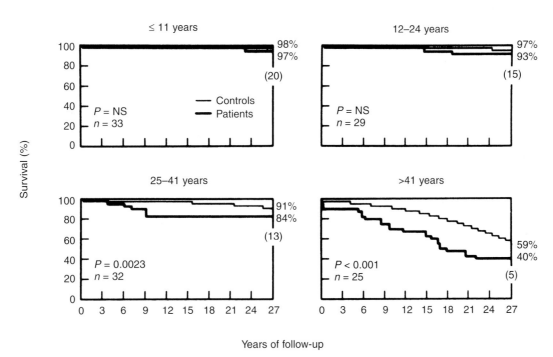

Figure 72.7. Acturial survival curves for patients after repair of atrial septal defect, grouped by age at operation. Survival is similar to that for age- and sex-matched controls in patients who were operated on at less that 25 years of age. Survival was significantly worse than control values, however, for those operated in later adult life.

decrease in size and closure is common for small or moderately sized perimembranous or muscular defects (Engle et al, 1987; Van Praagh et al, 1989). The spectrum of isolated defects seen in the adult is, therefore, limited to four groups of patients. The first is those with small restrictive defects that were either small to begin with or have partially closed. The second group includes the occasional patient with a moderately restrictive defect in whom the diagnosis has been overlooked, or the patient with a defect that has not been closed in childhood. The third group is those patients who have had their defects closed in childhood. The final group comprises patients with Eisenmenger's syndrome and a predominant right-to-left shunt with cyanosis (Wood, 1958). The last group needs to be distinguished from those who develop secondary infundibular pulmonary stenosis. This complication can also decrease the left-to-right shunt and may result in cyanosis with reversal of this shunt (Warnes et al, 1991b).

NATURAL HISTORY

The natural history of small restrictive ventricular septal defects is very favourable. Nevertheless, the risk of infective endocarditis persists, and lifelong prophylaxis is required. A subset of patients with perimembranous defects, or defects between the ventricular outlets, may develop prolapse of aortic valver leaflets and aortic regurgitation. This may be progressive and is often severe by the end of the second decade of life. As regurgitation increases, the ventricular septal defect may become 'closed' by the prolapsing leaflet. If ignored, the aortic valvar lesion may progress; however, the 'natural history' and indications for closure are still controversial (Tatsuno et al, 1973). These defects are associated with a high risk of infective endocarditis.

Severe and irreversible pulmonary vascular disease is a feature of older patients with non-restrictive and large defects. Eisenmenger's syndrome is compatible with survival into adult life, but the complications of right heart failure, paradoxical embolization and polycythaemia usually result in death by the third or fourth decade (Daliento et al, 1998). Occasionally, patients with ventricular septal defect and left-to-right shunts who did not develop pulmonary vascular disease may present in adolescence and young adult life with symptoms of fatigue, effort intolerance and respiratory infections.

MANAGEMENT

Patients with small ventricular septal defects are asymptomatic. They should be managed conservatively. Continued medical follow-up, however, is helpful to remind patients about the need for prophylaxis against infective endocarditis, and to minimize inappropriate discrimination during the search for employment and insurance. Ventricular septal defects associated with

aortic prolapse and regurgitation should be repaired, even when the shunt is small, in an effort to prevent progressive deterioration of the aortic valve (Trusler et al, 1992). Surgical repair is indicated in the rare adult with a significant left-to-right shunt, with a ratio of pulmonary to systemic flows greater than 2:1 and a low pulmonary vascular resistance.

Unfortunately, adults are still seen with a large ventricular septal defect and pulmonary vascular disease. Surgery may be attempted in those with borderline pulmonary vascular resistance, but the benefits are unpredictable as the pulmonary vascular disease may progress despite closure of the defect (Cartmill et al, 1966). Medical management, and eventual consideration for transplantation, are the only realistic options for patients with established pulmonary vascular disease.

LATE RESULTS

Late results of surgery are good, but life expectancy for the whole group is not normal (Figure 72.8). In a study of survivors from the Mayo Clinic undergoing surgery between 1956 and 1959, 30-year survival was 80%, compared with 97% in age- and sex-matched controls (Murphy et al, 1989). Only one quarter of patients were below 10 years of age at surgery, and their 30-year survival of 70% was substantially lower than the figure of 88% obtained in patients younger than 2 years at operation. Survival after 30 years was 83% for patients aged from 3 to 10 years at surgery. Older age at repair, and preoperative pulmonary vascular disease, were important predictors of late outcome. Postoperative conduction defects, especially right bundle branch block, are common; however, complete heart block, which was seen in the early surgical experience, is now rare. Late ventricular arrhythmia has been reported, as after repair of tetralogy of Fallot (Blake et al, 1982). The incidence of late sudden death, nonetheless, is extremely low. Prophylactic antiarrhythmic therapy in asymptomatic

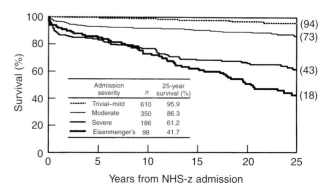

Figure 72.8. Actuarial survival curves for patients with ventricular septal defect followed in the Second Natural History Study of Congenital Heart Defects (NHS-2), according to admission severity. The numbers in parentheses indicate the number of patients remaining under observation 25 years after admission.

patients does not appear to be indicated. Certain ventricular septal defects can be closed by catheter devices, emphasizing the growing trend for collaboration between cardiologists and surgeons, especially in the management of complex defects.

In postoperative patients, the risk of late infective endocarditis is small providing the defect is completely closed. Antibiotic prophylaxis, however, is usually advised. Recommendations regarding physical activity and competitive sport require detailed evaluation. This may need to include exercise testing, cross-sectional echocardiography, and ambulatory electrocardiographic monitoring. The presence of abnormal left ventricular function, a more than trivial residual shunt, arrhythmia or any degree or pulmonary hypertension may mandate some restriction of physical activity.

PULMONARY STENOSIS

Isolated pulmonary valvar stenosis is a common lesion in adults and is typically characterized by a trifoliate valve with fused zones of apposition between the leaflets. Subvalvar stenosis caused by infundibular hypertrophy is usually a secondary phenomenon occurring in response to obstruction to right ventricular outflow, but it may occur as a rare isolated entity. Supravalvar or peripheral pulmonary arterial stenosis is also extremely uncommon as an isolated entity, but it may be associated with congenital rubella syndrome and with supravalvar aortic stenosis in William's syndrome.

NATURAL HISTORY

Prolonged survival into adult life is common and depends upon the severity of obstruction. In patients with severe stenosis, symptoms of right-sided failure increase with age owing to progressive obstruction and alteration in right ventricular compliance (Nugent et al, 1977). In the First Joint Study of the Natural History of Congenital Heart Disease, one-fifth of patients with severe stenosis aged between 2 and 11 years, and almost two fifths of those aged 12 to 21 years, were symptomatic (Nadas et al, 1977). Patients with mild or moderate stenosis, in contrast to those with aortic stenosis, rarely have symptoms when older than 2 years and rarely develop progressive obstruction.

MANAGEMENT

Patients with mild stenosis are asymptomatic. They require no intervention other than antibiotic prophylaxis against infective endocarditis. In patients with more severe stenosis, when the gradient between the right ventricle and pulmonary arteries is greater than 40 mm, intervention is warranted to reduce the severity even if the patient is asymptomatic.

Surgical valvotomy for isolated pulmonary stenosis has been successfully performed for over 40 years. Late results are excellent (Hayes et al, 1993). In a study from the Mayo Clinic of patients undergoing surgery between 1956 and 1957, late survival for those undergoing valvotomy was slightly worse than for a control population matched for age and sex (Figure 72.9) (Kopecky et al, 1988). Survival was similar to controls for patients undergoing surgery before the age of 21 years but significantly worse than normal in those having pulmonary valvotomy in adult life. Amongst patients undergoing surgery at an older age, late survival, although still good, was less than that for the control population. This effect of age on late outcome was independent of the use of ventriculotomy and outflow patches. Late functional results were excellent, and pulmonary regurgitation was well tolerated in the short and medium term. More important pulmonary regurgitation results when a pulmonary valvectomy or a transjunctional patch is required, as may be the case for a small or dysplastic valve. The long-term consequences of the regurgitation on the right ventricle and on functional capacity are not yet well documented but are likely to be of similar importance to the haemodynamics after repair of tetralogy of Fallot.

Surgical valvotomy is now rarely required because of the advent of balloon pulmonary valvotomy (Kan et al, 1982; Sullivan et al, 1985). This is the initial procedure of choice at all ages, even though most results thus far accumulated accrue from treatment of younger patients (McCrindle and Kan, 1991). In the largest series reported, of 822 patients in the Valvuloplasty and Angioplasty of Congenital Heart Abnormalities registry, balloon valvotomy was substantially less effective in patients with dysplastic valves (Mullins et al, 1990). Complications can occur, and intervention procedures should be confined to centres with experienced operators. It would appear that the excellent early results are maintained for at least 5 years, especially in older patients

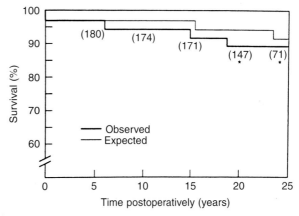

Figure 72.9. Long-term outcome of perioperative survivors following surgical repair of isolated pulmonary stenosis, and expected survival of an age- and sex-matched control population. Difference between expected and observed $P < 0.002$.

(Masura et al, 1993). The late effects of pulmonary regurgitation resulting from the use of large balloons remain to be determined, as after surgical relief.

The risk of infective endocarditis is less in patients with mild pulmonary stenosis, or in those with small gradients after surgical or balloon valvotomy. Long-term follow-up is recommended to evaluate not only gradients across the right ventricular outflow tract but also pulmonary regurgitation, right ventricular function and exercise performance. In patients with good relief of pulmonary stenosis, no restriction of physical activities is required. In those with moderate residual obstruction, or right ventricular dysfunction, exercise should be reduced as appropriate, or a further attempt should be considered to relieve the obstruction.

AORTIC STENOSIS

Aortic stenosis is a common abnormality amongst adults with congenital cardiac disease. It may be an isolated defect, or it may be associated with other lesions such as aortic coarctation or ventricular septal defect. It is usually found in the setting of a valve with two leaflets, seen in 1 to 2% of the overall adult population. This is three to four times more common in males than in females (Friedman and Johnson, 1987).

NATURAL HISTORY

The natural history of congenital aortic valvar stenosis is variable in adults but is characterized by progressive obstruction (Pellikka et al, 1990; Chizner et al, 1980; Beppu et al, 1993). By the age of 45 years, approximately half of all patients with bicuspid valves have some degree of narrowing (Mills et al, 1978). Slowly progressive aortic regurgitation may occur in young adulthood, but sudden deterioration is rare except as a sequel to infection (Donofrio et al, 1992).

MANAGEMENT

The development of symptoms, such as angina, exertional dyspnoea and syncope, mandates prompt intervention, either by surgery or balloon dilation. In asymptomatic younger individuals, the documentation of severe aortic stenosis, with valvar area of less than 1.0 cm² is an indication for intervention (Cohen et al, 1972). Milder aortic stenosis, with valvar area of more than 1.5 cm², or a gradient lower than 50 mmHg with good left ventricular function, warrants careful serial evaluation.

Surgery in the young adult with congenital aortic stenosis must be considered as palliative (Kugelmeier et al, 1982; Keane et al, 1996). In the absence of calcification, aortic valvotomy is the procedure of choice. Perioperative mortality in adolescents and adults is

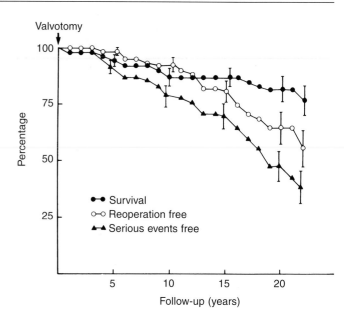

Figure 72.10. These three actuarial survival curves show the percentage of patients remaining free of reoperation and serious events in a study of 59 patients who underwent aortic valvotomy. Serious events included death, reoperation and endocarditis. The bars represent standard errors.

extremely low, and late survival is excellent. Up to half of the patients, however, will require reoperation over the following 25 years (Figure 72.10) (Presbitero et al, 1982; Heish et al, 1986). Balloon valvotomy is an important alternative approach for those with non-calcified valves. Its safety and efficacy are well documented, and restenosis is less of a problem than in patients with degenerative aortic stenosis (Sholler et al, 1988; Fields et al, 1989; Borghi et al, 1999). Severe aortic regurgitation requiring early surgical management is a complication in a small number of patients (Lock et al, 1991). Balloon valvotomy, however, is unlikely to be applicable to all patients because of the variable pathology of the aortic valve. It is difficult to compare the results of surgical and balloon valvotomy, as long-term follow-up data for the catheter technique are not yet available, and controlled trials have not been, and may never be, undertaken. Medical follow-up of patients who have undergone surgical or balloon valvotomy should focus on the development of restenosis, the severity and progression of aortic regurgitation and the constant hazard of infective endocarditis. Echocardiography has facilitated serial evaluation of gradients, valvar areas, dimension of the cardiac chambers and ventricular mass.

Replacement is the only option for those with valves unsuitable for valvotomy, such as those with significant calcification and regurgitation. The age, sex and size of the patient are major factors determining selection of the prosthesis, as are individual characteristics that determine the safety of anticoagulation, such as compliance and the desire for future pregnancies.

Insertion of the pulmonary autograft by means of the Ross procedure may be the operation of choice in many young adults, particularly in women of childbearing age (Chambers et al, 1997; Oswalt et al, 1999). Surgical mortality has fallen since its introduction, and results in the medium term are excellent. It is not possible, however, based on current available evidence, to determine the precise indications and timing of the Ross operation in the population of adolescents and young adults with congenitally stenotic aortic valves.

The acceptable level of physical activity in patients with aortic stenosis remains very controversial. It is debatable whether any patient who has had significant obstruction should be allowed to participate in competitive sport. We consider a residual gradient of greater than 50 mmHg, or persistent left ventricular hypertrophy, as contraindications (Cullen et al, 1991). Before sanctioning strenuous activity, evaluation should include electrocardiographic monitoring and maximal exercise testing.

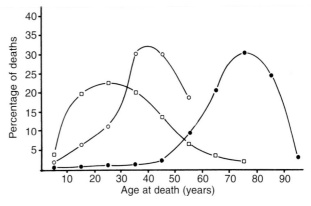

Figure 72.11. These curves illustrate the distribution of death by age in subjects with aortic coarctation that has remained unoperated (□), subjects who have undergone coarctation repair (○) and in a control population (●). In this series, most subjects were repaired in older childhood or young adult life.

AORTIC COARCTATION

Although aortic coarctation is a congenital malformation, it may be diagnosed in adolescence or adult life. Most commonly, coarctation diagnosed in older ages is discovered in asymptomatic patients in whom a routine physical examination has disclosed hypertension in the arms. In such cases, there are frequently large collateral arteries and/or aortic dilation proximal and distal to the narrowed segment.

NATURAL HISTORY

Many patients with undetected coarctation will remain free of symptoms until adolescence or early childhood. Symptoms, such as headaches related to hypertension, leg fatigue, or cramps may then develop. Endocarditis, or a major catastrophic event such as a cerebrovascular accident or rupture of the aorta, is occasionally the first recognized problem. An aortic valve with two leaflets is found in between one quarter and half of patients with coarctation. These abnormal valves have a recognized tendency to calcify in early or middle adult life, producing aortic stenosis. Calcific aortic stenosis may be the presenting condition, with subsequent investigation disclosing an additional aortic coarctation. In the era antedating surgical intervention, approximately half the patients with coarctation died within their first three decades, and three quarters were dead by the age of 50 (Figure 72.11) (Campbell, 1970b). Death was most frequently caused by one of the complications of hypertension, such as stroke or aortic dissection, but other causes included endocarditis or endarteritis and congestive heart failure.

MANAGEMENT

Coarctation may infrequently be sufficiently mild not to justify intervention. In the great majority of patients,

however, symptoms or the presence of significant hypertension in the upper body will mandate surgical repair. On occasion, an asymptomatic adolescent or adult will demonstrate severe coarctation but will be normotensive at rest because of well-developed collateral circulation around the site of coarctation. Such patients, nonetheless, have inappropriate hypertension with exercise and should be repaired. Repair should be undertaken soon after diagnosis, as there is evidence that residual hypertension, and late complications, are directly related to age at the time of repair (Cohen et al, 1989).

Surgery for coarctation has been available for over 50 years (Gross and Hufnagel, 1945). Various techniques have been used, including end-to-end anastomosis, patch grafting and the use of the subclavian flap technique (Waldhausen et al, 1981). Aneurysmal or atherosclerotic changes in the aorta found in adolescents or adults may occasionally require the use of an interposition prosthetic graft. Surgery is performed without cardiopulmonary bypass, and the risk of death from operation is small. Serious morbidity is rare, but occasionally paraplegia can occur secondary to ischaemia of the spinal cord (Keen, 1987). In a multicentric review, the incidence of such complications after repair of coarctation was less than 0.5% (Brewer et al, 1972). Some patients require antihypertensive medication for either transient or persistent postoperative hypertension. Balloon angioplasty of coarctation was first reported in 1983, but its role in treating native lesions remains controversial (Sperling et al, 1983). Immediate reduction of the degree of obstruction is usually possible but is achieved at the price of tearing both the aortic intima and media (Wren et al, 1987). Late formation of aneurysms, presumably secondary to the disruption of the media, has been observed (Ritter, 1989). Currently, most centres do not perform balloon angioplasty alone as the primary procedure for coarctation, even in the adolescent or adult. Instead, the technique is reserved for recoarctation, where it appears to have a much clearer role (Redington, 1998). The prevention of restenosis and support of the aortic wall by implantation of a stent may resolve some of the problems. Preliminary data in adults suggest that stenting may have a role, although clearly it is not a panacea (Bulbul et al, 1996; Magee et al, 1999).

LATE RESULTS

The Mayo Clinic has published late results of a large series of patients undergoing surgery between 1946 and 1981 (Cohen et al, 1989). Median age at operation was 16 years, with one tenth of patients aged over 35 years. Although survival was good, at 91% at 10 years and 72% at 30 years, the mean age at death was 38 years, confirming other reports that life expectancy is reduced even after repair. In this, and other, series reporting long-term follow-up, the most common cause of death was premature coronary arterial disease with secondary myocardial infarction (Maron et al, 1973; Presbitero et al, 1987). Other causes of death included congestive heart failure, stroke and ruptured aortic aneurysm. Age at operation was an important prognostic factor. The older the patient, the greater the probability of premature death. The duration of preoperative obstruction and hypertension, therefore, is important in the aetiology of arterial disease and subsequent cardiovascular events.

The incidence of recoarctation is low when surgical repairs have been performed after infancy, irrespective of technique, but surgery may be required in later years for associated abnormalities, such as aortic valvar disease. The majority of survivors are asymptomatic, but there is a high incidence of later hypertension, even in those who activate a satisfactory early postoperative fall in blood pressure and good relief of obstruction. Only one third of the patients followed-up by Presbitero et al (1987) were normotensive 30 years after repair, and one quarter were significantly hypertensive. Long-term surveillance of blood pressure, both at rest and on exercise, is, therefore, important. It is anticipated, however, that the incidence of late hypertension will decline in the years ahead, as most patients are now diagnosed and repaired during infancy or early childhood, but this remains to be demonstrated.

TETRALOGY OF FALLOT

Tetralogy of Fallot is the most common form of cyanotic congenital heart disease seen in the adult. The adult with unoperated tetralogy has fortunately become a rarity, since the overwhelming majority of patients will have undergone palliation, or more usually repair, in childhood. From an anatomical and pathophysiological standpoint, the manifestations of tetralogy of Fallot are similar at all ages, although hypercyanotic spells, often seen in infants and young children, are rare in adults. The devel-

opment of systemic hypertension with age is a problem, as this increases the afterload to both ventricles (Abraham et al, 1979). Although flow of blood to the lungs may improve, this occurs at the expense of right ventricular failure. Acquired calcific aortic stenosis has similar effects. Aortic regurgitation may occur as a result of prolapse of the valvar leaflets in those patients who have subarterial defects. If exacerbated by infective endocarditis, the burden of volume overload will be transmitted to both ventricles. The development of chronic obstructive lung disease may place the adult with tetralogy of Fallot at particular risk.

NATURAL HISTORY

Survival into the seventh decade is described (Phadke et al, 1977), but the natural history without surgery, which is determined by the severity of obstruction of the right ventricular outflow tract and the state of the pulmonary vasculature, is poor. Only one-quarter of patients reach the age of 10 years, one-tenth are alive at 20 years, just over one-twentieth at age 30 years and only 3% at 40 years (Bertranou et al, 1978). Complications of non-restrictive right-to-left shunting and polycythaemia, which include stroke and cerebral abscess, are common. These prove fatal in many instances. Patients are at continuing risk of infective endocarditis, and the development of congenital heart failure in adolescence or early adult life is a major cause of death, as is arrhythmia. Myocardial fibrosis resulting from long-standing pressure overload on the right ventricle and hypoxaemia are postulated predisposing factors (Deanfield et al, 1983). The clinical significance of arrhythmia may be determined by electromechanical associations in the right ventricle, and in particular by the consequence of pulmonary regurgitation (Gatzoulis et al, 1995a). Prior palliative surgery with a Waterston or Potts shunt can lead to the late development of pulmonary vascular disease or important distortions of the pulmonary arteries (Katz et al, 1982).

MANAGEMENT

The focus of medical treatment in patients who have not undergone surgery is on the management of an elevated haematocrit, bleeding disorders and the abnormal metabolism of uric acid, which occurs in all cyanotic patients. Repair is indicated in all suitable patients, with the principles and techniques not being significantly different in adults from those in children (Figure 72.12) (Kirklin and Barratt-Boyes, 1986). Most adults are suitable for complete repair, but the occasional patient with small pulmonary arteries may require a palliative procedure. In patients with an anomalous origin of the left anterior descending from the right coronary artery, a conduit may need to be placed between the right ventricle and the pulmonary trunk.

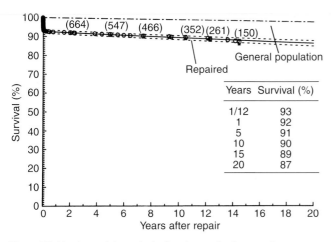

Figure 72.12. Actuarial survival of patients who have undergone repair of tetralogy of Fallot, with time 0 being the day of operation. Numbers refer to patients in follow-up.

LATE RESULTS

Late survival is excellent, even in patients who underwent repair during the very early years of open heart surgery (Figure 72.12) (Kirklin and Barratt-Boyes, 1986). Surgery, however, cannot be considered 'curative', as survival even in excellent series is slightly but significantly worse than for a matched control population (Murphy et al, 1993). At 30 years, over three quarters of an initial cohort of patients submitted to surgery between 1954 and 1960 were alive, including one patient who was at 45 years of age at the time of operation (Lillehei et al, 1986). The risk factors for an adverse late outcome include older age at surgery, preoperative congestive heart failure, a previous Potts shunt, persistent right ventricular systolic hypertension and a residual ventricular septal defect (Katz et al, 1982; Murphy et al, 1993). The risk of arrhythmia and late sudden death following repair

of tetralogy of Fallot has already been discussed. Ventricular failure owing to right ventricular pressure and volume overload or left ventricular volume overload are other important causes of late mortality in older patients.

The late functional outcome is excellent for the majority of patients. Most lead normal lives, but results appear to be better in those who have undergone surgery at a younger age (Wennevold et al, 1982). Persistent or recurrent symptoms are usually the result of pulmonary regurgitation, incomplete relief of right ventricular systolic hypertension or incomplete closure of the ventricular septal defect. These problems may require reoperation (Finck et al, 1988). An increasing number of patients who had transannular patch repair of tetralogy of Fallot require reoperations for symptomatic long-term pulmonary regurgitation. Homograft reconstruction of the right ventricular outflow tract will reduce right ventricular dilation and symptoms (d'Udekem et al, 1998)

Objective testing has emphasized the effects of older age at operation on subsequent exercise performance. This is essentially normal in children repaired before the age of 5 years but is usually impaired when surgery is undertaken in adolescence or adulthood (Bjarke, 1975). Before unrestricted physical activity can be recommended after repair of tetralogy of Fallot, careful evaluation, including cross-sectional echocardiography, electrocardiographic monitoring and exercise testing, should be undertaken. If surgery was performed at a young age, right and left ventricular size and function are normal, there is no significant residual ventricular septal defect or obstruction in the right ventricular outflow tract, and no worrisome arrhythmia, then normal activity including competitive sport seems reasonable. In others who do not fulfil these criterions, the degree to which physical activity should be restricted requires judgment, and the decision must be tailored to the individual.

COMPLETE TRANSPOSITION

Most adult survivors with complete transposition will have undergone an intra-atrial repair following the Mustard or Senning techniques. Approximately half will have had associated anomalies, such as ventricular septal defect in one-third, obstruction of the left ventricular outflow tract in one-tenth, a ventricular septal defect combined with obstruction in the left ventricular outflow tract in another tenth and, more rarely, aortic coarctation or atrioventricular valvar anomalies (Keith et al, 1978).

NATURAL HISTORY

Without treatment, actuarial survival at 1 month is 55% and is less than 10% at 1 year (Keith et al, 1953; Leibman et al, 1969). Death is usually from profound hypoxaemia. In those with a large ventricular septal

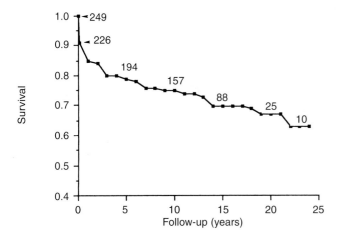

Figure 72.13. The actuarial survival of 249 patients who underwent Mustard operation for complete transposition with intact ventricular septum, including hospital deaths (time 0 being the day of Mustard operation). Numbers refer to the patients in follow-up.

defect, severe hypoxaemia is rare, but patients do badly as a result of heart failure from excessive pulmonary flow and early pulmonary vascular disease (Senning, 1959). Occasionally, prolonged survival into adult life may occur when a large communication between the pulmonary and systemic circulations is associated with Eisenmenger's syndrome, or when the combination of a ventricular septal defect with obstruction of the left ventricular outflow tract has resulted in well-balanced haemodynamics.

MANAGEMENT

In the late 1950s and early 1960s, the Senning and Mustard operations involving atrial redirection of the systemic and pulmonary venous returns were introduced. These operations transformed the outlook for patients. The age at surgery was gradually reduced to 3–12 months, and early mortality was much less than 10% in experienced centres. Survival into adult life was usual (Figure 72.13), and long-term follow-up for both procedures is now available. Outcome after the Senning operations appears better largely because of the lower incidence of baffle obstruction. Late problems, nonetheless, are now recognized after both procedures, with sudden death, arrhythmia, tricuspid regurgitation and morphologically right ventricular dysfunction being the major concerns (Deanfield, 1999). These have led to the general acceptance of the arterial switch procedure as the operation of choice (Jatene et al, 1975). The other common operation that has resulted in survival to adulthood is the repair activated by insertion of a conduit in those with a ventricular septal defect and obstruction of the left ventricular outflow tract (Rastelli et al, 1969). Long-term results are reasonable, but further surgery to replace the extracardiac conduit in adolescent and adult life is inevitable (Vouhe et al, 1992).

LATE RESULTS

Three specific problems occurring after atrial redirection have caused concern in long-term follow-up. These are arrhythmia (Figures 72.14 and 72.15), obstruction of the venous pathways and systemic ventricular dysfunction. Loss of sinus rhythm is progressive and is found in over half the adults who have had either a Mustard or a Senning operation (Flinn et al, 1984). In most cases, this is asymptomatic, but occasionally marked bradycardia may necessitate insertion of a pacemaker. There appears, however, to be no relation between loss of sinus rhythm and risk of sudden death (Deanfield et al, 1988). Most asymptomatic patients should not, therefore, require pacing. It has been argued that bradycardia may compromise right ventricular function in the long term, but this has not been proven. More worrying is the development of atrial flutter. This arrhythmia may have profound haemodynamic consequences. It is a risk factor for

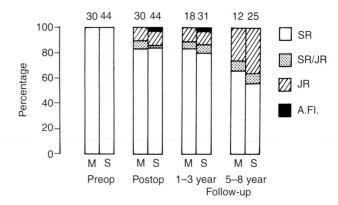

Figure 72.14. Cardiac rhythm on serial 24-hour Holter monitoring after Mustard (M) or Senning (S) operation for simple transposition of the great arteries. There is a decrease in sinus rhythm at late follow-up. A. Fl., atrial flutter; JR, junctional rhythm; SR, sinus rhythm; Preop, before operation; Postop, after operation.

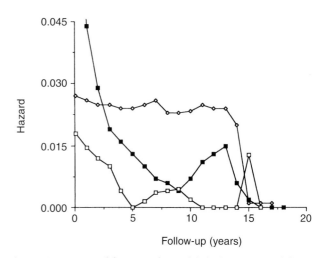

Figure 72.15. Hazard functions for nodal rhythm (◇), atrial flutter (□) and death (■). The risk for nodal rhythm is constant at 2.4% per year up to 15 years. The risk of both atrial flutter and death is bimodal.

sudden death, especially in the presence of obstructed venous pathways, or right ventricular dysfunction (Gewillig et al, 1991). Deteriorating performance of the morphologically right ventricle supporting the systemic circulation has been reported in some patients, but the precise aetiology of this problem remains unclear (Graham et al, 1975; Hagler et al, 1979). It is not yet known whether ventricular performance will deteriorate in the majority of patients and, if so, over what period (Graham et al, 1975). Current evidence indicates that cardiac performance may be limited not by systolic dysfunction of the morphologically right ventricle but rather by abnormal atrioventricular coupling, with restriction in ventricular preload to both ventricles (Redington, 1998). This has implications for assessment during follow-up, particularly in patients in whom atrial tachyarrhythmias have developed.

As most patients who have undergone intra-atrial repair are well, clinical follow-up is directed largely at attempts to stratify risk for sudden death. This is currently difficult. Late death cannot be predicted merely from serial electrocardiograms or ambulatory monitoring (Deanfield et al, 1988). This underscores the need for a more sophisticated approach. This should involve both electrophysiological and haemodynamic assessments, evaluation of cardiac performance on exercise and careful assessment of the systemic and pulmonary venous pathways. Transoesophageal echocardiography appears useful in this situation (Stumper et al, 1992). Treatment of unsuspected baffle obstruction by balloon dilation and stenting may then improve cardiac function. Cardiac transplantation should be considered in the patient who has severe right ventricular failure. An alternative approach has been to band the pulmonary trunk as preparation for conversion of the atrial repair to an arterial switch (Mee, 1986). The indications for this approach are uncertain. Current studies indicate that retraining of the left ventricle is less successful in older patients, and these constitute precisely the group who have clinical problems (Helvind et al, 1998).

The information so far available after the arterial switch operation suggests that late electrophysiological problems may be much less prevalent (Cochrane et al, 1993). The morphologically left ventricle, nonetheless, is at risk from the surgical procedure itself. This can potentially induce myocardial ischaemia through coronary arterial distortion or result in neo-aortic regurgitation. Furthermore, late problems clearly occur with the coronary arteries and may be progressive (Bonhoeffer et al, 1997). Early results are encouraging, although only a few patients have yet reached adult life (Colan et al, 1988).

CONGENITALLY CORRECTED TRANSPOSITION

NATURAL HISTORY

In a small proportion of patients, approximately one-tenth in one reported series but this is probably an underestimate, there are no associated cardiac defects (Allwork et al, 1976; Lundstrom et al, 1990). Such individuals are asymptomatic and may survive undiagnosed until adult life. The only specific abnormality in these patients is the tendency to develop atrioventricular block. This may be present from birth (Friedberg and Nades, 1970) and develops in about 2% of patients per year (Huhta et al, 1983). It is not clear whether the systemic morphologically right ventricle in patients with corrected transposition can maintain its normal function over extended periods, and whether this has an impact on outcome, as few studies have examined enough patients over a long enough period. The majority of patients have a ventricular septal defect and/or pulmonary stenosis (Allwork

et al, 1976). Abnormalities of the morphologically tricuspid valve, such as Ebstein's malformation, are common. These defects influence both the natural history and the optimal surgical strategy (Connelly et al, 1996).

MANAGEMENT

Indications for surgery differ from those in patients with concordant segmental connections because of the potential for the operation to aggravate systemic ventricular dysfunction, systemic atrioventricular valvar incompetence or conduction problems. Palliative surgery is sometimes performed in childhood, as definitive repair may involve insertion of an extracardiac conduit. These who have required a conduit or a prosthetic atrioventricular valve inserted in childhood inevitably require reoperation. Some patients may have a well-balanced circulation and survive to adult life without operation.

In patients with morphologically right ventricular failure and tricuspid regurgitation, banding of the pulmonary trunk, with resulting septal shift and improved left and right ventricular interaction, may produce marked improvement both in symptoms and haemodynamics. Appreciation of potential problems over the long term associated with a morphologically right ventricle supporting the systemic circulation have led to development of the 'double switch' approach in childhood (Connelly et al, 1996; Imai, 1997; Karl et al, 1997).

LATE RESULTS

Long-term follow-up is mandatory for assessment of ventricular function, especially in patients whose repair involved insertion of an extracardiac conduit, prosthetic atrioventricular valve and/or a pacemaker. Atrial arrhythmias are common in postoperative patients, particularly those with tricuspid regurgitation. Some patients in whom the repair has failed need to be considered for transplantation. Long-term results of the 'double switch' option are not yet available (Connelly et al, 1996).

EBSTEIN'S MALFORMATION OF THE TRICUSPID VALVE

Ebstein's malformation is characterized by displacement of the proximal hingepoints of the tricuspid valve from the atrioventricular junction into the right ventricle. The severity of the displacement is variable; this accounts for the broad clinical spectrum, from severe disease causing fetal or neonatal death to mild disease compatible with natural survival as late as the eighth decade of life (Celermajer et al, 1992). Ebstein's malformation is an uncommon defect, but it is disproportionately represented in the adult population with congenital cardiac disease because of its relatively favourable natural history.

NATURAL HISTORY

Diagnosis of Ebstein's malformation has become much easier with the advent of cross-sectional echocardiography. This has altered the understanding of the natural history. For example, in a large collaborative study reported in 1974, less than one tenth of patients included were younger than 1 year of age (Watson, 1974). Neonates presenting with Ebstein's malformation comprise, not surprisingly, the worst end of the spectrum. They have a severe anatomical defect and a high incidence of associated abnormalities, particularly obstruction of the right ventricular outflow tract. Their outcome is poor and is predictable from the echocardiographic findings (Celermajer et al, 1992). Those who survive the neonatal period with or without surgery may live into adult life, although there is a continued morbidity and mortality throughout childhood. Many other patients are clinically well, or only minimally symptomatic, in childhood. They do not present until adolescence or adult life. Ebstein's malformation is often associated with ventricular pre-excitation (Lev et al, 1995). Approximately one-quarter of adults will have symptomatic arrhythmias, which may be difficult to treat and may result in sudden death (Till et al, 1992). Symptoms and signs, when they develop, also include cyanosis owing to right-to-left shunting at atrial level, and dyspnoea secondary to heart failure. Progressive heart failure may be related not just to right-sided problems but also to left ventricular abnormalities. Excessive fibrosis has been reported in the left ventricle (Celermajer et al, 1992), and left ventricular dysfunction may be induced on exercise (Saxena et al, 1991).

MANAGEMENT

Outcome is poor in patients with increasing cyanosis, congestive cardiac failure, uncontrolled arrhythmias and in those in the more severe functional grades defined by the New York Heart Association. These features should, therefore, be taken as indications for surgery (Danielson et al, 1992). In their absence, medical follow-up is appropriate as the risk is low. Objective assessment of effort tolerance by stress testing and monitoring of cardiac rhythm and size, nonetheless, is advisable.

Surgery may consist of repair or replacement of the tricuspid valve, together with closure of the atrial septal defect to prevent cyanosis (Danielson et al, 1992). In the occasional patient, the atrial septal defect may be responsible for a left-to-right shunt and can be closed as the only procedure. In others, the non-atrialized right ventricle may be too small for a biventricular repair. A cavopulmonary circulation may then be the only surgical option.

The results of surgery are affected by the presence of arrhythmias (Smith et al, 1982; Gentles et al, 1992). Uncontrolled preoperative supraventricular arrhythmia is a risk factor for early postoperative rhythm problems, which may have serious haemodynamic consequences (Till et al, 1992). It is usually recommended that division of an accessory electrophysiological pathway be performed at the time of tricuspid valvar surgery, or it should be ablated at catheterization prior to surgery. The pathways are usually in the region posterior to the septum or in the right free wall. They may be multiple.

COMPLEX LESIONS

A number of complex malformations involve structural abnormalities that preclude the creation of a biventricular circulation. This group of patients includes those with double inlet ventricle, absent right or left atrioventricular connection, some cases of pulmonary atresia with intact ventricular septum, and those with hypoplastic left or right ventricles. The natural history of these defects is highly variable and depends to a large extent on the impact of the associated defects.

NATURAL HISTORY

Despite the complex morphological defects, prolonged natural survival is sometimes seen if the physiology is well balanced. The patients with double inlet left ventricle, discordant ventriculo-arterial connections and pulmonary stenosis with balanced pulmonary flow do best, with predicted actuarial survival of 96% at 1 year and 91% at 10 years. Such patients may continue to well past the third decade of life without intervention (Franklin et al, 1991).

For most patients with complex malformations, however, prolonged survival into adult life is only possible with one or more palliative operations, such as construction of systemic-to-pulmonary shunts, Glenn shunts, banding of the pulmonary trunk, relief of systemic outflow obstruction or a Fontan-type procedure (Driscoll et al, 1992; Gatzoulis et al, 2000). With palliative surgery alone, clinical deterioration usually begins in the second decade of life and is often a result of progressive ventricular dysfunction and/or atrioventricular valvar regurgitation (LaCorte et al, 1975; Moodie et al, 1984).

MANAGEMENT

The goals of management during childhood are often to maintain suitable anatomy and physiology for later conversion to a Fontan-type circulation. A number of modifications of Fontan's original operation (Fontan and Baudet, 1971) have been introduced, including the total cavopulmonary connection (de Leval et al, 1988) and 'fenestration' of the Fontan connection, with a defect being created between the right and left atriums to decompress the systemic venous atrium (Bridges et al, 1991; Laks et al, 1991). Operative risk, and postoperative status, are largely dependent on the suitability of the individual patient (Choussat et al, 1978). Most important features are a low pulmonary vascular resistance and adequate ventricular function, both systolic and diastolic (Gewillig et al, 1990b). Careful preoperative haemo-dynamic assessment is vital to optimize selection for surgery, and reported operative risks vary considerably between institutions.

LATE RESULTS

The early and medium-term results of the successful Fontan operation are excellent when compared with the preoperative status of the patients (Figures 72.16 and 72.17). Improvement in arterial saturation and exercise tolerance have been confirmed by objective testing (Fontan et al, 1983; Driscoll et al, 1992; Driscoll and Durongpisitkul, 1999). The patients with the best haemo-dynamics can perform well, achieving submaximal levels of exercise equivalent to most normal daily activities (Figure 72.18) (Gewillig et al, 1990a; Rosenthal et al, 1995).

Less encouraging data are now emerging over the longer term. An analysis of 334 patients revealed a pre-mature decline in survival and functional status, and a late rise in hazard for which no risk factors could be identified other than the Fontan circulation itself (Fontan et al, 1990). Late problems include supraventricular arrhythmia, thrombus in the atriums, protein-losing enteropathy and declining ventricular function (Matsuda et al, 1987; Driscoll et al, 1992). Another concern is the effect of non-pulsatile pulmonary flow favouring the development of pulmonary arterio-venous malform-ations, as seen after the Glenn anastomosis (Mathur and Glenn, 1973; Mainwaring et al, 1994).

The recently introduced surgical modifications to the Fontan procedure may improve both early and late

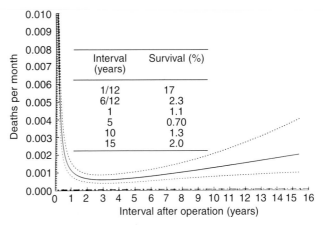

Figure 72.17. The hazard function for death after the 'perfect' Fontan operation. The dashed line shows the survival of age and sex-matched controls, and the dotted lines show 70% confidence intervals.

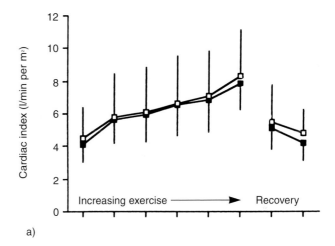

a)

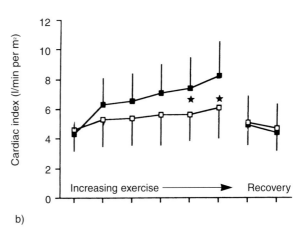

b)

Figure 72.18. Changes in cardiac index with increasing exercise and then on recovery in patients who have undergone the Fontan procedure. In this study, 42 patients underwent graded supine bicycle exercise tests and had serial measurement of cardiac index performed. (a) The 10 best performers (□) were compared with 10 age-matched control subjects (■) and there was no difference found in the cardiac index. (b) In contrast, the worst 10 subjects (□) had significantly lower rise in cardiac index at higher workloads compared with control subjects (■) (*P <0.05).

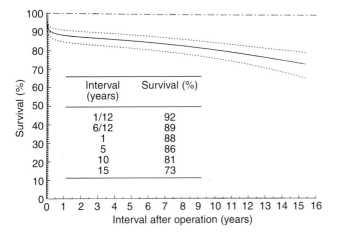

Figure 72.16. Actuarial survival curve showing predicted survival after a 'perfect' Fontan operation. The dashed line represents the survival of age- and sex-matched controls. The dotted lines indicate 70% confidence intervals.

haemodynamics and the functional results. Perforation of the patch at surgery can be performed safely, and with good outcome over the medium term (Bridges et al, 1992). Such holes may be closed later with a device inserted at catheterization if this is required. Data also suggest that a total cavopulmonary connection may result in improved flow and energy characteristics compared with the standard atriopulmonary connection. Fewer early supraventricular arrhythmias have been shown in one prospective study (Balaji et al, 1991).

Many of these young adults will have limited exercise tolerance, difficulty with obtaining employment and insurance and, often, important psychosocial problems. They present some of the greatest challenges. Several will eventually become candidates for heart transplantation.

RARE CONDITIONS WITH SURVIVAL INTO ADULT LIFE

A wide variety of other lesions may present to the clinic. Unoperated patients may be seen with subaortic stenosis, partially anomalous pulmonary venous connection, coronary arterial fistulas or congenitally complete heart block. Their management is similar to children with the same lesions. Postoperative patients may present with haemodynamic or electrophysiological problems late after surgery, sometimes during pregnancy. Examples include progressive left atrioventricular valvar regurgitation after repair of atrioventricular septal defect. This may require afterload reduction and/or valvar replacement. Palpitations caused by atrial fibrillation or flutter may become apparent later after repair of Ebstein's malformation. These should be investigated and managed according to the principles outlined above. Accurate definition of the cardiac anatomy is always essential.

WHO SHOULD LOOK AFTER THESE PATIENTS?

There is a major gap in care when children with heart disease become adolescents (Deanfield and Cullen, 2000). Many leave the care of a children's hospital with no arrangement for specialized follow-up. Which doctors should look after them? What training should these doctors have? In what setting should inpatient care take place? What do the patients themselves require? There are no easy answers to these questions. On the one hand, paediatric cardiologists are well versed in the problems created by congenital cardiac disease but are not trained in adult medicine. Adolescents or young adults may acquire cardiac problems, such as hypertension or coronary arterial disease, or extracardiac problems secondary to long-standing cyanosis. Paediatricians may be uncomfortable treating these entities. Furthermore, there may be political or financial reasons why adolescents and young

adults may not be allowed treatment in the setting of a children's hospital. The patients themselves may not wish the childhood image of the disease to be perpetuated by staying under the care of a paediatrician and may be anxious to shed their parental surveillance. The nursing staff, and even the size of the beds, may not be geared to accommodating an infant and an adult on the same ward.

On the other hand, most adult cardiologists have little or no training in congenital cardiac disease. Adult cardiologists treat large numbers of patients with ischaemic, hypertensive or valvar problems. They may feel inadequately prepared to deal with the very different problem of young adults with complex congenital cardiac malformations. The adolescents themselves may not wish to share a ward with much older people with degenerative or terminal problems. If an adolescent is treated at an adult hospital, this often involves separation from the parents. This may be difficult, especially for parents who have been very involved with the physical illness of their offspring as a child. At what age do parents stop attending consultations with their child, and who decides this? Many of these decisions must be made according to individual circumstances. Hard and fast rules based on a chronological 'cut-off point', determining the time at which a child becomes an adult, are unsuitable. The time of transfer must be as flexible as possible. The medical community needs to come to terms with the concept of adolescence and transitional care, rather than the sharp cut-off between child and adult on which provisions are currently based.

Different approaches to this problem can be found around the world. At some centres, patients with congenital cardiac disease stay at the children's hospital for as long as they live, even into the geriatric phase of life. Because of the increased numbers of young adults with congenital cardiac disease, this practice is not advisable. Specialized medical facilities for this new category of patients have now been established (Somerville et al, 1991). Patients enter these programmes when they are judged to have reached appropriate psychological and physical maturity. In many centres, unfortunately, children with cardiac disease are discharged from the children's hospital in mid-adolescence, and no organized follow-up is available for them. Many adolescents are happy to be free of medical and parental surveillance. They may 'disappear' for many years, only to reappear several years later when serious symptoms arise.

Progress in paediatric cardiology and surgery has produced a new population of adults with congenital cardiac disease who have complex medical and psychosocial needs. It is no longer sufficient to assess results of such disease in terms of survival or follow-up during childhood. A new type of cardiologist is required who can deal with both the underlying congenital defect and the problems of adulthood. The establishment of specialized centres, with inpatient and outpatient facilities for diagnosis and treatment of cardiac and non-cardiac problems, will enable training of the necessary group of cardiologists, surgeons and allied health professionals, as well as facilitating research. Routine referrals to such centres will result in a high level of care and will give each adult with congenital cardiac disease the best chance of achieving his or her full potential.

REFERENCES

Abraham K A, Cherian G, Rao V D, Sukumar I P, Krishnaswami S, John S 1979 Tetralogy of Fallot in adults: a report on 147 patients. American Journal of Medicine 66: 811–816

Ad-hoc Working Party of the American Heart Association 1998 Diagnosis and management of infective endocarditis and its complications. Circulation 98: 2936–2948

Allan L D, Crawford D C, Chita S K, Anderson R H, Tynan M J 1986 Familial recurrence of congenital heart disease in a prospective series of mothers referred for fetal echocardiography. American Journal of Cardiology 58: 334–337

Allan L D, Santos R, Pexieder T 1997 Anatomical and echocardiographic correlates of normal cardiac morphology in the late first trimester fetus. Heart 77: 68–72

Allen H D, Gersony W M, Taubert K A 1992 Insurability of the adolescent and young adult with heart disease. Circulation 86: 703–710

Allwork S P, Bentall H H, Becker A D et al 1976 Congenitally corrected transposition of the great arteries: morphologic study of 32 cases. American Journal of Cardiology 38: 910–923

Ammesh W H, Connolly H M, Abel M D, Warnes C A 1999 Non cardiac surgery in Eisenmenger syndrome. Journal of the American College of Cardiology 33: 222–277

Antunes M J, Myer I G, Santos L P 1984 Thrombosis of mitral valve replacement. British Journal of Obstetrics and Gynaecology 91: 716–718

Aram D M, Ekelman B L, Ben-Shachae G, Levinsohn M W 1985 Intelligence and hypoxaemia in children with congenital heart disease; fact or artifact? Journal of the American College of Cardiology 6: 889–893

Balaji S, Gewillig M, Bull C, de Leval M R, Deanfield J E 1991 Arrhythmias after the Fontan procedure: comparison of total cavopulmonary connection and atriopulmonary connection. Circulation 84(suppl III): 162–167

Benny P S, Prasao J, MacVicar J 1980 Pregnancy and coarctation of the aorta. Case Report. British Journal of Obstetrics and Gynaecology 87: 1159–1161

Beppu S, Suzuki S, Matsuda H, Ohmori F, Nagata S, Miyatake K 1993 Rapidity of progression of aortic stenosis in patients with congenital bicuspid aortic valves. American Journal of Cardiology 71: 322–327

Bertranou E G, Blackstone E H, Hazelrig J B, Turner M E, Kirklin J W 1978 Life expectancy without surgery in tetralogy of Fallot. American Journal of Cardiology 42: 458–466

Bjarke B 1975 Oxygen uptake and cardiac output during submaximal and maximal exercise in adult subjects with totally corrected tetralogy of fallot. Acta Medica Scandinavica 197: 177–186

Blake R S, Chung E E, Wesley H, Hallidie-Smith K A 1982 Conduction defects, ventricular arrhythmias and late death after surgical closure of ventricular septal defect. British Heart Journal 47: 305–315

Bonhoeffer P, Bonnet D, Piechaud J F et al 1997 Coronary artery obstruction after the arterial switch operation for transposition of the great arteries in newborns. Journal of the American College of Cardiology 29: 202–206

Bonnet D, Acar P, Aggoun Y et al 1998 Can partial cavo-pulmonary connection be considered an alternative to the Fontan procedure? Archives des Maladies du Coeut et des Vaisseaux 91: 569–573

Borghi A, Agnoletti G, Valsecchi O, Carminati M 1999 Aortic balloon dilatation for congenital aortic stenosis: report of 90 cases (1986–1998). Heart 82: 10

Borow K M, Braunwald E 1988 Congenital heart disease in the adult. In: Braunwald E (ed.) Heart disease, 3rd edn. Saunders, Philadelphia, PA, p 976–1002

Brandenburg R O Jr, Holmes D R Jr, Brandenburg R O, McGoon D C 1983 Clinical follow-up study of paroxysmal supraventricular arrhythmias after operative repair of a secundum type atrial septal defect in adults. American Journal of Cardiology 51: 273–276

Brewer L A, Fosburg R A, Mulder G A, Verska J J 1972 Spinal cord complications after surgery for coarctation of the aorta. Journal of Thoracic and Cardiovascular Surgery 64: 368–381

Bridges N D, Perry S B, Keane J F et al 1991 Preoperative transcatheter closure of congenital muscular ventricular septal defects. New England Journal of Medicine 324: 1312–1317

Bridges N D, Mayer J E, Lock J E et al 1992 Effect of baffle fenestration on outcome of the modified Fontan operation. Circulation 86: 1762–1769

Brookes C I, White P A, Bishop A J, Oldershaw P J, Redington A N, Moat N E 1998 Validation of a new intraoperative technique to evaluate load-independent indices of right ventricular performance in patients undergoing cardiac operations. Journal of Thoracic and Cardiovascular Surgery 116: 468–476

Bulbul Z R, Bruckheimer E, Love J C, Fahey J T, Hellenbrand W E 1996 Implantation of balloon-expandable stents for coarctation of the aorta: implantation data and short-term results. Catheterization and Cardiovascular Diagnosis 39: 36–42

Burn J 1987 The aetiology of congenital heart disease. In: Anderson R H, Macartney F J, Shinebourne E A, Tynan M (eds) Paediatric cardiology. Churchill Livingstone, Edinburgh, p 15–63

Campbell M 1970a Natural history of atrial septal defect. British Heart Journal 32: 820–826

Campbell M 1970b Natural history of coarctation of the aorta. British Heart Journal 32: 633–640

Canadian Cardiovascular Society 1996 Adult congenital heart disease. Report of a consensus conference of the Canadian Cardiovascular Society

Cartmill T B, DuShane J W, McGoon D C, Kirklin J W 1966 Results of repair of ventricular septal defect. Journal of Thoracic and Cardiovascular Surgery 52: 486–499

Celermajer D S, Deanfield J E 1993 Employment and insurance for young adults with congenital heart disease. British Heart Journal 69: 539–543

Celermajer D S, Dodd S M, Greenwald S E, Wyse R K, Deanfield J E 1992 Morbid anatomy in neonates with Ebstein's anomaly of the tricuspid valve: pathophysiologic and clinical implications. Journal of the American College of Cardiology 19: 1049–1053

Celermajer D S, Robinson J T C, Taylor J F N 1993 Vascular access in previously catheterised children and adolescents–a prospective study of 131 consecutive cases. British Heart Journal 70: 554–557

Chambers J C, Somerville J, Stone S, Ross D N 1997 Pulmonary autograft procedure for aortic valve disease: long-term results of the pioneer series. Circulation 96: 2206–2214

Chan K C, Godman M J, Walsh K, Wilson N, Redington A, Gibbs J L 1999 Transcatheter closure of atrial septal defect and interatrial communications with a new self expanding nitinol double disc device (Amplatzer septal occluder): multicentre UK experience. Heart 82: 300–306

Chaturvedi R R, Kilner P J, White P A, Bishop A, Szware R, Redington A N 1997 Increased airway pressure and simulated brach pulmonary artery stenosis increase pulmonary regurgitation after repair of tetralogy of Fallot. Real-time analysis with a conductance catheter technique. Circulation 95: 643–649

Child J S, Perloff J K 1991 Natural survival patterns. A narrowing base. In: Child J S, Perloff J K (eds) Congenital heart disease in adults. Saunders, Philadelphia, PA, p 24–26

Chizner M A, Pearle D L, deLeon A C 1980 The natural history of aortic stenosis in adults. American Heart Journal 99: 419–424

Choussat A, Fontan I, Besse P, Vallot F, Cahuve A, Bricand H 1978 Selection criteria for Fontan's procedure. In: Anderson R H, Shinebourne E A (eds) Paediatric cardiology. Churchill Livingstone, Edinburgh, p 559–566

Cochrane A D, Karl T R, Mee R B 1993 Staged conversion to arterial switch for late failure of the systemic right ventricle. Annals of Thoracic Surgery 56: 854–861

Cohen L S, Friedman W F, Braunwald E 1972 Natural history of mild congenital aortic stenosis elucidated by serial hemodynamic studies. American Journal of Cardiology 30: 1–5

Cohen M, Fuster V, Steele P M et al 1989 Coarctation of the aorta: long term follow-up and prediction of outcome after surgical correction. Circulation 80: 840–845

Colan S D, Trowitzsch E, Wernovsky G, Sholler G F, Sanders S P, Castaneda A 1988 Myocardial performance after arterial switch operation for transposition of the great arteries with intact ventricular septum. Circulation 78: 132–141

Connelly M S, Liu P P, Williams W G, Webb G D, Robertson P, McLaughlin P R 1996 Congenitally corrected transposition in the adult: functional status and complications. Journal of the American College of Cardiology 27: 1238–1243

Copeland W E, Wolley C F, Ryan J M, Runco V, Levin H S 1963 Pregnancy and congenital heart disease. American Journal of Obstetrics and Gynaecology 86: 107–110

Craig R J, Selzer A 1968 Natural history and prognosis of atrial septal defects. Circulation 37: 805–815

Cullen S, Celermajer D S, Deanfield J E 1991 Exercise in congenital heart disease. Cardiology in the Young 1: 129–135

Cullen S, Celermajer D S, Franklin R C G, Hallidie-Smith K A, Deanfield J E 1994 Prognostic significance of ventricular arrhythmia after repair of tetralogy of Fallot: a 12 year prospective study. Journal of the American College of Cardiology 23: 1151–1155

Dajani A S, Taubert K A, Wilson W et al 1997 Prevention of bacterial endocarditis. Recommendations by the American Heart Association. Journal of the American Medical Association 277: 1794–1801 [Circulation 96: 358–366]

Daliento L, Somerville J, Presbitero P et al 1998 Eisenmenger syndrome. Factors relating to deterioration and death. European Heart Journal 19: 1845–1855

Danielson G K, Driscoll D J, Mair D D, Warnes C A, Oliver W C, Jr 1992 Operative treatment of Ebstein's anomaly. Journal of Thoracic and Cardiovascular Surgery 104: 1195–1202

Deal K, Colley C F 1973 Coarctation of the aorta and pregnancy. Annals of Internal Medicine 78: 706–710

Deanfield J E 1992 Adult congenital heart disease with special reference to the data on long term follow-up of patients surviving to adulthood with or without surgical correction. European Heart Journal 13: 111–116

Deanfield J E 1999 Intra-atrial repair of transposition late results and management problems. Journal of Thoracic and Cardiovascular Surgery 117: 488–495

Deanfield J E, Cullen S 2000 Grown-up congenital heart and the general cardiologist. Current Medical Literature – Cardiology 19: 1–4

Deanfield J E, McKenna W J, Hallidie-Smith K A 1980 Detection of late arrhythmia and conduction disturbance after correction of tetralogy of Fallot. British Heart Journal 44: 577–583

Deanfield J E, Ho S-Y, Anderson R H, McKenna W J, Allwork S P, Hallidie-Smith K A 1983 Late sudden death after repair of tetralogy of Fallot: a clinico-pathological study. Circulation 67: 636–641

Deanfield J E, McKenna W J, Presbitero P, England D, Graham G R, Hallidie-Smith K 1984 Ventricular arrhythmia in unrepaired and repaired tetralogy of Fallot: relation to age, timing of repair and haemodynamic status. British Heart Journal 52: 77–81

Deanfield J E, McKenna W, Rowland E 1985 Local abnormalities of right ventricular depolarisation after repair of tetralogy of Fallot: a basis for ventricular arrhythmia. American Journal of Cardiology 55: 522–526

Deanfield J, Camm J, Macartney F et al 1988 Arrhythmia and late mortality after Mustard and Senning operation for transposition of the great arteries: an eight year prospective study. Journal of Thoracic and Cardiovascular Surgery 96: 569–576

de Leval M R, Kilner P, Gewillig M, Bull C 1988 Total cavopulmonary connection: a logical alternative to atriopulmonary connection for complex Fontan operations. Journal of Thoracic and Cardiovascular Surgery 96: 682–695

de Swiet M 1987 Management of congenital heart disease in pregnancy. In: Anderson R H, Macartney F J, Shinebourne

E A, Tynan M (eds) Paediatric cardiology. Churchill Livingstone, Edinburgh, p 1353–1361

de Swiet M, Ramsey I D, Rees G M 1975 Bacterial endocarditis after insertion of intrauterine contraceptive device. British Medical Journal 3: 76–77

di Carlo D, de Leval M R, Stark J 1984 'Fresh' antibiotic sterilized aortic homografts in extracardiac valved conduits. Long-term results. Thoracic and Cardiovascular Surgery 32: 10–14

Didier D, Ratib O, Beghetti M, Oberhaenasli, Friedli B 1999 Morphologic and functional evaluation of congenital heart disease by magnetic resonance imaging. Journal of Magnetic Resonance Imaging 10: 639–655

Dhillon R, Thanopoulos B, Tsausis G, Triposkiadis F, Kyriakidis M, Redington A N 1999 Transcatheter closure of atrial septal defects in adults with the Amplatzer septal occluder. Heart 82: 559–562

Dobell A R C, Jain A K 1984 Catastrophic hemorrhage during redo sternotomy. Annals of Thoracic Surgery 37: 273–278

Donofrio M T, Engle M A, O'Loughlin J E et al 1992 Congenital aortic regurgitation: natural history and management. Journal of the American College of Cardiology 20: 366–372

Dorostkar P C, Cheng J, Scheinman M M 1998 Electroanatomical mapping and ablation of the substrate supporting intraatrial re-entrant tachycardia after palliation for complex congenital heart disease. Pacing and Clinical Electrophysiology 21: 1810–1819

Driscoll D J, Durongpisitkul K 1999 Exercise testing after the Fontan operation. Pediatric Cardiology 20: 57–59

Driscoll D J, Offord K P, Felot R H, Schaff H V, Puga F J, Danielson G K 1992 Five to fifteen year follow-up after Fontan operation. Circulation 85: 469–496

d'Udekem Y, Rubay J, Shango-Lody P et al 1998 Late homograft valve insertion after transannular patch repair of tetralogy of Fallot. Journal of Heart and Valve Disease 7: 450–454

Ebert P A, Turley K, Stanger P, Hoffman J I E, Hyemann M A, Rudolph A M 1984 Surgical treatment of truncus arteriosus in the first 6 months of life. Annals of Surgery 200: 451–456

Elkayam U, Ostrzega E, Shotan A, Mehra A 1995 Cardiovascular problems in pregnant women with Marfan syndrome. Annals of Internal Medicine 123: 117–122

Engle M A, Kline S A, Borer J S 1987 Ventricular septal defect. In: Roberts W C (ed.) Adult congenital heart disease. Davis, Philadelphia PA, p 409–441

Fields C D, Rosenfield K, Losordo D W, Isner J M 1989 Percutaneous balloon valvuloplasty: current status. Current Opinion in Cardiology 4: 229–241

Finck S J, Puga F J, Danielson G K 1988 Pulmonary valve insertion during reoperation for tetralogy of Fallot. Annals of Thoracic Surgery 45: 610–613

Flinn C J, Wolff G S, Dick M et al 1984 Cardiac rhythm after the Mustard operation for complete transposition of the great arteries. New England Journal of Medicine 310: 1635–1638

Fontan F, Baudet E 1971 Surgical repair of tricuspid atresia. Thorax 26: 240–248

Fontan F, Deville C, Quagebeur J et al 1983 Repair of tricuspid atresia in 100 patients. Journal of Thoracic and Cardiovascular Surgery 85: 647–658

Fontan F, Kirklin J W, Fernandez G et al 1990 Outcome after a 'perfect' Fontan operation. Circulation 81: 1520–1536

Franklin R C, Spiegelhalter D J, Anderson R H et al 1991 Double inlet ventricle presenting in infancy: I. Survival without definitive repair. Journal of Thoracic and Cardiovascular Surgery 101: 767–776

Fraser I S 1988 Progestogens for contraception. Australian Family Physician 17: 882–885

Friedberg D Z, Nades A S 1970 Clinical profile of patients with congenitally corrected transposition of the great arteries. A study of 60 cases. New England Journal of Medicine 282: 1053–1059

Friedman W F, Johnson A D 1987 Congenital aortic stenosis. In: Roberts W C (ed.) Adult congenital heart disease. Davis, Philadelphia, PA, p 357–374

Fryda R J, Kaplan S, Helmsworth J A 1971 Postoperative complete heart block in children. British Heart Journal 33: 456–462

Gardiner H M, Dhillon R, Bull C, de Leval M R, Deanfield J E 1996 Prospective study of the incidence and determinants of arrhythmia after total cavopulmonary connection. Circulation 94 (suppl II): 17–21

Garson A Jr 1990 Chronic postoperative arrhythmia. In: Gillette P C, Garson A Jr (eds) Pediatric arrhythmia: electrophysiology and pacing. Saunders, Philadelphia, PA, p 667–678

Garson A, Nihill M R, McNamara D G, Cooley D A 1979 Status of the adult and adolescent after repair of tetralogy of Fallot. Circulation 59: 1232–1240

Garson A J, Bink-Boelkens M, Hesslein P S et al 1985 Atrial flutter in the young: a collaborative study of 380 cases. Journal of the American College of Cardiology 6: 871–878

Gatzoulis M A, Till J A, Somerville J, Redington A N 1995a Mechanolectrical interaction in tetralogy of Fallot. QRS prolongation relates to right ventricular size and predicts malignant ventricular arrhythmias and sudden death. Circulation 92: 231–237

Gatzoulis M A, Clark A L, Cullen S, Newman C G, Redington A N 1995b Right ventricular diastolic function 15 to 35 years after repair of tetralogy of Fallot. Restrictive physiology predicts superior exercise performance. Circulation 91: 175–181

Gatzoulis M A, Till J A, Redington A N 1997 Depolarization–repolarization inhomogeneity after repair of tetralogy of Fallot. The substrate for malignant ventricular tachycardia? Circulation 95: 401–404

Gatzoulis M A, Freeman M A, Siu S C, Webb G D, Harris L 1999 Atrial arrhythmias after surgical closure of ASD in adults. New England Journal of Medicine 340: 839–846

Gatzoulis M A, Munk M D, Williams W G, Webb G D 2000 Definitive palliation with cavopulmonary or aortopulmonary shunts for adults with single ventricle physiology. Heart 83: 51–57

Gelatt M, Hamilton R M, McCrindle B W et al 1997 Arrhythmia and mortality after the Mustard procedure: a 30 year single centre experience. Journal of the American College of Cardiology 29: 194–201

Gentles T L, Calder A L, Clarkson P M, Neutze J M 1992 Ebstein's anomaly of the tricuspid valve: a clinical review with long-term follow-up. American Journal of Cardiology 69: 377

Gentles T L, Mayer J T, Gauvreau K et al 1997 Fontan operation in 500 consecutive patients: factors influencing early and late outcome. Journal of Thoracic and Cardiovascular Surgery 114: 376–391

Gewillig M H, Lundstrom U R, Bull C, Wyse R K H, Deanfield J E 1990a Exercise responses in patients after Fontan repair: patterns and determinants of performance. Journal of the American College of Cardiology 15: 1424–1432

Gewillig M H, Lundstrom U R, Deanfield J E et al 1990b Impact of the Fontan operation on left ventricular size and contractility. Circulation 81: 118–127

Gewillig M, Cullen S, Mertens B, Lesaffre E, Deanfield J 1991 Risk factors for arrhythmia and death after Mustard operation for simple transposition of the great arteries. Circulation 83 (suppl III): 187–192

Gewillig M, Wyse R K, de Leval M R, Deanfield J E 1992 Early and late arrhythmia after the Fontan operation: predisposing factors and clinical consequences. British Heart Journal 67: 72–79

Gibbs J L 2000 Interventional catheterization. Opening up I: the ventricular outflow tracts and great arteries. Heart 83: 111–115

Godman M J, Roberts N K, Izukawa T 1974 Late postoperative conduction disturbances after repair of ventricular septal defect and tetralogy of Fallot. Circulation 49: 214–221

Gorge G, Erbel R, Henrichs J, Wensschel H, Werner J, Meyer J 1990 Positive blood cultures during transoesophageal echocardiography. Journal of the American College of Cardiology 15: 62A

Graham T P, Atwood G F, Boucek R J, Boerth R C, Bender H W 1975 Abnormalities of right ventricular function following Mustard's operation for transposition of the great arteries. Circulation 52: 678–684

Greene H L, Roden D M, Katz R J et al 1992 The Cardiac Arrhythmia Suppression Trial: first CAST ... then CAST II. Journal of the American College of Cardiology 19: 894–898

Gross R E, Hubbard J P 1939 Surgical ligation of a persistent ductus arteriosus. Journal of the American Medical Association 112: 729–731

Gross R E, Hufnagel C A 1945 Coarctation of the aorta. Experimental studies regarding its surgical correction. New England Journal of Medicine 233: 287–293

Hagler D J, Ritter D G, Mair D D et al 1979 Right and left ventricular function after the Mustard procedure for transposition of the great arteries. American Journal of Cardiology 44: 276–283

Hall J G 1981 Disorders of connective tissue and skeletal dysplasia. In: Simpson J L, Shulman J D (eds) Genetic disorders in pregnancy. Academic Press, New York, p 57–87

Hall J G, Pauli R M, Wilson K M 1980 Maternal and fetal sequelae of anticoagulation during pregnancy. American Journal of Medicine 68: 122–140

Harringer W, Wiebe K, Struber M et al 1999 Lung transplantation–10 year experience. European Journal of Cardiothoracic Surgery 16: 546–554

Hayes C J, Gersony W M, Driscoll D J et al 1993 Second natural history study of congenital heart defects. Results of treatment of patients with pulmonary valvar stenosis. Circulation 87 (suppl I): 28–37

Hegerty A, Anderson R H, Deanfield J E 1988 Myocardial fibrosis in tetralogy of Fallot: effect of surgery or part of the natural history? British Heart Journal 59: 123

Heish K, Keane J F, Nadas A S, Bernhard W F, Castañeda A R 1986 Long-term follow-up of valvulotomy before 1968 for congenital aortic stenosis. American Journal of Cardiology 58: 338–341

Hellenbrand W E, Fahey J T, McGowan F X, Welton G G, Kleinman C S 1990 Transophageal echocardiographic guidance of transcatheter closure of atrial septal defect. American Journal of Cardiology 66: 207–213

Helvind M H, McCarthy J F, Imamura M et al 1998 Ventriculo-arterial discordance: switching the morphologically left ventricle into the systemic circulation after 3 months of age. European Journal of Cardiothoracic Surgery 14: 173–178

Hirsch R, Kilner P J, Connelly M S, Redington A N, St John Sutton M G, Somerville J 1994 Diagnosis in adolescents and adults with congenital heart disease. Prospective assessment of individual and combined roles of magnetic resonance imaging and transesophageal echocardiography. Circulation 90: 2937–2951

Horowitz L N, Vetter V L, Harken A H, Josephson M E 1980 Electrophysiologic characteristics of sustained ventricular tachycardia after repair of tetralogy of Fallot. American Journal of Cardiology 46: 446–452

Hosenpud J A, Bennett L E, Keck B M, Fiol B, Boucek M M, Novick R J 1999 The Registry of the International Society for Heart and Lung Transplantation: 16th Official Report. Journal of Heart and Lung Transplantation 18: 611–626

Huffman J W 1981 Sex and the teenager. In: Huffman J W, Dewhurst J C, Capuaro V J (eds) The gynaecology of childhood and adolescence, 2nd edn. Saunders, Philadelphia, PA, p 527–542

Huhta J C, Maloney J E, Ritter D G, Ilstrup D M, Feldt R H 1983 Complete atrioventricular block in patients with atrioventricular discordance. Circulation 67: 1374–1377

Hurbe-Alessio I, Del Carmen Fonseca M, Mutchinik O, Santos M A, Zajarias A, Salazar E 1986 Risks of anticoagulant therapy in pregnant women with artificial heart valves. New England Journal of Medicine 315: 1390–1393

Ilbawi M N, Idriss F S, Muster A J, Wessel H U, Paul M H, de Leon S Y 1981 Tetralogy of Fallot with absent pulmonary valve. Should valve insertion be part of the intracardiac repair? Journal of Thoracic and Cardiovascular Surgery 81: 906–915

Imai Y 1997 Double-switch operation for congenitally corrected transposition. Advances in Cardiovascular Surgery 9: 65–86

Iyer R S, Jacobs J P, de Leval M R, Stark J, Elliott M J 1997 Outcomes after delayed sternal closure in paediatric heart operations: a 10 year experience. Annals of Thoracic Surgery 63: 489–491

Jatene A D, Fontes V F, Paulista P P et al 1975 Successful anatomic correction of transposition of the great vessels. A preliminary report. Archives of Brazilian Cardiology 28: 461–464

Jonas R A, Freed M D, Mayer J E Jr, Castañeda A R 1985 Long-term follow-up of patients with synthetic right heart conduits. Circulation 72(suppl II): 77–83

Jones M, Ferrans V J 1989 Myocardial degeneration in congenital heart disease: comparison of morphologic findings in young and old patients with congenital heart disease associated with muscular obstruction to right ventricular outflow. American Journal of Cardiology 61: 1050–1055

Jones P, Patel A 1996 Eisenmenger's syndrome and problems with anaesthesia. British Journal of Hospital Medicine 54: 214–219

Jordan C E, White R C Jr, Fischer K C, Neill C, Dorst J P 1972 The scoliosis of congenital heart disease. American Heart Journal 84: 463–469

Kan J S, White R I Jr, Mitchell S E, Gardner T J 1982 Percutaneous balloon valvuloplasty: a new method for treating congenital pulmonary valve stenosis. New England Journal of Medicine 307: 540–542

Kaplan E L, Rich H, Gersony W, Manning J 1979 A collaborative study of infective endocarditis in the 1970s: emphasis on patients who have undergone cardiovascular surgery. Circulation 59: 327–335

Karl T R, Weintraub R G, Brizard C P, Cochrane A D, Mee R B 1997 Senning plus arterial switch operation for discordant (congenitally corrected) transposition. Annals of Thoracic Surgery 64: 495–502

Katz N M, Blackstone E H, Kirklin J W, Pacifico A D, Bergeron L M Jr 1982 Late survival and symptoms after repair of tetralogy of Fallot. Circulation 65: 403–410

Kavey R E, Blackman M S, Sondheimer H M 1982 Incidence and severity of chronic ventricular dysrhythmia after repair of tetralogy of Fallot. American Heart Journal 103: 342–350

Keane J F, Driscoll D J, Gersony W M et al 1996 Second natural history study of congenital heart defects: results of treatment of patients with aortic valvar stenosis. Circulation 87: 16–27

Keen G 1987 Spinal cord damage and operations for coarctation of the aorta. Aetiology, practice and prospects. Thorax 42: 11–18

Keith J D, Neill C A, Vlad P, Rowe R D, Chute A L 1953 Transposition of the great vessels. Circulation 7: 830–838

Keith J D, Rowe R D, Vlad P 1978 Heart disease in infancy and childhood, 3rd edn. Macmillan, New York

Kellerman J, Zeltzer L, Ellenberg L, Dash J, Rigler D 1980 Psychological effects of illness in adolescence. I. Anxiety, self-esteem, and perception of control. Journal of Pediatrics 97: 126–131

Kirklin J W, Barratt-Boyes B G (eds) 1986 Cardiac surgery. John Wiley, New York, p 463–497

Kobayashi J, Hirose H, Nakano S, Matsuda H, Shirakura R, Kawashima Y 1984 Ambulatory electrocardiographic study of the frequency and cause of ventricular arrhythmia after correction of tetralogy of Fallot. American Journal of Cardiology 54: 1310–1313

Kopecky S L, Gersh B J, McGoon M D et al 1988 Long-term outcome of patients undergoing surgical repair of isolated pulmonary valve stenosis. Follow-up at 20 to 30 years. Circulation 78: 1150–1156

Kratz J M, Gillette P C, Crawford F A, Sade R M, Zeigler V L 1992 Atrioventricular pacing in congenital heart disease. Annals of Thoracic Surgery 54: 485–489

Kugelmeier J, Egloff L, Real F, Rothlin M, Turina M, Senning A 1982 Congenital aortic stenosis. Early and late results of aortic valvotomy. Thoracic Cardiovascular Surgery 30: 91–95

Kulbertus H E, Coyne J J, Hallidie-Smith K A 1969 Conduction disturbances before and after surgical closure of ventricular septal defect. American Heart Journal 77: 123–131

LaCorte M A, Dick M, Scheer G, LaFarge C G, Flyer D C 1975 Left ventricular function in tricuspid atresia. Angiographic analysis in 28 patients. Circulation 52: 996–1000

Laks H, Pearl J M, Haas G S et al 1991 Partial Fontan: advantages of an adjustable interatrial communication. Annals of Thoracic Surgery 52: 1084–1095

Leibman J, Cullum L, Belloc N B 1969 Natural history of transposition of the great arteries. Anatomy and birth and death characteristics. Circulation 40: 237–262

Lev M, Gibson S, Millar R A 1955 Ebstein's disease with Wolff–Parkinson–White syndrome: Report of a case with histopathologic study of possible conduction pathways. American Heart Journal 49: 724–741

Lillehei C W, Varco R L, Cohen M et al 1986 The first open heart corrections of tetralogy of Fallot: a 26–31 year follow-up of 106 patients. Annals of Surgery 204: 490–501

Limet R, Grondin C M 1977 Cardiac valve prosthesis, anticoagulation, and pregnancy. Annals of Thoracic Surgery 23: 337–341

Lock J E 1991 The adult with congenital heart disease. Cardiac catheterisation as a therapeutic intervention. Journal of the American College of Cardiology 18: 330–331

Lundstrom U, Bull C, Wyse R K H, Somerville J 1990 The natural and 'unnatural' history of congenitally corrected transposition. American Journal of Cardiology 65: 1222–1229

Lusher J M 1987 Diseases of coagulation: the fluid phase. In: Nathan D G, Oski F A (eds) Haematology in infancy and childhood, 3rd edn. Saunders, Philadelphia PA, p 1328–1329

Lutz D J, Noller K L, Spittell J A, Danielson G K, Fish C R 1978 Pregnancy and its complications following cardiac valve prothesis. American Journal of Obstetrics and Gynecology 131: 460–468

MacMahon B, McKeown T, Record R G 1953 The incidence and life expectation of children with congenital heart disease. British Heart Journal 15: 121–129

Magee A G, Brzezinska-Rajszys G, Qureshi S A et al 1999 Stent implantation for aortic coarctation and recoarctation Heart 82: 600–606

Mahoney L T, Truesdell S C, Hamburgen M, Skorton D J 1991 Insurability, employability, and psychosocial considerations. In: Perloff J K, Child J S (eds) Congenital heart disease in adults: Saunders, New York, p 178–189

Mainwaring P D, Lamberti J J, Uzark K 1994 The directional Glenn procedure: palliation of the univentricular heart. Advances in Cardiovascular Surgery 5: 115–140

Maron B J, Humphries J, Rowe R D et al 1973 Prognosis of surgically corrected coarctation of the aorta. A 20 year postoperative appraisal. Circulation 47: 119–126

Maron B J, Epstein S E, Mitchell J H 1985 Sixteenth Bethesda Conference. Cardiovascular abnormalities in the athlete: recommendations regarding eligibility for competition. Journal of the American College of Cardiology 6: 1189–1190

Massumi R A, Nutter D O et al 1966 The syndrome of familial defects of the heart and upper extremities (Holt–Oram syndrome). Circulation 34: 65–76

Masura J, Burch M, Deanfield J E, Sullivan I D 1993 Five-year follow-up after balloon pulmonary valvuloplasty. Journal of the American College of Cardiology 21: 132–136

Mathur M, Glenn W W L 1973 Long-term evaluation of cavopulmonary artery anastomosis. Surgery 74: 889–916

Matsuda H, Kawashima Y, Kishimoto H et al 1987 Problems with the modified Fontan operation for univentricular heart of the right ventricular type. Circulation 76(suppl III): 45–52

Mayer J A, Bullen B A 1974 Nutrition, weight control and exercise. In: Johnson W R, Buskurk E R (eds) Science and medicine of exercise and sport. Harper & Row, New York, p 259–275

McCrindle B W, Kan J S 1991 Long-term results after balloon pulmonary valvuloplasty. Circulation 83: 1915–22

McFaul P B, Dornan J C, Lam K I, Boyle D 1988 Pregnancy complicated by maternal heart disease: a review of 519 women. British Journal of Obstetrics and Gynaecology 95: 861–867

Mee R B B 1986 Severe right ventricular failure after Mustard or Senning operation. Two-stage repair: pulmonary artery banding and switch. Journal of Thoracic and Cardiovascular Surgery 92: 385–390

Mendelson C L 1940 Pregnancy and coarctation of the aorta. American Journal of Obstetrics and Gynaecology 39: 1014–1021

Merin G, McGoon D C 1973 Reoperation after insertion of aortic homograft as a right ventricular outflow tract. Annals of Thoracic Surgery 16: 122–126

Mills P, Leech G, Davies M, Leatham A 1978 The natural history of a non-stenotic bicuspid aortic valve. British Heart Journal 40: 951–957

Moodie D S, Ritter D G, Tajik A H, McGoon D C, Danielson G K, O'Fallon W M 1984 Long-term follow-up after palliative operation for univentricular heart. American Journal of Cardiology 53: 1648–1651

Morrison D, Sorenson S, Caldwell J et al 1983 The effect of pulmonary hypertension on systolic function of the right ventricle. Chest 84: 250–257

Mullins C E, Latson L A, Neches W H, Colvin E V, Kan J 1990 Balloon dilatation of miscellaneous lesions: results of valvuloplasty and angioplasty of the Congenital Anomalies Registry. American Journal of Cardiology 65: 802–803

Murphy J G, Gersh B J, Warnes C A et al 1989 The late survival after surgical repair of isolated ventricular septal defect (VSD). Circulation 80(suppl II): 490

Murphy J G, Gersh B J, McGoon M D 1990 Long term (30 year) survival of patients undergoing complete repair of tetralaogy of Fallot. Journal of the American College of Cardiology 15: 205A

Murphy J G, Gersh B J, Mair D D et al 1993 Long-term outcome in patients undergoing surgical repair of tetralogy of Fallot. New England Journal of Medicine 329: 593–599

Must A, Jacques P F, Dallal G E, Bajema C J, Dietz W H 1992 Long-term morbidity and mortality of overweight adolescents. New England Journal of Medicine 327: 1350–1355

Myers-Vando R, Steward M S, Folkins C H, Hines P 1979 The effects of congenital heart disease on cognitive development, illness causality concepts, and vulnerability. American Journal of Orthopsychiatry 49: 617–625

Nadas A S, Ellison R C, Weidman W H (eds) 1977 Pulmonary stenosis, aortic stenosis, ventricular septal defect: clinical course and indirect assessment. Circulation 56(suppl I): 1–87

Nathan A W, Davies D W 1992 Is VVI pacing outmoded: British Heart Journal 67: 285–288

Neilson G, Galea E G, Blunt A 1970 Congenital heart disease and pregnancy. Medical Journal of Australia 1: 1086–1088

Newburger J W, Silbert A R, Buckley L P, Fyler D C 1984 Cognitive function and age at repair of transposition of the great arteries in children. New England Journal of Medicine 310: 1495–1499

Nora J J, McNamara D, Fraser F C 1967 Hereditary factors in atrial septal defect. Circulation 35: 448–456

Nugent E W, Freedom R M, Nora J J, Ellison R C, Rowe R D, Nadas A S 1977 Clinical course in pulmonary stenosis. Circulation 56(suppl I): 38–47

Oakley C M 1995 Anticoagulants in pregnancy. British Heart Journal 74: 107–111

Oakley C, Somerville W 1981 Prevention of infective endocarditis. British Heart Journal 45: 233–235

Oechslin E N, Harrison D A, Harris L et al 1999 Reoperation in adults with repair of tetralogy of Fallot: indications and outcomes. Journal of Thoracic and Cardiovascular Surgery 118: 245–251

Oldershaw P J, St John Sutton M S 1980 Haemodynamic effects of haemocrit reduction in patients with polycythaemia secondary to cyanotic congenital heart disease. British Heart Journal 44: 584

Oswalt J D 1999 Acceptance and versatility of the Ross procedure. Current Opinions in Cardiology 14: 90–94

Packer M 1985a Therapeutic application of calcium channel antagonists for pulmonary hypertension. American Journal of Cardiology 55: 196–198

Packer M 1985b Vasodilation therapy for primary pulmonary hypertension. Limitations and hazards. Annals of Internal Medicine 103: 258–270

Park S C, Neches W H, Lenox C C, Zuberbuhler J R, Bahnson H T 1973 Massive calcification and obstruction in a homograft after the Rastelli procedure for transposition of the great arteries. American Journal of Cardiology 32: 860–864

Pellikka P A, Nishimura R A, Bailey K R, Takij A J 1990 The natural history of adults with assymptomatic, haemodynamically significant aortic stenosis. Journal of the American College of Cardiology 15: 1012–1017

Perloff J K 1984 Ostium secundum atrial septal defect–survival for 87–94 years. American Journal of Cardiology 53: 388–389

Perloff J K 1989 Congenital heart disease in adults. In: Kelly W N (ed.) Textbook of internal medicine, Lippincott Philadelphia, PA, p 223–235

Perloff J K 1991 Pregnancy in congenital heart disease. In: Perloff J K, Child J S (eds) Congenital heart disease in adults. Saunders, Philadelphia, PA, p 124–140

Perloff J K, Rosove M H, Child J S, Wright G B 1988 Adults with cyanotic congenital heart disease: haematological management. Annals of Internal Medicine 109: 406–413

Phadke A R, Phadke S A, Handy M, Junnarkar R V 1977 Acyanotic Fallot's tetralogy with survival to the age of 70 years: case report. Indian Heart Journal 29: 46–49

Poirier R A, McGoon D C, Danielson G K et al 1977 Late results after repair of tetralogy of Fallot. Journal of Thoracic and Cardiovascular Surgery 73: 900–908

Presbitero P, Somerville J, Revel-Chion R, Ross D 1982 Open aortic valvotomy for congenital aortic stenosis: late results. British Heart Journal 47: 26–34

Presbitero P, Demarie D, Villani M et al 1987 Long-term results (15–30 years) of surgical repair of aortic coarctation. British Heart Journal 57: 462–467

Presbitero P, Somerville J, Stone S, Aruta E, Spiegelhalter D 1992 Pregnancy in cyanotic congenital heart disease: maternal complications and factors influencing successful fetal outcome. Journal of the American College of Cardiology 19(suppl A): 288A

Puga F J, Leoni F E, Julsrud P R, Mair D D 1998 Complete repair of pulmonary atresia, ventricular septal defect and severe peripheral arborization abnormalities of the central pulmonary arteries. Experience with preliminary unifocalization procedures in 38 patients. Journal of Thoracic and Cardiovascular Surgery 6: 1018–1029

Quattlebaum T G, Varghese J, Neill C A, Donahoo J S 1976 Sudden death among postoperative patients with tetralogy of Fallot: a follow-up study of 243 patients for an average of twelve years. Circulation 54: 289–293

Rabajoli F, Aruta E, Presbitero P, Todros T 1992 Risks of contraception and pregnancy in patients with congenital cardiopathies. Retrospective study on 108 patients. Giornale Italiano di Cardiologia (Padua) 22: 1133–1137

Rao P S, Thapar M K, Wilson A D, Levy J M, Chopra P S 1989 Intermediate long-term follow-up results of balloon aortic valvuloplasty in infants and children with special reference to causes of restenosis. American Journal of Cardiology 64: 1356–1360

Rastelli G G, Wallace R B, Ongley P A 1969 Complete repair of transposition of the great arteries with pulmonary stenosis. A review and report of a case corrected by using a new surgical technique. Circualtion 39: 83–95

Rebergen S A, Ottenkamp J, Chin J G J, Doombos J, de Roos A, van der Wall E E 1992 Pulmonary regurgitation following Fallot surgery: volumetric quantitation using cine magnetic resonance velocity mapping. Circulation 86(suppl I): 774

Reddy V M, Liddicoat J R, Hanley F L 1995 Middle one-stage complete unifocalization and repair of pulmonary atresia with ventricular septal defect and major aortopulmonary collaterals. Journal of Thoracic and Cardiovascular Surgery 10: 832–845

Redington A N 1998 The Mustard and Senning procedures: assessment of right ventricular performance In: Redington A N, Brawn W J, Deanfield J E, Anderson R H (eds) The right heart in congenital heart disease. Greenwich Medical, London, p 157–161

Redington A N, Rigby M L, Oldershaw P, Gibson D G, Shinebourne E A 1989 Right ventricular function 10 years after the Mustard operation for transposition of the great arteries: analysis of size, shape, and wall motion. British Heart Journal 62: 455–461

Redington A N, Weil J, Somerville J 1994 Self expanding stents in congenital heart disease. British Heart Journal 72: 378–383

Rich S, Kaufmann E, Levy P S 1992 The effect of high doses of calcium-channel blockers in survival in primary pulmonary hypertension. New England Journal of Medicine 327: 76–81

Ritter S B 1989 Coarctation and balloons: inflated or realistic? Journal of the American College of Cardiology 13: 696–699

Rocchini A P, Katch V, Anderson J et al 1988 Blood pressure in obese adolescents: effects of weight loss. Paediatrics 82: 16–23

Roest A, Helbing W A, van der Wall E E, de Roos A 1999 Postoperative evaluation of congenital heart disease by magnetic resonance imaging. Journal of Magnetic Resonance Imaging 10: 656–666

Rosenthal M, Bush A, Deanfield J E, Redington A N 1995 Comparison of cardiopulmonary adaptation during exercise in children after the atriopulmonary and total cavopulmonary connection Fontan procedures. Circulation 91: 372–378

Ross D N, Somerville J 1966 Correction of pulmonary atresia with a homograft aortic valve. Lancet ii: 1446–1447

Rounds S, Hill N S 1984 Pulmonary hypertensive disease. Chest 85: 397–405

Rudolph A M, Nadas A S, Borges W H 1953 Hematologic adjustment to cyanotic congenital heart disease. Pediatrics 11: 454–464

Safian R D, Berman A D, Diver D J et al 1988 Balloon aortic valvuloplasty in 170 consecutive patients. New England Journal of Medicine 319: 125–130

Sande M A, Levison M E, Lukas D A, Kaye D 1969 Bacteremia associated with cardiac catheterisation. New England Journal of Medicine 281: 1104–1106

Saul J P, Alexander M E 1999 Preventing sudden death after repair of tetralogy of Fallot: complex therapy for complex patients. Journal Cardiovascular Electrophysiology 10: 1271–1287

Saxena A, Fong L V, Tristram M, Ackery D M, Keeton B R 1991 Late non-invasive evaluation of cardiac performance in mildly symptomatic older patients with Ebstein's anomaly of the tricuspid valve: role of radionuclide imaging. Journal of the American College of Cardiology 17: 182–186

Senning A 1959 Surgical correction of transposition of the great vessels. Surgery 45: 966–980

Shabbo F P, Wain W H, Ross D N 1980 Right ventricular outflow reconstruction with aortic homograft conduit: analysis of the long-term results. Thoracic Cardiovascular Surgery 28: 21–25

Sharples L D, Caine N, Mullins P et al 1991 Risk factor analysis for the major hazards following heart transplantation-rejection, infection and coronary occlusive disease. Transplantation 52: 244–252

Sholler G F, Keane J F, Perry S B, Sanders S P, Lock J E 1988 Balloon dilatation of congenital aortic valve stenosis. Circulation 78: 351–360

Shull H J Jr, Greene B M, Allen S D, Dunn G D, Schenker S 1975 Bacteremia with upper gastrointestinal endoscopy. Annals of Internal Medicine 83: 212–214

Shulman S T, Amren D P, Bisno A L et al 1984 Prevention of bacterial endocarditis: a statement for health professionals by the Committee on Rheumatic Fever and Infective Endocarditis of the Council on Cardiovascular Disease in the Young. Circulation 70: 1123A

Silbert A, Wolff P, Mayer B, Rosenthal A, Nadas A 1969 Cyanotic heart disease and psychological development. Pediatrics 43: 192–200

Smith W M, Gallagher J J, Kerr C R et al 1982 The electrophysiologic basis and management of symptomatic recurrent tachycardia in patients with Ebstein's anomaly of the tricuspid valve. American Journal of Cardiology 49: 1223–1234

Snabes M C, Poindexter A N 1991 Laparoscopic tubal sterilization under local anaesthesia in women with cyanotic heart disease. Obstetrics and Gynecology 78: 437–440

Somerville J, Webb G D, Skorton D J, Mahoney L T, Warnes C A, Perloff J K 1991 Medical center experiences. Journal of the American College of Cardiology 18: 315–318

Soni N R, Deanfield J E 1997 Assessment of cardiovascular fitness for competitive sport in high risk groups. Archives of Disease in Childhood 77: 386–388

Sperling D R, Dorsey T J, Rowen M, Gazzaniga A B 1983 Percutaneous transluminal angioplasty of congenital coarctation of the aorta. American Journal of Cardiology 51: 562–564

Stark J 1989a Do we really correct congenital heart defects? Journal of Thoracic and Cardiovascular Surgery 97: 1–9

Stark J 1989b Reoperations in patients with extracardiac valved conduits. In: Stark J, Pacifico A D (eds) Reoperations in cardiac surgery. Springer-Verlag, London, p 271–290

Stark J 1998 The use of valved conduits in paediatric cardiac surgery. Paediatric Cardiology 19: 282–288

Stark J, Pacifico A D (eds) 1989 Reoperations in cardiac surgery. Springer-Verlag, London, p 107–312

St John Sutton M G, Tajik A J, McGoon D C 1981 Atrial septal defect in patients aged 60 years or older: operative results and long-term postoperative follow-up. Circulation 64: 402–409

Stevenson W G, Klitzner T, Perloff J K 1991 Electrophysiologic abnormalities. Natural occurrence and postoperative residua and sequelae. In: Child J S, Perloff J K (eds) Congenital heart disease in adults. Saunders Philadelphia, PA, p 259–295

Stewart J R, Paton B C, Blunt S G Jr, Swan H 1978 Congenital aortic stenosis: ten to twenty years after valvulotomy. Archives of Surgery 113: 1248–1252

Studer M, Blackstone E H, Kirklin J W et al 1982 Determinants of early and late results of repair of atrioventricular septal (canal) defects. Journal of Thoracic and Cardiovascular Surgery 84: 523–542

Stumper O F W, Sutherland G R, Magee A, Burn J E, Godman M J 1992 Evaluation of Mustard procedures by transoesophageal ultrasound. Circulation 86(suppl I): 570

Sullivan I D, Robinson P J, Macartney F J et al 1985 Percutaneous balloon valvuloplasty for pulmonary valve stenosis in infants and children. British Heart Journal 54: 435–441

Sullivan I D, Presbitero P, Gooch V M, Aruta E, Deanfield J E 1987 Is ventricular arrhythmia in repaired tetralogy of Fallot an effect of operation or a consequence of the course of the disease? A prospective study. British Heart Journal 58: 40–44

Sullivan I D, Wren C, Stark J, de Leval M, Macartney F J, Deanfield J E 1988 Surgical unifocalisation in pulmonary atresia and ventricular septal defect. A realistic goal? Circulation 78(suppl III): 5–13

Sullivan N M, Sutter V L, Mims M M, Marsh V H, Finegold S M 1973 Clinical aspects of bacteremia after manipulation of the genitourinary tract. Journal of Infectious Diseases 127: 49

Tatsuno K, Konno S, Sakakibara S 1973 Ventricular septal defect with aortic insufficiency: Angiocardiographic aspects and a new classification. American Heart Journal 85: 13–21

Territo M C, Rosove M, Perloff J K 1991 Cyanotic congenital heart disease: haematologic management, renal function, and urate metabolism. In: Perloff J K, Child J S (eds) Congenital heart disease in adults. Saunders, Philadelphia, PA, p 94–95

Till J, Celermajer D, Deanfield J 1992 The natural history of arrhythmias in Ebstein's anomaly. Journal of American College of Cardiology 19(suppl A): 273A

Thorne S A 1998 Management of polycythaemia in adults with cyanotic congenital heart disease. Heart 79: 315–316

Thorne S A, Barnes I, Cullinan P, Somerville J 1999 Amiodarone-associated thyroid dysfunction: risk factors in adults with congenital heart disease. Circulation 100: 149–154

Truesdell S C, Skorton D J, Lauer R M 1986 Life insurance for children with cardiovascular disease. Pediatrics 77: 687–691

Trusler G A, Williams W G, Smallhorn J F, Freedom R M 1992 Late results after repair of aortic insufficiency associated with ventricular septal defect. Journal of Thoracic and Cardiovascular Surgery 103: 276–281

Tunstall-Pedoe H 1988 Acceptable risk in aircrew. European Heart Journal 9(suppl G): 9–11

Vaksmann G, Fournier A, Davignon A, Ducharme G, Houyel L, Fouron J-C 1990 Frequency and prognosis of arrhythmias after operation 'correction' or tetralogy of Fallot. American Journal of Cardiology 66: 346–349

Van Praagh R, Geva T, Kreutzer J 1989 Ventricular septal defects: a surgical viewpoint. Journal of the American College of Cardiology 14: 1298–1299

Vetter V L, Horowitz L N 1982 Electrophysiologic residua and sequelae of surgery for congenital heart defects. American Journal of Cardiology 50: 588–604

Vouhe P R, Tamisier D, Leca F, Ouaknine R, Vernant F, Neveux J Y 1992 Transposition of the great arteries, ventricular septal defect and pulmonary outflow tract obstruction: Rastelli or Lecompte procedure? Journal of Thoracic and Cardiovascular Surgery 103: 428–436

Waldhausen J A, Whitman V, Werner J C et al 1981 Surgical intervention in infants with coarctation of the aorta. Journal of Thoracic and Cardiovascular Surgery 81: 323–325

Walsh E D, Rockenmacher S, Keane J F, Hougen T J, Lock J E, Castañeda A R 1988 Late results in patients with tetralogy of Fallot repaired during infancy. Circulation 77: 1062–1067

Ward D E, Clarke B, Schofield P M, Jones S, Dawkins K, Bennett D 1983 Long-term transvenous ventricular pacing in adults with congenital abnormalities of the heart and great arteries. British Heart Journal 50: 325–329

Warnes C A, Fuster V, Driscoll D J, McGoon D C 1991a Atrial septal defect. In: Giuliani E R, Fuster V, Gersh B J,

McGoon M D, McGoon D C (eds) Cardiology fundamentals and practise, 2nd edn. Mosby Yearbook, St Louis, MO, p 1622–1638

Warnes C A, Fuster V, Driscoll D J, McGoon D C 1991b Ventricular septal defect. In: Giuliani E R, Fuster V, Gersh B J, McGoon M D, McGoon D C (eds) Cardiology: fundamentals and practice, 2nd edn, vol 2. Mosby Year Book, St Louis, MO, p 1639–1652

Watson H 1974. Natural history of Ebstein's anomaly of the tricuspid valve in childhood and adolescence: an international cooperative study of 505 cases. British Heart Journal 36: 417–427

Watterson K G, Wilkinson J L, Karl T R, Mee R B B 1991 Very small pulmonary arteries: the central end-to-side shunt. Annals of Thoracic Surgery 52: 1132–1137

Weber H S, Hellenbrand W E, Kleinmann C S, Perlmutter R A, Rosenfeld L E 1989 Predictors of rhythm disturbances and subsequent morbidity after the Fontan operation. American Journal of Cardiology 64: 762–767

Weidman W H, Lenfant C, Hayes C J et al 1988 Symposium: the Report of the Natural History Study of Congenital Heart Defects: A 20-year follow-up. Presented at 61st Scientific Session of the American Heart Association, Washington DC, 1988

Wennevold A, Rygg I, Lauridsen P, Efsen F, Jacobsen J R 1982 Fourteen to nineteen-year follow-up after corrective repair for tetralogy of Fallot. Scandinavian Journal of Thoracic and Cardiovascular Surgery 16: 41–45

Wessel H U, Cunningham W J, Paul M H, Nastanier C K, Muster A J, Idriss F S 1980 Exercise performance in tetralogy of Fallot after intracardiac repair. Journal of Thoracic and Cardiovascular Surgery 80: 582–593

White P A, Brookes C I, Ravn H B et al 1998 The effect of changing excitation frequency on parallel conductance in different sized hearts. Cardiovascular Research 38: 668–675

Whittemore R 1989 Pregnancy and congenital heart disease. In: Adams F H, Emmanoulides G C, Riemenschneider T A (eds), Heart disease in infants, children and adults, 4th edn. Williams & Wilkins, Baltimore MD, p 684–690

Wolff G S, Rowland T W, Ellison R C 1972 Surgically induced right bundle branch block with left anterior hemiblock. Circulation 46: 587–594

Wood P 1958 The Eisenmenger syndrome or pulmonary hypertension with reversed central shunt. British Medical Journal 2: 701–709

Wren C, Peart I, Bain H, Hunter S 1987 Balloon dilatation of unoperated coarctation: immediate results and one year follow-up. British Heart Journal 58: 369–373

Young D 1980 Hyperuricemia in cyanotic congenital heart disease. American Journal of Diseases in Children 134: 902–903

Zelter L, Kellerman J, Ellenberg L, Dash J, Rigler D 1980 Psychologic effects of illness in adolescence. II. Impact of illness in adolescents–crucial issues and coping styles. Journal of Pediatrics 97: 132–138

Zhao H, Miller D C, Reitz B A, Shumway N E 1985 Surgical repair of tetralogy of Fallot. Long-term follow-up with particular emphasis on late death and reoperation. Journal of Thoracic and Cardiovascular Surgery 89: 204–220

PART VIII

PSYCHOSOCIOLOGICAL PROBLEMS

73

Psychological aspects of congenital heart disease

D. Glaser

Heart disease in children exerts a powerful effect on the child and the family; it elicits a response so profound that this may, in turn, have a strong bearing on the child's ultimate health and wellbeing.

There are many strands that enter the complex inter-relationships in paediatric heart disease. The heart as the seat of the pathology, the fact that the subject is a dependent child, and the early age of onset of the condition, are all significant and immutable. The role of the medical, nursing and ancillary professions is crucial, but not independent of other multiple factors. The nature of the response of the parents and the family is variable and is related to these considerations.

At the centre is the child, whose own development is both a response to, and an ongoing influence on, the illness and network on which the child depends. This chapter traces the origin and course of these interdependent influences (Figure 73.1) and examines some effects and therapeutic interventions.

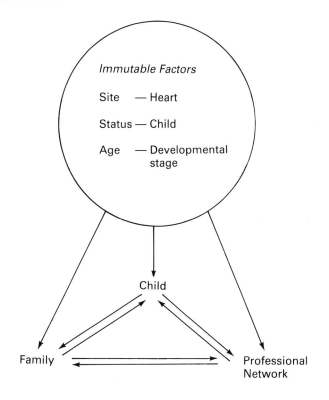

Figure 73.1. Interrelationships in paediatric heart disease.

MEANINGS AND INFLUENCES

THE HEART

The heart is the person's central organ, both physically and metaphorically. Allusions to its role as host to the soul and seat of the emotions are widespread in literature and folklore. In ancient Egyptian practice, the heart was mummified separately, and a cardiac amulet placed in the mummy (Toker, 1971). In Hindu writing, the heart and the soul are synonymous. The Upanishads, which are the secret teachings of the Brahmins (their priestly caste) as long ago as 1000–1500 BC stated 'Verily, this soul is in the heart ... therefore, it is the heart' (Hume, 1930). Shakespeare wrote in Othello (Act IV, scene ii, line 56),

'My heart, where either I must live or bear no life, the fountain from the which my current runs or else dries up'. Jewish writings and thought are replete with references to the centrality of the heart, exemplified by a quotation from Proverbs (4:23), 'Guard your heart with all vigilance, for from it flow the springs of life'.

PROFESSIONAL AND LAY PERCEPTIONS

It is common knowledge that life ends when the heart ceases to function. Furthermore, in adulthood, myocardial infarction is the most common cause of death and is, therefore, as a 'heart attack', a concept familiar to most people. But the distinctions between degenerative, congenital and acquired heart diseases are less familiar to many parents. Nor is there an awareness of a meaningful difference, in terms of complexity and prognosis, between different diagnoses. Rather, families often show global and undifferentiated responses to the presence of a paediatric cardiac illness. For example, a condition that is relatively simple cardiologically, such as a small ventricular septal defect, may be perceived by the family as a 'hole in the heart', a term ominously fraught with danger.

Heart disease in a child, therefore, carries very different connotations for the medical profession and the lay public. Both are aware of the potentially life-threatening nature of paediatric cardiac disease. For the medical profession, the complexity of its management may stand in the way of recognizing the less tangible but real emotional and psychological effects.

For the family, the anxiety engendered by the very fact of paediatric heart disease may, at times, cloud their capacity to differentiate between severe and less serious conditions.

It is important to remember that approximately one in ten children with congenital heart disease is also additionally affected by other conditions. The cumulative effect of multiple problems places a particularly heavy burden on parents. Furthermore, babies and children suffering from congenital heart disease are not immune to those adverse social circumstances that can affect many normal babies. A combination of these factors renders these young children vulnerable to abuse (Glaser and Bentovim, 1979).

The conception, or birth, of a congenitally affected child constitutes the loss of a normal child, for whom the family will need to mourn in some way before the affected child can be fully accepted (Bentovim, 1972, 1975; Lax, 1972; Solnit and Stark, 1961).

THE CHILD

For the child, when the defect is declared early on in life, it is incorporated as an intrinsic part of his or her existence (Goldberg, 1974). The child may, nevertheless, later come to question why he or she was 'chosen' to suffer this condition. When heart disease first manifests itself later on in childhood (for example, following discovery of a murmur, the onset of cardiac symptomatology or subacute bacterial endocarditis), the process of readjustment to the loss involved becomes as difficult for the child as for the family (Debuskey, 1970; Hofmann et al, 1976).

THE FAMILY

Both clinical experience and research (Linde et al, 1970; Goldberg, 1974) support the observation that the child's

psychological wellbeing is very directly related to the environment, of which the family is the most salient part. The parents' relationship with the child is governed in part by the child's characteristics. It is also conditioned by the parents' personalities and their conjugal relationship, and by their own past and current experiences and socioeconomic circumstances. Without question, family life will be pervasively affected by having a child with congenital heart disease (Gottesfeld, 1979).

THE MEDICAL AND CARING PROFESSIONS

The contact with the medical and caring professions, and the nature of the care that the child and the family have received, is an additional major component contributing to the psychological outcome.

While the medical and surgical treatment is directly related to the heart disease and the age of the child, the nature of the contact, explanation and support that the family receive is to some extent determined by factors characterizing the family, such as their level of anxiety, intelligence, social class (see Offord et al, 1972) and cooperation, as well as the style and approach of the professionals themselves. The physically complex (and emotionally charged) area of paediatric heart disease requires close cooperation within an integrated team (Rowe et al, 1974). This should include, in addition to the physicians, surgeons and nursing staff, the social worker, playleader or teacher, and a member of the child mental health service (child psychologist or psychiatrist) (Bingley et al, 1980). Figure 73.1 illustrates the complex pathways of interaction between these various factors.

SPECIFIC ASPECTS OF THE EXPERIENCE OF CONGENITAL HEART DISEASE

Congenital heart disease are discussed initially as these form several aspects of the orientating background to the subsequent discussion of the adjustment of the child and of the family to the disease and its treatment, to aspects of psychological management and to the effect of the condition on the child and family.

ANTENATAL DIAGNOSIS

With current technology, many parents now learn before the birth of their child about the existence of serious heart disease in the baby and are able to begin the process of adjustment very early. This period of preparation, while increasing the emotional stress of the pregnancy, reduces the trauma of a neonatal diagnosis, as well as helping the parents to know that the baby is being 'received' into a world that is prepared. The option of termination of the pregnancy, which is offered in very severe cases, allows those parents who decide to continue with the pregnancy to feel more in control of their sad reality.

HOSPITALIZATION

Although there is evidence to show that repeated or prolonged hospitalizations may be antecedents of later emotional problems (Rutter, 1976; Hall and Stacey, 1979), psychosocial disadvantage probably contributes to this. Recent, more child-centered practice, which is also sensitive to the needs of the family, has led to some reduction of the stress (Shannon et al, 1984). Difficulties experienced may, in part, be caused by the repeated separations from the family, and by disruption of an orderly pattern of development. Admission to hospital constitutes, for the child, an experience of meeting with institutional life and bureaucracy. The essence of such institutions is that they possess a life of their own, into which the needs of the individuals have to fit. While within the family, accommodation is invariably made to the needs of particular members, the reverse occurs in hospital. Practices that are part of the institution's routine (such as regular observations) or which afford little individual choice (such as food) may be perceived by the child as insensitive and intrusive. The child, therefore, needs the presence of an adult, who is familiar with the child and the child's life, to mediate between the child's reality and that of the hospital. Many families may have other young siblings with their own needs and may live far from the geographically centralized paediatric cardiological institutes. In the absence of a parent or close relative, and because of the necessary separation of the child from the family, the assignment of personal nurses is an important alternative (Menzies Lyth, 1976).

Within the experience of hospitalization, babies and children also undergo moves from paediatric ward to intensive care unit and back, as well as moves between a local district hospital and a cardiac centre. These are often perceived as disruptions rather than transitions, both for children who are old enough to be aware of the changes and for their families. Parents often find it difficult to move from intensively staffed and specialist care units and settings to more routine wards, perceiving these latter to afford less expert care and attention for their sick child (Emery, 1989).

Painful medical procedures have been shown to constitute an independent and significant source of distress during hospitalization (Saylor et al, 1987).

PROCEDURES: NON-INVASIVE AND INVASIVE INVESTIGATIONS AND SURGERY

The course of congenital heart disease is punctuated by outpatient attendances, investigative and monitoring procedures, and surgery. The procedures vary in the degree to which they provoke aversiveness and discomfort, fear and anxiety. Like the scars, they serve as constant fore- or background reminders of the existence of the heart disease (past or present). The cumulative effect of procedures, whatever their frequency, is more perceptible to the child and the parents than to the treating clinicians.

PACEMAKERS

It could be postulated that dependence on an inserted, physically tangible small piece of electronic equipment would be a source of anxiety for children and adolescents. Interestingly, Alpern et al (1989) reported that two groups of peers without a pacemaker (one healthy and the other with congenital heart disease) regarded children with a pacemaker as more anxious, fearful of death and socially compromised than did the children with pacemakers themselves. The children with pacemakers, aged from 7 to 19 years, were shown to feel less in control of their lives. This could be based on fears of battery depletion, pacemaker failure and the possibility of consequent sudden death.

CARDIAC TRANSPLANTATION

The advent of transplants has altered the prospect from a hopeless prognosis to one of hope. This has a significant impact, both on the family and the medical profession. In the light of the relatively early stage reached in the development of this treatment, however, the reality of outcome is less clear, and it often differs from the expectation. Indeed, it has been suggested that parents 'must adapt to the new disease called organ transplant' (Gold et al, 1986). There are many stages in the process, each carrying its individual stress, which affects children and families differently. These stages include the rigorous assessment, preparation, anxious wait against time on constant alert, the transplantation itself, the postoperative phase and the peri- and post-operative medication that is required for protection from rejection. Much of this will almost invariably take place in previously unfamiliar medical settings, far removed from home and the treating hospital. Although the process of transplantation is familiar to clinicians, the enumeration of its various stages helps to increase professional awareness about the cumulative impact of the whole experience on the patients and their families.

There are also the issues concerning the relationship to the donor, including their identity and mode of death, and the wish of some donor or recipient families to meet the other. This is particularly poignant, since the donor will often be a child. Feelings of guilt and sadness tinge the relief of the recipient family. This issue requires particular attention in discussion with the child, who, at the appropriate developmental stage either at the time of the transplant or later, will be preoccupied with feelings and questions about the meaning of surviving with the vital organ from another person.

For those patients where the transplant leads to several years of relatively good and fulfilling functioning for the child, the considerable emotional and physical toll of the procedure is likely to be gratefully borne, although this awaits further empirical substantiation. Uzark and Crowley (1989) evaluated the effect of cardiac transplantation on the family life of 10 children who survived the procedure. They showed continuing stressful effects on the parents, including uncertainty about the child's long-term prognosis, significant strain on the parenting role, and social isolation. They did not mention the effect upon siblings, who are often equally affected but may well, at times, feel neglected. A recent retrospective comparative study of 65 children who had undergone heart or heart–lung transplantations reported important psychological effects associated with transplantation for the children. These effects included cognitive, behavioural and emotional aspects (Wray et al, 1994). There has also been some concern about compliance with long-term medication in adolescent transplant recipients.

When the transplant fails, questions may arise retrospectively in the minds of parents about how worthwhile the procedure was, particularly in relation to the likely suffering that the child will have undergone in vain. Conversely, however, most parents would find great difficulty in refusing the prospect of survival for their child, particularly since the anticipated cost of the experience to the child and family, including siblings, will always be underestimated even with the best preparation.

DEATH

Despite considerable advances in early diagnosis and treatment, including transplantation and the decreasing need for open heart surgery, death continues to be the inevitable outcome for a proportion of children. The fear of this fact is experienced by most families at some stage, but it is an ever-present reality for those professionals medically involved with congenital heart disease. The death of a child contravenes all expectations of the order of survival in a society that increasingly regards longevity and medical cure as the norm.

THE PROCESS OF ADJUSTMENT TO CONGENITAL CARDIAC DISEASE

THE NEONATAL PERIOD

When cardiac disease is first diagnosed in a neonate, it is the family that undergoes a profound process of readjustment. The mother is, at this puerperal point, in an emotionally vulnerable state. The reality of a seriously affected child only slowly replaces the anticipated healthy one. At this stage, as will occur with later major episodes in the child's life, shock and fear felt by the parents render much of what is said to them inaudible (Garson et al, 1978). The perceived seriousness of the diagnosis will be predominantly related to the site of the pathology – the heart – but is often poignantly underlined by the intensive nature of the investigations and treatment, particularly when this includes early surgery. Garson et al (1978), reporting on interviews and discussions with parents of 260 babies born with congenital heart disease, were able to distinguish different parental concerns and mechanisms for coping, according to the nature of the condition. Difficulty in acceptance, or denial of, the diagnosis was common with asymptomatic lesions. Anger was more frequently expressed when the child was seriously and symptomatically ill. It has been further observed that, having accepted their baby as ill, parents often assume that their child will be permanently handicapped, with no potential for complete recovery. Successful corrective surgery may not, for some time, erase this notion of handicap.

Some mothers, deeply upset or angry at the disaster that has befallen them and in search of explanations, dwell on their pregnancy. They may attribute causality to particular events such as failure to pay attention to minor illnesses (Linde et al, 1966; Garson et al, 1978). Such beliefs can give rise to feelings of guilt for failing to take preventative steps and, therefore, of causing the handicap. Alternatively, they may now feel guilty about smoking or drinking alcohol during the pregnancy. There may be anger at the medical profession for providing inadequate surveillance, or for failing to warn the mother about possible feto-toxic effects of drugs. These feelings may not be expressed openly. They need to be explored if they are not to remain a burden and carry long-term consequences for the mother–child relationship.

Pre-existing marital discord may lead to damaging mutual recrimination at a point of stress (Goldberg et al, 1990) just when mutual support is essential. A process of rejection of the child may set in at this time (Glaser and Bentovim, 1979). Acute discomfort and fear may also be experienced by older siblings, who may well believe that they have, in some way, been responsible for bringing about the handicap of the baby (Black and Sturge, 1979).

It is while these acute anxieties are active and accessible in the parents' minds – at the point of crisis (Caplan, 1963; Parad, 1965) – that careful, patient and repeated acknowledgements and explanations by medical and social work staff are necessary.

EARLY FORMATION OF THE RELATIONSHIP BETWEEN MOTHER AND INFANT

As with other neonatal problems, congenital heart disease may well necessitate early hospitalization. When a new baby is, for medical reasons, separated from the mother, the result for her may be disbelief in the birth of a baby and feelings of unreality, which may adversely affect acceptance of her child (Brimblecome et al, 1978). Keeping baby and mother together will help to confirm to the mother that she has indeed given birth to a real, albeit unwell, baby. This points to the need to provide facilities for peri- and postnatal care in or near paediatric cardiology centres, which are often geographically far from the obstetric units or place of birth of the baby. Antenatal diagnosis enables appropriate plans to be made for the place of birth.

Early meaningful contact is established between mother and infant in the process of feeding. The difficulties encountered in feeding babies with heart disease (Lobo, 1992), and their slow growth, are often experienced by the mother as rejection of her and signs of her own failure as a competent mother (Gudermuth, 1975; D'Antonio, 1976). This can be particularly frustrating if timing of surgery is made contingent on sufficient weight gain. Constant watchfulness, prompted by fears of sudden death, especially during the infant's sleep, will become an additional burden to the parents.

There are currently unresolved questions about the degree of security of attachment between mothers and their sick infants; Ludman et al (1992) reporting secure attachment and good mother–child relationship at 1 year in children who underwent major neonatal surgery. This contrasts with Goldberg et al (1991), who found that significantly fewer infants suffering from congenital heart disease were securely attached to their mothers than were healthy controls. Importantly, these studies found that, at the ages of 2 and 3 years, respectively, there were difficulties in the children's interaction with the mother and in the children's behaviour. Although these difficulties are likely to be a result of multiple factors, including the response of the whole family to the illness, the relationship between mother and child is likely to be an important factor. This again highlights the need for support and guidance for parents in the care of their child, particularly in helping them to gauge the degree of protection required by the child.

The slow motor development, cyanosis and early fatiguability of those severely affected young children (Linde et al, 1970) who do not undergo early surgery continue as constant reminders to the parents of their child's illness. They encourage parents in their belief in the existence of permanent handicap. To experienced medical staff, these symptoms are acceptable manifestations of a well-understood familiar process. In order to facilitate supportive communication, there needs to be an awareness of the different perceptions held by parents and by staff.

OVERPROTECTION

As the child matures, one of the most potent factors determining the adjustment to his or her condition is the parents' attitude to the illness. Congenital heart disease is a potential source of parental anxiety and consequently of overprotection. This may be experienced by the child as compliant parental indulgence or as an irritating limitation of the natural instinct to explore and define the limits of their physical and emotional capabilities. It may also be interpreted by the child as confirming a sense of fragility, and it may give rise to great anxiety about survival.

Parents are well acquainted with the notion, acquired from experience in adults, that physical and emotional stress may adversely affect the heart. They are, however, often unaware of the fact that most children have a healthy sense of self-preservation and learn to limit their activities appropriately (Bergman and Stamm, 1967). In their anxiety to prolong and protect their child's life, they attempt to restrain the child and limit the exploration of the environment (Calzolari et al, 1991). This may include limiting peer contacts and attempting constant surveillance of the child. Greater, and more inappropriate, limitations are sometimes imposed on the child who is not being seen to limit his or herself. A particular area of difficulty is encountered where children have a recognized but asymptomatic lesion.

The attribution of cardiac causality to all physical symptoms, be they minor upper respiratory infections or otherwise unrelated to the heart, indicates the pervasive extent of some parents' and older children's anxiety. Landtman et al (1968) reported a study in which there were 56 children mislabelled as having congenital heart disease. Of these, 39 subsequently developed precordial pain, 14 dyspnoea, 10 palpitations, 10 headaches and 15 suffered emotional and behavioural problems. Following appropriate diagnosis, the majority of symptoms disappeared, and mothers reported positive behavioural changes in 36 of the 56 children.

In addition to the physical protection, there is often a well-intentioned attempt to limit the child's frustrations and grant his or her every desire. This arises, in part, out of the parents' wish to compensate for their child's loss of health and considerable suffering. Unresolved guilt, which many parents continue to experience in relation to their child's illness, will impel them to make up for their presumed wrongdoings. The guilt may originate from the belief of having, in some way, brought about the defect but may equally arise from feelings of anger, frustration and rejection, which many parents feel at some time and which may be self-perpetuating. Not uncommonly, parents who are concerned not to upset their child experience difficulties in managing his or her behaviour. The child often senses the power possessed in exerting will over the parents. Common battlegrounds are sleep, food and separations (D'Antonio, 1976). Children who are overprotected acquire a growing awareness of their special position in the family and in relation to their siblings.

An important finding has been that overprotection is unrelated to the severity of the cardiac defects (D'Antonio,

1976; Garson et al, 1974; DeMaso et al, 1991). It appears to be related more to the parents' perception of their child's condition. This will depend on their own experience of cardiac illness, level of education and anxiety. Overprotection has been found to be more common among the socioeconomically disadvantaged, who, in addition to having less knowledge and understanding of medical facts and physiology, feel themselves to be culturally and socially at a disadvantage in relation to the medical profession (Kennell et al, 1969). They have less opportunity, therefore, to become informed and thus establish a more reality-based view of their child.

Overprotection often leads to difficulty for parents in talking openly and appropriately with their children about the illness and its prognosis, and especially in preparing them for procedures. In their wish to spare their children further anxiety, parents may deny facts, or knowingly underplay the significance or nature of impending events.

IMPACT ON THE CHILD

The impact of congenital heart disease on the child results from a complex interaction between many variables. These include the child's innate constitution, the severity of the condition, the timing and success of surgery, the child's physical experiences of pain and discomfort, continuing physical limitations leading to less opportunities for exploration and learning, awareness of limited future functioning and indeed survival, the family's socioeconomic status, stressful life events and the family's capacity for coping with these factors (O'Dougherty et al, 1983).

Children who continue to experience physical symptomatology have been shown to have a lower intelligence quotient than asymptomatic children. Kramer et al (1989), studying a controlled sample of 128 children aged from 4 to 14 years, also showed that cardiologically symptomatic children suffered anxiety and low self-esteem. This is likely to be related to limited capacity to learn and explore and to the effects of chronic (O'Dougherty et al, 1985) or perisurgical anoxia.

As part of our sense of security, we carry implicit assumptions about the intactness and safety of our bodies. We perceive them as functioning adequately and without undue interference. These implicit assumptions are severely challenged for a child with heart disease. Procedures (including those considered minimal by medical staff) are often perceived by children as intrusions and attacks on their selves. Feelings of owning defective or violated and vulnerable bodies are well illustrated in children's drawings.

There are, however, different mediators of the effects of procedures on children. An interesting study, looking at the response of very young children (aged 1–4 years) with congenital heart disease to a routine X-ray procedure, found that behavioural distress was associated with stranger-wariness and negative parental styles of discipline. While these parental reactions may well have been independent of the cardiac condition, the children also had only limited social experiences, probably because of the severity of their heart disease, which would increase their wariness of strangers and new situations and lead to more distress during hospital procedures (Bradford, 1990).

Children's understanding of their illnesses varies with their age. They are always aware of the existence of pathology through limitation of their activity compared with others, cardiopulmonary symptomatology, the existence of a scar, visits to hospitals and parental surveillance and anxiety. Such awareness, if not accompanied by explanations coming from the caregiving adults, will be enveloped in the child's own mythology. This may include equating a leaking valve or hole in the heart with a leaking tap. They may imagine that it can lead to fatal blood loss, collapse or even cause the heart to cease beating. Such mythology bears little resemblance to reality and is more likely to be frightening than comforting. Children tend to assume that absence of open discussion by parents or professionals indicates a truth too awful to utter.

Like adults, children seek causes for events. In the absence of sufficient explanations, children will invent their own. Chance is a concept that is very difficult to accommodate. Younger children will often see their illness or painful experiences, lack of recovery, further procedures such as surgery and superimposed infections (such as endocarditis) as a punishment for some blameworthy thought, feeling or action (Peterson, 1989). These may include objectively minor incidents or natural feelings, such as sibling rivalry (Brewster, 1982). The burden of guilt, one of the most intolerable of human feelings, then compounds physical discomfort and fear. Only in later childhood do children begin to understand external causality.

There may be family circumstances, such as marital disharmony or break-up, that will predispose the child to emotional problems. These can be precipitated by cardiac surgery. In order to understand children's responses to their illness, there is a need to become acquainted with the context in which they live. The following case study illustrates this.

> Following major corrective cardiac surgery, a 12-year-old girl was found to be worryingly withdrawn and anxious. This reaction was initially perceived by staff as being entirely related to the surgery. When the impending break-up of her parents' marriage became apparent, staff were able to respond more appropriately to her distress.

Children employ a variety of cognitive and emotional mechanisms for coping and defence in overcoming the effects of cardiac illness. These include 'rationing' their anxieties to immediate concerns, seeking information from different sources, denying the seriousness of the condition and regressing to younger behaviour patterns (Graham, 1991a). Coping is undoubtedly enhanced by understanding the nature of the condition, and of the procedures, that the child undergoes.

ADOLESCENTS

Adolescents who suffer from congenital heart disease have very specific concerns and needs (Celermajer and Deanfield, 1993). Are they to be considered as young adults? Should they continue to be cared for by paediatric cardiologists or 'graduate' to the care of the adults' cardiological service? In what wards should they be hospitalized? They need, and usually wish to begin to assume, responsibility for their own health and, therefore, require careful individual and direct explanations about their condition, prognosis and any specific precautions that they might need to take, for instance antibiotic cover for dental treatment.

Adolescents increasingly enquire and seek information about lifestyles and plans, including recreation, exercise and sport. They require advice and counselling about issues of contraception and pregnancy (Uzark et al, 1989).

Further questions arise as the adolescent nears the time for employment. A condition that restricts physical activity is particularly handicapping when manual occupation is anticipated (Offord et al, 1972). There is evidence suggesting the need for specific vocational training programmes (Ferencz, 1976). The issue of restricted or unobtainable life insurance must also be faced (Weidman, 1976; Celermajer and Deanfield, 1993).

SIBLINGS

It is important to remember siblings. They may well share many of the feelings discussed above, including unarticulated fear of the patient's death and a sense of responsibility for the illness. Some brothers and sisters believe that their negative feelings towards the sick child, especially when the child has been receiving much positive attention, have been disastrously enacted and translated into reality. These fears, and consequent guilt, add to the inevitable discomfort that siblings undergo (Stewart et al, 1992). This may become intolerable if the sick child dies.

Following the death, from congenital heart disease, of her infant brother, an 11-year-old girl became irritable and unhappy and developed asthma. In talking with the family, the girl's intense motherly feelings towards her brother, to the extent of sensing rivalry with her mother, became clear. She had nursed her brother while she suffered from a respiratory infection and believed that she had thereby caused his death. She experienced great relief when open discussion dispelled her worst fear.

Other children may feel a burden of responsibility to succeed where they feel their ill siblings have failed in fulfilling the parents' aspirations. Many siblings feel neglected and their needs overlooked; during periods of extreme concern for the sick child, there may be a considerable element of reality here. They are usually unable to voice these feelings and may present at school with behaviours construed as problems.

A 7-year-old girl was found to be taking small objects from other children in her school, and an alarmed teacher reported this to the parents. The family context of a seriously ill younger sister, who was receiving much emotional and material attention during her current prolonged hospitalization, came to light. Both parents and teacher became more sensitively aware of the needs of the older girl.

MANAGEMENT

CONTACT AND COMMUNICATION WITH THE CHILD AND FAMILY

Many children and their parents continue to attend as outpatients regularly even if infrequently, and become quite attached to this important contact with specialists whom they trust. Continuity of care is, therefore, greatly valued and can often only be ensured by senior staff who themselves become well acquainted with these patients and families.

Communication with the children about their condition is a vitally important issue. Many questions arise in this context. Who should talk to the child, and when? How much should the child be told, and how should he or she be told? Children are owners of their bodies and, like adults, are entitled to explanations of disordered functions.

Explanations must be made in language and at a cognitive level that the particular child can comprehend. In chronic ill health, which congenital heart disease may become, there is a need for ongoing revision and development of explanations as the child matures. It is always very important to establish initially what the child knows and thinks about the condition. If the child's current understanding contains frightening elements and cognitive distortions, he or she will be unlikely to be receptive to rational concepts until the anxiety is dealt with. Then, building on the child's own ideas, explanations can be interwoven with what is already known, and the synthesis becomes unique to that particular child. A child may confidently talk of their valve not working. If care is taken to explore with the child their impression of the function of a valve, or what it looks like, it may be discovered that the ideas bear little resemblance to reality. It is, therefore, unsafe to assume that any real knowledge lies behind the correct use of terminology. Explanation through simple diagrams or plasticine models are helpful, and many parents are themselves relieved to receive explicit explanations, which they often feel too ashamed to request. It is, therefore, helpful to include the family in this activity, which will also prepare them for future and necessarily repeated questions. It enables the parents to know about their child's degree of awareness, and it reassures the child.

Some children refuse to be involved in discussion about their condition. This implies that natural curiosity has been overwhelmed by anxiety. It would be quite inappropriate to impose explanations, but one is alerted to a need to deal with the anxiety.

PREPARATION FOR PROCEDURES AND EVENTS —

In preparing children for future events, such as hospitalization, procedures and, especially, surgery, it is important to take into account their concept of time, which varies with age. The younger the child, the shorter is the timespan that is meaningful. The child requires sufficient time to become prepared for the event without redundant anticipation, which would lead to unnecessary anxiety. While it is unhelpful to burden a child with long-term plans, there remains a need to inform the child in simple and explicit terms in advance of events.

Preparation for procedures, including catheterization and surgery, through the use of guided play is now well recognized (Cassell and Paul, 1967). It allows children to enact their fantasies of procedures and to express some of their feelings. It further provides a vehicle for imparting information to a child who may not be at a developmental stage ready to comprehend abstract verbal explanations. Whatever the medium, the content and amount of information given in preparation for surgery or procedures will have to be suited to the particular child. Although there can be no standardly prepared packages, photograph albums prepared on the ward with past patients or tape-recorded accounts in simple language are examples of very helpful tools.

Levels of anxiety vary between different children of similar ages, as does their degree of understanding. It is important to gauge carefully the degree of detail in preparation. The aim is first to answer all the questions that the child will have, be they articulated or not. In addition, certain facts should always be mentioned, however sensitive and unpleasant they may appear for the particular child. These include the fact and site of incisions, the target organ for surgery and the inevitability of postoperative pain and discomfort. A visit to the intensive care area is usual, and a description of the postoperative experience, including the use of machinery, is important. Familiarity that follows good preparation gives the patient some sense of control in a situation in which he or she feels, and is, very powerless (Bergmann and Freud, 1965). In the name of kindness, important details are sometimes misguidedly omitted. At the other extreme, a comprehensive approach, which although factual and full may overwhelm the child by its magnitude and detail, should be avoided.

There has been some discussion concerning the person most suitable to prepare children. Some would argue that this lies within the province of nurses (Peterson, 1979) or doctors. Others see this as the task of the social worker or specialist playleader (Lindquist et al, 1977). In some settings, the help of psychologists or psychiatrists is enlisted, and parents sometimes will prepare their own children, with the help of written information such as booklets provided by the hospital. The decision should be based on the person's capacity for talking to children, being sensitive to anxiety, having awareness of language and cognitive levels at different ages, and being medically informed. Indeed, amid confusion of roles, children may occasionally not be prepared at all.

It is vital to ascertain, both from the child and the parents, what the child already knows and to ensure that parental agreement has been sought. Resistance to openness is met, at times, from parents who, in their wish not to upset their child, wish to withhold information about what is about to happen. This may well be an indication of the parents' own difficulty in facing and coming to terms with the very painful facts. It points to a need to provide help for the parents to overcome their denial or anxiety and to enable them to support their child. In this context, it is helpful to acquaint parents with experience, which has shown that even very fearful children are calmer before surgery if preparation has taken place (Peterson, 1989). It is also important to explain to them that an honest approach enables the child to continue to trust those who provide care, allowing the child to gain comfort from their support. A child who is actively involved in understanding the illness is able to contribute more fully to recovery.

An 8-year-old boy, seriously ill with subacute bacterial endocarditis, was highly irritable and extremely uncooperative with his treatment. He was described by his mother as a difficult, inflexible intelligent child, whom she had always found difficult to handle. Following exploration of the boy's own perception of his illness, and giving honest and explicit explanations of procedures, there was a lessening of his sense of being invaded and intruded upon. For instance, fears of fatal exanguination following the proposed removal of a central venous line, and mistrust of a battery-operated pump attached to him, were acknowledged and dispelled. He became quite cooperative and very knowledgeable.

Factual preparation for parents is a vital aspect of the process and as, increasingly, surgery is performed on very young babies, it is the parents who require the support. Parents may be too anxious or uninformed to ask about facts, the ignorance of which may lead them to pessimistic and frightening conclusions. Particularly pertinent here are the projected duration of surgery and the sight of the child postoperatively. Although no amount of preparation will wholly protect a parent from the shock of their child's postoperative appearance, prior acquaintance will help to lessen anxiety and enhance the parental cooperation in active rehabilitation of their child. It is also important to note that children rarely display the traumatic postcardiotomy reaction commonly met in adults (Danilowicz and Gabriel, 1971).

After surgery or other procedures it is, however, important to enable the child to describe their experiences, including those aspects that the child found unpleasant or frightening, in order to lessen later post-traumatic reactions such as nightmares and fears of return visits to the hospital.

POOR PROGNOSIS

There are circumstances where divulgence of the whole truth, insofar as it can be known, may be inappropriate. Parents are rightly very sensitive to these. Where prognosis is guarded or poor, how much and how to communicate this to a child requires much thought. This includes high-risk or unsuccessful surgery or inoperable conditions, although the advent of heart and heart–lung transplantation has, to some extent, altered this situation. Most children are naturally optimistic but are invariably sensitive to parental and professional gloom and despondency, however well masked. Questions should not be answered untruthfully, but uncertainty, openly discussed, is an acceptable compromise. This will allow the child to voice concerns, fears and anxieties about not getting better without feeling inhibited, and without fear of upsetting his parents overwhelmingly. The child may then feel freer to pursue other immediate issues of current life, such as peer friendships and school activities, within his or her physical limitations.

SPECIFIC ASPECTS OF COMMUNICATION WITH AND HELP FOR PARENTS

The details of the more complex conditions are difficult for lay people to comprehend, although not all parents are able to volunteer that they do not understand. The greater their anxiety, the less information they absorb but the more repeatedly do they seek it. Sometimes, this dilemma is eased by inviting the parents to voice openly their greatest fears.

Imparting bad news to parents about their child is always a most difficult and uncomfortable aspect of paediatrics. Even when the child is of a sufficient age to understand, the initial conversation needs to take place with the parents alone, the presence of both being highly desirable. Particular difficulties sometimes arise with parents from ethnic minorities, when one or both parents may not speak English (or the prevalent language). The choice of interpreter is very important, since issues of confidentiality may arise. An older sibling may not be suitable because of the nature of the subject matter. Occasionally, there are concerns that one partner may not fully translate the information for the other.

The medical information should be given by the senior and most experienced doctor in the team, who will be aware of the likelihood of an upset reaction by the parents and will be able to accept this. Indeed, it is very helpful to have a senior nurse or social worker present. Since the parents will be left with many unanswered questions, it is very important to record in the medical notes what has been told to them, so that other team members will not give different or conflicting information when subsequently approached by the parents.

When the prognosis is poor, or when seeking consent for procedures and surgery that carry a high risk, then the question arises of how to balance or temper the degree of honesty required with some optimism. A qualitative description of the risk is far more meaningful to parents than numerical values of percentage risks. When the ultimate outcome is bad, particularly if the child dies, then the fact of having been prepared for this possibility is very likely to soften the impact.

Particular difficulties may arise when the baby or child requires intensive care for prolonged periods with very uncertain prognosis. The hopefulness or otherwise of the prognosis given will, to a considerable extent, determine the parents' wishes for continuation of the treatment. How the ultimate decision is reached varies in different centres. Some parents would wish doctors to decide. Others feel too overawed to express their wishes. Frequent communication between family and medical staff is an integral part of the treatment.

During a baby's or child's hospitalization, a discussion group for parents is one useful way of allowing for exchange of information, expression of feelings and mutual support to occur.

The group can be convened by nursing or non-medical support staff such as a social worker.

DEALING WITH THE CHILD'S EMOTIONS

No amount of explanation will suffice unless accompanied by a capacity to receive and acknowledge the child's feelings. These will inevitably include anger, fear, insecurity and often guilt. The anger may be directed at the staff, who are perceived as the aggressor. It may not be directly expressed for fear of 'biting the hand that is feeding'. Children may also feel angry at their parents for not protecting them from pain and suffering. Young children may, indeed, express bewilderment and incomprehension at their parents' condoning of the trauma to which they feel subjected. From the child's vantage point, this anger is justified. An unconditional acceptance and uncritical open acknowledgement of these feelings will relieve the child. Parents who are not threatened, who are not too ridden with guilt and who do not attempt to silence the child or retaliate against a child's perceived attack on them are helping the child slowly to accept that those who are understandably blamed are not, in reality, culpable. Indeed, they can be trusted. Here, some parents require a great deal of support and guidance. In addition to pain, all children have their own particular fears. Some fear that they may not wake up from an anaesthetic. Others fear that their central wounds will not heal securely. Children have unarticulated fears of death. Allusions to these acute anxieties lie masked in drawings, stories and play.

> A 9-year-old boy was found to have a systolic murmur. Following an admission for cardiac catheterization, he became clinging, refused to go to school and was panic-stricken at the thought of returning for an out-patient appointment. On meeting with the family, the mother's anxiety was manifest. For fear of upsetting her son, questions had been avoided and answers not given. Following an open discussion, losses in mother's early life were mentioned and permitted the boy's fears of death to be acknowledged. His anxiety subsided with the knowledge that his parents were now emotionally available to him, receptive to his fears and able to reassure him meaningfully.

Some children develop very specific phobias, the commonest being related to needles. Here, the help of psychologists who are skilled at desensitization and relaxation training is very useful.

THE EXPERIENCE OF DEATH

Death of the child is a possibility that is integral to paediatric heart disease. When parents sense that a fatal outcome is likely, they find great relief in being able to name it, and total denial of impending death will make its acceptance far more difficult.

Dying children continue to respond to parental cues. The less anxiety and overprotection the child perceives, the less pessimistic will he or she feel. Some children die after a prolonged, slowly deteriorating illness. Their death may initially be a relief as well as a great loss to the family, but guilt associated with the relief may compound the pain.

While the child lives, the parents are faced with the difficult and delicately balanced task of neither withdrawing from their child (and thus confirming the child's overwhelming fear of abandonment) nor denying the reality they know, which would compromise their later adjustment.

In these situations, too, there is the vexed question of what, if anything, the child should be told. There can be no rules here. Some children would become unjustifiably distressed, others greatly relieved. It is likely that the parents' wishes will be guided by the comfort of their children, but it may be necessary for the staff to help parents recognize cues that their children may be giving them. The greater the opportunity for parents to share their grief with each other, and gain support for themselves, the more sensitive and receptive will they be to the feelings of the dying child.

Apprehensions of death in children are based on fears of suffocation and pain, separation and sadness, and loneliness and abandonment. Communication with children around the issue of impending death is possible. Having discovered, through informal and sensitive discussion, the source of the main fears of the child, it is usually possible to allay fears about his or her own suffering. As Howarth (1974) describes, the approach to the child must be highly personal, honest and informed. Younger children find even greater difficulty than adults in comprehending the irreversible nature of their own death. They are, therefore, primarily preoccupied with its physical and emotional discomfort. Some older children may want to broach the subject.

Ultimately, it is the survivors who carry the burden. As increasingly complex surgical procedures are available and carried out, more children die in hospital. The fact that the parents gave the consent for surgery may well later lead them to feel guilty. The inevitable, retrospective search for alternatives, together with doubts concerning the correctness of their decision, are problems that staff too sometimes experience.

The process of adjustment to a child's death has been comprehensively examined by Burton (1974). She describes how foreknowledge allows for anticipatory grief to occur. Initial denial may be the only mechanism available for coping. Searching for alternatives delays acceptance of the inevitable. Parents may blame themselves, or they may feel a deep sense of inadequacy in having produced a doomed child. The feelings may be displaced and expressed in different situations that affect their wider relationships with other family members or possibly at work. For families, the mourning process entails the 'letting go' of the dead child, adjusting to the environment in which the child is now missing and the formation of new relationships (Lindemann, 1944).

Having passed through the early mourning stages of shock, numbness, disbelief, distress and anger, parents slowly begin to realize the truth of their loss. A meeting with staff involved with their child is felt by many to be helpful. It affords an opportunity to examine the details of the course and causes of their child's illness and death. Parents also gain comfort from the knowledge that the attention and interest of the professionals has not immediately been removed from their dead child to another living one. Some parents continue to maintain contact with staff who cared for their child, by telephone, letters or visits to the hospital or ward for some time after the death.

PARENT SELF-HELP

As in other areas, the self-support movement has found an increasingly important place in the life of families with children affected by congenital heart disease. The groups fulfil several important functions. They serve to reduce the sense of isolation that many parents feel. This isolation is partly a consequence of the often great geographical distance between the families' homes and the treating centre. The sharing of experience and information, through telephone networks, meetings and newsletters, as well as detailed booklets are a valuable source of strength in bewildering and stressful situations.

A forum is also created in which parents and professionals can meet and exchange information and feelings in a way that may not be possible in individual contact between parents and staff.

This fosters work towards common goals, inevitably bringing about improvements in the social and emotional climate of medical care. Self-help groups are also able to continue to offer support if a child dies.

LONG-TERM ADJUSTMENT

The nature of adjustment in the longer term is significantly, but not entirely, related to the degree and nature of residual physical (cardiac and neurological) impairment and intelligence quotient. Encouraging results in terms of emotional development and personality have been reported by Kramer et al (1989) in children who no longer experience physical limitation to their activity. Similarly, DeMaso et al (1990) found that psychological adjustment was good in children who did not suffer neurological or intellectual impairment. Utens et al (1993), by contrast, in a large follow-up study, have reported residual behavioural, and especially emotional adjustment, problems in a controlled group of children and adolescents aged 9–17 years, even when physical limitation and lowered intelligence were controlled for. A similar, less good outcome in terms of psychological distress was reported by Brandhagen et al (1991), who followed up a large sample of former patients 25 years after the original diagnosis of congenital heart disease had been made. Their response rate was, however, only 30%. Interestingly, in this group, current stress was unrelated either to clinical severity of the original cardiac defect or to educational or occupational achievement.

Very early surgery is unlikely to be recalled by the child. When the surgery has been corrective, later effects will be mediated to the child by what he or she is subsequently told, through residual parental attitudes and because of the remaining physical aspects. The level of parental anxiety is often more predictive of a child's adjustment than the severity of the lesion (DeMaso, 1991). Some outstanding reminders continue with the child throughout their life, including the scar, the vulnerability to future infective endocarditis and possible difficulties in obtaining life insurance. The effect of the scar depends partly on the child's ability to have a clear explanation for it and on his or her emotional acceptance of the defect with which he or she was afflicted. Some children are troubled by peers who can be less than kind. In adolescence, young people may find the scar a source of embarrassment.

The need for antibiotic prophylaxis may continue as a focus of anxiety, as are annual 'check-ups', both of which contradict the message of a total correction. It is, therefore, important that cardiologists do not equate surgical corrections with cures.

Corrections during childhood may also lead to difficulties for the parents. Having hitherto regarded the child as sick or handicapped, the family now have to adjust to a new reality of a healthy child. Relief may be tinged by disbelief. There may be fear of future disappointments and caution in accepting the change (Myers-Vando et al, 1979). A previous fatalistic stance, which had enabled the family to accept their child's handicap, is now challenged (Carr, 1976).

Following successful aortic valvotomy, a 12-year-old boy became increasingly demanding, irritating and moody. On meeting with the family, it emerged that neither parent was able to believe in the good prognosis given to them. The family had experienced a series of deaths and disasters over previous years. Their attitude had become fatalistic and they had become accustomed to pessimism. In this climate, the parents were unable to set reassuring age-appropriate limits and goals for their son, who therefore believed that the surgery had been unsuccessful. Open acknowledgement of these feelings and attitudes led to a more normalizing relationship to the boy, and the disappearance of his difficulties.

Other difficulties affecting family members, such as marital discord, which had previously been ignored or avoided in the preoccupation with the child, may now intrude and come to the fore. Amid this confusion, the child (who now feels physically better) may be uncertain to what extent he is allowed to progress or is responsible for the parents' difficulties. A change for the better may require considerable adjustment in some families. Staff may interpret the response of the family as ingratitude. There is also evidence of continuing invalidism in adolescents many years after correction of cardiac defects (Garson et al, 1974).

STAFF STRESS, RELATIONSHIPS AND COMMUNICATION

Staff themselves are well aware of the painful, exacting and highly responsible nature of much of the treatment. They are often naturally upset by a baby's or child's condition, particularly when a child dies. For a profession that exists primarily to improve and save life, a death inevitably spells a degree of failure or a battle lost (Gordon, 1974). These feelings must be articulated, enabling staff to accommodate them in a more realistic context. This makes it possible to continue the work positively. If this does not occur, unrelated difficulties may be precipitated amongst staff by the death. Here, other members of an integrated team, such as the social worker, psychologist or psychiatrist, who have not been directly involved in the physical care of the child, have an important contribution to make. Staff, too, form attachments to their paediatric patients, whose death will need to be mourned in some way if the memory is not to continue to haunt them.

The expression of feelings of distress, repeated questioning to different members of staff or complaints by children and their families may be persecuting to staff. Parents are often more willing to complain to nurses than to doctors, of whom they are more apprehensive. In their distress, parents may blame some members of staff, causing inadvertent splits in staff relationships.

There are also times when differences arise among staff members in their opinions or feelings about the treatment being offered, particularly when a very chronic or prolonged, but probably terminal, phase is reached. Nurses are in the most vulnerable position, being the frontline workers who are also in constant contact with the babies, children and their families. This situation, at times, leads to a sense of failure or despondency, especially when wards are short-staffed and there are very sick children or babies being nursed for long periods of time with little apparent progress.

Mutual staff support and trust is vital in this very stressful situation. These can only be achieved by open communication between members of the professional team. One aspect of this is recording in the notes what parents have already been told, or how much a child knows about his condition. This avoids giving conflicting or inconsistent information, truth denied inappropriately, or unnecessarily distressing details divulged insensitively. Another aspect of good communication is the regular explanation of the reasons for medical decisions to non-medical staff members, with opportunities for discussion.

Regular weekly psychosocial meetings offer a further setting in which potential difficulties can be discussed and constructive solutions found (Graham, 1991b). Such meetings need to include representatives from all the professions involved in the treatment team, including play staff and ward teachers. Good functioning teams usually include also a social worker and a child psychologist or psychiatrist. During these meetings, the developmental and psychological needs of each child are discussed and communication with community agencies, such as schools, health visitors, social workers and family

doctors, can be planned. The meeting affords an opportunity for the team to review responses to, and the management of, the death of a child. Plans can also be made for dealing with particularly troubled children, parents or families who need additional support. In well-functioning teams, staff members are able to express the particular concerns that they feel and can gain understanding of the origins of conflicts into which they may have been drawn.

Although time-consuming, these meetings are necessary in order to provide an optimal service to children and families through healthy staff functioning.

THE COMMUNITY

In the hospital setting, it is all too often forgotten that children live in the community, even when patients. In this setting, attitudes of caution, if not fear, prevail in relation to children known to suffer from heart defects. Teachers, for instance, sometimes extend well-intentioned but possibly emotionally detrimental and physically unnecessary protection to these children, exacerbating any overprotection experienced at home. Peers, especially in adolescence, may also perceive these children with undue caution. General practitioners, school medical officers, and health visitors are often consulted by parents in relation to questions arising about development, surgery, prognosis and management.

More information and education about the nature of congenital heart disease, as well as full communication from the cardiac centre with all those involved in management of the child outside the hospital, is, therefore, vital if the child and family are to feel accepted and contained at all times (Emery, 1989).

SUMMARY

The theme presented in this chapter is the complex set of interrelating factors encountered by the professionals when a child suffers from congenital heart disease. The many psychological needs of the children and their families can be met by careful assessment, together with open and informative communication with them, and by offering both the children and their family opportunities for exploring and expressing their concerns and reactions. This approach enhances the healthy coping and adaptation of most of the children. It requires close and regular communication, cooperation and mutual support between medical, surgical, nursing, social work, child care, teaching and psychiatric/psychological staff. Attention may then be devoted to therapeutic changes, as well as to the immutable factors which together combine to produce the reality of congenital heart disease in children.

REFERENCES

Alpern D, Uzark D, Macdonald D 1989 Psychosocial responses of children to cardiac pacemakers. Journal of Pediatrics 114, 3: 494–501

Bentovim A 1972 Emotional disturbance of handicapped preschool children and their families. British Medical Journal 3: 579–581, 634–637

Bentovim A 1975 The impact of malformation on the emotional development of the child and his family. In: Barry C L, Poswilli D E (eds) Teratology. Springer-Verlag, Berlin, p 223–234

Bergman A B, Stamm SJ 1967 The morbidity of cardiac non-disease in school-children. New England Journal of Medicine 276: 1008–1013

Bergmann T, Freud A 1965 Children in the hospital. International University Press, New York

Bingley L, Leonard J, Hensman S, Lask B 1980 Comprehensive management of children on a paediatric ward. Archives of Disease in Childhood 55: 555–561

Black D, Sturge C 1979 The young child and his siblings. In: Howells JG (ed.) Modern perspectives in the psychiatry of infancy. Bruno Mazell, New York

Bradford R 1990 The importance of psychosocial factors in understanding child distress during routine X-ray procedures. Journal of Child Psychology and Psychiatry 31: 973–981

Brandhagen D, Feldt R, Williams D 1991 Long-term psychologic implications of congenital heart disease: a 25 year follow-up. Mayo Clinic Proceedings 66: 474–479

Brewster AB 1982 Chronically ill children's concept of their illness. Pediatrics 69: 355–362

Brimblecome F S W, Richards M P M, Roberton N R C 1978 Separation and special care baby units. Clinics in developmental medicine, No. 68. Spastics International Medical Publications, Heinemann, London

Burton L 1974 Tolerating the intolerable – the problems facing parents and children following diagnosis. In: Burton L (ed.) Care of the child facing death. Routledge & Kegan Paul, London

Calzolari A, Drago F, Turchetta A, Marcelletti C 1991 Rehabilitation of children after cardiac surgery. Bambino Gesu Children's Hospital Scientific Research Institute, Rome

Caplan G 1963 Prevention of mental disorders in children. Tavistock, London

Carr RP 1976 Psychological adaptation to cardiac surgery. In: Kidd B S L, Rose R D (eds) The child with congenital heart disease after surgery. Futura, Mount Kisco, NY, p 433–483

Cassell S, Paul M H 1967 The role of puppet therapy on the emotional responses of children hospitalised for cardiac catheterisation. Journal of Pediatrics 71: 233–239

Celemajer D, Deanfield J 1993 Cardiology. In: Brooke CGD (ed.) The practice of medicine in adolescence. Edward Arnold, London, p 92–107

Danilowicz D A, Gabriel H P 1971 Post-operative reactions in children. Normal and abnormal responses after cardiac surgery. American Journal of Psychiatry 128: 185–188

D'Antonio I J 1976 Mothers' responses to the functioning and behaviour of cardiac children in child-rearing situations. Maternal–Child Nursing Journal 5: 207–264

Debuskey M (ed.) 1970 The chronically ill child and his family. Charles Thomas, Springfield, I L

DeMaso D, Beardslee W, Silbert A, Fyler D 1990 Psychological functioning in children with cyanotic heart defects. Journal of Developmental and Behavioral Pediatrics 11: 289–294

DeMaso D, Campis L, Wupij D, Bertram S, Lipshitz M, Freed M 1991 The impact of maternal perceptions and medical severity on the adjustment of children with congenital heart disease. Journal of Pediatric Psychology 16: 137–149

Emery JL 1989 Families with congenital heart disease. Archives of Disease in Childhood 64: 150–154

Ferencz C 1976 Preventive habilitation of cardiac children. In: Kidd B S L, Rose R D (eds) The child with congenital heart disease after surgery. Futura, Mount Kisco, NY, p 401–408

Garson A, Williams R B, Reckless J 1974 Long-term follow-up of patients with tetralogy of Fallot: physical health and psychopathology. Behavioural Pediatrics 85: 429–433

Garson A, Benson R S, Ivler L, Patton C 1978 Parental reactions to children with congenital heart disease. Child Psychiatry and Human Development 9: 86–94

Glaser D, Bentovim A 1979 Abuse and risk to handicapped and chronically ill children. Child Abuse and Neglect 3: 565–576

Gold L M, Kirkpatrick P S, Fricker F J, Zitelli B J 1986 Psychological issues in pediatric organ transplantation: the parents' perspective. Pediatrics 77: 738–744

Goldberg R T 1974 Adjustment of children with invisible and visible handicaps: congenital heart disease and facial burns. Journal of Counselling Psychology 21, 5: 428–432

Goldberg S, Morris P, Simmons R J et al 1990 Chronic illness in infancy and parenting stress: a comparison of three groups of parents. Journal of Pediatric Psychology 15: 347–358

Goldberg S, Simmons R, Newman J, Campbell K, Fowler R 1991 Congenital heart disease, parental stress and infant–mother relationships. Journal of Pediatrics 119: 661–666

Gordon B 1974 An interdisciplinary approach to the dying child and his family. In: Burton L (ed.) Care of the child facing death. Routledge & Kegan Paul, London, p 142

Gottesfeld I B 1979 The family of the child with congenital heart disease. Maternal–Child Nursing Journal 2: 101–104

Graham P 1991a Psychological aspects of physical disorders in child psychiatry: a developmental approach. Oxford University Press, Oxford, p 271

Graham P 1991b Psychological aspects of physical disorders in child psychiatry: a developmental approach. Oxford University Press, Oxford, p 280

Gudermuth S 1975 Mothers' reports of early experiences of infants with congenital heart disease. Maternal–Child Nursing Journal, 4: 155–164

Hall D, Stacey M 1979 Beyond separation: further studies of children in hospital. Routledge & Kegan Paul, London

Hofmann AD, Becker R D, Gabriel H P (eds) 1976 The hospitalised adolescent. Free Press, New York

Howarth R 1974 The psychiatric care of children with life-threatening illnesses. In: Burton L (ed.) Care of the child facing death. Routledge & Kegan Paul, London

Hume R E (translator) 1930 Chandogya Upanishad. In: Hume R E, The thirteen principal Upanishads, part 8, 3.4, section 3, verse 4. Oxford University Press, Oxford

Kennel J E, Soroker E, Thomas P, Wasman M 1969 What parents of rheumatic fever patients don't understand about the disease and its prophylactic management. Pediatrics 43: 160–167

Kramer H, Awiszus D, Sterzel U, van Halteren A, Classen R 1989 Development of personality and intelligence in children with congenital heart disease. Journal of Child Psychology and Psychiatry 30: 299–308

Landtman B, Valanne E, Aukee M 1968 Emotional implications of heart disease. Annals of Paediatrics Finnland 14: 71–92

Lax R L 1972 Some aspects of the interactions between mother and the impaired child. Mother's narcissistic trauma. International Journal of Psycho-Analysis 53: 339–343

Linde L, Rasof B, Dunn O J, Rabb E 1966 Attitude factors in congenital heart disease. Paediatrics 38: 92–101

Linde L M, Rasof B, Dunn O J 1970 Longitudinal studies of intellectual and behavioural development in children with congenital heart disease. Acta Paediatrica Scandinavica 59: 167–175

Lindemann E 1944 Symptomatology and management of acute grief. American Journal of Psychiatry 101: 141

Lindquist I, Lind J, Harvey D 1977 Play in hospital. In: Tizard B, Harvey D (eds) The biology of play. Heinemann, London

Lobo M L 1992 Parent–infant interaction during feeding when the infant has congenital heart disease. Journal of Pediatric Nursing 7, 2: 97–105

Ludman L, Lansdown R, Spitz L 1992 Effects of early hospitalization and surgery on the emotional development of 3 year olds: an exploratory study. European Child and Adolescent Psychiatry 1: 186–195

Menzies Lyth I 1976 The psychological welfare of young children making long stays in hospital. Tavistock Institute of Human Relations, London

Myers-Vando R, Stewart M S, Folkins C H, Hines P 1979 The effects of congenital heart disease on cognitive development, illness causality concepts, and vulnerability. American Journal of Orthopsychiatry 49: 617–625

O'Dougherty M, Wright F 1983 Later competence and adaptation in infants who survive severe heart defects. Child Development 54: 1129–1142

O'Dougherty M, Wright F, Loewenson R, Torres F 1985 Cerebral dysfunction after chronic hypoxia in children. Neurology 35: 42–46

Offord D R, Cross L A, Andrews E J, Aponte J F 1972 Perceived and actual severity of congenital heart disease and effect on family life. Psychosomatics 13, 6: 390–396

Parad H J 1965 Crisis intervention – selected readings. Family Service Association of America, Washington, DC

Peterson L 1989 Coping by children undergoing stressful medical procedures: some conceptual, methodological and therapeutic issues. Journal of Consulting and Clinical Psychology 57: 380–387

Peterson M C 1979 Preparation of the cardiac child and the family for surgery. Issues in Comprehensive Pediatric Nursing 3: 161–171

Rowe R D, Kidd B S L, Fowler R S et al 1974 Long-term management of heart defects. Symposium on chronic disease in children. Pediatric Clinics of North America 21: 842–869

Rutter M 1976 Parent–child separation: psychological effects on the children. In: Clarke A M, Clarke A D B (eds) Early experience – myth and evidence. Open Books, London, p 184

Saylor C, Pallmeyer T, Finch A, Eason L, Trieber F, Folger C 1987 Predictors of psychological distress in hospitalized pediatric patients. Journal of the American Academy of Child and Adolescent Psychiatry 26: 232–236

Shannon F T, Fergusson D M, Dimond M E 1984 Early hospital admissions and subsequent behaviour problems in six year olds. Archives of Disease in Childhood 59: 815–819

Solnit A J, Stark M H 1961 Mourning and the birth of a defective child. Psychoanalytic Study of the Child 16: 523–537

Stewart D A, Stein A, Forrest G C, Clark D M 1992 Psychosocial adjustment in siblings of children with chronic life-threatening illness: a research note. Journal of Child Psychology and Psychiatry 33: 779–784

Toker E 1971 Psychiatric aspects of cardiac surgery. Journal of the American Academy of Child Psychiatry 10: 156–162

Utens E, Verhulst F, Meijboom F 1993 Behavioural and emotional problems in children and adolescents with congenital heart disease. Psychological Medicine 23: 415–424

Uzark K, Crowley D 1989 Family stresses after pediatric heart transplantation. Progress in Cardiovascular Nursing 4: 23–27

Uzark K, von Bargen-Mazza P, Messiter E 1989 Health education needs of adolescents with congenital heart disease. Journal of Pediatric Health Care 3: 137–143

Weidman W H 1976 Growth, development and habilitation after cardiac surgery. In: Kidd B S L, Rose R D (eds) The child with congenital heart disease after surgery. Futura, Mount Kisco, NY, p 393–399

Wray J, Pot-Mees C, Zeitlin H, Radley-Smith R, Yacoub M 1994 Cognitive function and behavioural status in paediatric heart and heart–lung transplant recipients: the Harefield experience. British Medical Journal 309: 837–841

74

Social aspects of congenital heart disease

P. Alderson

INTRODUCTION

Social aspects of congenital heart disease cover many topics. These include the effects of the disease and treatment on the child's and parents' daily life; ways in which understanding and treatment of the disease have developed in different cultures; varying methods of planning and providing health care for affected children; the role of all the relevant professionals, their relations with one another and with patients; and the influence of wider forces, such as the law, the media, economics and politics on public and professional responses to congenital heart disease. This chapter examines one theme, the meeting point between social and clinical aspects and touches on the range of social issues as they relate to the theme, mainly in British hospitals in the late 20th century.

The most obvious meeting point of the social and clinical aspects is when families and doctors discuss diagnoses, proposed treatment and the progress of the disease. Whereas doctors are mainly concerned with the child's physical state, children and parents mainly consider the social–personal implications. Yet there is an overlap of concerns as families acquire clinical knowledge and doctors take account of social aspects. The clinical–professional concerns of nurses and health service managers overlap more broadly with families' social concerns; their contribution to social aspects of care will be discussed, besides present trends and likely future developments. Ways of negotiating the clinical–social overlap will be considered in the following sections: information, decision-making and the growing child.

INFORMATION

Studies in the 1960s show how little information doctors routinely shared with adult patients (Roth, 1963) and with parents of child patients (Davis, 1963). Practice is now transformed, great efforts being made to explain to families the purpose and nature of proposed treatment, the hoped-for benefits, the risks and the possible alternatives. Medical explanations are supplemented by clear leaflets (Scott and Gerlis, 1984) and booklets (Rees et al, 1990). At a glance, coloured illustrations illuminate more about haemodynamics than long verbal explanations alone would achieve. Nurses and play specialists devise play preparation programmes using many visual aids, such as dolls and annotated photographic albums following children through each stage of investigation and treatment. Children from about 1 year onwards respond to the explanations with interest; older children and parents appreciate the simple, graphic explanations, which provide a clear basis for more detailed discussion. These and all later unreferenced comments and quotations are drawn from studies of parents' consent to paediatric cardiac treatment (Alderson, 1990) and of children's con-

sent to surgery (Alderson, 1993). The studies involved hundreds of interviews with parents, health professionals and, in the second study, with children.

REASONS FOR SHARING INFORMATION

Professionals' motives for informing families have expanded from the need to gain informed compliance to greater concern about medico-legal obligations to request informed consent, in particular following enquiries during 1998–1999 regarding children who had heart surgery at Bristol, United Kingdom. Beyond major risks, many professionals also warn and prepare patients for the inevitable harms and costs of surgery, such as pain, wounds and the time and effort required during treatment. Some ward staff believe that even children who are just beginning to talk accept and cooperate with treatment more fully if they have some idea of what to expect and the purpose of each intervention. Anger, resentment and high anxiety are expressed by children who have not had due warning and time to come to terms with their initial fears. A clinical nurse specialist commented:

> I think there can't be a greater shock to a child than to have all these invasive procedures done without any explanation or psychological preparation. Never tell lies. If you do you can't expect children to cooperate in future. Parents can be surprised if they are honest, how well their child reacts.

A ward sister described the hard task of balancing honesty with reassurance: 'Sometimes we try too hard to play down the difficulties, we're so keen to have the family feeling happy about it. Then wham – reality hits – pain, drips, restricted life-style, depression.'

CHILDREN'S UNDERSTANDING

Among the hospital staff we interviewed about parents' and children's capacity to understand medical information, the replies varied greatly. Some professionals believed that explaining details about surgery only served to frighten and confuse parents and children. Others who spent much time talking with them believed that young children can cope with complex information intellectually and emotionally. Psychologists gave us examples of understanding in young children.

> A 3-year old understood his liver biopsy as well as some adults. He knew that a piece would be taken from his liver, a little piece so it wouldn't matter. And it would be looked at under a glass (he didn't seem to know the word for microscope) to see if it was good or not. He seemed to understand that it was for investigation only, not for cure. He knew that his liver was near his stomach. His mother was a nurse and she spent ages preparing and explaining.

A limited vocabulary does not necessarily mean an inability to grasp key concepts. Young children are thoughtful and constantly questioning (Tizzard and Hughes, 1984); clear explanation can help to prevent them from developing alarming fantasies and misunderstandings. The importance of explaining to young patients the purpose of each intervention is illustrated by studies of children who have experienced disasters, such as famine, war or torture. Children who feel too betrayed to regain their trust in adults, even when the harm was unintentional, endure psychological havoc (Melzak, 1992). Two-year-old children who survive shipwreck are able to talk about their serious depression and to benefit from therapy (Yule, 1992). To adults treating children with cardiac defects, the child's need for treatment and the adults' compassion and excellent intentions may seem too obvious to need explanation. Yet to the child, painful and frightening treatment can logically appear to be deliberate torture unless continuing explanations and reassurance are given.

Information is now seen by many professionals as an integral part of therapy, increasing children's tolerance of anticipated harms and their confidence in their treatment. Some ward staff felt that parents who wanted to keep a child in ignorance were protecting themselves, rather than the child. A psychologist commented: 'Our policy is that children should know, and if their parents don't want them to know, children really worry and carry around secrets that they do know and they pretend that they don't.' Many professionals respected the parents' knowledge of how much worrying news their child could accept, but they also tried to persuade reluctant parents to inform their child honestly. 'I would discuss it very carefully with the parents and try to get them to think about how much their child already knows and worries about' said one sister. An orthopaedic surgeon commented, 'I would always try to bring the parents round to being open with the child. It has never happened to me that I have been in direct conflict with parents over this. Kids know much more than parents realise – parents are often unaware of their child's maturity. I think the child has every right to know – it's their back.' This comment applies equally to the heart. Yet orthopaedics can be easier to discuss with children than cardiology. Orthopaedics usually concerns visible, painful or disabling symptoms on which many children have strong views; heart disease is often invisible and asymptomatic, carries higher risks and can be more complicated and distressing to explain.

EXPLAINING RISKS

The health professionals we interviewed generally agreed that children should be warned about definite events, such as having tubes and drains inserted perioperatively. Yet explaining the purpose as well as the nature of surgery may involve discussing indefinite and contentious matters, such as risk and alarming prognoses. Can and should such matters be explained to young children? Some clinicians dismiss the suggestion that asymptomatic children can have any concept of a severe defect, or a condition that sooner or later could seriously deteriorate. Other clinicians believe that the only way to enable children to accept major surgery as potentially beneficial is to help the child to see the disease as worse than the treatment. This can entail comparing the high risks of surgery with the higher risks of untreated disease. Some doctors think that children have no idea of risk 'until they're about 17'. Others discuss high-risk surgery with young children in such terms as: 'You'd talk about the risk of crossing the road, and how you have to be careful, or very, very careful' and that 'the risk is rare or very rare'. Preventative treatment can similarly be explained. In one surgeon's words: 'I use the analogy sometimes that if you save money you can't spend it now, but you've got it in the future. You're treating the future, not the present. A lot of children can accept that, that it's going to make them better able to deal with things.'

The hardest risks to discuss concern severe neurological damage and mortality. Some young interviewees discussed risks openly with us; examples from orthopaedics as well as from cardiac surgery have been included because they consider similarly serious risks. Eleven-year-old Niki (interviewees' names have been changed) explained that her scoliosis was so severe that she must have a spinal fusion, 'Or else, my sister who's eight says I'll bend right over and I'll squash my heart and my lungs and I'll die'. Alison aged 14 years, also awaiting a spinal fusion, said that when the risk of paralysis was explained to her, she fainted. Alison said that, although very anxious, she preferred to be informed and to have time to come to terms with accepting the risks. Everyone who reported that they had been clearly warned said that they preferred to know. Yet we interviewed parents who said that risks had not been discussed and some of these said they were satisfied that they were adequately informed. Relating reported satisfaction levels to the quality of services is notoriously difficult, and rigorous research attempts to discover whether everyone wishes to be informed about risks present insuperable practical and ethical problems. Our interviews showed that clinicians who explained risks with great care appeared to increase the confidence of the parents and children we met. 'The best thing about being in hospital is seeing my marvellous surgeon' commented one girl about her much-praised consultant, after describing her alarm at his information. Many professionals agreed that information could increase trust, such as the senior sister who remarked, 'If everything is explained fully, the parents are happy and trust in the whole team.' Some surgeons explained risk to young children, for example:

Children vary enormously but a typical child will understand as well as an average adult can somewhere around the age of eight. But they'll understand the basic outline earlier, from about 18 months. I spend a lot of time talking to the children. I'd talk to an 8-year-old as though they are an adult, softening bits. I'm very unhappy if I don't think a child understands *why* I'm doing something and what I'm trying to do.

You can give children down to 5- or 6-years old having spinal surgery some idea of what spinal cord injury means. Even though the risks of paralysis are so small, if it happens it totally destroys a child's life … If we don't inform children, and they then have to face something they weren't expecting, that's something they carry with them for the rest of their lives. They're resentful, and rightly so.

High-risk surgery is considered when the risks to the child's survival or quality of life from an untreated con-

dition are expected to be even higher. As with adult patients, there is doubt concerning the merits of raising anxiety about indefinite and possibly remote risks. A social worker in a paediatric cardiac unit described her recent experience of talking about risk with Lisa, her 13-year-old daughter. Lisa did not have a heart condition, but her case illustrates the complexities of discussing life-threatening treatment with children, as experienced by someone who had spoken with many children with heart defects. Lisa has mucopolysaccharide disease, which has not affected her mentally but has caused many skeletal problems including very severe scoliosis. Spinal fusion was recommended. In Lisa's own words, 'I have a choice. Either I have this operation and I might die, or I might go on without it and I might be paralysed.' Lisa summed up this choice after weeks of discussion into which her mother was drawn, like many parents, suddenly and almost involuntarily. Lisa's mother said:

When we saw the surgeon, he dumbfounded us by saying he wasn't sure the surgery mightn't be too risky. Lisa is a bit deaf, so I started telling her afterwards that the surgery might be too risky, and she immediately said, 'What do you mean? I might die?' And I hesitated for a moment, but I knew I had to be honest because she would have understood my hesitation, and so I said, 'Yes', and she immediately burst into tears, and said, 'I never knew you could die from an operation', and was very, very upset.

In the following weeks, Lisa and her mother talked about risk and paralysis and death. Lisa, who used a wheelchair, already knew that people with her condition did not have a full lifespan. Her mother continued:

She wrote a story about going up into heaven and she was running (that was her idea so it was very real to her) and she got to the doors of heaven and she saw Granny and Granddad and they said, 'Come in', and an angel said, 'No, go back. It's not time. You have a bit more time before you come.'

A further complication was a possible clash of interests between Lisa and her parents. 'If she did not have surgery it would put an enormous strain on us. It would affect the whole family lifestyle,' as Lisa became more disabled. Lisa's mother worried that she was putting unfair pressure on her daughter to consider her parents' interests. When medical information is so heavily loaded with social implications, inevitably discussion is pervaded with hope and fear, and completely impartial presentation of the options is not possible.

Like many children, Lisa 'managed to go on at school quite cheerfully. It was only at intervals she wanted to talk and got upset.' The cheerful times can mislead adults into thinking that children are not deeply troubled or do not fully understand, or that they will 'be all right' if upsetting issues are not discussed with them. Lisa's way of coping was to be able to talk and be upset when she felt she needed to. Her mother did not tell her every detail, but she thought that

> Lisa's understanding is as good as many adults. But there are issues I'm not sure one gives to a 13-year-old, such as that she might die during the operation. Was that fair for her to have to take that on? She went through a lot of pain thinking about that. I could have saved her from that. As a parent, I feel my child has the right to know if she asks. From the professional view, unless parents go along with it we don't proactively tell children, but we tell parents. It's a grey area. We won't go behind parents' backs, but I do feel children are left with anxieties no one can reach because their parents can't face it. Lisa is so physically dependent I have to be more active in promoting her independence.
>
> The anaesthetist thought the risk wasn't all that high. So maybe we needn't have put her through all that. Whether it's right to share, I honestly don't know. Yet I think Lisa's survived it perfectly, and she's probably grown in having to think about it to that extent. But if she'd been a less emotionally robust child, perhaps it wouldn't have been right to share so much.

Doctors' and nurses' reluctance to explain serious treatment, risk and uncertainty (Taylor and Kelner, 1987) and the ways they evade questioning (Maguire, 1985) have been well documented. Professionals are constrained by seeing most patients briefly and seldom, by uncertainty about how children and parents can cope with bad news and by the stress of repeatedly caring for patients at risk. Lisa's mother was exceptionally well qualified to support her daughter while she came to terms with knowledge of risk; the example illustrates the stresses and complications of being honest in such circumstances, and the kinds of support that many families perhaps need. Some of the staff we interviewed took informing parents and children very seriously, offering emotional support as well as technical information. A senior registrar described preparing parents to accept a very poor prognosis for their son's heart condition by trying to sense how far they were still hopeful.

> What's important is to know how quickly you can be that honest ... It depends on how rapidly you can turn their attention to that degree of pessimism. So if the outlook is extremely pessimistic then you can sense that it comes as no surprise to them when you start to say he's not doing well.

A senior sister described her response to adolescent girls' fears.

> I usually say to the child, 'What do you want to be told?' Sometimes the teenagers say, 'Everything', but then you can see them edge away as if what I am saying is too much for them. I don't leave it at that. I say, 'What is it upsetting you?' I make sure that before the day of surgery they have an opportunity to voice their fears and uncertainties. These girls can be very protective of their mothers. They don't want to upset them by showing how worried they really are, and they put on a brave face when others are around.
>
> Sometimes it is important that they know more than they have asked for. I try to edge them forwards to accept a little more information each time we have a chat. I watch carefully to see how successful this is being – and I ration it out, particularly if they seem very anxious, only telling them one main thing at a time. It can become obvious that the child doesn't really want to have the operation done – they have been persuaded by the parents – and these children can just switch off and avoid getting involved. They just won't listen to the information, and rarely ask questions.

Some health professionals told us that young children have no real concept of death; others confirmed the research that has demonstrated that 5-year-old children can understand death as final and irrevocable (Clunies-Ross and Lansdown, 1988), although they may not share their knowledge with their parents (Bluebond-Langner, 1978). A sister in a heart–lung transplantation unit described talking with children about mortality. Families stay in the unit for four days of assessment and 'pretty horrendous' discussion. The sister thought children with cystic fibrosis have far more understanding, because of their experience of severe illness and arduous daily treatment, than the relatively asymptomatic children with heart defects have.

> I feel that when transplantation is being considered, it is the *only* time parents have the opportunity of true informed consent. With more conventional surgery parents are given enough information to sign the consent form, but I do not believe that parents are aware that they have the option to refuse. Transplantation is about choice; therefore you feel able to give families 100% information on which to *make* their decision. You include all the risks, complications and long-term difficulties – you spare nothing, you give them the lot, and you do exactly the same for children.
>
> Naturally you have to tailor your information to the individual child's age and cognitive development. You wouldn't discuss percentage risks with a 6-year-old. You'd probably say, 'Do you know why you're here? Do you know what is wrong with you? Are you taking any medicines? What are they for?' You would talk about the treatments they will need after they have a transplant, and that some may be unpleasant and you wish they weren't necessary. You talk about body changes, including the puffiness and possible hairiness.

The sister said that detailed information is given because 'transplantation is a limited resource', and it is important to treat the children most likely to benefit. Also, 'it's a luxury treatment in a way, commanding a lot of resources that aren't normally available', allowing time for thorough information, although severe illness could complicate this.

> The children we see are often very depressed and demotivated. Are they capable of taking in the information? How easy is it for them even to remember what it was like to feel well? Often they've had to go along with having lots of physio and taking lots of medicines to keep well but they haven't *felt* better. I think it's very hard for them to believe that any treatment is going to make them feel better.

Important reasons for informing children include the uncertainty of benefit and the very high risks.

> *Sister*: None of us know whether transplantation is an appropriate treatment. There's only what is right or wrong for individuals. We don't have the right to assume we know what's appropriate for a particular family. It's a major procedure, with so many built in uncertainties and difficulties, it's not routine.
> *Interviewer*: What if parents want information withheld from their child?
> *Sister*: No. Never, never, in the case of transplants.

Sometimes children with cystic fibrosis have been protected from recognizing how ill they are. The sister added: 'It isn't right for us in four days to take away that protection from them. It's their armour.' Instead, families can go home and talk more openly in their own time then return when the child is better prepared.

The alienating disaffection and sense of banality for health professionals when they treat patients simply as bodies have been graphically recorded (Zussman, 1992). Treating children as people, and sharing their 'wishes and feelings', as advocated in the Children Act 1989 of the United Kingdom, can be rewarding aspects of caring for them. Professionals who take time to talk with children need the practical support of health service managers who recognize the value of this stressful work and allow time and space for quiet discussion (Williamson, 1992). They also benefit from the cooperation of colleagues, which support group meetings for staff can encourage (Menzies Lyth, 1988). Children's understanding of medical information depends on far more than their age or ability. It is influenced by the care with which they are informed and supported while coming to terms with fear and risk, by their own knowledge and experience and by how much adults expect and encourage them to understand. Yet understanding the need for surgery differs from evaluating or accepting it, which are considered in the next section.

DECISION-MAKING

At clinical case conferences, cardiologists and surgeons aim to reach objective decisions based on medical evidence. They tend to avoid social issues, such as the wishes and feelings of the child and parents about proposed treatment, and they attempt to treat everyone justly by applying general clinical principles. Yet every reference to the magnitude of harm or benefit is inevitably relative and value-laden and carries some allusion to the present or hoped-for quality of the child's social life. Clinicians' difficulty, at times, in reaching consensus illustrates how varied their individual views can be. In contentious cases, some consultants believe that it is wrong to burden parents, let alone children, with the responsibility and potential guilt of sharing in decisions. Surgeons commented, for example: 'Children can't possibly decide whether they need an operation. They'll all say "no" because they're frightened.' 'Children have no idea about long-term goals. They live in the present.' One surgeon remarked,

> Don't you think we're going in for over-kill with this consent business? Adults don't have the knowledge to make decisions. People should take their surgeon's instructions. I make it clear to them. 'This is my opinion. If you don't like it then go elsewhere.'

A paediatric cardiologist commented:

> I consider that we are paid to make decisions, it's part of the job. If parents agree that their child should go to surgery and the child dies, they will blame themselves and it's a decision they have to live with for ever afterwards. Sometimes it helps if they can blame someone else. I think we have to accept this. I try to present the choices without bias, but that's impossible.

Yet can parents and children share in making decisions, and do they want to?

ABILITY TO SHARE IN DECISION-MAKING

Concepts of the patient's right to refuse or consent to surgery stem from the work of Locke in 1690 (reprinted 1959) and of Kant in the 1780s (quoted in Paton, 1972). They argued that rational men, capable of pure reason and knowing the correct answer to moral questions, must be able to control their own life without interference. Women and children were denied this right as they were assumed to be irrational. In the 1850s, Mill acknowledged that not all moral questions have 'correct' solutions. He advocated liberty as the greatest good, the individual's sovereign right 'over his own body and mind' to make wise or foolish decisions. No adult should be compelled into any decision unless this would prevent harm to others (reprinted, Mill, 1982). Children were again excluded. These two meanings of competence, wisdom to know the correct decision or else courage to make a best guess and to take responsibility for mistakes, contradict one another. Yet both are integral to modern meanings of competence. Asking adults when they think a child becomes competent is a kind of trick question that usually ends in contradictions; for example:

> *Interviewer*: When do you think your daughter was or will be able to decide for herself about the proposed operation?
> *Mother*: Well, now at 12 she is very sensible. I think she could decide now.
> *Interviewer*: What would you do if you disagreed with her decision?
> *Mother*: I don't think we would disagree, she's very sensible. But then, I suppose if it's life-threatening, I'd want to have the last say – just in case.

A child's mature independent judgement that happens to agree with the adults' views can seem like dependent compliance. It is only when the child and adults disagree that competence becomes a live issue, and then children can be dismissed as foolish simply because they disagree with adults. We asked 70 health professionals how they would define and assess competence and their replies varied widely. Competence is very hard to define positively; it is easier to define negatively, when it is obviously missing in bizarrely self-destructive decisions. Anthropologists argue that the vague concept of the competent person is mainly defined negatively, by classifying certain groups as 'incompetents' (Young, 1990). Then adults, for example, do not need to question their own abilities and rest assured that they fit comfortably within the status of competent adulthood. However, the assumption of competent adulthood depends on the contrasting state of incompetent childhood. Many of our interviewees accepted this dichotomy. They assumed that 'children can't possibly decide for themselves until they grow up/leave home/have done GCSE biology'. They dismissed the possibility of the competent child, or felt troubled or threatened by it. Others did not identify competence with age and believed that young children could be competent.

Many ethicists continue to accept simplistic status definitions of competence and assert that minors do not have the cognitive and moral maturity to evaluate complex decisions (Buchanan and Brock, 1989). The evidence challenges their theories. A sister in the transplantation unit reported children's evaluations of the risks and benefits of heart–lung transplants.

> *Sister*: A little girl of about seven with cystic fibrosis ended up by summing up what I had said beautifully. She said, 'You're telling me that with cystic fibrosis you can get very ill and die'. I said, 'We hope very much that won't happen, but that's why the doctors are thinking about *whether*, and it is only whether, a transplant might help you.' 'And you said that even if I say I want it, I might not live long enough to get one.' I said, 'Well not everyone does. We think you probably will because you're fairly well at the moment but people do die waiting.' 'And you're telling me that I could *die* when I have the operation.' 'We haven't had anyone die in the operating theatre, but yes it could happen.' Then she said, 'Even if I survive, you're not promising me that everything's going to be good, or that I will be able to do all the things I want to.' So I said, 'When we put new lungs inside somebody, you *should* be able to do a lot more, but it's not a promise that anyone's going to be able to give you.' She said, 'But, there is a chance that I could feel really good and I could come first in a race on my pony.' And I said, 'Yes'. Then she continued, 'All those other things are going to happen to me anyway, so please ask them to give me some new lungs.'
>
> I think for someone of seven or eight to say that illustrates how she had totally taken on board as well as I could, the consequences of transplantation. She had managed to set it all out and look at it very clearly. She had understood the uncertainties. Okay, on a child's level, but who could better it? I couldn't.
>
> I think it's very different when they have cystic fibrosis. Children who have been perfectly healthy don't have that perception of the value of life. Whereas these children were looking at certain death and exchanging that with the uncertainty of transplantation.
>
> *Interviewer*: So you think their suffering, rather than retarding their understanding, heightens it?
> *Sister*: They are the most sure, mature children. They're physically immature, but their understanding of life and death knocks spots off us. I think they're immature in some of their attitudes, but their understanding of their own wellbeing and what life is all about is mature. Of course they have temper tantrums. They've got this debilitating illness. They've done nothing to justify being sick day in, day out. It's awful for them. But they tell you it all. Why they have this nebulizer, what this tablet does, et cetera. They're very manipulative children. Knowing that food is a major issue, they'll have steak at 2 o'clock in the morning. But that's very different to their actually understanding.
> *Interviewer*: It seems that suffering and difficulty help some children to grow. The usual convention is that this holds them back.
> *Sister*: I think it often holds them back in some of the academic things because of missing school. They often have a poor concentration span, and their intelligence quotient may be lower.
> *Interviewer*: Some people have related intelligence to wisdom.
> *Sister*: I think it's totally, totally different. If I'd had this conversation with you 3 years ago, it would have been very different. Working with these children is a real eye opener. Previously I'd have said that some level of mature understanding of the medical information might be possible, say, for an 8-year-old, but I would not have felt comfortable involving a child in actual decision-making unless they were at least 12-years or 13-years old.

I remember one 10-year-old who said, 'I don't want it'. These children are given that right of choice. It's not a question are they capable of making a decision? If a child truly understands what is involved and the alternative outcome, then they are not forced into agreeing to a transplant. That causes a lot of problems for nursing staff when the present age of consent is what – 16? Certainly that's an age we are comfortable with.

Several other professionals agreed that certain very ill children have exceptional wisdom and maturity, and other nurses described how their respect for younger children increased through years of working with them. Protective adults who want to spare children the risk of making harmful decisions with ensuing blame and guilt, themselves risk making harmful decisions and being resentfully blamed by the child. Yet sincere attempts to listen can sometimes resolve deadlock. A girl aged 10 years whose brother had died of cystic fibrosis refused to consider having a transplant. The sister respected her refusal, but added, 'The next day she asked to go on the waiting list, because, "You listened. I don't like physio but I'm told, 'sorry you have to have it'. It's the same with medication. I just wanted to see what would happen if I said 'no'. If you would take any notice."'

The girl's change of decision meant that treatment could be given with her fairly willing cooperation, instead of being withheld or enforced. If children refuse, serious family discord and distress can ensue. Yet this may be a case of conflict being acknowledged and shared by the family, whereas if a child's protests are ignored and treatment is enforced, the repressed conflict remains as inner mental turmoil for the child to cope with alone. Families may need continuing support after refusal as well as after consent. Children are also assured that they will be on a provisional transplant list, in case they change their mind.

In England and Wales, people aged over 16 years can give valid consent to treatment (Family Law Reform Act, 1969, s.8). The consent of people under 16 years is legally valid if their doctor considers that they are competent to make an informed and wise decision (*Gillick v. West Norfolk & Wisbech HA*, 1985; Age of Legal Capacity (Scotland) Act, 1991 s2 (4)). The 1989 Children Act states that children deemed to be competent can 'refuse medical or psychiatric examination'. The United Nations 1989 Convention on the Rights of the Child, ratified by the British government in 1991, emphasizes the best interests and welfare of the child, which include adults listening respectfully to the child's views 'on all matters affecting the child' (United Nations, 1989; article 12). As discussed later, since 1991 English law has become more ambivalent about minors' consent. Yet among our interviewees in 1989–1991, the ages when certain children were believed to become competent varied from early childhood to adulthood. One way to

discover personal assessments of competence is to ask who decided about consent to surgery. We asked 120 children aged 8–15 years having major orthopaedic surgery, and their parents, who they thought was the 'main decider' about whether to accept or reject the proposed operation (Table 74.1). Ages of the 13 'main deciders' ranged from 8–15 years. Parents were more likely than children to say that the child was involved in the decision. The figures represent widely ranging comments, such as Julie aged 11, who said, 'I think everyone should give an opinion, and maybe the doctor put them together.'

Table 74.1. Views about who was the 'main decider' about proposed surgery

Main decider	Views of what did happen	
	Parent's view (n = 120)	Child's view (n = 120)
Child	13	13
Child + adults	62	44
Adults	32	60
Child accepted after persuasion	9	–
Don't know	4	3

WANTING TO SHARE IN DECISION-MAKING

The ability to decide differs from the desire and confidence to do so. We also asked the 120 children aged 8–15 years, before and about a week after their operation, who they thought 'should be the main decider' (Table 74.2). Like women interviewed about breast cancer decisions, most interviewees wanted to share decision-making with others; fewer children and women wanted to decide independently or to leave others to decide (Alderson et al, 1994). Although the proportion of replies from children having cardiac surgery may be very different, a similarly

Table 74.2. Views about who should be the 'main decider'

Preferred main decider	Views of what should happen[a]	
	Before operation	After operation
Child	18	21
Child + parents	3	5
Child + doctors	3	1
All together	49	41
Parents + doctors	19	13
Doctors	25	25
Parents	2	7
Don't know	1	7

[a] Views of 120 children.

wide range of opinions might be found among 120 children with heart defects.

The children showed more confidence in their doctors' than in their parents' judgement. The figures suggest that parents are seen as mediators rather than 'main deciders', and that joint decision-making is a major preference. Some children were unaware of the possibility of choice and consent. Examples from the youngest children include two girls aged 8 years who said, 'I don't care who decides about the operation, as long as I get better,' and 'My doctor and my mummy decided about my operation. They knew what I wanted. After all she is my mum and I do trust her.' Another girl said, 'When you are 8, I think you tell your parents when you need an operation. We all decided about my heart operation together, we knew we had to because I was so breathless.' Another 8-year-old child said that she was 'the main decider' about her surgical leg lengthening, and her mother agreed, believing that only her daughter had the necessary knowledge of the many social problems associated with her short stature and the right to decide about such long, painful treatment. Children and parents both thought that, on average, girls are able to make informed and wise decisions 2 years earlier than boys.

Although some people say that they wish to defer to doctors, many others want to have a small or large part in making decisions and may rely on doctors to ascertain how much they wish to be informed and involved. One mother who was thought by the nurses to be 'very simple, she doesn't really understand' insisting on staying during intensive care rounds, when parents were usually excluded. Talking about her son's heart surgery, she said:

> I'd feel more guilty and upset than the doctors would, because I'd signed the form. They're only doing their best, their job. But how would you feel if something went wrong with your child on the table? The doctors don't see it like that, that he's my child. They think I'm moaning. I'm not complaining, but I have a right to know what is happening, the good and the bad, and what his condition would be if he didn't have these operations. I feel really guilty when I look at his scars. I've got to have second thoughts about whether to say 'no'. Mothers really should have more say than doctors, because you have to carry it all.

This mother saw her rights not as property rights over her son, but as the means of fulfilling her parental responsibility. Through learning about the risks of non-treatment she came to accept the risks of surgery; working towards a decision is an important means of coming to accept it and differs from being presented with a ready-made medical conclusion. Through sharing in decisions, parents can feel that they have fulfilled their obligations, instead of feeling guilt and inadequacy that they allowed themselves to be excluded from making decisions that they still have to authorize by signing the consent form.

Reports in 1998 and 1999 about enquiries into children's heart surgery at Bristol, in the United Kingdom indicate that, when a child dies or is brain damaged, parents increasingly channel their protests through allegations of doctor's negligence to inform parents fully about the risks of surgery in order that parents will give informed consent or refusal. English legal cases during the 1990s will now briefly be reviewed. They show that, despite doctors' rising anxieties about litigation concerning consent, the courts have increased doctors' control over parents' and children's consent or refusal.

In 1991, Lord Donaldson, in the Court of Appeal, began the 'backlash against Gillick'. He ruled that R, aged almost 16 and refusing mental health treatment, could be forced to have medication (re R, 1991). In 1992, he ruled that W, aged 16, who had anorexia could be force-fed against her wishes (re W, 1992). This overturned the 1969 Act mentioned earlier that respected 16-year-olds as having adults' rights of consent. The 1989 Children Act increased the potential number of people with 'parental responsibility', and Lord Donaldson further ruled that if any one of these adults gave consent, this could overrule the refusal of everyone else concerned including the 'Gillick competent child' aged up to 18. (The details are discussed in Anderson and Montgomery (1996).)

Both rulings were criticized by lawyers on several grounds, including the point that mental illness affected one if not both cases, which would have been better dealt with using the Mental Health Act 1983. Lawyers warned against generalizing from these exceptional cases to all teenagers and children, but this has happened. Since 1992, doctors often mention that 'the law does not allow children to refuse'. Of course children can refuse, no law can stop them. The legal and also ethical questions are whether doctors should override refusal or should respect the informed decision of a child they deem to be competent.

It is likely that there are many unreported cases of doctors and parents gradually coming to accept the child's informed refusal, even with (almost certainly hopeless) attempts to prolong life with repeated surgery, chemotherapy or organ transplantation (such as Irwin, 1996). Yet professional and public attention is drawn to the series of reported court cases that have all authorized doctors either to treat or not to treat as they originally intended, and that have ruled against children's and parents' wishes. The sole exception was a very young boy whose parents refused a liver transplant for him (re T, 1997). These parents were intensive care nurses and it seems that, exceptionally, their views counterbalanced the expert medical views that the courts usually favour against the families' lay views. Court cases are based on precedent, and so each case confirms previous ones. Doctors have great power to shape legal judgements and individual patients' and parents' consent. When they wish to proceed with treatment they can emphasize the hoped-for benefits. When they consider it best to withhold or withdraw treatment, they can emphasize the pains, risks and uncertainties of treatment (Silverman, 1981; Zussman, 1992).

Medical authority was taken still further when doctors were authorized to transplant a new heart into M, aged almost 16, despite her refusal. Previously healthy, she had developed heart disease a few weeks earlier and a transplant was proposed a few days before the court hearing (Dyer, 1999a). M was quoted as saying, 'Death is final – I know I can't change my mind. I don't want to die, but I would rather die than have the transplant and have someone else's heart.' The judge, Mr Justice Johnson, said that he was 'very conscious of the great gravity' of overruling M's wishes, she might resent this for the rest of her life, and the already high risks of the surgery not being successful might be increased by M's unwillingness. Yet he concluded that M was 'over-whelmed by her circumstances and the decision she was being asked to make. Events have overtaken her so swiftly she has not been able to come to terms with her situation' to make a competent decision. Yet M's reactions are typical of the initial stages of consent to heart surgery. Consent involves a process, not simply an event. People begin with a dilemma between mutually incompatible ends, such as gaining health and avoiding surgery. Gradually they think and feel their way towards a resolution, such as preferring treatment to the untreated condition. They begin to let go of some desires and hold to others more strongly. At first, the dilemma is inevitably confusing, but the person is not necessarily confused.

The desperate urgency felt by M's parents and doctors and the judge is understandable. Yet it is unfortunate if such an exceptional case encourages the belief that, when an extreme procedure such as a heart transplant can be enforced, almost any other procedure can also be enforced on minors, whose views need not count. Adults' own refusal has to be respected in English law, to the extent of respecting women's refusal of Caesarean section even if the baby might die (re S, 1998). This case reversed and critized two earlier decisions in 1996, by M's judge Mr Justice Johnson, that Caesarean sections could be performed against the women's wishes. One of them said that she would 'rather die' than have a second Caesarean and the Judge commented, 'I concluded that a patient who could speak in terms which seemed to accept the inevitability of her own death was not a patient who was able to weigh up the considerations.' His view contrasts with those of the senior nurse quoted earlier who believed that it is only when young children accept the high possibility that they might die that they are able to give informed consent.

Newspapers compared M's case with cases of force-feeding girls with anorexia (Editorial, 1999a). They ignored the great differences between administering food and implanting a heart, and between patients with a physical condition and those with anorexia, which is linked to mental disorder. Most seriously, emergency court rulings undermine the respect for informed and willing consent, which, to many practitioners, is an integral part of therapy – even for young children as far as they can understand.

Despite the judge's report that he had considered M's views, her views were unlikely to influence the inevitable precedent-based legal outcome of supporting medical opinion. This inevitability was demonstrated in two further cases in the same month. David Glass's mother failed to obtain a court ruling that treatment should not be withheld from her severely disabled son, aged 13 (Dyer 1999b). The courts also upheld consultants' refusal to refer Katie Atkinson aged 9, who has Down's syndrome, to be assessed for a possible heart transplantation as her parents had requested.

Katie's case illustrates controversies about children with Down's syndrome. They have a high incidence of heart defects but not one so far in Britain has had a heart transplant. Although the Department of Health declared in news bulletins on 26 July 1999 'there is certainly no ban on people with Down's syndrome receiving organ transplants', politicians leave doctors to select the patients who they think will have the best chances. So far, clinicians have excluded children with Down's syndrome because, for example, of their shorter life expectancy. Yet since less than half the transplanted recipients survive for more than 10 years (Fraund et al, 1999), the expected survival time is well within the lifetime of children and teenagers with Down's syndrome. Many kinds of minor and major medical treatment are withheld from children with Down's syndome (Julian-Reynier et al, 1995), which partly accounts for their shorter average lifespan; consequently to deny treatment to children because of shorter life expectancy can be a circular argument. Children with Down's syndrome may be considered less worthy of costly care because of their average lower intelligence. Intelligence tests of children with Down's syndrome found a range from 10 to 92, the latter figure being near the centre of the normal range (Lorenz, 1984). As more children with Down's syndrome are educated in mainstream schools, their achievements and expectations about them are rising considerably, and in the future are likely to influence medical decisions about their treatment.

The sister in a transplantation unit quoted earlier discussed children's desire to share in decisions about transplants.

> All the children we see have demonstrated an ability to make their own decisions. Whether they do it or not is another matter. Many aren't autonomous enough. One mother said to her son after his brother had died, 'We owe it to your brother for you to have a transplant.' He was very distressed. I said to him, 'If you didn't want that operation would you tell us?' He said, 'No, because my mother would be so sad if I said that.'
> I would say that often as young as 4 or 5 they can understand a lot about a transplant. Of course, it varies

very much, and you can't generalize. I believe the child *always* has to be involved. We know that they literally have their life in their hands afterwards. If they stop taking their medications, for example, they will die. Children may find a way of keeping control. One, previously very active, little 7-year-old girl with cystic fibrosis became desperately ill. The family had been denying how ill she was. Our assessment indicated that she only had a few months to live. She cried desperately when she was told she needed a transplant. She died 2 weeks later. She had developed an infection, but medically there was no reason for her to deteriorate quite so dramatically. I think that if children don't want something, then they can give up, and I believe she gave up. A girl in another hospital on the transplant waiting list died and they found a bag of food in her locker. She hadn't been eating.

There have probably always been doctors who skilfully share decision-making with their patients, though this has only recently been recommended as routine practice with adult patients. The process can be still more complicated with children who have life-threatening disease. Sharing decisions with them can involve uncertainty and anguish about whether to respect children by involving them, or to protect them by excluding them from decision-making. A hospital chaplain and former headmaster asked:

But are you going to lay on children the weight of their future? Perhaps let them make a decision that could lead to their death? These are impossible questions, but hospital staff have to find the answers. Am I big enough to say, 'Whatever you choose will be valued, even if you decide against the tide; okay, you've made that decision, I'll do all I can to support you, and we'll go forward together.'? It's such a big step for the adult to surrender power to the child.

In the ethics literature, consent to surgery tends to be seen implicitly as an individual's decision made in lonely autonomy. In practice, many people prefer to share decisions about surgery. On the quite rare occasions when children and parents disagree, postponing surgery and continuing the discussion can resolve differences. If disagreement continued, some parents said that they came to accept their child's decision and the values it was based on, and to 'help them to make the best of it'. Our research found that many medical and nursing staff respect young children's views.

Competence, as understanding, wisdom and courage, continually develops. For example, Nigel, aged 13 years, agreed with his mother before his operation that he could not decide for himself until he was 18. An uncomfortable week later, not yet knowing if his operation was successful, he said spontaneously:

I think I'm changing from that idea that I have to be 18, for big things as well as little things. I've made sensible grown-up decisions before, and I can take care of myself. I see the others in here going through so much, so bravely. I think I can make difficult decisions and understand them now, at 13.

Apart from the possible emotional benefits of involving children and parents who wish to share in decision-making, there are practical advantages in taking account of the social issues they introduce, as discussed in the final sections.

THE GROWING CHILD

A few of the social aspects of treating children with heart disease at different ages will be considered from the care of babies to adolescents. Many of the points apply to every age group.

THE BABY

So far, this chapter has mainly considered information and decisions about treatment. Another social issue is the context in which decisions are made and carried out. This includes the professional teamwork, the design of paediatric cardiac units, funding and support for the staff and families. If parents are to be reasonably informed and involved in decisions about their child's treatment, they need to have ready access to their child, and somewhere to stay overnight nearby. Modern design of wards and intensive care units, with room for parents to sit beside the cot, quiet areas for discussion and overnight accommodation, all aid communication.

Parents are affected by psychological support as well as physical space, and the two are connected. In one cramped unit where parents used to be discouraged from being with their child, many of them spoke of their helplessness and shock. 'I still haven't come to terms with the awful shock of seeing him in the Intensive Care Unit. I feel that it's a dead body, plumbed into everything, immobile. There's nothing you can do.' 'I'd just be in the way. Things often go wrong and that would make me panic.' 'She's completely in other people's hands.' In a more welcoming unit, parents tended to thank nurses for helping them to overcome their initial fears, and to feel that they were contributing. 'I'm sure it's very important for him that I'm sitting here, stroking him and going through it with him.'

Parents who can stay near their child become knowledgeable by observing the daily treatment and are better qualified to share in discussions. They give their child continuing care, in contrast to professionals' changing shifts and rotas. During emergency admissions, often after long journeys to the tertiary centre, parents arrive shaken and bewildered. If told that there is nowhere for them to stay, they are further alarmed, and they need proper accommodation. When they feel welcomed, supported and respected as their child's primary carers, parents are in a better position to attend to complex clinical explanations and to take time to absorb them.

Shared decisions can affect the future wellbeing of the child within the family, as in this example given by a social worker.

> It's very important that this decision is discussed fully with both parents. It may relieve a lot of their enormous worries. Last time Mrs W had to consent without Mr W being there and he was very angry. It's vital that he is fully aware of what the next operation is going to be like so that Mrs W is protected in case something goes wrong.

Families also benefit when information is shared among all the relevant staff, so reducing anxiety about conflicting reports. A senior registrar described a staff meeting as 'useful because it became apparent that all of us had received bits of information from the parents that went unheeded'. He also believed that, 'We need to meet as a team to carry responsibility. It would make decision-making and anxiety less difficult' and would help to coordinate feelings of hope or reasonable pessimism among the staff. In one unit, some people felt 'frozen out', whereas parents tended to feel better informed and supported in another unit where the nurses had regular support meetings. The professional team's sense of being informed and committed to treatment decisions, and how this affects families' informed and willing consent, is worth researching further. Understanding their child's heart treatment is, for parents, more than a matter of passing around packets of information. It is growing awareness, encouraged in centres that value the give-and-take of open discussion. A sister commented:

> It is easier for nurses to talk in a unit where they don't exclude parents from the rounds, because there isn't the feeling, 'Should we tell them?' or 'Do they know this?' The atmosphere is very different. You're not frightened to tell parents what's going on, if everything is done in front of parents, nothing is hidden and they are actively encouraged to be there. How can you be at ease sitting with the parents for hours when you're apprehensive of them asking, perhaps, 'When's he going to come off the ventilator?' and you don't know if the parents are supposed to know?

This is not to argue for overwhelming families with many technical details or with dire, remote possibilities. Sometimes, parents are excluded from ward rounds in order to shield them from hearing about frightening possibilities. Yet such discussions should not be held near children from the second year upwards, who need someone familiar present during all discussions to prevent misunderstandings from alarming the child.

Usually the adults in closest continuing contact with their child, parents can contribute detailed reports of the changing effects of the heart disease and the treatment to clinical discussions. They carry out much of the everyday and nursing care, help to prevent and relieve distress and care for children at home much earlier during convalescence than used to be thought possible. They help to assess the need for pain relief (Cunningham Butler, 1989) and can practise methods of psychological pain relief with very young children (McGrath and Unruh, 1987). The campaign begun in the United States of America by the mother of a baby having ligation of patent arterial duct to improve analgesia for babies during surgery (Lawson, 1986) has changed Western neonatal policies on pain relief.

The discussions preceding informed consent can help doctors and parents to inform one another about children's best interests. It is argued that listening to parents benefits babies: 'In order to protect our children from abusive overtreatment [or] discriminatory under-treatment ... parents can take steps to enter the decision-making process ... by fully informing ourselves and others about the complex ethical problems created by neonatal medicine' (Harrison, 1985) and by drawing attention to social aspects of their baby's care.

THE CHILD AND TEENAGER

Although most paediatric cardiac surgery is performed on children less than 5 years of age, school-age surgical patients are a particularly important group. As they tend to have the more complicated conditions and keep returning for treatment, they gain knowledge through experience. If they feel unwillingly forced to undergo procedures, from X-ray examination to operations, they are likely to refuse to cooperate as they become more independent. Respecting them as early as possible as sensible people who can share in making decisions about their best interests encourages them to cooperate with their treatment and to assume responsibility, such as for taking medication (Eiser, 1990; Krementz, 1990).

Since the 1960s, there has been a growing awareness of the need of children and teenagers for parenting support in hospital, and to have their privacy and dignity protected. Recently, theories about clear-cut stages of childhood have been challenged. Very young children also want to be respected; many older teenagers want their parents' continuing care during crises such as surgery. Young children with chronic conditions can discuss their treatment in adult terms. Consequently, it is not helpful to stereotype children according to age. Over the decades, respect for children has increased. A surgeon, said approvingly:

> Today's teenagers are very competent, particularly girls. An 11-year-old girl will have very strong views on what she wants, what she'll tolerate, and what she won't.

> Attitudes have changed and children are given more freedom, and encouraged much more, not just to listen and do as they're told, but to have strong views.

Professionals mentioned teenagers who were more informed and sensible than their parents, or who spoke English much more fluently. Instead of imposing on children traditional beliefs about their immaturity and limitations, it can be more helpful to expect them to be mature and then adapt for the minority who are not (Alderson, 1999). The government of the United Kingdom advises that 'the consent of the child and the parent or guardian should be obtained to treat children under age 16 save in an emergency', and that 'young people should be kept as fully informed as possible about their condition and treatment to enable them to exercise their rights' (Department of Health, 1991). Children who prefer adults to make major decisions for them still have strong views on interim decisions, such as whether a parent goes with them to the anaesthetic room. They can only exercise choice when they are clearly informed about the options, and when cared for in units where the staff are willing to revise policies in the light of children's requests.

Chronically ill children often miss school and other events to attend hospital as inpatients and outpatients. They especially appreciate joint clinics shared by paediatric cardiologists with local paediatricians. These very much reduce travelling and waiting times for families, and the child's trapped sense of being a patient rather than a person, besides extending attention to social aspects of care through involving general paediatricians. By increasing local knowledge of paediatric cardiology, the clinics contribute to the tendency to encourage as much local care as possible, with shorter admissions to tertiary centres. Children who convalesce at home or in local hospitals can enjoy more contact with their friends and relatives, with less disruption to their everyday life; the trend is to admit them to tertiary centres for shorter periods of increasingly intensive care.

Heart defects can affect many social concerns, food (from feeding breathless babies to nausea related to medication), play and education, self-image, leisure activities, employment opportunities, contraception and childbearing. Medical support ranges from giving assurance that children can live a full, 'normal' life, to helping them to cope with limitations. Parents and children become expert in coping with difficulties and benefit from sharing their hard-won knowledge. Helpful channels for exchanging information and support include specialist nurses and self-help organizations and websites for children with heart defects and their parents and siblings. As many more children with serious defects survive into adolescence and young adulthood, services are slowly developing to meet their changing needs.

High-risk and innovative treatments are most likely to be considered for children with the most intractable conditions. If clear improvement cannot be ensured, it is important to involve them as much as they wish in decisions about whether to embark on treatment and the best means of providing it, taking into account their social concerns. Doctors increasingly offer choices rather than making them. As a psychologist asked, 'In the end, how much misery do you put people through, and for what pay-off?' The answer partly depends on the patient's views. 'Nothing clinical occurs in isolation'; therefore, when planning and evaluating treatment 'it is as important to know the person *with* the disease as it is to know the disease' (Meador, 1992).

Medical research increases clinicians' ability to classify, predict, control and generalize about the course of disease. In contrast, much social research demonstrates the variety, complexity and unpredictability of individuals and organizations. Health service structures and the status of children in society are just two social aspects of paediatric cardiology that constantly change. Amidst this change and variety, young patients' personal needs are effectively met when each one is approached as an individual, rather than a stereotype, by asking what they know and need instead of assuming the answers.

ACKNOWLEDGEMENTS

I thank all the children, parents and health professionals who helped in the consent research projects, and my co-researcher Jill Siddle.

REFERENCES

Age of Legal Capacity (Scotland) Act 1991 HMSO, London

Alderson P 1990 Choosing for children: parents' consent to surgery. Oxford University Press, Oxford

Alderson P 1993 Children's consent to surgery. Open University Press, Buckingham, UK

Alderson P 1999 The rights of young children: exploring beliefs, attitudes, principles and practice. Save the Children/Jessica Kingsley Publishers, London

Alderson P, Montgomery J 1996 Health care choices: making decisions with children. Institute for Public Policy Research, London

Alderson P, Madden M, Oakley A, Wilkins R 1994 Women's views of breast cancer treatment and research. Institute of Education/Cancer Research Campaign, London

Bluebond-Langner M 1978 The private worlds of dying children. Princeton University Press, Princeton, NJ

Buchanan A, Brock D 1989 Deciding for others: the ethics of surrogate decision making. Cambridge University Press, New York

Children Act 1989 HMSO, London

Clunies-Ross C, Lansdown R 1988 Concepts of death, illness and isolation found in children with leukaemia. Child Care, Health and Development 14: 373–386

Cunningham Butler N 1989 The issue of medically caused pain in infants. Children's Hospital Care 18, 2: 70–74

Davis F 1963 Passage through crisis. Bobbs-Merrill, New York

Delight E, Goodall J 1990 Love and loss: conversations with parents of babies with spina bifida manage without surgery, 1971–1981. Developmental Medicine & Child Neurology, Supp. 61, 32: 8

Department of Health 1991 Welfare of children and young people in hospital. HMSO London

Dyer C 1999a English teenager given heart transplant against her will. British Medical Journal 319: 209

Dyer C 1999b Mother fails to win right to control treatment for son. British Medical Journal 319: 278

Editorial 1999a London Metro, Daily Mail, 17 June

Editorial 1999b Heart 82: 47–51

Eiser C 1990 Chronic childhood disease: an introduction to psychological theory and research. Cambridge University Press, Cambridge, UK

Fraund S, Pethig K, Fronbe U et al 1999 A ten year survival after heart transplantation: palliative or successful long term treatment? Heart 82; 1: 47–51

Family Law Reform Act 1969 HMSO, London

Gillick v. West Norfolk & Wisbech HA [1985] 3 All ER 402, 432

Harrison H 1985 Neonatal intensive care: parents' role in ethical decision-making. Birth 13, 3: 172–173

Irwin C 1996 Samantha's wish. Nursing Times, 92, 36: 29–30

Julian-Reynier C, Aurran Y, Dunmaret A, Chabal F, Giraud F, Ayrne S 1995 Attitudes towards Down's syndrome: follow up of a cohort of 280 cases. Journal of Medical Genetics 32, 8: 597–599

Paton H (ed.) 1972 The moral law. Hutchinson, London

Krementz J 1990 How it feels to fight for your life. Gollancz, New York

Lawson J 1986 Letter to the editor. Birth 13: 124–125

Locke J 1690 (reprinted 1959) An essay concerning human understanding. Dover, New York

Lorenz 1984 Long term effects of early interventions in children with Down's syndrome. Unpublished PhD thesis, University of Manchester, quoted in Wolfendale S (ed.) 1997 Meeting special needs in the early years. Paul Chapman, London p 73

Maguire P 1985 Barriers to psychological care of the dying. British Medical Journal 291: 178–183

McGrath P, Unruh A 1987 Pain in children and adolescents. Elsevier, New York

Meador C 1992 The person with the disease. Journal of American Medical Association 268, 1: 35

Melzak S 1992 Secrecy, privacy, survival, repressive regimes, and growing up. Bulletin of the Anna Freud Centre 15: 205–224

Mental Health Act 1983 HMSO, London

Menzies Lyth I 1988 Containing anxiety in institutions. Free Association Book, London

Mill J 1858 (reprinted 1982) On liberty. Penguin, Harmondsworth, UK

Rees P, Tunstill A, Pope T, Kinnear D, Rees S 1990 Heart children: a practical handbook for parents. Heartline Association, Biggleswade

re R [1991] 4 All ER 177

re W [1992] 4 All ER 627

re T [1997] I (a minor) All ER 74 906

re S [1998] Dyer C Judge misled over call for caesarean operation. British Medical Journal 316: 574

Roth J 1963 Timetables. Bobbs-Merrill, New York

Scott O, Gerlis L 1984 Sheets on congenital heart defects. British Heart Foundation, London

Silverman D 1981 The child as a social object: Down's syndrome children in the paediatric cardiology clinic. Sociology of health and illness 3: 4

Solberg A 1997 Negotiating childhood. In: James A, Prout A (eds) Constructing and reconstructing childhood. Falmer Press, Basingstoke, UK

Taylor K, Kelner M 1987 Informed consent: the physicians' perspective. Social Science and Medicine 24, 2: 135–143

Tizzard B, Hughes M 1984 Young children learning. Fontana, Glasgow, UK

United Nation 1989 Convention on the Rights of the Child. UN, Geneva

Williamson C 1992 Whose standards? consumer and professional standards in health care. Open University Press, Buckingham, UK

Young A 1990 Moral conflicts in a psychiatric hospital. In: Weisz G (ed.) Social science perspectives on medical ethics. Kluwer, Dordrecht p 65–82

Yule W 1992 Post traumatic stress disorders in children. Current Opinion in Paediatrics 4: 4

Zussman R 1992 Intensive care: medical ethics and the medical profession. University of Chicago Press, Chicago, IL

75

Ethics in paediatric cardiology

G. R. Dunstan

THE NEW ABSORPTION WITH ETHICS

When the first edition of this work was published in 1987, the final chapter was on ethical issues in paediatric cardiology. Its inclusion may have surprised some readers. Today, it is usual to find a session on ethics in medical conferences, and articles or chapters on ethics abound in professional journals and publications. New specialties may be expected to generate ethical discussions. Transplant surgery has done so since the 1960s, in vitro fertilization and embryology since the 1970s. It is more surprising to find an ethical analysis accompanying what appears to be no more than technical advances within a specialty, like micromanipulation of sperm and ova within in vitro fertilization (Fishel and Symonds, 1993). A textbook on paediatric cardiology would seem to fall into this latter category. The editorial justification for inclusion of ethics in the 1987 edition lay in technical advance: the new means to study in three dimensions by cross-sectional echocardiology had become 'the cornerstone of diagnosis'. Technical refinements since then have made possible the study of the function of organs – like blood flow velocity – as well as their volume and structure by means virtually devoid of hazard; this is possible in the fetal as well as in the infant heart. Genetic and biochemical screening add clues to predictive patterns. More knowledge widens opportunities in prognosis, as well as in diagnosis. Opportunities demand decisions, and those choices are not always determinable only from the observable features. When doctors, having concluded what technically they can do in a particular case, ask themselves also 'What ought we to do?', they are asking an ethical question. Ethics is, for them, the discipline of deciding action appropriate to the facts of each case within the tension exerted by a cluster of principles or human obligations and constraints.

The constraints are not only those of principle; they are also economic and financial, and even political. Doctors in a long tradition have accepted an obligation, in the words of a Tudor physician, to 'do their diligence aswel to the poore as to the riche', and 'of the riche to take liberally for bothe' (Vicary, 1548). But once a nation resolves that the health care of its population shall be funded primarily by national insurance and from taxation – leaving open the extra option of commercial insurance and private fee – the allocation of resources to the Health Service becomes a matter for political decision. Medical decisions, therefore, have to take account of resources available. These include hospital beds and equipment; nursing, medical and support staff; screening; and other services. In the new millennium, these pressures are severe and subject to political controversy. While clinical decisions are, in principle, still insulated from politics, the non-availability of resources has already begun to intrude into the simple weighing of what can be done medically and what ought to be done ethically (Kennedy, 1991, p 287–299).

Sensitivity to these factors has grown since the 1960s, although the principles themselves have been longer in development and varied in application. Scientific and technical advance has invested medicine with new power: power over patients, over people. An awareness, common to the profession and patients, that power has been abused – at the dictate of an evil politics, of excessive zeal in research or of sheer financial gain – has resulted in a common determination to erect safeguards against abuse. More respect is required for people's capacity and wish to make responsible decisions for themselves, and for their need to be given information apt to enable them so to do. Consent has assumed a new importance in the doctor–patient relationship, with stricter legal definition and requirement. Medical secrecy, the duty to preserve medical confidences, calls for stricter attention. More can now be known about people, more can be recorded or stored in databanks and more people may have administrative access to that knowledge. Fear of disclosure lessens willingness to confide. Permitted access by patients to their own records may tax medical discretion. Genetic information, or reasons for a decision not to operate, if not disclosed to patients or to parents at the time may evoke resentment if discovered later. In reverse, a patient's refusal to disclose genetic inheritance to, for example, a sister at serious risk may strain the doctor's duty of confidence to that patient.

Safeguards have been mounted against exploiting patients or putting them to undue discomfort or risk in the name of research. The freedom with which doctors could impose experimental treatments, unresearched, upon patients at will is no longer acceptable. Above all, a new quality of relationship is sought between doctor and patient in which the respect and courtesy long evident in the best is now to be evident in all. Whatever may or may not be exaggerated in the portrayal of an authoritarian past, doctors are now required to try to bring patients into an intelligent and responsible partnership in which aims are common and duties are reciprocal. Irritation with the rhetoric and slogans of polemics – 'autonomy', 'paternalism', 'consumerism', 'defensive medicine' and the rest – need not blind us to these simple truths.

WHEN THE PATIENT IS A CHILD

These truths are not special to paediatric cardiology, of course, but common to the practice of medicine. Special claims are made, however, when the patient is a child. Here, writers on ethics face an initial difficulty. How do they distinguish an ethical from a medical decision? Within the medical literature, chapter after chapter contains material on which the cardiologist has to make decisions: mostly technical decisions on the means most effective to an immediate goal, the next stage on to the optimal end-point and the course with the least risk. Even the assessment of benefit and risk is primarily a technical matter. It is possible that a doctor only finds himself asking ethical as well as medical questions when he considers when means are related to the end pursued, leading to the question, *ought* this end to be pursued. Generally he will ask, 'How shall we help this baby to live?' Sometimes he must ask, 'Ought we to help this baby to live, given the means we have and the predictable outcome?' (Royal College of Paediatricians and Child Health, 1997).

RELATIONS WITH PARENTS

Whatever the question, the first factor special to paediatrics is that, although the child is the patient, the conscious, deliberative professional relationship is with the parents, and, for various reasons, chiefly with the mother. Parents have a duty of care for their children. They are the primary agents of care. Doctors are their surrogates and helpers. The only 'rights' parents enjoy are those necessary to perform their parental obligations, as trustees of the interests of their child (Kennedy, 1991, p 61–62). As children attain years of discretion – the capacity to decide and determine for themselves – so parental rights over the child diminish. But, until that stage is reached, parents must be consulted, and a medical intervention upon a child without parental consent would be a breach of duty and of the law.

In good present-day practice, parents are brought firmly into the decision to be made concerning treatment. Care is taken to minimize separation and to interfere as little as possible with bonding. Parents are in hospital, at critical periods, with their children. The *rapport* normally necessary with an adult patient for the conveying of information and the winning of cooperation must here be established with the parents. They also have their own emotional needs, which claim respect and sympathetic attention. Their consent, grounded in understanding, must be sought not exacted. There may be difficulties. The line between the mother's welfare and that of the fetus is sometimes fine, but it is always real. Echocardiography is now a routine part of antenatal care. It is performed, with consent, as a diagnostic procedure in the interest of the fetus. It may prove to be for the mother's benefit also in freeing her from anxiety if it reveals no defect. But, if it should yield a bad prognosis, it sets before her choices in which her interest and those of the fetus may conflict. These choices include whether or not to terminate the pregnancy. This occurs equally with other new techniques. The detection of dominant autosomal genetic defects by chromosomal analysis is now established and advancing. Familial clustering is also now found in some conditions such as hypertrophic cardiomyopathy and systemic hypertension. Advances in penetration and precision in echocardiography and Doppler scanning make possible the diagnosis of defects in the fetal heart. For some conditions diagnosed, treatment is not yet possible, but for others it is. Fetal surgery requires maternal consent. Within a good professional relationship, it may be given. But, if it is refused, no power exists in English law to compel the mother to accept intervention (Royal College of Obstetricians and Gynaecologists, 1994, 1996). Her body is inviolable without her consent, and wardship cannot be extended to a fetus, as it might be to a child, as a means of dispensing with her consent (Kennedy, 1991, p 364–384). The welfare of the future child depends on the quality of the ethical relationship established between the paediatrician or obstetrician and the mother. The judgement of the English Court of Appeal in *re T (Refusal of consent)* (CA July 10 1992) that the refusal of a blood transfusion by a woman 34 weeks pregnant could be overruled did not alter this doctrine. It was not delivered on the ground that the claim of the fetus overrode that of the mother but on the grounds that, at the time of her refusal, the mother's physical and mental condition was such that she lacked the capacity to refuse, that she was subjected to undue influence in her refusal and that she had been misled as to the anticipated circumstances in which her refusal would operate (Grubb, 1992).

This factor is relevant to the question whether screening for congenital heart disease in the fetus should be a routine procedure for all mothers at about 18 weeks of pregnancy. Given the relative ease of the procedure, and the absence of known risk, the proposition looks attractive, especially to minds eager to maximize the benefits of advancing technology. In practice, the issue is less clear. The fetal heart, even though less obstructed by the sternum, rib cage and unaerated lungs than after birth, remains a little less easy to study. Maternal consent to universal screening is by no means certain. Only a widely assured beneficial outcome could justify the allocation of straitened resources. While the first remedy of popular resort remains the termination of pregnancy, even for defects for which treatment might be or might become available, there is little ground for confidence that a convincingly wide benefit is assured. On examination, the case for routine screening of the fetal heart looks less persuasive.

Even after birth, parental consent is not confined to treatment: it extends to diagnosis also. Accurate diagnosis is a strict prerequisite to treatment. Pursuit of diagnostic accuracy may involve extra risk. Cardiac catheterization is an obvious example. Exercise testing may be helpful in assessing the need for surgery or may be required as a means of assessing the results of treatment or for advice on whether activity should be restricted. It need not be frightening or painful, but it may incur risk. It may not be undertaken without parental consent. The doctor who believes that he would be negligent not to undertake it (particularly cardiac catheterization) is, therefore, faced with the ethics of exposition and persuasion. A relationship must be established in which risk and uncertainty can be appreciated and weighed, and the good can be agreed upon and chosen. It cannot be imposed. But first the doctor must be confident that the intervention is justified; that is, it is so required by necessity as to outweigh risk.

There is, inevitably, a distance between a physician and a parent in the impact made upon them by heart disease in a child, especially a very young child. Maternal feelings are deeply involved. A mother may need time, and help, to assuage her disappointment, grief or even self-imputed guilt for the birth. Present understanding lays upon the paediatric unit the duty of caring for such a parent, whether by the responsible physician or nurse or by a social worker or counsellor. The essential art is to convey the assurance both that the burden is shared and that the parent is respected as one accepting responsibility. There are tendencies in the now fashionable ethics by slogan to exalt the 'autonomy' of the parent and so to denigrate the 'paternalism' of the doctor in a way that can deny the parent some of the help she may need and to which she is justly entitled. Because she lacks the doctor's medical knowledge, her assessment of risk must be even less certain than the professional view. The doctor's duty is not done when a factual explanation has been provided and a request made for her consent or decision. Should things not turn out well, her burden of regret or loss will be heavier than that of the professional. It is not for her good if she adds to it a burden of guilt. Guilt may be lessened or avoided if she can feel that her decision had the warrant of her doctor's approval or

support. Certainty cannot be required. It is unattainable. But if a doctor feels sufficiently encouraged by the data to suggest the procedure in the first place, there seems to be no reason why, without over-reaching, that encouragement cannot be shared with a responsible parent. The same consideration is apt – although it is not the only one – in discussing the option of terminating a pregnancy after the detection of grave fetal abnormality. It has even stronger force when a medical decision is taken, as licitly it may be in ethics and in law, to desist from further efforts to keep alive a severely ill baby. Doctors have to learn to live with such decisions. Parents need not be obliged to. When a heart–lung transplant is offered or performed, there is a double claim on understanding. The loss to the parents of the baby who has died may weigh heavily on the parents of the baby who may live because of that death. It would be an inhumane ethical theory which distanced those parents from apt medical concern.

RISK

It is an axiom of practice that accurate diagnosis must precede treatment. It would be an error, for instance, to begin anti-inflammatory or suppressive drug treatment for signs of rheumatic heart disease before the condition had been definitely established. It is another axiom that, before any diagnostic procedure is undertaken, the question to be answered or the objective sought must be clearly defined, and that the procedure proposed is right for that end. Otherwise, an investigation may be prolonged, altered in mid-course, cumulatively hazardous and ultimately futile. These obligations are higher for patients seen as infants than for adults because infants are more vulnerable and because the time available for making decisions may be shorter. Extrapolation from adults to infants is not always valid, even from the findings of research that are valid for adults. In addition, children present conditions specific to themselves for which experience with adults gives no guidance. Normal values also vary and must be known for comparative purposes.

Yet, in very young babies, some diagnostic procedures, like cardiac catheterization and angiocardiography, can incur risk. In the first edition (p 391) of this book it was stated that 'cardiac catheterization, done well, is of enormous value in decision making, therapy and research. Done badly it is a menace'.

Risk can be justified, in diagnosis and in treatment, when the benefit sought is substantial and a less-hazardous course is not available. Surgery in infancy to correct ventricular septal defect can be life saving. There is some risk, but most infants survive to live normal lives. Necessity may justify the taking of high risk. An operation for severe aortic stenosis in a neonate shows poorer results than in older children. Yet it may be required because the progressive consequences of the obstruction do not permit delay or further palliative treatment. Innovative surgery may carry a high risk, which falls with experience. Surgery for double outlet right ventricle had a chequered history with 'some operative tragedies' yet it is now usually successful, despite complications, for most patients. Long-term prospective studies may be necessary for a conclusive interpretation of results.

It would follow that high-risk innovative measures should be introduced, time permitting, only after the most careful deliberation and consultation. Apparent success in initial attempts does not, by itself, justify continuance or extension. Verification is required, when possible, from a formally mounted clinical trial, approved by a research ethics committee as well as by peer review. Here another difficulty is encountered with children. A parent may lawfully consent to an experimental procedure on a child provided that it is potentially for that child's benefit. At the extreme limit of permissibility stands the rule that the procedure must not be potentially adverse to the child's interests. Proxy consent may not be given, in contrast, for a research commonly called 'non-therapeutic', where the intention is not to serve the child's interest. This rule would limit the use of children as 'controls' for the trial of a new procedure, unless the trial was compared with the best known procedure already indicated for those children. If the trial were proving successful, fine judgement would be required to decide at what point it was no longer ethical to deny those serving as controls the benefit of the new procedure. A final judgement may not be possible without prolonged clinical observation of progress. Research ethics committees are required to be particularly vigilant in their scrutiny of proposals involving children, and not only of the formalities about consent (Nicholson, 1986; Royal College of Physicians, 1990, 1996; Department of Health, 1991; Medical Research Council, 1991; British Paediatric Association, 1993).

Not all research is so clinically related. Some may be epidemiological. Some may involve linkage studies: establishing a relationship between a newly isolated gene and a clinical condition. In these, children and parents may be hurt by insensitivity in scientific pursuit. Information from a database may mark out a child for recall. It is important, first, that the approach to the family be made through one who knows its constitution and circumstances. This is more likely to be the general practitioner or the original consultant. Second, the subsequent interview should be conducted by someone able to relate acceptably with a rather frightened parent and child. Follow-up studies, when required, should also be conducted with the least possible intrusion into the life of the family and of the child.

----------- SPECIAL CASES -----------

The paediatric cardiologist, like the obstetrician before him or her, works with a presumption in favour of life. The objective is to enable patients to live, and to live with the minimum impairment and the utmost capacity for the enjoyment of life. The ethics of practice recognize a continuity of claim to protection and care, progressing from early embryonic existence through gestation and birth into infancy. The law has a demarcation point at birth. Birth confers upon the child the status of legal personality, a bearer of rights, which the fetus does not enjoy. The law permits the interests of the fetus to be subordinated, for serious cause, to those of the mother. The right of the born child, in contrast, is equal to that of the mother and is not to be subordinated. The courts can intervene to protect that right, by care or institution of wardship proceedings. Even so, neither the claim of the fetus nor the right to life of the child is absolute, in the sense that the doctor is under strict duty, regardless of any other consideration, to prolong life by all possible means. For sufficient reason, under the law common or statute, fetal life may be taken by termination of pregnancy. A child, for whom further active intervention would be against his or her interests, may lawfully be offered nursing care only until the intervention of death. No action may be taken, however, intentionally to kill the child (Royal College of Paediatricians and Child Health, 1997). These considerations must govern practice in paediatric cardiology in rare cases. They demand of the doctor sensitivity and moral insight plus the capacity for moral analysis and for decision. Insofar as the outcome has deep personal significance for parents, they demand from the physician human empathy and a capacity to communicate.

The new refinements in fetal scanning and echocardiography give the cardiologist higher diagnostic precision, whether for attempting fetal cardiac surgery or other intervention, for preparing for intervention after birth or for recognizing indications for a possible termination of pregnancy. Responsibility for management during pregnancy is shared between the obstetrician and the cardiologist (Robinson, 1992). Accurate diagnosis is an essential prerequisite of management. The presence of Eisenmenger's syndrome, or primary pulmonary hypertension, in the mother has been set down as 'the only absolute indication for termination' (de Swiet, 1987) because of the high risk of maternal death. Echocardiography may reveal conditions that, though rare, are life threatening and virtually irremediable. An external location of the heart ('ectopia cordis') is, to our knowledge, uniformly fatal, with one documented exception. For twins conjoined at the chest, with hearts separate or conjoined in a common thoracic cavity, successful surgery is remarkably rare. Before it became possible to recognize such conditions in the fetus, decision waited upon birth. Now earlier knowledge invites earlier decision. Termination of pregnancy becomes a valid option when conditions are foreseen to be serious and the likelihood of operational success low. For Down's syndrome, the issue is less clear. Chromosomal analysis may confirm the condition antenatally. Echocardiography may disclose severe impairment of the heart. The degree of neurological impairment is not yet predictable. A heart transplant may be offered to replace the defective heart; but the question whether this is in the child's interest remains unanswered while severe neural damage remains a possibility.

It is not open to a moralist to prescribe clinical decisions in such cases. At most, the moralist may open out principles by which clinicians will make decisions proper to each case.

Given an adverse condition, the doctor's prima facie duty is to intervene to preserve and ameliorate life whenever possible. That is the essence of the profession. Practitioners might say, they will *try* what can be done. The verb *try* is of critical ethical importance. There are Latin words for it, from which we can learn. One is *tentare*, from which we derive the adjective 'tentative'. Another is *attemptare*, from which we derive 'attempt'. Yet another is *experiri*, which gives us both 'experiment' and 'experience' which is gained by experiment, by trying. It follows, by simple logic, that a prima facie or presumptive duty to try does not commit the clinician to an absolute duty to persist if it becomes evident that his intervention is proving adverse to the interest of the patient. Each such intervention is a 'trial', an experiment, varying in the degree of its tentativeness with the condition of the patient, the status of the operation from novel to routine and the experience of the operator. The attempt may be abandoned if it does not succeed. In some circumstances, it must be abandoned, even though, for professional reasons, it would seem preferable to continue. It would be unethical to continue any experiment, to the detriment of the patient, to satisfy a research interest or for mere curiosity or determination not to be beaten. The physician is, indeed, not bound to intervene, to try, at all if the clinical conviction, well evidenced, exists that to do so would be pointless in terms of the child's continuing condition. This principle is defensible in law (Kennedy, 1991, p 296). The decision must rest finally with the clinician in charge. It will, of course, be taken only after professional consultation and having done the best to take along the parents and the child, if old enough, in reaching the decision. The decision is not one to abandon care; it is to change the management to nursing care, when any other regimen would be wrong.

These considerations are relevant also during pregnancy when termination is an option, though with one significant exception. The decision to request termination must come from the mother. The clinician may only decline to recommend it, or to operate, if it seems that the indications are not within the terms of the Abortion Act – or, of course, if there is a personal objection in conscience, when the mother must be offered the opportunity for consultation elsewhere.

The principles may be clear, but their application may be far from clear. The more variants and uncertainties there are, the more difficult is decision and the more demanding is the duty laid on the clinician. The unborn child with Down's syndrome has been mentioned. In this context, the condition of the heart, and what may be done for it before and after birth, will be first to be considered. But other systemic factors are relevant, for example the lungs, the brain and the immune defences. Environment conditions the welfare of this child. Given a secure relationship where there is affection, consistency and a firm emotional and mental commitment to the task, the child may well have such prospects as to make termination an unwarranted interruption of life. The attitude and capacity of the parents are in the forefront of consideration. Parents must decide, but they require help in their decision, with apt information and advice and (a different service) counselling to enable them to absorb what they hear and to make the decision their own. That there may be a call to shield them from the added burden of guilt has already been suggested.

Stereotypes are not to be relied on. Not all Roman Catholic women accept the prohibition of abortion in all circumstances, as now pronounced by the Vatican authorities. And many women who are not Roman Catholics have scruples about abortion. Each must be listened to and enabled to open and explore their own minds. Genuine conscientious conviction may not be lightly brushed aside.

INTUITION: PERSONAL AND CORPORATE

Decision is a day-to-day, hour-to-hour reality in practice. Decisions are taken at every step: first presentation and examination, tentative initial diagnosis, choice of routes and modes of investigation, prognosis, choice of management (palliative or corrective), timing of intervention, and discharge or allocation to long-term or short-term nursing care. The material for decision is the information derived by systematic examination of the patient and from the literature, interpreted by the canons of established medical science and practice. The doctor is trained to gather this information, to interpret it and to frame his duty accordingly. But reflection and an elementary self-awareness teach that the strictly scientific element in reaching decisions is sometimes limited.

The scientific data – readings from scans, dials, graphs, assays of biochemical values and the like – do not themselves dictate decision. They may paralyse decision, for they may pull in different directions. Recorded experience warns that an early operation to correct a pulmonary venous abnormality or stenosis may carry a higher risk than an operation postponed. Yet necessity may require such early intervention because of the baby's condition. Only a personal decision can resolve the conflict. Scientific logic might argue that, given one gap in a particular pattern of knowledge, experiment or research in one direction might fill it. If the research would require the violation of some vulnerable interest, however, it cannot be undertaken. Scientific logic cannot have the last word.

Decisions, therefore, though grounded as they are in medical science, contain a large intuitive element. And the acquisition and sharpening of a disciplined intuition is part of a wholesome medical and social training. Medical intuition is essential to the humane practice of medicine. When autonomous, it can be a menace.

There is, therefore, another ethical demand. It is for what might be called a corporate intuition, a community of minds working together by which personal intuitions, subjective judgements, may be checked, validated or countermanded. Paediatric cardiology requires work in a team, within which consultation precedes decision. The physician and surgeon are obvious members as is the obstetrician in fetal cardiology. Other specialists are drawn on as each case requires: echocardiographers, neurologists, endocrinologists, haematologists. Nurses contribute from their continuing contact with parents as well as with the neonatal and infant patient. The development of a corporate conscience, a facility in moral reasoning together, is a necessary condition if decisions are to be made that, on the one hand, take the empirical data into account, and, on the other, amount to the best apparent choice possible among the available options, none of which may be ideal. Such a common possession is not acquired without discipline. The present organization of specialist hospital medicine should, in theory, favour it.

The group of consultants and senior nurses provide continuity in the longer term. The training posts attached to them bring a succession of younger doctors for set terms of years. Between them there is an interchange not only in terms of science and technical education but also in values, in those tensions that constrain the transmission of ethics from generation to generation.

Medical ethics is first a corporate possession, that of a profession. It is embodied personally as each member makes it his or her own. Codes like the Helsinki Declaration governing medical research are markers of minimum demand and social expectation. The living practice of the ethics, and its necessary development, is ideally an activity of the small group or team, as just described. The individual works best as a moral agent in small, tangible *societies*. The Latin root of that word is *societas*, for which the old English translation is 'fellowship' (as old, incidentally, as the translation of *mores*, morals, as 'manners'). Models of collegiate fellowship exist, within the common experience, in which knowledge is valued, pursued, ordered and transmitted. Standards, intellectual and professional, are set, acquired and maintained. Members are disciplined. Persons are fulfilled. Ethics is an activity proper to humans as rational and social beings. This is what William of Wykeham meant when, out of Aristotle, he devised the motto for his college at Winchester: 'Manners makyth man'.

REFERENCES

British Paediatric Association 1993 Guidelines for the ethical conduct of medical research involving children. British Paediatric Association, London

de Swiet M 1987 Management of congenital heart disease in pregnancy. In: Anderson R H, Macartney F J, Shinebourne E A, Tynan M (eds) Paediatric cardiology. Churchill Livingstone, Edinburgh, p 1355

Department of Health 1991 Report of Local Research Ethics Committees. Department of Health, London, p 16

Fishel S, Symonds E M 1993 Gamete and embryo micromanipulation. In: Human reproduction. Edward Arnold, London

Grubb A 1992 Refusal of medical treatment. Dispatches of King's College London Centre of Medical Law and Ethics 3.1 (Autumn)

Kennedy I 1991 Treat me right: essays in medical law and ethics. Clarendon Press, Oxford

Medical Research Council 1991 The ethical conduct of research on children. Medical Research Council, London

Nicholson R H 1986 Medical research with children: ethics, law and practice. Oxford University Press, Oxford

Royal College of Obstetricians and Gynaecologists 1994 A consideration of the law and ethics in relation to court-authorized obstetric intervention. RCOG

Guidelines, Ethics, No 1. Royal College of Obstetricians and Gynaecologists, London

Royal College of Obstetricians and Gynaecologists 1996 A consideration of the law and ethics in relation to court-authorized obstetric intervention. RCOG Guidelines, Ethics, Supplement on Advance Directives. Royal College of Obstetricians and Gynaecologists, London

Royal College of Paediatricians and Child Health 1997 Witholding and withdrawing treatment in children. A framework for practice. Royal College of Paediatricians, London

Royal College of Physicians 1990 Research involving patients. Royal College of Physicians, London p 19–20

Royal College of Physicians 1996 Guidelines on the practice of ethics committees in medical research involving human subjects, 3rd edn. Royal College of Physicians, London, p 36–37

Robinson S 1992 The physician in the antenatal clinic. Journal of the Royal College of Physicians, London 26: 226–230

Vicary T 1548 The anatomy of the body of man. The text of 1577, Furnival F J, Furnivall P (eds), for the Early English Text Society 1880. Oxford University Press, Oxford

INDEX